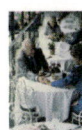

SECTION 8

PROBLEMS OF INGESTION, DIGESTION, ABSORPTION, AND ELIMINATION

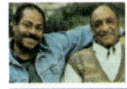

SECTION 9

PROBLEMS OF URINARY FUNCTION

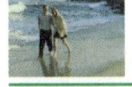

SECTION 10

PROBLEMS RELATED TO REGULATORY MECHANISMS

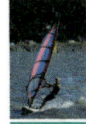

SECTION 11

PROBLEMS RELATED TO MOVEMENT AND COORDINATION

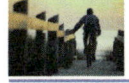

SECTION 12

NURSING CARE IN SPECIALIZED SETTINGS

APPENDIXES

CONGRATULATIONS
You now have access to Mosby's "Get Smart" Bonus Package!

Here's what's included to help you "Get Smart"

sign on at:

http://www.mosby.com/MERLIN/medsurg_lewis/

A Web site just for you as you learn medical-surgical nursing with the new 5th edition of **Medical-Surgical Nursing: Assessment and Management of Clinical Problems**

what you will receive:

Whether you're a student, an instructor, or a clinician, you'll find information just for you. Things like:
- Content Updates • Links to Related Products
- Author Information . . . and more

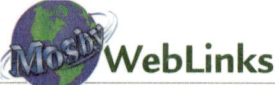 **WebLinks**

An exciting new program that allows you to directly access hundreds of active Web sites keyed specifically to the content of this book. The WebLinks are continually updated, with new ones added as they develop.

Free CD-ROM

with every copy of **Medical-Surgical Nursing**, 5th Edition

This valuable CD-ROM Features:

Overviews of Common Diseases
Key Terms
Case Studies
Review Questions

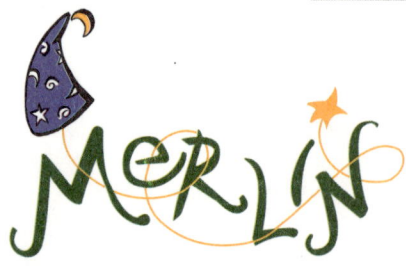

Mosby's Electronic Resource Links & Information Network

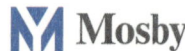 Mosby

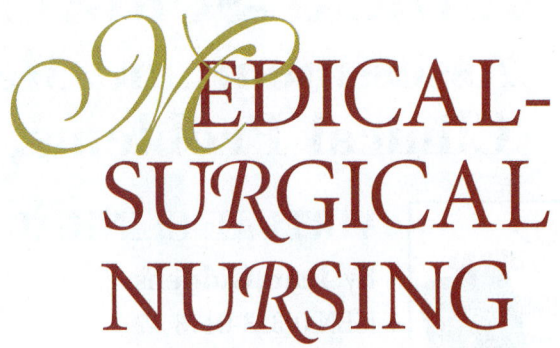

MEDICAL-SURGICAL NURSING

ASSESSMENT and MANAGEMENT of CLINICAL PROBLEMS

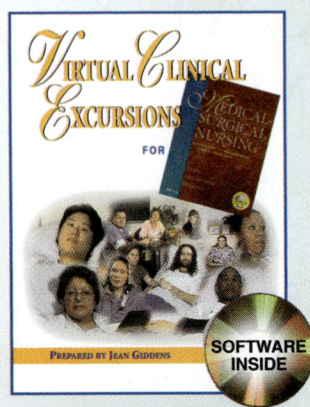
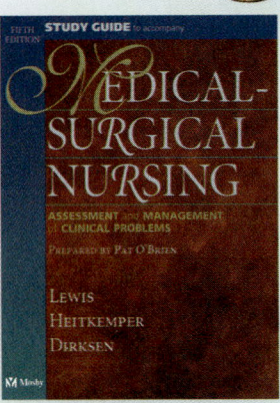
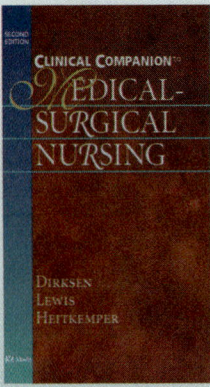

VOLUME 2
CHAPTERS 37-64
PAGES 1011-1998

FIFTH EDITION

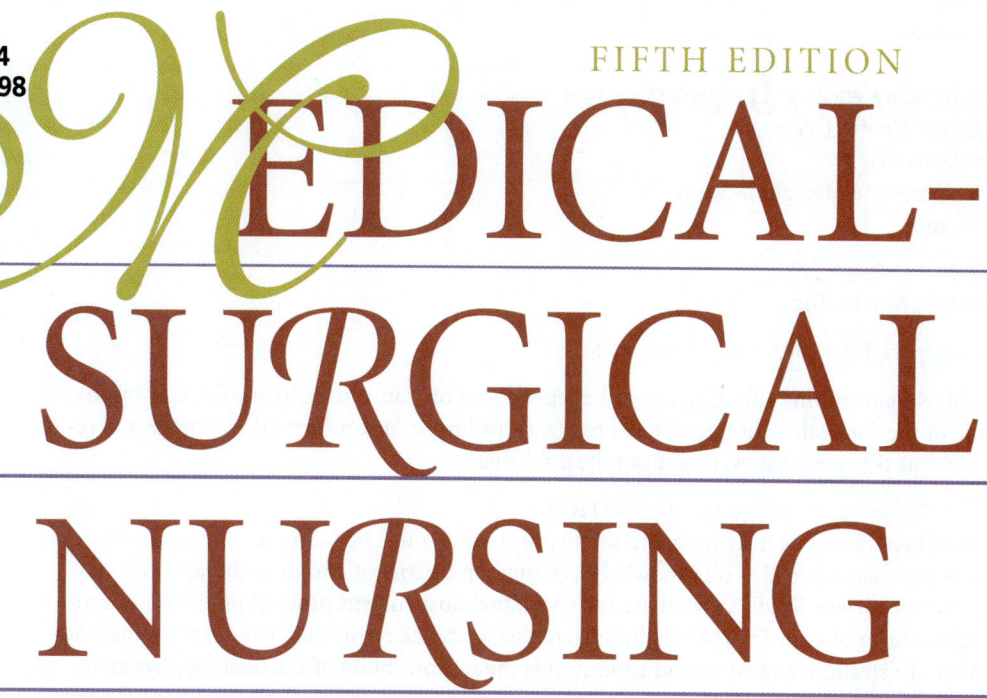

MEDICAL-SURGICAL NURSING

ASSESSMENT and MANAGEMENT of CLINICAL PROBLEMS

SHARON MANTIK LEWIS, RN, PhD, FAAN
Professor, College of Nursing
Research Associate Professor, Department of Pathology
University of New Mexico
Albuquerque, New Mexico

MARGARET McLEAN HEITKEMPER, RN, PhD, FAAN
Professor, Biobehavioral Nursing and Health Systems
School of Nursing
University of Washington
Seattle, Washington

SHANNON RUFF DIRKSEN, RN, PhD
Associate Professor, College of Nursing
Arizona State University
Tempe, Arizona

with 845 illustrations

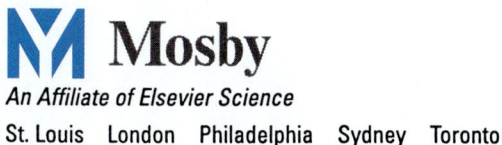
Mosby
An Affiliate of Elsevier Science
St. Louis   London   Philadelphia   Sydney   Toronto

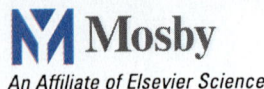

Mosby
An Affiliate of Elsevier Science

Editor-in-Chief Sally Schrefer
Developmental Editor Kristin Geen
Project Manager Dana Peick
Project Specialist Catherine Albright Jackson
Designer Amy Buxton

FIFTH EDITION
Copyright © 2000 by Mosby, Inc.

Previous editions copyrighted 1983, 1987, 1992, 1996.

NOTICE

Pharmacology is an ever-changing field. Standard safety precautions must be followed, but as new research and clinical experience broaden our knowledge, changes in treatment and drug therapy may become necessary or appropriate. Readers are advised to check the most current product information provided by the manufacturer of each drug to be administered to verify the recommended dose, the method and duration of administration, and contraindications. It is the responsibility of the treating physician, relying on experience and knowledge of the patient, to determine dosages and the best treatment for each individual patient. Neither the Publisher nor the editor assume any liability for any injury and/or damage to persons or property arising from this publication.

Mosby, Inc.
An Affiliate of Elsevier Science
11830 Westline Industrial Drive
St. Louis, Missouri 63146

Printed in the United States of America.

ISBN 0-323-01048-2

02 03 / 9 8 7 6 5

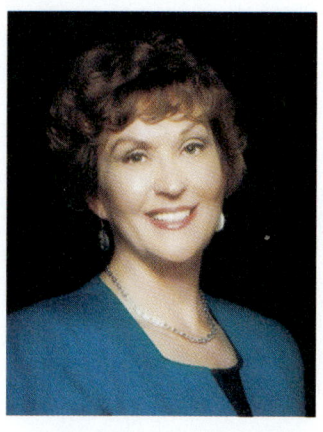

Sharon Mantik Lewis, RN, PhD, FAAN

Sharon Lewis received her Bachelor of Science in nursing from the University of Wisconsin-Madison, Master of Science in nursing with a minor in biological sciences from the University of Colorado, and PhD in immunology from the Department of Pathology at the University of New Mexico School of Medicine. She had a 2-year postdoctoral fellowship from the National Kidney Foundation. Her more than 25 years of teaching experience include inservice education and teaching in associate, baccalaureate, and master's degree programs in Maryland, Illinois, Wisconsin, and New Mexico. Favorite teaching areas are pathophysiology, immunology, and renal failure. She has been actively involved in clinical research for the last 18 years, investigating altered immune responses in patients with chronic renal failure and other chronic illnesses. Currently she is using biofeedback and immune parameters to study the effects of relaxation therapy for caregivers of Alzheimer's patients.

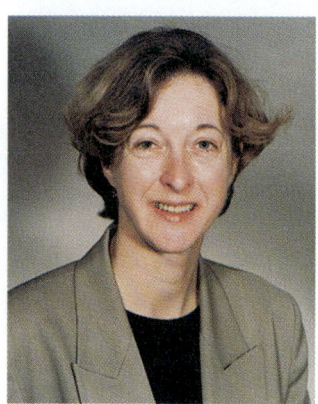

Margaret McLean Heitkemper, RN, PhD, FAAN

Margaret Heitkemper received her Bachelor of Science in nursing from Seattle University, Master of Science in gerontologic nursing from the University of Washington, and PhD in physiology and biophysics from the University of Illinois. She was a research associate on an NIH research grant project related to problems with enteral nutrition where she developed an interest in gastrointestinal problems. She has experience as a staff nurse and has worked in an acute geriatric care facility associated with Rush-St. Luke's Presbyterian Medical Center. Since 1981, she has been on the faculty at the University of Washington where she is department chairperson and teaches at all levels—undergraduate and graduate. She currently teaches medical-surgical nursing theory and pharmacology for nurses.

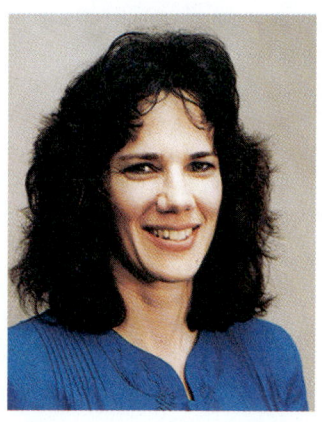

Shannon Ruff Dirksen, RN, PhD

Shannon Dirksen received her Bachelor of Science in nursing from Arizona State University and Master of Science and PhD in nursing from the University of Arizona. In her 12 years of teaching at the graduate and undergraduate levels, she has taught at Edith Cowan University (Western Australia), Intercollegiate Center for Nursing Education (Spokane, Washington), University of New Mexico, and Arizona State University. She currently teaches nursing research and management and leadership. For the past 14 years, she has been actively involved in oncology research, focusing on adjustment in Caucasian and Hispanic patients with melanoma and breast cancer and cancer prevention in the community. She is the primary author of the *Clinical Companion to Medical-Surgical Nursing,* which accompanies this book.

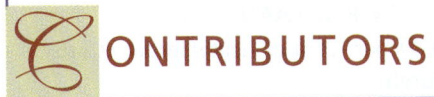

CONTRIBUTORS

CHARLOTTE R. ABBINK, RN, PhD
Professor Emeritus
University of New Mexico College of Nursing
Albuquerque, New Mexico

ELIZABETH A. AYELLO, RN, PhD, CS, CETN
Clinical Assistant Professor
Division of Nursing
New York University
New York, New York

MARILYN ROSSMAN BARTUCCI, MSN, RN, CS, CCTC
Head Nurse Manager, Transplant Center
University Hospitals of Cleveland
Cleveland, Ohio

PATRICIA BATES, RN, BSN, CURN
Staff Nurse, Urology
Kaiser Permanente
Portland, Oregon

CATHERINE M. BENDER, RN, PhD
Assistant Professor
University of Pittsburgh School of Nursing/
University of Pittsburgh Cancer Institute
Pittsburgh, Pennsylvania

CHUCK BIDDLE, RN, CRNA, PhD
Associate Professor
Department of Anesthesiology
Dartmouth Hitchcock Medical Center
Lebanon, New Hampshire

DONNA ZIMMARO BLISS, PhD, RN, CCRN
Assistant Professor, School of Nursing
University of Minnesota
Minneapolis, Minnesota

ELEANOR F. BOND, PhD, RN
Associate Professor, School of Nursing
University of Washington
Seattle, Washington

LUCY A. BRADLEY-SPRINGER, RN, PhD
Co-Director, New Mexico AIDS Education and
Training Center
Assistant Professor
University of New Mexico School of Medicine
Albuquerque, New Mexico

BARBARA BRILLHART, RN, PhD, CRRN, FNP-C
Associate Professor, College of Nursing
Arizona State University
Tempe, Arizona

GILLIAN BRUNIER, RN, MScN, CNEPH(C)
Clinical Nurse Specialist/Nurse Practitioner, Nephrology
Sunnybrook and Women's College Health Science Centre
Toronto, Ontario
Canada

MELISSA BUSH, RN, MSN
Nurse Practitioner
Dr. Gary J. Silverman
Scottsdale, Arizona

KATHRYN ANN CAUDELL, RN, PhD, OCN
Assistant Professor
University of New Mexico College of Nursing
Albuquerque, New Mexico

CECILIA C. DAIL, BS, MT (ASCP)
Instructor, Medical Laboratory Sciences
Department of Pathology, School of Medicine
University of New Mexico
Albuquerque, New Mexico

LEE DANIELSON, BS, MT (ASCP)
Instructor, Medical Laboratory Sciences
Department of Pathology, School of Medicine
University of New Mexico
Albuquerque, New Mexico

JENNIE DAUGHERTY, MSN, RN, CS
Clinical Nurse Specialist
Edwards Eve Clinic
Nashville, Tennessee

PATRICIA J. DAVIES, RN, MSN
Pulmonary Clinical Nurse Specialist
Primary Teacher/Instructor
University of Pittsburgh School of Nursing
Pittsburgh, Pennsylvania

JULIE M. DAX, MSN, RN
Critical Care Nurse Educator
University Hospital
Albuquerque, New Mexico

ANNE M. DEVNEY, EdD, RN
Director, Health Services
College of Lake County
Grayslake, Illinois

SHANNON RUFF DIRKSEN, RN, PhD
Associate Professor
College of Nursing
Arizona State University
Tempe, Arizona

ELLEN STOETZNER DUKE, RN, MSN
Nursing Instructor
Angelina College Nursing Program
Lufkin, Texas

LAURA DULSKI, RN, MSN
Staff Nurse
Rush-Presbyterian St. Luke's Medical Center
Chicago, Illinois

PATSY ORTH DUPHORNE, RN, MN
Assistant Professor
College of Nursing
University of New Mexico
Albuquerque, New Mexico

TANA DURNBAUGH, RNCS, EdD
Professor of Nursing
College of Lake County
Grayslake, Illinois

RACHEL ELROD, RN, MS
Professor of Nursing
Front Range Community College
Westminster, Colorado
University of Phoenix-Colorado Campus
Aurora, Colorado

SUSAN FLAGLER, DNS, RNC (WHCNP)
Associate Professor
School of Nursing
University of Washington
Seattle, Washington

LINDA B. HAAS, PhC, RN, CDE
Endocrinology Clinical Nurse Specialist
VA Puget Sound HCS, Seattle Division
Seattle, Washington

MARGARET MCLEAN HEITKEMPER, RN, PhD, FAAN
Professor, Biobehavioral Nursing and Health Systems
School of Nursing
University of Washington
Seattle, Washington

PATRICIA ROBERTSON HERCULES, RN, MS
Director, Nursing Support and Patient Education Department
The Methodist Hospital
Houston, Texas

CYNTHIA L. HERMEY, RN, MN, CCRN
Manager of Cardiac and Intensive Care Services
Oconee Memorial Hosptial
Seneca, South Carolina

MARGARET M. HICKEY, RN, MSN, MS, OCN, CORLN
Clinical Director
Tulane University Comprehensive Cancer Center
New Orleans, Louisiana

LESLIE A. HOFFMAN, RN, PhD, FAAN
Professor and Chair, Department of Acute/Tertiary Care
University of Pittsburgh
Pittsburgh, Pennsylvania

MIMA M. HORNE, RN, MSN, CDE
Diabetes Clinical Nurse Specialist
New Hanover Regional Medical Center
Wilmington, North Carolina

MARY ANN HOUSE-FANCHER, RN, ARNP, MSN
Nurse Practitioner, Cardiothoracic Surgery
University of Florida
Gainesville, Florida

BETTYANN HUTCHISSON, RN, BSN, CNOR
Nurse Clinician, Perioperative Education
The Methodist Hospital
Houston, Texas

LINDA WITEK JANUSEK, RN, PhD
Professor, School of Nursing
Loyola University of Chicago
Chicago, Illinois

CAROLYN I. JOHNS, RN, CANP, MS
Adult Nurse Practitioner, Cardiology
Lovelace Health Systems
Albuquerque, New Mexico

ANNE M. JONES, MN, RNC
Medical Surgical Clinical Nurse Specialist
Providence Saint Joseph Medical Center
Burbank, California

THE REVEREND BARBARA GAIL JORELMAN, BA, MDIV
President, New Mexico Health Decisions
Albuquerque, New Mexico

MARY KERR, RN, PhD, FAAN
Associate Professor, School of Nursing
Director for Center for Nursing Research
University of Pittsburgh
Pittsburgh, Pennsylvania

CINDY J. KNIPE, RN
Care Delivery Director
Wishard Regional Burn Center
Wishard Memorial Hospital
Indianapolis, Indiana

NANCY STOETZNER KUPPER, RN, MSN
Associate Professor
Tarrant County Junior College
Fort Worth, Texas

BARBARA S. LEVINE, PhD, RN, CRNP, CS
Clinical Director
Gerontological Nursing
Assistant Professor
School of Nursing
University of Pennsylvania Health System
Philadelphia, Pennsylvania

SHARON MANTIK LEWIS, RN, PhD, FAAN
Professor, College of Nursing
Research Associate Professor, Department of Pathology
University of New Mexico
Albuquerque, New Mexico

KATHLEEN OARE LINDELL, RN, MSN
Pulmonary Clinical Nurse Specialist
University of Pennsylvania Health System
Philadelphia, Pennsylvania

PHYLLIS LISANTI, RN, PhD
Undergraduate Program Director
Clinical Associate Professor
New York University-Division of Nursing
New York, New York

KIM LITWACK, PhD, RN, FAAN, CFNP
Associate Professor
University of New Mexico College of Nursing
Albuquerque, New Mexico

CAROL O. LONG, RN, PhD
Assistant Professor
College of Nursing
Arizona State University
Tempe, Arizona

JANIS LUFT, RN, MSN
UCSF/Stanford Women's Health
San Francisco, California

NANCY J. MACMULLEN, RNC, PhD
Associate Professor
Rush University College of Nursing
Chicago, Illinois

LINDA C. GRIEGO MARTINEZ, MSN, RN, CS, CCRN
Cardiology Care Manager
Presbyterian Heart Group
Albuquerque, New Mexico

KATHERYN E. MCCASH, RNC, MSN
Instructor
University of New Mexico College of Nursing
Albuquerque, NM

CINDY MEREDITH, RN, MSN
Adjunct Lecturer in Nursing
Jackson Community College
Jackson, Michigan

DIANE H. MICHALEC, RN, MSN, CCRN, CNRN
Clinical Systems Analyst IV
University of Pittsburgh Medical Center
Pittsburgh, Pennsylvania

LORENE NEWBERRY, RN, MS, CEN
Clinical Nurse Specialist—Emergency Services
WellStar Health System
Marietta, Georgia

NOREEN HEER NICOL, RN, MS, FNP
Director of Nursing
Dermatology Clinical Specialist/Nurse Practitioner
National Jewish Medical and Research Center;
Clinical Senior Instructor
University of Colorado, School of Nursing
Denver, Colorado

ANN M. O'MARA, RN, PhD, AOCN
Fellow, Division of Cancer Prevention and Control
National Cancer Institute, National Institutes of Health
Bethesda, Maryland;
Assistant Professor, University of Maryland School of Nursing
Baltimore, Maryland

JUDY OZUNA, RN, MN, ARNP, CNRN
Clinical Nurse Specialist in Neurology
Veterans Affairs Medical Center
Clinical Assistant Professor
Biobehavioral Nursing and Health Systems
University of Washington School of Nursing
Seattle, Washington

ANITA M. RALSTIN, RN, MS, CS, CNP
Family Nurse Practitioner
New Mexico Heart Institute, Surgery Division
Albuquerque, New Mexico

LYNN F. REINKE, RN-CS, MSN
Adult Nurse Practitioner, Pulmonary
VA Medical Center
Milwaukee, Wisconsin

SUSAN C. RUDA, RN, MS, ONC
Clinical Nurse Specialist
Parkview Musculoskeletal Institute
Palos Heights, Illinois

ANNE MARIE RUSZKOWSKI, RN, BSN
Director of Nursing
Deparment of Dermatology
Columbia University
New York, New York

LINDA SAWCHUK, RN, ARNP, CETN
Enterostomal Therapy Nurse
Virginia Mason Medical Center
Seattle, Washington

SARAH C. SMITH, RN, MA, CRNO
Educational Associate/Advanced Practice Nurse
Department of Ophthalmology
The University of Iowa Hospitals and Clinics
Iowa City, Iowa

LAURIE A. SOINE, RN, MN, ARNP
Clinical Nurse Specialist/Nurse Practitioner
University of Washington Medical Center
Seattle, Washington

KATHLEEN C. SOLOTKIN, RN, MSN
Trauma Nurse Coordinator
Wishard Memorial Hospital
Indianapolis, Indiana

SALLY SPERRY STEEN, BS, MT (ASCP)
Instructor, Medical Laboratory Sciences
Department of Pathology, School of Medicine
University of New Mexico
Albuquerque, New Mexico

ROBERTA A. STROHL, RN, MN, AOCN
Clinical Associate Professor
Department of Radiation Oncology
University of Maryland at Baltimore
Baltimore, Maryland

VIRGINIA VALENTINE, RN, MSN, CDE
CEO and Clinical Specialist
Diabetes Network, Inc.
Albuquerque, New Mexico

TRISCH VAN SCIVER, RN, MS, PCNS, CFNP, DOM
Nurse Practitioner
Lovelace Health Systems
Albuquerque, New Mexico

JOAN STEHLE WERNER, RN, DNS
Professor, Department of Adult Health and Illness
Oregon Health Sciences University
School of Nursing
Portland, Oregon

UNA E. WESTFALL, PhD, RN
Professor, School of Nursing
Oregon Health Sciences University
Portland, Oregon

MARIE BAKITAS WHEDON, RN, MS, AOCN, FAAN
Research Assistant Professor
Norris Cotton Cancer Center
Dartmouth-Hitchcock Medical Center
Lebanon, New Hampshire

MARY E. WILBUR, RN, MSN
Continuum of Care Manager
Medical University of South Carolina
Charleston, South Carolina

DIANA J. WILKIE, PhD, RN, AOCN, FAAN
Associate Professor
School of Nursing
University of Washington
Seattle, Washington

JOYCE M. YASKO, RN, PhD, FAAN
Associate Director for Clinical Network Administration
University of Pittsburgh Cancer Institute
Professor of Oncology Nursing
University of Pittsburgh School of Nursing
Pittsburgh, Pennsylvania

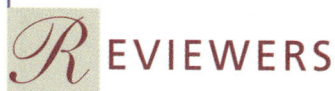

REVIEWERS

ARIS ANDREWS, RN, MS
Hastings, Nebraska

KATHLEEN C. ASHTON, RN, PhD, CS
Camden, New Jersey

MARY BAIRD, RN, MN, ARNP
Seattle, Washington

DEBRA A. BANCROFT, RN, MSN, FNP-C
Milwaukee, Wisconsin

LINDA BERNARD, RN, MS
Chicago, Illinois

DONNA BERRY, RN, PhD, AOCN
Seattle, Washington

CAROL BLAINEY, RN, MN
Seattle, Washington

PATRICIA A. BLISSITT, RN, MSN, CCRN, CNRN, CCM
Seattle, Washington

DIANE BRITT, RN, MN, CS, CDE
Seattle, Washington

GILLIAN BRUNIER, MScN, RN, CNeph (C)
Toronto, Ontario, Canada

KATHRYN ANN CAUDELL, RN, PhD, OCN
Albuquerque, New Mexico

ANN TYLER CHADWICK, MN, RN, CCRN
Seattle, Washington

ELIZABETH CHAPMAN, RN, MS, CCRN
Long Beach, Mississippi

KERRY H. CHEEVER, RN, PhD, CEN
Milwaukee, Wisconsin

SHARON G. CHILDS, RN, MS, CRNP, CS, CEN, ONC
Baltimore, Maryland

CHRISTINE CHMIELEWSKI, RN, MS, CRNP
Philadelphia, Pennsylvania

EVELYN M. CLINGERMAN, RN, MS
Rochester, Michigan

REBECCA CRANE, RN, PhD, AOCN
Santa Monica, California

JANET T. CRIMLISK, RN, MS, NP, CS
Boston, Massachusetts

MARJORIE CYPRESS, C-ANP, CDE, RN
Albuquerque, New Mexico

DEBORAH K. DRUMMONDS, RN, MN, CCRN, CEN
Milledgeville, Georgia

SHEILA A. DUNN, RN, MSN, C-ANP
St. Louis, Missouri

SHEENA FERGUSON, RN, MSN, CCRN
Albuquerque, New Mexico

DIANE M. FESLER, RN, MSN, PhD Candidate
DeKalb, Illinois

LINDA MONFORE FLUKE, RN, MN, ARNP
Seattle, Washington

REBECCA FRUGE, RN, MN
San Juan, Puerto Rico

MICHELE GEIGER-BRONSKY, RN, MSN, CS, FAACVPR
Manitowoc, Wisconsin

MARGARET GRADY, RN, MS
Albuquerque, New Mexico

MIKEL GRAY, RN, PhD, CUNP, CCCN, FAAN
Charlottesville, Virginia

PAULINE MCKINNEY GREEN, RN, PhD
Washington, DC

SHIRLEY M. GULLO, RN, MSN, OCN
Cleveland, Ohio

JAMES P. HALLORAN, RN, MSN, OCN, ANP
Houston, Texas

SUSAN HARRINGTON, RN, MN, ARNP
Seattle, Washington

STEPHINE HEITKEMPER, RN, ARNP
Olympia, Washington

KATHRYN HENNESSY, RN, MS, CNSN
Deerfield, Illinois

MARY JO HOLECHEK, RN, MS, CRNP, CS, CNN
Baltimore, Maryland

ALICIA M. HORKAN, RN, MSN, CEN
Moultrie, Georgia

KATHERINE A. HOWE, RN, MSN, MEd
Toledo, Ohio

MARGUERITE JACKSON, RN, PhD, CIC, FAAN
San Diego, California

MONICA JARRETT, RN, PhD
Seattle, Washington

JANET KATZ, RNC, MSN
Spokane, Washington

JUDY KAYE, RN, CNRN, CCRN, ANP, GNP, CS, PhDc
Augusta, Georgia

JUDY KNIGHTON, RN, MScN
Toronto, Ontario, Canada

JOY KNOPP, RN, MN, ARNP
Seattle, Washington

BARBARA S. LEVINE, RN, PhD, CRNP, CS
Philadelphia, Pennsylvania

KIM LITWACK, PhD, RN, FAAN, CFNP
Albuquerque, New Mexico

CAROL O. LONG, RN, PhD
Tempe, Arizona

MARCI LOVETT, RN, MN, FNP, CS
Los Angeles, California

MARGARET LUNNEY, PhD, RN, CS
Staten Island, New York

HOLLY EVANS MADISON, RN, MS
Manchester, Vermont

ELYSE B. MANDELL, MSN, RNCS
Boston, Massachusetts

KAREN MARCH, RN, MN, CNRN, CCRN
Seattle, Washington

DEBORAH L. MARTIN, RN, MN
Austin, Texas

KATHERINE E. MATAS, RN, PhD
Kalamazoo, Michigan

MARTHA A. MELCHER, RN, GNP
Port Angeles, Washington

MARY S. MERCHANT, RN, MSN, FNP
Charleston, South Carolina

CARMELLA MORAN, RN, MSN
Naperville, Illinois

MARY LOU MUWASWES, RN, MS
San Francisco, California

BETSY NIELSEN-OMEIS, RN, BSN
San Antonio, Texas

JANE PARKS, RN, MSN
Hastings, Nebraska

JILL H. PENDARVIS, RNC, MA, CNOR
Fort Walton Beach, Florida

JANICE POST-WHITE, RN, PhD
Minneapolis, Minnesota

VIRGINIA PRINTZ-FEDDERSEN, RNC, MSN, CNS, CNOR, CNRN
Albuquerque, New Mexico

KIMBERLY L. QUINN, RN, MS, CCRN
Baltimore, Maryland

DENNIS ROSS, RN, PhD
Castleton, Vermont

DEBORAH L. ROUSH, RN, MSN
Valdosta, Georgia

PAUL RUSTON, RN, BS
Warrenville, Illinois

LINDA SCHAKENBACH, RN, MSN, CS, CCRN, CETN
Annandale, Virginia

DARLENE F. SCHELPER, RN, MSN, CEN, RNC
Hershey, Pennsylvania

SUZANNE SHAFFER, MN, RN, AOCN
Kansas City, Kansas

LISA ANDERSON SHAW, RNC, MSN, MA
Chicago, Illinois

GEOFF SHUSTER, RN, PhD
Albuquerque, New Mexico

SANDRA SOMMA, RN, BSN
New Haven, Connecticut

SUSAN B. STILLWELL, RN, MSN
Tempe, Arizona

PRISCILLA ANN TAYLOR, RN, MN, CGRN
Tacoma, Washington

TRISCH VAN SCIVER, RN, MS, PCNS, CFNP, DOM
Albuquerque, New Mexico

KATHLEEN DORMAN WAGNER, RN, MSN, CS
Lexington, Kentucky

EILEEN WALSH, RN, MSN, CVN
Toledo, Ohio

JOYCE S. WILLENS, PhD, RN
Villanova, Pennsylvania

To the profession of nursing
and
to the important people in our lives

PREFACE TO THE INSTRUCTOR

The fifth edition of *Medical-Surgical Nursing: Assessment and Management of Clinical Problems* has been extensively revised to incorporate the most recent medical-surgical nursing information in an attractive, easy-to-use format. More than just a textbook, this is a comprehensive resource containing essential information that students need to prepare for lectures, classroom activities, examinations, clinical assignments, and comprehensive care of patients. In addition to the readable writing style and full-color illustrations, the text includes many special features to help students learn the most important medical-surgical nursing content. This edition highlights this content for today's nursing students, including patient teaching, gerontology, collaborative care, cultural and ethnic considerations, nutrition, community and home care, nursing research, and much more.

The comprehensive and accurate content, special features, attractive layout, and student-friendly writing style have combined to make this the number one medical-surgical nursing textbook used in more nursing schools around the country than any other medical-surgical textbook.

The strengths of the first four editions have been retained, including the use of the nursing process as an organizational theme for nursing management and a commitment to support the role of nurses on the home health care team. Numerous new features have been added to address some of the rapid changes in practice. Contributors have again been selected for their acknowledged excellence in specific content areas; one or more specialists in the subject area have thoroughly reviewed each chapter to increase accuracy. The editors have undertaken final rewriting and editing to achieve internal consistency. All efforts were directed toward building on the strengths of the previous edition while preparing an even more effective new edition.

ORGANIZATION

Content is organized into two major divisions. The first division, Section One (Chapters 1 through 10), discusses general concepts related to adult patients. The second division, Sections Two through Twelve (Chapters 11 through 64), presents nursing assessment and nursing management of medical-surgical problems.

The various body systems are grouped to reflect their interrelated functions. Each section is organized around two central themes: assessment and management. Chapters dealing with assessment of a body system include a discussion of the following:

1. A brief review of anatomy and physiology, focusing on information that will promote understanding of nursing care

2. Health history and noninvasive physical assessment skills to expand the knowledge base on which decisions are made

3. Common diagnostic studies, expected results, and related nursing responsibilities to provide easily accessible information

Chapters dealing with management of the various diseases and disorders focus on the etiology and pathophysiologic bases, clinical manifestations, diagnostic study results, collaborative care, and nursing management of diseases and disorders. The nursing management sections are organized into nursing assessment, nursing diagnoses, planning, nursing implementation, and evaluation. To emphasize the importance of patient care in various clinical settings, nursing implementation of all major health problems is organized by the following levels of care:

1. Health Promotion

2. Acute Intervention

3. Ambulatory and Home Care

SPECIAL FEATURES

- **Home health care/community-based care** is an ongoing theme throughout the text. Coverage has been significantly increased in the fifth edition, including a new chapter (Chapter 2: Community-Based Nursing and Home Health Care) and Patient and Family Home Care Guides appearing throughout the text. Ambulatory and Home Care headings appear in Nursing Implementation sections. In addition, there are examples of clinical pathways—home care of diabetes mellitus and ostomy—that focus specifically on home health care.

- **Patient teaching** has also been emphasized in this edition. Coverage includes a new chapter (Chapter 6: Patient Teaching) and more than 50 Patient Teaching Guides and Patient and Family Teaching Guides throughout the text.

- **Collaborative care** is highlighted in this revision, including new Collaborative Care sections in all management chapters and more than 80 Collaborative Care tables throughout the text.

- **Gerontology** coverage includes Chapter 3: Adult Development and Chapter 4: Gerontologic Considerations and appears throughout the text under Gerontologic Considerations headings and in Gerontologic Differences in Assessment and Effects of Aging tables.

- **Nutrition** is highlighted throughout the book. Nutritional Therapy tables summarize nutritional interventions and promote healthy lifestyles in patients with various conditions.

■ **Nursing management** is presented in a consistent and comprehensive format, which now includes Evaluation headings where appropriate. In addition, 78 Nursing Care Plans appear in management chapters. These are thoroughly updated to incorporate (1) current NANDA nursing diagnoses, including the problem, etiologic statement, and defining characteristics; (2) specific nursing interventions with rationales; (3) expected patient outcomes; and (4) collaborative problems.

■ A new chapter on **alternative and complementary therapies** addresses timely issues in today's health care settings related to nontraditional therapies.

■ **Nursing research** encourages application of research into clinical practice. Research Implications for Nursing Practice boxes appear throughout the text, and Nursing Research Issues at the end of management chapters present possible research questions to be used for research studies.

■ **Cultural and ethnic considerations** information is integrated into the text and appears in special boxes highlighting important issues related to the nursing care of various ethnic populations.

■ **Ethical Dilemmas** boxes appear in management chapters to promote critical thinking for timely and sensitive issues that nursing students may deal with in practice. Each box contains a discussion of ethical and legal principles.

■ **Clinical Pathways** for selected medical-surgical disorders show how hospitals and home health agencies are implementing collaborative care.

■ **Emergency Management** tables outline the emergency treatment of health problems most likely to require emergency intervention.

■ **Common Assessment Abnormalities** tables in assessment chapters alert the nurse to frequently encountered abnormalities and their possible etiologies.

■ **Nursing Assessment** tables summarize the key subjective and objective data related to common diseases. Subjective data are organized by functional health patterns.

■ **Health History** tables in assessment chapters present key questions to ask patients related to a specific disease or disorder.

LEARNING AIDS

✔ Learning Objectives beginning each chapter help students focus on the key information for that body system or disorder.

✔ Review Questions at the end of each chapter help students learn the important points in the chapter. Answers are provided in an appendix so that the review questions serve as a self-study tool.

✔ Critical Thinking Exercises appearing at the end of nursing management chapters include Case Studies with Critical Thinking Questions for clinical application, as well as Nursing Research Issues.

✔ Resources at the end of each chapter contain information about nursing and health care organizations that provide patient teaching and disease and disorder information. Resources include Internet sites to help students find current information online.

Media learning tools provided free with the text include the following:

✔ The CD-ROM packaged with this text contains overviews of common diseases and disorders, key terms, case studies, and review questions to help students apply this challenging content. This special icon 🌐 appears in the margin of the text to designate content areas where students are encouraged to use their free CD-ROM for further self-study.

✔ MERLIN The MERLIN website customized for this book features WebLinks for each chapter of the book and Content Updates by the authors to keep students and instructors informed on the most current medical-surgical nursing information. Be sure to visit the site at www.mosby.com/MERLIN/medsurg_lewis

ANCILLARIES

The fifth edition ancillary package has been extensively revised to include even more creative and comprehensive materials to aid instructors and students.

■ **Clinical Companion to Medical-Surgical Nursing,** 2nd edition, presents more than 300 common medical-surgical conditions and procedures in a concise, alphabetical format for quick clinical reference. Designed for portability, this valuable reference includes the essential, need-to-know information for medical-surgical nursing practice. This edition features an attractive and functional two-color internal design, as well as an increased emphasis on patient teaching.

■ **Instructor's Resource Kit** remains the most comprehensive set of instructor's materials available, containing suggested lecture strategies, case studies with critical thinking questions, answers to worksheets included in the *Study Guide*, a test bank with more than 1000 questions with coded answers, and worksheets to accompany *Mosby's Medical-Surgical Nursing Video Series*.

■ **Test Bank** includes more than 1200 questions with NCLEX-coded answers.

■ **Electronic Image Collection** is a CD-ROM containing hundreds of full-color images from the text for use in lectures and to import into PowerPoint.

■ **Study Guide** contains extensive review and testing material that has been thoroughly updated to reflect the revision of the textbook. It features a wide variety of clinically relevant exercises and activities, including fill-in-the-blank worksheets, anatomy identification review, true-false questions, critical thinking activities, crossword puzzles, case studies, matching exercises, word scrambles, and multiple-choice questions in NCLEX format. Answers to all questions are included in the back of the *Study Guide* to provide students with immediate feedback as they study.

■ **Virtual Clinical Excursions** is an exciting and innovative new teaching and learning tool. The dynamic CD-ROM presents true-to-life simulations of clinical practice in a "virtual hospital" setting. The accompanying workbook contains case-based activities prepared specifically for this text. This is an excellent way for students to apply what they learn from the text and to foster critical thinking skills.

ACKNOWLEDGMENTS

The editors are especially grateful to many people at Mosby who assisted with this major revision effort. In particular, we wish to thank the team of Sally Schrefer, Jeanne Allison, Kristin Geen, Dana Peick, Catherine Albright, and Amy Buxton. In addition, we want to thank the marketing team of Janet Blanner and Tom Wilhelm.

We would like to thank Idolia Cox Collier for her ideas, creativity, and hard work as co-editor on the first four editions of this book.

Our persevering typists have earned our special thanks and include Christa Cooper and Elizabeth Miller. Kay McCash provided invaluable assistance as a consultant on nursing diagnoses and revision of the nursing care plans. Pat O'Brien worked diligently on the *Study Guide* and provided excellent new material for the *Test Bank, Instructor's Resource Kit,* and CD-ROM to accompany the text.

We are particularly indebted to the nurses and student nurses who have put their faith in our book to assist them on their path to excellence. The increasing use of this book throughout the United States and Canada has been gratifying. We appreciate the many users who have shared their comments and suggestions on the previous editions.

We also wish to thank our contributors and reviewers for their conscientious attention to detail throughout the revision process. We sincerely hope that this book will assist both students and clinicians in practicing truly professional nursing.

Sharon Lewis

Margaret McLean Heitkemper

Shannon Ruff Dirksen

PREFACE TO THE STUDENT

Medical-Surgical Nursing: Assessment and Management of Clinical Problems was developed to provide you, today's busy nursing student, with the most important medical-surgical nursing information in an attractive, easy-to-use format. The authors know how important it is that you have a resource containing the essential information you need to prepare for lectures, classroom activities, examinations, clinical assignments, and overall care of your patients. This bestselling text is carefully designed to meet these needs.

Not only will this book help you to succeed in your studies, it will also prepare you for advanced study and practice in clinical settings. In addition to the readable writing style and full-color illustrations, it includes many special features to help you study and learn the most important medical-surgical nursing concepts. Some of these features include:

✔ **Learning Objectives** beginning each chapter to help you focus on the key information.

✔ **Review Questions** at the end of each chapter to help you learn the important points in the chapter. Answers are provided in an appendix so that the review questions serve as a self-study tool.

✔ **Critical Thinking Exercises** at the end of nursing management chapters include Case Studies with Critical Thinking Questions useful for clinical application and Nursing Research Issues useful for research projects.

✔ **Special tables and boxes** summarizing information that is key to understanding disease management and providing effective patient care. These features include:

- **Patient Teaching Guides**
- **Patient & Family Home Care Guides**
- **Ethical Dilemmas**
- **Research Implications for Nursing Practice**
- **Cultural & Ethnic Considerations**
- **Nursing Care Plans** and many others.

✔ **Resources at the end of each chapter** containing information about nursing and health care organizations that provide patient teaching and disease and disorder information. Resources include Internet sites to help you find current information online.

In addition to the text, here are some additional learning tools provided free:

✔ **CD-ROM** packaged with this text containing overviews of common diseases, key terms, case studies, and review questions to help you apply this challenging content. This special icon appears in the margins of the text to indicate areas where you may want to access your CD-ROM for further content review.

✔ **MERLIN website** customized for this book featuring WebLinks for each chapter of the book and Content Updates by the authors to keep you informed on the most current medical-surgical nursing information. Be sure to visit the site at www.mosby.com/MERLIN/medsurg_lewis

And do not forget the **Study Guide** to accompany this book. This valuable study tool contains extensive review and testing material that has been thoroughly updated to reflect the revision of the book. It features a wide variety of clinically relevant exercises and activities, including:

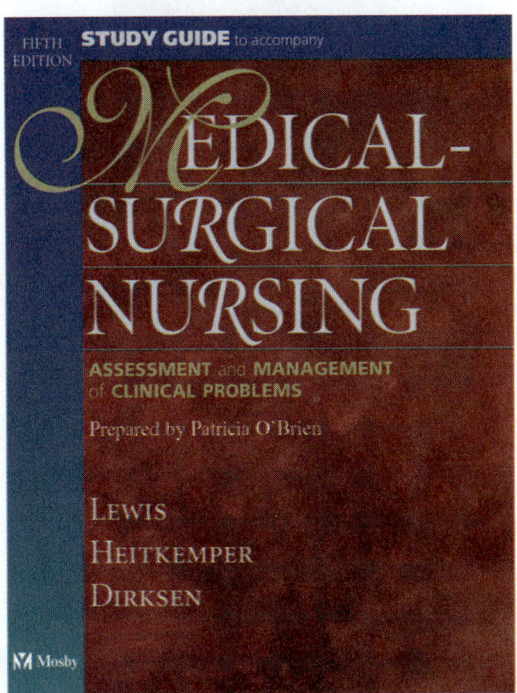

✔ Fill-in-the-blank worksheets

✔ Anatomy identification review

✔ True-false questions

✔ Critical thinking activities

✔ Crossword puzzles

✔ Case studies

✔ Matching exercises

✔ Word scrambles

✔ Multiple-choice questions in NCLEX format

Answers to all questions are included in the back of the *Study Guide* to provide immediate feedback as you study.

Also accompanying this text is the *Clinical Companion to Medical-Surgical Nursing,* 2nd edition. This handy reference presents more than 300 common medical-surgical conditions and procedures in a concise, alphabetical format for quick clinical reference. Designed for portability, it includes the essential, need-to-know information for medical-surgical nursing practice.

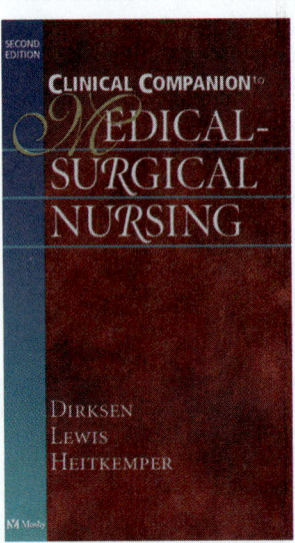

Be sure to check out **Virtual Clinical Excursions,** an exciting and innovative new study tool. The CD-ROM presents true-to-life simulations of clinical practice in a "virtual hospital" setting. The accompanying workbook contains case-based activities prepared specifically for this text. This is an excellent way to practice what you are learning in the text, and to apply your knowledge to clinical settings.

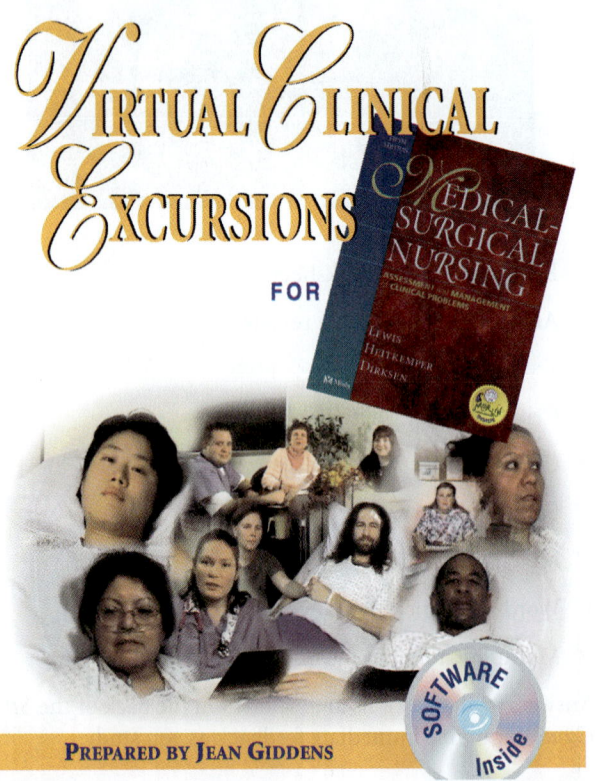

The authors and Mosby hope that you find this book helpful as you continue your nursing education! Please feel free to contact us anytime with feedback about the book.

DETAILED CONTENTS

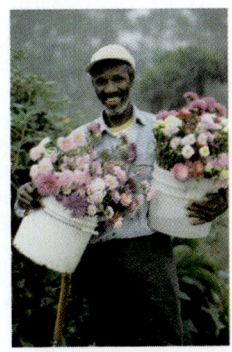

SECTION 1

GENERAL CONCEPTS OF NURSING PRACTICE

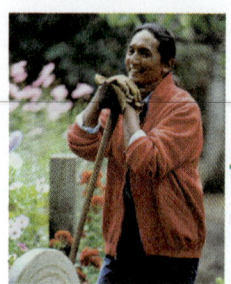

SECTION 2

PATHOPHYSIOLOGIC MECHANISMS OF DISEASE

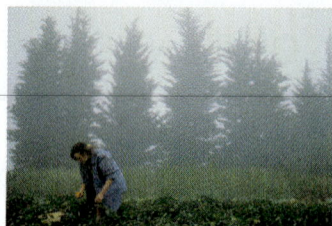

SECTION 3

THE SURGICAL EXPERIENCE

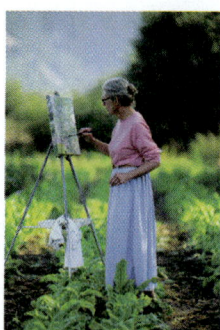

SECTION 4

PROBLEMS RELATED TO ALTERED SENSORY INPUT

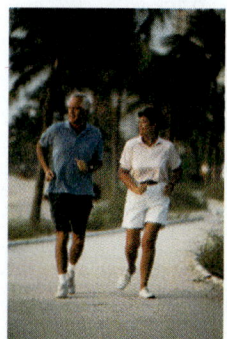

SECTION **5**

PROBLEMS OF OXYGENATION: VENTILATION

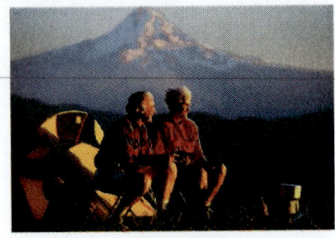

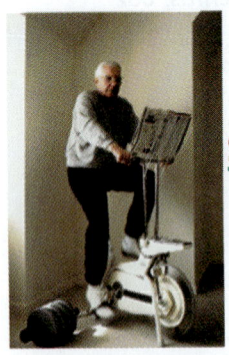

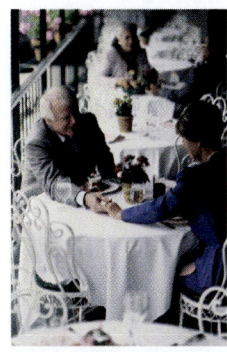

SECTION 8

PROBLEMS OF INGESTION, DIGESTION, ABSORPTION, AND ELIMINATION

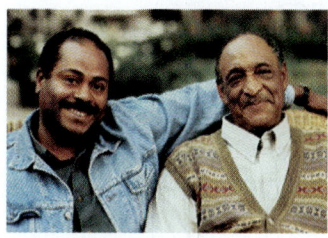

SECTION 9

PROBLEMS OF URINARY FUNCTION

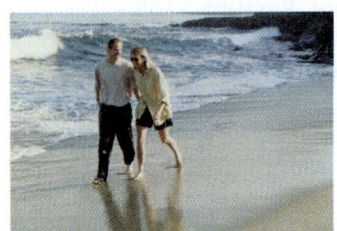

SECTION 10

PROBLEMS RELATED TO REGULATORY MECHANISMS

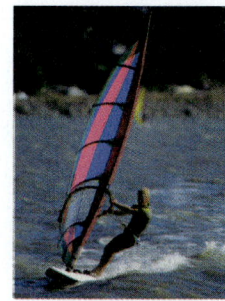

SECTION 11

PROBLEMS RELATED TO MOVEMENT AND COORDINATION

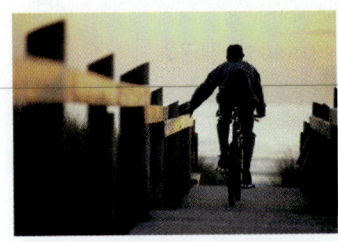

NURSING CARE IN SPECIALIZED SETTINGS

NURSING CARE PLANS

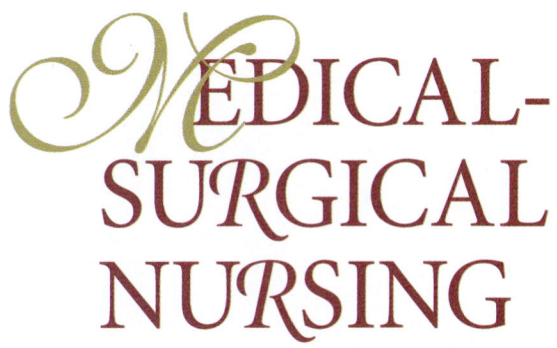

MEDICAL-SURGICAL NURSING

ASSESSMENT and MANAGEMENT of
CLINICAL PROBLEMS

PROBLEMS OF INGESTION, DIGESTION, ABSORPTION, AND ELIMINATION

SECTION OUTLINE

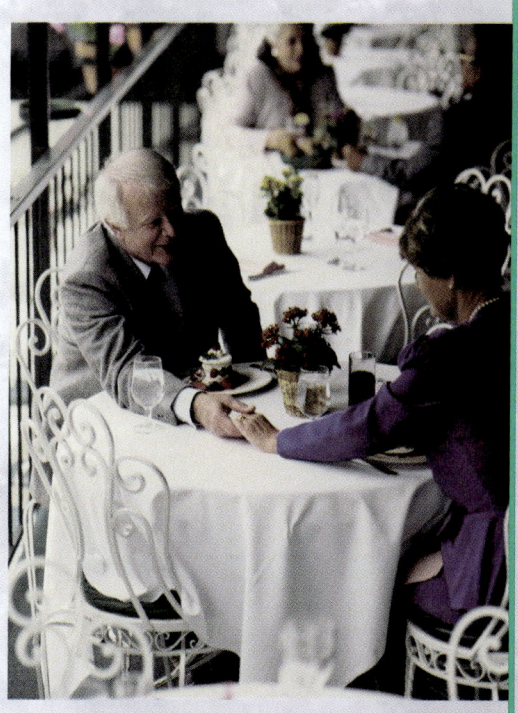

PROBLEMS OF INGESTION, DIGESTION, ABSORPTION AND ELIMINATION

SECTION OUTLINE

37 NURSING ASSESSMENT
Gastrointestinal System

Rachel Elrod

www.mosby.com/MERLIN/medsurg_lewis

LEARNING OBJECTIVES

1. Describe the structures and functions of the organs of the gastrointestinal tract.
2. Describe the structures and functions of the liver, gallbladder, biliary tract, and pancreas.
3. Explain the processes of ingestion, digestion, absorption, and elimination.
4. Explain the processes of biliary metabolism, bile production, and bile excretion.
5. Describe age-related changes in the gastrointestinal system and differences in assessment findings.
6. Identify the significant subjective and objective data related to the gastrointestinal system that should be obtained from a patient.
7. Describe the appropriate techniques used in the physical assessment of the gastrointestinal system.
8. Differentiate normal from common abnormal findings of a physical assessment of the gastrointestinal system.
9. Describe the purpose, significance of results, and nursing responsibilities related to diagnostic studies of the gastrointestinal system.

The main function of the gastrointestinal (GI) system is to supply nutrients to body cells. This is accomplished through the processes of *ingestion* (taking in food), *digestion* (breakdown of food), and *absorption* (transfer of food products into circulation). *Elimination* is the process of excreting the waste products of digestion.

The GI system (also called the *digestive system*) consists of the GI tract and its associated organs and glands. Included in the GI tract are the mouth, esophagus, stomach, small intestine, large intestine, rectum, and anus. The associated organs are the liver, pancreas, and gallbladder (Fig. 37-1).

Psychologic or emotional factors, such as stress and anxiety, influence GI functioning in many people. Stress may be manifested as anorexia, epigastric and abdominal pain, or diarrhea. However, GI problems should never be solely attributed to psychologic factors. Organic and psychologically based problems can exist independently or concurrently. Physical factors, such as dietary intake, ingestion of alcohol and caffeine-containing products, cigarette smoking, and fatigue, may also affect GI function. Some organic diseases of the GI system, such as peptic ulcer disease and ulcerative colitis, may be aggravated by stress. Thus both physical and emotional factors affect GI function.

STRUCTURES AND FUNCTIONS OF THE GASTROINTESTINAL SYSTEM

The GI tract is a tube approximately 30 feet (9 m) long extending from the mouth to the anus. The entire tract is composed of four common layers. From the inside to the outside, these layers are (1) mucosa, (2) submucosa, (3) muscle, and (4) serosa (Fig. 37-2). In the esophagus the outer coat is fibrous tissue rather than serosa. The muscular coat consists of two layers: the circular (inner) and the longitudinal (outer).

The GI tract is innervated by the parasympathetic and the sympathetic branches of the autonomic nervous system. The parasympathetic system is mainly excitatory, and the sympathetic system is mainly inhibitory. For example, peristalsis is increased by parasympathetic stimulation and decreased by sympathetic stimulation. Pain is relayed through sensory fibers of the sympathetic nervous system.

The GI tract also has its own nervous system: the enteric, or intrinsic, nervous system. The enteric nervous system is composed of two nerve layers that lie between the mucosa and the circular muscle layer and the circular and longitudinal muscle layers. These neurons contribute to the coordination of GI motor and secretory activities. The enteric nervous system is also known as the "gut brain." It contains 10^8 neurons (about as many as the spinal cord) and has the ability to control movement and secretion of the GI tract.

The GI tract and accessory organs receive approximately 25% to 30% of the cardiac output. Circulation in the GI system is unique in that venous blood draining the GI tract organs empties into the portal vein, which then perfuses the liver. The upper portion of the GI tract receives its blood supply from the splanchnic artery. The small intestine receives its blood supply from branches of the hepatic and superior mesenteric artery. The large intestine receives its blood supply mainly from the superior and inferior mesenteric arteries. Because such a large percentage of the cardiac output perfuses these organs, the GI tract is a major source from which blood flow can be diverted during exercise or stress.

Reviewed by Linda Monfore Fluke, RN, MN, ARNP, Adult and Geriatric Nurse Practitioner, State of Washington, Seattle, Wash.

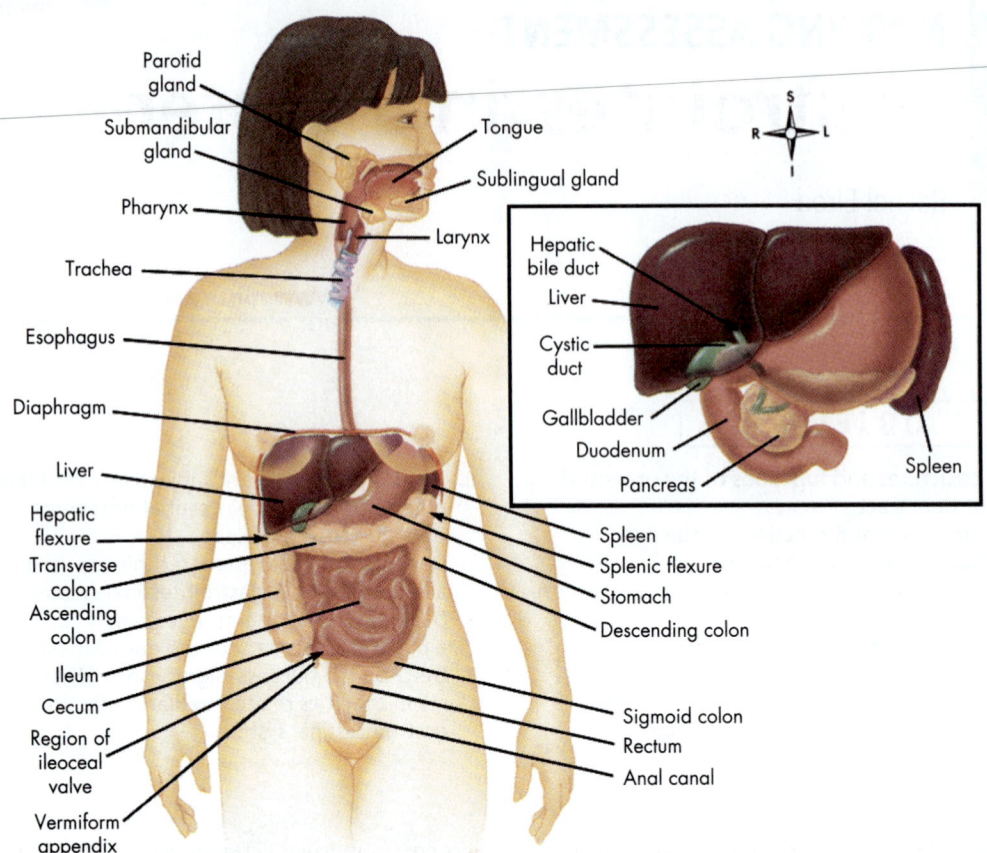

Fig. 37-1 Location of organs of the gastrointestinal system.

The two types of movement of the GI tract are mixing and propulsion. These movements are accomplished by segmentation and peristalsis. The secretions of the GI system consist of enzymes and hormones for digestion, mucus to provide protection and lubrication, and water and electrolytes.

The abdominal organs are almost completely covered by the peritoneum. The two layers of the peritoneum are the parietal, which lines the abdominal cavity wall, and the visceral, which covers the abdominal organs. The peritoneal cavity is the potential space between the parietal and visceral layers. The two folds of the peritoneum are the mesentery and omentum. The mesentery attaches the small intestine and part of the large intestine to the posterior abdominal wall and contains blood and lymph vessels. The lesser omentum goes from the lesser curvature of the stomach and upper duodenum to the liver, and the greater omentum hangs from the stomach over the intestines like an apron. The omentum contains fat and lymph nodes.

The primary functions of the GI system are (1) ingestion and propulsion (movement) of food, (2) digestion, (3) absorption, and (4) elimination. Each part of the GI system performs different activities to accomplish these functions.

Ingestion and Propulsion of Food

Ingestion is the intake of food. A person's appetite or desire to ingest food is a significant factor in how much food is eaten. Multiple factors are involved in the control of appetite. An appetite center is located in the hypothalamus. It is directly or indirectly stimulated by hypoglycemia, an empty stomach, de-

crease in body temperature, and input from higher brain centers. The sight, smell, and taste of food frequently stimulate appetite. Appetite may be inhibited by stomach distention, illness (especially accompanied by fever), hyperglycemia, nausea and vomiting, and certain drugs (e.g., amphetamines).

Deglutition (swallowing) is the mechanical component of ingestion. The organs involved in the deglutition of food are the mouth, pharynx, and esophagus.

Mouth. The mouth consists of the lips and oral (buccal) cavity. The lips surround the orifice of the mouth and function in speech. The roof of the oral cavity is formed by the hard and soft palate. The oral cavity contains the teeth, used in mastication (chewing), and the tongue. The tongue is a solid muscle mass and assists in mastication by keeping food between the teeth during chewing and moving the food to the back of the throat for swallowing (deglutition). Taste receptors are found on the sides and tip of the tongue. The tongue is also important in speech.

Within the oral cavity are three pairs of salivary glands: the parotid, submaxillary, and sublingual. These glands produce saliva, which consists of water, protein, mucin, inorganic salts, and salivary amylase. Approximately 1 liter of saliva is produced each day.

Pharynx. The pharynx is a musculomembranous tube that may be divided into the nasopharynx, oropharynx, and laryngeal pharynx. The mucous membrane of the pharynx is continuous with the nasal cavity, mouth, auditory tubes, and larynx. The oropharynx secretes mucus, which aids in swal-

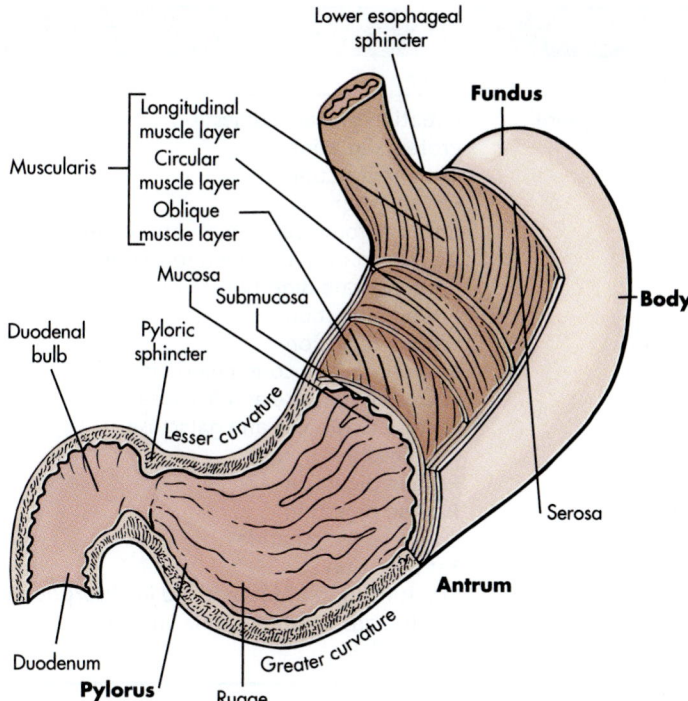

Fig. 37-2   Parts of the stomach.

lowing. The *epiglottis* is a lid of fibrocartilage that closes over the larynx during swallowing. During ingestion the oropharynx provides a route for the food from the mouth to the esophagus. When receptors in the oropharynx are stimulated by food or liquid, the swallowing reflex is initiated.

Esophagus.   The esophagus is a hollow, muscular tube that receives food from the pharynx and moves it to the stomach by peristaltic contractions. It is 9.2 to 10.0 inches (23 to 25 cm) long and 0.8 inches (2 cm) in diameter. The esophagus is located in the thoracic cavity and starts behind the trachea at the lower end of the pharynx and extends to the stomach. The upper one third of the esophagus is composed of striated skeletal muscle and the distal two thirds is composed of smooth muscle.

With swallowing, the upper esophageal sphincter (cricopharyngeal muscle) relaxes and a peristaltic wave moves the bolus into the esophagus. The muscular layers contract (peristalsis) and propel the food to the stomach. The lower esophageal sphincter (LES) at the distal end of the esophagus remains contracted except during swallowing, belching, or vomiting. The LES is an important barrier that prevents reflux of acidic gastric contents into the esophagus.

Digestion and Absorption

Mouth.   Digestion begins in the mouth. It involves both mechanical (mastication) and chemical digestion. Saliva is the first secretion involved in digestion, and its main function is to lubricate and soften the food mass, thus facilitating swallowing. Saliva contains amylase (ptyalin), which hydrolyzes starches to maltose. However, salivary amylase is not necessary for the digestion of carbohydrates.

Stomach.   The functions of the stomach are to store food, mix the food with gastric secretions, and empty contents into the small intestine at a rate at which digestion can occur. The stomach absorbs only small amounts of water, alcohol, electrolytes, and certain drugs.

The stomach lies obliquely in the epigastric, umbilical, and left hypochondriac regions of the abdomen (see Fig. 37-7). The shape and position of the stomach change based on the degree of gastric distention. It always contains gastric fluid and mucus. The three main parts of the stomach are the fundus, body, and antrum (see Fig. 37-2). The pylorus is a small portion of the antrum that lies proximal to the pyloric sphincter. Sphincter muscles (the LES and the pyloric sphincter) guard the entrance to and exit from the stomach. The cardiac orifice is the opening between the esophagus and the stomach.

The serous (outer) layer of the stomach is formed by the peritoneum. The muscular layer consists of the longitudinal (outer) layer, circular (middle) layer, and oblique (inner) layer. The mucosal layer forms folds called *rugae* that contain many small glands. In response to nutrient intake, these glands secrete most of the gastric juice. In the fundus the glands contain chief cells, which secrete pepsinogen, and parietal cells, which secrete hydrochloric acid, water, and intrinsic factor. The secretion of hydrochloric acid makes gastric juice acidic in comparison to other body fluids. This acidic pH aids in the protection against ingested organisms. Intrinsic factor promotes cobalamin absorption in the small intestine. Mucus is secreted by glands in the cardiac and pyloric areas.

Small Intestine.   The two primary functions of the small intestine are digestion and absorption. The small intestine is a coiled tube approximately 23 feet (7 m) in length and from 1 to 1.1 inch (2.5 cm to 2.8 cm) in diameter, diminishing in diameter at the lower end. It extends from the pylorus to the ileocecal valve. The small intestine is composed of the duodenum, jejunum, and ileum. The ileocecal valve, which separates the small intestine from the large intestine, prevents reflux of large intestine contents into the small intestine.

Table **37-1**	Gastrointestinal Secretions Related to Digestion		
Location	**Daily Amount (ml)**	**Secretion/Enzymes**	**Action**
Salivary glands	1000-1500	Salivary amylase (ptyalin)	Initiation of starch digestion
Stomach	2500	Pepsinogen	Protein digestion
		HCl	Protein digestion
		Lipase	Fat digestion
		Intrinsic factor	Essential for cobalamin absorption in ileum
Small intestine	3000	Enterokinase	Activation of trypsinogen to trypsin
		Amylase	Carbohydrate digestion
		Peptidases	Protein digestion
		Aminopeptidase	Protein digestion
		Maltase	Maltose to 2 glucose molecules
		Sucrase	Sucrose to glucose and fructose
		Lactase	Lactose to glucose and galactose
		Lipase	Fat digestion
Pancreas	700	Trypsinogen	Protein digestion
		Chymotrypsin	Protein digestion
		Amylase	Starch to disaccharides
		Lipase	Fat digestion
Liver and gallbladder	1000	Bile	Emulsification of fats and aid in absorption of fatty acids and fat-soluble vitamins (A, D, E, K)

The serous coat of the small intestine is formed by the peritoneum. The mucosa is thick, vascular, and glandular. The circular folds in the mucous and submucous layers provide a greater surface area for digestion and absorption.

The functional units of the small intestine are *villi.* They are present in the entire small intestine. Villi are minute, finger-like projections in the mucous membrane. They contain goblet cells that secrete mucus and epithelial cells that produce the intestinal digestive enzymes. The epithelial cells on the villi also have microvilli, which compose the brush border. Thus the presence of villi and microvilli greatly increases the surface area for absorption.

The digestive enzymes on the brush border of the microvilli chemically break down nutrients so that they can be absorbed. The villi are surrounded by the crypts of Lieberkühn, which contain the base columnar cells that are the stem cells for the other epithelial cell types. Brunner's glands in the submucosa of the duodenum secrete mucus.

Physiology of Digestion. *Digestion* is the physical and chemical breakdown of food into absorbable substances. Digestion in the GI tract is facilitated by the timely movement of food through the various organs and the secretion of specific enzymes. These enzymes break down foodstuffs to appropriate size particles for absorption (Table 37-1).

The process of digestion begins in the mouth, where the food is chewed, mechanically broken down, and mixed with saliva. The saliva lubricates the food. In addition, salivary amylase begins the breakdown of starch. Salivary gland secretion is stimulated by chewing movements and the sight, smell, thought, and taste of food. The food is swallowed and passes into the esophagus where peristaltic waves propel it to the stomach. No digestion or absorption occurs in the esophagus.

In the stomach the digestion of proteins begins with the release of pepsinogen from chief cells. The acidic environment of the stomach results in the conversion of pepsinogen to its active form, pepsin. Pepsin begins the initial breakdown of proteins.

In the stomach there is minimal digestion of starches and fats. The food is mixed with gastric secretions, which are under neural and hormonal control (Tables 37-2 and 37-3). The stomach also serves as a reservoir for food, which is slowly expelled into the small intestine. The length of time food remains in the stomach depends on the composition of the food, but average meals remain from 3 to 4 hours.

Digestion is completed in the small intestine, where carbohydrates are hydrolyzed to monosaccharides, fats to glycerol and fatty acids, and proteins to amino acids. The physical presence of chyme (food mixed with gastric secretions), along with its chemical nature in the small intestine, stimulates motility and secretion. Secretions involved in digestion include enzymes from the pancreas, bile from the liver (see Table 37-1), and intestinal secretions from glands in the small intestine. Both secretion and motility are under neural and hormonal control.

When food enters the stomach and small intestine, hormones are released into the bloodstream (see Table 37-3). The hormone secretin stimulates the pancreas to secrete fluid with a high concentration of bicarbonate. This alkaline secretion enters the duodenum and neutralizes acid in the chyme. The duodenal mucosa also secretes mucus to protect against the hydrochloric acid. In response to the presence of chyme, the hormone cholecystokinin (CCK), produced by the duodenal mucosa, enters the bloodstream and stimulates contraction of the gallbladder and relaxation of the sphincter of Oddi. These actions permit bile to flow from the common bile duct into the duodenum. Bile is necessary for the digestion of fats. CCK also stimulates the pancreas to synthesize and secrete enzymes for enzymatic digestion of carbohydrates, fats, and proteins.

Enzymes present on the brush border of the microvilli complete the digestion process. These enzymes hydrolyze disaccharides to monosaccharides and peptides to amino acids for absorption.

Absorption is the transfer of the end products of digestion across the intestinal wall to the circulation. Most absorption oc-

Table 37-2 Phases of Gastric Secretion

Phase	Stimulus to Secretion	Secretion
Cephalic (nervous)	Sight, smell, taste of food (before food enters stomach); initiated in the CNS and mediated by the vagus nerve	Hydrochloric acid, pepsinogen, mucus
Gastric (hormonal and nervous)	Food in antrum of stomach, vagal stimulation	Release of gastrin hormone from antrum into circulation to stimulate gastric secretions and motility
Intestinal (hormonal)	Presence of chyme in small intestine	Acidic chyme (pH <2) release of secretin, gastric inhibitory polypeptide, cholecystokinin into circulation to decrease acid secretion
		Chyme (pH >3) release of duodenal gastrin to increase acid secretion

CNS, central nervous system.

Table 37-3 Major Hormones Controlling Gastrointestinal Secretion and Motility

Hormone	Source	Activating Stimuli	Function
Gastrin	Gastric and duodenal mucosa	Stomach distention, partially digested proteins in pylorus	Gastric acid secretion, increased motility, maintenance of lower esophageal sphincter tone
Secretin	Duodenal mucosa	Acid entering small intestine	Inhibition of gastric motility and acid secretion, pancreatic bicarbonate secretion
Cholecystokinin	Duodenal mucosa	Fatty acids and amino acids in small intestine	Contraction of gallbladder and relaxation of sphincter of Oddi, allowing increased flow of bile into duodenum; release of pancreatic digestive enzymes
Gastric inhibitory peptide	Duodenal mucosa	Fatty acids and lipids in the small intestine	Inhibition of gastric acid secretion and gastric motility

curs in the small intestine. The surface area of the small intestine is greatly increased by its circular folds, villi, and microvilli. The movement of the villi provides for exposure of the end products of digestion to be in contact with the absorbing membrane. Monosaccharides (from carbohydrates), fatty acids (from fats), amino acids (from proteins), water, electrolytes, and vitamins are absorbed.

Elimination

Large Intestine. The large intestine is a hollow muscular tube approximately 5 to 6 feet (1.5 to 2 m) long and 2 inches (5 cm) in diameter. The four parts of the large intestine are (1) the cecum and appendix, a narrow tube at the end of the cecum; (2) the colon (ascending colon on the right side, transverse colon across the abdomen, descending colon on the left side, and the sigmoid colon); (3) the rectum; and (4) the anus, the terminal portion of the large intestine (Fig. 37-3).

The most important function of the large intestine is the absorption of water and electrolytes. It also forms feces and serves as a reservoir for the fecal mass until defecation occurs. Feces is composed of water (75%), bacteria, unabsorbed minerals, undigested foodstuffs, bile pigments, and desquamated epithelial cells. The large intestine secretes mucus, which acts as a lubricant and protects the mucosa.

Microorganisms in the colon are responsible for the breakdown of proteins not digested or absorbed in the small intestine. These amino acids are deaminated by the bacteria, leaving ammonia, which is carried to the liver and converted to urea. Bacteria in the colon also synthesize vitamin K and some of the B vitamins. Bacteria also play a part in the production of flatus.

The movements of the large intestine are usually slow. When the circular muscles contract, they produce a kneading action termed *haustral churning.* Propulsive (mass movements) peristalsis also occurs. When food enters the stomach and duodenum, the gastrocolic and duodenocolic reflexes are initiated, resulting in peristalsis in the colon. These reflexes are more active after the first daily meal and frequently result in bowel evacuation.

Defecation is a reflex action involving voluntary and involuntary control. Feces in the rectum stimulate sensory nerve endings that produce the desire to defecate. The reflex center for defecation is in the sacral portion of the spinal cord (parasympathetic nerve fibers). These fibers produce contraction of the rectum and relaxation of the internal anal sphincter. Defecation is controlled voluntarily by relaxing the external anal sphincter when the desire to defecate is felt. An acceptable environment for defecation is usually necessary or the urge to defecate will be ignored. If defecation is suppressed over long

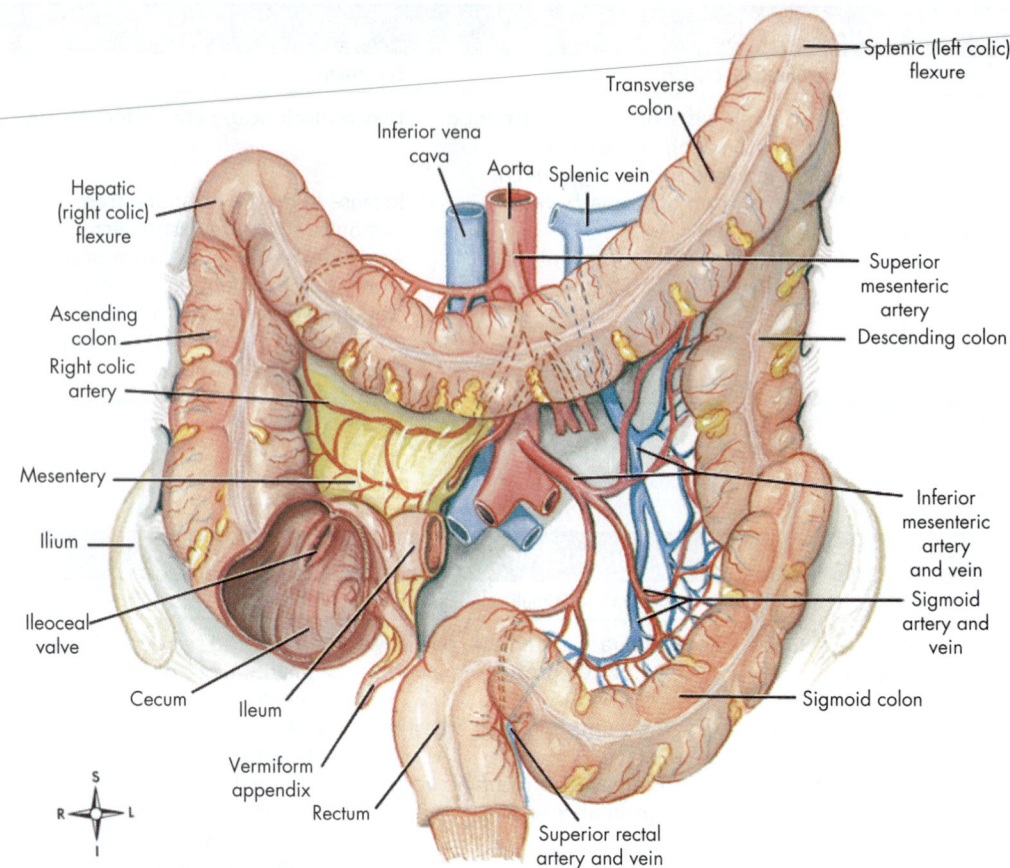

Fig. 37-3   Anatomic locations of the large intestine.

periods of time, problems can occur, such as constipation or stool impaction.

Defecation can be facilitated by Valsalva's maneuver. This maneuver involves contraction of the chest muscles on a closed glottis with simultaneous contraction of the abdominal muscles. These actions result in increased intraabdominal pressure. Valsalva's maneuver is contraindicated in the patient with a head injury, eye surgery, cardiac problems, hemorrhoids, abdominal surgery, or liver cirrhosis with portal hypertension. Constipation is common in the older adult and is due to many factors, including slower peristalsis, inactivity, decreased dietary fiber, decreased fluids, depression, constipating medications, and laxative abuse.[1] (Constipation is discussed in Chapter 40.)

Liver, Biliary Tract, and Pancreas

Liver.   The liver is the largest internal organ in the body, weighing approximately 3 lb (1.37 kg) in the adult. It lies in the right hypochondriac and epigastric regions (see Fig. 37-7). Most of the liver is enclosed in peritoneum. It has a fibrous capsule that divides it into the right and left lobes (Fig. 37-4).

The functional units of the liver are lobules (Fig. 37-5). The lobule consists of rows of hepatic cells (hepatocytes) arranged around a central vein. The capillaries (sinusoids) are located between the rows of hepatocytes and are lined with Kupffer cells, which carry out phagocytic activity (removal of bacteria

and toxins from the blood). Interlobular bile ducts form from bile capillaries (canaliculi). The hepatic cells secrete bile into the canaliculi.

The nerve supply to the liver is from the left vagus and sympathetic celiac plexus. About one third of the blood supply comes from the hepatic artery (branch of the celiac artery), and two thirds comes from the portal vein.

The portal circulatory system (enterohepatic) brings blood to the liver from the stomach, intestines, spleen, and pancreas. This blood enters the liver through the portal vein. The portal vein carries absorbed products of digestion directly to the liver. In the liver the portal vein branches and comes in contact with each lobule. The blood in the sinusoids is a mixture of arterial and venous blood.

The liver is essential for life. It functions in the manufacture, storage, transformation, and excretion of a number of substances involved in metabolism. The functions of the liver are numerous but can be classified into four main areas, as identified in Table 37-4.

Biliary Tract.   The biliary tract consists of the gallbladder and the duct system. The gallbladder is a pear-shaped sac located below the liver. The function of the gallbladder is to concentrate and store bile. It can hold approximately 45 ml of bile.

Bile is produced by the hepatic cells and secreted into the biliary canaliculi of the lobules. Bile then drains into the interlobular bile ducts, which unite into the two main left and right

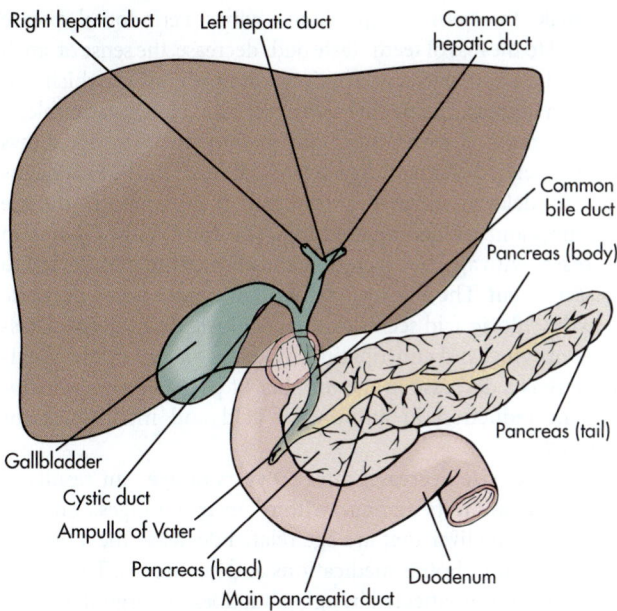

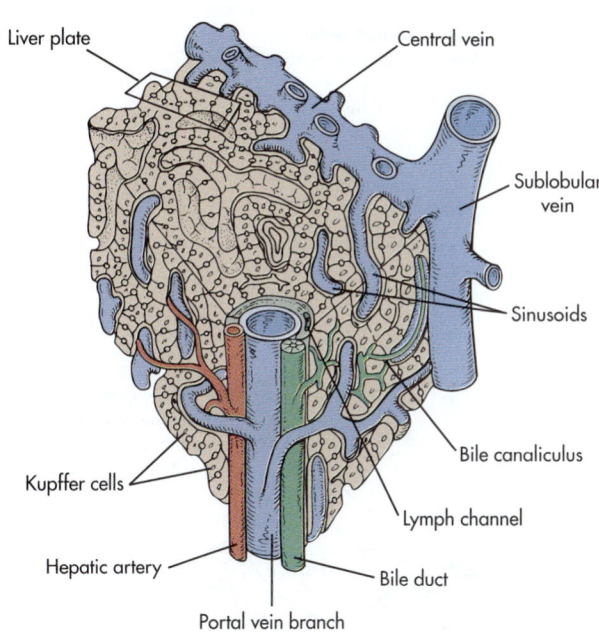

Fig. 37-4   Gross structure of the liver, gallbladder, and pancreas and the duct system.

Fig. 37-5   Microscopic structure of liver lobule.

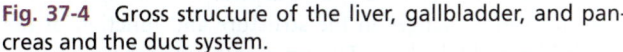

Table **37-4**	**Major Functions of the Liver**
Function	**Description**
Metabolic functions	
Carbohydrate metabolism	Glycogenesis (conversion of glucose to glycogen), glycogenolysis (process of breaking down glycogen to glucose), gluconeogenesis (formation of glucose from amino acids and fatty acids)
Protein metabolism	Synthesis of nonessential amino acids, synthesis of plasma proteins (except γ-globulin), synthesis of clotting factors, urea formation from NH_3 (NH_3 formed from deamination of amino acids by action of bacteria on proteins in colon)
Fat metabolism	Synthesis of lipoproteins, breakdown of triglycerides into fatty acids and glycerol, formation of ketone bodies, synthesis of fatty acids from amino acids and glucose, synthesis and breakdown of cholesterol
Detoxification	Inactivation of drugs and harmful substances and excretion of their breakdown products
Steroid metabolism	Conjugation and excretion of gonadal and adrenal steroids
Bile synthesis	
Bile production	Formation of bile, containing bile salts, bile pigments (mainly bilirubin), and cholesterol
Bile excretion	Bile excretion by liver about 1 L/day
Storage	Glucose in form of glycogen; vitamins, including fat soluble (A, D, E, K) and water soluble (B_1, B_2, cobalamin, and folic acid); fatty acids; minerals (iron and copper); amino acids in form of albumin and β-globulins
Mononuclear phagocyte system	Breakdown of old RBCs, WBCs, bacteria, and other particles, breakdown of hemoglobin
Kupffer cells	from old RBCs to bilirubin and biliverdin

RBC, red blood cell; *WBC*, white blood cell.

hepatic ducts. The hepatic ducts merge with the cystic duct from the gallbladder to form the common bile duct (see Fig. 37-4). This duct enters the duodenum at the ampulla of Vater. The sphincter of Oddi keeps the ampulla closed except when stimulated by the presence of food in the GI tract.

Bilirubin metabolism. Bilirubin, a pigment derived from the breakdown of hemoglobin, is constantly produced (Fig. 37-6). Because it is insoluble in water, it is bound to albumin for its transport to the liver. This form of bilirubin is referred to as *unconjugated*. In the liver bilirubin is conjugated with glu-

curonic acid. Conjugated bilirubin is soluble and is excreted in bile. Bile also consists of water, cholesterol, bile salts, electrolytes, and phospholipids. Bile salts are needed for fat emulsification and digestion.

Bile initially enters the duct system in the canaliculi and flows through the interlobular ducts to the hepatic ducts. From the hepatic duct it can move to the cystic duct or down the common bile duct. Most bile is stored and concentrated in the gallbladder. It is then released into the cystic duct and moves down the common bile duct to enter the duodenum at the ampulla of Vater. In

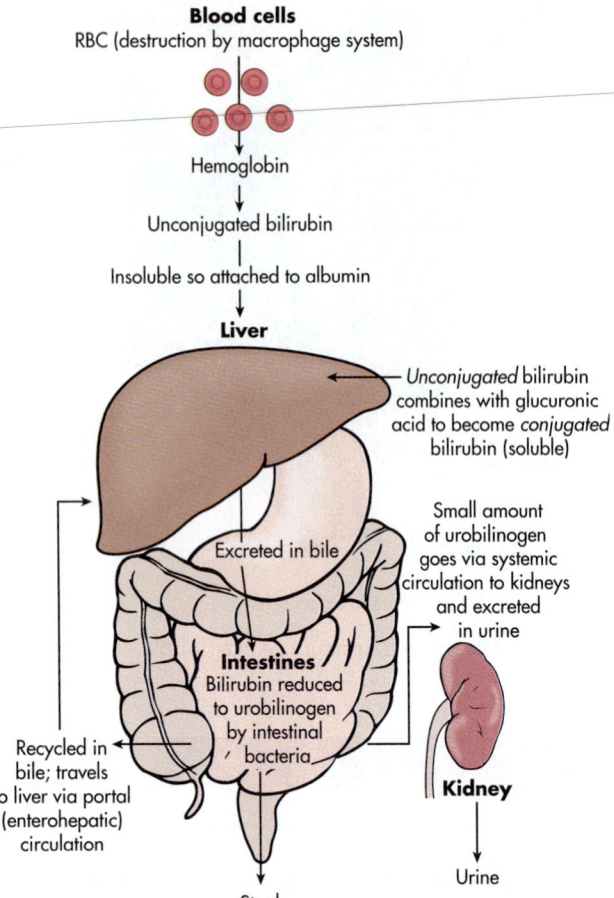

Blood cells
RBC (destruction by macrophage system)

Hemoglobin

Unconjugated bilirubin

Insoluble so attached to albumin

Liver

Unconjugated bilirubin combines with glucuronic acid to become *conjugated* bilirubin (soluble)

Excreted in bile

Small amount of urobilinogen goes via systemic circulation to kidneys and excreted in urine

Intestines
Bilirubin reduced to urobilinogen by intestinal bacteria

Recycled in bile; travels to liver via portal (enterohepatic) circulation

Kidney

Stool

Urine

Fig. 37-6   Bilirubin metabolism and conjugation.

the intestines, most of the bilirubin is reduced to stercobilinogen and urobilinogen by bacterial action. Stercobilinogen accounts for the brown color of stool. A small amount of conjugated bilirubin is reabsorbed by the blood. Some urobilinogen is reabsorbed by the blood and returned to the liver through the portal circulation (enterohepatic) and excreted in the bile. An insignificant amount of urobilinogen is excreted in the urine.[2]

Pancreas.   The pancreas is a long, slender gland lying behind the stomach and in front of the first and second lumbar vertebrae. It consists of the head, body, and tail. The anterior surface is covered by peritoneum. The pancreas contains lobes and lobules. The pancreatic duct extends along the gland and enters the duodenum through the common bile duct (see Fig. 37-4). The pancreas has both exocrine and endocrine functions. It is the exocrine function of the pancreas that contributes to the process of digestion. Exocrine cells in the pancreas secrete pancreatic enzymes (see Table 37-1). The endocrine function occurs in the islets of Langerhans, whose beta cells secrete insulin; alpha cells secrete glucagon; delta cells secrete somatostatin; and F cells secrete pancreatic polypeptide (see Chapter 45).

■ GERONTOLOGIC CONSIDERATIONS ■

Effects of Aging on the Gastrointestinal System

The process of aging causes changes in the functional ability of the GI system (Table 37-5). Tooth enamel and dentin wear down

and make the teeth susceptible to cavities. Periodontal disease can lead to the loss of teeth. Taste buds decrease, the sense of smell diminishes, and salivary secretions diminish, all of which can lead to a decrease in appetite and make eating less pleasurable.

As compared with other body systems the GI tract shows few age-related changes. Age-related changes in the esophagus include delayed emptying resulting from smooth muscle weakness and an incompetent LES.[1] Motility of the GI system decreases with age, but secretion and absorption are affected to a lesser extent. The elderly patient often experiences a decrease in hydrochloric acid secretion (hypochlorhydria), delayed gastric emptying, and constipation. With chronic atrophic gastritis there is a decrease in the number of parietal cells and subsequent reduction in amount of acid and intrinsic factor secreted.

The liver size decreases after 50 years of age, but results of liver function tests remain within normal ranges. Enzyme changes in the liver that are age related decrease the ability of the liver to metabolize medications and hormones. The size of the pancreas is unaffected by aging but does undergo structural changes such as fibrosis, fatty acid deposits, and atrophy. Aging does not cause changes in the structure and function of the gallbladder and bile ducts. However, with aging there is an increase in the incidence of gallstones.[3]

The economic inability to purchase food supplies may affect nutritional intake, especially in the older adult. Economic constraints may also reduce the number of fresh fruits and vegetables consumed and thus the amount of fiber. A reduction in dietary fiber, along with reduced fluid intake and decreased physical activity, contributes to constipation. Age-related changes in the GI system and differences in assessment findings are presented in Table 37-5.

ASSESSMENT OF THE GASTROINTESTINAL SYSTEM

Subjective Data

Important Health Information

Past health history.   Information should be gathered from the patient about the history or existence of the following diseases or problems related to GI functioning: abdominal pain, gastritis, nausea and vomiting, diarrhea and constipation, hepatitis, colitis, peptic ulcer, abdominal distention, jaundice, anemia, hiatal hernia, gallbladder disease, dysphagia, heartburn, dyspepsia, changes in appetite, hematemesis, food intolerance, indigestion, excessive gas, bloating, melena, hemorrhoids, hernia, or rectal bleeding.

The patient should be questioned about weight history. Any unexplained or unplanned weight loss or weight gain within the past 12 months should be explored in detail. A history of chronic dieting and repeated weight loss and gain should be documented.

Medications.   The health history should include an assessment of the patient's past and current use of medications. This is an important part of the assessment, particularly in relation to liver problems. It should include over-the-counter and prescription drugs. Many chemicals and drugs are potentially hepatotoxic (Table 37-6). The nurse should ask the patient if laxatives or antacids are taken, including the kind and frequency. Some people take baking soda (sodium bicarbonate) for an

GERONTOLOGIC DIFFERENCES IN ASSESSMENT

Table 37-5 Gastrointestinal System

Changes	Differences in Assessment Findings
Mouth	
Loss of teeth	Presence of dentures, difficulty chewing
Decreased taste buds, decreased sense of smell	Diminished sense of taste (especially salty and sweet)
Decreased volume of saliva	Dry oral mucosa
Atrophy of gingival tissue	Poor-fitting dentures
Esophagus	
Decreased tone and motility	Complaints of pyrosis (heartburn), dysphagia, eructation
Abdominal Wall	
Thinner and less taut	More visible peristalsis, easier palpation of organs
Decrease in number and sensitivity of sensory receptors	Less sensitivity to surface pain
Stomach	
Decreased acid secretion, atrophy of gastric mucosa	Food intolerances, signs of anemia as result of cobalamin malabsorption
Small Intestines	
Decreased secretion of most digestive enzymes, decreased motility	Complaints of indigestion
Liver	
Decreased size and lowered in position	Easier palpation
Large Intestine, Anus, Rectum	
Decreased anal sphincter tone and nerve supply to rectal area	Fecal incontinence
Decreased muscular tone, decreased motility	Flatulence, abdominal distention, relaxed perineal musculature
Increase in transit time	Constipation, fecal impaction

Table 37-6 Hepatotoxic Chemicals and Drugs

Alcohol	Halothane
Arsenic	Isoniazid
Carbon tetrachloride	Propylthiouracil
Chloroform	Sulfonamides
Gold compounds	Thiazide diuretics
Mercury	6-Mercaptopurine
Phosphorus	Methotrexate
Anabolic steroids	Acetaminophen

Table 37-7 Surgeries of the Gastrointestinal System

Antrectomy: Removal of antrum portion of stomach
Cecostomy: Opening into cecum
Cholecystectomy: Removal of gallbladder
Cholecystostomy: Opening into gallbladder
Choledochojejunostomy: Opening between common bile duct and jejunum
Choledocholithotomy: Opening into common bile duct for removal of stones
Colostomy: Opening into colon
Esophagoenterostomy: Removal of portion of esophgus with segment of colon attached to remaining portion
Esophagogastrostomy: Removal of esophagus and anastomosis of remaining portion to stomach
Gastrectomy: Removal of stomach
Gastrostomy: Opening into stomach
Glossectomy: Removal of tongue
Hemiglossectomy: Removal of half of tongue
Ileostomy: Opening into ileum
Mandibulectomy: Removal of mandible
Pyloroplasty: Enlargement and repair of pyloric sphincter area
Vagotomy: Resection of branch of vagus nerve

upset stomach. This can be dangerous because it is a systemic antacid that is readily absorbed and can cause metabolic alkalosis. Sodium bicarbonate is also in many over-the-counter effervescent drugs, such as Alka-Seltzer.

The use of prescription or over-the-counter appetite suppressant medication should be noted. The names of drugs and frequency and duration of use are also important. The patient should also be asked about herbal medicines that may be used to relieve GI symptoms such as nausea and constipation.

Surgery or other treatments. Information should be obtained about hospitalizations for any problems related to the GI system. Data should also be obtained related to any abdominal or rectal surgery, including year, reason for surgery, postoperative course, and possible blood transfusions. Terminology related to surgery of the GI system is presented in Table 37-7.

Functional Health Patterns. Key questions to ask a patient with a GI problem are presented in Table 37-8.

Health perception–health management pattern. The nurse should ask about the patient's health practices related to the GI system, such as maintenance of normal body weight, attention to proper dental care, maintenance of adequate nutrition, and effective elimination habits.

HEALTH HISTORY

Table 37-8 | Gastrointestinal System

Health Perception–Health Management Pattern
- Describe any measures used to treat gastrointestinal symptoms such as diarrhea or vomiting.
- Do you smoke?* Do you drink alcohol?*
- Are you exposed to any chemicals on a regular basis?* Have you been exposed in the past?*
- Have you recently traveled outside the United States?*

Nutritional-Metabolic Pattern
- Describe your usual daily food and fluid intake.
- Do you take any supplemental vitamins or minerals?*
- Have you experienced any changes in appetite or food tolerance?*
- Has there been a weight change in the past?*
- Are you allergic to any foods?*

Elimination Pattern
- Describe the frequency and time of day you have bowel movements. What is the consistency of the bowel movement?
- Do you use laxatives or enemas?* If so, how often?
- Have there been any recent changes in your bowel pattern?*
- Describe any skin problems caused by gastrointestinal problems.
- Do you need any assistive equipment, such as ostomy equipment?

Activity-Exercise Pattern
- Do you have limitations in mobility that make it difficult for you to procure and prepare food?*
- Are you able to feed yourself?
- Do you have any gastrointestinal symptoms, such as vomiting or diarrhea, that affect your activity?*
- Do you have any difficulty accessing a toilet when needed?*
- Is a safe and comfortable environment for elimination available?

Sleep-Rest Pattern
- Do you experience any difficulty sleeping because of a gastrointestinal problem?*
- Are you awakened by symptoms such as gas or esophageal burning?*

Cognitive-Perceptual Pattern
- Have you experienced any change in taste or smell that has affected your appetite?*
- Do you have any heat or cold sensitivity that affects eating?*
- Does pain interfere with food preparation, appetite, or chewing?*
- Do pain medications cause constipation or appetite suppression?*

Self-Perception–Self-Concept Pattern
- Describe any changes in your weight that have affected how you feel about yourself.
- Have you had any changes in normal elimination that have affected how you feel about yourself?*
- Have any symptoms of gastrointestinal disease caused physical changes that are a problem for you?*

Role-Relationship Pattern
- Describe the impact of any gastrointestinal problem on your usual roles and relationships.
- Have any changes in elimination affected your relationships?*
- Do you live alone? Describe how your family or others assist you with your gastrointestinal problems.

Sexuality-Reproductive Pattern
- Describe the effect of your gastrointestinal problem on your sexual activity.

Coping–Stress Tolerance Pattern
- Do you experience gastrointestinal symptoms in response to stressful or emotional situations?*
- Describe how you deal with any gastrointestinal symptoms that result.

Value-Belief Pattern
- Describe any culturally specific health beliefs regarding food and food preparation that may influence the treatment of this gastrointestinal problem.

*If yes, describe.

The patient should be asked about exposure to hepatotoxic chemicals such as arsenic, phosphorus, and mercury. The nurse should also ask about foreign travel with possible exposure to hepatitis or parasitic infestation.

The patient should be assessed in relation to certain habits that have a direct effect on GI functioning. The consumption of alcohol in large quantities has detrimental effects on the mucosa of the stomach and also increases the secretion of hydrochloric acid and pepsinogen. Chronic alcohol exposure causes fatty infiltration of the liver. The nurse should obtain a history of cigarette smoking. Nicotine is irritating to the entire GI tract mucosa. Cigarette smoking is related to various GI cancers (especially mouth and esophageal cancers), esophagitis, and ulcers. Smoking will also delay the healing of ulcers.

Nutritional-metabolic pattern. A thorough nutritional assessment is essential. A dietary history should be taken and compared with the food pyramid (Fig. 38-1). The nurse should ask open-ended questions that will allow the patient to express beliefs and feelings about the diet. The nurse may need to ask the patient to do a 24-hour dietary recall to analyze the adequacy of the diet. The nurse should assist the patient in recalling the preceding day's food intake, including early-morning and nighttime intake. The nurse should find out about the intake of snacks, liquids, and vitamin supplements. The nurse must then evaluate the diet in terms of the recommended groups and servings on the food pyramid and try to determine whether the 24-hour recall is typical of the patient's usual eating habits. If weekend eating habits vary greatly, the nurse should obtain a separate weekend diet history and assess the patient's intake for both quality and quantity of food.

The nurse should ask the patient about the use of sugar and salt substitutes, caffeine, and amount of fluid and fiber intake. The patient should be questioned about any changes in appetite, food tolerance, and weight. Anorexia and weight loss may indicate carcinoma. The nurse should ask the patient about allergies to any food and determine what GI symptoms such allergic responses cause.

Elimination pattern. A detailed account of the patient's bowel elimination pattern should be elicited. The frequency, time of day, and usual consistency of stool should be noted. The use of laxatives and enemas, including type, frequency, and results, should be documented. Any recent change in bowel patterns should be investigated.

The amount and type of fluid and fiber intake should be determined because they have an important effect on the frequency and consistency of stools. Inadequate intake of fiber can be associated with constipation. Analysis of fluid intake and output could indicate the presence of a urinary problem and the possibility of fluid retention.

Skin problems can be associated with GI problems. Food allergies can cause lesions, pruritus, and edema. Diarrhea can result in redness, irritation, and pain in the perianal area. External drainage systems such as an ileostomy or ileal conduit can cause local skin irritation. The possible association between a skin problem and a GI problem should be investigated.

Activity-exercise pattern. The patient's ambulatory status should be assessed to determine if the patient is capable of securing and preparing food. If the patient is unable to do these tasks, it should be determined if family or an outside agency is meeting this need. Any limitation in the patient's ability to feed self independently should be noted. Any difficulty accessing a safe environment of elimination should be assessed. Use of and access to elimination supplies should be assessed, such as commode or ostomy supplies. Activity and exercise may affect GI motility. Immobility is a risk factor for constipation.

Sleep-rest pattern. Many food-related events can interrupt and interfere with the quality of sleep. Nausea, vomiting, diarrhea, indigestion, bloating, and hunger can produce sleep problems and should be investigated. The patient should be asked if GI symptoms affect sleep or rest. For example, a patient with a hiatal hernia may be awakened because of burning pain; sleep may be improved by elevating the head of the bed for this patient.

A patient often has a bedtime ritual that involves the use of a particular food or beverage. Warm milk is known to induce sleep through the effect of the serotonin precursor L-tryptophan. Herbal teas and melatonin are often sleep inducing. Individual routines should be noted and complied with whenever possible to avoid sleeplessness. Hunger can prevent sleep and should be relieved by a light, easily digested snack unless contraindicated.

Cognitive-perceptual pattern. Decreases in sensory adequacy can result in problems related to the acquisition, preparation, and ingestion of food. Changes in taste or smell can affect appetite and eating pleasure. Vertigo can make shopping and standing at a stove difficult and dangerous. Heat or cold sensitivity could make certain foods painful to eat. Problems in expressive communication could make it difficult and frustrat-

ing for the patient to make personal desires and preferences known. The nurse should assess the patient in this pattern to judge the effect of deficiencies on adequate nutritional intake. If the patient has been diagnosed as having a GI disorder, the nurse should ask questions to determine the patient's understanding of the illness and its treatment.

Pain is another area that requires careful assessment related to its effect on the GI system and nutrition. Relevant behaviors associated with chronic pain include avoidance of activity, fatigue, and disruption of eating patterns. The possible effects of pain medication related to constipation, sedation, and appetite suppression should be assessed.

Self-perception–self-concept pattern. Many GI and nutritional problems can have serious effects on the patient's self-perception. Overweight and underweight persons often have problems related to self-esteem and body image. Repeated attempts to achieve a personally acceptable weight can be discouraging and depressing for the patient. The manner in which a person recounts a weight history can alert the nurse to potential problems in this area.

Another potentially problematic area is the need for external devices to manage elimination, such as a colostomy or an ileostomy. The patient's willingness to engage in self-care and to discuss this situation should provide the nurse with valuable information related to body image and self-esteem.

The altered physical changes often associated with liver disease can be problematic for the patient. Jaundice and ascites cause significant changes in external appearance. The patient's attitude toward these changes should be assessed.

Role-relationship pattern. Problems related to the GI system such as cirrhosis, alcoholism, hepatitis, ostomies, obesity, and carcinoma can have a major impact on the patient's ability to maintain usual roles and relationships. A chronic illness may necessitate leaving a job or reducing the number of hours worked. Changes in body image and self-esteem can affect relationships. The availability of and satisfaction with support should be determined. It is important that the nurse be aware of these possible consequences and assess for their presence.

Sexuality-reproductive pattern. Changes related to sexuality and reproductive status can result from problems of the GI system. For example, obesity, jaundice, anorexia, and ascites could decrease the acceptance of a potential sexual partner. The presence of an ostomy could affect the patient's confidence related to sexual activity. Chronic alcoholism could discourage a meaningful relationship that could develop into a sexual relationship. Sensitive questioning by the nurse could determine the presence of potential problems.

Anorexia can affect the reproductive status of a female patient. Alcoholism can affect the reproductive status of both men and women. A poor nutritional intake before and during pregnancy can result in a low-birth-weight infant. The nurse should determine the patient's desires in the area of reproduction and direct the assessment based on the patient's responses.

Coping–stress tolerance pattern. The nurse should try to determine what is a stressor for the patient and what coping mechanisms the patient uses to function with these stressors. GI symptoms such as epigastric pain, nausea, and diarrhea develop in many people in response to stressful or emotional situations. Some organic GI problems such as peptic ulcers are aggravated by stress.

Value-belief pattern. The patient's spiritual and cultural beliefs regarding food and food preparation should be assessed. Whenever possible, these preferences should be respected by the health care provider. In addition, it should be determined if any value or belief could interfere with planned interventions. For example, if the patient with anemia is a vegetarian, the prescription of a high-meat diet would be met with patient resistance. Likewise, the recovering alcoholic could not take an alcohol-based cough medicine. Thoughtful

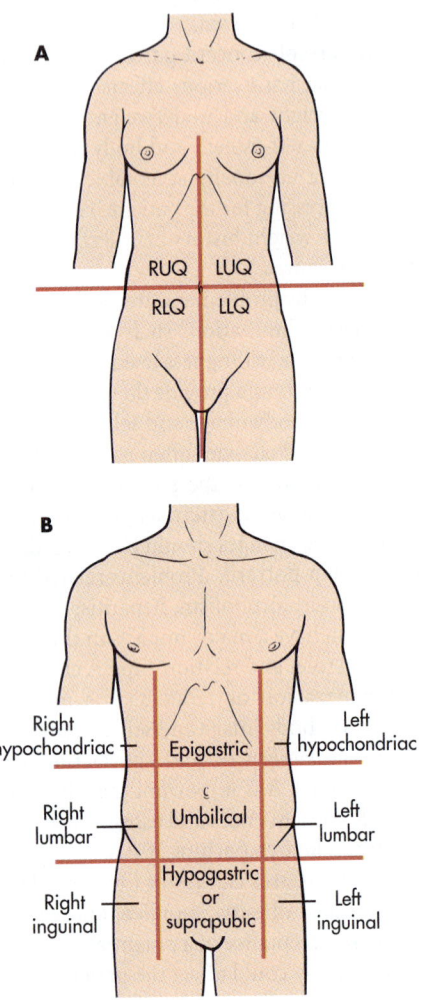

Fig. 37-7 **A,** Abdominal quadrants. **B,** Abdominal regions.

assessment and consideration of the patient's beliefs and values will usually increase patient compliance and satisfaction.

Objective Data

In addition to collecting subjective data related to a diet history and functional health patterns, objective data related to a nutritional assessment should be collected. Anthropometric measurements (height, weight, skinfold thickness) and blood studies such as serum protein, albumin, and hemoglobin are examples of important objective data related to the GI system. A physical examination also adds valuable information.

Physical Examination

Mouth

Inspection. The lips should be inspected for symmetry, color, and size. They should be observed for abnormalities such as pallor or cyanosis, cracking, ulcers, or fissures. The dorsum (top) of the tongue should have a thin white coating; the undersurface should be smooth. The nurse should observe for any lesions. Using a tongue blade, the nurse should inspect the buccal mucosa and note the color, any areas of pigmentation, and any lesions. Dark-skinned individuals normally have patchy areas of pigmentation. In assessing the teeth and gums, the nurse should look for caries; loose teeth; abnormal shape and position of teeth; and swelling, bleeding, discoloration, or inflammation of the gingivae. Any distinctive breath odor should be noted.

The pharynx is inspected by tilting the patient's head back and depressing the tongue with a tongue blade. The tonsils, uvula, soft palate, and anterior and posterior pillars should be observed. The nurse should have the patient say "ah." The uvula and soft palate should rise and remain in the midline.

Palpation. The nurse should palpate any suspicious areas in the mouth. Ulcers, nodules, indurations, and areas of tenderness should be palpated.

The mouth of the older adult requires careful assessment. Particular attention should be given to dentures (e.g., fit, condition), ability to swallow, and lesions. The patient who has dentures must remove the dentures during an oral examination to allow for good visualization and palpation of the area.

Abdomen. Two systems are used to anatomically describe the surface of the abdomen. One system divides the abdomen into four quadrants by a perpendicular line from the sternum to the pubic bone and a horizontal line across the abdomen at the umbilicus (Fig. 37-7, *A*, and Table 37-9). The other system divides the abdomen into nine regions (Fig. 37-7, *B*), but only

Table 37-9	Abdominal Structures in Regions of the Abdomen		
Right Upper Quadrant	**Left Upper Quadrant**	**Right Lower Quadrant**	**Left Lower Quadrant**
Liver and gallbladder	Left lobe of liver	Lower pole of right kidney	Lower pole of left kidney
Pylorus	Spleen	Cecum and appendix	Sigmoid flexure
Duodenum	Stomach	Portion of ascending colon	Portion of descending colon
Head of pancreas	Body of pancreas	Bladder (if distended)	Bladder (if distended)
Right adrenal gland	Left adrenal gland	Right ovary and salpinx	Left ovary and salpinx
Portion of right kidney	Portion of left kidney	Uterus (if enlarged)	Uterus (if enlarged)
Hepatic flexure of colon	Splenic flexure of colon	Right spermatic cord	Left spermatic cord
Portion of ascending and transverse colon	Portion of transverse and descending colon	Right ureter	Left ureter

the epigastrium, umbilical, and suprapubic or hypogastric regions are commonly addressed.

For the abdominal examination, good lighting should shine across the abdomen. The patient should be in the supine position and as relaxed as possible. To help relax the abdominal muscles, the patient should slightly flex the knees and the head of the bed should be raised slightly. The patient should have an empty bladder. The examiner should use warm hands when doing the abdominal examination to avoid eliciting muscle guarding. The patient should be asked to breathe slowly through the mouth.

Inspection. The nurse should assess the abdomen for skin changes (color, texture, scars, striae, dilated veins, rashes, and lesions), umbilicus (location and contour), symmetry, contour (flat, rounded [convex], concave, protuberant, distention), observable masses (hernias or other masses), and movement (pulsations and peristalsis). A normal aortic pulsation may be seen in the epigastric area. The nurse should look across the abdomen tangentially (across the abdomen in a line) for peristalsis. Peristalsis is not normally visible in an adult but may be visible in a thin person.

Auscultation. During examination of the abdomen, auscultation is done before percussion and palpation because these latter procedures may alter the bowel sounds. Auscultation of the abdomen includes listening for increased or decreased bowel sounds and vascular sounds. The diaphragm of the stethoscope is used to auscultate bowel sounds because they are relatively high pitched. The bell of the stethoscope is used to detect lower-pitched sounds. Normal bowel sounds occur 5 to 35 times per minute and sound like high-pitched clicks or gurgles.[4] Before auscultation, warming the stethoscope in the hands helps prevent abdominal muscle contraction. The nurse should listen in the epigastrium and in all four quadrants. The nurse should listen for bowel sounds for 2 to 5 minutes. Bowel sounds cannot be described as absent until no sound is heard for 5 minutes (in each quadrant).[5] The frequency and intensity of bowel sounds will vary, depending on the phase of digestion. Normally they will sound relatively high pitched and gurgling. Loud gurgles indicate hyperperistalsis and are termed *borborygmi* (stomach growling). The bowel sounds will be more high pitched (rushes and tinkling) when the intestines are under tension, such as in intestinal obstruction. The nurse should listen for decreased or absent bowel sounds. Terms used to describe bowel sounds include *present, absent, increased, decreased, high pitched, tinkling, gurgling,* and *rushing.* Normally no aortic bruits should be heard. A *bruit,* best heard with the bell of the stethoscope, is a swishing or buzzing sound and indicates turbulent blood flow.

Percussion. The purpose of percussion of the abdomen is to determine the presence of fluid, distention, and masses. Sound waves vary according to the density of underlying tissues; the presence of air produces a higher-pitched, hollow sound termed *tympany;* the presence of fluid or masses produces a short, high-pitched sound with little resonance termed *dullness.* The nurse should lightly percuss all four quadrants of the abdomen and assess the distribution of tympany and dullness. Tympany is the predominant percussion sound of the abdomen.

To percuss the liver, the nurse should start below the umbilicus in the right midclavicular line and percuss lightly up-

ward until dullness is heard, thus determining the lower border of liver dullness. After the lower border of the liver has been determined, the nurse should start at the nipple line in the right midclavicular line and percuss downward between ribs to the area of dullness indicating the upper border of the liver. The height or vertical space between the two areas should be measured to determine the size of the liver. The normal range of liver height in the right midclavicular line is 2.4 to 5 inches (6 to 12 cm).

Palpation. Light palpation is used to detect tenderness or cutaneous hypersensitivity, muscular resistance, masses, and swelling. It also helps in relaxation for deeper palpation. The nurse should keep fingers together and press gently with the pads of the fingertips, depressing the abdominal wall about 0.4 inches (1 cm). Smooth movements should be used and all quadrants palpated (Fig. 37-8, *A*).

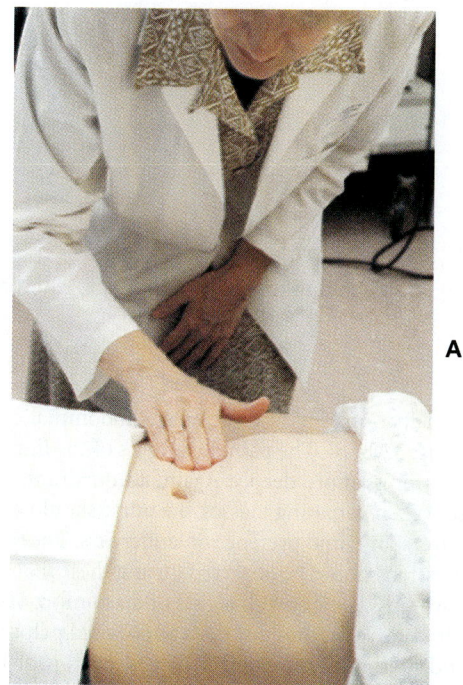

A

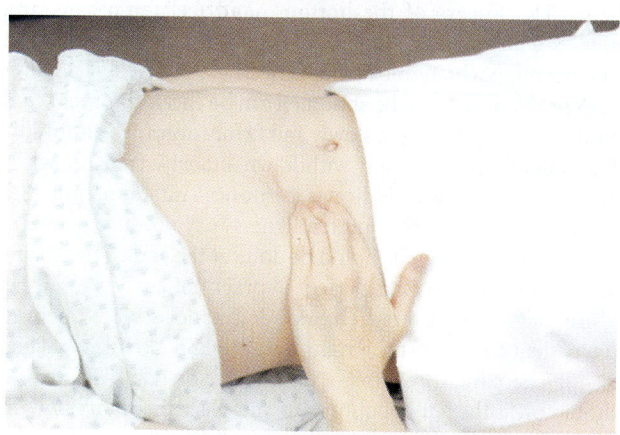

B

Fig. 37-8 **A,** Technique for light palpation of the abdomen. **B,** Technique for deep palpation.

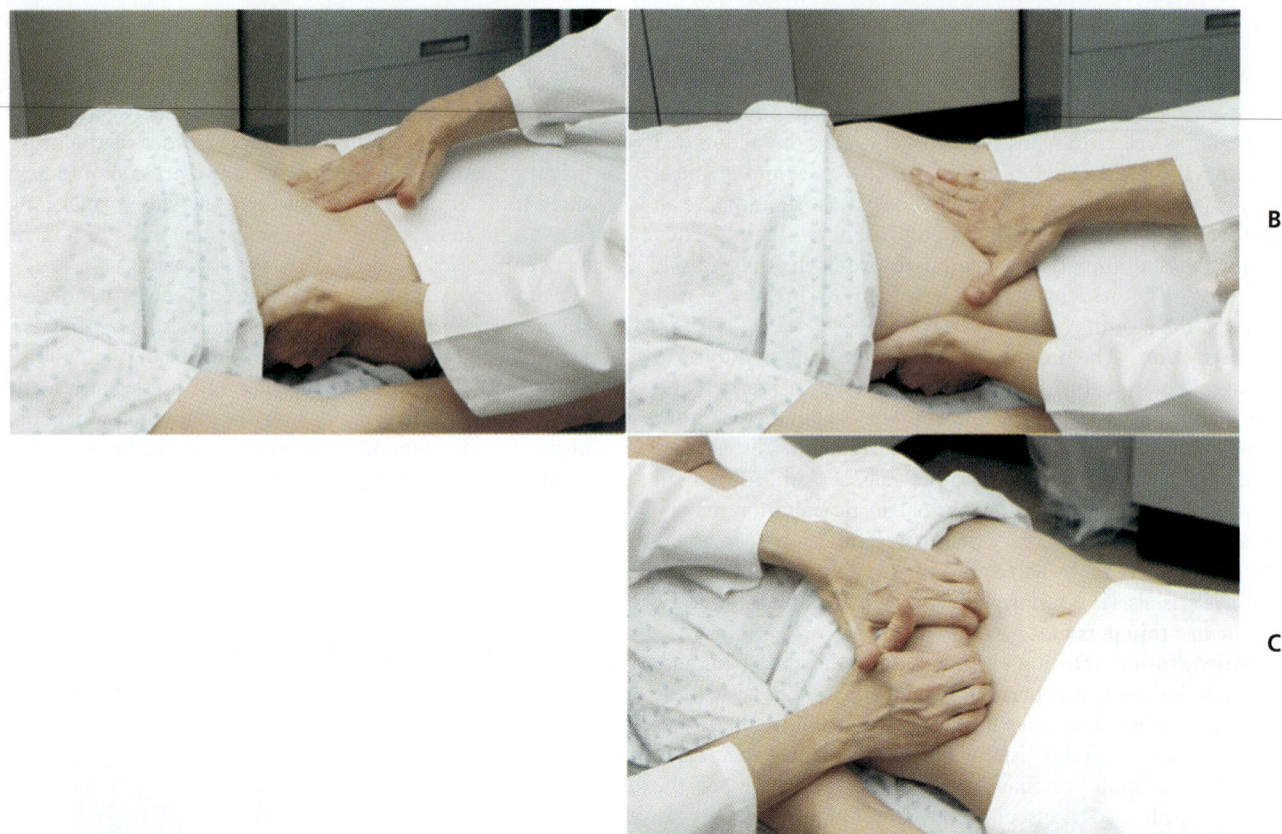

Fig. 37-9   A, Technique for liver palpation. **B,** Alternative technique. **C,** Palpating liver with fingers hooked over the costal margin.

Deep palpation is used to delineate abdominal organs and masses (Fig. 37-8, *B*). The palmar surfaces of the fingers should be used to press more deeply. Again, all quadrants should be palpated. When palpating masses, the nurse should note the location, size, shape, and presence of tenderness. The patient's facial expression should be observed during these maneuvers because it will provide nonverbal cues of discomfort or pain.

An alternative method for deep abdominal palpation is the two-hand method. One hand is placed on top of the other. The fingers of the top hand apply pressure to the bottom hand. The fingers of the bottom hand feel for organs and masses. The nurse should practice both methods of palpation to determine which one is most effective.

A problem area on the abdomen can be checked for rebound tenderness by pressing in slowly and firmly over the painful site. The palpating fingers are withdrawn quickly. Pain on withdrawal of the fingers indicates peritoneal inflammation. Because assessing for rebound tenderness may produce pain and severe muscle spasm, it should be done at the end of the examination and only by an experienced practitioner.

To palpate the liver, the nurse's left hand is placed behind the patient to support the right eleventh and twelfth ribs (Fig. 37-9). The patient may relax on the nurse's hand. The nurse should press the left hand forward and place the right hand on the patient's right abdomen lateral to the rectus muscle. The fingertips should be below the lower border of liver dullness

Table **37-10**	Normal Physical Assessment of the Gastrointestinal System

Mouth
Moist and pink lips; pink and moist buccal mucosa and gingivae without plaques or lesions; teeth in good repair; protrusion of tongue in midline without deviation or fasciculations; pink uvula midline; soft palate, tonsils, and posterior pharynx; swallows smoothly without coughing or gagging

Abdomen
Flat without masses or scars, no abdominal tenderness, no bruises, bowel sounds in all quadrants, nonpalpable liver and spleen, liver 10 cm in right midclavicular line, generalized tympany

Rectum/Anus
Absence of lesions, fissures, hemorrhoids; good sphincter tone; rectal walls smooth/soft; no masses; stool soft, brown, and heme-negative

and pointed toward the right costal margin. The nurse should gently press in and up. The patient should take a deep breath with the abdomen so that the liver drops and is in a better position to be palpated. The nurse should try to feel the liver edge as it comes down to the fingertips. The liver edge should feel

COMMON ASSESSMENT ABNORMALITIES

Table 37-11 Gastrointestinal System

Finding	Description	Possible Etiology and Significance
Mouth		
Ulcer, plaque on lips or in mouth	Sore or lesion	Carcinoma, viral infections
Cheilosis	Softening, fissuring, and cracking of lips at angles of mouth	Riboflavin deficiency
Cheilitis	Inflammation of lips (usually lower) with fissuring, scaling, crusting	Often unknown
Geographic tongue	Scattered red, smooth (loss of papillae) areas on dorsum of tongue	Unknown
Smooth tongue	Red, slick appearance	Cobalamin deficiency
Leukoplakia	Thickened white patches	Premalignant lesion
Pyorrhea	Recessed gums, purulent pockets	Periodontitis
Herpes simplex	Benign vesicular lesion	Herpesvirus
Candidiasis	White, curdlike lesions surrounded by erythematous mucosa	*Candida albicans*
Glossitis	Reddened, ulcerated, swollen tongue	Exposure to streptococci, irritation, injury, vitamin B deficiency, anemia
Acute marginal gingivitis	Friable, edematous, painful, bleeding gingivae	Irritation from ill-fitting dentures, calcium deposits on teeth, food impaction
Esophagus and Stomach		
Dysphagia	Difficulty in swallowing, sensation of food sticking in esophagus	Esophageal problems, cancer of esophagus
Hematemesis	Vomiting of blood	Esophageal varices, bleeding peptic ulcer
Pyrosis	Heartburn, burning in epigastric or substernal area	Hiatal hernia, esophagitis, incompetent lower esophageal sphincter
Dyspepsia	Burning or indigestion	Peptic ulcer, gallbladder disease
Odynophagia	Painful swallowing	Cancer of esophagus, esophagitis
Eructation	Belching	Gallbladder disease
Nausea and vomiting	Feeling of impending vomiting, expulsion of gastric contents through mouth	GI infections, common manifestation of many GI diseases; stress, fear, and pathologic conditions

Continued

firm, sharp, and smooth. The surface and contour and any tenderness should be described.

To palpate the spleen, the nurse moves to the left side of the patient. The nurse places the left hand under the patient and supports and presses the patient's left lower rib cage forward. The right hand is placed below the left costal margin and presses it in toward the spleen. The nurse should ask the patient to breathe deeply. The tip or edge of an enlarged spleen will be felt by the fingertips. The spleen is normally not palpable. If it is palpable, the nurse should not continue because manual compression of an enlarged spleen may cause it to rupture.

The standard approach for examining the abdomen can be used on the older adult. Palpation is important because it may reveal a tumor. The abdomen may be thinner and more lax unless the patient is obese. If the patient has chronic obstructive pulmonary disease, large lungs, or a low diaphragm, the liver may be palpated 0.4 to 0.8 inches (1 to 2 cm) below the right costal margin.

Rectum and anus. The perianal and anal area should be inspected for color, texture, lumps, rashes, scars, erythema, fissures, and external hemorrhoids. Any lumps or unusual areas should be palpated with a gloved hand.

For the digital examination of the rectum the gloved, lubricated index finger is placed against the anus while the patient strains (Valsalva's maneuver). Then, as the sphincter relaxes, the finger is inserted. The finger is pointed toward the umbilicus. The nurse should try to get the patient to relax. The finger is inserted into the rectum as far as possible, and all surfaces are palpated. Nodules, tenderness, or any irregularities should be assessed. A sample of stool can be removed with the gloved finger and should be checked for occult blood.

Recording of the normal physical assessment of the GI system is found in Table 37-10. Gerontologic differences in the GI system and differences in assessment findings are described in Table 37-5. Common assessment abnormalities are presented in Table 37-11.

COMMON ASSESSMENT ABNORMALITIES

Table 37-11   Gastrointestinal System—cont'd

Finding	Description	Possible Etiology and Significance
Abdomen		
Distention	Excessive gas accumulation, enlarged abdomen; generalized tympany	Obstruction, paralytic ileus
Ascites	Accumulated fluid within abdominal cavity; eversion of umbilicus (usually)	Peritoneal inflammation, congestive heart failure, metastatic carcinoma, cirrhosis
Bruit	Humming or swishing sound heard through stethoscope over vessel	Partial arterial obstruction (narrowing of vessel), turbulent flow (aneurysm)
Hyperresonance	Loud, tinkling rushes	Intestinal obstruction
Borborygmi	Waves of loud, gurgling sounds	Hyperactive bowel as result of eating
Absent bowel sounds	No auscultation of bowel sounds	Peritonitis, paralytic ileus, obstruction
Absence of liver dullness	Tympany on percussion	Air from viscus (e.g., perforated ulcer)
Masses	Lump on palpation	Tumors, cysts
Rebound tenderness	Sudden pain when fingers withdrawn quickly	Peritoneal inflammation, appendicitis
Nodular liver	Enlarged, hard liver with irregular edge or surface	Cirrhosis, carcinoma
Hepatomegaly	Enlargement of liver, liver edge >1-2 cm below costal margin	Metastatic carcinoma, hepatitis, venous congestion
Splenomegaly	Enlargement of spleen	Chronic leukemia, hemolytic states, portal hypertension, some infections
Hernia	Bulge or nodule in abdomen, usually appearing on straining	Inguinal (in inguinal canal), femoral (in femoral canal), umbilical (herniation of umbilicus), or incisional (defect in muscles after surgery)
Rectum and Anus		
Hemorrhoids	Thrombosed veins in rectum and anus (internal or external)	Portal hypertension, chronic constipation, prolonged sitting or standing, pregnancy
Mass	Firm, nodular edge	Tumor, carcinoma
Pilonidal cyst	Opening of sinus tract, cyst in midline just above coccyx	Probably congenital
Fissure	Ulceration in anal canal	Straining, irritation
Melena	Abnormal, black, tarry stool containing digested blood	Cancer, bleeding in upper GI tract from ulcers, varices
Tenesmus	Painful and ineffective straining at stool	Ulcerative colitis, diarrhea secondary to GI infection such as food poisoning
Steatorrhea	Fatty, frothy, foul-smelling stool	Chronic pancreatitis, biliary obstruction, malabsorption problems

DIAGNOSTIC STUDIES OF THE GASTROINTESTINAL SYSTEM

Diagnostic studies provide important information to the nurse in monitoring the patient's condition and planning appropriate interventions. These studies are considered to be objective data. Table 37-12 presents diagnostic studies common to the GI system. For most diagnostic studies nurses should make sure a signed consent form for the procedure has been completed and is in the medical record. It is the responsibility of the health care provider doing the procedure to explain the procedure and obtain the written consent. However, nurses play an important role in educating patients regarding the procedures.

Many of the diagnostic procedures of the GI system require measures to cleanse the GI tract, as well as the ingestion or injection of a contrast medium or a radiopaque dye. Often the patient has a series of GI diagnostic tests done. The nurse must monitor the patient closely to ensure adequate hydration and nutrition during the tests. Some diagnostic studies of the GI system are especially difficult and uncomfortable for the older adult. It may be necessary to individualize and make adjustments. It is particularly important to prevent diarrhea from bowel cleansing procedures and dehydration from prolonged fluid restriction.

Many radiologic studies use either barium sulfate or meglumine diatrizoate (Gastrografin) as a contrast medium. Barium sulfate is more effective for visualizing mucosal detail. Gastrografin is water soluble and rapidly absorbed, so it is preferred when a perforation is suspected. Spillage of barium into the peritoneal cavity can result in peritonitis, which is difficult to manage.[6] Under other circumstances in a person at high risk for aspiration, water-soluble media are contraindicated and barium is preferred.

Text continued on p. 1033

DIAGNOSTIC STUDIES

Table 37-12 Gastrointestinal System

Study	Description and Purpose	Nursing Responsibility
Radiologic		
Upper GI or Barium Swallow	X-ray study with fluoroscopy with contrast medium. Study is used to diagnose structural abnormalities of the esophagus, stomach, and duodenal bulb.	Explain procedure to patient and that patient will need to drink contrast medium and assume various positions on x-ray table. Keep patient NPO for 8-12 hr before procedure. Tell patient to avoid smoking after midnight the night before the study. After x-ray test, take measures to prevent contrast medium impaction (fluids, laxatives). Tell patient that stool may be white up to 72 hr after test.
Small Bowel Series	Contrast medium is ingested and flat film taken q20min until medium reaches terminal ileum.	Same as for upper GI.
Lower GI or Barium Enema	Fluoroscopic x-ray examination of colon uses contrast medium, which is administered rectally (enema). Double contrast or air contrast barium enema is test of choice. Air is infused after barium is evacuated.	Before the procedure, administer laxatives and enemas until colon is clear of stool evening before procedure. Administer clear liquid diet evening before procedure. Keep patient NPO for 8 hr before test. Instruct patient about being given barium by enema. Explain that cramping and urge to defecate may occur during procedure and that patient may be placed in various positions on tilt table. After the procedure, give fluids, laxatives, or suppositories to assist in expelling barium. Observe stool for passage of contrast medium.
Oral Cholecystogram (GB Series)	X-ray examination visualizes GB after radiopaque dye such as iopanoic acid (Telepaque) has been ingested orally. Study determines GB's ability to concentrate and store dye and patency of biliary duct system.	Assess patient for sensitivity to iodine. Administer radiopaque dye evening before test. Give 6 tablets (3 g), 1 q5min. Explain that patient may need 2 consecutive days of dye ingestion. Keep patient NPO after ingestion of dye. Observe for side effects of dye such as nausea, vomiting, diarrhea. May give fatty test meal after x-ray test to check for GB emptying. Assess patient's medication for possible contraindications, precautions, or complications with the use of dye.
Cholangiography ■ IV Cholangiogram	X-rays are used to visualize biliary duct system after IV injection of radiopaque dye.	Keep patient NPO for 8 hr. Assess sensitivity to iodine dye. During injection of dye, assess for urticaria, extreme flushing, respiratory distress. Assess patient's medication for possible contraindications, precautions, or complications with the use of dye.
■ Percutaneous transhepatic cholangiogram	After local anesthesia, liver is entered with long needle (under fluoroscopy), bile duct is entered, bile withdrawn, and radiopaque dye injected. Fluoroscopy is used to determine filling of hepatic and biliary ducts.	Observe patient for signs of hemorrhage or bile leakage. Assess patient's medication for possible contraindications, precautions, or complications with the use of dye.
■ Surgical cholangiogram	Study is performed during surgery on biliary structures, such as GB. Contrast medium is injected into common bile duct.	Explain to patient that anesthetic will be used. Assess patient's medication for possible contraindications, precautions, or complications with the use of dye.

Continued

DIAGNOSTIC STUDIES

Table 37-12 Gastrointestinal System—cont'd

Study	Description and Purpose	Nursing Responsibility
Radiologic—continued		
Ultrasound	This noninvasive procedure uses high-frequency sound waves (ultrasound waves), which are passed into body structures and recorded as they are reflected (bounded). A conductive gel (lubricant jelly) is applied to the skin and a transducer is placed on the area.	Be aware that bowel must be cleansed because presence of solid material in GI tract causes changes in reflected sounds and that ultrasound is not transmitted well through gas or air. Schedule test before upper GI or barium enema.
▪ Abdominal ultrasound	Study detects abdominal masses (tumors and cysts) and is also used to assess ascites.	Same as above.
▪ Hepatobiliary ultrasound	Study detects subphrenic abscesses, cysts, tumors, cirrhosis and is used to visualize biliary ducts.	Be aware that bowel must be cleansed. Explain procedure to patient.
▪ GB ultrasound	Study detects gallstones (high degree of accuracy) and can be used for a patient with jaundice or allergic reaction to GB contrast media.	Administer clear liquids for 24 hr before examination. Give laxative evening before and cleansing enema morning of examination. Keep patient NPO 8 hr before procedure.
Nuclear Imaging Scans	Purpose is to show size, shape, and position of organ. Functional disorders and structural defects may be identified. Radionuclide (radioactive isotope) is injected IV and a counter (scanning) device picks up radioactive emission, which is recorded on paper. Only tracer doses of radioactive isotopes are used.	Tell patient that substances contain only traces of radioactivity and pose little to no danger. Schedule no more than one radionuclide test on the same day. Explain to patient need to lie flat during scanning.
▪ Gastric emptying studies	Radionuclide study is used to assess ability of stomach to empty solids or liquids. In solid-emptying study, cooked egg white containing Tc-99m is eaten. In liquid-emptying study, orange juice with Tc-99m is drunk. Sequential images from gamma camera are recorded q2min for up to 60 min. Study is used in patients with emptying disorders from peptic ulcer, ulcer surgery, diabetes, or gastric malignancies.	Same as above.
▪ Liver and spleen scans	Patient is given IV injection of Tc-99m and positioned under camera to record distribution of radioactivity in liver and spleen. In normal person, intensity of liver and spleen images is equal. Test is useful in detecting hepatomegaly, hepatocellular diseases, hepatic malignancies, and splenomegaly.	Same as above.
Computed Tomography (CT)	Noninvasive radiologic examination combines special x-ray machine used for CT (exposures at different depths) with computer. Study detects mainly biliary tract, liver, and pancreatic disorders. Use of contrast medium accentuates density differences and helps detect biliary problems.	Explain procedures to patient. Determine sensitivity to iodine if contrast material used.
Magnetic Resonance Imaging (MRI)	Noninvasive procedure using radiofrequency waves and a magnetic field. Procedure is used to detect hepatic metastases, sources of GI bleeding, and to stage colorectal cancer.	Patient is NPO for 6 hr before procedure. Explain procedure to patient. Contraindicated in patient with metal implants (e.g., pacemaker) or who is pregnant.

Continued

DIAGNOSTIC STUDIES

Table 37-12   Gastrointestinal System—cont'd

Study	Description and Purpose	Nursing Responsibility
Endoscopic		
Upper GI Endoscopy ■ Esophagogastro- duodenoscopy	Technique directly visualizes mucosal lining of esophagus, stomach, and duodenum with flexible, fiberoptic endoscope. Test may use video imaging to visualize stomach motility. Inflammations, ulcerations, tumors, varices, or Mallory-Weiss tear may be detected.	Before the procedure, keep patient NPO for 8 hr. Make sure signed consent is on chart. Give preoperative medication if ordered (diazepam, midazolam, or meperidine). Explain to patient that local anesthetic may be sprayed on throat before insertion of scope, and that patient will be sedated during the procedure. After the procedure, keep patient NPO until gag reflex returns. Gently tickle back of throat to determine reflex. Use warm saline gargles for relief of sore throat. Check temperature q15-30min for 1-2 hr (sudden temperature spike is sign of perforation).
Colonoscopy	Study directly visualizes entire colon up to ileocecal valve with flexible fiberoptic scope. Patient's position is changed frequently during procedure to assist with advancement of scope to cecum. Test is used to diagnose inflammatory bowel disease, detect tumors, and dilate strictures. Procedure allows for removal of colonic polyps without laparotomy.	Before the procedure, keep patient on clear liquids 1-3 days and NPO for 8 hr. Administer laxatives 1-3 days before and enemas night before. Explain to patient same information regarding insertion of scope as for sigmodoscopy. Explain to patient that sedation will be given. Administer alternate preparation of 1 gal of Golytely or Colyte evening before (8 oz glass q10min). On morning of procedure, allow clear liquids. After the procedure, be aware that patient may experience abdominal cramps caused by stimulation of peristalsis because the patient's bowel is constantly inflated with air during procedure. Observe for rectal bleeding and signs of perforation (e.g., malaise, abdominal distention, tenesmus). Check vital signs.
Proctosigmoidoscopy	Study directly visualizes rectum and sigmoid colon with lighted endoscope. It is usually done with rigid metal scope but may be done with flexible fiberscope. Sometimes special table is used to tilt patient into knee-chest position. Test may detect tumors, polyps, inflammatory and infectious diseases, fissures, hemorrhoids.	Administer enemas evening before and morning of procedure. Be aware that patient may have clear liquids day before or that no dietary restrictions may be necessary. Explain to patient knee-chest position (unless patient is older or very ill), need to take deep breaths during insertion of scope, and possible urge to defecate as scope is passed. Encourage patient to relax—let abdomen go limp. Observe for rectal bleeding after polypectomy or biopsy.
Endoscopic Retrograde Cholangiopancreatography (ERCP)	Fiberoptic endoscope is inserted through the oral cavity into descending duodenum, then common bile and pancreatic ducts are cannulated. Contrast medium is injected into ducts and allows for direct visualization of structures. Technique can also be used to retrieve a gallstone from distal CBD, dilate strictures, biopsy tumors, diagnose pseudocysts.	Before the procedure, explain procedure to patient, including patient role. Keep patient NPO 8 hr before procedure. Ensure consent form signed. Administer sedation immediately before and during procedure. Administer antibiotics if ordered. After the procedure, check vital signs. Check for signs of perforation or infection. Be aware that pancreatitis is most common complication. Check for return of gag reflex.

Continued

DIAGNOSTIC STUDIES

Table 37-12	Gastrointestinal System—cont'd	
Study	**Description and Purpose**	**Nursing Responsibility**
Endoscopic—continued		
Peritoneoscopy (Laparoscopy)	Peritoneal cavity and contents are visualized with laparoscope. Biopsy specimen may also be taken. Double-puncture peritoneoscopy permits better visualization of abdominal cavity, especially liver. Technique can eliminate need for exploratory laparotomy in many patients.	Make sure signed permit is on chart. Keep patient NPO 8 hr before study. Administer preoperative sedative medication. Ensure that bladder and bowel are emptied. Instruct patient that local anesthetic is used before scope insertion. Observe for possible complications of bleeding and bowel perforation after the procedure.
Blood Chemistries		
▪ Serum amylase	Study measures secretion of amylase by pancreas and is important in diagnosing acute pancreatitis. Level of amylase peaks in 24 hr and then drops to normal in 48-72 hr. Depending on method, *normal finding* is 0-130 U/L (0-2.17 μkat/L).	Obtain blood sample in acute attack of pancreatitis. Explain procedure to patient.
▪ Serum lipase	Study measures secretion of lipase by pancreas. Level stays elevated longer than serum amylase. *Normal finding* is 0-160 U/L (0-2.66 μkat/L).	Explain procedure to patient.
Liver Biopsy	Invasive procedure uses needle inserted between sixth and seventh or eighth and ninth intercostal spaces on the right side to obtain specimen of hepatic tissue.	Before the procedure, check patient's coagulation status (PT, clotting or bleeding time). Ensure that patient is typed and crossmatched. Take vital signs as baseline data. Explain holding of breath after expiration when needle is inserted. Ensure that informed consent has been signed. After the procedure, check vital signs to detect internal bleeding q15min × 2, q30min × 4, q1hr × 4. Keep patient lying on right side for minimum of 2 hr to splint puncture site. Keep patient in bed in flat position for 12-14 hr. Assess patient for complications such as bile peritonitis, shock, pneumothorax.
Miscellaneous Tests		
▪ Gastric analysis	Purpose is to analyze gastric contents for acidity and volume. NG tube is inserted and gastric contents are aspirated. Contents are analyzed mainly for hydrochloric acid, but pH, pepsin, and electrolytes may be determined. Histalog and pentagastrin may be used to stimulate hydrochloric acid secretion. Exfoliative cytology may be done to determine whether malignant cells are present. With fasting, *normal acidity* is 2.5 mEq/L (2.5 mmol/L) and *normal volume* is 62 ml/hr; 30 min after Histalog or pentagastrin administration, normal acidity is 1.5 mEq/L (1.5 mmol/L) and normal volume is 110 ml/hr.	Keep patient NPO for 8-12 hr. Explain insertion of NG tube. Withhold drugs affecting gastric secretions 24-48 hr before test. Ensure no smoking morning of test (nicotine increases gastric secretion).
▪ Fecal analysis	Form, consistency, color are noted. Specimen examined for mucus, blood, pus, parasites, and fat content. Tests for occult blood (guaiac test, Hemoccult, Hematest) are done.	Observe patient's stools. Collect stool specimens. Check stools for blood with Hemoccult or Hematest. Keep diet free of red meat for 24-48 hr before guaiac test.

Continued

DIAGNOSTIC STUDIES

Table 37-12   Gastrointestinal System—cont'd

Study	Description and Purpose	Nursing Responsibility
Miscellaneous Tests—continued		
■ D-Xylose	Absorption test involves xylose, a monosaccharide, given orally in water. All urine is collected for 5 hr and amount of D-Xylose excreted is measured. *Normal finding* is 20% of xylose excreted in 5 hr. Blood levels of xylose may also be obtained 1 hr after ingestion (especially in elderly).	Keep patient NPO for 10-12 hr before test. Ensure that patient empties bladder before xylose given orally.
■ Duodenal drainage	Duodenal contents are aspirated by double-lumen NG tube—one lumen in stomach, the other in duodenum. Stimulant IV drug is given (usually CCK). Duodenal contents are analyzed for enzymes, blood, bile, malignant cells, cholesterol crystals, and volume.	Explain procedure to patient. Insert NG tube. Keep patient on NPO status.

CBD, common bile duct; *CCK,* cholecystokinin; *GB,* gallbladder; *NG,* nasogastric; *Tc-99m,* technetium-99m.

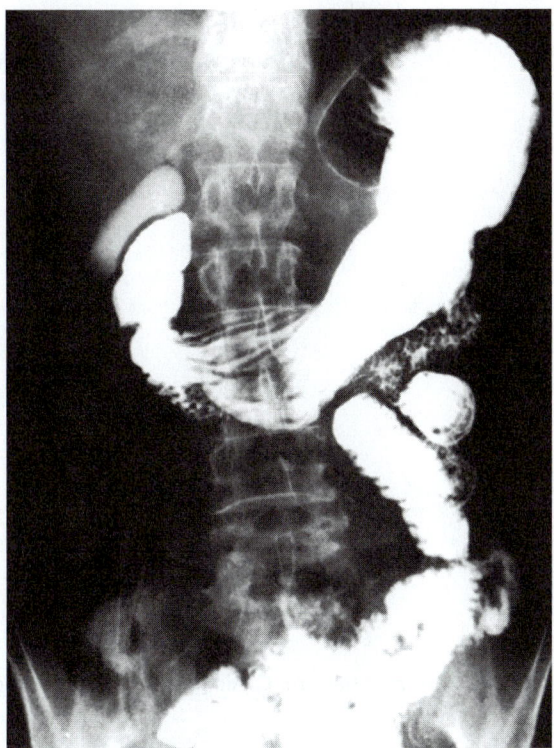

Fig. 37-10   Upper gastrointestinal tract x-ray.

Radiologic Studies

Upper Gastrointestinal Series. The purpose of an upper GI series (barium swallow) is to observe the movement of a contrast medium through the esophagus and into the stomach by means of fluoroscopy and x-ray examination. It is used to identify esophageal and stomach disorders such as esophageal strictures, varices, polyps, tumors, hiatal hernia, and peptic ulcers in the stomach or duodenum (Fig. 37-10).

The procedure consists of the patient swallowing contrast medium and then assuming different positions on the x-ray table. The movement of the contrast medium is observed with fluoroscopy, and several x-rays are taken (see Table 37-12).

Lower Gastrointestinal Series. The purpose of a lower GI series (barium enema) x-ray examination is to observe by means of fluoroscopy the filling of the colon with contrast medium and to observe by x-ray the filled colon. This procedure identifies polyps, tumors, and other lesions in the colon. It consists of administering an enema of contrast medium to the patient. The air-contrast barium enema provides better visualization of an inflammatory bowel disease, polyps, and tumors (Fig. 37-11). It is not tolerated as well in an older or immobile patient.

Oral Cholecystogram. The purpose of an oral cholecystogram (gallbladder series) is to visualize the gallbladder. It is used to determine the gallbladder's ability to concentrate and store dye and to observe the patency of the biliary duct system. It may be used to detect gallstones, obstructions of the biliary tract, and other gallbladder disorders.

The procedure consists of an x-ray examination after the oral ingestion of a radiopaque dye. The radiopaque dye used is an organic-insoluble iodide such as iopanoic acid (Telepaque, Priodax, or Oragrafin) (see Table 37-12).

Endoscopy

Endoscopy refers to the direct visualization of a body structure through a lighted instrument (scope). Most of the GI tract can be visualized by endoscopy, especially with the flexible fiberoptic scopes. The GI structures that can be examined by fiberoptic endoscopy include the esophagus, stomach, duodenum, colon, and, with the aid of fluoroscopy and x-rays, the pancreas and biliary tree. It is now possible to visualize the pancreatic, hepatic, and common bile ducts with sideviewing flexible endoscopes.[5]

The fiberscope is an instrument channel through which biopsy forceps and cytology brushes may be passed. Cameras may be attached and pictures taken. Endoscopy of the GI tract

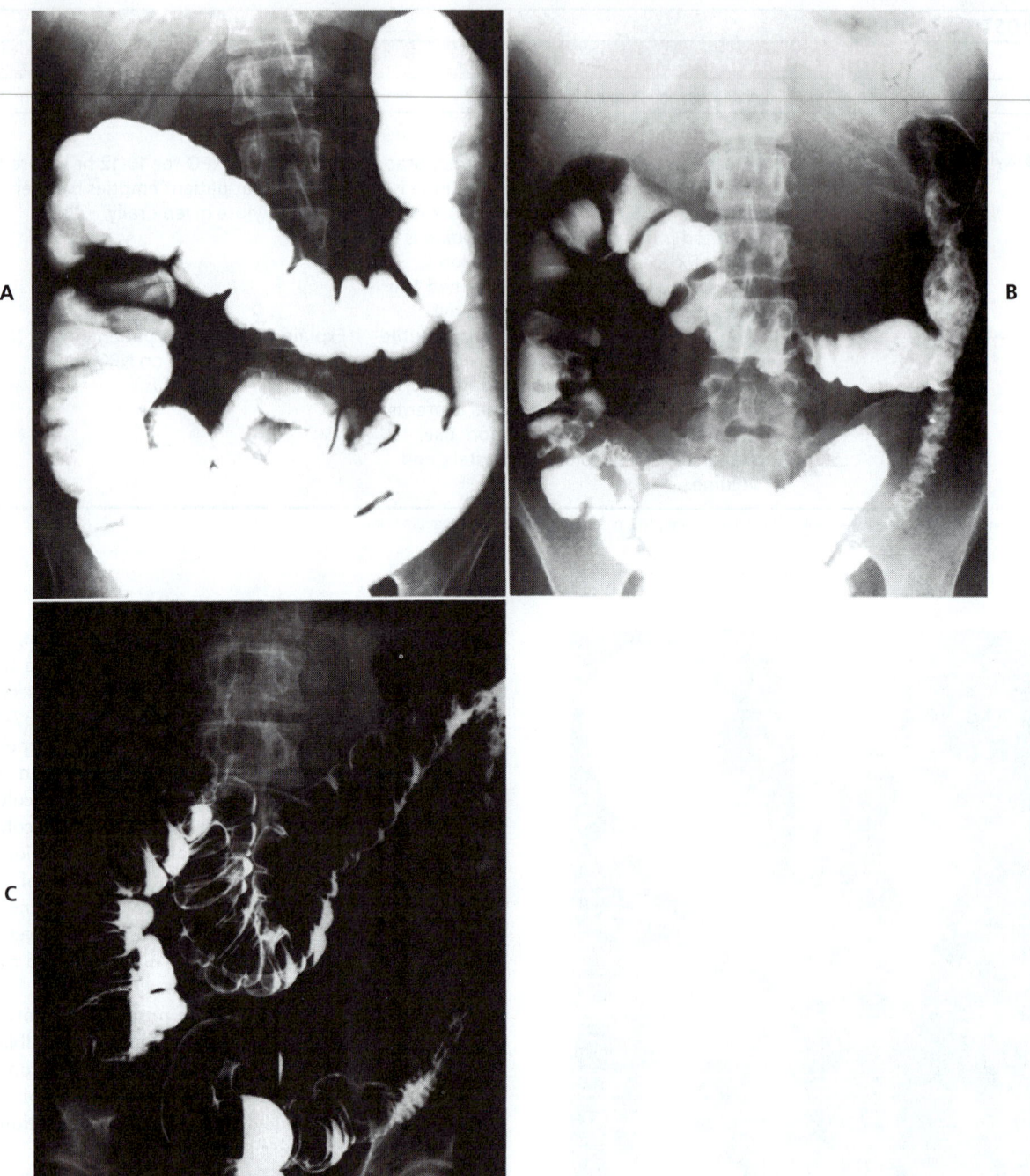

Fig. 37-11 Barium enema x-ray. **A,** Colon filled with barium. **B,** Colon after evacuation of barium. **C,** Air-contrast study of colon.

is frequently done in combination with biopsy and cytologic studies. The major complication of GI endoscopy is perforation through the structure being scoped. This complication is decreased with the use of the flexible fiberoptic scopes. All endoscopic procedures require informed, written consent. Specific endoscopy procedures are discussed in Table 37-12. In addition to diagnostic procedures, many invasive and therapeutic procedures may be done with endoscopes. These include procedures such as polypectomy, sclerosis of varices, laser treatment, cauterization of bleeding sites, papillotomy, common bile duct

stone removal, and balloon dilations. A new and valuable diagnostic procedure is video endoscopy. In this procedure an electronic video endoscope converts electronic signals that can be seen on a television screen.

Liver Biopsy

The purpose of a liver biopsy is to obtain hepatic tissue to be used in establishing a diagnosis such as cirrhosis, hepatitis, and neoplasms. It may also be useful for following the progress of liver disease.

Table 37-13	Liver Function Tests

Test	Description and Purpose
Bile Formation and Excretion	
■ Serum bilirubin	Measurement of ability of liver to conjugate and excrete bilirubin, allowing differentiation between unconjugated (indirect) and conjugated (direct) bilirubin in plasma
Total	Measurement of direct and indirect total bilirubin *Normal finding* of 0.2-1.3 mg/dl (3.4-22.0 μmol/L)
Direct	Measurement of conjugated bilirubin, elevation in obstructive jaundice *Normal finding* of 0.1-0.3 mg/dl (1.7-5.1 μmol/L)
Indirect	Measurement of unconjugated bilirubin, elevation in hepatocellular and hemolytic conditions *Normal finding* of 0.1-1.0 mg/dl (1.7-17 μmol/L)
■ Urinary bilirubin	Measurement of urinary excretion of conjugated bilirubin *Normal finding* of 0
■ Urinary urobilinogen	Measurement of urinary excretion of urobilinogen; maximum excretion midafternoon to early evening, collection of total urinary output for 2 hr in afternoon, sent to laboratory in dark container immediately because of oxidation of urobilinogen to urobilin on exposure to air *Normal finding* of 0.5-4 mg/day (0.8-6.8 μmol/day)
■ Fecal urobilinogen	Measurement of fecal urobilinogen in stool specimen *Normal finding* of 30-220 mg/100 g stool (55-372 μmol/100 g of stool)
Dye Excretion Tests (Detoxification)	
■ Indocyanine green	Determination of liver's ability to take up and excrete dye given IV, drawing of blood samples every 5 min for 20-30 min *Normal finding* of 500-800 ml/m^2 of body surface/min
Protein Metabolism	
■ Serum protein levels	Measurement of serum proteins that are manufactured by the liver; measurement of albumin, *normal finding* of 3.5-5.0 g/dl (35-50 g/L); measurement of globulin, *normal finding* of 2.0-3.5 g/dl (20-35 g/L) *Normal total protein* of 6-8 g/dl (60-80 g/L) *Normal A/G ratio* of 1.5:1-2.5:1
■ α-Fetoprotein	Indication of hepatic cancer *Normal finding* of <25 ng/ml (<25 μg/L)
■ Blood ammonia levels	Conversion of ammonia to urea normally occurs in the liver, elevation can result in hepatic encephalopathy secondary to liver cirrhosis *Normal finding* of 30-70 μg/dl (17.6-41.1 μmol/L)
Hemostatic Functions	
■ Prothrombin	Determination of prothrombin activity *Normal finding* of 12-15 sec
■ Vitamin K production	Determination of response of liver to vitamin K, checking of PT necessary 24 hr after injection of vitamin K

Continued

The two types of liver biopsy are open and closed. The open method involves making an incision and removing a wedge of tissue. It is done in the operating room with the patient under general anesthesia, often concurrently with another surgical procedure. The closed, or needle, biopsy is an invasive procedure in which the site is infiltrated with a local anesthetic and a needle is inserted between the sixth and seventh or eighth and ninth intercostal spaces on the right side. The patient lies supine with the right arm over the head. The patient should be instructed to expire fully and not breathe while the needle is inserted. Nursing assessment before and after a liver biopsy is important (see Table 37-12).

Liver Function Studies

Liver function tests are usually described separately from other GI diagnostic studies. Liver function tests are basically biochemical determinations that reflect hepatic disease. Table 37-13 describes some common liver function tests.

Table **37-13**	**Liver Function Tests—cont'd**
Test	**Description and Purpose**

Serum Enzyme Tests

- Alkaline phosphatase (ALP) — Originating in bone and liver. Serum levels rise when excretion is impaired as a result of obstruction in the biliary tract.
  Normal finding of 30-120 U/L (0.5-2.0 μkat/L), depending on method and age
- Aspartate aminotransferase (AST) or serum glutamic-oxaloacetic transaminase (SGOT) — Elevation in liver damage and inflammation
  Normal finding of 7-40 U/L (0.12-0.67 μkat/L)
- Alanine aminotransferase (ALT) or serum glutamic-pyruvic transaminase (SGPT) — Elevation in liver damage and inflammation
  Normal finding of 5-36 U/L (0.08-0.6 μkat/L)
- δ-Glutamyl transpeptidase (GGT) — Present in biliary tract (not in skeletal muscle or cardiac), increase in hepatitis and alcoholic liver disease. More sensitive for liver dysfunction than ALP.
  Normal finding of 0-30 U/L (0-.5 μkat/L)

Lipid Metabolism

- Serum cholesterol — Synthesis and excretion by liver, increase in biliary obstruction, decrease in extensive liver disease and malnutrition
  Normal finding of 140-200 mg/dl (3.6-5.2 mmol/L), varying with age

REVIEW QUESTIONS

The number of the question corresponds to the same-numbered objective at the beginning of the chapter.

1. A patient is admitted to the hospital with a diagnosis of diarrhea with dehydration. The nurse recognizes that increased peristalsis resulting in diarrhea can be related to
   a. sympathetic inhibition.
   b. mixing and propulsion.
   c. sympathetic stimulation.
   d. parasympathetic stimulation.

2. A patient has an elevated blood level of indirect bilirubin. One cause of this finding is that
   a. the gallbladder is unable to contract to release stored bile.
   b. bilirubin is not being conjugated and excreted into the bile by the liver.
   c. the Kuppfer cells in the liver are unable to remove bilirubin from the blood.
   d. there is an obstruction in the biliary tract preventing flow of bile into the small intestine.

3. As gastric contents move into the small intestine the bowel is normally protected from the acidity of gastric contents by the
   a. inhibition of secretin release.
   b. release of bicarbonate by the pancreas.
   c. release of pancreatic digestive enzymes.
   d. release of gastrin by the duodenal mucosa.

4. A patient is jaundiced and her stools are clay colored (gray). This is most likely related to
   a. decreased bile flow into the intestine.
   b. increased production of urobilinogen.
   c. increased production of cholecystokinin.
   d. increased bile and bilirubin in the blood.

5. An 80-year-old man states that although he adds a lot of salt to his food it still does not have much taste. The nurse's response is based on the knowledge that the older adult
   a. should not experience changes in taste.
   b. has some loss of taste but no difficulty chewing food.
   c. has a loss of taste buds, especially for sweet and salt.
   d. loses the sense of taste because the ability to smell is decreased.

6. When assessing the health promotion–health maintenance pattern as related to GI function an appropriate question by the nurse is,
   a. "What is your usual bowel elimination pattern?"
   b. "What percentage of your income is spent on food?"
   c. "Have you traveled to a foreign country in the last year?"
   d. "Do you have diarrhea when you are under a lot of stress?"

7. During an examination of the abdomen the nurse should
   a. position the patient in the supine position with the bed flat and knees straight.
   b. listen in the epigastrium and all four quadrants for 2 to 5 minutes for bowel sounds.
   c. use the following order of techniques: inspection, palpation, percussion, auscultation.
   d. describe bowel sounds as absent if no sound is heard in the lower right quadrant after 2 minutes.

8. A normal physical assessment finding of the GI system is
   a. tympany on percussion of the abdomen.
   b. liver edge (1-2 cm below the costal margin).
   c. finding of a firm, nodular edge on the rectal examination.
   d. easy palpation of the spleen edges with moderate pressure.

9. In preparing a patient for a colonoscopy the nurse explains that
   a. a signed permit is not necessary.
   b. sedation may be used during the procedure.
   c. only one cleansing enema is necessary for preparation.
   d. a light meal should be eaten the day before the procedure.

References

1. Eliopoulos C: *Gerontological nursing,* ed 4, Philadelphia, 1997, Lippincott.
2. Porth CM: *Pathophysiology concepts of altered health states,* ed 5, Philadelphia, 1999, Lippincott.
3. Burke MM, Walsh MB: *Gerontologic nursing: wholistic care of the older adult,* ed 2, St Louis, 1997, Mosby.
4. Bates B: *A guide to physical examination and history taking,* ed 7, Philadelphia, 1999, Lippincott.
5. Seidel HM and others: *Mosby's guide to physical examination,* ed 4, St Louis, 1999, Mosby.
6. Karanikas ID and others: Barium peritonitis: a rare complication of upper gastrointestinal contrast investigation, *Postgrad Med J* 73:297, 1997.
7. Thibodeau G, Patton KT: *Anatomy and physiology,* ed 4, St. Louis, 1999, Mosby.
8. Barkausus V and others: *Health and physical assessment,* ed 2, St Louis, 1998, Mosby.
9. Ebersole P, Hess P: *Toward healthy aging,* ed 5, St Louis, 1998, Mosby.
10. McCance KL, Huether SE: *Pathophysiology: the biologic basis for disease in adults and children,* ed 3, St Louis, 1998, Mosby.

Resources

Resources for this chapter are listed after Chapter 38 on p. 1079.

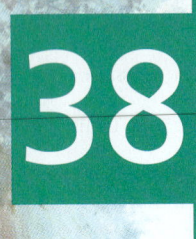

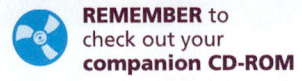
38 NURSING MANAGEMENT
Nutritional Problems

Una Elizabeth Westfall

www.mosby.com/MERLIN/medsurg_lewis

LEARNING OBJECTIVES

1. Describe the essential components of a nutritionally sound diet and their importance to good health.
2. Describe possible adverse interactions between drugs and various foods.
3. Describe the common etiologic factors, clinical manifestations, and management of malnutrition.
4. Compare the etiologic factors, clinical manifestations, and collaborative and nursing management of bulimia and anorexia nervosa.
5. Differentiate between central and peripheral total parenteral nutrition administration and tube feedings,

including the indications for use, complications, and collaborative and nursing management.
6. Describe the types of gastrostomy tubes and related nursing care.
7. Discuss the multiple etiologies, complications, and collaborative care approaches to the management of obesity.
8. Describe the nursing care related to conservative and surgical management of obesity.

The focus of this chapter is on problems related to nutrition. The primary nutritional problems discussed are malnutrition and obesity.

NUTRITIONAL PROBLEMS

Nutritional problems are present in all age-groups, cultures, ethnic groups, and socioeconomic classes in all parts of the world. Intelligence and wealth do not necessarily preclude the development of poor nutritional habits. The nurse in the roles of caregiver, teacher, and resource person can have a profound influence on the nutritional practices of patients and their families. A strong foundation in the principles of sound nutrition is essential. Together with the physician and the registered dietician, the nurse is in a strategic position to assess the dietary practices of the patient and provide important information, as well as link an individual with nutritional resources within and outside the institutional setting.

The nutritional state of a person or a family may be influenced by many factors. Attitudes toward the importance of food and eating habits are established early. Cultural or religious preferences and requirements are frequently reflected in dietary intake. The financial condition of a family or an individual often determines the type and amount of nutritionally sound food that can be purchased. Findings support that, generally, the lower the socioeconomic status, the poorer the nutritional state.[1] The availability of food sources also contributes to

the nutritional state of people. This is usually not a problem in developed countries in which agriculture is well established and productive, but it may be a problem in underdeveloped countries.

NORMAL NUTRITION

Nutrition is the process by which the body uses food for energy, growth, and maintenance and repair of body tissues. Good nutrition in the absence of any underlying disease process results from the ingestion of a balanced diet. The United States Department of Agriculture (USDA) has adopted the food guide pyramid, which consists of food groups that are presented in proportions appropriate for a healthful diet. Figure 38-1 and Table 38-1 show these food groups with the recommended daily requirements and examples of common sources.

The essential components of the basic food groups are carbohydrates, fats, proteins, vitamins, and minerals. Carbohydrates, the body's primary source of energy, yield approximately 4 kilocalories per gram. (Kilocalorie is the correct unit to designate caloric intake and expenditure. However, calorie is more commonly used.) Carbohydrates are either simple or complex. Simple carbohydrates come in two forms: monosaccharides (e.g., glucose and fructose), found in fruits and honey; and disaccharides (e.g., sucrose, maltose, and lactose), found in such substances as table sugar, malted cereal, and milk, respectively. Complex carbohydrates or polysaccharides commonly appear in the diet as starches, such as cereal grains, potatoes, and legumes. Carbohydrates are the chief protein-sparing ingredient in a nutritionally sound diet and compose approximately 47% of the daily caloric needs of the body. The National Research Council recommends that, after infancy, at least half

Reviewed by Kathryn Hennessy, RN, MS, CNSN, Adult Nurse Practitioner, Manager, Clinical and Nursing Services, Nestle Clinical Nutrition, Deerfield, Ill.

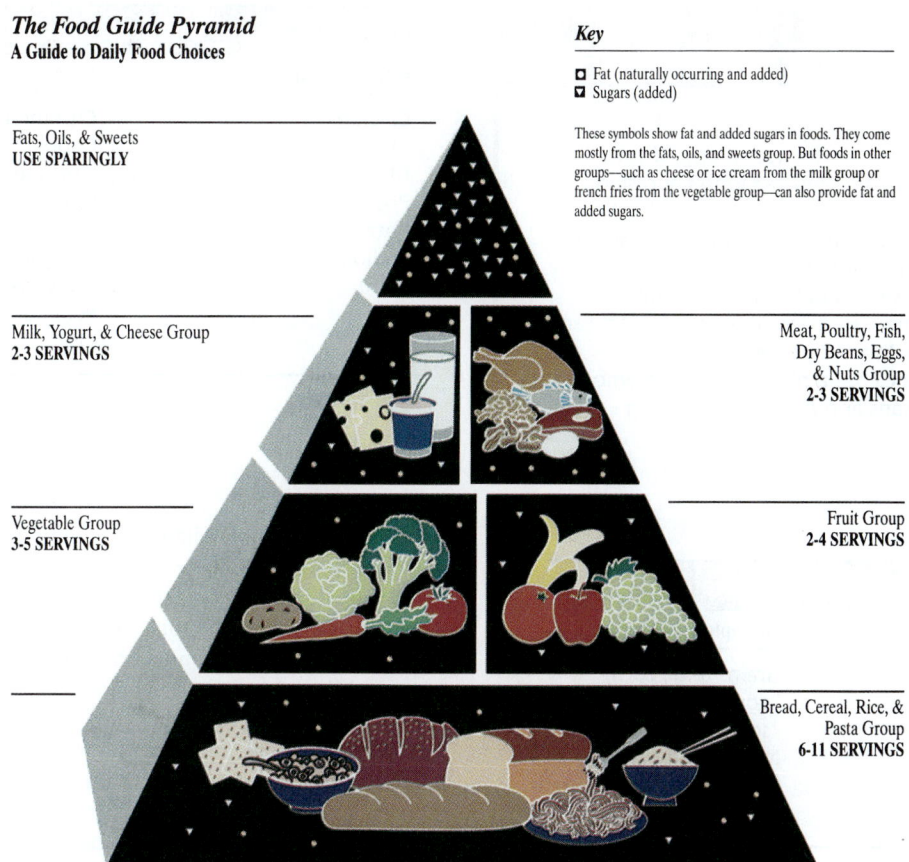

The Food Guide Pyramid
A Guide to Daily Food Choices

Key

☐ Fat (naturally occurring and added)
▼ Sugars (added)

These symbols show fat and added sugars in foods. They come mostly from the fats, oils, and sweets group. But foods in other groups—such as cheese or ice cream from the milk group or french fries from the vegetable group—can also provide fat and added sugars.

Fats, Oils, & Sweets
USE SPARINGLY

Milk, Yogurt, & Cheese Group
2-3 SERVINGS

Meat, Poultry, Fish,
Dry Beans, Eggs,
& Nuts Group
2-3 SERVINGS

Vegetable Group
3-5 SERVINGS

Fruit Group
2-4 SERVINGS

Bread, Cereal, Rice, &
Pasta Group
6-11 SERVINGS

Fig. 38-1   Food guide pyramid: a guide to daily food choices and number of servings.

Table 38-1   Pyramid Food Groups and Recommended Number of Servings

Group	Nutrients Provided	Number of Servings Daily	Serving Size
■ Bread, cereal, rice, pasta	Thiamine, niacin, iron, protein	6-11	1 slice of bread 1 oz ready-to-eat cereal ½ cup of cooked cereal, rice, or pasta
■ Vegetable	Vitamins A and C, folic acid	3-5	1 cup of raw leafy vegetables ½ cup of other vegetables, cooked or raw ¾ cup of vegetable juice
■ Fruit	Vitamins A and C	2-4	1 medium apple, banana, or orange ½ cup of chopped, cooked, or canned fruit ¾ cup of fruit juice
■ Milk, yogurt, cheese	Calcium, protein, riboflavin, vitamin B_6, and cobalamin	2-3	1 cup of milk or yogurt 1½ oz of natural cheese 2 oz of processed cheese
■ Meat, poultry, fish, dry beans, eggs, nuts	Protein, niacin, thiamine, iron, zinc, cobalamin, folic acid	2-3	2-3 oz of cooked lean meat, poultry, or fish ½ cup of cooked dry beans, 1 egg, or 2 tbsp of peanut butter (count as 1 oz lean meat)

From Human Nutrition Information Service: *Food guide pyramid*, Hyattsville, Md, 1992, USDA.

of the body's energy needs should come from carbohydrates, especially complex carbohydrates.[2]

Approximately 36% of the daily caloric intake in current American diets is derived from fat.[2] This level is considerably higher than that found in many other societies and is a cause for national concern. The Food and Nutrition Board's Com-

mittee on Diet and Health recommends that people reduce their fat intake to 30% of their total daily caloric intake.[3] One gram of fat yields 9 calories. Fats are stored in adipose tissue and in the abdominal cavity. Besides being a major source of energy, fats act as insulation, which reduces loss of body heat in cold environments and provides padding and protection for

Table **38-3**	Major Minerals and Trace Elements
Major Minerals	**Trace Elements**
Calcium	Chromium
Chloride	Copper
Magnesium	Fluoride
Phosphorus	Iodine
Potassium	Iron
Sodium	Manganese
Sulfur	Molybdenum
	Selenium
	Zinc

Table **38-2**	Good Sources of Protein
Complete Proteins	**Incomplete Proteins**
Milk and milk products (e.g., cheese)	Grains (e.g., corn)
	Legumes (e.g., navy beans, soybeans, peas)
Eggs	Nuts (e.g., peanuts)
Fish	Seeds (e.g., sesame seeds, sunflower seeds)
Meats	
Poultry	

vital organs. Fats also act as carriers of essential fatty acids and fat-soluble vitamins. Fats provide a feeling of satiety after eating, partly from the flavor added and partly from their slow rate of digestion, which delays hunger.

Proteins, another essential component of a well-balanced diet, are obtained from both animal and plant sources. Ideally, proteins provide 15% to 20% of daily caloric needs of the body. The recommended daily maintenance protein intake is 0.8 to 1.0 g/kg of body weight. One gram of protein yields 4 calories. Proteins are complex nitrogenous organic compounds, of which amino acids are the fundamental units of structure. The 22 amino acids can be classified as essential and nonessential. The body is capable of synthesizing nonessential amino acids if an adequate supply of nitrogen is available. However, the nine essential amino acids cannot be synthesized, and their availability depends totally on dietary sources. Protein sources containing all the essential amino acids are called complete proteins. Proteins that lack one or more of the essential amino acids are called incomplete proteins. Table 38-2 lists good sources of protein. Proteins are essential for tissue growth, repair, and maintenance; body regulatory functions; and energy production.

Vitamins are organic compounds required in small amounts by the body for normal metabolism. Vitamins function primarily in enzyme reactions that facilitate the metabolism of amino acids, fats, and carbohydrates. The body must rely on a dietary source to meet requirements for some vitamins, such as cobalamin (vitamin B_{12}). Vitamins are divided into two cate-gories: water-soluble vitamins (vitamin C and the B-complex vitamins) and fat-soluble vitamins (vitamins A, D, E, and K).

Mineral salts (e.g., magnesium, iron, calcium) make up approximately 4% of the total body weight. When minerals are present in minute amounts, they are referred to as trace elements. Minerals required in amounts greater than 100 mg per day are called major minerals. Table 38-3 lists the major minerals and trace elements. Minerals are necessary for the body to build tissues, regulate body fluids, and assist in various body functions. Some minerals are stored in a manner similar to that of the fat-soluble vitamins and can be toxic if taken in excess amounts. The amount of minerals needed in the daily diet varies greatly from a few micrograms of trace minerals to 1 g or more of the major minerals, such as calcium, phosphorus, and sodium. A well-balanced diet can usually meet the daily requirements of needed minerals. However, deficiency states can occur.

The daily caloric requirements of a person are influenced by body build, age, gender, physical activity, and level of physical and emotional health. Adjustments in caloric intake are necessary, depending on changes in health status and daily activity level. Table 38-4 summarizes the recommended daily caloric and protein intake. Table 38-5 gives an example of caloric and protein needs under normal and stress conditions.

NUTRITIONAL NEEDS
Children and Adolescents

Parents are responsible for setting an example of good nutritional habits for their children. Parental eating habits and attitudes toward food are readily passed on to their children. Parents who have little understanding of what constitutes a well-balanced diet or who cannot or will not learn good nutritional habits influence their children to follow the same poor dietary practices. The nurse is in a good position to help parents understand the changing food requirements of their children from infancy through adolescence.

Infants and children differ from adults in several ways. In the first months of life, the infant's gastrointestinal (GI) tract and kidneys are not functionally mature and therefore are limited in the kinds and quantities of nutrients that should be given. The metabolic rate of infants is higher and they have smaller nutritional reserve as compared with adults.

Table **38-4**	Recommended Daily Protein and Caloric Intake by Median Heights and Weights						
Category	Age (yr)	Weight (lb)	(kg)	Height (in)	(cm)	Protein (g)	Average Daily Energy Allowance* (calories)
■ Men	19-24	160	72	70	177	58	2900
	25-50	174	79	70	176	63	2900
	51 and over	170	77	68	173	68	2300
■ Women	19-24	128	58	65	164	46	2200
	25-50	138	63	64	163	50	2200
	51 and over	143	65	63	160	50	1900

Modified from Food and Nutrition Board, National Research Council, National Academy of Sciences: *Recommended dietary allowances,* ed 10, Washington, DC, 1989, National Academy Press.
*For light to moderate activity.

Table **38-5**	Caloric and Protein Needs of a 150 lb (68 kg) Man	
Activity	Calories	Protein (g)
Basal	1400	49
Moderate activity (activities of daily living)	2500	70
Postoperative (no complications)	3150	105
Stress response (e.g., to chemotherapy, radiation therapy)	3500	140
Infection	>4500	>175

Table **38-6**	Low-Cost Protein Supplements
Brewer's yeast	2⅓ tbs
Cheese	1-in cube
Cottage cheese	¼ cup
Egg	1
Milk (whole, low fat, or skim)	⅞ cup
Peanut butter	2 tbs
Pinto beans	¼ cup
Poultry	1 oz
Soybeans (cooked)	1 cup and 2 tsp
Split peas, lentils (cooked)	½ cup

Adolescence is a particularly vulnerable time for the development of nutritional deficiencies because this is a time of rapid growth and bodily changes. It is a period during which there is extreme concern with body appearance and social acceptability. Teenage girls are often attracted to fad diets as a means of weight control. Unfortunately, fad diets are often nutritionally unsound. Unless good nutritional habits are encouraged and supervised by peers and parents during this developmental period, poor nutritional patterns may become established as a way of life. A state of chronic inadequate nutrition may result.

Socioeconomic Status

Because individuals and families from the lower socioeconomic class spend a greater percentage of their limited income on food, there is a tendency to seek out cheaper foods as the cost of food increases. These foods may not provide adequate or balanced nutrition. In contrast, some lower-income persons may prefer to select foods that are more expensive, but only marginally nutritious, because of their prestige value. The nurse and the registered dietician can assist the poor in making food choices that meet nutritional requirements while staying within their limited resources. Table 38-6 lists low-cost protein supplements.

Older Adults

The unique nutritional requirements of an older adult are often overlooked. It is more common to find an undernourished older person than an obese one. As a person grows older there are decreases in lean body mass (the metabolically active tissue), basal metabolic rate, and physical activity. Combined, these factors decrease the caloric needs for energy. The older person frequently reduces the consumption of needed protein, vitamins, and minerals and may take in "empty calories," such as candy and pastries. The reasons given for such alterations are varied. Table 38-7 outlines factors affecting nutritional intake in older adults.

As a group, older adults may be less well informed about what constitutes a well-balanced diet. The older adult may be induced to purchase more costly "health foods" at specialty stores under mistaken assumptions, such as that these foods offer more nutrients than foods bought at the local market, or that the food supply is nutritionally inadequate.[4]

When these factors are added to already existing medical problems, it is easy to see why poor dietary practices develop. In addition, poor dentition, ill-fitting dentures, anorexia, multiple losses affecting the social setting of meals, low income, and medical conditions involving the GI tract contribute to the type and amount of foods that is eaten. The nurse, working with the registered dietician, must be aware of common medical and psychosocial factors in the older adult and should incorporate interventions for overcoming these problems in the plan of care.

Patients with Physical Illnesses

Regardless of the cause of the illness, the sick person has increased nutritional needs. Pathologic conditions are frequently aggravated by undernutrition, and an existing deficiency state is

Table **38-7**	Factors Affecting Nutritional Intake in Older Adults
Age	Feelings of being
Anorexia	valued
Availability of	Food fads
desired foods	Food intolerance
Availability of	Gender
transportation to	Health status
food stores	Importance of food in the past
Available time for	Income level
preparation and	Lack of food preparation
eating	equipment
Chronic conditions	Loneliness or loss
Decrease in number	Mental awareness
of taste buds	Physical disability
Degree of physical	Prescribed diets
activity	Prescribed or over-the-counter
Dental problems	medicines
Education level	Social isolation
and nutritional	
knowledge	

likely to become more severe during illness. Malnutrition is not an uncommon consequence of illness, surgery, injury, or hospitalization. Anorexia, nausea, vomiting, diarrhea, abdominal distention, and abdominal cramping may accompany diseases of the GI system. Any combination of these symptoms interferes with normal food consumption and metabolism. Additionally, a patient may restrict the dietary intake to a few foods or fluids that may not be nutritionally sound out of fear of aggravating the already disturbed GI function.

Malabsorption syndrome is defined as the impaired absorption of nutrients from the GI tract. It may result from decreased amounts of necessary enzymes or a reduced bowel surface area and can quickly lead to a deficiency state. Many pharmacologic agents may result in undesirable GI side effects, as well as alter normal digestive and absorptive processes. For example, antibiotics change the normal flora of the intestines, decreasing the body's ability to synthesize biotin.

Fever accompanies many illnesses, injuries, and infections, with a concomitant increase in the body's basal metabolic rate (BMR). Each degree of temperature increase on the Fahrenheit scale raises the BMR by 7%.[2] Without an increase in the amount of calories ingested in the diet, body protein stores will be used to supply calories, and protein depletion can become a problem.

The hospitalized patient, especially the older adult, is at risk of becoming malnourished. Prolonged illness, major surgery, sepsis, draining wounds, burns, hemorrhage, fractures, and immobilization can all contribute to malnutrition. The nurse must assume responsibility, along with the physician and the dietician, for meeting the patient's nutritional needs. The nurse must also be knowledgeable of the requirements of a patient who is not overtly ill but who is undergoing diagnostic studies. This patient may be nutritionally fit on entering the hospital but can develop nutritional problems because of the dietary restrictions imposed by multiple diagnostic studies.

The role of nutrition in the development of diseases has long been studied. Studies of the association of personal dietary habits with the development of selected cancers and cardiovascular diseases have been widely published in recent years. There now appear to be links between some types of cancers and dietary intake; for example, high ingestion of fatty foods is linked with breast and endometrial cancer, and a low fiber intake may be linked with colon cancer (see Chapter 40). Further research in this area is needed for a better understanding of diet and the development of disease, especially cancer.

VITAMIN IMBALANCES

Vitamin deficiencies are rare in most of the developed countries of the world. When vitamin deficiencies are present, several vitamins are usually involved rather than a single vitamin deficiency. The recommended dietary allowance (RDA) for essential vitamins and minerals can be obtained by eating a diet consisting of foods from the basic five food groups. RDAs from the Food and Nutrition Board have a safety margin because the levels exceed minimum daily requirements for most people. When vitamin imbalances do occur, they are usually found among persons with a pattern of alcohol and drug abuse, persons who are chronically ill, and individuals who follow poor dietary practices. Followers of fad diets or poorly planned vegetarian diets are also subject to a potential deficiency state. Clinical manifestations of vitamin imbalances are most commonly exhibited as neurologic manifestations (Table 38-8). In the growing child, the central nervous system (CNS) is primarily involved, while the peripheral nervous system is most affected in the adult.

Vegetarian Diets

The common element among all vegetarians is the exclusion of red meat from the diet. Vegetarianism cannot be considered a nutritional fad because it is found in all age-groups, occupations, and lifestyles. A variety of reasons have been given for following this type of dietary practice, including religious or cultural beliefs that it is a better way of attaining total health, respect for all living beings, ethical-ecologic ideals, and economics.

The two large classes of vegetarians are *vegans*, who are pure or total vegetarians and use only plant food, and *lacto-ovo-vegetarians*, who use plant foods and sometimes dairy products and eggs. There are several other types, including the fruitarians, but they constitute only a small percentage of the total group.

Vegetarian diets can result in a potential vitamin deficiency state. In well-planned vegetarian diets the essential vitamins and minerals are easily obtained. Plant protein, although of a lesser quality than that of animal origin, fulfills most of the protein requirements. Combinations of vegetable protein foods (e.g., cornmeal, kidney beans) can increase the nutritional value. Lacto-ovo-vegetarians obtain additional protein sources from dairy products and eggs. Milk made from soybeans is an excellent protein source, especially for the true vegan. The primary deficiency of a strict vegan is lack of cobalamin (vitamin B_{12}). This vitamin can be obtained only from animal protein, special supplements, or foods that have been fortified with the

Table **38-8**	**Recommended Dietary Vitamin Allowances and Signs of Imbalance**		
Vitamin	**Recommended Dietary Allowances**	**Symptoms of Overdose**	**Manifestations of Deficiencies**
Fat Soluble			
▪ A	Men: 1000 μg/Retinol equivalents* Women: 800 μg/Retinol equivalents	Hair loss, dry skin; headaches; dry mucous membranes; liver damage; bone and joint pain; blurred vision; nausea and vomiting	Dry, scaly skin; increased susceptibility to infection; night blindness; anorexia; eye irritation; xerosis; keratinization of respiratory and GI mucosa; bladder stones; anemia; retarded growth
▪ D	Adults 5-10 μg of cholecalciferol†	Deposits of calcium and phosphorus in soft tissue; kidney and heart damage; bone fragility; constipation; anorexia, nausea, vomiting; headache	Muscular weakness; excessive sweating; diarrhea and other GI disturbances; bone pain; active rickets; healed rickets; osteomalacia
▪ E	Men: 10 mg Women: 8 mg	Relatively nontoxic	Neurologic defects; hemolytic anemia (only in newborns)
▪ K	Men: 70-80 μg Women: 60-65 μg	Anemia	Defective blood coagulation
Water Soluble			
▪ B_1	Men: 1.2-1.5 mg Women: 1.0-1.1 mg	Not stored in body, therefore overdose does not occur	Loss of appetite; fatigue; nervous irritability; constipation; paresthesias; insomnia
▪ B_6	Men: 1.7-2.0 mg Women: 1.4-1.6 mg	Not stored in body, therefore overdose does not occur	Seizures; dermatitis; anemia; neuropathy with motor weakness; anorexia
▪ Cobalamin (B_{12})	Adults: 2-10 μg	Not stored in body, therefore overdose does not occur	Megaloblastic anemia; inadequate myelin synthesis; anorexia; glossitis; sore mouth and tongue; pallor; neurologic problems such as depression and dizziness; weight loss; nausea; constipation
▪ C	Adults: 50-60 mg	Not stored in body, therefore overdose does not occur	Bleeding gums; loose teeth; easy bruising; poor wound healing; scurvy; dry, itchy skin
▪ Folic acid	Men: 200 μg Women: 180 μg	Not stored in body, therefore overdose does not occur	Impaired cell division and protein synthesis; megaloblastic anemia; anorexia; fatigue; sore tongue; diarrhea; forgetfulness

Modified from Food and Nutrition Board, National Academy of Sciences, National Research Council: *Recommended dietary allowances,* ed 10, Washington DC, 1989, National Academy Press.
*1 Retinol Equivalent = 10 IU vitamin A activity from β-carotene or 3.33 IU vitamin A activity from retinol.
†1 μg of cholecalciferol = 40 IU vitamin D.
GI, gastrointestinal.

vitamin. Vegans not using cobalamin supplements are susceptible to the development of megaloblastic anemia and the neurologic signs of cobalamin deficiency. Strict vegetarians and lacto-ovo-vegetarians are also at risk for iron deficiency. Iron-enriched foods or iron supplements are often prescribed during pregnancy, early childhood, adolescence, and after major blood loss. Table 38-9 lists examples of foods high in iron. Other deficiencies that may be present in a vegan include calcium, zinc, vitamins A and D, and protein.

Megavitamin Therapy

Megavitamin therapy refers to the administration of high doses of one or more vitamins, usually 10 to 20 times the RDA. Unless there are serious vitamin deficiencies, megavitamin therapy has a limited place in maintaining nutrition. The beneficial effects derived from the ingestion of commercially prepared daily vitamins are negligible if a balanced diet is eaten.

The water-soluble vitamins (vitamins C and B complex) are absorbed only as needed by the body, and the excess is excreted rapidly in the urine. Toxicity from overdoses is rare. However, because the excess is excreted through the kidney and urinary tract, detrimental effects may occur. Vitamin C is uricosuric (increases the renal excretion of uric acid) and may cause the formation of urinary tract stones (uric acid stones) in susceptible persons when taken in megadoses. When taken in large doses, vitamins can function as drugs rather than as nutrients and can cause toxic manifestations.

The fat-soluble vitamins (vitamins A, D, E, and K) are readily stored and can accumulate to toxic levels. Because most vitamins can be purchased without a prescription, high doses of

NUTRITIONAL THERAPY

Table 38-9 Foods High in Iron

Food	Selected Serving Size	% of U.S. RDA
Breads, Cereals, and Grain Products		
Farina, regular or quick cooked (enriched)	⅔ cup	25-39
Oatmeal, instant, fortified, prepared (enriched)	⅔ cup	25-39
Ready-to-eat cereals, fortified (enriched)	1 oz	25-39
Meat, Poultry, Fish, and Alternatives		
Beef liver, braised	3 oz	25-39
Pork liver, braised	3 oz	>39
Chicken or turkey liver, braised	½ cup diced	25-39
Clams; steamed, boiled, or canned, drained	3 oz	>39
Oysters; baked, broiled, steamed or canned, undrained	3 oz	25-39
Soybeans, cooked	½ cup	25-39

From Human Nutrition Information Service: *Good sources of nutrients,* Washington, DC, 1990, USDA.
NOTE: Vitamin C improves iron absorption.
RDA, recommended dietary allowance.

vitamins A, D, and E can result in serious health hazards because the excess is not eliminated (see Table 38-8). Toxic levels of the fat-soluble vitamins can be reached within a matter of weeks, especially in infants and children.

DRUG-FOOD INTERACTIONS

When health conditions require drug therapy, drug and food or nutrient interactions may not be explored before starting a prescription. Adverse interactions can include incompatibilities, altered drug effectiveness, and impaired nutritional status. Table 38-10 outlines examples of common drug and food-nutrient interactions. As members of the health team, nurses have a responsibility for monitoring and preventing potential interactions for patients while in the hospital and at home.

EATING DISORDERS

Anorexia Nervosa

Anorexia nervosa, sometimes called anorexia, is a specific psychiatric diagnosis. Anorexia nervosa is characterized by refusal to maintain body weight to greater than 85% of that expected for age and height.[5] This condition results in a severely malnourished state characterized by the vigorous pursuit of thinness and a morbid fear of becoming fat. Restricted intake occurs even in the presence of hunger.

The two subgroups of anorexia nervosa are termed the *bulimic type* and the *restrictive type*, depending on whether there are cycles of binging and purging. This condition is found predominantly in adolescent girls. The disorder was first recorded in England in 1684 and was misnamed anorexia nervosa because it was thought to be secondary to severe sadness and anxiety. The name has persisted to the present day even though current research indicates a different cause. Anorexia nervosa usually begins during adolescence or early adulthood. It is a chronic illness that can place the patient at high risk for serious complications, affecting multiple organ systems. Life-threatening cardiac complications include hypotension, bradycardia, and malignant arrhythmias. It is rare for the illness to occur for the first time in a woman who is more than 25 years old.

Anorexia nervosa is now recognized as occurring more often among persons whose sisters and mothers have the disorder than among the general population. Patients usually come from a middle- or upper-class background.[6] They often are perfectionists and tend to be high achievers. At the same time, they may be dependent and experience insecurity in social situations. In some patients the disorder is associated with stressful life situations with which they are unable to cope. In addition, many patients are somewhat overweight at the onset of their illness.

Common physical signs and symptoms of anorexia nervosa include amenorrhea, bradycardia, orthostatic hypotension, cold intolerance, breast atrophy, lanugo (soft, downlike hair normally associated with a fetus), dry skin, hair loss, severe constipation, and edema with altered fluid balance. Diagnostic studies often show iron deficiency anemia and an elevated blood urea nitrogen that is reflective of marked intravascular volume depletion and prerenal azotemia. Lack of potassium in the diet and loss of potassium in the urine lead to potassium deficiency in blood and tissues, leading to weakness, cardiac arrhythmias, and renal failure. If the eating pattern is permitted to continue for a prolonged time, body wasting and signs of severe malnutrition are evident.

Once anorexia nervosa has developed, the person will go to almost any extreme to hide the eating behavior from parents or peers. Eating habits are severely disturbed. If purging is present, it is often accomplished by self-induced vomiting or the use of cathartics or enemas.

Multidisciplinary treatment must involve a combination of nutrition support and psychiatric care. Hospitalization may be necessary if there are severe physical complications that cannot be managed in an outpatient therapy program. Nutritional replenishment must be closely supervised to ensure consistent and ongoing weight gains. The use of tube or parenteral feedings may be necessary. Improved nutrition, however, is not a cure for anorexia nervosa. The underlying psychiatric problem must be addressed by identification of the disturbed patterns of individual and family interactions, followed by individual and family counseling.

Table 38-10	Common Drug and Food/Nutrient Interactions	
Drug Category/Drug	**Food/Nutrient**	**Drug-Food Effects or Cautions**
Anticoagulants	Dietary vitamin K (e.g., green leafy vegetables, green tea, dairy products/meats)	Decrease or loss of anticoagulant effect
Antiseizure agents • Phenytoin (Dilantin)	Folic acid	Long-term drug use may increase folic acid requirement
Antidepressants • Trazodone (Desyrel) • Tricyclic antidepressants	Food Riboflavin	Food slows drug absorption Riboflavin requirements may increase with amitriptyline (Elavil) or imipramine (Tofranil)
Antidiabetic agents • Glyburide (Micronase, DiaBeta)	High fat diet	Drug should not be taken with high fat diet
Antithyroid agents • Methimazole (Tapazole)	Food	Foods may inconsistently alter bioavailability of methimzaole
Barbiturates • Phenobarbital • Mephobarbitol (Mebaral)	Folic acid	Drugs may increase folic acid requirements; long-term therapy may require vitamin D supplements for osteomalacia
β-adrenergic blocking agents • Labetalol (Normodyne) • Metaproterenol (Alupent) • Carteolol (Cartrol) • Sotalol (Betapace)	Food	Bioavailability of drug may be enhanced when taken with food
Bronchodilators • Theophylline • Oxtriphylline (Choledyl) • Dyphylline (Lufyllin)	High-carbohydrate, low-protein diets Caffeine-containing foods and fluids	Decrease drug elimination Caffeine may increase CNS stimulant effects of xanthine-derivative bronchodilators
Cholestyramine (Questran)	Fat-soluble vitamins	Drug may interfere with their absorption
Corticosteroids (prolonged therapy)	Salt seasonings	May require sodium limits and/or potassium supplements
Erythropoietin	Folic acid and/or cobalamin	Nutrient deficiencies may reduce/delay drug response
Etidronate (Didronel)	Foods, fluids, or drugs high in calcium	May prevent drug absorption
Furazolidone (Furoxone)	Food and fluids containing tyramine (e.g., aged cheese, smoked or pickled meats or poultry, fermented meat, overripe fruit, beer, wine, liqueurs)	MAO-inhibiting effects may last at least 2 wk after stopping drug. Dietary restrictions need to continue for at least 2 wk after MAO inhibitors discontinued if received large doses or prolonged therapy
Isoniazid (INH)	Cheese (e.g., Swiss or Cheshire) or fish (e.g., tuna, skipjack)	Concurrent ingestion may lead to redness or itching, HR changes, sweating, chills or clammy feeling, headache or light-headedness; thought to be related to altered metabolism of tyramine in foods
Parkinson's drug • Selegiline (Eldepryl)	Food and fluids containing tyramine (e.g., aged cheese, smoked or pickled meats or poultry, fermented meat, overripe fruit, beer, wine, liqueurs)	When used concurrently, may cause sudden and severe hypertensive reactions; dietary restrictions need to continue for at least 2 wk after MAO inhibitors discontinued
Phenothiazines	Riboflavin	Drugs may increase riboflavin requirements
Procarbazine (Matulane)	Food and fluids containing tyramine or other high pressor amines (e.g., aged cheese, smoked or pickled meats or poultry, fermented meat, overripe fruit, beer, wine, liqueurs)	When used concurrently, may cause sudden and severe hypertensive reactions; dietary restrictions need to continue for at least 2 wk after MAO inhibitors discontinued
Ticlopidine (Ticlid)	Food	Drug absorption increased when taken after a meal
Zafirlukast (Accolate)	High-fat and high protein meal	When taken concurrently drug bioavailability reduced by about 40%
Zinc supplements	Foods	Many foods impair zinc absorption

MAO, monoamine oxidase.

Bulimia

Bulimia is a chronic disorder that is often confused with anorexia nervosa. Concern about body image is a key feature in both bulimia and anorexia nervosa; however, the syndrome of bulimia is different from anorexia nervosa. Bulimia is characterized by compulsive binge eating and purging (through self-induced vomiting, laxative abuse, excessive exercise, and diuretics). Food becomes an obsession and an addiction—an escape from the pressures of life. Unlike the person with anorexia, the patient caught up in the syndrome of bulimia usually maintains a normal or near-normal body weight, and the primary symptom is gorging rather than starvation.

Bulimia is increasing in incidence and may be even more prevalent than anorexia nervosa. Female college students seem to be susceptible to this syndrome. The cause remains unclear but is thought to be similar to that of anorexia nervosa. Substance abuse, anxiety, affective disorders, and personality disturbances have been reported among persons with bulimia.

In addition to the psychologic considerations, bulimia may lead to some physical effects in those persons who binge and purge on a daily basis. Characteristic skin lesions on the back of the hand, which are often over the metacarpophalangeal joint and called Russell's sign, can result from repeated trauma to the skin from self-induced vomiting. In addition, dental problems may develop from constant vomiting. Swollen glands or salivary gland hypertrophy, sore throat, facial puffiness, chronic indigestion, irregular menstrual periods, electrolyte imbalances, and dehydration can also occur. Sudden death from cardiac arrest or a fatal arrhythmia is not uncommon. Although rare, esophageal tears and gastric rupture secondary to overdistention can occur. However, most bulimics have few, if any, noticeable signs of the illness.[7]

The patient with bulimia, similar to the one with anorexia nervosa, goes to great lengths to conceal abnormal eating habits. As the behavior persists, many problems associated with the condition become increasingly hard to deal with effectively.

Treatment of bulimia is similar to that described for anorexia nervosa. The multidisciplinary approach consists of strategies that include individual psychotherapy, nutritional counseling (including discussion of the dangers involved in binge eating and purging), cognitive behavior therapy, and drug therapy. Antidepressants (e.g., fluoxetine [Prozac], amitriptyline [Elavil]) are useful for the depression associated with both anorexia nervosa and bulimia. Vitamin, mineral, and iron supplements may be prescribed. However, iron supplementation is not generally required if amenorrhea is present. The return to normal eating habits may take several months to years to accomplish because relapses are frequent. Recovery is difficult; the abnormal eating behavior is hard to change because binge eating and purging provide the person with a feeling of satisfaction and of control over the body. For help and support, several organizations for eating disorders have been formed, including American Anorexia/Bulimia Association; Anorexia Nervosa and Related Eating Disorders, Inc.; National Eating Disorders Organization; National Association of Anorexia Nervosa and Associated Disorders, Inc.; and Overeaters Anonymous. (See Resources at end of chapter.)

MALNUTRITION

Malnutrition may be defined as an excess, a deficit, or an imbalance in the essential components of a balanced diet. Terms such as *undernutrition* and *overnutrition* are also used to describe malnutrition. Undernutrition describes a state of poor nourishment as a result of inadequate diet or diseases that interfere with normal appetite and assimilation of ingested food. Overnutrition refers to the ingestion of more food than is required for body needs, as in obesity.

Malnutrition is most prevalent in developing countries in which adequate food sources do not exist, the inhabitants are not well educated about their nutritional needs, and economic conditions often preclude the purchase of a balanced diet. Undernutrition does exist in scattered parts of the United States, and it is usually found in individuals or groups from the lower socioeconomic class.

Types of Malnutrition

Protein-Calorie Malnutrition. Protein-calorie malnutrition (PCM) is the most common form of undernutrition and can result from either primary or secondary factors. Primary PCM is present when nutritional needs are not met as a result of poor eating habits. Secondary PCM is the result of an alteration or defect in ingestion, digestion, absorption, or metabolism. In this type of malnutrition, tissue needs are not met even though the dietary intake would be satisfactory under normal conditions. Secondary malnutrition may occur as a result of GI obstruction, surgical treatment (e.g., after peptic ulcer surgery), cancer, malabsorption syndromes, medications, and infectious diseases.

PCM may also be due to the ingestion of foods deficient in protein. In addition to decreased quantities of protein, the diet is generally low in necessary vitamins and minerals. PCM is a serious nutritional problem common throughout the world, affecting every socioeconomic group and age-group. In the United States and Canada, where protein intake is high and of good quality, severe malnutrition is less of a problem, but it can occur in high-risk groups.

Marasmus and Kwashiorkor. Malnutrition has long been recognized in infants and children throughout the world by the terms *marasmus* and *kwashiorkor*. Malnutrition in adults may also be classified by this terminology. Marasmus is the result of a concomitant deficiency of both caloric and protein intake leading to generalized loss of body fat and muscle. Kwashiorkor is caused by a deficiency of protein intake that is superimposed on a catabolic stress event, such as a GI obstruction, a surgical procedure, cancer, a malabsorption syndrome, or an infectious disease.

Etiology and Pathophysiology

The following factors increase the potential for the development of malnutrition:

1. Major surgery, radiation therapy, or chemotherapy
2. Severe burns with exudate high in protein
3. Draining wounds, including pressure ulcers
4. Chronic renal or liver diseases
5. Hemorrhage

6. Bone fractures with prolonged immobilization
7. Malabsorption syndrome
8. Presence of infectious diseases such as tuberculosis or acquired immunodeficiency syndrome (AIDS)

The nitrogen loss after severe injury or major surgery may be as much as 20 g per day, excreted as urea, creatinine, and creatine.

Knowledge of the phases of the starvation process is essential to better understand the physiologic changes that occur in PCM. Initially, the body selectively uses carbohydrates (glycogen) rather than fat and protein to maintain metabolic function. These carbohydrate stores, found in the liver and muscles, are minimal and may be totally depleted within 18 hours. During this early phase of starvation, the only use of protein is in its obligatory participation in cellular metabolism. However, once carbohydrate stores are depleted, protein begins to be converted to glucose for energy. Alanine and glutamine are the first amino acids to be used by the liver for the formation of glucose in a process termed *gluconeogenesis*. The resulting available plasma glucose allows the metabolic processes to continue. With these amino acids being used as energy sources, the person is in negative nitrogen balance (greater nitrogen excretion). However, within 5 to 9 days, body fat is fully mobilized to supply much of the needed energy.

In prolonged starvation up to 97% of calories are provided by fat, and protein is conserved. Depletion of fat stores depends on the amount available, but fat stores are generally used up in 4 to 6 weeks. Once fat stores are used, body proteins, including those in internal organs and plasma, can no longer be spared and rapidly decrease because they are the only remaining body source of energy available.

If the malnourished patient has surgery, experiences bodily trauma, or has an infection, the stress response with concomitant increase in energy expenditure is superimposed on the starvation response. These body insults cause an increase in the metabolic rate, with a subsequent increase in energy requirements. Protein stores are no longer spared and are used with increasing frequency for body energy because of the increased metabolic energy needs.

As the protein depletion continues, liver function is impaired, and synthesis of proteins is diminished. The plasma oncotic pressure is decreased because of decreased protein synthesis. A major function of plasma proteins, primarily of albumin, is the maintenance of the osmotic pressure of the blood. Because of this decreased pressure, a shift in body fluids occurs from the vascular space into the interstitial compartment. As protein ingestion decreases and body stores are depleted, albumin eventually leaks into the interstitial space along with the fluid. Edema becomes clinically observable. Often the edema present in the face and legs of the patient masks the muscle wasting that occurs. Ascites (abnormal intraperitoneal accumulation of fluid containing large amounts of protein and electrolytes) is a classic manifestation of kwashiorkor.

As the total blood volume is reduced, the skin appears dry and wrinkled. Along with the shift of fluids to the interstitial space, ions also move. Sodium (a predominant extracellular ion) is found in increased amounts within the cell, and potassium (a predominant intracellular ion) and magnesium are shifted to the extracellular space. The sodium-potassium exchange pump, which is dependent on adenosine triphosphatase (ATPase), has high energy needs, using 20% to 50% of all calories ingested. When the diet is extremely deficient in calories and essential proteins, the pump will fail, leaving sodium inside the cell (along with water), and the cell will expand.

The liver is the body organ that loses the most mass during protein deprivation. It gradually becomes infiltrated with fat secondary to decreased synthesis of lipoproteins. Immediate restoration to the diet of protein and other necessary constituents must be instituted or death will rapidly ensue. The most serious problem associated with PCM in the young is the probability of mental retardation. In severe malnutrition the development of brain cells is greatly slowed down. Brain cells increase most rapidly during fetal life and in the first 5 to 6 months after birth. Once this critical time for brain development has passed, improvement in the nutritional state of the infant will not correct any mental deficiency already incurred.

Clinical Manifestations

The adult who is deprived of adequate protein and calories will have many of the clinical manifestations presented in Table 38-11. The most obvious clinical signs on physical examination are apparent in the skin, eyes, mouth, muscles, and CNS. The speed at which the protein deficiency develops depends on the quantity and quality of the protein intake, caloric value, and the age of the person.

Clinical manifestations of malnutrition are the result of numerous interactions occurring at the cellular level. As protein intake is severely reduced, the muscles, which make up the largest reservoir of protein in the body, become wasted and flabby, leading to weakness, fatigability, and decreased endurance. There is decreased protein available for repair, and as a result, wound healing may be delayed. Malnutrition in the hospitalized patient may result in delayed recovery and prolonged hospitalization. The person is more susceptible to all types of infections. Both humoral and cell-mediated immunity are deficient in PCM. There is a decrease in leukocytes in the peripheral blood. Phagocytosis is altered as a result of the lack of energy (ATP) necessary to drive the process. Most malnourished persons are anemic. Anemia resulting from PCM is usually caused by nutritional deficiencies such as iron and folic acid, the necessary building blocks for red blood cells (RBCs).

Complications

The severity of complications ranges from mild to emaciation and death. Major complications center around delayed wound healing and increased susceptibility to infection from decreased immune function.

Diagnostic Studies

The diagnosis of PCM can be determined by a variety of laboratory studies used in conjunction with physical examination. Serum albumin is useful in the diagnosis of malnutrition. The degree of protein depletion can be identified with the use of the scale in Table 38-12. Serum albumin has a half-life of

Table 38-11	Signs of Protein-Calorie Malnutrition	
Body System	**Subclinical Signs**	**Clinical Signs**
Integumentary	Slowed tissue turnover rate, surface temperature 1° F-2° F cooler	Brittle nails, decreased tone and elasticity of skin, xeroderma (dry skin), pigment changes (brown-gray), erythematous seborrheic dermatitis, scrotal dermatitis
Visual	Night blindness	Hair: easy loss of hair, color changes, lack of luster Blood vessel growth in cornea, Bitot's spots (gray keratinized epithelium on conjunctiva), dryness of conjunctiva and cornea, pale to red conjunctiva
Gastrointestinal		
Mouth and lips	Reduction in saliva production	Cheilosis (crusting and ulceration at angle of mouth)
Tongue	Mucosa more permeable to bacteria	Raw and beefy red, edematous and smooth, atrophy or hypertrophy of papillae
Teeth	Improper development, delayed eruption	Caries, loose teeth, discolored enamel
Gingivae		Periodontal disease, tendency to bleed easily, receding, pale, and soft
Stomach	Decreased gastric acidity, delayed gastric emptying	Constant hunger, increased incidence of ulcers
Intestines	Decreased motility and absorption, normal flora causing infection from increased permeability of mucosa	Diarrhea and flatulence, protruding abdomen, increased incidence of parasitic diseases
Liver-biliary	Fatty liver, decreased absorption of fat-soluble vitamins	Hepatomegaly
Cardiovascular	Decreased cardiac output, decreased hemoglobin, shift in heart position, increased risk of thrombophlebitis	Decreased blood pressure and pulse, slight cyanosis, anemia, body edema
Endocrine	Decreased insulin production	Thyroid enlargement, polydipsia, polyuria, increased sensitivity to cold
Immunologic	Decreased lymphocyte proliferation, decreased albumin levels, decreased antibody production, decreased total protein, diminished febrile response to infection, delayed immune response	Increased number of infections, decreased response to skin tests
Musculoskeletal	Decreased growth rate, decreased body stature with chronic PCM, decreased muscle mass	Prominence of bony structures such as face, clavicle, scapula, ribs, iliac crests, and spinal vertebrae, due to subcutaneous tissue loss, weak and spindly arms and legs, flat buttocks, weak and flabby muscles, decreased physical activity and ability to work, severe weight loss
Neurologic	Loss of ambition, feeling of being tired	Depression, confusion, decreased reflexes in legs and ankles, decreased position sense, decreased vibratory sense, paresthesias of hands and feet, syncope, motor weakness
Renal	Negative nitrogen balance, decreased BUN and creatinine levels	Nocturia, decreased urinary output
Reproductive	Decreased gonadotropin levels	Amenorrhea, impotence, atrophied breasts
Respiratory	Pulmonary edema, decreased strength of respiratory muscles	Increased susceptibility to respiratory infection, decreased respiratory rate, decreased vital capacity

BUN, blood urea nitrogen; *PCM,* protein-calorie malnutrition.

approximately 20 to 22 days. In the absence of marked fluid loss, such as from hemorrhage or burns, the serum albumin value lags behind actual protein changes by more than 2 weeks and therefore is not a good indicator of acute changes in nutrition status. Prealbumin, which has a half-life of 2 days, is a better indicator of recent or current nutritional status. Serum transferrin level is another indicator of protein status. Transferrin, a protein synthesized by the liver and used to transport iron, decreases during states of protein deficiency. Serum electrolyte levels reflect changes taking place between the intracellular and the extracellular spaces. The serum potassium level is often elevated. The RBC count and the hemoglobin level will indicate the presence and degree of anemia. The total lymphocyte count decreases during malnutrition states. The total lymphocyte count is calculated by multiplying the percent of lymphocytes times total white blood cell (WBC) count.

Liver enzyme levels, a reflection of liver function, may be elevated during malnutrition. Serum levels of both fat-soluble

Table 38-12	Serum Albumin and Prealbumin Levels
Albumin	
Normal value	3.5-5.0 g/dl (35-50 g/L)
Mild depletion	3.0-3.4 g/dl (30-34 g/L)
Moderate depletion	2.5-2.9 g/dl (25-29 g/L)
Severe depletion	<2.5 g/dl (<25 g/L)
Prealbumin	
Normal value	20 mg/dl (200 mg/L)
Mild depletion	10-15 mg/dl (100-150 mg/L)
Moderate depletion	5-10 mg/dl (50-100 mg/L)
Severe depletion	<5 mg/dl (<50 mg/L)

and water-soluble vitamins are usually diminished in malnutrition. The lowered levels of the fat-soluble vitamins correlate with the clinical signs of steatorrhea (fatty stools).

Collaborative Care

The patient with PCM is often below the ideal on weight-for-height scales according to age and gender. Inspection of the unclothed body reveals loss of muscle mass, muscle wasting, and marked reduction in body fat. Diagnosis may be masked, however, when edema is present. The management of early uncomplicated PCM can be achieved without hospitalization by means of a diet high in calories and protein and by close supervision. Table 38-13 gives an example of a high-calorie, high-protein diet.

In severe PCM the patient may be hospitalized for correction of fluid and electrolyte imbalances and for treatment of infections secondary to a compromised immune system. Enteral feeding, both oral and tube feedings, can be used to provide total nutrition or to supplement calories and protein. In cases of severe PCM, total parenteral nutrition (TPN) may be initiated if enteral feedings are not feasible.

NURSING MANAGEMENT: MALNUTRITION
■ Nursing Assessment

Across all settings of care delivery, the nurse must be aware of the nutritional status of the patient. Nursing assessment of the patient with malnutrition is presented in Table 38-14. The recording of the patient's height and weight is an important component of this assessment. The patient's current weight relative to usual body weight and ideal body weight such as the Metropolitan Life Insurance tables (see Table 38-22 later in this chapter) are determined. The percent change in body weight over time provides information on the degree of weight loss. In addition, the nurse should get a record of the complete diet history from the patient or the family. The patient's nutritional state may not be the reason medical assistance was sought. However, it may well be a major factor in the outcome and perhaps may be the underlying reason for the patient's illness. A registered dietician should also be involved in the planning of care. However, the nurse, as the first health care professional dealing with the patient, should take the initiative in determining the seriousness of the nutritional problems.

The nurse should be aware that psychosocial problems have a direct effect on appetite. This is often overlooked as a cause of undernourishment. A diet history of foods eaten over the past week will reveal a great deal about the patient's dietary habits and knowledge of good nutrition. In addition to the height and weight and vital signs, the patient's physical state should be thoroughly assessed and documented. Each body system should be assessed. Table 38-15 summarizes conditions that can predispose persons to malnutrition.

Anthropometric measurements may be ordered. These measurements tend to be most beneficial in evaluating long-term effects of malnutrition or responses to nutritional interventions. Serial measures of skinfold thickness at various sites, an indicator of subcutaneous fat stores, and midarm muscle circumference, an indicator of protein stores, are compared with standards for healthy persons of the same age and gender. Training and practice are required to perform these measurements accurately and reliably. To provide information on the patient's nutritional status in response to treatment, serial measurements are needed. Sites most reflective of body fat are those over the biceps and the triceps, below the scapula, above the iliac crest, and the upper thigh. Both skinfold thickness and midarm muscle circumference measurements are decreased in chronic PCM and acute protein malnutrition. These measurements may also be influenced by shifts in hydration status. The exact relationship of the midarm circumference measure to body composition of functional protein, both muscle and nonmuscle, remains to be established.

■ Nursing Diagnoses

Nursing diagnoses for the patient with malnutrition include, but are not limited to, the following:

- Altered nutrition: less than body requirements *related to* decreased access, ingestion, digestion, or absorption of food or to anorexia
- Self-care deficits *related to* decreased strength and endurance, fatigue, and apathy
- Constipation or diarrhea *related to* poor eating patterns, immobility, or medication effects
- Risk for fluid volume deficit *related to* factors affecting access to or absorption of fluids
- Risk for impaired skin integrity *related to* poor nutritional state
- Noncompliance *related to* alteration in perception, lack of motivation, or incompatibility of regimen with lifestyle or resources
- Activity intolerance *related to* weakness, fatigue, and inadequate caloric intake or iron stores

■ Planning

The overall goals are that the patient with malnutrition will (1) achieve weight gain, (2) consume a specified number of calories per day (with a diet individualized for the patient), and (3) have no adverse consequences related to malnutrition.

■ Nursing Implementation

Health Promotion. The nurse is in a good position to teach and reinforce healthy eating habits with individuals and groups of persons throughout their life span. In the 1990s the

NUTRITIONAL THERAPY

Table 38-13   High-Caloric, High-Protein Diet

General Principles

1. A normal diet is supplemented with larger portions to increase the protein and caloric content. It is used for patients with hypermetabolism, burns, excessive stress, and cancer.
2. It is important to eat regularly and not to skip meals or snacks.

Meal	Protein Content (g)	Sample Menu Plan 1	Sample Menu Plan 2	Sample Menu Plan 3
Breakfast				
Fruit	2	Large orange juice	Large apple juice	½ grapefruit
Starch, fat		1 toast with butter or jelly	Flour tortilla with butter	Biscuits and gravy
Starch, protein supplement	4	Cream of wheat with 2 tbs skim milk powder	Atole with 2 tbs skim milk powder	Grits with 2 tbs margarine
2 meat		2 poached eggs	2 fried eggs	Omelet with 2 eggs
Milk, protein supplement	14 10	High-protein milk shake (2 tbs skim milk powder added)	High-protein milk shake	High-protein milk shake
Lunch				
4 meat	28	Cheeseburger on bun with double meat patty, lettuce, tomato	2 burritos with extra cheese, meat	Split pea soup with ham hocks
4 starches	8			Grilled cheese sandwich
Vegetable	2		Lettuce and tomato salad with dressing	Watermelon wedge
4 fats	10	French fried potatoes	Biscochitos	Sugar cookies
Milk, protein supplement		High-protein milk shake	High-protein milk shake	High-protein milk shake
Dinner				
4 meat	28	Spaghetti with 4 oz meat sauce, Parmesan cheese	2 tamales with red chili sauce	4 oz fried chicken
3 starches	6			Sweet potato
Vegetable	2	Green beans with 2 tbs margarine	Spanish rice	Mustard greens with 2 tbs butter
7 fats		Bread with butter	Peas with 2 tbs butter	Biscuit
		Tapioca pudding	Custard	Vanilla ice cream
Milk, protein supplement	10	High-protein milk shake	High-protein milk shake	High-protein milk shake
Snack				
Milk		Fruit yogurt	Cottage cheese with fruit	½ sandwich with peanut butter
Fruit	8			Banana
	Total 132			

gap between perceived importance of nutrition and care in selecting foods has widened.[8] To assist in these efforts are the mandatory food labels that are now on all packaged food. These provide more useful and accurate nutritional information than labeling before 1994. The latest *Surgeon General's Report on Nutrition and Health* offers key recommendations for improving nutrition that are useful points for a teaching program.[9] The following recommendations are applicable to most people:

1. Reduce consumption of fat and cholesterol
2. Achieve and maintain a desirable weight
3. Increase energy expenditure through regular and sustained physical activity
4. Increase consumption of whole grain foods and cereal products, vegetables, and fruits
5. Reduce intake of sodium
6. Take alcohol only in moderation, if at all

Acute Intervention.   The nurse must assess the patient's nutritional state, as well as focus on the other physical problems of the patient. The incidence of nutritional deficiency, especially PCM, is high in hospitalized patients. A number of nutritional studies have indicated that PCM may develop in as many as 50% of medical and surgical patients.[10] As a direct consequence of these findings, the nurse must become more aware of who is at risk, why, and how to intervene appropriately. In states of increased stress, such as surgery, severe trauma, and sepsis, more calories and protein are required. Wound healing requires increased protein synthesis. In cases of cancer, there may be additional demands made by tumor growth at the same time that appetite is reduced. When fever is present, the metabolic rate is increased and nitrogen loss is accelerated. Despite the return of body temperature to normal, the rate of protein breakdown and resynthesis may be accelerated for several weeks. After major surgery several weeks of

NURSING ASSESSMENT

Table 38-14   Malnutrition

Subjective Data

Important Health Information

Past health history: Severe burns, major trauma, hemorrhage, draining wounds, bone fractures with prolonged immobility, chronic renal or liver disease, cancer, malabsorption syndrome, GI obstruction, infectious diseases (TB, AIDS)

Medications: Corticosteroids, chemotherapeutic agents, diet pills

Surgery or other treatments: Recent surgery, radiation

Functional Health Patterns

Health perception–health management: Alcohol or drug abuse; malaise, apathy

Nutritional-metabolic: Increase or decrease in weight, weight problems; increase or decrease in appetite, typical dietary intake; food preferences and aversions; food allergies or intolerance; ill-fitting or absent dentures; dry mouth, difficulty in chewing or swallowing; bloating or gas; increased sensitivity to cold; delayed wound healing

Elimination: Constipation; diarrhea; nocturia, decreased urinary output

Activity-exercise: Increase or decrease in activity patterns; weakness, fatigue, decreased endurance

Cognitive-perceptual: Pain in mouth; paresthesias; loss of position and vibratory sense

Role-relationship: Change in family (e.g., loss of a spouse); financial resources

Sexual-reproductive: Amenorrhea, impotence, decreased libido

Objective Data

General

Listless; cachectic; underweight for height

Integumentary

Dry, brittle, sparse hair with color changes and lack of luster, alopecia; dry, scaly lips, fever blisters, angular crusts and lesions at corners of mouth (cheilosis); brittle, ridged nails; decreased tone and elasticity of skin; cool, rough, dry, scaly skin with brown-gray pigment changes; reddened, scaly dermatitis, scrotal dermatitis; slight cyanosis; peripheral edema

Eyes

Pale or red conjunctivae, gray keratinized epithelium on conjunctiva (Bitot's spots); dryness and dull appearance of conjunctiva and cornea, soft cornea; blood vessel growth in cornea; redness and fissuring of eyelid corners

Respiratory

Decreased respiratory rate, decreased vital capacity, crackles, weak cough

Cardiovascular

Increase or decrease in heart rate, decreased blood pressure, arrhythmias

Gastrointestinal

Swollen, smooth, raw, beefy red tongue (glossitis), hypertrophic or atrophic papillae; dental caries, absent or loose teeth, discolored tooth enamel; spongy, pale, receded gums with a tendency to bleed easily, periodontal disease; ulcerations, white patches or plaques, redness, swelling of oral mucosa; distended, tympanic abdomen, ascites, hepatomegaly, decreased bowel sounds; steatorrhea

Neurologic

Decreased or loss of reflexes, tremor; inattention, irritability, confusion, syncope

Musculoskeletal

Decreased muscle mass with poor tone, "wasted" appearance; bowlegs, knock-knees, beaded ribs, chest deformity, prominent bony structures

Possible Findings

Decreased hemoglobin and hematocrit; decreased MCV, MCH, or MCHC (iron deficiency); increased MCV or MCHC (folic acid or cobalamin deficiency); altered serum electrolyte levels, especially hyperkalemia; decreased BUN and creatinine; decreased serum albumin, transferrin, and prealbumin; decreased lymphocytes; increased liver enzymes; decreased serum vitamin levels

AIDS, acquired immunodeficiency syndrome; *MCH,* mean corpuscular hemoglobin; *MCHC,* mean corpuscular hemoglobin concentration; *MCV,* mean corpuscular volume; *TB,* tuberculosis.

Table 38-15   Conditions That Increase the Risk for Malnutrition

- Chronic alcoholism
- Drugs with antinutrient or catabolic properties, such as corticosteroids and oral antibiotics
- Gross underweight or overweight with recent weight loss exceeding 5% of usual body weight or 10 lb (4.5 kg) per month for several months
- No oral intake or receiving standard intravenous solutions (5% dextrose) for 10 days or in older adults for 5 days
- Extreme need for nutrients because of hypermetabolism or stresses such as infection, burns, trauma, or fever
- Nutrient losses from malabsorption, dialysis, fistulas, or wounds
- Decreased mobility that limits access to food and its preparation

Table 38-16	Commonly Used Elemental Diets					
Product	Protein (g/L)	Carbohydrates (% total kcal)	Lipids (% total kcal)	Protein (% total kcal)	kcal/ml	Osmolarity (mOsm/kg)
Criticare HN	38.0	81.5	4.5	14.0	1.1	650
Reabilan	31.5	52.5	35.0	12.5	1.0	350
Reabilan HN	58.5	47.5	35.0	17.5	1.3	490
Tolerex	21.0	91.0	1.0	8.0	1.0	550
Vital HN	41.7	73.6	9.7	16.7	1.0	500
Vivonex TEN	38.0	82.0	3.0	15.0	1.0	630
Peptamen	40.0	51.0	33.0	16.0	1.0	270
Crucial	93.8	36.0	39.0	25.0	1.5	490

increased protein and calorie intake are needed to promote healing and replenish body stores.

The nurse must have a thorough understanding of nutritional support and the rationale for recording the daily weight, intake, and output. Daily weights can give an ongoing record of body weight gain or loss. However, rapid gains and losses are usually the result of shifts in fluid balance. The body weight, in conjunction with accurate recording of food and fluid intake, provides a clearer picture of the patient's fluid and nutritional state. To obtain an accurate weight, the nurse should weigh the patient at the same time each day, on the same scale, with the same type or amount of clothing, and preferably with the bladder recently emptied.

The protein and calorie intake required in the malnourished patient depends on the cause of the malnutrition, the treatment being employed, and other stressors affecting the patient. If the patient is able to take food by mouth, a daily calorie count and diet diary can be obtained to give an accurate record of food intake.

The nurse and the dietician working with the patient and family can assist in the selection of high-caloric and high-protein foods (unless medically contraindicated). Preparation of foods preferred by the patient enhances the daily intake. Discussion with the patient and family about foods that should be eaten to provide high-protein, high-calorie content is important. The family can be encouraged to bring the patient's favorite foods from home while the patient is still hospitalized.

The undernourished patient usually receives between-meal supplements. These may consist of items prepared in the dietary department or commercially prepared products. Eating these items between meals increases the total daily intake and provides extra calories, proteins, fluids, and nutrients. In addition, multiple small feedings improve the tolerance for food intake by distributing the amount more evenly throughout the day.

Elemental diets are chemically defined, nutritionally sound diets that contain glucose, glucose derivatives, dextrin, amino acids, peptides, essential fatty acids, vitamins, and minerals. They are lactose free and easily absorbed in the small intestine. The nurse should be familiar with the commercial products being used in the particular setting, their ingredients, and whether the products can be used as complete meal replacements or only as dietary supplements. (See Table 38-16 for information about sample elemental formulas.) Disease-specific elemental formulas are also available for spe-cial patient groups (e.g., Amin-Aid for patients with renal failure).

Ambulatory and Home Care. With shortened hospital stays, many patients are discharged home on a therapeutic diet. Discharge preparation for both the patient and the family is important. They must be carefully instructed on the cause of the undernourished state and ways to avoid the problem in the future. The patient must be made aware that undernourishment, whatever the cause, can recur and that adhering to a diet high in protein and calories for a few weeks cannot restore a normal nutritional state. Many months are needed to reach this goal. Diet instruction is usually carried out by the dietician, but it is important for the nurse to assess the patient's understanding and reinforce the information whenever possible. The patient's ability to comply with the dietary instructions must be examined in light of past eating habits, religious and ethnic preferences, age, income, other resources, and state of health.

Unless the patient and the family can be convinced of the necessity for dietary change and have the resources to effect change, it is likely that no long-term benefits will be achieved. Ways should be found in which the patient can become involved in the recovery. The need for continuous follow-up care must be strongly emphasized if rehabilitation is to be accomplished and maintained.

The nurse is in an ideal position to determine the need for nutritious meals and snacks after discharge from the hospital. In addition, it is important to consider the availability and acceptability of nutritionally based community resources. Such aspects can be integrated into discharge planning and follow-up home visits by the nurse.

Keeping a diet diary or a calorie count for 3 days at a time is one way to analyze and reinforce healthful eating patterns. These records are also helpful to the health care team in the follow-up care. Self-assessment of progress can be encouraged by having the patient weighed once or twice a week and keeping a weight record.

■ Evaluation

The expected outcomes are that the patient who is malnourished will

- achieve and maintain body weight
- consume a well-balanced diet
- experience no adverse outcomes related to malnutrition

Malnutrition

The eating patterns established in youth and earlier years usually extend into old age. However, adjustments in the type of food ingested may be made as adaptations to age-related physiologic changes. These changes can result either in obesity or loss of weight depending on individual circumstances.

Some of the physiologic changes associated with aging affect the nutritional status of older adults. The following changes are of particular interest:

1. Changes in the oral cavity (e.g., change in bite surfaces of the teeth, periodontal disease, drying of the mucous membrane of the mouth and tongue, poorly fitting dentures, decreased muscle strength for chewing, decreased number of taste buds, decreased saliva production)
2. Changes in digestion and motility (e.g., decreased absorption of cobalamin, vitamin A, and folic acid and decreased GI motility)
3. Changes in the endocrine system (e.g., decreased tolerance to glucose)
4. Changes in the musculoskeletal system (e.g., decreased bone density, degenerative joint changes)
5. Decrease in vision and hearing (e.g., procurement and preparation of food are more difficult)

Certain illnesses that are more prevalent in the older population are considered to be diet related. These include atherosclerosis, osteoporosis, diabetes mellitus, and diverticulosis. The need to treat these and other common chronic illnesses of the older patient often requires the use of multiple medications. These medications often have an adverse effect on the appetite of older adults, increasing the possibility of inadequate intake caused by anorexia.

To date, with the exception of calories, it has not been determined that older adults have requirements for specific nutrients that are different from those of middle-aged adults. Caloric intake should be decreased with age because there is a progressive loss of lean body mass and a decrease in basal metabolic rate. Therefore fewer calories are needed to meet nutritional needs. Unless caloric intake is decreased by careful attention to food intake, or energy expenditure is increased through greater physical activity and exercise, obesity will result.

Socioeconomic factors are important variables when assessing the nutritional status of an older adult. Because more than one third of older adults have incomes below the poverty level, it would follow that obtaining adequate and nutritious food can be an ongoing problem. In many cases the older person cannot afford to purchase meat, fresh vegetables, and fruits that provide many necessary nutrients.

Lifestyle changes such as relocation to a nursing home or retirement can have a significant impact on the eating habits of the older adult. Other important considerations that should be assessed when evaluating the nutritional status of an older adult include the ethnic background, previous dietary practices, food preferences, knowledge of proper diet, availability and accessibility of food stores, transportation, and health status. Problems related to any or all of these areas can alert the nurse to the possibility of a nutritional problem.

Malnutrition can occur in an older person even though the caloric requirements decrease with age. If malnutrition is present, few malnourished older persons are able to ingest enough food to correct the malnourished state. Special strategies, such as adaptive devices (e.g., large-handled eating utensils), often are helpful in increasing dietary intake. Some older persons may require nutritional support therapies until their strength and general health are improved.

Many community nutritional programs are available to the older person to make mealtime a pleasant, social event. Improving the social setting of a meal often improves the dietary intake. Home-delivered meals and meal sites in a central location are popular meal alternatives for many older adults. The use of food stamps is another alternative that allows low-income households, regardless of age, to buy more food of a greater variety.

TYPES OF SUPPLEMENTAL NUTRITION

ORAL FEEDING

High-calorie supplemental oral feedings may be used in the patient whose nutritional intake is deficient. This may include dietary items such as milk shakes, puddings, eggnogs, or commercially available products (e.g., Ensure, Sustacal, NuBasics).

TUBE FEEDING

Tube feedings may be ordered for the patient who has a functioning GI tract but is unable to take oral nourishment. Indications for tube feeding, besides PCM, may include those persons with anorexia, orofacial fractures, head and neck cancer, neurologic or psychiatric conditions that prevent oral intake, extensive burns, and those who are receiving chemotherapy or radiation therapy. Tube feedings are easily administered, safer, more physiologically efficient, and less expensive than parenteral nutrition. They are used to provide nutrients by way of the GI tract (alone or as a supplement to oral or parenteral nutrition) or as a treatment for malnutrition.

Common delivery options are continuous infusion by pump, intermittent by gravity, intermittent bolus by syringe, and cyclic intermittent by infusion pump.[11] Continuous infusion is most often used with critically ill patients and feedings into the small intestine. Intermittent feeding may be preferred as the patient improves or is receiving such feedings at home.

A nasogastric (NG) tube is most commonly used for short-term feeding problems. If the feedings are necessary for an extended time, other means of feeding may be used, such as an esophagostomy tube, a gastrostomy tube (placed surgically, endoscopically, or percutaneously), or a jejunostomy tube that empties directly into the jejunum. Transpyloric (nasointestinal) tube placement or placement into the jejunum is used when physiologic conditions warrant feeding the patient below the pyloric sphincter. (Figure 38-2 shows the locations of commonly used enteral feeding tubes.)

Nasogastric and Nasointestinal Tubes

Feeding tubes made of polyurethane or silicone materials have added to the comfort level of the patient in tolerating extended periods of feeding. These tubes are long, small in diameter, soft, and flexible, thereby decreasing the risk of mucosal damage from prolonged placement. The older tubes made of rubber or polyvinyl chloride tend to stiffen with time. Polyurethane and

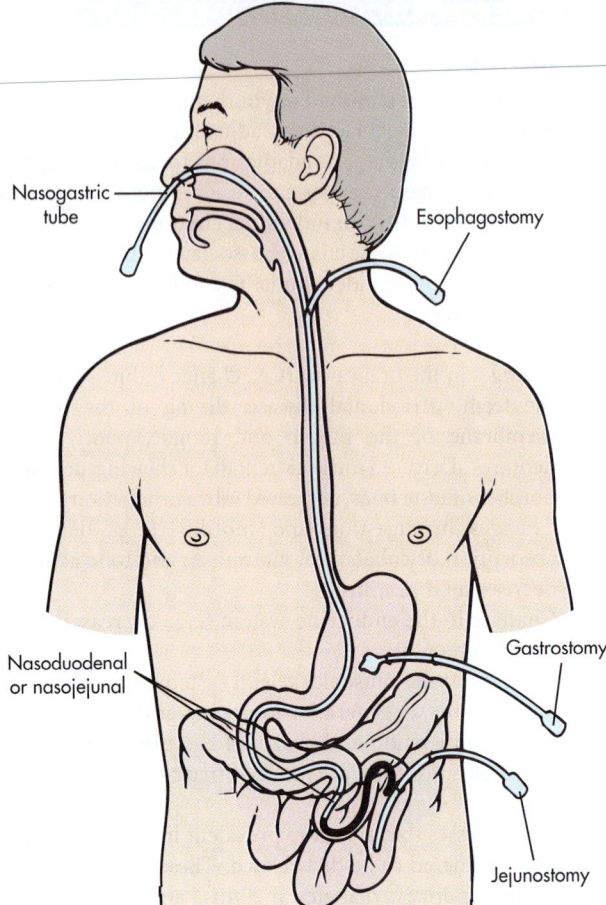

Fig. 38-2   Common enteral feeding tube placement locations.

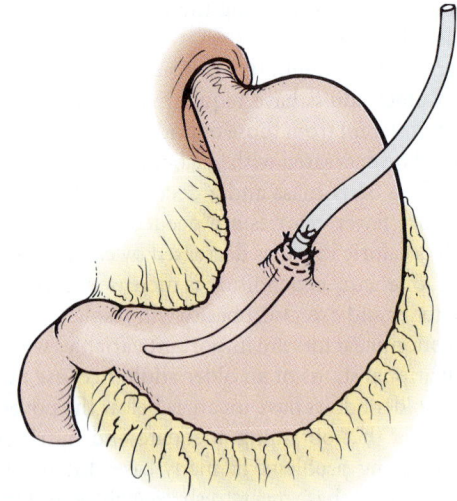

Fig. 38-3   Placement of a gastrostomy tube.

silicone tubes are radiopaque, making their position readily identified by x-ray. Many of these tubes also have weighted tips, allowing for easier passage of the tube through the pylorus into the duodenum. Placement into the intestine decreases the likelihood of regurgitation of contents into the esophagus and subsequent aspiration. With the use of a stylet these tubes can be placed in an uncooperative or comatose patient because the ability to swallow is not essential during insertion.

Although the smaller feeding tubes have many advantages over wider-lumen tubes, such as the Levine tube, there are some disadvantages that the nurse must keep in mind. Because of the small diameter, these tubes are more easily clogged when feedings are thick and are more difficult to use for checking residual volumes. They are particularly prone to obstruction when oral medications have not been thoroughly crushed and dissolved in water before administration. They can become dislodged by vomiting or coughing and can also become knotted or kinked in the GI tract. Failure to flush the tubing after both medication administration and residual volume determinations can result in tube clogging. When the tube becomes clogged, it may necessitate removal and insertion of a new tube, adding to cost and patient discomfort.

Gastrostomy and Jejunostomy

A permanent gastrostomy, such as a Janeway gastrostomy, may be used for a patient who requires tube feedings over an extended time (Figs. 38-3 and 38-4). A tunnel of gastric tissue is formed and brought out to form a stoma at the skin surface. A small catheter (5F to 10F) is inserted at the skin surface. The

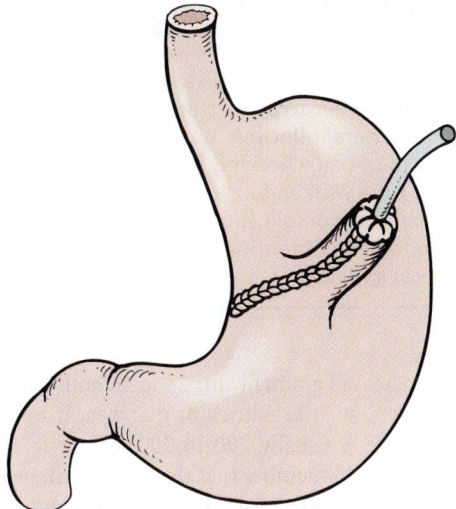

Fig. 38-4 Janeway gastrostomy.

stoma closes when the catheter is removed. Problems of leakage and skin irritation are decreased or eliminated.[12]

A gastrostomy tube may be placed by means of percutaneous endoscopic gastrostomy (PEG) (Fig. 38-5). The patient must have an intact, unobstructed GI tract, and the esophageal lumen must be wide enough to pass the endoscope. A PEG has several advantages. The procedure itself has fewer risks (no general anesthesia or laparotomy), it can be done at a lower cost, and it requires minimum or no sedation of the patient who is severely compromised. The most common complications of gastrostomy feedings include aspiration, pneumonia, accidental tube removal, wound cellulitis, and clogged tubes.[12]

Feedings can usually be started when bowel sounds are present, usually within 24 hours after catheter placement. Immediately after tube insertion, the tube length from the insertion site to the distal end should be measured and recorded. The tube is then marked at the skin insertion site.[12] At regular intervals the tube insertion length should be rechecked. The catheter is frequently connected to a pump for continuous feeding. Tap water may be infused within 2 hours after placement. For the patient with chronic reflux, a jejunostomy tube with jejunostomy feedings may be necessary to reduce reflux. Some important nursing implications for care and feeding of patients with PEGs are listed in Table 38-17.

Procedures for Tube Feedings

The procedure for the administration of tube feeding through an NG tube is standard. The following principles apply:

1. *Patient position.* The patient should be sitting or lying with the head of the bed elevated 30 to 45 degrees to prevent aspiration. If intermittent delivery, the head should remain elevated for 30 to 60 minutes after feeding.
2. *Patency of tube.* If feedings are intermittent, the tube should be irrigated with water before and after each feeding to ensure that the tube is patent and to prevent blockage of the tube. If the feedings are continuous, they should be administered by using an electric or a battery-operated feeding pump with a built-in alarm that will sound if the tubing becomes occluded. If no

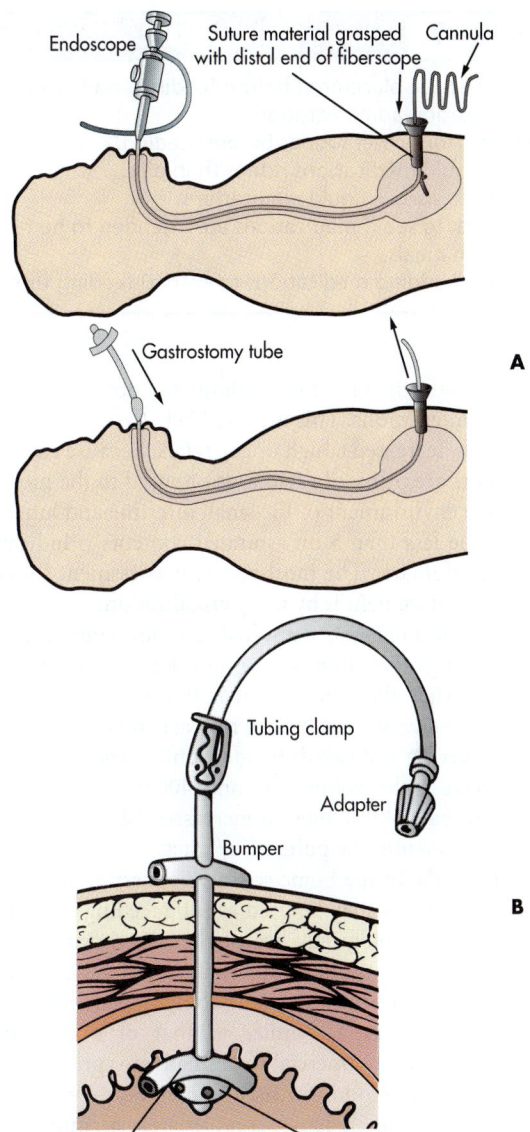

Fig. 38-5 Percutaneous endoscopic gastrostomy. **A,** Gastrostomy tube placement via percutaneous endoscopy. Using endoscopy, a gastrostomy tube is inserted through the esophagus into the stomach and then pulled through a stab wound made in the abdominal wall. **B,** A retention disk and bumper secure the tube.

pump is available, the feedings require frequent monitoring of the drip rate so that blockage does not occur from the patient lying on the tubing inadvertently or from too slow a drip rate.
3. *Tube position.* Proper placement of the tube in the stomach should be checked before each feeding or every 4 hours with continuous feedings. Methods used to check for tube placement can include aspiration of stomach contents and checking the pH of contents using a pH meter or pH paper. Two advantages of a pH meter over pH paper are that neither the formula nor the added food coloring affect the pH meter results, and the smaller feeding tubes may be passed directly into the bronchus on insertion or may become dislodged and

| Table **38-17** | **Nursing Management: Percutaneous Endoscopic Gastrostomy** |

- Check tube placement before feeding and before each medication administration.
- Assess for bowel sounds before feeding.
- Use liquid medications rather than pills.
  Dilute viscous liquid medications.
  Check to see if medications are intended to be taken with meals.
  Avoid adding medications to enteral feeding formula.

- If it is necessary to use tablets, be sure to crush medications to a fine powder to avoid clogging feeding tubes.
- Follow other general principles of tube feeding such as elevating head of bed, checking for residual volumes, and flushing tube with water.
- Assess regularly for complications, such as aspiration, diarrhea, abdominal distention, hyperglycemia, constipation, and fecal impaction.

slip into the bronchus without any obvious respiratory manifestations. This is more likely to occur in a patient with decreased cough or gag reflex. Because gastric contents are primarily acidic, as opposed to the more alkaline environment of the small intestine and lungs, a pH value less than 5 on aspirated contents is indicative of the stomach. The most accurate assessment for correct tube placement is by x-ray visualization.

Checking gastric residual volumes is important when feedings are administered into the stomach. For example, when the infusion rate is 100 ml per hour, the total infused volume of 400 ml may accumulate when gastric emptying is delayed. In addition, gastric secretions can increase the volume beyond 400 ml. With increased residual volume there is increased risk for aspiration of formula into the pulmonary tract.

4. *Formula.* In the home setting blenderized foods from a normal diet may be used as tube feedings. The patient may psychologically accept these feedings better than commercial products. Normal bowel function is promoted by fiber and residue content, which, in blenderized feedings, is similar to that of a normal diet. However, commercial formulas are preferable over blenderized foods for small-lumen tubes because of the risk of tube clogging, completeness of nutrition, and decreased risk of formula contamination.

The feeding should be given at room or body temperature to decrease the likelihood of diarrhea and other GI complaints. The pleasurable aspects of eating, such as smelling, seeing, tasting, and chewing the food, are frequently denied the tube-fed patient. If clinical condition permits, the patient may be allowed to smell, taste, and even chew small amounts of food before the feeding, and then the chewed food must be spit out. The patient may hesitate to do this because it is not esthetic, but it stimulates salivary and gastric secretions and provides the pleasurable sensations associated with oral intake. Before initiating the feeding, the nurse should aspirate gastric contents and measure the amount. If greater than 100 ml and there are clinical signs of intolerance, including report of nausea or increase in abdominal girth, the next feeding is held for 1 hour and then the residual volume is rechecked. The aspirate should be reinstilled.

5. *Administration of feeding.* Feedings are administered either by gravity drip method or by feeding pump. Applying pressure to force the feeding can damage the gastric mucosa. If the feedings have been refrigerated, they should be warmed to room temperature. The feed-

ing is increased gradually for 24 to 48 hours to minimize side effects, such as nausea or diarrhea. If intermittent, the volume is usually 200 to 500 ml per feeding. It is important to remember that the patient still needs water replacement of 30 ml/kg body weight per day.

6. *General nursing considerations.* The patient should be weighed daily or several times a week, and accurate intake and output records should be maintained. These measures provide information on weight gain or loss, as well as tolerance of the feedings. Initially blood glucose checks to assess glucose tolerance are performed at the bedside. An older patient who has glucose intolerance is particularly vulnerable. Feedings that have been opened and not refrigerated or feedings that have been infusing longer than 8 hours should be discarded to minimize bacterial growth and to prevent the administration of contaminated feeding. Feedings should, therefore, be labeled with the date and time they are initially used. If a pump is used, pump tubing should be changed every 24 hours or per manufacturer's guideline. See NCP 38-1 for care of the patient receiving enteral nutrition.

Complications Related to Tubes and Feedings

The types of problems encountered in patients receiving tube feedings and corrective measures are presented in Table 38-18.

When commercial products are used, the concentration, taste, osmolarity, and amounts of protein, sodium, and fat vary according to the manufacturer. Most if not all commercial formulas are lactose free. The concentrations range from 0.5 to 2.0 kcal/ml, with most between 1.0 and 1.5 kcal/ml. A limited number of flavors are available, and the overuse of one or two flavors, even in tube feedings, can lead to dislike and less tolerance with time.

The osmolality of the solution is determined by the number and size of particles in solution. With regard to feeding formulas, the more hydrolyzed the nutrients, the greater the osmolality. Many tube feeding formulas are isotonic, although some are hypertonic. The more calorically dense the formula, the less water it contains. Protein content greater than 16% can lead to dehydration unless the patient is given supplemental fluids or is sufficiently alert to request additional fluids. The nurse must be aware of this potential problem and must provide extra fluids through the feeding tube or, if permitted, by mouth. Tube feedings with high sodium content are contraindicated in the patient with cardiovascular problems, such as congestive heart failure. High fat content is not advocated for a patient suffering from short bowel syndrome or ileocecal resections because of impaired fat absorption.

38-1   NURSING CARE PLAN   PATIENT RECEIVING ENTERAL NUTRITION

Expected Patient Outcomes	Nursing Interventions and *Rationales*

NURSING DIAGNOSIS   Altered nutrition: less than body requirements *related to* enteral feeding problems *as manifested by* body weight ≤10% less than ideal, diarrhea, abdominal distention.

- Stable or gain in weight.
- No diarrhea or abdominal distention.

- Monitor weight and compare with baseline *to make adjustments as needed in calorie intake.*
- Progress the patient slowly from clear liquids to blenderized foods that are added to clear liquids *to prevent gastric distention.*
- Gradually add high-calorie foods to patient's blenderized foods *to maintain body weight while preventing distention.*

NURSING DIAGNOSIS   Impaired skin integrity *related to* enzymatic action of gastric juices, which may leak around tube *as manifested by* red, irritated tissue around the tube.

- No skin breakdown around gastrostomy tube.
- Daily inspections of skin performed and problems reported.

- Assess skin daily for signs of irritation or redness *so that early treatment is provided.*
- Wash skin around the tube with soap and water daily; apply a protective skin barrier such as zinc oxide or petrolatum or a Stomahesive wafer *to maintain skin integrity.*
- Teach patient and family to assess and provide care *to ensure involvement in self-care and early detection of problems.*

NURSING DIAGNOSIS   Body image disturbance *related to* presence of feeding tube *as manifested by* refusal to participate in own feeding, verbalization of fear of rejection by family and friends, avoidance of any social activities associated with food and eating.

- Participation in self-care related to feedings.
- Verbalization of acceptance of enteral feeding.
- Support systems established.

- Encourage patient to express feelings about the enteral feedings *to increase the patient's self-awareness.*
- Provide information about the tube, feedings, purpose, and patient progress *so that the patient makes decisions based on correct information.*
- Acknowledge the patient's fears *to establish a trusting nurse-patient relationship.*
- Incorporate the patient in care of operative site; gradually encourage patient to assume full self-care responsibility *to promote positive coping with the change.*

NURSING DIAGNOSIS   Risk for fluid volume deficit *related to* diarrhea or inadequate fluid intake.

- No signs of fluid volume deficit.
- Adequate fluid intake.

- Monitor patient for poor skin turgor, decreased blood pressure, tachycardia, decreased urine output, and dry mucous membranes *to identify signs of fluid volume deficit.*
- Provide adequate fluid intake, including water, as determined by intake records.
- Monitor urine output for osmotic diuresis, *which may occur secondary to high glucose load of feedings or too rapid infusion.*
- Identify possible cause of diarrhea *so that appropriate treatment is started.*

NURSING DIAGNOSIS   Ineffective management of therapeutic regimen *related to* care required for skin around tubing and tube feedings *as manifested by* questioning about self-care.

- Demonstration of skin care and tube feeding before discharge.

- Assess the patient's home environment and lifestyle *to make teaching relevant to individual requirements.*
- Provide detailed information about how to prepare the formula and manage the tube feeding *to facilitate self-care.*
- Use return demonstration technique *to validate patient's and family's learning of the necessary skills.*

NURSING DIAGNOSIS   Risk for aspiration *related to* enteral tube with tube feedings.

- No aspiration.
- Able to describe measures to prevent aspiration.

- During feeding have the patient's head elevated at least 30 degrees; remain in this position 30 minutes after feeding *to prevent aspiration.*
- Aspirate gastric contents before feeding *to validate gastric emptying.*
- Reinstill the residual gastric contents *to prevent excessive fluid and electrolyte losses.*

Table 38-18	Common Problems of Patients Receiving Tube Feedings
Problems and Possible Causes	**Corrective Measures**

Vomiting or Aspiration

Improper placement of tube	Replace tube in proper position. Check tube position before beginning feeding and every 4 hr if continuous feedings.
Delayed gastric emptying, increased residual volume	Hold feeding 1 hr; then, if residual volume is less than previous rate, resume feeding.
Potential for aspiration	Keep head of bed elevated to 30° to 45° angle. Have patient lie on right side for ½ hr after feeding. Have patient sit up on side of bed or in chair. Encourage ambulation unless contraindicated.
Contamination of formula	Refrigerate unused formula and record date opened. Discard outdated formula every 24 hr. Discard formula left standing for longer than manufacturer's guidelines: 8-12 hr for ready-to-feed formulas (cans), or 4 hr for reconstituted formula. Use closed system to prevent contamination.
Air in stomach	Clear tubing of air before feeding. Keep tube feeding container filled so air does not enter through feeding set.

Diarrhea

Feeding too fast, hypertonic formula	Decrease rate of feeding. Change to continuous-drip feedings. Check for drugs that may cause diarrhea (e.g., antibiotics, sorbitol).
Lactose intolerance	Consult physician for change in formula to lactose-free solution.
Contamination of formula or tubing	Change tubing every 24 hr. Hang 8 hr formula at a time. Do not exceed manufacturer's guidelines.
Low-fiber formula	Change to formula with more fiber.
Tube moving distally	Properly secure tube before beginning to feed. Check before each feeding or at least every 24 hr if receiving continuous feedings.

Constipation

Formula components	Consult physician for change in formula to one with more fiber content. Obtain laxative order.
Poor fluid intake	Increase fluid intake if not contraindicated. Give free water as well as formula. Total fluid 30 ml/kg body weight.
Drugs	Check for drugs that may be constipating.
Impaction	Rectal examination to check and manually remove feces if present.

Dehydration

Excessive diarrhea, vomiting	Decrease rate or change formula. Check drugs patient is receiving, especially antibiotics. Take care to prevent bacterial contamination of formula and equipment.
Poor fluid intake	Increase intake and check amount and number of feedings. Increase amount of intake if appropriate.
High-protein formula	Change formula
Hyperosmotic diuresis	Frequent blood glucose checks. Change formula.

The registered dietician can be of considerable assistance to the nursing staff. When close consultation with the nursing staff occurs, existing problems with tube feedings can be quickly and efficiently addressed and resolved. Some institutions have nutrition support teams composed of a physician, nurse, dietician, and pharmacist whose function is to oversee the nutrition support of select inpatients and outpatients.

In patients receiving gastrostomy feeding, the nurse is alert to two possible problems: (1) skin irritation and (2) pulling out of the tube. Skin care around the gastrostomy opening is important because the action of the gastric juice is irritating to the skin. The skin around the gastrostomy should be assessed daily for signs of redness and maceration. To keep the skin clean and dry, initially it should be rinsed with sterile water and dried. Once the site has healed, it can be washed with mild soap and water. A protective ointment (zinc oxide, petroleum gauze) or a skin barrier (karaya, Stomahesive) may be used on the skin around the gastrostomy. A small dressing may be placed around the tube until the site is healed. It must be changed promptly if it gets wet. Other types of drain or tube pouches may be used if there is a problem with skin irritation. The patient and family members can be taught how to care for the gastrostomy. Teaching should include skin care, care of the tube, and complete information about feedings.

■ **GERONTOLOGIC CONSIDERATIONS** ■

Enteral Nutrition

Enteral nutrition strategies, including nasogastric, nasointestinal, and gastrostomy feedings, are frequently used in the older patient to improve nutritional status. Because of physiologic changes associated with aging, the older adult is more vulnerable to complications associated with these interventions, especially fluid and electrolyte imbalances. Complications such as diarrhea can leave the patient dehydrated and saline depleted. Decreased thirst perception or impaired cognitive function de-

ETHICAL DILEMMAS

Withholding Treatment

SITUATION

A 26-year-old patient in a permanent vegetative state is diagnosed with her fifteenth bladder infection. Her home care nurse must determine whether or not to seek antibiotics for this infection. The family members have expressed a concern that no *heroic* measures be used to extend the biologic life of their daughter and sister, but they have been unwilling to withdraw the existing treatment, which is enteral nutrition. Should antibiotics be withheld?

DISCUSSION

The questions that arise when discussing heroic measures are of degree and intent. Is the intent not to prolong the patient's life or not to extend any suffering that the patient might experience? Does antibiotic treatment constitute treatment above and beyond the normal care of the patient, or is it simply appropriate treatment of a manageable condition? The family's resistance to the withdrawal of enteral nutrition may stem from discomfort and revulsion about starving the patient to death, or from strong beliefs about the importance of maintaining her biologic existence. The nurse must clarify what the patient's wishes were, if they are known. The family's values and their concerns about the patient, especially about her ability to feel pain or discomfort and about her quality of life, also should be discussed.

ETHICAL AND LEGAL PRINCIPLES

- Medical treatment may be withheld if a competent patient refuses to consent to it, if it is medically futile treatment, or if the burden of its provision outweighs its benefit.
- If withholding treatment or support leads to death, the underlying disease or condition is the cause. Technologic intervention simply prolongs life.
- Patients in a permanent vegetative state cannot be cured of that brain damage. Any treatable comorbidities related to this condition will not lead to a recovery from the permanent vegetative state.

RESEARCH
IMPLICATIONS FOR NURSING PRACTICE

Fiber and Tube Feeding

Citation Bass DJ, Forman LP, Abrams SE, Hsueh AM: The effect of dietary fiber in tube-fed elderly patients, *J Gerontol Nurs* 22:37, 1996.

Purpose To describe the pattern of stools in patients receiving tube feeding with or without fiber-containing formula.

Methods Retrospective chart review of 50 (29 males and 21 females) tube-fed long-term care patients. The number and consistency of each bowel movement were recorded. Antibiotic use was monitored.

Results and Conclusions Patients on fiber-containing formula had a lower frequency of liquid or loose stools and a higher frequency of formed stools as compared with those on the fiber-free formula. There was no correlation between stool characteristics and antibiotic use.

Implications for Nursing Practice Patients receiving long-term tube feedings may be at risk for constipation as a result of the low fiber content of most formulas. These patients may benefit from the inclusion of fiber in their enteral feeding formula.

TOTAL PARENTERAL NUTRITION

When the GI tract cannot be used for the ingestion, digestion, and absorption of essential nutrients, TPN may be substituted. Parenteral nutrition has become a relatively safe and practical method of delivering total nutritional needs by an IV route.

The goal of using TPN is to meet the patient's nutritional needs and to allow for growth of new body tissue. Regular IV solutions of 5% dextrose (5 g dextrose/100 ml) in water (D_5W) or 5% dextrose in lactated Ringer's solution (D_5LR) contain no protein and have approximately 170 calories per liter. The normal adult requires a minimum of 1200 to 1500 calories per day to carry out normal physiologic functions. Patients who sustain severe injury, surgery, or burns, and those who are malnourished as a result of medical treatment or disease processes, have greatly increased nutritional needs. The volume of regular dextrose solutions needed to meet these high caloric requirements could exceed the capacity of the cardiovascular system. Table 38-19 lists common indications for the use of TPN.

Composition

Commercially prepared TPN base solutions are available for both central and peripheral use (explained on p. 1060). These base solutions contain dextrose and nitrogen in the form of amino acids or protein hydrolysates. The hospital pharmacy adds the prescribed electrolytes (e.g., sodium, potassium, chloride, calcium, magnesium, and phosphate), vitamins, and trace elements (e.g., zinc, copper, chromium, and manganese) to customize the solution for the patient. A three-in-one, or total nutrient, mixture containing an IV fat emulsion, dextrose, and amino acids has become widely available, especially in the

creases the ability of the patient to seek additional fluids. With aging there is decreased ability to handle glucose loads (glucose intolerance). As a result, the older patient may be more susceptible to problems of hyperglycemia in response to the high carbohydrate load of some enteral feeding formulas. If the older adult has compromised cardiovascular function (e.g., congestive heart failure) there will be a decreased ability to handle large volumes of formula, in which case the use of more concentrated formulas may be warranted. The older adult also is at increased risk for aspiration caused by gastroesophageal reflux disease, hiatal hernia, or diminished gag reflex. Physical mobility, fine motor movement, and visual system changes associated with aging may contribute to difficulties in managing enteral nutrition equipment at home. In addition, age-related changes such as a decrease in lean muscle mass influence the reliability of measures used for nutritional assessment.

Table 38-19	Common Indications for Total Parenteral Nutrition

Acute or chronic renal failure*
Gastrointestinal tract anomalies and fistula
Burns
Chronic diarrhea and vomiting
Complicated surgery or trauma
Diverticulitis
Failure to thrive
Gastrointestinal obstruction
Granulomatous enterocolitis
Hepatic failure (reversible)*
Hypermetabolic states (sepsis, fractures)
Inflammatory bowel disease (Crohn's disease and
  ulcerative colitis)
Malabsorption
Malnutrition
Pancreatitis
Severe anorexia nervosa
Severe peptic ulcer disease
Short bowel syndrome

*Total parenteral nutrition should be used with extreme caution in this situation.

home setting. In hospital settings this total nutrient mixture is less likely to be used.

Calories. Calories in TPN are supplied primarily by carbohydrates in the form of dextrose (20% to 50% of total calories). The administration of between 100 and 150 g of dextrose (1 g provides approximately 3.4 calories, as opposed to oral carbohydrates, which provide 4 calories) daily has a protein-sparing effect. Protein should be provided at the rate of 1.0 to 1.5 g/kg per day depending on the patient's needs. Adequate nonprotein calories in the form of glucose and lipids must be provided to allow metabolism of amino acids for wound healing and not as energy. However, overfeeding can lead to multiple organ failure. To minimize these problems, an energy intake of 25 to 30 calories per kilogram per day in a nonobese patient is often recommended. Providing both lipid and amino acid components meets the energy requirement while minimizing problems of overfeeding.

Nitrogen. The normal healthy person of average body size needs approximately 45 to 65 g of protein daily (see Table 38-4). In a nutritionally depleted patient under the stress of illness or surgery, requirements can exceed 150 g per day to ensure a positive nitrogen balance. However, in the most recent guidelines, protein intake levels of 1.5 to 2.0 g per kilogram per day are suggested for most patients with moderate to severe stress.[13]

Electrolytes. The assessment of individual requirements should take place daily at the beginning of therapy and then several times a week as the treatment progresses. The following are ranges for average daily electrolyte requirements for adult patients:

Sodium: 60 to 200 mEq
Potassium: 50 to 160 mEq
Chloride: 100 to 200 mEq
Magnesium: 20 to 30 mEq
Calcium: 5 to 15 mEq
Phosphate: 30 to 100 mEq

The exact amount needed depends on the patient's health problem and on electrolyte levels as determined by blood testing.

Trace Elements. Zinc, copper, manganese, cobalt, selenium, and iodine supplements must be ordered according to the patient's condition and needs. Levels of these elements are monitored in the patient receiving TPN. The physician may order additional amounts of these elements to be added to the solutions according to the patient's requirements.

Vitamins. The daily addition of a multivitamin preparation to 1 L of TPN generally meets the vitamin requirements. If multivitamin infusion is used, the cobalamin (vitamin B_{12}) requirement may be met without the need for supplemental injections. It is necessary for the physician to order vitamin K and folic acid separately. Folic acid 500 µg is given daily. Intramuscular (IM) vitamin K may be ordered depending on the results of the prothrombin time.

Methods of Administration

TPN may be administered by central or peripheral veins. Central parenteral nutrition is given through a catheter whose tip lies in the superior vena cava. The central catheter often originates at the subclavian vein. More recently single- or double-lumen peripherally inserted central catheters (PICCs) are being placed, usually into the basilic or cephalic vein and then advanced into the central circulation. Such catheters are made of soft, flexible material (silicon, polymer) and are 20 to 24 inches long. Ease of placement, cost, and limited complications make this an attractive alternative to a centrally placed line. Central TPN is indicated when long-term nutritional support is necessary, when the patient has high protein and caloric requirements, and when suitable peripheral veins are not available.

Peripheral parenteral nutrition (PPN) is administered through a peripherally inserted catheter or vascular access device (VAD), which uses a large peripheral vein. PPN is used when (1) nutritional support is needed for only a short time (up to 2 weeks), (2) protein and caloric requirements are not excessively high, (3) the risk of a central catheter is too great, or (4) nutritional support is used to supplement inadequate oral intake. Both central and peripheral TPN are used in a patient who is not a candidate for enteral support.

Central and peripheral parenteral nutrition differ in tonicity, which is measured in milliosmoles (mOsm), the concentration of particles in a fluid. Blood is isotonic and measures approximately 280 mOsm per liter. The standard IV solutions of D_5W and normal saline are essentially isotonic. Central TPN solutions are hypertonic, measuring approximately 1600 mOsm per liter. The high glucose content ranges from 20% to 50%. Thus nutrients can be infused using smaller fluid volumes than PPN. Central TPN must be infused in a large central vein so that rapid dilution can occur. The use of a peripheral vein causes irritation and thrombophlebitis. PPN is less hypertonic (using as much as 20% glucose) and can be safely administered through a large peripheral vein, although phlebitis can occur. Another potential complication is fluid overload.

All TPN solutions should be prepared by a pharmacist or a trained technician using strict aseptic techniques under a laminar flow hood. Nothing should be added to parenteral nutrition solutions after they are prepared in the pharmacy. The danger of drug incompatibilities and contamination is high.

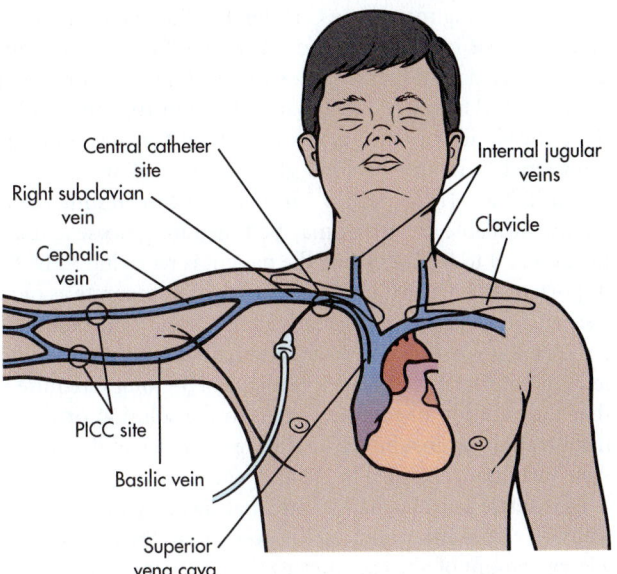

Fig. 38-6 Placement of a catheter for total parenteral nutrition using subclavian vein. Peripherally inserted central catheters (PICC) inserted using the basilic or cephalic veins.

Table **38-20**	Complications of Total Parenteral Nutrition

Infection
Fungus
Gram-positive bacteria
Gram-negative bacteria

Metabolic Problems
Glucose metabolism
  Hyperglycemia, hypoglycemia, and hyperosmolar nonketotic coma
  Glycosuria
  Osmotic diuresis
  Ketoacidosis
Amino acid metabolism
  Serum amino acid imbalances
  Elevated serum ammonia
  Prerenal azotemia
Essential fatty acid deficiency
Electrolyte and vitamin excesses and deficiencies
Trace mineral deficiencies

Mechanical Problems
Insertion
  Air embolus
  Pneumothorax, hemothorax, and hydrothorax
  Hemorrhage
Dislodgement
Thrombosis of great vein
Phlebitis

The fewer the personnel involved in the preparation and administration of TPN, the lower the risk of infection for the patient. In most hospitals the physician must order the TPN solution daily. In this way the solution and additives can be adjusted to the patient's current needs. Each bottle of solution indicates the glucose and protein content, all additives, the time mixed, and the date and time of expiration. In general, solutions are good for 24 to 36 hours and must be refrigerated until one-half hour before use.

Catheter Placement

The central placement of the catheter into a large main vein for TPN is performed by the physician or a specially trained advanced practice nurse. The vein most commonly used is the subclavian, although the innominate or the jugular vein may be used. The procedure is the same as for the insertion of a central venous pressure line and should be done under strict aseptic conditions.

A standard isotonic IV solution is infused through the central line until x-ray confirms proper placement of the catheter tip in the superior vena cava and not in the jugular vein or the heart. The catheter insertion site is covered with an iodine ointment, and an occlusive dressing is placed over it. The date is marked on the dressing.

Placement of a PICC catheter is done under sterile conditions, often by a specially trained nurse. A baseline measurement of the upper arm circumference is recommended. A tourniquet is then placed around the upper arm near the axilla to allow examination of the antecubital fossa and selection of a vein. If possible, the patient should be supine with the arm straight and at a 90-degree angle. Preparation of the insertion site should be done according to institutional policy. The sterile catheter will need to be cut to the predetermined length, depending on the vein selected.

A local anesthetic is usually used at the insertion site. This site should be cleaned, protected, and maintained according to institutional policy. As with the centrally placed line, chest x-ray is needed to verify proper tip placement before administering any TPN solution.

Proper placement of a catheter for central TPN is illustrated in Fig. 38-6. Once established for TPN, a single-lumen central catheter should not be used for the administration of blood or antibiotics, the drawing of blood samples, or the monitoring of central venous pressure.

Administration of Solution

Because TPN solutions are excellent media for microbial growth, it is essential that proper aseptic techniques be followed. The Food and Drug Administration (FDA) recommends that 0.22 μm millipore filters be placed on all parenteral lines. When the filter is used, it should be placed proximal to the catheter hub. Filters are changed every 24 hours, and new IV tubing is changed with each new bottle of TPN. The tubing and the filter should be clearly labeled with the date and the time they are put into use.

Complications

Complications of TPN can be divided into three categories: (1) infectious, (2) metabolic, and (3) mechanical. The major complications of each category are presented in Table 38-20.

NURSING MANAGEMENT: TOTAL PARENTERAL NUTRITION

PPN is a form of IV nutrition that may be given concurrently with oral nourishment. A large peripheral vein can be used because the solution is less hypertonic and therefore less irritating. The peripheral injection site should be observed for signs of phlebitis (redness and swelling). The insertion site dressing is changed at least every 48 hours, depending on established hospital policy and type of peripheral access device. The preparation and administration of PPN follow the same criteria as outlined for central TPN (see NCP 38-2).

Vital signs should be monitored every 2 to 4 hours in the patient receiving TPN. Daily weights give an indication of the patient's hydration status as therapy progresses. Body weight is considered the sum of the changes in protein, fat, and water. On a daily basis, body water fluctuates more than protein or fat. Analysis must be made of whether gains or losses in weight are caused by fluid gained from edema, fluid lost through diuresis, or actual increase or decrease in tissue weight. Blood levels of glucose, electrolytes, protein, a complete blood count, and enzyme studies are followed daily until stable and then weekly as the patient's condition warrants. Assessment of these important values assists the nurse in assessing the patient's tolerance of parenteral nutrition.

Dressings covering the catheter site are changed according to institutional protocol, ranging from every other day to once a week. Frequently, specially trained nurses from the IV team or the nutritional support team are responsible for these dressing changes. Some institutions allow a staff nurse to do the dressing changes after special instruction. The procedure for changing the dressing is similar to that followed after catheter insertion. The institutional routine should be followed with respect to the appropriate use of solutions for the dressing change. The site is carefully observed for signs of inflammation and infection. Phlebitis can readily occur in the vein as a result of the hypertonic infusion, and the area can become infected. The patient receiving central TPN may be immunosuppressed and thus more susceptible to opportunistic infections. In this patient signs of inflammation or infection can be subtle, if present at all. Many patients receiving TPN are receiving chemotherapy, corticosteroids, or antibiotics, which can mask signs of infection.

If sutures are used to anchor the catheter, they may become infected. If an infection is suspected during dressing change, a culture specimen of the site and drainage should be sent for analysis, and the physician should be notified immediately. The use of an occlusive dressing protects the wound from contamination.

Complications frequently associated with catheter placement are hemorrhage, hydrothorax and pneumothorax, hemothorax, air embolus, and venous thrombosis. It is important that the tip of the catheter not lie within the right atrium. The TPN solution is hyperosmolar, and the catheter tip can cause erosions of the atrial tissue with subsequent infection.

Hyperglycemia is a metabolic complication of parenteral nutrition. At the beginning of TPN therapy, the solution is infused at a gradually increasing rate for 24 to 48 hours. This allows the pancreas to adapt to the increased amount of glucose in the circulation by producing more insulin. Blood glucose levels should be checked at the bedside every 4 to 6 hours with a glucose-testing meter (see Chapter 46). Some increase in the blood glucose level is expected during the first few days after TPN is started. A sliding scale dose of insulin may be ordered to keep the level below 180 to 200 mg/dl (9.8 to 10.9 mmol/L). In the critically ill patient it is recommended that insulin be administered to maintain blood glucose level below 150 to 200 mg/dl (8.3 to 11.1 mmol/L).[14] If blood glucose–testing meters are not available, the urine may be tested for glucose and acetone every 4 to 6 hours while the patient is receiving TPN. It is important to note that urine testing is not as accurate as blood testing and thus is not frequently done. As with the blood glucose level, glycosuria of 1+ or 2+ is expected during the first few days of therapy. However, readings of 3+ or 4+ require either the addition of regular insulin to the solution or the administration of insulin on a sliding-scale schedule. (Sliding scale insulin is explained in Chapter 46.)

The nurse must be made aware that speeding or slowing the infusion rate is contraindicated. Speeding up the rate results in a large amount of glucose entering the circulation. Endogenous insulin levels often are not adequate to handle this increase in glucose, and a hyperglycemic state results. The renal tubules are unable to reabsorb the glucose and it spills into the urine. Conversely, slowing the rate may result in a hypoglycemic state because it takes time for the pancreatic islet cells to adjust to a reduced glucose level. Checking the amount infused and the rate every 30 minutes to 1 hour is recommended. An infusion pump should be used during administration of TPN so that the infusion rate can be maintained, and an alarm will sound if the tubing becomes obstructed. Even when using an infusion pump, the nurse should periodically check the volume infused because pump malfunctions can alter the rate.

Before setting up and administering TPN, the nurse must check the label and ingredients in the solution to see that they are what the physician ordered. Solutions must also be examined for signs of contamination, such as a cloudy appearance. If contamination is suspected, the solution should be promptly returned to the pharmacy for replacement. It is the nurse's responsibility to ensure that the TPN solution is discontinued and replaced with a new solution if it is still infusing at the end of 24 hours. At room temperature, the solution is an excellent medium for microorganism growth.

Catheter-related infection and septicemia can occur in patients receiving TPN through both peripherally and centrally placed lines. Local manifestations of infection include erythema, tenderness, and exudate at the catheter insertion site. Systemically the patient may have fever, chills, nausea, vomiting, and malaise. If no other causes can be identified, a catheter-related infection is suspected. Because of the risk of infection, catheters with antibiotic or antiseptic surfaces are frequently used. To diagnose the presence of infection and to determine the causative organism, cultures are performed of the catheter tip if the catheter has been removed or the blood in the catheter if still in place. Blood cultures are drawn simultaneously from the catheter and a peripheral vein. A chest x-ray is taken to detect changes in pulmonary status. The current bottle of TPN solution with tubing and filter should also be cultured and replaced with an entirely new setup. When the catheter tip is the source of infection, antibiotic therapy is generally not necessary because removal of the catheter will eliminate the problem. A

38-2 | **NURSING CARE PLAN** | **PATIENT RECEIVING TOTAL PARENTERAL NUTRITION**

Expected Patient Outcomes	Nursing Interventions and *Rationales*

NURSING DIAGNOSIS | **Risk for infection** *related to* placement of a central venous access catheter, inadequate aseptic practices, and decreased defense mechanisms.

- No manifestations of infection.
- Normal body temperature.
- Negative blood cultures.

- Assess for altered defense mechanisms caused by inadequate nutrition, compromised health status, open wound for TPN line *to plan for prevention of infection.*
- Refrigerate solution until 30 minutes before using *to prevent bacterial growth in the solution.*
- Use protocols for tubing and filter changes; change dressing over catheter site according to institution policy *to minimize the possibility of infection.*
- Observe for signs of inflammation and infection; monitor vital signs q4hr *to ensure early detection of infection.*

NURSING DIAGNOSIS | **Impaired physical mobility** *related to* muscle or nerve trauma *as manifested by* decreased muscle strength and control, neuromuscular impairment (e.g., brachial plexus injury).

- Satisfactory movement of upper body.
- Satisfactory pain control.

- Observe patient for pain in shoulder and sensory changes *to determine possible nerve damage or faulty catheter placement.*
- Assist with range of motion within position restrictions *to maintain normal range of motion of shoulder.*
- Administer pain medication as ordered *to maintain patient's comfort.*

NURSING DIAGNOSIS | **Anxiety** *related to* inability to ingest food and fluids; lack of knowledge regarding catheter, benefits and management of TPN *as manifested by* restlessness and apprehension; frequent questioning regarding care of catheter and TPN line.

- Statement of rationale for and demonstration of care of TPN line.

- Instruct patient on rationale and benefits of TPN and care of line *because knowledge and facts may reduce anxiety.*
- Illustrate catheter position by drawings and pictures *to increase patient understanding.*

COLLABORATIVE PROBLEMS

Nursing Goals	Nursing Interventions and *Rationales*

POTENTIAL COMPLICATION | **Hyperglycemia, hypoglycemia, and electrolyte imbalances** *related to* administration of TPN.

- Monitor blood glucose and serum electrolytes.
- Report deviations from acceptable parameters.
- Carry out medical and nursing interventions.

- Monitor for signs of hyperglycemia such as thirst, polyuria, confusion, elevated fasting blood glucose, blurred vision, dizziness, nausea and vomiting, dehydration, and deep labored breathing *to plan appropriate treatment.*
- Monitor for signs of hypoglycemia such as sweating, hunger, weakness, and tremors *to ensure early intervention.*
- Monitor serum electrolyte levels daily *to identify and treat complications early.*
- Check for symptoms of hyperkalemia (e.g., muscle weakness, flaccid paralysis, cardiac arrhythmias, abdominal cramps, diarrhea) and hypokalemia (e.g., general weakness, decreased muscle tone, weak or irregular pulse, low blood pressure, shallow respirations, abdominal distention, and ileus). (Other manifestations of electrolyte imbalances are discussed in Chapter 15.)
- Check blood glucose q4hr. Notify physician of increased levels *so that regular insulin may be added to the solution or administered on a sliding scale basis.*
- Maintain accurate infusion rate *to control the amount of glucose administered and prevent fluctuations in blood glucose levels.*
- Check every 30 minutes or use an infusion pump *to ensure accurate administration.*
- Never increase or decrease flow rate by more than 10% *to prevent fluctuations in blood glucose levels.*
- Never stop TPN abruptly unless it is replaced by another glucose source *to prevent hypoglycemia.*

Continued

38-2 NURSING CARE PLAN PATIENT RECEIVING TOTAL PARENTERAL NUTRITION—continued

Expected Patient Outcomes	Nursing Interventions and *Rationales*
POTENTIAL COMPLICATION ■ Monitor for and report signs of air embolus. ■ Carry out medical and nursing interventions.	**Air embolus** *related to* incorrect position of TPN catheter. ■ On catheter insertion, place patient in Trendelenburg's position with rolled towel between scapulae *to distend subclavian vein by increasing venous pressure.* ■ Instruct patient to take a deep breath (Valsalva's maneuver) and hold while needle is inserted into subclavian vein. ■ Use same position and Valsalva's maneuver when changing tubing *to prevent air from being sucked into vein.* ■ If air embolism is suspected, place patient in Trendelenburg's position with left side down *to trap "air" in right atria.* ■ Continue to observe for shock, cough, and shortness of breath. ■ Notify physician immediately *so definitive diagnosis and treatment can be initiated.* ■ Monitor for signs of air embolus such as abnormal blood gases, cough, cyanosis, pain, anxiety, fatigue, respiratory rate and depth changes, altered chest excursion, shortness of breath *to ensure early identification and treatment.*

Table **38-21**	Common Characteristics of a 20% Intralipid Fat Emulsion in Water*
Soybean triglycerides	20%*
Egg yolk phospholipids	1.20%
Glycerin	2.25%
Electrolytes	1.50 mm phosphorus/100 ml
Total kilocalories	2 cal/ml
Typical pH	8
Osmolarity	260 mOsm/L

*Other stock lipids are 10% and 30%.

new central line may be immediately established or replaced by a peripheral route. It is important that a glucose source be maintained to prevent rebound hypoglycemia.

Weaning. The same precautions should be followed in weaning from TPN as when therapy is being initiated, except in the reverse order. The flow rate must be gradually decreased for 4 to 6 hours, while oral intake is increased. If an emergency situation precludes a slow weaning process, other dextrose-containing fluids should be administered without interruption. When the catheter is removed, the dressing should be changed daily until the wound heals. Oral nourishment should be encouraged, and a careful record of intake should be maintained. Body weight recording and laboratory analysis of serum electrolyte and glucose levels may continue.

Home Parenteral Nutrition. Home parenteral nutrition is an accepted mode of nutritional therapy for the person who does not require hospitalization but who benefits from continued nutritional support. Some patients have been successfully treated at home for many months and even years. It is important to educate the patient or the family about catheter care, aseptic technique in mixing and handling of the IV solutions and tubing, and side effects.

Intravenous Fat Emulsion

The first infusion of fat emulsions occurred during the 1920s in Japan. Further research was delayed until after World War II. The FDA has currently approved the use of 10%, 20%, and 30% intralipid fat emulsion solutions. These lipid emulsions provide approximately 1 calorie per milliliter (10% solution) or 2 calories per milliliter (20% solution). The contents of intralipid fat emulsion are listed in Table 38-21. The use of IV fat emulsions is indicated for the following patients:

1. Those receiving peripheral parenteral nutrition who require an additional source of calories
2. Those receiving long-term (more than 5 days) parenteral nutrition who require a source of essential fatty acids
3. Those receiving central TPN who have high caloric needs

Using daily IV fat emulsions provides another nonprotein energy source. In practice, the conservative approach is IV-administered fat emulsions providing not more than 20% to 30% of the total energy to minimize possible linoleic acid immunosuppressive effects. The maximum fat emulsion amount should not exceed a dose of 2.5 g/kg per day.[15] It is administered slowly over 12 to 24 hours to minimize immune suppression. Nausea, vomiting, and elevated temperature have been reported, especially when lipids are infused quickly.

The administration of fat emulsion is contraindicated in the patient with a disturbance in fat metabolism. It should also be used with caution in the patient who is in danger of fat embolism (e.g., fractured femur) and the patient with an allergy to eggs.

Intralipid solution (10%) is isotonic and in balanced combination with other proteins and carbohydrates contributes to complete peripheral TPN solutions. It can be infused separately. When it is used with TPN, the fat emulsion provides essential fatty acids that are not included in the standard dextrose–amino acid preparations of TPN. Prolonged use of TPN can lead to a fatty acid deficiency, which is manifested by dermatitis and loss of hair. Recent pharmacologic advances now permit the direct mixing of lipid emulsion with dextrose and amino acids in a single bag suitable for infusion in some situations.

Unopened intralipid solutions do not require refrigeration. However, those that have been opened or mixed with other nutrients do require refrigeration and should be refrigerated until 1 hour before administration. Special tubing is provided by the manufacturer, and new tubing is used with each bottle. Nothing is to be added to the solution before administration. Lipid solutions can be filtered but require a 1.2 μm filter. When PPN is being run concurrently, the fat emulsion should be connected below the filter through a Y-injection site as close as possible to the injection site. The preferred delivery method is a continuous low volume, such as 20% lipids delivered at 10 to 30 ml per hour depending on patient needs. Adverse reactions that can occur are allergic manifestations, dyspnea, cyanosis, fever, flushing, phlebitis, chest and back pain, and pain at the IV site. A major benefit derived from IV fat administration is that a large number of calories can be provided in a relatively small amount of fluid. This is especially beneficial when the patient is at risk for fluid overload.

OBESITY

Obesity has reached epidemic proportions in our society.[16] In the United States obesity is the most common nutritional problem. Among adults age 20 years and older, 33% of men and 36% of women are overweight.[17] The prevalence of overweight increases with age, for both men and women, but to a greater degree in women. African-American and Hispanic women have a higher prevalence of being overweight than do Caucasian women.[17]

The calculated body mass index (BMI) is a common clinical index of obesity or altered body fat distribution. A well-accepted scale has been developed to calculate BMI by gender using weight-to-height ratios (Fig. 38-7).[18] Individuals with a BMI of 25 to 29.9 kg/m^2 are classified as being overweight, and those with values of 30 kg/m^2 or more are classified as obese.

The waist-to-hip ratio is another way to define obesity. This ratio is a method of describing the distribution of both subcutaneous and intraabdominal adipose tissue. The waist measurement is divided by the hip measurement to calculate the ratio. A number greater than 1.0 in men and 0.8 in women indicates overweight. This ratio increases with age and excessive weight.[18]

Anthropometric measurements can also be used to define the different levels of overweight. A patient with body weight 10% above the ideal for height and frame is considered overweight. A patient with body weight 20% above the ideal for height and frame is considered obese. Triceps skinfold greater than 15 mm in men and 25 mm in women would classify the person as overweight. When body weight exceeds 100% of the ideal body weight it is classified as morbid obesity.

In obese persons a variety of problems occur at a rate higher than the expected rate. These include hypertension, hyperlipidemia, type 2 diabetes mellitus, degenerative joint disease, gout, insulin resistance with hyperinsulinemia, cardiovascular disease, gallbladder disease, stroke, some kinds of cancer (breast,

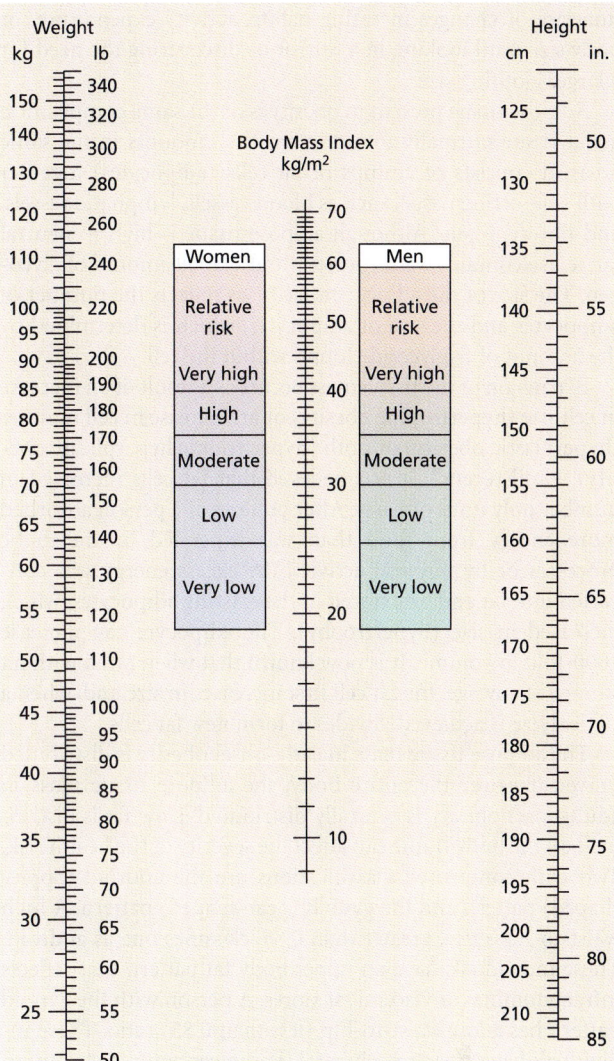

Fig. 38-7 A nomogram for determining body mass index (BMI). To use this nomogram, place a rule or other edge between the column for height and the column for weight connecting an individual's numbers for these two variables. Read the BMI in kg/m^2 where the straight line crosses the middle lines when the height and weight are connected. Overweight: BMI of 25 to 29.9 kg/m^2; obesity: BMI 30 kg/m^2 or more. Heights and weights are without shoes or clothes. Relative risk for health problems associated with obesity are shown.

colon), and menstrual irregularities.[19] These conditions generally improve if weight loss occurs.

Formation of Adipose Tissue

The formation of adipose tissue, unless determined to be secondary to an organic cause, can occur only when a person consumes more food than is required to carry out normal physiologic functions and growth. The excess energy is converted to fat and is stored in adipose tissue in layers beneath the skin surface, the omentum, the mesentery, and in fat pads that normally surround the kidneys and the heart. The process of reaching an obese state is usually insidious. The person may be completely unaware of changes in eating habits, activity expenditure, or body size until looking in a mirror or discovering the need for a larger clothing size.

Adipose tissue present in obesity is of the same composition as fat tissue normally found in smaller amounts in the same areas. It consists of clumps of fat cells (adipocytes) together with supporting tissue, such as blood vessels, lymphatic vessels, and fibrous tissue. Although adipose tissue is high in neutral fat, it also contains water, protein, and a small amount of glycogen. The size of the adipose tissue mass reflects the number of adipocytes and the size of adipocytes, which is determined by the amount of triglyceride found within the cell.

Expansion of the tissue mass occurs as a result of an increase in cell size (hypertrophic obesity) or an increase in cell number (hyperplastic obesity) or both (hypertrophic hyperplastic obesity). Until recently it was believed that fat cells increased in number only until puberty. After puberty, if a person absorbed more energy from food than was expended by metabolic processes or by physical activity, the excess energy was converted into fat and was stored in the existing adipocytes, which increased in size (hypertrophy). The adipocyte can increase 1000-fold in volume. It is now known that when faced with fat storage at any age, the fat cell first increases in size and, when a critical size is achieved, divides to form new fat cells.

The adipose tissue mass in early-onset obesity is distributed universally over the entire body; the adipose tissue mass in adult-onset obesity is centrally distributed. How fat is distributed on the body frame can affect the severity of the health risk. Two commonly used classifications are the android (apple-shaped) pattern and the gynoid (pear-shaped) pattern. A high waist-to-hip ratio, greater than 0.85, classifies one as android. These individuals have an upper body fat pattern that reflects intraabdominal or visceral fat stores. A person with the gynoid pattern has a low waist-to-hip (less than 0.85) ratio. These individuals have greater peripheral (i.e., lower body) distribution of fat, including gluteal and femoral prominence. The android pattern is associated with a higher risk of coronary artery disease, hypertension, and disorders of glucose tolerance and hyperlipidemia.

An understanding of how adipose tissue is formed has considerable impact on methods of weight loss and of reduction of the adipose tissue mass in the adult. Severe dietary restrictions do not decrease the number of fat adipocytes present but do result in a decrease in the size of the cells.

Etiology and Pathophysiology

Many factors have been investigated in an effort to identify the critical elements in the development and maintenance of obesity. Once obesity is present, the number of calories consumed must exceed the energy expended for the condition to continue. However, there is debate about processes leading to obesity.[20] When assessing the obese patient, the nurse should consider several different types of questions, such as the following:

1. What is the psychologic importance of food to the patient?
2. Is the patient's food intake influenced by hunger?
3. Do the taste and appearance of food or other physical factors in the environment stimulate the patient to eat?
4. Is there an emotional problem that stimulates the patient to eat?
5. Are there any stressors influencing the patient's eating patterns?
6. Is there a tendency in the patient's family for members to be overweight?

The nurse must recognize that environmental and genetic factors are important. The children of obese parents tend to be obese. Obesity tends to affect several persons within a family. Evidence of a genetic component is suggested in twin and adoptive children studies.[21] More recently, obesity genes have been identified in rodents. Further research is needed to determine whether similar genes are involved in human obesity.[22,23]

There are a growing number of theories related to etiology of obesity.[24] It is likely that the human obesity genotypes will be complex multigenic systems with networks of gene-gene and gene-environment interactions. The etiology of obesity is complex. The body fat content and, more specifically, an excess of body fat result from an intricate network of additive and interactive causes that may be related to DNA sequence variation but may also be associated with behavior and lifestyle. Obesity is a heterogeneous phenotype, and evidence is growing that each phenotypic entity is modulated by a different set of causal factors. These factors include energy intake, resting metabolic rate, level of habitual physical activity, chemical signals, and nutrient partitioning (tendency to store ingested energy in the form of fat or lean tissue).

Research on the pathophysiology of obesity has focused on multiple factors, including genetics and the role of the hypothalamus and energy balance. The lateral and ventral-medial parts of the hypothalamus control appetite and, as a result, influence eating behavior. It is hypothesized that the hypothalamus has a set point for energy balance, above which energy conservation becomes increasingly less efficient and below which energy conservation becomes increasingly more efficient. This homeostatic mechanism accounts for the fact that most adults keep their weight remarkably constant, despite large swings in energy input and expenditure.

This ability of the body to conserve energy as dieting continues may account for the failure of sustained weight loss to occur even though caloric intake is drastically curtailed. It could also account for why the obese person, no matter what dietary regimen is followed, tends to remain overweight.

A sedentary lifestyle including a nonstrenuous indoor occupation and engagement in few, if any, spirited recreational activities is associated with the development of excess body weight and obesity. Thus an obese person with sedentary habits only adds to an already positive energy balance by not engaging in activities that burn off some excess fatty tissue through energy-consuming exercises.

The emotional component of the tendency to overeat is powerful. People use food for many reasons, including comfort and reward. Some people are triggered by specific foods to continue eating beyond satiety. The social component of eating develops early in life when food is associated with pleasure and fun at such events as birthday parties, Thanksgiving, and religious holidays. All of these factors must be included when considering the etiology of obesity.

Complications

The medical and social problems associated with obesity are numerous. These problems are more common in a patient who exceeds ideal body weight by greater than 20%. The medical problems associated with obesity may be a direct result of too much fat. In addition, medical problems such as hypothyroidism can have an adverse effect on energy balance and result in excess body weight gain. Cardiovascular and respiratory problems are common in the obese person. Many patients experience dyspnea on exertion, orthopnea, paroxysmal nocturnal dyspnea, drowsiness, and somnolence. Obstructive sleep apnea is more prevalent in overweight or obese older men.

In addition, the obese patient is prone to the development of polycythemia secondary to low oxygenation of arterial blood. Polycythemia results in an increased viscosity of the circulating blood and sluggish flow through all vessels and capillaries. As a result, an obese patient may have occluded vessels and clotting abnormalities. Varicose veins, as well as venous leg ulcers, are common partly because of increased back pressure on the venous return from the lower limbs by excess intraabdominal adipose tissue. Heart size increases as body weight increases because the heart must work harder to maintain adequate circulation. Hypertension is the most common cardiovascular problem associated with obesity. The presence of polycythemia creates considerable strain on the heart because of the increased RBC count and plasma volume. Therefore obesity can precipitate hypertrophy of the heart, especially of the left ventricle.

The pickwickian syndrome, which is known as obesity hypoventilation, has long been recognized as a result of morbid obesity. The bellows action of the chest wall is compromised, and there is dysfunction of the central respiratory control center. The movement of the muscles of the chest wall and the diaphragm is reduced because of the weight of the fatty tissue mass. Hypoventilation results in a state of chronic hypercapnia manifested by cyanosis, dyspnea, edema, and somnolence. In addition, most patients have a reduced vital capacity and polycythemia. Blood gas exchange is also directly affected. Although the pickwickian syndrome is rare, caution should always be used when sedatives are used for the morbidly obese person because these drugs can precipitate severe respiratory complications.

Impaired glucose tolerance is common with obesity. The incidence of type 2 diabetes mellitus is high in obese persons. Excessive food intake stimulates hyperinsulinemia. Through a negative-feedback mechanism, excessive insulin levels decrease the number of insulin-receptor sites on the cell membrane. The loss of insulin-receptor sites decreases the amount of glucose that can enter the cells. This promotes high levels of blood glucose. Thus the obese patient is often hyperglycemic and hyperinsulinemic. Weight reduction appears to reverse these effects by increasing insulin receptors and enhancing the movement of glucose into cells.

Gallstone formation in the obese patient is also common. The incidence of gallstones rises as the body weight increases. There is a concomitant rise in the serum cholesterol and triglyceride levels, as well as an increase in body weight. These substances precipitate in the gallbladder, resulting in cholelithiasis and cholecystitis. With weight loss, cholesterol and triglyceride levels often decrease, resulting in decreased risk of gallstone formation. The high levels of cholesterol and triglycerides can also contribute to the development of coronary artery disease (see Chapter 32).

Excessive weight on the weight-bearing joints (hips and knees) and the lower spine can cause pain and discomfort. Although obesity has not been implicated as a cause of degenerative joint disease, it is a predisposing factor. Obesity may contribute to the pathogenesis of osteoarthritis in multiple joints when the disease process has already started.

Other complications associated with obesity are menstrual irregularities, infertility, endometrial cancer, and fatty liver infiltration. Understandably, the life expectancy of an obese person can be shortened as a result of the medical problems.

In addition to the many physical complications associated with obesity, the person may suffer from long-standing emotional and social problems. Society today puts great emphasis on attaining and maintaining a slim and vigorous look. Those who deviate from this prescribed standard often meet with discrimination and disdain. The morbidly obese person may find it difficult to obtain a desired job, social acceptance, or membership in organizations. Choice of clothing is often limited in style, color, size, and quantity. These socioemotional problems may be manifested in poor self-esteem and body image.

Diagnostic Studies

The overwhelming majority of obese persons have primary obesity, that is, excess calorie intake for the body's metabolic demands. Others have secondary obesity, which can result from various congenital anomalies, chromosomal anomalies, metabolic lesions, or CNS lesions and disorders. A first step in the treatment process is to determine whether any such physical conditions are present. A thorough history and physical examination are necessary and will reveal the extent and duration of the obese state.

There is no definite agreement on a technique for determining who is obese. Several methods are currently in use. One widely used method is to compare the patient's weight to a standardized weight-for-height chart and then designate the patient to be overweight by a certain percentage. Table 38-22 provides a standardized weight-for-height chart. Normal weight depends largely on body build. A limitation of this method of assessing obesity can be seen from the following example: A person who inherits a medium frame and develops a bulky muscle mass may be considered 20% overweight according to the standardized chart and yet not be obese.

A more sensitive approach to determine the presence of obesity is the BMI discussed earlier in this chapter. The BMI (see Fig. 38-7) is not dependent on frame size. Because the BMI value rises with age, it has been suggested that age-specific guidelines for older adults be established. A more individualized method of determining the amount of body fat is by measuring skinfold thickness with special calipers at one or more of four body sites: the biceps, the triceps, the subscapular site, or the suprailiac site. Estimates of body fat are then derived as a result of correlations established with body density from anthropometric charts. Although considered a more exact technique, this method also has limitations. The disadvantage of this method of calculating the degree of obesity is that the standards for the skinfold thickness are generally obtained from healthy young men and women, 20 to 30 years of age, and do not consider age-related changes. As a person ages, the percent of total body fat increases, as does the skinfold thickness for the fatty tissue at each site.[25] This measure is not as reliable in an obese individual as in midrange body weights. These measurements should be performed by trained clinicians. The

| Table **38-22** | Desirable Weights for Men and Women* | | |

Height	Frame Size		
	Small	Medium	Large
Men			
5'2"	128-134	131-141	138-150
5'3"	130-136	133-143	140-153
5'4"	132-138	135-145	142-156
5'5"	134-140	137-148	144-160
5'6"	136-142	139-151	146-164
5'7"	138-145	142-154	149-168
5'8"	140-148	145-157	152-172
5'9"	142-151	148-160	155-176
5'10"	144-154	151-163	158-180
5'11"	146-157	154-166	161-184
6'	149-160	157-170	164-188
6'1"	152-164	160-174	168-192
6'2"	155-168	164-178	172-197
6'3"	158-172	167-182	176-202
6'4"	162-176	171-187	181-207
Women			
4'10"	102-111	109-121	118-131
4'11"	103-113	111-123	120-134
5'	104-115	113-126	122-137
5'1"	106-118	115-129	125-140
5'2"	108-121	118-132	128-143
5'3"	111-124	121-135	131-147
5'4"	114-127	124-138	134-151
5'5"	117-130	127-141	137-155
5'6"	120-133	130-144	140-159
5'7"	123-136	133-147	143-163
5'8"	126-139	136-150	146-167
5'9"	129-142	139-153	149-170
5'10"	132-145	142-156	152-173
5'11"	135-148	145-159	155-176
6'	138-151	148-162	158-179

*From 1983 Metropolitan Life Insurance Company weight tables by height and size of frame for people aged 25 to 59, in 1-inch shoes and wearing 5 pounds of indoor clothing for men or 3 pounds for women.

hip-to-waist ratio described earlier is another useful assessment technique.

The least reliable technique and yet perhaps the most frequently used is direct observation of the patient. A subjective assessment of total body fat is made. The ideal body is one that has only a thin layer of adipose tissue covering the skeletal frame. When a roll of excess subcutaneous adipose tissue is seen, the patient is often considered obese.

More sophisticated measures of obesity utilize densitometry, dual photon absorption, magnetic resonance imaging, and ultrasonography. However, such measures are generally used only for research purposes.

The physician explores genetic and endocrine factors in the workup. Etiologic factors such as hypothyroidism, hypothalamic tumors, Cushing's syndrome, hypogonadism in men, or polycystic ovarian disease in women are studied. Laboratory tests of liver function, fasting glucose level, triglyceride level, and low- and high-density lipoprotein cholesterol levels assist in evaluating the cause and effects of obesity.

Collaborative Conservative Care

When no organic cause can be found for obesity, it should be considered a chronic, complex illness. Any supervised plan of care should be directed at (1) successful weight loss, requiring a short-term energy deficit, and (2) successful weight control, requiring long-term behavior changes. These are two different processes. A multipronged approach ought to be used with attention to multiple elements in the fat cycle, such as dietary intake, physical activity, behavioral-cognitive modification, and perhaps drug therapy. Focusing on more than one aspect will likely give better balance to weight-loss and weight-control efforts.

Nutritional Therapy. Restricted food intake is a cornerstone for any weight loss or maintenance program. A good weight loss plan should contain foods from the basic food groups. Diets may be classified as low calorie (800 to 1200 calories per day) or very low calorie (less than 800 calories per day). Persons on low and very low calorie diets need frequent professional monitoring because the severe energy restriction places them at risk for multiple nutrient deficiencies. A diet that includes adequate amounts of fruits and vegetables provides enough bulk to prevent constipation and meets daily vitamin A and vitamin C requirements. Lean meat, fish, and eggs provide sufficient protein, as well as the B-complex vitamins. The caloric intake may need to be restricted to 800 to 1200 calories per day, depending on the patient's age, weight, nutritional status, activity level, and length of time estimated for the ideal weight to be achieved. Table 38-23 contains a sample 1200-calorie reducing diet.

The only effective method of treating primary obesity is to restrict dietary intake so that it is below energy requirements. It is rare to find an overweight person who has not at some time attempted to lose weight. Some have met with limited and temporary success, and others have met only with failure. It is likely that the great majority of these persons attempted weight loss by trying out at least one of the many fad diets that offer the enticement to eat and get slim. Fad diets in general claim weight loss quickly, easily, and inexpensively. Although it is true that initially weight is lost, it is not fat but body water that is lost. The normal fat cell is composed of approximately 80% fat, 18% water, and 2% protein. It is also a storage area for small amounts of glycogen. Glycogen is known to bind with water. When reducing diets severely restrict carbohydrates, the body's glycogen stores become depleted within a few days. It is only when the glycogen-water pool is almost depleted of energy that protein and adipose tissue are burned to release energy for bodily functions.

An obese patient must understand that following a well-balanced, low-calorie diet is an essential part of weight loss. Continuing to follow a well-balanced food plan will have a more satisfying and long-lasting result than fad diets.

The degree of success of any reducing diet depends in part on the amount of weight to be lost. A moderately obese person will obviously attain the goal more easily than will a massively obese person. Men are able to lose weight more quickly than women. Women have a higher percentage of metabolically less active body fat, whereas men have a higher percentage of metabolically more active lean body mass. Adult-onset obesity is often more amenable to successful treatment than the obesity of juvenile onset. In juvenile-onset obesity, the eating patterns

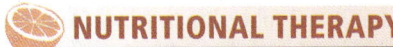

NUTRITIONAL THERAPY

Table 38-23 | 1200-Calorie-Restricted Weight-Reduction Diet*

General Principles
1. Eat regularly. Do not skip meals.
2. Measure foods to determine the correct portion size.
3. Avoid concentrated sweets, such as sugar, candy, honey, pies, cakes, cookies, and regular sodas.
4. Reduce fat intake by baking, broiling, or steaming foods.
5. Maintain a regular exercise program for successful weight loss.

Meal	Exchanges	Meal Plan 1	Meal Plan 2	Meal Plan 3
Breakfast	1 meat	1 scrambled egg	1 hard-boiled egg	1 oz ham
	2 bread	1 slice toast	1 flour tortilla	2 griddle cakes with
		¾ cup dry cereal (unsweetened)	½ cup Cream of Wheat	diet syrup
	1 fruit	½ small banana	⅓ cup orange juice	⅓ cup pineapple juice
	1 fat	1 tsp margarine	1 slice bacon	1 tsp margarine
	1 dairy	1 cup low-fat milk	1 cup low-fat milk	1 cup low-fat milk
	Beverage	Coffee	Coffee	Coffee
Lunch	2 meat	1 slice bologna	Cheese enchiladas (made with 2 oz cheese, 2 corn tortillas, chili sauce)	2 oz baked breaded pork chop
		1 slice cheese		
	2 bread	2 slices bread		1 corn muffin
	Vegetable	Lettuce, pickles	Tomato wedges	Spinach
	1 fruit	Fresh grapes (12)	2 canned peach halves (packed in water)	Fresh orange
	Beverage	Diet soda	Artificially sweetened lemonade	Unsweetened iced tea
Dinner	2 meat	1 oz roast beef	Chili con carne (made with ½ cup ground beef, ½ cup pinto beans, and chili powder)	2 oz baked chicken
	1 bread	Baked potato (with 1 tsp margarine†)		Corn on the cob with 1 tsp margarine
	Vegetable	Cooked carrots	Tossed salad and 1 tbs salad dressing†	Okra
	1 fruit	¾ cup strawberries	Fresh apple	Fruit cocktail (packed in water)
	1 milk	1 cup low-fat milk	1 cup low-fat milk	1 cup low-fat milk

*For 1000 calories, omit 1 fruit exchange and change low-fat milk to skim milk. For 1500 calories, add 1 meat, 1 fruit, and 2 fat exchanges; change low-fat milk to whole milk. For 1800 calories, add 2 bread, 3 meat, 3 fat, and 1 fruit exchanges; change low-fat milk to whole milk.
†One extra fat exchange allowed for each cup of 2% low-fat milk; 2 extra fat exchanges allowed for each cup of skim milk.

have been present longer, and the number of fat cells is often higher. As a result, more drastic dieting efforts and perseverance are necessary to achieve weight reduction.

Motivation is an essential ingredient for achievement of success. The obese patient must see the need for weight loss and weight control and the advantages that will accrue. The nurse can assist by helping the patient track eating patterns by keeping a diet diary. A frank discussion of eating habits helps the patient realize that often eating is the result of bad habits picked up with time and not of hunger. The bad habits must be changed, or weight loss will be only temporary.

Setting a realistic goal, such as losing 1 to 2 pounds per week, must be mutually agreed on at the outset. Trying to lose too much too fast usually results in a sense of frustration and failure for the patient. The nurse can help the patient understand that losing large amounts of weight in a short period of time causes skin and underlying tissue to lose elasticity and tone and become unsightly folds of flabby tissue. Slower weight loss offers better cosmetic results. Inevitably, the patient reaches plateau periods

during which no weight is lost. These plateaus may last from several days to several weeks. It is especially important that the patient realize that these are normal occurrences during weight reduction, so that discouragement, frustration, and giving up of the prescribed dietary plan is prevented. A weekly check of body weight is a good method of monitoring progress. Daily weighing is not recommended because of the frequent fluctuations resulting from retained water (including urine) and elimination of feces. The patient should be instructed to record the weight at the same time each day, wearing the same type of clothing.

There is no firm agreement on the number of meals to be eaten when a person is on a diet. Some nutritionists advocate several small meals per day because the body's metabolic rate is temporarily increased immediately after eating. When several small meals a day are ingested, more calories are used. There seems to be general agreement that consumption of most of the daily caloric intake at a large evening meal results in less weight loss than when the calories are evenly distributed throughout the day.

When a person is first starting on a weight reduction program, food portions should be weighed in order to stay within the dietary guidelines. After a time, weighing may not be necessary because the patient can make more accurate judgments of size and weight. A list of permitted foods serves as a good reference and permits an occasional meal to be eaten at a restaurant. The patient who carefully follows the prescribed diet will not need to take vitamin supplements. Appropriate fluid intake should be encouraged. Alcoholic beverages are usually not permitted on a reducing diet because they increase the caloric intake and are low in nutritional value.

Exercise. Exercise is an essential part of a weight control program. There is no evidence that increased activity promotes an increase in appetite or leads to dietary excess. In fact, exercise frequently has the opposite effect.

The addition of exercise to diet intervention produces more weight loss than does dieting alone. Exercise has a favorable effect on body fat distribution, with a reduction in waist-to-hip ratio with increased exercise.

Exercise is especially important in maintaining weight loss in overweight persons. Overweight men and women who are active and fit have lower rates of morbidity and mortality than overweight persons who are sedentary and unfit. Therefore exercise is of benefit to overweight persons even if it does not make them lean.

Behavior-Cognitive Modification. For successful long-term weight loss management, behavior modification or cognitive therapy should be integrated into the management plan. Useful basic techniques include (1) self-monitoring, (2) stimulus control, and (3) rewards. Self-monitoring can focus on a record that shows what and when foods are eaten, as well as how the person was feeling when the foods were consumed. Stimulus control is aimed at separating events that trigger eating from the act of eating. Rewards may be used as incentive for weight loss. Short- and long-term goals are useful benchmarks for earning rewards. It is important that the reward for a specified weight loss not be associated with food, such as dinner out or a favorite treat. Reward items do not have to have a monetary component. For instance, time for a hot bath or an hour of pleasure reading would be an enjoyable reward for many people. People may participate in group or individual sessions, or both, as they work toward their goals.

Drug Therapy. Medications have been used in the treatment of obesity but only as adjuncts to a good diet and exercise program. Although effective and safe drugs are available for obesity treatment, multiple barriers exist to their proper and effective use. Adverse experiences with "diet drugs" such as amphetamines and fenfluramine have contributed to reluctance by health care providers and many in the public to explore newer pharmacologic agents that could be part of obesity treatment.

Appetite suppressant drugs reduce food intake through noradrenergic (drugs that mimic norepinephrine) or serotonergic mechanisms. Abuse of noradrenergic agents such as amphetamine, methamphetamine, and phenmetrazine has given the entire group of drugs a bad name. These drugs have been replaced by newer drugs, although no perfect drug currently exists. The chemical manipulation of amphetamine has resulted in drugs that have less risk for CNS stimulation and abuse but that have retained the appetite-suppressing effects. Drugs such as benzphetamine (Didrex) and phendimetrazine (Anorex, Obalan) are examples of this type of drug. Adverse effects of these drugs include palpitations, tachycardia, overstimulation, restlessness, dizziness, insomnia, weakness, and fatigue.

In 1998 the FDA approved sibutramine (Meridia) for use in management of obesity, including weight loss and maintenance of weight loss. This agent works by blocking the uptake of norepinephrine, serotonin, and dopamine centrally. These actions ultimately decrease appetite. Its use is recommended in conjunction with reduced calorie intake. Because this drug has been shown to increase blood pressure in some patients, blood pressure must be monitored in patients taking the drug. This drug should not be taken by patients with congestive heart failure, arrhythmias, or coronary artery disease.

In 1997 fenfluramine (Pondimin) and d-fenfluramine (Redux), serotonergic drugs that act as appetite suppressants, were recalled by the FDA after reported cardiac side effects, especially valvular heart disease. They are mentioned to advise patients that their use is dangerous.

Orlistat (Xenical), a new drug that was developed for weight loss and maintenance, works by blocking fat absorption in the intestine. It inhibits the action of pancreatic and gastric lipases. The undigested fat is excreted in the feces.

Because drugs will not cure obesity without substantial changes in food intake and increased physical activity, weight gain will occur when short-term drug therapy is stopped. Supervised long-term drug therapy with safe compounds can contribute to weight management, as well as loss. As with any pharmacologic treatment, there are side effects. Careful evaluation for the presence of other medical conditions can help determine which drugs, if any, would be advisable for a given patient.

The role of the nurse in relation to drug therapy should center around teaching the patient about proper administration and side effects and how the drugs fit into the larger weight loss plan. The modification of dosage without consultation with the physician or the nurse can have detrimental effects. The nurse should reemphasize that the diet and exercise regimens are the cornerstones of permanent weight loss. Medications may be helpful, but they do not help the patient change eating behavior. The purchase of over-the-counter diet aids should be discouraged. Emphasis here should be on the dangers of drug dependence and tolerance.

Even with a comprehensive action plan, there is a high rate of recidivism (weight regain) among all age-groups. For successful management of obesity, it helps if obesity is viewed as a chronic condition that needs day-to-day attention to maintain weight loss.

Collaborative Surgical Care

Many different types of surgical techniques have been described for treating obesity. These techniques can be classified as physical or mechanical (e.g., lipectomy), malabsorptive (e.g., gastric bypass), and regulator (e.g., banding gastroplasty). Though used in the past, jaw wiring and placement of an intragastric balloon are being used less frequently, if at all. Disappointing long-term results, complications from these techniques, and improved effectiveness of other surgical approaches, especially gastric bypasses, have made bypass surgeries the techniques of choice for morbid obesity.

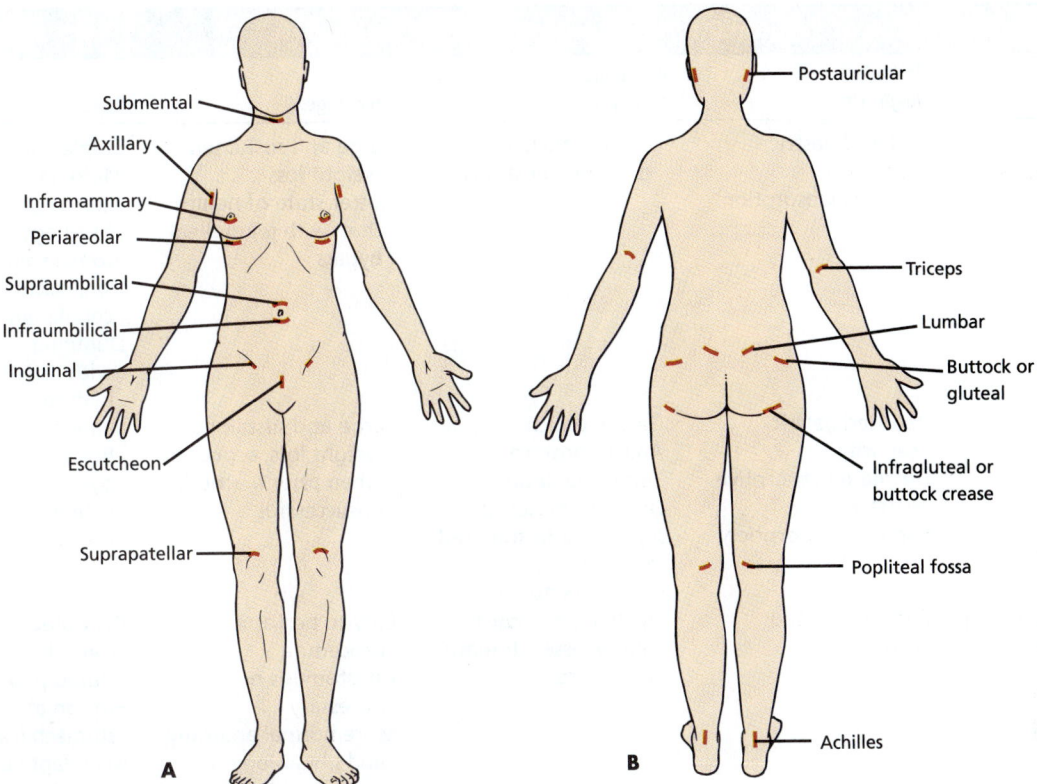

Fig. 38-8   Incision area for suction-assisted lipectomy.

For a patient to be selected for any of the operations for morbid obesity, the following criteria are considered:

1. Gross obesity for 5 years
2. Failure to reduce weight with other forms of therapy
3. Body weight 100% above the ideal for age, gender, and height
4. No serious endocrine problem causing the obesity
5. Absence of other medical conditions (liver disease, alcoholism, cardiovascular or pulmonary disease, inflammatory bowel disease, cancer)
6. Psychiatric and social stability and willingness to cooperate with long-term follow-up
7. Availability of a team of health care providers (nurses, physicians, dieticians) to provide immediate and long-term care
8. Presence of a high-risk condition (degenerative joint disease) that weight loss would ameliorate

Patients older than age 50 are frequently discouraged from seeking surgical treatment because the complications that accompany these procedures are more devastating with age.

Lipectomy. Lipectomy (adipectomy) is performed to remove unsightly flabby folds of adipose tissue. The patient who chooses adipectomies does so for cosmetic reasons. In some patients, up to 15% of the total fat cells are removed from the breasts, abdomen, and lumbar and femoral areas. There is no evidence that a regeneration of adipose tissue occurs at the surgical sites. However, it must be emphasized to the patient that surgical removal does not prevent obesity from recurring, especially if lifetime eating habits remain the same. Al-

though body image and self-esteem may be enhanced by such procedures, these operations are not without complications. The dangerous effects of general anesthesia and the potential for poor wound healing in the obese patient cannot be overemphasized. It is more useful for the majority of patients contemplating adipectomy to be instructed in preventive health measures, such as slow weight reduction to maintain and preserve tissue integrity, the value of exercise, and behavior-modification techniques.

Liposuction. Another surgical procedure is liposuction, or suction-assisted lipectomy. The current use is for cosmetic purposes and not for weight reduction. This surgical intervention helps improve facial appearance or body contours. A candidate for this type of surgery is one who has achieved weight reduction but who has excess fat under the chin, along the jawline, in the nasolabial folds, over the abdomen, or around the waist and upper thighs. The procedure is relatively easy to perform and generally free of major complications; Fig. 38-8 shows incision areas for this procedure. A long, hollow, stainless steel cannula is inserted through a small incision over the fatty tissue to be suctioned. The purpose of this type of surgery is to improve body appearance, thereby enhancing body image and self-concept. It is not usually recommended for the older person because the skin is less elastic and will not accommodate to the new underlying shape.

Gastrointestinal Surgeries. Many different types of GI surgery have been tried for severe obesity and rejected primarily because of complications or because they were not effective. However, three procedures endorsed for clinical use are vertical banded gastroplasty, Roux-en-Y gastric bypass,[26] and

Table **38-24**   Comparison of Surgical Interventions for Morbid Obesity

Procedure	Method of Weight Loss	Anatomic Changes	Advantages	Risks
■ Roux-en-Y gastric bypass*	Reduced gastric capacity Some malabsorption	Gastric pouch and gastrojejunostomy	Large and sustained weight loss Better state of health than with jejunoileal bypass	Staple line dehiscence Marginal ulceration Altered gastric histology Stomal stenosis Iron, calcium, and cobalamin deficiency Dumping syndrome with refined carbo-hydrates
■ Biliopancreatic diversion*	Reduced gastric capacity Decreased absorptive surface Some malabsorption	Gastric pouch Anastomosis to Y intestinal loop Duodenum closed Jejunum anastomosed to ileum cholecystectomy	Large and sustained weight loss, especially when prior methods unsuccessful	Same as above, for Roux-en-Y gastric bypass Protein-calorie malnutrition
■ Vertical banding gastroplasty*	Reduced gastric capacity	Small gastric pouch along lesser stomach curvature	Easy to perform procedure Anastomosis not necessary More normal anatomy and physiology maintained	Disrupted staple line Stomach stenosis Dilated pouch Erosion at band into stomach (rare) Maladaptive eating (calorically dense food intake)

*See Fig. 38-9.

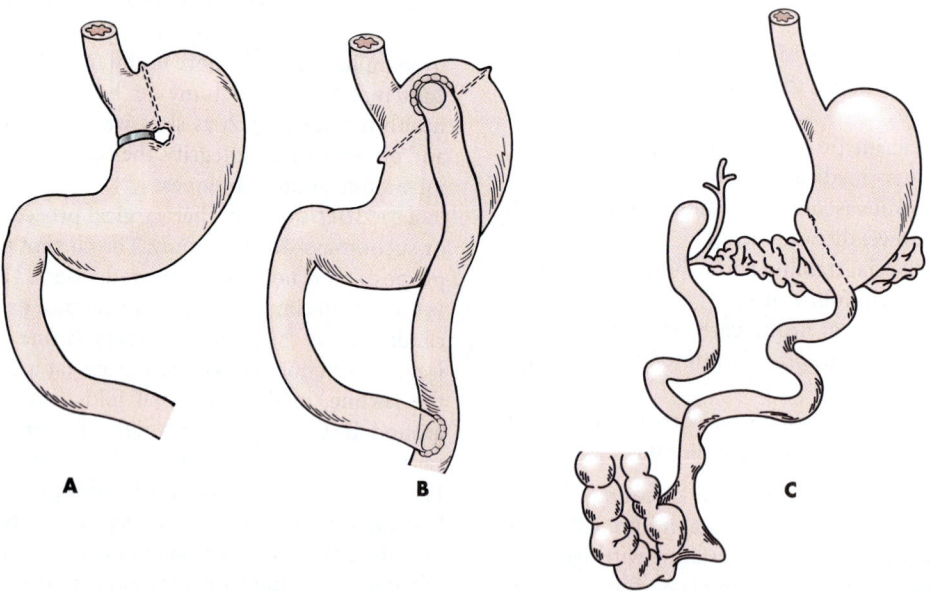

A   **B**   **C**

Fig. 38-9   Three gastrointestinal surgical procedures currently being used in the treatment of morbid obesity. **A,** Vertical banded gastroplasty consists of constructing a small pouch with a restricted outlet along the lesser curvature of the stomach. This outlet may be externally reinforced to prevent disruption or dilation. **B,** Roux-en-Y gastric bypass procedure involves constructing a proximal gastric pouch whose outlet is a Y-shaped limb of small bowel. **C,** Biliopancreatic diversion in addition to a proximal gastric pouch involves removal of gallbladder, closure of duodenum, and anastomosis of jejunum to the ileum.

biliopancreatic diversion[27] (Table 38-24 and Fig. 38-9). For these procedures, weight loss results depend more on the patient's motivation and behavior than on metabolic, GI, or technical factors.[27]

Surgical approaches within the GI tract have been directed toward either limiting food intake or producing malabsorption. An early surgery that led to malabsorption was the jejunoileal bypass.[27] This procedure resulted in excellent weight loss. However, because of frequent serious health-related complications, including electrolyte imbalance, osteoporosis, bypass enteritis, and liver failure, this surgery is no longer performed. Many patients had surgical procedures done to reverse the bypass. Nonetheless, a group of patients may still have a jejunoileal bypass in place.

Gastric bypass. The gastric bypass operation now being performed leads to weight loss by reducing food intake. Some malabsorption results. With the Roux-en-Y surgical procedure, the stomach size is decreased with a gastric pouch anastomosis emptying directly into the jejunum. Variations of this procedure include (1) stapling the stomach without transection to create a small, 30 to 45 ml gastric pouch; (2) creating an upper and a lower gastric pouch and totally disconnecting the pouches; and (3) creating an upper gastric pouch and completely removing the lower pouch. In the first two variations, the surgical changes can be reversed. The greatest rate of weight loss is usually achieved during the first year after surgery. Weight tends to stabilize after 18 months.[27] The chief contraindications to this surgical procedure are a history of peptic ulcer disease, coronary artery disease, malignant lesions, drug dependence, alcohol abuse, or psychiatric problems. A complication of this procedure is dumping syndrome, in which gastric contents empty too rapidly into the small intestine, overwhelming its ability to digest nutrients. This operation is more likely to cause iron or calcium deficiency and cobalamin hypovitaminosis, which can require lifelong supplementation.

Biliopancreatic diversion. Biliopancreatic diversion, introduced in 1968 by Scopinaro, is a more severe operation that may be used if other procedures are not successful.[28] In addition to a partial gastric resection, the gallbladder is removed, and bile and pancreatic juices are diverted into the ileum. With this surgery, there is greater potential for metabolic complications and nutritional deficiencies, including protein malnutrition.[28]

Vertical banded gastroplasty. Vertical banded gastroplasty is not used frequently to induce weight loss in the morbidly obese person. This approach leads to physical restriction of food intake. Previously, horizontal banding procedures were also done. However, lack of long-term weight loss coupled with complications such as disrupted staple lines and dilated pouch and stoma led to discontinuing the use of horizontal banding in the treatment of morbid obesity. In vertical banded gastroplasty, the stomach is partitioned into a small (usually about 30 ml) upper portion along the lesser curvature of the stomach. This small pouch drastically limits capacity. Additionally the stoma opening to the rest of the stomach is banded to delay emptying of solid food from the proximal pouch. This procedure has achieved considerable success in management of weight loss. Problems associated with gastric restriction operations include intractable vomiting from too rapid intake of solids,[29] distention of the wall of the proximal pouch, rupture of the staple line, and erosion of the band into the stomach.

Gastroplasty has some advantages over the gastric bypass operation for acceptable candidates. It is technically easier to perform, especially when stapling is used. If reversal of the procedure is required, removal of the staples is easier than the difficult procedure of converting the gastric bypass. In addition, symptoms of the dumping syndrome and malabsorption are eliminated. However, the weight loss record is often disappointing.[30]

NURSING MANAGEMENT: OBESE PATIENT

■ Nursing Assessment

The nurse, working closely with the physician and dietician, plays a major role in the planning and management of the obese patient. To be effective, the nurse must be aware of perceptions of and beliefs about obesity. If a care provider associates this condition with lack of will power and gluttony, the patient can experience shame in a setting that claims to be a caring one. By being sensitive when asking specific and leading questions, the nurse can often obtain information that the patient may withhold out of embarrassment or shyness or because of being a poor historian. Information that can assist the nurse in understanding an obese patient and provide a basis for intervention is presented in Table 38-25. The nurse must provide acceptable reasons for such personally intrusive questions, respond to the patient's concerns about diagnostic tests, and interpret test outcomes. The patient's answers to questions must be treated with respect, understanding, and a nonjudgmental attitude, regardless of negative personal feelings the nurse may have about obesity and working with "fat" people.

Anthropometric measurements are an integral part of the assessment of an obese person. The nurse may perform these measurements and explain their significance to the patient. Measurements used with the obese person include skinfold thickness, height, weight, and BMI. Accumulation of fat cells in the gluteal-femoral area may be metabolically inert, except during the latter part of pregnancy and during lactation. Android obesity, in which fat is distributed over the abdomen and upper body (neck, arms, and shoulders), is associated with a greater cardiovascular risk of hypertension, type 2 diabetes mellitus, dyslipidemia, ischemic heart disease, stroke, and death. The nurse should emphasize the importance of vigorous treatment of this type of obesity. The patient should be informed that gynecoid obesity carries a better prognosis but may be more difficult to reduce.

As part of the initial nursing physical assessment, each body system should be examined with particular attention to the organ system in which the patient has expressed a problem or concern. Providing specific documentation on these areas assists the physician with a more in-depth history and physical examination.

■ Nursing Diagnoses

Nursing diagnoses for the patient with obesity include, but are not limited to, the following:

- Altered nutrition: more than body requirements *related to* excessive intake in relation to metabolic need and decreased activity
- Impaired physical mobility *related to* excessive body weight

NURSING ASSESSMENT

Table 38-25   Obese Patient

Subjective Data

Important Health Information

Past health history: Time of obesity onset; diseases related to metabolism and obesity such as hypertension, cardiovascular problems, stroke, cancer, chronic joint pain, respiratory problems, diabetes mellitus, cholelithiasis

Medications: Thyroid preparations, diet pills

Surgery or other treatments: Weight reduction procedures

Functional Health Patterns

Health perception–health management: Family history of obesity; perception of problem; methods of weight loss attempted

Nutritional-metabolic: Amount and frequency of eating; overeating in response to boredom, stress, specific times or activities

Elimination: Constipation

Activity-exercise: Typical physical activity; drowsiness, somnolence; dyspnea on exertion, orthopnea, paroxysmal noctural dyspnea

Sleep-rest: Sleep apnea

Cognitive-perceptual: Feelings of rejection, isolation, guilt, or shame; meaning or value of food, compliance with prescribed reducing diets, degree of long-term commitment to a weight-loss program

Role-relationship: Change in financial status or family; personal, social, and financial resources to support a reducing diet

Sexuality-Reproductive: Menstrual irregularity, heavy menstrual flow in women, infertility; effect of obesity on sexual activity

Objective Data

General

Body mass index ≥ 30 kg/m^2; waist-to-hip ratio greater than 0.8 (women) or 1.0 (men), body weight 20% above ideal for height and frame, triceps skinfold greater than 25 (women) or 15 (men)

Respiratory

Hypoventilation

Cardiovascular

Hypertension

Musculoskeletal

Decreased joint mobility

Possible Findings

Elevated serum glucose, cholesterol, triglycerides; polycythemia

---

- Social isolation *related to* alterations in physical appearance and perceived unattractiveness
- Risk for impaired skin integrity *related to* alterations in nutritional state (obesity), immobility, excess moisture, and multiple skinfolds
- Ineffective breathing pattern *related to* decreased lung expansion from obesity
- Noncompliance *related to* alteration in perception or lack of motivation
- Body image disturbance *related to* deviation from usual or expected body size and inability to lose or retain weight loss

■ Planning

The overall goals are that the obese patient will (1) achieve weight loss to a specified level, (2) maintain weight loss at a specified level, (3) modify eating levels, and (4) participate in a regular physical activity program.

■ Nursing Implementation

Health Promotion. In collaboration with nutritionists, the nurse is in a prime position to participate in formal and informal health and nutritional teaching activities. This teaching can span the entire life span, including prenatal instruction. Targeting groups in the work setting is one way health promotion activities can be conducted and reinforced. Group competition within the work environment has been reported to offer moderate success for participants. Intterrelated key factors are group support coupled with competition.

Acute Intervention

Preoperative care. Special considerations are necessary in the care of the patient who is admitted to the hospital for surgical treatment of obesity, especially the morbidly obese. Most nursing units are not prepared to meet the needs of a patient who is often too large for a typical hospital or recovery room bed or who has arms or legs that even a large-size blood pressure cuff will not fit. To eliminate embarrassment for the patient and frustration for the staff, plans for these special needs should be made before the patient's admission. Oversized blood pressure cuffs should be ready for use when the patient arrives. A private room may be necessary for privacy of the patient and to accommodate the bed and sitting arrangements. A strongly reinforced trapeze bar should be placed over the bed to facilitate movement and positioning. In some cases a specially constructed chair may have to be built and beds joined together to allow the patient to sit and sleep in comfort.

A care-planning conference should be a priority so that even simple nursing care measures do not become impossible tasks. Consideration should be given to questions such as how the patient will be weighed, how the patient will be transported throughout the hospital, and how simple physical assessment strategies may have to be adjusted to accommodate the morbidly obese patient. Anticipation of the need to use the hospital's meat or freight scales saves time and energy later for both the staff and the patient. Another need is a wheelchair with removable arms that is large enough to safely accommodate the patient and that will pass easily through doorways. Strategies for bathing, turning, and ambulating the patient, including the number of extra hands needed to carry out these measures, are invaluable when the actual need arises. Special gowns are also needed for the patient. Routine physical assessment strategies do not work well with a morbidly obese female patient who has numerous layers of skinfolds covering the chest and abdomen in addition to huge, pendulous breasts obscuring the area to be assessed. Without identifying alternatives or unique methods of dealing with this problem, assessment of respiratory status and bowel sounds or even wound inspection could be awkward for the nurse and embarrassing for the patient.

Wound infection is one of the most common complications after surgery. Because of the many layers of flabby skinfolds, especially in the abdominal area, preoperative skin preparation is important. Frequently the patient is instructed to take several showers a day for several days before admission to the hospital. Careful cleansing with soap and warm water of the abdominal area from the breasts to below the waist is emphasized.

The patient must be instructed in the proper coughing technique, deep breathing, and methods of turning and positioning to prevent pulmonary complications after surgery. The use of a spirometer may be introduced before surgery. Because most obese patients breathe shallowly, use of the spirometer helps prevent and alleviate postoperative lung congestion. Practicing these strategies preoperatively can aid in performing them correctly postoperatively.

All patients admitted for major bypass surgery, gastroplasty, or partitioning procedures have an NG tube inserted during surgery and attached to low suction after surgery. Allowing the patient to see a typical tube and explaining why it is necessary is a good method of involving the patient in the plan of care. The patient should know that oral nourishment will be impossible for a few days after the surgery and that IV fluids will be the main source of intake. Parenteral nutrition support may be necessary for some patients.

Early ambulation is mandatory for the obese patient. It is essential that the patient know that it is usually necessary to get out of bed soon after surgery and with increasing frequency thereafter, generally three to four times each day. The dangers of thrombophlebitis and measures to counteract its development are a routine part of preoperative teaching. The patient should know that elastic stockings, elastic compression stockings, or elastic wraps will be applied to the legs and that active and passive range-of-motion exercises will be a frequent part of daily care. Low-dose heparin often will be ordered. (General preoperative nursing care is discussed in Chapter 16.)

Postoperative care. The patient experiences considerable abdominal pain after surgery. Administration of pain medications should be given as frequently as necessary during the immediate postoperative period. If pain medication is not given by patient-controlled analgesia (PCA), the nurse must remember that IM medications must be given with an extra-long needle, such as a spinal needle, so that the medication is administered into the muscle and not into the adipose or subcutaneous tissue, which will delay absorption. Because prevention of pulmonary complications is a major nursing goal, it can be anticipated that the patient will not fully cooperate with respiratory strategies. In addition, the large amount of truncal adipose tissue, especially on the abdomen and chest, compromises respiratory ability. Keeping the head of the bed elevated at a 30-degree angle at all times facilitates ventilatory efforts. Encouraging and assisting the patient to turn, cough, and deep breathe at least every 1 to 2 hours minimizes the risk for atelectasis and pneumonia. Frequent mouth and nose care also helps breathing efforts because the NG tube is inserted through one nostril.

Position changes and range-of-motion exercises are instituted immediately after surgery and carried out every 1 to 2 hours. Ambulatory efforts generally are begun on the evening of surgery. For patient safety, the nurse should enlist the assistance of other staff members during these initial efforts, while encouraging the patient to help.

The abdominal wound requires frequent observation for the amount and type of drainage, condition of the sutures, and signs of infection. The incision must be protected against undue straining that accompanies turning and coughing. Wound dehiscence and wound healing are potential problems for all obese patients. Monitoring the vital signs assists in identifying problems such as infection.

It is important that the NG tube be kept patent and in the correct position. Vomiting is common following gastroplasty, gastric bypass, and gastric partitioning procedures. If patency is blocked or the tube requires repositioning, the physician should be notified at once. The upper gastric pouch is small (usually 15 to 40 ml), and irrigating the tube with too much solution or manipulating tube position can lead to disruption of the anastomosis or staple line. In most cases the NG tube can be removed in approximately 48 hours, or when bowel sounds have resumed.

Skin care should be carried out several times each shift. Perspiration may be excessive at times. The many layers of flabby skin should be kept clean and dry so that this source of irritation is eliminated. The patient who has gastric bypass may experience severe diarrhea early in the postoperative period. This is caused by malabsorption created by surgical shortening of the small intestine. Meticulous care should be taken of the skin around the anal area, and antidiarrheal medications should be administered immediately. For the patient who has an indwelling catheter, perineal care is important so that a urinary tract infection can be avoided.

Clear liquids are given orally when tolerance is established. The amount offered at first is necessarily limited to approximately 1 ounce, which is to be sipped slowly. More solid types of food are given to the patient who has had bypass surgery as progress is made through the postoperative recovery period. The patient who has had gastroplasty surgery is kept on a fluid diet for a longer time. The need for a liquid diet only is based on the rationale that the ingestion of too much fluid or foods can cause disruption of the staple or suture line, leading to leakage and possible peritonitis.

Discharge teaching. The patient who has undergone major surgical treatment for obesity has not, in the past, been successful in following or maintaining a prescribed diet. Now the patient is forced to reduce the oral intake as a result of the anatomic changes brought about by the operation. This patient finds that adherence to a reduced intake is necessary because of the concern for abdominal distention, cramping abdominal pain, increased and foul-smelling flatus, and frequent diarrhea.

Weight loss is considerable during the first 6 to 12 months. More weight is lost by those who have bypass surgery than by those who undergo gastric partitioning procedures. It is during this time that the patient must learn to adjust intake sufficiently to maintain a stable weight. Although behavior modification was not an intended outcome when these surgical procedures were devised, it becomes an unexpected secondary gain. The diet generally prescribed should be high in protein and low in carbohydrates, fat, and roughage and consist of six small feedings daily. Fluids should not be ingested with the meal, and in some cases, fluids should be restricted to less than 1000 ml per day. Fluids and foods high in carbohydrate tend to promote diarrhea and symptoms of the dumping syndrome. Generally calorically dense foods (foods high in fat) should be avoided to permit more nutritionally sound food to be consumed.

Vitamin deficiencies are a long-term concern after bypass surgery because of the induced malabsorption and the body's inability to absorb important vitamins such as vitamins A, C, and D. Parenteral cobalamin supplements are usually prescribed on a permanent basis because absorption of this vitamin takes place in the ileum. Ileal absorption capacity is drastically reduced by the surgical intestinal bypass. The patient should be aware of the signs and symptoms of vitamin deficiencies, as well as of electrolyte imbalances (see Table 38-8). It is often necessary to replace iron, calcium, and potassium to maintain required physiologic levels.

Proper diet and use of antidiarrheal medications must be clearly understood by the patient. Late complications can be anticipated after gastric bypass or gastroplasty, including anemia, vitamin deficiencies, diarrhea, and psychiatric problems. Failure to lose weight or loss of too much weight may be caused by the surgical formation of too large a stomach pouch or of an outlet that is much too small, respectively. Peptic ulcer formation, dumping syndrome, and small bowel obstruction may be seen late in the recovery and rehabilitative stage.

Long-term follow-up care must be stressed, in part because of complications late in the recovery period. The patient must be encouraged to adhere strictly to the prescribed diet and to keep the physician informed of any changes in physical or emotional condition. Some patients have been known to overeat when they return home and to gain rather than lose weight.

Reversal of the surgical procedures may be required for some patients. Reversal of the gastric bypass may be difficult because of the technical nature of the procedure. Reasons for revisional surgery include hepatic failure, weight loss below ideal weight, debilitating weakness, severe psychiatric problems, intractable electrolyte deficiencies, pulmonary tuberculosis, and renal failure.

The nurse must anticipate and recognize several potential psychologic problems after surgery. Some patients express guilt feelings concerning the fact that the only way they could lose weight was by surgical means rather than by the "sheer will power" of reduced dietary intake. The nurse should be ready to provide support so that this patient does not dwell on negative feelings.

Many morbidly obese patients who blamed their feelings of social inferiority or inadequacies on their appearance before bypass surgery may suffer from episodes of depression. By 6 to 8 months after surgery, considerable weight loss has occurred, and they are able to see clearly how much their appearance has changed. Massive weight loss often leaves the patient with large quantities of flabby skin that result in problems of both body image and hygiene. Reconstructive surgery at least 1 full year after the initial surgery may alleviate this unsightly situation. Reduction of the breasts, upper arms, thighs, and excess abdominal skinfolds are possible solutions. Discussion of this possible outcome with the patient before surgery and again during the rehabilitation phase of recovery helps facilitate the patient's adjustment to a new body image and social reintegration.

Ambulatory and Home Care

Physical activity teaching. Once a physical activity program has been outlined for the patient, the nurse can reinforce instruction and help individualize it to the patient's time schedule and physical limitations. The nurse should point out that engaging in weekend exercise only or in spurts of strenuous activity is not advantageous and can actually be dangerous. Joining a health club can be one mechanism of getting exercise. However, sitting in a sauna and trying to spot-reduce a specific part of the body do not constitute an appropriate daily physical activity program. Walking, swimming, and cycling are more sensible forms of exercise and have more long-term benefits. The combination of a good reducing diet and an increased physical activity program can have profound effects on the patient's achievement of weight loss. When large muscles are involved in the exercise program, a primary benefit is cardiovascular conditioning.

Many psychologic benefits can be derived from an increased physical activity program. Reduction in tension and stress, better-quality sleep and rest, decreased desire to eat excessively, increased stamina and energy, improved self-concept and self-confidence, better attitudes toward work and play, and increased optimism about the future can be achieved.

Behavior-modification and cognitive training. The person who is on any type of restrictive dietary program is often encouraged to join a group of other obese persons who are receiving professional counseling to help them modify their eating habits. The assumption behind behavior modification is that obesity is a learned disorder caused by overeating, and that the critical difference between an obese person and a nonobese person are the cues that stimulate eating behavior. Therefore most behavior-modification programs deemphasize the diet and focus on how and when the person eats. Participants often are taught to restrict their eating to designated meals and to increase the amount of physical activity in their lives. Persons who have undergone behavior therapy are more successful in maintaining their losses over an extended time than those who do not participate in such training.

Many self-help groups are available to the person who wants to learn more about successful dieting and who likes the support of others having the same problems and experiences. Take Off Pounds Sensibly (TOPS) is the oldest nonprofit organization of this type. Behavioral modification is an integral part of the program, along with nutrition education. Weight Watchers International, Inc., is probably the most successful commercial weight-reduction enterprise. Weight Watchers offers a food plan that is nutritionally balanced and practical to follow, and it has used behavior-modification techniques since 1974. Other self-help groups and organizations are Overeaters Anonymous; Weight Losers; Trim Clubs, Inc.; and the Diet Workshop, Inc. These groups offer diet education, exercise plans, and behavior modification.

There has been a proliferation of commercial weight-reduction centers across the nation. Many of these programs are staffed by nurses or nutritionists, or both, and require an initial physical examination by a physician before a candidate is accepted for weight reduction. These weight-reduction centers are costly and therefore are cost prohibitive for those with limited financial resources. Many of these programs also offer special prepackaged foods and supplements that must be purchased as part of the weight-reduction plan. Only these prescribed foods and drinks are to be consumed until an agreed-on amount of weight is lost. The patient is encouraged to buy the same type of foods for the maintenance phase of the program, lasting from 6 months to 1 year. Behavior-modification training is incorporated within these programs as well. Research has shown that, regardless of the commercial products used, successful weight loss and control were limited and required individualized programs consisting of restricted caloric intake, behavior modification, and exercise.[29] Although persons who follow this type of program are likely to lose weight,

once they leave the program the weight is usually regained because they tend to resume previous eating behaviors and return to the foods previously eaten.

A new concept of influencing health behavior and better employee health has occurred recently. Programs on health teaching and maintenance have been started at places of employment. The rationale for such programs is that better health repays the cost of the programs through improved work performance, decreased absenteeism, and eventually less hospitalization. Weight-reduction and hypertension-reduction programs have been instituted and are popular with employees.

■ **Evaluation**

The expected outcomes are that the obese patient will

- experience long-term weight loss
- have improvement in obesity-related comorbidities
- integrate healthy practices into daily routines
- monitor for adverse side effects of surgical therapy

CRITICAL THINKING EXERCISES

CASE STUDY

Obesity

Patient Profile

Mrs. R. is a 60-year old woman who is 5' 4" tall and weighs 190 pounds.

Subjective Data

- Reports gradual weight gain during past 40 years
- Spends most of her free time watching television
- Reports health problems related to type 2 diabetes mellitus, shortness of breath, hypertension, and chest pressure
- Had knee replacement surgery at age 56

Objective Data

Physical Examination

- Has obese, nontender, soft abdomen
- BP is 150/90

Laboratory Results

- Fasting blood glucose 250 mg/dl (13.9 mmol/L)
- Total cholesterol 205 mg/dl (5.3 mmol/L)
- Triglyceride 298 mg/dl (3.36 mmol/L)
- HDL cholesterol 31 mg/dl (0.8 mmol/L)

Critical Thinking Questions

1. What are Mrs. R.'s obesity risk factors?
2. What is her estimated BMI (use Fig. 38-7)?
3. What are the primary types of body fat distribution? Which type do you think Mrs. R. has, and why?
4. Of the possible complications of obesity, which ones does Mrs. R. have? What is the pathophysiology of Mrs.

R.'s type 2 diabetes mellitus? Of her cardiovascular symptoms? Of her knee replacement surgery?
5. What would you, as the nurse, include in a successful weight loss and weight management program for Mrs. R.?
6. Is Mrs. R. a candidate for surgical intervention for obesity? If so, why? If not, why not?
7. Based on the assessment data presented, write one or more appropriate nursing diagnoses. Are there any collaborative problems?

NURSING RESEARCH ISSUES

1. What impact does rapid gastric emptying of protein have on protein absorption, protein utilization, and subsequent nutritional status?
2. What mechanisms beyond physical activity maintain body weight in obese people when they generally consume fewer carbohydrates than do slender people?
3. How can fat-soluble vitamins be maintained within the RDA when population groups increase their use of fat substitutes in dietary patterns?
4. What happens to serum calcium and bone density in vegetarian patients over time?
5. What is the effect of surgical procedures for obesity on the quality of life or on functional abilities?
6. Does early enteral feeding reduce the risk of sepsis in critically ill patients?
7. Are there valid and reliable bedside methods for determining NG and NI tube placement?
8. What are the ways to reduce the risk of catheter sepsis in a patient receiving TPN?
9. What characteristics (medical condition, antibiotic therapy) are associated with diarrhea in the patient receiving tube feeding?

REVIEW QUESTIONS

The number of the question corresponds to the same-numbered objective at the beginning of the chapter.

1. The nurse identifies a need for dietary teaching for the patient whose daily intake of food groups consists of
   a. 2 to 4 servings of the fruit group.
   b. 2 to 3 servings of the milk, yogurt, and cheese group.
   c. 4 to 5 servings of the bread, cereal, rice, and pasta group.
   d. 2 to 3 servings of the meat, poultry, fish, beans, egg, and nut group.

2. In general, nutrient or food interactions with medications can result in all of the following except
   a. enhancing drug absorption.
   b. retarding drug bioavailability.
   c. increasing a nutrient requirement.
   d. all of the above can happen.

3. During the first 24 hours of starvation the order in which the body obtains substrate for energy is
   a. glycogen, skeletal protein.
   b. visceral protein, fat stores, glycogen.
   c. fat stores, skeletal protein, visceral protein.
   d. liver protein, muscle protein, visceral protein.

4. The nurse recognizes that the major goal of treatment for a patient with anorexia nervosa is being met when the patient
   a. demonstrates a rapid weight gain.
   b. consumes the required daily intake of nutrients.
   c. commits to long-term individual and family counseling.
   d. verbalizes feelings regarding self-image and fears of becoming obese.

5. A nutritionally stressed patient weighing 60 kg is receiving nothing by mouth (NPO) and total parenteral nutrition (TPN). In evaluating the patient's nutritional intake the nurse calculates that the daily TPN solution should provide
   a. 40 g fat.
   b. 80 g protein.
   c. 20 calories per kilogram.
   d. 1000 calories from carbohydrate.

6. One advantage of a percutaneous endoscopic gastrostomy tube placement relative to nasogastric feedings for the patient receiving long-term enteral nutrition is that
   a. it increases patient comfort.
   b. it eliminates the risk of aspiration.
   c. feedings can be initiated before bowel sounds are present.
   d. more calories can be delivered as compared with nasogastric feeding.

7. The obesity aspect that is most often associated with cardiovascular health problems is
   a. primary obesity.
   b. secondary obesity.
   c. gynoid fat distribution.
   d. android fat distribution.

8. A morbidly obese patient has undergone Roux-en-Y gastric bypass surgery. In planning postoperative care the nurse anticipates that the patient
   a. may have severe diarrhea early in the postoperative period.
   b. will not be allowed to ambulate for 5 to 7 days postoperatively.
   c. will require nasogastric suction until healing of the site occurs.
   d. may have only liquids orally, and in very limited amounts, during the postoperative period.

References

1. VanItallie TB: Prevalence of obesity, *Endocrinol Metab Clin North Am* 25:887, 1996.
2. Townsend CD: *Nutrition and diet therapy*, Albany, NY, 1994, Delmar.
3. Food and Nutrition Board, National Research Council, National Academy of Sciences: *Recommended dietary allowances*, ed 10, Washington DC, 1989, National Academy Press.
4. Barrett S: Nutrition quackery, *Sci Med* 4:6, 1997.
5. Garfinkel P, Kennedy S, Kaplan A: Views on classification and diagnosis of eating disorders, *Can J Psychiatry* 40:445, 1995.
6. Gard M, Freeman C: The dismantling of a myth: a review of eating disorders, *Int J Eat Disord* 20:1, 1996.
7. Rock C, Curran-Celentano J: Nutritional management of eating disorders, *Psychiatr Clin North Am* 19:701, 1996.
8. Morreale SJ, Schwartz NE: Helping Americans eat right: developing practical and actionable public nutrition education messages based on the ADA survey of American dietary habits, *J Am Diet Assoc* 95:305,1995.
9. *Surgeon General's report on nutrition and health*, Rocklin, Calif, 1989, Prima Publishing and Communications.
10. McWhirter JP, Pennington CR: Incidence and recognition of malnutrition in hospital patients, *BMJ* 308:945, 1994.
11. Forloines-Lynn S: How to smooth the way for cyclic tube feedings, *Nursing* 50:57, 1996.
12. Caring for a gastrostomy: guidelines and troubleshooting tips, *Nursing* 24:48, 1994.
13. ASPEN Board of Directors: Guidelines for the use of parenteral and enteral nutrition in adult and pediatric patients, *JPEN J Parenter Enteral Nutr* 17:21SA, 1993.
14. Shuster MH: Parenteral nutrition. In Hennessey KA, Orr ME, editors: *Nutrition support nursing core curriculum*, ed 3, Silver Spring, Md, 1996, ASPEN.
15. Bradford S: Method of nutritional support. In Mahan LK, Escott-Stump S, editors: *Krause's food, nutrition, and diet*, ed 9, Philadelphia, 1996, Saunders.
16. Dwyer J: Policy and healthy weight, *Prev Med* 25:30, 1996.
17. Update: prevalence of overweight among children, adolescents, and adults—United States, 1988-1994, *MMWR Morb Mortal Wkly Rep* 46:199, 1997.
18. Bray G: Obesity: part 1—pathogenesis, *West J Med* 149:431, 1988.
19. Dwyer J: Medical evaluation and class of obesity. In Blackburn GL, Kanders BS, editors: *Obesity pathophysiology, psychology and treatment*, New York, 1994, Chapman & Hall.
20. Trayburn P: Socratic debate: obesity is predominantly a problem of food intake—the case against. In Angel A and others, editors: *Progress in obesity research*, London, 1996, John Libbey.
21. Allison DB and others: A genetic analysis of relative weight among 4020 twin pairs with an emphasis on sex effects, *Health Psychol* 13:362, 1994.
22. Roberts S, Greenberg A: The new obesity genes, *Nutr Rev* 54:41, 1996.
23. Weigle DS, Kuijoer J: Obesity genes and the regulation of body fat content, *Bioessays* 18:867, 1996.
24. Angel A and others, editors: *Progress in obesity research*, London, 1996, John Libbey.
25. Heshka S, Buhl K, Heymsfield SB: Obesity: clinical evaluation of body composition and energy expenditure. In Blackburn GL, Kanders BS, editors: *Obesity pathophysiology, psychology, and treatment*, New York, 1994, Chapman & Hall.
26. NIH, NHLBI: *Clinical guidelines on the identification of overweight and obesity in adults: the evidence report*, 1998, NIH, Bethesda, MD.
27. Benotti PN, Forse RA: The role of gastric surgery in the multidisciplinary management of severe obesity, *Am J Surg* 169:361, 1995.
28. Scopinaro N and others: Biolipopancreatic diversion for obesity at 18 years, *Surgery* 119:261, 1996.
29. Kolanowski J: Surgical treatment for morbid obesity, *Br Med Bull* 53:433, 1997.
30. Brolin RE: Update: NIH consensus conference. Gastrointestinal surgery for severe obesity, *Nutrition* 12:403, 1996.

Resources

American Society for Parenteral and Enteral Nutrition
8630 Fenton Street, Suite 412
Silver Spring, MD 20910
301-587-6215
http://www.clinnutr.org/

American Association of Family and Consumer Sciences
1555 King Street
Alexandria, VA 22314
703-706-4600
fax: 703-706-4663
http://www.aafcs.org

American Dietetic Association—Government Affairs
The American Dietetic Association
216 W. Jackson Blvd.
Chicago, IL 60606-6995
312-899-0040
fax: 312-899-1979
http://www.eatright.org

American Society for Clinical Nutrition/American Society for
  Nutritional Sciences and *The American Journal of Clinical Nutrition*
9650 Rockville Pike
Bethesda, MD 20814-3998
301-530-7110
fax: 301-571-1863
http://www.faseb.org/ascn/

Food and Nutrition Information Center
Agricultural Research Service, USDA
National Agricultural Library, Room 304
10301 Baltimore Avenue
Beltsville, MD 20705-2351
301-504-5719
fax: 301-504-6409
http://www.nal.usda.gov/fnic

FDA Center for Food Safety and Applied Nutrition
200 C Street SW
Washington, DC 20204
http://vm.cfsan.fda.gov/index.html

Nutrition Links—Kansas State University
http://www.oznet.ksu.edu/ext_f&n/nutlink/n2.htm

For additional Internet resources, see the website for this book at
www.mosby.com/MERLIN/medsurg_lewis

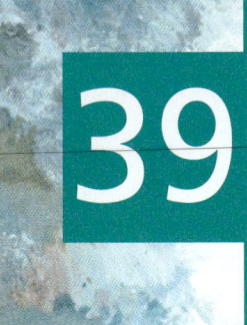
NURSING MANAGEMENT

39 Upper Gastrointestinal Problems

Margaret M. Heitkemper

www.mosby.com/MERLIN/medsurg_lewis

LEARNING OBJECTIVES

1. Describe the etiology, prevention, and treatment of common dental problems.
2. Describe the etiology, clinical manifestations, and treatment of common oral inflammations and infections.
3. Describe the etiology, clinical manifestations, complications, collaborative care, and nursing management of carcinoma of the oral cavity.
4. Describe the nursing management after surgical stabilization of a mandibular fracture.
5. Explain the types, pathophysiology, clinical manifestations, complications, and collaborative care, including surgical therapy, of gastroesophageal reflux disease and hiatal hernia.
6. Describe the nursing management of the patient with gastroesophageal reflux disease and hiatal hernia.
7. Explain the pathophysiology, clinical manifestations, complications, collaborative care, and nursing management of cancer of the esophagus.
8. Describe the clinical manifestations, complications, and management of esophageal diverticula, achalasia, esophageal strictures, and esophagitis.
9. Describe the pathogenesis, complications, collaborative care, and nursing management of nausea and vomiting.
10. Differentiate between acute and chronic gastritis, including the causes, pathophysiology, collaborative care, and nursing management.
11. Explain the common causes, clinical manifestations, collaborative care, and nursing management of upper gastrointestinal bleeding.
12. Compare and contrast gastric and duodenal ulcers, including pathogenesis, clinical manifestations, complications, and collaborative and nursing management.
13. Explain the anatomic and physiologic changes and the common complications that result from surgical procedures for gastric and duodenal ulcers.
14. Describe the clinical manifestations and collaborative, surgical, and nursing management of cancer of the stomach.
15. Identify the common types of food poisoning and the nursing responsibilities related to food poisoning.

Ingestion is the process of taking food and fluids into the body via the gastrointestinal (GI) tract. It begins in the mouth with mastication of food by the teeth. Food then passes down the esophagus and into the stomach. It is important that sufficient nutrients be ingested to meet bodily needs. Oral problems, such as poor dental health, infections and inflammations, and cancer, interfere with ingestion. Esophageal problems may also interfere with swallowing food and fluids and with passage of food to the stomach.

Digestion is the breakdown of foodstuffs to smaller components so that absorption of nutrients can occur. Problems with the stomach and, to a greater extent, the small intestine can profoundly impact the nutritional status of the patient. The older individual is particularly vulnerable to problems related to alterations in both ingestion and digestion.

Reviewed by Diane Britt, RN, MN, CS, CDE, Medical-Surgical Clinical Nurse Specialist, University of Washington Medical Center, Seattle, Wash.

DENTAL PROBLEMS

Dental Caries

Dental caries (decay of teeth) is a general term applied to the decalcification of the mineral components and dissolution of the organic matrix of the teeth. Cavity formation is the clinical evidence of the progression of this process. Although there has been a marked decline in dental caries in recent years, it remains a problem that affects millions of individuals, particularly those from lower socioeconomic groups.[1]

Caries development starts when *plaque* builds up and adheres to the teeth. Plaque is a gelatinous substance consisting of bacteria, saliva, and epithelial cells. The tight adherence of plaque to the teeth provides protection for the bacteria (usually *lactobacilli* and *Streptococcus mutans*). Within 30 minutes after eating, these bacteria produce acids from the breakdown of sugars in food deposits on the teeth. The acids destroy the outer enamel and, later, the underlying dentin of the tooth (Fig. 39-1). The decay proceeds and can progress to the pulp of the tooth.

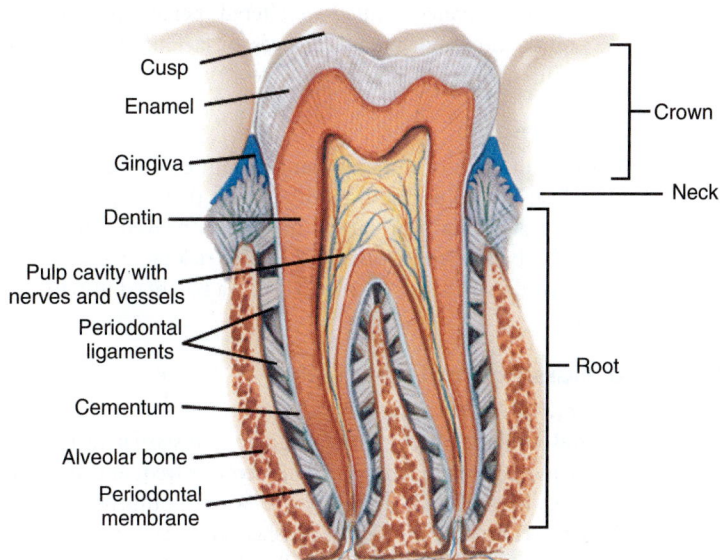

Fig. 39-1   Normal tooth structure.

If the decay is not treated, a *pulpitis* develops and extends to the alveolar bone, forming an abscess. This results in pain, facial edema, and sometimes malaise and fever. During the early stages of pulpitis, pain may be induced by temperature changes, especially cold drinks. In the later stages of pulpitis, heat or reclining may stimulate the onset of severe pain. At this stage, damage to the pulp is irreversible. Treatment consists of tooth removal or root canal therapy (removal of the pulp and filling of the pulp canal with inert material).

Periodontal Disease

The *periodontium* is the tissue surrounding and supporting the teeth. It is composed of the gingivae (gums), cementum, alveolar bone, and the periodontal ligament, which helps to fix the tooth firmly in its bony socket. Periodontal disease is the major cause of tooth loss in adults. The majority of adults have some form of periodontal disease.[1] Periodontal disease begins with gingivitis and eventually involves the periodontal ligament and the alveolar bone. Periodontal disease is the clinical result of a complex interplay between bacterial infection and host response often modified by bacterial factors.[2]

Dental plaque is the most important etiologic factor in periodontal disease. When plaque calcifies, it forms *calculus,* which is a hard, tenacious mass on the crowns of teeth. *Malocclusion* (faulty relationships between the teeth when the jaws are closed), margins of overextended fillings, and impacted food are other etiologic factors that can cause local irritation to the gingivae. Systemic conditions such as poorly controlled diabetes mellitus, thyroid diseases, pregnancy, HIV infection, and vitamin and nutritional deficiencies may modify the person's response to the local etiologic factors and make them more susceptible to periodontal disease. The exact role of systemic conditions is unknown.

Certain drugs cause changes, such as inflammation and hyperplasia of the gingiva, which may be related to periodontal disease. A common drug known to produce these effects is phenytoin (Dilantin). Smoking is a known risk factor for periodontal disease.[2]

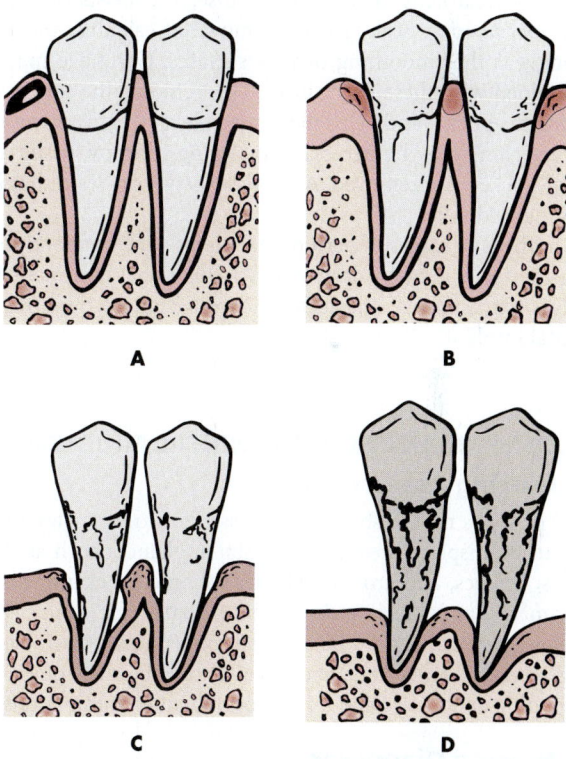

Fig. 39-2   Progression of periodontal disease. **A,** Calculus deposits on teeth at gingival line, causing gingivitis. **B,** Gingivae become swollen and tender with spread of inflammation. **C,** Inflammation spreads and pockets develop between teeth and gingivae, which are receding. **D,** The alveolar bone is destroyed and teeth become loose.

When the gingivae are irritated, they become inflamed (Fig. 39-2). The inflammation causes the gingiva to separate from the surface of the tooth. Pockets created between the teeth and the gingivae can collect pus and bacteria (periodontitis). At this stage, bleeding occurs easily, and pus may ooze from the gingiva. Gradually the bone supporting the teeth is destroyed, and

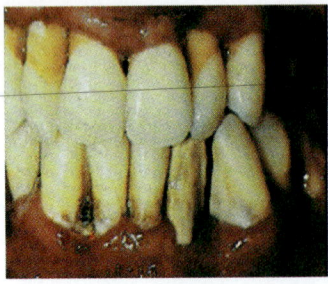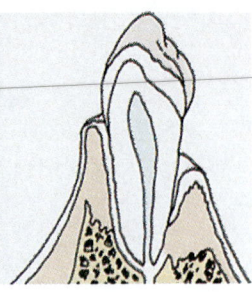

Fig. 39-3 Periodontitis. Signs include edema, periodontal abscess, hemorrhage on slight pressure, tissue recession with retraction of gingival margin, color change from light pink to deep red, loss of tissue in interdental area, horizontal bone loss, and widening of periodontal space.

the teeth become loose. As the periodontal pockets deepen and seal themselves off, periodontal abscesses may occur (Fig. 39-3). At this stage the usual treatment is extraction of the involved tooth or teeth.

Early treatment of periodontal disease consists of *scaling* and *root planing*. Scaling is the removal of calculus, and root planing is the smoothing of root surfaces. Curettage may be combined with these procedures. This removes the soft tissue lining the pocket and helps the gums to heal. *Gingivectomy* and *gingivoplasty* may be necessary. In a gingivectomy, tissue and deep pockets are removed. A gingivoplasty involves reshaping of gingival tissue.

In the later stages of periodontal disease, the bone supporting the teeth is often destroyed. At this stage, treatment involves extraction of the teeth and provision of dentures or dental implants.

NURSING MANAGEMENT: DENTAL PROBLEMS
■ Nursing Assessment

The patient's mouth should be assessed for tooth caries, missing teeth, displaced teeth, and dental appliances such as dentures, bridges, and crowns. The face should be examined for symmetry, and the jaw should be palpated for lumps. The gingivae (gums) should be assessed for redness, pallor, bleeding, recession, and ulcers. The patient should be asked questions regarding dental care and frequency of dental examinations.

■ Nursing Diagnoses

Nursing diagnoses for the patient with dental problems include, but are not limited to, the following:

- Altered oral mucous membrane *related to* caries, ineffective oral hygiene, periodontal disease, or ill-fitting dentures
- Altered nutrition: less than body requirements *related to* inability to ingest adequate nutrients because of ill-fitting dentures, displaced teeth, gingival disease, dental caries, sensitive teeth, edentulous condition, or oral pain
- Body image disturbance *related to* change in appearance of or unattractive teeth, difficulty with eating, or halitosis

- Noncompliance *related to* altered perception, lack of motivation, inadequate finances, or lack of knowledge of consequences of noncompliance

■ Planning

The overall goals of nursing management of the patient with dental caries and periodontal disease are that the patient will (1) have a decrease in caries through improved dental hygiene, (2) be able to identify and reduce risk factors for caries and periodontal diseases, and (3) have a balanced nutritional intake.

■ Nursing Implementation
Health Promotion

Oral hygiene. Proper oral hygiene is essential to prevent caries and periodontal disease. This involves frequent complete cleaning of the teeth and gingivae with toothbrushing and flossing. The teeth should be brushed after each meal with a soft, rounded-bristle toothbrush. Brushing the teeth should remove food debris and plaque and stimulate the gingivae. The teeth should be brushed by first placing the bristles of the toothbrush next to the gum line and then brushing with a motion away from the gum line.

Flossing should be done at least once a day. It is an important measure to remove plaque between teeth, an area that is not easily accessible when brushing. Flossing is done by gently forcing the floss between the teeth and moving the floss up and down the tooth surface a few times until it reaches the gum line.

During illness the patient may not salivate as usual, thereby reducing the natural cleaning process of the teeth and mouth. The nurse may need to assume responsibility for dental care and oral hygiene. Swabbing the patient's mouth and rinsing it with mouthwash are inadequate measures. Mechanical cleansing is essential to remove the plaque. Either a regular or an electric toothbrush should be used on all surfaces to remove plaque and mechanically stimulate the gingivae to increase blood supply. The patient's mouth should be assessed each time oral care is given.

Dental examinations. Regular, periodic dental examinations are important to maintain a healthy mouth and teeth. At the time of a dental examination a thorough cleaning with removal of plaque and calculus is done. Caries and early signs of periodontal disease can be detected and treated. The mouth is examined for any signs of oral cancer. For most adults, an examination every 6 to 12 months is adequate. Some persons may require more frequent visits. Persons at risk for infective endocarditis (e.g., those with prolapsed mitral valve) require prophylactic antibiotics for dental procedures such as teeth cleaning that may provoke bleeding (see Chapter 35).

Nutrition. Caries develop with increasing frequency in persons who ingest diets high in refined carbohydrates. In addition, the cariogenicity (caries promotion) of diet is also related to the frequency of carbohydrate ingestion and eating patterns.[3] A prevention program should, therefore, include reduction in sugar intake. If sugars are eaten, the teeth should be brushed within 30 minutes of eating. Another aspect of diet therapy that seems to reduce plaque formation is increased vitamin C intake. There has been increasing interest in the development of sugar substitutes that are noncariogenic.

Fluoride. Fluoridation makes tooth enamel more resistant to the acids produced from the action of bacteria on sugars in the mouth. In drinking water, one part fluoride per million parts water results in a significant decrease in the decay rate.[1] Many communities consider the fluoridation of drinking water a municipal responsibility and have enacted the necessary legislation. Currently 56% of the U.S. population lives in fluoridated communities.[4] A fluoride solution can be applied topically on the teeth during a dental office visit. In addition, many toothpastes have fluoride added to them, and the American Dental Association recommends them. Fluoride rinses and tablets are also available for at-home use.

Sealants. In addition to fluoride, sealants can be applied to the pits and fissures of teeth in children following the eruption of the teeth or in young adults to reduce caries. Sealant is a coating material that is applied directly to teeth surfaces in the dentist's office. Sealants reduce the attachment of plaque and have been found to be effective in reducing caries.[5]

New techniques. Some chemical methods to inhibit plaque formation and accumulation offer promise. Antimicrobial agents such as chlorhexidine have been used in mouthwashes and varnishes to reduce the *S. mutans* bacterial count in high-risk individuals.[6,7]

Acute Intervention. The nurse may need to refer the patient for intervention and care of an acute dental problem. Local manifestations of dental problems include pain that is intermittent and caused by sensitivity to heat or cold stimulation, dull and continuous pain, facial swelling, halitosis, and bleeding or drainage of pus from the mouth. Systemic manifestations include fever, nausea, vomiting, and malaise.

If pulpitis and abscess develop, immediate dental care is needed to prevent further spread of infection to the bone. An opening may be drilled into the pulp chamber, or the gingivae may be incised to provide drainage for the abscess. Sometimes a root canal procedure or extraction of a tooth is necessary. After treatment of an abscess, the patient can use warm saline rinses. Analgesics may also be required to alleviate the pain.

A damaged or defective tooth or a tooth that has a severe abscess may need to be extracted. After the extraction, the patient should apply cold compresses (e.g., ice bag, cold washcloth) to the side of the face to reduce swelling and relieve discomfort. Some oozing of blood is expected the first 1 to 2 days. If there is loss of large amounts of bright-red blood, direct pressure should be applied to the bleeding site by the patient biting on a gauze pad, and the dentist should be notified. During the first 24 hours the patient should not suck (e.g., smoke or use a straw) because this increases the risk of clot disruption.

Ambulatory and Home Care. Day surgery is used for the extraction of several teeth, such as when impacted molars are excised or when dentures are required. Postoperatively the patient will experience pain and soreness. Ice packs and analgesics are used to relieve the discomfort. Nutrients should be liquid or semisoft for a few days. The dentist or oral surgeon may order mouthwashes for cleansing and relief of soreness.

Dentures. There are approximately 17 million Americans who are edentulous and 10 million of these are more than 65 years of age.[1] The decision to obtain dentures is not easy for most people. They are concerned about changes in cosmetic appearance and the ability to chew food. They must be assured that dentures usually decrease the spread of infection, improve nutritional intake, and improve appearance, especially if they have had multiple dental problems preceding the decision to obtain dentures.

Patience must be stressed in the adjustment phase to dentures. It takes time to get used to a different feel and way of chewing. The gingivae should be checked for proper fit and for any signs of gingival irritation. Dentures should be cleaned at least twice a day with salt and sodium bicarbonate or a dentifrice. When the dentures are removed, the patient should massage the gums for a few minutes. Some patients prefer to wear their dentures at all times, and there are generally no contraindications to this. In fact, facial contour is better maintained by this practice. If dentures are removed at night, they should be covered with water (especially if they are made of vulcanite) and stored in a safe place.

The patient who wears dentures should be encouraged to obtain regular dental care. Dentures will need to be modified because tissue changes occur from aging, weight changes, or disease processes. Poorly fitting dentures can cause pain and oral ulceration leading to poor nutrition.

Dental implants are being used in some patients who require tooth extractions. An implant involves insertion of a titanium post into the bone. The bone fuses with the post and then techniques of restorative dentistry are used to create a crown that is attached to the post. An advantage of dental implants is that the patient experiences less mandibular bone loss compared with dentures.[8]

■ Evaluation

The expected outcomes for the patient with dental problems are that the patient will

- have a decrease in incidence of active disease
- comply with dental hygiene measures including regular dental examinations
- have balanced nutritional intake

Table 39-1	Infections and Inflammations of the Mouth		
Condition	**Etiology**	**Clinical Manifestations**	**Treatment**
▪ Gingivitis	Neglected oral hygiene, malocclusion, missing or irregular teeth, faulty dentistry, eating of soft rather than fibrous foods	Inflamed gingivae and interdental papillae; bleeding during toothbrushing; development of pus, formation of abscess with loosening of teeth (periodontitis)	Prevention through health teaching, dental care, gingival massage, professional cleaning of teeth, fibrous foods, conscientious brushing habits with flossing
▪ Vincent's infection (acute necrotizing ulcerative gingivitis, trench mouth)	Fusiform bacteria; Vincent spirochetes; predisposing factors of stress, excessive fatigue, poor oral hygiene, nutritional deficiencies (B and C vitamins)	Painful, bleeding gingivae; eroding necrotic lesions of interdental papillae; ulcerations that bleed; increased saliva with metallic taste; fetid mouth odor; anorexia, fever, and general malaise	Rest (physical and mental); avoidance of smoking and alcoholic beverages; soft, nutritious diet; correct oral hygiene habits; topical applications of antibiotics; mouth irrigations with hydrogen peroxide and saline solutions
▪ Oral candidiasis (moniliasis or thrush)	*Candida albicans* (a yeastlike fungus), debilitation, prolonged high-dose antibiotic or corticosteroid therapy	Pearly, bluish white "milk-curd" membranous lesions on mucosa of mouth and larynx; sore mouth; yeasty halitosis	Nystatin or amphotericin B as oral suspension or buccal tablets, good oral hygiene
▪ Herpes simplex (cold sore, fever blister)	Herpes simplex virus, type I or II; predisposing factors of upper respiratory infections, excessive exposure to sunlight, food allergies, emotional tension, onset of menstruation	Lip lesions, mouth lesions, vesicle formation (single or clustered), shallow, painful ulcers	Spirits of camphor, corticosteroid cream, mild antiseptic mouthwash, viscous lidocaine; removal or control of predisposing factors, antiviral agents (e.g., acyclovir [Zovirax])
▪ Aphthous stomatitis (canker sore)	Recurrent and chronic form of infection secondary to systemic disease, trauma, stress, or unknown causes	Ulcers of mouth and lips, causing extreme pain; ulcers surrounded by erythematous base	Corticosteroids (topical or systemic), tetracycline oral suspension
▪ Parotitis (inflammation of parotid gland, surgical mumps)	Usually *Staphylococcus* species, *Streptococcus* species occasionally, debilitation and dehydration with poor oral hygiene, NPO status for an extended time	Pain in area of gland and ear, absence of salivation, purulent exudate from duct of gland	Antibiotics, mouthwashes, warm compresses; preventive measures such as chewing gum, sucking on hard candy (lemon drops), adequate fluid intake
▪ Stomatitis (inflammation of mouth)	Trauma; pathogens; irritants (tobacco, alcohol); renal, liver, and hematologic diseases; side effect of many cancer chemotherapy drugs	Excessive salivation, halitosis, sore mouth	Removal or treatment of cause, oral hygiene with soothing solutions, topical medications; soft, bland diet

ORAL INFLAMMATIONS AND INFECTIONS

Oral infections and inflammations may be specific mouth diseases, or they may occur in the presence of some systemic diseases such as leukemia or vitamin deficiency. When oral inflammations and infections are present, they can severely impair the ingestion of food and fluids. Common inflammations and infections of the oral cavity are presented in Table 39-1. The patient who is immunosuppressed (patient with acquired immunodeficiency syndrome or receiving chemotherapy) is most susceptible to oral infections.

CARCINOMA OF THE ORAL CAVITY

Carcinoma of the oral cavity may occur on the lips or anywhere within the mouth (e.g., tongue, floor of the mouth, buccal mucosa, hard palate, soft palate, pharyngeal walls, and tonsils). Oropharyngeal cancer is diagnosed in 30,300 Americans annually, and it is estimated that 8000 persons a year die from the disease.[9] It is more common after 40 years of age, with 60 years being the average age at onset. Carcinoma of the oral cavity occurs in all ethnic groups. It is more common in men (male-to-female ratio of 2:1). Squamous cell carcinoma is the most common oral malignant tumor (more than 90%). The 5-year survival for all stages of cancer of the oral cavity and pharynx combined is 53% and the 10-year rate is 43%.[9]

Most of the malignant lesions occur on the lower lip in men. Other common sites are the lateral border and undersurface of the tongue, the labial commissure, and the buccal mucosa. Carcinoma of the lip has the most favorable prognosis of any of the oral tumors. This is probably because lip lesions are more ap-

Table 39-2	Oral Tumors		
Location	**Predisposing Factors**	**Clinical Manifestations**	**Treatment**
■ Lip	Constant overexposure to sun, ruddy and fair complexion, recurrent herpetic lesions, irritation from pipe stem, syphilis, immunosuppression	Indurated, painless ulcer	Surgical excision, radiation
■ Tongue	Tobacco, alcohol, chronic irritation, syphilis	Ulcer or area of thickening; soreness or pain; increased salivation, slurred speech, dsyphagia, toothache, earache (later signs)	Surgery (hemiglossectomy or glossectomy), radiation
■ Oral cavity	Poor oral hygiene, tobacco usage (pipe and cigar smoking, snuff, chewing tobacco), chronic alcohol intake, chronic irritation (jagged tooth, ill-fitting prosthesis, chemical or mechanical irritants)	Leukoplakia; erythroplakia; ulcerations; sore spot; rough area; pain, dysphagia, difficulty in chewing and speaking (later signs)	Surgery (mandibulectomy, radical neck dissection, resections of buccal mucosa), internal and external radiation

parent to the patient than other oral lesions and are usually diagnosed earlier.

Etiology and Pathophysiology

Although the cause of carcinoma of the oral cavity is not definitive, there are a number of predisposing factors (Table 39-2). Constant overexposure to ultraviolet radiation from the sun is also a factor in the development of cancer of the lip. Irritation from the pipe stem resting on the lip is a factor in pipe smokers. Factors that influence intraoral cancer include tobacco use (cigar, cigarette, pipe, snuff), excessive alcohol intake, and chronic irritation such as from a jagged tooth or poor dental care. A positive history of tobacco and alcohol use, in the past or currently, is the most significant etiologic factor in oral cancer.[10]

Clinical Manifestations

The common manifestations of carcinoma of the oral cavity are leukoplakia, erythroplakia, ulcerations, a sore spot, and a rough area (felt with the tongue). Later symptoms are pain, dysphagia, and difficulty in chewing and speaking. *Leukoplakia*, called "white patch" or "smoker's patch," is frequently considered a precancerous lesion, although less than 5% of these lesions actually transform into malignant cells. It is a whitish patch on the mucosa of the mouth or tongue. The patch becomes keratinized (hard and leathery) and is sometimes described as hyperkeratosis. Leukoplakia is the result of chronic irritation, especially from smoking. *Erythroplasia* (erythroplakia), which is seen as a red velvety patch on the mouth or tongue, is also considered a precancerous lesion. Areas of erythroplakia have a 90% chance of becoming malignant.

Cancer of the lip usually appears as an indurated, painless ulcer on the lip. The first sign of carcinoma of the tongue is an ulcer or area of thickening. Soreness or pain of the tongue may occur, especially on eating hot or highly seasoned foods. Cancerous lesions are most likely to develop in the proximal half of the tongue. Some patients experience limitation of movement of the tongue. Later symptoms of cancer of the tongue include increased salivation, slurred speech, dysphagia, toothache, and

COLLABORATIVE CARE

Table 39-3	Oral Carcinoma

Diagnostic
Biopsy
Oral exfoliative cytology
CT and MRI scans (for metastases)

Collaborative Therapy*
Surgical excision of the tumor
Radical neck dissection
Radiation (internal or external)
Combined surgical resection with radiation
Chemotherapy

*Any of the following approaches may be used, depending on the primary lesion and the extent of metastasis.
CT, computed tomography; *MRI*, magnetic resonance imaging.

earache. Approximately 30% of patients with oral cancer present with an asymptomatic neck mass.

Diagnostic Studies

Biopsy of the suspected lesion with cytologic examination is the best definitive diagnostic measure for oral cancer. Oral exfoliative cytology involves scraping of a suspicious lesion and spreading this scraping on a slide. Unlike biopsy, a negative cytologic smear does not reliably rule out the possibility of a malignant condition, but it may be used as a screening test. The toluidine blue test may also be used as a screening test for oral cancer. Toluidine blue is applied topically to stain an area of carcinoma.[11]

Collaborative Care

Collaborative care of oral carcinoma usually consists of surgery, radiation, chemotherapy, or a combination of these (Table 39-3).

Surgical Therapy. Surgery remains the most effective treatment, especially for removing the central core of the tumor. Many of the operations are radical procedures involving extensive resections. Various surgical procedures may be performed, depending on the location and extent of the tumor. Some examples are partial *mandibulectomy* (removal of the mandible), *hemiglossectomy* (removal of half of the tongue), *glossectomy* (removal of the tongue), resections of the buccal mucosa and floor of the mouth, and radical neck dissection. Composite resections, which are combinations of the various surgical procedures, may be performed.

Because cancers of the oral cavity metastasize early to the cervical lymph nodes, a *radical neck dissection* is commonly performed. It includes wide excision of the involved primary lesion with removal of the regional lymph nodes, the deep cervical lymph nodes, and their lymphatic channels. In addition, the following structures may also be removed or transected (depending on the extent of the primary lesion): the sternocleidomastoid muscle and other closely associated muscles, the internal jugular vein, the mandible, the submaxillary gland, part of the thyroid and parathyroid glands, and the spinal accessory nerve. A tracheostomy is commonly performed along with the radical neck dissection. Drainage tubes are inserted into the surgical area and connected to suction to remove fluid and blood.

Chemotherapy and radiation therapy are used together when the lesions are more advanced or involve several structures of the oral cavity. Chemotherapy may also be used when surgery and radiation therapy fail or as the initial therapy for smaller tumors. Chemotherapeutic agents used include 5-fluorouracil (5-FU), cyclophosphamide (Cytoxan), bleomycin (Blenoxane), vinblastine (Velban), hydroxyurea (Hydrea), and cisplatin (Platinol) (see Chapter 14).

Palliative treatment may be the best management when the prognosis is poor, the cancer is inoperable, or the patient decides against surgery. Palliation aims to treat the symptoms and make the patient more comfortable. If it becomes difficult for the patient to swallow, a gastrostomy may be performed to allow for adequate nutritional intake (see Gastrostomy, Chapter 38). Analgesic medication should be given freely to this patient. Frequent suctioning of the oral cavity becomes necessary when swallowing becomes difficult. (Other nursing measures for the terminally ill patient are discussed in Chapter 14.)

Nutritional Therapy. Because of depression, alcoholism, or presurgery radiation treatment, patients may be malnourished even before surgery. After radical neck surgery, the patient may be unable to take in nutrients through the normal route of ingestion because of swelling, the location of sutures, or difficulty with swallowing. Parenteral fluids will be given for the first 24 to 48 hours. After this time, tube feedings are usually given via a nasogastric (NG) or nasointestinal tube that was placed during surgery. Sometimes a temporary feeding gastrostomy may be used. (Nasogastric and gastrostomy feedings are described in Chapter 38.) Cervical esophagostomy and pharyngostomy have also been used. The nurse must observe for tolerance of the feedings and adjust the amount, time, and formula if nausea, vomiting, diarrhea, or distention occurs. The patient is usually instructed about the tube feedings. When the patient can swallow, small amounts of water are given. Close observation for choking is essential. Suctioning may be necessary to prevent aspiration.

NURSING MANAGEMENT: CARCINOMA OF THE ORAL CAVITY

■ Nursing Assessment

Subjective and objective data that should be obtained from a patient with carcinoma of the oral cavity are presented in Table 39-4.

■ Nursing Diagnoses

Nursing diagnoses for the patient with carcinoma of the oral cavity may include, but are not limited to, the following:

- Altered nutrition: less than body requirements *related to* oral pain, difficulty chewing and swallowing, surgical resection, and radiation treatment
- Pain *related to* the tumor and surgical radiation
- Anxiety *related to* diagnosis of cancer, uncertain future, potential for disfiguring surgery, potential for recurrence, and prognosis
- Ineffective individual coping *related to* body image change, smoking, and alcohol cessation
- Altered health maintenance *related to* lack of knowledge of disease process and therapeutic regimen, and unavailability of a support system

■ Planning

The overall goals are that the patient with carcinoma of the oral cavity will (1) have a patent airway, (2) be able to communicate, (3) have adequate nutritional intake to promote wound healing, and (4) have relief of pain and discomfort.

■ Nursing Implementation

Health Promotion. The nurse has a significant role in early detection and treatment of carcinoma of the oral cavity. The nurse should provide the patient with information regarding predisposing factors, such as constant overexposure to the sun, tobacco, and other irritants. Smoking and the long-term use of smokeless tobacco are the major risk factors for oral cancer. A patient identified as a smoker should be informed about smoking cessation programs available in the community. (Smoking cessation is discussed in the section on lung cancer in Chapter 26 and in Table 26-19.)

It is important that adolescents and teenagers be informed about the danger of using "snuff" and chewing tobacco. In addition, oral cancers have an increased chance of recurrence if risk factors are not reduced. The nurse should also teach correct oral hygiene and dental care and encourage the patient to seek preventive dental care. Risk factors must be identified. Because early detection of oral carcinoma is important, the patient should be taught to examine the mouth and to recognize danger signals of oral cancer. If any of these signals are present, the patient should be instructed to visit a doctor. Danger signals are as follows:

- Unexplained pain or soreness in the mouth
- Unusual bleeding from the oral cavity
- Dysphagia
- Swelling or lump in the neck

NURSING ASSESSMENT
Table 39-4   Cancer of the Mouth

Subjective Data

Important Health Information

Past health history: Recurrent herpetic lesions, syphilis, exposure to sunlight

Medications: Immunosuppressants

Surgery or other treatments: Removal of prior tumors or lesions

Functional Health Patterns

Health perception–health management: Use of alcohol and tobacco, pipe smoking; poor oral hygiene

Nutritional-metabolic: Reductions in oral intake, weight loss; difficulty in chewing food; increased salivation; intolerance to certain foods or temperatures of food

Cognitive-perceptual: Mouth or tongue soreness or pain, toothache, earache, neck stiffness, dysphagia, difficulty speaking

Objective Data

Integumentary

Indurated, painless ulcer on lip; painless neck mass

Gastrointestinal

Areas of thickening or roughness, ulcers, leukoplakia, or erythroplakia on the tongue or oral mucosa; limited movement of the tongue; increased salivation, drooling; slurred speech, foul breath odor

Possible Findings

Positive exfoliative smear cytology; positive biopsy

Any individual with an ulcerative lesion that does not heal within 2 to 3 weeks should be referred to a physician, and a biopsy of the lesion should probably be performed. The nurse should inspect the patient's oral cavity to detect suspicious lesions.

Acute Intervention. Preoperative care for the patient who is having a radical neck dissection involves consideration of the patient's physical and psychosocial needs (see the nursing care plan for the patient with a radical neck dissection on p. 604, NCP 25-6). Physical preparation is the same as for any major surgery, with special emphasis on oral hygiene. Thorough assessment of alcohol intake should be done and measures to assess and treat withdrawal, if it occurs, should be implemented early. Explanations and emotional support are of special significance and should include postoperative measures relating to communication and feeding. The surgical procedure should be explained to the patient, and the nurse should make sure that the patient understands the information.

Care of the patient following radical neck dissection is presented in Chapter 25 and NCP 25-6.

■ Evaluation

The expected outcomes are that the patient with oral carcinoma will

- maintain a patent airway
- be able to communicate
- have adequate nutritional intake to promote wound healing
- have relief of pain and discomfort

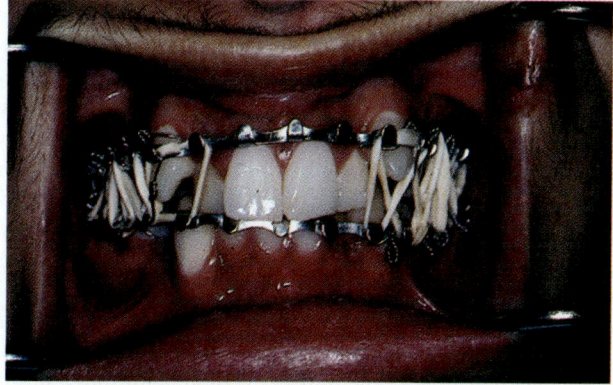

Fig. 39-4   Intermaxillary fixation.

MANDIBULAR FRACTURE

Fracture of the mandible may result from trauma to the face or jaws. Maxillary fractures may also occur, but they are less common than mandibular fractures. The fracture may be simple, with no bone displacement, or it may involve loss of tissue and bone. The fracture may require immediate and sometimes long-term treatment to ensure survival and restore satisfactory appearance and function. Mandibular fracture may also be therapeutically performed to correct an underlying malocclusion problem that cannot be corrected by orthodontic procedures alone. In these conditions, the mandible is split during surgery and moved forward or backward depending on the occlusion problem. For this patient, the procedure is performed on an elective basis.

Surgery consists of immobilization, usually by wiring the jaws (intermaxillary fixation). Internal fixation may be accomplished with screws and plates. In a simple fracture with no loss of teeth, the lower jaw is wired to the upper jaw. First, wires are placed around the teeth; then cross-wires or rubber bands are used to hold the lower jaw tight against the upper jaw (Fig. 39-4). Arch bars may be used and placed on the maxillary and mandibular arches of the teeth. Vertical wires are placed between the arch bars holding the jaws together. When teeth are missing or if there is bone displacement, other forms of fixation such as metal arch bars in the mouth or insertion of a pin in the bone may be used. The immobilization is usually necessary for only 4 to 6 weeks because the fractures heal rapidly.

NURSING MANAGEMENT: MANDIBULAR FRACTURE

■ Preoperative Care

The patient should be told preoperatively about the surgical procedure, including what it involves, how the face will look, and alterations the surgery will cause. The patient must be reassured about the ability to breathe normally, speak, and swallow liquids. Usually hospitalization is brief unless there are other injuries or problems.

■ Postoperative Care

Postoperative care should focus on a patent airway, oral hygiene, communication, and adequate nutrition. Two major potential problems in the immediate postoperative period are airway obstruction and aspiration of vomitus. Because the patient cannot open the jaws, measures to ensure an airway are essential. The nurse must observe for signs of respiratory distress. The patient should be placed on the side with the head slightly elevated immediately after surgery. A wire cutter or scissors (for rubber bands) must be taped to the head of the bed. These may be used to cut the wires or elastic bands in case of an emergency. The wires should be cut only as a last resort. Once the patient is awake the wires should be cut only in case of cardiac or respiratory arrest.

The physician should explain, by using a picture, the appropriate wire or wires to cut, and this should be included in the care plan. In some cases, cutting the wires may cause the entire facial and upper jaw structure to collapse and worsen the problem. A tracheostomy or an endotracheal tray should always be available.

If the patient begins to vomit or choke, the nurse should try to clear the mouth and airway. Suctioning may be necessary and may be done by the nasopharyngeal or oral route, depending on the extent of injury and the type of repair. An NG tube may be used for decompression to remove fluids and gas from the stomach to help prevent aspiration. It also helps prevent vomiting. Antiemetics may also be used. The NG tube can later be used as a feeding tube. The nurse should teach the patient to clear secretions and vomitus.

Oral hygiene is an important part of the nursing care. The mouth should be rinsed frequently, particularly after meals and snacks, to remove food debris. Warm normal saline solution, water, or alkaline mouthwashes may be used. A soft rubber catheter or a Water-Pik is effective for a thorough oral cleansing. The nurse should inspect the mouth several times a day to see that it is clean. A flashlight is necessary, and a tongue depressor is used to retract the cheeks. The lips and corners of the mouth should be kept moist.

Communication may be a problem, particularly in the early postoperative period. An effective way of communication must be established preoperatively (e.g., use of picture board, pad and pencil, small chalkboard). Usually the patient can speak well enough to be understood, especially after the first few postoperative days.

Ingestion of sufficient nutrients poses a challenge because the diet must be liquid. The patient easily tires of sucking through a straw or laboriously using a spoon. The diet must be planned to include adequate calories, protein, and fluids. Liquid protein supplements may be helpful for improving the nutritional status. The nurse works with the dietician and the patient to ensure adequate nutrition. The low-bulk, high-carbohydrate diet and the intake of air through the straw create a problem with flatus and constipation. Ambulation, prune juice, and bulk-forming laxatives may help relieve these problems.

The patient is usually discharged with the wires in place. The nurse should allow the patient to verbalize feelings about the altered appearance. Discharge teaching should include oral care, techniques of handling secretions, diet, and how and when to use wire cutters.

NAUSEA AND VOMITING

Nausea and vomiting are the most common manifestations of GI diseases. Although each symptom can occur independently, they are usually closely related and usually treated as one problem. They are also found in a wide variety of conditions that are unrelated to GI disease. These include pregnancy, infectious diseases, central nervous system (CNS) disorders (e.g., meningitis, CNS lesion), cardiovascular problems (e.g., myocardial infarction, congestive heart failure), side effects of drugs (e.g., digitalis, antibiotics), metabolic disorders (e.g., uremia), and psychologic factors (e.g., stress, fear).

Nausea is a feeling of discomfort in the epigastrium with a conscious desire to vomit. Anorexia usually accompanies nausea and is brought on by unpleasant stimulation involving any of the five senses. Generally, nausea occurs before vomiting and is characterized by contraction of the duodenum and by slowing of gastric motility and emptying. A single episode of nausea accompanied by vomiting in an adult may not be significant. However, if vomiting occurs several times it is important that the cause be identified.

Vomiting is the forceful ejection of partially digested food and secretions from the upper GI tract. It occurs when the gut becomes overly irritated, excited, or distended. It can be a protective mechanism to rid the body of spoiled or irritating foods and liquids. Immediately before the act of vomiting, the person becomes aware of the need to vomit. The autonomic nervous system is activated resulting in both parasympathetic and sympathetic nervous system stimulation. Sympathetic activation produces tachycardia, tachypnea, and diaphoresis. Parasympathetic stimulation causes relaxation of the lower esophageal (cardiac) sphincter, an increase in gastric motility, and a pronounced increase in salivation. These manifestations are experienced immediately before vomiting.

Vomiting is a complex act that requires the coordinated activities of several structures: closure of the glottis, deep inspiration with contraction of the diaphragm in the inspiratory position, closure of the pylorus, relaxation of the stomach and lower esophageal sphincter, and contraction of the abdominal muscles with increasing intraabdominal pressure. These simultaneous activities force the stomach contents up through the esophagus, into the pharynx, and out the mouth.

Etiology and Pathophysiology

There is a vomiting center in the brainstem that coordinates the multiple components involved in vomiting. This center receives input from various stimuli. Neural impulses reach the vomiting center via afferent pathways through branches of the autonomic nervous system. Visceral receptors for these afferent fibers are located in the GI tract, kidneys, heart, and uterus. When stimulated, these receptors relay information to the vomiting center, which then initiates the vomiting reflex (Fig. 39-5).

In addition, the chemoreceptor trigger zone (CTZ) located on the floor of the fourth ventricle in the brain responds to chemical stimuli of drugs and toxins. The CTZ also plays a role in vomiting when it is due to labyrinthine stimulation (e.g., motion sickness). Once stimulated, the CTZ transmits impulses directly to the vomiting center. Emotions, stress, unpleasant sights

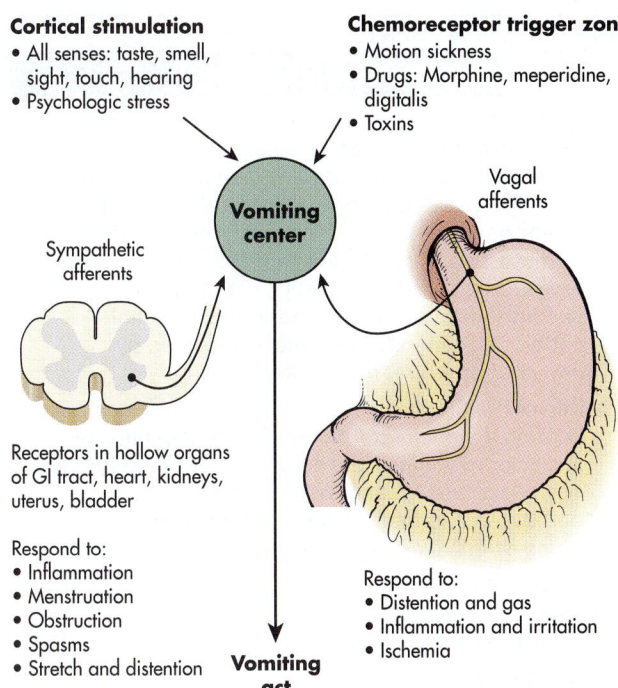

Cortical stimulation
- All senses: taste, smell, sight, touch, hearing
- Psychologic stress

Chemoreceptor trigger zone
- Motion sickness
- Drugs: Morphine, meperidine, digitalis
- Toxins

Vomiting center

Vagal afferents

Sympathetic afferents

Receptors in hollow organs of GI tract, heart, kidneys, uterus, bladder

Respond to:
- Inflammation
- Menstruation
- Obstruction
- Spasms
- Stretch and distention

Respond to:
- Distention and gas
- Inflammation and irritation
- Ischemia

Vomiting act

Fig. 39-5   Stimuli involved in the act of vomiting.

and odors, and pain are all capable of triggering vomiting. Nausea and vomiting are frequently associated with uremia, hyperthyroidism, hyperparathyroidism and hypoparathyroidism, diabetic acidosis, Addison's disease, and hypertensive crisis.

When nausea and vomiting are prolonged, dehydration can rapidly occur. In addition to water, essential electrolytes (e.g., potassium) are also lost. As vomiting persists, there may be severe electrolyte imbalances, loss of extracellular fluid (ECF) volume, decreased plasma volume, and eventually circulatory failure. Metabolic alkalosis can result from loss of gastric hydrochloric acid. Metabolic acidosis can occur because of the loss of bicarbonate when contents from the small intestine are vomited. However, metabolic acidosis as a result of severe vomiting is less common than metabolic alkalosis. Weight loss is evident in a short time when vomiting is severe.

The threat of aspiration is a constant concern when vomiting is severe. Aspiration is especially a risk in the older adult and in the patient who is weak and debilitated. The patient who cannot adequately manage self-care should be put in a semi-Fowler's or side-lying position to prevent aspiration.

Collaborative Care

The goals of collaborative care are to determine and treat the underlying cause of the nausea and vomiting and to provide symptomatic relief of nausea and vomiting. Determining the cause is often difficult because nausea and vomiting are manifestations of many conditions of the GI tract and of disorders of other body systems.

A careful history elicits important information regarding times when the vomiting occurs, precipitating factors, and a description of the contents of the vomitus. Differentiation must be made between vomiting, regurgitation, and projectile vomiting. *Regurgitation* is a process in which partially digested food is slowly brought up from the stomach. Retching or vomiting seldom precedes it. *Projectile vomiting* is a very forceful projection of stomach contents without nausea and is characteristic of CNS lesions.

The presence of fecal odor and bile after prolonged vomiting is indicative of intestinal obstruction beyond the pylorus. A functioning ileocecal valve ordinarily prevents the backflow of fecal contents from the colon into the small intestine. The presence of bile may suggest obstruction below the ampulla of Vater or bile reflux gastritis. The presence of partially digested food several hours after a meal is indicative of gastric outlet obstruction or delay in gastric emptying.

The color of the emesis aids in determining the presence and source of bleeding. Vomitus with a "coffee ground" appearance is associated with bleeding in the stomach, where blood changes to dark brown as a result of its interaction with gastric acid. Bright red blood indicates active bleeding suggestive of a tear in the mucosal lining of the lower esophagus or fundus of stomach, bleeding gastric or duodenal ulcer or neoplasm, or bleeding esophageal varices.

The time of day at which the vomiting occurs is often helpful in determining the cause. Early morning vomiting is a frequent occurrence in pregnancy and in uremia associated with renal disease. Emotional stressors with no evident functional disorder may elicit vomiting during or immediately after the ingestion of a meal.

Drug Therapy. The use of drugs in the treatment of nausea and vomiting depends on the cause of the problem. Many different drugs can be used (Table 39-5). Because the cause cannot always be readily determined, medications must be used with caution. The use of antiemetics before the cause of the vomiting is established can lead to masking of the underlying disease process and delay of diagnosis and treatment. Many of the antiemetic drugs act on the CNS at the level of the CTZ. In general, they block the neurochemicals that appear to trigger nausea and vomiting. Drugs that control nausea and vomiting include antimuscarinics (e.g., scopolamine), antihistamines (e.g., diphenhydramine), and phenothiazines (e.g., chlorpromazine, prochlorperazine). Because many of these drugs have anticholinergic actions, they are contraindicated for the patient with glaucoma, prostatic hyperplasia, pyloric or bladder neck obstruction, or biliary obstruction. They share many common side effects, which include dry mouth, hypotension, sedative effects, rashes, and GI disturbances such as constipation. Consultation with a clinical pharmacist may be indicated before administering these medications to the patient with multiple medical problems. Other drugs with antiemetic properties include metoclopramide (Reglan) and ondansetron (Zofran), which act peripherally to block serotonin receptors. These drugs are considered prokinetic agents because they stimulate gastric emptying and are used prophylactically to reduce nausea and vomiting associated with cancer chemotherapy and postanesthesia.

Nutritional Therapy. The patient with severe vomiting requires intravenous (IV) fluid therapy with electrolyte replacement until able to tolerate oral intake. In some cases an

Table 39-5 Nausea and Vomiting

Classification	Generic Name	Trade Name
■ Antiemetic and antipsychotic	Chlorpromazine	Thorazine
	Haloperidol	Haldol
	Perphenazine	Trilafon
	Prochlorperazine	Compazine
	Promazine	Sparine
	Trifluoperazine	Stelazine
	Triflupromazine	Vesprin
■ Antihistamine	Buclizine	Bucladin-S
	Cyclizine	Marezine, meclizine
	Dimenhydrinate	Dramamine
	Diphenhydramine	Benadryl
	Promethazine	Phenergan
■ Prokinetics	Metoclopramide	Reglan
	Ondansetron	Zofran
	Granisetron	Kytril
	Dolasetron	Anzemet
■ Antimuscarinic	Scopolamine transdermal	Transderm-Scop
■ Others	Benzquinamide	Emete-Con
	Diphenidol	Vontrol
	Thiethylperazine	Torecan
	Trimethobenzamide	Tigan

Table 39-6 Nausea and Vomiting

Subjective Data

Important Health Information

Past health history: GI disorders, chronic indigestion, food allergies, pregnancy, infection, CNS disorders, recent travel, bulimia, metabolic disorders, cancer, cardiovascular disease, renal disease

Medications: Use of antiemetics, digitalis, opiates, ferrous sulfate, aspirin, aminophylline, alcohol, antibiotics; general anesthesia, chemotherapy

Surgery or other treatments: Recent surgery

Functional Health Patterns

Nutritional-metabolic: Amount, frequency, character, and color of vomitus; dry heaves; anorexia; weight loss

Activity-exercise: Weakness, fatigue

Cognitive-perceptual: Abdominal tenderness

Coping–stress tolerance: Stress, fear

Objective Data

General

Lethargy, sunken eyeballs

Integumentary

Pallor, dry mucous membranes, poor skin turgor

Gastrointestinal

Amount, frequency, character (e.g., projectile), content (undigested food, blood, bile, feces), and color of vomitus (red, "coffee ground," green-yellow)

Urinary

Decreased output, concentrated urine

Possible Findings

Altered serum electrolytes (especially hypokalemia), metabolic alkalosis, abnormal upper GI findings or abdominal x-rays

CNS, central nervous system.

NG tube and suction are used to decompress the stomach. Once the symptoms have subsided, oral nourishment beginning with clear liquids is started. Extremely hot or cold liquids are not usually well tolerated. Carbonated beverages at room temperature and with the carbonation gone and warm tea are more easily tolerated. The addition of dry toast or crackers may alleviate the feeling of nausea and help prevent vomiting. Although broth and Gatorade have been used widely for the patient with severe vomiting, these substances are high in sodium and should be administered with caution. Water is the fluid of choice for rehydration by mouth.

As the patient's condition improves, a diet high in carbohydrates and low in fatty foods should be provided. Items such as a baked potato, plain gelatin, cereal with milk and sugar, and hard candy may be added. Foods that are known to be poorly tolerated include coffee, spicy foods, and highly acidic foods. Food should be eaten slowly and in small amounts so that overdistention of the stomach is avoided. When solid foods have been reintroduced, fluids should be taken between meals rather than with meals. It is advised that the patient remain quietly relaxed for approximately 1 hour after meals. A registered dietician may be consulted regarding appropriate foods that have nutritional value and are well tolerated by the patient during the recovery process.

NURSING MANAGEMENT: NAUSEA AND VOMITING

■ Nursing Assessment

Each patient with a history of prolonged and persistent nausea or vomiting requires a thorough nursing assessment before a specific plan of care is developed. Although the conditions associated with nausea and vomiting are numerous, the nurse should have a basic understanding of the more common conditions and should be able to identify the patient who is at high risk. Knowledge of the physiologic mechanisms involved in nausea and vomiting and the demonstration of a genuine regard for the patient are essential. Table 39-6 presents subjective and objective data that should be obtained from a patient with nausea and vomiting, regardless of the underlying cause.

■ Nursing Diagnoses

Nursing diagnoses for the patient with nausea and vomiting may include, but are not limited to, those presented in NCP 39-1. Additional nursing diagnoses may include the following:

- Self-care deficits *related to* fatigue and discomfort of prolonged nausea and vomiting
- Altered oral mucous membrane *related to* persistent vomiting and inadequate oral hygiene

■ Planning

The overall goals are that the patient with nausea and vomiting will (1) experience minimal or no nausea and vomiting, (2) have

39-1 NURSING CARE PLAN   PATIENT WITH NAUSEA AND VOMITING

Expected Patient Outcomes	Nursing Interventions and *Rationales*

NURSING DIAGNOSIS Vomiting *related to* multiple etiologies *as manifested by* episodes of nausea and vomiting.

- Minimal or no nausea or vomiting.
- Verbalization of satisfaction with care.

- Assess duration, frequency, and nature of vomitus, and aggravating and alleviating factors *to plan appropriate interventions.*
- Offer reassurance and explanations *to increase patient cooperation.*
- Remove visual stimuli and source of odors *to avoid precipitating factors of nausea and/or vomiting.*
- Provide mouth care; change soiled gown and linens *to ensure patient comfort.*
- Use diversional activities (if appropriate) *to decrease awareness of nausea.*
- Maintain quiet environment, restrict visitors, and avoid unnecessary procedures or activities *to minimize triggers of vomiting.*
- Administer antiemetics as ordered.
- Instruct patient to take several deep breaths; prevent sudden changes in position; keep head of bed elevated *to decrease stimulation of the vomiting center.*
- Instruct patient to avoid foods and beverages *that stimulate nausea and vomiting.*

NURSING DIAGNOSIS Fluid volume deficit *related to* prolonged vomiting and inability to ingest, digest, or absorb food and fluids *as manifested by* decreased urine output and increased urine concentration, increased pulse rate, hypotension (postural), decreased intake, decreased skin turgor, dry skin and mucous membranes.

- No signs of dehydration.

- Assess for signs of dehydration *to plan appropriate care.*
- Administer and monitor amount and type of IV fluid *to maintain fluid and electrolyte balance.*
- Administer antiemetic as prescribed.
- Provide small amounts of clear liquids when vomiting stops *to maintain hydration.*
- Record amount and frequency of vomitus; maintain accurate intake and output records; weigh daily in acute phase *to accurately monitor fluid balance.*
- Monitor laboratory results of serum sodium, potassium, and chloride *as indicators of electrolyte balance.*

NURSING DIAGNOSIS Anxiety *related to* lack of knowledge of cause of problem, treatment plan, and follow-up care *as manifested by* verbalization of lack of knowledge, apprehension.

- Decrease in anxiety.
- Verbalization of understanding of causative factors and therapeutic interventions.

- Explain rationale for plan of care and diagnostic tests *to increase patient's understanding and reduce anxiety.*
- Teach about relationship between nausea and vomiting and foods, medications, treatment regimens, and psychosocial factors *to elicit patient's cooperation in avoiding potential causative factors.*

NURSING DIAGNOSIS Altered nutrition: less than body requirements *related to* nausea and vomiting *as manifested by* lack of interest in or aversion to food, perceived or actual inability to ingest food, weight loss.

- Gradual return to usual weight and eating habits.

- Assess patient's interest in food, ability to ingest food, and weight *to determine if a problem is present.*
- Assure patient that appetite will return when nausea and vomiting are controlled.
- Maintain IV feedings or total parenteral nutrition until oral intake is possible *to provide necessary fluids, electrolytes, calories, and protein intake.*
- Instruct patient to resume eating cautiously with bland, nonirritating foods *to avoid irritating the stomach and initiating recurrence of nausea and vomiting.*

normal electrolyte levels and hydration status, and (3) return to a normal pattern of fluid balance and nutrient intake.

■ Nursing Implementation

Acute Intervention.   The majority of individuals with nausea and vomiting can be managed at home. However, when nausea and vomiting persist regardless of home treatment strategies, hospitalization may be necessary for diagnosis of the underlying problem. Until a diagnosis is confirmed, the patient is kept on NPO status and given IV fluids. An NG tube connected to suction may be necessary for the patient with persistent vomiting as well as for the patient in whom the possible diagnosis may be bowel obstruction or paralytic ileus. Keeping the stomach empty reduces the stimulus to vomit. The NG tube should be stabilized to eliminate its movement in the nose and back of the throat because this can stimulate nausea and vomiting.

With prolonged vomiting, there is a possibility of dehydration and electrolyte imbalances. The nurse plans care that includes accurate recording of intake and output, monitoring vital signs, assessing for signs of dehydration, proper positioning to prevent possible aspiration in the susceptible patient, and observing for changes in the patient's general physical comfort and mentation. The nurse must take responsibility for providing physical and emotional support, maintaining a quiet, odor-free environment, and giving explanations regarding any diagnostic tests or procedures performed.

Those who are already hospitalized for other health problems are also prone to episodes of nausea and vomiting. These individuals include the postoperative patient who is recovering from the effects of a surgical procedure, anesthesia, and pain, and who is experiencing adverse reactions to medications and treatment. Nausea and vomiting are common side effects in the cancer patient receiving chemotherapeutic drugs or radiation therapy. (Nursing care for the patient who is receiving chemotherapy and radiation therapy is found in Chapter 14.)

Ambulatory and Home Care.   The patient and family may need instructions on how to deal successfully with the unpleasant sensations of nausea, discussion of methods of preventing nausea and vomiting, and strategies to maintain fluid and nutritional intake during periods of nausea. The occurrence of nausea or vomiting may be minimized if measures are taken to keep the immediate environment quiet, free of noxious odors, and well ventilated. The avoidance of sudden changes of position and unnecessary activity is also helpful. Use of relaxation techniques, frequent rest periods, and diversional tactics help prevent nausea and vomiting or facilitate a more rapid recovery from their effects. Cleansing the face and hands with a cool washcloth and mouth care between episodes increase the person's comfort level. When the symptoms occur, all foods and medications should be stopped until the acute phase is past.

If a medication is suspected as the cause, the physician should be notified immediately so that either the dosage can be altered or a new medication can be prescribed. The patient should be reminded that stopping the drug without consulting the physician may eliminate the immediate cause of the nausea and vomiting but that omission of the prescribed medication may have detrimental effects on health or the disease state.

When food is identified as the precipitating cause of nausea and vomiting, the nurse should help the patient solve the problem. What food was it? When was it eaten? Has this food caused problems in the past? Is anyone else in the family sick?

When the patient believes some foods and fluids can be tolerated, the nurse might suggest that it would be helpful to begin with clear liquids or warm cola beverages, Gatorade, tea or broth, dry crackers or toast, and then plain gelatin. Bland foods, such as pasta, rice, and cooked chicken, are generally well tolerated in small amounts. An antiemetic drug should be taken only if prescribed by the physician. Taking over-the-counter (OTC) drugs for relief of symptoms may make the condition worse.

■ Evaluation

The expected outcomes are that the patient with nausea and vomiting will

- experience minimal or no nausea and vomiting
- have normal electrolyte levels and hydration status
- return to a normal pattern of fluid balance and nutrient intake

■ GERONTOLOGIC CONSIDERATIONS

Nausea and Vomiting

The older patient experiencing nausea and vomiting requires careful assessment and monitoring, particularly during periods of fluid loss and subsequent rehydration therapy. The older patient is at increased risk for preexisting conditions, such as cardiac or renal failure, and may experience a sudden compromise in renal or cardiac system functioning during episodes of fluid volume deficit.[12] In addition, the electrolyte imbalances that often accompany dehydration may result in life-threatening consequences for the elderly person who is already experiencing conditions such as congestive heart failure. Finally, the older adult with a decreased level of consciousness may be at high risk for aspiration of vomitus. Close monitoring of the patient's physical status and level of consciousness during episodes of nausea and vomiting must be a primary concern for the nurse.

In addition, the elderly are particularly susceptible to the CNS side effects of antiemetic medications; these medications may produce confusion. Dosages should be reduced and efficacy closely evaluated. Safety precautions should be instituted for frail patients taking these medications.

GASTROESOPHAGEAL REFLUX DISEASE

Etiology and Pathophysiology

Gastroesophageal reflux disease (GERD) is not a disease but a syndrome produced by conditions that result in reflux of gastric secretions into the esophagus. More than 60 million Amer-

Table 39-7	Factors Affecting Lower Esophogeal Sphincter Pressure

Increase Pressure
Bethanechol (Urecholine)
Cisapride (Propulsid)
Metoclopramide (Reglan)

Decrease Pressure

Fatty foods	Theophylline
Chocolate (theobromine, caffeine)	Diazepam (Valium)
Peppermint, spearmint	Morphine sulfate
Alcohol	β-Adrenergic blocking drugs
Nicotine	Calcium channel blockers
Anticholinergics	Nitrates
Progesterone	
Tea, coffee (caffeine)	

COLLABORATIVE CARE

Table 39-8	Gastroesophageal Reflux Disease and Hiatal Hernia

Diagnostic
Barium swallow
Radionuclide tests
Esophagoscopy with biopsy and cytologic analysis
Motility (manometry) studies
pH monitoring (laboratory or 24 hr ambulatory)

Collaborative Therapy
Conservative
Elevation of head of bed on 4- to 6-inch blocks
High-protein, low-fat diet with avoidance of foods that decrease LES pressure or irritate acid-sensitive esophagus
Antacids/Gaviscon
Cholinergic drugs
Antisecretory agents
  Histamine H_2-receptor antagonists (cimetidine, ranitidine)
  Proton pump inhibitors (omeprazole)
Prokinetic drug therapy
  Metoclopramide (Reglan)
Surgical
Nissen fundoplication
Hill gastropexy
Belsey fundoplication
Antireflux prosthesis

LES, lower esophageal sphincter.

icans periodically experience symptoms of gastroesophageal reflux and approximately 17.5 million (or 7%) experience symptoms daily.[13] Predisposing conditions include hiatal hernia, incompetent lower esophageal sphincter (LES), decreased esophageal clearance, and decreased gastric emptying. In GERD there is reflux of gastric contents into the lower portion of the esophagus. The acidity of the gastric secretion results in esophageal irritation and inflammation (esophagitis). In addition, the presence of intestinal secretions such as trypsin and bile salts are also corrosive to the esophageal mucosa. The degree of inflammation is dependent on the amount of acid refluxed as well as on the ability of the esophagus to clear the acid (esophageal clearance).

One of the primary factors in GERD is an incompetent LES. An incompetent LES results in a decrease in pressure in the distal portion of the esophagus. As a result, gastric contents are able to move from an area of higher pressure (stomach) to an area of lower pressure (esophagus) when the patient is in a supine position or there is an increase in intraabdominal pressure. A common cause of GERD is a hiatal hernia, which is discussed in the next section.

Clinical Manifestations

Heartburn (*pyrosis*) from gastroesophageal reflux is the most common clinical manifestation. It is caused by irritation of the esophagus by the gastric secretions. Heartburn is described as a burning, tight sensation that appears intermittently beneath the lower sternum and spreads upward to the throat or jaw. Heartburn occurs following ingestion of substances that decrease the LES pressure (Table 39-7). Heartburn is relieved with milk, alkaline substances, or water. Pulmonary symptoms including wheezing, coughing, and dyspnea are secondary to microaspiration of gastric contents into the pulmonary system. Otolaryngologic symptoms include hoarseness, sore throat, a globus sensation, and choking. Gastric symptoms including early satiety, posteating bloating, nausea, and vomiting are related to gastric stasis, which is common in patients with GERD.[13]

Regurgitation (effortless return of material from stomach into esophagus or mouth) is a fairly common manifestation of an incompetent LES. It is often described as hot, bitter, or sour liquid coming into the throat or mouth. Other symptoms include feelings of a lump in the throat or of food stopping, *dysphagia* (difficulty in swallowing), painful swallowing, and bleeding. An individual with GERD may also experience respiratory complications including bronchospasm, laryngospasm, and cricopharyngeal spasm because of movement of gastric contents into the upper airway.[14]

Complications

Complications of GERD are related to the direct local effects of gastric acid on the esophageal mucosa. As a result of repeated exposure, there may be scar tissue formation and decreased distensibility (esophageal stricture) of the esophagus. This may result in dysphagia. In addition, esophageal metaplasia (Barrett's esophagus, which is a precancerous lesion) may occur. There is also the potential for pulmonary complications (pneumonia) as a result of aspiration of gastric contents into the pulmonary system.

Diagnostic Studies

Diagnostic studies are performed to determine the cause of the GERD (e.g., hiatal hernia) (Table 39-8). Barium swallow is done to determine if there is protrusion of the upper part of the stomach (called the gastric cardia). Radionuclide tests may also

Table **39-9**	**Gastroesophageal Reflux Disease (GERD)**
Mechanism of Action	**Examples**
Increase LES Pressure	
Cholinergic	Bethanechol (Urecholine)
Dopamine antagonist	Metoclopramide (Reglan)
Acid Neutralizing	
Antacids	Gelusil, Maalox, Mylanta
Antisecretory	
Histamine H$_2$-receptor antagonists	Ranitidine (Zantac)
	Cimetidine (Tagamet)
	Famotidine (Pepcid)
	Nizatidine (Axid)
Proton pump inhibitors	Omeprazole (Prilosec)
	Lansoprazole (Prevacid)
	Pantoprazole (Pantoloc)
Cytoprotective	
Alginic acid-antacid	Gaviscon
Antacids	Gelusil, Maalox, Mylanta
Acid-protective	Sucralfate (Carafate)

LES, lower esophageal sphincter.

be performed to detect reflux of gastric contents and the rate of esophageal clearance. Esophagoscopy is useful in determining the incompetence of the LES and the extent of inflammation, potential scarring, and strictures. Biopsy and cytologic specimens can be taken to differentiate hiatal hernia from carcinoma of the stomach or esophagus and Barrett's esophagus. Esophageal motility studies are performed to measure pressure in the esophagus as well as the LES. The determination of pH using specially designed probes in the laboratory or using ambulatory monitoring systems may demonstrate the presence of acid in the normally alkaline esophagus.

Collaborative Care

A four-phase management approach is often used. Phase 1 is lifestyle modification (see Tables 39-7 and 39-8); Phase 2 involves drug therapy; Phase 3 is intensified drug therapy; and Phase 4 is antireflux surgery.[14]

Drug Therapy. Pharmacologic management is focused on improving LES function, increasing esophageal clearance, decreasing volume and acidity of reflux, and protecting esophageal mucosa. Antacids are used to relieve heartburn by their neutralizing effect on hydrochloric acid. They should be taken 1 to 3 hours after meals and at bedtime. Alginic acid and an antacid (Gaviscon) are sometimes given together. The alginic acid reacts with sodium bicarbonate and forms a viscous solution that floats to the surface of the gastric contents and coats the esophagus, acting as a mechanical barrier to reflux. However, antacids alone are often not effective in relieving symptoms or healing erosive lesions.[14]

In Phase 2, agents that decrease gastric hydrochloric acid secretion are used in the management of reflux esophagitis. Histamine H$_2$-receptor blockers (e.g., ranitidine [Zantac] or cimetidine [Tagamet]) have no effect on LES pressure but do decrease

gastric acid production. They are particularly helpful for the patient with high acid outputs. Prokinetic drugs, such as cisapride (Propulsid), facilitate gastric emptying and thus reduce the volume of reflux. Prokinetic agents are often administered with antisecretory agents to promote esophageal healing.

If Phase 2 drug therapy is ineffective, patients may begin Phase 3 antisecretory drugs such as omeprazole (Prilosec) and lansoprazole (Prevacid).[15] These agents act by inhibiting the proton pump mechanism responsible for the secretion of H$^+$ ions, decreasing acid secretion, and facilitating the healing of erosive reflux esophagitis.

Other agents that may be used in both Phase 2 and 3 include sucralfate (Carafate), an antiulcer drug used for its cytoprotective properties, and cholinergic drugs, such as bethanechol (Urecholine), which may be used to increase LES pressure, improve esophageal emptying in the supine position, and increase gastric emptying. A summary of the drug therapy is shown in Table 39-9.

The nurse should observe for and instruct the patient about side effects of the medications being taken. Antacids have minimal side effects. Antacids that contain aluminum tend to cause constipation, whereas those that contain magnesium tend to cause diarrhea. Several of the antacids are combinations of aluminum and magnesium designed to minimize these side effects. If the patient is taking bethanechol, side effects to observe for include urinary urgency, increased salivation, abdominal cramping with diarrhea, nausea, vomiting, and hypotension. Such side effects often limit the effectiveness of cholinergic agents in the treatment of GERD. Side effects of metoclopramide, a prokinetic drug, include restlessness, anxiety, and insomnia. Side effects of metoclopramide (Reglan) a prokinetic agent that increases gastric emptying, include restlessness, anxiety, and insomnia. Side effects of sucralfate include drowsiness, dizziness, nausea, vomiting, constipation, urticaria, and rash.

Nutritional Therapy. A diet high in protein and low in fats is recommended for GERD. Fatty foods stimulate the release of cholecystokinin, which decreases LES pressure. Foods that decrease LES pressure, such as chocolate, peppermint, coffee, and tea (see Table 39-7), should be avoided because they cause reflux. Milk products should be avoided, especially at bedtime, because milk increases gastric acid secretion. Small, frequent meals are advised to prevent overdistention of the stomach. The patient should avoid late meals and nocturnal snacking. Fluids should be taken between rather than with meals to reduce distention. Certain foods (e.g., spicy tomato juice and orange juice) may irritate the acid-sensitive esophagus and thus may have to be avoided. No specific diet is necessary, but foods that cause reflux should be avoided. Weight reduction is recommended if the patient is obese.

NURSING MANAGEMENT: GASTROESOPHAGEAL REFLUX DISEASE

Patients with GERD must avoid factors that cause reflux. A patient teaching guide is provided in Table 39-10. The patient who is a smoker should stop smoking. Smoking causes an almost immediate drop in LES pressure. The patient may need to be referred to other members of the health care team or to community resources for assistance in stopping smoking. Substances

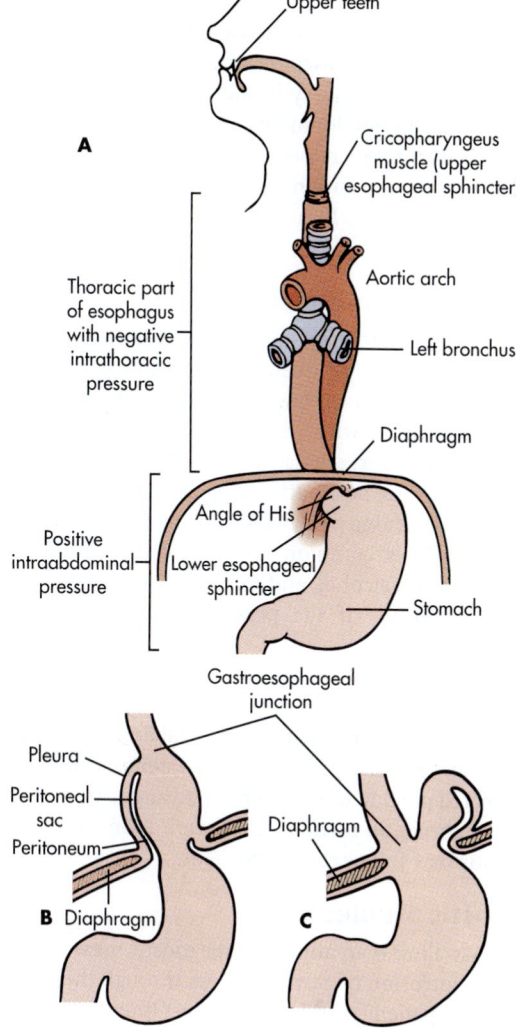

Fig. 39-6 **A,** Normal esophagus. **B,** Sliding hiatal hernia. **C,** Rolling or paraesophageal hernia.

that decrease LES pressure and tone should be avoided (see Table 39-7). If stress seems to bring on symptoms, measures to cope with stress should be discussed.

Nursing care for the patient who is having acute symptoms consists mainly of teaching and encouraging the patient to follow the necessary regimen. The nurse should ensure that the head of the bed is elevated to approximately 30 degrees (usually on 4- to 6-inch blocks) and that the patient does not lie down during the first 2 to 3 hours after eating. Teaching the patient to avoid food and activities that cause reflux is important (e.g., late-night eating should be avoided). The patient may be taking medications to relieve heartburn, so the nurse must observe for side effects and evaluate whether the medications are relieving symptoms. The patient should also be taught possible side effects of medications.

Surgical therapy (antireflux surgery) may be necessary if conservative therapy fails, if a hiatal hernia is present, or if complications, such as stenosis, chronic esophagitis, and bleeding exist. The objective of surgery is to restore gastroesophageal integrity. Procedures used for the management of hiatal hernia including surgery are discussed below.

HIATAL HERNIA

Hiatal hernia is herniation of a portion of the stomach into the esophagus through an opening, or hiatus, in the diaphragm. It is also referred to as *diaphragmatic hernia* and *esophageal hernia.*

The incidence of hiatal hernia is difficult to determine. Although it is said to be the most common abnormality found on x-ray examination of the upper GI tract, the hernia is often asymptomatic. Hiatal hernias are common in older adults and occur more frequently in women than in men.

Types

Hiatal hernias are classified into two types (Fig. 39-6):

1. *Sliding:* The junction of the stomach and esophagus is above the hiatus of the diaphragm, and a part of the stomach slides through the hiatal opening in the diaphragm. It "slides" into the thoracic cavity when the patient is supine and usually goes back into the abdominal cavity when the patient is standing upright. This is the most common type.
2. *Paraesophageal or rolling:* The esophagogastric junction remains in the normal position, but the fundus and the greater curvature of the stomach roll up through the diaphragm, forming a pocket alongside the esophagus.

Etiology and Pathophysiology

The actual cause of hiatal hernia is unknown. Many factors contribute to the development of hiatal hernia. Structural changes, such as weakening of the muscles in the diaphragm around the esophagogastric opening, are usually contributing factors. Factors that increase intraabdominal pressure, including obesity, pregnancy, ascites, tumors, tight corsets, intense physical exertion, and heavy lifting on a continual basis, may also predispose to development of a hiatal hernia. Other predisposing factors are increased age, trauma, poor nutrition, and a forced recumbent position, as when a prolonged illness confines the person to bed. In some cases, congenital weakness is a contributing factor.

Clinical Manifestations

The signs and symptoms of hiatal hernia are similar to that described under GERD. Frequently the symptoms of hiatal hernia mimic gallbladder disease, peptic ulcer, and angina. However, some patients with hiatal hernia have no symptoms. Reflux and discomfort are also associated with position, occurring soon or several hours after lying down. Bending over may cause a severe burning pain, which is usually relieved by sitting or standing. Other common precipitating factors of pain include large meals, alcohol, and smoking. Nocturnal attacks are common, especially if the person has eaten before going to sleep.

Complications

Complications that may occur with hiatal hernia include problems such as hemorrhage from erosion, stenosis, ulcerations of the herniated portion of the stomach, strangulation of the hernia, and regurgitation with tracheal aspiration. Severe chronic esophagitis may follow reflux problems.

Diagnostic Studies

A barium swallow is an important diagnostic measure that may show the protrusion of gastric mucosa through the esophageal hiatus in the patient with hiatal hernia. Other tests are similar to those described in Table 39-8.

Collaborative Care

Conservative Therapy. Conservative therapy of hiatal hernia includes administration of antacids and antisecretory agents, elimination of constricting garments, avoidance of lifting and straining, elimination of alcohol and smoking, and elevation of the head of the bed. Elevation of the bed on 4- to 6-inch blocks assists gravity in maintaining the stomach in the abdominal cavity and also helps prevent reflux and tracheal aspiration. If obese, the patient is encouraged to lose weight.

Surgical Therapy. The objective of surgical interventions for hiatal hernia is to reduce reflux by enhancing the integrity of the LES. Surgical procedures are termed *valvuloplasties* or *antireflux* procedures. There are three slightly varied procedures: the Nissen fundoplication, the Hill gastropexy, and the Belsey's fundoplication. These three surgical procedures are all variations of fundoplication, which involves "wrapping" the fundus of the stomach around the lower portion of the esophagus in varying degrees. These procedures reduce the hernia, provide an acceptable LES pressure, and prevent movement of the gastroesophageal junction. The Nissen fundoplication is shown in Fig. 39-7. The Nissen fundoplication procedure is being performed laparoscopically with increasing frequency. The use of laparoscopic techniques has re-

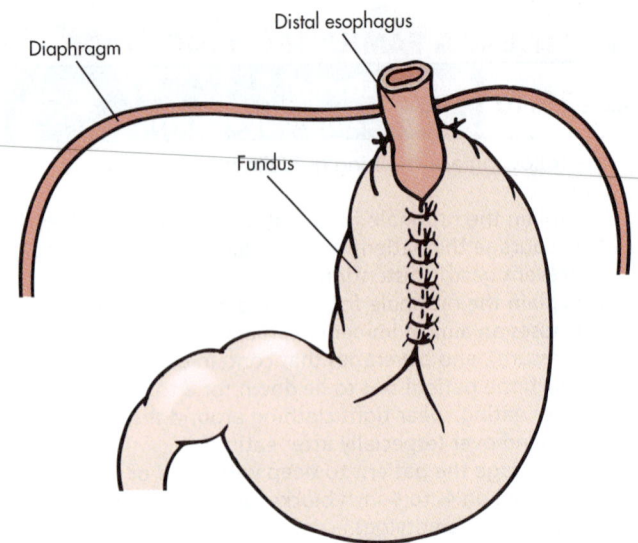

Fig. 39-7 Nissen fundoplication for repair of hiatal hernia. Fundus of stomach is wrapped around distal esophagus and sutured to itself.

duced the overall morbidity associated with abdominal surgery.[14] A thoracic or open abdominal approach may also be used.

Fundoplication prevents reflux in 90% of the patients. The success of fundoplication depends on achieving correct tightness of the fundal wrap. If it is too loose, reflux is not prevented. If it is too tight, dysphagia and the gas-bloat syndrome are problems.

NURSING MANAGEMENT: SURGICAL INTERVENTIONS FOR HIATAL HERNIA

Postoperative care focuses on concerns related to prevention of respiratory complications, maintenance of fluid and electrolyte balance, and prevention of infection. If a thoracic approach is used, a chest tube is inserted. Assessment and management related to closed chest drainage are important (see Chapter 26).

Respiratory complications can occur in a patient treated by an abdominal approach because of the high abdominal incision. Respiratory assessment should include respiratory rate and rhythm, chest reexpansion, pulse rate and rhythm, and signs of pneumothorax (e.g., dyspnea, chest pain, and cyanosis). Deep breathing is essential to fully expand the lungs.

The patient receives IV fluids and electrolytes until the return of peristalsis. Care should be taken to maintain patency of the NG tube (if present) to prevent the need to reinsert the tube. It is dangerous to attempt to replace the tube because of the possibility of perforation of the surgical repair. When peristalsis returns, only fluids are initially given. Solids are added gradually so that the stomach is not overdistended. The nurse must maintain an accurate recording of intake and output and observe for fluid and electrolyte imbalances (see Chapter 15). (Care of the patient undergoing a laparotomy procedure is described in the NCP 40-2 on p. 1147.)

After surgical intervention, there should be no symptoms of gastric reflux. The patient should be instructed to report symptoms such as heartburn and regurgitation. In the early postoperative period there is usually mild dysphagia caused by edema, but it should resolve. The patient should report persistent dysphagia, epigastric fullness, and bloating. Immediately after the surgical procedure, the patient cannot voluntarily vomit or belch, and this may cause the bloating and abdominal discomfort. A normal diet can be resumed within 6 weeks. The patient should avoid foods that are gas forming and should try to prevent gastric distention. Food should be thoroughly chewed.

GERONTOLOGIC CONSIDERATIONS

Gastroesophageal Reflux Disease and Hiatal Hernia

The incidence of hiatal hernia increases with age. It is associated with weakening of the diaphragm, obesity, kyphosis, and use of corsets or other factors that increase intraabdominal pressure. Some older adults with hiatal hernia are asymptomatic. The first indications may include esophageal bleeding secondary to esophagitis or pulmonary complications (e.g., aspiration, pneumonia) related to aspiration of gastric contents. The lower esophageal sphincter may become less competent with aging in some individuals.

The clinical course and management of these problems are similar to that for the younger adult. With the increased use of laparoscopic procedures, surgical risks have been reduced. However, an older adult with cardiovascular and pulmonary problems may not be a good candidate for surgical intervention. In addition, changes in lifestyle, including elimination of dietary factors, such as caffeine-containing beverages and chocolate, and elevating the head of the bed on blocks, may be more difficult.

ESOPHAGEAL CANCER

Carcinoma of the esophagus is unique in its geographic distribution. There are portions of Asia in which the rate of esophageal cancer is extremely high while in Western societies the incidence is relatively low. For example, esophageal cancer is the second most common type of cancer in China.[16] In the United States it is estimated that there will be 12,300 new cases of esophageal cancer (9300 will be men) and that 11,900 Americans will die in 1998 from esophageal cancer.

The incidence of squamous cell esophageal cancer is currently decreasing in the United States, whereas the incidence of adenocarcinoma of the distal esophagus is increasing. However, squamous cell carcinoma remains the most common form of esophageal cancer. The incidence of esophageal cancer increases with age. There is a higher incidence of squamous cell carcinoma in African-Americans and in men. The incidence of esophageal cancer is higher in Alaska Native men and women compared with Caucasians.[17] Because esophageal cancer is rarely diagnosed in early stages, the 5-year prognosis is poor.

A condition called *Barrett's esophagus* is considered a metaplastic change that may progress to adenocarcinoma of the esophagus. This syndrome is characterized by replacement of areas of the normal squamous epithelium of the esophagus with columnar epithelium. It may result from severe reflux esophagitis and is considered an important complication of GERD. Signs and symptoms of Barrett's esophagus can range from none to mild to bleeding and perforation.[14] Because patients with Barrett's esophagus are at risk for adenocarcinoma, they must be monitored on an annual basis by endoscopy and biopsy.

Etiology and Pathophysiology

The cause of cancer of the esophagus is unknown. Possible predisposing factors are cigarette smoking, excessive alcohol intake, chronic trauma, poor oral hygiene, and spicy foods. The two most important risk factors are smoking and excessive alcohol intake. Other risk factors include exposure to asbestos and metal and low intake of fresh fruits and vegetables.[18]

The majority of tumors are located in the middle and lower portions of the esophagus. The malignant tumor usually appears as an ulcerated lesion. It may have advanced to this stage before the appearance of symptoms. The tumor may penetrate the muscular layer and even extend outside the wall of the esophagus. Obstruction of the esophagus occurs in the later stages.

Clinical Manifestations

The onset of symptoms is usually late in relation to the extent of the tumor. Progressive dysphagia is the most common symptom and may be expressed as a substernal feeling as if food is not passing. Initially the dysphagia occurs only with meat, then with soft foods, and eventually with liquids.

Pain develops late and is described as occurring in the substernal, epigastric, or back areas and usually increases with swallowing. The pain may radiate to the neck, jaw, ears, and shoulders. If the tumor is in the upper third of the esophagus, symptoms such as sore throat, choking, and hoarseness may occur. Weight loss is fairly common. When esophageal stenosis is severe, regurgitation of blood-flecked esophageal contents is common.

Complications

Hemorrhage may occur if the cancer erodes through the esophagus and into the aorta. Esophageal perforation with fistula formation into the lung or trachea sometimes develops. The tumor may enlarge enough to cause esophageal obstruction. Esophageal carcinoma has a poor prognosis because of early lymphatic spread and late development of symptoms. The liver and lung are common metastatic sites.

Diagnostic Studies

Barium swallow with fluoroscopy may demonstrate a narrowing of the esophagus at the site of the tumor (Table 39-11). Sometimes a crater is visible. Esophagoscopy with biopsy is necessary to make a definitive diagnosis of carcinoma by identification of malignant cells. Endoscopic ultrasonography is also used to detect tumor invasion into the muscle layer. A bronchoscopic examination may be performed to detect malignant involvement of the trachea. Computerized tomography (CT) scanning and magnetic resonance imaging (MRI) are also used to assess the extent of the disease.

Collaborative Care

The treatment of carcinoma of the esophagus depends on the location of the tumor and whether invasion or metastasis has

COLLABORATIVE CARE

Table **39-11**   Esophageal Cancer

Diagnostic
Barium swallow
Esophagoscopy with biopsy
CT and MRI
Ultrasonography
Bronchoscopy

Collaborative Therapy
Surgical resection
  Esophagectomy
  Esophagogastrostomy
  Esophagoenterostomy
Radiation
Palliative
  Dilation
  Stent or prosthesis
  Gastrostomy
  Laser therapy

occurred (see Table 39-11). Surgical removal and radiation are the two methods used. Cancer of the esophagus has a poor prognosis, mainly because in most cases it is not diagnosed until the disease is advanced. Relatively few people are cured. The best results have been obtained with a combination of surgery and radiation. Chemotherapeutic agents, cisplatin (Platinol), and 5-FU in combination with radiation are currently under investigation.[19]

If the tumor is in the cervical section (upper third) of the esophagus, radiation is usually indicated. A tumor in the lower third of the esophagus is usually resected surgically. In addition, radiation may be used either before or after surgery.

The types of surgical procedures that can be performed are (1) removal of part or all of the esophagus (*esophagectomy*) with use of a Dacron graft to replace the resected part, (2) resection of a portion of the esophagus and anastomosis of the remaining portion to the stomach (*esophagogastrostomy*), and (3) resection of a portion of the esophagus and anastomosis of a segment of colon to the remaining portion (*esophagoenterostomy*). The surgical approaches may be thoracic or both abdominal and thoracic.

Surgery may not be performed if the patient is an older adult or in poor physical health. Palliative therapy consists of restoration of the swallowing function and maintenance of nutrition and hydration. Dilation, stent placement, or both can relieve obstruction. Laser therapy or vaporization of the tumor by means of endoscopy may be used in combination with dilation. Obstruction recurs as the tumor grows, but laser therapy can be repeated. Sometimes these procedures are combined with radiation therapy. Other measures for palliation include gastrostomy or esophagostomy tube placements for nutrition support and pain management.

Dilation is done with various types of dilators (e.g., Celestin tube). Dilation often relieves dysphagia and allows for improved nutrition. Placement of a stent or prosthesis may help when dilation is no longer effective. The prostheses are composed of silicone rubber or nylon-reinforced latex tubes with distal and proximal collars. The prosthesis is placed in the esophagus so that food and fluids can pass through the stenotic segment of the esophagus. The prosthesis can be placed endoscopically.

Nutritional Therapy. After esophageal surgery, parenteral fluids are given. When fluids are allowed after bowel sounds have returned, 30 to 60 ml of water are given hourly, with gradual progression to small, frequent bland meals. The patient should be in an upright position to prevent regurgitation of the fluid. The patient is observed for signs of intolerance to the feeding or leakage of the feeding into the mediastinum. Symptoms that indicate leakage are pain, increased temperature, and dyspnea. Symptoms of food intolerance include vomiting and abdominal distention. A gastrostomy may be performed for the purpose of feeding the patient. (Gastrostomy tubes are discussed in Chapter 38.)

NURSING MANAGEMENT: ESOPHAGEAL CANCER

■ Nursing Assessment

The patient should be assessed for progressive dysphagia and odynophagia (burning, squeezing pain while swallowing). The nurse should question the patient regarding the type of substances ingested that cause dysphagia, such as meat, soft foods, and liquids. The patient should also be assessed for pain (substernal, epigastric, or back areas), choking, hoarseness, cough, anorexia, weight loss, and regurgitation (sometimes bloody). The patient should also be questioned regarding tobacco and alcohol use.

■ Nursing Diagnoses

Nursing diagnoses for the patient with esophageal cancer include, but are not limited to, the following:

- Altered nutrition: less than body requirements *related to* dysphagia, odynophagia, weakness, and radiation therapy
- Pain *related to* tumor
- Fluid volume deficit *related to* inadequate intake
- Risk for aspiration *related to* impaired esophageal function
- Anxiety *related to* diagnosis of cancer, uncertain future, and poor prognosis
- Anticipatory grieving *related to* diagnosis of life-threatening malignancy
- Altered health maintenance *related to* lack of knowledge of disease process and therapeutic regimen, unavailability of a support system, and chronic debilitating disease

■ Planning

The overall goals are that the patient with esophageal cancer will (1) have relief of symptoms including pain and dysphagia, (2) achieve optimal nutritional intake, (3) understand the prognosis of the disease, and (4) experience a quality of life appropriate to disease progression.

■ Nursing Implementation

Health Promotion. Because the cause of esophageal cancer is not definitive, it is difficult to identify preventive measures. Health counseling should focus on elimination of smoking and excessive alcohol intake. Maintenance of good oral hygiene and dietary habits (intake of fresh fruits and vegetables) may also be helpful.

Having the patient obtain treatment of esophageal problems, such as Barrett's esophagus, is helpful because this is considered a premalignant condition. Early diagnosis of esophageal tumors is important but difficult because the onset of symptoms is usually late. The patient should be encouraged to have regular physical examinations and to seek medical attention for any esophageal problems, especially dysphagia. The patient who is at risk of esophageal adenocarcinoma, such as those with Barrett's esophagus, need regular (yearly) endoscopic screening with biopsy and cytologic study.

Acute Intervention

Preoperative care. In addition to general preoperative teaching and preparation, particular attention to the patient's nutritional needs and oral care is important. Many patients are poorly nourished because of the inability to ingest adequate amounts of food and fluids before surgery. A high-calorie, high protein diet is recommended. It may have to be in liquid form. Some patients may need IV fluid replacement or total parenteral nutrition. The patient and or family member is instructed on how to keep an intake and output record and assess for signs of fluid and electrolyte imbalance.

Meticulous oral care is essential. A thorough cleaning of the mouth, including tongue, gingivae, and teeth or dentures, is necessary. It may be necessary to use swabs or a gauze pad and to really scrub the mouth, including the tongue. Milk of magnesia with mineral oil may be used to remove crust formation. A mixture of mouthwash, ice, and water makes a refreshing rinse for the patient.

Teaching should include information about chest tubes (if a thoracic approach is used), IV lines, NG tube, gastrostomy feeding, turning, coughing, and deep breathing. (General preoperative care is presented in Chapter 16.)

Postoperative care. The patient usually has an NG tube in place, and there may be bloody drainage for 8 to 12 hours. The drainage gradually changes to greenish yellow. Assessment of the drainage, maintenance of the tube, and oral and nasal care are nursing responsibilities. The NG tube should not be repositioned or reinserted without consulting with the surgeon.

Because of the location of the incision and the general condition of the patient, special emphasis must be placed on prevention of respiratory complications. Turning and deep breathing should be done every 2 hours. Use of an incentive spirometer helps in preventing respiratory complications.

The patient should be positioned in a semi-Fowler's or Fowler's position to prevent reflux and aspiration of gastric secretions. When the patient can drink fluids or eat, the upright position should be maintained for at least 2 hours after eating to assist the movement of food through the GI tract.

Ambulatory and Home Care.
Many patients require long-term follow-up care after surgery for esophageal cancer. The patient may undergo radiation treatment following surgery. The patient needs encouragement and assistance in maintaining adequate nutrition. The patient may need a permanent feeding gastrostomy. The patient usually has fears and anxieties about a diagnosis of cancer. The nurse should know what the doctor has told the patient regarding the prognosis and then provide appropriate counseling. Some communities have resource groups consisting of persons with cancer who

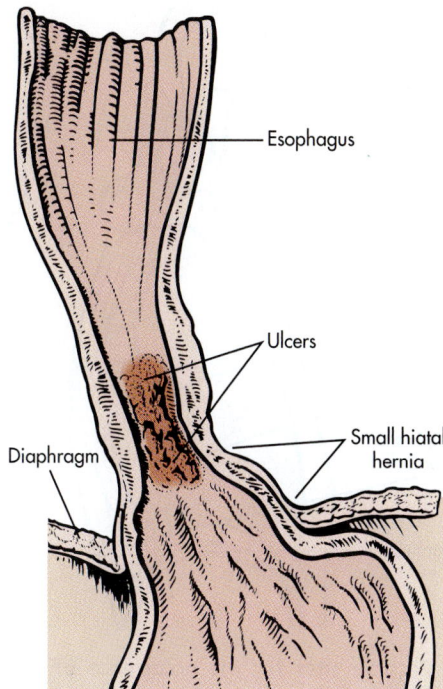

Fig. 39-8 Esophagitis with esophageal ulcerations.

can serve as support systems. Groups can usually be contacted through the local chapter of the American Cancer Society.

Referral to a home health nurse may be necessary for continued care of the patient (e.g., gastrostomy teaching and follow-up wound care). (Management of the terminally ill cancer patient is discussed in Chapter 14.)

■ Evaluation

The expected outcomes are that the patient with esophageal cancer will

- have relief of symptoms including pain and dysphagia
- achieve optimal nutritional intake
- understand the prognosis of the disease
- experience quality of life appropriate to disease progression

OTHER ESOPHAGEAL DISORDERS

Esophagitis

Esophagitis (inflammation of the esophagus) is a frequent condition and may occur as a result of chemical irritation from lye or dust or physical irritants such as smoking, cold or hot liquids, and excessive alcoholic intake. Trauma to the esophagus may also produce inflammation. *Achalasia* (cardiospasm) and carcinoma may lead to esophagitis. Esophagitis with esophageal ulcerations is shown in Fig. 39-8.

Reflux esophagitis is common. It results from the reflux of gastric contents into the esophagus (see section on Gastroesophageal Reflux Disease). A sliding hiatal hernia is a common cause of reflux esophagitis (see section on Hiatal Hernia),

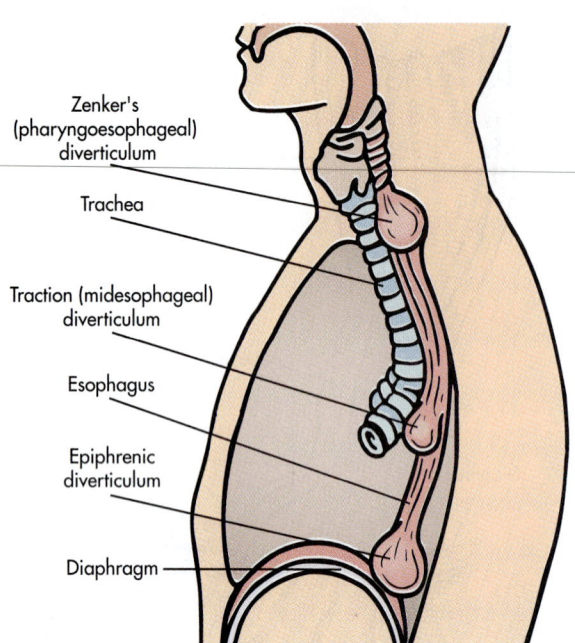

Fig. 39-9 Possible sites for the occurrence of esophageal diverticula. These hollow outpouchings may occur just above the upper esophageal sphincter (Zenker's, the most common type of pulsion diverticulum), near the midpoint of the esophagus (traction), and just above the lower esophageal sphincter (epiphrenic).

although it occurs in many patients without hiatal hernia. Esophagitis results from an incompetent LES.

Treatment of esophagitis depends on the cause. If strong alkalis or acids cause acute esophagitis, prompt, vigorous treatment is necessary. The treatment of chronic esophagitis includes oral antacids, agents that decrease acid secretion (histamine H_2-antagonists, proton pump inhibitors), dietary alterations (Table 39-8), and sleeping with the head of the bed elevated. The goal of treatment is to prevent gastric juices from damaging the esophageal mucosa.

Diverticula

Diverticula are saclike outpouchings of one or more layers of the esophagus. They occur in three main areas: (1) above the upper esophageal sphincter (Zenker's diverticulum), which is the most common location; (2) near the esophageal midpoint (traction); and (3) above the LES (epiphrenic) (Fig. 39-9). The main symptoms are dysphagia and regurgitation, especially with Zenker's diverticulum. Traction diverticula may not cause signs and symptoms. The patient frequently complains of tasting sour food and smelling a foul odor caused by the stagnant food. Complications include malnutrition, aspiration, and perforation.

There is no specific treatment for diverticula. Some patients find they can empty the pocket of food that collects by applying pressure at a point on the neck. The diet may have to be limited to foods that pass more readily (e.g., blenderized foods). Surgical removal of the diverticulum may be necessary if nutrition becomes disrupted. An alternative to surgery is endoscopic division of the septum between the diverticulum and the esophagus.

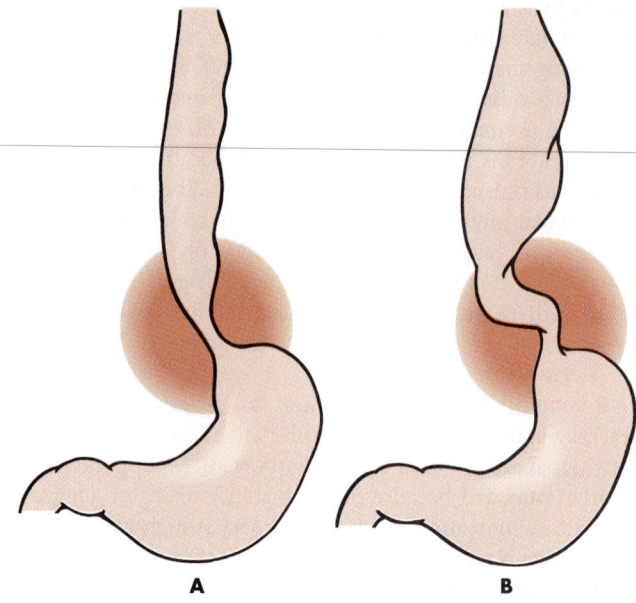

Fig. 39-10 Esophageal achalasia. **A,** Early stage, showing tapering of lower esophagus. **B,** Advanced stage, showing dilated, tortuous esophagus.

Esophageal Strictures

The most common causes of esophageal strictures are strong acids or alkalis that have been ingested and reflux or peptic strictures. Trauma such as throat lacerations and gunshot wounds may also lead to strictures as a result of scar formation from healing. The strictures usually develop over a long period of time. Strictures can be dilated endoscopically using bougies (dilating instruments). Another technique is balloon dilation, which is done under endoscopy and does not require fluoroscopy. Surgical excision with anastomosis is sometimes necessary. The patient may have a temporary or permanent gastrostomy.

Achalasia

In achalasia (*cardiospasm*), peristalsis of the lower two-thirds (smooth muscle) of the esophagus is absent. Pressure in the LES is increased, along with incomplete relaxation of the LES. Obstruction of the esophagus at or near the diaphragm occurs. Food and fluid accumulate in the lower esophagus. The result of this condition is dilation of the lower esophagus (Fig. 39-10). The altered peristalsis is a result of impairment of the autonomic nervous system innervating the esophagus. Achalasia affects all ages and both genders. The course of the disease is chronic.

Dysphagia is the most common symptom and occurs more frequently with liquids. Substernal chest pain (similar to the pain of angina) occurs during or immediately after a meal. Halitosis and the inability to eructate are other symptoms. Another common symptom is regurgitation of sour-tasting food and liquids, especially when the patient is in a horizontal position. Weight loss is typical.

Treatment consists of dilation, surgery, and use of drugs. All these therapies are directed at relieving the stasis caused by the increased LES pressure, nonrelaxing LES, and aperistaltic esophagus. The aim of management is to relieve symptoms.

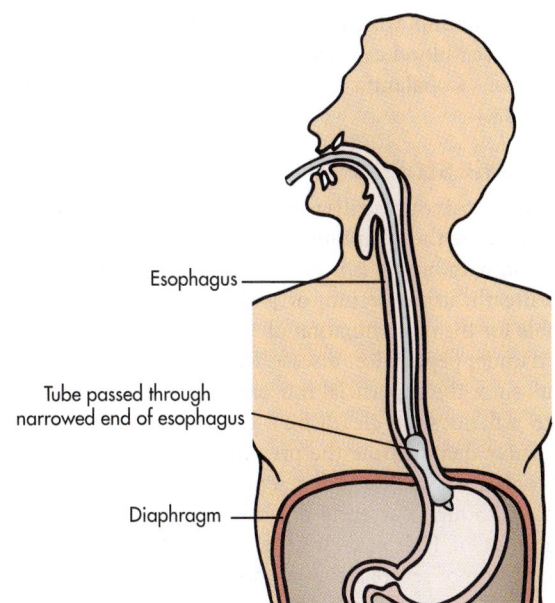

Fig. 39-11 Pneumatic dilation attempts to treat achalasia by maintaining an adequate lumen and decreasing lower esophageal sphincter (LES) tone.

Symptomatic treatment consists of a semisoft bland diet, eating slowly and drinking fluid with meals, and sleeping with the head elevated.

Esophageal dilation (*bougienage*) is an effective treatment measure for many patients. Pneumatic dilation of the LES with a balloon-tipped dilator passed orally is usually used. Commonly used dilators for pneumatic dilation are the Mosher bag, the Tucker mercury dilator, and the Browne-McHardy dilator. They all depend on forcible expansion of a balloon in the LES (Fig. 39-11). The forceful dilation does not restore normal esophageal motility, but it does provide for emptying of the esophagus into the stomach.

Surgical intervention may become necessary. An *esophagomyotomy* may be performed. In this procedure the muscle fibers that enclose the narrowed area of the esophagus are divided. This allows the mucosa to pouch out through the division in the muscle layer to allow food to be swallowed without obstruction.

A similar procedure is Heller's myotomy (cardiomyotomy), which disrupts the LES in a similar manner and reduces LES pressure. An antireflux procedure is frequently done with the myotomy. This procedure can be performed laparoscopically, reducing the potential for postoperative complications.

Classes of drugs used in the treatment of achalasia include anticholinergics, calcium channel blockers (e.g., nifedipine [Procardia]), and long-acting nitrates. Recent studies indicate a role for botulinum toxin injection, which relaxes esophageal muscle, delivered endoscopically in the management of achalasia.[20]

Esophageal Varices

Esophageal varices are dilated, tortuous veins occurring in the lower portion of the esophagus as a result of portal hypertension. Esophageal varices are a common complication of liver cirrhosis and are discussed in Chapter 41.

Table **39-12**	**Causes of Gastritis**
Aspirin	Smoking
Nonsteroidal anti-inflammatory drugs	Physiologic stress
	Shock
Corticosteroid drugs	Sepsis
Alcohol	Burns
Radiation	Psychologic stress
Helicobacter pylori	Renal failure (uremia)
Staphylococcus organisms	Spicy, irritating food
	Trauma
Salmonella	Nasogastric suction
Reflux of bile and pancreatic secretions	Large hiatal hernia
	Endoscopic techniques

GASTRITIS

Types

Gastritis, an inflammation of the gastric mucosa, is one of the most common problems affecting the stomach. Gastritis may be *acute* or *chronic* and may be diffuse or localized. Chronic gastritis can be further classified as type A (fundal) and type B (antral). Presently, the causes of gastritis and its relationship to other gastric disorders, such as gastric cancer, are the focuses of intensive research.

Etiology and Pathophysiology

Gastritis occurs as the result of a breakdown in the normal gastric mucosal barrier. This mucosal barrier normally protects the stomach tissue from autodigestion by acid and the enzyme pepsin. When the barrier is broken, acid can diffuse back into the mucosa. This allows hydrochloric (HCl) acid to enter. The HCl acid stimulates the conversion of pepsinogen to pepsin and stimulates the release of histamine from mast cells. The combined result of these occurrences is tissue edema, disruption of capillary walls with loss of plasma into the gastric lumen, and possible hemorrhage.

Causes of gastritis are listed in Table 39-12. Corticosteroids and nonsteroidal antiinflammatory drugs (NSAIDs) are known to inhibit the synthesis of prostaglandins, which then results in increased HCl acid secretion. Drugs such as aspirin, digitalis, and NSAIDs are directly irritating to the gastric mucosa. The ingestion of even small amounts of aspirin by the susceptible person is known to result in asymptomatic GI bleeding manifested by positive stool tests for occult blood. After an alcoholic drinking binge, acute damage to the gastric mucosa can range from local destruction of superficial epithelial cells to desquamation and destruction of the mucosa, with mucosal congestion, edema, and hemorrhage. Eating large quantities of spicy, irritating foods and metabolic conditions such as uremia can also cause acute gastritis.

Gastritis can occur from reflux of bile salts from the duodenum into the stomach as a result of anatomic changes following surgical procedures such as gastroduodenostomy and gastrojejunostomy. Prolonged vomiting may also cause reflux of bile salts. Intense emotional responses and CNS lesions may also produce inflammation of the mucosal lining as a result of hypersecretion of HCl acid.

Chronic exposure to the factors previously described (e.g., chronic alcohol abuse, excess ingestion of aspirin, reflux of duodenal contents after gastric surgery, uremia) will result in inflammation and eventual loss of viable mucosal tissue. This form of chronic gastritis can result from repeated episodes of acute gastritis.

Chronic gastritis, type A, is likely to be an autoimmune disorder. Approximately 95% of patients with pernicious anemia and 60% of patients with chronic atrophic gastritis have antibodies to parietal cells in their serum. Autoimmune atrophic gastritis affects both the fundus and body of the stomach and is associated with an increased risk of gastric malignancy.

Chronic gastritis, Type B, is related to the presence of *Helicobacter pylori* (*H. pylori*). Type B gastritis primarily involves the antrum of the stomach and is a common problem in adults.[21]

The presence of *H. pylori* also has been correlated with the presence of other gastric disorders, including gastric and duodenal ulcers and gastric cancer. A description of the epidemiology of *H. pylori* and its proposed role in the promotion of gastric disorders is discussed in the sections on peptic ulcers and gastric cancer. This section describes the current understanding of the mechanism by which *H. pylori* functions as a causative agent in chronic gastritis.

It is currently thought that *H. pylori* is acquired in childhood and is able to survive in the hostile environment of the gastric lumen. For reasons not clearly understood, *H. pylori* are capable of promoting the breakdown of the gastric mucosal barrier, given certain "triggers" or conditions. Thus given time, *H. pylori* will eventually have a destructive effect on its host environment. This is congruent with the finding that the incidence of chronic gastritis increases with age. However, studies also have shown that not all persons infected with *H. pylori* go on to develop chronic gastritis. Thus it may be that a combination of factors is at work to "turn on" the virulent process by which *H. pylori* damages the gastric mucosal barrier.

Progressive gastric atrophy from chronic alterations in the protective mucosal barrier causes the chief and parietal cells to eventually die. As the number of the acid-secreting parietal cells decreases with atrophy of the gastric mucosa, *hypochlorhydria* (decreased acid secretion) or *achlorhydria* (lack of acid secretion) occurs.

Clinical Manifestations

The symptoms of acute gastritis include anorexia, nausea and vomiting, epigastric tenderness, and a feeling of fullness. Hemorrhage is commonly associated with alcohol abuse and at times may be the only symptom. Acute gastritis is self-limiting, lasting from a few hours to a few days, with complete healing of the mucosa expected.

The manifestations of chronic gastritis are similar to those described for acute gastritis. Some patients have no symptoms directly associated with the gastric lesion. However, when the acid-secreting cells are lost or do not function as a result of atrophy, the source of intrinsic factor is also lost. Intrinsic factor, which normally combines with cobalamin (vitamin B_{12}), is unavailable, and thus cobalamin cannot be absorbed in the ileum. The intrinsic factor protects cobalamin from digestion by the GI enzymes. Eventually the body's storage of cobalamin in the liver is depleted and a deficiency state exists. Lack of this important vitamin, which is essential for the growth and maturation of red blood cells (RBCs), results in the development of anemia. (Cobalamin deficiency anemia is discussed in Chapter 28.)

Diagnostic Studies

Proper diagnosis of gastritis is frequently delayed or completely missed because the symptoms are nonspecific. Endoscopic examination with biopsy is necessary to obtain a definitive diagnosis. Breath, urine, serum, or gastric tissue biopsy tests are available for the determination of *H. pylori*. These tests are described under peptic ulcer disease. Radiographic studies are not helpful, since the superficial mucosa is generally involved, and changes will not show clearly on x-ray. A complete blood count (CBC) may demonstrate the presence of anemia from blood loss. Stools are tested for the presence of occult blood. A gastric analysis, although currently not used as much, demonstrates the amount of HCl acid present, with achlorhydria being a common sign of severe atrophic gastritis. Serum tests for antibodies to parietal cells and intrinsic factor may be performed. Cytologic examination is needed to rule out gastric carcinoma.

Collaborative Care

Elimination of the cause and preventing or avoiding it in the future are generally all that is needed to treat acute gastritis. The plan of care is supportive and similar to that described for nausea and vomiting. During the acute phase, bed rest, NPO status, and IV fluids may be prescribed. Fluids and electrolytes lost through vomiting and, occasionally, diarrhea are replaced. In severe cases an NG tube may be used, either for lavage of the precipitating agent from the stomach or in conjunction with suction to keep the stomach empty and free of noxious stimuli. Antiemetics are given for nausea and vomiting. Antacids have proved beneficial in the relief of abdominal discomfort by raising intragastric pH to above 6. H_2 antagonists, such as ranitidine (Zantac) or cimetidine (Tagamet), or proton pump inhibitors, such as omeprazole (Prilosec) or lansoprazole (Prevacid), may be prescribed to reduce gastric HCl acid secretion. Once *H. pylori* has been diagnosed, antibiotic therapy is initiated. Clear liquids are resumed when acute symptoms have subsided, with gradual reintroduction of solid, bland foods. Acute gastritis with hemorrhage is treated with blood transfusion and fluid replacement. Surgical intervention with partial gastrectomy, vagotomy, or pyloroplasty may be necessary if treatment fails.

The treatment of chronic gastritis focuses on evaluating and eliminating the specific cause (e.g., cessation of alcoholic intake, abstinence from drugs). Currently, double and triple antibiotic combinations are used to eradicate infection with *H. pylori* (Table 39-13). Triple therapy containing lansoprazole, clarithromycin, and amoxicillin is now available as Prevpac in one convenient package. For the patient with pernicious anemia, regular injections of cobalamin are needed (see Chapter 29). An individualized bland diet and use of antacids are recommended. Smoking is contraindicated in all forms of gastritis. The patient undergoing treatment for gastritis may have to adapt to many lifestyle changes and adopt a strict adherence to a medication regimen. An interdisciplinary team approach in which the physician, nurse, dietician, and pharmacist provide consistent information and support may increase the patient's success in making these alterations.

DRUG THERAPY

Table 39-13 *Helicobacter Pylori* Infection

Treatment	Duration	Eradication Rate
Original Triple Therapy		
Tetracycline		
Metronidazole (Flagyl)	14 days	>90%
Bismuth subsalicylate		
New Triple Therapy		
Amoxicillin		
Clarithromycin (Biaxin)	7 days	>90%
Omeprazole (Prilosec)		
Dual Therapy		
Amoxicillin or clarithromycin (Biaxin)		
Omeprazole (Prilosec)	14 days	60 - 80%

Table 39-14 Types of Upper Gastrointestinal Bleeding

Type	Clinical Manifestations
Obvious bleeding	
■ Hematemesis	Bloody vomitus appearing as fresh, bright red blood or "coffee ground" appearance (dark, grainy digested blood)
■ Melena	Black, tarry stools (often foul smelling) caused by digestion of blood in the GI tract. The black appearance is from the presence of iron
Occult bleeding	Small amounts of blood in gastric secretions, vomitus, or stools not apparent by appearance; detectable by guaiac test

NURSING MANAGEMENT: ACUTE GASTRITIS

■ Nursing Assessment

Dehydration can occur rapidly in severe gastritis that is accompanied by vomiting. Keeping the patient quiet, maintaining NPO status, and monitoring IV fluids are essential. If hemorrhage is considered likely, frequent checking of vital signs and testing the vomitus for blood are indicated. Elimination of the cause of the gastritis results in rapid improvement in the patient's condition. Identification of the causative agent is important to prevent future gastric irritation.

■ Nursing Diagnoses

The nursing diagnoses for the patient with nausea and vomiting (see NCP 39-1) are also applicable to the patient with gastritis.

■ Planning

The overall goals are that the patient with gastritis will (1) experience minimal or no symptoms of gastritis, (2) have no recurrent episodes of acute gastritis, and (3) achieve an optimal pattern of gastric function relative to the stage of the disease.

■ Nursing Implementation

The patient with gastritis should be encouraged to avoid causative factors and to follow the prescribed diet and medication regimen. Because the incidence of gastric cancer is higher in the patient who has a history of chronic gastritis, especially atrophic gastritis, close medical follow-up should be stressed.

Most patients with gastritis receive care in the home, and chronic management may be necessary for extended periods of time. A bland diet consisting of six small feedings a day and the use of an antacid after meals may help provide symptomatic relief. It is essential that the nurse have knowledge of the action and therapeutic effects of antisecretory and H_2 antagonists to teach the patient and to monitor drug effects. The care of the patient with chronic atrophic gastritis and gastric atrophy is also supportive. With advanced gastric atrophy, cobalamin injections may be necessary for the lifetime of the patient. Discussion of the continued need for this essential vitamin must be included in the plan of care.

The patient with severe dehydration and gastric bleeding may require acute intervention. All of the management strategies discussed in the section on gastric bleeding are also applicable to the patient with severe gastritis.

UPPER GASTROINTESTINAL BLEEDING

Etiology and Pathophysiology

Although the most serious loss of blood from the upper GI tract is characterized by a sudden onset, insidious occult bleeding can also be a major problem. The severity of bleeding depends on whether the origin is venous, capillary, or arterial. (Types of upper GI bleeding are presented in Table 39-14.) Bleeding from an arterial source is profuse, and the blood is bright red. The bright red color indicates that the blood has not been in contact with the stomach's acid secretions. In contrast, "coffee ground" vomitus reveals that the blood and other contents have been in the stomach for some time and have been changed by contact with gastric secretions. A massive upper GI hemorrhage is generally defined as a loss of more than 1500 ml of blood or a loss of 25% of intravascular blood volume. Despite improvements in detection and treatment of acute upper GI bleeding, the mortality rate remains around 10%. *Melena* (black, tarry stools) indicates slow bleeding from an upper GI source. The longer the passage of blood through the intestines, the darker the color of the stool as a result of the degradation of hemoglobin and the release of iron.

Discovering the cause of the bleeding is not always an easy task. A variety of areas in the GI tract may be involved, and there may be many different reasons for the blood loss. Table 39-15 lists the common causes of bleeding.

Esophageal Origin. Bleeding from an esophageal source is most likely the result of chronic esophagitis, bleeding from a tear in the mucosa near the esophagogastric junction (Mallory-Weiss tear or syndrome), or esophageal varices. Chronic esophagitis can be caused by the ingestion of chemicals including medications irritating to the mucosa or hot, spicy, irritating foods. Alcohol and cigarettes are known irritants of the esophageal mucosa. An incompetent lower

Table **39-15**	Common Causes of Upper Gastrointestinal Bleeding

Drug Induced	**Stomach and Duodenum**
Salicylates	Peptic ulcer disease
Corticosteroids	Stress ulcer
Nonsteroidal	Hemorrhagic gastritis
antiinflammatory agents	Carcinoma
Esophagus	Polyps
Esophageal varices	**Systemic Diseases**
Esophagitis	Blood dyscrasias
Mallory-Weiss syndrome	Leukemia
	Uremia

esophageal sphincter, which permits reflux of the acidic stomach contents into the esophagus, can lead to chronic irritation and erosion. Severe retching and vomiting can cause a tear in the esophageal mucosa resulting in severe bleeding.

Esophageal varices usually occur secondary to cirrhosis of the liver. Branches of the vena cava and the azygos vein from the systemic circulation converge with the smaller vessels of the lower esophagus. These vessels are inelastic and become engorged and tortuous because of increased pressure exerted on them secondary to portal hypertension. Anything that may increase the pressure (e.g., coughing, sneezing, trauma) or result in mechanical irritation (e.g., vomiting, irritation, erosion) may result in sudden, massive bleeding. (Esophageal varices are discussed in Chapter 41.)

Stomach and Duodenal Origin. Erosion of a blood vessel by a peptic ulcer located in the stomach or duodenum must always be considered as a possible cause of upper GI bleeding. Peptic ulcers account for more than 50% of cases of upper GI bleeding.[22] Ulcers frequently penetrate blood vessels. A gastric ulcer may penetrate the left gastric artery, and a duodenal ulcer may penetrate the superior pancreaticoduodenal artery.

Some medications, either prescribed by the physician or self-administered, have been implicated as a cause of upper GI bleeding. The patient who regularly takes aspirin or aspirin-containing compounds may be at risk for bleeding episodes. Aspirin, NSAIDs (e.g., ibuprofen), and corticosteroids, can cause irritation and disruption of the gastric mucosal barrier.[23] Aspirin-containing products are sold without prescriptions as OTC drugs (see Table 29-15). It is not unusual for a patient to deny the use of aspirin yet be self-medicating with aspirin-containing drugs, such as Alka-Seltzer, Bufferin, and Excedrin. A careful history of all commonly used medications is therefore necessary whenever upper GI bleeding is suspected.

Stress ulcers, which may occur after severe burn, trauma, or major surgery, erode more superficial blood vessels than does a peptic ulcer. They may also cause bleeding from erosion of a larger blood vessel. Gastritis produced by ingestion of drugs or alcohol or the reflux of bile from the small intestine can result in bleeding. Gastric carcinoma can be the cause of a steady blood loss as it grows and ulcerates through the mucosa and blood vessels located in its path. Hematemesis and melena are commonly associated with cancer of the stomach.

Systemic Diseases. Systemic diseases (e.g., leukemia, blood dyscrasias) that interfere with normal blood clotting must be considered whenever upper GI bleeding occurs.

Emergency Assessment and Management

Although approximately 80% of patients who have massive hemorrhage spontaneously stop bleeding, the cause must be identified and treatment initiated immediately. In spite of advances in intensive care, hemodynamic monitoring, and fiberoptic endoscopy, there has been little change in the mortality rate for upper GI bleeding, which has remained approximately 10% for the past 40 years. This is due in part to the greater incidence of upper GI bleeding in older adults, especially women, related to the use of NSAIDs agents.

Although a complete history of events leading to the bleeding episode is important in discovering the cause of the blood loss, it should be deferred until emergency care has been initiated. The immediate physical examination must include a systemic evaluation of the patient's condition with emphasis on blood pressure, rate and character of pulse, peripheral perfusion with capillary refill, and observation for the presence or absence of neck vein distention. Vital signs should be monitored every 15 to 30 minutes. Signs and symptoms of shock must be evaluated, and treatment should be started as soon as possible (see Chapter 61). The patient's respiratory status is carefully assessed, along with a thorough abdominal examination. The presence or absence of bowel sounds should be assessed and noted. A tense, rigid, boardlike abdomen may indicate a perforation and peritonitis.

Once the immediate interventions have begun, the patient or family should answer the following questions. Is there a history of previous bleeding episodes? Has weight loss been a recent problem? Has the patient received blood transfusions in the past, and were there any transfusion reactions? Is there a religious preference that prohibits the use of blood or blood products? Are there any other illnesses that may contribute to bleeding or interfere with treatment (e.g., congestive heart failure, diabetes mellitus)?

Laboratory studies are ordered, including a CBC, blood urea nitrogen (BUN), serum electrolytes, blood glucose, prothrombin time, liver enzymes, arterial blood gases (ABGs), and a type and cross-match for possible blood transfusions. All vomitus and stools should be tested for the presence of gross and occult blood. A urinalysis provides information on the presence of blood in the urine, and the specific gravity gives an immediate indication of the patient's hydration status.

IV lines, preferably two, with a 16- or 18-gauge needle should be established for fluid and blood replacement. The type and amount of fluids infused are dictated by physical and laboratory findings. It is generally best to begin with an isotonic crystalloid solution (e.g., lactated Ringer's solution). Whole blood, packed RBCs, and fresh frozen plasma may be used for replacement of lost volume in massive hemorrhage. Because of the potential for fluid overload and immunologic reactions, packed RBCs are often preferred over whole blood.[24] (The use of blood transfusions and volume expanders is discussed in Chapter 29.) The hemoglobin and hematocrit values are not of immediate assistance in estimating the degree of blood loss, but they provide a baseline for guiding further treatment. The initial hematocrit may be normal and may not reflect the loss until 4 to 6 hours after fluid replacement has taken place, since initially the loss of plasma and RBCs is equal. When upper GI bleeding is less profuse, infusion of isotonic saline solution followed by packed RBCs permits restoration of the hematocrit more quickly and does not create complications related to fluid volume overload. The use of supplemental oxygen delivered by face mask or nasal cannula may help increase blood oxygen saturation.[24]

For most patients who are bleeding profusely, an indwelling urinary catheter is inserted so that urine volume can be accurately assessed hourly. A central venous pressure line may be inserted so that the patient's fluid volume status can be monitored easily. A central venous pressure line is capable of monitoring right-sided heart pressure and function but does not reflect accurate left ventricular function. When a history of valvular heart disease, coronary artery disease, or congestive heart failure is elicited or when pulmonary edema is a factor, a pulmonary artery catheter may be necessary. An NG tube is indicated when the patient is vomiting blood. A large tube passed through the mouth may be more beneficial than a small one passed through the nose. Passage through the mouth is easier, but no tube should ever be advanced against resistance because of the likelihood of damaging the gastric mucosa or causing perforation. Aspiration of stomach contents through a large bore tube such as an Ewald tube facilitates the removal of clots from the stomach and alleviates the patient's need to vomit. In addition, the removal of gastric contents allows the stomach wall to collapse, contributing to hemostasis.

In 80% of cases, bleeding ceases spontaneously without any intervention. However, for many years it has been common practice to lavage the stomach with cool or ice water or saline solution through an NG tube to induce local vasoconstriction of the bleeding vessel. The value of lavage is now in question. Recent studies indicate that ice water lavage has no effect on the rate of bleeding from gastric ulcers and may actually impede the body's normal coagulation mechanism by inhibiting platelet function.[24] The major use for lavage is to ensure that blood will not interfere with emergency endoscopic visualization of the gastric mucosa. If used, the usual procedure for gastric lavage is to instill approximately 50 to 100 ml of tap water or saline solution each time, leave it in place for several minutes, and then allow drainage by gravity or low suction. This procedure may be repeated every 30 to 45 minutes.

Diagnostic Studies

Fiberoptic Panendoscopy. In addition to using endoscopic procedures to stop bleeding, these procedures also allow for direct visualization of the bleeding site. Fiberoptic panendoscopy, which should be used before either angiography or barium studies, is quite accurate in identifying the specific source of the bleeding. When a skilled practitioner performs the procedure, bleeding from severe gastritis can be easily distinguished from that of a gastric or duodenal ulcer.

Angiography. Angiography is used in diagnosing upper GI bleeding. It is used most commonly when the bleeding site is not seen by endoscopic procedures.[25] The procedure requires preparation and setup time and may not be appropriate for a high risk, unstable patient. In this procedure a catheter is placed into the left gastric or superior mesenteric artery and advanced until the site of bleeding is discovered.

Angiography is an invasive procedure and should be undertaken only if the patient has no allergies to the contrast medium, has adequate hydration and urinary output, and has no cardiovascular contraindications.

Barium Contrast Studies. Barium contrast studies have less immediate value in the identification of major bleeding sites during the acute phase of treatment. These studies are of little value if the bleeding is the result of gastritis or a shallow superficial ulcer. Barium studies can document an actual lesion but cannot verify that it is the bleeding source. If barium is used initially as a diagnostic tool and the bleeding intensifies, the barium will obscure and delay endoscopy and angiography until it has been cleared from the stomach.

Collaborative Care

Endoscopic Therapy. The goal of endoscopic hemostasis is to coagulate or thrombose the bleeding artery and then reduce the necessity of a surgical procedure. This procedure has proved useful in stopping the bleeding of gastritis, Mallory-Weiss syndrome, esophageal and gastric varices, bleeding peptic ulcers, and polyps. Several techniques are used including (1) thermal (heat) probe, (2) electrocoagulation probe, and (3) neodymium: yttrium-aluminum-garnet (Nd-YAG) laser. The heat probe is considered faster, safer, and more effective than the laser. It coagulates tissue by directly applying a heating element to the bleeding site. Endoscopic therapy is more effective than medical management alone in reducing bleeding episodes.[26]

Surgical Therapy. Surgical intervention is indicated when bleeding continues regardless of the therapy provided and when the site of the bleeding has been identified. A high percentage of patients are known to have another massive hemorrhage within 5 years after the first bleeding episode. Some physicians regard surgical therapy as necessary when the patient continues to bleed after rapid transfusion of up to 2000 ml of whole blood or remains in shock after 24 hours. The site of the hemorrhage determines the choice of operation. In addition, the surgeon must consider the age of the patient, since mortality rates increase considerably over the age of 60 years. It is essential that the operation be performed as soon as the need has been established.

Drug Therapy. During the acute phase, drugs are used to decrease bleeding, decrease HCl acid secretion, and neutralize the HCl acid that is present. Table 39-16 reviews their mechanism of action in relation to upper GI bleeding. Histamine H_2-receptor antagonists cimetidine (Tagamet), ranitidine (Zantac), famotidine (Pepcid), and nizatidine (Axid) and the proton pump inhibitors (e.g., omeprazole [Prilosec]) are well established in the treatment of peptic ulcer disease and in the prophylactic treatment of the patient at risk of stress-related upper GI hemorrhage. Although these drugs have no proven ability to control active bleeding, they have become part of standard treatment protocols. H_2-receptor antagonists inhibit the action of histamine at the H_2 receptors of parietal cells and thereby decrease acid secretion. Omeprazole inhibits the pump that is necessary for the secretion of HCl acid. The neutralizing effects of each of these medications are much longer than those of antacid therapy.

Vasopressin (Pitressin), which is posterior pituitary extract, can produce vasoconstriction and has been used to treat upper

DRUG THERAPY

Table 39-16 Gastrointestinal Bleeding

Drug	Source of GI Bleeding	Mechanism of Action
Antacids*	Duodenal ulcer, gastric ulcer, acute gastritis (corrosive, erosive, and hemorrhagic)	Neutralizes acid and maintains gastric pH above 5.5, elevated pH inhibits activation of pepsinogen
Histamine H_2-receptor antagonists Cimetidine (Tagamet), ranitidine (Zantac), famotidine (Pepcid), nizatidine (Axid)	Duodenal ulcer, gastric ulcer, esophagitis, acute gastritis (especially hemorrhagic)	Inhibits action of histamine at H_2-receptors of parietal cells and decreases acid secretion
Proton pump inhibitors Omeprazole (Prilosec), lansoprazole (Prevacid), pantoprazole (Pantoloc)	Same as above	Inhibits the cellular pump that is necessary for secretion of HCl acid
Vasopressin (Pitressin)	Acute gastritis (corrosive, erosive, and hemorrhagic), esophageal varices	Causes vasoconstriction and increases smooth muscle activity of the GI tract, reduces pressure in the portal circulation and arrests bleeding
Somatostatin analogue octreotide (Sandostatin)	Upper GI bleeding, esophageal varices	Decreases splanchnic blood flow, decreases acid secretion via decrease in release of gastrin

*See Table 39-21.

GI bleeding, especially in those patients who do not respond to other therapies and are poor surgical risks. It is administered systemically through a vein or intraarterially at the local site of actual bleeding. However, vasopressin should be used with caution in the patient with a known history of vascular disease. Other side effects of intravenously administered vasopressin include decreased myocardial contractility and decreased coronary blood flow. The patient undergoing vasopressin therapy must be closely monitored for its myocardial, visceral, and peripheral ischemic side effects.[27]

Early administration of the somatostatin analog octreotide (Sandostatin) has been shown to reduce upper GI bleeding related to esophageal varices and nonvariceal upper GI hemorrhage. This drug is given in IV boluses up to 5 to 6 days after the initiation of bleeding. Octreotide reduces splanchnic blood flow as well as inhibits the release of GI hormones such as gastrin, thereby decreasing HCl secretion.[28]

The injection of a vasoconstricting agent into the bleeding site has provided limited improvement in controlling upper GI bleeding. It is a simple procedure that requires little patient preparation. An agent such as epinephrine or norepinephrine (vasoconstrictors) is diluted and injected through the biopsy portal of the endoscope, causing the formation of submucosal deposits around the bleeding site. The resultant vasoconstriction and local inflammation compress the site, and bleeding is controlled.

Antacids have long been known to neutralize HCl acid and are used prophylactically in the management of peptic ulcer disease. Antacids are also beneficial to the healing process as well. Because antacids neutralize HCl acid and increase the pH of gastric contents to above 5, there is inhibition of the conversion of pepsinogen to its active form pepsin. The most frequently used antacid preparations are magnesium hydroxide, magnesium trisilicate, aluminum hydroxide, calcium carbonate, and sodium bicarbonate (see Table 39-21 later in this chapter). Aluminum hydroxide and magnesium trisilicates are the

most useful because they are nonabsorbable. Calcium carbonate and sodium bicarbonate are absorbable, and prolonged use can lead to systemic alkalosis.

The neutralizing effects of antacids taken on an empty stomach last only 20 to 30 minutes. When antacids are taken after meals, the effects may last as long as 3 to 4 hours. After the acute phase of bleeding has diminished, antacids are generally administered hourly, either orally or through the NG tube. If the tube is in place, the stomach contents should be aspirated and tested periodically for pH. If pH is less than 5, intermittent suction may be used, or the frequency or dosage of the antacid may be increased.

Sedatives to control agitation and restlessness should be administered cautiously. They make accurate assessment of the patient's condition more difficult. Anticholinergic drugs are contraindicated in acute upper GI bleeding episodes.

NURSING MANAGEMENT: UPPER GASTROINTESTINAL BLEEDING

■ Nursing Assessment

As the nurse begins care of the patient admitted with upper GI bleeding, a thorough and accurate nursing assessment is an essential first step. Subjective and objective data that should be obtained from the patient or significant others are presented in Table 39-17.

The patient experiencing upper GI bleeding may not be able to provide specific information about the cause of the bleeding until the immediate physical needs are met. An immediate nursing assessment should be performed while getting the patient ready for initial treatment. The assessment should include the patient's level of consciousness, vital signs, appearance of neck veins, skin color, and capillary refill. The abdomen should be checked for distention, guarding, and peristalsis. Immediate determination of vital signs indicates whether the patient is in

NURSING ASSESSMENT

Table 39-17 | Upper Gastrointestinal Bleeding

Subjective Data

Important Health Information

Past health history: Precipitating events before bleeding episode, previous bleeding episodes and treatment, peptic ulcer disease, esophageal varices, esophagitis, chronic gastritis, stress ulcers

Medications: Use of aspirin, nonsteroidal antiinflammatory drugs, corticosteroids, anticoagulants

Functional Health Patterns

Health perception–health management: Family history of bleeding, smoking, alcohol use

Nutritional-metabolic: Nausea, vomiting, weight loss; thirst

Elimination: Diarrhea; black, tarry stools; decreased urinary output; sweating

Activity-exercise: Weakness, dizziness, fainting

Cognitive-perceptual: Epigastric pain, abdominal cramps

Coping–stress tolerance: Acute or chronic stressors

Objective Data

General

Fever

Integumentary

Clammy, cool, pale skin; pale mucous membranes, nailbeds, and conjunctivae; spider angiomas; jaundice; peripheral edema

Respiratory

Rapid, shallow respirations

Cardiovascular

Tachycardia, weak pulse, orthostatic hypotension, slow capillary refill

Gastrointestinal

Red or coffee-ground vomitus; tense, rigid abdomen, ascites; hypoactive or hyperactive bowel sounds; black, tarry stools

Urinary

Decreased urinary output, concentrated urine

Neurologic

Agitation, restlessness; decreasing level of consciousness

Possible Findings

Decreased hematocrit and hemoglobin; hematuria; guaiac-positive stools, emesis, or gastric aspirate; decreased levels of clotting factors; elevated liver enzymes; abnormal upper GI studies or endoscopy results

---

shock from blood loss and also provides a baseline blood pressure and pulse by which to monitor the progress of treatment. Signs and symptoms of shock include low blood pressure; rapid, weak pulse; increased thirst; cold, clammy skin; and restlessness. Vital signs should be monitored every 15 to 30 minutes, and the physician should be informed of any significant changes.

When obtaining vital signs, the nurse should consider the patient's age and physical condition. Taking the blood pressure and pulse with the patient lying down and then sitting will indicate postural changes that occur after acute blood loss. The older the patient, the more changes in vital signs should be expected.

■ Nursing Diagnoses

Nursing diagnoses for the patient with upper GI bleeding include, but are not limited to, the following:

- Fluid volume deficit *related to* acute loss of blood
- Altered peripheral tissue perfusion *related to* loss of circulatory volume
- Altered renal and cerebral tissue perfusion *related to* decreased blood volume
- Anxiety *related to* upper GI bleeding, hospitalization, uncertain outcome, source of bleeding
- Ineffective individual coping *related to* situational crisis and personal vulnerability
- Risk for aspiration *related to* active bleeding and altered level of consciousness
- Potential complication: hypovolemic shock *related to* loss of blood

■ Planning

The overall goals are that the patient with upper GI bleeding will (1) have no further GI bleeding, (2) have the cause of the bleeding identified and treated, (3) experience a return to a normal hemodynamic state, and (4) experience minimal or no symptoms of pain or anxiety.

■ Nursing Implementation

Health Promotion. Although not all cases of upper GI bleeding can be anticipated and prevented, the nurse shares responsibility with the physician in trying to identify the patient who is at high risk. The patient with a history of chronic gastritis or peptic ulcer disease should always be considered in the high-risk category because of the increased incidence of bleeding associated with chronic irritation or chronic ulcers. The patient who has had one major bleeding episode is likely to have another within 5 years. This patient must be instructed to avoid irritating foods, prevent or decrease stress-inducing situations at home or at work, and take only prescribed medications. OTC medications can be harmful, since their contents may include drugs that are contraindicated because of their potentially irritating effects on the mucosa. This patient should be instructed in the methods of testing vomitus or stools for the presence of occult blood. Positive results should be promptly reported to the physician or the nurse. Close and frequent follow-up care is very important for all patients with ulcers because recurrence rates are high.

The patient who requires regular administration of ulcerogenic drugs, such as aspirin, corticosteroids, or NSAIDs, should receive instructions regarding the potential adverse effects these agents may have on the GI mucosa. These drugs should be avoided if at all possible. However, if aspirin must be prescribed, enteric-coated tablets can be substituted for regular tablets. Taking the medications with meals or snacks lessens the potential irritating effects. The use of an antacid along with the prescribed medication is usually beneficial.

For the patient at risk for gastric ulcers because of NSAID use, misoprostol (Cytotec) may be prescribed. In addition to inhibiting acid secretion, this prostaglandin analog may have a protective effect on the gastric mucosal barrier. This drug may reduce upper GI bleeding episodes associated with NSAID use. However, the drug has several important side effects including uterine cramping and diarrhea. Because of its effects on the uterus, it is contraindicated in women of childbearing age.[23]

When the nurse is working with the patient who has a history of cirrhosis of the liver with esophageal varices, the instructions must be specific regarding the importance of avoiding known irritants, such as alcohol and hot, spicy, irritating foods. The prompt treatment of an upper respiratory tract infection should be stressed. Severe coughing or sneezing can create increased pressure on the already fragile varices and may result in massive hemorrhage.

The patient who is known to have blood dyscrasias or liver dysfunction or who is taking cancer chemotherapeutic drugs has a potential bleeding problem because of altered hemostasis caused by a decrease in clotting factors and platelets. When these patients also have a history of ulcer disease, gastritis, varices, or drug and alcohol abuse, they should be carefully instructed regarding their disease process and medications, and they should be closely observed for bleeding.

Acute Intervention. The patient should be approached in a calm and assured manner to help decrease the level of anxiety. Caution should be used before administering sedatives for restlessness because it is one of the warning signs of shock and may be masked by the medication.

Once an infusion has been started, the IV line must be maintained for fluid or blood replacement. An accurate intake and output record is essential so that the patient's hydration status can be assessed. Urine output should be measured hourly. A rate of at least 0.5 ml/kg per hour indicates adequate renal perfusion. Lesser amounts may indicate renal ischemia secondary to loss of blood volume. Urine specific gravity should be measured because it gives additional information regarding the patient's hydration status. Consistent readings greater than 1.025 (normal is 1.005 to 1.025) indicate that the urine is extremely concentrated and that there is probably a low blood volume. The physician must be kept informed of these important parameters so that the IV solutions can be increased or decreased accordingly. If the patient has a central venous pressure line or pulmonary artery catheter in place, readings should be recorded every 1 to 2 hours. Hemodynamic monitoring provides an accurate and quick assessment of blood flow and pressure within the cardiovascular system (see Chapter 63).

The older adult or the patient with a history of cardiovascular problems should be observed closely for signs of fluid overload. However, the threat of volume overload and pulmonary edema must be a constant concern in all patients who are receiving large amounts of IV fluids within a short time. Therefore, auscultation of breath sounds and close observation of respiratory effort are important. Electrocardiographic (ECG) monitoring can also be used to evaluate cardiac function.

Foods such as beets or even swallowed mouthwash can give vomitus a bloody appearance. Unless the contents of the vomitus are checked for occult blood, false information may be recorded. Swallowed blood from a nosebleed must also be accurately noted to avoid misdiagnosis of an upper GI bleeding episode. When an NG tube is inserted, the nurse must pay special attention to keeping it in proper position and observing the aspirate for blood.

The majority of upper GI bleeding episodes cease spontaneously, even without intervention. Although the use of cool or iced gastric lavage is used in some institutions, its effectiveness is of questionable value. Therefore the nurse must understand the rationale for this therapy and the results that are anticipated. Either cool or iced tap water or saline solution may be used. Water has the advantage of being able to break up large clots more easily than saline solution, is less expensive, and is always available. A disadvantage of tap water is that it may create more electrolyte imbalance than would an isotonic saline solution.

When lavage is used, approximately 50 to 100 ml of fluid is instilled at a time into the stomach. The lavage fluid may be aspirated from the stomach or drained by gravity. When aspiration is the method used, it is important not to aspirate if resistance is felt. The tip of the NG tube may be up against the gastric mucosal lining. The constant pressure from attempts to aspirate the lavage fluid may cause erosion of the mucosa. When resistance is a factor, the nurse should use gravity as the alternative method of gastric drainage. Close monitoring of vital signs, especially in the patient with a heart problem, is important because arrhythmias may occur. Keeping the patient warm and the head of the bed elevated provide comfort and prevent possible aspiration problems.

The nurse caring for a patient with upper GI bleeding should be well informed as to what constitutes blood in the stools. Black, tarry stools are not usually associated with a brisk hemorrhage but are indicative of the presence of bleeding of prolonged duration. Bright red blood in the stool is usually from a source in the lower bowel. When vomitus contains blood but the stool contains no gross or occult blood, the hemorrhage is considered to have been of short duration. Menses and bleeding hemorrhoids should be ruled out as possible sources of blood in the stools.

Monitoring the patient's laboratory studies enables the nurse to estimate the effectiveness of therapy. The hemoglobin and hematocrit are usually evaluated about every 4 to 6 hours if the patient is actively bleeding. At first the hematocrit may not accurately reflect the amount of blood lost or the amount of blood replaced and will appear falsely high or low. The patient's BUN level is assessed. It is generally elevated with a significant hemorrhage, since blood proteins are subjected to bacterial breakdown in the GI tract. However, renal disease may also result in an elevated BUN level. Many patients receive oxygen by mask or nasally so that the circulating blood is ensured of an adequate oxygen content.

When oral nourishment is begun, the patient is observed for symptoms of nausea and vomiting and a recurrence of bleeding. Feedings initially consist of clear fluids or milk and are given hourly until tolerance is determined. These feedings help neutralize the gastric secretions and assist in the mucosal repair. Gradual introduction of bland foods follows if the patient exhibits no signs of discomfort.

Antacids are sometimes used after upper GI bleeding to reduce the acidity of gastric contents. Anticipating the effects of the prescribed preparations can be helpful in providing better care. The nurse should know that preparations containing calcium or aluminum may result in constipation, whereas those

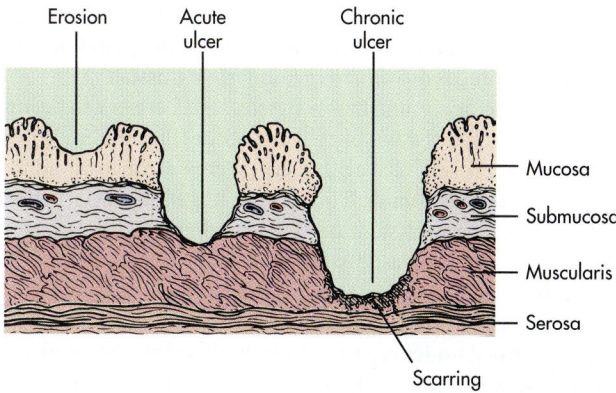

Fig. 39-12 Peptic ulcers, including an erosion, acute ulcer, and chronic ulcer. Both the acute and chronic ulcer may penetrate the entire wall of the stomach.

with magnesium cause diarrhea. Although these preparations are generally nonabsorbable and result in fewer systemic problems, magnesium products must be used cautiously in the patient with renal insufficiency. Administering the antacid preparation accurately and on schedule is important if the stomach pH is to be maintained at a level no lower than 5.

The patient in whom hemorrhage was the result of chronic alcohol abuse requires close observation for the beginning of delirium tremens as withdrawal from alcohol takes place. Symptoms indicating the beginning of delirium tremens are agitation, uncontrolled shaking, sweating, and vivid hallucinations. (Alcohol withdrawal is discussed in Chapter 10.)

Ambulatory and Home Care. The patient and family must be taught how to avoid future bleeding episodes. Ulcer disease, drug or alcohol abuse, and liver and respiratory diseases can all result in upper GI bleeding. The patient and family must be made aware of the consequences of noncompliance with diet and drug therapy. It must be emphasized that no medications (especially aspirin) other than those prescribed by the physician should be taken. Smoking and alcohol should be eliminated because they are sources of irritation and interfere with tissue repair. The need for long-term follow-up care may be necessary because of the possibility of another bleeding episode. The patient and family should be instructed on what to do if an acute hemorrhage occurs in the future.

■ Evaluation

The expected outcomes are that the patient with upper GI bleeding will

- have no further GI bleeding
- have the cause of the bleeding identified and treated
- experience a return to a normal hemodynamic state
- experience minimal or no symptoms of pain or anxiety

PEPTIC ULCERS

Peptic ulcer is an erosion of the GI mucosa resulting from the digestive action of HCl acid and pepsin. Any portion of the GI tract that comes into contact with gastric secretions is susceptible to ulcer development, including the lower esophagus, stomach, duodenum, and margin of gastrojejunal anastomosis after

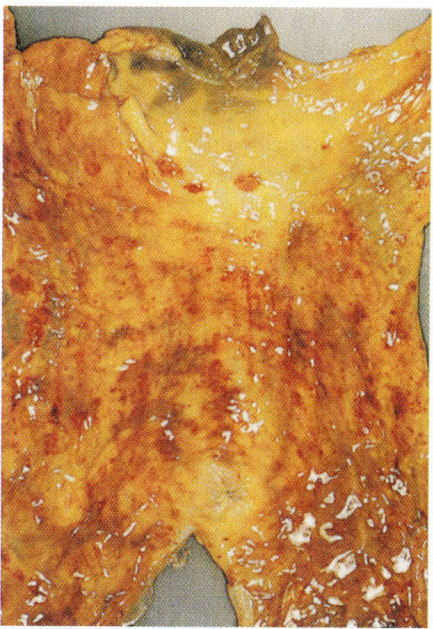

Fig. 39-13 Acute erosive gastritis. Acute erosive gastritis is shown in the opened stomach. The mucosa appears hyperemic, and the foci of superficial ulceration are manifest as scattered, small, red areas termed erosions.

surgical procedures. It is estimated that approximately 10% of men and 4% of women in the United States will have duodenal ulcers during their lifetimes.

Types

Peptic ulcers can be classified as *acute* or *chronic,* depending on the degree of mucosal involvement (Fig. 39-12), and *gastric* or *duodenal,* according to the location. The acute ulcer (Fig. 39-13) is associated with superficial erosion and minimal inflammation. It is of short duration and resolves quickly when the cause is identified and removed. A chronic ulcer (Fig. 39-14) is one of long duration, eroding through the muscular wall with the formation of fibrous tissue. It is present continuously for many months or intermittently throughout the person's lifetime. A chronic ulcer is at least four times as common as acute erosion. Gastric and duodenal ulcers, although defined as peptic ulcers, are distinctly different in their etiology and incidence (Table 39-18). Generally, the treatment of all types of ulcers is quite similar.

Etiology and Pathophysiology

Pepsinogen, the precursor of pepsin, is activated to pepsin in the presence of HCl acid and a pH of 2 to 3. HCl acid is secreted by the parietal cells at a pH of 0.8. After mixing with the stomach contents, the pH reaches 2 to 3, a highly favorable range of acidity for pepsin activity. When the stomach acid level is neutralized by the presence of food or antacids, the pH is increased to 3.5 or more. At a pH of 3.5 or more, pepsin has little or no proteolytic activity.

Peptic ulcers develop only in the presence of an acid environment. It has been well established that the patient with pernicious anemia and achlorhydria rarely has gastric ulcers. An excess of gastric acid may not be necessary for ulcer development.

The typical person with a gastric ulcer has normal to less than normal gastric acidity compared with the person with a duodenal ulcer. However, some intraluminal acid does seem to be essential for a gastric ulcer to occur.

The stomach is normally protected from autodigestion by the gastric mucosal barrier. The GI tract has a high cell turnover rate, and the surface mucosa of the stomach is renewed about every 3 days. As a result of this high turnover rate, the mucosa can continually repair itself except in extreme instances when the cell breakdown surpasses the cell renewal rate. Normally, water, electrolytes, and water-soluble substances (e.g., glucose)

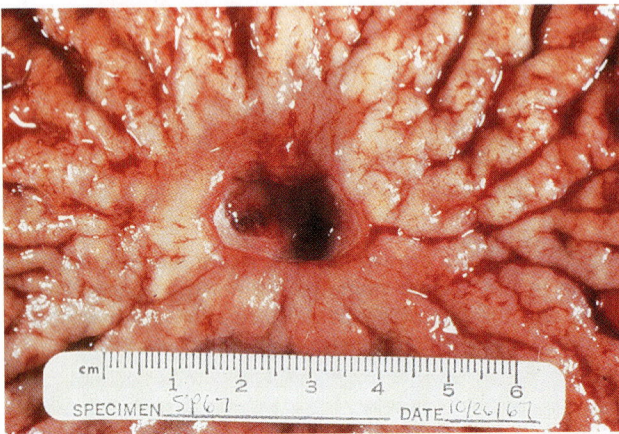

Fig. 39-14 Photograph of a chronic peptic ulcer located in lesser curvature of stomach.

can easily pass through the barrier. However, the mucosal barrier prevents the back diffusion of acid from the gastric lumen through the mucosal layers to the underlying tissue.

Under specific circumstances the mucosal barrier can be impaired and back-diffusion of acid can occur (Fig. 39-15). When the barrier is broken, HCl acid freely enters the mucosa and injury to the tissues occurs. This results in cellular destruction and inflammation. Histamine is released from the damaged mucosa, resulting in vasodilation and increased capillary permeability. The released histamine is then capable of stimulating further secretion of acid and pepsin.

As described under gastritis, a variety of agents are known to destroy the mucosal barrier. By generating ammonia in the mucous layer, *H. pylori* may create a condition of chronic inflammation, rendering the mucosa especially vulnerable to other noxious substances.[10] Ulcerogenic drugs, such as aspirin and aspirin-like agents, inhibit synthesis of mucus and prostaglandins and cause abnormal permeability. Corticosteroids have the ability to decrease the rate of mucous cell renewal and thereby decrease its protective effects. Lipid-soluble cytotoxic drugs can pass through the barrier and destroy it.

When the mucosal barrier is disrupted, there is a compensatory increase in blood flow. This phenomenon can occur in several ways. Prostaglandin-like substances and histamine act as vasodilators, thus increasing capillary blood flow. As blood flow increases within the affected mucosa, hydrogen ions are rapidly removed from the area, buffers are delivered to help neutralize the hydrogen ions present, nutrients necessary for cell function arrive, and the rate of mucosal cell replication increases. When blood flow is not sufficient to carry out these events, tissue in-

Table **39-18** Comparison of Gastric and Duodenal Ulcers		
	Gastric Ulcers	**Duodenal Ulcers**
Lesion	Superficial; smooth margins; round, oval, or cone-shaped	Penetrating (associated with deformity of duodenal bulb from healing of recurrent ulcers)
Location of lesion	Predominantly antrum, also in body and fundus of stomach	First 1-2 cm of duodenum
Gastric secretion	Normal to decreased	Increased
Incidence	▪ Greater in women ▪ Peak age fifth to sixth decade ▪ More common in persons of lower socioeconomic status and in unskilled laborers ▪ Increased with smoking, drug, and alcohol use ▪ Increased with incompetent pyloric sphincter ▪ Increased with stress ulcers after severe burns, head trauma, and major surgery	▪ Greater in men, but increasing in women especially postmenopausal ▪ Peak age 35-45 yr ▪ Associated with psychologic stress ▪ Increased with smoking, drug, and alcohol use ▪ Associated with other diseases (e.g., chronic obstructive pulmonary disease, pancreatic disease, hyperparathyroidism, Zollinger-Ellison syndrome, chronic renal failure)
Clinical manifestations	▪ Burning or gaseous pressure in high left epigastrium and back and upper abdomen ▪ Pain 1-2 hr after meals; if penetrating ulcer, aggravation of discomfort with food ▪ Occasional nausea and vomiting, weight loss	▪ Burning, cramping, pressurelike pain across midepigastrium and upper abdomen; back pain with posterior ulcers ▪ Pain 2-4 hr after meals and midmorning, midafternoon, middle of night, periodic and episodic ▪ Pain relief with antacids and food; occasional nausea and vomiting
Recurrence rate	High	High
Complications	Hemorrhage, perforation, outlet obstruction, intractability	Hemorrhage, perforation, obstruction

jury results. When the increase is sufficient to dilute, buffer, and remove the excess hydrogen ions, tissue damage may be minimal or may result in no injury at all. Figure 39-16 shows a representation of the interrelationship between the mucosal blood flow and disruption of the gastric mucosal barrier.

Although gastric ulcers are characterized by a normal to low secretion of gastric acid, the back-diffusion of acid is greater with chronic gastric ulcers than with duodenal ulcers or in the normal person. Therefore the critical pathologic process in gastric ulcer formation may not be the amount of acid that is secreted but the amount that is able to penetrate the mucosal barrier.

The gastric mucosa is also protected from the damage of ulceration by two other mechanisms. First, mucus is secreted by superficial mucous cells and forms a layer that can entrap or slow the diffusion of hydrogen ions across the mucosal barrier. Second, bicarbonate is secreted by the gastric and duodenal mucosa, and this helps neutralize HCl acid in the lumen of the GI tract.

Increased vagal nerve stimulation from a variety of causes (e.g., emotions) causes hypersecretion of HCl acid. Increased concentrations of HCl acid can alter the mucosal barrier. Duodenal ulcers are associated with high acid content. The fact that the person with duodenal ulcers is more vulnerable to the effects of emotional stressors may be one reason acid levels are above normal. It has been suggested that the continual response of the parietal cells to maximal stimulation results in hyperplasia of the cell mass. There is also an increase in gastrin levels in most persons with duodenal ulcers.

Gastric Ulcers. Although gastric ulcers can occur in any portion of the stomach, they are most commonly found on the lesser curvature in close proximity to the antral junction.

Before 1900, gastric ulcers were more common than duodenal ulcers, and they were found predominantly in young women. Since the turn of the century, the incidence of gastric ulcers has decreased, and they are now surpassed in incidence by duodenal ulcers by a ratio of 4:1. Gastric ulcers remain more prevalent in women and in older adults.

The mortality rate from gastric ulcers is greater than that from duodenal ulcers because the peak incidence of gastric ulcers occurs in persons over 50 years of age. Contrary to common belief, gastric ulcers are not more prevalent among those in executive or managerial positions. Persons from the lower socioeconomic class and manual or unskilled workers are more prone to gastric ulcers.

The understanding of the factors that contribute to ulcer formation is developing rapidly at the present time. As described previously in the section concerning gastritis (p. 1102), the discovery of the bacterium *H. pylori* provides a new understanding of ulcer formation. *H. pylori* are thought to be a dominant factor in the promotion of peptic ulcer formation. Although many questions remain to be answered regarding *H. pylori*, it survives in the human upper GI tract for long periods of time as a result of its ability to move in mucus and attach to mucosal cells. In addition, it secretes a substance called urease, which buffers the area around the bacterium and protects it from destruction in an acidic environment. Infection with *H. pylori* is highest in underdeveloped countries and in persons of low socioeconomic status. Although the routes of transmission are largely unknown, it is thought that infection occurs during childhood via transmission from family members to the child, possibly through an oral-oral route. In the United States and Canada, persons born before 1940 have a significantly higher risk of carrying *H. pylori* than persons in younger age groups.[29] This enhanced prevalence in older persons has been attributed to the presence of crowded living conditions and poor sanitation practices, which were more common in the earlier part of the 1900s.

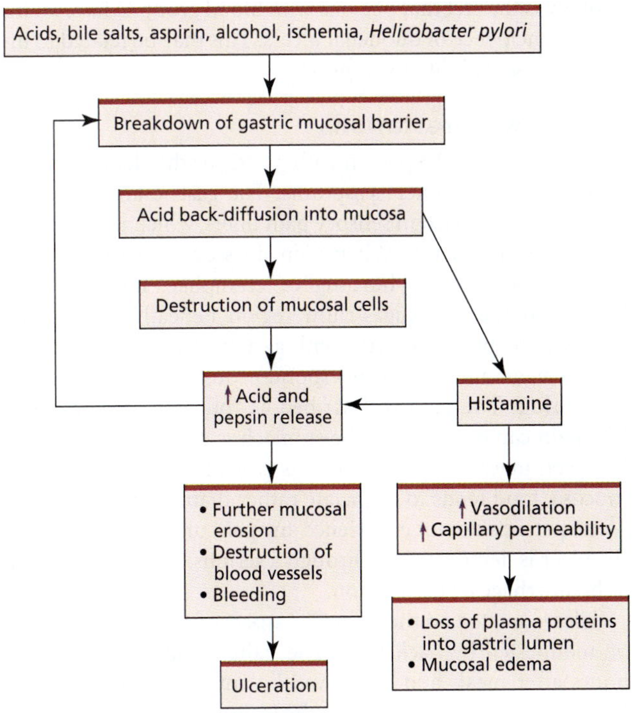

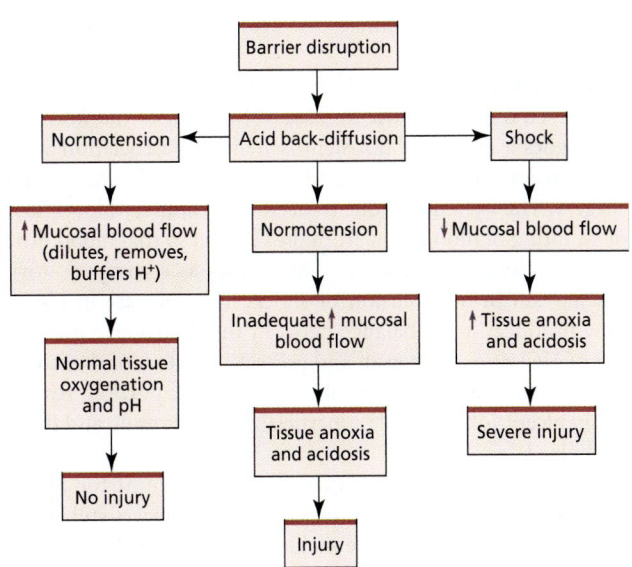

Fig. 39-15 Disruption of gastric mucosa and pathophysiologic consequences of back diffusion of acids.

Fig. 39-16 The relationship between mucosal blood flow and disruption of the gastric mucosal barrier.

Research into a genetic cause for ulcers has shown that some members of the same family are more prone to develop gastric or duodenal ulcers. Evidence is not complete, however, and the ulcer development could just as well be due to the sharing of the same environment. For example, the transmission of *H. pylori* may be increased by crowded living conditions. Gastric ulcer personality has not been demonstrated, yet ulcer-prone persons do appear to react to stress with more frustration, fear, anxiety, and guilt than do those who are less predisposed to ulcer formation. It is thought that destruction of the gastric mucosa by noxious agents such as drugs or smoking may be enhanced by the presence of *H. pylori*, which further promotes gastric mucosal destruction as described in the previous section on gastritis.

It is rare for gastric ulcers to become malignant, but transformation may occur in about 1% of all cases. When there is any doubt, a biopsy of the gastric mucosa should be performed during endoscopy to differentiate between a benign ulcer and a malignant neoplasm.

Gastric ulcers have also been attributed to various factors that can lead to acute episodes or to chronic involvement. Drugs and physiologically stressful situations can precipitate acute gastric lesions.

Medication-induced ulcers. Medications can cause acute gastric ulcers and in some cases can lead to the development of chronic ulcers. The drugs most often implicated include aspirin, corticosteroids, NSAIDs (e.g., ibuprofen), and reserpine. It is estimated that 2% to 4% of patients taking NSAIDs for 1 year experience serious GI complications including gastric ulcer, upper GI hemorrhage, or perforation.[22] Other known causative factors of gastric ulcer formation are chronic alcohol abuse, gastritis, and bile reflux gastritis from an incompetent pyloric sphincter. Caffeine is known to stimulate gastric acid secretion. Cigarette smoking is positively linked with gastric ulcer. One proposed theory is that smoking causes a reduction of pancreatic bicarbonate secretion, thus creating a decreased pH in the duodenum. In addition, nicotine seems to enhance reflux of duodenal contents into the antrum of the stomach. The ingestion of hot, rough, or spicy foods has been suggested as a causative factor, but there is no evidence to substantiate this claim.

Stress ulcers. A *stress ulcer* is a form of erosive gastritis. It is believed that the gastric mucosa of the body of the stomach undergoes a period of transient ischemia in association with hypotension, severe injury, extensive burns, and complicated surgery. The ischemia is due to decreased capillary blood flow or shunting of blood away from the GI tract so that blood flow bypasses the gastric mucosa. This occurs as a compensatory mechanism in hypotension or shock. The decrease in blood flow produces an imbalance between the destructive properties of HCl acid and pepsin and protective factors of the stomach's mucosal barrier, especially in the fundic portion, resulting in ulceration. Multiple superficial erosions result, and these may bleed.

Duodenal Ulcers. Duodenal ulcers account for about 80% of all peptic ulcers. Although duodenal ulcers still affect more men than women, the incidence of duodenal ulcers has followed a downward trend in men and a steady increase in women. The explanation for this change has not been clearly identified. However, it is possible that the overuse of aspirin

and NSAIDs and increased consumption of alcohol by women may partially account for this increased incidence. Duodenal ulcers may occur at any age, but the incidence is especially high between the ages of 35 and 45 years.

Whereas many factors are thought to contribute to the formation of duodenal ulcers, *H. pylori* has been identified as playing a key role. The prevalence of *H. pylori* infection in duodenal ulcer patients has consistently been found to be between 95% and 100%. However, a clear-cut direct causal relationship between *H. pylori* and duodenal ulcer formation has not yet been proven. Although duodenal ulcers often occur in persons susceptible to psychologic pressures and anxieties, this theory of causation requires more study. It is known that a duodenal ulcer can develop in anyone, regardless of occupation or socioeconomic group. The development of duodenal ulcers is associated with a high HCl acid secretion. Several diseases have been identified with a high risk of duodenal ulcer development, including chronic obstructive pulmonary disease, cirrhosis of the liver, chronic pancreatitis, hyperparathyroidism, chronic renal failure, and the Zollinger-Ellison syndrome. A high HCl acid concentration is believed to be the factor common to all these conditions. It is possible that the treatment of these conditions may also have detrimental effects on the gastric mucosa. Alcohol ingestion and heavy smoking habits are also associated with duodenal ulcer formation, since both are known irritants to the GI mucosa.

Pregnancy appears to protect women from developing ulcers. Estrogen and progesterone have demonstrated positive effects on ulcer healing. Progesterone has also been noted to lower acid secretion to a small degree. There is evidence that women past menopause, who no longer have this endocrine protection, develop ulcers at the same rate as men.

As with gastric ulcers, some persons in certain families are more prone to duodenal ulcer formation. Supporting a genetic etiology is the fact that persons with blood group O have an increased incidence of duodenal ulcers. This may be related to increased susceptibility to *H. pylori*.

Clinical Manifestations

It is common for the person with gastric or duodenal ulcers to have no pain or other symptoms. The gastric and duodenal mucosas are not rich in sensory pain fibers, which may account for this phenomenon. When pain does occur with duodenal ulcer, it is described as "burning" or "cramplike." It is most often located in the midepigastrium region beneath the xiphoid process. The pain associated with gastric ulcers is located high in the epigastrium and occurs spontaneously about 1 to 2 hours after meals. The pain is described as "burning" or "gaseous." The pain can occur when the stomach is empty or when food has been ingested. If the ulcer has eroded through the gastric mucosa, food tends to aggravate rather than alleviate the pain. Some persons do not experience any pain until the presence of the ulcer is demonstrated through a serious complication such as hemorrhage or perforation.

Ulcers located on the posterior aspect of the duodenum can be manifested by back pain. The pain usually occurs 2 to 4 hours after meals and is relieved by antacids and sometimes foods that neutralize and dilute the HCl acid. A characteristic of duodenal ulcer is its tendency to occur continuously for a few weeks or months and then disappear for a time, only to recur

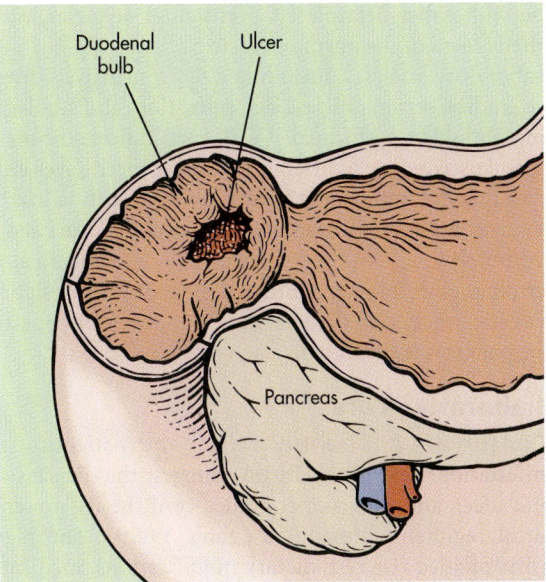

Fig. 39-17   Duodenal ulcer of the posterior wall penetrating into the head of the pancreas, resulting in walled-off perforation.

some months later. Some patients claim their symptoms worsen in the spring and fall of the year, thus strengthening the concept of a seasonal trend in occurrence. This course of events usually lasts throughout the entire life span of the ulcer.

Complications

The three major complications of chronic peptic ulcer disease are hemorrhage, perforation, and gastric outlet obstruction. All are considered emergency situations and are initially treated conservatively. However, surgery may become necessary at any time during the course of the therapy.

Hemorrhage. Hemorrhage is the most common complication of peptic ulcer disease. It develops from erosion of the granulation tissue found at the base of the ulcer during healing or from erosion of the ulcer through a major blood vessel. Duodenal ulcers account for a greater percentage of upper GI bleeding episodes than gastric ulcers.

Perforation. Perforation is considered the most lethal complication of peptic ulcer. Perforation is commonly seen in large penetrating duodenal ulcers that have not healed and are located on the posterior mucosal wall (Fig. 39-17). Perforated gastric ulcers are most frequently located on the lesser curvature of the stomach. Even though duodenal ulcers are more prevalent and perforate more frequently, mortality rates associated with perforation of gastric ulcers are higher. The older age of the patient with gastric ulcers, who often has other concurrent medical problems, is thought to be the crucial factor.

Perforation of a peptic ulcer occurs when the ulcer penetrates the serosal surface, with spillage of either gastric or duodenal contents into the peritoneal cavity. The size of the perforation is directly proportional to the length of time the patient has had the ulcer. The larger the perforation, the longer the history of the ulcer. Small perforations seal themselves and result in a cessation of symptoms; larger perforations require immediate surgical closure. Spontaneous sealing occurs as a result of large amounts of fibrin being produced in

response to the perforation. This leads to fibrinous fusion of the duodenum or gastric curvature to adjacent tissue, mainly the liver.

The clinical manifestations of perforation are characterized by their sudden and dramatic onset. The patient experiences sudden, severe upper abdominal pain that quickly spreads throughout the abdomen. The visceral and parietal layers of the peritoneum have an abundance of pain receptors, and this contributes to the abrupt, intense pain experienced. There may be shoulder pain if the spillage causes irritation to the phrenic nerve. The abdominal muscles contract, appearing rigid and boardlike as they attempt to protect the abdomen from further injury. The patient's respirations become shallow and rapid. Bowel sounds are usually absent. Nausea and vomiting may occur but are generally absent. Many patients report a history of ulcer disease or recent symptoms of indigestion.

The contents entering the peritoneal cavity from the stomach or duodenum contain a variety of ingredients that include air, saliva, food particles, HCl acid, pepsin, bacteria, bile, and pancreatic fluid and enzymes. A bacterial peritonitis may occur within 6 to 12 hours, followed by paralytic ileus. The intensity of the peritonitis is proportional to the amount and duration of the spillage through the perforation. It is difficult to determine from the sudden onset of symptoms whether gastric or duodenal ulcer is the cause, since the clinical characteristics of intestinal perforation are the same (see Chapter 40).

Gastric Outlet Obstruction. Ulcers located in the antrum and the prepyloric and pyloric areas of the stomach and the duodenum are predisposed to obstruction. In the early phase of obstruction (often referred to as the *compensated phase*), gastric emptying is normal to near normal. This phase may be associated with large peristaltic waves. Over time, excessive peristalsis creates hypertrophy of the stomach wall. After long-standing obstruction the stomach enters the *decompensated phase*, which results in dilation and atony. The obstruction is not totally due to fibrous scar tissue because active ulcer formation is associated with edema, inflammation, and pylorospasm, all of which contribute to the narrowing of the pylorus.

The patient with gastric outlet obstruction generally has a long history of ulcer pain. Ulcerlike pain of short duration or complete absence of pain is more indicative of a malignant obstruction. The pain progresses to a more generalized upper abdominal discomfort that becomes worse toward the end of the day as the stomach fills and dilates. Relief may be obtained by belching or by self-induced vomiting. Vomiting is common and often projectile. The vomitus contains food particles that were ingested many hours or even a day or two before the vomiting episode. There is often an offensive odor if the contents have been dormant in the stomach for a time. The patient who vomits frequently will be anorectic, with evident weight loss, and will complain of thirst and an unpleasant taste in the mouth. Constipation is a common complaint that usually results from dehydration and lack of roughage in the diet.

The patient with gastric outlet obstruction may show a swelling in the upper abdomen indicating dilation of the stomach. Loud peristalsis can be heard, and visible peristaltic waves are often observed passing across the abdomen from left to right. If the stomach is grossly dilated, it is possible to palpate it as well.

An upper GI examination with barium as contrast medium is helpful in making a diagnosis, and it demonstrates the presence of an active ulcer crater or scarring from previously healed ulcers. Barium normally should pass from the stomach within 2 hours, but with gastric outlet obstruction, 50% of the barium remains on follow-up films up to 6 hours later.

Diagnostic Studies

The diagnostic measures used to determine the presence and location of a peptic ulcer are similar to those with acute upper GI bleeding. *Fiberoptic endoscopy* is the procedure most often used. It is more reliable than barium contrast studies because of the maneuverability of fiberoptic scopes for viewing the entire gastric and duodenal mucosa. This procedure can also be used to determine the degree of ulcer healing after treatment. During endoscopy, specimens can be obtained for identification of *H. pylori*. When gastric malignancy is a possibility, the endoscope also can be used in obtaining tissue specimens for biopsy.

There are currently four diagnostic tests available to confirm *H. pylori* infection: serologic (blood) test,[13] C-urea breath test, histology of mucosa, and the Campylobacter-like organism test.[28] The blood test measures anti–*H. pylori* IgG, IgA, and IgM and is useful in patients who have not been treated with antibiotics. However, because of the length of time that IgG levels remain elevated in the blood after the infection, the serologic tests will not distinguish active from recently treated disease. The breath test determines the presence of active infection. The invasive tests (Campylobacter-like organism, culture, and histology) require endoscopy. The Campylobacter-like organism test is a rapid test that can determine the presence of active infection. The mucosa histology examination remains the most sensitive test.

Barium contrast studies, although widely used, are not accurate in identifying shallow, superficial ulcers because of failure of the barium to properly fill the ulcer crater. X-ray studies are also ineffective in differentiating a peptic ulcer from a malignant tumor. In addition, x-rays do not as readily demonstrate the degree of healing that can be visually determined with the endoscope. Barium studies are of benefit in the diagnosis of pyloric obstruction caused by recurrent ulcers.

Gastric analysis has questionable value in the diagnosis of peptic ulcer disease because in many patients gastric secretions are normal in amount and composition. However, it can provide important data in (1) identifying a possible gastrinoma (Zollinger-Ellison syndrome), (2) determining the degree of gastric hyperacidity, and (3) evaluating the results of therapy such as vagotomy and antisecretory drug therapy. Several methods may be used to determine the amount of gastric secretions. An NG tube can be placed into the antrum with the use of fluoroscopy, and the secretions can be collected overnight for a 12-hour period. The HCl acid concentration is calculated and compared with equivalents already established for persons who do not have ulcers, those with gastric and duodenal ulcers, and those with Zollinger-Ellison syndrome. This method is not extremely accurate because the NG tube may become plugged or aspiration methods may be inconsistent. Augmented histamine or pentagastrin stimulation may be more accurate in estimating the degree of acid secretion. In these tests the stomach's ability to secrete HCl acid is studied after stimulation with either betazole HCl (Histalog) or pentagastrin (a synthetic form of the hormone gastrin).

Laboratory analyses, including a CBC, urinalysis, liver enzyme studies, serum amylase determination, and stool examination, should be performed. A CBC may indicate the presence of anemia secondary to bleeding from the ulcer. Liver enzyme studies help determine any liver problems, such as cirrhosis, that may complicate the treatment of the ulcer. Urine and stool are routinely tested for the presence of blood. A serum amylase determination is frequently ordered to provide information on pancreatic function in patients in whom posterior penetration of the pancreas is suspected.

Collaborative Care

Conservative Therapy. When the patient's clinical manifestations and health history suggest the diagnosis of a peptic ulcer and diagnostic studies confirm its presence, a medical regimen is instituted (Table 39-19). The regimen consists of adequate rest, dietary modifications, medications, elimination of smoking, and long-term follow-up care. The aim of the treatment program is to decrease the degree of gastric acidity, enhance mucosal defense mechanisms, and minimize the harmful effects on the mucosa. Patients are often treated in ambulatory care clinics.

Adequate rest, both physical and emotional, is important in the treatment process. A quiet, calm environment at home or on the job is not easy to achieve and may require some modifications in the patient's daily routine. The benefits derived from the elimination of stressors help decrease the stimulus for overproduction of HCl acid. Moderation in daily activity is essential.

Dietary modifications may be necessary so that foods and beverages irritating to the patient can be avoided or eliminated. A bland diet consisting of six small meals a day may be recommended to the patient during the symptomatic phase. However, there is considerable controversy over the actual therapeutic benefits derived from a bland diet, since the rationale is not supported by scientific evidence. Each patient should be instructed to eat and drink foods and fluids that do not cause any distressing or harmful side effects. Alcohol and caffeine-containing products should be eliminated because of their irritating effects.

Smoking has an irritating effect on the mucosa, increases gastric motility, and delays mucosal healing. It should be eliminated completely or severely reduced. The combination of adequate rest and abstinence from smoking accelerates ulcer healing.

Medications are a vital part of therapy. The patient must be well informed about each drug prescribed, why it is ordered, and the expected benefits. Strict adherence to the prescribed regimen of drugs is mandatory. Drug therapy that includes the use of antacids, histamine H_2-receptor antagonists, antisecretory agents, antibiotics, and anticholinergics is presented in Tables 39-19, 39-20, 39-21, and 39-22. Aspirin and NSAIDs should be discontinued. When these medications must be continued, enteric-coated or highly buffered preparations are more suitable.

Antibiotics to eradicate *H. pylori* infection are prescribed. When *H. pylori* is present, ulcer recurrence rates with H_2-receptor antagonists alone can be as high as 75% to 90% while

COLLABORATIVE CARE
Table 39-19 Peptic Ulcer Disease

Diagnostic
Complete blood count
Urinalysis
Liver enzymes
Serum electrolytes
Fiberoptic endoscopy with biopsy
Upper GI barium-contrast study
Gastric analysis
Exfoliative cytology
H. pylori testing of breath, urine, blood, stool

Collaborative Therapy
Conservative Therapy
Adequate rest
Bland diet (six small meals a day)
Cessation of smoking
Medications
  Antacids (Table 39-21)
  H_2-receptor blocking agents (Table 39-20)
  Anticholinergics (Table 39-20)
  Cytoprotective drugs (Table 39-20)
  Proton pump inhibitors (Table 39-20)
  Misoprostol (Cytotec)
  Antibiotics for *H. pylori* (Table 39-13)
Stress reduction

Acute Exacerbation Without Complications
NPO
NG suction
Bed rest to moderate light activity
Cessation of smoking
IV fluid replacement
Medications
  Antacids
  H_2-receptor antagonist
  Proton pump inhibitor (omeprazole)
  Anticholinergics
  Sedatives

Acute Exacerbation with Complications (Hemorrhage, Perforation, Obstruction)
NPO
NG suction
Bed rest
IV fluid replacement (lactated Ringer's solution)
Blood transfusions
Stomach lavage (possible)

Surgical Therapy
Perforation—simple closure with omentum graft
Gastric outlet obstruction—pyloroplasty and vagotomy
Ulcer cure
  Billroth I and II
  Vagotomy and pyloroplasty

NG, nasogastric; *NPO,* nothing by mouth.

DRUG THERAPY
Table 39-20 Peptic Ulcer Disease

Antisecretory
H_2-receptor antagonists
  Cimetidine (Tagamet)
  Ranitidine (Zantac)
  Famotidine (Pepcid)
  Nizatidine (Axid)
Proton pump inhibitors
  Omeprazole (Prilosec)
  Lansoprazole (Prevacid)
  Pantoprazole (Pantoloc)
Anticholinergics

Antisecretory and Cytoprotective
Misoprostol (Cytotec)

Cytoprotective
Sucralfate (Carafate)
Bismuth subsalicylate (Pepto-Bismol)

Neutralizing
Antacids*

Antibiotics for *H. pylori*†
Amoxicillin
Metronidazole
Tetracycline

Others
Tricyclic antidepressants
  Imipramine (Tofranil)
  Doxepin (Sinequan)

*See Table 39-21.
†See Table 39-13.

ulcer should be assessed by means of x-rays or endoscopic examination. Barium-contrast films can be used to provide a rough estimate of the degree of gastric ulcer healing. However, it should be noted that endoscopic examination is the only accurate method to monitor for duodenal ulcer healing.

Because recurrence of peptic ulcer is frequent, interruption or discontinuation of therapy can have detrimental results. The patient must be encouraged to comply with therapy and continue with follow-up care for at least 1 year. If changes in lifestyle were part of the prescribed therapy, they should be maintained. Antacids, H_2-receptor antagonists, and proton pump inhibitors may be stopped after the ulcer has healed or may be prescribed in the form of low-dose maintenance therapy. No other medications, unless prescribed by the physician, should be taken because they may have an ulcerogenic effect. Finally, the patient and family should be told what to do in the event pain and discomfort recur or blood is noted in the vomitus or stools.

Acute Exacerbation. The patient with an acute exacerbation of peptic ulcer can usually be treated with the same regimen used for conservative management. However, the situation is considered more serious because of the possible complications of perforation, hemorrhage, and obstruction.

An acute exacerbation is frequently accompanied by bleeding, increased pain and discomfort, and nausea and vomiting. If the patient experiences recurrent vomiting or pyloric outlet obstruction, an NG tube is placed into the stomach with intermittent suction for about 24 to 48 hours.

with antibiotic treatment the recurrence rate may be as low as 2%. Antibiotic therapy for *H. pylori* is shown in Table 39-13.[30]

The healing of a peptic ulcer requires many weeks of therapy. Pain disappears after 3 to 6 days, but ulcer healing is much slower. Complete healing may take 3 to 9 weeks, depending on ulcer size and treatment regimen employed. Healing of the

Table **39-21**   **Antacid Preparations**

Ingredient	Trade Name
Single Substance	
Aluminum carbonate	Basaljel
Aluminum hydroxide gel tablets	Amphojel, Alu-Cap
Aluminum phosphate	Phosphaljel
Calcium carbonate	Alka-2, Tums
Dihydroxyaluminum aminoacetate	Robalate
Dihydroxyaluminum sodium carbonate	Rolaids
Magaldrate	Riopan
Magnesium hydroxide	Mag-Ox
Sodium bicarbonate	Alka-Seltzer
Mixtures of Aluminum Hydroxide and Magnesium Salts	
	Aludrox
	A-M-T
	Cremalin
	Delcid
	Gaviscon
	Gelusil and Gelusil M
	Maalox
	Mylanta
	WinGel
Mixtures of Calcium Carbonate and Aluminum and Magnesium Hydroxides	
	Camalox
	Ducon
Mixtures of Calcium Carbonate, Magnesium Carbonate, and Magnesium Oxide	
	Alkets

Table **39-22**   **Side Effects of Antacid Therapy**

Antacid	Reactions
Aluminum hydroxide gels	Constipation, phosphorus depletion with chronic use
Calcium carbonate	Constipation or diarrhea, hypercalcemia, milk-alkali syndrome, renal calculi
Magnesium preparations	Diarrhea, hypermagnesemia
Sodium preparations	Milk-alkali syndrome if used with large amounts of calcium; used with caution in patients on sodium restrictions

If there is a history of an incompetent pyloric sphincter allowing reflux of duodenal contents into the stomach, an NG tube will remove intestinal contents from the stomach. The maintenance of an empty stomach decreases the stimulus for pancreatic enzyme secretion as well. This period of stomach rest eliminates any causative factors that may have precipitated the acute exacerbation and permits the resolution of edema and inflammation of the mucosa. Fluids and electrolytes are replaced by IV infusion until the patient is able to tolerate oral feedings without distress.

Blood or blood products may be administered, depending on the amount of blood loss. Careful monitoring of the vital signs, intake and output, laboratory studies, and signs of impending shock are important during this acute episode.

Endoscopic evaluation is performed to reveal the degree of inflammation or bleeding, as well as the ulcer location. It is important to ascertain the presence of a prepyloric or pyloric ulcer that can cause gastric outlet obstruction. When endoscopic examination reveals no major problems and the patient's physical condition stabilizes, the plan of care for the patient should follow the same regimen of diet, activity, and medications used in conservative therapy. A 5-year follow-up program is recommended after acute exacerbation. An increase in the healing rate is achieved after conservative treatment, but the treatment plan cannot prevent the scar formation that can result in gastric outlet obstruction. Approximately 42% to 88% of ulcers recur.

Perforation.   The immediate focus of management of a patient with a perforation is to stop the spillage of gastric or duodenal contents into the peritoneal cavity and restore blood volume. An NG tube is inserted into the stomach to provide continuous aspiration and gastric decompression to halt spillage through the perforation. Although duodenal aspiration is not achieved as promptly, placement of the tube as near to the perforation site as possible facilitates decompression.

Circulating blood volume must be replaced with lactated Ringer's and albumin solutions. These solutions substitute for the fluids lost from the vascular and interstitial space as the peritonitis develops. Blood replacement in the form of packed RBCs may be necessary. Unless contraindicated, a central venous pressure line and an indwelling urinary catheter should be inserted and monitored hourly. The patient with a history of cardiac disease requires ECG monitoring or placement of a pulmonary artery catheter for more accurate assessment of left ventricular function. Broad-spectrum antibiotic therapy should be started immediately to treat bacterial peritonitis. Administration of pain medications provides comfort.

The operative procedure involving the least risk to the patient is simple oversewing of the perforation and reinforcement of the area with a graft of omentum. The excess gastric contents are suctioned from the peritoneal cavity during the surgical procedure. Before surgical closure some surgeons irrigate with warm lactated Ringer's solution or instill an antibiotic solution into the abdominal cavity to help counteract the peritonitis.

There is controversy regarding the need for more definitive surgical treatment of a perforated ulcer than can be achieved with simple closure. Other types of surgical procedures depend on the location of the peptic ulcer and the surgeon's preference. If cure of the ulcer is the ultimate goal, the surgical procedures may include gastric resection or vagotomy and pyloroplasty.

Gastric Outlet Obstruction.   The aim of therapy for gastric outlet obstruction is to decompress the stomach, correct any existing fluid and electrolyte imbalances, and improve the patient's general state of health. An NG tube is inserted into the stomach and attached to continuous suction to remove excess fluids and undigested food particles. With continuous decompression for several days the stomach has the opportunity to regain its normal muscle tone, the ulcer can begin healing, and the inflammation and edema will subside.

The tube is clamped after several days of suction, and gastric residue is measured periodically. The frequency and amount of time the tube remains clamped are proportional to the amount of aspirate obtained and the comfort level of the patient. A method commonly followed is to clamp the tube overnight for approximately 8 to 12 hours and to measure the gastric residue in the morning. When the aspirate falls below 200 ml, it is considered to be within a normal range and the patient can begin oral intake of clear liquids. Initially, oral fluids are begun at 30 ml per hour and then gradually increased in amount. The patient must be watched carefully for signs of distress or vomiting. As the amount of gastric residue decreases, solid foods are added and the tube is removed.

IV fluids and electrolytes are administered according to the degree of dehydration, vomiting, and electrolyte imbalance indicated by laboratory studies. Pain relief results from the decompression measures, and analgesics are usually not necessary. Antacid and antisecretory drug therapy (i.e., histamine H_2-receptor antagonists, proton pump inhibitors) is an integral part of treatment if the obstruction has been determined on endoscopic examination to be the result of an active ulcer. Pyloric obstruction may be removed nonsurgically by balloon dilations performed through the endoscope. Surgical intervention may be necessary to remove scar tissue.

Drug Therapy

Drug therapy for peptic ulcer disease is outlined in Table 39-20.

Antacids. Antacids are one of the initial drugs of choice in the treatment of peptic ulcers.[14] They decrease gastric acidity and the acid content of chyme reaching the duodenum. By raising the pH level to above 3.5, antacids effectively block the conversion of pepsinogen to its active form pepsin. In addition to their neutralizing effects, some antacids, such as aluminum hydroxide, can bind to bile salts, thus decreasing the salts' detrimental effects on the gastric mucosa.

Antacids consist of systemic and nonsystemic types. Systemic antacids, such as sodium bicarbonate, are extremely soluble and are absorbed into the circulation. Their long-term use can lead to systemic alkalosis; therefore they are rarely used in ulcer treatment. The nonsystemic antacids are insoluble and poorly absorbed. The common commercial nonsystemic antacids consist of magnesium hydroxide or aluminum hydroxide as single preparations or in various combinations (see Table 39-21).

The antacid preparation may be in liquid or tablet form. A large number of tablets may be required to equal the same dose of a liquid preparation. Since the tablets are chewable, some of the medication is left coating the teeth and gingivae instead of the stomach.

It has long been recognized that antacids ingested on an empty stomach are quickly evacuated and only partially used. Because the duration of action is only about 30 minutes, best results are obtained when they are prescribed 1 and 3 hours after meals and at bedtime. More frequent administration has resulted in poor tolerance and reduced long-term compliance. Acid secretion is also known to occur with higher doses and frequency by maintaining a high antral pH, which in turn stimulates release of gastrin.

The type and dosage of antacid prescribed depends on the adverse effects some of these preparations have on the health status or on other medications the patient may be taking (see Table 39-22). Preparations high in sodium, such as Titralac, Di-Gel, and Amphojel, should be used with caution in older adults and in the patient with cirrhosis of the liver, hypertension, congestive heart failure, and renal disease. Magnesium preparations should not be prescribed for the patient in renal failure because of the risk of magnesium toxicity. The most frequent side effect experienced with magnesium antacids is diarrhea. Aluminum hydroxide causes constipation. An antacid combination of aluminum and magnesium salts seems to lessen the side effects of both. Side effects of antacids are shown in Table 39-22.

Antacids have the capacity to interact unfavorably with some medications. They can enhance the absorption of drugs such as dicumarol and amphetamines. The action of digitalis preparations can be potentiated when taken in combination with calcium or magnesium antacids. In some instances, antacids may decrease the absorption rates of prescribed drugs, such as tetracycline. Therefore it is important to inform the physician of any drugs that are being taken before antacid therapy is begun.

The physician must often adjust the dosage of antacid so that the amount prescribed has the capacity of neutralizing the acid present. It is generally recommended that each dose of an antacid be capable of neutralizing 100 mEq of HCl acid. Any alteration in dosage should be carefully communicated to the patient and family, along with the rationale for the change so that compliance is more likely. The adjustment of antacids by the patient must be avoided. Taking too much or too little of an antacid can compromise its effectiveness and may lead to unpleasant side effects or an increase in ulcer discomfort.

For active gastric and duodenal ulcers, the prescribed treatment period varies from 4 to 8 weeks or until healing is demonstrated through endoscopic or barium-contrast studies. Many physicians recommend daily maintenance doses of an antacid to minimize ulcer recurrence.

Compliance with long-term antacid therapy seems to diminish with time. The patient fails to take the correct dose or stops taking the drug altogether. Many persons stop therapy because they find it inconvenient to keep the necessary daily supply at work, when traveling, or at home. For some patients it is embarrassing to be seen taking medications generally known to be prescribed for people with ulcers.

Histamine H_2-receptor Antagonists. The use of the histamine H_2-receptor antagonists cimetidine (Tagamet), ranitidine (Zantac), famotidine (Pepcid), and nizatidine (Axid) is now a standard component of most ulcer treatment regimens. Histamine is believed to be the final intracellular activator of HCl acid secretion. These drugs block the action of histamine on the H_2 receptors and thus reduce HCl acid secretion and accelerate ulcer healing. Antihistamine drugs used to treat allergies are H_1-receptor antagonists and thus have no effect on gastric acid secretion.

Histamine H_2-blocker drugs may be administered orally or IV. Their therapeutic effects are considerably longer than are those of antacids, some lasting for up to 12 hours. However, the onset of action (i.e., symptom relief) is longer than antacids. In addition, the drugs have demonstrated capabilities in the healing of gastric and duodenal ulcers. When the oldest of the H$_2$ blockers, cimetidine and ranitidine, are compared, the latter clearly has several advantages: (1) it is 5 to 12 times more potent and therefore has a longer duration of action; (2) optimal dosage can be achieved on a bid (twice a day) schedule versus qid (four times a day) schedule for cimetidine; (3) it inhibits nocturnal acid secretion for a longer time period; and (4) it has fewer side effects (headache, dizziness, malaise, neutropenia, thrombocytopenia, and elevated liver enzyme levels) than cimetidine (granulocytopenia, gynecomastia, diarrhea, fatigue, dizziness, rash, and mental confusion in the older adult).

Famotidine (Pepcid) and nizatidine (Axid) are the most recently available of these drugs. They are considered more potent at reduced dosage levels. Side effects appear to be minimal. Muscle cramps, headache, and constipation have been associated with the use of famotidine. Somnolence, sweating, and urticaria have occurred with nizatidine. Both drugs can be administered with antacids. Several of these preparations (e.g., Pepcid-AC, Tagamet) are now available as OTC drugs.

Proton Pump Inhibitors. Proton pump inhibitors, such as omeprazole (Prilosec), lansoprazole (Prevacid), and pantoprazole (Pantoloc), block the ATPase enzyme that is important for the secretion of gastric acid. These agents tend to be more effective than H$_2$-receptor antagonists are in reducing gastric acid secretion and promoting ulcer healing. Proton pump inhibitors are also used in combination with antibiotics to treat ulcers caused by *H. pylori*.

Antibiotic Therapy. Once the presence of *H. pylori* has been determined, antibiotic treatment is instituted. It has been recommended that only those patients with verified *H. pylori* be treated with antibiotics to reduce the potential for drug resistance. As shown in Table 39-13 triple and double drug therapies are used because no single agent has been found effective in eliminating *H. pylori*.

Anticholinergic Drugs. Anticholinergic drugs are only occasionally ordered in the treatment of peptic ulcer disease. These drugs decrease cholinergic stimulation of HCl acid. There is divided opinion concerning their efficacy in preventing recurrences and their therapeutic effectiveness in alleviating symptoms and preventing complications. Because of their tendency to decrease gastric motility, they should be avoided in gastric ulcers in which stasis of secretions increases the patient's pain and discomfort. Anticholinergics are associated with a high number of side effects, such as dry mouth and skin, flushing, thirst, tachycardia, dilated pupils, blurred vision, and urine retention. Anticholinergics must be prescribed with caution in the patient with narrow-angle glaucoma, prostatic hyperplasia, and gastric outlet obstruction. The use of anticholinergics has decreased as a result of histamine H$_2$-receptor antagonists and proton pump inhibitors.

Other Drug Therapy. Several other medications are used in the management of ulcers. Sucralfate (Carafate) is used for the short-term treatment of ulcers. It has proven to be cytoprotective of the esophagus, stomach, and duodenum. Its ability to accelerate ulcer healing is thought to be a result of the formation of an ulcer-adherent complex covering the ulcer and thereby protecting it from erosion caused by pepsin, acid, and bile salts. Sucralfate does not have acid-neutralizing capabilities. Its action is most effective at a low pH, and it should be given at least 30 minutes before or after an antacid.

Adverse side effects are minimal. However, it does bind with cimetidine, digoxin, warfarin (Coumadin), phenytoin (Dilantin), and tetracycline, causing reduced bioavailability of these drugs.

Colloidal bismuth or bismuth subsalicylate (Pepto-Bismol) has demonstrated the ability to facilitate healing of peptic ulcer. It is thought to be partially effective against *H. pylori* infection. This drug is nonabsorbable and causes black stools.

Misoprostol (Cytotec) is a synthetic prostaglandin analog. It has protective and some antisecretory effects on gastric mucosa. Misoprostol is the only drug approved in the United States for the prevention of gastric ulcers induced by NSAIDs and aspirin. A major advantage of misoprostol is that it does not interfere with the therapeutic effects of aspirin and NSAIDs. It is believed that persons who require chronic NSAID therapy, such as those with osteoarthritis, benefit from the use of misoprostol because it reduces the risk of gastric ulcers and their complications.

Tricyclic antidepressants (e.g., imipramine, doxepin) have duodenal ulcer healing rates close to those obtained with cimetidine. The mode of action is not fully understood but appears similar to that of anticholinergic agents.

Nutritional Therapy
Related to Conservative Therapy

Food acts as a buffer for gastric secretions. The buffering action of food lasts about 60 minutes and is then followed by an increase in the concentration of acid in the secretions. There are no specific diets or foods that are totally effective in treating peptic ulcer disease. The patient is encouraged to eat as normally as possible. If certain foods result in pain or discomfort, they should be avoided. The critical aspect is individualization of the dietary plan. Dietary orders may also vary according to the preference of the physician. Small, frequent meals (six per day) may be recommended. The rationale for ingesting six meals a day instead of three large ones is that the stomach should never be totally empty. In this way, gastric acid is neutralized.

Dietary instructions should include a sample diet with a list of foods that usually cause distress and should therefore be eliminated from the diet. Foods known to irritate the gastric mucosa include hot, spicy foods and pepper, alcohol, carbonated beverages, tea, coffee, and broth (meat extract). These foods also have limited buffering ability in addition to stimulating gastric acid secretion. Foods high in roughage, such as raw fruit, salads, and vegetables, may irritate an inflamed mucosa. If these foods are well chewed, this seems to be less of a problem.

Protein is considered the best neutralizing food, but it also stimulates gastric secretions. Carbohydrates and fats are the least stimulating to HCl acid secretion, but they do not neutralize well. The patient must determine a suitable combination of these essential nutrients without causing undue distress.

Historically, milk was an essential part of ulcer therapy until it was learned that milk proteins and calcium stimulate gastric acid production. For this reason, milk as part of diet therapy for ulcers was out of favor for a time. However, milk is again used as part of the diet plan because it can neutralize gastric acidity and contains prostaglandins and growth factors, both of which are known to protect the GI mucosa from injury.

NURSING MANAGEMENT: PEPTIC ULCER

■ Nursing Assessment

Subjective and objective data that should be obtained from a patient with peptic ulcer disease are presented in Table 39-23.

■ Nursing Diagnoses

Nursing diagnoses related to peptic ulcer may include, but are not limited to, those presented in NCP 39-2.

■ Planning

Overall goals are that the patient with peptic ulcer disease will (1) experience a reduction or absence of discomfort related to peptic ulcer disease, (2) exhibit no signs of GI complications related to the ulcerative process, (3) have complete healing of the peptic ulcer, (4) make appropriate lifestyle changes to prevent recurrence, and (5) comply with the prescribed therapeutic regimen.

■ Nursing Implementation

Health Promotion. Nurses are involved in identifying patients at risk for ulcer development. Early detection and treatment of ulcers are important aspects of reducing morbidity associated with ulcers. Patients who are taking ulcerogenic medications such as aspirin and NSAIDs are at risk for ulcer development. Patients are encouraged to take these medications with food or milk. Patients are also taught to report symptoms related to gastric irritation including epigastric pain to their care provider.

Acute Intervention. During the acute exacerbation of an ulcer, the patient generally complains of increased pain and nausea and vomiting, and some may have evidence of bleeding. Initially many patients attempt to cope with the symptoms at home before seeking medical assistance.

Very often during this acute phase all that is necessary for the patient's immediate recovery is to maintain NPO status for a few days, have an NG tube inserted and connected to intermittent suction, and replace fluids intravenously. The rationale for this therapy must be conveyed to the anxious patient and family. They must understand that the advantages far outweigh any temporary discomfort imposed by the presence of the tube. Regular mouth care alleviates the dry mouth. Cleansing and lubrication of the nares facilitates breathing and decreases soreness. Gastric contents should be analyzed for pH, blood, bile, or other irritating substances. When the stomach is kept empty of gastric secretions, the ulcer pain diminishes and ulcer healing begins. Usually this form of intervention is effective.

Because the patient is on NPO status, IV fluids are ordered. The type and amount administered are directly related to the fluid lost, the manifestations exhibited by the patient, and the results of the hemoglobin, hematocrit, and electrolyte determinations. The nurse should be aware of any other current health problem that could be adversely affected by the type of fluid used or the rate of the infusion. Repeated monitoring of these parameters provides information on the hydration status and the effectiveness of treatment. Vital signs are initially taken at least hourly so that shock can be detected and treated.

Physical and emotional rest are conducive to ulcer healing. The patient's immediate environment should be quiet and restful, and visitors should be restricted. The use of a mild sedative

NURSING ASSESSMENT

Table 39-23 Peptic Ulcer

Subjective Data

Important Health Information

Past health history: Chronic renal failure, pancreatic disease, chronic obstructive pulmonary disease, serious illness or trauma, hyperparathyroidism, cirrhosis of the liver, Zollinger-Ellison syndrome

Medications: Use of aspirin, corticosteroids, nonsteroidal antiinflammatory drugs, reserpine

Surgery or other treatments: Complicated or prolonged surgery

Functional Health Patterns

Health perception–health management: Chronic alcohol abuse, smoking, caffeine use; family history of peptic ulcer disease

Nutritional-metabolic: Weight loss, anorexia; nausea and vomiting, hematemesis; dyspepsia, heartburn, belching

Elimination: Black, tarry stools

Cognitive–perceptual: **Duodenal ulcers**—Burning, mid-epigastric or back pain occurring 2 to 4 hours after meals and relieved by food; nocturnal pain common; **Gastric ulcers**—High epigastric pain occurring 1 to 2 hours after meals; pain may be precipitated or aggravated by food

Coping-stress tolerance: Acute or chronic stress

Objective Data

General

Anxiety, irritability

Gastrointestinal

Epigastric tenderness

Possible Findings

Anemia; guaiac-positive stools; gastric analysis indicating high gastric acid secretion; positive *H. pylori* culture from gastric tissue, abnormal upper gastrointestinal endoscopic and barium studies

---

or tranquilizer has beneficial effects when the patient is anxious and apprehensive. The nurse must use good judgment before sedating a person who is becoming increasingly restless. There is danger that the medication will mask the signs of shock secondary to upper GI bleeding.

If the patient's condition improves without progression of symptoms (e.g., increased pain, vomiting, and hemorrhage), the regimen outlined for conservative therapy is followed. All too frequently an acute exacerbation is accompanied by one or more complications, especially hemorrhage and perforation and, to a lesser extent, obstruction.

Hemorrhage. Changes in the vital signs and an increase in the amount and redness of the aspirate often signal massive upper GI bleeding. When there is an increased amount of blood in the gastric contents, the patient's pain is often decreased because the blood helps to neutralize the acidic gastric contents. It is important to maintain the patency of the NG tube so that blood clots do not obstruct the tube. If the tube becomes blocked, the patient can develop abdominal distention.

39-2 NURSING CARE PLAN PATIENT WITH PEPTIC ULCER

Expected Patient Outcomes	Nursing Interventions and *Rationales*

CONSERVATIVE MANAGEMENT

NURSING DIAGNOSIS **Pain** *related to* increased gastric secretions, decreased mucosal protection, and ingestion of gastric irritants *as manifested by* burning cramplike pain in epigastrium and abdomen; pain onset 1 to 2 hr after meals with gastric ulcer; pain onset 2 to 4 hr after meals (midmorning, midafternoon) and middle of night with duodenal ulcer.

- Verbalization of satisfaction with pain control.

- Determine pain characteristics from verbal description and physical assessment data *so appropriate interventions can be planned.*
- Administer antacids, H_2 antagonists, proton pump inhibitors, anticholinergics, and protective agents as ordered *to reduce pain.*
- Teach patient to avoid smoking and ingesting spicy, hot or cold foods, coffee, tea and cola drinks, and alcoholic beverages *to prevent increasing acid production.*
- Teach patient stress reduction *as relaxation results in decreased acid production and reduction in pain.*

NURSING DIAGNOSIS **Ineffective management of therapeutic regimen** *related to* lack of knowledge of long-term management of peptic ulcer disease, not following treatment plan, and unwillingness to modify lifestyle *as manifested by* frequent questions about home care, incorrect responses to questions about peptic ulcer disease, noncompliance with medical regimen.

- Verbalization of plan to modify lifestyle and incorporate therapeutic regimen into lifestyle.

- Explain ulcer disease process at patient's level *to foster understanding.*
- Help patient identify stressors and initiate modifications in daily routine *as stress causes hypersecretion of HCl acid and pepsin, which can alter the mucosal barrier.*
- Discuss diet plan and assist with implementation at home and in work setting.
- Explain rationale for the elimination of alcohol, spicy foods, coffee, tea, and colas from diet; explain the harmful effects of smoking *as these agents increase acid production and directly irritate gastric mucosa.*
- Provide information on medication actions and side effects *to ensure safe self-administration.*
- Inform patient what to do if symptoms related to ulcers reoccur *to ensure early initiation of treatment.*

EXACERBATION MANAGEMENT

NURSING DIAGNOSIS **Pain** *related to* acute exacerbation of disease process and inadequate comfort measures *as manifested by* verbalization of increase in pain, nonverbal indicators of pain (e.g., moaning, crying, doubling up).

- Expression of satisfaction with pain management.

- Encourage bed rest or light activity *to conserve energy and promote comfort.*
- Provide quiet, relaxed environment and limit visitors *to decrease stress and other factors that increase acid secretion.*
- Administer medications as ordered *to relieve pain.*

NURSING DIAGNOSIS **Vomiting** *related to* acute exacerbation of disease process and inadequate comfort measures *as manifested by* increase in nausea and/or vomiting.

- Decrease in or absence of nausea and vomiting.

- Maintain NPO status *to prevent irritation of GI mucosa.*
- Maintain NG tube to suction *to keep stomach empty and remove any stimulus for HCl acid and pepsin secretion.*
- Check vomitus or aspirate for occult blood *to assess for hemorrhage.*

Continued

39-2 NURSING CARE PLAN PATIENT WITH PEPTIC ULCER—continued

Expected Patient Outcomes	Nursing Interventions and *Rationales*

COLLABORATIVE PROBLEMS

POTENTIAL COMPLICATION **Hemorrhage** *related to* eroded mucosal tissue.

Nursing Goals	Nursing Interventions and *Rationales*
■ Monitor for signs of hemorrhage. ■ Carry out medical and nursing interventions if hemorrhage occurs.	■ Assess for evidence of hematemesis, bright red or melena stool, abdominal pain or discomfort, symptoms of shock (e.g., decreased blood pressure; cool, clammy skin; cyanosis; dyspnea; tachycardia; decreased urine output); *to plan appropriate interventions.* ■ If ulcer is actively bleeding, observe NG tube aspirate or emesis for amount and color *to assess degree of bleeding.* ■ Take vital signs every 15 to 30 min *to determine patient's hemodynamic status and as indicators of shock.* ■ Maintain IV infusion line *to provide ready access for blood and fluid replacement.* ■ If RBC transfusion is given, observe for transfusion reaction *so appropriate actions can be taken immediately.* ■ Monitor hematocrit and hemoglobin *as indicators of severity of hemorrhage and need for fluid and blood replacement.* ■ Record intake and output *to monitor fluid balance.* ■ Reassure patient and family *to decrease their anxiety.* ■ Remain calm and confident in plan of care *to foster calm and confidence in patient and family.*

POTENTIAL COMPLICATION **Perforation of GI mucosa** *related to* impaired mucosal tissue integrity.

Nursing Goals	Nursing Interventions and *Rationales*
■ Monitor for signs of perforation. ■ Report deviations from expected parameters. ■ Carry out appropriate medical and nursing interventions.	■ Observe for manifestations of perforation (e.g., sudden, severe abdominal pain; rigid, boardlike abdomen; pain to shoulders; increasing distention; decreasing bowel sounds) *to ensure early recognition and intervention.* ■ Monitor vital signs every 15 to 30 min *as indicators of shock.* ■ Maintain NG tube to suction *to provide continuous aspiration and gastric decompression to prevent further leakage of gastric fluid through the perforation.* ■ Administer pain medication *to promote comfort and reduce anxiety.* ■ Prepare patient for emergency diagnostic tests and possible surgical intervention *to foster timely intervention.*

The nurse must monitor the results of the hemoglobin and hematocrit determinations. Awareness of the significance of these laboratory results and ability to correlate the data to the patient's signs and symptoms can be lifesaving.

Perforation. When there is sudden, severe abdominal pain unrelated in intensity and location to the pain that brought the patient to the hospital, the nurse must recognize the possibility of ulcer perforation. When any person with an ulcer, particularly a chronic duodenal ulcer, demonstrates these manifestations, perforation should be suspected and the physician notified immediately.

Perforation is indicated by a rigid, boardlike abdomen; severe generalized abdominal and shoulder pain; drawing up of the knees; and shallow, grunting respirations. The bowel sounds that may have been previously normal or hyperactive may diminish and become absent.

Vital signs are important parameters and should be promptly recorded and taken every 15 to 30 minutes. The nurse should temporarily stop all oral or NG medications and feedings until the physician can be notified and a definitive diagnosis made. If perforation does exist, anything taken internally can add to the spillage into the peritoneal cavity and increase discomfort. If IV fluids are being administered at the time of the perforation, the rate should be maintained or increased to replace the depleted plasma volume.

The symptoms experienced by the patient are very frightening. The reaction of the nursing staff must be one of calm reassurance in spite of the seriousness of the situation. Simple explanations of the need for chest and abdominal x-rays help diminish the patient's anxiety and give some insight into the diagnostic plan. Indicating why frequent samples of blood are necessary lessens confusion and resistance.

When perforation is confirmed, the nurse should ensure that any known allergies the patient has have been recorded on the chart. This is important because antibiotic therapy is usually started, and careful observation for allergic reactions must

PATIENT & FAMILY TEACHING GUIDE
Table 39-24 Peptic Ulcer Disease

The following are teaching guidelines for patient and family:

1. Explain dietary modifications, including avoidance of foods that cause epigastric distress. This may include black pepper, spicy foods, and acidic foods. Small frequent meals may be better tolerated than large meals.
2. Explain the rationale for avoiding cigarettes. In addition to promoting ulcer development, smoking will delay ulcer healing.
3. Encourage the need to reduce or eliminate alcohol ingestion.
4. Explain the rationale for avoiding OTC medications unless approved by the patient's care provider. Many preparations contain ingredients, such as aspirin, that should not be taken unless approved by the physician. Check with the care provider regarding the use of nonsteroidal antiinflammatory drugs.
5. Explain the rationale for not interchanging brands of antacids and H_2-antagonists that can be purchased without a prescription without checking with the physician or nurse. This can lead to harmful side effects.
6. Teach the need to take all medications as prescribed. This includes both antisecretory and antibiotic medications. Failure to take medications as prescribed can result in relapse.
7. Explain the importance of reporting any of the following:
   - increased nausea and/or vomiting
   - increase in epigastric pain
   - bloody emesis or tarry stools
8. Explain the relationship between symptoms and stress. Stress-reducing activities or relaxation strategies are encouraged.
9. Encourage patient and family to share concerns about lifestyle changes and living with a chronic illness.

OTC, over-the-counter.

be made. When the perforation fails to seal spontaneously, surgical closure is necessary and is performed as soon as possible. There is often little time to prepare the patient and family thoroughly for the surgical intervention, yet some instructions can be carried out while the immediate therapy is begun. If major reconstructive surgery is anticipated, the patient and family may question the need when the problem is only a small hole. To answer this type of question, the nurse must first have an understanding of the usual operative procedures being used and, in addition, must know that unless the surgery can cure the ulcer that caused the perforation, the patient may need more surgery in the future. (Nursing management of peritonitis is discussed in Chapter 40.)

Gastric outlet obstruction. Gastric outlet obstruction is a complication of peptic ulcer disease that can occur at any time. Obstruction is a possible complication, particularly in the patient whose ulcer is located close to the pylorus. Because the onset of symptoms is usually gradual, the condition is not generally as serious an emergency as hemorrhage or perforation. Relief of symptoms may be achieved by constant NG aspiration of stomach contents. This allows edema and inflammation to subside and then permits normal flow of gastric contents through the pylorus.

Obstruction can also occur during the treatment of an acute episode of peptic ulcer exacerbation. If these symptoms are experienced while the patient is still on NPO status, the patency of the NG tube should be suspected. Regular irrigation of the tube with a saline solution facilitates proper functioning. It may be helpful to reposition the patient from side to side so that the tube tip is not constantly lying against the mucosal surface.

When oral feedings have been resumed and symptoms of obstruction are observed, the physician should be promptly informed. Generally, all that is necessary to treat the problem is to resume gastric aspiration so that the edema and inflammation resulting from the acute episode have time to resolve. IV fluids with electrolyte replacement keep the patient hydrated during this period. The NG tube can be clamped and gastric fluids can be aspirated to check for retention. It is important to maintain accurate intake and output records, especially of the gastric aspirate. The patient should be kept aware of why these symptoms are being experienced. In some instances in which treatment is not successful, surgery may be performed after the acute phase has passed.

Ambulatory and Home Care. The patient in whom peptic ulcer disease has been diagnosed has specific needs that must be met to prevent and avoid recurrence or complications. General instructions should cover aspects of the disease process itself, medications, possible changes in lifestyle (including diet), and regular follow-up care. Table 39-24 provides a patient teaching guide for the patient with peptic ulcer disease.

Knowing the cause of the ulcer and understanding the disease process may motivate the patient to become more involved in care and increase compliance with therapy. The patient must understand the dietary modifications and why they are important for recovery and health maintenance. The nurse and the dietician should elicit a dietary history from the patient and plan for ways that dietary modifications can be easily incorporated into the patient's home and work setting. The patient who is following a diet prescribed for another illness needs to know how to balance the two so that neither condition is harmed by dietary interventions.

The patient does not always provide the physician with accurate information regarding habitual use of alcohol or cigarettes. The nurse may be looked on as less threatening and more understanding of these habits than the physician may be. The nurse should provide useful information about the detrimental effects of alcohol and cigarettes on ulcer disease and ulcer healing.

The nurse should instruct the patient about prescribed medications, including their actions, side effects, and inherent dangers if omitted for any reason. The patient should know why OTC medications (e.g., aspirin) should not be taken unless approved by the physician. Because antacids and some H_2-receptor antagonists may be bought without a prescription, the patient must be informed that interchanging brands without checking with the physician or nurse can lead to harmful side effects.

Efforts should be made to obtain more information about the patient's psychosocial status. Knowledge of lifestyle, occupation, and coping behaviors can be helpful to the plan of care. The patient may be reluctant to talk about personal subjects, the stress experienced at home or on the job, the usual methods of coping, or dependence on drugs or alcohol. Unfortunately, the patient does not often see the relationship between lifestyle or occupation and ulcer disease. It is important to listen for subtle clues from the patient's statements and to observe for behaviors that broaden this database.

When the occupation, related work habits, home, or environment have been implicated as factors in peptic ulcer development, the patient must be made aware of these stressors, how to avoid them in the future, or how to cope with them successfully if they cannot be altered. Vocational or psychologic counseling may be necessary so that fatigue and repeated emotional upsets can be avoided when possible.

The need for long-term follow-up care must be stressed. Because successful treatment is frequently followed by a recurrence of the ulcer disease, the patient should be encouraged to seek immediate intervention if symptoms of the disease recur. The patient who has recurrence of ulcer disease following initial healing must learn to live with a disease that is chronic. The patient may be angry and frustrated, especially if the prescribed mode of therapy has been faithfully followed yet has failed to prevent the recurrence or extension of the disease process.

Unfortunately, many patients do not comply with the plan of care originally designed, and they experience repeated exacerbations. Patients quickly learn that they often experience no discomfort when they omit prescribed medications or indulge in occasional dietary indiscretions. Consequently they make no or little alteration in lifestyle. After an acute exacerbation the patient is often more amenable to following the plan of care and open to suggestions for changes in lifestyle. Changes are difficult for most people and may be met with resistance. If the patient has been instructed to stop smoking or to avoid the use of alcohol, this request may be met with resistance. The patient may fare better from a reduction in his or her use of these substances rather than from total elimination. Although alcohol and smoking are known to interfere with ulcer healing, they frequently serve as coping mechanisms. From the patient's point of view, the distress caused by their total elimination may outweigh the benefits to be gained from abstention. The goal, however, should always be total cessation. A patient with chronic ulcers must be aware of the complications that may result from the disease, the clinical manifestations indicating their presence, and what to do until the physician can be seen.

■ Evaluation

Expected outcomes for the patient with a peptic ulcer are addressed in NCP 39-2 on p. 1120.

Surgical Therapy for Peptic Ulcers

Approximately 20% of patients with ulcers need surgical intervention. Because there is a high recurrence rate for both duodenal and gastric ulcers and complications increase with the duration of the ulcer, many physicians believe that surgery is necessary after therapy has been tried and proved unsuccessful. The following criteria are used as general indications for surgical intervention:

1. Intractability: failure of the ulcer to heal or recurrence of the ulcer after therapy

2. History of hemorrhage or increased risk of bleeding during treatment
3. Prepyloric or pyloric ulcers (both have high recurrence rates)
4. Concurrent condition, such as severe burns, trauma, or sepsis
5. Multiple ulcer sites
6. Drug-induced ulcers, especially when withdrawal from the drug may put the person at risk
7. Possible existence of a malignant ulcer
8. Obstruction

A variety of surgical procedures are used to treat ulcer disease. They usually involve a partial gastrectomy, vagotomy, or pyloroplasty. Partial gastrectomy with removal of the distal two thirds of the stomach and anastomosis of the gastric stump to the duodenum is called a *gastroduodenostomy* or *Billroth I operation* (Fig. 39-18). Partial gastrectomy with removal of the distal two thirds of the stomach and anastomosis of the gastric stump to the jejunum is called a *gastrojejunostomy* or *Billroth II operation.* In both procedures the antrum and the pylorus are removed. Because the duodenum is bypassed, the Billroth II operation is the preferred surgical procedure to prevent recurrence of duodenal ulcers.

Vagotomy is the severing of the vagus nerve, either totally (truncal) or selectively at some point in its innervation to the stomach. In a truncal vagotomy the nerve is severed bilaterally in both the anterior and the posterior trunk. Selective vagotomy consists of cutting the nerve at a particular branch of the vagus nerve, resulting in denervation of only a portion of the stomach, such as the antrum or the parietal cell mass.

Pyloroplasty consists of surgical enlargement of the pyloric sphincter to facilitate the easy passage of contents from the stomach. It is most commonly done after vagotomy or to enlarge an opening that has been constricted from scar tissue. A vagotomy causes decreased gastric motility. A pyloroplasty accompanying vagotomy increases gastric emptying.

The combination of a Billroth I or II procedure with vagotomy has the advantage of eliminating the ulcer and the stimulus for acid secretion. Surgical removal of the antrum results in removal of the source of gastrin secretion. (Gastrin normally stimulates parietal and chief cells.) Vagotomy eliminates the stimulus of HCl acid and gastrin hormone secretion caused by vagal stimulation.

Postoperative Complications. The most common postoperative complications from peptic ulcer surgery are (1) dumping syndrome, (2) postprandial hypoglycemia, and (3) bile reflux gastritis.

Dumping syndrome. Dumping syndrome is the direct result of surgical removal of a large portion of the stomach and the pyloric sphincter. These changes drastically reduce the reservoir capacity of the stomach. Although dumping syndrome is more commonly experienced after a Billroth II procedure, it can occur after any gastric reconstruction and vagotomy.

Dumping syndrome is associated with meals having a hyperosmolar composition. Normally, gastric chyme enters the small intestine in small amounts, and shifts in fluid from the extracellular space are minimal. After surgery, however, the stomach no longer has control over the amount of gastric chyme entering the small intestine. Consequently a large bolus

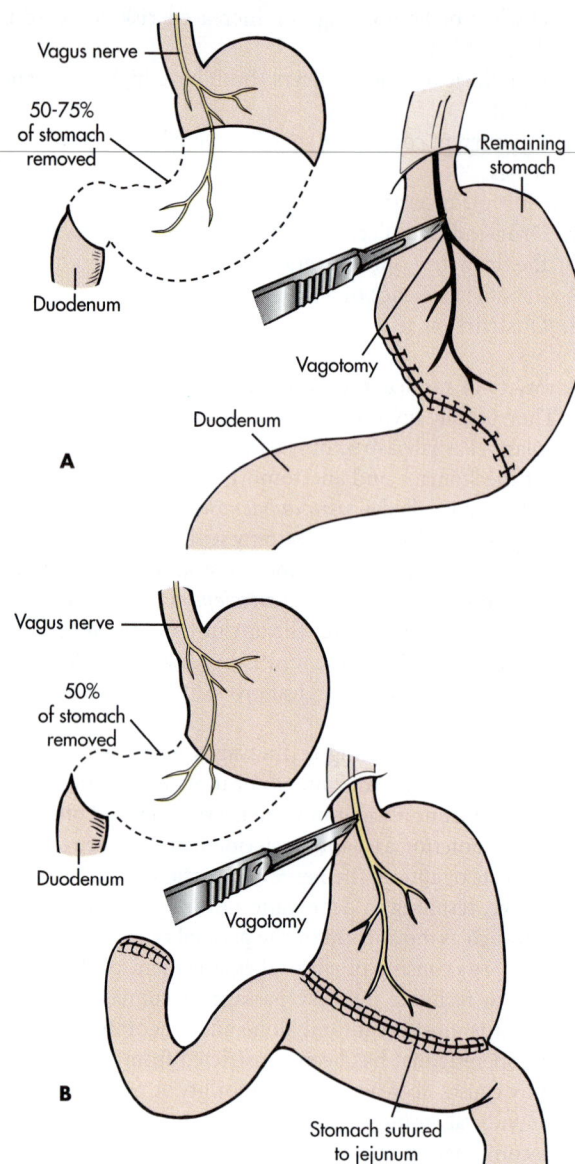

Fig. 39-18   **A,** Billroth I procedure (subtotal gastric resection with gastroduodenostomy anastomosis). **B,** Billroth II procedure (subtotal gastric resection with gastrojejunostomy anastomosis).

of hypertonic fluid enters the intestine and results in fluid being drawn into the bowel lumen. This creates a decrease in plasma volume. A secondary consequence of this fluid shift is distention of the bowel lumen, which stimulates intestinal motility and the urge to defecate.

Approximately one third to one half of patients experience dumping syndrome after peptic ulcer surgery. The onset of symptoms occurs at the end of a meal or within 15 to 30 minutes after eating. The patient usually describes feelings of generalized weakness, sweating, palpitations, and dizziness. These symptoms are attributed to the sudden decrease in plasma volume. The patient complains of abdominal cramps, borborygmi, and the urge to defecate. These manifestations usually last for no longer than an hour after meals.

Postprandial hypoglycemia. Postprandial hypoglycemia is considered a variant of the dumping syndrome, since it is the result of uncontrolled gastric emptying of a bolus of fluid high in carbohydrate into the small intestine. The bolus of concentrated carbohydrate results in hyperglycemia and the release of excessive amounts of insulin into the circulation. A secondary hypoglycemia then occurs, with symptoms appearing about 2 hours after meals. The symptoms experienced are the ones observed in any hypoglycemic reaction and include sweating, weakness, mental confusion, palpitations, tachycardia, and anxiety.

The immediate ingestion of sugared fluids or candy relieves the hypoglycemic symptoms. The treatment of this type of hypoglycemia is similar to that of the dumping syndrome. To avoid similar occurrences the patient should be instructed to limit the amount of sugar consumed with each meal and to eat small, frequent meals with moderate amounts of protein and fat.

Bile reflux gastritis. Gastric surgery that involves the pylorus, either reconstruction or removal, can result in reflux alkaline gastritis. Prolonged contact of bile, especially bile salts, causes damage to the gastric mucosa. Chronic gastritis of this form may result in the back-diffusion of hydrogen ions through the gastric mucosa. Paradoxically, peptic ulcer may recur after surgical treatment that was intended as a cure.

The symptoms associated with reflux alkaline gastritis are continuous epigastric distress that increases after meals. Vomiting relieves the distress but only temporarily. The administration of cholestyramine (Questran), either before or with meals, has met with considerable success. Cholestyramine binds with the bile salts that are the source of irritation in this condition. Aluminum hydroxide antacids have also been used in the treatment of this condition.

Nutritional Therapy Related to Surgical Therapy. Discharge planning and instruction should be started as soon as the immediate postoperative period is successfully passed. Dietary instructions may be given by the dietician and reinforced by the nursing staff. Because the stomach's reservoir has been greatly diminished after gastric resection, the meal size must be reduced accordingly. The patient must be advised to eliminate drinking fluids with meals as had been done in the past. Dry foods with a low-carbohydrate content and moderate protein and fat content are better tolerated initially. These dietary changes, with the incorporation of a short rest period after each meal, reduce the likelihood of dumping syndrome. Reassurance that following these dietary measures will result in cessation of these symptoms within a few months is essential to long-term compliance.

Postprandial hypoglycemic reaction can be avoided if these dietary instructions are followed with special emphasis on eating foods low in sugar content. Although only a small percentage of patients experience bile reflux gastritis, the patient must be cautioned to notify the physician of any continuous epigastric distress after meals that is similar to that felt before surgery.

With regard to dumping syndrome, the symptoms are self-limiting and frequently disappear within several months to a year after surgery. Interventions prescribed for the patient are diet instruction, rest, and reassurance. The diet should consist of small dry feedings daily that are low in carbohydrate, restricted in refined sugars, and contain moderate amounts of protein and fat. Sample menu plans are presented in

NUTRITIONAL THERAPY

Table 39-25   Postgastrectomy Dumping Syndrome

Purpose

To slow the rapid passage of food into the intestine; to control symptoms of the dumping syndrome (dizziness, sense of fullness, diarrhea, tachycardia), which sometimes occur following a partial or total gastrectomy

Diet Principles

1. Meals are divided into six small feedings to avoid overloading intestines at mealtimes.
2. Fluids should not be taken with meals but at least 30 to 45 minutes before or after meals; this helps prevent distention or a feeling of fullness.
3. Concentrated sweets (e.g., honey, sugar, jelly, jam, candies, sweet pastries, sweetened fruit) are avoided because they sometimes cause dizziness, diarrhea, and a sense of fullness.
4. Protein and fats are increased to promote rebuilding of body tissues and to meet energy needs. Meat, cheese, eggs, and milk products are specific foods to increase in the diet.
5. Amount of time these restrictions should be followed varies. The health care provider decides the proper amount of time to remain on this prescribed diet according to the patient's clinical condition and progress.

Exchanges	Sample Menu 1	Sample Menu 2	Sample Menu 3
Breakfast			
1 meat	1 poached egg	1 fried egg	1 oz ham
1 starch	1 slice toast	1 corn tortilla	2 biscuits with 2 tsp gravy
Fat	2 sausage	2 slices bacon	
	Margarine	Margarine	
10 AM snack			
1 starch	¾ cup dry cereal	½ cup atole	½ cup grits with 2 tbs
½ cup milk	½ cup milk	½ cup milk	margarine added
1 fruit	½ fresh banana	2 unsweetened canned	⅓ cantaloupe
	Sugar substitute	peach halves	½ cup buttermilk
		Sugar substitute	
Lunch			
2 meat	Grilled cheese sandwich with	1 burrito with 1 oz meat, 1	2 oz fried fish
2 starch	2 oz cheese, lettuce	oz cheese, ½ cup pinto	½ cup buttered rice
1 vegetable	2 unsweetened pear halves	beans, 1 flour tortilla	½ cup mustard greens
1 fruit		½ diet gelatin dessert with	1 fresh apple
Fat		fruit cocktail added	1 slice bread
2 PM snack			
1 meat or substitute	½ cup plain yogurt	½ cup cottage cheese	2 tsp peanut butter
1 starch	2 graham crackers	5 soda crackers	1 slice bread
Dinner			
2 meat	2 oz tomato meatloaf	2 tamales	2 oz fried pork chop
1 starch	½ cup mashed potatoes with	½ cup buttered corn	½ cup black-eyed peas
Vegetable	gravy	1 fresh orange	½ cup buttered carrots
1 fruit	½ cup buttered green beans		1 fresh plum
Fat	½ cup unsweetened apple		
	sauce		
8 PM snack			
1 meat	½ sandwich with 1 slice	1 corn tortilla with 1 oz	½ sandwich with 1 slice
1 starch	bread, 1 oz roast beef,	melted cheese and green	bread, 1 slice salami, let-
Vegetable	lettuce, mayonnaise	chili	tuce, mayonnaise
Fat			

Table 39-25. Fluids should be taken between meals but not with the meal and the patient should plan rest periods of at least 30 minutes after each meal. The recumbent position is the most beneficial if the patient can arrange for it. Reassuring the patient that the unpleasant symptoms are usually of short duration is helpful in gaining cooperation. A small percentage of patients experience long-term problems and may require further reconstructive surgery.

NURSING MANAGEMENT: SURGICAL THERAPY FOR PEPTIC ULCERS

■ Preoperative Care

When surgery is planned with the goal of curing the ulcer disease, the surgeon should provide necessary information about the procedure and the expected outcome so that the patient can make an informed decision. The nurse can help the patient and family by clarifying and interpreting their questions. A discussion of the surgical procedure accompanied by a diagram or picture showing the anatomical changes that will result should be incorporated into the preoperative teaching plan. Instructions should be clear on what to expect after surgery, including comfort measures, pain relief, coughing and breathing exercises, use of an NG tube, and IV fluid administration (see Chapter 16).

■ Postoperative Care

Care of the patient after major abdominal surgery is similar to the postoperative care after abdominal laparotomy (see Chapter 40). An NG tube is used to decompress the remaining portion of the stomach to decrease pressure on the suture line and to allow for resolution of edema and inflammation resulting from surgical trauma.

The gastric aspirate must be carefully observed for color, amount, and odor during the immediate postoperative period. The color of the aspirate is expected to be bright red at first, with a gradual darkening within the first 24 hours after surgery. Normally the color changes to yellow-green within 36 to 48 hours. If the tube becomes clogged during this period, the physician may order periodic gentle irrigations with normal saline solution. It is essential that the NG suction is working and that the tube remains patent so that accumulated gastric secretions do not put a strain on the anastomosis. This can lead to distention of the remaining portion of the stomach and result in (1) rupture of the sutures, (2) leakage of gastric contents into the peritoneal cavity, (3) hemorrhage, and (4) possible abscess formation. If the tube must be replaced or repositioned, the physician must be called to perform this task because of the danger of perforating the gastric mucosa or disrupting the suture line.

The nurse should observe the patient for signs of decreased peristalsis and lower abdominal discomfort that may indicate impending intestinal obstruction. Accurate intake and output records must be kept. Vital signs are monitored and recorded every 4 hours.

The patient should be kept comfortable and free of pain by the administration of the prescribed medications and by frequent changes in position. The incision is relatively high in the epigastrium and may interfere with deep-breathing and coughing measures. Splinting the area with a pillow while gently and persistently encouraging the patient to put forth the best efforts possible helps prevent pulmonary complications. Splinting also protects the abdominal suture line from rupturing during coughing. The dressing must be observed for signs of bleeding or odor and drainage indicative of an infection. Ambulation is encouraged and is increased daily.

While the NG tube is connected to suction, IV therapy is maintained. Potassium and vitamin supplements are added to the infusion until oral feedings are resumed. Before the NG tube is removed, the patient is started on oral feedings of clear liquids to determine the tolerance level. The stomach is aspirated within 1 or 2 hours to assess the amount remaining and its color and consistency. When fluids are well tolerated, the tube is removed and fluids are increased in frequency with a slow progression to regular foods. The regimen of six small meals a day is begun.

Pernicious anemia is a long-term complication that may occur after partial gastrectomy. However, it is seen more often when the entire stomach is surgically removed. Pernicious anemia is caused by the loss of intrinsic factor, which is produced by the parietal cells. Depending on the amount of parietal cell mass removed in surgery, the patient may eventually require regular injections of cobalamin. (Cobalamin deficiency and pernicious anemia are discussed in Chapter 29.)

Because the patient is generally returning to the same home and work environment, there is always the danger of ulcer redevelopment, especially at the site of the anastomosis. Adequate rest, nutrition, and avoidance of known stressors are keys to complete recovery. Avoiding the use of medications not prescribed by the physician should be reemphasized, along with restrictions on smoking and alcohol use. If the patient is willing to make these kinds of adjustment in lifestyle, a successful rehabilitation is more likely.

■ GERONTOLOGIC CONSIDERATIONS

Peptic Ulcer Disease

The incidence of gastric ulcers in patients over 60 years of age is increasing. This is related to the increased use of NSAIDs. In the elderly patient pain may not be the first symptom associated with an ulcer. For some patients the first indication may be frank gastric bleeding (e.g., hematemesis, melena) or a subtle decrease in hematocrit. The morbidity and mortality rates associated with gastric ulcers in the elderly patient are higher than younger adults because of concomitant health problems (e.g., cardiovascular, pulmonary) and a decreased ability to withstand hypovolemia. The treatment and management of gastric ulcers in the older adult are similar to that in younger adults. An emphasis is placed on prevention of gastritis and gastric ulcers. This includes teaching the patient to take NSAIDs and other gastric-irritating medications with food, milk, or antacids. If necessary, the patient may be treated with antisecretory agents (i.e., proton pump inhibitors or H_2-receptor antagonists). The patient should be instructed to avoid irritating substances, such as alcohol and smoking, and to report abdominal pain or discomfort to his or her health care provider.

CANCER OF THE STOMACH

Although the rate of stomach cancer has been steadily declining in the United States since the 1930s, it is the seventh leading cause of cancer mortality in the United States, accounting for more than 13,700 deaths and 22,600 new cases annually.[9] Worldwide gastric adenocarcinoma is the second most common malignant growth. Costa Rica and Japan have the highest incidence rates in the world. Cancer of the stomach is more prevalent in men of the lower socioeconomic class, primarily those living in urban areas. Stomach cancer is typically at an advanced stage when diagnosed and is not usually amenable to surgical resection. Only 10% to 20% of patients develop disease confined to the stomach. Survival of patients with nonlocalized gastric cancer is less than 10% 5 years after diagnosis.

Etiology and Pathophysiology

Many factors have been implicated in the development of gastric cancer, yet no single causative agent has been identified. It is believed that a diet of smoked, highly salted, or spiced foods may have a carcinogenic effect. A genetic etiology has been postulated because of the greater than normal occurrence of stomach cancer in immediate family members. Persons with blood group A have a greater incidence of gastric cancer than the general population. At the present time there is no universally accepted genetic connection.

Gastric carcinogenesis probably begins with a nonspecific mucosal injury as a result of aging, autoimmunity, or repeated exposure to irritants such as bile, antiinflammatory agents, or alcohol. Nutritional or other undetermined genetic deficiencies may impede mucosal repair, resulting in chronic gastritis and subsequent proliferation of *H. pylori*. It is possible that *H. pylori* and resulting metabolic changes can induce a sequence of transitions from dysplasia to carcinoma *in situ*.

Other predisposing factors associated with a high incidence of gastric cancer are atrophic gastritis, pernicious anemia, benign gastric polyps, and achlorhydria. The relationship between chronic peptic ulcers of the stomach and the development of gastric cancer is still controversial. Malignant transformation of a benign chronic ulcer does occur but accounts for less than 5% of all gastric cancers. It is known that the person with achlorhydria or pernicious anemia is more likely to develop gastric cancer than is the person with normal gastric acid production.

Malignant tumors of the stomach may be present for a long time and may have spread to adjacent organs before any distressing symptoms occur. The tumor may grow to large dimensions without obstructing the lumen of the stomach simply because the lumen itself is so large. The mean interval from onset of symptoms to consultation with a physician may be as long as 6 months. This long delay is largely attributed to the vague, intermittent abdominal distress experienced by the patient. Unfortunately, most healthy persons at one time or another experience this type of early symptom as a result of dietary indiscretions, nervous tension, and anxiety.

Gastric cancer can occur in any portion of the stomach. In the past, cancers of the pyloric antral region were most common. Recently there has been an increase in the incidence of proximal gastric cancer. Tumors located at the cardia and fundus are associated with a poor prognosis. These tumors typically infiltrate rapidly to the surrounding tissue, the regional lymph nodes, and the liver. The patient with tumor growth along the lesser curvature has a better survival rate. Adenocarcinomas account for more than 95% of the cancers, and sarcomas (comprising lymphomas and leiomyomas) make up the rest.

The tumor growth is insidious and follows a pattern of continuous infiltration. Cancer of the stomach may spread by direct extension along the mucosal surface and infiltrate through the gastric wall. The rich lymphatic plexuses in the stomach wall facilitate distant metastasis. Seeding of tumor cells into the peritoneal cavity may occur late in the course of the disease. Evidence of spread to the peritoneal cavity is manifested by ascites and by spread to the ovaries.

Clinical Manifestations

The clinical manifestations exhibited by persons with gastric cancer can be categorized by signs and symptoms of anemia, peptic ulcer disease, or indigestion. Anemia is a common occurrence with stomach cancer. It is caused by chronic blood loss as the lesion erodes through the mucosa or as a direct result of pernicious anemia, which develops when intrinsic factor is lost. The person appears pale and weak and complains of fatigue, weakness, dizziness, and, in extreme cases, shortness of breath. The stool may be positive for occult blood.

The symptoms of gastric malignancy are sometimes identical to those of peptic ulcer disease. The pain and discomfort may be alleviated by belching and by the use of antacids, antisecretory agents and diet modifications.

Manifestations related to indigestion include vague epigastric fullness with feelings of early satiety after meals. Weight loss, dysphagia, and constipation frequently accompany epigastric distress. When nausea, vomiting, and hematemesis occur, they may indicate obstruction at the gastric outlet or may be a warning of impending hemorrhage.

The early detection of gastric cancer is difficult because of the vagueness of the symptoms. On physical examination the patient may be pale and lethargic if anemia is present. When the appetite has been poor and weight loss has been considerable, the patient may appear cachectic. A mass can often be detected beneath the abdominal wall and is seen to move with each inspiration. On palpation the mass may be felt in the epigastrium. Masses that are predominantly in the antrum of the stomach are generally found to the left of the midline. Masses located to the right of midline usually tend to be metastases to the liver or indicate involvement of the perigastric lymph nodes. Supraclavicular lymph nodes that are hard and enlarged and located on the left side are suggestive of metastasis via the thoracic duct from the stomach lesion. The presence of ascites is a poor prognostic sign.

Diagnostic Studies

The diagnostic studies for gastric malignancy include laboratory analysis of blood, stool, and gastric secretions (Table 39-26). Blood chemistry studies assist in the determination of anemia and its severity. Liver enzymes and serum amylase may indicate liver and pancreatic involvement or other abnormalities related to their dysfunction. Stool examination provides evidence of occult or gross bleeding. A gastric analysis indicates the level of HCl acid present in the stomach after fasting. Washings obtained during the gastric analysis can be used for the exfoliative cytologic examination. The test demonstrates the histologic changes indicative of malignancy. However, this test should never be used as the sole diagnostic criterion because false readings are sometimes obtained.

The carcinoembryonic antigen (CEA) test is used as an adjunctive diagnostic tool for cancer of the GI tract. CEA is a glycoprotein that is found in significant amounts in embryonic life, especially in the large intestine. It is also found in some adult patients with GI carcinomas. Elevated levels of CEA may indicate malignancy, yet CEA may be elevated in persons who smoke and also in those with benign lesions. Therefore, whereas the CEA test may be of some use in the preoperative workup of a patient with suspected cancer of the stomach, it

COLLABORATIVE CARE

Table 39-26   Gastric Cancer

Diagnostic
History and physical examination
Complete blood count
Urinalysis
Stool examination
Liver enzymes
Serum amylase
Upper gastrointestinal barium study
Carcinoembryonic antigen
Exfoliative cytology
Fiberoptic endoscopy and biopsy
Gastric analysis

Collaborative Therapy
Surgery
  Subtotal gastrectomy—Billroth I or II procedure
  Total gastrectomy with esophagojejunostomy
Adjuvant therapy
  Radiation therapy
  Chemotherapy
  Combination radiation therapy and chemotherapy

RESEARCH
IMPLICATIONS FOR NURSING PRACTICE

Patients with Colorectal and Gastric Cancer

Citation   Forsberg C, Bjovell H, Cedermark B: Well-being and its relation to coping ability in patients with colorectal and gastric cancer before and after surgery, *Scand J Caring Sci* 10:35-44, 1996.

Purpose   To describe and compare the perceived well-being and general health, symptoms, and coping ability of a group of patients with colorectal and gastric cancer before and after surgery. In addition, to describe the patients' perceptions of their postoperative recovery and to determine the relationship between sense of coherence and well-being.

Methods   The sample included 79 patients diagnosed with either colorectal or gastric cancer. The Health Index, symptom checklist, and Sense of Coherence Scale were used to measure responses before surgery and 6 weeks after surgery.

Results and Conclusions   Compared with presurgery, patients experienced a decrease in pain and improvement in bowel function postoperatively. However, patients had greater problems related to energy level, sleep, and mobility postoperatively. Patients living with relatives rated their well-being as better than those who lived alone did. A stronger sense of coherence was related to sense of well-being.

Implications for Nursing Practice   Patients undergoing surgery for GI malignancies have a number of postoperative care needs. Instruments used in this study may be helpful when used in the preoperative period to plan nursing care and in particular patient teaching during the postoperative period.

should never be used as the only diagnostic tool. (CEA is also discussed in Chapters 14 and 40.) Another more promising tumor marker for gastric cancer is carbohydrate antigen 19-9 (CA 19-9), which correlates with advanced stages and poorer prognosis.[31]

Upper GI barium studies may demonstrate defects in tone, secretion, motility, and spasm of the stomach. On x-ray examination the malignant ulcer crater is more irregular around the edges and more elevated than the craters found with benign peptic ulcers. Barium studies do not always detect small lesions of the cardia and fundus.

Endoscopic examination of the stomach remains the best diagnostic tool. Lesions that go undetected on x-ray can be more easily viewed and biopsied when the fiberoptic scope is used. The stomach can be distended with air during the procedure so that the mucosal folds can be stretched. Fixation of the mucosa is indicative of malignancy.

Collaborative Care

When the diagnosis of gastric malignancy has been confirmed, the treatment of choice is surgical removal of the tumor. The preoperative management of the patient with gastric cancer focuses on the correction of nutritional deficits, treatment of anemia, and replacement of blood volume.

Transfusions of packed RBCs correct the anemia. If a gastric lesion has been located at or near the pylorus and is causing gastric outlet obstruction, gastric decompression may be necessary before surgery. When the tumor has extended into the transverse colon and partial colon resection is also required, special preparation of the bowel is necessary. This preparation may include a low-residue diet, enemas to cleanse the bowel, and the use of antibiotics to reduce the intestinal bacteria. Correction of malnutrition is important if surgery is planned. Malnutrition is associated with increased postoperative complications and mortality rates.

Surgical Therapy.   The surgical intervention used in the treatment of stomach cancer may be the same surgical procedures used for peptic ulcer disease. The location and extent of the lesion, the patient's physical condition, and preference of the surgeon determine the specific surgery employed. When metastasis is widespread at the time of diagnosis, surgical intervention may be only palliative.

The surgical aim is to remove as much of the stomach as necessary to remove the tumor and a margin of normal tissue. When the lesion is located in the cardia or high in the fundus, a total gastrectomy with esophagojejunostomy is performed. This procedure involves anastomosis of the lower end of the esophagus to the jejunum (Fig. 39-19). Lesions located in the antrum or the pyloric region are generally treated by either a Billroth I or Billroth II procedure. When metastasis has occurred to adjacent organs, such as the spleen, ovaries, or bowel, the surgical procedures must be modified and extended as necessary.

The chance of a complete cure by surgical means is decreased considerably when the lymph nodes are involved. Sur-

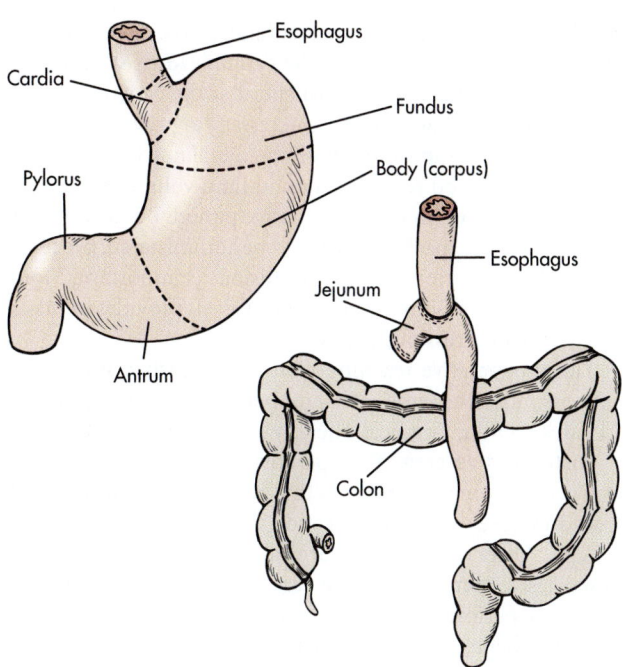

Fig. 39-19   A total gastrectomy for gastric cancer (total gastrectomy with esophagojejunostomy).

vival rates are considerably shortened when organs adjacent to the stomach show evidence of invasion at the time of surgery.

Adjuvant Therapy.   Surgery is the only definitive means of achieving a cure. However, when the patient cannot physically withstand a surgical procedure or when surgical cure is not feasible, radiation or chemotherapy alone or in combination may be used. Neither radiation therapy nor chemotherapeutic agents have been very successful when used as the primary mode of treatment. Because the radiosensitivity of gastric cancers is low, radiation therapy has proved to be of little value.

When radiation is used as a palliative measure, the tumor mass can be decreased, with temporary relief of the cardia or pyloric obstruction. The combination of chemotherapy and radiation is now being used for patients who are not candidates for surgical excision. Combination chemotherapy only causes a temporary relief of symptoms, and long-term survival rates have not shown significant improvement.

Until recently, single-agent chemotherapy for gastric cancer has proved of little value. Agents that have been identified as having some effect on gastric cancer are 5-FU, BCNU, methyl CCNU, doxorubicin (Adriamycin), and triazinate (TZT). A better response rate in patients with advanced gastric cancer is now found when chemotherapeutic agents are used in combination, such as FAT (5-FU, doxorubicin, and triazinate). The hope for better outcomes with the use of chemotherapy depends on finding new ways of administering old drugs, finding new drugs, and determining new drug combinations. The hope for the ultimate cure of patients with gastric cancer now seems to lie in the combined efforts of surgery, radiation, and chemotherapy. The role of biologic therapy is still under investigation for use in gastric cancer. (These therapies are discussed in Chapter 14.)

NURSING MANAGEMENT: GASTRIC CANCER

■ Nursing Assessment

The assessment of a person with possible gastric cancer is similar to that for one with peptic ulcer disease (see Table 39-23). Important data to be obtained from the patient and the family should include a nutritional assessment, a psychosocial history, the patient's perceptions of the health problem and need for hospitalization, and the physical examination of the patient.

The nutritional assessment must elicit information regarding appetite, changes in eating patterns over the previous 6 months, and the role of highly seasoned or salty foods as a regular part of the diet. It is necessary to determine the patient's normal weight and any changes that may have occurred in the past few months. Unexplained weight loss is common in many types of cancer before diagnosis. A history of vague symptoms of dyspepsia, early satiety, feeling full after consuming even a small amount of food, or reporting symptoms of gas pain should help the nurse differentiate these typical gastric cancer symptoms from those of peptic ulcer. As with peptic ulcer patients, the nurse should determine whether pain is present, where and when it occurs, and how it is relieved. When the pain has been controlled with ingestion of foods, fluids, or antacids for a period of time but now continues or worsens regardless of interventions, gastric cancer may be the underlying cause.

Psychosocial and demographic data include age, present or previous occupation, and financial status. Gastric cancer can occur at any age, but the risk is more prevalent in men in the fifth to the sixth decade of life. A family history of cancer, especially gastric cancer, puts a person at greater than normal risk.

It is important to determine the patient's personal perception of the health problem and method of coping with hospitalization, diagnostic tests, and procedures. The possibility of a diagnosis of cancer and a treatment regimen that may include surgery, chemotherapy, or radiation treatment forecasts a prolonged stressful period and a possibly fatal outcome. Therefore it is important for the nurse to support the patient and family if tests result in an unfavorable diagnosis and complex treatment interventions are planned. If surgery is probable, the nurse should assess what the patient expects from surgery (cure or palliation) and how that patient has responded to any previous surgical procedures.

A complete physical examination reveals the patient's current functional abilities, the presence of other health problems, and an estimate on how well the patient may respond to therapy. Cachexia may be evident if the nutritional state has been compromised for an extended time. A malnourished patient does not respond well to chemotherapy or radiation therapy and is a poor surgical risk.

■ Nursing Diagnoses

Nursing diagnoses for the patient with gastric cancer include, but are not limited to, the following:

- Altered nutrition: less than body requirements *related to* inability to ingest, digest, or absorb nutrients
- Activity intolerance *related to* generalized weakness, abdominal discomfort, and nutritional deficits

- Anxiety *related to* lack of knowledge of diagnostic tests, unknown diagnostic outcome, disease process, and therapeutic regimen
- Pain *related to* underlying disease process and side effects of surgery, chemotherapy, or radiation therapy
- Anticipatory grieving *related to* perceived unfavorable diagnosis and impending death

■ Planning

The overall goals are that the patient with gastric cancer will (1) experience minimal discomfort, (2) achieve optimal nutritional status, and (3) maintain a degree of spiritual and psychologic well-being appropriate to the disease stage.

■ Nursing Implementation

Health Promotion. The nursing role in the early detection of cancer of the stomach is focused primarily on identification of the patient at risk because of specific disorders such as pernicious anemia and achlorhydria. The nurse should be aware of symptoms associated with gastric cancer, method of spread, and the significant findings on physical examination. The nurse should understand that the cure rate is often quite dismal because symptoms arise late in the course of the disease process, are vague, and often mimic other conditions, such as peptic ulcers.

The nurse must be alert to problems suggesting gastric cancer, such as poor appetite, weight loss, fatigue, and persistent gastric distress. If any of these manifestations are present, medical attention should be obtained and the necessary diagnostic tests performed.

In addition, any patient with a positive family history of gastric cancer should be encouraged to undergo diagnostic evaluation if manifestations of anemia, peptic ulcer, or vague epigastric distress are present. It is important that the nurse recognize the possible existence of stomach cancer in a patient who is treated for peptic ulcer and who fails to gain relief after 3 weeks of diet and prescribed medications. The ulcer, if it is benign, should show signs of healing on x-ray examination.

Acute Intervention

Preoperative care. When the diagnostic tests confirm the presence of a malignancy, the patient and the family generally react with shock, disbelief, and depression, regardless of how thoroughly they may have been prepared for this possible outcome. Throughout this period the nurse must give emotional and physical support, provide information, clarify test results, and maintain a positive attitude with respect to the patient's immediate recovery and long-term survival.

On admission to the hospital, the patient may be in poor physical condition. Surgery may have to be delayed while the patient becomes more physically able to withstand the strain of major surgery. A positive nutritional state enhances wound healing as well as the ability to withstand infection and other possible postoperative complications. Often the patient is better able to tolerate several small meals a day rather than three regular meals. The diet may be supplemented by a variety of commercial liquid supplements (see Chapter 38) and vitamins. The nurse is challenged to find innovative ways of persuading the patient to eat when lack of appetite and state of mind make eating difficult and unrewarding. Getting the patient's family to assist with meals and encourage intake may be beneficial. If the patient is unable to ingest oral feedings, it may be necessary to provide for nutritional needs with tube feedings or parenteral nutrition.

If needed, blood replacement and fluid volume restoration may be carried out in the preoperative period. Because anemia is usually present, packed RBCs may be administered. Close observation for reactions to the transfusions is important. Monitoring the hemoglobin and hematocrit levels provides information on the progress of therapy.

The preoperative teaching plan before gastric surgery for cancer is much the same as that for peptic ulcer surgery (see the previous section, "Surgical Therapy Related to Peptic Ulcer").

Postoperative care. Postoperative care of the patient with gastric carcinoma is similar to that following a Billroth I or II procedure (see the previous section, "Surgical Therapy Related to Peptic Ulcer"). When the surgical intervention has involved a total gastrectomy, the plan of care is somewhat different. The operation performed usually requires some resecting of the lower esophagus along with the removal of the entire stomach and anastomosis of the esophagus to the jejunum. The chest cavity must be entered, and drainage is accomplished by the insertion of chest tubes. (Chest surgery and drainage tubes are discussed in Chapter 26.) After total gastrectomy, the NG tube does not drain a large quantity of secretions because removal of the stomach has eliminated the reservoir capacity. The NG tube is removed after several days, when peristalsis has resumed. Small amounts of clear fluid may then be started. The patient requires close observation for signs of leakage of the fluids at the anastomosis as evidenced by an elevation in the temperature and increasing dyspnea. When fluids are well tolerated without distress, the amount may be increased along with the addition of some solid foods.

As a consequence of a total gastrectomy, a patient experiences the symptoms of the dumping syndrome. Unfortunately, weight loss is very common, and poor nutritional intake often contributes. Postoperative wound healing may be impaired because of inadequate dietary intake. This necessitates the IV or oral replacement of vitamins C, D, K, and the B complex vitamins and IM or intranasal administration of cobalamin. Because these vitamins are absorbed primarily in the upper part of the small intestine, they must be replaced, since the duodenum has been bypassed in the surgical procedure.

A patient who has a Billroth I or II operative procedure should receive the same postoperative care as one who has had peptic ulcer surgery. This patient is also subject to the same type of postoperative complications as dumping syndrome and postprandial hypoglycemia.

The patient with advanced malignant disease can be offered only palliative treatment. The chemotherapy agent found most useful for controlling symptoms of gastric cancer is 5-FU. When this medication or any of the combination drugs is prescribed, the nurse must have current information regarding the action and side effects of the drugs. The patient should be made aware of the potential benefits and hazards that can result from the chemotherapy. (The care of the patient receiving chemotherapy is discussed in detail in Chapter 14.)

Radiation therapy can be used as an adjuvant to surgery or for palliation. A patient is generally quite fearful of radiation and may develop many misconceptions regarding its value and dangers. To reassure the patient and ensure completion of the designated number of treatments, the nurse must provide detailed instruction. Because most therapy is completed on an outpatient basis, the nurse should assess the patient's knowledge of radiation, care of the skin, the need for good nutrition and fluid intake during therapy, and the appropriate use of antiemetic drugs. (Specific care of the patient receiving radiation therapy is discussed in Chapter 14.)

Ambulatory and Home Care. Before the patient is discharged, the need for teaching should be reviewed. Most dietary measures useful after peptic ulcer surgery are applicable after surgery for gastric carcinoma. Plans should be made for the relief of pain, including comfort measures and the judicious use of analgesics. Wound care, if needed, must be taught to the primary caregiver in the home situation. Dressings, special equipment, or special services may be required for the patient's continued care at home. A list of community agencies that are available for assistance can be provided before the patient goes home. The services of the American Cancer Society are especially helpful.

When treatment in the form of chemotherapy or radiation therapy is to be continued after discharge, a referral to the home health nurse may be beneficial. The home health nurse can assist with recovery, determine the degree of patient compliance, and be a sympathetic health care provider with whom the patient can consult.

Long-term follow-up must be stressed. The patient must be encouraged to comply with the prescribed dietary and medication regimens, keep appointments for chemotherapy administration or radiation treatments, and keep the physician informed of changes in physical condition. (Long-term management of the cancer patient is discussed in Chapter 14.)

■ **Evaluation**

Expected outcomes are that the patient with gastric cancer will

- experience minimal discomfort
- achieve optimal nutritional status
- maintain a degree of spiritual and psychologic well-being appropriate to the disease stage

FOOD POISONING

Food poisoning is a nonspecific term that describes acute GI symptoms such as nausea, vomiting, diarrhea, and colicky abdominal pain caused by the intake of contaminated food. Food most commonly causes illness if it is contaminated with microorganisms or their products. The GI tract is frequently the portal of entry for the microorganisms. The epidemiology of food-borne illness is changing. There are new organisms and many have spread worldwide. The two main types of food poisoning are (1) acute gastroenteritis from bacteria and (2) neurologic symptoms from botulism. The most common bacterial food poisonings are presented in Table 39-27.

Poisonous chemicals, such as mercury, arsenic, zinc, and potassium chlorate may contaminate foods. Poisoning can also occur from ingestion of poisonous plants (e.g., certain mushroom species).

Prevention of occurrence is the focus of interventions. Teaching should include correct food preparation and cleanliness, adequate cooking, and refrigeration. If the patient is hospitalized, care focuses on correction of fluid and electrolyte imbalance from diarrhea and vomiting. With botulism, additional assessment and care relative to neurologic symptoms are indicated (see Chapter 57).

Escherichia Coli Food Poisoning

Of recent importance is the increase in number of cases of hemorrhagic colitis caused by the presence of the bacterial strain *Escherichia coli* 0157:H7. Widespread outbreaks in the United States and Japan have increased the public's awareness of this organism. *E. coli* 0157:H7 is found primarily in undercooked meats, such as roast beef, ham, and turkey. However, other sources include cheese sandwiches, apple cider, and unpasteurized milk. *E. coli* can also be transmitted from person to person, particularly in settings such as nursing homes and day care centers. Recent studies suggest that *E. coli* 0157:H7 may be responsible for 0.6% to 2.4% of all nonbloody diarrhea and 15% to 36% of all cases of bloody diarrhea.[32]

The clinical manifestations of *E. coli* 0157:H7 vary from mild diarrhea to bloody diarrhea and systemic complications including hemolytic uremia and thrombocytopenic purpura and even death. The diarrhea may start out as watery but may progress to bloody. Treatment involves use of antibiotics and supportive care to maintain intravascular volume.

Table 39-27 Bacterial Food Poisoning

Type	Causative Agent	Sources	Onset of Symptoms (hr)	Symptoms	Treatment	Prevention
Staphylococcal	Toxin from *Staphylococcus aureus*	Meat, bakery products, cream fillings, salad dressings, milk; skin and respiratory tract of food handlers	30 min–7 hr	Vomiting, nausea, abdominal cramping, diarrhea	Symptomatic, fluid and electrolyte replacement, antiemetics	Immediate refrigeration of foods, monitoring of food handlers
Clostridial	*Clostridium perfringens*	Meat or poultry dishes cooked at lower temperature (stew or pot pie), rewarmed meat dishes, gravies, improperly canned vegetables	8–24 hr	Diarrhea, nausea, abdominal cramps, vomiting (rare); midepigastrium pain	Symptomatic, fluid replacement	Correct preparation of meat dishes, serving of food immediately after cooking or rapid cooling of food
Salmonella	*Salmonella typhimurium* (grows in gut)	Improperly cooked poultry, pork, beef, lamb, and eggs	8 hr–several days	Nausea and vomiting, diarrhea, abdominal cramps, fever and chills	Symptomatic, fluid and electrolyte replacement	Correct preparation of food
Botulism	Toxin from *Clostridium botulinum*, ingested from gut and blocks acetylcholine at neuromuscular junction	Improperly canned or preserved food, home-preserved vegetables (most common), preserved fruits and fish, canned commercial products	12–36 hr	GI symptoms of nausea, vomiting, abdominal pain, constipation, distention Central nervous system symptoms of headache, dizziness, muscular incoordination, weakness, inability to talk or swallow, diplopia, breathing difficulties, paralysis, delirium, coma	Maintenance of ventilation, polyvalent antitoxin, guanidine hydrochloric acid (enhances acetylcholine release)	Correct processing of canned foods, boiling of suspected canned foods for 15 min before serving
Escherichia coli	*E. coli* serotype 0157:H7	Contaminated beef, pork, milk, cheese, fish	Varies by strain: 8 hr–1 wk	Bloody stools, hemolytic uremic syndrome, abdominal cramping, profuse diarrhea	Symptomatic, fluid and electrolyte replacement	Correct preparation of food

CRITICAL THINKING EXERCISES

CASE STUDY

Hiatal Hernia

Patient Profile

Mary, 63 years old, has had a sliding hiatal hernia for 10 years. Mary is admitted to the hospital for a hiatal hernia repair.

Subjective Data

- Reports increasing heartburn, especially at night
- Is currently on a bland diet and taking antacids
- Complains of substernal pain and heartburn
- Reports some problems with regurgitation

Objective Data

Physical Examination
- 5 feet 2 inches tall and weighs 195 pounds

Diagnostic Study
- Barium swallow and an esophagoscopy revealed a large sliding hiatal hernia.

Collaborative Care

- Mary had a Nissen fundoplication through a laparoscopic approach.

Critical Thinking Questions

1. Explain the pathophysiology of a hiatal hernia. What is the difference between a sliding and a paraesophageal hiatal hernia?
2. What are the characteristic symptoms of a hiatal hernia? Which of these did Mary have?
3. Describe a Nissen fundoplication procedure. What is the objective of this surgical procedure?
4. What are potential postoperative complications, and what nursing measures prevent them?
5. What should be included in a teaching plan for Mary?
6. Based on the assessment data presented, write one or more nursing diagnoses. Are there any collaborative problems?

NURSING RESEARCH ISSUES

1. What are the most effective methods to get an individual to comply with dental and oral hygiene care?
2. What are the most effective topical methods to relieve pain related to stomatitis secondary to infection?
3. Are dietary interventions successful in improving symptoms in the patient with gastroesophageal reflux disease?
4. What are optimal strategies to promote multiple lifestyle changes in a patient with peptic ulcer disease?
5. What are environmental manipulations that could be used to promote decreased nausea in patients receiving chemotherapy?
6. What sensory stimuli in the environment, including sight, smell, and sound, could promote optimal nutrient intake in the chemotherapy patient who is experiencing nausea?
7. What is the most effective way to obtain a nutritional assessment from a patient with gastric carcinoma?

REVIEW QUESTIONS

The number of the question corresponds to the same-numbered objective at the beginning of the chapter.

1. The most appropriate nursing intervention to provide oral care for a patient unable to do this for himself or herself involves
   a. brushing and flossing the patient's teeth.
   b. applying a fluoride solution to the surface of the teeth.
   c. using oral antimicrobial agents to reduce local bacterial counts.
   d. swabbing the patient's mouth with soft foam applicators soaked with mouthwash.
2. The nurse explains to the patient with Vincent's infection that treatment will include
   a. smallpox vaccinations.
   b. viscous lidocaine rinses.
   c. amphotericin B suspension.
   d. topical application of antibiotics.
3. A patient with oral cancer returns from the postanesthesia care unit awake and alert following a partial mandibulectomy and radical neck resection. An appropriate nursing intervention to facilitate the patient's respiratory function at this time is to
   a. elevate the head of the bed.
   b. assess chest expansion and symmetry.
   c. perform oral hygiene with half-strength hydrogen peroxide.
   d. position the patient supine with the head turned to one side.
4. A patient with wired intermaxillary fixation to stabilize a fractured mandible vomits following removal of the NG tube on the second postoperative day. The nurse should
   a. cut the wires to allow the patient to open the mouth.
   b. teach the patient to clear the vomitus from the mouth.
   c. turn the patient's head to the side and suction the vomitus.
   d. notify the physician and prepare the patient for a tracheostomy.
5. The nurse explains to the patient with gastroesophageal reflux disease that this disorder
   a. will require surgical wrapping or repair of the pyloric sphincter to control the symptoms.
   b. results in acid erosion and ulceration of the esophagus caused by the frequent vomiting.
   c. is the protrusion of a portion of the stomach into the esophagus through an opening in the diaphragm.
   d. often involves relaxation of the lower esophageal sphincter allowing stomach contents to back up into the esophagus.

6. To help the patient with a hiatal hernia control the symptoms of this disorder the nurse teaches the patient to
   a. drink a glass of milk at bedtime to coat the esophagus.
   b. lie down after eating to promote relaxation of the GI tract.
   c. avoid tight clothing and bending to decrease intraabdominal pressure.
   d. drink several glasses of liquids with meals to promote stomach emptying.

7. A patient who has undergone an esophagectomy for esophageal cancer develops increasing pain, fever, and dyspnea when a full liquid diet is started postoperatively. The nurse recognizes that these symptoms are most indicative of
   a. an intolerance to the feedings.
   b. extension of the tumor into the aorta.
   c. leakage of fluid or foods into the mediastinum.
   d. esophageal perforation with fistula formation into the lung.

8. During assessment of the patient with esophageal achalasia the nurse would expect the patient to report
   a. a history of alcohol use.
   b. a sore throat and hoarseness.
   c. dysphagia, especially with liquids.
   d. relief of pyrosis with the use of antacids.

9. Mrs. J. calls to tell you that her elderly mother, who is 85 years of age, has been nauseated all day and has vomited twice. Before you hang up and telephone the physician to communicate your assessment data, you instruct Mrs. Jones to
   a. administer antispasmodic medications and observe skin turgor.
   b. give her mother sips of water and elevate the head of her bed to prevent aspiration.
   c. offer her mother a high-protein liquid supplement to drink to maintain her nutritional needs.
   d. offer her mother large quantities of Gatorade to drink, since elderly people are at risk for sodium depletion.

10. The pernicious anemia that may accompany gastritis is due to which of the following?
    a. Chronic autoimmune destruction of cobalamin stores in the body
    b. Progressive gastric atrophy from chronic breakage in the mucosal barrier and blood loss
    c. A lack of intrinsic factor normally produced by acid-secreting cells of the gastric mucosa
    d. Hyperchlorhydria resulting from an increase in acid-secreting parietal cells and degradation of RBCs

11. Your teaching plan for the patient being discharged following an acute episode of GI bleeding will include information concerning the importance of
    a. taking only medications prescribed by the physician.
    b. avoiding taking aspirin with acidic beverages such as orange juice.
    c. taking all medications 1 hour before mealtime to prevent further bleeding.
    d. reading all OTC medication labels to avoid medications containing stearic acid and calcium.

12. You are teaching your patient and her family about possible causative factors for peptic ulcers. You explain that ulcer formation is
    a. caused by a stressful lifestyle and other acid-producing factors such as *C. pylori*.
    b. inherited within families and reinforced by bacterial spread of *Staphylococcus aureus* in childhood.

c. promoted by factors that tend to cause oversecretion of acid, such as excess dietary fats, smoking, and *B. pylori*.
d. promoted by a combination of possible factors that may result in erosion of the gastric mucosa, including certain medications, and alcohol.

13. The dumping syndrome is associated with large
    a. hyperosmolar volumes emptying rapidly into the intestine.
    b. isotonic volumes stimulating increased GI motility.
    c. hypertonic volumes promoting third-spacing in the intestinal cavity.
    d. hyposmolar volumes drawing fluid out of the plasma space and into the bowel.

14. An optimal teaching plan for an outpatient with gastric carcinoma receiving radiation therapy should include information about
    a. cancer support groups, alopecia, and stomatitis.
    b. avitaminosis, ostomy care, and community resources.
    c. prosthetic devices, skin conductance, and grief counseling.
    d. wound and skin care, nutrition, medications, and community resources.

15. Several patients are seen at an urgent care center with symptoms of nausea, vomiting, and diarrhea that began while attending a large family reunion potluck dinner. The nurse questions the patients specifically about foods they ingested containing
    a. beef.
    b. meat and milk.
    c. poultry and eggs.
    d. home-preserved vegetables.

References

1. Brown LJ, Brunelle JA, Kingman A: Periodontal status in the United States, 1988-1991: prevalence, extent, and demographic variation, *J Dent Res*, 75:672, 1996.
2. Position paper: Epidemiology of periodontal diseases, American Academy of Periodontology, *J Periodontol* 67:935, 1996.
3. Kandelman D: Sugar, alternative sweeteners and meal frequency in relation to caries prevention: new perspectives, *Brit J Nutr* 77 (suppl 1):S121, 1997.
4. Horowitz HS: The effectiveness of community water fluoridation in the United States, *J Public Health Dent* 56:253, 1996.
5. Brown LJ, Selwitz RH: The impact of recent changes in the epidemiology of dental caries on guidelines for the use of dental sealants, *J Public Health Dent* 55:274, 1995.
6. Twetman S, Peterson LG: Effect of different chlorhexidine varnish regimens on mutans streptococci levels in interdental plaque and saliva, *Caries Res* 31:189, 1997.
7. Anderson GB and others: Clinical effects of chlorhexidine mouthwashes on patients undergoing orthodontic treatment, *Am J Orthod Dentofacial Orthop* 111:606, 1997.
8. Cosci F, Cosci B: A 7-year retrospective study of 423 immediate implants, *Compend Contin Educ Dent* 18:940, 1997.
9. Cancer Facts and Figures-1998, American Cancer Society.
10. NIH Consensus Conference. *Helicobacter pylori* in peptic ulcer disease, *JAMA* 272:65, 1994.
11. Epstein JB and others: The utility of toluidine blue application as a diagnostic aid in patients previously treated for upper oropharyngeal carcinoma, *Oral Surgery, Oral Medicine, Oral Pathology, Oral Radiology and Endodontics* 83:537, 1997.
12. Hampton JK, Craven R, Heitkemper MM: *The biology of human aging*, ed 2, Dubuque, Iowa, 1996, Brown Publishers.
13. Greenberger NJ: *Helicobacter pylori* and peptic ulcer disease: current status, *Hosp Pract* 30:11, 1995.
14. Horwitz BJ, Fisher RS: Intervening in GERD: the phases of management, *Hosp Pract* 30:43, 1995.

15. Johnson DA: Medical therapy of GERD: current state of the art, *Hosp Pract*, 31:135, 1996.

16. Dawsey SM, Shen Q, Neiberg RK: Studies of esophageal balloon cytology in Linxian, China, *Cancer Epidemiology, Biomarkers and Prevention* 6:121, 1997.

17. Miller BA and others: Human papillomavirus type 16 DNA in esophageal cancer from Alaska Natives, *Int J Cancer* 71:218, 1997.

18. Kang SK and others: Gastrointestinal cancer mortality of workers in occupations with high asbestos exposures, *Am J Industrial Med* 31:713, 1997.

19. Ilson DH, Kelsen CP: Management of esophageal cancer, *Oncology* 10:1385, 1996.

20. Birgisson S, Richter JE: Achalasia: what's new in diagnosis and treatment? *Dig Dis* 15 (suppl 1): 1, 1997.

21. McQuaid KR: Dyspepsia and nonulcer dyspepsia. In *Current diagnosis and treatment in gastroenterology,* Stamford, Conn, 1996, Appleton & Lange.

22. Peura DA and others: The American College of Gastroenterology Bleeding Registry: Preliminary findings. 92:924, 1997.

23. Wolfe MM: NSAIDs and the gastrointestinal mucosa, *Hosp Pract* 32:37, 1997.

24. Lichtenstein DR, Berman MD, Wolfe MM: Approach to the patient with acute upper gastrointestinal hemorrhage. In Taylor MB: *Gastrointestinal emergencies,* ed 2, Baltimore, 1997, Williams & Wilkins.

25. Porter DH, Ducksoo K: Angiographic intervention in upper gastrointestinal bleeding. In Taylor MB: *Gastrointestinal emergencies,* ed 2, Baltimore, 1997, Williams & Wilkins.

26. Savides TJ, Jensen DM: Severe gastrointestinal hemorrhage. In Ayres SM and others: *Textbook of critical care,* ed 3, Philadelphia, 1995, WB Saunders.

27. Bracy W, Peterson WL: Medical therapy of nonvariceal upper gastrointestinal hemorrhage. In Taylor MB: *Gastrointestinal emergencies,* ed 2, Baltimore, 1997, Williams & Wilkins.

28. Imperiale TF, Birgisson S: Somatostatin or octreotide compared with H_2 antagonists and placebo in the management of acute nonvariceal upper gastrointestinal hemorrhage: a meta-analysis, *Ann Intern Med* 127:1062, 1998.

29. Cave DR, Hoffman JS: Management of *Helicobacter pylori* infection in ulcer disease, *Hosp Pract* 31:63, 1996.

30. Greenberger NR: *Helicobacter pylori* and peptic ulcer disease: current status, *Hosp Pract* 30:11, 1995.

31. Grem J: The prognostic importance of tumor markers in adenocarcinomas of the gastrointestinal tract, *Curr Opin Oncol* 9:380, 1997.

32. Greenwald DA, Brandt LJ: Recognizing *E. coli* 0157:H7 infection, *Hosp Pract* 32:123, 1997.

Resources

American College of Gastroenterology
4900 B South 31st Street
Arlington, VA 22206
703-820-7400
fax: 703-931-4520
http://www.acg.gi.org/

American Gastroenterological Association
7910 Woodmont Ave., 7th Floor
Bethesda, MD 20814
301-654-2055
fax: 301-652-3890
http://www.gastro.org/

American Society for Gastrointestinal Endoscopy
13 Elm Street
Manchester, MA 01944-1314
978-526-8330
fax: 978-526-4018
http://www.asge.org/

Digestive Disease National Coalition
711 2nd Street, NE, Suite 200
Washington, DC 20002
202-544-7497
fax: 202-546-7105

National Digestive Diseases Information Clearinghouse
2 Information Way
Bethesda, MD 20892-3570
301-654-3810
fax: 301-907-8906
http://www.niddk.nih.gov/health/digest/nddic.htm

National Institute of Diabetes & Digestive & Kidney Diseases (NIDDK)
Building 31, Room 9A-52
Bethesda, MD 20892
301-496-5877
http://www.niddk.nih.gov/index.htm

Society of Gastroenterology Nurses & Associates, Inc.
401 North Michigan Avenue
Chicago, IL 60611-4267
800-245-7462
In Illinois: 312-321-5165
fax: 312-321-51941070
http://www.sgna.org

For additional Internet resources, see the website for this book at **www.mosby.com/MERLIN/medsurg_lewis**

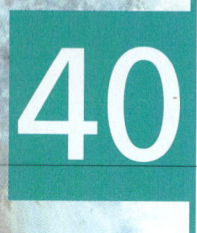

NURSING MANAGEMENT

40 Lower Gastrointestinal Problems

Donna Zimmaro Bliss & Linda Sawchuk

www.mosby.com/MERLIN/medsurg_lewis

LEARNING OBJECTIVES

1. Explain the common etiologies, collaborative care, and nursing management of diarrhea, fecal incontinence, and constipation.
2. Formulate a teaching plan for the patient with constipation.
3. Describe common causes of acute abdominal pain and nursing care of the patient following an exploratory laparotomy.
4. Describe the nursing management of a patient with acute appendicitis.
5. Describe the collaborative care and nursing management of peritonitis.
6. Describe the common etiologies, clinical manifestations, and nursing management of gastroenteritis.
7. Compare and contrast ulcerative colitis and Crohn's disease, including pathophysiology, clinical manifestations, complications, collaborative care, and nursing management.
8. Differentiate among mechanical, neurogenic, and vascular bowel obstructions, including causes and collaborative care and nursing management.

9. Describe the clinical manifestations and surgical and nursing management of cancer of the colon and rectum.
10. Explain the anatomic and physiologic changes that result from a sigmoid colostomy, a transverse colostomy, and an ileostomy.
11. Describe the preoperative and postoperative nursing management of a patient having bowel surgery.
12. Compare and contrast a colostomy and an ileostomy in relation to nursing care and patient teaching.
13. Differentiate between diverticulosis and diverticulitis, including clinical manifestations, collaborative care, and nursing management.
14. Compare and contrast the types of hernias, including etiology and surgical and nursing management.
15. Describe the types of malabsorption syndrome and appropriate management of sprue syndrome, lactase deficiency, and short bowel syndrome.
16. Describe the types, clinical manifestations, collaborative care, and nursing management of anorectal conditions.

DIARRHEA, FECAL INCONTINENCE, AND CONSTIPATION

Diarrhea is not a disease but a symptom. The term *diarrhea* may mean different things to different patients. It is commonly used to denote an increase in stool frequency or volume and an increase in the looseness of stool.

DIARRHEA
Etiology

Causes of diarrhea can be divided into the general classifications of decreased fluid absorption, increased fluid secretion, motility disturbances, or a combination of these (Table 40-1). Causes of acute infectious diarrhea are listed in Table 40-2.

Clinical Manifestations and Complications

Diarrhea may be acute or chronic. *Acute* diarrhea most commonly results from infection. Bacterial or viral infection of

the intestine may result in explosive watery diarrhea, *tenesmus* (spasmodic contraction of anal sphincter with pain and persistent desire to defecate), and abdominal cramping pain. Perianal skin irritation may also develop. Systemic manifestations include fever, nausea, vomiting, and malaise. Leukocytes, blood, and mucus may be present in the stool, depending on the causative agent (see Table 40-2). Acute diarrhea is often self-limiting in the adult. Symptoms continue until the irritant or causative agent is excreted. The mucous membrane lining of the gastrointestinal (GI) tract is composed of epithelial cells, which regenerate following the inflammatory response.

Diarrhea is considered *chronic* when it persists for at least 2 weeks or when it subsides and returns more than 2 to 4 weeks after the initial episode. Severe diarrhea may be debilitating and life threatening. A patient may have severe dehydration (water and sodium loss) and electrolyte disturbances. Malabsorption and malnutrition are also sequelae of chronic diarrhea. Throughout the world diarrhea is one of the major causes of death, especially in infants.

Reviewed by Priscilla Ann Taylor, RN, MN, CGRN, Clinical Nurse Specialist in Gastroenterology, Tacoma, Wash.

Table 40-1   Causes of Diarrhea

Decreased Fluid Absorption
Oral intake of poorly absorbable solutes (e.g., laxatives)
Maldigestion and malabsorption
  Mucosal damage: tropical sprue, Crohn's disease, radiation injury, ulcerative colitis, ischemic bowel disease
  Pancreatic insufficiency
  Intestinal enzyme deficiencies (e.g., lactase)
  Bile salt deficiency
  Decreased surface area (e.g., intestinal resection)

Increased Fluid Secretion
Infectious: bacterial endotoxins (e.g., *Cholera, Escherichia coli, Shigella, Salmonella, Staphylococcus, Clostridium difficile,* viral agents [rotavirus], and parasitic agents *[Giardia lamblia]*)
Drugs: laxatives, antibiotics, suspensions or elixirs containing sorbitol (e.g., acetaminophen)
Hormonal: vasoactive intestinal polypeptide secretion from adenoma of the pancreas; gastrin secretion caused by Zollinger-Ellison's syndrome; calcitonin secretion from carcinoma of the thyroid
Tumor: villous adenoma

Motility Disturbances
Irritable bowel syndrome
Diabetic enteropathy
Visceral scleroderma
Carcinoid syndrome
Vagotomy

Diagnostic Studies

Accurate diagnosis and management require a thorough history, physical examination, and, when indicated, laboratory tests. A history of travel, medication use, diet, previous surgery, interpersonal contacts, and family history should be obtained. Blood tests may identify anemia, elevated white blood cell (WBC) count, iron and folate deficiencies, elevated liver enzyme levels, and electrolyte disturbances. Stools may be examined for the presence of blood, mucus, WBCs, and parasites. Stool cultures help in identifying infectious organisms.

In a patient with chronic diarrhea, measurement of stool electrolytes, pH, and osmolality may help determine whether the diarrhea is related to decreased fluid absorption or increased fluid secretion (secretory diarrhea). Measurement of stool fat and undigested muscle fibers may indicate fat and protein malabsorption conditions, including pancreatic insufficiency. Elevated serum levels of GI peptides such as vasoactive intestinal polypeptide (VIP) and gastrin may be present in some patients with secretory diarrhea. Endoscopy may be used to examine the mucosa and to obtain specimens for examination. Upper and lower barium studies may be helpful in detecting mucosal disease.

Collaborative Care

The treatment of diarrhea is based on the cause and is aimed at replacement of fluid and electrolytes and decreasing the number, volume, and frequency of stools. Oral solutions containing glucose and electrolytes (e.g., Gatorade, Pedialyte) may be sufficient to replace losses from mild diarrhea. In situations

Table 40-2   Causes of Acute Infectious Diarrhea

	Onset	Duration	Symptoms and Signs
Viral			
Rotavirus, Norwalk	18-24 hr	24-48 hr	Explosive, watery diarrhea; nausea; vomiting; abdominal cramps
Bacterial			
Escherichia coli	4-24 hr	3-4 days	Four or five loose stools per day, nausea, malaise, low-grade fever
Enterohemorrhagic *E. coli* (0157:H7)	4-24 hr	4-9 days	Bloody diarrhea, severe cramping, fever
Shigella	24 hr	7 days	Watery stools containing blood and mucus, tenesmus, urgency, severe cramping, fever
Salmonellae	6-48 hr	2-5 days	Watery diarrhea, nausea, vomiting, abdominal cramps, fever
Campylobacter species	24 hr	<7 days	Profuse, watery diarrhea; malaise, nausea, abdominal cramps, low-grade fever
Clostridium perfringens	8-12 hr	24 hr	Watery diarrhea, abdominal cramps, vomiting
Clostridium difficile	4-9 days after start of antibiotics	24 hr	Associated with antibiotic treatment; symptoms range from mild, watery diarrhea to severe abdominal pain, fever, leukocytosis, leukocytes in stool
Parasitic			
Giardia lamblia	1-3 wk	Few days to 3 months	Sudden onset; malodorous, explosive, watery diarrhea; flatulence, epigastric pain and cramping, nausea
Entamoeba histolytica	4 days	Weeks to months	Frequent soft stools with blood and mucus (in severe cases, watery stools), flatulence, distention, abdominal cramps, fever, leukocytes in stool
Cryptosporidium	2-10 days	1-6 months	Watery diarrhea, nausea, vomiting, abdominal cramps, weight loss in AIDS

AIDS, acquired immunodeficiency syndrome.

DRUG THERAPY

Table 40-3 Antidiarrheal Drugs

Type	Mechanism of Action	Examples
Demulcent	Soothes, coats, and protects mucous membranes	Bismuth subsalicylate* (Pepto-Bismol); calcium polycarbophil (Mitrolan-OTC); activated charcoal; kaolin[†], pectin, hyoscyamine sulfate, and hyoscine hydrobromide (Donnagel)*[†]; Donnagel and opium (Donnagel-PG)*[†]
Anticholinergic	Inhibits GI motility	Donnagel*[†], Donnagel-PG*[†], diphenoxylate with atropine sulfate (Lomotil, Colonaid), loperamide (Imodium)[†‡]
Antisecretory	Decreases intestinal secretion	Octreotide (Sandostatin), a synthetic analog of somatostatin
Narcotic	Decreases CNS stimulation of GI tract motility and secretion	Camphorated tincture of opium (paregoric); Donnagel-PG[†]; paregoric, pectin, and kaolin (Parepectolin)[†]; tincture of opium, homatropine methylbromide, and pectin (Dia-Quel liquid OTC)[§]

*Also inhibits bacterial activity.
[†]Also absorbent, which contributes to the adhesiveness of the stool.
[‡]Has cholinergic and noncholinergic actions.
[§]Also an anticholinergic.
CNS, central nervous system; *GI,* gastrointestinal.

NURSING ASSESSMENT

Table 40-4 Diarrhea

Subjective Data

Important Health Information
Past health history: Recent travel, infections, stress; diverticulitis or malabsorption; metabolic disorders; inflammatory bowel disease; irritable bowel syndrome
Medications: Use of laxatives, magnesium-containing antacids, sorbitol-containing suspensions or elixirs, antibiotics, methyldopa, digitalis, colchicine; OTC antidiarrheal medications
Surgery or other treatments: Stomach or bowel surgery, radiation

Functional Health Patterns
Health perception–health management: Chronic laxative abuse, malaise
Nutritional-metabolic: Ingestion of coarse and spicy foods, food intolerances; anorexia, nausea, vomiting; weight loss; thirst
Elimination: Increased stool frequency, volume, and looseness; change in color and character of stools; abdominal bloating; decreased urinary output
Cognitive-perceptual: Abdominal tenderness, abdominal pain and cramping; tenesmus

Objective Data

General
Lethargy, sunken eyeballs, fever, malnutrition

Integumentary
Pallor, dry mucous membranes, poor skin turgor, perianal irritation

Gastrointestinal
Frequent soft to liquid stools that may alternate with constipation; altered stool color; abdominal distention, hyperactive bowel sounds; presence of pus, blood, mucus, or fat in stools; fecal impaction

Urinary Tract
Decreased output, concentrated urine

Possible Findings
Abnormal serum electrolyte levels; anemia; leukocytosis; eosinophila, hypoalbuminemia; positive stool cultures; presence of ova, parasites, leukocytes, blood, or fat in stools; abnormal sigmoidoscopic or colonoscopic findings; abnormal lower GI series

OTC, over-the-counter.

of severe diarrhea, parenteral administration of fluids, electrolytes, vitamins, and, potentially, nutrition is warranted.

Once the cause of the diarrhea has been determined, antidiarrheal agents may be given to coat and protect mucous membranes, absorb irritating substances, inhibit GI motility, decrease intestinal secretions, and decrease central nervous system (CNS) stimulation of the GI tract (Table 40-3). Antiperistaltic agents are not given to a patient who has infectious diarrheal syndromes because of the potential of prolonging exposure to the infectious agent. Antidiarrheal medications should not be given for a prolonged time.

Antibiotics are reserved for treating specific bacterial organisms. Antibiotics can cause diarrhea by altering the normal bowel flora. Patients receiving antibiotics (e.g., clindamycin [Cleocin]), are susceptible to *Clostridium difficile* infection. Health care workers who do not adhere to infection control pre-

cautions can transmit *C. difficile* from patient to patient. Some strains of *C. difficile* release a toxin that causes mucosal damage resulting in cramps, pain, and diarrhea that may be bloody. *C. difficile* infection can lead to mucosal damage, pseudomembranous enterocolitis, and intestinal perforation.[1] Vancomycin (Vancocin) or metronidazole (Flagyl) is used to treat *C. difficile.*

NURSING MANAGEMENT: ACUTE INFECTIOUS DIARRHEA

■ Nursing Assessment

Nursing assessment should begin with a thorough history and physical examination (Table 40-4). The patient should be asked to describe the stool pattern and associated symptoms. Questions should focus on the duration, frequency, character,

40-1 NURSING CARE PLAN PATIENT WITH ACUTE INFECTIOUS DIARRHEA

Expected Patient Outcomes	Nursing Interventions and *Rationales*

NURSING DIAGNOSIS Diarrhea *related to* acute infectious process *as manifested by* frequent loose, watery stools.

- Normal bowel elimination.
- Afebrile.

- Monitor frequency, amount, color, consistency of stools *to determine severity of diarrhea and need for intervention.*
- Record intake and output *to monitor fluid balance.*
- Follow hospital procedure for infection control precautions; use strict medical asepsis when handling bedpan, linens, or patient *to prevent spread of infection.*
- Monitor vital signs q4hr *as changes can indicate development of hypovolemia.*
- Administer antiinfective and antidiarrheal medications as ordered *to treat bacterial infection and relieve diarrhea.*

NURSING DIAGNOSIS Fluid volume deficit *related to* excessive fluid loss and decreased fluid intake secondary to diarrhea *as manifested by* dry skin and mucous membranes, poor skin turgor, hypotension, tachycardia, decreased urine output, electrolyte imbalance.

- Normal vital signs.
- Normal skin turgor.
- Moist mucous membranes.
- Urine output >0.5 ml/kg/hr.
- Normal serum electrolytes.

- Assess for skin turgor changes, sunken eyes, rapid pulse, and anorexia *as indicators of fluid volume deficit.*
- Monitor intake and output *to determine fluid balance.*
- Monitor serum sodium and potassium levels *so abnormalities can be reported to physician.*
- Monitor vital signs q4hr.
- Weigh patient daily *to monitor fluid loss.*
- Administer IV fluids as ordered and increase intake of fluids as tolerated to at least 3000 ml/day *to replace fluids and electrolytes lost in stools.*
- Assess mouth for dryness and note patient's complaints of thirst *as dry mucous membranes and thirst are indicators of dehydration.*
- If patient is not vomiting, administer fluids, such as Gatorade or Pedialyte *to replace electrolytes lost in stools.*
- Medicate with antidiarrheals as ordered *to decrease diarrhea.*

NURSING DIAGNOSIS Impaired skin integrity *related to* perianal contact with diarrheal stools and inadequate perianal hygiene *as manifested by* redness, irritation, swelling, possible ulceration of skin, pain during elimination.

- No evidence of skin breakdown in perianal area.

- Assess skin of perianal area *to plan appropriate interventions.*
- Cleanse area with warm water after each bowel movement, rinse well and dry with a soft towel *to prevent skin excoriation and promote patient comfort.*
- Apply ointment (e.g., A and D, zinc oxide) *to protect skin and promote healing.*
- Use an anesthetic ointment or spray foam *to decrease local discomfort.*

NURSING DIAGNOSIS Risk for infection transmission *related to* lack of knowledge about prevention of reinfection or transmission of infectious disease.

- No recurrence of symptoms.
- Knowledgeable about disease process and preventive measures.

- Teach patient to be alert for recurrence of diarrhea, fever, and other presenting symptoms; evidence of same symptoms in family members *as signs of possible infection transmission.*
- Assist patient in identifying factors that precipitated diarrhea *to avoid causing reinfection of self or transmission to others.*
- Stress importance of good hand-washing techniques *to prevent spread of diarrhea to others.*
- Explain importance of seeking medical care when diarrhea and other symptoms begin *so early treatment can be initiated.*

and consistency of stool. A medication history should include use of antibiotics, laxatives, and other drugs known to cause diarrhea. Recent travel, stress, and health and family history should be discussed. Dietary history should include questions about eating habits, appetite, and food intolerances, especially milk and dairy products, and food preparation practices.

Physical examination begins with obtaining vital signs, height, and weight. The patient's skin should be inspected for decreased turgor, dryness, and areas of breakdown. The abdomen should be inspected for distention, auscultated for bowel sounds, and palpated for tenderness.

■ Nursing Diagnoses

Nursing diagnoses for the patient with acute infectious diarrhea may include, but are not limited to, those presented in NCP 40-1 on p. 1139.

■ Planning

The overall goals are that the patient with diarrhea will (1) not transmit the microorganism causing the infectious diarrhea, (2) cease having diarrhea and resume normal bowel patterns, (3) have normal fluid and electrolyte and acid-base balance, (4) have normal nutritional intake, and (5) have no perianal skin breakdown.

■ Nursing Implementation

Adherence to infection control precautions for infectious diseases (see Table 11-19) is important because some cases of acute diarrhea are infectious. All cases of acute diarrhea should be considered infectious until the cause is determined. The use of precautions is effective in reducing the spread of infectious diarrhea.

Hand washing is the most important measure in prevention of the transfer of microorganisms. Hands should be washed before and after contact with each patient and when body fluids of any kind are handled. The patient should be taught the principles of hygiene, infectious control precautions, and the potential dangers of an illness that is infectious to themselves and others. Proper handling, cooking, and storage of food should be discussed with the patient suspected of having infectious diarrhea.

FECAL INCONTINENCE
Etiology and Pathophysiology

Fecal incontinence, or the involuntary passage of stool, may be due to multiple causes (Table 40-5). Knowledge of the mechanisms involved in fecal continence is helpful in understanding fecal incontinence. Normally, fecal contents pass from the sigmoid colon into the rectum, causing rectal distention. Sensory (stretch) receptors in the muscles surrounding the rectum provide the sensation of rectal filling. This causes a reflex relaxation of the internal anal sphincter and contraction of the external anal sphincter. Sensory receptors in the epithelium of the anal canal can usually distinguish among solid, liquid, and gas. The combination of contraction of the abdominal muscles, relaxation of the pelvic muscles, squatting (which straightens the

Table **40-5**	Causes of Fecal Incontinence
Traumatic	**Inflammatory**
Obstetric	Infection
Postsurgical	Trauma
Hemorrhoidectomy	Radiation
Anterior resection	**Other**
Fistulectomy	Pelvic floor relaxation
Anorectal surgery	Perineal descent
Spinal cord injuries	Loss of elasticity of rectum
Neurologic	Decreased sphincter tone (age-related)
Stroke	Rectal prolapse
Tumor	Fecal impaction
Degenerative diseases	Diarrhea
Iatrogenic drug intoxication	Medications
Multiple sclerosis	
Diabetes mellitus	
Dementia	

anorectal angle), and voluntary relaxation of the external anal sphincter allows for elimination of feces.

Diagnostic Studies and Collaborative Care

The diagnosis and effective management of fecal incontinence require a thorough health history and physical examination with appropriate diagnostic studies. In all cases a rectal examination should be performed, followed by examination with a flexible sigmoidoscope. Fecal impaction, internal prolapse, increased perineal descent, and rectocele may be identified by rectal examination. If the impaction is higher in the colon, an abdominal x-ray may be helpful. Flexible sigmoidoscopy may identify inflammation, tumors, fissures, and other sigmoid-rectum pathology. Other studies may include barium enema, colonoscopy, and anorectal manometry.

Treatment of incontinence depends on the underlying cause. If fecal incontinence is related to noninfectious diarrhea, antidiarrheal agents may be prescribed. For example, loperamide (Imodium) may be useful in reducing diarrhea and increasing sphincter tone.

Fecal incontinence caused by fecal impaction can be a common problem in the older adult. Fecal impaction usually resolves after manual disimpaction and cleansing enemas. To prevent recurrence, a high-fiber diet (see Table 40-9 later in this chapter), along with increased fluid intake, should be given unless contraindicated. Dietary fiber supplements (e.g., psyllium in Metamucil) can improve continence by increasing stool bulk and promoting sensation of rectal filling.

Biofeedback therapy is aimed at improving awareness of rectal sensation and coordination of the internal and external anal sphincters and increasing the strength of contraction of the external sphincter.[2] Biofeedback training requires adequate mental status and motivation to learn. Components of biofeedback include education, reinforcement, and concentration. It is a safe, painless, and inexpensive treatment for fecal incontinence. (Biofeedback is discussed further in Chapter 8.)

Surgery (e.g., sphincter repair procedures) should be considered only when conservative treatment fails, in cases of full-thickness prolapse, and when the sphincter needs repair.

NURSING MANAGEMENT: FECAL INCONTINENCE

■ Nursing Assessment

Fecal incontinence is not only an embarrassment to the patient but also a potential hazard to normal skin integrity. It is necessary to make an assessment of the patient's general condition to identify the best alternative for managing the patient with fecal incontinence. The nurse should identify normal bowel habits and current symptoms, including frequency and nature of the stools.

A neurologic assessment that includes evaluation of mental status can be helpful in identifying the most effective treatment for the patient. Assessment should also include history of multiple or traumatic childbirths, previous anorectal surgery, and injury.

■ Nursing Diagnoses

Nursing diagnoses for the patient with fecal incontinence include, but are not limited to, the following:

- Impaired skin integrity *related to* incontinence of stool and irritation of perianal area
- Social isolation *related to* embarrassment and odor
- Self-esteem disturbance *related to* inability to control bowel functions
- Self-care deficits *related to* inability to manage bowel evacuation independently

■ Planning

The overall goals are that the patient with fecal incontinence will (1) have normal bowel control, (2) maintain perianal skin integrity, and (3) not suffer any self-esteem problems related to problems with bowel control.

■ Nursing Implementation

Prevention and treatment of fecal incontinence may be managed by implementing a bowel-training program. The patient should be put on a bedpan, assisted to a bedside commode, or walked to the bathroom at a regular time daily to assist with reestablishment of bowel regularity. A good time to establish this pattern is within 30 minutes after breakfast. Most individuals experience an urge to defecate following the first meal of the day because of the gastrocolic reflex. If the usual bowel habits differ from this pattern, efforts should be made to adhere to the patient's individual timing.

If these techniques are ineffective in reestablishing bowel regularity, a bisacodyl (Dulcolax) or glycerin suppository or "mini-enema" may be given 15 to 30 minutes before the usual evacuation time. A mini-enema is a small (4 ml) gelatin capsule with an enema tip for instilling its contents (e.g., Therevac Plus contains docusate, soft-soap, and xylocaine).[3] These preparations stimulate the anorectal reflex and often can be discontinued when a regular pattern is reestablished.

Maintenance of skin integrity is of utmost importance, especially in the bedridden and older adult patient. Nursing management may necessitate drainage tubes or catheters, use of incontinence briefs, and meticulous skin care. Tubes and catheters are usually not recommended because their use for an extended period may decrease responsiveness of the rectal sphincter and cause ulceration of the rectal mucosa. Use of incontinence briefs may be helpful in maintaining skin integrity if changed frequently, but this can be demeaning and humiliating to the patient. Meticulous cleaning after each stool is required. Washing, rinsing, thorough drying, and application of a protective barrier are essential to the maintenance of skin integrity. Because the patient may have several stools each day, maintaining skin integrity is a time-consuming task for the nurse and the family.

Perianal pouching is an alternative in the management of fecal incontinence. Pouching provides skin protection and fecal containment as well as comfort and dignity. Because odor is often a problem, deodorant sprays and room deodorizers may be used. For the patient who is ambulatory, a chair (regular or special commode wheelchair) may be used. Regardless of the patient's mobility, the nurse must make sure the skin is clean, odorless, and intact.

CONSTIPATION

Constipation may be defined as a decrease in frequency of bowel movements from what is "normal" for the individual, hard, difficult-to-pass stools, a decrease in stool volume, and retention of feces in the rectum. Normal bowel elimination may vary from three times a day to once every 3 days.[4] Because of this variability, it is important to determine the severity of constipation on the basis of the patient's normal pattern of elimination. It is important to remember that changes in bowel habits may also indicate bowel obstruction produced by a tumor. Millions of people suffer from constipation.

Etiology

Frequently constipation may be due to insufficient dietary fiber, inadequate fluid intake, medication use, and lack of exercise. If proper preventive measures are subsequently taken, constipation should not recur. Constipation may also be due to sociocultural beliefs, environmental constraints, ignoring the urge to defecate, chronic laxative abuse, and multiple organic causes (Table 40-6). Changes in diet, in mealtime, or in daily routines are a few environmental factors that may cause constipation. Depression and stress can also result in constipation. For many patients with constipation, however, it is not possible to identify the underlying cause.[4]

Some patients believe that they are constipated if they do not have a daily bowel movement. This can result in chronic laxative use and subsequent *cathartic colon syndrome*. In this condition, the colon becomes dilated and atonic.

Ignoring the urge to defecate for a period of time causes the muscles and mucosa in the rectal area to become insensitive to the presence of feces. In addition, the prolonged retention of feces in the rectum results in drying of stool because of the absorption of water. The harder and drier the feces, the more difficult it is to expel.

Clinical Manifestations and Complications

The clinical presentation of constipation may vary from a chronic discomfort to an acute event mimicking an "acute abdomen." Other clinical manifestations are presented in Table 40-7.

Table 40-6	Causes of Constipation

Colonic Disorders	Systemic Disorders
Luminal or extra-luminal obstructing lesions	**Metabolic/Endocrine**
	Diabetes mellitus
Inflammatory strictures	Hypothyroidism
Volvulus	Pregnancy
Intussusception	Hypercalcemia/hyper-parathyroidism
Irritable bowel syndrome	Pheochromocytoma
Diverticular disease	**Collagen Vascular Disease**
Rectocele	Scleroderma
Drug Induced	Amyloidosis
Antacids (calcium and aluminum)	**Neurogenic Disorders**
Antidepressants	Hirschsprung's megacolon
Anticholinergics	Neurofibromatosis
Antipsychotics	Autonomic neuropathy (pseudoobstruction)
Antihypertensives	Multiple sclerosis
Barium sulfate	Parkinson's disease
Iron supplements	Spinal cord lesions or injury
Bismuth	Cerebrovascular accident
Calcium supplements	
Laxative abuse	

Hemorrhoids are the most common complication of chronic constipation. They result from venous engorgement caused by repeated *Valsalva's maneuvers* (straining) and venous compression from hard impacted stool.

Valsalva's maneuver, which occurs during straining to pass a hardened stool, may cause serious problems in patients with congestive heart failure, cerebral edema, hypertension, and coronary artery disease. During straining, the patient takes a deep inspiration, the breath is held, and the glottis closes and traps the air. The abdominal muscles contract and try to push against the colon. Increases in intraabdominal pressure and intrathoracic pressure occur, reducing venous return to the heart. The heart slows temporarily (bradycardia), the cardiac output is decreased, and there is a transient drop in arterial pressure. When the patient relaxes, there is decreased thoracic pressure and a sudden flow of blood into the heart, causing distention and an increase in heart rate. Immediately the arterial pressure rises momentarily. These changes may be fatal for the patient who cannot compensate for sudden overload of blood flow returning to the heart.

Diverticulosis is another potential complication of chronic constipation. This is a relatively common complication in an older adult. Diverticuli or outpouchings of the colon wall are thought to be due to the increased intraluminal pressure

DRUG THERAPY

Table 40-8	Cathartic Agents

Category	Mechanisms of Action	Example	Onset of Action	Comments
■ Bulk forming	Absorbs water; increases bulk, thereby stimulating peristalsis	Metamucil, Perdiem, Konsyl, Hydrocil, Citrucil, Fibercon	Usually within 24 hr	Contraindicated in patients with abdominal pain, nausea, and vomiting and in patients suspected of having appendicitis, biliary tract obstruction, or acute hepatitis; needs to be taken with fluids
■ Stimulants	Increase peristalsis by irritating colon wall and stimulating enteric nerves	Antraquinone drugs: Cascara sagrada, senna Phenolphthalein drugs Ex-Lax, Correctol, Feen-a-Mint, Bisacodyl, Dulcolax	Usually within 12 hr	Cause melanosis coli (brown or black pigmentation of colon); are most widely abused laxatives; should not be used in patients with impaction or obstipation
■ Stool softeners and lubricants	Lubricate intestinal tract and soften feces, making hard stools easier to pass; do not affect peristalsis	Mineral oil, dioctyl sodium, sulfosuccinate, Colace, Peri-Colace, Doxidan	Softeners up to 72 hr, lubricants up to 8 hr	Can block absorption of fat-soluble vitamins such as vitamin K, which may increase risk of bleeding in patients on anticoagulants
■ Saline and osmotic solutions	Cause retention of fluid in intestinal lumen caused by osmotic effect	Magnesium salts: Magnesium citrate, Milk of Magnesia Sodium phosphates: Fleets enema, Phospho-soda Lactulose Polyethylene glycolsaline solutions Go-Lytely, Colyte	15 min to 3 hr	Magnesium-containing products may cause hypermagnesemia in patients with renal insufficiency

Table 40-7	Clinical Manifestations of Constipation

Hard, dry stool	Increased flatulence
Abdominal distention	Nausea
Abdominal pain	Anorexia
Decreased frequency of bowel movements	Headache
	Palpable mass
Straining	Stool with blood
Rectal pressure	Dizziness
Tenesmus	Urinary retention

needed to expel hard stool. Diverticulosis and diverticulitis are described later in this chapter.

In the presence of *obstipation,* or fecal impaction secondary to constipation, colonic perforation may occur. Perforation, which is life threatening, causes abdominal pain, nausea, vomiting, fever, and an elevated WBC count. An abdominal x-ray shows the presence of free air, which is diagnostic of perforation. Rectal mucosal ulcers may also occur as a result of stool stasis or straining. These complications are most common in older patients.

Diagnostic Studies and Collaborative Care

A thorough history and physical examination should be performed so that the underlying cause of constipation can be identified and treatment started. Abdominal x-rays, barium enema, colonoscopy, sigmoidoscopy, and anorectal manometry may be helpful in the diagnosis. Most cases of constipation can be managed with diet therapy including fiber and fluids and an exercise program. Laxatives (Table 40-8) should always be used cautiously because with chronic overuse they may become a cause of constipation. Enemas are fast acting and are beneficial in the immediate treatment of constipation but should be limited in their use for long-term treatment of constipation. Soapsuds enemas should be avoided because they may lead to inflammation of colon mucosa. Oil-retention enemas may be used to soften fecal impactions. Biofeedback therapy may benefit patients who are constipated as a result of *anismus* (uncoordinated contraction of the anal sphincter during straining).[5]

For the patient in whom perceived constipation is related to rigid beliefs regarding bowel function, the nurse should initiate a discussion about these beliefs with the patient. Appropriate information on normal bowel function is given and discussed along with the adverse consequences of excessive use of laxatives and enemas.

A patient with severe constipation related to motility or mechanical disorders may require more intensive treatment. Studies such as anorectal manometry, GI tract transit studies, and sigmoidoscopic rectal biopsies should be performed before treatment. In a patient with unrelenting constipation, a subtotal colectomy with ileorectal anastomosis is the procedure of choice.[4]

Nutritional Therapy. Diet is an important factor in the prevention of constipation. Many patients experience an improvement in their symptoms when they simply increase their intake of dietary fiber and fluids. Dietary fiber is found in two forms: insoluble and soluble in water. Both are contained in most foods, but some foods are higher in soluble fiber (Table 40-9).

NUTRITIONAL THERAPY
Table 40-9	High Fiber Foods*		
	Fiber Per Serving (g)	Size of Serving	Calories Per Serving
Vegetables			
Asparagus	3.5	½ cup	18
Beans			
Navy	8.4	½ cup	80
Kidney	9.7	½ cup	94
Lima	8.3	½ cup	63
Pinto	8.9	½ cup	78
String	2.1	½ cup	18
Broccoli	3.5	½ cup	18
Carrots, raw	1.8	½ cup	15
Corn	2.6	½ medium ear	72
Peas, canned	6.7	½ cup	63
Potatoes			
Baked	1.9	½ medium	72
Sweet	2.1	½ medium	79
Squash			
Acorn	7.0	1 cup	82
Tomato, raw	1.5	1 small	18
Fruits			
Apple	2.0	½ large	42
Banana	1.5	½ medium	48
Blackberries	6.7	¾ cup	40
Orange	1.6	1 small	35
Peach	2.3	1 medium	38
Pear	2.0	½ medium	44
Raspberries	9.2	1 cup	42
Strawberries	3.1	1 cup	45
Grain Products			
Bread			
Rye	0.8	1 slice	62
White	0.7	1 slice	64
Whole wheat	1.3	1 slice	59
Cereal			
All Bran (100%)	8.4	⅓ cup	70
Corn Flakes	2.6	¾ cup	70
Shredded Wheat	2.8	1 biscuit	70
Crackers			
Graham	1.4	2 squares	53
Popcorn	3.0	3 cups	62
Rice			
Brown	1.6	⅓ cup	72
White	0.5	⅓ cup	76

*Recommended for patients with diverticulosis, irritable bowel syndrome, constipation, hemorrhoids, colon cancer, atherosclerosis, hyperlipidemia, and diabetes mellitus.

Insoluble fiber remains essentially unchanged by the time it reaches the colon, and it is found in higher concentrations in whole wheat and bran. *Soluble fibers* form gel-like substances that add viscosity to the digested contents, causing decreased gastric emptying and increased transit in the small intestine. When these fibers are fermented, they increase stool bulk,

NURSING ASSESSMENT

Table 40-10   Constipation

Subjective Data	Objective Data
Important Health Information	**General**
Past health history: Colorectal disease, neurologic dysfunction, bowel obstruction, environmental changes, cancer	Lethargy
	Integumentary
Medications: Use of aluminum antacids, anticholinergics, antidepressants, antihistamines, antipsychotics, diuretics, narcotics, iron, laxatives, enemas	Anorectal fissures, hemorrhoids, abscesses
	Gastrointestinal
Functional Health Patterns	Abdominal distention; hypoactive or absent bowel sounds; palpable abdominal mass; fecal impaction, small, hard, dry stool, stool with blood
Health perception–health management: Chronic laxative or enema abuse; rigid beliefs regarding bowel function; malaise	**Possible Findings**
Nutritional-metabolic: Changes in diet or mealtime; inadequate fiber and fluid intake; anorexia, nausea	Guaiac-positive stools, abdominal x-ray demonstrating stool in lower colon
Elimination: Change in usual elimination patterns; hard, difficult to pass stool, decrease in frequency and amount of stools; flatus, abdominal distention; tenesmus, rectal pressure; fecal incontinence (if impacted)	
Activity-exercise: Change in daily activity routines; immobility; sedentary lifestyle	
Cognitive-perceptual: Dizziness, headache, anorectal pain; abdominal pain on defecation	
Coping–stress tolerance: Acute or chronic stress	

promoting defecation and sequestering fluid, which softens stools. Soluble fiber is found in oat bran, fruits, vegetables, and psyllium. Patients should be told that initially fiber will increase gas production but that this effect decreases with time.

The diet should also include a fluid intake of at least 3000 ml per day, unless contraindicated by cardiac or renal disease. Increasing fiber intake without increasing fluids may predispose the patient to impaction or obstruction. The nurse should encourage the selection of foods that the patient likes, is able to prepare, and can afford. The patient's understanding of the diet and the importance of dietary fiber is important to ensure compliance.

NURSING MANAGEMENT: CONSTIPATION

■ Nursing Assessment

Subjective and objective data that should be obtained from a patient with constipation are presented in Table 40-10.

■ Nursing Diagnoses

Nursing diagnosis for the patient with constipation includes, but is not limited to, the following:

- Constipation *related to* inadequate intake of dietary fiber and fluid and decreased physical activity

■ Planning

The overall goals are that the patient with constipation will (1) increase dietary intake of fiber and fluids; (2) have the passage of soft, formed stools; and (3) not have any complications, such as bleeding hemorrhoids.

■ Nursing Implementation

Nursing management should be based on the patient's symptoms (see Table 40-7) and the assessment of the patient (see Table 40-10). An important role of the nurse is teaching the patient the importance of dietary measures to prevent constipation. A patient teaching guide for constipation is presented in Table 40-11. Emphasis should be placed on maintenance of a high-fiber diet, increasing fluid intake, and a regular exercise program. The patient should be taught to establish a regular time to defecate and not to suppress the urge to defecate. In many persons the urge to defecate occurs after breakfast because of the stimulation of the gastrocolic reflex. The patient should be discouraged from using laxatives and enemas to achieve fecal elimination.

Proper position is important when defecating. For a patient in bed, the bedpan should be placed and the head of the bed should be elevated as high as the patient can tolerate. For the person who can sit on a toilet, a footstool may be placed in front of the toilet. Placing the feet on the footstool promotes flexion of the thighs, which assists in defecation.

The patient with poor muscle tone should be encouraged to exercise the abdominal muscles and can be taught to contract the abdominal muscles several times a day. Sit-ups and straight leg raises can also be used to improve abdominal muscle tone.

Some patients may have to be encouraged to increase their social activities, as well as their physical activity. This is especially true for older adults who may become depressed and socially isolated because of multiple factors. Inactivity can lead to constipation. This patient should be encouraged and assisted in establishing social contacts and activities outside the home.

PATIENT TEACHING GUIDE
Table 40-11 | Constipation

The following are teaching guidelines for the patient:

1. **Eat dietary fiber**

   Eat 20 to 30 g of fiber per day. Gradually increase amount of fiber eaten over 1 to 2 weeks. Fiber softens hard stools and adds bulk to stool, promoting evacuation.
   - Foods high in fiber: raw vegetables and fruits, beans, breakfast cereals (All Bran, oatmeal)
   - Fiber supplements: Metamucil, Citrucel, and FiberCon

2. **Drink fluids**

   Drink 3 quarts per day. Drink water or fruit juices; avoid caffeinated coffee, tea, and cola. Fluid softens hard stools; caffeine stimulates fluid loss through urination.

3. **Exercise regularly**

   Walk, swim, or bike at least three times per week. Contract and relax abdominal muscles when standing or by doing sit-ups to strengthen muscles and prevent straining. Exercise stimulates bowel motility and moves stool through the intestine.

4. **Establish a regular time to defecate**

5. **Do not delay defecation**

   Respond to the urge to have a bowel movement as soon as possible. Delaying defecation results in hard stools and a decreased "urge" to defecate. Water is absorbed from stool by the intestine over time. The intestine becomes less sensitive to the presence of stool in the rectum.

6. **Record your bowel elimination pattern**

   Develop a habit of recording when you have a bowel movement on your calendar. Regular monitoring of bowel movement will assist in early problem identification.

7. **Avoid laxatives and enemas**

   Do not overuse laxatives and enemas as they can actually cause constipation. The normal motility of the bowel is interrupted and bowel movements slow or stop.

ABDOMINAL PAIN

ACUTE ABDOMINAL PAIN

Etiology

The patient with an *acute abdomen* has an acute onset of abdominal pain requiring prompt decision making. Causes of an acute abdomen are varied (Table 40-12). Many disorders must be ruled out before a diagnosis is confirmed.

Clinical Manifestations

Pain is the most common presenting symptom. The patient may also complain of abdominal tenderness, vomiting, diarrhea, constipation, flatulence, fatigue, fever, and an increase in abdominal girth.

Diagnostic Studies and Collaborative Care

Diagnosis begins with a complete history and physical examination. Physical examination should include a rectal and pelvic examination. A complete blood count (CBC), urinalysis, abdominal x-ray, and an electrocardiogram (ECG) are done initially. Pregnancy tests should be performed in women of childbearing age who have acute abdominal pain. The findings of these studies may provide some information as to the cause of the acute abdomen.

Emergency management of the patient with an acute abdomen is presented in Table 40-13. The goal of management is to identify and treat the cause. The physician attempts to make a differential diagnosis when the patient is seen with an acute abdomen because many causes of abdominal pain do not require surgery (see Table 40-12). It was previously thought that pain medication should be withheld because analgesics might obscure progression of clinical manifestations and impede diagnosis. Appropriate pain management that does not result in

Table 40-12 | Causes of Acute Abdomen

Abdominal penetrating trauma	Peptic ulcer
Acute ischemic bowel	Perforated gastro-intestinal malignancy
Appendicitis	Peritonitis
Bowel obstruction with perforation or necrosis	Ruptured abdominal aneurysm
Cholecystitis	Ruptured ectopic pregnancy
Crohn's disease	Ruptured ovarian cyst
Diverticulitis with peritonitis	Ulcerative colitis
Foreign body perforation	Uterine rupture
Gastritis	Volvulus
Gastroenteritis	
Mesenteric adenitis	
Pancreatitis	
Pelvic inflammatory disease	

altered consciousness (e.g., ketorolac [Toradol]) can decrease diffuse pain and abdominal rigidity and help localize the pain. This can lead to earlier diagnosis and treatment.[6]

In addition to being a therapeutic measure, surgery can also be diagnostic. Operative exploration is usually done after a careful examination of the patient and is justified when "look and see" is better than "wait and see." The surgical procedure is an *exploratory laparotomy*, in which an opening is made through the abdominal wall into the peritoneal cavity to determine the cause of an acute abdomen. If the cause of the acute abdomen can be surgically removed (e.g., inflamed appendix) or surgically repaired (e.g., ruptured abdominal aneurysm), surgery is considered definitive therapy.

✚**EMERGENCY MANAGEMENT**

Table **40-13** **Acute Abdomen**

Etiology	Assessment Findings	Interventions

Inflammation
  Appendicitis
  Cholecystitis
  Pancreatitis
  Ulcerative colitis/Crohn's disease
  Gastritis
  Pyelonephritis
 	
Vascular Problems
  Ruptured aortic aneurysm
  Mesenteric vascular occlusion
 	
Gynecologic Problems
  Ruptured ectopic pregnancy
  Ruptured ovarian cyst
  Pelvic inflammatory disease
 	
Infectious Disease
  Giardia
  Salmonella
 	
Other
  Obstruction or perforation of
    abdominal organ
  Gastrointestinal bleeding
	Abdominal/Gastrointestinal Findings
	■ Diffuse, localized, dull, burning, or
	  sharp abdominal pain or tenderness
	■ Rebound tenderness
	■ Abdominal distention
	■ Abdominal rigidity
	■ Nausea, vomiting
	■ Diarrhea
	■ Hematemesis
	■ Melena
	
	Hypovolemic Shock
	■ Decreased blood pressure
	■ Decreased pulse pressure
	■ Tachycardia
	■ Cool, clammy skin
	■ Decreased level of consciousness
		Initial
		■ Ensure patent airway.
		■ Administer oxygen via nasal cannu-
		  la or nonrebreather mask.
		■ Establish IV access with large bore
		  catheter and infuse warm normal
		  saline or lactated Ringer's solution.
		  Insert additional large bore
		  catheter if shock present.
		■ Obtain blood for CBC, electrolytes.
		■ Anticipate order for amylase, preg-
		  nancy tests, clotting studies, and
		  type and crossmatch as appropriate.
		■ Insert indwelling urinary catheter.
		■ Obtain urinalysis.
		■ Insert NG tube as needed.
		
		Ongoing Monitoring
		■ Monitor vital signs, level of con-
		  sciousness, oxygen saturation, and
		  intake and output.
		■ Assess quality and amount of pain.
		■ Assess amount and character of
		  emesis.
		■ Anticipate surgical intervention.
		■ Keep NPO.

NG, nasogastric.

NURSING MANAGEMENT: ACUTE ABDOMEN

■ Nursing Assessment

Vital signs should be taken immediately. Blood pressure and pulse rate should be obtained to determine hypovolemic changes. An elevated temperature may indicate an inflammatory or infectious process. The abdomen should be inspected for distention, masses, abnormal pulsation, rashes, scars, and pigmentation changes. Bowel sounds should be auscultated. Bowel sounds that are diminished or absent in a quadrant may indicate a complete bowel obstruction, acute peritonitis, or paralytic ileus. Palpation should be gentle.

A thorough assessment of the patient's symptoms should be made to determine the onset, location, intensity, duration, frequency, and character of pain. The nurse should determine whether the pain has spread or moved to new locations (quadrants), as well as what makes the pain worse or better. It should also be determined whether the pain is associated with other symptoms, such as nausea, vomiting, changes in bowel and bladder habits, or vaginal discharge in women. Assessment of vomiting should include the amount, color, consistency, and odor of the vomitus. Bowel patterns and habits should also be carefully assessed.

■ Nursing Diagnoses

Nursing diagnoses for the patient with acute abdomen peritonitis include, but are not limited to, the following:

■ Pain *related to* inflammation of the peritoneum and abdominal distention
■ Risk for fluid volume deficit *related to* collection of fluid in peritoneal cavity secondary to inflammation or infection
■ Altered nutrition: less than body requirements *related to* anorexia, nausea, and vomiting
■ Anxiety *related to* uncertainty of cause or outcome of condition and pain

■ Planning

The overall goals are that the patient with acute abdomen will have (1) resolution of inflammation, (2) relief of abdominal pain, (3) freedom from complications (especially hypovolemic shock), and (4) normal nutritional status.

■ Nursing Implementation

Nursing interventions are based on the diagnosis and medical or surgical management of the patient. General care for the patient involves management of fluid and electrolyte imbalances, pain, and anxiety.

Preoperative Care. Emergency preparation of the patient with an acute abdomen is usually limited to a CBC, typing and crossmatching of blood, and clotting studies. Catheterization, preparation of the abdominal skin, and the passage of a nasogastric (NG) tube may be done in the emergency department or operating room. (General care of the preoperative patient is discussed in Chapter 16.)

40-2 NURSING CARE PLAN PATIENT FOLLOWING LAPAROTOMY

Expected Patient Outcomes	Nursing Interventions and *Rationales*

NURSING DIAGNOSIS **Pain** *related to* surgical incision and inadequate pain control measures *as manifested by* complaints of pain, body posturing, unwillingness to move in bed or to ambulate.

■ Satisfactory level of pain control.	■ Assess for pain and give pain medication every 3 to 4 hr as ordered for first 72 hr *to treat pain appropriately.* ■ Splint incision with pillows during coughing, deep breathing, and moving *to relieve pain while performing these activities.* ■ Position patient comfortably *to relieve pain.*

NURSING DIAGNOSIS **Nausea and vomiting** *related to* decreased GI motility, GI distention, and narcotics *as manifested by* nausea, vomiting, lack of or diminished bowel sounds, abdominal distention.

■ Relief of nausea and vomiting.	■ Administer antiemetic medications (as ordered) *to relieve nausea and vomiting.* ■ Assess response to pain medications *to determine if this is a possible cause of nausea and vomiting.* ■ Maintain patency of NG tube (if present) *to prevent accumulation of gastric juices and subsequent vomiting.* ■ Assess for bowel sounds and abdominal distention *to determine return of peristalsis.* ■ Keep patient on NPO status until bowel sounds return *to prevent vomiting.* ■ Limit unpleasant sights, smells, and stimuli *to prevent initiating episodes of nausea and vomiting.*

NURSING DIAGNOSIS **Constipation** *related to* immobility, pain, medication, and decreased GI motility *as manifested by* decreased or absent bowel sounds, abdominal pain, abdominal distention, inability to pass flatus or stool.

■ Normal bowel sounds within 72 hr after surgery. ■ Soft, formed bowel movement within 4 days.	■ Assess abdomen for distention and bowel sounds every shift *to determine need for intervention.* ■ Administer cathartic as ordered if patient has not had bowel movement in 4 days *to soften fecal mass or promote elimination.* ■ Encourage frequent position changes and ambulation as tolerated *to increase peristalsis.* ■ Encourage increased fluid intake as tolerated *to soften fecal material.*

*General nursing care for the postoperative patient is presented in NCP 18-1 in Chapter 18 on p. 401.

Postoperative Care. Postoperative care depends on the type of surgical procedure performed. The increased use of laparoscopic procedures has reduced the risk of postoperative complications related to wound care and altered GI motility. These procedures generally result in shorter hospital stays.

A general nursing care plan for the postoperative patient is presented in Chapter 18. Nursing care for the patient following a laparotomy is presented in NCP 40-2.

An NG tube may or may not be present in the patient returning from surgery. If present, the NG tube is connected to suction as ordered. The purpose of the NG tube is to empty the stomach of secretions and gas to prevent gastric dilation. GI peristaltic activity is often impaired because of the manipulative procedures of the surgery and anesthesia. Low intermittent suctioning is ordered to prevent trauma to the gastric mucosa.

Drainage from the NG tube may be dark brown to dark red for the first 12 hours. Later it should be light yellowish brown, or it may have a greenish tinge because of the presence of bile. If a dark red color continues or if bright red blood is observed, the physician should be notified at once of the possibility of hemorrhage. "Coffee ground" granules in the drainage are due to the presence of small amounts of blood that have been chemically acted on by gastric secretions.

The NG tube is checked frequently for patency. The tube may become obstructed with mucus, sediment, or old blood. An order is usually written to irrigate the tube with 20 to 30 ml of normal saline solution if needed. Repositioning the tube may facilitate drainage.

An accurate record of intake and output, including emesis and gastric drainage, is essential. The nurse should assess serum electrolyte values and acid-base balance because prolonged gastric suctioning results in loss of sodium, chloride, potassium, water, and hydrochloric acid.

The NG tube is removed when intestinal peristalsis returns, usually 24 to 72 hours after surgery. Motility of the stomach normally returns within 24 to 48 hours. Motility of the small intestine usually resumes within 24 hours, whereas return of large intestine motility may take as long as 3 to 5 days. Peristaltic activity is assessed by auscultation for bowel sounds.

Mouth care and nasal care are essential. The patient tends to breathe through the mouth while the NG tube is in place. In addition, increased nasal secretions and crusting result from mechanical stimulation of the NG tube.

Parenteral fluids are administered to provide the patient with fluids and electrolytes until bowel sounds return. Occasionally, ice chips may be ordered because they aid in the flow of saliva and prevent dry mouth. When bowel sounds return, fluids and food are increased gradually. The diet may be supplemented with multivitamins and iron.

Nausea and vomiting are not uncommon after abdominal surgery. These problems are often self-limiting. Observation is important in determining the cause. Antiemetics such as promethazine (Phenergan), hydroxyzine (Vistaril), prochlorperazine (Compazine), or trimethobenzamide (Tigan) may be ordered.

Abdominal distention and gas pains are also common after surgery; these are due to swallowed air and impaired peristalsis resulting from immobility, manipulation of abdominal contents during surgery, and side effects of anesthesia. The pain can be so uncomfortable that medications to stimulate peristalsis, such as bethanechol (Urecholine) or neostigmine methylsulfate (Prostigmin), may be given. A rectal tube or moist heat on the abdomen may be effective in relieving distention. The physician should be informed of abdominal distention and rigidity. Gradually, as intestinal activity increases, distention and gas pains decrease.

Emotional support from the nursing staff is important. Honest, clear, concise explanations of all procedures in language the patient and the family can understand may assist in allaying anxiety.

Ambulatory and Home Care. Preparation for discharge begins when the patient returns from the operating room. Instructions to the patient and the family should include any modifications in activity, care of the incision, diet, and drug therapy. Small, frequent meals high in calories should be taken initially, with a gradual increase in intake of food as tolerated.

Normal activities should be resumed gradually, with planned rest periods. The patient should be aware of possible complications after surgery and should notify the physician immediately if vomiting, pain, weight loss, incisional drainage, or changes in bowel functions occur.

■ Evaluation

The expected outcomes are that the patient with acute abdomen will have

- resolution of inflammation
- relief of abdominal pain
- freedom from complications (especially hypovolemic shock)
- normal nutritional status

CHRONIC ABDOMINAL PAIN

Chronic abdominal pain may originate from abdominal structures or may be referred from a site with the same or a similar nerve supply. Some common causes are irritable bowel syndrome (IBS), peptic ulcer disease, diverticulitis, chronic pancreatitis, hepatitis, cholecystitis, pelvic inflammatory disease, and vascular insufficiency. Psychogenic pain should also be considered.

Diagnosis of chronic abdominal pain presents a challenge. Assessment should begin with a thorough history and identification of the specific pain pattern. Character and severity of pain, location, duration, and onset should be determined. The assessment should also include the relationship of pain to meals, defecation, activity, and factors that increase or decrease the pain. Chronic abdominal pain is often described as dull, aching, or diffuse.

Endoscopy, computed tomography (CT) scans, magnetic resonance imaging (MRI), laparoscopy, and radiographic barium studies have decreased the need for exploratory laparotomy. Treatment for chronic abdominal pain is comprehensive and directed toward palliation of symptoms using analgesics and antiemetics as well as psychologic or behavioral therapies (e.g., relaxation).[7]

ABDOMINAL TRAUMA

Etiology

Injuries to the abdominal area most often occur as a result of *blunt trauma* (e.g., motor vehicle accident) or *penetration injuries,* primarily gunshot wounds or stab wounds to the abdomen. Blunt trauma is most common. Regardless of whether it is a blunt or penetration injury, the result is often the same damage to or alteration of the internal organs.

Common injuries of the abdomen include lacerated liver, ruptured spleen, pancreatic trauma, mesenteric artery tears, diaphragmatic rupture, urinary bladder rupture, great vessel tears, renal injury, and stomach or intestinal rupture. These injuries may result in massive blood loss and hypovolemic shock. Surgery must be performed as early as possible to repair the damaged organs and to stop the bleeding. Common sequelae of intraabdominal trauma are peritonitis and massive infection, particularly when the bowel is perforated.

Clinical Manifestations

Clinical manifestations of abdominal trauma are (1) guarding and splinting of the abdominal wall; (2) a hard, distended abdomen (indicating intraabdominal bleeding); (3) decreased or absent bowel sounds; (4) contusions, abrasions, or bruising over the abdomen; (5) abdominal pain; (6) pain over the scapula caused by irritation of the phrenic nerve by free blood in the abdomen; (7) hematemesis or hematuria; and (8) signs of hypovolemic shock (Table 40-14). An ecchymotic discoloration around the umbilicus (Cullen's sign) can indicate intraabdominal or retroperitoneal hemorrhage.

Intraabdominal injuries are often associated with low rib fractures, fractured femur, fractured pelvis, and thoracic injury. If any of these injuries are present, the patient should be observed for abdominal trauma.

✚ EMERGENCY MANAGEMENT

Table **40-14**   Abdominal Trauma

Etiology	Assessment Findings	Interventions
Blunt Falls Motor vehicle collisions Pedestrian event Assault with blunt object Crush injuries Explosions **Penetrating** Knife Gunshot wounds Other missiles	**Hypovolemic Shock** ■ Decreased level of consciousness ■ Tachypnea ■ Tachycardia ■ Decreased blood pressure ■ Decreased pulse pressure **Surface Findings** ■ Abrasions or ecchymoses on abdominal wall, flank, or peritoneum. ■ Open wounds—lacerations, eviscerations, puncture wounds, gunshot wounds ■ Impaled object ■ Healed incisions or old scars **Abdominal/Gastrointestinal Findings** ■ Nausea and vomiting ■ Bloody urine ■ Abdominal distention ■ Abdominal rigidity ■ Abdominal pain with palpation ■ Rebound tenderness ■ Pain radiation to shoulder and back	**Initial** ■ Ensure patent airway. ■ Administer oxygen via non-rebreather mask. ■ Control external bleeding with direct pressure or sterile pressure dressing. ■ Establish IV access with two large bore catheters and infuse warm normal saline or lactated Ringer's solution. ■ Obtain blood for type and cross-match and CBC. ■ Remove clothing. ■ Stabilize impaled objects with bulky dressing—*do not remove.* ■ Cover protruding organs or tissue with sterile, saline dressing. ■ Insert indwelling urinary catheter if there is no blood at the meatus, pelvic fracture, or boggy prostate. ■ Obtain urine for urinalysis. ■ Insert NG tube if no evidence of facial trauma. ■ Anticipate diagnostic peritoneal lavage. **Ongoing Monitoring** ■ Monitor vital signs, level of consciousness, oxygen saturation, and urine output. ■ Maintain patient warmth using blankets, warm IV fluids, or warm humidified oxygen.

Diagnostic Studies

Specific diagnostic procedures include CBC, urinalysis, x-ray of the abdomen, CT scan, and peritoneal lavage. In peritoneal lavage the abdomen below the umbilicus is locally anesthetized, and a large angiocatheter or peritoneal dialysis catheter is inserted into the abdomen. A syringe is attached to the catheter, and an attempt is made to gently aspirate any blood. If less than 10 ml of blood is aspirated, a liter of saline solution is then infused into the abdomen and drained. The fluid is observed for gross abnormalities, especially blood, and is sent to the laboratory for microscopic evaluation. Positive findings may include (1) RBC count greater than $100,000/\mu l$, (2) WBC count greater than $500/\mu l$, (3) high amylase level, and (4) presence of bacteria, bile, or fecal material. If the results are positive, immediate surgery is indicated. If the results are negative, continued observation of the patient is warranted. An impaled object should never be removed until skilled care is available. Removal may cause further injury and bleeding.

NURSING AND COLLABORATIVE MANAGEMENT: ABDOMINAL TRAUMA

Emergency management of abdominal trauma focuses on establishing a patent airway and adequate breathing, fluid replacement, and prevention of hypovolemic shock (see Table 40-14). IV lines are inserted, and volume expanders or blood is given if the patient is hypotensive. An NG tube is inserted to decompress the stomach and prevent the aspiration of vomitus.

Regardless of the mechanism of injury, physical evidence of abdominal trauma in a patient who is hemodynamically unstable mandates immediate laparotomy. In other cases the indications for laparotomy must be correlated with the mechanism of injury. For example, if an individual has a gunshot wound or impaled object, surgery is usually indicated. If surgery is performed, the postoperative nursing care is for the patient after laparotomy (see NCP 40-2).

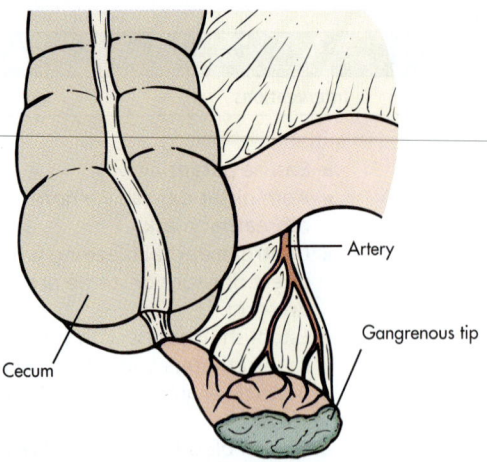

Fig. 40-1   In appendicitis the blood supply of the appendix is impaired by inflammation and bacterial infection in the wall of the appendix, which may result in gangrene.

INFLAMMATION

APPENDICITIS

Appendicitis is an inflammation of the appendix, a narrow blind tube that extends from the inferior part of the cecum. It occurs in 6% of the general population. Peak incidence is between the ages of 11 and 30 years, and the condition occurs equally in both sexes.[8]

Etiology

The most common causes of appendicitis are obstruction of the lumen by a *fecalith* (accumulated feces) (Fig. 40-1), foreign bodies, tumor of the cecum or appendix, or intramural thickening caused by lymphoid hyperplasia. After age 30 years, the number of appendicular lymph follicles declines until they are nearly absent at age 60 years.[8] Obstruction results in distention, venous engorgement, and the accumulation of mucus and bacteria, which can lead to gangrene and perforation.

Clinical Manifestations

Appendicitis typically begins with periumbilical pain, followed by anorexia, nausea, and vomiting. The pain is persistent and continuous, eventually shifting to the right lower quadrant and localizing at McBurney's point (located halfway between the umbilicus and the right iliac crest). Further assessment of the patient reveals localized tenderness, rebound tenderness, and muscle guarding. The patient usually prefers to lie still, often with the right leg flexed. Low-grade fever may or may not be present, and coughing aggravates pain. Rovsing's sign may be elicited by palpation of the left lower quadrant, causing pain to be felt in the right lower quadrant. Complications of acute appendicitis are perforation, peritonitis, and abscesses.

Diagnostic Studies and Collaborative Care

Examination of the patient includes a complete history and physical examination (particularly palpation of the abdomen) and a differential WBC count. A urinalysis may be done to rule out genitourinary (GU) conditions that mimic the manifestations of appendicitis.

   The treatment of appendicitis is immediate surgical removal (*appendectomy*) if the inflammation is localized. If the appendix

Table **40-15**	Causes of Peritonitis
Primary	**Secondary**
Blood-borne organisms	Appendicitis with rupture
Genital tract organisms	Blunt or penetrating
Cirrhosis with ascites	trauma to abdominal
	organs
	Diverticulitis with rupture
	Ischemic bowel disorders
	Obstruction in the
	gastrointestinal tract
	Pancreatitis
	Perforated peptic ulcer
	Peritoneal dialysis
	Postoperative (breakage
	of anastomosis)

has ruptured and there is evidence of peritonitis or an abscess, conservative treatment, consisting of antibiotic therapy and parenteral fluids, may be used to prevent sepsis and dehydration for 6 to 8 hours before an appendectomy is performed.

NURSING MANAGEMENT: APPENDICITIS

The patient with abdominal pain is encouraged to see a physician and to avoid self-treatment, particularly the use of laxatives and enemas. The increased peristalsis from these procedures may cause perforation of the appendix. Until the patient is seen by a physician, nothing should be taken by mouth (NPO) to ensure that the stomach is empty in the event surgery is needed. An ice bag may be applied to the right lower quadrant to decrease the flow of blood to the area and impede the inflammatory process. Heat is never used because it may cause the appendix to rupture. Surgery is usually performed as soon as a diagnosis is made.

   Postoperative nursing management is similar to postoperative care of the patient after laparotomy (see NCP 40-2). In addition, the patient should be observed for evidence of peritonitis. Ambulation begins the day of surgery or the first postoperative day. The diet is advanced as tolerated. The patient is usually discharged on the first or second postoperative day, and normal activities are resumed 2 to 3 weeks after surgery.

PERITONITIS

Peritonitis results from a localized or generalized inflammatory process of the peritoneum.

Etiology and Pathophysiology

Causes of peritonitis are listed in Table 40-15. Peritonitis may appear in acute and chronic forms, and trauma or rupture of an organ containing chemical irritants or bacteria (which are released into the peritoneal cavity) may cause it. Examples of a chemical peritonitis include gastric ulcer perforation and ruptured ectopic pregnancy. A chemical peritonitis is commonly followed by bacterial invasion. Bacterial peritonitis can be caused by a traumatic injury (e.g., gunshot wound, ruptured appendix), or it can be secondary to other diseases or conditions (e.g., pancreatitis, peritoneal dialysis).

COLLABORATIVE CARE

Table 40-16 Peritonitis

Diagnostic
CBC
Serum electrolytes
Abdominal x-ray
Abdominal paracentesis and culture of fluid
CT scan or ultrasound
Peritoneoscopy

Collaborative Therapy
Preoperative or Nonoperative
NPO status
Fluid replacement
Antibiotic therapy
NG suction
Analgesics
Preparation for surgery to include the above and total parenteral nutrition

Postoperative
NPO status
NG tube to low-intermittent suction
Semi-Fowler's position
IV fluids with electrolyte replacement
Total parenteral nutrition as needed
Antibiotic therapy
Blood transfusions as needed
Sedatives and narcotics

CBC, complete blood count; *CT*, computed tomography; *IV*, intravenous; *NPO*, nothing by mouth.

The response of the peritoneum to the leakage of GI contents is localization of the offending agent by attempting to "wall it off" by exuding fibrin-containing fluids and swelling. Adhesions may form. These adhesions may shrink and disappear when the infection is eliminated. Normally, peritoneal injuries heal without formation of adhesions unless other factors, such as infection, ischemia, or foreign substances, are present.

Clinical Manifestations

Abdominal pain is the most common symptom of peritonitis.[9] A universal sign of peritonitis is tenderness over the involved area. Rebound tenderness, muscular rigidity, and spasm are other major signs of irritation of the peritoneum. Abdominal distention or ascites, fever, tachycardia, tachypnea, nausea, vomiting, and altered bowel habits may also be present. These manifestations vary, depending on severity and acuteness of the underlying cause. Complications of peritonitis include hypovolemic shock, septicemia, intraabdominal abscess formation, paralytic ileus, and organ failure.

Diagnostic Studies

A CBC is done to determine leukocytosis and hemoconcentration (Table 40-16). Peritoneal aspiration may be performed and the fluid analyzed for blood, bile, pus, bacteria, fungus, and amylase content. An x-ray of the abdomen may show dilated loops of bowel consistent with paralytic ileus, free air if perforation has occurred, or air and fluid levels if an obstruction is present. Ultrasound and CT scans may be useful in identifying the presence of ascites and abscesses. Perito-

neoscopy may be helpful in the patient without ascites. Direct examination of the peritoneum can be obtained, along with biopsy specimens for diagnosis.

Collaborative Care

The goals of management of peritonitis are to identify and eliminate the cause, combat infection, and prevent complications. Patients with milder cases of peritonitis or those who are poor surgical risks may be managed nonsurgically. Treatment consists of antibiotics, NG suction, analgesics, and IV fluid administration. Patients who require surgery need preoperative preparation as previously described. Those patients may be placed on total parenteral nutrition (TPN) because of increased nutritional requirements.

NURSING MANAGEMENT: PERITONITIS

■ Nursing Assessment

Assessment of the patient's pain, including the location, is important and may help in determining the cause of peritonitis. The patient should be assessed for the presence and quality of bowel sounds, increasing abdominal distention, abdominal guarding, nausea, fever, and manifestations of hypovolemic shock.

■ Nursing Diagnoses

Nursing diagnoses for the patient with peritonitis include, but are not limited to, the following:

- Pain *related to* inflammation of the peritoneum and abdominal distention
- Risk for fluid volume deficit *related to* collection of fluid in peritoneal cavity secondary to trauma, infection, or ischemia
- Altered nutrition: less than body requirements *related to* anorexia, nausea, and vomiting
- Anxiety *related to* uncertainty of cause or outcome of condition and pain
- Potential complication: hypovolemic shock *related to* loss of circulatory volume

■ Planning

The overall goals are that the patient with peritonitis will have (1) resolution of inflammation, (2) relief of abdominal pain, (3) freedom from complications (especially hypovolemic shock), and (4) normal nutritional status.

■ Nursing Implementation

The patient with peritonitis is extremely ill and needs skilled supportive care. The patient is monitored for pain and response to analgesic therapy. The patient may be positioned with knees flexed to increase comfort. The nurse should provide rest and a quiet environment. Sedatives may be given to allay anxiety.

Accurate monitoring of fluid intake and output and electrolyte status is necessary to determine replacement therapy. Vital signs are monitored frequently. Antiemetics may be administered to decrease nausea and vomiting and further fluid losses. The patient is on NPO status and may have an NG tube in place to decrease gastric distention.

If the patient has an open surgical procedure, drains are inserted to remove purulent drainage and excessive fluid. Postoperative care of the patient is similar to the care of the patient with an exploratory laparotomy (see NCP 40-2).

GASTROENTERITIS

Gastroenteritis is an inflammation of the mucosa of the stomach and small intestine. Clinical manifestations include nausea, vomiting, diarrhea, abdominal cramping, and distention. Fever, leukocytosis, and blood or mucus in the stool may be present. Causative agents are varied (see Table 40-2). Most cases are self-limiting and do not require hospitalization. However, older adults and chronically ill patients may be unable to consume sufficient fluids orally to compensate for fluid loss. Until vomiting has ceased, the patient should be on NPO status. If dehydration has occurred, IV replacement of fluids may be necessary. As soon as tolerated, fluids containing glucose and electrolytes (e.g., Pedialyte) should be given. If the causative agent is identified, appropriate antibiotic, antimicrobial, or antiinfective medication is given.

NURSING MANAGEMENT: GASTROENTERITIS

Accurate monitoring of intake and output is important for successful replacement of lost fluid. Strict medical asepsis and infection control precautions should be instituted when indicated. The patient should be instructed in the importance of proper food handling and preparation of food to prevent infections such as salmonellosis and trichinosis (see Chapter 39).

Symptomatic nursing care is given for nausea, vomiting, and diarrhea. The importance of rest and increased fluid intake should be stressed. The nurse should assess complaints of pain, vomiting, and diarrhea because gastroenteritis is often confused with appendicitis. To allay the patient's apprehension, the nurse should explain that gastroenteritis usually runs an acute course with no sequelae.

IRRITABLE BOWEL SYNDROME

Irritable bowel syndrome (IBS) is a symptom complex characterized by intermittent and recurrent abdominal pain associated with an alteration in bowel function (diarrhea or constipation). Other symptoms commonly found include abdominal distention, excessive flatulence, urge to defecate, and sensation of incomplete evacuation. IBS is a common problem affecting approximately 10% to 17% of the population in the United States.[10] In western societies, approximately two times as many women as men seek health care services for IBS. Stress, psychologic factors, and specific food intolerances have been identified as major factors that precipitate IBS symptoms.

The key to accurate diagnosis is a thorough health history and physical examination. Emphasis should be on symptoms, past health history (including psychosocial aspects including physical or sexual abuse), family history, and drug and dietary history. Diagnostic tests should be selectively used to rule out more serious life-threatening disorders with symptoms similar to those of IBS, such as colon cancer, peptic ulcer disease, and malabsorption disorders.

The health care provider should establish a trusting relationship with the patient at the onset of treatment. The patient needs reassurance that the symptoms are functional. The patient should be encouraged to verbalize concerns and anxiety. A diet containing at least 20 g per day of dietary fiber should be

initiated (see Table 40-9). This may also include the addition of psyllium-containing products (e.g., Metamucil).

The patient whose primary symptoms are abdominal distention and increased flatulence should be advised to eliminate common gas-producing foods such as broccoli and cabbage from the diet and to substitute yogurt for milk products if there is lactose intolerance. Anticholinergic agents, such as dicyclomine (Bentyl), may be helpful if taken before meals to alleviate the pain associated with ingestion of food. For the patient with a high level of anxiety, a mild sedative or tranquilizer may be ordered but should be prescribed for only a short time. Additional therapies include relaxation and stress management techniques, although no single therapy has been found to be effective for all patients with IBS.

INFLAMMATORY BOWEL DISEASE

Crohn's disease and *ulcerative colitis* are immunologically related disorders that are referred to as *inflammatory bowel disease* (IBD). These disorders are characterized by chronic, recurrent inflammation of the intestinal tract. For both conditions, the clinical manifestations are varied, with long periods of remission interspersed with episodes of acute inflammation. Both diseases can be debilitating.

Although there has been extensive research on the etiology of IBD, the cause of both ulcerative colitis and Crohn's disease remains unknown. Possible causes include (1) an infectious agent (e.g., virus, bacteria) because IBD produces mucosal changes in the colon similar to those of infectious diarrhea, although no consistent pathogen has been identified; (2) an autoimmune reaction from the presence of other immune-related disorders, such as systemic lupus erythematosus, ankylosing spondylitis, and erythema nodosum in patients with IBD; (3) food allergies (although this has not been substantiated); and (4) heredity. (Both Crohn's disease and ulcerative colitis occur more commonly in related families.[11]) In one study, 84% of identical twins of patients who had Crohn's disease also had the disorder.[12] For years IBD (especially ulcerative colitis) was thought to be due to psychosomatic factors, such as severe emotional stress. It is now believed that these emotional changes result from and are not the cause of the disease.

ULCERATIVE COLITIS

Ulcerative colitis is characterized by inflammation and ulceration of the colon and rectum. It may occur at any age but peaks

Table **40-17**   **Comparison of Ulcerative Colitis and Crohn's Disease**

Characteristic	Ulcerative colitis	Crohn's disease
Clinical		
Age at onset	Young to middle age	Young
Diarrhea	Common	Common
Abdominal crampy pain	Possible	Common
Fever (intermittent)	During acute attacks	Common
Weight loss	Common	Severe
Rectal bleeding	Common	Infrequent
Tenesmus	Severe	Rare
Malabsorption and nutritional deficiencies	Minimal incidence	Common
Pathologic		
Location	Starts distally and spreads in a continuous pattern up the colon	Occurs anywhere along GI tract in characteristic skip lesions; most frequent site is terminal ileum
Distribution	Continuous	Segmental
Depth of involvement	Mucosa and submucosa	Entire thickness of bowel wall (transmural)
Granulomas	Absent	Common
Cobblestoning of mucosa	Rare	Common
Pseudopolyps	Common	Rare
Small-bowel involvement	Minimal	Common
Complications		
Fistulas	Rare	Common
Strictures	Rare	Common
Anal abscesses	Rare	Common
Perforation	Common	Common
Toxic megacolon	Common	Rare
Carcinoma	Increased incidence after 10 yr of disease	Slightly greater than general population
Recurrence after surgery	Cure with colectomy	70% or more recurrence after segmental resections of small or large intestine

between the ages of 15 and 25 years. There is a second, smaller peak onset between 50 and 80 years of age. Ulcerative colitis affects both sexes but has a higher incidence in women. It is more common in Jewish and upper-middle-class urban populations.

Etiology and Pathophysiology

The inflammation of ulcerative colitis is diffuse and involves the mucosa and submucosa, with alternate periods of exacerbations and remissions (Table 40-17). The disease usually begins in the rectum and sigmoid colon and spreads up the colon in a continuous pattern.

The mucosa of the colon is hyperemic and edematous in the affected area (Fig. 40-2). Multiple abscesses develop in the crypts of Lieberkühn (intestinal glands). As the disease advances, the abscesses break through the crypts into the submucosa, leaving ulcerations. These ulcerations also destroy the mucosal epithelium, causing bleeding and diarrhea. Losses of fluid and electrolytes occur because of the decreased mucosal surface area for absorption. Breakdown of cells results in protein loss through the stool. Areas of inflamed mucosa form *pseudopolyps*, tonguelike projections into the bowel lumen. Granulation tissue develops, and the mucosa musculature becomes thickened, shortening the colon.

Clinical Manifestations

Ulcerative colitis may appear as an acute fulminating crisis or, more commonly, as a chronic disorder with mild to severe acute exacerbations that occur at unpredictable intervals over many

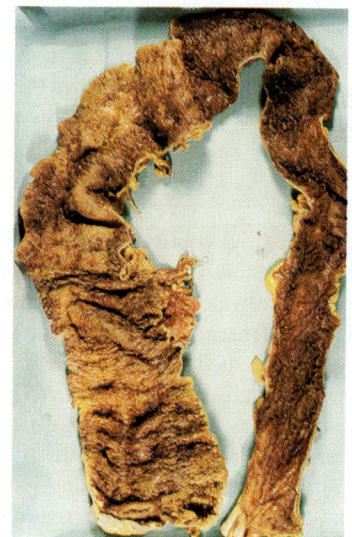

Fig. 40-2 Acute ulcerative colitis. Colitis with extensive mucosal ulceration involving the entire colon.

years. The major symptoms of ulcerative colitis are bloody diarrhea and abdominal pain. Pain may vary from the mild lower-abdominal cramping associated with diarrhea to the severe, constant abdominal pain associated with acute perforations. With mild disease, diarrhea may consist of one or two semiformed stools containing small amounts of blood per day.

Table **40-18** | **Extraintestinal Complications of Ulcerative Colitis**

Colitis Related
Joints
- Peripheral arthritis (colitic)
- Ankylosing spondylitis
- Sacroiliitis
- Finger clubbing

Skin
- Erythema nodosum
- Pyoderma gangrenosum

Mouth
- Aphthous ulcers

Eye
- Conjunctivitis
- Uveitis
- Episcleritis

Related to Small Bowel Pathology
- Malabsorption
- Gallstones
- Kidney stones

Nonspecific
- Liver disease—primary sclerosing cholangitis
- Osteoporosis
- Amyloidosis
- Peptic ulcer disease

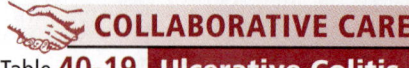

COLLABORATIVE CARE

Table **40-19** | **Ulcerative Colitis**

Diagnostic
- Fiberoptic colonoscopy
- Sigmoidoscopy
- Barium enema
- CBC
- Stool for blood, culture and sensitivity

Collaborative Therapy
Mild and Moderate Disease
- Low-roughage diet and no milk or milk products
- Antimicrobial therapy*
- Corticosteroids
- Anticholinergic therapy*
- Antidiarrheal agents*

Severe (Fulminant) Disease
- IV fluids with electrolytes
- Blood transfusions
- NPO status
- NG tube to low suction
- Antimicrobial therapy*
- Corticosteroids
- Parenteral nutritional therapy
- Surgery if no improvement (colon resection with ileostomy)

*See Table 40-20.

The patient may have no other systemic manifestations. In moderate ulcerative colitis there is increased stool output (4 to 5 stools per day), increased bleeding, and systemic symptoms (fever, malaise, anorexia). In severe cases, diarrhea is bloody, contains mucus, and occurs 10 to 20 times a day. In addition, fever, weight loss greater than 10% of total body weight, anemia, tachycardia, and dehydration are present. Acute fulminant colitis is present in only 6% to 10% of patients with severe ulcerative colitis.[11]

Complications

Complications of ulcerative colitis may be classified into those that are *intestinal* and those that are *extraintestinal*. Intestinal complications of ulcerative colitis include hemorrhage, strictures, perforation, toxic megacolon, and colonic dilation. Hemorrhage is a result of inflamed, ulcerated mucosa and is usually controlled with conservative therapy. Massive hemorrhage is unusual and requires emergency surgery. Strictures are less common in ulcerative colitis than in Crohn's disease and are seen most often in patients with severe, long-standing disease. *Toxic megacolon* (dilation and paralysis of the colon) occurs in approximately 5% of patients with ulcerative colitis.[13] Colonic dilation, most often in the transverse colon, occurs as a result of severe acute inflammation of the entire colon wall. Perforation is most often associated with toxic megacolon but may occur alone. Most cases of perforation occur in the left side of the colon.

A patient who has had ulcerative colitis for more than 10 years is at greater risk of colon cancer. The risk of cancer depends on age at onset, duration, and extent of disease. The patient should be periodically screened with surveillance colonoscopy.

During this procedure, biopsy specimens should be taken every 10 cm throughout the entire colon.

Extraintestinal complications may be directly related to the colitis and small intestine pathology (malabsorption), or they may be nonspecific complications mediated by a disturbance in the immune system (Table 40-18). Colitis-related complications are associated with active inflammation and often respond to treatment of the underlying bowel disease. These manifestations can involve the joints, skin, mouth, and eyes as well as disturbances of the hematologic system including anemia, leukocytosis, and thrombocytosis.[14] Skin lesions such as erythema nodosum and pyoderma gangrenosum are among the most frequently seen extraintestinal manifestations. Uveitis is the most common eye problem.

Diagnostic Studies

Several studies are appropriate for diagnosis of ulcerative colitis (Table 40-19). Blood studies should include a CBC, serum electrolyte levels, and serum protein levels. A CBC typically shows iron deficiency anemia from blood loss. An elevated WBC count may indicate toxic megacolon or perforation. Decreases in serum electrolytes, such as sodium, potassium, chloride, bicarbonate, and magnesium, are due to fluid and electrolyte losses from diarrhea and vomiting. Hypoalbuminemia is present with severe disease and is due to protein loss from the bowel. The stool should be examined for blood, pus, and mucus. Stool cultures should be obtained to rule out infectious causes of inflammation.

Examinations with a flexible sigmoidoscope and a colonoscope allow direct examination of the mucosa of the large

DRUG THERAPY

Table 40-20 Ulcerative Colitis

Category	Action	Examples
■ Antimicrobial	Prevention or treatment of secondary infection	Cephalothin sodium (Keflin) Sulfasalazine (Azulfidine)* Mesalamine (Rowasa)* Olsalazine (Dipentum)
■ Corticosteroids	Antiinflammatory	Corticosteroids (cortisone, prednisone)
■ Anticholinergic	Decrease in GI motility and secretions and relief of smooth muscle spasms†	Methantheline bromide (Banthine) Propantheline (Pro-Banthine) Oxyphencyclimine (Daricon)
■ Sedatives	Quieting of CNS without inducing sleep or analgesia	Diazepam (Valium) Flurazepam (Dalmane)
■ Antidiarrheal	Decrease in GI motility†	Diphenoxylate (Lomotil)
■ Immunosuppressives	Suppression of immune response	Azathioprine (Imuran), cyclosporine
■ Hematinics and vitamins	Correction of iron deficiency anemia and promotion of healing	Iron dextran injection (Imferon) Cobalamin, zinc

*Mechanism of action unknown, likely to be antiinflammatory as well as antimicrobial.
†Used with caution during severe disease because of potential to produce toxic megacolon.
CNS, central nervous system; GI, gastrointestinal.

intestine. Using a sigmoidoscope the physician can view the rectum, the sigmoid colon, and the descending colon. The colonoscope allows for examination of the entire large intestine. The extent of inflammation, ulcerations, pseudopolyps, strictures, and lesions may be identified. Biopsy specimens should be taken for definitive diagnosis.

A double-contrast barium enema may show areas of granular inflammation with ulcerations. The colon may appear narrow and shortened, and pseudopolyps may be present. A double-contrast study (in which air is introduced into the bowel after the expulsion of barium) is effective in detecting mucosal abnormalities in ulcerative colitis.

Collaborative Care

The goals of treatment are to (1) rest the bowel, (2) control the inflammation, (3) combat infection, (4) correct malnutrition, (5) alleviate stress, and (6) provide symptomatic relief using drug therapy (see Table 40-20). The mainstays of drug therapy are sulfasalazine (Azulfidine) and corticosteroids. Hospitalization is indicated if the patient fails to respond to corticosteroid therapy or if complications are suspected.

Drug Therapy. Drug therapy is an extremely important aspect of treatment (see Table 40-20).[15] Sulfasalazine, a combination of sulfapyridine and 5-aminosalicylic acid (5-ASA), is the principal drug used. It is effective in the maintenance of clinical remission and in the treatment of mild to moderately severe attacks. After remission is obtained, therapy is continued with a gradual reduction over several months. The maintenance dose is usually continued for at least 1 year.

During active disease 5-ASA (the active form of sulfasalazine) and 4-ASA, given as retention enemas, are effective in the treatment of left-sided ulcerative colitis and proctitis. Topical salicylate therapy is the treatment of choice in patients with localized disease. 5-ASA (mesalamine [Rowasa]) can also be administered orally. The acrylic-coated tablets provide delivery of the drug more distally in the intestine.

Corticosteroids are of proven benefit in the management of active ulcerative colitis. Oral prednisone or prednisolone is effective in treatment of mild to moderate disease without systemic manifestations. If remission is not achieved, the patient requires hospitalization and IV corticosteroid therapy. The patient is placed on a regimen of bowel rest. Fluids and electrolytes are administered intravenously. Hydrocortisone enemas and foams are effective in the treatment of colitis limited to the rectosigmoid area. Rectal foams are usually administered in 5 ml volumes and are generally preferred over enemas because of the ease of administration. However, enemas are the preferred choice if the disease spreads beyond the sigmoid colon. Retention enemas have been shown to deliver medication into the descending colon and beyond in patients with active disease. Although corticosteroids are reported to bring remission in 60% to 89% of cases, they do not necessarily prolong remission.[15] The patient on corticosteroids is to be monitored for signs of Cushing's syndrome, hypertension, hirsutism, and mood swings. In some cases, psychosis may develop.[16]

Immunosuppressive drugs (e.g., 6-mercaptopurine [6-MP]) have been used in severe cases of ulcerative colitis when a patient has failed to respond to any of the usual medications and before surgery is considered. Side effects of 6-MP, including bone marrow suppression and increased risk of infection, necessitate that it be used cautiously in these patients. Patients receiving this medication need to maintain an adequate fluid intake of 1800 to 2400 ml to reduce the risk of nephrotoxicity.[15] The drug should be taken with food and milk to reduce gastric irritation. Cyclosporine (discussed in Chapter 44) and methotrexate have been evaluated for their effectiveness in the treatment of severe ulcerative colitis that is unresponsive to corticosteroid treatment. New therapies such as monoclonal antibodies against tumor necrosis factor [TNF] or the antiinflammatory cytokine interleukin-10 [IL-10] that are used to modify the inflammatory response in IBD are under investigation.[17]

Epidemiologic studies showing a low incidence of ulcerative colitis among smokers has led to investigation of nicotine transdermal patches or gum to induce remission.[18] For distal ulcerative colitis, rectal enemas containing short chain fatty acids

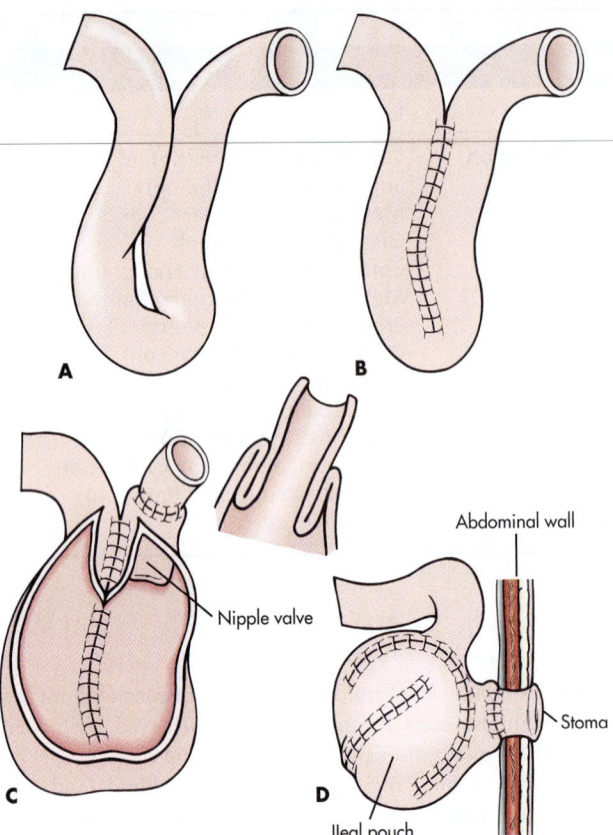

Fig. 40-3 Surgical formation of continent ileostomy (Kock pouch). **A,** Loop of terminal ileum. **B,** Both limbs sutured together and incised in a *U shape.* **C,** Pouch created with nipple valve. **D,** Pouch sutured to abdominal wall.

have been evaluated for their antiinflammatory effects. Short chain fatty acids are important fuels supporting colonic cell function and are naturally produced from fiber fermentation.[19]

Surgical Therapy. Approximately 85% of patients with ulcerative colitis go into remission with conservative therapy and nursing care, but 15% to 20% require surgery. Surgery is indicated if (1) the patient fails to respond to treatment; (2) exacerbations are frequent and debilitating; (3) massive bleeding, perforation, strictures, or obstruction occur; (4) changes that suggest dysplasia are occurring; or (5) carcinoma develops.

Surgical procedures used to treat chronic ulcerative colitis include (1) total proctocolectomy with permanent ileostomy, (2) total proctocolectomy with continent ileostomy (Kock pouch), and (3) total colectomy with rectal mucosal stripping and ileoanal reservoir.

Total proctocolectomy with permanent ileostomy. Total proctocolectomy with an ileostomy, is a one-stage operation involving the removal of the colon, rectum, and anus with closure of the anus. The end of the terminal ileum is brought out through the abdominal wall and forms a stoma, or ostomy. The stoma is usually placed in the right lower quadrant below the belt line.

Total proctocolectomy with continent ileostomy. Kock pouch is a continent ileostomy, which is a variation from the traditional ileostomy (Fig. 40-3). This method eliminates the need for the patient to wear an external pouch over the stoma. The stoma is usually covered with a cap or dressing in case of mucus leakage. This procedure is considered curative for ulcerative colitis but has a higher complication rate than the traditional ileostomy.

In this procedure an internal pouch in the distal segment of the ileum is made surgically, the intestine is split, a fold is made, and a one-way nipple valve is created and sutured into place on the abdomen. The pouch acts as a reservoir and is drained at regular intervals on insertion of a catheter. During surgery, a catheter is inserted into the pouch to allow suture lines to heal and to allow fixation of scar tissue around the valve to prevent slippage. Postoperative irrigations are performed every 2 to 4 hours to rinse mucus from the pouch. The catheter may stay in place for up to 3 to 4 weeks. Once the catheter is removed, insertion of a catheter to remove contents begins every 2 hours and is gradually decreased until it is needed only three to six times a day. The patient eventually determines the frequency by the changes in sensation of pressure in the pouch. A continuous leakage of fluid is prevented by the one-way valve created at the internal end of the ileum from the stoma to the ileal pouch. Pressure created when the pouch fills with feces forces the valve to close. The majority of complications that arise are a result of valve failure, which has been reported to be as high as 40%.

The primary late complications of the procedure include pouchitis, fistula development, and nipple valve extrusion. These complications affect function by increasing intubation frequency and compromising pouch continence. Manifestations of pouchitis are fever, malaise, and watery diarrhea. The lining appears red and inflamed, and biopsy shows nonspecific inflammation. Patients usually respond to treatment with metronidazole (Flagyl).

Total colectomy and ileal reservoir. A more widely performed procedure involves total colectomy and ileoanal anastomosis with the formation of an ileal reservoir (Fig. 40-4). The ileoanal surgical procedure is usually a combination of two procedures performed approximately 8 to 12 weeks apart. The initial procedure includes colectomy, rectal mucosectomy, ileal reservoir construction, ileoanal anastomosis, and temporary ileostomy. The second surgery involves closure of the ileostomy, which functionalizes the reservoir. Adaptation of the reservoir occurs over the next 3 to 6 months, which usually results in the ability to control and have decreased numbers of bowel movements over a 24-hour period.

Patient selection criteria include absence of colon cancer, small intestine free of disease (e.g., Crohn's), competent anorectal sphincter, and physical status adequate to permit lengthy surgery. In addition, the patient needs to be motivated and capable of understanding self-care instructions.

Postoperative Care. Postoperative care following surgical procedures to treat ulcerative colitis includes routine observations for patients who have had abdominal surgery. Stoma viability, mucocutaneous juncture, and peristomal skin integrity must be monitored. Because a more proximal portion of the bowel is used to create the ileostomy, output initially may be as high as 1500 to 2000 ml per 24 hours. The patient must be observed for signs of hemorrhage, abdominal abscess, small bowel obstruction, dehydration, and other related complications. If an NG tube is used, it will be removed

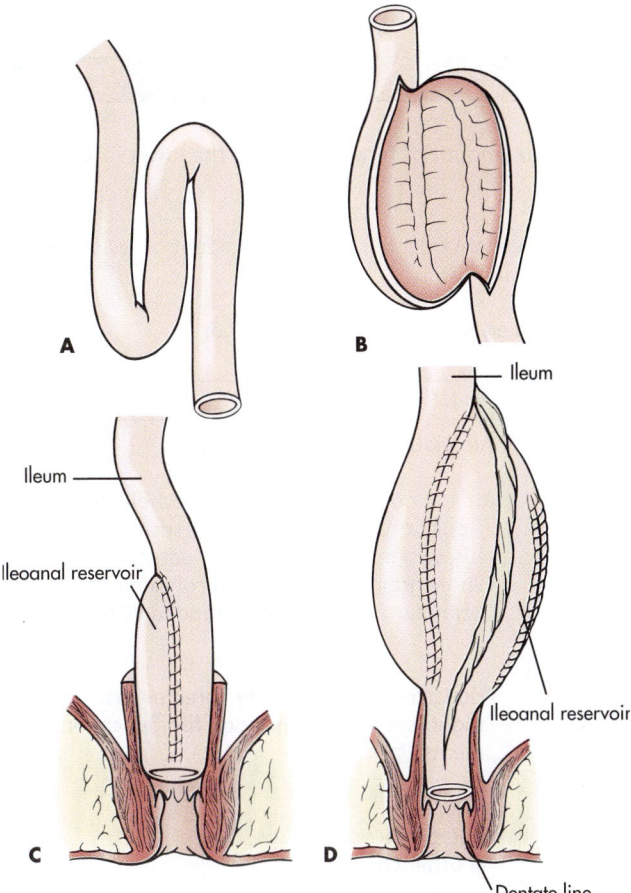

Fig. 40-4   Ileoanal reservoir. **A,** Formation of a reservoir. **B,** Posterior suture lines completed. **C,** J-shaped configuration for ileoanal reservoir. **D,** S-shaped configuration for ileoanal reservoir.

when bowel function returns and oral intake is instituted. Drainage of serosanguineous fluid from the abdominal drain site may vary from 100 to 150 ml per 24 hours. The drain is usually removed within 4 days of surgery. The urinary catheter is removed 2 to 5 days after surgery. Systemic antibiotics are discontinued within 24 hours of the operation and corticosteroids, if used, are tapered.

Transient incontinence of mucus is a result of intraoperative manipulation of the anal canal. The patient should be reassured before the operation regarding this potential transient problem. Kegel exercises are recommended later on (several weeks postoperatively) to strengthen the pelvic floor and sphincter muscles. They are not recommended in the immediate postoperative period. Perianal skin care must be implemented to protect the epidermis from mucous drainage and maceration. The patient should be instructed to gently rinse the skin with water and dry thoroughly. A moisture barrier ointment may be used, and a perineal pad may be required.

The most frequent type of ileostomy that is constructed is a loop. This frequently presents a pouching challenge because it retracts or drains inferiorly, resulting in effluent contact with the skin and predisposing to a denuded epidermis. An enterostomal therapy nurse is an appropriate referral for these chal-

lenging problems. Self-care instructions should be reviewed and written information provided before discharge. Stoma care is presented later in this chapter (see p. 1174).

Nutritional Therapy.   An important component in the treatment of ulcerative colitis is diet. The dietician is an important member of the team and should be consulted regarding dietary recommendations. The goals of diet management are to provide adequate nutrition without exacerbating symptoms, to correct and prevent malnutrition, to replace fluid and electrolyte losses, and to prevent weight loss. The diet for each patient must be individualized.

Traditionally during the acute phase the patient may be on NPO status. When food is permitted, a high-calorie, high-protein, low-residue diet with vitamin and iron supplements is frequently prescribed. (A low-residue diet is presented in Table 40-21.) Special dietary restrictions are not usually necessary. Some physicians allow the patient to eat anything that does not cause symptoms. Cold foods, high-residue foods (whole-wheat bread, cereal with bran, nuts, raw fruit), and smoking increase GI motility and should be avoided.

Often enteral supplements and parenteral nutrition are necessary. Patients with systemic manifestations, significant fluid and electrolyte losses, or malabsorption may need parenteral nutrition or enteral feedings, such as elemental diets. Elemental diets are high in calories and nutrients, lactose-free, and absorbed in the proximal small intestine, which allows the more distal bowel to rest. (Elemental diets are discussed in Chapter 38.)

Parenteral nutrition allows for a positive nitrogen balance while resting the bowel. Vitamins, minerals, electrolytes, and other important nutrients can be administered to promote healing and correct nutritional deficiencies.

Iron dextran (Imferon) intramuscularly (IM) by Z-track or IV may be necessary if anemia is severe. In patients receiving long-term sulfasalazine therapy, folic acid deficiency may develop and supplementation may be necessary. Patients with small bowel disease, ileal resection, or malabsorption, which affects the absorption of cobalamin (vitamin B_{12}), may need monthly injections of cobalamin. Potassium supplements may be necessary if corticosteroid therapy is used because hypokalemia can lead to toxic megacolon. Zinc deficiency can result from severe or chronic diarrhea and supplementation may be necessary.

NURSING MANAGEMENT: ULCERATIVE COLITIS
■ Nursing Assessment
Subjective and objective data that should be obtained from a person with ulcerative colitis are presented in Table 40-22.

■ Nursing Diagnoses
Nursing diagnoses for the patient with ulcerative colitis include, but are not limited to, those presented in NCP 40-3.

■ Planning
The overall goals are that the patient with ulcerative colitis will (1) experience a decrease in number and severity of acute exacerbations, (2) maintain normal fluid and electrolyte balance, (3) be free from pain or discomfort, (4) comply with medical regimens, and (5) maintain nutritional balance.

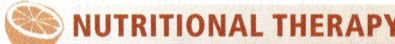

NUTRITIONAL THERAPY

Table **40-21**   Low-Residue Diet

Purpose

Low-residue diet provides foods low in fiber, which will result in a reduced amount of fecal material in the lower intestinal tract.

General Principles

1. This diet eliminates foods that are indigestible or stimulating to the intestinal tract to reduce the amount of residue in the colon. Foods should be included or excluded according to the following list.
2. Hot and cold foods should be eaten slowly.
3. Milk products are limited to 2 cups daily. For a more restricted-residue diet, milk should be eliminated.

Food	Foods Included	Foods Excluded
Beverages	Carbonated drinks, coffee, tea, cocoa, strained fruit juices	Alcohol, fruit juices with pulp
Bread	White bread, rolls, rusk, melba toast, crackers	Bread and crackers containing whole grain flour or bran; any hot breads such as biscuits, muffins, waffles, or pancakes
Cereals	Cooked, refined, or strained cereals: Cream of Wheat, Cream of Rice, farina, grits, dry cereals without bran, noodles, spaghetti, and macaroni	Whole grain cereals; cereals containing bran, nuts, and raisins; Shredded Wheat
Meat	Lean, tender ground beef, lamb, pork, veal or fish, broiled, stewed, or baked; canned tuna or salmon; shellfish; crisp bacon, chicken or turkey without skin, liver; creamy peanut butter	Fried, smoked, pickled, or cured meats, highly seasoned ham, fried fish, luncheon meats
Egg	All but fried	Fried or uncooked eggs
Cheese	Milk, cheese (American, cheddar), cottage cheese	All other cheeses
Milk	Limit to 1-2 cups (if tolerated), including that used in cooking; plain yogurt	Fruit yogurt
Fats	Butter, margarine, cream, oil, crisp bacon, mayonnaise, plain gravy	Any other; rich or spiced gravies
Soup	Cream and vegetable soups made from foods allowed and with milk allowed, bouillon, broth; strained vegetable juices	Cream and vegetable soups from foods not allowed (peas and dried beans)
Vegetables	Tender carrots, beets, or asparagus; strained vegetables; potatoes without skins; vegetable juices	Raw vegetables, all vegetables not strained, dried beans, peas, and legumes
Fruits	Strained fruit juices, ripe bananas, applesauce, pears, peaches, peeled apricots, Napoleon cherries, baked apple (no skin)	Raw fruits, fruits with skins, seeds
Desserts	Plain desserts (custards and puddings, plain ice cream from milk allowance), sherbet, plain gelatin desserts, angel food cake, sponge cake, plain butter cake, plain cookies	Nuts, coconut, raisins, rich desserts (pies, rich cakes, cobblers)
Condiments	Allspice, cinnamon, mace, paprika, salt, ground thyme, sugar, vinegar, lemon juice	All others

Breakfast	Lunch	Dinner

Sample Menu Plan

Breakfast	Lunch	Dinner
½ cup applesauce	Roast beef sandwich on 2 slices white bread (no lettuce or tomato)	Baked chicken
½ cup Cream of Wheat	1 tbs mayonnaise	Mashed potato
Scrambled egg	2 sugar cookies	Cooked carrots
White toast	Canned peach halves	White bread
Butter or jelly	Coffee	Butter
1 cup milk		Angel food cake
Coffee		1 cup milk
		Coffee

NURSING ASSESSMENT
Table 40-22 Ulcerative Colitis

Subjective Data

Important Health Information
Past health history: Infection, autoimmune disorders
Medications: Use of antidiarrheal medications

Functional Health Patterns
Health perception–health management: Family history of ulcerative colitis; fatigue, malaise
Nutritional-metabolic: Nausea, vomiting; anorexia; weight loss
Elimination: Frequent bloody stools containing mucus and pus
Cognitive-perceptual: Lower abdominal pain (worse before defecation), cramping, tenesmus

Objective Data

General
Intermittent fever; emaciated appearance

Integumentary
Pale skin with poor turgor, dry mucous membranes; rash, nodules, or blisters; anorectal excoriation

Gastrointestinal
Abdominal distention, hyperactive bowel sounds

Cardiovascular
Tachycardia, hypotension

Possible Findings
Anemia; leukocytosis; electrolyte imbalance; hypoalbuminemia; vitamin and trace metal deficiencies; guaiac-positive stool; abnormal proctosigmoidoscopic, colonoscopic, and barium enema findings

■ Nursing Implementation

During the acute phase, attention is focused on hemodynamic stability, pain control, fluid and electrolyte balance, and nutritional support. Accurate intake and output records must be maintained. The number and appearance of stools are monitored. Nursing care of the patient with ulcerative colitis is directed toward an intensive therapeutic and supportive program (see NCP 40-3). Emotional support is important because the patient with ulcerative colitis may feel insecure, dependent, and sensitive. It is important that the nurse establishes a good working relationship and encourages the patient to talk about self and daily activities. Honesty, patience, and understanding are crucial in the relationship with the patient. An explanation of all procedures and treatment is necessary and may allay some apprehension.

Appropriate diversional activity should be used to move the patient's attention away from the intestinal tract. Psychotherapy may be indicated if the patient is experiencing emotional problems, but the nurse must recognize that the patient's behavior may result from factors other than emotional ones. Any person who has 10 to 20 bowel movements a day and has rectal discomfort may be anxious, frustrated, discouraged, and depressed. Along with other team members, the nurse can assist the patient to accept the chronic condition and have an optimistic view with the possibility of cure after surgery. The nurse may find that inadequate coping mechanisms in the patient with ulcerative colitis are due to early onset of the disease (often at 10 to 15 years of age), which may have interfered with usual growth, development, and maturation.

Bed rest may be ordered if the patient has a severe exacerbation. Nursing interventions to prevent complications of immobility should be instituted. A sedative or tranquilizer may be prescribed to ensure rest. In addition to teaching related to treatment, medications, diet, diagnostic tests, and the disease and its management, discussion of everyday topics should also be a part of diversional therapy.

Rest is important in the management of ulcerative colitis. Patients may lose much sleep because of frequent episodes of diarrhea and abdominal pain. Nutritional deficiencies and anemia leave the patient feeling weak and listless. Activities should be scheduled around rest periods. The nurse should also set limits and follow through because the patient can be demanding. The patient needs to know and understand that the nurse wants to help and does not consider the care repugnant.

Until diarrhea is controlled, the patient must be kept clean, dry, and free of odor. A bedpan and wipes should be kept within reach of the patient. The bedpan should be emptied as soon as possible. A deodorizer should be placed in the room. Antidiarrheal agents should be administered as ordered. If the patient has continuous diarrhea, the enterostomal therapy nurse may give helpful suggestions. Meticulous perianal skin care using plain water (no harsh soap) is necessary to treat and prevent skin breakdown. Dibucaine (Nupercaine), witch hazel, or other soothing compresses or prescribed ointment and sitz baths may reduce irritation and relieve discomfort of the anus.

■ Evaluation

The expected outcomes for the patient with ulcerative colitis are presented in NCP 40-3.

CROHN'S DISEASE

Crohn's disease is a chronic, nonspecific inflammatory bowel disorder of unknown origin that can affect any part of the GI tract. It was once thought to be a disease specific to the small intestine and was called *regional enteritis.*

Crohn's disease may occur at any age but occurs most often between the ages of 15 and 30 years. When it occurs in older adults, the morbidity and mortality rates are higher because of other chronic problems that may be present. Both sexes are affected, with a slightly higher incidence in women. Similar to ulcerative colitis, it occurs more often in Jewish and upper-middle-class urban populations. The incidence of Crohn's disease is slightly lower than that of ulcerative colitis.

40-3   NURSING CARE PLAN   PATIENT WITH ULCERATIVE COLITIS

| Expected Patient Outcomes | Nursing Interventions and *Rationales* |

NURSING DIAGNOSIS   **Diarrhea** *related to* irritated bowel and intestinal hyperactivity *as manifested by* frequent diarrheal stools (>10 per day).

- Fewer, firmer stools.

- Monitor frequency and character of stools *to evaluate effectiveness of antidiarrheal agents and dietary restrictions.*
- Maintain food and fluid restrictions *to rest bowel during exacerbations.*
- Teach patient to avoid caffeine and foods or fluids that are *irritating to bowel or cause increased motility.*
- Rarely administer antidiarrheal medications *as they may precipitate colonic dilation.*

NURSING DIAGNOSIS   **Anxiety** *related to* possible social embarrassment, unfamiliar environment, diagnostic tests, and treatment *as manifested by* expression of concerns about effect of disease on social relationships, questions about disease and treatment.

- Less anxious feelings.

- Monitor signs of anxiety *to plan appropriate interventions.*
- Encourage open discussion of feelings about diagnosis *to demonstrate acceptance and concern for patient and allow verbalization of concerns.*
- Explain disease treatments, diagnostic tests, and medications *as understanding may reduce anxiety.*
- Provide privacy *to reduce embarrassment and anxiety associated with frequent bowel movements.*

NURSING DIAGNOSIS   **Altered nutrition: less than body requirements** *related to* decreased intake, increased nutrient loss through diarrhea and decreased absorption *as manifested by* anorexia, weight loss, weakness, lethargy, anemia.

- Maintenance of body weight within normal range.
- Adequate nutritional intake.
- Increased strength and activity tolerance.

- Assess and document signs of malnutrition (e.g., hair loss, dry skin, bleeding, fatigue) *to direct plan for treating the problem.*
- Record daily weights *to evaluate nutritional status and response to treatment.*
- Perform ongoing calorie counts *to determine adequacy of caloric intake.*
- Administer IV fluids and TPN as ordered *to provide nutrients for healing* and *promote fluid balance while resting the bowel.*
- Administer and instruct patient on high-calorie, nonspicy, caffeine-free, low-residue diet with small, frequent feedings *to reduce the amount of fecal material in the lower intestinal tract.*
- Administer nutritional supplements (as ordered) *to provide additional calories, protein, and fluid.*
- Teach patient to take small bites, eat slowly, and chew well *to facilitate digestion by slowing GI activity and breaking food down first in the mouth.*

NURSING DIAGNOSIS   **Impaired skin integrity** *related to* diarrhea and altered nutritional status *as manifested by* erythema of perianal area, discomfort around perianal area during and after evacuation, poor nutritional intake.

- No evidence of skin breakdown.

- Assess skin for signs of breakdown *to ensure early intervention.*
- Cleanse perianal area after each bowel movement with mild soap and warm water and dry thoroughly *to remove bacteria, provide comfort, and stimulate circulation to treat and prevent skin breakdown.*
- Provide sitz baths for comfort and hygiene and apply protective ointment.
- Encourage increased intake of proteins *to promote healing.*
- Instruct patient and family on proper skin care techniques *to enable them to participate fully in treatment plan.*

Continued

40-3 NURSING CARE PLAN PATIENT WITH ULCERATIVE COLITIS—continued

Expected Patient Outcomes	Nursing Interventions and *Rationales*

NURSING DIAGNOSIS Ineffective individual coping *related to* chronic disease, lifestyle changes, stress, and pain *as manifested by* inability to express feelings and concerns; display of dependent, attention-getting behavior.

- Development of healthy coping behaviors.

- Identify ineffective behaviors and institute plan *to assist patient in learning more effective behaviors.*
- Include other staff members and family in setting limits *to provide a consistent approach.*
- Encourage patient's expression of feelings *to provide support as patient explores areas of concern and add to patient's feelings of self-worth.*
- Offer reassurance and psychologic support *to demonstrate caring and concern.*
- Know limitations and refer to counseling when appropriate *as more intensive treatment may be required to deal with specific stress or problem areas.*

NURSING DIAGNOSIS Ineffective management of therapeutic regimen *related to* lack of knowledge of course of disease, appropriate lifestyle adjustments, and nutritional and drug interventions *as manifested by* questioning about disease and treatment, poor decisions about activities of daily living.

- Able to repeat correct information about disease and treatment.

- Provide information about the disease *to ensure patient has adequate knowledge about the disease and treatment.*
- Refer to dietician if complex dietary changes are necessary *to provide patient with expert counseling.*
- Teach about the relationship of stress to the disease *as stress may stimulate hyperreactivity of the colon in susceptible persons.*
- Teach stress-reduction techniques *to assist patient in developing positive ways to reduce stress.*
- Recommend regular appointments for colon cancer screening *as there is an increased risk of colon cancer.*

COLLABORATIVE PROBLEMS

POTENTIAL COMPLICATION Hypovolemia and electrolyte imbalances *related to* fluid and electrolyte losses from diarrhea.

Nursing Goals	Nursing Interventions and *Rationales*

- Monitor for signs of hypovolemia and electrolyte imbalances.
- Report deviations from acceptable parameters.
- Carry out medical and nursing interventions.

- Monitor for tachycardia, hypotension, weakness, dizziness, poor skin turgor, pallor, sunken eyes, rectal bleeding, abnormal serum electrolytes, urine output <0.5 ml/kg/hr *to identify hypovolemia and electrolyte imbalances and guide treatment.*
- Maintain accurate intake and output records; include stool volumes *to enable appropriate fluid replacement.*
- Administer IV fluids as ordered *to restore fluid volume.*
- Encourage oral intake (at least 3000 ml/day) when tolerated *to maintain fluid balance.*

TPN, total parenteral nutrition.

Etiology and Pathophysiology

Crohn's disease is characterized by inflammation of segments of the GI tract. It can affect any part of the GI tract but is most often seen in the terminal ileum, jejunum, and colon. Involvement of the esophagus, stomach, and duodenum is rare. The inflammation involves all layers of the bowel wall (i.e., transmural). Areas of involvement are usually discontinuous, with segments of normal bowel occurring between diseased portions (Table 40-17). Typically, ulcerations are deep and longitudinal and penetrate between islands of inflamed edematous mucosa, causing the classic cobblestone appearance (Fig. 40-5). Thickening of the bowel wall occurs, as well as narrowing of the lumen with stricture development. Abscesses or fistula tracts that communicate with other loops of bowel, skin, bladder, rectum, or vagina may develop. Histologically, granulomas are present in 50% of patients and may be located in any layer of the bowel wall.

Clinical Manifestations

The manifestations depend largely on the anatomical site of involvement, extent of the disease process, and presence or absence of complications. The onset of Crohn's disease is usually insidious, with nonspecific complaints such as diarrhea, fatigue, abdominal pain, weight loss, and fever. Early diagnosis

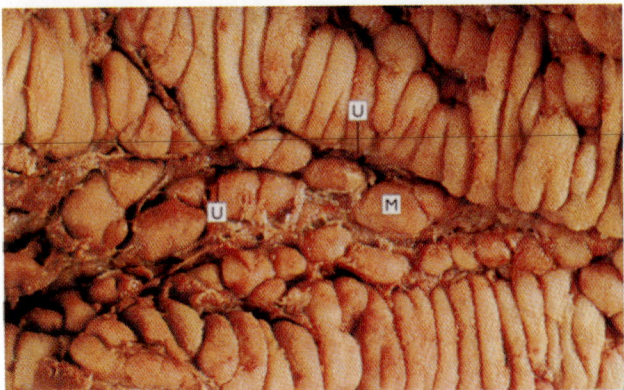

Fig. 40-5 Crohn's disease. The mucosa in Crohn's disease demonstrates a cobblestone pattern as a result of fissured ulcers (U) with intervening areas of edematous mucosa (M).

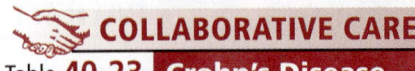

COLLABORATIVE CARE

Table 40-23 | **Crohn's Disease**

Diagnostic
- Complete blood cell count
- Serum chemistries
- Stool for occult blood
- Barium enema of small and large intestine
- Proctosigmoidoscopic examination
- Sigmoidoscopy and colonoscopy with biopsy

Collaborative Therapy
- High-calorie, high-vitamin, high-protein, low-residue, milk-free diet
- Antimicrobial agents*
- Corticosteroid drugs
- Supplementary parenteral nutrition
- Elemental diet
- Physical and emotional rest
- Surgery†

*See Table 40-20.
†See Table 40-24.

may be more difficult than for ulcerative colitis. The principal symptoms of Crohn's disease are diarrhea and abdominal pain. Diarrhea is usually nonbloody and is a result of the inflammatory process or malabsorption. Pain may be severe and intermittent or constant, depending on the cause. Other manifestations include abdominal cramping and tenderness, abdominal distention, fever, and fatigue. Extraintestinal manifestations, such as arthritis and finger clubbing, may precede the onset of bowel disease. As the disease progresses, there is weight loss, malnutrition, dehydration, electrolyte imbalances, anemia, increased peristalsis, and pain around the umbilicus and right lower quadrant.

Crohn's disease is a chronic disorder with unpredictable periods of recurrence and remission. Attacks are intermittent, usually recurring over a period of several weeks to months, with diarrhea and abdominal pain subsiding spontaneously.

Complications

Complications, both gastrointestinal and extragastrointestinal, are common in Crohn's disease. Scar tissue from the inflammation narrows the lumen of the intestine and may cause strictures and obstruction, a frequent complication. *Fistulas* are a cardinal feature and may develop between segments of bowel. Cutaneous fistulas, common in the perianal area, and rectovaginal fistulas also occur. Fistulas communicating with the urinary tract may cause urinary tract infections. Inflammation of the intestines may involve all layers, predisposing the patient to perforation and the formation of intraabdominal abscesses and peritonitis.

Impaired absorption causing various nutritional abnormalities may occur as a result of damage to areas of the intestinal mucosa. Fat malabsorption causes a deficiency in the fat-soluble vitamins (A, D, E, and K). The patient may have an intolerance to gluten (a protein found in barley, rye, and wheat).

Systemic complications are similar to those of ulcerative colitis and include arthritis, liver disease, cholelithiasis (especially with ileal involvement), ankylosing spondylitis, pyoderma gangrenosum, erythema nodosum, and uveitis. Renal disorders are common, especially nephrolithiasis (kidney stones) secondary to increased oxalate absorption.

Diagnostic Studies

Diagnosis of Crohn's disease can be made by means of a thorough history and physical examination to establish clinical signs and symptoms, barium studies, and endoscopy with biopsy (Table 40-23). Laboratory studies may determine electrolyte disturbances and the presence of anemia. Barium studies are useful in determining location and extent of the disease and may reveal classic findings, such as stricturing of the ileum (string sign), cobblestoning of the mucosa, fistulas, and areas of abnormal and normal mucosa. Endoscopic studies, such as colonoscopy and sigmoidoscopy, are useful in detecting such early mucosal changes as patchy inflammation, small ulcerations, and skip areas that may not be seen radiographically. Biopsies may be performed to determine the presence of granulomas. A small-bowel barium enema is preferred over an upper GI x-ray series with small bowel follow-through for defining mucosal abnormalities.

Collaborative Care

The goal of collaborative care is to control the inflammatory process, relieve symptoms, correct metabolic and nutritional problems, and promote healing. Drug therapy and nutritional support are the mainstays of treatment.

Drug Therapy. Sulfasalazine is effective when the disease involves the large intestine but is much less effective when only the small intestine is involved. Corticosteroid therapy is effective in reducing inflammation and suppressing disease. The dosage and the route of administration depend on the severity of the illness and the area involved. Once clinical symptoms subside, the dosage should be tapered. Immunosuppressive agents (6-MP, azathioprine) may be tried if repeated trials with corticosteroids fail. Patients require close monitoring because of the serious side effects of these drugs.

Table 40-24	Indications for Surgical Management of Crohn's Disease
Drainage of abdominal abscess	Intestinal obstruction
Failure to respond to conservative therapy	Massive hemorrhage
Fistulas	Perforation
Growth retardation	Secondary hydronephrosis
Inability to decrease corticosteroids	Severe anorectal disease
	Suspicion of carcinoma

Metronidazole (Flagyl) is useful in treating Crohn's disease of the perianal area. Marked exacerbations have been reported when the drug is stopped. Fish oil preparations have been evaluated for their ability to prevent recurrence of inflammation in Crohn's patients in remission; however, their palatability has been low.[20]

Balloon dilation of strictures may be effective in relieving symptoms in some patients. This is usually performed through a colonoscope or under fluoroscopic guidance. Strictures most often dilated are those in the colon or small bowel.

Nutritional Therapy. Elemental diets and parenteral nutrition may be used in the patient with Crohn's disease (see Chapter 38). Parenteral nutrition may be given to patients with severe disease, small-bowel fistulas, or short bowel syndrome (described later in this chapter). It is given before and after surgery to promote wound healing, reduce complications, and hasten recovery. The elemental diet provides a high-calorie, high-nitrogen, fat-free, no-residue substrate that is absorbed in the proximal small bowel. This diet can be given to most patients with Crohn's disease, even during acute exacerbations.

The diet should otherwise be low in residue, roughage, and fat but high in calories and protein. It may be difficult to maintain adequate absorption during periods of disease exacerbation and even during periods of remission. Milk and milk products may need to be excluded from the diet. Lactose, the primary disaccharide found in milk, may not be adequately absorbed because of the inability of the damaged mucosa of the intestine to produce adequate amounts of lactase. High-fat diets are poorly tolerated because of the loss of absorbing mucosa and altered bile salt metabolism and absorption.

Vitamin deficiencies may develop as a result of malabsorption. Cobalamin (vitamin B_{12}) injections every month may be needed because of the inability of the terminal ileum (if affected) to absorb this vitamin.

Surgical Therapy. Surgery is used in patients with severe symptoms that are unresponsive to therapy and in those with life-threatening complications. The majority of patients with Crohn's disease eventually require surgery at least once in the course of their disease. Indications for surgery are outlined in Table 40-24. Unlike ulcerative colitis, which can be cured by total proctocolectomy, Crohn's disease is not cured by surgery. The recurrence rate after surgery is high. The surgical procedure depends on the affected area and the condition of the patient. Conservative intestinal resection with anastomosis of healthy bowel is the procedure of choice.

NURSING MANAGEMENT: CROHN'S DISEASE

Care of the patient is similar to that of the patient with ulcerative colitis (see NCP 40-3 and p. 1160). As the patient's condition improves, the nurse should allow for more self-care, provide frequent rest periods, and advise the patient of the importance of rest and avoidance or control of emotional stress. Initially this may be difficult for the patient when told the nature of the disease and the limitations of the treatment. Patients who have perianal fistulas or abscesses may need special skin care. Postoperative care should be the same as for exploratory laparotomy.

In the majority of patients with Crohn's disease the course is chronic and intermittent, regardless of the site of involvement. The patient and significant others may need help in setting realistic short-term and long-term goals. Teaching is important and should include (1) the importance of rest and diet management, (2) perianal care, (3) action and side effects of medications, (4) symptoms of recurrence of disease, (5) when to seek medical care, and (6) use of diversional activities to reduce stress.

GERONTOLOGIC CONSIDERATIONS

Inflammatory Bowel Disease

Although inflammatory bowel diseases (i.e., ulcerative colitis and Crohn's disease) are considered diseases of young adults, a second peak in the distribution of these inflammatory conditions occurs around the age of 70 years. The pathogenesis, natural history, and clinical course of ulcerative colitis and Crohn's disease in older adults are similar to those observed in younger patients. However, the distribution of the inflammation appears to be somewhat different. In the older patient with ulcerative colitis the distal colon (proctitis) is usually involved. In the older patient with Crohn's disease the colon rather than the small intestine tends to be involved. There tends to be less recurrence of Crohn's disease in older patients treated with surgical resection. The degree of inflammation associated with both conditions tends to be less in the older adult than in the younger patient.

Collaborative care of the older patient with one of these conditions is similar to the younger patient. However, because of increased risk of cardiovascular and pulmonary complications, older adults tend to have increased morbidity associated with surgical procedures.

In addition to Crohn's disease and ulcerative colitis, older adults are also vulnerable to inflammation of the colon (colitis) from medication use and systemic vascular disease. Drugs such as nonsteroidal antiinflammatory drugs (NSAIDs), digitalis, vasopressin, estrogen, and allopurinol (Zyloprim) have been associated with colitis development in the elderly patient. Colitis may also be secondary to ischemic bowel disease related to atherosclerosis and congestive heart failure.

Inflammation of the colon as a result of IBD or colitis results in diarrhea, which may be bloody. The loss of fluid and electrolytes and possibly blood may leave the older adult more vulnerable to problems related to volume depletion and dehydration. This may be particularly problematic in the patient with diminished renal and cardiovascular function. Thus

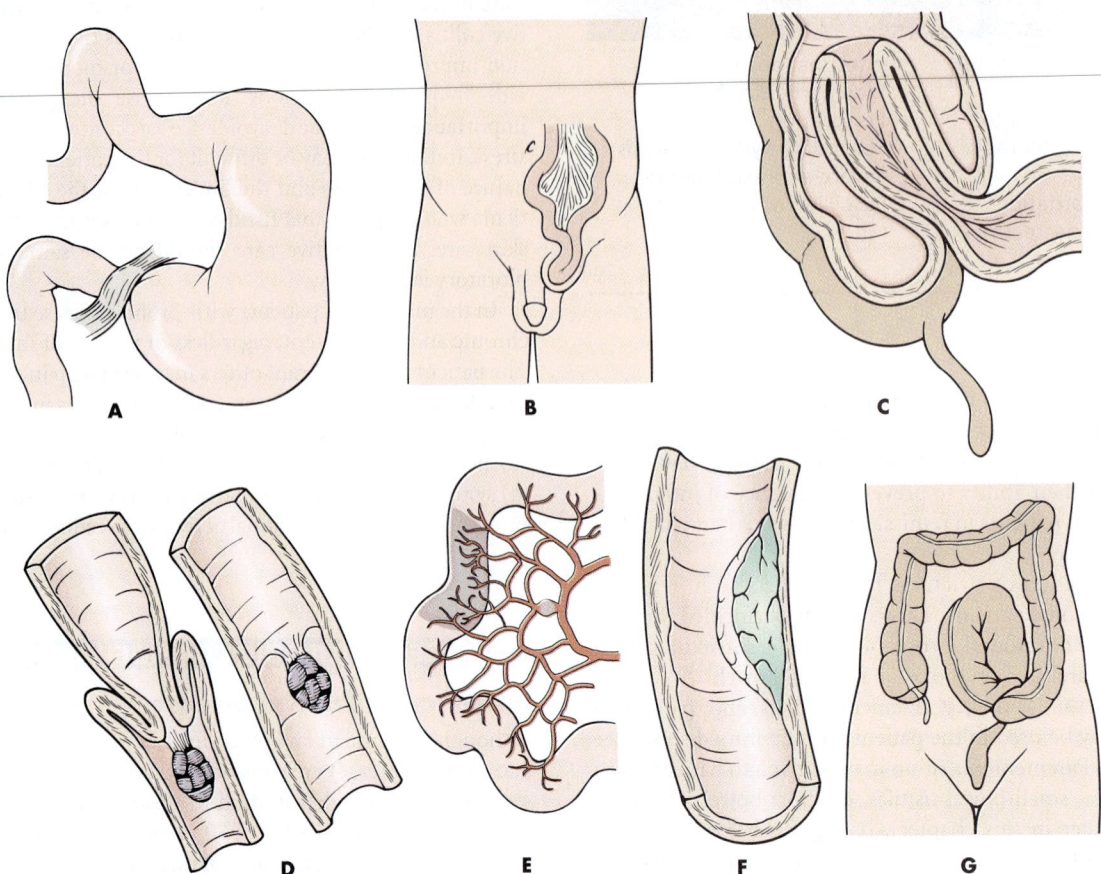

Fig. 40-6 Bowel obstructions. **A,** Adhesions. **B,** Strangulated inguinal hernia. **C,** Ileocecal intussusception. **D,** Intussusception from polyps. **E,** Mesenteric occlusion. **F,** Neoplasm. **G,** Volvulus of the sigmoid colon.

nursing management is focused on careful assessment of fluid and electrolyte status and evaluation of the replacement therapies.

INTESTINAL OBSTRUCTION

Intestinal obstruction occurs when intestinal contents cannot pass through the GI tract, and it requires prompt treatment. The obstruction may be partial or complete. The causes of intestinal obstruction can be classified as *mechanical* or *nonmechanical.*

Types of Intestinal Obstruction

Mechanical. Mechanical obstruction may be caused by an occlusion of the lumen of the intestinal tract. Most intestinal obstructions occur in the small intestine, most often in the ileum. Mechanical obstruction accounts for 90% of all intestinal obstructions (Fig. 40-6).[21] Adhesions account for 50%, hernias for 15%, and neoplasms for 15% of obstructions of the small intestine. Adhesions can develop after abdominal surgery. Obstruction can occur within days of surgery or years later. Carcinoma is the most common cause of large bowel obstruction, followed by volvulus and diverticular disease.

Nonmechanical. A nonmechanical obstruction may result from a neuromuscular or vascular disorder. *Paralytic (adynamic) ileus* is the most common form of nonmechanical obstruction. It occurs to some degree after any abdominal

surgery. Other causes of paralytic ileus include inflammatory responses (e.g., acute pancreatitis, acute appendicitis), electrolyte abnormalities, and thoracic or lumbar spinal fractures.

Pseudoobstruction is an apparent mechanical obstruction of the intestine without demonstration of obstruction by radiographic methods. Collagen vascular diseases and neurologic and endocrine disorders may cause pseudoobstruction, but mostly it is found to be idiopathic.

Vascular obstructions are rare and are due to an interference with the blood supply to a portion of the intestines. The most common causes are emboli and atherosclerosis of the mesenteric arteries. The celiac, inferior, and superior mesenteric arteries supply blood to the bowel. Emboli may originate from thrombi in patients with chronic atrial fibrillation, diseased heart valves, and prosthetic valves. Venous thrombosis may be seen in low-blood-flow states, such as heart failure and shock.

Etiology and Pathophysiology

Normally 6 to 8 L of fluid enters the small bowel daily. Most of the fluid is absorbed before it reaches the colon. Approximately 75% of intestinal gas is swallowed air. Bacterial metabolism produces methane and hydrogen gases. Fluid, gas, and intestinal contents accumulate proximal to the intestinal obstruction. This causes distention, and the distal bowel may collapse. The distention reduces the absorption of fluids and

Table 40-25	Clinical Manifestations of Small and Large Intestinal Obstructions	
Clinical Manifestation	**Small Intestine**	**Large Intestine**
Onset	Rapid	Gradual
Vomiting	Frequent and copious	Rare
Pain	Colicky, cramplike, intermittent	Low-grade, crampy abdominal pain
Bowel movement	Feces for a short time	Absolute constipation
Abdominal distention	Minimally increased	Greatly increased

stimulates intestinal secretions. As the fluid increases, so does the pressure in the lumen of the bowel. The increased pressure leads to an increase in capillary permeability and extravasation of fluids and electrolytes into the peritoneal cavity. Edema, congestion, and necrosis from impaired blood supply and possible rupture of the bowel may occur. The retention of fluid in the intestine and peritoneal cavity can lead to a severe reduction in circulating blood volume and result in hypotension and hypovolemic shock.

The electrolyte-rich fluids, which are normally absorbed in the bowel, are retained in the bowel and subsequently lost into the peritoneal cavity. The location of the obstruction determines the extent of fluid, electrolyte, and acid-base imbalances. If the obstruction is high, as in the pylorus, metabolic alkalosis may result from the loss of hydrochloric acid from the stomach through vomiting or NG intubation.

When the obstruction is located in the small bowel, dehydration occurs rapidly. Dehydration and electrolyte imbalances do not occur early in large bowel obstruction. If the obstruction is below the proximal colon, most GI fluids have been absorbed before reaching the point of the obstruction. Solid fecal material accumulates until symptoms of discomfort appear. Reverse peristalsis may cause vomiting of fecal material very late in the bowel obstruction.

Simple obstructions of the intestine involve blockage of the lumen in one spot. A closed-loop obstruction occurs when the lumen is blocked in two different spots (e.g., volvulus). This results in an isolated segment of bowel and obstruction proximal to that segment. Strangulation and gangrene are likely to develop if treatment is not immediate. A strangulated obstruction occurs when the circulation to the obstructed intestine is impaired. This is the most dangerous form of obstruction because it may lead to necrosis of the intestine (incarcerated). Volvulus, hernias, or adhesions are the most common causes.

Clinical Manifestations

The clinical manifestations of intestinal obstruction vary, depending on the location of the obstruction, and include nausea, vomiting, abdominal pain, distention, inability to pass flatus, and obstipation (Table 40-25). Obstruction located high in the small intestine produces rapid-onset, sometimes projectile vomiting with bile-containing vomitus. Vomiting from more distal obstructions of the small intestine is more gradual in onset. The vomitus may be orange-brown and foul smelling because of bacterial overgrowth. Vomiting may be entirely absent in large bowel obstruction if the ileocecal valve is competent; otherwise, the patient may eventually vomit feculent material.

Vomiting usually relieves abdominal pain in high intestinal obstructions. Persistent, colicky abdominal pain is seen with lower intestinal obstruction. A characteristic sign of mechanical obstruction is pain that comes and goes in waves. This is due to intestinal peristalsis trying to move bowel contents past the obstructed area. In contrast, paralytic ileus produces a more constant generalized discomfort. Strangulation causes severe, constant pain that is rapid in onset. Abdominal distention is a common manifestation of intestinal obstructions. It is usually absent or minimally noticeable in high obstructions of the small intestine and greatly increased in lower intestinal obstructions. Abdominal tenderness and rigidity are usually absent unless strangulation or peritonitis has occurred.

Auscultation of bowel sounds reveals high-pitched sounds above the area of obstruction. The patient often notes audible borborygmi. The patient's temperature rarely rises above 100° F (37.8° C) unless strangulation or peritonitis has occurred.

Diagnostic Studies

A thorough history and physical examination should be performed. Abdominal x-rays are the most useful diagnostic aids. Upright and lateral abdominal x-rays show the presence of gas and fluid in the intestines. The presence of intraperitoneal air indicates perforation. Barium enemas are helpful in locating large intestinal obstructions. However, barium is not used if perforation is suspected. If the location is unknown, a lower GI tract study is done before an upper GI series. Sigmoidoscopy or colonoscopy may provide direct visualization of an obstruction in the colon.

Laboratory tests are important and provide essential information. A CBC and serum electrolyte, amylase, and blood urea nitrogen (BUN) determinations should be performed. An elevated WBC count may indicate strangulation or perforation; elevated hematocrit values may reflect hemoconcentration. Decreased hemoglobin and hematocrit values may indicate bleeding from a neoplasm or strangulation with necrosis. Serum electrolytes should be monitored frequently. They provide essential information on the patient's fluid and electrolyte balance. Serum sodium, potassium, and chloride concentrations are decreased in small bowel obstruction. The BUN value may be increased because of dehydration. The stool should be checked for occult blood.

Collaborative Care

Treatment is directed toward decompression of the intestine by removal of gas and fluid, correction and maintenance of fluid and electrolyte balance, and relief or removal of the obstruction. NG or intestinal tubes (Fig. 40-7) may be used to decompress the bowel. NG tubes should be inserted before surgery to empty the stomach and relieve distention. They are also used instead of nasointestinal tubes to treat partial or complete small-bowel obstruction. Intestinal tubes, such as the Cantor or Miller-Abbott tubes, are passed into the small intestine. They are 10 feet (300 cm) long and mercury weighted.

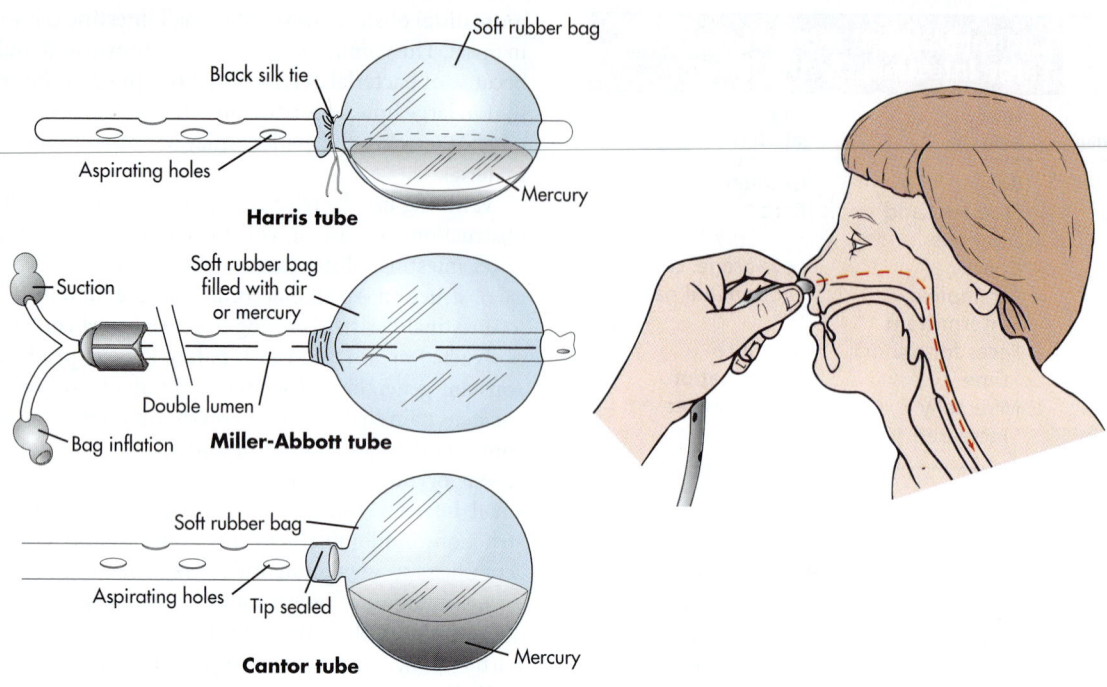

Fig. 40-7   Intestinal tubes used for decompression.

Insertion of an intestinal tube is controversial. Use of a long intestinal tube is difficult and time consuming. Some clinicians believe there is inadequate gastric decompression once the tube is in the small intestine. NG or intestinal tubes are effective in the treatment of patients with neurogenic obstruction who do not require surgery.

Sigmoidoscopy may successfully reduce a sigmoid volvulus. Colon-decompression catheters may be passed through partially obstructed areas via a colonoscope to decompress the bowel before surgery.

IV infusions that contain normal saline solution and potassium should be given to maintain fluid and electrolyte balance. Total parenteral nutrition may be necessary in some cases to correct nutritional deficiencies, improve the patient's nutritional status before surgery, and promote postoperative healing.

Most mechanical obstructions are treated surgically. They may involve simply resecting the obstructed segment of bowel and anastomosing the remaining healthy bowel. Partial or total colectomy, colostomy, or ileostomy may be required when extensive obstruction or necrosis is present. Occasionally obstructions can be removed nonsurgically. A colonoscope can be used to remove polyps, dilate strictures, and remove and necrose tumors with a laser.

NURSING MANAGEMENT: INTESTINAL OBSTRUCTION

■ Nursing Assessment

Intestinal obstruction is a potentially life-threatening condition. Signs and symptoms are varied. Nursing assessment must begin with a detailed patient history and physical examination. The type and location of obstruction usually cause characteristic symptoms. The nurse should determine the location, duration, intensity, and frequency of abdominal pain and whether abdominal tenderness or rigidity is present. Onset, frequency, color, odor, and amount of vomitus should be recorded. Bowel function, including passage of flatus, should be determined. The nurse should auscultate for bowel sounds and document character and location; inspect the abdomen for scars, palpable masses, and distention; and observe for muscle guarding and tenderness.

■ Nursing Diagnoses

Nursing diagnoses for the patient with intestinal obstructions include, but are not limited to, the following:

- Pain *related to* abdominal distention and increased peristalsis
- Fluid volume deficit *related to* decrease in intestinal fluid absorption and loss of fluids secondary to vomiting
- Altered nutrition: less than body requirements *related to* intestinal obstruction and vomiting

■ Planning

The overall goals are that the patient with an intestinal obstruction will have (1) relief of the obstruction and return to normal bowel function, (2) minimal to no discomfort, and (3) normal fluid and electrolyte status.

■ Nursing Implementation

The patient should be monitored closely for signs of dehydration and electrolyte imbalance. A strict intake and output record should be maintained. All vomitus and tube drainage should be included. IV fluids should be administered as ordered. Serum electrolyte levels should be monitored closely. A patient with a high obstruction is more likely to have metabolic alkalosis; a patient with a low obstruction is at greater risk of

Table **40-26**	Types of Polyps of the Large Intestine

Neoplastic	Nonneoplastic
Epithelial polyps (adenomatous)	Epithelial polyps (hyperplastic)
Tubular adenoma	Hereditary polyposis syndromes (hamartomatous polyposis syndrome)
Tubular villous adenoma	Familial juvenile polyposis
Villous adenoma	Peutz-Jeghers syndrome
Hereditary polyposis syndromes (adenomatous polyposis syndrome)	Inflammatory polyps
	Pseudopolyps
	Benign lymphoid polyp
Familial adenomatous polyposis	Submucosal polyps
Gardner syndrome	Lipomas
	Leiomyomas
	Fibromas

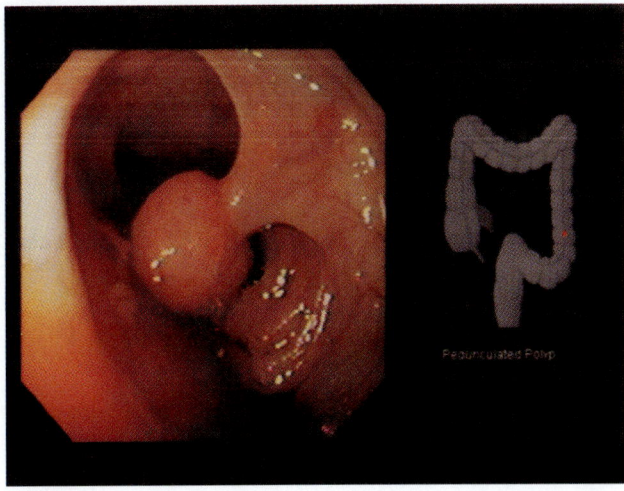

Fig. 40-8 Endoscopic image of pedunculated polyp in descending colon.

metabolic acidosis. The patient is often restless and constantly changes position to relieve the pain. Analgesics may be withheld until the obstruction is diagnosed because they may mask other signs and symptoms and decrease intestinal motility. The nurse should provide comfort measures, promote a restful environment, and keep distractions and visitors to a minimum. Nursing care of the patient after surgery for an intestinal obstruction is similar to care of the patient after a laparotomy (see NCP 40-2).

Care of Nasogastric and Intestinal Tubes. Although the physician usually inserts intestinal tubes, the nurse assists with the procedure. Insertion is easier if the patient relaxes, takes deep breaths, and swallows when instructed. If insertion of the tube to the small intestine is desired, the patient may be instructed or positioned to lie on the right side to facilitate tube passage through the pylorus. In some situations a prokinetic drug such as metoclopramide (Reglan) may be used to facilitate tube movement.

Once the tube is in place, mouth care is extremely important. Vomiting leaves a terrible taste in the patient's mouth, and fecal odor may be present. When an NG tube is in place, the patient breathes through the mouth, drying the mouth and lips. The nurse should encourage and assist the patient to brush the teeth frequently. Mouthwash and water for the patient to use in rinsing the mouth and petroleum jelly or water-soluble lubricant for the lips should be provided at the bedside.

The patient's nose should be checked for signs of irritation from the NG tube. This area should be cleaned and dried daily with application of a water-soluble lubricant and retaping of the tube. NG and intestinal tubes should be checked every 4 hours for patency. The patient may be placed on a schedule to clamp the tube for 1 hour out of every 3 hours or for 3 out of every 4 hours before removal of the tube.

POLYPS OF THE LARGE INTESTINE

Colonic polyps arise from the mucosal surface of the colon and project into the lumen. They may be *sessile* (flat, broad-based, and attached directly to the intestinal wall) or *pedunculated* (at-

tached to the intestinal wall by a thin stalk). Polyps tend to be sessile when small and become pedunculated as they enlarge, especially if they are in the left or descending colon (Fig. 40-8).[22] They may be found anywhere in the large intestine but are most commonly found in the rectosigmoid area. Although most polyps are asymptomatic, rectal bleeding or occult blood in the stool are the most common symptoms.

TYPES OF POLYPS

The most common types of polyp are *hyperplastic* and *adenomatous*. Hyperplastic polyps originate from the epithelium and are nonneoplastic growths. They rarely grow larger than 5 mm in size and never cause clinical symptoms. Other benign (nonneoplastic) polyps include inflammatory polyps, lipomas, and juvenile polyps (Table 40-26).

Adenomatous polyps are characterized by neoplastic changes in the epithelium. They are closely linked to colorectal adenocarcinoma. Structurally, there are three types, with tubular adenomas being the most prevalent. The risk of cancer in the polyp increases with polyp size and villous structure. Villous adenomas have a higher risk of turning cancerous than tubular adenomas.[22]

Although there are several polyposis syndromes, they are relatively rare. Of these, *familial adenomatous polyposis* (FAP) is the most common. This disorder is characterized by multiple polyps that at times number in the thousands and that are located in the large intestine and sometimes in other areas of the GI tract. Patients with a history of FAP have lifetime risk of developing colorectal cancer that approaches 100%. They also develop cancer at an earlier age (i.e., 40 years of age) than patients with non-FAP colon cancer. For children of patients with FAP, screening must be initiated at puberty and then conducted annually. There is a 50% risk for these children to develop FAP. When there is indication of disease, total colectomy with ileostomy is the treatment of choice.[22]

Diagnostic Studies and Collaborative Care

Barium enema, sigmoidoscopy, and colonoscopy are used to make diagnosis of polyps. All polyps are considered abnormal

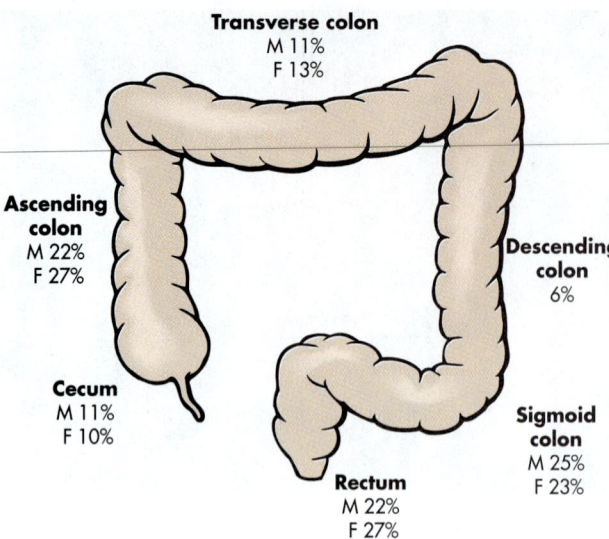

Fig. 40-9 Incidence of cancer. Approximately one half of all colon cancers occur in the rectosigmoid area. Percentages are listed for men and women.

Table **40-27**	**Risk Factors for Colorectal Cancer**
Age	
Familial polyposis	
Colorectal polyps	
Chronic IBD	
Family history of colorectal cancer or adenomas	
Previous history of colorectal cancer	
History of genital or breast cancer (women)	
High-fat and/or low-fiber diet	

IBD, inflammatory bowel disease.

and should be removed. In patients whose polyps are identified through barium enema, removal (polypectomy) should be done through a colonoscope or a sigmoidoscope. If the polyp is not removable, a biopsy specimen should be taken for tissue examination. Surgery is not indicated unless carcinoma is present or in certain cases of polyposis syndromes. The patient should be observed for rectal bleeding, fever, severe abdominal pain, and abdominal distention, which may indicate hemorrhage or perforation.

CANCER OF THE COLON AND RECTUM

Colorectal cancer is the second most common cause of cancer death in the United States.[23] Death rates from colorectal cancer in the United States and Canada are approximately 16.5 per 100,000 males and 11 per 100,000 females, accounting for approximately 56,500 deaths.[24] In 1998, there were approximately 131,600 new cases of colorectal cancer in the United States.[24] Cancer of the colon and rectum may occur at any age but is most prevalent over the age of 50 years. The 5-year survival rate for early, localized colorectal cancers is 91% and 63% for cancer spread to adjacent organs and lymph nodes.[24]

The incidence of cancer at specific sites in the colon varies (Fig. 40-9). In both sexes, the incidence of right colon cancers

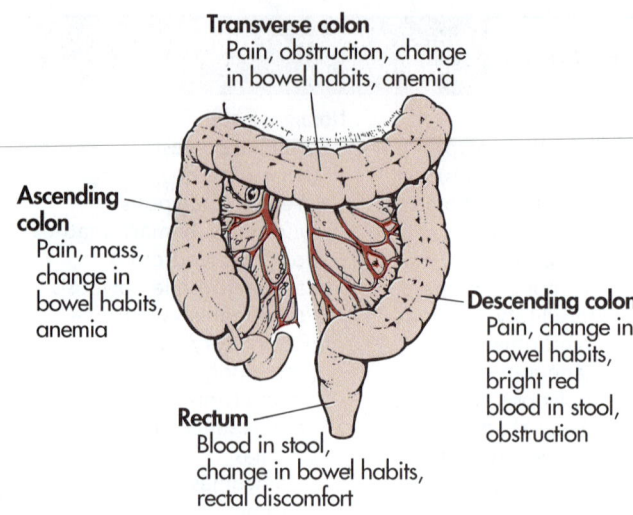

Fig. 40-10 Signs and symptoms of colorectal cancer by location of primary lesion.

has increased and cancers in the rectum have decreased. The highest percentages of colorectal cancers in the United States are currently located in the cecum, ascending colon, and sigmoid colon. Approximately 20% of colorectal cancers are within reach of the examining finger, and 50% are within reach of the sigmoidoscope.

Etiology and Pathophysiology

The causes of colorectal cancer remain unclear. Groups at high risk of colorectal cancer have been identified (Table 40-27). Age is a risk factor in both men and women. The risk for development in the general population increases slightly after the age of 40 years and then rises rapidly in the following decades. Diet is the most important environmental factor associated with colorectal cancer. The high-calorie, high-fat Western diet has been closely associated with development of colon cancer.

Adenocarcinoma is the most common type of colon cancer. Most colorectal cancers appear to arise from adenomatous polyps. All tumors tend to spread through the walls of the intestine and into the lymphatic system. Tumors commonly spread to the liver because the venous blood flow from the colorectal tumor is through the portal vein.

Clinical Manifestations

Clinical manifestations of colon cancer are usually nonspecific or do not appear until the disease is advanced. Cancer on the right side of the colon gives rise to clinical manifestations that are different from those on the left side of the colon.[25] Rectal bleeding, the most common symptom of colorectal cancer, is most often seen with left-sided lesions. Other commonly seen manifestations of left-sided lesions include alternating constipation and diarrhea, change in stool caliber (narrow, ribbonlike), and sensation of incomplete evacuation. Obstruction symptoms appear earlier with left-sided lesions because of the smaller lumen size (Fig. 40-10).

Cancers of the right side of the colon are usually asymptomatic. Vague abdominal discomfort or crampy, colicky abdominal pain may be present. Iron deficiency anemia and occult bleeding dictate further investigation. Weakness and fatigue result from anemia.

COLLABORATIVE CARE
Table 40-28   Cancer of the Colon

Diagnostic
Rectal examination
Sigmoidoscopy
Colonoscopy
Barium enema
CBC
Liver function tests
Testing of stools for occult blood
Carcinoembryonic antigen test
CT scan of abdomen
Ultrasound

Collaborative Therapy
Surgery
    Right hemicolectomy
    Left hemicolectomy
    Abdominal-perineal resection
    Laparoscopic colectomy
Radiation
Chemotherapy
    5-FU
    Methotrexate
    Levamisole (Ergamisol)
    Irinotecan (Camptosar)

Table 40-29   Dukes' Staging System for Colorectal Carcinoma

Classification	Description
A	Negative nodes, limitation of lesion to mucosa
B_1	Negative nodes, extension of lesion through mucosa but still within bowel wall
B_2	Negative nodes, extension through entire bowel wall
C_1	Positive nodes, limitation of lesion to bowel wall
C_2	Positive nodes, extension of lesion through entire bowel wall
D	Presence of distant, unresectable metastases

Diagnostic Studies

A thorough history with close attention to family history should be obtained, and a physical examination should be performed initially (Table 40-28). The digital rectal examination is the most important aspect of the physical examination because many rectal cancers are within reach of the finger. In the asymptomatic person who is 50 years or older with no risk factors (other than age), fecal occult blood testing once a year and flexible sigmoidoscopy every 5 years beginning at age 50 years are important aspects of the examination.[26] If colorectal cancer is suspected, examinations with the flexible sigmoidoscope and an air-contrast barium enema (in combination) are often performed. Colonoscopy is the procedure of choice if a questionable lesion is seen on barium enema or sigmoidoscopy. Other procedures include endorectal ultrasonography and a CT scan of the abdomen and pelvis to localize the lesion or determine its size. Synchronous lesions may be present at other sites in the colon, and tissue diagnosis may be made by brushing or biopsy during the procedure.

Laboratory studies should include a CBC to check for anemia, clotting studies, and liver function tests. A CT scan of the abdomen may be helpful in detecting liver metastases, retroperitoneal and pelvic disease, and depth of penetration of tumor into the bowel wall. A CT scan should be done before surgery. Liver function tests are performed to determine liver metastases.

A carcinoembryonic antigen (CEA) test is often performed, although it is not specific for colon cancer. A normal level of CEA does not exclude the possibility of a malignant condition. This test is used most effectively in following the progress of a patient after surgery. Return to normal of a previously elevated CEA indicates successful removal of the tumor. In contrast, persistent postoperative elevated or increasing CEA levels suggest residual tumor or tumor spread.

Collaborative Care

Prognosis and treatment correlate with pathologic staging of the disease. Several methods of staging are currently being used. The most widely known is Dukes' classification (Table 40-29). Surgical removal of the primary lesion is the treatment for Dukes' stages A, B, and C. Prognosis for Dukes' stage A is 90% to 100% 5-year survival compared with less than 15% with Dukes' stage D.

The most recent classification of colorectal cancer is the TNM system (Table 40-30), which is based on pathologic assessment and includes data from the history and physical examination and presurgical endoscopic and laboratory evaluations. Cancer of the colon can also be divided into stages, with stage 0 representing cancer in situ, stage I corresponding to Dukes' A and B_1, stage II corresponding to B_2, stage III corresponding to C_1 and C_2, and stage IV corresponding to Dukes' D.

Several noninvasive procedures may be performed through a colonoscope to effectively treat certain types of colorectal cancer. Endoscopic polypectomy is a highly effective and safe procedure. Adequate treatment is thought to be obtained if the resected margin of the polyp is free of cancer, the cancer is well differentiated, and there is no apparent lymphatic or blood vessel involvement. Laser therapy may be used to ablate nonresectable tumors. This is usually used only as palliative therapy in patients with obstructive symptoms.

Surgical Therapy. Surgery is the only curative treatment of colorectal cancer. The location and extent of the cancer determine the type of surgery performed. Success of surgery depends on resection of the tumor with an adequate margin of healthy bowel and resection of the regional lymph nodes.

Right hemicolectomy is performed when the cancer is located in the cecum, ascending colon, hepatic flexure, or transverse colon to the right of the middle colic artery. A portion of the terminal ileum, the ileocecal valve, and the appendix are removed, and an ileotransverse anastomosis is performed. A *left hemicolectomy* involves resection of the left transverse colon, the splenic flexure, the descending colon, the sigmoid colon, and the upper portion of the rectum.

Table **40-30**	**Tumor-Node-Metastasis (TNM) Classification of Colon and Rectal Cancer**	
T	**Primary Tumor**	
TX	Primary tumor cannot be assessed	
TO	No evidence of primary tumor	
Tis	Carcinoma in situ	
T1	Tumor invades submucosa	
T2	Tumor invades muscularis propria	
T3	Tumor invades through the muscularis propria into the subserosa, or into nonperitonealized pericolic or perirectal tissues	
T4	Tumor perforates the visceral peritoneum, or directly invades other organs or structures	
N	**Regional Lymph Node Involvement**	
NX	Regional lymph node cannot be assessed	
NO	No regional lymph node metastasis	
N1	Metastasis in 1 to 3 pericolic or perirectal lymph nodes	
N2	Metastasis in 4 or more pericolic or perirectal lymph nodes	
N3	Metastasis in any lymph node along the course of a named vascular trunk	
M	**Distant Metastasis**	
MX	Presence of distant metastasis cannot be assessed	
MO	No distant metastasis	
MI	Distant metastasis	

RESEARCH
IMPLICATIONS FOR NURSING PRACTICE

Patient Education Needs
Following Colon Cancer Surgery

Citation Galloway SC, Graydon JE: Uncertainty, symptom distress, and information needs after surgery for cancer of the colon, *Cancer Nurs* 19:112, 1996.

Purpose To determine the relationships among uncertainty, symptom distress, and information needs in people with a first-time diagnosis of cancer who had a colon resection.

Methods Twenty male and twenty female patients from three Canadian hospitals were interviewed and asked to complete questionnaires. The tools asked about uncertainty related to illness; amount of distress caused by symptoms of fatigue, pain, anorexia, constipation, and diarrhea; and discharge information needs. Patients were interviewed initially less than 72 hours before discharge and then 13 to 60 days after discharge.

Results and Conclusions The results indicated that patients after surgery for colon cancer had moderate levels of uncertainty and low levels of symptom distress. The most distressing symptom was fatigue followed by pain. As uncertainty increased, patients had a greater need for discharge information. Patients perceived information related to treatment, actions to take if a complication occurred, guidelines about diet and activity, and management of symptoms as important.

Implications for Nursing Practice Information about the impact of cancer on physical functioning appears to take priority over information about community resources and how to handle feelings about cancer in the early postoperative period. Discharge teaching should include explanations of follow-up treatments, possible complications, and how to manage symptoms such as pain and fatigue. Discharge teaching should be individualized, since many patients can predict their needs for information at the time of discharge.

Clear margins are most difficult to obtain with rectal carcinoma. Location of the rectal lesion determines the surgical procedure to be performed. There must be enough rectum left to ensure a secure anastomosis, or an abdominal-perineal resection is indicated. *Abdominal-perineal resection* is most often performed when the cancer is located within 5 cm of the anus.

In the abdominal-perineal resection, an abdominal incision is made and the proximal sigmoid is brought through the abdominal wall in a permanent colostomy. The distal sigmoid, rectum, and anus are removed through a perineal incision. The perineal wound may be closed around a drain or left open with packing to allow healing by granulation. Complications that can occur are delayed wound healing, hemorrhage, persistent perineal sinus tracts, infections, and urinary tract and sexual dysfunctions.

Low anterior resection may be indicated for tumors of the rectosigmoid and the mid-to-upper rectum. The use of EEA (end-to-end anastomosis) staplers has allowed lower and more secure anastomoses. The stapler is passed through the anus, where the colon is stapled to the rectum. This technique has made it possible to resect lesions as low as 5 cm from the anus.

Sphincter-sparing procedures are being performed on the patient who is a poor operative risk and for the patient with early disease. The number of these procedures may increase with continued early detection and surveillance. In these procedures a local resection is performed and the anal sphincters are left intact.

Laparoscopic colectomy is being evaluated for its effectiveness in eliminating cancer and improving survival. Potential benefits are reduced pain, shortened hospital stay, and improved cosmetic appearance.[27]

Radiation Therapy and Chemotherapy. Radiation may be used preoperatively or as a palliative measure for patients with advanced lesions. As a palliative measure, its primary objective is to reduce tumor size and provide symptomatic relief. (For discussion on radiation therapy, see Chapter 14.) Chemotherapy is recommended when a patient has positive lymph nodes at the time of surgery or has metastatic disease. No drug is available that can cure malignant colon or rectal tumors. The most commonly used drugs are 5-fluorouracil (5-FU) and methotrexate. Levamisole (Ergamisol), BCNU, and MeCCNU are sometimes used in combination with 5-FU. Irinotecan (Camptosar) is used for the treatment of metastatic colorectal cancer. New agents being examined for adjuvant therapy of colorectal cancer include leucovorin, monoclonal antibody to epithelial antigen 17-1A, and tegafur-4M uracil (UFT).[28]

NURSING ASSESSMENT

Table 40-31   Colorectal Cancer

Subjective Data

Important Health Information

Past health history: Previous breast or gynecologic cancer; familial polyposis; villous adenoma; adenomatous polyps; inflammatory bowel disease

Medications: Use of any medications affecting bowel function (e.g., cathartics, antidiarrheal medication)

Functional Health Patterns

Health perception–health management: Family history of cancer, especially colon or breast; weakness, fatigue

Nutritional-metabolic: High-calorie, high-fat, low-fiber diet; anorexia, weight loss; nausea and vomiting

Elimination: Change in bowel habits; alternating diarrhea and constipation, defecation urgency; rectal bleeding; mucoid stools; black, tarry stools; increased flatus, decrease in stool caliber; feelings of incomplete evacuation

Cognitive-perceptual: Abdominal and low back pain, tenesmus

Objective Data

General

Pallor, cachexia, lymphadenopathy (later signs)

Gastrointestinal

Palpable abdominal mass, distention, ascites and hepatomegaly (liver metastasis)

Possible Findings

Anemia; guaiac-positive stools, palpable mass on digital rectal examination; positive proctosigmoidoscopy, colonoscopy, barium enema, or CT scan; positive biopsy

NURSING MANAGEMENT: COLON AND RECTAL CANCER

■ Nursing Assessment

Subjective and objective data that should be obtained from a patient with cancer of the colon or rectum are presented in Table 40-31.

■ Nursing Diagnoses

Nursing diagnoses for the patient with cancer of the colon or rectum include, but are not limited to, the following:

- Diarrhea or constipation *related to* altered bowel elimination patterns
- Pain *related to* difficulty in passing stools because of partial or complete obstruction from tumor
- Fear *related to* diagnosis of colon cancer, surgical or therapeutic interventions, and possible terminal illness
- Ineffective individual coping *related to* diagnosis of cancer and side effects of treatment

■ Planning

The overall goals are that the patient with cancer of the colon or rectum will have (1) no metastasis or recurrence of the cancer, (2) normal bowel elimination patterns, (3) quality of life appropriate to disease progression, (4) relief of pain, and (5) feelings of comfort and well-being.

■ Nursing Implementation

Health Promotion. The current recommendations from the American Cancer Society for colorectal cancer screening in patients who are not at high risk include annual digital rectal examination beginning at the age of 40 years. Starting at the age of 50 years, fecal testing for occult blood should be done every year, and flexible sigmoidoscopy should be performed every 5 years. Positive findings should be followed with colonoscopy or air-contrast barium enema.[26]

Screening for high-risk patients usually begins with colonoscopy and continues at more frequent intervals that vary according to risk factors.[29] Participation in early cancer screening is effective in decreasing mortality, but barriers exist including lack of information and fear of diagnosis.[30]

Recent epidemiology studies reported that use of nonsteroidal antiinflammatory drugs (e.g., sulindac [Clinoril])[31] or long-term use of aspirin (four to six tablets per day)[32] may reduce the risk of colorectal cancer.

Acute Intervention

Preoperative care. Acute nursing care for the patient with a colon resection is similar to care of the patient having a laparotomy (see NCP 40-2). In addition to general preoperative teaching and ostomy care instructions, the patient undergoing abdominal-perineal resection should be informed of the extent of the surgical procedure and the amount of care necessary to facilitate complete wound healing. The patient should be taught side-to-side positioning and made to understand that short walks are better than sitting. The nurse should teach and assist the patient in proper positioning for taking a sitz bath. The patient may not know that the sitz bath and positioning are sources of comfort. The patient may experience phantom rectal sensation because the sympathetic nerves responsible for rectal control are not severed during the surgery. The nurse must be astute in distinguishing phantom sensations from perineal abscess pain.

A well-developed, consistent nursing care plan should be coordinated early. The implementation of this plan will facilitate the healing process and hasten the patient's rehabilitation.

Postoperative care. After an abdominal-perineal resection, there are two wounds and a stoma is surgically constructed in the left lower quadrant. There is an abdominal incision through which the colon is resected and an incision is made in the perineum. The management of a perineal incision differs depending on the type of wound. Three techniques are used: (1) packing of the entire open wound; (2) partial closure with Penrose drains for open drainage; and (3) primary closure of the perineal wound with closed-suction drainage of the pelvic cavity. The type of management of the perineal wound is individualized. The open and packed method is used in patients with extensive surgery or uncontrollable bleeding in the pelvic wound. When infection or contamination is minimal, a partial closure with drains is used. Wound sites connected to low intermittent suction or a Jackson Pratt or Hemovac suction placed in the perineal wound is commonly used to provide drainage of the operative site during the early postoperative period. This usually remains until drainage is less than 50 ml per 24 hours, which occurs after approximately 3 to 5 days.

A patient who has open and packed wounds requires meticulous postoperative care. During the immediate postoperative period the perineal dressing is reinforced and changed frequently because drainage can be profuse for several hours after surgery. All drainage is carefully assessed for amount, color, and consistency. The drainage is usually serosanguineous.

The packing is usually left in place for 2 to 3 days. Packing the pelvic cavity for prolonged periods may result in sepsis and rigidity of the cavity wall and thus impede the healing process. The nurse should examine the wound regularly and record bleeding, excessive drainage, and unusual odor. The perineal wound is usually irrigated with a normal saline solution when the dressings are changed. Dressings are changed several times a day, and aseptic technique is always used.

If the wound is partially closed and drains are in place, the nurse assesses the incision for suture integrity and signs and symptoms of wound inflammation and infection. The drainage is examined for amount, color, and characteristics. When the primary closure technique is used, the catheters are left in place for approximately 3 to 5 days, and during this time the drainage is examined and observations recorded. The area around the catheter is observed for signs of inflammation and kept clean and dry. The nurse should observe for signs of edema, erythema, drainage around the suture line, fever, and elevated WBC count. If the perineal wound was not closed, warm sitz baths at 100.4° to 106° F (38° to 41° C) for 10 to 20 minutes three to four times a day assist in tissue debridement, provide comfort, and increase circulation to the area. Moist heat causes vasodilation, which allows more oxygen to flow to the affected area. Sitz baths of more than 20 minutes may result in too much vasodilation, causing congestion and discomfort.

The patient may complain of pain and itching in and around the wound. There is no physiologic explanation of sensations that are felt, but a careful examination should be made to rule out delayed wound healing. Antipruritic agents and sitz baths are usually ordered. Use of a pressure-reducing chair cushion provides comfort when sitting. Sitting on a toilet for prolonged periods is discouraged until the perineal wound is well healed.

Sexual dysfunction is a possible complication of an abdominal-perineal resection and should be included in the plan of care. Although the effect of the procedure depends on the technique used, the surgeon should discuss the subject intelligently and tactfully, with follow-up as necessary by other members of the health care team. The nurse should understand that erection, ejaculation, and orgasm involve different nerve pathways and that a dysfunction of one does not mean total sexual dysfunction. The enterostomal therapy nurse is an important member of the team and can often provide correct and factual information concerning sexual dysfunction resulting from an abdominal-perineal resection.

Ambulatory and Home Care. Psychologic support for the patient and family is important. The recovery period is long, and the possibility of recurrence of cancer is always present. The overall 5-year survival rate for all patients undergoing resection for colon cancer is less than 50%. This presents a problem for the patient and health care providers because of the often painful, debilitating, and demoralizing manifestations produced by the recurrent disease and the lack of any effective palliative therapy. Chemotherapy may be used as an adjuvant measure for the patient with evidence of local or distant metastasis. (The special needs of the cancer patient are discussed in Chapter 14.)

The perineal wound may not be completely healed before discharge. After discharge the physician, the home health nurse, and the enterostomal therapist in an outpatient clinic usually see the patient. The wound is usually irrigated and debrided. The skin around the wound should be assessed for loose hair. Shaving may be necessary to prevent the development of a chronic draining sinus. The nurse should report the drainage because it may also indicate the presence of a foreign body, fistula, osteomyelitis, or rectal tissue not removed during surgery. The patient and significant others are taught management of the wound and the procedure to take a sitz bath at home. The patient and the family should be aware of all community services available for assistance.

■ Evaluation

The expected outcomes for the patient with cancer of the colon or rectum are that the patient will have

- no alterations in bowel elimination patterns
- relief of pain
- balanced nutritional intake
- quality of life appropriate to disease progression
- feelings of comfort and well-being

OSTOMY SURGERY

TYPES

An *ostomy* is a surgical procedure in which an opening is made to allow the passage of intestinal contents from the bowel to an incision or *stoma*. The stoma, which is the opening on the surface of the abdomen is created when the intestine is brought through the abdominal wall and sutured to the skin. It may be permanent or temporary. Fecal matter is diverted through the stoma to the outside of the abdominal wall.

An *ileostomy* is an opening from the ileum through the abdominal wall and is also referred to as a *conventional* or *Brooke* ileostomy (Fig. 40-11). It is most commonly used in surgical treatment of ulcerative colitis, Crohn's disease, and familial polyposis.

A *cecostomy* is an opening between the cecum and the abdominal wall. Both cecostomies and ascending colostomies are uncommon. They are usually temporary and most often are used for fecal diversion before surgery or for palliation.

A *colostomy* is an opening between the colon and the abdominal wall. The proximal end of the colon is sutured to the skin. Locations for colostomies are shown in Fig. 40-11. A

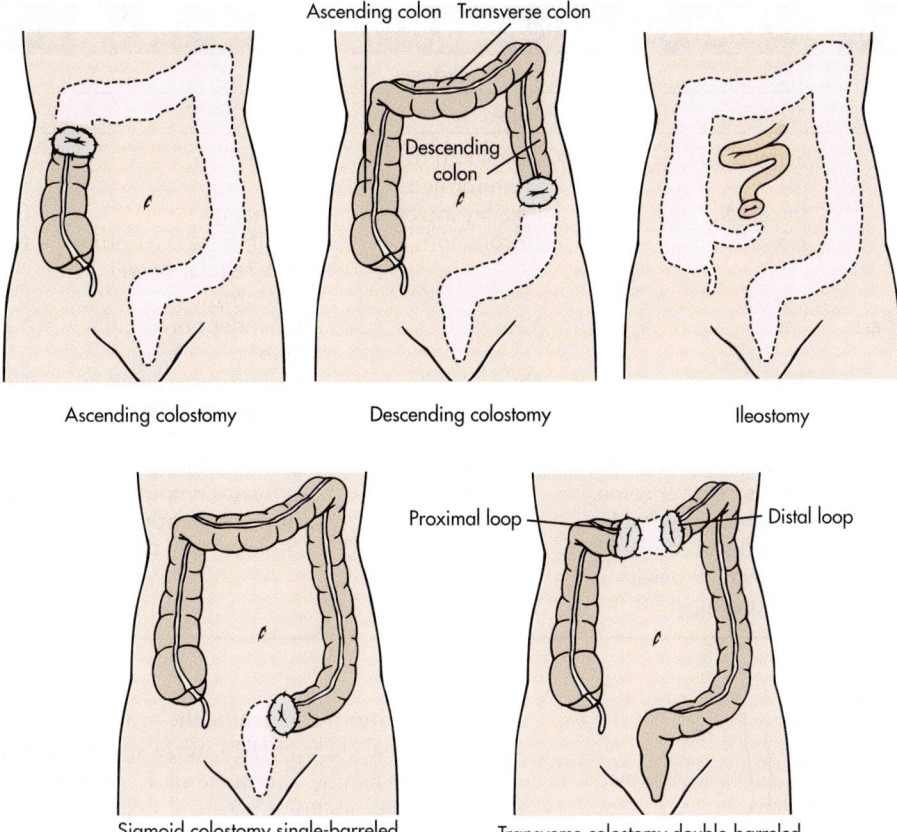

Ascending colon   Transverse colon

Descending colon

Ascending colostomy   Descending colostomy   Ileostomy

Proximal loop   Distal loop

Sigmoid colostomy single-barreled   Transverse colostomy double-barreled

Fig. 40-11   Types of ostomies.

temporary colostomy is usually performed to protect an end-to-end anastomosis after a bowel resection or is an emergency measure following bowel obstruction (e.g., malignant tumor), abdominal trauma (e.g., gunshot wound), or a perforated diverticulum. Temporary colostomies are usually located in the transverse colon. *Loop colostomy* (Fig. 40-12) and *double-barrel colostomy* (see Fig. 40-11) are most commonly performed as temporary colostomies, but they may be permanent. A comparison of colostomies and ileostomy is shown in Table 40-32.

Surgical Therapy

End stoma. An end stoma is surgically constructed by dividing the bowel and bringing out the proximal end as a single stoma. The distal portion of the GI tract is surgically removed, or the distal segment is oversewn and left in the abdominal cavity with its mesentery intact. An end colostomy or ileostomy is then constructed. When the distal bowel is oversewn rather than removed, the procedure is known as a *Hartmann's pouch* (Fig. 40-13). If the distal bowel is removed, the stoma is permanent; if the distal bowel remains intact and oversewn, the potential exists for the bowel to be reanastomosed and the stoma to be closed (referred to as a *takedown*).

Loop stoma. A loop stoma is constructed by bringing a loop of bowel to the abdominal surface and then opening the anterior wall of the bowel to provide fecal diversion. This results in one stoma with a proximal and distal opening and an intact posterior wall that separates the two openings. The loop of bowel is frequently held in place with a plastic rod for 7 to 10 days after surgery to prevent it from slipping back into the abdominal cavity (see Fig. 40-12). A loop stoma is usually temporary.

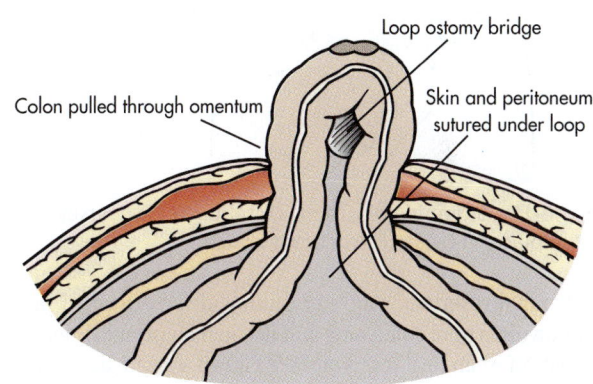

Loop ostomy bridge

Colon pulled through omentum

Skin and peritoneum sutured under loop

Fig. 40-12   Loop colostomy.

Double-barrel stoma. When the bowel is divided, both the proximal and distal ends are brought through the abdominal wall as two separate stomas (see Fig. 40-11). The proximal one is the functioning stoma; the distal, nonfunctioning stoma is referred to as the *mucus fistula*. The double-barrel stoma is usually temporary.

Kock pouch. As described previously in this chapter the *Kock pouch* is a continent ileostomy, which is a variation from the traditional ileostomy (see Fig. 40-3). This method eliminates the need for the patient to wear an external pouch over the stoma. The stoma is usually covered with a cap or dressing in case of mucus leakage. Additional information is provided on p. 1156.

Table **40-32** **Comparison of Colostomies and Ileostomy**

	Colostomy			
	Ascending	Transverse	Sigmoid	Ileostomy
Stool consistency	Semiliquid	Semiliquid to semiformed	Formed	Liquid to semiliquid
Fluid requirement	Increased	Possibly increased	No change	Increased
Bowel regulation	No	Uncommon	Yes (if there is a history of a regular bowel pattern)	No
Pouch and skin barriers	Yes	Yes	Dependent on regulation	Yes
Irrigation	No	No	Possible every 24-48 hr (if patient meets criteria)	No
Indications for surgery	Perforating diverticulitis in lower colon; trauma; inoperable tumors of colon, rectum, or pelvis; rectovaginal fistula	Same as for ascending; birth defect	Cancer of the rectum or rectosigmoidal area; perforating diverticulum; trauma	Ulcerative colitis, Crohn's disease, diseased or injured colon, birth defect, familial polyposis, trauma, cancer

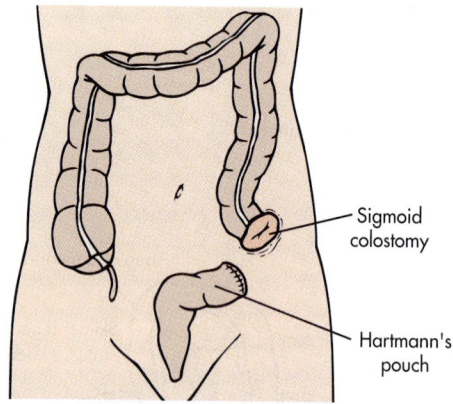

Sigmoid colostomy

Hartmann's pouch

Fig. 40-13 Sigmoid colostomy. Distal bowel is oversewn and left in place to create Hartmann's pouch.

Ileoanal reservoir. Another more widely performed procedure involves total colectomy and ileoanal anastomosis with the formation of an ileal reservoir (see Fig. 40-4). The ileoanal surgical procedure is usually a combination of two procedures performed approximately 8 to 12 weeks apart. The initial procedure includes colectomy, rectal mucosectomy, ileal reservoir construction, ileoanal anastomosis, and temporary ileostomy. The second surgery involves closure of the ileostomy, which functionalizes the reservoir. Adaptation of the reservoir occurs over the next 3 to 6 months, which usually results in the ability to control and have decreased numbers of bowel movements over a 24-hour period. Additional information is provided on p. 1156.

NURSING MANAGEMENT: OSTOMY SURGERY

■ Preoperative Care

It is important to review the information the patient has received from the physician. Psychologic preparation is very important. The family and the patient usually have many questions concerning the procedures. If available, an enterostomal therapy (ET) nurse should visit with the patient and the family. The nurse or ET nurse must determine the patient's ability to perform self-care, identify support systems, and determine potential adverse factors that could be modified to facilitate learning during rehabilitation. Preoperative assessment must be comprehensive and include physical, psychologic, social, cultural, and educational components. Assessment is ongoing, including both the patient and family. The ET nurse marks the stoma site before surgery. An improperly placed stoma complicates rehabilitation by increasing time and expense of pouch change routine. It can also contribute to skin irritation and poor adaptation. The patient and the family should understand the extent of surgery and the type of stoma and its care.

If the patient desires a referral and the physician agrees, a trained ostomy visitor from the United Ostomy Association can provide meaningful psychologic support. The patient has the opportunity to see a person who has adjusted well and who has experienced some of the same feelings and concerns. The family will also benefit from the visit.

Bowel preparation before surgery decreases the chance of a postoperative infection by cleansing the bowel of feces and bacteria. Orally administered osmotic lavages (e.g., Go-Lytely) have shortened the classic 72-hour preparation with clear liquids, cathartics, and enemas. IV and oral antibiotics are given. Nonabsorbable neomycin and erythromycin are given orally to decrease the number of intracolonic bacteria.

■ Colostomy Care

Postoperative nursing care should focus on assessing the stoma, protecting the skin, selecting the pouch, and assisting the patient to adapt psychologically to a changed body. Nursing care for the patient with a colostomy is presented in NCP 40-4.

40-4 NURSING CARE PLAN PATIENT WITH A COLOSTOMY/ILEOSTOMY

| Expected Patient Outcomes | Nursing Interventions and *Rationales* |

NURSING DIAGNOSIS **Risk for impaired skin integrity** *related to* irritation from fecal drainage, irritation of pouch, and lack of knowledge of skin care.

- Normal skin integrity.
- Intact pouch seal.

- Have enterostomal therapy nurse see patient before surgery *to mark stoma site in area free of creases and folds for better seal of appliance.*
- After surgery assess peristomal skin for erythema with burning and itching, poorly fitting appliance with leakage, lack of adequate skin care, and failure to use skin barrier *to initiate treatment if indicated.*
- During pouch change assess skin for signs of breakdown *to initiate treatment if indicated.*
- Clean area with mild soap and water and dry thoroughly *to prevent irritation from intestinal contents or pouch adhesive.*
- Apply skin barrier *to protect skin and prevent direct contact with intestinal contents.*
- Teach patient proper skin and pouch care *to ensure proper technique for long-term care.*
- Plan for outpatient or home visit *for continued teaching and monitoring.*
- Empty pouch when it is one-third full *to prevent seal from leaking.*

NURSING DIAGNOSIS **Body-image disturbance** *related to* presence of stoma and malodor *as manifested by* verbalization of embarrassment or shame due to malodor or presence of stoma.

- Adjustment to altered body image.
- Satisfactory plan for control of odor.

- Assess patient's attitude toward stoma *to determine if problem is present* and, if indicated, *plan appropriate intervention.*
- Instruct patient on measures for odor control, use of odor-proof pouch, pouch deodorants, and use of room deodorants when pouch is emptied *to minimize embarrassing odors from drainage.*
- Teach patient to use loose clothing *to conceal pouch.*
- Discuss normal emotional response to stoma and encourage patient to express feelings *to assist patient in adjusting to change in body.*
- Encourage family members to participate in care *to foster patient's support system.*
- Provide patient with information on local United Ostomy Association *to offer patient and family an opportunity for education and support.*
- Prepare patient to do own stoma and pouch care *to increase independence and enhance self-esteem.*

NURSING DIAGNOSIS **Altered nutrition: less than body requirements** *related to* lack of knowledge of appropriate foods and decreased appetite *as manifested by* weight loss, vitamin and mineral deficiencies, inability to tolerate certain foods.

- Dietary intake to maintain weight at optimum level.

- Assess nutritional intake *to determine need for intervention.*
- Gradually introduce foods one at a time *to identify individual foods that may be problematic* and begin with low-residue diet, *which is usually well-tolerated.*
- Teach patient to chew food slowly and thoroughly *to facilitate digestion and prevent gas.*
- Give list of foods to avoid *so patient has a ready source of referral.*
- Arrange visit with dietician if indicated.

NURSING DIAGNOSIS **Altered sexuality patterns** *related to* perceived loss of sexual appeal and possibility of accidental seepage of fecal material during sexual activity *as manifested by* verbalization of concern about intimate relations with spouse or significant other.

- Confidence in ability to resume previous sexual activity.

- Assess patient's attitude about impact of ostomy on sexual functioning *to determine if a problem exists and if there is a need to plan interventions.*
- Encourage discussion of meaning of sexuality to patient and significant other *to allow patient opportunity to discuss sensitive topic in a nonthreatening situation.*

Continued

40-4   NURSING CARE PLAN   PATIENT WITH A COLOSTOMY/ILEOSTOMY
—continued

| Expected Patient Outcomes | Nursing Interventions and *Rationales* |

NURSING DIAGNOSIS   Altered sexuality patterns —*continued*

- Discuss ways to avoid seepage and conceal stoma and/or pouch during intimate relations *to decrease fear of embarrassment or withdrawal from intimate situations because of anxiety over "accidents."*
- If appropriate, arrange visit with person of same sex and condition *to discuss sexual concerns and share potential solutions, to provide an opportunity to ask questions, and get practical, realistic answers from a supportive, understanding other.*

NURSING DIAGNOSIS   **Risk for fluid volume deficit** *related to* excess fluid loss from ileostomy or diarrhea with a colostomy and inadequate oral intake.

■ Normal serum electrolytes. ■ Normal vital signs. ■ Good skin turgor. ■ Urine output >0.5 ml/kg/hr.	■ Assess for signs of weakness, poor skin turgor, sunken eyes, hypotension, tachycardia, hypokalemia, hyponatremia, oliguria *to determine presence of fluid volume deficit and, if present, plan appropriate interventions.* ■ Record intake and output and include ileostomy drainage *to have an accurate record of fluid balance.* ■ Ensure fluid intake of at least 3000 ml/day in the initial postoperative period *to prevent dehydration.* ■ Instruct patient to maintain high fluid intake and to increase it during hot weather, when patient is perspiring excessively, and during episodes of diarrhea *to ensure adequate fluid intake in various situations.* ■ Monitor serum electrolytes *as inadequate fluid volume will be reflected in changed electrolyte values.* ■ Instruct patient on signs and symptoms of sodium, potassium, and fluid deficits *to ensure early reporting and correction of underlying electrolyte problem.*

The stoma should be pink. A dusky-blue stoma indicates ischemia, and a brown-black stoma indicates necrosis. The nurse should assess and document stoma color every 8 hours. There is mild to moderate swelling of the stoma the first 2 to 3 weeks after surgery (Table 40-33). A skin barrier should be applied to protect the peristomal suture line and skin surrounding the stoma. Solid skin barriers include Stomahesive (Convatec), Coloplast, and Hollister skin barriers. The skin should be washed with warm water and dried thoroughly before the barrier is applied.

With an open-ended, transparent, plastic, odor-proof pouch it is easy to protect the skin and to observe and collect the drainage. The pouch must fit snugly to prevent leakage around the stoma. The size of the stoma is determined with a stoma-measuring card. Although the pouch is applied after surgery, the colostomy functions when peristalsis has been adequately restored. When a temporary colostomy is performed and the stoma is opened in the operating room with no bowel preparation being done previously the stoma functions immediately.

The volume, color, and consistency of the drainage are recorded. Each time the pouch is changed, the condition of the skin is observed for irritation. A pouch should *never* be placed directly on irritated skin without the use of a skin barrier.

A colostomy in the ascending and transverse colon has semi-liquid stools. The patient needs to be instructed to use a drainable pouch. A colostomy in the sigmoid or descending colon has semiformed or formed stools and can sometimes be regulated by the irrigation method. The patient may or may not wear a drainage pouch. A nondrainable pouch should have a gas filter.

For most patients with colostomies, there are few, if any, dietary restrictions. A well-balanced diet and adequate fluid in-

Table **40-33**	**Characteristics of Stoma**
Characteristic	**Description or Cause**
Color*	
Rose to brick red	Viable stoma mucosa
Pale	May indicate anemia
Blanching, dark red to purple	Indicates inadequate blood supply to the stoma or bowel from adhesions, low flow state, or excessive tension on the bowel at the time of construction
Edema†	
Mild to moderate edema	Normal in the initial postoperative period
	Trauma to the stoma
	Any medical condition that results in edema
Moderate to severe edema	Obstruction of the stoma
	Allergic reaction to food
	Gastroenteritis
Bleeding	
Small amount	Oozing from the stoma mucosa when touched is normal because of its high vascularity
Moderate to large amount‡	Moderate to large amount‡ of bleeding from the stoma mucosa could indicate coagulation factor deficiency; stomal varices secondary to portal hypertension
	Moderate to large amount from intestinal stoma opening could indicate lower gastrointestinal bleeding

*Sustained color changes must be reported to surgeon.
†Closely observe and report to the surgeon and adjust the stoma opening size in the pouch.
‡Report moderate to large amounts of bleeding to surgeon.

NUTRITIONAL THERAPY

Table **40-34**	**Effects of Food on Stoma Output**		
Odor Producing*		**Diarrhea Causing***	
Eggs		Alcohol	
Garlic		Beer	
Onions		Cabbage family	
Fish		Spinach	
Asparagus		Green beans	
Cabbage		Coffee	
Broccoli		Spicy foods	
Alcohol		Fruits (raw)	
Gas Forming*		**Potential Obstruction in Ileostomy****	
Beans		Nuts	
Cabbage family		Raisins	
Onions		Popcorn	
Beer		Seeds	
Carbonated beverages		Vegetables (raw)	
Cheeses, strong		Celery	
Sprouts		Corn	

*The effect of food on stoma output is individual. Patients are not discouraged from eating the above listed foods and beverages.
**Patients are encouraged to chew high roughage food well, drink increased fluids, and initially limit the amount.

ment needed. The nurse should encourage the patient to watch the procedure and should explain each step to the patient. The cone tip on the tubing controls the depth of insertion and prevents the water from coming out from the stoma and not going into the colon. If resistance is met, force should not be used because perforation of the intestine can result. However, this is unlikely when using a stoma cone. A hard plastic catheter is not recommended because of the risk of intestinal perforation. The procedure should not be rushed; the patient should feel relaxed. The patient or family member must be instructed in the procedure and must be able to demonstrate the ability to irrigate before being independent. This can be done in the outpatient setting.

The patient should be able to perform skin care, control odor, care for the stoma, and identify signs and symptoms of complications. The patient should know the importance of fluids and food in the diet, have names and addresses of the United Ostomy Association, and know when to seek medical care. Home care and outpatient follow-up by an ET nurse is highly recommended. Patients should be discharged with written pouch change instructions, teaching literature relevant to the type of stoma they have, a list of equipment they use, a list of equipment retailers (including names and phone numbers), outpatient follow-up appointments with the surgeon and ET nurse, and the phone numbers of the surgeon and nurse. The patient and family teaching guidelines are included in Table 40-36.

take is important. The patient's medical and surgical history must be considered when individualizing dietary instructions. Table 40-34 lists foods and their effects on stoma output.

■ Colostomy Irrigations

Colostomy irrigations are intended to regulate bowel function, treat constipation, or prepare the bowel for surgery. When irrigating to achieve a regular bowel pattern, the irrigations stimulate the bowel to function at a specific time every day or every other day. If control is achieved, there should be little or no spillage between irrigations. The patient who establishes regularity may need to wear only a pad or cover over the stoma. The patient who cannot or chooses not to establish regularity by irrigations must wear a pouch at all times. The procedure for colostomy irrigation is presented in Table 40-35.

All equipment should be assembled before the irrigation. A commercially obtained irrigation set usually has all the equip-

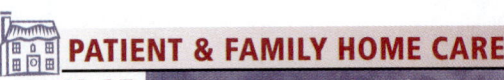

PATIENT & FAMILY HOME CARE GUIDE

Table **40-35** Colostomy Irrigation

Equipment
Lubricant
Irrigation set (1000-2000 ml container, tubing with irrigating cone, clamp)
Irrigating sleeve with adhesive or belt
Toilet tissue to clean around the stoma
Disposal sack for soiled dressing

Procedure
1. Place 500-1000 ml of lukewarm water (not to exceed 105° F) [40.5° C] in container. The volume is titrated for the individual; use enough irrigant to distend the bowel but not enough to cause cramping pain. Most adults use 500-1000 ml of water.
2. Ensure comfortable position. Patient may sit in chair in front of toilet or on the toilet if the perineal wound is healed.
3. Clear tubing of all air by flushing it with fluid.
4. Hang container on hook or IV pole (18-24 in) above stoma (about shoulder height).
5. Apply irrigating sleeve and place bottom end in toilet bowl.
6. Lubricate cone and insert cone tip gently into the stoma and hold tip securely in place.
7. Allow irrigation solution to flow in steadily for 5-10 min.
8. If cramping occurs, stop the flow of solution for a few seconds, leaving the cone in place.
9. Clamp the tubing and remove irrigating cone when the desired amount of irrigant has been delivered or when the patient senses colonic distention.
10. Allow 30-45 minutes for the solution and feces to be expelled. Initial evacuation is usually complete in 10-15 min. Close off the irrigating sleeve at the bottom to allow ambulation.
11. Clean, rinse, and dry peristomal skin well.
12. Replace the colostomy drainage pouch or desired stoma covering.
13. Wash and rinse all equipment and hang to dry.

PATIENT & FAMILY TEACHING GUIDE

Table **40-36** Ostomy Self-Care

The following are guidelines to include for patient and family teaching:
1. Explain the following principles of ostomy and pouch care:
   - Apply and change pouch to collect intestinal drainage.
   - Empty pouch before it is full to prevent leakage.
   - Cleanse skin and use skin barriers and deodorizers to prevent skin breakdown and malodor.
   - Irrigate colostomy to regulate bowel elimination (optional).
   - Explain how to contact enterostomal therapist with questions.
   - Explain how to obtain additional supplies.
2. Instruct the following dietary and fluid intake guidelines:
   - Identify a well-balanced diet and dietary supplements to prevent nutrition deficiencies.
   - Identify foods to avoid to reduce diarrhea, gas, malodor, or obstruction.
   - Drink at least 3000 ml/day of fluid to prevent dehydration (unless contraindicated).
   - Increase fluid intake during hot weather, excessive perspiration, and diarrhea to replace losses and prevent dehydration.
   - Explain how to contact registered dietitian with questions.
3. Describe potential resources to assist with emotional and psychologic adjustment:
   - Identify persons available to provide emotional support.
   - Identify community resources for psychologic counseling.
   - Contact United Ostomy Association for information or peer support.
   - Inform that treatment for potential depression is available if needed.
4. Explain the importance of follow-up care:
   Report signs and symptoms of:
   - Fluid and electrolyte deficits
   - Fever
   - Diarrhea
   - Skin irritation
   - Other stoma problems including inversion, eversion, discoloration, abscess, or infection

Ileostomy Care

Care of the ileostomy is presented in NCP 40-4. An ileostomy stoma protrusion of at least 1 to 1.5 cm makes care easier. When the stoma is flat, seepage occurs resulting in altered skin integrity. Drainage is constant and extremely irritating to the skin. Regularity cannot be established. A pouch must be worn at all times. An open-ended, drainable pouch is worn by the patient so that drainage can be emptied when one-third full. The drainable pouch is usually worn for 4 to 7 days before being changed as long as leakage does not occur around the stoma. If pouch leakage occurs, the pouch should be promptly removed and the skin should be cleansed and a new pouch placed. A solid skin barrier should always be used. A transparent pouch should be used in the initial postoperative period to facilitate assessment of stoma viability.

Immediately after surgery, intake and output must be accurately monitored. The patient should be observed for signs and symptoms of fluid and electrolyte imbalance, particularly potassium, sodium, and fluid deficits. In the first 24 to 48 hours after surgery the amount of drainage from the stoma may be negligible. A person with an ileostomy has lost the absorptive functions provided by the colon, as well as the delay feature provided by the ileocecal valve. Once peristalsis returns, the patient may experience a period of high-volume output of 1000 to 1800 ml per day. Later on, the average amount can be 800 ml daily because the proximal small bowel adapts. If the small bowel has been shortened as a result of surgical resections in Crohn's or other disease, the drainage from the ileostomy may be greater. The patient must understand the importance of fluid and electrolyte balance.

The patient should be instructed to drink at least 2 to 3 L of fluid daily; more may be necessary when diarrhea occurs and in the summer, when perspiration is increased. Diarrhea from an ileostomy produces acidosis from the loss of bicarbonate. The physician may instruct the patient to take an electrolyte solution at home (e.g., 1 teaspoon of salt and 1 teaspoon of baking soda in 1 quart of water). Fluids rich in electrolytes should be encouraged.

Usually a low-roughage diet is ordered initially. Fiber-containing foods are reintroduced gradually. Later there are no dietary restrictions except for foods that are troublesome (e.g., high-roughage popcorn). The goal for the patient is a return to a normal, presurgical diet.

The stoma often bleeds easily when it is touched because it has a high vascular supply. The patient should be told that minimal oozing of blood is normal. If the terminal ileum has been removed, the patient may need cobalamin injections or use intranasal cobalamin.

■ Adaptation to an Ostomy

Adaptation to the ostomy is a gradual process. The patient experiences a grief reaction to the loss of a body part and an alteration in body image. Each person uses different coping mechanisms. The adjustment period for the person depends on the individual. Psychologic support during the grieving process is needed. There are concerns about body image, sexual activity, family responsibilities, and changes in lifestyle. The patient may become resentful and have fears of odor or soiling. Supportive measures by nurses include helping the patient acquire knowledge, providing or recommending support services, and identifying coping mechanisms that are effective. The nurse provides support by responding to the physiologic needs of stoma care and the psychosocial needs of self-esteem.

The patient should not be forced to learn to care for the stoma. The nurse should watch for clues that the patient is ready. Teaching at the appropriate time is an important part of the care and can contribute to a smooth adjustment process.

Activities of daily living are resumed within 6 to 8 weeks. Heavy lifting should be avoided. The patient's physical condition determines when sports may be resumed. Bathing and swimming are not prohibited. Water does not harm the stoma.

A clinical pathway for home care of the patient with an ostomy is provided on p. 1180.

■ Sexual Dysfunction After Ostomy Surgery

Discussion of sexuality and sexual function must be incorporated in the plan of care. The nurse can help the patient understand that sexual function or sexual activity may be affected, but sexuality does not have to be altered.

Pelvic surgery can disrupt nerve and vascular supply to the genitals. Radiation, chemotherapy, and medications can also alter sexual function. Hormones and overall physical health of the patient influence desire. Certain pain medications and antiemetics can lower the sex drive. Generalized fatigue caused by illness can also influence desire. By communicating this information to patients, they can plan sexual activity around a medication schedule and energy levels. Any pelvic surgery that removes the rectum has the potential of damaging the parasympathetic nerve plexus. Erection in men depends on the parasympathetic nerves that control blood flow and vascular supply to the pelvis and the pudendal nerves that transmit sensory responses from the genital area. Nerve-sparing surgical techniques are used when possible to preserve sexual function. Radiation therapy to the pelvis can reduce blood vascularity to the pelvis by causing scarring in the small blood vessels. A woman's sexual functioning after healing includes expansion and lubrication of the vagina. Pelvic surgery usually does not affect a woman's arousal unless part or the entire vagina is removed. Radiation therapy can affect the small blood vessels, which reduces available blood supply and can affect vaginal expansion and lubrication.

Muscular contraction and genital pleasure that occur during orgasm are not disrupted by pelvic surgery. If the sympathetic nerves in the presacral area are damaged, the male mechanism of emission can be disrupted. This can occur in an abdominal-perineal resection. Orgasms can occur in both men and women with stoma surgery, although other aspects of the response cycle may be affected.

The psychologic impact of the stoma and how it affects the patient's body image and self-esteem must be discussed. Emotional factors can contribute to sexual problems. A life-threatening illness can override concerns about sexual function. The nurse can assist a patient to identify ways of coping with depression and anxiety resulting from illness, surgery, or postoperative problems.

The social impact of the stoma is interrelated with the psychologic, physical, and sexual aspects. Concerns of people with stomas include the ability to resume sexual activity, altering clothing styles, the effect on daily activities, sleeping while wearing a pouch, passing gas, the presence of odor, cleanliness, and deciding when or if to tell others about the stoma. The fear of rejection from a partner or the fear that others will not find them desirable as a sexual partner can be a concern. The nurse should encourage open communication about feelings and should realize that the patient needs time to adjust to the pouch and to body changes before feeling secure in his or her sexual functioning.

Although pregnancy is possible, the physician may recommend a limited number of pregnancies on the basis of the patient's physical condition. The person with an ostomy who becomes pregnant should have regular medical care.

CLINICAL PATHWAY   Home Care of Ostomy (attention to colostomy)

ICD-9 Code(s) **V55.3**

Patient Name _____   Pt. ID No. _____   SOC Date _____   Discharge Date _____

Date Noted	Expected Outcomes	Achieved Y	N	Date	Variance Codes	Date Noted	Nursing/Functional Diagnoses	Date Closed
	1. Wound site stabilized with no signs of infection (per agency clinical parameters) by visit no. ____ .						Body image disturbance Outcome(s) no. ____ :	
	2. Patient/caregiver/family demonstrates compliance with ostomy therapeutic care plan, as evidenced by clinical assessment of patient, by visit no. ____ .						Knowledge deficit: self-management, observation skills. Outcome(s) no. ____ :	
	3. Patient demonstrates skills needed to cope with lifestyle adjustment by visit no. ____ .						Skin integrity, impaired Outcome(s) no. ____ :	
	4. Other:						Social interaction, impaired Outcome(s) no. ____ :	
	5. Other:						Other: Outcome(s) no. ____ :	
	6. Other:						Other: Outcome(s) no. ____ :	

Assessments/Instructions/Interventions

	VS No. _	VS No. _	VS No. _	VS No. _	VS No. _	VS No. _	VS No. _	VS No. _	VS No. _	VS No. _
Explain patient rights and responsibilities.										
Assess for home safety management.										
Assess ostomy/wound.										
Assess gastrointestinal status.										
Assess vital signs.										
Assess skin integrity.										
Assess hydration and nutrition status.										
Assess coping skills of patient and caregiver.										
Assess patient/caregiver's willingness and ability to provide home therapeutic regimen.										
Assess patient/caregiver's strengths/weaknesses related to therapeutic regimen.										
Assess patient/caregiver's need for personal care assistance.										
Refer to: Enterostomal nurse for ostomy and wound care.										
Refer to: Dietitian for nutritional assessment (especially if receiving tube feedings).										
Refer to: Social worker for linkage to appropriate community resources.										
Instruct patient/caregiver on home safety.										
Instruct patient/caregiver on use of ostomy supplies and lifestyle adjustment.										

Medical Supplies/Home Medical Equipment Needs
1. Ostomy supplies
2. Wound care supplies
3. Other _____

Variance codes

1. Patient related   Team member signature _____   Initials _____
2. Situation related   Team member signature _____   Initials _____
3. Systems related   Team member signature _____   Initials _____

Case manager name_____

_____
Patient signature
(involved in care planning)

From Marrelli TM, Hilliard LS: *Home care and clinical paths: effective care across the continuum,* St Louis, 1996, Mosby.

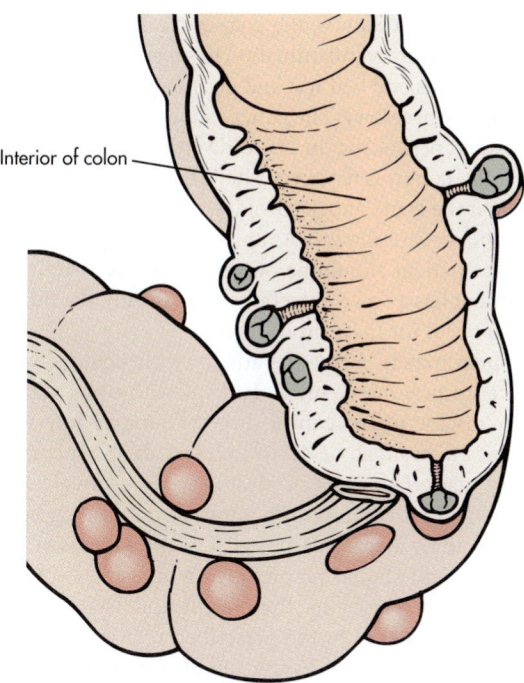

Fig. 40-14   Diverticula are outpouchings of the colon. When they become inflamed, the condition is diverticulitis. The inflammatory process can spread to the surrounding area in the intestine.

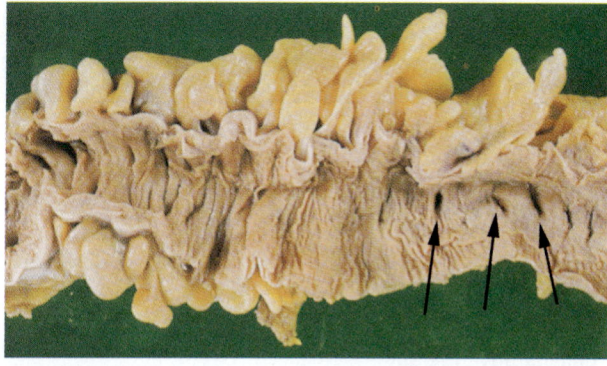

Fig. 40-15   In diverticular disease, the outpouches (arrows) of mucosa appear as slitlike openings from the mucosal surface of the open bowel.

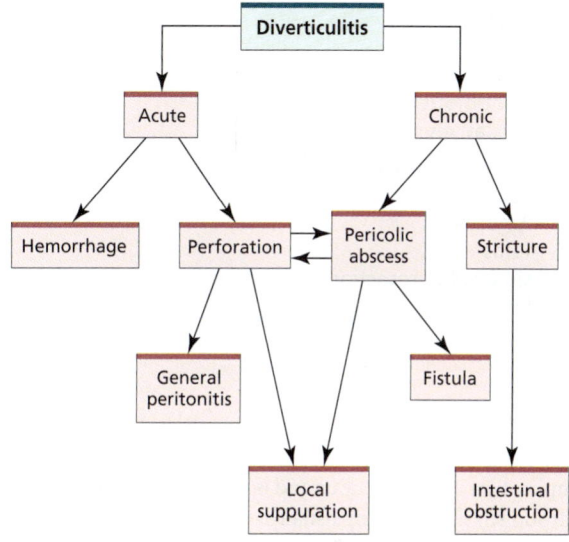

Fig. 40-16   Complications of diverticulitis.

DIVERTICULOSIS AND DIVERTICULITIS

A *diverticulum* is a saccular dilation or outpouching of the mucosa through the circular smooth muscle of the intestinal wall. Clinically, diverticular disease occurs in two forms: diverticulosis and diverticulitis. Multiple noninflamed diverticula are present with diverticulosis. The patient is most often free of symptoms but may have some abdominal discomfort. In diverticulitis, inflammation of the diverticula occurs (Fig. 40-14). Diverticula may occur at any point within the GI tract but are most commonly found in the sigmoid colon.

Etiology and Pathophysiology

Diverticular disease is a common GI disorder that affects 5% of the population by the age of 40 years, and 50% are affected by the age of 80 years.[33] It affects men and women equally, but men seem to have a higher complication rate. Although it affects almost 30 million Americans, most are asymptomatic.

There is no known cause of diverticular disease, but deficiency in dietary fiber has been associated with it. The disease is more prevalent in Western populations that consume diets low in fiber and high in refined carbohydrates, and it is virtually unknown in areas of the world, such as rural Africa, where high-fiber diets are consumed.

When diverticula form, the smooth muscle of the colon wall becomes thickened (Fig. 40-15). Lack of dietary fiber slows transit time and more water is absorbed from the stool, making it more difficult to pass through the lumen. Decreased bulk of the stool, combined with a more narrowed lumen in the sigmoid colon, causes high intraluminal pressures. These factors are believed to contribute to the formation of diverticula.

The cause of diverticulitis is related to the retention of stool and bacteria in the diverticulum, forming a hardened mass called a *fecalith*. This causes inflammation and usually small perforations. Inflammation of the diverticulum spreads to the surrounding area in the intestines (Fig. 40-16), causing the tissue to become edematous. Abscesses may form, or complete perforation with peritonitis may occur.

Clinical Manifestations

The majority of patients with diverticulosis have no symptoms. Those with symptoms typically have crampy abdominal pain located in the left lower quadrant that is usually relieved by passage of flatus or bowel movement. Alternating constipation and diarrhea may be present.

Approximately 15% of patients with diverticulosis progress to acute diverticulitis. In patients with diverticulitis, abdominal pain is localized over the involved area of the colon. A tender, left lower quadrant mass may be felt on palpation of the abdomen. Fever, chills, nausea, anorexia, and leukocytosis may be present. Elderly patients with diverticulitis are frequently afebrile, with a normal WBC, and little, if any, abdominal tenderness.

Complications of diverticulitis include perforation with peritonitis, abscess and fistula formation, bowel obstruction, ureteral obstruction, and bleeding. Bleeding is a common

COLLABORATIVE CARE

Table 40-37   Diverticulosis and Diverticulitis

Diagnostic
- Stool for occult blood
- Barium enema
- Sigmoidoscopy
- Colonoscopy
- CBC
- Urinalysis
- Blood culture

Collaborative Therapy

Ambulatory and Home Care
- High-residue diet
- Dietary fiber supplements
- Stool softeners
- Anticholinergics
- Mineral oil
- Bed rest
- Clear liquid diet
- Oral antibiotics
- Bulk laxatives

Acute Care: Diverticulitis
- Antibiotics
- NPO status
- IV fluids
- Possible colon resection for obstruction or hemorrhage
- Bed rest
- NG suction

complication of diverticulitis and is manifested by *hematochezia* (maroon stools). Bleeding usually stops spontaneously.

Diagnostic Studies

A barium enema is typically used to diagnose diverticular disease. A CBC, urinalysis, and fecal occult blood test should be performed (Table 40-37). A colonoscopy should be performed on patients with symptoms to rule out possible hidden polyps or lesions. A patient with acute diverticulitis should not have a barium enema or colonoscopy because of the possibility of perforation and peritonitis.

NURSING AND COLLABORATIVE MANAGEMENT: DIVERTICULOSIS AND DIVERTICULITIS

Uncomplicated diverticular disease is treated with a high-fiber diet (see Table 40-9) and bulk laxatives, such as psyllium hydrophilic mucilloid (Metamucil). Anticholinergic drugs such as dicyclomine (Bentyl) and Donnatal may be used to relieve discomfort from spasm of the bowel (see Table 40-37).

Fluids should be increased because fibers retain water, thus decreasing the amount absorbed by the body. If the patient is obese, a reduction in weight is needed. Increased intraabdominal pressure should be avoided because it may precipitate an attack. Factors that increase intraabdominal pressure are straining at stool, vomiting, bending, lifting, and tight, restrictive clothing.

In acute diverticulitis, the goal of treatment is to allow the colon to rest and the inflammation to subside. The patient is kept on NPO status and bed rest and given parenteral fluids. An NG tube may be necessary. The patient should be observed for signs of possible peritonitis. In acute diverticulitis, broad-spectrum antibiotic therapy is required. The WBC count is monitored.

When the acute attack subsides, oral fluids progressing to a semisolid diet are allowed. Ambulation is also permitted. At this stage the patient should be observed for a recurrent attack. If the patient has a bowel resection or colostomy, the nursing care is the same as for these procedures.

Approximately 30% of patients with acute diverticulitis require surgical intervention. Patients with complicated diverticular disease often require surgery. Surgical intervention is necessary to drain abscesses or to resect an obstructing inflammatory mass. The usual surgical procedures involve resection of the involved colon with a temporary diverting colostomy. The colostomy is reanastomosed after the colon is healed.

The patient should be provided with a full explanation of the condition. The better the patient understands the disease process and adheres to the prescribed regimen, the less likely the exacerbation of the disease and the onset of complications.

HERNIAS

A hernia is a protrusion of a viscus through an abnormal opening or a weakened area in the wall of the cavity in which it is normally contained. A hernia may occur in any part of the body, but it usually occurs within the abdominal cavity. If the hernia can be placed back into the abdominal cavity, it is known as *reducible*. The hernia can be reduced by manipulation, or it can occur without manipulation when the person lies down. If the hernia cannot be placed back into the abdominal cavity, it is known as *irreducible,* or *incarcerated.* In this situation the intestinal flow may be obstructed. When the hernia is irreducible and the intestinal flow and blood supply are obstructed, the hernia is *strangulated.* The result is an acute intestinal obstruction.

Types

The *inguinal* hernia is the most common type of hernia and occurs at the point of weakness in the abdominal wall where the spermatic cord in men and the round ligament in women emerge (Fig. 40-17). When the protrusion escapes through the inguinal ring and follows the spermatic cord or the round ligament, it is termed an *indirect* hernia. When it escapes through the posterior inguinal wall, it is a *direct* hernia. An inguinal hernia is more frequent in men.

A *femoral* hernia occurs when there is a protrusion through the femoral ring into the femoral canal. It occurs below the inguinal (Poupart's) ligament as a bulge. It becomes strangulated easily and occurs more frequently in women. The *umbilical* hernia occurs when the rectus muscle is weak or the umbilical opening fails to close after birth. This type is found most commonly in children.

Ventral, or *incisional,* hernia is due to weakness of the abdominal wall at the site of a previous incision. It is found most commonly in patients who are obese, who have had multiple surgical procedures in the same area, and who have had inadequate wound healing because of poor nutrition or infection.

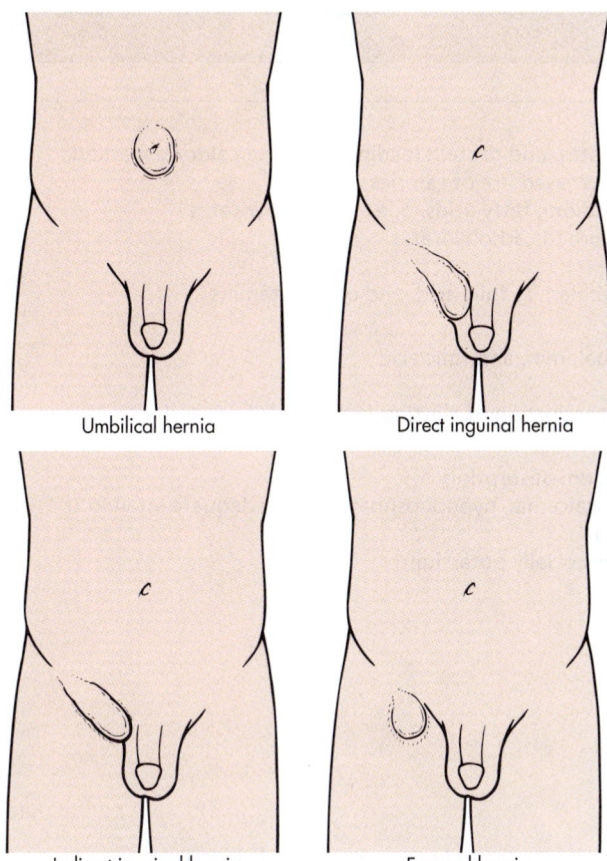

Fig. 40-17   Types of hernias.

Table **40-38**	**Common Causes of Malabsorption**

Biochemical or Enzyme Deficiencies
Lactase deficiency
Biliary tract obstruction
Pancreatic insufficiency
   Cystic fibrosis
   Chronic pancreatitis
   Zollinger-Ellison syndrome

Bacterial Proliferation
Tropical sprue
Parasitic infection

Small Intestinal Mucosal Disruption
Celiac disease
Whipple's disease
Crohn's disease

Disturbed Lymphatic and Vascular Circulation
Lymphoma
Ischemia
Lymphangiectasia
Heart failure

Surface Area Loss
Billroth II gastrectomy
Short bowel syndrome
Distal ileal resection, disease, or bypass

Clinical Manifestations

A hernia commonly occurs over the involved area when the patient stands or strains. There may be some discomfort as a result of tension. Severe pain is caused if the hernia becomes strangulated. In this situation the clinical manifestations of a bowel obstruction, such as vomiting, crampy abdominal pain, and distention, are found.

NURSING MANAGEMENT: HERNIAS

Diagnosis is based on history and physical examination findings. Surgery is the treatment of choice for hernias to prevent the possible complication of strangulation. An umbilical hernia is not usually repaired surgically because it may reduce itself if left alone until the child gets older. The surgical repair of a hernia is known as a *herniorrhaphy*. The reinforcement of the weakened area with wire, fascia, or mesh is known as a *hernioplasty*. When there is strangulation, necrosis and gangrene may develop if immediate care is not given. A bowel resection of the involved area or a temporary colostomy may be needed to treat a strangulated hernia.

Some patients with hernias wear a *truss,* a pad placed over the hernia and held in place with a belt. The truss is worn to keep the hernia from protruding. If a patient wears a truss, the nurse should check for skin irritation caused by the continual rubbing of the truss.

After a hernia repair, the patient may have difficulty voiding. Therefore the nurse should observe for a distended bladder. An accurate intake and output record is important. Scrotal edema is a painful complication after an inguinal hernia repair. A scrotal support with application of an ice bag may help relieve pain and edema. Coughing is not encouraged, but deep breathing and turning should be done. If the patient needs to cough or sneeze, the incision should be splinted during coughing, and sneezing should be done with the mouth open.

After discharge the patient may be restricted from heavy lifting for 6 to 8 weeks. Some surgeons do not put any limitations on physical activities.

MALABSORPTION SYNDROME

Malabsorption results from impaired absorption of fats, carbohydrates, proteins, minerals, and vitamins. The stomach, small intestine, liver, and pancreas regulate normal digestion and absorption. Digestive enzymes ordinarily break down nutrients so that absorption can take place through the intestinal mucosa and nutrients can get into the bloodstream. If there is an interruption in this process at any point, malabsorption may occur. Several problems can cause malabsorption (Table 40-38). They can be classified into malabsorptions caused by (1) biochemical or enzyme deficiencies, (2) bacterial proliferation, (3) disruption of small intestine mucosa, (4) disturbed lymphatic and vascular circulation, or (5) surface area loss. Lactose intolerance is the most common malabsorption disorder, followed by inflammatory bowel disease, nontropical (celiac) and tropical sprue, and cystic fibrosis.

Table 40-39　Clinical Manifestations of Malabsorption

Manifestations	Pathophysiology
Gastrointestinal	
Weight loss	Malabsorption of fat, carbohydrates, and protein leading to loss of calories; marked reduction in caloric intake or increased use of calories
Diarrhea	Impaired absorption of water, sodium, fatty acids, bile, or carbohydrates
Flatulence	Bacterial fermentation of unabsorbed carbohydrates
Steatorrhea	Undigested and unabsorbed fat
Glossitis, cheilosis, stomatitis	Deficiency of iron, riboflavin, cobalamin, folic acid, and other vitamins
Hematologic	
Anemia	Impaired absorption of iron, cobalamin, and folic acid
Hemorrhagic tendency	Vitamin C deficiency
	Vitamin K deficiency inhibiting production of clotting factors II, VII, IX, and X
Musculoskeletal	
Bone pain	Osteoporosis from impaired calcium absorption
	Osteomalacia secondary to hypocalcemia, hypophosphatemia, inadequate vitamin D
Tetany	Hypocalcemia, hypomagnesemia
Weakness, muscle cramps	Anemia, electrolyte depletion (especially potassium)
Muscle wasting	Protein malabsorption
Neurologic	
Altered mental status	Dehydration
Paresthesias	Cobalamin deficiency
Peripheral neuropathy	Cobalamin deficiency
Night blindness	Thiamine deficiency
	Vitamin A deficiency
Integumentary	
Bruising	Vitamin K deficiency
Dermatitis	Fatty acid deficiency, zinc deficiency, niacin and other vitamin deficiencies
Brittle nails	Iron deficiency
Hair thinning and loss	Protein deficiency
Cardiovascular	
Hypotension	Dehydration
Tachycardia	Hypovolemia, anemia
Peripheral edema	Protein malabsorption, protein loss in diarrhea

The most common clinical manifestation of malabsorption is *steatorrhea* (fatty stools). Bulky, foul-smelling stools that float in water and are difficult to flush are characteristic of steatorrhea (Table 40-39). However, steatorrhea does not occur with lactose intolerance.

Screening tests available for malabsorption include qualitative examination of stool for fat (Sudan stain), a 72-hour stool collection for quantitative measurement of fecal fat, and the d-xylose absorption-excretion test, which is a good screening test for carbohydrate absorption (see Table 37-11). Other diagnostic studies include three different kinds of breath tests: (1) the bile acid breath test, which is used to evaluate bile salt malabsorption or malabsorption from bacterial overgrowth; (2) the triolein breath test, which measures carbon dioxide excretion after ingestion of a radioactive triglyceride; and (3) the excretion of breath hydrogen after ingestion of lactose, which is a sensitive, specific, and noninvasive test for detection of lactase deficiency. The rationale for the hydrogen breath test is that bacterial metabolism is the only source of hydrogen production in humans, and most of this occurs in the colon.

A pancreatic secretion test using secretion may be performed to rule out pancreatic insufficiency. Endoscopy may be used to obtain a small bowel biopsy specimen for diagnosis. Radiographic studies of the esophagus, stomach, and small intestine may be indicated. A small bowel barium enema is frequently performed to identify abnormal mucosal patterns.

Laboratory studies that are frequently ordered include a CBC, determination of prothrombin time, serum vitamin A and carotene levels, serum electrolytes, cholesterol, and calcium.

SPRUE

Two closely related malabsorption conditions are *nontropical sprue* and *tropical sprue*. Tropical and nontropical sprue are found in adults. Nontropical sprue is most commonly referred to as *celiac sprue* (especially in children) but is also called *adult celiac disease* and *gluten-induced enteropathy.*

Etiology and Pathophysiology

In celiac disease there is marked atrophy and flattening of the villi. As a result, absorption within the small intestine is reduced. The proposed reason for the injury to the villi is a hypersensitivity response initiated by gluten and gliadin (a breakdown product of gluten). Gluten is a protein found in wheat, rye, barley, and oats. The hypersensitivity leads to an inflammatory response of the mucosa.

Tropical sprue is a chronic disorder acquired in endemic tropical areas. The exact cause is unknown, but the disorder has been linked to an infectious agent. Folate deficiency is also believed to play a role in the development of this disease. Clinically, it resembles nontropical sprue.

Clinical Manifestations

A patient may become symptomatic at any age with celiac sprue, but the incidence peaks in childhood when gluten is first introduced and then during the fourth and fifth decades.[34] Symptoms include steatorrhea (bulky, foul-smelling, yellow-gray, greasy stools with puttylike consistency), diarrhea, weight loss, abdominal distention, and excessive flatulence. There may also be signs of multiple vitamin deficiencies (e.g., glossitis, cheilosis).

Diagnostic Studies and Collaborative Care

Diagnosis of sprue may be made by stool content analyses or intestinal biopsy. Barium enema may demonstrate abnormalities, including obliteration of intestinal folds. Treatment of sprue syndrome is based on the underlying cause. In nontropical sprue, a gluten-free diet usually leads to clinical recovery. Wheat, barley, oats, and rye products should be avoided. Soybean flours may be used. Foods must be scrutinized for the gluten content. Additives such as hydrolyzed vegetable proteins are often derived from cereal grains, including wheat. For those patients who are unresponsive to dietary exclusion therapy (gluten-free diet), corticosteroids may be used to treat nontropical sprue. The basis for this treatment is that the inflammatory response is mediated by an immunologic response.

Tropical sprue is treated with broad-spectrum antibiotics (e.g., tetracycline) in conjunction with folic acid therapy. The patient who responds to this therapy and achieves a remission is usually maintained on folic acid.

LACTASE DEFICIENCY

Lactase deficiency is a condition in which the lactase enzyme is deficient or absent. Lactase is the enzyme that breaks down lactose into two simple sugars—glucose and galactose. Although primary lactase deficiency seems to be hereditary, milk intolerance may not become clinically evident until late adolescence or early adulthood. About 5% of the adult population have primary lactase deficiency. The highest incidence is found in African-Americans, Native-Americans, Mexican-Americans, and persons of Jewish descent. Acquired lactase deficiency is often seen in other GI diseases in which the mucosa has been damaged, including ulcerative colitis, Crohn's disease, gastroenteritis, and sprue syndrome.

Clinical Manifestations

The symptoms of lactose intolerance include bloating, flatulence, crampy abdominal pain, and diarrhea. They may occur within one half hour to several hours after drinking a glass of milk or ingesting a milk product. The diarrhea of lactose intolerance results from fluid secretion into the small intestines, responding to the osmotic action of undigested lactose.

NURSING AND COLLABORATIVE MANAGEMENT: LACTASE DEFICIENCY

Many lactose-intolerant persons are aware of their milk intolerance and avoid milk. A lactose intolerance test can be performed to rule out milk allergies. The patient is given 50 g of lactose orally. Blood samples are drawn before the consumption of lactose and at 15-, 30-, 60-, and 90-minute intervals. Failure of the blood glucose level to increase more than 20 mg/dl is suggestive of lactase deficiency. Results of the hydrogen breath test after ingestion of lactose are abnormal.

Treatment consists of eliminating lactose from the diet by avoiding milk and milk products. A lactose-free diet is given initially and is gradually advanced to a low-lactose diet as tolerated by the patient. The objective of care is to teach the importance of adherence to the diet. Many lactose-intolerant persons may not exhibit symptoms if lactose is taken in small amounts. In some persons, lactose may be tolerated better if taken with meals.

The patient needs to be aware that milk, ice cream, cottage cheese, and cheese have a high lactose content. If the milk has been fermented (e.g., cultured buttermilk, yogurt, sour cream), the patient with low lactase levels may tolerate it better.

Lactase enzyme (Lactaid) is available commercially as an over-the-counter (OTC) product. It is mixed with milk and breaks down the lactose before the milk is ingested.

SHORT BOWEL SYNDROME

Short bowel syndrome (SBS) results from extensive resection of the small intestine. Rapid intestinal transit, impaired digestive and absorption processes, and fluid and electrolyte losses characterize the syndrome. In adults, resection of the small intestine may be necessary for bowel infarction because of vascular thrombosis or insufficiency, abdominal trauma, cancer, radiation enteritis, or Crohn's disease.

The amount and portions of small bowel resected are associated with the number and severity of symptoms. Resections of up to 50% of the small intestine cause little disturbance of bowel function, especially if the terminal ileum and ileocecal valve remain intact. After large resections, the remaining intestine undergoes adaptive changes that are more pronounced in the ileum. The villi and crypts increase in size, and absorptive capacity of the remaining intestine increases. Intestinal adaptation is enhanced by the presence of food, fiber, bile, and pancreatic secretions in the lumen and continues for up to 2 years. Resection of the ileum, ileocecal valve, or colon results in a rapid intestinal transit, decreasing absorption time. Ileal resection causes malabsorption of cobalamin, bile salts, and fat, resulting in steatorrhea.

Clinical Manifestations

The predominant manifestations of SBS are diarrhea or steatorrhea.[35] There may be signs of malnutrition and multiple vitamin and mineral deficiencies (e.g., weight loss, cobalamin, and zinc deficiency, hypocalcemia). The patient may develop lactase deficiency and bacterial overgrowth. Oxalate kidney stones may form from increased colonic absorption of oxalate.

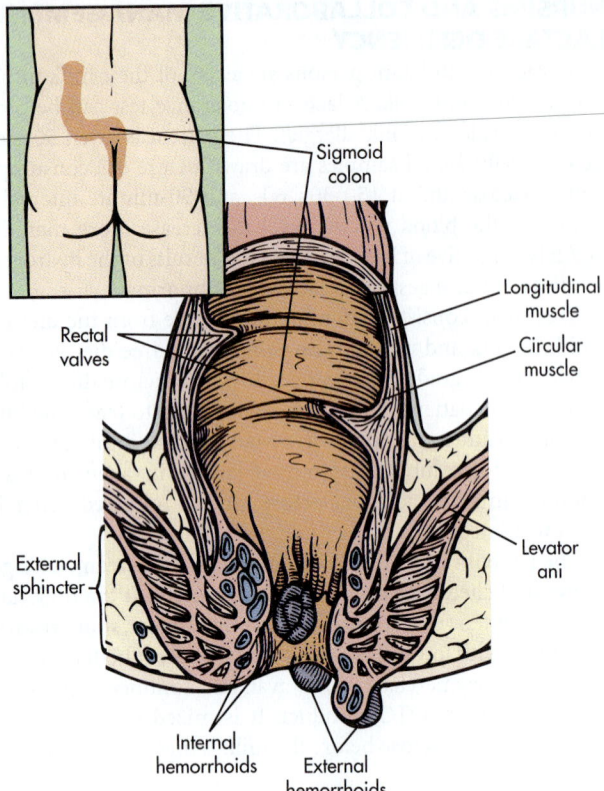

Sigmoid colon

Longitudinal muscle

Circular muscle

Rectal valves

Levator ani

External sphincter

Internal hemorrhoids

External hemorrhoids

Fig. 40-18 Anatomic structures of the rectum and anus with external and internal hemorrhoids.

Collaborative Care

The overall goals are that the patient with SBS will have fluid and electrolyte balance, normal nutritional status, and control of diarrhea. In the period immediately following massive bowel resection, patients receive total parenteral nutrition to replace fluid, electrolyte, and nutrient losses and to rest the bowel. Hypersecretion of gastric acid, whose cause is unknown, is reduced by H_2-receptor antagonists (e.g., cimetidine [Tagamet]).

A diet high in carbohydrate and low in fat is recommended. A high-carbohydrate, low-fat diet supplemented with soluble fiber, pectin, the amino acid glutamine, and parenteral growth hormone improved nutrient absorption, decreased stool output, and enabled patients to wean off parenteral nutrition.[35] The patient with SBS is encouraged to eat at least six meals per day to increase the time of contact between food and the intestine. Oral intake can be supplemented with elemental nutrient formulas and tube feeding during the night. For patients with severe malabsorption, total parenteral nutrition may be reinstituted. Intestinal transplantation is an experimental procedure primarily used for patients with severe SBS complicated by liver failure.[36]

Narcotic antidiarrheal drugs are the most effective in decreasing intestinal motility (see Table 40-3). For patients with limited ileal resections (<100 cm), cholestyramine (Questran) reduces diarrhea resulting from unabsorbed bile acids and increasing their excretion in feces. Bile acids stimulate intestinal fluid secretion and reduce colonic fluid absorption.

ANORECTAL PROBLEMS

HEMORRHOIDS

Hemorrhoids are dilated hemorrhoidal veins. They may be *internal* (occurring above the internal sphincter) or *external* (occurring outside the external sphincter) (Fig. 40-18). Symptoms of hemorrhoids, including bleeding, pruritus, prolapse, and pain, are common in all age groups. In affected persons, hemorrhoids appear periodically, depending on amount of anorectal pressure.

Etiology and Pathophysiology

Hemorrhoids develop when the flow of blood through the veins of the hemorrhoidal plexus is impaired. Internal hemorrhoids may become constricted and painful. They are the most common cause of bleeding with defecation. The amount of blood lost at one time may be small but may lead to iron deficiency anemia over time. External hemorrhoids are reddish blue and seldom bleed or cause pain unless a vein ruptures. If the blood clots in external hemorrhoids, they become inflamed, painful, and are said to be *thrombosed.*

Hemorrhoids may be caused by many factors, including pregnancy, prolonged constipation, straining in an effort to defecate, heavy lifting, prolonged standing and sitting, and portal hypertension (as found in cirrhosis).

Collaborative Care

Hemorrhoids are diagnosed by inspection, digital examination, proctoscopy, or examination with the flexible sigmoidoscope. Therapy should be directed toward the causes and the patient's symptoms. A high-fiber diet and increased fluid intake prevents constipation and reduces straining, which allows engorgement of the veins to subside. Ointments such as Nupercaine; creams, suppositories, and impregnated pads that contain antiinflammatory agents (e.g., hydrocortisone); or astringents and anesthetics (e.g., witch hazel, pramoxine, and benzocaine) may be used to shrink the mucous membranes and relieve discomfort. Stool softeners may be ordered to keep the stools soft, and sitz baths may be ordered to relieve pain.

Application of ice packs for a few hours, followed by warm packs, may be used for thrombosed hemorrhoids. Another conservative treatment involves use of a sclerosing solution, such as 5% phenol in oil, or a combined solution of quinine and urea may be injected into the submucous tissue surrounding the hemorrhoids, causing a fibrosing and shrinking of the supporting tissues.

Internal hemorrhoids may be ligated with a rubber band. The constrictive effect impairs circulation, and the tissue becomes necrotic, separates, and sloughs off. There is some local discomfort with this procedure, but no anesthetic is required. Aspirin or propoxyphene (Darvon) is usually given for discomfort. Anal dilation and lateral sphincterotomy may be performed to reduce vascular engorgement by reducing sphincter pressure. Other methods, such as infrared photocoagulation, bipolar diathermy, and cryotherapy, are used to treat the mucosa.

A *hemorrhoidectomy* is the surgical excision of hemorrhoids. Surgery is indicated when there is prolapse, excessive pain or bleeding, or large hemorrhoids. In general, hemorrhoidectomy is reserved for patients with severe symptoms related to multiple thrombosed hemorrhoids or marked protrusion. Surgical removal may be done by cautery, clamp, or excision. One surgical approach is to leave the area open so that healing takes place by secondary intention. In another approach the hemorrhoids are removed, the tissue is sutured, and healing takes place by primary-intention wound healing.

NURSING MANAGEMENT: HEMORRHOIDS

Conservative nursing management for the patient with hemorrhoids includes teaching measures to prevent constipation, avoidance of prolonged standing or sitting, proper use of OTC medications available for hemorrhoidal symptoms, and the need to seek medical care for severe symptoms of hemorrhoids (e.g., excessive pain and bleeding, prolapsed hemorrhoids) when necessary.

Pain is a common problem after a hemorrhoidectomy. The nurse must be aware that although the procedure is minor the pain is severe, and narcotics are usually given initially.

Sitz baths are started 1 to 2 days after surgery. A warm sitz bath provides comfort and keeps the anal area clean. A sponge ring in the sitz bath helps relieve pressure on the area. Initially the patient should not be left alone because of the possibility of weakness or fainting.

Packing may be inserted into the rectum to absorb drainage. A T-binder may hold the dressing in place. If packing is inserted, it usually is removed the first or second postoperative day. The nurse should assess for rectal bleeding. The patient may be embarrassed when the dressing is changed, and privacy should be provided. The patient usually dreads the first bowel movement and often resists the urge to defecate. Pain medication may be given before the bowel movement to reduce discomfort.

A stool softener such as docusate (Colace) is usually ordered the first few postoperative days. If the patient does not have a bowel movement within 2 to 3 days, an oil retention enema is given.

Discharge teaching includes the importance of the diet, care of the anal area, symptoms of complications (especially bleeding), and avoidance of constipation and straining. Sitz baths are recommended for 1 to 2 weeks. The physician may order a stool softener to be taken for a time. Hemorrhoids may recur. Occasionally anal strictures develop and dilation is necessary. Regular checkups are important in the prevention of any further problems.

ANAL FISSURE

An *anal fissure* (*fissura in ano*) is a skin ulcer or a crack in the lining of the anal wall that is caused by trauma or local infection. It is frequently associated with constipation and subsequent stretching of the anus from hard feces. The most common clinical manifestations are painful spasms of the anal sphincter and severe, burning pain during defecation. Some bleeding may occur, and constipation results because of fear of pain associated with bowel movements.

Conservative treatment consists of bowel regulation with mineral oil and stool softeners. Sitz baths and anal anesthetic

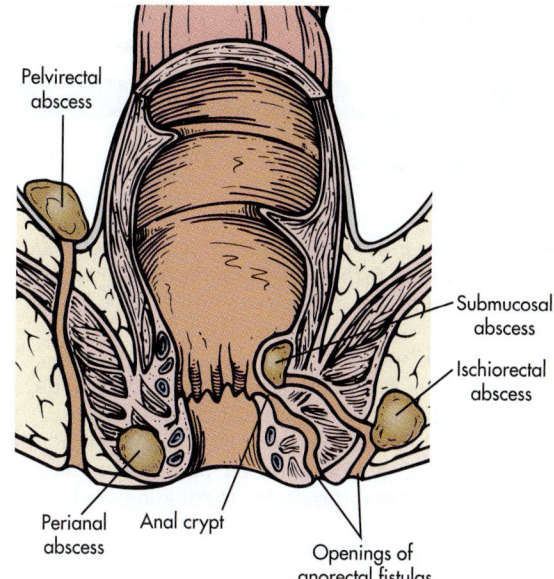

Pelvirectal abscess

Submucosal abscess

Ischiorectal abscess

Perianal abscess   Anal crypt

Openings of anorectal fistulas

Fig. 40-19 Common sites of anorectal abscesses and fistula formation.

suppositories (Anusol) are also ordered. Surgical treatment usually consists of excision of the fissure. Postoperative nursing care is the same as the care for the patient who has had a hemorrhoidectomy.

ANORECTAL ABSCESS

Anorectal abscesses are defined as undrained collections of perianal pus (Fig. 40-19). They are due to perirectal infections in patients who have compromised local circulation or active inflammatory disease. The most common causative organisms are *Escherichia coli*, staphylococci, and streptococci. Clinical manifestations include local pain and swelling, foul-smelling drainage, tenderness, and elevated temperature. Sepsis can occur as a complication.

Surgical therapy consists of drainage of abscesses. If packing is used, it should be impregnated with petroleum jelly and the area should be allowed to heal by granulation. The packing is changed every day, and moist, hot compresses are applied to the area. Care must be taken to avoid soiling the dressing during urination or defecation. A low-residue diet is given. The patient may leave the hospital with the area open. Discharge teaching should include wound care, the importance of sitz baths, thorough cleaning after bowel movements, and follow-up visits to the physician.

ANORECTAL FISTULA

An anal fistula is an abnormal tunnel leading out from the anus or rectum. It may extend to the outside of the skin, vagina, or buttocks. Anorectal fistulas are a complication of Crohn's disease. This condition often precedes an anorectal abscess.

Feces may enter the fistula and cause an infection. There may be persistent, bloodstained, purulent discharge or stool leakage from the fistula. The patient may have to wear a pad to prevent staining of clothes.

CRITICAL THINKING EXERCISES

CASE STUDY

Ulcerative Colitis

Patient Profile

Marie, a 37-year-old mother to two school-aged children, is admitted for the fifth time in 11 months with acute ulcerative colitis.

Subjective Data

- Complains of severe diarrhea (10 to 15 stools a day with blood and mucous) and intestinal cramping.
- States she has lost 8 lb (3.6 kg) in the past 11 months.
- Complains of fatigue, anorexia, nausea, vomiting.
- States she takes sulfasalazine (Azulfidine) and prednisone.
- Has not taken any medication in past 72 hours because of nausea and vomiting.
- Tearfully states she is "tired of this disease interfering with her life."

Objective Data

Physical Examination
- Temperature of 100.4°F (38°C)
- Heart rate of 110 beats per minute; BP of 115/70 mm Hg
- Weight 109 lb (50 kg)
- Palpation over the colon reveals abdominal tenderness.

Laboratory Tests
Hct 26%
Hb 9 g/dl (90 g/L)
Serum albumin 2.3 g/dl (23 g/L)

Critical Thinking Questions

1. How do the pathophysiologic changes of ulcerative colitis differ from those of Crohn's disease?
2. Explain the reason for Marie's anemia and low serum albumin.
3. What is the significance of Marie's tachycardia?
4. What nursing interventions are indicated for Marie at this stage of her illness?
5. Explain the actions of sulfasalazine and prednisone in treating ulcerative colitis.
6. What are complications of ulcerative colitis and the role of the nurse in preventing their occurrence?
7. Based on the assessment data, write one or more nursing diagnoses. Are there any collaborative problems?

NURSING RESEARCH ISSUES

1. What are the primary problems related to sexuality and sexual function in patients with an ostomy?
2. Are the psychologic responses and coping strategies of younger patients "receiving" an ostomy different from those of older patients?
3. What can a nurse do to help improve the self-image of patients with ostomies?
4. Do psychosocial factors have a significant role in the exacerbation of IBD?
5. Do nonpharmacologic, complementary therapies alleviate the symptoms of a patient with IBS?
6. Which sources of dietary fiber are most effective in treating fecal incontinence and IBS?
7. Which strategies can increase screening behaviors for colorectal cancer, especially among minority groups?
8. How can a nurse facilitate self-care among older adults with chronic IBD?

Surgical therapy involves a fistulotomy or a fistulectomy. In a fistulotomy the fistula is opened and healthy tissue is allowed to granulate. A fistulectomy is an excision of the entire fistulous tract. Gauze packing is inserted and the wound is allowed to heal by granulation. Care is the same as after a hemorrhoidectomy.

PILONIDAL SINUS

A *pilonidal sinus* is a small tract under the skin between the buttocks in the sacrococcygeal area. It is thought to be of congenital origin. It may have several openings and is lined with epithelium and hair, thus the name pilonidal ("a nest of hair").

The skin is moist, and movement of the buttocks causes the short, wiry hair to penetrate the skin. The irritated skin becomes infected and forms a pilonidal cyst or abscess. There are no symptoms unless there is an infection. If it becomes infected, the patient complains of pain and swelling at the base of the spine.

The formed abscess requires incision and drainage. The wound may be closed or left open to heal by secondary intention. The wound is packed and sitz baths are ordered.

Nursing care includes hot, moist heat applications when an abscess is present. The patient is usually more comfortable lying on the abdomen or side. The patient should be instructed to avoid contaminating the dressing when urinating or defecating and to avoid straining whenever possible.

REVIEW QUESTIONS

The number of the question corresponds to the same-numbered objective at the beginning of the chapter.

1. Common treatment measures for the patient with constipation include
   a. enemas and high fluid intake.
   b. anticholinergic drugs and low fiber diet.
   c. antiemetics and high fluid intake.
   d. stool softeners and high fiber diet.
2. In teaching the patient with chronic constipation, the nurse instructs the patient to
   a. drink at least 3 quarts of liquids daily.
   b. avoid intake of insoluble fiber to prevent gas production.
   c. use laxatives until the bowel establishes a regular emptying pattern.
   d. schedule enemas three to four times a week to completely empty the large bowel.

3. During the first 12 hours following an exploratory laparotomy for an acute abdomen the nurse anticipates that drainage from the NG tube will be
   a. yellowish in color.
   b. clear gastric secretion.
   c. dark brown to dark red.
   d. bright red with blood clots.

4. The nurse notifies the physician, suspecting a possible ruptured appendix when the patient has
   a. a low-grade fever with a leukocytosis.
   b. a distended, rigid abdomen and muscle spasms.
   c. right lower quadrant pain on palpation of the left lower quadrant.
   d. localized abdominal pain halfway between the umbilicus and the right iliac crest.

5. A patient is admitted to the emergency department with right lower abdominal pain of 6 hours duration. During the examination of the patient to establish a diagnosis the nurse would expect medical orders to include
   a. application of a heating pad to relax the abdominal muscles.
   b. obtaining a urine specimen to rule out genitourinary conditions.
   c. encouraging oral fluids to prevent dehydration and hypovolemia.
   d. administration of cleansing enemas in preparation for colonoscopy.

6. On assessment of the patient with gastroenteritis the nurse would expect to find
   a. fever, diarrhea, and leukopenia.
   b. anorexia, pain, and constipation.
   c. vomiting, fever, and constipation.
   d. abdominal cramps, nausea, and vomiting.

7. In planning care for the patient with ulcerative colitis the nurse recognizes that a major difference between ulcerative colitis and Crohn's disease is that ulcerative colitis
   a. causes more nutritional deficiencies than does Crohn's disease.
   b. causes more abdominal pain and cramping than does Crohn's disease.
   c. is curable with a colectomy while Crohn's disease often recurs after surgery.
   d. is more highly associated with a familial relationship than is Crohn's disease.

8. The nurse performs a detailed assessment of the abdomen of a patient with a possible bowel obstruction knowing that a manifestation of an obstruction high in the small intestine is
   a. orange-brown, feculent vomitus.
   b. widespread abdominal distention.
   c. persistent, colicky abdominal pain.
   d. projectile vomiting that relieves abdominal pain.

9. A patient with cancer of the rectum is scheduled for an abdominal-perineal resection. Preoperatively the nurse teaches the patient that postoperative measures will include
   a. positioning from side-to-side to prevent perineal pressure.
   b. care of an abdominal ileostomy site that drains fecal material.
   c. administration of medicated enemas to prevent anal infections.
   d. maintenance of portable suctions draining the abdominal incision.

10. The nurse explains to the patient undergoing ostomy surgery that the procedure that maintains the most normal functioning of the bowel is
    a. a sigmoid colostomy.
    b. a transverse colostomy.
    c. a descending colostomy.
    d. an ascending colostomy.

11. The use of nonabsorbable antibiotics as preparation for bowel surgery is done primarily to
    a. reduce the bacterial flora in the colon.
    b. prevent additional formation of ammonia.
    c. prevent postoperative formation of intestinal gas.
    d. stimulate bowel bacteria to increase production of Vitamin K.

12. The patient with an ileostomy is more likely than a patient with transverse colostomy to require
    a. ostomy irrigations.
    b. solid skin barriers.
    c. drainable pouches.
    d. increased fluid intake.

13. In contrast to diverticulitis, the patient with diverticulosis
    a. has rectal bleeding.
    b. often has no symptoms.
    c. has localized crampy pain.
    d. frequently develops peritonitis.

14. A nursing intervention that is most appropriate to decrease postoperative edema and pain following an inguinal herniorrhaphy is
    a. applying a truss to the hernia site.
    b. allowing the patient to stand to void.
    c. elevation of the scrotum with a support or small pillow.
    d. supporting the incision during routine coughing and deep breathing.

15. The nurse determines that the goals of dietary teaching have been met when the patient with nontropical sprue selects from the menu
    a. cornmeal mush and sausage.
    b. yogurt, fresh fruit, and rye toast.
    c. oatmeal, skim milk, and orange juice.
    d. pancakes with syrup and scrambled eggs.

16. A patient undergoes a hemorrhoidectomy in a day surgery unit. To promote bowel movements the first several days postoperatively the nurse teaches the patient to
    a. take a sitz bath in the morning before defecating.
    b. administer an oil-retention enema to empty the bowel.
    c. use prescribed pain medication before the bowel movement.
    d. avoid straining and increasing abdominal pressure during defecation.

References

1. Kelly CP, LaMont JT: *Clostridium difficile* infection, *Ann Rev Med* 49:375, 1998.
2. Bentsen D, Braun JW: Controlling fecal incontinence with sensory retraining managed by advanced practice nurses, *Clin Nurs Specialist* 10:171, 1996.
3. Doughty D: A physiologic approach to bowel training, *J WOCN* 23:46, 1996.
4. Norton C: The causes and nursing management of constipation, *Br J Nurs* 5:1252, 1996.
5. Storrie JB: Biofeedback: a first line treatment for idiopathic constipation, *Br J Nurs* 6:152, 1997.
6. Town J: Bringing acute abdomen into focus, *Nursing* 27:52, 1997.
7. Drossman DA: Diagnosing and treating patients with refractory functional gastrointestinal disorders, *Ann Intern Med* 123:688, 1995.
8. Sabiston DC: Appendicitis. In Sabiston DC, editor: *Textbook of surgery: the biological basis of modern surgical practice*, ed 15, Philadelphia, 1997, WB Saunders.
9. Hau T: Biology and treatment of peritonitis: the historic development of current concepts, *J Am Coll Surg* 186:475, 1998.

10. Drossman DA and others: US householder survey of functional gastrointestinal disorders: prevalence, sociodemography, and health impact, *Dig Dis Sci* 38:1569, 1993.
11. Moses PL and others: Inflammatory bowel disease: 1. Origins, presentation, and course, *Postgrad Med* 103:77, 1998.
12. Tayoda H and others: Distinct associations of HLA class II genes with inflammatory bowel disease, *Gastroenterology* 104:741, 1993.
13. Jewell DP: Ulcerative colitis. In Feldman M and others, editors: *Sleisenger and Fardtran's gastrointestinal and liver disease,* ed 6, Philadelphia, 1998, WB Saunders.
14. Zlatanic J and others: Inflammatory bowel disease and immune thrombocytopenic purpura: is there a correlation? *Am J Gastroenterol* 92:2285, 1997.
15. Hanauer SB: Drug therapy: inflammatory bowel disease, *N Engl J Med* 334:841, 1996.
16. Rogler G, Andus T: Cytokines in inflammatory bowel disease, *World J Surg*, 22:382, 1998.
17. Sachar DB: Maintenance strategies in Crohn's disease, *Hosp Prac* 31:99, 1996.
18. Birtwistle J, Hall K: Does nicotine have beneficial effects in the treatment of certain diseases? *Br J Nurs* 5:1195, 1996.
19. Cummings JH: Short-chain fatty acid enemas in the treatment of distal ulcerative colitis, *Europ J Gastroenterol Hepatol* 9:149, 1997.
20. Belluzzi A and others: Effect of an enteric-coated fish-oil preparation on relapses in Crohn's disease, *N Engl J Med* 334:1557, 1996.
21. McCloy C and others: The etiology of intestinal obstruction in patients without prior laparotomy or hernia, *Am Surg* 64:19, 1998.
22. Markowitz A, Winawer SJ: Management of colorectal polyps, *CA-A Cancer Journal for Clinicians* 47:93, 1997.
23. American Cancer Society: Cancer facts and figures—1998, Atlanta, 1998, American Cancer Society.
24. Parker SL and others: Cancer statistics 1997, *CA-A Cancer Journal for Clinicians* 47:5, 1997.
25. Meissner JE: Caring for patients with colorectal cancer, *Nursing* 26:60, 1996.
26. Bond JH: Screening for colorectal cancer, *Hosp Prac* 32:59, 1997.
27. Hammerhofer-Jereb A: Laparoscopic bowel resection? *RN* 59:22, 1996.
28. Diaz-Canton E, Pazdur R: Adjuvant medical therapy for colorectal cancer, *Surg Clin North Am* 77:211, 1997.
29. Byers T and others. American Cancer Society guidelines for screening and surveillance for early detection of colorectal polyps and cancer: update 1997, *CA-A Cancer Journal for Clinicians* 47:154, 1997.
30. Powe BD: Fatalism among elderly African-Americans. Effects on colorectal cancer screening, *Cancer* 18:385, 1995.
31. Vainio H, Morgan G, Kleihues P: An international evaluation of the cancer-preventive potential of nonsteroidal antiinflammatory drugs, *Cancer Epidemiol Biomarkers Prev* 6:749, 1997.
32. Sandler RS and others: Aspirin and nonsteroidal antiinflammatory agents and risk for colorectal adenomas, *Gastroenterology* 114:441, 1998.
33. Roberts P and others: Practice parameters for sigmoid diverticulitis-supporting documentation, *Dis Colon Rectum* 38:126, 1995.
34. Murphy D: Celiac sprue, *Gastroenterology Nursing* 18:133, 1995.
35. Thompson JS: Management of the short bowel syndrome, *Postsurgical Syndromes* 23:403, 1994.
36. Byrne TA and others: Growth hormone, glutamine and a modified diet enhance nutrient absorption in patients with severe short bowel syndrome, *JPEN* 19:296, 1995.

Resources

American Cancer Society
1599 Clifton Rd NE
Atlanta, GA 30329
404-320-3333
http://www.acs.org

American Gastroenterological Association
7910 Woodmont Ave, 7th Floor,
Bethesda, MD 20814
301-654-2055
fax: 301-652-3890
http://www.gastro.org/

American Society for Gastrointestinal Endoscopy
13 Elm Street
Manchester, MA 01944-1314
978-526-8330
fax: 978-526-4018
http://www.asge.org/

Crohn's & Colitis Foundation of America (CCFA)
386 Park Avenue South, 17th Floor
New York, NY 10016-8804
212-685-3440
800-932-2423
fax: 212-779-4098
http://www.ccfa.org

Crohn's & Colitis Foundation of Canada (CCFC)
21 St. Clair Avenue East, Suite 301
Toronto, Ontario M4T 1L9 CANADA
416-920-5035
800-387-1479
fax: 416-929-0364
http://www.ccfc.org

United Ostomy Association (UOA)
19772 MacArthur Blvd, Suite 200
Irvine, CA 92612-2405
800-826-0826
http://www.uoa.org/

Wound, Ostomy & Continence Nurses Society
2755 Bristol Street, Suite 110
Costa Mesa, CA 92626
714-476-0268
fax: 714-545-3643

For additional Internet resources, see the website for this book at www.mosby.com/MERLIN/medsurg_lewis/

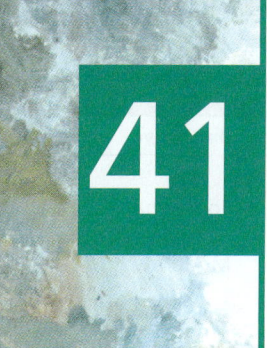
41

NURSING MANAGEMENT
Liver, Biliary Tract, and Pancreas Problems

Rachel Elrod

www.mosby.com/MERLIN/medsurg_lewis

LEARNING OBJECTIVES

1. Define jaundice and describe signs and symptoms that may occur with the different types of jaundice.
2. Differentiate among the types of viral hepatitis, including etiology, pathophysiology, clinical manifestations, complications, and collaborative care.
3. Describe the nursing management of the patient with viral hepatitis.
4. Explain the etiology, pathophysiology, clinical manifestations, complications, and collaborative care of the patient with cirrhosis of the liver.
5. Describe the nursing management of the patient with cirrhosis.
6. Describe the clinical manifestations and management of carcinoma of the liver.

7. Describe the pathophysiology, clinical manifestations, complications, and collaborative care of acute and chronic pancreatitis.
8. Describe the nursing management of the patient with pancreatitis.
9. Explain the clinical manifestations and collaborative care of the patient with carcinoma of the pancreas.
10. Explain the pathophysiology, clinical manifestations, complications, and collaborative care including surgical therapy of gallbladder disorders.
11. Describe the nursing management of the patient undergoing conservative or surgical treatment of cholecystitis and cholelithiasis.

JAUNDICE

Jaundice, a yellowish discoloration of body tissues, results from an alteration in normal bilirubin metabolism or flow of bile into the hepatic or biliary duct systems. It is a symptom rather than a disease. Jaundice results when the concentration of bilirubin in the blood becomes abnormally increased. The bilirubin level has to be approximately three times normal levels (2 to 3 mg/dl [34 to 51 mol/L]) for jaundice to occur. Jaundice can usually first be detected in the sclera and skin (Fig. 41-1).

Most of the body's bilirubin is formed from the breakdown of hemoglobin (from erythrocytes) by macrophages (see Fig. 37-6). This unconjugated (indirect) bilirubin is released into the circulation bound to albumin and is not water soluble. Because unconjugated bilirubin is not water soluble and cannot be filtered in the kidneys, it is not excreted in the urine. In the liver the unconjugated bilirubin is conjugated with glucuronic acid to form conjugated (direct) bilirubin, which is water soluble. Conjugated bilirubin is secreted into bile, which flows through the hepatic and biliary duct system into the small intestine. In the large intestine, bilirubin is converted to stercobilinogen and urobilinogen by bacterial action. Stercobilinogen gives the char-

acteristic brown color to feces. Some urobilinogen is reabsorbed into the portal circulation and returned to the liver. Normally a very small amount of urobilinogen is excreted in urine.

The three types of jaundice are classified as hemolytic, hepatocellular, and obstructive. Diagnostic findings associated with these types of jaundice are shown in Table 41-1.

Hemolytic Jaundice

Hemolytic (prehepatic) jaundice is due to an increased breakdown of red blood cells (RBCs), which produces an increased amount of unconjugated bilirubin in the blood (see Table 41-1). The liver is unable to handle this increased load. Causes of hemolytic jaundice include blood transfusion reactions, sickle cell crisis, and hemolytic anemia.

Hepatocellular Jaundice

Hepatocellular (hepatic) jaundice results from the liver's altered ability to take up bilirubin from the blood or to conjugate or excrete it. Both unconjugated and conjugated bilirubin serum levels increase (see Table 41-1). Because conjugated bilirubin is water soluble, it is excreted in the urine. The most common causes of hepatocellular jaundice are hepatitis, cirrhosis, and hepatic carcinoma.

Obstructive Jaundice

Obstructive (posthepatic) jaundice is due to impeded or obstructed flow of bile through the liver or biliary duct system.

Reviewed by Deborah L. Martin, RN, MN, Chief Executive Officer, Infection Control and Prevention Analysis, Inc., Austin, Tex.

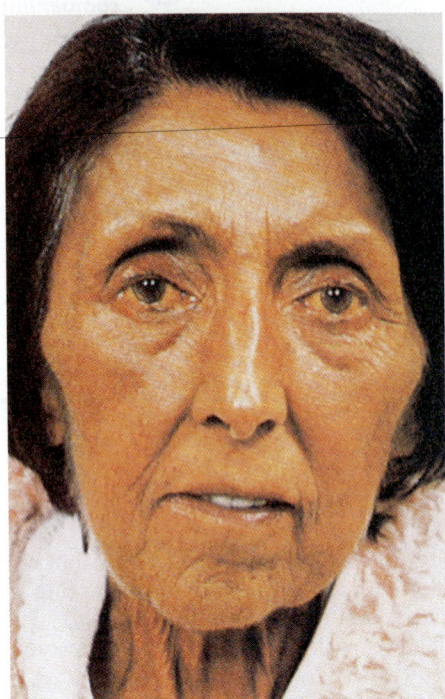

Fig. 41-1   Severe jaundice.

Table **41-1**	Diagnostic Findings in Jaundice		
	Hemolytic	Hepatocellular	Obstructive
Serum bilirubin			
Unconjugated (indirect)	↑	↑	Somewhat ↑
Conjugated (direct)	Normal	↑	Moderately ↑
Urine bilirubin	Negative	↑	↑
Urobilinogen			
Stool	↑	Normal to ↓	Negative
Urine	↑	Normal to ↑	Negative

CULTURAL & ETHNIC CONSIDERATIONS

Disorders of the Liver, Pancreas, and Gallbladder

- Mortality from cirrhosis occurs more frequently among African-Americans than in other ethnic groups.
- Primary hepatic cancer has a higher incidence among African-Americans, Asian-Americans, and Eskimos than Caucasians.
- Pancreatic cancer occurs more frequently among African-Americans and Asian-Americans than Caucasians.
- Caucasians and Native-Americans have a higher incidence of gallbladder disease than African-Americans or Asian-Americans.

The obstruction may be intrahepatic or extrahepatic. Intrahepatic obstructions are due to swelling or fibrosis of the liver's canaliculi and bile ducts. This can be caused by damage from liver tumors, hepatitis, or cirrhosis. Causes of extrahepatic obstruction include common bile duct obstruction from a stone, sclerosing cholangitis, and carcinoma of the head of the pancreas. Laboratory findings show an elevation of both unconjugated and conjugated bilirubin and urine bilirubin (see Table 41-1). Because bilirubin does not enter the intestines, there is decreased to no fecal or urinary urobilinogen. With complete obstruction, the stools are clay colored.

VIRAL HEPATITIS

Hepatitis is an inflammation of the liver. Acute viral hepatitis is the most common cause of hepatitis. The types of infectious viral hepatitis are A, B, C (formerly called post-transfusion non-A, non-B), D, E, and G. Noninfectious hepatitis may also be caused by drugs and other chemicals (see Table 37-6). Rarely, hepatitis is caused by bacteria, such as streptococci, salmonellae, and *Escherichia coli.*

Viral hepatitis is a major public health concern in the United States. Approximately 152,000 cases of hepatitis A occur annually in the United States and 10 million worldwide. It is nearly universal during childhood in developing countries. There is an estimated 140,000 cases of hepatitis B annually in the United States. In the 1990s the incidence of hepatitis B decreased overall, partly because of the hepatitis B vaccine. However, since 1993 there has been an increase in the incidence of hepatitis B in homosexual men, injecting drug users, and sexually active heterosexuals.

Approximately 35,000 Americans contract hepatitis C annually.[1] Each year 8000 to 12,000 persons chronically infected with hepatitis C die of a liver-related complication of their infection.[2,3] Chronic hepatitis C infection is now the most common liver disease in the United States.[3] Fortunately, there has been a decline in the incidence of hepatitis C in recent years, which is due in part to screening of the blood supply for anti-HCV (antibody to hepatitis C virus) and safer needle-using practices by injecting drug users.

Etiology

Viral hepatitis can be caused by one of five major viruses: A, B, C, D, and E. Hepatitis G has recently been described. Approximately 90% of post-transfusion and community-acquired hepatitis cases are due to viruses A to E.[1] Other viruses known to damage the liver include cytomegalovirus, Epstein-Barr virus, herpes virus, coxsackievirus, and rubella virus.

The only definitive way to distinguish the various forms of viral hepatitis is by the presence of the antigens and antigenic subtypes and the subsequent development of antibodies to them. Outbreaks of hepatitis are consistently caused by hepatitis A virus. Approximately 50% of viral hepatitis cases in adults in the United States are hepatitis B, 20% are hepatitis C, and 30% are hepatitis A.[4] Infection with each virus provides immunity to that virus (homologous immunity). However, the patient can still develop another type of viral hepatitis. Characteristics of hepatitis viruses are summarized in Table 41-2.

Hepatitis A Virus. The hepatitis A virus (HAV) is an RNA virus that is transmitted through the fecal-oral route. It

Table 41-2 Characteristics of Hepatitis Viruses

	Incubation Period	Mode of Transmission	Sources of Infection and Spread of Disease	Infectivity
Hepatitis A virus (HAV)	15-50 days (average 28)	Fecal-oral (fecal contamination and oral ingestion)	Crowded conditions; poor personal hygiene; poor sanitation; contaminated food, milk, water, and shellfish; persons with subclinical infections; infected food handlers; sexual contact	Most infectious during 2 weeks before onset of symptoms; infectious until 1-2 weeks after symptoms start
Hepatitis B virus (HBV)	45-180 days (average 56-96)	Percutaneous (parenteral)/permucosal exposure to blood or blood products Sexual contact Perinatal transmission Human bile	Contaminated needles, syringes, and blood products; sexual activity with infected partners; asymptomatic carriers Tattoo/body piercing, bites	Before and after symptoms appear; infectious for 4-6 months; in carriers continues for patient's lifetime
Hepatitis C virus (HCV)	14-180 days (average 56)	Percutaneous (parenteral)/permucosal exposure to blood or blood products High-risk sexual contact Perinatal contact	Blood and blood products, needles and syringes, sexual activity with infected partners	1-2 weeks before symptoms; continues during clinical course; indefinitely with carriers
Hepatitis D virus (HDV)	2-26 weeks HBV must precede HDV; chronic carriers of HBV are always at risk	Can cause infection only together with HBV; routes of transmission same as for HBV	Same as HBV	Blood is infectious at all stages of HDV infection
Hepatitis E virus (HEV)	15-64 days (average 26-42 days in different epidemics)	Fecal-oral Outbreaks associated with contaminated water supply in developing countries	Contaminated water; poor sanitation; found in Asia, Africa, and Mexico; not common in the United States and Canada	Not known; may be similar to HAV

frequently occurs in small outbreaks caused by fecal contamination of food or drinking water. It is found in feces 2 or more weeks before the onset of symptoms and up to 1 week after the onset of jaundice (Fig. 41-2). It is present in the blood only briefly. Anti-HAV (antibody to hepatitis A virus) IgM appears in the serum as the stool becomes negative for the virus. Detection of IgM anti-HAV indicates acute hepatitis, and IgG anti-HAV is an indicator of past infection. The presence of IgG antibody provides lifelong immunity.

The mode of transmission of HAV is predominantly fecal-oral (mainly by ingestion of food or liquid infected with the virus) and rarely parenteral. Poor hygiene, crowded situations, and poor sanitary conditions are all factors related to hepatitis A. Transmission occurs between family members, institutionalized individuals, and from common-source outbreaks. The disease occurs more frequently in underdeveloped countries. The eating of raw shellfish from contaminated waters can also be a

source of infection. Food-borne hepatitis A outbreaks are usually due to contamination of food during preparation by an infected food handler.

There is no chronic carrier state for HAV. The virus is present in feces during the incubation period, so it can be carried by persons who have undetectable, subclinical infections. The greatest risk of transmission occurs before clinical symptoms are apparent. It can also be transmitted by patients with anicteric (nonjaundice) hepatitis A.

Hepatitis B Virus. Hepatitis B virus (HBV) is a DNA virus that is transmitted by percutaneous (IV drug use, accidental needle-stick punctures) or permucosal exposure to infectious blood, blood products, or other body fluids (semen, vaginal secretions, saliva). Perinatal transmission is also possible. In persons who have HBV, hepatitis B surface antigen (HBsAg) has been detected in almost every body fluid, including vaginal secretions, menstrual fluids, semen, saliva,

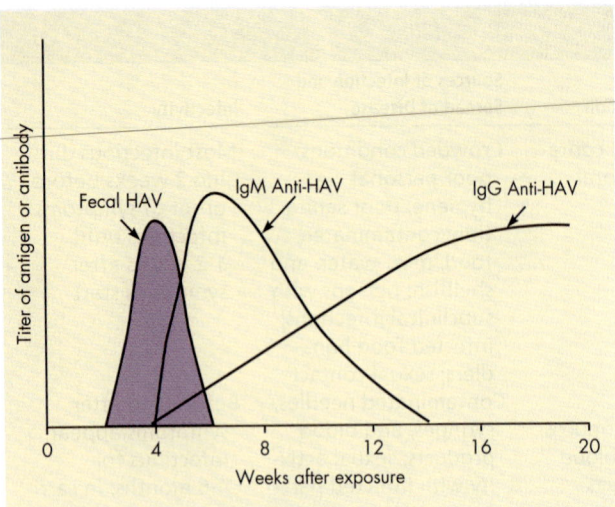

Fig. 41-2 Clinical and serologic events of a typical patient infected with hepatitis A virus (HAV). Elevated alanine aminotransferase (ALT) levels are present by 4 weeks and jaundice appears by about 5 weeks after exposure to the virus.

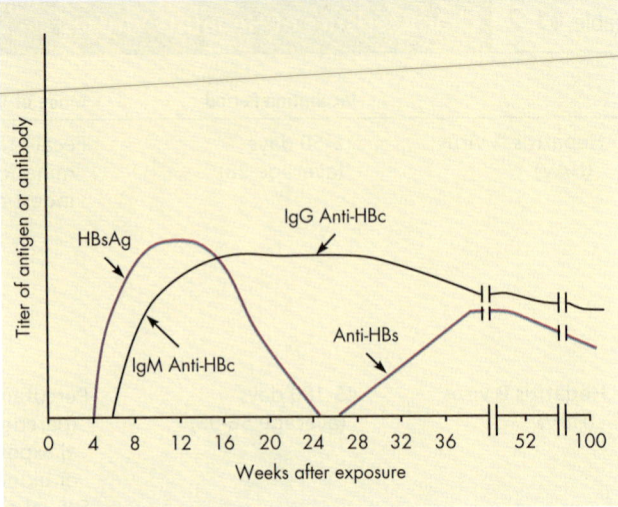

Fig. 41-3 Clinical and serologic events of a typical patient infected with acute hepatitis B virus (HBV). Elevated alanine aminotransferase (ALT) levels are present by about 8 weeks and jaundice appears by about 10 weeks after exposure to the virus. *HBc,* hepatitis B core antigen; *HBsAg,* hepatitis B surface antigen.

respiratory secretions, tears, gastric juice, synovial fluid, and cerebrospinal fluid. Infected semen and saliva contain much lower concentrations of HBV than blood, but the virus can be transmitted via these secretions. If GI bleeding occurs, feces can be contaminated with the virus from the blood. There is no evidence that urine, feces, breast milk, tears, and sweat are infective. Sometimes HBV is transmitted by unidentified means. In 20% to 30% of patients with acute hepatitis B there are no readily identifiable risk factors.[5]

Hepatitis B is a sexually transmitted disease. Approximately 30% of HBV cases are related to heterosexual activity, either with multiple sexual partners or unprotected sex with an infected person.[6] Male homosexuals (especially those practicing anal intercourse) are at risk for HBV infection. Although there is a much lower risk of transmission, kissing and sharing of food items may spread the virus via saliva. The hepatitis B virus can live on a dry surface for at least 7 days. HBV is considered to be 100 times more infectious than human immunodeficiency virus (HIV).[6]

HBV is a complex structure with three distinct antigens: the surface antigen (HBsAg), the core antigen (HBcAg), and the e antigen (HBeAg). The persistence of HBsAg in the serum for 6 to 12 months or longer indicates a carrier state of hepatitis B. Each antigen has a corresponding antibody that may be elicited during an attack of acute viral hepatitis B. These antibodies can be detected in the serum of persons with prior exposure to the antigenic virus (Fig. 41-3). The presence of anti-HBsAg indicates immunity to hepatitis B.

From 2% to 10% of adults who become infected with HBV become chronic HBV carriers and may transmit the virus.[6] The HBsAg level remains elevated in carriers (HBsAg-positive on at least two occasions at least 6 months apart). With carrier status, liver enzyme values may be normal. The carriers of hepatitis B may have low-grade disease, a normal liver, or severe chronic active liver disease. α-Interferon is now being used to try to eliminate the chronic HBV carrier state. A positive test

for anti-HBsAg in adults indicates that they have had hepatitis B or the vaccine.

Hepatitis C Virus. Hepatitis C virus (HCV) is an RNA virus that is primarily transmitted percutaneously. Thus the major risk factor for infection is direct percutaneous exposure, such as injecting drugs, transfusion of blood products, hemodialysis, tattooing, high-risk sexual behavior, organ transplants, and exposure to blood and blood products by health care workers. Less frequent routes of transmission are sexual and perinatal. However, 40% to 50% of patients with HCV have no known source of infection.[7]

Hepatitis D Virus. Hepatitis D virus (HDV), also called delta virus, is a defective RNA virus that cannot survive on its own. The importance of HDV relates to its clinical virulence. It can transform asymptomatic or mild chronic hepatitis B infection to severe, progressive chronic active hepatitis and cirrhosis and can accelerate the course of chronic active hepatitis B. Delta virus is also a contributing factor in a substantial number of cases of fulminant hepatitis B. Delta hepatitis can occur as a primary infection along with HBV (coinfection) or in a carrier of hepatitis B (superinfection). HDV is transmitted percutaneously.

Hepatitis E Virus. Hepatitis E virus (HEV) is an RNA virus that is transmitted by the fecal-oral route. The most common mode of transmission is drinking contaminated water. Hepatitis E is also called enteric non-A, non-B hepatitis. Hepatitis E occurs primarily in developing countries. There have been reported epidemics in India, Asia, Mexico, and Africa. Only a few cases have been reported in the United States. Occurrence in the United States is almost always in persons who have recently traveled to HEV-endemic areas.[8] Although not yet commercially available, there is an assay test to determine the antibody to HEV.

Hepatitis G Virus. Recently hepatitis G virus (HGV), an RNA virus, has been discovered. HGV has been found in some

Table 41-3	Clinical Manifestations of the Phases of Hepatitis	
Preicteric	Icteric	Posticteric
Anorexia	Jaundice	Malaise
Nausea, vomiting	Pruritus	Easy fatigability
Right upper quadrant discomfort	Dark urine	Hepatomegaly
Constipation or diarrhea	Bilirubinuria	
Decreased sense of taste and smell	Light stools	
Malaise	Fatigue	
Headache	Continued hepatomegaly with tenderness	
Fever	Weight loss	
Arthralgias		
Urticaria		
Hepatomegaly		
Splenomegaly		
Weight loss		

blood donors and can be transmitted by transfusion.[9,10] It frequently coexists with other hepatitis viruses, such as HCV. However, most HGV infections are not associated with chronic hepatitis.[9] Thus at this time HGV association with liver disease is uncertain.

Pathophysiology

Liver. The pathophysiologic changes in the various types of viral hepatitis are similar. Hepatitis involves widespread inflammation of liver tissue. Liver cell damage consists of hepatic cell degeneration and necrosis. There is proliferation and enlargement of the Kupffer cells. Inflammation of the periportal areas may interrupt bile flow. Cholestasis may occur. The liver cells regenerate in an orderly manner, and if no complications occur, they should resume their normal appearance and function during convalescence.

Systemic Effects. The antigen-antibody complexes between the virus and its corresponding antibody form a circulating immune complex in the early phases of hepatitis. The presence of circulating immune complexes activates the complement system (see Chapter 12). The clinical manifestations of this activation are rash, angioedema, arthritis, fever, and malaise. Glomerulonephritis and vasculitis have also been found secondary to immune complex disease.

Clinical Manifestations

A large number of patients, especially the younger ones, have no symptoms. The clinical manifestations of viral hepatitis may be classified into three phases: (1) preicteric or prodromal phase, (2) icteric phase, and (3) posticteric or convalescent phase (Table 41-3).

Preicteric Phase. The preicteric phase precedes jaundice and lasts from 1 to 21 days. This is the period of maximal infectivity for hepatitis A. Hepatitis B patients who are HBcAg positive can be infective for years. Gastrointestinal (GI) symptoms include anorexia, nausea, abdominal (right upper quad-

rant) discomfort, and sometimes vomiting, constipation, or diarrhea. The anorexia is frequently severe and is thought to be caused by a toxin produced by the diseased liver. The patient may find food repugnant and, if a smoker, may have a distaste for cigarettes. There is also a decreased sense of smell. Weight loss occurs during the preicteric phase. Other symptoms during this phase are malaise, headache, low-grade fever, arthralgias, and skin rashes. Physical examination reveals hepatomegaly, lymphadenopathy, and sometimes splenomegaly.

Icteric Phase. The icteric phase lasts 2 to 4 weeks and is characterized by jaundice. Jaundice results when bilirubin diffuses into the tissues. The urine may darken because of excess bilirubin being excreted by the kidneys. If conjugated bilirubin cannot flow out of the liver because of obstruction or inflammation of the bile ducts, the stools will be light or clay colored. Pruritus sometimes accompanies the jaundice, especially if cholestasis is present. The pruritus occurs as a result of the accumulation of bile salts beneath the skin.

When jaundice occurs, the fever usually subsides. The GI symptoms usually remain, and some fatigue may continue. The liver is usually enlarged and tender.

Posticteric Phase. The convalescent stage of the posticteric phase begins as jaundice is disappearing and lasts weeks to months, with an average of 2 to 4 months. During this period the patient's major complaint is malaise and easy fatigability. Hepatomegaly remains for several weeks, but splenomegaly subsides during this period. Relapses may occur, and the disappearance of jaundice does not mean the patient has totally recovered.

General Considerations

Not all patients with viral hepatitis have jaundice. This is termed *anicteric hepatitis* and occurs more frequently in children. A high percentage of persons with HAV are anicteric and do not have symptoms.

There is some slight variation in manifestations between the types of hepatitis. In hepatitis A the onset is more acute and the symptoms are usually mild, flulike manifestations. In hepatitis B the onset is more insidious and the symptoms are usually more severe. There may be fewer GI symptoms. In hepatitis C, although the majority of cases are asymptomatic or mild, HCV has a high rate of persistence and can induce chronic liver disease.

Complications

Most patients with acute HAV and HBV hepatitis recover completely with no complications. The overall mortality rate for hepatitis is less than 1%. The mortality rate is higher in older adults and those with underlying debilitating diseases. Complications that can occur include chronic persistent hepatitis, chronic active hepatitis, fulminant viral hepatitis, and cirrhosis of the liver.

Chronic Persistent Hepatitis. The most common complication of viral hepatitis is chronic persistent hepatitis in which there is a delayed convalescent period. It is usually benign and is characterized by fatigue and hepatomegaly. However, no treatment is required. Liver function tests may remain abnormal for several years.

Table **41-4**	Tests for Viral Hepatitis	
Virus	**Tests**	**Significance**
A	Anti-HAV IgM	Acute infection
	Anti-HAV IgG	Previous infection and long-term immunity
B	HBsAg (hepatitis B surface antigen)	Current infection (but not necessarily acute)*
		Positive in chronic carriers
	Anti-HBs (antibody to surface antigen)	Indicates previous infection with hepatitis B or immunization
		Marker for response to vaccine
	HBeAg (hepatitis B e antigen)	Indicates high infectivity; present in acute, active infection
	Anti-HBe (antibody to e antigen)	Indicates previous infection
	HBcAg	Ongoing infection with hepatitis B
	Anti-HBc IgM	Acute infection*
	Anti-HBc IgG (antibody to HB core antigen)	Indicates previous infection or ongoing infection with hepatitis B
		Does not appear after vaccination
	HBV-DNA	Indicates active ongoing viral replication
		Best indicator of viral replication
C	Anti-HCV (antibody to hepatitis C)	Marker for acute or chronic infection with HCV
		Coexisting infection with HBV
	HCV RNA	Indicates active ongoing viral replication
D	Anti-HDV	Present in past or current infection with hepatitis D

*If positive HBsAg and anti-HBc IgM, it indicates the presence of acute infection.
DNA, deoxyribonucleic acid.

Chronic Active Hepatitis. Chronic active hepatitis is characterized by the persistence of signs and symptoms of hepatitis and abnormal liver function tests for more than 6 months. Chronic active hepatitis is seen in hepatitis B and C but not in hepatitis A or E. It is seen in patients with hepatitis D only if they also have hepatitis B. A high percentage of persons with HCV infection (at least 85%) become chronically infected.[11] HBsAg persists longer than 6 months in approximately 10% of patients with hepatitis B. It is distinguished from chronic persistent hepatitis by liver biopsy. The ongoing process of liver necrosis may progress to cirrhosis.

The HBsAg-positive patient whose serum remains positive for HBeAg is more likely to have chronic active hepatitis. In addition, alteration in the patient's cellular immune response may be important in the development of the chronic HBsAg carrier state and consequent progression from acute hepatitis B to chronic active hepatitis. This finding may explain why the patient with chronic renal failure who is undergoing dialysis when hepatitis B develops is more at risk for chronic active hepatitis. (Persons with chronic renal failure are known to have a depressed cellular immune response.)

There is a greater risk for HCV infection to become chronic as compared with HBV. Approximately 85% of patients who have acute HCV will go on to develop chronic infection.[3]

Fulminant Hepatitis. Fulminant viral hepatitis is a clinical syndrome that results in severe impairment or necrosis of liver cells and potential liver failure. Fulminant viral hepatitis develops in a small percentage of patients. The disorder may occur as a complication of hepatitis B, particularly hepatitis B accompanied by infection with delta virus (HDV). Fulminant hepatitis occurs much less frequently with hepatitis C. Toxic reactions to drugs and congenital metabolic disorders may also cause fulminant hepatitis and fulminant liver failure. Hepatocellular failure with death usually occurs.

Diagnostic Studies

Tests for the different types of viral hepatitis are presented in Table 41-4. In viral hepatitis many of the liver function tests show significant abnormalities. The common abnormalities are identified in Table 41-5.

Antibodies to HCV are not protective and are often an indication of active disease. For the patient who has a positive anti-HCV test by enzyme immunoassay (EIA) or if HCV is suspected and there is a false HCV antibody test (only 90% of patients with hepatitis C are positive for anti-HCV), the hepatitis C virus recombinant immunoblot assay (HCV-RIBA) is used to make the diagnosis. There are tests to detect HCV RNA (the virus); however, because of their expense and the possibility of false-negative results, they are not used as the primary tests to confirm or rule out a diagnosis.[12]

Physical assessment reveals hepatic tenderness, hepatomegaly, and splenomegaly. The liver is palpable. A liver biopsy is not indicated unless the diagnosis is in doubt or a more severe form of hepatitis is suspected.

Collaborative Care

There is no specific treatment or therapy for viral hepatitis. Most patients can be managed at home. Emphasis is on measures to rest the body and assist the liver in regenerating (Table 41-6). Adequate nutrients and rest seem to be most beneficial for healing and liver cell (hepatocyte) regeneration. Dietary emphasis is on a well-balanced diet that the patient can tolerate.

Rest reduces the metabolic demands on the liver and promotes cell regeneration. Bed rest may be indicated while the patient is symptomatic. The degree of rest ordered depends on the severity of symptoms, but usually alternating periods of activity and rest are adequate.

Drug Therapy. There are no specific drug therapies for the treatment of acute viral hepatitis. Corticosteroid therapy

Table **41-5**	Diagnostic Findings in Hepatitis	
Test	**Abnormal Finding**	**Etiology**
Transaminases (aminotransferases)		
Aspartate aminotransferase (AST) or serum glutamic-oxaloacetic transaminase (SGOT)	Elevation in preicteric phase; decrease as jaundice disappears	Liver cell injury
Alanine aminotransferase (ALT) or serum glutamic-pyruvic transaminase (SGPT)	Elevation in preicteric phase; decrease as jaundice disappears	Liver cell injury
γ-Glutamyl transpeptidase (GGT)	Elevation	Liver cell injury
Alkaline phosphatase	Some elevation	Impaired excretory function of the liver
Serum proteins		
γ-Globulin	Normal or increased	Impaired clearance of the liver
Albumin	Normal or decreased	Liver damage
Serum bilirubin (total)	Elevation to about 8-15 mg/dl (137-257 μmol/L)	Hepatocellular damage
Urinary bilirubin	Elevation	Conjugated hyperbilirubinemia
Urinary urobilinogen	Elevation 2-5 days before jaundice	Diminished reabsorption of urobilinogen
Prothrombin time	Prolonged	Decreased absorption of vitamin K in intestine with decreased production of prothrombin by liver

COLLABORATIVE CARE

Table **41-6**	**Viral Hepatitis**

Diagnostic
Liver function studies
Hepatitis serology
  HBsAg (HBeAg in some cases)
  Anti-HBs
  Anti-HBc—IgM and IgG
  Anti-HAV—IgM and IgG
  Anti-HCV

Collaborative Therapy
High-calorie, high-protein, high-carbohydrate, low-fat diet
Vitamin supplements
Rest—degree of strictness varying
Avoid alcohol intake and drugs detoxified by the liver
α-Interferon

is controversial. Supportive drug therapy may include antiemetics, such as dimenhydrinate (Dramamine) or trimethobenzamide (Tigan). Phenothiazines should not be used because of their possible cholestatic and hepatotoxic effects. If the patient requires a sedative or hypnotic drug, diphenhydramine (Benadryl) or chloral hydrate may be used.

α-**Interferon.** α-Interferon (antiviral or immune-modulating drug) has been approved to treat hepatitis B and C. It is primarily used in the treatment of chronic hepatitis. The efficacy of α-interferon is greater in the treatment of HBV than in HCV

infections. α-Interferon is considered effective if the patient with HBV becomes negative for HBsAg. Ribavirin (Virazole), given in combination with α-interferon, has a synergistic effect.

Treatment protocols for hepatitis B and C using α-interferon are variable. In approximately 30% to 40% of patients with HBV treated with α-interferon 5 million units per day for 16 weeks, there will be loss of HBeAg and undetectable HBV DNA levels. In patients with chronic HCV a typical treatment protocol might include 3 million units three times weekly for 6 months. Approximately 40% to 50% of these patients will initially respond with a decrease in HCV DNA. However, 50% of these patients will relapse in 6 months, indicating that interferon therapy is effective in less than 25% of patients with chronic HCV.[13] Combination therapy using ribavirin with α-interferon is used in some medical centers to reduce the rate of relapse following α-interferon therapy for hepatitis C. Although not as high as with hepatitis C, relapse is also a problem in patients with chronic hepatitis B receiving α-interferon.

α-Interferon treatment is associated with a number of side effects (Table 41-7). These side effects are dose related and tend to decrease in severity with continued treatment. Newer antiviral drugs such as lamivudine (3TC) and famciclovir may be used to inhibit HBV replication.[14]

Hepatitis A vaccine and immune globulin. Immune globulin is used in the prevention and modification of viral hepatitis. Immune globulin (IG) is effective for hepatitis A if given up to 2 weeks after exposure. It provides temporary passive immunity. IG is recommended in cases of exposure to hepatitis A from close (household, day care center) contact in persons who are not positive for anti-HAV and for travelers to countries with high endemic levels of hepatitis A.

DRUG THERAPY

Table 41-7 Side Effects of α-Interferon

Flulike symptoms
  Myalgia
  Arthralgia
  Headache
  Nausea
  Fatigue
Other effects
  Decline in platelet and neutrophil counts
  Weight loss
  Hair loss
  Thyroid disease
Less common effects
  Diarrhea
  Seizures
  Severe depression
  Vasculitis
  Retinopathy
  Peripheral neuropathy

Both IG and hepatitis A vaccine are used for prevention of hepatitis A. The vaccine is used for preexposure prophylaxis, and IG can be used either before or after exposure. Because patients with hepatitis A are most infectious just before the onset of symptoms, those exposed through household contact or food-borne outbreaks should be given IG within 1 to 2 weeks of exposure. If the exposed person has anti-HAV antibodies, the IG is not necessary. When given within 2 weeks of exposure, IG can prevent infection in most people. Although IG may not prevent infection in all persons, it may modify the illness to a subclinical infection. IG provides 6 to 8 weeks of passive protection. It may also be used as a prophylactic measure for travelers to countries that have a high incidence of hepatitis A.

There are currently three hepatitis A vaccines, Havrix, Vaqta, and Avaxim. This active immunization can be a means to control the disease from a public health perspective. Primary immunization consists of a single dose administered intramuscularly in the deltoid. A booster is recommended any time between 6 and 12 months after the initiation of the primary dose to ensure adequate antibody titers and long-term protection. However, a primary immunization provides immunity within 30 days after a single dose. The vaccine may be administered concomitantly with IG, although the ultimate antibody titer obtained is likely to be lower than if the vaccine is given alone.

The side effects of the vaccine are mild and are usually limited to soreness and redness at the injection site. It is recommended that until routine vaccination of children is feasible, the following persons who are at risk for infection be vaccinated for hepatitis A: persons traveling to countries where hepatitis A is endemic; sexually active homosexual and bisexual men; injecting drug users; patients with chronic liver disease; and persons at risk for occupational infection, suchas those who work with hepatitis A in research laboratory settings.[15]

Hepatitis B vaccine and immune globulin. The first line of defense against hepatitis B is the hepatitis B vaccine. Immunization with hepatitis B vaccine is the most effective method of preventing HBV infection. Recommendations of the Centers for Disease Control and Prevention (CDC) Immunization Practices Advisory Committee include making hepatitis B vaccine a part of routine vaccination schedules for all newborns and adolescents.

In addition to immunizing newborns and adolescents, it is important to vaccinate adolescents and adults in the major risk groups. It may be helpful to screen for the antibody before vaccination because past infection is high in sexually active homosexual men and injecting drug users. It is hoped that universal vaccination will lead to eventual prevention and control of hepatitis B.

Hepatitis B vaccine is produced through recombinant DNA technology (see Fig. 12-12). The vaccines are Recombivax HB and Engerix-B. The vaccine is given in a series of three intramuscular (in the deltoid) injections. The second dose is administered within 1 month of the first one, and the third one within 6 months of the first. The cost is about $150 for the series. The vaccine is greater than 95% effective.[1] Successful vaccination should result in anti-HBsAg titers of 10 mIU/ml or greater. Only minor adverse reactions have been reported with vaccination, including transient fever and soreness at the injection site. The vaccine is not contraindicated in pregnancy.

It has not been definitely determined what level of antibody is required to provide protection. Therefore it remains to be determined how frequently boosters (additional doses) are necessary. For postexposure prophylaxis, the vaccine and hepatitis B immune globulin (HBIG) are used. HBIG contains antibodies to HBV and confers temporary passive immunity. HBIG is given to persons who have been exposed to HBV (needle stick, sexual exposure, infants born to mothers who are positive for HBsAg) and who have not been vaccinated. It should be given after exposure, preferably within 24 hours. The vaccine series should also be started.

For acute one-time exposure to the virus in individuals who have been vaccinated against HBV, HBIG plus the vaccine can be administered. HBIG is prepared from plasma of donors with a high titer of anti-HBsAg and is expensive. HBIG provides temporary passive immunity and is recommended for postexposure prophylaxis in cases of needle stick, mucous membrane contact, or sexual exposure.

Hepatitis C vaccine and immune globulin. Currently there are no products to prevent hepatitis C; however, several vaccines are in development. The CDC does not recommend immune globulin or antiviral agents such as α-interferon for postexposure prophylaxis (e.g., needle-stick exposure from an infected patient) for HCV infection.[16] Immune globulin is of no proven benefit for hepatitis C postexposure prevention.[17] Instead the exposed person should have baseline and 6-month follow-up testing for antibodies to HCV.

Nutritional Therapy. An important measure in assisting hepatocytes to regenerate is adequate nutrition. No special diet is required in the treatment of viral hepatitis. However, a diet high in carbohydrates and proteins with low fat content is usually recommended. Adequate calories are important because the patient usually loses weight. If fat content is poorly tolerated because of decreased bile production, it should be reduced. Basically the specific foods in the diet are dictated by the patient. Vitamin supplements, particularly B-complex vitamins and vitamin K, are frequently used. If anorexia, nausea, and vomiting are severe, intravenous (IV) solutions of glucose or supplemental tube feedings may be used. Fluid and electrolyte balance must be maintained.

NURSING ASSESSMENT

Table 41-8 Hepatitis

Subjective Data

Important Health Information

Past health history: Hemophilia; exposure to infected persons; ingestion of contaminated food or water; sexual promiscuity; exposure to benzene, carbon tetrachloride, or other hepatotoxic agents; crowded, hepatotoxic, unsanitary living conditions; exposure to contaminated needles; recent travel; organ transplant recipient; exposure to new drug regimens

Medications: Use and misuse of acetaminophen, phenytoin, halothane, methyldopa

Functional Health Patterns

Health perception–health management: IV drug and alcohol abuse; malaise, distaste for cigarettes (in smokers)

Nutritional-metabolic: Weight loss, anorexia, nausea, vomiting; feeling of fullness in right upper quadrant

Elimination: Dark urine; light-colored stools, constipation or diarrhea; skin rashes, hives

Activity-exercise: Fatigue, arthralgias, myalgias

Cognitive-perceptual: Right upper quadrant pain and liver tenderness, headache; pruritis

Role-relationship: Exposure as health care worker, chronic care institution resident

Objective Data

General

Low-grade fever, lethargy, lymphadenopathy

Integumentary

Rash, angioedema, jaundice, icteric sclera, injection sites

Gastrointestinal

Hepatomegaly, splenomegaly

Possible Findings

Abnormal liver enzyme studies; elevated serum bilirubin, hypoalbuminemia, anemia, bilirubin in urine and increased urobilinogen, prolonged prothrombin time, serologic tests positive for hepatitis, including anti-HAV IgM, HBsAg, HBeAg, anti-HBc IgM, anti-HCV, anti-HDV, abnormal liver scan, positive liver biopsy

NURSING MANAGEMENT: HEPATITIS

■ Nursing Assessment

Subjective and objective data that should be obtained from a person with hepatitis are presented in Table 41-8.

■ Nursing Diagnoses

Nursing diagnoses for the patient with hepatitis may include, but are not limited to, those presented in NCP 41-1.

■ Planning

The overall goals are that the patient with viral hepatitis will (1) have relief of discomfort, (2) be able to resume normal activities, and (3) return to normal liver function without complications.

■ Nursing Implementation

Health Promotion. Viral hepatitis is a community health problem. The nurse must assume a significant role in the control and prevention of this disease. It is helpful to first understand the epidemiology of the different types of viral hepatitis before considering appropriate control measures.

Hepatitis A. Outbreaks of viral hepatitis are usually due to HAV. Preventive measures include personal and environmental hygiene and health education to promote good sanitation (see Table 41-9). Hand washing is essential and is probably the most important precaution. Health teaching should include careful hand washing after bowel movements and before eating. When hepatitis A occurs in a food handler, IG should be administered to all other food handlers at the establishment. Patrons may also need to be given IG.

Isolation is not required for hepatitis A. For a patient with hepatitis A, infection control precautions should be used (see Table 11-19). A private room is indicated if the patient is incontinent of stool or has poor personal hygiene. Hand washing is essential.

Hepatitis B. Control and prevention of hepatitis B focuses on identification of possible exposure via percutaneous and sexual transmission (Table 41-9). The nurse must be aware of the individuals at high risk of contracting hepatitis B and teach methods to reduce risks. These include patients receiving frequent transfusions or hemodialysis, workers in hemodialysis units and blood chemistry laboratories, IV drug users, persons with multiple sexual partners, prison inmates, and household members and sexual partners of HBV carriers.

Good hygienic practices, including hand washing and the use of gloves when expecting contact with blood, are important. A condom is advised for sexual intercourse, and the partner should be vaccinated. Razors, toothbrushes, and other personal items should not be shared. Close contacts of the patient with hepatitis B who are HBsAg negative and antibody negative should be vaccinated.

According to CDC guidelines, infection control precautions should be followed for the patient with hepatitis B. This includes the use of disposable needles and syringes, which should be disposed of in puncture-resistant disposal units without recapping, bending, or breaking. (See Table 11-19 for various types of infection control precautions.) Preventive and control measures for hepatitis A and B are summarized in Table 41-9.

Hepatitis C. The primary measures to prevent hepatitis C are screening of blood, organ, and tissue donors; use of infection control precautions; and modification of high-risk behavior (see Table 41-9).

Acute Intervention

Jaundice. The nurse should assess for the degree of jaundice. In light-skinned persons the jaundice is usually observed first in the sclera of the eyes and later in the skin. In dark-skinned persons, jaundice is observed in the hard palate of the mouth and inner canthus of the eyes. Ictotest reagent tablets may be used to detect urinary bilirubin. The urine may be cola colored or mahogany because of the presence of bilirubin. Comfort measures to relieve pruritus (if present), headache, and arthralgias are helpful (see NCP 41-1).

Ensuring that the patient receives adequate nutrients is not always easy. The anorexia and extreme distaste for food cause nutritional problems. Dietary assessment must be considered. The nurse should try to determine whether there is something that appeals to the patient in spite of the anorexia. Small,

41-1   NURSING CARE PLAN   PATIENT WITH VIRAL HEPATITIS

| Expected Patient Outcomes | Nursing Interventions and *Rationales* |

NURSING DIAGNOSIS **Altered nutrition: less than body requirements** *related to* anorexia, nausea, and altered metabolism of nutrients by liver *as manifested by* inadequate food intake; aversion to eating; actual or potential metabolic needs in excess of intake.

- Adequate nutritional intake.
- Maintenance of normal body weight.

- Assess patient's appetite and adequacy of intake *so appropriate interventions can be planned.*
- Offer frequent small feedings, provide oral care before meals *to enhance patient's dietary intake.*
- Allow patient to choose food items; serve high-carbohydrate and high-protein foods at time of day patient feels most like eating *to increase likelihood of adequate intake.*
- Provide attractively served meals in pleasant surroundings *to stimulate patient's appetite.*
- Take weight daily on same scale, at same time, with same clothing *to monitor weight loss secondary to poor appetite.*

NURSING DIAGNOSIS **Activity intolerance** *related to* fatigue and weakness *as manifested by* verbal report of fatigue or weakness, altered response to activity (as measured by BP, pulse, respiratory rate).

- Increased tolerance for activity.

- Provide rest periods.
- Increase patient's activity gradually as allowed and tolerated *so previous activity pattern can be resumed.*
- Conserve patient's strength by careful monitoring activity *to prevent increasing weakness and fatigue.*
- Teach patient to monitor and control activities that provoke fatigue *so patient can be an active participant in plan.*

NURSING DIAGNOSIS **Body image disturbance** *related to* stigma of having a communicable disease, change in appearance (jaundice), and possible alterations in lifestyle and roles (alcohol consumption, drug use, restriction of sexual activity) *as manifested by* negative verbal or nonverbal response to actual or perceived changes.

- Positive adaptation to changes in appearance.
- Verbalization of understanding of body changes.

- Assist patient in expressing feelings and assess patient's feelings about disease process and appearance *to plan appropriate interventions.*
- Clarify misconceptions regarding limitations *to avoid unnecessary restrictions on patient's activities.*
- Encourage participation in self-care *to foster independence and self-esteem.*
- Instruct patient in ways to prevent spread of hepatitis *to reduce fear and guilt associated with potential for infecting others.*
- Encourage patient to ask questions *because accurate information fosters good decision making.*

NURSING DIAGNOSIS **Ineffective management of therapeutic regimen** *related to* lack of knowledge of follow-up care *as manifested by* frequent questions about transmission of disease, activities allowed, and general follow-up care.

- Verbalization of understanding of follow-up care.
- Plan for follow-up visit with health care provider.

- Teach patient basic facts about illness, modes of transmission, diet, activities allowed, avoidance of alcohol, and need for follow-up care *so appropriate follow-up care will be planned and carried out.*
- Teach patient to watch for and report signs of complications such as bleeding gums or bloody stools, worsening of symptoms *to enable prompt intervention.* Emphasize the importance of adequate rest *to enable liver to repair itself and to prevent relapse.*

NURSING DIAGNOSIS **Risk for infection transmission** *related to* lack of knowledge about source of and prevention of infection.

- Able to explain methods of disease transmission and methods of preventing transmission to others.

- Teach about the causative agent *because teaching varies depending on the specific cause.*
- Teach use of infection control precautions *to reduce risk of cross-contamination.*
- Explain the mode of infection transmission *to enable patient to prevent spread of hepatitis.*
- Depending on type of hepatitis, for example, encourage possible hepatitis A contact to have immune globulin *to prevent infection from hepatitis A virus.*

Table 41-9   Preventive Measures for Viral Hepatitis

Hepatitis A	Hepatitis B and C

General Measures
Hand washing
Proper personal hygiene
Environmental sanitation
Control and screening (signs, symptoms) of food handlers
Serologic screening while carrying virus
Active immunization: HAV vaccine to anyone over age 2
 	
Use of Immune Globulin
Early administration (1-2 wk after exposure) to those exposed
Use of prophylaxis for travelers to areas where hepatitis A is common
	Percutaneous Transmission
	Screening of donated blood
	  B—HBsAg
	  C—anti-HCV
	Use of disposable needles and syringes
	
	Sexual Transmission
	Acute exposure: HBIG administration to sexual partner of HBsAg-positive person
	Administer hepatitis B vaccine series to uninfected sexual partners
	Use condoms for sexual intercourse
	
	General Measures
	Hand washing
	Avoid sharing toothbrushes and razors
	HBIG administration for one-time exposure (needle stick, contact of mucous membranes with infectious material)
	Active immunization: HBV vaccine

Table 41-10   Measures to Prevent Transmission of Hepatitis Viruses from Patients to Health Care Personnel*

Hepatitis A	Hepatitis B	Hepatitis C
Always maintain good personal hygiene. Wash hands after contact with a patient or removal of gloves. Use infection control precautions.[†]	Use infection control precautions.[†] Wash hands. Reduce contact with blood or blood-containing secretions. Handle the blood of patients as potentially infective. Dispose of needles properly. Administer HBV vaccine to all health care personnel. Use needleless IV access devices when available.	Use infection control precautions.[†] Wash hands. Reduce contact with blood or blood-contaminated secretions. Handle the blood of patients as potentially infective. Dispose of needles properly. Use needleless IV access devices when available.

*A suggested guideline for general practice to prevent the nurse from contracting viral hepatitis from diagnosed and undiagnosed patients and carriers is for the nurse to wear disposable gloves, goggles, gowns (sometimes) when fecal or blood contamination is likely in handling (1) soiled bedpans, urinals, and catheters and (2) patient's bed linens soiled by body excreta or secretions.

[†]See Table 11-19.

frequent meals may be preferable to three large ones and may also help prevent nausea. Frequently, a patient with hepatitis finds that anorexia is not as severe in the morning, so it is easier to eat a good breakfast than a large dinner. Measures to stimulate the appetite, such as mouth care, antiemetics, and attractively served meals in pleasant surroundings, should be included in the nursing care plan. Other measures that may be tried to counteract the anorexia are carbonated beverages and avoidance of very hot or very cold foods. Adequate fluid intake is important (2500 to 3000 ml per day).

Rest.   Rest is essential and is an important factor in promoting liver cell regeneration. The nurse must assess the patient's response to the rest and activity plan and modify it accordingly. The care plan should include appropriate time schedules for rest and activity, with scheduled rest periods uninterrupted by visitors or nursing staff. If the patient is on strict bed rest, measures to prevent respiratory and circulatory complications should be initiated. Assessment of the liver function tests and symptoms should continue as a guide to activity.

Psychologic and emotional rest are as essential as physical rest. Strict bed rest may produce anxiety and extreme restlessness in some patients and may be more damaging than reasonable ambulation. Diversional activities, such as reading and hobbies (e.g., knitting, stamp collecting), may help the patient. The patient should be assisted to understand the temporary nature of symptoms during the period of communicability.

Ambulatory and Home Care.   Most patients with viral hepatitis will be cared for at home, so the nurse must assess the patient's knowledge of nutrition and provide the necessary dietary teaching. Rest and adequate nutrition are especially important until studies show that liver function has returned to normal. The patient must be cautioned about overexertion and the need to follow the physician's advice about when it is safe to return to work. The nurse must also teach the patient and family about preventive measures and how to prevent transmission to other family members. The patient should know what symptoms need to be reported to the physician.

The patient should be assessed for any manifestations indicative of complications. Bleeding tendencies with increasing prothrombin time values, symptoms of encephalopathy, or abnormal liver function tests indicate problems, and the patient should be assessed and treated promptly.

The patient should be instructed to have regular follow-up for at least 1 year after the diagnosis of hepatitis. Because relapses are fairly common with hepatitis B and C, the patient should be instructed about symptoms of recurrence. Alcohol should be avoided for 1 year because it is detoxified in the liver and may interfere with recovery.

A patient who remains positive for HBsAg is a carrier and should never be a blood donor. The patient with hepatitis B should also be instructed to use condoms when engaging in sexual intercourse until tests for HBsAg are negative.

The patient who is receiving α-interferon for the treatment of hepatitis B or C requires education regarding the medication. α-Interferon is administered intramuscularly or subcutaneously, and thus the patient or family member needs to be taught how to administer the drug. There are numerous side effects with the therapy, including flulike symptoms (fever, malaise, fatigue, chills). The physician may recommend that acetaminophen be administered 30 to 60 minutes before injection to reduce these symptoms. Other significant side effects include thrombocytopenia, neutropenia, psychologic disturbances (mood swings, depression) and limited alopecia (see Table 41-7). (Additional information on α-interferon is presented in Chapters 10 and 12.)

■ Evaluation

Expected outcomes for the patient with hepatitis are addressed in NCP 41-1.

Control of Hepatitis in Health Care Personnel

Hepatitis A. Hepatitis A is rarely transmitted from patients to health care personnel. When this does occur, it is associated with patients with undiagnosed hepatitis A who are treated for other problems. Usually these patients are incontinent of feces. The use of infection control precautions should prevent transmission of HAV to health care personnel.

Hepatitis B. Health care workers may be exposed to HBV from needle sticks or blood contamination to mucous membranes or nonintact skin. If a health care worker is exposed to HBV through a needle stick and does not receive the vaccine, there is a 6% to 30% chance of infection with hepatitis B.[1] Vaccination is the most effective method to prevent hepatitis B in health care workers. Employers are required by the Occupational Safety and Health Administration (OSHA) to provide free HBV immunization to employees at risk for infection.

The principal mode of transmission of HBV for health care personnel is parenteral. Examples of parenteral transmission include accidental needle sticks and, rarely, transfusion of contaminated blood or blood products. Because all blood and blood products are tested for HBV and anti-HCV, there is diminishing risk of this latter mode of transmission. Other forms of transmission include contamination of fresh cutaneous scratches or abrasions, burns, and contamination of mucosal surfaces with infective blood, blood products, saliva, or semen.

Hepatitis C. Transmission is usually due to percutaneous needle exposure or other blood exposure and undetected parenteral transmission. Measures to prevent transmission of the viruses from patients to health care personnel are presented in Table 41-10. Very rarely do health care workers infect patient contacts.

TOXIC AND DRUG-INDUCED HEPATITIS

Liver injury and death may occur after the inhalation, parenteral injection, or ingestion of certain chemical substances (see Table 37-6). The two major types of chemical hepatotoxicity are toxic and drug-induced hepatitis. Agents producing toxic hepatitis are generally systemic poisons (e.g., carbon tetrachloride, gold compounds) or are converted in the liver to toxic metabolites (e.g., acetaminophen). Liver necrosis generally occurs within 2 to 3 days of acute exposure to a toxic substance.

Idiosyncratic drug reactions produce drug-induced hepatitis. Such agents as halothane, isoniazid (INH), chlorothiazides (e.g., Diuril), methotrexate, and methyldopa (Aldomet) may produce idiosyncratic reactions because of patient susceptibility (metabolic reactivity) to these agents or immunologically mediated hypersensitivity responses. Liver injury may occur at any time during or shortly after exposure. Some responses occur 2 to 5 weeks after exposure.

Older patients are particularly vulnerable to drug-induced hepatitis. This is due to several factors, including increased use of prescription and over-the-counter drugs, which can lead to drug interactions and potential drug toxicity. Age-related decreases in liver function caused by decreased liver blood flow and enzyme activity result in decreased drug metabolism. In addition, with aging there is a decreased ability of the liver to recover from drug-induced injury.

Toxic and drug-induced hepatitis are similar to viral hepatitis in the pathophysiologic changes in the liver and the clinical manifestations. The usual presenting clinical findings are anorexia, nausea, vomiting, hepatomegaly, splenomegaly, and abnormal liver function studies. Treatment is largely supportive as in acute viral hepatitis. Recovery may be rapid if the hepatotoxin is identified and removed. Liver transplantation may be necessary.

IDIOPATHIC HEPATITIS

Chronic active hepatitis may also occur in a number of patients who have no known risk factors for the development of viral hepatitis. The cause of this form of hepatitis is idiopathic. However, because many of these patients often have a number of systemic problems, including glomerulonephritis and arthritis, the disease is thought to be autoimmune. The presenting signs and symptoms are variable and similar to viral hepatitis. Laboratory tests (elevation of liver enzymes) reveal liver inflammation without evidence of viral antigens. The majority (70% to 80%) of patients who are diagnosed with autoimmune hepatitis are women. The course of the disease is also variable, with the majority of the patients exhibiting chronic active hepatitis.

Unlike viral hepatitis, autoimmune hepatitis (in which there is evidence of necrosis and cirrhosis) is treated with cortico-

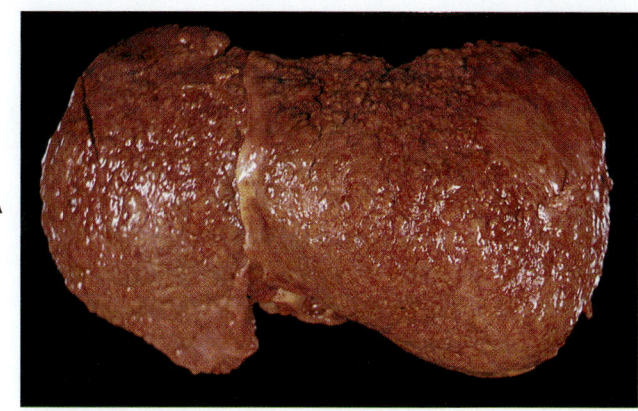

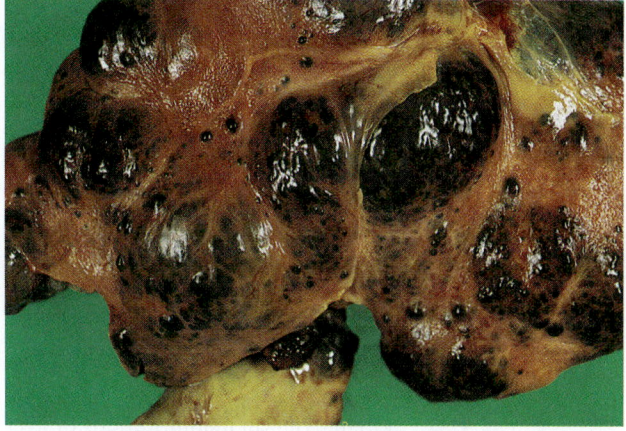

Fig. 41-4 Cirrhosis. **A,** Micronodular cirrhosis. **B,** Macronodular cirrhosis.

steroids or other immunosuppressive agents. Daily treatment with methylprednisolone is the first line of therapy for nonviral chronic active hepatitis. Azathioprine (Imuran) may also be used to treat the disease.

CIRRHOSIS OF THE LIVER

Cirrhosis is a chronic progressive disease of the liver characterized by extensive degeneration and destruction of the liver parenchymal cells (Fig. 41-4). The liver cells attempt to regenerate, but the regenerative process is disorganized, resulting in abnormal blood vessel and bile duct relationships from the fibrosis. The overgrowth of new and fibrous connective tissue distorts the liver's normal lobular structure, resulting in lobules of irregular size and shape with impeded vascular flow. Cirrhosis may have an insidious, prolonged course.

Cirrhosis is ranked as the ninth leading cause of death in the United States and the fourth leading cause of death in persons between 35 and 54 years of age. The highest incidence occurs between the ages of 40 and 60, and it is twice as common in men as in women. Excessive alcohol ingestion is the single most common cause of cirrhosis.

Etiology and Pathophysiology

The four types of cirrhosis, in order of incidence, are as follows:

1. *Alcoholic* (previously called *Laënnec's*), also called portal or nutritional cirrhosis, is usually associated with alcohol abuse. The first change in the liver from excessive alcohol intake is an accumulation of fat in the liver cells. Uncomplicated fatty changes in the liver are potentially reversible if the person stops drinking alcohol. If the alcohol abuse continues, widespread scar formation occurs throughout the liver.
2. *Postnecrotic cirrhosis* is a complication of viral, toxic, or idiopathic (autoimmune) hepatitis. Broad bands of scar tissue form within the liver.
3. *Biliary cirrhosis* is associated with chronic biliary obstruction and infection. There is diffuse fibrosis of the liver with jaundice as the main feature.
4. *Cardiac cirrhosis* results from long-standing, severe right-sided heart failure in patients with cor pulmonale, constrictive pericarditis, and tricuspid insufficiency.

In cirrhosis, cell necrosis occurs, and the destroyed liver cells are replaced by scar tissue. The normal lobular architecture becomes nodular. Eventually irregular, disorganized regeneration; poor cellular nutrition; and hypoxia caused by inadequate blood flow and scar tissue result in decreased functioning of the liver.

The specific cause of cirrhosis may not be determined in all patients. It is known that cirrhosis occurs with greatest frequency among alcoholics. There continues to be some controversy as to whether the cause is the alcohol or the malnutrition that frequently coexists with chronic ingestion of alcohol. A common problem in alcoholics is protein malnutrition. There have been cases of nutritional cirrhosis resulting from extreme dieting or malnutrition. It is believed that the combined impact of malnutrition and alcohol is especially damaging to hepatocytes. Alcohol alone has a direct hepatotoxic effect. It is known to produce necrosis of cells and fatty infiltration with formation of fibrous septa. Some persons seem to have a predisposition to cirrhosis, regardless of their dietary or alcohol intake.

Clinical Manifestations

Early Manifestations. The onset of cirrhosis is usually insidious. Occasionally there is an abrupt onset of symptoms. GI disturbances are common early symptoms and include anorexia, dyspepsia, flatulence, nausea and vomiting, and change in bowel habits (diarrhea or constipation). These symptoms occur as a result of the liver's altered metabolism of carbohydrates, fats, and proteins. The patient may complain of abdominal pain described as a dull, heavy feeling in the right upper quadrant or epigastrium. The pain may be due to swelling and stretching of the liver capsule, spasm of the biliary ducts, and intermittent vascular spasm. Other early manifestations are fever, lassitude, slight weight loss, and enlargement of the liver and spleen. The liver is palpable in many patients with cirrhosis.

Later Manifestations. Later symptoms may be severe and result from liver failure and portal hypertension. Jaundice, peripheral edema, and ascites develop gradually. Other late symptoms include skin lesions, hematologic disorders, endocrine disturbances, and peripheral neuropathies (Fig. 41-5). In the advanced stages the liver becomes small and nodular.

Jaundice. Jaundice results from the functional derangement of liver cells and compression of bile ducts by connective tissue overgrowth. Jaundice occurs as a result of the decreased

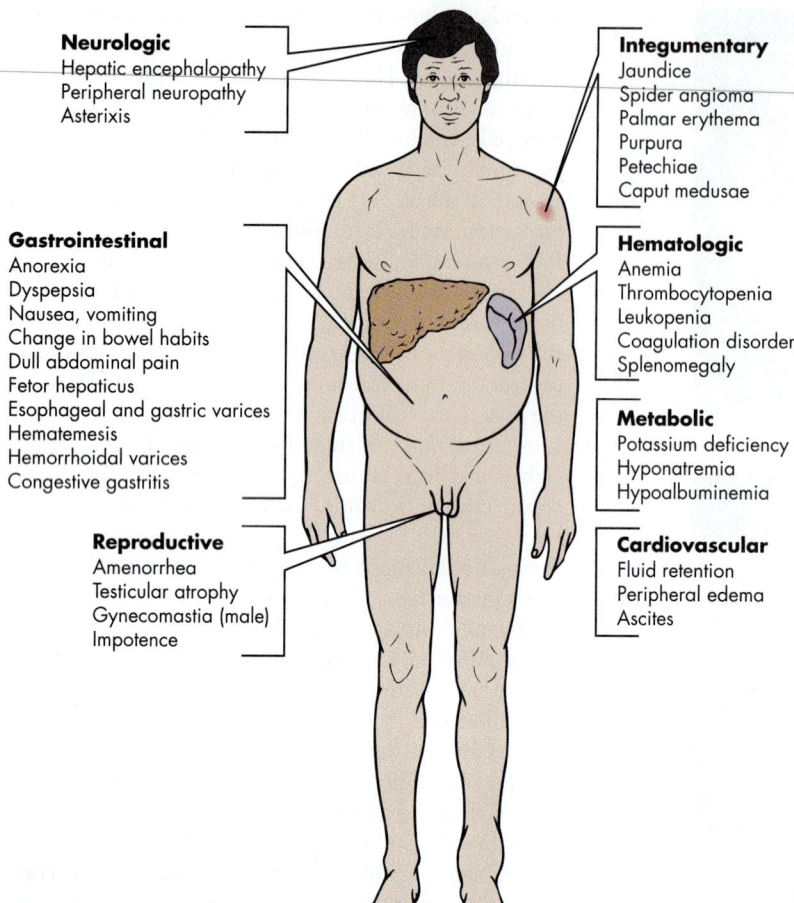

Neurologic
Hepatic encephalopathy
Peripheral neuropathy
Asterixis

Gastrointestinal
Anorexia
Dyspepsia
Nausea, vomiting
Change in bowel habits
Dull abdominal pain
Fetor hepaticus
Esophageal and gastric varices
Hematemesis
Hemorrhoidal varices
Congestive gastritis

Reproductive
Amenorrhea
Testicular atrophy
Gynecomastia (male)
Impotence

Integumentary
Jaundice
Spider angioma
Palmar erythema
Purpura
Petechiae
Caput medusae

Hematologic
Anemia
Thrombocytopenia
Leukopenia
Coagulation disorders
Splenomegaly

Metabolic
Potassium deficiency
Hyponatremia
Hypoalbuminemia

Cardiovascular
Fluid retention
Peripheral edema
Ascites

Fig. 41-5   Systemic clinical manifestations of liver cirrhosis.

ability to conjugate and excrete bilirubin (hepatocellular jaundice). The jaundice may be minimal or severe, depending on the degree of liver damage. If obstruction of the biliary tract occurs, obstructive jaundice may also occur and is usually accompanied by pruritus. The pruritus is due to an accumulation of bile salts underneath the skin.

Skin lesions. Various skin manifestations are commonly seen in cirrhosis. *Spider angiomas* (*telangiectasia* or *spider nevi*) are small, dilated blood vessels with a bright-red center point and spider-like branches. They occur on the nose, cheeks, upper trunk, neck, and shoulders. *Palmar erythema* (a red area that blanches with pressure) is located on the palms of the hands. Both of these lesions are attributed to an increase in circulating estrogen as a result of the damaged liver's inability to metabolize steroids.

Hematologic problems. Hematologic problems include thrombocytopenia, leukopenia, anemia, and coagulation disorders. Thrombocytopenia, leukopenia, and anemia are probably caused by the splenomegaly. Splenomegaly results from backup of blood from the portal vein into the spleen. Overactivity of the enlarged spleen results in increased removal of blood cells from circulation. The anemia is also due to inadequate red blood cell production and survival. Other factors involved in the anemia relate to poor diet, poor absorption of folic acid, and bleeding from varices.

The coagulation problems result from the liver's inability to produce prothrombin and other factors essential for blood clotting. Coagulation problems are manifested by hemorrhagic phenomena or bleeding tendencies, such as epistaxis, purpura, petechiae, easy bruising, gingival bleeding, and heavy menstrual bleeding.

Endocrine disturbances. Several signs and symptoms relating to the metabolism and inactivation of adrenocortical hormones, estrogen, and testosterone occur in cirrhosis. Normally the liver metabolizes these hormones. When the damaged liver is unable to do this, various manifestations occur. In men, gynecomastia, loss of axillary and pubic hair, testicular atrophy, and impotence with loss of libido may occur as a result of estrogen accumulation. In younger women amenorrhea may occur, and in older females there may be vaginal bleeding. The liver fails to metabolize aldosterone adequately, and this results in hyperaldosteronism with subsequent sodium and water retention and potassium loss.

Peripheral neuropathy. Peripheral neuropathy is a common finding in alcoholic cirrhosis. It is probably due to a dietary deficiency of thiamine, folic acid, and cobalamin (vitamin B_{12}). The neuropathy usually results in mixed nervous system symptoms, but sensory symptoms may predominate. Clinical manifestations of cirrhosis of the liver are numerous and may eventually involve the total body (see Fig. 41-5).

Complications

Major complications of cirrhosis are portal hypertension with resultant esophageal varices, peripheral edema and ascites, hepatic encephalopathy (coma), and hepatorenal syndrome.

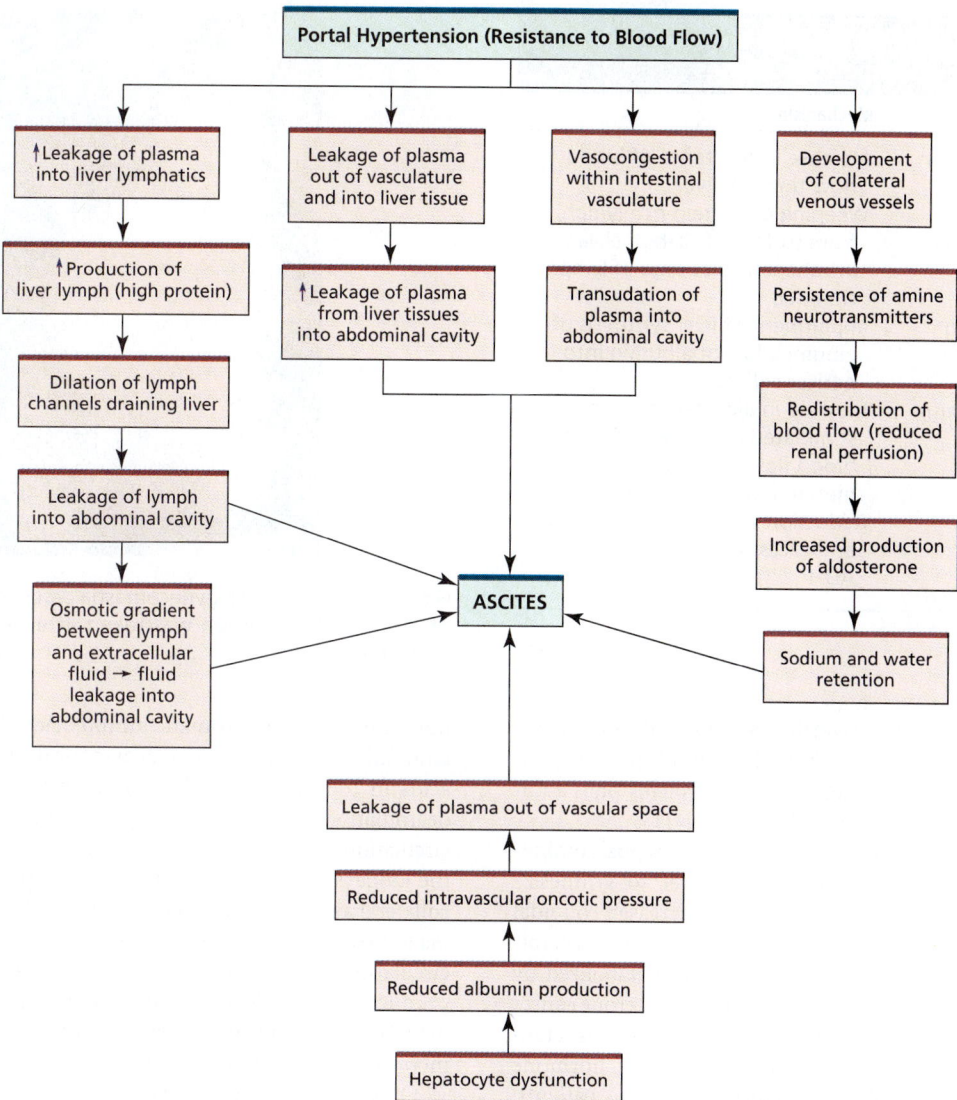

Fig. 41-6   Mechanisms for development of ascites.

Portal Hypertension and Esophageal Varices. Because of the structural changes in the liver from the cirrhotic process, there is compression and destruction of the portal and hepatic veins and sinusoids. These changes result in obstruction to the normal flow of blood through the portal system, resulting in portal hypertension. Many pathophysiologic changes result from portal hypertension. Collateral circulation develops in an attempt to reduce this high portal pressure and also to reduce the increased plasma volume and lymphatic flow. The common areas where the collateral channels form are in the lower esophagus (the anastomosis of the left gastric vein and the azygos veins), the anterior abdominal wall, the parietal peritoneum, and the rectum. Varicosities may develop in areas where the collateral and systemic circulations communicate, resulting in esophageal and gastric varices, caput medusae (ring of varices around the umbilicus), and hemorrhoids.

Esophageal varices are a common complication, occurring in two thirds to three fourths of patients with cirrhosis. These collateral vessels contain little elastic tissue and are quite fragile. They tolerate the high pressure poorly, and the result is distended, tortuous veins that bleed easily. Large varices are more likely to bleed.

Bleeding esophageal varices are the most life-threatening complication of cirrhosis. The mortality rate for hemorrhage of esophageal varices is 30% to 60%.[18] The varices rupture and bleed in response to ulceration and irritation. Factors producing ulceration and irritation include alcohol ingestion; swallowing of poorly masticated food; ingestion of coarse food; acid regurgitation from the stomach; and increased intraabdominal pressure caused by nausea, vomiting, straining at stool, coughing, sneezing, or lifting heavy objects. The patient may have melena or hematemesis. There may be slow oozing or massive hemorrhage. Massive hemorrhage is a medical emergency.

Peripheral Edema and Ascites. Peripheral edema sometimes precedes ascites, but in some patients its development coincides with or occurs after ascites. Edema results from decreased colloidal osmotic pressure from impaired liver synthesis of albumin and increased portocaval pressure from portal hypertension. Peripheral edema occurs as ankle and presacral edema.

Ascites is the accumulation of serous fluid in the peritoneal or abdominal cavity. It is a common manifestation of cirrhosis. When the blood pressure is elevated in the liver, as occurs in portal cirrhosis, proteins move from the blood vessels via the larger pores of the sinusoids (capillaries) into the lymph space (Fig. 41-6).

Table **41-11**	Factors Involved in the Development of Ascites
Factor	**Mechanism**
Portal hypertension	Increase in resistance of blood flow through liver
Increased flow of hepatic lymph	Weeping of protein-rich lymph from surface of cirrhotic liver, intrahepatic blockage of lymph channels
Decreased serum colloidal oncotic pressure	Impairment of liver synthesis of albumin, loss of albumin into peritoneal cavity
Hyperaldosteronism	Increase in aldosterone secretion stimulated by decreased renal blood flow, impairment of liver metabolism of aldosterone
Impaired water excretion	Reduction in renal vascular flow and excessive serum levels of ADH

ADH, antidiuretic hormone.

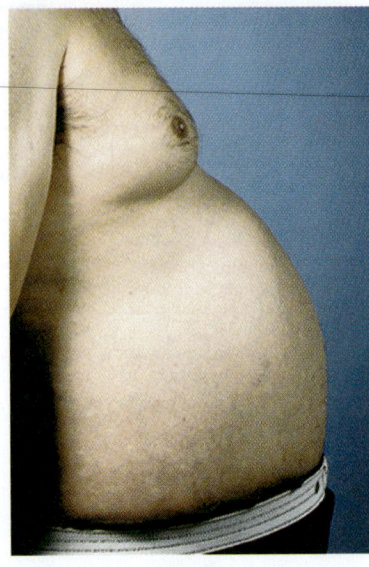

Fig. 41-7   Ascites and gynecomastia associated with cirrhosis of the liver. Photograph was taken after a paracentesis was performed.

When the lymphatic system is unable to carry off the excess proteins and water, they leak through the liver capsule into the peritoneal cavity. The osmotic pressure of the proteins pulls additional fluid into the peritoneal cavity (Table 41-11).

A second mechanism of ascites formation is hypoalbuminemia resulting from the inability of the liver to synthesize albumin. The hypoalbuminemia results in decreased colloidal osmotic pressure. A third mechanism of ascites, hyperaldosteronism, results when aldosterone is not metabolized by damaged hepatocytes. The increased level of aldosterone causes increased sodium reabsorption by the renal tubules. This retention of sodium, as well as an increase in antidiuretic hormone (ADH), causes additional water retention in these patients. Because of edema formation there is decreased intravascular volume and subsequently decreased renal blood flow and glomerular filtration.

Ascites is manifested by abdominal distention with weight gain (Fig. 41-7). If the ascites is severe, the umbilicus may be everted. Abdominal striae with distended abdominal wall veins may be present. The patient has signs of dehydration (e.g., dry tongue and skin, sunken eyeballs, muscle weakness). There is also a decrease in urinary output. Hypokalemia is common and is due to an excessive loss of potassium because of the effects of aldosterone. Low potassium levels can also result from diuretic therapy used to treat the ascites.

Hepatic Encephalopathy. Hepatic encephalopathy, or coma, is a frequent terminal complication in liver disease. *Encephalopathy* is a more descriptive term than *coma*. Hepatic encephalopathy can occur in any condition in which liver damage causes ammonia to enter the systemic circulation without liver detoxification. There is a high mortality rate associated with hepatic encephalopathy.

The pathogenesis of hepatic encephalopathy is incompletely understood at this time. A number of etiologic factors may be involved. It is basically a disorder of protein metabolism and excretion. The main pathogenic agents appear to be nitrogenous ammonia and aromatic amino acids. A major source of ammonia is the bacterial and enzymatic deamination of amino acids in the intestines. The ammonia that results from this deamination process normally goes to the liver via the portal circulation and is converted to urea, which is then excreted by the kidneys. When the blood is shunted past the liver via the collateral anastomoses or the liver is unable to convert ammonia to urea, large quantities of ammonia remain in the systemic circulation. The ammonia crosses the blood-brain barrier and produces neurologic toxic manifestations. A number of factors may precipitate hepatic encephalopathy, mostly because they increase the amount of circulating ammonia (Table 41-12).

Other metabolic products that may contribute to hepatic encephalopathy are mercaptans (such as methionine) and short-chain fatty acids. Another theory is that the liver may produce substances necessary for normal brain functioning. When the diseased liver can no longer produce these substances, encephalopathy may result.

Clinical manifestations of encephalopathy are changes in neurologic and mental responsiveness, ranging from lethargy to deep coma. Changes may occur suddenly because of an increase in ammonia in response to bleeding varices or gradually as blood ammonia levels slowly increase. In the early stages, manifestations include euphoria, depression, apathy, irritability, memory loss, confusion, yawning, drowsiness, insomnia, agitation, slow and slurred speech, emotional lability, impaired judgment, hiccups, slow and deep respirations, hyperactive reflexes, and a positive Babinski's reflex.

Clinical manifestations of impending coma include disorientation as to time, place, or person. A characteristic symptom is *asterixis,* or flapping tremors (liver flap). This may take several forms, the most common involving the arms and hands. When asked to hold the arms and hands stretched out, the patient is unable to hold this position and there will be a series of rapid flexion and extension movements of the hands. Other signs of asterixis are rhythmic movements of the legs with dorsiflexion

Table 41-12	Factors Precipitating Hepatic Encephalopathy
Factor	**Mechanism**
GI hemorrhage	Increase in ammonia in GI tract
Constipation	Increase in ammonia from bacterial action on feces
Hypokalemia	Potassium ions are needed by brain to metabolize ammonia
Hypovolemia	Increase in blood ammonia by causing hepatic hypoxia; impairment of cerebral, hepatic, and renal function because of decreased blood flow
Infection	Increase in catabolism, increase in cerebral sensitivity to toxins
Cerebral depressants (e.g., narcotics)	No detoxification by liver, causing increase in cerebral depression
Metabolic alkalosis	Facilitation of transport of ammonia across blood-brain barrier, increase in renal production of ammonia
Paracentesis	Loss of sodium and potassium ions, decrease in blood volume
Dehydration	Potentiation of ammonia toxicity
Increased metabolism	Increase in workload of liver
Diuretics	Increase in renal formation of ammonia, possibly resulting in azotemia, which increases endogenous ammonia production; hypokalemia also possible
Uremia (renal failure)	Retention of nitrogenous metabolites

Table 41-13	Bilirubin Metabolism Abnormalities in Cirrhosis*	
Type		**Finding**
Serum bilirubin		
Unconjugated		↑↓
Conjugated		↑↓
Urine bilirubin		↑↓
Urobilinogen		
Stool		Normal, ↓↑
Urine		Normal, ↑↓

*These are bilirubin metabolism abnormalities occurring with hepatocellular jaundice, the most frequent type of jaundice with cirrhosis.

Diagnostic Studies

A liver profile in cirrhosis demonstrates abnormalities in most of the liver function studies (see Table 37-13). Enzyme levels, including alkaline phosphatase, aspartate aminotransferase (AST) (serum glutamic-oxaloacetic transaminase [SGOT]), alanine aminotransferase (ALT) (serum glutamate pyruvate transaminase [SGPT]), and γ-glutamyltransferase (GGT), are elevated because of the release of these enzymes from damaged liver cells. Protein metabolism tests show decreased total protein, decreased albumin, and increased globulin levels. The liver does not synthesize γ-globulins but does synthesize albumin. γ-Globulins (antibodies) are produced by B lymphocytes in the lymphatic system and spleen. The globulin level often increases in cirrhosis and indicates increased synthesis or decreased removal. Fat metabolism abnormalities are reflected by decreased cholesterol levels. The prothrombin time is prolonged, and bilirubin metabolism is altered (Table 41-13). Liver biopsy may be performed to identify liver cell changes and alterations in the lobular structure. Differential analysis of ascitic fluid may be helpful in establishing a diagnosis.

Collaborative Care

Rest. Although there is no specific therapy for cirrhosis, certain measures can be taken to promote liver cell regeneration and prevent or treat complications (Table 41-14). Rest is significant in reducing metabolic demands of the liver and allowing for recovery of liver cells. At various times during the progress of cirrhosis the rest may have to take the form of complete bed rest.

Ascites. Management of ascites is focused on sodium restriction, diuretics, and fluid removal. A low-sodium diet is prescribed (250 to 500 mg per day). The patient is usually not on restricted fluids unless severe ascites develops. There should be accurate assessment and control of fluid and electrolyte balance. Bed rest initially produces diuresis, which increases fluid excretion. Salt-poor albumin may be used to help maintain intravascular volume and adequate urinary output by increasing plasma colloid osmotic pressure.

Diuretic therapy is an important part of management. Frequently a combination of drugs that work at multiple sites in the nephron is more effective. Spironolactone (Aldactone) is an effective diuretic, even in patients with severe sodium retention. Spironolactone is an antagonist of aldosterone and is

of the foot and rhythmic movements in the face with strong closure of the eyelids. Impairments in writing involve difficulty in moving the pen or pencil from left to right and apraxia (the inability to construct simple figures). Other signs include hyperventilation, hypothermia, and grimacing and grasping reflexes.

Fetor hepaticus occurs in some patients with encephalopathy. It is a musty, sweet odor of the patient's breath. This odor is from the accumulation of digestive by-products that the liver is unable to degrade.

Hepatorenal Syndrome. Hepatorenal syndrome is a serious complication of cirrhosis. It is characterized by functional renal failure with advancing azotemia, oliguria, and intractable ascites. There is no structural abnormality of the kidneys. The exact cause of the decreased renal function is unknown but is thought to be related to a redistribution of blood flow from the kidneys to peripheral and splanchnic circulations or hypovolemia secondary to ascites. In the patient with cirrhosis the syndrome frequently follows diuretic therapy, GI hemorrhage, or paracentesis. Hepatic encephalopathy is also associated with the deterioration in renal function. Treatment measures include salt-poor albumin, salt and water restrictions, and diuretic therapy. However, treatment is usually unsuccessful.

COLLABORATIVE CARE

Table 41-14   Cirrhosis of the Liver

Diagnostic
- Liver function studies
- Liver biopsy (percutaneous needle)
- Esophagogastroduodenoscopy
- Angiography (percutaneous transhepatic portography)
- Liver scan
- Serum electrolytes
- Prothrombin time
- Serum albumin
- CBC
- Stool for occult blood
- Upper GI barium swallow

Collaborative Therapy

Conservative Therapy
- Administration of B-complex vitamins
- Rest
- Avoidance of alcohol and aspirin

Ascites
- Administration of 3000-calorie, high-carbohydrate, protein (depends on stage), low-fat diet, low sodium for ascites
- Diuretics
  - Spironolactone (Aldactone)
  - Amiloride (Midamor)
  - Triamterene (Dyrenium)
  - Furosemide (Lasix)
- Paracentesis (if indicated)
- Peritoneovenous shunt (if indicated)

Esophageal Varices
- β-adrenergic blockers
- Vasopressin (Pitressin)
- Endoscopic sclerotherapy or ligation
- Balloon tamponade
- Somatostatin
- Surgical shunting procedure
- Transjugular intrahepatic portosystemic shunt

Hepatic Encephalopathy
- Sterilization of GI tract with antibiotics
- Lactulose (Cephulac)
- Levodopa

CBC, complete blood count.

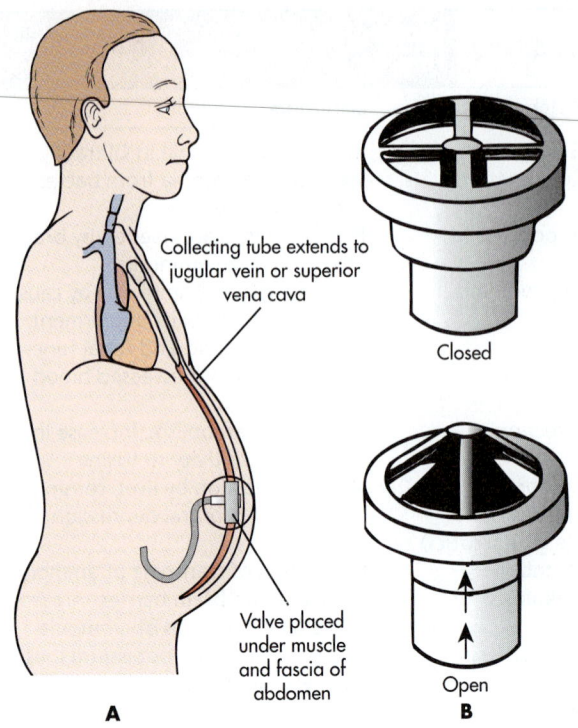

Fig. 41-8   LaVeen continuous peritoneovenous shunt. **A,** Collecting tube. **B,** Valve in closed and open positions.

fluid into the venous system. One type, the LaVeen peritoneovenous shunt, consists of a tube and a one-way valve. The tube runs from the abdominal cavity through the peritoneum, under the subcutaneous tissue, and into the jugular vein or superior vena cava (Fig. 41-8). The valve opens when the pressure in the peritoneal cavity is 3 to 5 cm H_2O higher than that in the superior vena cava. This allows the ascitic fluid to flow into the venous system. The patient's inspiration increases the intraperitoneal pressure, causing the valve to open. Another shunt, the Denver shunt, has a subcutaneous pump that irrigates the tubing when manually compressed. This shunting of the ascitic fluid causes an improvement in hemodynamic factors and increases sodium and fluid excretion. Urine output is also increased.

Esophageal Varices.   The main therapeutic goal related to esophageal varices is avoidance of bleeding and hemorrhage. The patient who has esophageal varices should avoid ingesting alcohol, aspirin, and irritating foods. Upper respiratory infections should be treated promptly, and coughing should be controlled.

Management related to bleeding esophageal varices includes emergency, therapeutic, and prophylactic interventions. Management measures used are vasopressin (VP) and nitroglycerin (NTG), β-adrenergic blockers, balloon tamponade, sclerotherapy, ligation of varices, and shunt therapy.

When esophageal variceal bleeding occurs, the first step is to stabilize the patient and manage the airway. IV therapy is initiated and may include administration of blood products. The next step is to make a definitive diagnosis. This is important because patients with cirrhosis can also bleed from erosive

potassium sparing. Other potassium-sparing diuretics are amiloride (Midamor) and triamterene (Dyrenium). A high-potency loop diuretic, such as furosemide (Lasix), is frequently used in combination with a potassium-sparing drug. Chlorothiazide (Diuril) or hydrochlorothiazide may also be used, but the thiazide diuretics are not as potent as the loop diuretics.

A paracentesis (needle puncture of the abdominal cavity) may be performed to remove ascitic fluid. However, it is reserved for the patient with impaired respiration or abdominal pain caused by severe ascites. It is only a temporary measure because the fluid tends to reaccumulate.

Peritoneovenous shunt.   A surgical procedure, peritoneovenous shunt, provides for the continuous reinfusion of ascitic

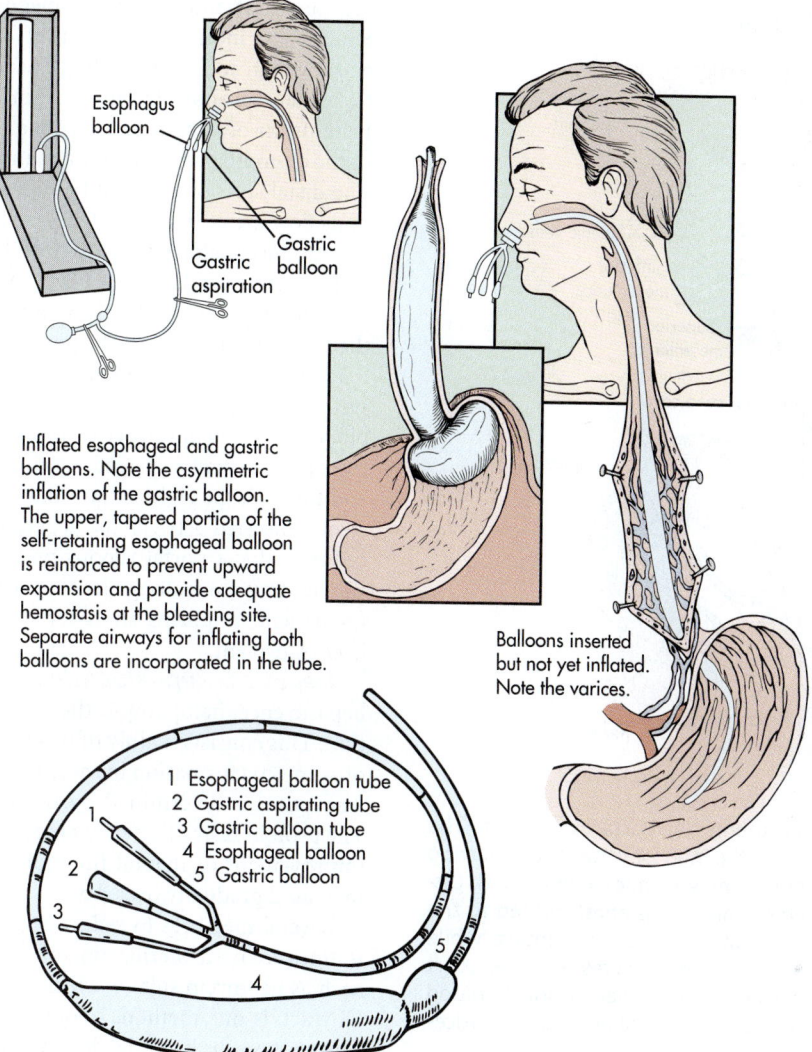

Esophagus balloon

Gastric aspiration

Gastric balloon

Inflated esophageal and gastric balloons. Note the asymmetric inflation of the gastric balloon. The upper, tapered portion of the self-retaining esophageal balloon is reinforced to prevent upward expansion and provide adequate hemostasis at the bleeding site. Separate airways for inflating both balloons are incorporated in the tube.

Balloons inserted but not yet inflated. Note the varices.

1 Esophageal balloon tube
2 Gastric aspirating tube
3 Gastric balloon tube
4 Esophageal balloon
5 Gastric balloon

Fig. 41-9 Esophageal tamponade accomplished with Sengstaken-Blakemore tube.

gastritis, peptic ulcers, and Mallory-Weiss tears. The diagnosis is made by endoscopic examination as soon as possible. Lavage with a wide-bore nasogastric (NG) tube (e.g., Ewald) may be done to remove blood and clots to prepare the patient for endoscopy.

The main goal of drug therapy is to stop bleeding so treatment measures can be done. The initial measures to stop the bleeding include IV administration of VP. VP produces vasoconstriction of the splanchnic arterial bed, decreased portal blood flow, and decreased portal hypertension. It has many side effects, including decreased coronary blood flow and heart rate and increased blood pressure. Current drug therapy in some institutions is a combination of VP and NTG. The NTG reduces the detrimental effects of the VP while enhancing its beneficial effect.

Endoscopic sclerotherapy is a treatment method for both acute and chronic bleeding varices in many institutions. The sclerosing agent, introduced via endoscopy, thromboses and obliterates the distended veins.

Another procedure for managing acute variceal bleeding is endoscopic ligation or banding of the varices. A small rubber band (elastic O-ring) is slipped around the base of the varix.

Endoscopic variceal ligation can be done using clips instead of the O-rings (endoscopic clipping). Endoscopic ligation is as effective as endoscopic sclerotherapy with fewer complications. A combination of endoscopic sclerotherapy and ligation may be used and seems to be more effective than either treatment alone.[19]

Balloon tamponade may be used if sclerotherapy or ligation is unsuccessful. Balloon tamponade controls the hemorrhage by mechanical compression of the varices. The Minnesota or Sengstaken-Blakemore tube is used for this purpose (Fig. 41-9). These tubes have two balloons: gastric and esophageal. The Sengstaken-Blakemore has three lumens: one for the gastric balloon, one for the esophageal balloon, and one for gastric aspiration. The Minnesota tube has an esophageal aspiration port. When inflated, the gastric and esophageal balloons put mechanical compression on the varices. The gastric balloon anchors the tube in position and also applies pressure to any bleeding gastric varices.

Supportive measures during an acute variceal bleed include administration of fresh frozen plasma and packed RBCs, vitamin K (Aquamephyton), and histamine (H_2)

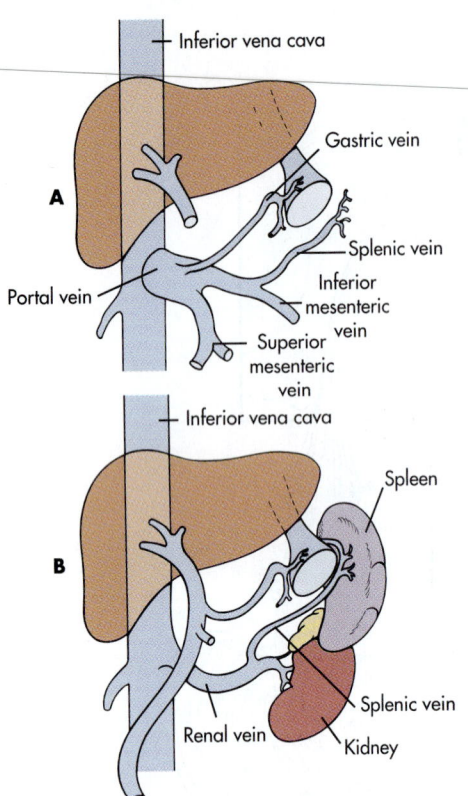

Fig. 41-10 Portosystemic shunts. **A,** Portacaval shunt. The portal vein is anastomosed to the inferior vena cava, diverting blood from the portal vein to the systemic circulation. **B,** Distal splenorenal shunt. The splenic vein is anastomosed to the renal vein. The portal venous flow remains intact while esophageal varices are selectively decompressed. (The short gastric veins are decompressed.) The spleen conducts blood from the high pressure of the esophageal and gastric varices to the low-pressure renal vein.

blockers such as cimetidine (Tagamet). Neomycin administration may be started to prevent hepatic encephalopathy from breakdown of blood and the release of ammonia in the intestine.

Long-term management. Long-term management of patients who have had an episode of bleeding includes β-adrenergic blockers, repeated sclerotherapy, endoscopic ligation, and portosystemic shunts. There is a high incidence of recurrent bleeding with a high mortality risk with each bleeding episode, so continued therapy is necessary. Repeated endoscopic sclerotherapy and ligation is commonly used.

Propranolol (Inderal), a β-adrenergic blocker, can be given orally to prevent recurrent GI bleeding. It reduces portal venous pressure. This effect is due to reduced cardiac output and possibly constriction of splanchnic vessels. However, because it reduces hepatic blood flow, it can enhance the possibility of hepatic encephalopathy.

Various surgical shunting procedures may be used to decrease portal hypertension by diverting some of the portal blood flow while at the same time allowing adequate liver perfusion. Currently, the shunts most commonly used are the por-

tacaval shunt and the distal splenorenal shunt (Fig. 41-10). Shunts are indicated more after a second major bleeding episode than an initial bleeding episode. Although a prophylactic portacaval shunt lessens bleeding, it does not prolong life. Patients die of hepatic encephalopathy caused by the diversion of the ammonia past the liver and into the systemic circulation. The distal splenorenal shunt (Warren shunt) leaves portal venous flow intact (see Fig. 41-10), so it has a lower incidence of hepatic encephalopathy. With time, however, the flow of blood through the liver decreases.

Another procedure for the treatment of esophageal varices is the transjugular intrahepatic portosystemic shunt (TIPS). TIPS is a nonsurgical procedure in which a tract (shunt) between the systemic and portal venous systems is created to redirect portal blood flow. A stent is inserted to support the tract. Under fluoroscopy, the stent is passed via the right internal jugular vein and through the right atrium into the inferior vena cava. The stent is inserted between the hepatic and portal veins. This procedure reduces portal venous pressure and decompresses the varices, thus controlling bleeding. This procedure is used more for patients requiring short-term control while waiting for a liver transplant.

Hepatic Encephalopathy. The goal of management of hepatic encephalopathy is the reduction of ammonia formation. This consists mainly of protein restriction and reduction of ammonia formation in the intestines. The degree of protein restriction is determined by the severity of mental change. The protein restriction may range from 0 to 40 g per day. With improvement of mental function, dietary protein content is increased gradually over days.

Several measures to reduce ammonia formation in the intestines are used. Sterilization of the intestines with antibiotics such as neomycin sulfate, which are poorly absorbed from the GI tract, is one method. Neomycin is given orally or rectally. This reduces the bacterial flora of the colon. Bacterial action on protein in the feces results in ammonia production. Cathartics and enemas are also used to decrease bacterial action. Constipation should be prevented.

Lactulose (Cephulac) may also be used to treat hepatic encephalopathy. This is a synthetic keto-analog of lactose. In the colon, it is split into lactic acid and acetic acid, which decreases the pH from 7.0 to 5.0. The acidic environment discourages bacterial growth. The lactulose traps the ammonia in the gut, and the laxative effect of the drug expels the ammonia from the colon. It is usually given orally but may be given as a retention enema or via NG tube. Because neomycin may cause renal toxicity and hearing impairments, lactulose is frequently the preferred drug.

Levodopa has been used in the treatment of hepatic encephalopathy. It is a precursor of dopamine and norepinephrine. Use of levodopa is based on the theory that there is a deficiency of dopamine and norepinephrine in encephalopathy because they are replaced by false transmitters (amines from breakdown of dietary proteins). Normally these false transmitters are destroyed by liver enzymes, but when the liver is diseased, this no longer happens. The use of levodopa prolongs the lives of patients with coma resistant to other measures.

Control of hepatic encephalopathy also involves treatment of precipitating causes (see Table 41-12). This involves control-

DRUG THERAPY

Table 41-15 Cirrhosis

Medication	Mechanism of Action
Vasopressin (Pitressin)	Hemostasis and control of bleeding in esophageal varices, constriction of splanchnic arterial bed
Propranolol (Inderal)	Reduction of portal venous pressure, prevention of gastrointestinal bleeding
Neomycin sulfate	Decrease in bacterial flora, decreasing formation of ammonia
Lactulose (Cephulac)	Acidification of feces in bowel and trapping of ammonia, causing its elimination in feces
Levodopa	Conversion to dopamine, which has been displaced with amines from protein breakdown, to increase vascular resistance
Cimetidine (Tagamet)	Decrease in gastric acidity
Diuretics	
Spironolactone (Aldactone)	Blocking of action of aldosterone, potassium sparing
Amiloride (Midamor)	Inhibits reabsorption of sodium and secretion of potassium
Chlorothiazide (Diuril)	Thiazide that acts on proximal tubule to decrease reabsorption of sodium and water
Furosemide (Lasix)	Rapid action on distal tubule and loop of Henle to prevent reabsorption of sodium and water
Triamterene (Dyrenium)	Inhibits reabsorption of sodium and secretion of potassium
Magnesium sulfate	Magnesium replacement; hypomagnesemia occurs with liver dysfunction
Vitamin K (Synkavite)	Correction of clotting abnormalities

ling GI hemorrhage and removing the blood from the GI tract to decrease the protein in the intestine. Electrolyte and acid-base imbalances and infections should also be treated.

Liver transplantation should be considered in patients with recurring hepatic encephalopathy and end-stage liver disease. The use of liver transplantation depends on a number of factors, including the cause of the cirrhosis and other systemic medical problems.

Drug Therapy. There is no specific drug therapy for cirrhosis. However, a number of medications are used to treat symptoms and complications of advanced liver disease (Table 41-15). Some drug therapies are being used in the treatment of cirrhosis to try to prevent or reverse the fibrosis that occurs in the liver. The use of Colbenemid (combination of colchicine and probenecid) has shown an improvement in survival in cirrhotic patients. Propylthiouracil (PTU) has been used to reduce hepatic hypermetabolism, which occurs in alcoholic liver disease. More studies are needed before PTU can be recommended for routine use in these patients.[20]

Nutritional Therapy. The diet for the patient with cirrhosis without complications is high in calories (3000 kcal per day) with high carbohydrate content and moderate to low fat levels. The amount of protein varies depending on the degree of liver damage and the danger of encephalopathy. When the patient is symptomatic (e.g., ascites, edema, mental changes), a low-protein diet is indicated. When there is reduced risk of encephalopathy, 1.5 g of protein per kilogram of body weight may be ordered to maintain plasma osmotic balance and promote liver cell regeneration. Vitamin supplements are usually given. Foods high in protein include meat, fish, poultry, eggs, and dairy products. High-protein nourishment in the form of eggnogs, milkshakes, or protein supplements may be used, particularly for the patient who is malnourished.

The patient with hepatic encephalopathy is on a very-low-protein to no-protein diet (Table 41-16). Foods allowed include toast, cereal, rice, tea, fruit juices, and hard candies. Sufficient carbohydrate intake must be provided to maintain an intake of 1500 to 2000 calories to prevent hypoglycemia and catabolism. Glucose polymer (Polycose) is protein free and can be used as a source of calories. It can be given orally or via NG tube. A patient with alcoholic cirrhosis frequently has protein-calorie malnutrition. For the patient with protein malnutrition, enteral formulas such as Travasorb Hepatic or Hepatic-Aid may be used. These supplements contain protein from branched-chain amino acids that are metabolized by the muscles. They provide protein but put less burden on the liver. IV or tube feedings may be required.

The patient with ascites and edema is on a low-sodium diet. The degree of sodium restriction varies depending on the patient's condition. The patient needs instruction regarding the degree of restriction. Table salt is the most common source of sodium. Sodium is also present in baking soda and baking powder. Foods that are high in sodium content include canned soups and vegetables, salted snacks such as potato chips, nuts, smoked meats and fish, crackers, breads, olives, pickles, ketchup, and beer.

Sodium is also present in many over-the-counter medications (e.g., antacids). However, most antacids are now lower in sodium than previously. Carbonated beverages tend to be high in sodium, and low-sodium and sodium-free carbonated drinks are available. The patient should be advised to read labels. Foods high in protein usually have large amounts of sodium. Alternative protein supplements that are low in sodium may have to be used. The patient and the family need assistance to make the diet more palatable by the use of seasonings such as garlic, parsley, onion, lemon juice, and spices.

NUTRITIONAL THERAPY

Table 41-16 **Low-Protein Diet for Hepatic Failure***

General Principles

Limit protein to 20 g per day at onset of severe hepatic failure.
Protein must be from protein sources with high biologic value.
Diet must be high in calories.
Fat is limited only to prevent early satiety.
Protein is increased in diet by 10 g increments as tolerated without causing signs and symptoms of hepatic encephalopathy.
Sodium is also usually restricted as well as fluid when edema and ascites are present.

Meal	Menu Plan 1	Menu Plan 2	Menu Plan 3
Breakfast 1 fruit, calorie supplement 1 low-protein bread 1 egg (protein) Fat, calorie supplement ¼ cup milk (2 g protein)	½ cup grape juice with 2 tbs Polycose powder† French toast made with low-protein bread, 1 egg, 3 tsp salt-free butter and syrup ¼ cup milk	¼ cup cranberry juice with 2 tbs Polycose powder Low-protein toast with 3 tsp salt-free butter and 2 tsp jelly 1-egg omelet with 3 tsp salt-free butter ¼ cup milk	¼ cup prune juice with 2 tbs Polycose powder Low-protein toast with 3 tsp salt-free butter 1 egg fried in 3 tsp salt-free butter ¼ cup milk
Snack Calorie supplement	Jelly beans	Hard candy	Sugar mints
Lunch 2 starch (4 g protein) 1 vegetable (2 g protein) 1 fruit, calorie supplement Fat, calorie supplement	¼ cup half and half ½ cup Cream of Wheat with 3 tsp salt-free butter Applesauce with whipped topping or Lipomul‡ Small tossed salad with 3 tbs oil and vinegar§ Peas with 3 tsp salt-free butter	¼ cup half and half ½ cup cornmeal (atole) with 3 tsp salt-free butter Small guacamole salad Gelatin with whipped topping or Lipomul Corn with 3 tsp salt-free butter	¼ cup half and half ½ cup grits with 3 tsp salt-free butter Cucumbers in sour cream Peaches with whipped topping or Lipomul Sweet potatoes with brown sugar and 3 tsp salt-free butter
Snack Calorie supplement	Low-protein cookies	Low-protein bread cubes with whipped cream and strawberries	Popsicles made with Polycose
Dinner 1 starch (2 g protein) 1 vegetable (2 g protein) 1 low-protein bread ¼ cup milk (2 g protein) Fat, calorie supplement	½ baked potato 3 tsp salt-free butter Low-protein bread ¼ cup sour cream ½ cup green beans with 3 tsp salt-free butter and 2 tsp jelly ¼ cup milk	½ cup fried potatoes with 1 tsp melted salt-free butter ½ cup zucchini with 3 tsp salt-free butter Low-protein toast with 3 tsp salt-free butter and 2 tsp marmalade ¼ cup milk	½ cup mashed potatoes ½ cup fried okra Low-protein toast with 3 tsp salt-free butter and 2 tsp jam ¼ cup milk

*The diet plan contains approximately 20 g protein.
†Polycose is a brand-name product made by Ross Laboratories.
‡Lipomul is a fat emulsion made by Upjohn.
§Crisp food should be avoided because of the possibility of esophageal varices.

NURSING MANAGEMENT: CIRRHOSIS

■ Nursing Assessment

Subjective and objective data that should be obtained from an individual with cirrhosis are presented in Table 41-17.

■ Nursing Diagnoses

Nursing diagnoses for the patient with cirrhosis include, but are not limited to, those presented in NCP 41-2.

■ Planning

The overall goals are that the patient with cirrhosis will (1) have relief of discomfort; (2) have minimal to no complications (ascites, esophageal varices, hepatic encephalopathy); and (3) return to as normal a lifestyle as possible.

■ Nursing Implementation

Health Promotion. The common etiologies of cirrhosis are alcohol, malnutrition, hepatitis, biliary obstruction, and

NURSING ASSESSMENT

Table 41-17 Cirrhosis

Subjective Data

Important Health Information

Past health history: Previous viral, toxic or idiopathic hepatitis; chronic biliary obstruction and infection; severe right-sided heart failure

Medications: Adverse reaction to any medication; use of anticoagulants, aspirin, acetaminophen

Functional Health Patterns

Health perception–health management: Chronic alcoholism; weakness, fatigue

Nutritional-metabolic: Anorexia, weight loss, dyspepsia, nausea and vomiting; gingival bleeding

Elimination: Dark urine, decreased urinary output; light-colored or black stools, flatulence, change in bowel habits; dry, yellow skin, bruising

Cognitive-perceptual: Dull, right upper quadrant or epigastric pain; numbness, tingling of extremities; pruritis

Sexuality-reproductive: Impotence, amenorrhea

Objective Data

General

Fever, cachexia, wasting of extremities

Integumentary

Icteric sclera, jaundice, petechiae, ecchymoses, spider angiomas, palmar erythema, alopecia, loss of axillary and pubic hair; peripheral edema

Respiratory

Shallow, rapid respirations; epistaxis

Gastrointestinal

Abdominal distention, ascites, distended abdominal wall veins, palpable liver and spleen, foul breath; hematemesis; black, tarry stools; hemorrhoids

Neurologic

Altered mentation, asterixis

Reproductive

Gynecomastia and testicular atrophy (men), impotence (men), loss of libido (men and women), amenorrhea or heavy menstrual bleeding (women)

Possible Findings

Anemia, thrombocytopenia; leukopenia; decreased serum albumin, potassium; abnormal liver function studies; elevated coagulation studies, ammonia, and bilirubin levels; abnormal abdominal ultrasound and liver scan; positive liver biopsy

---

right-sided heart failure. Prevention and early treatment of cirrhosis must focus on the primary etiology. Alcoholism must be treated (see Chapter 10). Patients should be urged to avoid alcohol ingestion, and their efforts should be supported. Adequate nutrition, especially for the alcoholic and other individuals at risk for cirrhosis, is essential to promote liver regeneration. Hepatitis must be identified and treated early so that it does not progress to chronic hepatitis. Biliary disease must be treated so that the stones do not cause obstruction and infection. The underlying cause (e.g., chronic lung disease) of right-sided heart failure must be treated so that the heart failure does not lead to cirrhosis.

Acute Intervention. The focus of nursing care for the patient with cirrhosis is on conserving the patient's strength (see NCP 41-2). Rest enables the liver to restore itself. Complete bed rest may not always be necessary. When the patient requires complete bed rest, measures to prevent pneumonia, thromboembolic problems, and pressure ulcers should be taken. The activity and rest schedule may be modified according to signs of clinical improvement (e.g., decreasing jaundice, improvement in liver function studies). Major concerns of the nurse in determining appropriate nursing care measures to meet the need for rest involve regulation of the physical, emotional, and social climate.

Anorexia, nausea and vomiting, pressure from ascites, and poor eating habits all create problems in maintenance of an adequate intake of nutrients. The nursing measures relating to nutrition for patients with hepatitis also apply here. Oral hygiene before meals may improve the patient's taste sensation.

Between-meal nourishments should be available so that they can be provided at times when the patient can best tolerate them. Food preferences should be provided whenever possible. Explanations to the patient and the family of the reason for any dietary restrictions should be provided.

Nursing assessment and care should include the patient's physiologic response to cirrhosis. Is jaundice present? Where is it observed—sclera, skin, hard palate? What is the progression of jaundice? If the jaundice is accompanied by pruritus, measures to relieve itching should be carried out. Cholestyramine (Questran) may be ordered to help relieve the pruritus. The color of the urine and stools should be noted. With jaundice the urine is often cola colored or mahogany and the stool gray or tan.

Edema and ascites are frequent manifestations of cirrhosis and require nursing assessments and interventions. Accurate calculation and recordings of intake and output, daily weights, and measurements of extremities and abdominal girth help in the ongoing assessment of the location and extent of the edema. If the patient can assume a kneeling position when abdominal girth measurement is taken, the abdominal fluid will go to the most dependent part of the abdomen. This gives the best measurement of abdominal girth. For many patients, girth must be measured in the standing or lying position. Where the measurements are taken should be recorded and should be a part of the nursing care plan.

When a paracentesis is done, the nurse must have the patient void immediately before the procedure to prevent puncture of the bladder. The patient should sit on the side of the bed or be placed in high Fowler's position. Following the procedure the

41-2   NURSING CARE PLAN   PATIENT WITH CIRRHOSIS

| Expected Patient Outcomes | Nursing Interventions and *Rationales* |

NURSING DIAGNOSIS **Altered nutrition: less than body requirements** *related to* anorexia, impaired utilization and storage of nutrients, nausea, and vomiting *as manifested by* lack of interest in food, aversion to eating, reported inadequate food intake.

■ Adequate intake of nutrients. ■ Maintenance of normal body weight.	■ Monitor weight *to evaluate nitrogen balance.* ■ Provide oral care before meals *to remove foul tastes and improve taste of food.* ■ Administer antiemetics as ordered *to relieve nausea and vomiting.* ■ Provide small, frequent meals with nourishments *to prevent feeling of fullness and maintain nutritional status.* ■ Determine food preferences and allow these whenever possible *to increase nutritional appeal for patient, since a low- or no-protein diet is not very palatable.*

NURSING DIAGNOSIS **Impaired skin integrity** *related to* edema, ascites, and pruritus *as manifested by* complaints of itching; areas of excoriation from scratching; taut, shiny skin over edematous areas; areas of skin breakdown.

■ Maintenance of skin integrity. ■ Relief of pruritus.	■ Restrict sodium intake and fluids as ordered *to reduce fluid retention.* ■ Administer prescribed diuretics *to prevent fluid retention and promote diuresis.* ■ Monitor intake and output *to assess fluid balance and renal function.* ■ Assess location and extent of edema by weighing patient at the same time each day, taking daily measurements of extremities and of abdominal girth (same location each time) *to determine patient's response to treatment.* ■ Provide meticulous skin care *because edematous tissues are easily traumatized and subject to breakdown.* ■ Reposition patient at least q2hr *to relieve pressure over bony prominences.* ■ Elevate edematous areas *to promote venous drainage.* ■ Have patient use special mattress, such as alternating-air pressure mattress or egg crate mattress, *to reduce the risk of skin breakdown from prolonged pressure.* ■ Clip patient's nails short and keep clean *to prevent excoriation from pruritus secondary to deposit of bile salts on skin.* ■ Administer antipruritic medication as ordered *to relieve itching.* ■ Provide diversions and distractions *to assist patient in coping with the discomfort of itching and edema.*

NURSING DIAGNOSIS **Ineffective breathing pattern** *related to* pressure on diaphragm and reduced lung volume secondary to ascites *as manifested by* dyspnea, cyanosis, cough, changes in pulse or respiratory rate, depth, or pattern.

■ Able to breathe with minimal difficulty. ■ Effective breathing pattern. ■ Absence of cyanosis and other signs and symptoms of hypoxia.	■ Place patient in semi-Fowler's or Fowler's position; support the arms and chest with pillows *to facilitate breathing by relieving pressure on diaphragm.* ■ Auscultate chest for crackles *to identify fluid in lungs.* ■ Assess respiratory rate and rhythm *to identify increasing dyspnea.*

NURSING DIAGNOSIS **Risk for injury** *related to* diminished sensory perception secondary to peripheral neuropathy.

■ No injury due to decreased sensory perception.	■ Assess for numbness and tingling of lower extremities, decreased sensation in lower extremities *to determine risk of injury.* ■ Prevent excess stimulation or trauma to extremities *because patient may not be able to detect harmful stimuli.* ■ Do not use restrictive bed linens *because they reduce circulation and place pressure on edematous tissue.* ■ Instruct patient to avoid tight clothing *because it impedes circulation.* ■ Use care with heat and cold applications *because patient's ability to perceive temperature is impaired.* ■ Assist with ambulation *to assess patient's ability to safely ambulate and to prevent injury.*

Continued

41-2 NURSING CARE PLAN PATIENT WITH CIRRHOSIS—continued

Expected Patient Outcomes   Nursing Interventions and *Rationales*

NURSING DIAGNOSIS Activity intolerance *related to* fatigue, anemia, ascites, dyspnea, treatment schedule, and cardiac deconditioning *as manifested by* fatigue or weakness, abnormal heart rate or blood pressure, altered response to activity and weakness.

- Increased tolerance for activity.

- Assess patient's ability to perform activities *to plan appropriate interventions.*
- Conserve patient's strength *to minimize cardiac and respiratory work.*
- Provide activity and rest as required *to reduce metabolic demands on the liver, reduce hepatic blood flow, and allow for recovery of liver cells.*
- Monitor hemoglobin and hematocrit levels *to detect GI hemorrhage.*
- Assist with ADLs as needed *to ensure patient's needs are met.*

NURSING DIAGNOSIS Risk for infection *related to* leukopenia and increased susceptibility to environmental pathogens.

- No signs or symptoms of infections.

- Use appropriate infection control measures.
- Assess patient for evidence of risk factors, including leukopenia, and altered circulation *to ensure early identification of infection.*
- Monitor patient's temperature every 2 to 4 hr *because fever is an indicator of infection.*
- Observe for any local and systemic manifestations of infection *to enable early diagnosis and treatment.*
- Protect patient from others with infections *to reduce the risk of infection secondary to decreased resistance.*
- Monitor white blood cell count *to assess patient's response to treatment.*

NURSING DIAGNOSIS Ineffective airway clearance *related to* inability to remove and swallow secretions and bleeding from esophageal varices *as manifested by* ineffective cough; inability to remove airway secretions; abnormal breath sounds; abnormal respiratory rate, rhythm, depth.

- Patent airway.
- Normal breath sounds.

- Suction patient (oral and pharyngeal areas) frequently *to reduce risk of aspiration because patient is unable to swallow with Sengstaken-Blakemore (S-B) tube in place.*
- Place in semi-Fowler's position *to facilitate drainage from mouth and ease breathing by reducing intraabdominal pressure.*
- Have scissors near bed to cut S-B tube (if necessary) *to prevent a displaced esophageal balloon from obstructing the airway.*
- Encourage patient to expectorate, *since the patient is unable to swallow saliva because the inflated esophageal balloon occludes the esophagus.*
- Offer frequent oral and nasal care *to provide relief from taste of blood and irritation from mouth bleeding.*

COLLABORATIVE PROBLEMS

Nursing Goals   Nursing Interventions and *Rationales*

POTENTIAL COMPLICATION Hepatic encephalopathy *related to* increased formation of ammonia and aromatic amino acids.

- Monitor for signs of hepatic encephalopathy.
- Report deviation from acceptable parameters.
- Carry out appropriate medical and nursing interventions.

- Monitor for encephalopathy by assessing patient's general behavior, orientation to time and place, speech, blood pH, and ammonia levels *because liver is unable to convert accumulating ammonia to urea for renal excretion.*
- Encourage fluids (if not restricted) and give laxatives and enemas as ordered *to decrease production of ammonia.*
- Provide low-protein or no-protein diet as ordered *because ammonia (a breakdown product of protein) is responsible for mental changes.*
- Limit physical activity *because exercise produces ammonia as a by-product of metabolism.*

Continued

41-2 NURSING CARE PLAN PATIENT WITH CIRRHOSIS—continued

Expected Patient Outcomes	Nursing Interventions and *Rationales*
POTENTIAL COMPLICATION • Monitor for signs of hemorrhage. • Initiate appropriate medical and nursing interventions.	**Hemorrhage** *related to* bleeding tendency secondary to liver's inability to make clotting factors. • Monitor for hemorrhage by assessing for epistaxis, purpura, petechiae, easy bruising, gingival bleeding, heavy menstrual bleeding, hematuria, melena *because liver disease results in impaired synthesis of clotting factors.* • Provide gentle nursing care *to minimize the risk of tissue trauma.* • Observe for bleeding from body orifices, urine, and stool *to detect bleeding early and allow prompt intervention.* • Use smallest-gauge needle possible when giving injection and apply gentle but prolonged pressure after injection *to minimize risk of bleeding into tissue.* • Advise use of soft-bristle toothbrush *to reduce trauma to mouth because mucous membranes have increased risk of injury.* • Teach patient to avoid straining at stool, vigorous blowing of nose, and coughing *to reduce risk of hemorrhage from these areas.* • Observe for bruising on the forearms, axillae, and skin. • Monitor laboratory results (hematocrit, hemoglobin, and prothrombin time) *as indicators of anemia, active bleeding, or impending complications.*

nurse should monitor for hypovolemia and electrolyte imbalances and check the dressing for bleeding and leakage.

Dyspnea is a frequent problem for the patient with ascites. A semi-Fowler's or Fowler's position allows for maximal respiratory efficiency. Pillows can be used to support the arms and chest and may increase the patient's comfort and ability to breathe.

Meticulous skin care is essential because the edematous tissues are subject to breakdown. An alternating–air pressure mattress or other special mattress should be used. A turning schedule (minimum of every 2 hours) must be adhered to rigidly. The abdomen may be supported with pillows. If the abdomen is taut, cleansing must be done very gently. This patient tends to move very little because of the abdominal discomfort and dyspnea. Therefore range-of-motion exercises are helpful, and measures such as coughing and deep breathing to prevent respiratory problems should be implemented. The lower extremities may be elevated. If scrotal edema is present, a scrotal support provides some comfort.

When the patient is taking diuretics, the serum levels of sodium, potassium, chloride, and bicarbonate should be monitored. The patient should be observed for signs of fluid and electrolyte imbalance, especially hypokalemia. Hypokalemia may be manifested by cardiac arrhythmias, hypotension, tachycardia, and generalized muscle weakness. Water excess is manifested by muscle cramping, weakness, lethargy, and confusion.

Observations and nursing care in relation to hematologic disorders (bleeding tendencies, anemia, increased susceptibility to infection) are the same as for the patient with advanced liver disease (see NCP 41-2).

The nurse must assess the patient's response to altered body image resulting from jaundice, spider angiomas, palmar erythema, ascites, and gynecomastia. The patient may experience a great deal of anxiety regarding these changes. The nurse should explain these phenomena and should be a supportive listener. Nursing care with concern and warmth regardless of physical changes helps the patient maintain self-esteem.

Bleeding esophageal varices. If the patient has esophageal varices in addition to cirrhosis, the nurse must be observant of any signs of bleeding from the varices, such as hematemesis and melena. If hematemesis occurs, the nurse should assess the patient for hemorrhage, call the physician, and be ready to assist with whatever treatment is used to control the bleeding. The patient will be admitted to the intensive care unit (ICU). The patient's airway must be maintained.

When balloon tamponade is used, the initial nursing task related to insertion of the tube is to explain the use of the tube and how it will be inserted. The balloons should be checked for patency. Sometimes the stomach is lavaged with saline solution before insertion of the tube. It is usually the physician's responsibility to insert the tube. It may be inserted via the nose or the mouth (see Fig. 41-9). The placement of the tube is ascertained by x-ray. Then the gastric balloon is inflated with approximately 250 ml of air and the tube is retracted until resistance (gastroesophageal junction) is felt. The tube is secured by placement of a piece of sponge or foam rubber at the nostrils (nasal cuff). This protects the mucosal surfaces from irritation and injury. For continued bleeding the esophageal balloon is then inflated. A sphygmomanometer is used to measure and maintain the desired pressure at 20 to 40 mm Hg. The position of the balloons is verified by x-ray. Sometimes it is helpful to have the patient wear a football helmet with the tube secured to the mouth guard. This stabilizes the tube and applies traction. Traction may also be applied (0.75 to 1.25 pounds [0.3 to 0.6 kg]) to hold the tube securely in place and prevent downward movement. Traction causes ulceration of the nasal mucosa and can be used only for short intervals (2 to 3 hours) at a time.

ETHICAL DILEMMAS

Rationing

SITUATION

A 43-year-old patient with cirrhosis of the liver is frequently admitted to the hospital. She has been told that her continued drinking will inevitably lead to her death. Now she has been admitted for GI bleeding and needs blood transfusions. She has a rare blood type and it is frequently difficult to get compatible blood. Should the nurse call an ethics consultation?

DISCUSSION

A noncompliant patient whose behavior has led to a worsening of the disease process raises difficult ethical problems regarding rationing care. Rationing treatment of a manageable presenting problem probably would not be discussed for a cancer or a trauma patient. However, since alcoholism is understood as a disease with a behavioral component, this patient could be seen to be both noncompliant and unworthy of additional treatment. If the GI problem can be treated and transfusions are integral to that treatment, will that change the overall condition of the patient in regard to her cirrhosis? Will it extend her life or improve the quality of her life? If her underlying disease and quality of life cannot be treated or improved, this treatment could be seen as medically futile and therefore not required. Rationing decisions should be made based on triage, when necessary, rather than assessments of compliance or moral weakness. If the blood supply is very low and desperately needed by a patient whose disease or condition *can* be effectively treated by transfusions, rationing treatment to the patient with cirrhosis might be appropriate. However, if the blood supply is sufficient and no other patients are in competition for it, this is not a rationing decision. Regardless of the availability of resources, this continues to be a medical futility issue, and that may eventually be the basis for decisions about which treatments can be withheld for the greater benefit of all patients.

ETHICAL AND LEGAL DECISIONS

- Rationing is the distribution of scarce resources to an individual patient or a class of patients and the denial of those resources to others. It is based on a limited amount of technology, specific resources (e.g., blood, organs, ICU beds), or financing allocated at the societal level.
- Triage is the priority of care given to patients in an emergency or disaster situation based on the utility of providing the greatest good for the greatest number of patients.
- Prior noncompliant behavior should not be grounds for denying care of the present, acute problem. If the noncompliance is expected to continue and will affect the goals of this medical treatment, it can be grounds for decisions about whether or how to treat the presenting problem.

Sometimes saline lavage is used to remove blood from the stomach. (Nursing care of upper GI bleeding is discussed in Chapter 39.) This helps prevent the blood from degrading to ammonia, leading to encephalopathy. The nurse must ensure that the right amount of pressure is maintained for the correct time. Constant tension and an upward pull on the stomach initiate contraction of the stomach, which may lead to retching and increased portal pressures. The esophageal balloon should be deflated every 8 to 12 hours to avoid necrosis. Each lumen must be labeled to avoid confusion. The NG lumen may be connected to suction to remove blood and keep the stomach empty to reduce the risk of aspiration. The most common complication of balloon tamponade therapy is aspiration pneumonia.

Nursing care includes monitoring for complications of rupture or erosion of the esophagus, regurgitation and aspiration of gastric contents, and occlusion of the airway by the balloon. If the gastric balloon breaks or is deflated, the esophageal balloon will slip upward, obstructing the airway and causing asphyxiation. If this happens, the nurse must cut the tube or deflate the esophageal balloon. Scissors should be kept at the bedside. Regurgitation can be minimized by oral and pharyngeal suctioning and by keeping the patient in a semi-Fowler's position.

The patient is unable to swallow saliva because of the inflated esophageal balloon occluding the esophagus. With the Minnesota tube, which has an esophageal aspiration lumen, this problem can be alleviated. The nurse should encourage the patient to expectorate and should provide an emesis basin and tissues. Frequent oral and nasal care provides relief from the taste of blood and irritation from mouth breathing.

The patient is extremely ill at this stage. The crisis of the bleeding and the ordeal of the tube create a great deal of psychologic trauma. Emotional support and gentle caring must be provided.

Hepatic encephalopathy. The focus of nursing care of the patient with hepatic encephalopathy is on sustaining life and assisting with measures to reduce the formation of ammonia. The nurse should assess (1) the patient's level of responsiveness (e.g., reflexes, pupillary reactions, orientation); (2) sensory and motor abnormalities (e.g., hyperreflexia, asterixis, motor coordination); (3) fluid and electrolyte imbalances; (4) acid-base imbalances; and (5) the effect of treatment measures.

The neurologic status, including an exact description of the patient's behavior, should be assessed and recorded at least every 2 hours. Care of the patient with neurologic problems should be based on the severity of the encephalopathy.

Nursing measures to prevent constipation should be instituted to decrease ammonia production. Drugs, laxatives, and enemas should be given as ordered. Encouragement of fluids may also help if not contraindicated. The patient should not strain at stool because this may cause bleeding of hemorrhoidal varices. Any GI bleeding may worsen the coma. The patient who is taking lactulose should be assessed for diarrhea. Some physicians have diarrhea as a goal when treating with lactulose. The drug's laxative action expels the ammonia from the colon. Because lactulose can cause severe purging, the nurse should observe the patient for excessive fluid and electrolyte loss.

Factors that are known to precipitate coma should be controlled as much as possible (see Table 41-12). Because exercise

Table 41-18 | **Cirrhosis**

1. Explain to the patient and family the importance of continuous health care so they understand that cirrhosis is a chronic illness.
2. Teach the patient and family symptoms of complications and when to seek medical attention to enable prompt treatment of complications.
3. Teach proper diet because a low-protein, high-carbohydrate diet is usually indicated and can be difficult to follow.
4. Teach the patient to avoid potentially hepatotoxic over-the-counter drugs since the diseased liver is unable to metabolize these medications.
5. Encourage abstinence from alcohol because continued use of alcohol will increase the risk of liver complications.
6. Instruct the patient to avoid aspirin and control cough to prevent hemorrhage when esophageal or gastric varices are present.
7. Teach the patient to avoid spicy and rough foods and activities that increase portal pressure, such as straining at stool, coughing, sneezing, and retching and vomiting because hemorrhage is a danger due to inability of the liver to produce clotting factors.

produces ammonia as a by-product of metabolism, the physical activity of the patient must be limited. Hypokalemia should be controlled.

The patient is on either a very low-protein or a no-protein diet, neither of which is very palatable. Vegetable protein is better tolerated than meat protein. Foods and fluids high in carbohydrate should be given because the liver is not synthesizing and storing glucose. The patient may require tube feedings if an adequate diet cannot be ingested.

Ambulatory and Home Care. The patient with cirrhosis may be faced with a prolonged course and the possibility of serious, life-threatening problems and complications. The nurse should be a resource person in helping the patient achieve the highest level of wellness. The patient and the family need to understand the importance of continuous health care and medical supervision. They should be taught symptoms of complications and when to seek medical attention. Patients with cirrhosis should refrain from eating raw shellfish and avoid activities that place them at risk for contracting viral hepatitis.

Measures to achieve and maintain a remission should be encouraged. These include proper diet, rest, avoidance of potentially hepatotoxic over-the-counter drugs such as acetaminophen, and abstinence from alcohol. Abstinence from alcohol is important and results in improvement in most patients. The nurse must realize the difficulty this poses for some patients. The nurse's own attitude regarding the patient whose cirrhosis is attributed to alcohol abuse should be explored. Care should be given without rejection and moralizing. The alcoholic patient should be treated with a caring attitude.

Cirrhosis is a chronic disease. The patient is affected not only physically but also psychologically, socially, and economically. Major adjustments may be required to make lifestyle changes, especially if alcohol abuse is the primary etiologic factor. The nurse should provide information regarding community support programs, such as Alcoholics Anonymous, for help with alcohol abuse.

Adequate explanations, along with written instructions, related to fluid or dietary restrictions should be given to the patient and the family (Table 41-18). Other health teaching should include instruction about adequate rest periods, how to detect early signs of complications, skin care, drug therapy precautions, observation for bleeding, and protection from infection. Counseling information regarding sexual problems may be needed. Referral to a community or home health nurse may be helpful to ensure adequate patient compliance with prescribed therapy. The emphasis of home care for the patient with cirrhosis should be on helping the patient maintain the highest level of wellness possible and initiate and maintain necessary lifestyle changes.

■ Evaluation

Expected outcomes for the patient with cirrhosis are addressed in NCP 41-2.

FULMINANT HEPATIC FAILURE

Fulminant hepatic failure is a clinical syndrome characterized by severe impairment of liver function associated with hepatic encephalopathy. In fulminant hepatic failure the encephalopathy occurs within 8 weeks of the first symptoms. The most common cause is viral hepatitis, in particular HBV, but it may also occur with HAV and less frequently with HCV.

Medications are the second most common cause of fulminant hepatic failure. Acetaminophen (Tylenol) in combination with alcohol is a common offending agent. Persons who abuse alcohol are particularly susceptible to detrimental effects of acetaminophen on the liver. Other drugs include INH, halothane, sulfa-containing drugs, and nonsteroidal antiinflammatory drugs.

The patient has jaundice and signs of encephalopathy. Laboratory tests reveal elevated liver function tests and increased bilirubin. Depending on the degree of liver failure, treatment may involve liver transplantation.

CARCINOMA OF THE LIVER

Primary carcinoma (originating in the liver) is rare. Metastatic carcinoma of the liver is more common. Hepatocellular carcinoma is the most common malignant tumor of the liver. The remaining primary tumors are cholangiomas or bile duct carcinomas. A high percentage of patients with primary cell carcinoma have cirrhosis of the liver. Some cases of hepatocellular carcinoma are associated with chronic hepatitis B or C.[21] Men have a higher incidence of primary liver cancer than women.

The liver is a common site of metastatic growth because of its high rate of blood flow and extensive capillary network. Cancer cells in other parts of the body are commonly carried to the liver via the portal circulation.

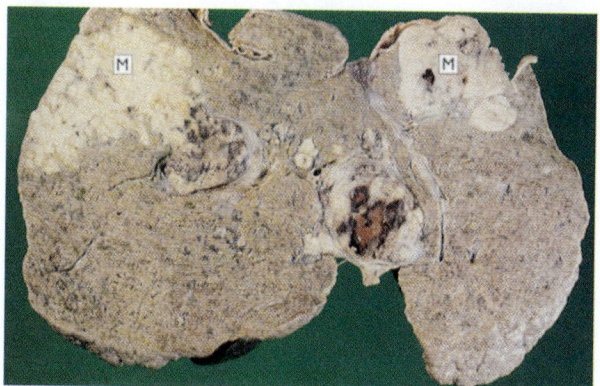

Fig. 41-11 Hepatocellular carcinoma. Macroscopically hepatocellular carcinoma may be single or multifocal. They usually develop in a liver already affected by cirrhosis. Tumor appears as an abnormal mass *(M)* within the liver.

The malignant cells cause the liver to be enlarged and misshapen. Hemorrhage and necrosis in the liver are common (Fig. 41-11). Lesions may be singular or numerous and nodular or diffusely spread over the entire liver. Some tumors infiltrate into other organs such as the gallbladder or into the peritoneum or diaphragm. Primary liver tumors commonly metastasize to the lung.

Clinical Manifestations

It is difficult to diagnose carcinoma of the liver. It is particularly difficult to differentiate it from cirrhosis in its early stages because many of the clinical manifestations (e.g., hepatomegaly, weight loss, peripheral edema, ascites, portal hypertension) are similar. Other common manifestations include dull abdominal pain in the epigastric or right upper quadrant region, jaundice, anorexia, nausea and vomiting, and extreme weakness. Patients frequently have pulmonary emboli. Tests used to assist in the diagnosis are a liver scan, hepatic arteriography, endoscopic retrograde cholangiopancreatography (ERCP), and a liver biopsy. The test for α-fetoprotein (AFP) may be positive in hepatocellular carcinoma. AFP helps distinguish primary cancer from metastatic cancer.

NURSING AND COLLABORATIVE MANAGEMENT: CANCER OF THE LIVER

Treatment of cancer of the liver is largely palliative. Surgical excision (lobectomy) is sometimes performed if the tumor is localized to one portion of the liver. Only 30% to 40% of patients have surgically resectable disease. Usually surgery is not feasible because the cancer is too far advanced when it is detected. Surgical excision offers the only chance for cure of liver cancer. Management is similar to that for cirrhosis. Chemotherapy may be used, but there is usually a poor response. Portal vein or hepatic artery perfusion with 5-fluorouracil (5-FU) may be attempted.

Nursing intervention for the patient with liver carcinoma focuses on keeping the patient as comfortable as possible. Because this patient manifests the same problems as any patient with advanced liver disease, the nursing interventions discussed

RESEARCH
IMPLICATIONS FOR NURSING PRACTICE

Sexual Functioning After Transplant Surgery

Citation Hart LK and others: Survey of sexual concerns among organ transplant recipients, *J Transpl Coord* 7:82, 1997.

Purpose To identify the frequency of sexual dysfunction, degree of satisfaction, overall satisfaction, and life quality in desire for and receipt of instruction regarding sexual dysfunction in organ transplant recipients.

Methods A survey was mailed to 768 adult liver, kidney, and pancreas/kidney recipients (39% responded) to determine satisfaction, quality of life, and sexual functioning among transplant recipients.

Results and Conclusions Of those who responded there were no differences among the transplant groups with respect to satisfaction, quality of life, or sexual functioning. The degree of relationship satisfaction was related to frequency of intercourse, sexual desire, orgasm, and acceptance of partners' advances. Sixty-seven percent of the patients received no instruction related to sexuality or fertility.

Implications for Nursing Practice The results of this survey indicate that many transplant recipients receive little or no information related to sexuality and fertility. This is an important area for nursing intervention. In addition, efforts should be made to validate and support sexual identity in this patient population.

for cirrhosis of the liver apply. (See Chapter 14 for care of the patient with cancer.)

The prognosis for cancer of the liver is poor. The cancer grows rapidly, and death may occur within 4 to 7 months as a result of hepatic encephalopathy or massive blood loss from GI bleeding.

LIVER TRANSPLANTATION

The first human liver transplant was performed in 1963 at the University of Colorado by Thomas Starzl. In the last decade, liver transplantation has become a practical therapeutic option for many adults and children with irreversible liver disease. It improves the quality of life for end-stage liver patients and is an accepted treatment modality for these patients. Indications for liver transplantation include congenital biliary abnormalities, inborn errors of metabolism, hepatic malignancy (confined to the liver), sclerosing cholangitis, and chronic end-stage liver disease.[23] Cirrhosis of the liver, primarily as a result of hepatitis viruses, is a major indication for transplantation in adults. Liver transplants are not recommended for the patient with widespread malignant disease.

The major postoperative complications are rejection and infection. Rejection is not as major a problem as in kidney transplants. The liver seems to be less susceptible to severe

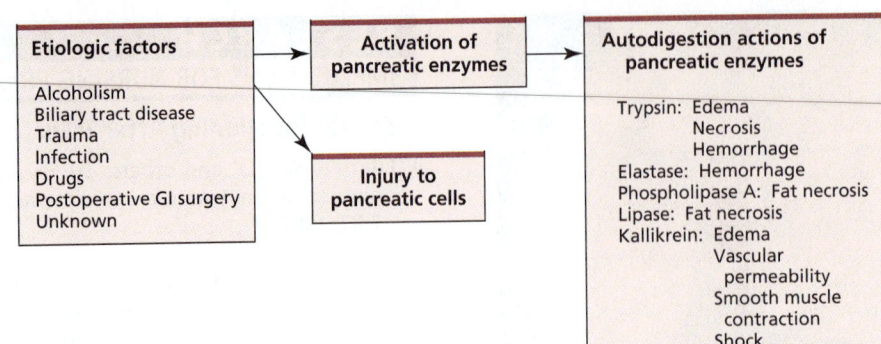

Fig. 41-12 Pathogenic process of acute pancreatitis.

rejection than the kidney. Cyclosporine is an effective immunosuppressant drug. The use of cyclosporine has been a major factor in the success rates of liver transplantation. The mechanism of action and side effects of cyclosporine are discussed in Chapter 44 and Table 44-12. It does not cause bone marrow suppression and does not impede wound healing. Other immunosuppressants used include azathioprine (Imuran), corticosteroids, and the monoclonal antibody OKT3 (see Table 44-12). Other factors in the improved success rate are advances in surgical techniques, better selection of potential recipients, and improved management of the underlying liver disease before surgery.

Patients who have liver disease secondary to viral hepatitis often experience reinfection of the graft with hepatitis C or B following transplantation. Despite this, the 5-year survival rate of patients with hepatitis C undergoing transplantation is 78%.[22]

The patient who has had a liver transplant requires competent and highly skilled nursing care, either in an ICU or in some other specialized unit. Postoperative nursing care includes assessing neurologic status; monitoring for signs of hemorrhage; preventing pulmonary complications; monitoring drainage, electrolytes, and urinary output; and monitoring for signs and symptoms of infection and rejection. Common respiratory problems are pneumonia, atelectasis, and pleural effusions. The nurse should have the patient use measures such as coughing, deep breathing, incentive spirometry, and repositioning to prevent these complications. Drainage from the Jackson-Pratt drain, NG tube, and T-tube should be measured and the color and consistency of drainage noted. A critical aspect of nursing care following liver transplantation is monitoring for infection. The first 2 months after the surgery are critical. Infection can be viral, fungal, or bacterial. Fever may be the only sign of infection. Emotional support and teaching the patient and family are essential.

ACUTE PANCREATITIS

Acute pancreatitis is an acute inflammatory process of the pancreas. The degree of inflammation varies from mild edema to severe hemorrhagic necrosis.

Acute pancreatitis is most common in middle-aged men and women, but it affects more men than women. The severity of the disease varies according to the extent of pancreatic destruction. Some patients recover completely, others have recurring attacks, and chronic pancreatitis develops in others. Acute pancreatitis can be life threatening.

Etiology and Pathophysiology

Many factors can cause injury to the pancreas. The primary etiologic factors are biliary tract disease and alcoholism. In the United States the most common cause is alcoholism, followed by gallbladder disease. Other, less common, causes of acute pancreatitis include trauma (postsurgical, abdominal); viral infections (mumps, coxsackievirus B); penetrating duodenal ulcer; cysts; abscesses; cystic fibrosis; Kaposi's sarcoma; certain drugs (corticosteroids, thiazide diuretics, oral contraceptives, sulfonamides, nonsteroidal antiinflammatory drugs); and metabolic disorders (hyperparathyroidism, hyperlipidemia, renal failure). Pancreatitis may occur after surgical procedures on the pancreas, stomach, duodenum, or biliary tract. Pancreatitis can also occur after ERCP. In some cases the cause is not known (idiopathic).

The most common pathogenic mechanism is believed to be autodigestion of the pancreas (Fig. 41-12). The etiologic factors cause injury to pancreatic cells or activation of the pancreatic enzymes in the pancreas rather than in the intestine. It is not clear how the activation of pancreatic enzymes occurs. One possible cause is believed to be the reflux of bile acids into the pancreatic ducts through an open or distended sphincter of Oddi. This reflux may occur because of gallstones impacted at the ampulla of Vater, atony and edema of the sphincter, or obstruction of pancreatic ducts and pancreatic ischemia.

Trypsinogen is an inactive proteolytic enzyme produced by the pancreas. Normally it is released into the small intestine via the pancreatic duct. In the intestine it is activated to trypsin by enterokinase. Normally, trypsin inhibitors in the pancreas and plasma bind and inactivate any trypsin that is inadvertently produced. In pancreatitis, activated trypsin is present in the pancreas. This enzyme can digest the pancreas and can activate other proteolytic enzymes such as elastase and phospholipase.

Elastase and phospholipase A play a major role in autodigestion of the pancreas. Elastase is activated by trypsin and causes hemorrhage by producing dissolution of the elastic fibers of blood vessels. Phospholipase A is probably activated by trypsin and bile acids and causes fat necrosis.

It is not entirely clear how alcohol causes acute pancreatitis. One theory is that it stimulates secretion and excess production of hydrochloric acid. A decrease in the gastric pH results in the release of the hormone secretin from the intestinal mucosa.

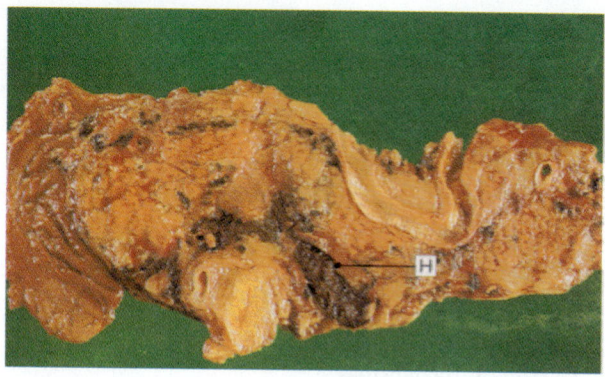

Fig. 41-13 In acute pancreatitis the pancreas appears edematous and is commonly hemorrhagic (H).

This hormone then stimulates pancreatic secretions. Alcohol may also cause regurgitation of duodenal contents into the pancreatic duct, resulting in inflammation.

The pathophysiologic involvement of acute pancreatitis ranges from edematous pancreatitis (which is mild and self-limiting) to necrotizing pancreatitis (in which the degree of necrosis correlates with the severity of manifestations) (Fig. 41-13).

Clinical Manifestations

Abdominal pain is the predominant symptom of acute pancreatitis. The pain is usually located in the left upper quadrant but may be in the mid-epigastrium. It commonly radiates to the back because of the retroperitoneal location of the pancreas. The pain has a sudden onset and is described as severe, deep, piercing, and continuous or steady. It is aggravated by eating and frequently has its onset when the patient is recumbent; it is not relieved by vomiting. The pain may be accompanied by flushing, cyanosis, and dyspnea. The patient may assume various positions involving flexion of the spine in an attempt to relieve the severe pain. The pain is due to distention of the pancreas, peritoneal irritation, and obstruction of the biliary tract.

Other manifestations of acute pancreatitis include nausea and vomiting, low-grade fever, leukocytosis, hypotension, tachycardia, and jaundice. Abdominal tenderness with muscle guarding is common. Bowel sounds may be decreased or absent. Ileus may occur and causes marked abdominal distention. The lungs are frequently involved, with crackles present. Intravascular damage from circulating trypsin may cause areas of cyanosis or greenish to yellow-brown discoloration of the abdominal wall. Other areas of ecchymoses are the flanks (Grey Turner's spots or sign, a bluish flank discoloration) and the periumbilical area (Cullen's sign, a bluish periumbilical discoloration). These result from seepage of blood-stained exudate from the pancreas and may occur in severe cases.

Shock may occur because of hemorrhage into the pancreas or toxemia from the activated pancreatic enzymes. The increased formation of kinin peptides (activated by trypsin), such as kallikrein and bradykinin, causes vasodilation, increased capillary permeability, and altered vasomotor tone. Hypovolemia also occurs as a result of exudation of blood and plasma proteins into the retroperitoneal space (massive fluid shifts).

Complications

Two significant local complications of acute pancreatitis are pseudocyst and abscess. A pancreatic pseudocyst is a cavity continuous with or surrounding the outside of the pancreas. The pseudocyst is filled with necrotic products and liquid secretions, such as plasma, pancreatic enzymes, and inflammatory exudates. As pancreatic enzymes escape from the pseudocyst, the serosal surfaces next to the pancreas become inflamed, with subsequent formation of granulation tissue leading to encapsulation of the exudate. Symptoms of pseudocyst are abdominal pain, palpable epigastric mass, nausea, vomiting, and anorexia. The serum amylase level frequently remains elevated. These cysts usually resolve spontaneously within a few weeks but may perforate, causing peritonitis, or rupture into the stomach or duodenum. Treatment consists of an internal drainage procedure with a Roux-en-Y anastomosis between the pancreatic duct and the jejunum.

A pancreatic abscess is a large fluid-containing cavity within the pancreas. It results from extensive necrosis in the pancreas. It may become infected or perforate into adjacent organs. Manifestations of an abscess include upper abdominal pain, abdominal mass, high fever, and leukocytosis. Pancreatic abscesses require prompt surgical drainage to prevent sepsis.

The main systemic complications of acute pancreatitis are pulmonary complications (pleural effusion, atelectasis, and pneumonia) and tetany caused by hypocalcemia. The pulmonary complications are probably caused by the passage of the exudate containing pancreatic enzymes from the peritoneal cavity through transdiaphragmatic lymph channels. When hypocalcemia occurs, it is a sign of severe disease. It is due in part to the combining of calcium and fatty acids during fat necrosis. The exact mechanisms of how or why hypocalcemia occurs are not well understood.

Diagnostic Studies

The primary diagnostic tests for acute pancreatitis are serum amylase (pancreatic isoamylase) and lipase and urinary amylase levels (Table 41-19). The serum amylase level is the criterion most commonly used. It may elevate to levels greater than 200 U/L (3.34 μkat/L). The serum amylase is usually elevated early and remains elevated for 24 to 72 hours.

The serum lipase is also elevated in acute pancreatitis and is a helpful complementary test because other disorders (e.g., mumps, cerebral trauma, renal transplantation) may also cause an increase in serum amylase.

There is an increase in urinary amylase, which may persist several days beyond the elevation of serum amylase. Urinary amylase may be increased to more than 3600 U per day. Normally a timed collection (e.g., a 2-hour collection) is a more dependable measure than a randomly collected urinary specimen.

The renal amylase-creatinine clearance test estimates the amount of blood cleared of amylase by the kidney per minute. The finding that the renal clearance of amylase is higher than the creatinine clearance in acute pancreatitis has led to the suggestion that the amylase-creatinine clearance ratio is a more specific test than urinary amylase levels alone.

Other laboratory abnormalities include hyperglycemia, hyperlipidemia, and hypocalcemia (see Table 41-19). There is a high incidence of hyperlipidemia with recurrent pancreatitis.

DIAGNOSTIC STUDIES

Table 41-19 Acute Pancreatitis

Laboratory Test	Abnormal Finding	Etiology
Primary Tests		
Serum amylase	Increased (>200 U/L [3.34 μkat/L])	Pancreatic cell injury
Serum lipase	Elevated	Pancreatic cell injury
Urinary amylase	Elevated	Pancreatic cell injury
Secondary Tests		
Blood glucose	Hyperglycemia	Impairment of carbohydrate metabolism due to β-cell damage and release of glucagon
Serum calcium	Hypocalcemia	Saponification of calcium by fatty acids in areas of fat necrosis
Serum triglycerides	Hyperlipidemia	Release of free fatty acids by lipase

COLLABORATIVE CARE

Table 41-20 Acute Pancreatitis

Diagnostic
- Serum amylase
- Serum lipase
- 2-hour urinary amylase and renal amylase clearance
- Blood glucose
- Serum calcium
- Triglycerides
- Flat plate of the abdomen
- Pancreatic ultrasound scan
- CT scan of the pancreas
- ERCP

Collaborative Therapy
- Meperidine
- NPO with NG tube to suction
- Cimetidine (Tagamet) or ranitidine (Zantac) IV
- Albumin (if shock present)
- IV calcium gluconate (10%) (if tetany present)
- Lactated Ringer's solution

CT, computed tomography; *ERCP*, endoscopic retrograde cholangiopancreatography; *NPO*, nothing by mouth.

ERCP is the definitive diagnostic test for gallstones, pancreatic cysts, and abscesses. A combination of laboratory studies and ERCP is usually used to help make the diagnosis. Abdominal x-ray and ultrasound scan of the pancreas may also be performed.

Collaborative Care

Objectives of collaborative care for acute pancreatitis include (1) relief of pain; (2) prevention or alleviation of shock; (3) reduction of pancreatic secretions; (4) control of fluid and electrolyte imbalance; (5) prevention or treatment of infections; and (6) removal of the precipitating cause, if possible (Table 41-20).

Conservative Therapy. A primary consideration in the treatment of acute pancreatitis is the relief and control of pain. Meperidine (Demerol) is preferred because it causes less spasm of the smooth muscles of the ducts than morphine. It may be combined with an antispasmodic. However, atropine-like drugs should be avoided when paralytic ileus is present because they may contribute to the problem. Other medications that relax smooth muscles (spasmolytics), such as nitroglycerin or papaverine, may be used.

If shock is present, blood volume replacements are used. Plasma or plasma volume expanders such as dextran or albumin may be given. Fluid and electrolyte imbalances are corrected with lactated Ringer's solution or other electrolyte solutions. Central venous pressure readings may be used to assist in determination of fluid-replacement requirements.

It is important to reduce or suppress pancreatic enzymes to decrease stimulation of the pancreas and allow it to rest. This is accomplished in several ways. First, the patient is allowed to take nothing by mouth (NPO). Second, NG suction may be used to reduce vomiting and gastric distention and to prevent gastric acidic contents from entering the duodenum. These measures suppress pancreatic secretion. Certain drugs may also be used for this purpose (Table 41-21).

The inflamed and necrotic pancreatic tissue is a good medium for bacterial growth. Therefore it is important to prevent infections. There is some controversy about the prophylactic use of antibiotics. It is important to monitor the patient closely so that antibiotic therapy can be instituted early if infection occurs.

Peritoneal lavage or dialysis has been used to remove the kinin and phospholipase A–containing exudate from the peritoneal cavity. This has proved beneficial in some cases of severe acute pancreatitis. It prevents early death but has little effect on overall mortality rate. Endoscopic papillotomy may be used to remove an impacted gallstone from the common bile duct when the pancreatitis is due to the stone.

Surgical Therapy. Surgical intervention may be indicated when the diagnosis is uncertain and in patients who do not respond to conservative therapy. Surgery is necessary for an abscess, acute pseudocyst, and severe peritonitis. Percutaneous drainage of a pseudocyst can be performed, and a drainage tube is left in place. Surgical treatment of associated biliary tract disease may be necessary.

Drug Therapy. Several different drugs may be used in the treatment of both acute and chronic pancreatitis (see Table 41-21). A number of drugs are used in an effort to suppress pancreatic secretion, but these drugs have not proved effective in the management of pancreatitis.

Nutritional Therapy. Initially the patient with acute pancreatitis is on NPO status to reduce pancreatic secretion. When food is allowed, small, frequent feedings are given. The

DRUG THERAPY

Table 41-21   Acute and Chronic Pancreatitis

Drug	Mechanisms of Action
Acute Pancreatitis	
Meperidine (Demerol)	Relief of pain
Nitroglycerin or papaverine	Relaxation of smooth muscles and relief of pain
Antispasmodics (e.g., dicyclomine [Bentyl], propantheline bromide [Pro-Banthine])	Decrease of vagal stimulation, motility, pancreatic outflow (inhibition of volume and concentration of bicarbonate and enzymatic secretion); contraindicated in paralytic ileus
Carbonic anhydrase inhibitor (acetazolamide [Diamox])	Reduction in volume and bicarbonate concentration of pancreatic secretion
Antacids	Neutralization of gastric secretions; decrease in hydrochloric acid stimulation of secretin, which stimulates production and secretion of pancreatic secretions
Histamine H_2-receptor antagonists (cimetidine [Tagamet], ranitidine [Zantac])	Decrease in hydrochloric acid by inhibiting histamine (hydrochloric acid stimulates pancreatic activity)
Calcium gluconate	Treatment of hypocalcemia to prevent or treat tetany
Corticosteroids	Use only for seriously ill patients with hypotension or shock
Aprotinin (Trasylol)	Antitryptic and antikallikreinic actions
Glucagon	Reduction in pancreatic inflammation and decrease in serum amylase, suppression of pancreatic secretions
Somatostatin	Inhibition of pancreatic secretions
Chronic Pancreatitis	
Pancreatin (Viokase), pancrelipase (Cotazym)	Replacement therapy for pancreatic enzymes
Insulin	Treatment for diabetes mellitus if it occurs or for hyperglycemia

diet is usually high in carbohydrate content because that is the least stimulating to the exocrine portion of the pancreas. The diet combines high carbohydrate intake with low fat and high protein intake. It is bland, with no stimulants (e.g., caffeine) or alcohol. Supplemental fat-soluble vitamins may be given. The patient may require supplemental commercial liquid preparations. If severe nutritional deficiencies exist, total parenteral nutrition (TPN) may be used (see Chapter 38).

NURSING MANAGEMENT: ACUTE PANCREATITIS

■ Nursing Assessment

Subjective and objective data that should be obtained from a person with acute pancreatitis are presented in Table 41-22.

■ Nursing Diagnoses

Nursing diagnoses for the patient with acute pancreatitis may include, but are not limited to, those presented in NCP 41-3.

■ Planning

The overall goals are that the patient with acute pancreatitis will have (1) relief of pain, (2) return of fluid and electrolyte balance, (3) minimal to no complications, and (4) no recurrent attacks.

■ Nursing Implementation

Health Promotion. The major factors involved in health promotion are assessment of the patient for predisposing and etiologic factors of pancreatitis and encouragement of early treatment of these factors to prevent occurrence of acute

pancreatitis. The nurse should encourage the early diagnosis and treatment of biliary tract disease, such as cholelithiasis. The patient should be encouraged to eliminate alcohol intake, especially if there have been any previous episodes of pancreatitis. Attacks of pancreatitis become milder or disappear with the discontinuance of alcohol use.

Acute Intervention. During the acute phase, it is important to monitor vital signs. Hemodynamic stability may be compromised by hypotension, fever, and tachypnea, which may result in fluid volume deficit. IV fluids are ordered and the response to therapy is monitored. A vital part of the nursing care plan for this patient is observation for electrolyte imbalances. Frequent vomiting, along with gastric suction, may result in decreased chloride, sodium, and potassium levels.

Respiratory failure may develop in the patient with severe acute pancreatitis. It is important that respiratory function be assessed (e.g., lung sounds). If acute respiratory distress syndrome develops, the patient may require intubation and mechanical ventilatory support.

Because hypocalcemia can also occur, the nurse must observe for symptoms of tetany, such as jerking, irritability, and muscular twitching. Numbness or tingling around the lips and in the fingers is an early indicator of hypocalcemia. The patient should be assessed for a positive Chvostek's or Trousseau's sign (see Chapter 15). Calcium gluconate as ordered should be given to treat symptomatic hypocalcemia. In addition, hypomagnesemia may develop, necessitating the observation of serum magnesium levels.

Because abdominal pain is a prominent symptom of pancreatitis, a major focus of nursing care is the relief of pain (see NCP 41-3). Giving the prescribed medications before the

NURSING ASSESSMENT

Table 41-22   Acute Pancreatitis

Subjective Data	Objective Data
Important Health Information	**General**
Past health history: Biliary tract disease, abdominal trauma, duodenal ulcers, infection, metabolic disorders	Restlessness, anxiety, low-grade fever
Medications: Use of thiazides, estrogens, corticosteroids, azathioprine, sulfonamides, nonsteroidal antiinflammatory agents	**Integumentary**
	Flushing, diaphoresis, discoloration of abdomen and flanks, cyanosis, jaundice; decreased skin turgor, dry mucous membranes
Surgery and other treatments: Surgical procedures on the pancreas, stomach, duodenum, or biliary tract; endoscopic retrograde cholangiopancreatography	**Respiratory**
	Tachypnea, basilar crackles
Functional Health Patterns	**Cardiovascular**
Health perception–health management: Alcohol abuse; weakness	Tachycardia, hypotension
Nutritional-metabolic: Nausea and vomiting; anorexia	**Gastrointestinal**
Activity-exercise: Dyspnea	Abdominal distention, tenderness, and muscle guarding; diminished bowel sounds
Cognitive-perceptual: Severe midepigastric or left upper quadrant pain that may radiate to the back, aggravated by food and alcohol intake and unrelieved by vomiting	**Possible Findings**
	Elevated serum amylase and lipase, leukocytosis, hyperglycemia, elevated urine amylase, hyperlipidemia, hypocalcemia, abnormal ultrasound and CT scans of pancreas

pain becomes too severe makes the medication more effective. Meperidine (Demerol) or pentazocine (Talwin) may be used for pain relief because morphine may cause spasm of the sphincter of Oddi. The nurse should ascertain how long the pain medication provides relief. Measures such as comfortable positioning, frequent changes in position, and relief of nausea and vomiting assist in reducing the restlessness that usually accompanies the pain. Some patients experience lessened pain by assuming positions that flex the trunk and draw the knees up to the abdomen. A side-lying position with the head elevated 45 degrees decreases tension on the abdomen and may help ease the pain. It is important to control the pain and restlessness because they increase body metabolism and subsequent stimulation of pancreatic secretions.

Nursing measures for the patient who is on NPO status or has an NG tube should be employed. Frequent oral and nasal care to relieve the dryness of the mouth and nose is comforting to the patient. Oral care is essential to prevent parotitis. If the patient is taking anticholinergics to decrease GI secretions, there will be additional dryness of the mouth caused by the side effects of the drug. If the patient is taking antacids to suppress secretions, they should be sipped slowly or inserted in the NG tube. The nurse must regularly assess the functioning of the suction.

The patient with acute pancreatitis is susceptible to infections. The nurse should observe for fever and other manifestations of infection. Respiratory infections are common because the retroperitoneal fluid raises the diaphragm, which causes the patient to take shallow, guarded abdominal breaths. Measures to prevent respiratory infections include turning, coughing, deep breathing, and assuming a semi-Fowler's position.

Other important assessments are observation for signs of paralytic ileus, renal failure, and mental changes. Determination of the blood glucose level should be done to assess damage to the β-cells of the islets of Langerhans in the pancreas.

After pancreatic surgery the patient may require special wound care for an anastomotic leak or a fistula. Measures to prevent skin irritation should be used. These include skin barriers such as Stomahesive, karaya paste, or Colley-Seel; pouching; and drains. In addition to protecting the skin, pouching also provides a more accurate determination of fluid and electrolyte losses and increases patient comfort. Sterile pouching systems are available. The nurse may want to consult with a clinical specialist or an enterostomal therapist, if available.

Ambulatory and Home Care. After acute pancreatitis most patients will need home care follow-up. The patient may have lost physical reserve and muscle strength. Physical therapy may be needed. Continued care to prevent infection and detect any complications is important. Because frequent doses of narcotics may be required for this patient during the acute stage, follow-up for assessment of possible narcotic addiction may be indicated. This is a more likely problem with chronic pancreatitis than in the patient with acute pancreatitis. Counseling regarding abstinence from alcohol is important to prevent the patient from experiencing future attacks of acute pancreatitis and development of chronic pancreatitis. Beverages with caffeine should not be consumed. Because smoking and stressful situations can overstimulate the pancreas, they should be avoided.

Dietary teaching should include restriction of fats because they stimulate the secretion of cholecystokinin, which then stimulates the pancreas. Carbohydrates are less stimulating to the pancreas, so they should be encouraged. The patient should be instructed to avoid crash dieting and bingeing because these can precipitate attacks.

Early detection makes it possible to correct neurologic changes by treating the cause before overt psychotic behavior is manifested. Possible causes of neurologic changes include sepsis, anorexia, toxicity from cellular breakdown products, and withdrawal from alcohol.

41-3   NURSING CARE PLAN   PATIENT WITH ACUTE PANCREATITIS

| Expected Patient Outcomes | Nursing Interventions and *Rationales* |

NURSING DIAGNOSIS **Pain** *related to* inflammation of pancreas, peritoneal irritation, and ineffective pain and comfort measures *as manifested by* communication of pain descriptors, guarding behavior, behaviors indicative of pain (e.g., moaning), diaphoresis, changes in blood pressure, pulse, and respiratory rate.

- Minimal to no pain.

- Assess degree and nature of pain *to plan appropriate interventions.*
- Give ordered analgesic and antispasmodic medications before pain becomes severe *to ensure more effective relief of pain.*
- Ascertain how long the medication provides relief *to adjust pain medication administration in order to provide ongoing relief of pain.*
- Provide comfort measures, such as positioning patient comfortably with frequent changes in position, and diversional activities *to assist in reducing the restlessness that usually accompanies the pain and to demonstrate caring behaviors by the nurse.*

NURSING DIAGNOSIS **Fluid volume deficit** *related to* nausea, vomiting, nasogastric suction, and restricted oral intake *as manifested by* thirst, increased fluid output, altered intake, dry skin and mucous membranes, decreased skin turgor, decreased oral intake.

- Adequate intake of fluids and electrolytes as evidenced by normal skin turgor.
- Moist mucous membranes.
- Stable weight.
- Normal serum electrolyte levels.

- Give antiemetics as ordered *to reduce fluid loss by preventing vomiting.*
- Measure and describe emesis *as indicators of replacement needs and effectiveness of treatment.*
- Observe for manifestations of metabolic alkalosis such as confusion, irritability, tachycardia, nausea, vomiting, muscle cramps, and tetany due to loss of chloride, sodium, and potassium with severe vomiting *so appropriate replacements can be started promptly.*

NURSING DIAGNOSIS **Altered nutrition: less than body requirements** *related to* anorexia, dietary restrictions, nausea, loss of nutrients from vomiting, and impaired digestion *as manifested by* weight loss, weakness, fatigue, weight below normal for height and age.

- Weight appropriate for height.
- No further weight loss.

- Monitor weight and laboratory values *as indicators of patient's response to treatment.*
- Observe stools for steatorrhea, *which may develop from incomplete digestion of fats.*
- Administer total parenteral nutrition if ordered *to provide carbohydrates and amino acids to prevent negative nitrogen balance.*
- Implement measures to reduce pain and nausea *to increase patient's desire to eat.*
- Provide oral care before and after meals *to decrease foul taste and odor that inhibit appetite.*
- If oral intake is allowed, provide small portions of high-carbohydrate, low-protein, low-fat foods.

NURSING DIAGNOSIS **Ineffective management of therapeutic regimen** *related to* lack of knowledge of preventive measures, diet restrictions, restriction of alcohol intake, and follow-up care *as manifested by* verbalization of the problem, request for information, inaccurate follow-through on instructions.

- Verbalization of understanding of condition or disease process and treatment.
- Initiation of lifestyle changes.
- Participation in treatment regimen.

- Teach patient to (1) abstain from alcohol *to prevent the patient from experiencing future attacks of acute pancreatitis and development of chronic pancreatitis;* (2) restrict fats and avoid rich, rough, and stimulating foods *to decrease stimulation of the pancreas and allow it to rest;* (3) use more carbohydrates in diet *because these are less stimulating to pancreas;* and (4) correctly measure blood glucose levels and observe for steatorrhea *because high blood glucose and fatty stools indicate destruction of pancreatic tissue.*
- Assess patient's understanding of prescribed regimen; provide details on follow-up care *to increase likelihood of successful convalescence and to minimize the possibility of recurrence.*
- Suggest follow-up if alcohol use is problematic *because continued use of alcohol will result in additional attacks of acute pancreatitis and eventual chronic pancreatitis.*

Continued

41-3 NURSING CARE PLAN PATIENT WITH ACUTE PANCREATITIS—continued

Expected Patient Outcomes	Nursing Interventions and *Rationales*

COLLABORATIVE PROBLEMS

Nursing Goals	Nursing Interventions and *Rationales*
POTENTIAL COMPLICATION ■ Monitor for signs of hypokalemia, hyponatremia, hypocalcemia, and hypochloremia. ■ Report deviations from acceptable parameters. ■ Carry out medical and nursing interventions.	**Fluid and electrolyte imbalance** *related to* loss of fluids into peritoneal cavity. ■ Observe for signs of fluid and electrolyte imbalance such as confusion, anorexia, diarrhea, seizures, muscle weakness, paralytic ileus, arrhythmias, metabolic alkalosis, muscle cramps, mental changes, tetany; monitor serum laboratory reports *to aid in early detection and prompt intervention.* ■ Give calcium gluconate as ordered *to treat symptomatic hypocalcemia.*
POTENTIAL COMPLICATION ■ Monitor for signs of hemorrhagic shock. ■ Report deviations from acceptable parameters. ■ Carry out appropriate medical and nursing interventions.	**Hemorrhagic shock** *related to* destruction of blood vessel walls by proteolytic enzymes. ■ Assess for continuing or increasing signs of shock such as pallor; cool, clammy skin; hypotension; tachycardia; increased respirations *to ensure prompt detection and intervention.* ■ Monitor vital signs every 1-2 hr *to evaluate patient's response to treatment.* ■ Assess hourly for decreased urinary output *as an indicator of circulating blood volume and renal perfusion.*

The patient and the family should be given instructions regarding the recognition and reporting of symptoms of infection, diabetes mellitus, or steatorrhea (foul-smelling, frothy stools). These changes indicate possible destruction of pancreatic tissue. The nurse should make sure the patient fully understands the prescribed regimen. Each aspect must be explained. The importance of taking the required medications and following the recommended diet should be stressed.

■ Evaluation

Expected outcomes for the patient with acute pancreatitis are presented in NCP 41-3.

CHRONIC PANCREATITIS

Etiology and Pathophysiology

Chronic pancreatitis is progressive destruction of the pancreas with fibrotic replacement of pancreatic tissue. Strictures and calcifications may also occur in the pancreas. There are several types of chronic pancreatitis, but they all have a common underlying pathophysiologic disorder. The two major types are chronic obstructive pancreatitis and chronic calcifying pancreatitis. Chronic pancreatitis may follow acute pancreatitis, but it may also occur in the absence of any history of an acute condition.

Chronic obstructive pancreatitis is associated with biliary disease. The most common cause is inflammation of the sphincter of Oddi associated with cholelithiasis. Cancer of the ampulla of Vater, duodenum, or pancreas can also cause this type of chronic pancreatitis.

In chronic calcifying pancreatitis there is inflammation and sclerosis, mainly in the head of the pancreas and around the pancreatic duct. This type of chronic pancreatitis is the most common form. It is also called alcohol-induced pancreatitis. Increases in heavy social drinking have produced a higher incidence in countries in which the disease was previously considered rare. In the United States chronic pancreatitis is found almost exclusively in alcoholics. As with cirrhosis there seems to be a metabolic abnormality that predisposes a person who drinks to the direct toxic effect of the alcohol on the pancreas.

In chronic calcifying pancreatitis the ducts are obstructed with protein precipitates. These precipitates block the pancreatic duct and eventually calcify. This is followed by fibrosis and glandular atrophy. Pseudocysts and abscesses commonly develop.

Clinical Manifestations

As with acute pancreatitis, a major manifestation of chronic pancreatitis is abdominal pain. The patient may have episodes of acute pain, but it usually is chronic (recurrent attacks at intervals of months or years). The attacks may become more and more frequent until they are almost constant, or they may diminish as the pancreatic fibrosis develops. The pain is located in the same areas as in acute pancreatitis but is usually described as a heavy, gnawing feeling or sometimes as burning and cramplike. The pain is not relieved with food or antacids.

Other clinical manifestations include symptoms of pancreatic insufficiency, including malabsorption with weight loss, constipation, mild jaundice with dark urine, steatorrhea, and diabetes mellitus. The steatorrhea may become severe, with voluminous, foul, fatty stools. Urine and stool may be frothy. Some abdominal tenderness may be present.

Diagnostic Studies

Laboratory findings in chronic pancreatitis include increased serum amylase (200 to 600 U/L [3.34 to 10.0 μkat/L]), increased serum bilirubin, and increased alkaline phosphatase levels. There is usually mild leukocytosis and an elevated sedimentation rate.

The secretin stimulation test is probably the most useful test in diagnosing chronic pancreatitis. Secretin is given IV, and gastric-duodenal secretions are collected with a double-lumen tube for separate gastric and duodenal aspiration. In chronic pancreatitis there is reduced volume of secretions and reduced bicarbonate concentration (less than 90 mEq/L). Normally, secretin stimulates the production of pancreatic fluid high in bicarbonate content.

Other abnormal diagnostic findings are hyperglycemia and fatty stools (steatorrhea) found in fecal fat determination. Neutral fat indicates maldigestion. Arteriography and x-rays may demonstrate fibrosis and calcification.

ERCP involves cannulation and visualization of the pancreatic and common bile ducts through a fiberoptic endoscope that is inserted into the esophagus and then into the duodenum. The common bile duct and the pancreatic duct are then cannulated. Contrast dye can be injected into the ducts for visualization. Changes in the pancreatic ductal system, such as gross dilation and microcysts, can be visualized through the use of ERCP.

Collaborative Care

When the patient with chronic pancreatitis is experiencing an acute attack, the therapy is identical to that for acute pancreatitis. At other times the focus is on prevention of further attacks, relief of pain, and control of pancreatic exocrine and endocrine insufficiency. It sometimes takes large, frequent doses of analgesics to relieve the pain.

Diet, pancreatic enzyme replacement, and control of the diabetes are measures used to control the pancreatic insufficiency. The diet is a bland, low-fat, high-carbohydrate, and high-protein diet. The patient does not tolerate fatty, rich, and stimulating foods, and these should be avoided to decrease pancreatic secretions and demands on the pancreas. Alcohol must be totally eliminated.

Antacids and anticholinergic drugs may be given to decrease hydrochloric acid, which stimulates pancreatic activity. Cimetidine (Tagamet) and ranitidine (Zantac), which block histamine receptors and thus decrease hydrochloric acid secretion, may be used for the same purpose. Pancreatic enzymes such as pancreatin (Viokase) and pancrelipase (Cotazym) contain amylase, lipase, and trypsin and are used to replace the deficient pancreatic enzymes. They are usually enteric coated to prevent their breakdown or inactivation by gastric acid. Bile salts are sometimes given to facilitate the absorption of the fat-soluble vitamins (A, D, E, and K) and prevent further fat loss. If diabetes develops, it is controlled with insulin or oral drugs.

Treatment of chronic pancreatitis sometimes requires surgery. When biliary disease is present or if obstruction or pseudocyst develops, surgery may be indicated. Operations performed are procedures to divert bile flow or relieve ductal obstruction. A choledochojejunostomy diverts bile around the ampulla of Vater, where there may be spasm or hypertrophy of the sphincter. In this procedure the common bile duct is anastomosed into the jejunum. If the pancreatic sphincter is fibrotic, a sphincterotomy enlarges it. Pancreatic drainage procedures relieve ductal obstruction. One type is the Roux-en-Y pancreatojejunostomy, in which the pancreatic duct is opened and an anastomosis is made with the jejunum.

NURSING MANAGEMENT: CHRONIC PANCREATITIS

Except during an acute episode, the focus of nursing management is on chronic care and health promotion. The patient should be instructed to take measures to prevent further attacks. Dietary control, along with consistency of other treatment measures, such as taking pancreatic enzymes, is essential. The pancreatic extracts are usually given with meals or can be given with a snack. The nurse should observe the patient's stools for steatorrhea to help determine the effectiveness of the enzymes. The patient and the family need instructions regarding observation of stools.

If diabetes has developed, the patient will need instruction regarding testing of blood glucose levels and medications (see Chapter 46). The patient who is taking liquid antacids should be instructed to sip the medication slowly, and the nurse should make certain it is taken as ordered to help control gastric acidity. Antacids should be taken after meals. Both the antacid and the pancreatic enzymes may be left at the bedside to prepare the patient for self-management at home.

Alcohol must be avoided, and the patient may need assistance with this problem. If the patient has developed a dependence on alcohol or narcotics, referral to other agencies or resources may be necessary (see Chapter 10).

CARCINOMA OF THE PANCREAS

In the United States more than 29,000 people are diagnosed with cancer of the pancreas each year.[23] It is the fifth leading cause of death from cancer. It is more common in men and more common in African-Americans than Caucasians. The risk increases with age, with the peak incidence occurring between 65 and 80 years of age.[24]

Most of the tumors are adenocarcinomas originating from the epithelium of the ductal system. More than half the tumors occur in the head of the pancreas. As the tumor grows, the common bile duct becomes obstructed and obstructive jaundice develops. Tumors starting in the body or tail often remain silent until their growth is advanced. The majority of cancers have metastasized at the time of diagnosis. The signs and symptoms of pancreatic cancer are often similar to chronic pancreatitis. The prognosis of a patient with cancer of the pancreas is poor. Most patients die within 5 to 12 months of the initial diagnosis, and the 5-year survival rate is only about 10%.[25] The prognosis is related to the location of the tumor.

Etiology and Pathophysiology

The cause of cancer of the pancreas remains unknown. There may be some relationship between cancer, diabetes mellitus, and chronic pancreatitis. However, it is not clear whether the cancer follows these diseases or whether these diseases occur as a result of pancreatic cancer. It is known that pancreatic cancer can be induced with chemicals such as nitrosoureas. Major risk factors seem to be cigarette smoking, high-fat diet, diabetes, and exposure to chemicals such as benzidine and coke. The most firmly established risk factor is cigarette smoking. Pancreatic cancer develops twice as frequently in persons with a history of heavy cigarette use (more than two packs a day) than in nonsmokers. The carcinogens from the tobacco probably reach the pancreatic ducts by bile reflux or via the bloodstream. Another risk factor is the Western diet, particularly the high fat content. High consumption of meat has also been implicated. Methods of processing foodstuffs may also be involved as a possible risk factor for cancer of the pancreas.

Clinical Manifestations

Common manifestations of pancreatic cancer include abdominal pain (dull, aching), anorexia, rapid and progressive weight loss, nausea, and jaundice. Pain is common and is related to the location of malignancy. Extreme, unrelenting pain is related to extension of the cancer into the retroperitoneal tissues and nerve plexuses. The pain is frequently located in the upper abdomen or left hypochondrium and frequently radiates to the back. It is commonly related to eating, and it also occurs at night. Weight loss is due to poor digestion and absorption caused by lack of digestive juices from the pancreas.

Diagnostic Studies

Better diagnostic measures are needed for detection of pancreatic cancer because most of the current methods detect only advanced stages. Cytologic examination of the pancreatic juice may reveal malignant cells. The secretin test frequently indicates a decreased volume of pancreatic juice with normal bicarbonate and enzyme production. Carcinoembryonic antigen (CEA) is elevated in a high percentage of patients with advanced disease, but it is also increased with other types of cancers and even some benign conditions. The CEA plasma level is therefore probably more useful in assessing the patient's response to treatment than in diagnosis. CA19-9 is a more specific tumor marker because it is associated with pancreatic cancer in particular.

Ultrasonography detects abnormalities of the pancreas but cannot distinguish cancer from other pancreatic disorders such as pancreatitis. Since this is a noninvasive procedure, it may be used in some situations. Computed tomography scans are effective in identifying a solid tumor mass and changes such as lymph node spread. Pancreatic arteriography demonstrates occlusion of the celiac axis and the superior mesenteric artery.

With ERCP it is possible to get excellent x-ray visualization of the pancreatic ducts. In pancreatic cancer, findings include obstruction or narrowing of a major duct and, frequently, saccular dilations of smaller peripheral ducts. Material for cytology and biopsy may show malignant cells. ERCP is usually considered to be the best diagnostic test.

Collaborative Care

Surgery provides the most effective treatment of cancer of the pancreas. The classic surgery is a radical pancreaticoduodenectomy, or Whipple's procedure (Fig. 41-14). This entails resection of the proximal pancreas (proximal pancreatectomy), the adjoining duodenum (duodenectomy), the distal portion of the stomach (partial gastrectomy), and the distal segment of

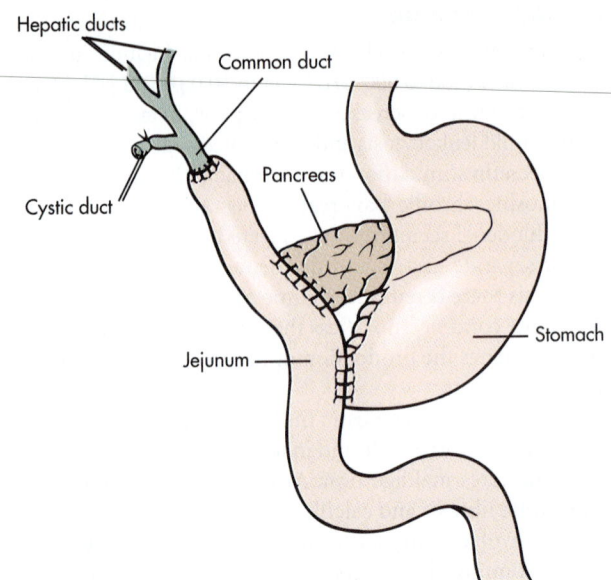

Fig. 41-14 Whipple procedure or radical pancreaticoduodenectomy. This surgical procedure involves resection of the proximal pancreas, adjoining duodenum, distal portion of the stomach, and distal portion of the common bile duct. An anastomosis of the pancreatic duct, common bile duct, and stomach to the jejunum is done.

the common bile duct. An anastomosis of the pancreatic duct, common bile duct, and stomach to the jejunum is done. A total pancreatectomy is performed in some institutions for cancers of the head of the pancreas. Sometimes a simple bypass procedure, such as a cholecystojejunostomy to relieve biliary obstruction, may be used as a palliative measure. Some surgeons suggest a more radical resection, such as a total pancreaticoduodenectomy with splenectomy. Biliary stents (e.g., Cotton-Leung stent) can be used as a palliative measure when tumors compress the bile duct.

Radiation therapy alters survival rates little but is effective for pain relief. External radiation is usually used, but implantation of internal radiation seeds into the tumor has also been used. Chemotherapy has limited success. Combinations of drugs such as 5-FU and carmustine (BCNU) produce a better response than single chemotherapeutic agents. Gemcitabine (Gemzar) is used in advanced pancreatic cancer. Biologic therapy is sometimes attempted (see Chapter 14). Adjuvant therapy, which uses surgical resection, radiation, and chemotherapy, is believed by some to be the most effective way to manage the almost always fatal cancer of the pancreas.

NURSING MANAGEMENT: CARCINOMA OF THE PANCREAS

Because the patient with carcinoma of the pancreas has many of the same problems as the patient with pancreatitis, nursing care includes the same measures (see NCP 41-3). The nurse should provide symptomatic and supportive nursing care. Medications and comfort measures to relieve pain should be provided before the patient reaches the peak of pain. Psycho-

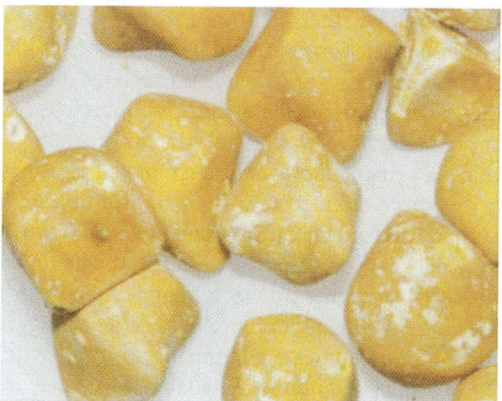

Fig. 41-15   Gallstones.

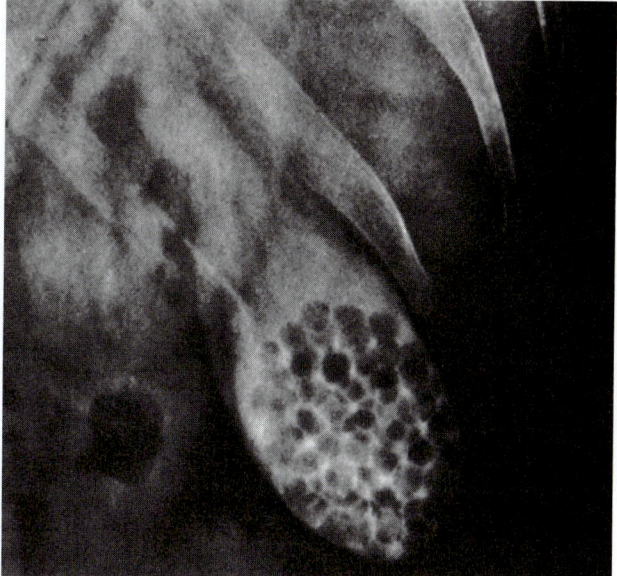

Fig. 41-16   X-ray of a gallbladder with gallstones.

logic support is essential, especially during times of anxiety or depression, which seem to occur frequently in these patients.

Adequate nutrition is an important part of the nursing care plan. Frequent and supplemental feedings may be necessary. Measures to stimulate the appetite as much as possible and to overcome anorexia, nausea, and vomiting should be included in the nursing care. Because bleeding can result from impaired vitamin K production, the nurse should assess for bleeding from body orifices and mucous membranes. If the patient is undergoing radiation therapy, the nurse must observe for adverse reactions, such as anorexia, nausea, vomiting, and skin irritation.

The prognosis for a patient with pancreatic cancer is not good. A significant component of the nursing care is helping the patient and the family or significant others through the grieving process.

DISORDERS OF THE BILIARY TRACT

The most common disorder of the biliary system is cholelithiasis (stones in the gallbladder) (Figs. 41-15 and 41-16). Cholecystitis (inflammation of the gallbladder) is usually associated with cholelithiasis. The stones may be lodged in the neck of the gallbladder or in the cystic duct. Cholecystitis may be acute or chronic. These conditions usually occur together.

Gallbladder disease is a common health problem in the United States. It is estimated that 8% to 10% of the adults in the United States have cholelithiasis. The actual number is not known because many persons are asymptomatic with stones. Cholecystectomy (removal of the gallbladder) ranks among the most common surgical procedures performed in the United States. The incidence of cholelithiasis is higher in women, multiparous women, and persons over 40 years of age. Postmenopausal women on estrogen therapy are at somewhat greater risk of having gallbladder disease than are women who are taking birth control pills. Oral contraceptives alter the character of bile, resulting in increased cholesterol saturation. Other factors that seem to increase the occurrence of gallbladder disease are a sedentary lifestyle, a familial tendency, and obesity. Obesity causes increased secretion of cholesterol in bile. Gallbladder disease is more common in Caucasians than in Asians and African-Americans. There is an especially high incidence in

the Native-American population, particularly in the Navajo and Pima tribes.

Etiology and Pathophysiology

Cholecystitis. Cholecystitis is most commonly associated with stones. When it occurs in the absence of stones, it is thought to be caused by bacteria reaching the gallbladder via the vascular or lymphatic route or chemical irritants in the bile. *Escherichia coli* is the most common bacterium involved. Streptococci and salmonellae are also common causative bacteria. Other etiologic factors include adhesions, neoplasms, extensive fasting, frequent weight fluctuations, anesthesia, and narcotics.

Inflammation is the major pathophysiologic condition and may be confined to the mucous lining or involve the entire wall of the gallbladder. During an acute attack of cholecystitis the gallbladder is edematous and hyperemic. It may be distended with bile or pus. The cystic duct is also involved and may become occluded. The wall of the gallbladder becomes scarred after an acute attack. Decreased functioning occurs if large amounts of tissue are fibrosed.

Cholelithiasis. The actual cause of gallstones is unknown. Basically, cholelithiasis develops when the balance that keeps cholesterol, bile salts, and calcium in solution is altered so that precipitation of these substances occurs. Conditions that upset this balance include infection and disturbances in the metabolism of cholesterol.

It is known that in patients with cholelithiasis the bile secreted by the liver is supersaturated with cholesterol (lithogenic bile). The bile in the gallbladder also becomes supersaturated with cholesterol. Whenever bile is supersaturated with cholesterol, precipitation of cholesterol will occur.

A high percentage of gallstones are precipitates of cholesterol. Other components of bile that precipitate into stones are bile salts, bilirubin, calcium, and protein. The stones sometimes have a mixed consistency. Mixed cholesterol stones, which are predominantly cholesterol, are the most common gallstones.

Table **41-23**	Clinical Manifestations Caused by Obstructed Bile Flow
Clinical Manifestation	**Etiology**
Obstructive jaundice	No bile flow into duodenum
Dark amber urine, which foams when shaken	Soluble bilirubin in urine
No urobilinogen in urine	No bilirubin reaching small intestine to be converted to urobilinogen
Clay-colored stools	Same as above
Pruritus	Deposition of bile salts in skin tissues
Intolerance for fatty foods (nausea, sensation of fullness, anorexia)	No bile in small intestine for fat digestion
Bleeding tendencies	Lack of or decreased absorption of vitamin K, resulting in decreased production of prothrombin
Steatorrhea	No bile salts in duodenum, preventing fat emulsion and digestion

The changes in the composition of bile are probably significant in the formation of gallstones. Stasis of bile leads to progression of the supersaturation and changes in the chemical composition of the bile. Immobility, pregnancy, and inflammatory or obstructive lesions of the biliary system decrease bile flow. Hormonal factors during pregnancy may cause delayed emptying of the gallbladder.

The stones may remain in the gallbladder or migrate to the cystic duct or to the common bile duct. They cause pain as they pass through the ducts and may lodge in the ducts and produce an obstruction. Small stones are more likely to move into a duct and cause obstruction. Table 41-23 depicts the changes and manifestations that occur when the stones obstruct the common bile duct. If the blockage occurs in the cystic duct, the bile can continue to flow into the duodenum directly from the liver. When the bile in the gallbladder cannot escape, however, this stasis of bile may lead to cholecystitis.

Clinical Manifestations

Manifestations of cholecystitis vary from indigestion to moderate to severe pain, fever, and jaundice. Initial symptoms of acute cholecystitis include indigestion and pain and tenderness in the right upper quadrant, which may be referred to the right shoulder and scapula. The pain may be acute and be accompanied by nausea and vomiting, restlessness, and diaphoresis. Manifestations of inflammation, such as leukocytosis and fever, occur. Physical findings include right upper quadrant tenderness and abdominal rigidity. Symptoms of chronic cholecystitis include a history of fat intolerance, dyspepsia, heartburn, and flatulence.

Cholelithiasis may produce severe symptoms or none at all. Many patients have "silent cholelithiasis." The severity of symptoms depends on whether the stones are stationary or mobile and whether obstruction is present. When a stone is lodged in the ducts or when stones are moving through the ducts, spasms may result. The spasms are the tissues' responses to the stone in an attempt to move it forward. This sometimes produces severe pain, which is termed *biliary colic* even though the pain is rarely colicky; it is more often steady. The pain can be excruciating and accompanied by tachycardia, diaphoresis, and prostration. The severe pain may last up to an hour, and when it subsides there is residual tenderness in the right upper quadrant. The attacks of pain frequently occur 3 to 6 hours after a heavy meal or when the patient assumes a recumbent position. When total obstruction occurs, symptoms related to bile blockage are manifested (see Table 41-23).

Complications

Complications of cholecystitis include subphrenic abscess, pancreatitis, cholangitis (inflammation of biliary ducts), biliary cirrhosis, fistulas, and rupture of the gallbladder, which can produce bile peritonitis.

Many of the same complications can occur from cholelithiasis, including cholangitis, biliary cirrhosis, carcinoma, and peritonitis. Choledocholithiasis (stone in the common bile duct) may occur, producing symptoms of obstruction.

Diagnostic Studies

Ultrasonography is probably the best means of diagnosing gallstones (see Table 37-12). It is 90% to 95% accurate in detecting stones. It is especially useful for patients with jaundice (because it does not depend on liver function) and for patients who are allergic to contrast medium.

An oral cholecystogram allows for the detection of stones when they are radiopaque. An IV cholangiogram outlines both the gallbladder and the ducts, so gallstones that have moved into the ductal system can be detected. Percutaneous transhepatic cholangiography may be used to diagnose obstructive jaundice and to locate stones within the bile ducts. Bile taken during ERCP is sent for culture to identify any possible infecting organism.

Laboratory tests may demonstrate abnormalities in some of the liver function tests and an increased WBC count as a result of inflammation. Both the direct and indirect bilirubin levels are elevated, as is the urinary bilirubin level if there is an obstructive process present. If the common bile duct is obstructed, no bilirubin will reach the small intestine to be converted to urobilinogen. Serum enzymes, such as alkaline phosphatase and AST (SGOT), may be elevated. The serum amylase is increased if there is pancreatic involvement.

Collaborative Care
Conservative Therapy

Cholecystitis. During an acute episode of cholecystitis the focus of treatment is on control of pain, control of possible infection with antibiotics, and maintenance of fluid and electrolyte balance (Table 41-24). Treatment is mainly supportive and symptomatic. If nausea and vomiting are severe, gastric decompression may be used to prevent further gallbladder stimulation. Anticholinergics to decrease secretions (which prevents

Table **41-24** **Cholelithiasis**

Diagnostic
Ultrasound
Cholecystogram or IV cholangiogram
Liver function studies
WBC count
Serum bilirubin

Collaborative Therapy
Conservative Therapy
IV fluid
NPO with NG tube, later progressing to low-fat diet
Antiemetics
Analgesics (e.g., meperidine)
Fat-soluble vitamins (A, D, E, and K)
Anticholinergics (antispasmodics)
Hydrocholetic drugs
   Dehydrocholic acid (Decholin)
   Florantyrone (Zanchol)
Antibiotics
ERCP with sphincterotomy (papillotomy)
Cholesterol solvents
Extracorporeal shock-wave lithotripsy

Dissolution Therapy
Ursodeoxycholic acid (UDCA)
Ursodiol (Actigall)
Chenodeoxycholic acid (CDCA)

Surgical Therapy
Laparoscopic cholecystectomy
Incisional cholecystectomy
See Table 41-25

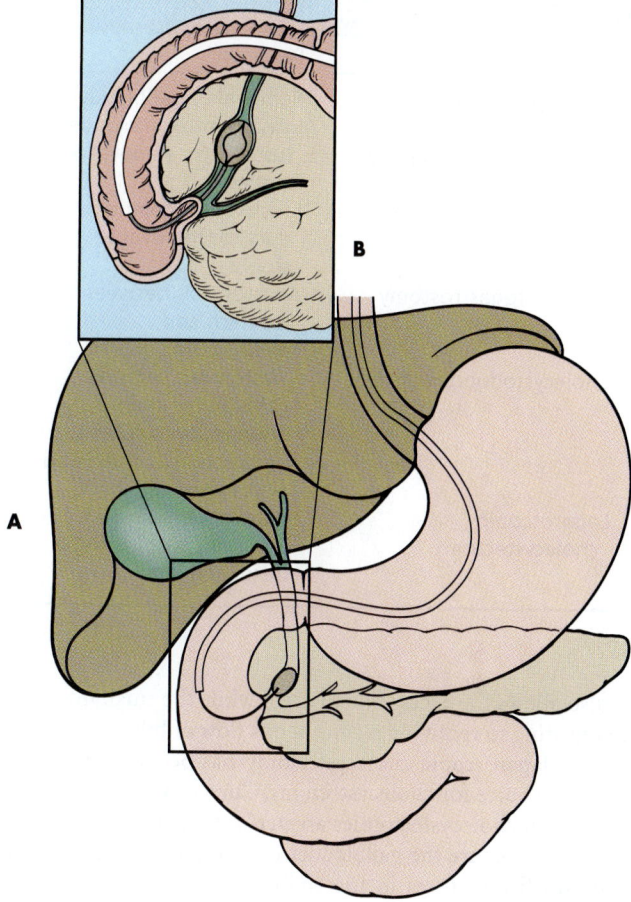

Fig. 41-17 **A,** During endoscopic sphincterotomy, a flexible endoscope is advanced through the mouth and stomach until its tip sits in the duodenum opposite the common bile duct. **B,** After widening the duct mouth by incising the sphincter muscle, the physician advances a basket attachment into the duct and snags the stone.

biliary contraction) and counteract smooth muscle spasms may be administered. Analgesics are given to decrease the pain.

Cholelithiasis. There are currently several options for management of cholelithiasis. These include cholesterol solvents such as methyl tertiary terbutyl ether (MTBE), oral drugs that dissolve stones, endoscopic sphincterotomy, extracorporeal shock-wave lithotripsy (ESWL), and surgery. Supportive treatment, similar to that given for cholecystitis, may also be necessary. If the stones cause an obstruction, additional treatment consists of replacement of fat-soluble vitamins, administration of bile salts to facilitate digestion and vitamin absorption, and a low-fat diet.

A direct-contact dissolving agent such as MTBE can be instilled into the gallbladder via a percutaneous catheter. MTBE dissolves cholesterol stones within hours. The gallstones may recur. Oral bile acids are also used to dissolve stones.

Endoscopic sphincterotomy (papillotomy) is especially effective in removing common bile duct stones (Fig. 41-17). The endoscope is passed to the duodenum. With an electrodiathermy knife attached to the endoscope, the sphincter of Oddi is widened by incision of the sphincter muscle (sphincterotomy). A basket is used to retrieve the stone. The stone may be removed in the basket, but more commonly it is left in the duodenum and will be passed naturally in the stool.

In ESWL a biliary lithotriptor uses high-energy shock waves to disintegrate gallstones. The patient must have a functioning gallbladder. An ultrasound scan is first done to locate the stones and to determine where to direct the shock waves. The shock waves are directed through the abdomen as a water-filled cushion is pressed against the area. It usually takes 1 to 2 hours to disintegrate the stones. After they are broken up, the fragments pass through the common bile duct and into the small intestine. There has been mixed success with ESWL.

Surgical Therapy. Surgical intervention for cholelithiasis is frequently indicated and may consist of any one of several procedures (Table 41-25). The procedure of choice for most patients is still a cholecystectomy. This is a safe procedure with minimal morbidity, and it requires only a brief hospitalization. One procedure is removal of the gallbladder through a right subcostal incision. A T-tube is inserted into the common bile duct during surgery when a common bile duct exploration is part of the surgical procedure (Fig. 41-18). This ensures patency of the duct until the edema produced by the trauma of exploring and probing the duct has subsided.

Table **41-25**	Gallbladder Surgery Procedures
Name	**Description**
Cholecystectomy	Removal of gallbladder
Cholecystostomy (usually an emergency)	Incision into gallbladder (usually for removal of stones)
Choledocholithotomy	Incision into common bile duct for removal of stones
Cholecystogastrostomy	Anastomosis between stomach and gallbladder
Cholecystoduodenostomy	Anastomosis between gallbladder and duodenum to relieve obstruction at distal end of common bile duct
Laparoscopic cholecystectomy	Removal of gallbladder via laparoscopy using a dissecting laser

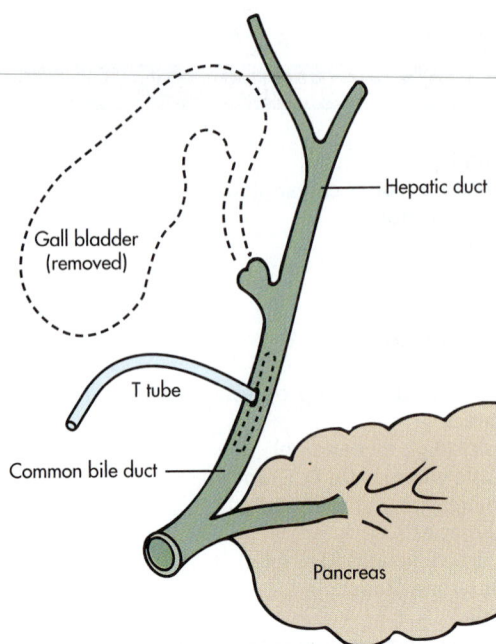

Fig. 41-18 Placement of T tube. Dotted lines indicate parts removed.

It also allows the excess bile to drain while the small intestine is adjusting to receiving a continuous flow of bile.

The laparoscopic cholecystectomy has become the treatment of choice for cholecystectomy. Currently approximately 90% of all cholecystectomies are performed laparoscopically. In this procedure the gallbladder is removed through one of four small punctures in the abdomen. A 1 cm puncture is made slightly above the umbilicus, and the surgeon inflates the abdominal cavity with 3 to 4 L of carbon dioxide to improve visibility. A laparoscope, which has a camera attached, is then inserted into the abdomen. Two additional punctures are made just below the ribs, one on the right anterior axillary line and the other on the right midclavicular line. These punctures are used for insertion of grasping forceps. A dissection laser is inserted into the fourth puncture, which is made just right of the midsection. (The incision sites may vary.) Using closed-circuit monitors to view the abdominal cavity, the surgeon retracts and dissects the gallbladder and removes it with grasping forceps.

This procedure is relatively minor with few complications. Most patients experience minimal postoperative pain and are discharged the day of surgery or the day after. In most cases they are able to resume normal activities and return to work after 2 or 3 days.

Advantages to the laparoscopic cholecystectomy include decreased postoperative pain, shorter hospital stay, and earlier return to work and full activity. The main complication is injury to the common bile duct. There are few contraindications to laparoscopic cholecystectomy. The primary ones are peritonitis, cholangitis, gangrene or perforation of the gallbladder, portal hypertension, and serious bleeding disorders.

Transhepatic Biliary Catheter. The transhepatic biliary catheter can be used preoperatively in biliary obstruction and in hepatic dysfunction secondary to obstructive jaundice. It can also be inserted when inoperable liver, pancreatic, or bile duct carcinoma obstructs bile flow. The catheter is in-

serted under fluoroscopy and involves percutaneous insertion across the liver parenchyma into the common bile duct and duodenum. It decompresses obstructed extrahepatic bile ducts so that bile can flow freely. After insertion, the catheter is connected to a drainage bag. The skin around the catheter insertion site has to be cleansed daily with an antiseptic. It is important to observe for bile leakage at the insertion site. Depending on the reason the catheter was inserted, the patient may be discharged with it in place.

Drug Therapy. The most common drugs used in the treatment of gallbladder disease are analgesics, anticholinergics (antispasmodics), fat-soluble vitamins, and bile salts. Meperidine (Demerol) is used if a narcotic analgesic is required. This causes less spasm in the ducts than opiates such as morphine sulfate. Anticholinergics such as atropine and other antispasmodics may be used to relax the smooth muscle and decrease ductal tone.

If the patient has chronic gallbladder disease or any biliary tract obstruction, fat-soluble vitamins (A, D, E, and K) will probably be given. Bile salts may be administered to facilitate digestion and vitamin absorption.

Hydrocholeretic drugs, which stimulate the production of bile with a low specific gravity, may be administered following gallbladder surgery when a T-tube is in place or with conservative therapy as long as there is no obstruction. These drugs stimulate the production of bile of a low specific gravity. Examples are bile salts such as dehydrocholic acid (Decholin) and florantyrone (Zanchol).

For treatment of pruritus, cholestyramine (Questran) may provide relief. This is a resin that binds bile salts in the intestine, increasing their excretion in the feces. Cholestyramine is administered in powder form and should be mixed with milk or

NURSING ASSESSMENT

Table 41-26 | Cholecystitis or Cholelithiasis

Subjective Data	Objective Data
Important Health Information	**General**
Past health history: Obesity, multiparity, infection, cancer, extensive fasting, pregnancy	Fever, restlessness
Medications: Use of estrogen or oral contraceptives	**Integumentary**
Surgery and other treatments: Previous abdominal surgery	Jaundice, icteric sclera; diaphoresis
Functional Health Patterns	**Respiratory**
Health perception–health management: Positive family history; sedentary lifestyle	Tachypnea, splinting during respirations
Nutritional-metabolic: Weight loss, anorexia; indigestion, fat intolerance, nausea and vomiting, dyspepsia; chills	**Cardiovascular**
	Tachycardia
Elimination: Clay-colored stools, steatorrhea, flatulence; dark urine	**Gastrointestinal**
	Palpable gallbladder, abdominal guarding and distention
Cognitive-perceptual: Moderate to severe pain in right upper quadrant that may radiate to the back or scapula; pruritus	**Possible Findings**
	Elevated serum liver enzymes and bilirubin, absence of urobilinogen in urine, increased urinary bilirubin; leukocytosis, abnormal gallbladder ultrasound, positive oral cholecystogram or IV cholangiogram

juice. Side effects include nausea, vomiting, diarrhea or constipation, and skin reactions.

Medical dissolution therapy is recommended for patients with small radiolucent stones who are mildly symptomatic and are poor surgical risks. Ursodeoxycholic acid (UDCA), ursodiol (Actigall), and chenodeoxycholic acid (CDCA, chenodiol, Chenix) may be used to dissolve the stones. The main side effects of CDCA are cramps and diarrhea, but these are usually not severe. A more serious side effect is hepatotoxicity. UDCA has fewer side effects than CDCA. Dissolution therapy may take anywhere from 6 months to 2 years for dissolution of the stones, and low-dose therapy is recommended to prevent recurrence. Results are often better in nonobese patients. These drugs may be used after ESWL to prevent formation of other stones. The drugs to dissolve the gallstones are not used as much currently because of high use of laparoscopic cholecystectomy.

Nutritional Therapy. The major dietary modification for a patient with cholelithiasis and cholecystitis is a low-fat diet (see Table 32-5). If obesity is a problem, a reduced-calorie diet is indicated. The low-fat diet decreases stimulation of the gallbladder. Foods that are avoided include dairy products such as whole milk, cream, butter, whole milk cheese, and ice cream; fried foods; rich pastries; gravies; and nuts. Many patients have fewer problems if they eat smaller, more frequent meals.

After a laparoscopic cholecystectomy the patient is instructed to have liquids for the rest of the day and eat light meals for a few days. If an incisional cholecystectomy is done, the patient will progress from liquids to a bland diet once bowel sounds have returned. The amount of fat in the postoperative diet depends on the patient's tolerance of fat. A low-fat diet may be helpful if the flow of bile is reduced (usually only in the early postoperative period) or if the patient is overweight. Sometimes the patient is instructed to restrict fats for 4 to 6 weeks. Otherwise no special dietary instructions are needed other than to eat nutritious meals and avoid excessive fat intake.

NURSING MANAGEMENT: GALLBLADDER DISEASE

■ Nursing Assessment

Subjective and objective data that should be obtained from a person with gallbladder disease are presented in Table 41-26.

■ Nursing Diagnoses

Nursing diagnoses for the patient with gallbladder disease treated surgically include, but are not limited to, the following:

- Pain *related to* surgical procedure
- Ineffective management of therapeutic regimen *related to* lack of knowledge of diet and postoperative management

■ Planning

The overall goals are that the patient with gallbladder disease will have (1) relief of pain and discomfort, (2) no complications postoperatively, and (3) no recurrent attacks of cholecystitis or cholelithiasis.

■ Nursing Implementation

Health Promotion. The nurse should assume responsibility for recognition of predisposing factors of gallbladder disease in general health screening. Ethnic groups in which the disease is more common, such as Native-Americans, should be taught initial manifestations and instructed to seek medical care if these manifestations occur. The patient with chronic cholecystitis does not have acute symptoms and may not seek help until jaundice and biliary obstruction occur. Earlier detection in these patients is beneficial so that they can be treated with a low-fat diet and monitored more closely.

Acute Intervention. Nursing objectives for the patient undergoing conservative therapy include relieving pain, relieving nausea and vomiting, providing comfort and emotional support, maintaining fluid and electrolyte balance and nutrition, making accurate assessments for effectiveness of treatment, and observing for complications.

The patient with cholecystitis or cholelithiasis is frequently experiencing severe pain. The medications ordered to relieve the pain should be given as required by the patient and before the pain becomes more severe. The nurse should assess what medications relieve the pain and how much medication is required. Observations for side effects of the medications must be part of the continued assessment. Nursing comfort measures, such as a clean bed, comfortable positioning, and oral care, are appropriate.

Some patients have more severe nausea and vomiting than others. For these patients it may be necessary to use gastric decompression. The elimination of intake of food and fluids also prevents further stimulation of the gallbladder. Oral hygiene, care of nares, accurate intake and output measurements, and maintenance of suction should be a part of the nursing care plan for this patient. For patients with less severe nausea and vomiting, antiemetics are usually adequate. When the patient is vomiting, comfort measures such as frequent mouth rinses should be provided. Any vomitus should be immediately removed from the patient's view.

If pruritus occurs with jaundice, measures to relieve itching are necessary. Such measures include baking soda or Alpha Keri baths; lotions, such as those containing calamine; antihistamines; soft, old linen; and control of the temperature (not too hot and not too cold). The patient's nails should be kept short and clean. Patients should be taught to rub with their knuckles rather than scratch with their nails when they cannot resist scratching.

A significant portion of the nursing care plan for this patient centers on accurate assessment of progression of the symptoms and development of complications. The nurse must be knowledgeable of and observe for signs of obstruction of the ducts by stones. These include jaundice; clay-colored stools; dark, foamy urine; steatorrhea; fever; and increased WBC count.

When symptoms of obstruction are present (see Table 41-23), the nurse must be aware of the possibility of bleeding as a result of decreased prothrombin production. Common sites to observe for bleeding are the mucous membranes of the mouth, nose, gingivae, and injection sites. If injections are given, a small-gauge needle should be used and gentle pressure applied after the injection. The nurse should know what the patient's prothrombin time is and use this as a guide in the assessment process.

Assessment for infections includes monitoring of vital signs. A temperature elevation with chills and jaundice may indicate choledocholithiasis.

Nursing care of the patient after endoscopic papillotomy includes assessment to detect complications such as pancreatitis, perforation, infection, and bleeding. The patient's vital signs should be monitored. Abdominal pain and fever may indicate pancreatitis. The patient should be on bed rest for several hours and should have nothing by mouth until the gag reflex returns.

Postoperative care. Postoperative nursing care following a laparoscopic cholecystectomy includes monitoring for complications such as bleeding, making the patient comfortable,

---

🖊 **PATIENT & FAMILY TEACHING GUIDE**

Table 41-27 **Postoperative Laparoscopic Cholecystectomy**

1. Instruct patient to remove the bandages on the puncture site the day after surgery and bathe or shower.
2. Explain the need to report the following signs and symptoms:
   - Redness, swelling, bile-colored drainage or pus from any incision
   - Severe abdominal pain, nausea, vomiting, fever, chills
3. Explain that normal activities can be resumed gradually.
4. Instruct that returning to work can occur within 1 week of surgery.
5. Instruct to resume usual diet; may need to be a low-fat diet for several weeks following surgery.

---

and preparing the patient for discharge. A common postoperative problem is referred pain to the shoulder because of the CO_2 that was not released or absorbed by the body. The CO_2 can irritate the phrenic nerve and the diaphragm, causing some difficulty breathing. Placing the patient in Sim's position (left side with right knee flexed) helps move the gas pocket away from the diaphragm. Deep breathing should be encouraged, along with movement and ambulation. There is usually minimal pain that can be relieved by narcotic analgesics such as oxycodone and acetaminophen with codeine. The patient is allowed clear liquids and can walk to the bathroom to void. Many patients go home the same day, but some will stay overnight.

Postoperative nursing care for incisional surgery (cholecystectomy) focuses on adequate ventilation and prevention of respiratory complications. Other nursing care is the same as general postoperative nursing care (see Chapter 18).

If the patient has a T-tube, part of the nursing care plan is related to maintaining bile drainage and observation of the T-tube functioning and drainage. The T-tube is connected to a closed gravity drainage system. If the Penrose or Jackson-Pratt drain or the T-tube is draining large amounts, it is helpful to use a sterile pouching system to protect the skin.

Ambulatory and Home Care. When the patient has conservative therapy, long-term nursing management depends on symptoms and on whether surgical intervention is being planned. Dietary teaching is usually necessary. The diet is usually low in fat, and sometimes a weight-reduction diet is also recommended. The patient may need to take fat-soluble vitamin supplements. The nurse should provide instructions regarding observations the patient should make indicating obstruction (stool and urine changes, jaundice, and pruritus). Continued health care is important, and its significance should be explained and stressed.

The patient who undergoes a laparoscopic cholecystectomy is discharged soon after the surgery, so home care is important. Teaching is essential (Table 41-27).

CRITICAL THINKING EXERCISES

CASE STUDY

Cirrhosis of the Liver

Patient Profile
Mr. R. is a 55-year-old man admitted with a diagnosis of cirrhosis of the liver.

Subjective Data
- Has had cirrhosis for 12 years
- Acknowledges that he had been drinking heavily for 20 years but has been sober for the past 2 years
- Complains of anorexia, nausea, and abdominal discomfort

Objective Data

Physical Examination
- Thin and malnourished
- Has moderate ascites
- Has jaundice of sclera and skin
- Has 4+ pitting edema of the lower extremities
- Liver and spleen are palpable

Laboratory Values
- Total bilirubin 15 mg/dl (257 μmol/L)
- Serum ammonia 220 μg/dl (122 μmol/L)
- AST 190 U/L (3.2 μkat/L)
- ALT 210 U/L (3.5 μkat/L)

Critical Thinking Questions

1. What are possible causes of cirrhosis? What type of cirrhosis does Mr. R. probably have?
2. Describe the pathophysiologic changes that occur in the liver as cirrhosis develops.
3. List Mr. R.'s clinical manifestations of liver failure. For each manifestation, explain the pathophysiologic bases.
4. Explain the significance of the results of his laboratory values.
5. If Mr. R. begins to manifest signs and symptoms of hepatic encephalopathy, what would you monitor? What measures should be instituted to control or decrease the ammonia level?
6. Mr. R. was being closely observed for the possibility of gastrointestinal bleeding. Why is this considered a possible complication?
7. In the early stages of cirrhosis, what can be done to control the disease?
8. Based on the assessment data presented, write one or more nursing diagnoses. Are there any collaborative problems?

NURSING RESEARCH ISSUES

1. What is the most effective way to assess jaundice in a dark-skinned person?
2. What are the most significant psychosocial problems experienced by a patient with viral hepatitis?
3. What are the best ways to treat pruritus associated with jaundice in patients with hepatitis?
4. What is the quality of life for a patient after a liver transplant?
5. Can nutritional support improve outcomes in patients with alcohol-related cirrhosis?
6. What support resources are needed by the family of a patient with pancreatic cancer?

After an open-incision cholecystectomy, the patient may be discharged as soon as 3 to 5 days. The patient should be instructed to avoid heavy lifting for 4 to 6 weeks. Usual sexual activities, including intercourse, can be resumed as soon as the patient feels ready unless given other instructions by the physician.

Sometimes the patient is required to remain on a low-fat diet for 4 to 6 weeks. If so, a dietary teaching plan is necessary. A weight-reduction program may be helpful if the patient is overweight. Most patients tolerate a regular diet with no difficulties but should avoid excessive fats.

■ Evaluation
The overall expected outcomes are that the patient with gallbladder disease will

- appear comfortable and verbalize pain relief
- verbalize knowledge of activity level and dietary restrictions

CANCER OF THE GALLBLADDER

Primary cancer of the gallbladder is uncommon. The majority of gallbladder carcinomas are adenocarcinomas. There seems to be a definite relationship between cancer of the gallbladder and chronic cholecystitis and cholelithiasis.

The early symptoms of carcinoma of the gallbladder are insidious and are similar to those of chronic cholecystitis and cholelithiasis, which makes diagnosis difficult. Later symptoms are usually those of biliary obstruction. Cancer of the gallbladder has a poor prognosis.

Treatment is mainly symptomatic and supportive. Sometimes the tumor is resected. Chemotherapy and radiotherapy are seldom used because they are neither curative nor palliative.

Nursing management involves supportive care with special attention to nutrition, hydration, skin care, and pain relief. Many of the nursing care measures used for patients with cholecystitis and cholelithiasis are frequently applied, as well as nursing care measures for the patient with cancer (see Chapter 14).

REVIEW QUESTIONS

The number of the question corresponds to the same-numbered objective at the beginning of the chapter.

1. During assessment of a patient with obstructive jaundice the nurse would expect to find
   a. serum bilirubin of 1 mg/dl.
   b. pyrexia and severe pruritus.
   c. elevated urinary urobilinogen.
   d. dark urine and clay-colored stools.

2. A patient with hepatitis A is in the prodromal (preicteric) phase. The nurse plans care for the patient based on the knowledge that
   a. pruritus is a common problem with the jaundice of this phase.
   b. the patient is most likely to transmit the disease during this phase.
   c. gastrointestinal symptoms are not as severe in hepatitis A as they are in hepatitis B.
   d. extrahepatic manifestations of glomerulonephritis and polyarteritis are common in this phase.

3. A patient with hepatitis B is being discharged in 2 days. The nurse includes in his discharge teaching plan instructions to
   a. avoid alcohol for 3 weeks.
   b. use a condom during sexual intercourse.
   c. have family members get an injection of immunoglobulin.
   d. follow a low-protein, moderate-carbohydrate, moderate-fat diet.

4. The patient with advanced cirrhosis asks the nurse why his abdomen is so swollen. The nurse's response to the patient is based on the knowledge that
   a. a lack of clotting factors promotes the collection of blood in the abdominal cavity.
   b. portal hypertension and hypoalbuminemia cause a fluid shift into the peritoneal space.
   c. decreased peristalsis in the GI tract contributes to gas formation and distention of the bowel.
   d. bile salts in the blood irritate the peritoneal membranes, causing edema and pocketing of fluid.

5. When caring for a patient with hepatic encephalopathy the nurse may give enemas, provide a low-protein diet, and limit physical activity. These measures are done to
   a. promote fluid loss.
   b. eliminate potassium ions.
   c. decrease portal pressure.
   d. decrease the production of ammonia.

6. In planning care for a patient with metastatic cancer of the liver the nurse includes interventions that
   a. focus primarily on symptomatic and comfort measures.
   b. reassure the patient that chemotherapy offers a good prognosis for recovery.
   c. promote the patient's confidence that surgical excision of the tumor will be successful.
   d. provide information necessary for the patient to make decisions regarding liver transplantation.

7. The nurse explains to the patient with acute pancreatitis that the most common pathogenic mechanism of the disorder is
   a. cellular disorganization.
   b. overproduction of enzymes.
   c. lack of secretion of enzymes.
   d. autodigestion of the pancreas.

8. Nursing management of the patient with acute pancreatitis includes
   a. checking for signs of hypercalcemia.
   b. observing stools for signs of steatorrhea.
   c. providing a diet low in carbohydrates with moderate fat.
   d. monitoring for infection, particularly respiratory infection.

9. A patient with pancreatic cancer is admitted to the hospital for evaluation for treatment. The patient asks the nurse to explain the Whipple procedure the surgeon has described. The nurse's explanation includes the information that a Whipple procedure involves
   a. creating a bypass around the obstruction caused by the tumor by joining the gallbladder to the jejunum.
   b. resection of the entire pancreas and the distal portion of the stomach, with anastomosis of the common bile duct and stomach into the duodenum.
   c. removal of part of the pancreas, part of the stomach, the duodenum, and the gallbladder, with joining of the pancreatic duct, common bile duct, and stomach into the jejunum.
   d. radical removal of the pancreas, duodenum, and spleen, attaching the stomach to the jejunum, which requires oral supplementation of pancreatic digestive enzymes and insulin replacement therapy.

10. The nursing management of the patient with cholecystitis associated with cholelithiasis is based on the knowledge that
    a. the disorder can be successfully treated with oral bile salts that dissolve gallstones.
    b. morphine is the drug of choice to relieve the pain of bile duct spasms during an acute attack.
    c. a heavy meal with a high fat content may precipitate the signs and symptoms of the disease.
    d. a low-cholesterol diet is indicated to reduce the availability of cholesterol for gallstone formation.

11. Teaching in relation to home management following a laparoscopic cholecystectomy should include
    a. keeping the bandages on the puncture sites for 48 hours.
    b. reporting any bile-colored drainage or pus from any incision.
    c. using over-the-counter antiemetics if nausea and vomiting occur.
    d. emptying and measuring the contents of the bile bag from the T-tube every day.

References

1. *Hepatitis statistics,* 1997, Hepatitis Foundation International. http://www.hepsi.org/stats.htm
2. Idilman R and others: Interferon treatment of cirrhotic patients with chronic hepatitis C, *J Viral Hepatitis* 4:81, 1997.
3. Koff RS: Chronic hepatitis C: early intervention, *Hosp Pract* 33:101, 1998.
4. Seeff LB: Acute viral hepatitis. In Kaplowtiz N, editor: *Liver and biliary diseases,* ed 2, Baltimore, 1996, Williams & Wilkins.
5. Lee WK: Hepatitis B virus infection, *N Engl J Med* 337:1733, 1997.
6. Bryan JP and others: Hepatitis B vaccine booster dose: low-dose recombinant hepatitis B vaccines as a booster dose, *Am J Infect Control* 25:215, 1997.
7. Sharara AI, Hunt CM, Hamilton JD: Hepatitis C, *Ann Intern Med* 125:658, 1996.
8. Hepatitis Branch, Centers for Disease Control and Prevention: Epidemiology and prevention of viral hepatitis A to E: an overview. http://www.cdc.gov/httoc.htm

9. Alter HJ and others: The incidence of transfusion-associated hepatitis G virus infection and its relation to liver disease, *N Engl J Med* 336:747, 1997.

10. Tacke M and others: Detection of antibodies to a putative hepatitis G virus envelope protein, *Lancet* 349:318, 1997.

11. Centers for Disease Control and Prevention: Notice to readers. Recommendations for follow-up of health-care workers after occupational exposure to hepatitis C virus, *MMWR* 46:26, 1997.

12. The hepatitis place. http://www.hepplace.com/tests/html

13. Woo MH, Burnakis TG: Interferon alpha in the treatment of chronic viral hepatitis B and C, *Ann Pharmacol* 31:330, 1997.

14. Perrillo RP: Mechanisms of anti-viral therapy for HBV: interferons; nucleoside analogues; immunomodulators. Internet: http://www.hepnet.com/boca/perrillo.html.

15. Centers for Disease Control and Prevention: Prevention of hepatitis A through active or passive immunization, *MMWR* 45(no. RR-15):1, 1996.

16. Centers for Disease Control and Prevention: Notice to readers. Interferon may be used in the treatment of chronic hepatitis C, *MMWR* 46:26, 1997.

17. Freitag-Koontz MJ: Prevention of hepatitis B and C transmission during pregnancy and the first year of life, *J Perinat Neonat Nurs* 10:40, 1996.

18. O'Hanlon-Nichols T: Clinical snapshot: portal hypertension, *AJN* 95:38, 1995.

19. Koutsomanis D: Endoscopic clipping for bleeding varices, *Gastrointest Endosc* 40:126, 1994.

20. Sogni P and others: Acute effects of propylthiouracil on hemodynamics and oxygen content in patients with alcoholic cirrhosis, *J Hepatol* 26:628, 1997.

21. Holland JF and others, editors: *Cancer medicine*, vol II, ed 4, Baltimore, 1997, Williams & Wilkins.

22. Feray SD, Bismuth H: HCV infection and liver transplantation, *Acta Gastroenterol Belg* 60:214, 1997.

23. *Cancer facts and figures—1998*, American Cancer Society, Atlanta, Ga.

24. Holland JF and others, editors: *Cancer medicine*, vol II, ed 4, Baltimore, 1997, Williams & Wilkins.

25. DeVita VT and others: *Cancer principles and practice of oncology*, ed 5, Philadelphia, 1997, Lippincott-Raven.

Resources

American Association for the Study of Liver Diseases (AASLD)
c/o American Gastroenterological Association
7910 Woodmont Ave, 7th Floor
Bethesda, MD 20814
301-654-2055
Fax: 301-652-3890

American Liver Foundation
1425 Pompton Avenue
Cedar Grove, NJ 07009
800-GO-LIVER (465-4837)
http://sadieo.ucsf.edu/alf/alffinal/homepagealf.html

United Ostomy Association
19772 MacArthur Boulevard, Suite 200
Irvine, CA 92612-2405
800-826-0826
http://www.uoa.org/

For additional Internet resources, see the website for this book at www.mosby.com/MERLIN/medsurg_lewis

PROBLEMS OF URINARY FUNCTION

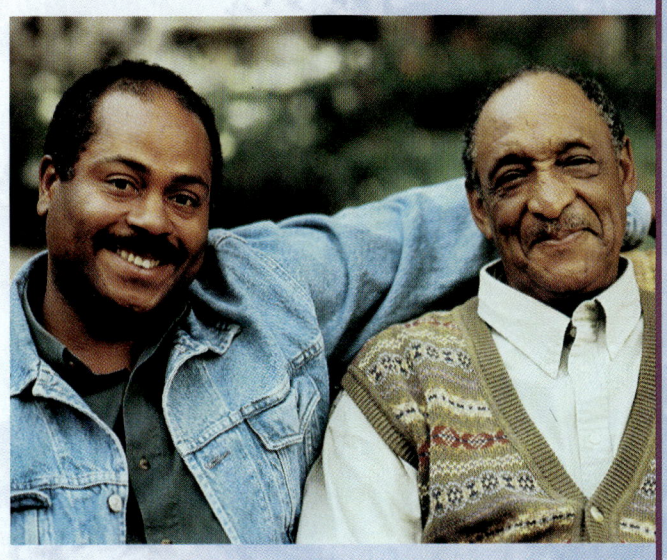

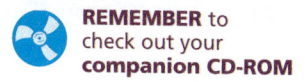

42 NURSING ASSESSMENT
Urinary System

Patricia Bates

LEARNING OBJECTIVES

1. Describe the anatomic location and functions of the kidneys, ureters, bladder, and urethra.
2. Explain the physiologic events involved in the formation and passage of urine from glomerular filtration to voiding.
3. Identify the significant subjective and objective data related to the urinary system that should be obtained from a patient.
4. Describe age-related changes in the urinary system and differences in assessment findings.
5. Describe the appropriate techniques used in the physical assessment of the urinary system.
6. Differentiate normal from common abnormal findings of a physical assessment of the urinary system.
7. Describe the purpose, significance of results, and nursing responsibilities related to diagnostic studies of the urinary system.
8. Describe the normal physical and chemical characteristics of urine.

"Bones can break, muscles can atrophy, glands can loaf, even the brain can go to sleep without immediate danger to survival. But should the kidneys fail . . . neither bone, muscle, gland, nor brain could carry on."[1] This statement underlines the importance of kidneys to our lives. Adequate functioning of the kidneys is essential to the maintenance of a healthy body. If there is complete kidney failure and treatment is not given, death is inevitable.

The kidneys are the principal organs of the urinary system. Besides the two kidneys, there are two ureters, a urinary bladder, and a urethra in the urinary system (Fig. 42-1). The other organs can be thought of as storage and drainage channels for the urine after it is formed by the kidneys.

The primary function of the kidneys is to regulate the volume and composition of extracellular fluid (ECF). The excretory function of kidneys is secondary to this regulatory function. Other major functions of the kidneys include renin secretion and blood pressure control, erythropoietin production, vitamin D activation, and acid-base balance regulation.

STRUCTURES AND FUNCTIONS OF THE URINARY SYSTEM

Kidneys

Macrostructure. The kidneys are bean-shaped organs that are retroperitoneal (behind the peritoneum) on either side of the vertebral column at about the level of the twelfth thoracic (T12) vertebra to the third lumbar (L3) vertebra.

Each kidney weighs 4 to 6 ounces (120 to 170 g) and is about 5 inches (12 cm) long. The right kidney, with the liver above it, is lower than the left. The right kidney is at the level of the twelfth rib. An adrenal gland lies on top of each kidney.

Each kidney is surrounded by a considerable amount of fat and connective tissue that serves to support and maintain its position. The surface of the kidney is covered by a thin, smooth layer of fibrous membrane called the *capsule.* The *hilus* on the medial side of the kidney serves as the entry site for the renal artery and nerves, as well as the exit site for the vein and ureter.

On a longitudinal section of the kidney (Fig. 42-2), the internal structures can be visualized. The outer layer is termed the *cortex,* and the inner layer is called the *medulla.* The medulla consists of a number of *pyramids.* The apices of these pyramids are called *papillae,* through which urine passes to enter the *calyces.* The minor calyces widen and merge to form major calyces, which form a funnel-shaped sac called the *renal pelvis.* The minor and major calyces and the renal pelvis are holding areas for urine before it exits the kidney via the ureter. The capacity of the renal pelvis is about 3 to 5 ml. The lumen of the renal pelvis decreases to form the ureter.

Microstructure. The functional unit of the kidney is termed the *nephron.* Each kidney has more than 1 million nephrons. A nephron is composed of a glomerulus, Bowman's capsule, and tubular system. The tubular system consists of the proximal convoluted tubule, the loop of Henle, and the distal convoluted tubule (Fig. 42-3). Several nephrons converge into a collecting duct, which eventually merges into a pyramid and empties via the papilla into a minor calyx.

The glomeruli, Bowman's capsule, proximal tubule, and distal tubule are located in the cortex of the kidney. The loop of Henle and the collecting ducts are located in the medulla.

Reviewed by Diane M. Fesler, RN, MSN, PhD Candidate, Assistant Professor, Northern Illinois University, Dekalb, Ill.

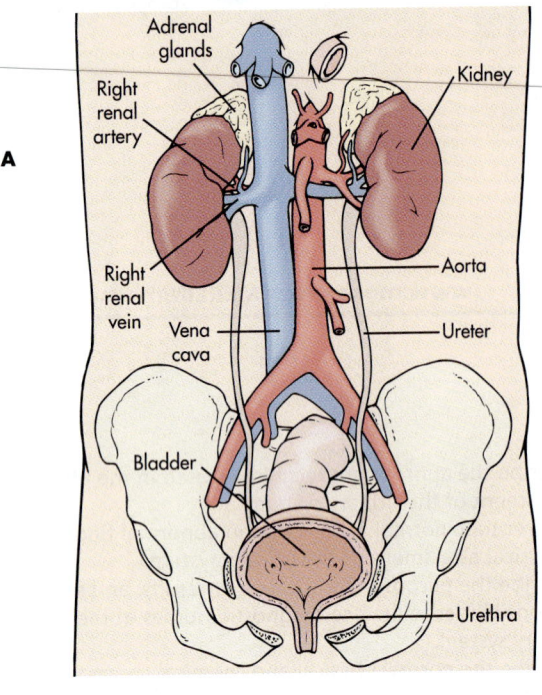

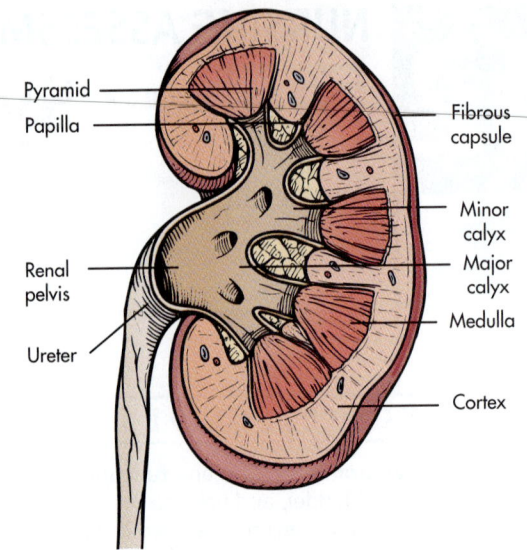

Fig. 42-2 Longitudinal section of the kidney.

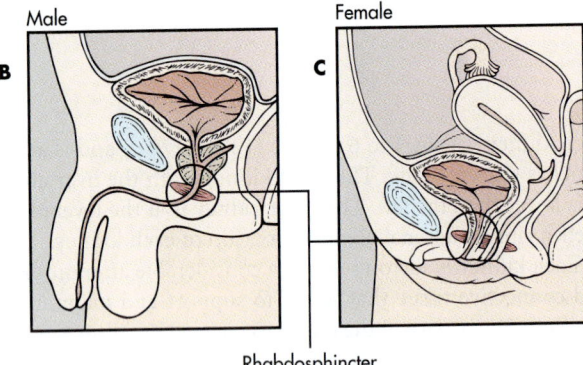

Fig. 42-1 Organs of the urinary system. **A,** Upper urinary tract in relation to other anatomic structures. **B,** Male urethra in relation to other pelvic structures. **C,** Female urethra.

Blood Supply. A blood supply of about 1200 ml/min, which is 20% to 25% of the cardiac output, flows to the two kidneys. Blood reaches the kidneys via the renal artery, which arises from the aorta and enters the kidney through the hilus. The renal artery divides into secondary branches and then into still smaller branches, each of which eventually forms an *afferent arteriole* (Fig. 42-4). The afferent arteriole divides into a capillary network termed the *glomerulus,* which is a tuft of up to 50 capillaries. The capillaries of the glomerulus eventually unite in the *efferent arteriole.* This arteriole splits to form a capillary network called the *peritubular capillaries,* which, as the name suggests, surround the tubular system. All peritubular capillaries eventually drain into the venous system. The renal vein empties into the inferior vena cava.

Physiology of Urine Formation

Normal Glomerular Function. Urine formation starts at the glomerulus where blood is filtered. The glomerulus, which is a semipermeable membrane, allows for filtration (see

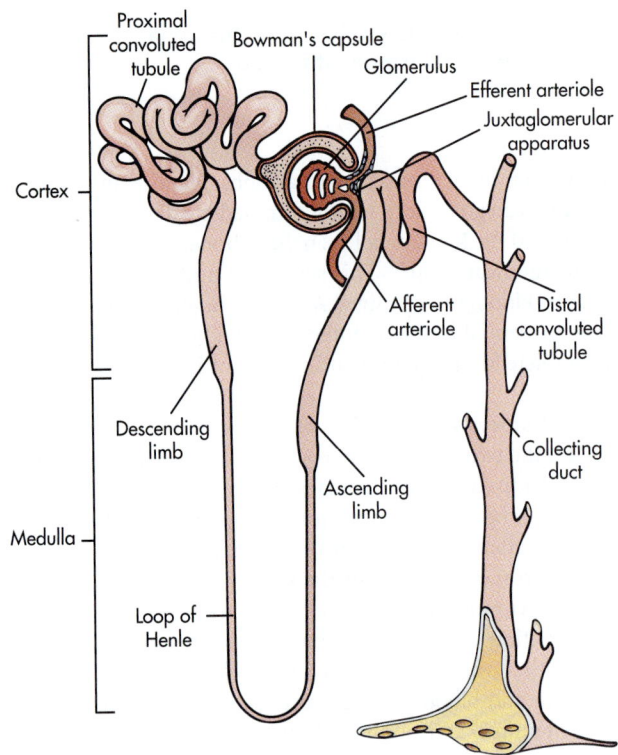

Fig. 42-3 Nephron of the kidney.

Fig. 42-3). The hydrostatic pressure of the blood within the glomerular capillaries causes a portion of blood to be filtered across the semipermeable membrane into Bowman's capsule, where the filtered portion of the blood called the *glomerular filtrate* begins to pass down to the tubule. Filtration is more rapid in the glomerulus than in ordinary tissue capillaries because of the porosity of the glomerular membrane. The ultrafiltrate is similar in composition to blood except that it lacks blood cells, platelets, and large plasma proteins. Under normal conditions the capillary pores are too small to allow the

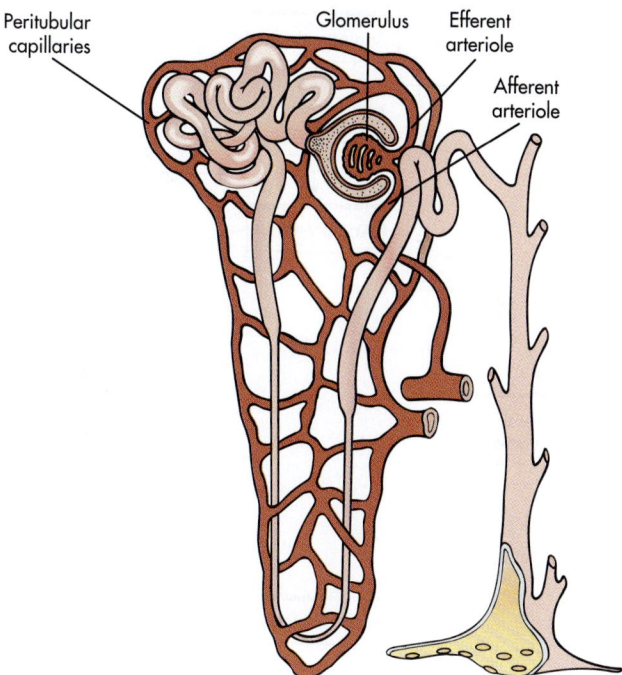

Peritubular capillaries   Glomerulus   Efferent arteriole   Afferent arteriole

Fig. 42-4 Blood supply of the nephron.

Table **42-1**	Functions of the Segments of the Nephron
Component	**Function**
■ Glomerulus	Selective filtration
■ Proximal tubule	Reabsorption of 80% of electrolytes and water, reabsorption of all glucose and amino acids, reabsorption of HCO_3^-, secretion of H^+ and creatinine
■ Loop of Henle	Reabsorption of Na^+ and Cl^- in ascending limb, reabsorption of water in descending loop, concentration of filtrate
■ Distal tubule	Secretion of K^+, H^+, ammonia; reabsorption of water (regulated by ADH); reabsorption of HCO_3^-; regulation of Ca^{2+} and PO_4^{2-} by parathyroid hormone, regulation of Na^+ and K^+ by aldosterone
■ Collecting duct	Reabsorption of water (ADH required)

ADH, antidiuretic hormone; *Ca^{2+}*, calcium ions; *Cl^-*, chloride ions; *H^+*, hydrogen ions; *HCO_3^-*, bicarbonate ions; *K^+*, potassium ions; *Na^+*, sodium ions; *PO_4^{2-}*, phosphate ions.

loss of these large blood components. Capillary permeability is increased in many renal diseases, permitting plasma proteins to pass into the urine.

The amount of blood filtered by the glomeruli in a given time is termed the *glomerular filtration rate* (GFR). The normal GFR is about 125 ml per minute. However, on the average only 1 ml per minute is excreted as urine because most glomerular filtrate is reabsorbed by the peritubular capillary network before it reaches the end of the collecting duct.

Tubular Function. Because the glomerular membrane is a selective filtration membrane that filters primarily by size, provision is made for the reabsorption of essential materials and the excretion of nonessential ones (Table 42-1). The tubules and collecting ducts carry out these functions by means of reabsorption and secretion (Fig. 42-5). *Reabsorption* is the passage of a substance from the lumen of the tubules through the tubule cells and into the capillaries. This process involves both active and passive transport. *Tubular secretion* is the passage of a substance from the capillaries through the tubular cells into the lumen of the tubule. Reabsorption and secretion occur along the entire length of the tubule, causing numerous changes in the composition of the glomerular filtrate as it moves through the tubules.

In the proximal convoluted tubule, about 80% of the electrolytes are reabsorbed. Normally, all the glucose, amino acids, and protein are reabsorbed. For the most part reabsorption occurs by active transport. Hydrogen ions (H^+) and creatinine are secreted into the filtrate.[2]

The loop of Henle is important in conserving water and thus concentrating the filtrate. In the loop of Henle, reabsorption continues. The descending loop is permeable to water and moderately permeable to sodium, urea, and other solutes. In the ascending limb, chloride ions (Cl^-) are actively reabsorbed,

followed passively by sodium ions (Na^+). About 25% of the filtered sodium is reabsorbed here.

Two important functions of the distal convoluted tubules are final regulation of water balance and acid-base balance. Antidiuretic hormone (ADH), released by the posterior pituitary gland, is required for water reabsorption. The stimuli for ADH release is increased serum osmolality and decreased blood volume. ADH makes the distal convoluted tubules and the collecting ducts permeable to water, allowing it to be reabsorbed into the peritubular capillaries and to be eventually returned to circulation. In the absence of ADH the tubules are practically impermeable to water, and any water in the tubules leaves the body as urine.

In the presence of aldosterone (released from the adrenal cortex) acting on the distal tubule, reabsorption of Na^+ and water occurs. In exchange for Na^+, potassium ions (K^+) are excreted. The secretion of aldosterone is influenced by both circulating blood volume and plasma concentrations of Na^+ and K^+.

Acid-base regulation involves reabsorbing and conserving most of the bicarbonate (HCO_3^-) and secreting excess H^+. The distal tubule functions in different ways to maintain the pH of ECF within a range of 7.35 to 7.45 (see Chapter 15).

Atrial natriuretic factor (ANF) is a hormone secreted from cells in the right atrium when right atrial blood pressure increases. ANF inhibits the secretion and effect of ADH and results in a large volume of dilute urine (see Chapter 45).

Parathyroid hormone (parathormone) is released from the parathyroid gland in response to low serum calcium levels. It causes increased tubular reabsorption of calcium ions (Ca^{2+}) and decreased tubular reabsorption of phosphate ions (PO_4^{-2}). Therefore serum Ca^{2+} levels are increased.

The basic function of nephrons is to clean or clear blood plasma of unnecessary substances. After the glomerulus has

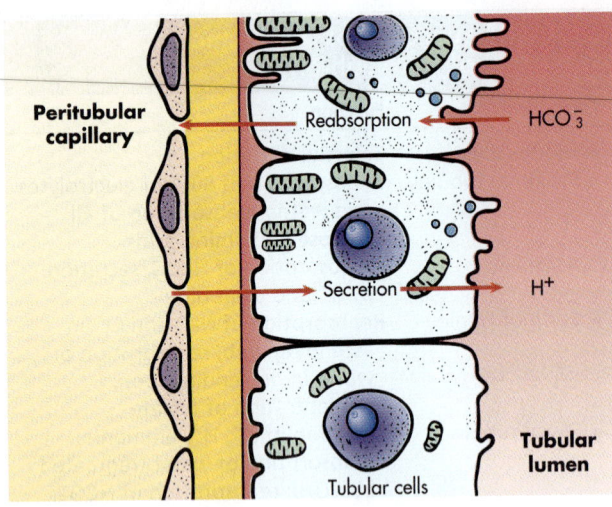

Fig. 42-5 Reabsorption and secretion in the tubules.

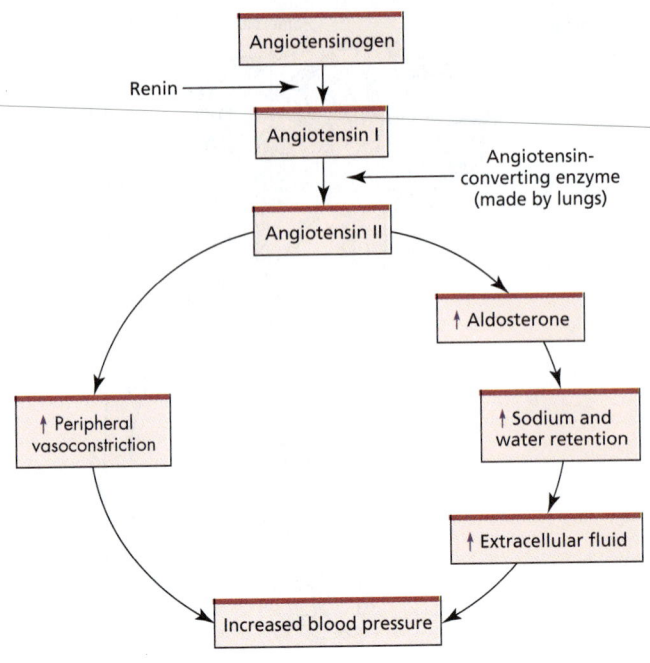

Fig. 42-6 Renin-angiotensin mechanism.

filtered the blood, the tubules separate the unwanted from the wanted portions of tubular fluid. The necessary portions are returned to the blood, and the unnecessary portions pass into urine.

Other Renal Functions

In addition to their function in regulating the volume and composition of ECF, the kidneys also have other vital functions, including the production of erythropoietin, production and secretion of renin, and activation of vitamin D.

Erythropoietin is produced and released in response to decreased oxygen tension in the renal blood supply, which is usually caused by a loss of red blood cells (RBCs). Erythropoietin stimulates the production of RBCs in the bone marrow. A deficiency of erythropoietin leads to anemia in renal failure.

Vitamin D is a hormone that can be obtained in the diet or synthesized by the action of ultraviolet radiation on cholesterol in the skin. These forms of vitamin D are inactive and require two more steps to become metabolically active. The first step in activation occurs in the liver. The second step occurs in the kidneys. Active vitamin D is essential for the absorption of calcium from the gastrointestinal (GI) tract. The patient with renal failure has a deficiency of the active metabolite of vitamin D and manifests problems of altered calcium and phosphate balance (see Chapter 44).

Renin is important in the regulation of blood pressure (Fig. 42-6). It is released from the granular cells of the afferent arteriole. These cells, together with the macula densa cells of the distal convoluted tubule and the mesangial cells, form the juxtaglomerular apparatus. Renin is released in response to decreased arterial blood pressure, renal ischemia, ECF depletion, increased norepinephrine, and increased urinary Na^+ concentration. Renin catalyzes the splitting of the plasma protein angiotensinogen into angiotensin I, which is subsequently converted to angiotensin II by a converting enzyme made in the lungs. Angiotensin II stimulates the release of aldosterone from the adrenal cortex, which causes Na^+ and water retention, leading to an increased ECF volume. Angiotensin II also causes increased peripheral vasoconstriction. The increase in ECF and vasoconstriction causes an elevation in blood pressure, which

should inhibit renin release. Excessive renin production caused by impaired renal perfusion may be a contributing factor in the etiology of hypertension (see Chapters 31 and 44).

Prostaglandins. Prostaglandins (PGs) are synthesized by most body tissues from the precursor, arachidonic acid, in response to appropriate stimuli. PGs, which are involved in the regulation of cell function and host defenses, exert their influence primarily on cells or tissues that are close to the site where they are synthesized. (See Chapter 11 and Fig. 11-7 for a more detailed discussion of PGs.)

In the kidney, PG synthesis (primarily PGE_2 and PGI_2) occurs primarily in the medulla. These PGs have a vasodilating action in addition to increasing renal blood flow and promoting Na^+ excretion. They counteract the vasoconstrictor effect of substances such as angiotensin and norepinephrine. Renal PGs may have a systemic effect in lowering blood pressure by decreasing systemic vascular resistance.[3]

The significance of these PGs is related to the role of the kidneys in causing hypertension. In renal failure with a loss of functioning tissue, these renal vasodilator factors are also lost. This may be one factor that contributes to the common finding of hypertension in renal failure (see Chapter 44).

Ureters

The ureters are tubes approximately 10 to 12 inches (25 to 35 cm) long and 0.08 to 0.3 inch (0.2 to 0.8 cm) in diameter that carry urine from the renal pelvis to the bladder. The narrow area where the ureter joins the renal pelvis is termed the *ureteropelvic junction* (UPJ). After coursing down along the psoas muscle, the ureter crosses over the pelvic brim and iliac artery and inserts into the base of the bladder at the *ureterovesical junction* (UVJ). The ureteral lumen is narrowest at these junctions; consequently, they are often the sites of urinary stone (calculi) obstruction. Since the lumen of the ureter is narrow, it can be easily occluded internally (e.g., calculi) or externally (e.g., tumors, adhesions, inflammation).

Sympathetic and parasympathetic nerves, along with the vascular supply, surround the mucosal lining of the ureter. Circular and longitudinal smooth muscle fibers are arranged in a meshlike outer layer and contract to promote the peristaltic one-way flow of urine. These muscle contractions can be affected by distention and neurologic, endocrine, and pharmacologic factors. Stimulation of these nerves during passage of a stone or clot may cause acute, severe pain termed *renal colic.*

Because the renal pelvis holds only 3 to 5 ml of urine, kidney damage can result from a backflow of more than that amount of urine. The UVJ relies on the ureter's angle of bladder penetration and muscle fiber attachments with the bladder to prevent the backflow of urine (reflux) and ascending infection. The distal ureter entering the bladder has more longitudinal muscle fibers than the upper ureter. This segment enters the bladder laterally at its base, courses along obliquely through the bladder wall for about 1.5 cm, and intermingles with muscle fibers of the bladder base. Circular and longitudinal bladder muscle fibers adjacent to the imbedded ureter help secure it. When bladder pressure rises (e.g., during voiding or coughing), muscle fibers that the ureter shares with the bladder base contract first to help promote ureteral lumen closure. The bladder then contracts against its base to further close the UVJ and prevent urine from moving back through the junction.

Bladder

The urinary bladder is a distendible organ positioned behind the symphysis pubis and anterior to the vagina and rectum. Its primary functions are to serve as a reservoir for urine and to help the body eliminate waste products. Normal adult urine output is approximately 1500 ml per day, which varies with food and fluid intake. The volume of urine produced at night is less than half of that formed during the day because of hormonal influences (e.g., ADH). This diurnal pattern of urination is normal. Most persons urinate five to six times during the day and occasionally at night.

The triangular area formed by the two ureteral openings and the bladder neck at the base of the bladder is termed the *trigone.* It is affixed to the pelvis by many ligaments, and it does not change its shape during bladder filling or emptying. The bladder muscle, termed the *detrusor,* is composed of layers of intertwined smooth muscle fibers and is capable of considerable distention during bladder filling and contraction during emptying. It is affixed to the abdominal wall by an umbilical ligament. Consequently, as the bladder fills, it rises toward the umbilicus. The dome, anterior, and lateral aspects of the bladder expand and contract. When the bladder is empty, it appears as multiple folds within the pelvis.

On the average, 200 to 250 ml of urine in the bladder causes moderate distention and the urge to urinate. When the quantity of urine reaches about 400 to 600 ml, the person feels uncomfortable. Bladder capacity varies with the individual, usually ranging from 600 to 1000 ml. Evacuation of urine is termed *urination, micturition,* or *voiding.*

The bladder has the same mucosal lining as that of the renal pelvis, ureter, and bladder neck. It is called *transitional cell epithelium* or *urothelium* and is unique to the urinary tract. Transitional cell epithelium is resistant to absorption of urine. Therefore urinary wastes produced by the kidneys do not leak out of the urinary system after they leave the kidneys. Microscopically, transitional cell epithelium is several cells deep.

These cells stretch out in the bladder to only a few cells deep as it accommodates filling. As the bladder empties, the epithelium resumes its multicellular layer formation.

Because the lining is the same, transitional cell tumors that occur in one section of the urinary tract can easily metastasize to other urinary tract areas. Malignant cells may move down from upper urinary tract tumors and imbed in the bladder, or large bladder tumors can invade the ureter. Tumor recurrence within the bladder is common. Intact urothelium also has phagocytic properties, although the exact mechanism is unknown.

Interstitial cystitis, a syndrome unique to the bladder, causes chronic inflammation of the bladder lining and wall. Histologic changes may be evident in the bladder epithelium. (Interstitial cystitis is discussed in Chapter 43.)

Urethra

The urethra is a small muscular tube that leads from the bladder neck to the external meatus. Its primary function is to serve as a conduit for urine to the bladder and then to the outside of the body.

The urothelium and submucosal layers are the same as that of the bladder. Smooth muscle fibers extend from the bladder neck down into the urethra and are further supported by circular smooth muscle fibers around the urethra. Special C-shaped striated muscle fibers (the rhabdosphincter, or external sphincter) surround a portion of the urethra and voluntarily contract and prevent leaking when bladder pressure increases.

The female urethra is 1 to 2 inches (3 to 5 cm) long and lies behind the symphysis pubis but anterior to the vagina. The rhabdosphincter encircles the middle third of the urethra. The short urethra is a contributing factor to the increased incidence of urinary tract infections in women.

The male urethra, which is about 8 to 10 inches (20 to 25 cm) long, originates at the bladder neck and extends the length of the penis. It is often separated into three parts. The prostatic urethra extends from the bladder neck through the prostate to the urogenital diaphragm. The membranous urethra passes through the urogenital diaphragm. The rhabdosphincter encircles this portion. Because of the concentrated muscular support, this short portion is not as expandable; consequently, stricture formation in this area after instrumentation is common. The penile urethra continues through the corpora spongiosum, a cavernous penile body, from the urogenital diaphragm to a distal dilated area, the fossa navicularis, before terminating at the meatus.

Urethrovesical Unit Function

Together, the bladder, bladder neck, urethra, and pelvic floor muscles form what is called the *urethrovesical unit.* Normal voluntary control of this unit is defined as continence. Various areas of the brain send stimulating and inhibiting impulses to the thoracolumbar (T11–L2) and sacral (S2–S4) areas of the spinal cord to control voiding. Distention of the bladder stimulates stretch receptors within the bladder wall. Impulses are transmitted to the sacral spinal cord and then to the brain, causing a desire to urinate. If the time to void is not appropriate, inhibitor impulses in the brain are stimulated and transmitted back to the thoracolumbar and sacral nerves innervating the bladder. In a coordinated fashion, the detrusor accommodates to the pressure (does not contract) while the sphincter and pelvic floor muscles tighten to resist bladder

GERONTOLOGIC DIFFERENCES IN ASSESSMENT

Table **42-2** **Urinary System**

Changes	Differences in Assessment Findings
Kidney	
Decrease in amount of renal tissue	Less palpable
Decrease in number of nephrons and renal vascular bed; thickened basement membrane of Bowman's capsule and glomeruli	Decrease in creatinine clearance, increase in BUN level
Decrease in function of loop of Henle and tubules	Alterations in drug excretion; nocturia; loss of normal diurnal excretory pattern because of decreased ability to concentrate urine; less concentrated urine
Ureter, Bladder, and Urethra	
Decrease in elasticity and muscle tone	Palpable bladder after urination because of retention
Weakening of urinary sphincter	Stress incontinence (especially during Valsalva maneuver), dribbling of urine after urination
Decrease in bladder capacity and sensory receptors	Frequency, urgency, nocturia, overflow incontinence
Estrogen deficiency leading to thin, dry vaginal tissue	Stress or urge incontinence, dysuria, positive urine culture
Uninhibited bladder contractions	Urge incontinence
Prostatic enlargement	Hesitancy, frequency, urgency, nocturia, straining to urinate, retention, dribbling

BUN, blood urea nitrogen.

pressure. If voiding is appropriate, cerebral inhibition is voluntarily suppressed, and impulses are transmitted via the spinal cord for the bladder neck, sphincter, and pelvic floor muscles to relax and for the bladder to contract. The sphincter closes and the detrusor muscle relaxes when the bladder is empty.

Any disease or trauma that affects function of the brain, spinal cord, or nerves that directly innervate the bladder, bladder neck, external sphincter, or pelvic floor can affect bladder function. These conditions include diabetes mellitus, paraplegia, and quadriplegia. Medications affecting nerve transmission also can affect bladder function.

GERONTOLOGIC CONSIDERATIONS

Effects of Aging on the Urinary System

Anatomic changes in the aging kidney include a 20% to 30% decrease in size and weight between the ages of 30 and 90 years. This loss in renal mass is predominantly in the cortex. The aging nephron fails as a unit because glomerular and tubular function appear to decrease at the same rate. By the seventh decade of life, 30% to 50% of glomeruli have lost their function because of sclerosis or other abnormalities. Despite losing this original kidney volume, older individuals maintain body fluid homeostasis unless they encounter diseases or other physiologic stressors.[4]

Blood flow to and within the kidneys also decreases. There is no evidence that atherosclerotic vascular disease is primarily responsible for the age-related changes in the kidneys.

Physiologic changes in the aging kidney include decreased renal blood flow; decreased GFR; and decreased ability to conserve Na^+, dilute or concentrate urine, and excrete an acid load. Under normal conditions, the aging kidney is able to maintain homeostasis, but after abrupt changes in blood volume, acid load, or other insults, the kidneys may not be able to function effectively because much of its renal reserve has been lost.

Physiologic changes also occur in the aging bladder and urethra.[5,6] Estrogen receptors exist in the female urethra, bladder, vagina, and pelvic floor. As estrogen levels decrease with age, tissues become less elastic, thin, and less vascular.[7] Periurethral striated muscle fibers and muscles supporting the bladder relax. Consequently, older women are more prone to urethral irritation, urethral and bladder infections, and urinary incontinence.

Men's prostates enlarge as they age, and since the prostate surrounds the proximal urethra, increasing prostate size may affect urinary patterns in men, causing hesitancy, retention, slow stream, and bladder infections.

Constipation, a complaint often expressed by the elderly, can also affect urination. Partial urethral obstruction may occur because of the rectum's close proximity to the urethra.

Age-related changes in the urinary system and differences in assessment findings are presented in Table 42-2.

ASSESSMENT OF THE URINARY SYSTEM

Subjective Data

Important Health Information

Past health history. The patient should be questioned about the presence or history of diseases that are known to be related to renal or other urologic problems. Some of these diseases are hypertension, diabetes mellitus, gout and other metabolic problems, connective tissue disorders (e.g., systemic lupus erythematosus, scleroderma), skin or upper respiratory infections of streptococcal origin, tuberculosis, viral hepatitis, congenital disorders, neurologic conditions (e.g., stroke, back injury), or trauma. Specific urinary problems such as cancer, infections, benign prostatic hyperplasia, and calculi should be noted.

Medications. An assessment of the patient's current and past use of medications is important. This should include over-the-counter drugs, as well as prescription medications and

Table 42-3   Nephrotoxic Agents

Antibiotics	Other Agents
Amikacin	Captopril
Amphotericin B	Cimetidine
Bacitracin	Cisplatin
Cephalosporins	Cocaine
Colistin	Contrast medium
Gentamicin	Cyclosporine
Kanamycin	Ethylene glycol
Neomycin	Gold
Polymyxin B	Heavy metals
Streptomycin	Heroin
Sulfonamides	Lithium
Tobramycin	Methotrexate
Vancomycin	Nitrosoureas (e.g., carmustine)
	Nonsteroidal antiinflammatory agents (e.g., ibuprofen, indomethacin)
	Phenacetin
	Quinine
	Rifampin
	Salicylate (large quantities)

herbs. Drugs affect the urinary tract in several ways. Many drugs are known to be nephrotoxic (Table 42-3). Certain drugs may alter the quantity and character of urine output (e.g., diuretics). Numerous drugs such as phenazopyridine (Pyridium) and nitrofurantoin (Macrodantin) change its color. Anticoagulants may cause hematuria. Many antidepressants, calcium channel blockers, antihistamines, and medications used for neurologic and musculoskeletal disorders affect the ability of the bladder or sphincter to contract or relax normally.

Surgery or other treatments. The patient should also be questioned about any previous hospitalizations related to renal or urologic diseases and all urinary problems during past pregnancies. The duration, severity, and patient's perception of any problem and its treatment should be elicited. Past surgeries, particularly pelvic surgeries, or urinary tract instrumentation should be documented. Information should be obtained from the patient about any radiation or chemotherapy treatment for cancer.

Functional Health Patterns. Key questions to ask a patient with problems related to the urinary system are listed in Table 42-4.

HEALTH HISTORY

Table 42-4   Urinary System

Health Perception–Health Management Pattern
- How is your energy level compared with a year ago?
- Do you notice any visual changes?*
- Have you ever smoked? If yes, how much?

Nutritional-Metabolic Pattern
- How is your appetite?
- Has your weight changed over the past year?*
- Do you take vitamin or mineral supplements?*
- How much and what kinds of fluids do you drink daily?
- How much dairy products or meat do you eat?
- Do you drink coffee? Colas?
- Do you eat chocolate?
- Do you spice your food heavily?*

Elimination Pattern
- How often do you urinate during the day and night?
- Is the color normal for you?
- Do you ever notice blood in your urine?* If so, at what point in the urination does it occur?
- Do you find it difficult to postpone urination when you feel the urge to urinate?*
- Do you ever leak urine? If so, when does it occur?
- Do you ever have pain when you urinate?*
- Have you ever experienced urinary incontinence? If so, please describe specifically.
- Do you use special devices or supplies for urine elimination or control?*
- Do your bowels move regularly?

Activity-Exercise Pattern
- Have you noticed any changes in your ability to do your usual daily activities?*
- Do certain activities aggravate your urinary problem?*
- Has your urinary problem caused you to alter or stop any activity or exercise?*
- Do you require assistance in moving or getting to the bathroom?*

Cognitive-Perceptual Pattern
- Describe any pain you have in relation to urination.

Self-Perception–Self-Concept Pattern
- How does your urinary problem make you feel about yourself?
- Do you perceive your body differently since you have developed a urinary problem?

Role-Relationship Pattern
- Does your urinary problem interfere with your relationships with family or friends?*
- Has your urinary problem caused a change in your job status or affected your ability to carry out job-related responsibilities?*

Sexuality-Reproductive Pattern
- Has your urinary problem caused any change in your sexual pleasure or performance?*
- Do you have hygiene problems related to sexual activities that cause you concern?*

Coping–Stress Tolerance Pattern
- Do you feel able to manage the problems associated with your urinary problem? If not, explain.
- What strategies are you using to cope with your urinary problem?

Values-Beliefs Pattern
- Has your present illness affected your belief system?*
- Are your treatment decisions related to your urinary problem in conflict with your value system?*

*If yes, describe.

Table **42-5**	**Clinical Manifestations of Disorders of the Urinary System**

General Manifestations

Fatigue	Itching
Headaches	Excess thirst
Blurred vision	Chills
Elevated blood pressure	Change in body weight
Anorexia	Change in mentation
Nausea and vomiting	

Related to Urinary System

Pain	**Changes in Urine Output**
Dysuria	Polyuria
Flank or costovertebral	Oliguria
angle	Anuria
Groin	
Suprapubic	**Changes in Urine**
	Consistency
Changes in Patterns of	Hematuria
Urination	Pyuria
Frequency	Concentrated
Nocturia	Dilute
Dysuria	Color (red, brown,
Hesitancy of stream	yellowish green)
Change in stream	
Urgency	**Edema**
Retention	Facial (periorbital)
Incontinence	Ankle
Stress incontinence	Ascites
Enuresis	Anasarca
Dribbling	Sacral

Health perception–health management pattern. The nurse may want to ask about the patient's general health. Sometimes responses such as "feeling tired all of the time," changes in weight or appetite, excess thirst, fluid retention, and complaints of headache, pruritus, or blurred vision may be related to abnormal kidney function.

An occupational history should be taken. Exposure to certain chemicals can affect the kidneys and urinary tract system. Phenol and ethylene glycol are examples of nephrotoxic chemicals. Aromatic amines and certain organic chemicals may increase the risk of bladder cancers. Textile workers, painters, hairdressers, and industrial workers have a high incidence of bladder tumors.[8]

A smoking history should be obtained. Cigarette smoking is a major factor in the risk for bladder cancer. Tumors occur four times more frequently in cigarette smokers than in nonsmokers.[8]

Places where a patient has lived may be important information to obtain. It has been shown that persons living in certain parts of the United States (Great Lakes, Southwest, Southeast) have a higher than normal incidence of urinary calculi. This may be caused by the higher mineral content of the soil and water. A person living in Middle Eastern countries or Africa can acquire certain parasites that can cause cystitis or bladder cancer.

The presence of certain renal or urologic problems in a family history increases the likelihood of similar problems occurring in the patient. The nurse should ask about family members who have had any of the diseases referred to in the past health history, as well as polycystic renal disease, congenital urinary tract abnormalities, and Alport's syndrome (hereditary nephritis).

Nutritional-metabolic pattern. The usual quantity and types of fluid a patient drinks are important information related to urinary tract disease. Dehydration may contribute to urinary infections, calculi formation, and renal failure. Large intake of particular foods, such as dairy products or foods high in proteins, may also lead to calculi formation. Coffee, alcohol, carbonated beverages, or spicy foods often aggravate urinary inflammatory diseases. An unexplained weight gain may be the result of fluid retention secondary to a renal problem. Anorexia and nausea and vomiting can dramatically affect fluid status and require careful assessment. Information on vitamin and mineral supplements and herbal therapies should be obtained. The patient may not think of these supplements and therapies when listing over-the-counter drugs; supplements are often considered part of nutritional intake.

Elimination pattern. The patient should be questioned about urinary patterns such as frequency or urgency and the amount of urine output. Table 42-5 lists some of the common clinical manifestations of urinary tract disorders. Changes in the color and appearance of urine are often significant and should be evaluated. If blood is visible in the urine, it should be determined if it occurs at the beginning, throughout, or at the end of urination.

Bowel function should also be investigated. Problems with fecal incontinence may signal neurologic causes for bladder problems because of shared nerve pathways. Constipation and fecal impaction can partially obstruct the urethra, causing inadequate bladder emptying and overflow incontinence.

The nurse should find out the patient's method of handling a urinary problem. A patient may already be using a catheter or collection device. Sometimes a patient has to assume a particular position to urinate or perform such maneuvers as pressing on the abdomen (Valsalva's maneuver), straining, or stretching the rectum to empty the bladder.

Activity-exercise pattern. The patient's level of activity should be assessed. A sedentary person is more likely than an active one to have stasis of urine, which can predispose to infection and calculi. Demineralization of bones in a person with limited physical activity causes increased urine calcium precipitation.

An active person may find that increasing activity aggravates the urinary problem. The patient who has had prostate surgery or who has weakened pelvic floor muscles may leak urine when attempting particular activities such as running. Some men may develop chronic inflammatory prostatitis or epididymitis after heavy lifting or long-distance driving.

Sleep-rest pattern. Lower urinary tract disorders, such as infections, neurologic conditions, or bladder outlet obstructions, often necessitate a person getting up as much as every hour at night. This situation can lead to sleep deprivation. Sleep problems associated with a urinary disorder should be documented. The older adult may awaken many times during the night to urinate and may need to be assured that this may be normal. However, a complete assessment should be made to rule out any problem.

Cognitive-perceptual pattern. Level of mobility, visual acuity, and dexterity are important factors to determine for a patient with urologic problems when managing his or her own care at home, particularly when bladder retention or inconti-

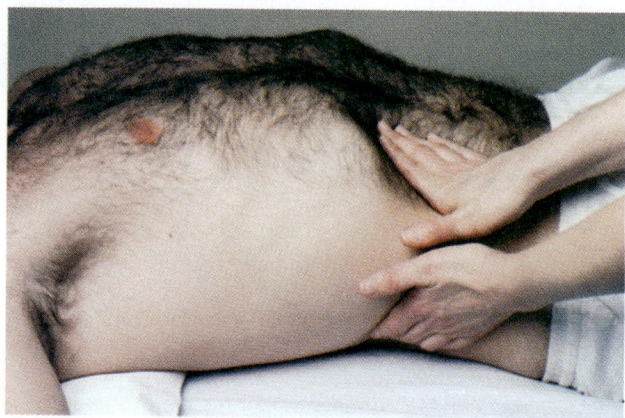

Fig. 42-7   Palpating the right kidney.

Table **42-6**	**Normal Physical Assessment of the Urinary System**

No costovertebral angle tenderness
Nonpalpable kidney and bladder
No palpable masses

Skin: pallor, yellow-gray cast, excoriations, changes in turgor, bruises, texture (e.g., rough, dry skin)
Mouth: stomatitis, ammonia breath odor
Face, abdomen, and extremities: generalized edema, peripheral edema, bladder distention, masses, enlarged kidneys
Weight gain: secondary to edema
General state of health: fatigue, lethargy, and diminished alertness

Palpation. The kidneys are posterior organs protected by the abdominal organs, the ribs, and the heavy back muscles. A landmark useful in locating the kidneys is the costovertebral angle (CVA) formed by the rib cage and the vertebral column. The normal-sized left kidney is rarely palpable because the spleen lies directly on top of it. Occasionally the lower pole of the right kidney is palpable.

To palpate the right kidney, the examiner's left hand is placed behind and supports the patient's right side between the rib cage and the iliac crest (Fig. 42-7). The right flank is elevated with the left hand, and the right hand is used to palpate deeply for the right kidney. The lower pole of the right kidney may be felt as a smooth, rounded mass that descends on inspiration. If the kidney is palpable, its size, contour, and tenderness should be noted. Kidney enlargement is suggestive of neoplasm or other serious renal pathology.

The urinary bladder is normally not palpable unless it is distended with urine. If the bladder is full, it may be felt as a smooth, round, firm organ and is sensitive to palpation.

Percussion. Tenderness in the flank area may be detected by fist percussion. This technique is performed by striking the fist (kidney punch) of one hand against the dorsal surface of the other hand, which is placed flat along the posterior CVA margin. Normally a firm blow in the flank area should not elicit pain. If CVA tenderness and pain are present, it may indicate a kidney infection or polycystic kidney disease.

Normally a bladder is not percussible until it contains 150 ml of urine. If the bladder is full, dullness is heard above the symphysis pubis. A distended bladder may be percussed as high as the umbilicus.

Auscultation. The diaphragm of the stethoscope may be used to auscultate over both CVAs and in the upper abdominal quadrants. With this technique, the abdominal aorta and renal arteries are auscultated for a bruit (an abnormal murmur), which indicates impaired blood flow to the kidneys.

Table 42-6 shows how to record the normal physical assessment findings of the urinary system. Table 42-7 presents common assessment abnormalities of the urinary system. Normally, assessment findings may vary in the older adult. Table 42-2 shows the age-related changes in the urinary system and differences in assessment findings.

nence is a problem. It should be determined if the patient is alert, is able to understand instructions, and can recall the instructions when necessary.

If urinary incontinence is present, a thorough history of the problem should be elicited to assist in determining the type of incontinence. It is important to document what the patient has tried in order to manage the problem. Incontinence is a distressing problem and calls for great sensitivity on the part of the nurse if accurate information is to be obtained.

Pain is a frequent symptom of urinary tract disease. Types of pain associated with renal and urologic problems include dysuria, groin pain, costovertebral pain, and suprapubic pain. If present, the location, character, and duration should be assessed. The absence of pain when other urinary symptoms exist is also significant. Many urinary tract tumors are painless in the early stages.

Self-perception–self-concept pattern. Problems associated with the urinary system, such as incontinence, urinary diversion procedures, and chronic fatigue, can result in loss of self-esteem and a negative body image. Sensitive questioning may elicit cues to problems in this area.

Role-relationship pattern. Urinary problems can affect many aspects of a person's life, including the ability to work and relationships with others. These factors will have important implications on future treatment and management. The nurse must be aware of cues from the patient.

Urinary system problems may be serious enough to cause problems in job- and social-related situations. Chronic dialysis therapy often makes regular employment or full-time homemaking difficult. Also, the concurrent poor health and negative body image can seriously alter existing roles. The nurse should assess this area to plan appropriate interventions.

Sexuality-reproductive pattern. The patient should be questioned about the effect of a renal or urologic problem on her or his sexual patterns and satisfaction. Problems related to personal hygiene and fatigue can seriously affect a sexual relationship. Counseling of both the patient and partner may be indicated.

Objective Data
Physical Examination

Inspection. The nurse should assess for changes in the following:

COMMON ASSESSMENT ABNORMALITIES

Table 42-7 Urinary System

Finding	Description	Possible Etiology and Significance
■ Dysuria	Painful or difficult urination	Sign of urinary tract infection and wide variety of pathologic conditions
■ Frequency	Increased incidence of urinating	Acutely inflamed bladder, retention with overflow, excess fluid intake
■ Enuresis	Involuntary nocturnal urinating	Symptomatic of lower urinary tract disorder
■ Hesitancy	Delay or difficulty in initiating urination	Partial urethral obstruction
■ Urgency	Strong desire to urinate	Inflammatory lesions in bladder or urethra, acute bacterial infections
■ Hematuria	Blood in the urine	Cancer of genitourinary tract, blood dyscrasias, renal disease, urinary tract infection, stones in kidney or ureter, medications (anticoagulants)
■ Burning on urination	Stinging pain in urethral area	Urethral irritation, urinary tract infection
■ Pneumaturia	Passage of urine containing gas	Fistula connections between bowel and bladder, gas-forming urinary tract infections
■ Retention	Inability to urinate, even though bladder contains excessive amount of urine	Finding after pelvic surgery, childbirth, catheter removal; urethral stricture or obstruction; neurogenic bladder; postanesthesia
■ Pain	Presence over suprapubic area (related to bladder), urethral pain (irritation of bladder neck), flank (CVA) pain	Infection, urinary retention, foreign body in urinary tract, urethritis, pyelonephritis, renal colic or stones
■ Incontinence	Inability to voluntarily control discharge of urine	Neurogenic bladder, bladder infection, injury to external sphincter
■ Stress incontinence	Involuntary urination with increased pressure (sneezing or coughing)	Weakness of sphincter control
■ Nocturia	Frequency of urination at night	Renal disease with impaired concentrating ability, bladder obstruction, congestive heart failure, diabetes mellitus, finding after renal transplant
■ Polyuria	Large volume of urine in a given time	Diabetes mellitus, diabetes insipidus, chronic renal failure, diuretics, excess fluid intake
■ Anuria	Technically no urination (24 hr urine output <100 ml)	Acute renal failure, end-stage renal disease, bilateral ureteral obstruction
■ Oliguria	Diminished amount of urine in a given time (24 hr urine output of 100-400 ml)	Severe dehydration, shock, transfusion reaction, kidney disease, end-stage renal disease

CVA, costovertebral angle.

DIAGNOSTIC STUDIES OF THE URINARY SYSTEM

Table 42-8 contains diagnostic studies common to the urinary system. Diagnostic studies are important in locating and understanding problems of the urinary system. The accuracy of the results is influenced by (1) adherence to the proper procedures related to the study and (2) cooperation of the patient in restricting fluids, collecting urine specimens, lying quietly on the examination table, or following other instructions.

Many radiologic studies require the use of a bowel preparation the evening before the study to clear the lower GI tract of feces and flatus. Because the kidneys lie in a retroperitoneal location, the contents of the colon may obstruct visualization of the urinary tract. If a bowel preparation is not properly done, the study may be unsuccessful and have to be rescheduled. Commonly used bowel preparations include enemas, castor oil, magnesium citrate, and bisacodyl (Dulcolax) tablets or suppositories. Sometimes a further bowel preparation is required the morning of the study. Some bowel preparations, such as magnesium citrate and Fleet Enema, are contraindicated in the patient with renal failure. Magnesium cannot be excreted by patients with renal failure (see Chapter 44).

When a patient has repeated diagnostic studies on consecutive days, it is important to prevent dehydration. It is not uncommon to have a patient take nothing by mouth (NPO) after midnight, spend all morning in the x-ray department, return too late for lunch or too tired to eat, sleep all afternoon, and be on NPO status after midnight again because of studies the next day. Severe dehydration, especially in a diabetic, debilitated, or older patient, may lead to acute renal failure. The nurse is responsible for ensuring that a patient undergoing diagnostic studies is properly hydrated and given adequate nourishment between studies. The nurse should also check with the physician regarding the insulin dose for the diabetic patient who is NPO.

Another important nursing responsibility related to diagnostic studies is providing the patient with an adequate explanation of the procedure. The period during a diagnostic workup is typically a time of anxiety for most patients. The fear inherent in not knowing what is wrong is often worse than the diagnosis itself. Additional anxiety is caused by the unknown

DIAGNOSTIC STUDIES

Table **42-8** | **Urinary System**

Study	Description and Purpose	Nursing Responsibility
Urine Studies		
■ Urinalysis	Study is a general examination of urine to establish baseline information or provide data to establish a tentative diagnosis and determine whether further studies are to be ordered. (See Table 42-9)	Try to obtain first urinated morning specimen. Ensure that specimen is examined within 1 hr of urinating. Wash perineal area if soiled with menses or fecal material.
■ Creatinine clearance	Creatinine is a waste product of protein breakdown (primarily body muscle mass). Clearance of creatinine by the kidney approximates the GFR. *Normal finding* is 85-135 ml/min.	Collect 24 hr urine specimen. Discard first urination when test is started. Save urine from all subsequent urinations for 24 hr. Instruct patient to urinate at end of 24 hr, and add specimen to collection. Ensure that serum creatinine is determined during 24 hr period.
■ Urine culture ("clean catch," "midstream")	Study is done to confirm suspected urinary tract infection and identify causative organisms. *Normally,* bladder is sterile, but urethra contains bacteria and a few WBCs. If properly collected, stored, and handled: <10,000 organisms/ml usually indicates no infection; 10,000-100,000/ml is usually not diagnostic, and test may have to be repeated; >100,000/ml indicates infection.	Use sterile container for collection of urine. Touch only outside of container. For women, separate labia with one hand and clean meatus with other hand, using at least three sponges (saturated with cleansing solution) in a front-to-back motion. For men, retract foreskin (if present) and cleanse glans with at least three cleansing sponges. After cleaning, instruct patient to start urinating and then continue voiding in sterile container. (The initial voided urine flushes out most contaminants in the urethra and perineal area.) Inform physician of need for catheterization if patient is unable to cooperate with this procedure.
■ Concentration test	Study evaluates renal concentration ability. Concentration is measured by specific gravity readings. *Normal finding* is 1.020-1.035.	Instruct patient to fast after given time in evening (in usual procedure). Collect three urine specimens at hourly intervals in morning.
■ Residual urine	Study determines amount of urine left in bladder after urinating. Finding may be abnormal in problems with bladder innervation, sphincter impairment, BPH, or urethral strictures. *Normal finding* is ≤50 ml urine (increases with age).	If residual urine test is ordered, catheterize patient immediately after urinating or use bladder ultrasound equipment. If a large amount of residual urine is obtained, physician may want catheter left in bladder.
■ Protein determination—Dipstick (Albustix, Combistix)	Test detects protein (primarily albumin) in urine. *Normal finding* is 0-trace.	Dip end of stick in urine, and read result by comparison with color chart on label as directed. Grading is from 0 to 4+. Interpret with caution. A positive result may not indicate significant proteinuria; some medications may give false-positive readings.
Quantitative test for protein	A 12- or 24-hr collection gives a more accurate indication of the amount of protein in urine. Persistent proteinuria usually indicates glomerular renal disease. *Normal finding* is <150 mg/24 hr (<0.15 g/24 hr), consisting mainly of albumin.	Perform 12 or 24 hr urine collection.
■ Urine cytology	Study is used to identify changes in cellular structure indicative of malignancy, especially bladder cancer.	Obtain urine and send immediately to lab. The first morning specimen should *not* be used.
Blood Chemistries		
■ BUN	Study is most commonly used to identify presence of renal problems. Concentration of urea in blood is regulated by rate at which kidney excretes urea. *Normal finding* is 10-30 mg/dl (1.8-7.1 mmol/L).	Be aware that when interpreting BUN, nonrenal factors may cause increase (e.g., rapid cell destruction from infections, fever, GI bleeding, trauma, athletic activity with excessive muscle breakdown, corticosteroid therapy).

Continued

DIAGNOSTIC STUDIES

Table 42-8 Urinary System—cont'd

Study	Description and Purpose	Nursing Responsibility
Blood Chemistries—cont'd		
■ Creatinine	Study is more reliable than BUN as a determinant of renal function. Creatinine is end-product of muscle and protein metabolism and is liberated at a constant rate. *Normal finding* is 0.5-1.5 mg/dl (44-133 μmol/L). Results are higher in men.	Explain test, and watch for postpuncture bleeding.
■ BUN/creatinine ratio	*Normal finding* is 10:1.	
■ Uric acid	Study is used as a screening test primarily for disorders of purine metabolism but can indicate kidney disease as well. Values depend on renal function and rate of purine metabolism and dietary intake of food rich in purines. *Normal finding* is 2.5-5.5 mg/dl (149-327 μmol/L) for women and 4.5-6.5 mg/dl (268-387 μmol/L) for men.	Explain test, and watch for postpuncture bleeding.
■ Sodium	Sodium is main extracellular electrolyte determining blood volume. Usually, values stay within normal range until late stages of renal failure. *Normal finding* is 135-145 mEq/L (135-145 mmol/L).	Explain test, and watch for postpuncture bleeding.
■ Potassium	Kidneys are responsible for excreting majority of body's potassium. In renal disease, K^+ determinations are critical because K^+ is one of the first electrolytes to become abnormal. Elevated K^+ levels of >6 mEq/L can lead to muscle weakness and cardiac arrhythmias. *Normal finding* is 3.5-5.5 mEq/L (3.5-5.5 mmol/L).	Explain test, and watch for postpuncture bleeding.
■ Calcium	Calcium is main mineral in bone and aids in muscular contraction, neurotransmission, and clotting. In renal disease, decreased absorption of Ca^{2+} leads to renal osteodystrophy. *Normal finding* is 9-11 mg/dl (4.5-5.5 mEq/L, 2.25-2.74 mmol/L).	Explain test, and watch for postpuncture bleeding.
■ Phosphorus	Phosphorus balance is inversely related to Ca^{2+} balance. In renal disease, phosphorus levels are elevated because the kidney is the primary excretory organ. Soft tissue calcification may occur if both Ca^{2+} and phosphorus are elevated. *Normal finding* is 2.8-4.5 mg/dl (0.9-1.45 mmol/L).	Explain test, and watch for postpuncture bleeding.
■ Bicarbonate	Most patients in renal failure have metabolic acidosis and low serum HCO_3^- levels. *Normal finding* is 20-30 mEq/L (20-30 mmol/L).	Explain test, and watch for postpuncture bleeding.
Radiologic Procedures		
■ Kidneys, ureters, bladder (KUB)	Study involves flat-plate x-ray examination of abdomen and pelvis and delineates size, shape, and position of kidneys.	Perform bowel preparation (if ordered).
■ IVP or excretory urogram	X-ray examination visualizes urinary tract after IV injection of contrast material.	Evening before procedure, give cathartic or enema to empty colon of feces and gas. Keep patient on NPO status 8 hr before procedure. Before procedure, assess patient for iodine sensitivity to avoid anaphylactic reaction. Inform patient that procedure involves lying on table and having serial x-rays taken. After procedure, force fluids (if permitted) to flush out contrast material.

Continued

DIAGNOSTIC STUDIES

Table 42-8 Urinary System—cont'd

Study	Description and Purpose	Nursing Responsibility
Radiologic Procedures—cont'd		
■ Nephrotomogram	X-ray is taken with rotating tubes. Test delineates segments of the kidney at different levels. Multiple exposures are taken to visualize specific sections of the kidney after IV injection of contrast material.	Explain procedure, and prepare patient as for IVP.
■ Retrograde pyelogram	X-ray of urinary tract is taken after injection of contrast material into kidneys. Cystoscope is inserted, and ureteral catheters are inserted through it into renal pelvis. Contrast material is injected through catheters.	Prepare patient as for IVP. Inform patient that pain may be experienced from distention of pelvis and discomfort from cystoscope. Inform patient that general anesthesia may be given for procedure.
■ Cystogram	Contrast material is instilled into bladder via cystoscope or catheter. Purpose is to visualize bladder and evaluate vesicoureteral reflux.	Explain procedure to patient. If done via cystoscope, follow nursing care related to cystoscopy.
■ Renal arteriogram (angiogram)	Study is performed by injecting contrast material into renal artery via catheter inserted into femoral artery. Purpose is to visualize renal blood vessels.	Prepare patient evening before procedure by giving cathartic or enema. Before injection of contrast material, test for iodine sensitivity. After procedure, check insertion site for bleeding, and take peripheral pulses in involved leg every 30-60 min to detect occluded blood flow.
■ Ultrasound	Small external ultrasound probe is placed on patient's skin. Conductive gel is applied to the skin. Noninvasive procedure involves passing sound waves into body structures and recording images as they are reflected back. Computer interprets tissue density based on sound waves and displays it in picture form. Study is most valuable in detection of renal or perirenal masses, differential diagnosis of renal cysts, solid masses, and identification of obstructions. It can be used safely in patients with renal failure.	Explain procedure to patient.
■ CT scan	Study provides excellent visualization of kidneys. Kidney size can be evaluated; tumors, abscesses, suprarenal masses (e.g., adrenal tumors, pheochromocytomas), and obstructions can be detected. Advantage of CT over ultrasound is its ability to distinguish subtle differences in density. Use of IV-administered contrast material during CT accentuates density of renal tissue and helps differentiate masses.	Explain procedure to patient.
■ MRI	Computer-generated films rely on radio waves and alteration in magnetic field. Useful for visualization of kidneys. Not proven useful for detecting urinary calculi or calcified tumors.	Explain procedure to patient. Have patient remove all metal objects. Patients with a history of claustrophobia may need to be sedated.
Renal Radionuclide Imaging		
■ Renal scan	Radioactive isotopes are injected IV. Radiation detector probes are placed over kidney, and scintillation counter monitors radioactive material in kidney. Purpose is to show blood flow, glomerular filtration, tubular function, and excretion. Radioisotope distribution in kidney is scanned and mapped. Test is useful in showing location, size, and shape of kidney and, in general, assessing blood perfusion and its ability to secrete urine. Abscesses, cysts, and tumors may appear as cold spots because of presence of nonfunctioning tissue.	Requires no dietary or activity restriction. Inform patient that no pain or discomfort should be felt during test.

Continued

DIAGNOSTIC STUDIES

Table 42-8   Urinary System—cont'd

Study	Description and Purpose	Nursing Responsibility
Endoscopy ■ Cystoscopy	Study involves use of tubular lighted scope to inspect bladder. Lithotomy position is used. It may be done using local or general anesthesia.	Before procedure, force fluids or give IV fluids if general anesthesia is to be used. Ensure consent form is signed. Explain procedure to patient. Give preoperative medication. After procedure, explain that burning on urination, pink-tinged urine, and urinary frequency are expected effects after cystoscopy. Do not let patient walk alone immediately after procedure because orthostatic hypotension may occur. Offer warm sitz baths, heat, mild analgesics to relieve discomfort.
Urodynamics ■ Cystometrogram	Study involves insertion of catheter and instillation of water or saline solution into bladder. Measurements of pressure exerted against bladder wall are recorded. Purpose is to evaluate bladder tone, sensations of filling, and bladder (detrusor) stability.	Explain procedure to patient. Observe patient for manifestations of urinary infection after procedure.
Invasive Procedure ■ Renal biopsy	Technique is usually done as a skin (percutaneous) biopsy through needle insertion into lower lobe of kidney. Purpose is to obtain renal tissue for examination to determine type of renal disease or to follow progress of renal disease.	Before procedure, ascertain coagulation status through patient history, medication history, CBC, hematocrit, prothrombin time, and bleeding and clotting time. Type and crossmatch patient for blood. Ensure consent form is signed. Be aware that IVP or ultrasound study is done before biopsy. After procedure, apply pressure dressing to biopsy site, and check frequently for bleeding. Keep patient on bed rest up to 24 hr. Take vital signs frequently. Observe urine for gross bleeding. Determine microscopic bleeding by use of dipstick. Assess patient for flank pain. Monitor hematocrit levels.

†See Chapter 44.

BPH, benign prostatic hyperplasia; *CBC,* complete blood count; *CT,* computed tomography; *GFR,* glomerular filtration rate; *IVP,* intravenous pyelogram; *KUB,* kidneys, ureters, bladder; *MRI,* magnetic resonance imaging; *NPO,* nothing by mouth; *WBC,* white blood cell.

nature of the procedure. The patient needs to know what the procedure involves and its basic purpose, where it will be done, how long it will take, and whether it will hurt. These things should be explained at a level appropriate to the patient's understanding. The patient should also be instructed on personal responsibility during a particular study (e.g., to lie flat on the table or to keep the legs straight).

Diagnostic studies of the urinary system often cause embarrassment and emotional stress. Examination of the urinary system may be perceived as an intrusion on a personal body area. The nurse should alleviate anxiety by providing privacy and protecting the patient's modesty.

Urine Studies

Urinalysis.   In evaluating disorders of the urinary tract, one of the first studies done is a urinalysis (Tables 42-8 and 42-9). This test may provide information about possible abnormalities, indicate what further studies need to be done, and supply information on the progression of a diagnosed disorder.

For a routine urinalysis, a specimen may be collected at any time of the day. However, it is best to obtain the first specimen urinated in the morning. This concentrated specimen is more likely to contain abnormal constituents if they are present in the urine. The specimen should be examined within 1 hour of urinating. If it is not, bacteria multiply rapidly, RBCs hemolyze, casts disintegrate, and the urine becomes alkaline as a result of urea-splitting bacteria. If it is not possible to send the specimen to the laboratory immediately, it should be refrigerated. However, to obtain the best results, the nurse should coordinate specimen collection with routine laboratory hours.

Multiple reagent strips (also called urine dipsticks) are commonly used by laboratories and in outpatient settings to provide chemical analysis of urine along with a microscopic interpretation. The results of a urinalysis usually include a description of the appearance, specific gravity (mass and density), pH, glucose, ketones, and protein in the urine and a microscopic examination of urine sediment for white blood cells (WBCs), RBCs, crystals, and casts (see Table 42-9).

Table 42-9   Urinalysis Findings

Test	Normal	Abnormal Finding and Significance
Color	Amber yellow	■ Dark, smoky color suggests hematuria. Yellow brown to olive green indicates excessive bilirubin. Orange red or orange brown caused by phenazopyridine (Pyridium) or urobilin in excess. Cloudiness of freshly voided urine indicates infection. Colorless urine indicates excessive fluid intake, renal disease, or diabetes insipidus.
Smell	Aromatic	■ On standing, urine becomes more ammonia-like in smell. In urinary tract infections, urine smells unpleasant.
Protein	0-150 mg/24 hr 0-18 mg/dl	■ Persistent proteinuria is characteristic of acute and chronic renal disease, especially involving glomeruli. In absence of disease, positive reading may be caused by high-protein diet, strenuous exercise, dehydration, fever, or emotional stress. Vaginal secretions may contaminate urine specimen and give positive reading.
Glucose	None	■ Glycosuria indicates diabetes mellitus or low renal threshold for glucose reabsorption (if blood glucose level is normal). Small amounts may be found after glucose loading (e.g., glucose tolerance test).
Ketones	None	■ Altered carbohydrate and fat metabolism indicates diabetes mellitus and starvation. Findings can also be seen in dehydration, vomiting, and severe diarrhea.
Bilirubin	None	■ Presence of bilirubinuria is as significant as jaundice in detection of liver disorders. Bilirubin may appear in urine before jaundice becomes visible or may be present in persons with hepatic disorders who do not have recognizable jaundice.*
Nitrite	None	■ Gram-negative bacteria commonly cause urinary infection and have an enzyme that produces nitrite in the urine. When nitrite is positive and WBCs are present, the probability of urinary infection is high. A negative nitrite, however, does not rule out infection because gram-positive organisms and yeast do not contain the converting enzyme.
Specific gravity	1.003-1.030	■ Specific gravity of morning urine specimen reflects maximum concentrating ability of kidney and is 1.025-1.030. Low specific gravity indicates dilute urine and possibly excessive diuresis. High specific gravity indicates dehydration. If it becomes fixed at about 1.010, this indicates renal inability to concentrate urine, suggesting that kidney is progressing to end-stage renal disease.
Osmolality	300-1300 mOsm/kg (300-1300 mmol/kg)	■ Measurement is a more accurate method than specific gravity for determining diluting and concentrating ability of kidneys. Deviations from normal indicate tubular dysfunction. Findings indicate if kidney has lost ability to concentrate or dilute urine. (Not part of routine urinalysis.)
pH	4.0-8.0 (average, 6.0)	■ If >8.0, finding may be the result of standing of urine or urinary tract infections because bacteria decompose urea to form ammonia. If <4.0, may indicate respiratory or metabolic acidosis.
RBC	0-4/hpf	■ Bleeding in urinary tract is caused by calculi, cystitis, neoplasm, glomerulonephritis, tuberculosis, kidney biopsy, or trauma.
WBC	0-5/hpf	■ Increased number of WBCs in urine (pyuria) indicates urinary tract infection or inflammation.
Casts	None-occasional hyaline	■ Casts are molds of the renal tubules and may contain protein, WBCs, RBCs, or bacteria. Noncellular casts are hyaline in appearance, and a few may be found in normal urine. Casts indicate renal dysfunction or urinary tract infections.
Culture for organisms	No organisms in bladder, <10⁴ organisms/ml result of normal urethral flora	■ Bacteria counts >10⁵/ml indicate urinary tract infection. Organisms most commonly found in urinary tract infections are *Escherichia coli,* enterococci, *Klebsiella, Proteus,* and streptococci.

*See Chapter 41 for further discussion.
hpf, high-powered field.

Composite Urine Collections. Composite urine specimens are collected over a period that may range from 2 to 24 hours. The purpose of a composite specimen is to examine or measure specific components, such as electrolytes, sugar, protein, 17-ketosteroids, catecholamines, creatinine, and minerals. These specimens may have to be refrigerated, or preservatives may have to be added to the container used for collecting urine.

For collection of a composite urine specimen, the patient is instructed to urinate and discard this first urine specimen. This time is noted as the start of the test. All urine from subsequent urinations is saved in a container for the designated period. Finally, at the end of the period, the patient is asked to urinate and this urine is added to the container. Incomplete collections do not provide valid results. Reminding the patient to save all urine during the study period is critical.

Creatinine Clearance. One of the most common composite indicators used to analyze urinary system disorders is creatinine clearance. Creatinine is a waste product produced by muscle breakdown. Urinary excretion of creatinine is a measure of the amount of active muscle tissue in the body, not of body weight. Therefore people with larger muscle mass have higher values. Because almost all creatinine in the blood is normally excreted by the kidneys, creatinine clearance is the most accurate indicator of renal function. The result of a creatinine clearance closely approximates that of the GFR. A blood specimen for serum creatinine determination should be obtained during the period of urine collection. Creatinine clearance is calculated as follows:

Creatinine clearance (ml/min) =

$$\frac{\text{Urine creatinine (mg/ml)} \times \text{Urine volume (ml/min)}}{\text{Serum creatinine (mg/ml)}}$$

Creatinine levels remain remarkably constant for each person because they are not significantly affected by protein ingestion, muscular exercise, water intake, or rate of urine production. Normal creatinine clearance values range from 85 to 135 ml per minute. After age 40, the creatinine clearance rate decreases at a rate of about 1 ml per minute per year.

Urine Cytology. Urine can be checked for abnormal cellular structures that occur with bladder cancer. Specimens may be obtained by voiding, catheterization, or bladder irrigation (bladder washing). The first morning's voided specimen should not be used because epithelial cells may change in appearance in urine held in the bladder overnight. As with urinalysis, the specimen should be fresh or brought to the lab within the hour. An alcohol-based fixative is then added to preserve the cellular structure. Urine cytology is currently being used for detection of and following the prognosis of bladder cancer.[9,10]

Radiologic Studies

Kidney, Ureter, and Bladder Film. The kidney, ureter, and bladder (KUB) film is an abdominal view taken without using a contrast medium to show the renal outline, psoas shadow, and the bladder, if full. Radiopaque stones and foreign bodies can be seen on this x-ray. The form, size, and position of the kidneys can also be seen. Abscesses, tumors, and cysts may distort anatomic relationships on the KUB. Sometimes tomograms (sectional views that focus on a single plane of the kidney) are ordered at the same time as the KUB x-ray.

Intravenous Pyelogram. The purpose of an intravenous pyelogram (IVP), or excretory urogram, is to visualize the urinary tract. The presence, position, size, and shape of the kidneys, ureters, and bladder can be evaluated. Cysts, tumors, lesions, and obstructions cause a distortion in the normal appearance of these structures. The IVP also gives clues to renal function since sequential films are taken, but other tests (discussed later) are more accurate for this purpose.

The procedure consists of injecting an IV dose of contrast material, which circulates in the blood and is excreted by the kidneys into the urine. During injection, the patient may experience warmth, a flushed face, and a salty taste. After injection, films are taken sequentially. (A rapid-sequence IVP has x-ray films taken every minute for the first 5 minutes.) The sequencing of films is planned so that contrast excretion can be followed from the cortex of the kidney to the bladder. A film taken at 45 minutes allows visualization of the bladder. The presence of bladder atony or outlet obstruction also can be detected by a film taken after urination, which shows the residual volume of urine in the bladder.

Preparation of the patient the evening before the test includes giving a cathartic or an enema to eliminate feces and air from the colon. The patient with neurologic bowel dysfunction may require more vigorous routines. Fluids are withheld for 8 hours before testing to produce slight dehydration so that the contrast material will concentrate and therefore improve visualization. The patient with significantly decreased renal function should not have an IVP because the contrast material will not be properly excreted by the kidneys. Contrast medium can also be nephrotoxic and can worsen renal function. An IVP should be avoided on a pregnant patient, particularly in the first trimester, because of radiation exposure and harm to the fetus.

The patient should be assessed for any possible allergic reactions to the contrast material. The contrast medium is typically an iodine derivative of shellfish. A person with iodine sensitivity may have an anaphylactic reaction after contrast material is injected. If known to have an allergy to iodine or seafood, the patient should not have an IVP, or it can be done using prophylactic diphenhydramine (Benadryl) and corticosteroids.

During contrast material injection, the patient should be observed for signs of respiratory distress, urticaria, decrease in blood pressure, and other signs of anaphylaxis. Emergency drugs such as diphenhydramine (Benadryl), corticosteroids, and epinephrine (Adrenalin) and cardiopulmonary resuscitation equipment should be available. A patient may experience transient hypersensitivity reactions (e.g., nausea, itching), but these are not considered serious reactions contraindicating future IVPs.

After the procedure, the nurse should encourage the patient to force fluids to dilute and flush out the contrast material. Dilution of the contrast medium makes it less nephrotoxic. The patient should be monitored for delayed reactions such as itching, nausea, respiratory problems, and decreased urine output.

Retrograde Pyelogram. A retrograde pyelogram evaluates the same structures as an IVP. This is an x-ray visualization of the kidneys, ureter, and bladder after direct injection of a contrast material into the kidney via a ureteral catheter introduced through a cystoscope. It may be done if an IVP does not visualize the urinary tract or if the patient is allergic to the contrast material or has decreased renal function. The dangers associated with a retrograde pyelogram are similar to those related to cystoscopy, including the risk of infection and the use of anesthesia.

Antegrade Pyelogram. Sometimes an antegrade pyelogram is done to evaluate the upper urinary tract when there is allergy to contrast material or decreased renal function and when abnormalities prevent passage of a ureteral catheter. Contrast may be injected percutaneously into the renal pelvis or via a nephrostomy tube that is already in place (also called a nephrostogram) when determining tube function or ureteral integrity after trauma or surgery. Complications of an antegrade pyelogram include hematuria, infection, and hematoma.

Renal Ultrasound. A renal ultrasound uses high-frequency waves to image the kidneys, ureter, and bladder. Because radiation exposure is avoided, a number of images can be obtained, and repeat studies over a brief period of time can be done. Images can be obtained from both the prone and supine positions. A bowel preparation is not required for a renal ultrasound.

Computed Tomography Scan. Computed tomography (CT) of the abdomen and pelvis may be done to detect tumors and possible metastases. The CT scan can differentiate these from cysts or abscesses. Contrast material may be used to help visualize urinary structures more clearly in the computer-generated images produced by the machine. The patient is instructed to lie very still during the procedure while the machine takes precise transaxial images. Sedation may be required if the patient is unable to cooperate.

Magnetic Resonance Imaging. Specific structures such as the kidney or prostate can be visualized by disturbing the electromagnetic fields generated by different body tissues and converting this to computer-generated images. This is done using radiofrequency waves. Magnetic resonance imaging (MRI) helps evaluate genitourinary tumors and abdominal or pelvic masses. The patient must lie still in an enclosed cylinder while these images are being produced. Some patients cannot tolerate being in the small MRI chamber, and sedation may be required. All metal objects must be removed because they interfere with the radiofrequency. The MRI is contraindicated in a patient with a pacemaker or with certain kinds of internal metallic vascular surgical clips.

Cystogram. The purpose of a cystogram is to outline and visualize the bladder and evaluate the UVJ for reflux. In addition to suspected vesicoureteral reflux, indications for a cystogram include a neurogenic bladder and recurrent urinary tract infections. A cystogram can also delineate abnormalities of the bladder, such as diverticuli, calculi, and tumors. The procedure involves instillation of a contrast material into the bladder, which may be done via a cystoscope or catheter.

A voiding cystourethrogram is a voiding study of the bladder opening and urethra. The bladder is filled with contrast material. During urination, films are taken to visualize the bladder and urethra. After urination, another film is taken to assess for residual urine. A voiding cystourethrogram can detect abnormalities of the lower urinary tract, urethral stenosis, bladder neck obstruction, and prostatic enlargement.

Urethrogram. A urethrogram is similar to a cystogram. Contrast material is injected retrograde into the urethra to identify strictures, diverticula, or other urethral pathology. When urethral trauma is suspected, a urethrogram is done before catheterization.

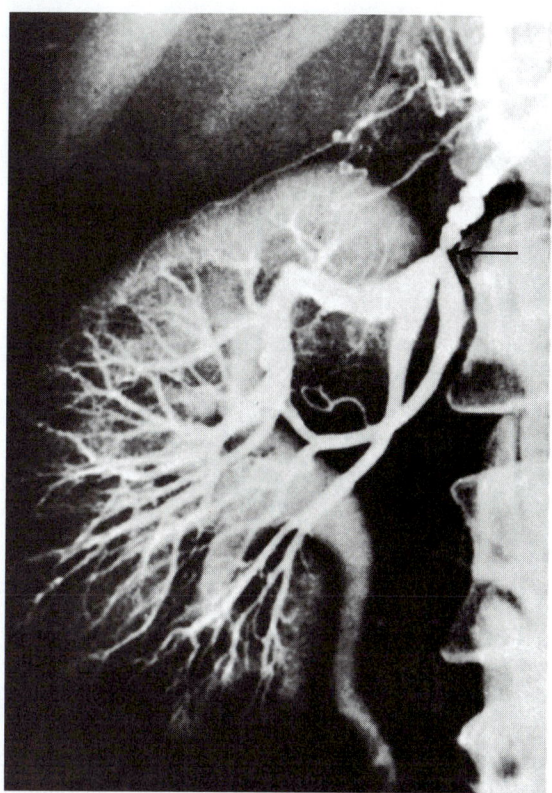

Fig. 42-8   Renal arteriogram showing stenosis of the right renal artery.

Loopogram. A loopogram is used to detect obstructions, anastomotic leaks, stones, reflux, and other uropathology when a patient has a urinary pouch or ileal conduit. Since urinary diversions are created with bowel, there is risk of contrast absorption. The patient should be closely monitored for contrast reactions.

Renal Arteriogram. The purpose of a renal arteriogram (angiogram) is to visualize the renal blood vessels. The findings of an arteriogram can assist in diagnosing renal artery stenosis (Fig. 42-8), additional or missing renal blood vessels, and renovascular hypertension and can assist in differentiating between a renal cyst and a renal tumor. Renal arteriograms are also included in the workup of a potential renal transplant donor.

The evening before the procedure, the patient is given a cathartic to eliminate fecal material from the colon. The morning of the procedure, a preoperative medication is given to relax and sedate the patient.

Most arteriograms are done in the x-ray department by a specially trained physician. The patient is given a local anesthetic at the site of catheter insertion. A catheter is usually inserted into the femoral artery and passed up the aorta to the level of the renal arteries (Fig. 42-9). Contrast material is then injected to outline the renal blood supply, and x-rays are taken. The patient may experience a transient warm feeling along the course of the blood vessel when the contrast material is injected. As with all contrast studies, possible iodine and shellfish allergies should be determined before the study.

After the catheter is removed, a pressure dressing is placed over the femoral injection site. It is important to observe the

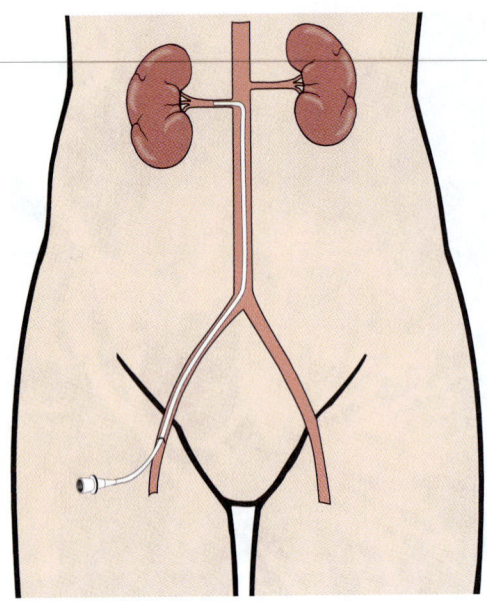

Fig. 42-9 Catheter insertion for a renal arteriogram.

site for bleeding. Bed rest is usually prescribed with the affected leg straight. Peripheral pulses in the involved leg should be taken at least every 30 to 60 minutes to detect occlusion of blood flow caused by a thrombus. Complications that may result from a renal arteriogram include thrombus, embolus, local inflammation, and hematoma. The patient with baseline renal insufficiency may experience a decrease in renal function secondary to the nephrotoxic contrast material.

Digital Subtraction Angiography. Because of potential complications, the renal arteriogram is sometimes replaced by digital subtraction angiography (DSA) in many hospitals that have the facilities to perform this procedure. Using computer technology, this procedure permits visualization of the arteries after an IV injection of contrast material. A primary advantage of DSA is that it requires small peripheral venous injections of contrast medium compared with the relatively large doses that must be injected via arterial cannulation for a renal arteriogram. (See Table 30-7 for a further description of DSA.)

Renal Radionuclide Imaging. Renal scans involving the use of radionuclides are useful in evaluating the anatomic structures, perfusion, and function of the kidneys. Different institutions use different imaging techniques. In general, the following radionuclides are used for these purposes:

Anatomic structures: technetium 99m (^{99m}Tc)–labeled compounds such as dimercaptosuccinic acid (DMSA) or glucoheptonate
Perfusion and function: iodine 131 (^{131}I)–labeled orthoiodohippurate (Hippuran) and ^{99m}Tc-labeled diethylenetriamine pentaacetic acid (DTPA)
Infection or abscesses: gallium 67 citrate

For this procedure a radioactive isotope is injected intravenously. Radiation detector probes are placed over the kidneys, and a scintillation counter monitors the appearance and disappearance of the radioactive material in the kidney.

The results reveal the difference between the two kidneys with respect to blood flow, tubular function, and excretion. A normal scan shows symmetric functioning of both kidneys. Normally the distribution of activity is recorded throughout the kidneys. A lesion (e.g., a tumor) is indicated by the absence of radioactivity in the involved area and the appearance of the resultant defect on the scan. In renovascular disease, an area with decreased blood flow can be readily visualized. This study is particularly useful in detecting renal vascular disease, acute renal failure, and upper urinary tract obstruction, as well as useful in monitoring the function of a transplanted kidney.

Usually there are no dietary or activity restrictions related to preparation of the patient. During the test the patient should feel no pain or discomfort. No special precautions are needed in the use of radioactive material since only tracer doses are used.

Renal Biopsy. The purpose of a renal biopsy is to determine the nature and extent of renal disease. This information can be used in establishing a diagnosis and following the progress of a disease, as well as determining the treatment. Biopsy material can be obtained through an open biopsy or a closed percutaneous needle biopsy. An open biopsy is rarely performed because it requires a surgical procedure with anesthesia. A percutaneous needle biopsy is more common. It is usually done in the x-ray department or in the patient's room, although it may be done in the operating room.

Absolute contraindications to a percutaneous renal biopsy are bleeding disorders, the presence of a single kidney, and uncontrolled hypertension. Relative contraindications include suspected renal infection, hydronephrosis, and possible vascular lesions.

Because hemorrhage is one danger of biopsy, the patient's coagulation status should be assessed before the procedure. This includes a health history, complete blood count, hematocrit, prothrombin time, and bleeding or clotting time determinations. The patient may also be typed and crossmatched for blood. The patient who is to be biopsied should not be taking aspirin or warfarin (Coumadin) before the procedure.

An IVP or ultrasound examination is done to determine the position and location of the kidneys as a guide to needle insertion. Preparation also includes explaining the procedure to the patient and discussing all concerns. A signed consent form is required before a biopsy is performed.

The procedure consists of having the patient lie prone with a pillow or sandbag to elevate the abdomen and kidneys. Using the IVP or ultrasound findings as a guide, the position of the kidney is marked on the body. Local anesthesia is used, and a biopsy needle is inserted into the kidney just below the twelfth rib. The patient is instructed to hold his or her breath while the biopsy specimen is being taken.

After the procedure, a pressure dressing is applied, and the patient is kept prone for 30 to 60 minutes. Usually bed rest is prescribed for 24 hours. Vital signs should be taken every 5 to 10 minutes during the first hour and then with decreasing frequency, if no problems are noted. The biopsy site should be inspected frequently for bleeding. Serial urine specimens should be assessed for gross and microscopic hematuria. A dipstick can be used to test for bleeding, even when hematuria is not obvious. The physician may order all urine sent for laboratory analysis to detect possible hematuria. The patient should also

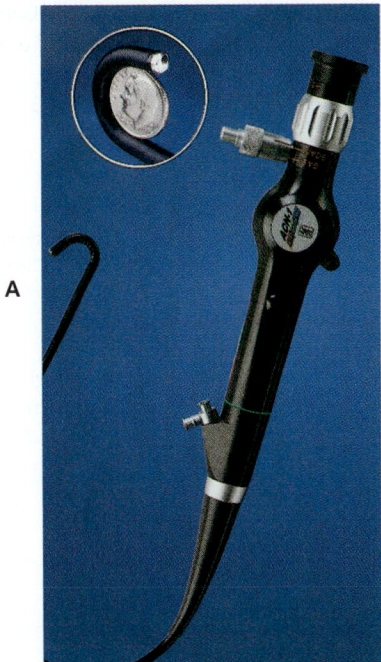

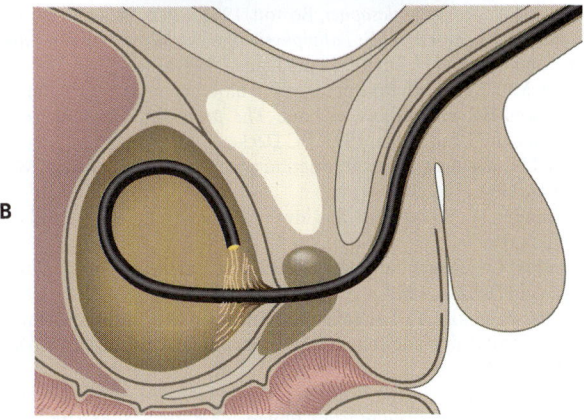

Fig. 42-10   Cystoscopic examination of the bladder in a man. **A,** Flexible Cysto Nephroscope. **B,** Scope inserted into bladder.

be assessed for flank pain, hypotension, decreasing hematocrit, and temperature elevation. The patient should be observed for chills, urinary frequency, and dysuria.

Complications of a renal biopsy include renal hemorrhage, hematoma, and infection. Even if no complications occur, the patient should be instructed to avoid lifting heavy objects for 5 to 7 days. The patient should be instructed not to take any anticoagulant medication until permission is given by the physician who performed the biopsy.

Endoscopy

Cystoscopy.   The main purpose of cystoscopy is to inspect the interior of the bladder with a tubular lighted scope called a *cystoscope* (Fig. 42-10). Cystoscopes can be used to insert ureteral catheters, remove calculi, obtain biopsy specimens of bladder lesions, and treat bleeding lesions. In most cases, bladder disorders can be determined by cystoscopic examination. Although rigid instruments still are used, newer

flexible cystoscopes (and ureteroscopes) make visualization easier for the urologist and the procedure more comfortable for the patient.

Cystoscopy is usually done in a cystoscopy room in the x-ray department, in urology clinics, or in the operating room. A signed consent form may be required. The cystoscopic examination may be performed with local or general anesthesia, depending on the needs and condition of the patient. The patient may be put in a lithotomy position. Most of the pain associated with cystoscopy results from spasms and contractions of bladder and sphincter. Relaxation and deep breathing by the patient alleviate some of the bladder and sphincter spasms. A local anesthetic is instilled into the urethra before scope insertion. During the examination, saline solution is inserted slowly to distend the bladder. This allows better visualization but causes an urge to urinate.

After the procedure the patient can expect to have some burning on urination, blood-tinged urine, and urinary frequency from the irritation of scope insertion and manipulation. The nurse should observe for bright-red bleeding, which is not normal. The patient should not be allowed to walk without assistance immediately after the procedure because postural hypotension may result from blood flow back to the legs after the patient has been in a lithotomy position. After the procedure the nurse is responsible for keeping the patient well hydrated, administering mild analgesics, providing sitz baths, and applying heat to decrease the patient's discomfort. Complications that may result from cystoscopy include urinary retention, urinary tract hemorrhage, bladder infection, and perforation of the bladder.

Urodynamics

Urodynamics can involve many tests that are used to evaluate voiding problems. The extent of testing depends on the patient's problems and access to urodynamic laboratories. Complex urodynamics are done in special clinics. Two common urodynamic tests done in hospitals or clinics are the urinary flow rate and cystometrogram.

Urinary Flow Rate.   The urinary flow rate study measures urine volume in a single voiding expelled in a period of time and is expressed as milliliters per second. As the patient voids, the stream pattern is depicted graphically on a printout.

The patient is asked to start the test with a full bladder, urinate into a special container, and try to empty completely. This test is used to (1) assess the degree of outflow obstruction caused by such conditions as benign prostatic hyperplasia or stricture, (2) assess bladder or sphincter dysfunction effects on voiding such as occurs with neuropathology, and (3) evaluate the effects of treatment for lower urinary tract problems. A residual urine volume may be obtained after a urinary flow rate using ultrasound or catheterization.

A normal maximum flow rate for men is about 20 to 25 ml/sec and about 25 to 30 ml/sec for women. However, the volume voided and the patient's age can affect the flow rate, so normal variations are common. Graphic displays can illustrate straining and intermittent flow patterns or other abnormal voiding disorders.[11]

Cystometrogram.   The purpose of a cystometrogram is to evaluate bladder tone and neurologic bladder dysfunction. It is usually ordered if a patient has incontinence or neurogenic dysfunction of the bladder.

The procedure consists of insertion of a retention catheter while the patient is in a supine position. A liter bottle of saline solution or water and a cystometer are connected to the catheter and taped to an IV pole for measurement. Fluid is instilled at a constant rate, and the pressure exerted against the bladder wall is measured. The patient is asked to indicate when the urge to void is first experienced (usually after 100 to 200 ml has been instilled). Fluids are instilled until urgency occurs (350 to 450 ml) or until it is determined that this sensation is absent. After the catheter is withdrawn the patient is asked to empty the bladder, and the amount of residual urine is determined. During the study a cholinergic drug such as bethanechol (Urecholine) may be given to determine whether it will enhance the tone of a flaccid bladder. However, an anticholinergic drug may be given to promote relaxation of a hyperactive bladder. Water or carbon dioxide gas may be used for this examination. Complete urodynamic studies are often done simultaneously using specialized equipment and catheters.

REVIEW QUESTIONS

The number of the question corresponds to the same-numbered objective at the beginning of the chapter.

1. A renal stone in the pelvis of the kidney will alter the function of the kidney by interfering with
   a. the structural support of the kidney.
   b. regulation of the concentration of urine.
   c. the entry and exit of blood vessels at the kidney.
   d. collection and drainage of urine from the kidney.
2. A patient with renal disease has oliguria and a creatinine clearance of 40 ml/min. The nurse recognizes that these findings most directly reflect abnormal function of
   a. tubular secretion.
   b. glomerular filtration.
   c. capillary permeability.
   d. concentration of filtrate.
3. The nurse identifies a risk for urinary calculi in a patient who relates a past health history that includes
   a. measles.
   b. gastric ulcer.
   c. diabetes mellitus.
   d. hyperparathyroidism.
4. Normal changes associated with aging of the urinary system that the nurse expects to find include
   a. decreased levels of BUN.
   b. postvoiding urine residual.
   c. increased bladder capacity.
   d. more easily palpable kidneys.
5. During physical assessment of the urinary system the nurse
   a. percusses the flank area with a firm blow.
   b. palpates an empty bladder as a small nodule.
   c. positions the patient prone to palpate the kidneys.
   d. uses auscultation to determine the level of urine in the bladder.
6. Normal findings expected by the nurse on physical assessment of the urinary system include
   a. nonpalpable left kidney.
   b. auscultation of renal artery bruit.
   c. CVA tenderness elicited by a kidney punch.
   d. palpable bladder to the level of the pubic symphysis.
7. An important nursing responsibility after an intravenous pyelogram is to
   a. assess the patient for flank pain.
   b. encourage extra oral fluid intake.
   c. observe urine for remaining contrast material.
   d. encourage ambulation 2 to 3 hours after the study.
8. On reading the urinalysis results of a dehydrated patient the nurse would expect to find
   a. a pH of 8.4.
   b. RBC of 4/hpf.
   c. color: yellow, cloudy.
   d. specific gravity of 1.035.

References

1. Smith HW: *Fish to philosopher,* Boston, 1953, Little, Brown.
2. McCance KL, Huether SE: *Pathophysiology: the biologic basis for disease in adults and children,* ed 3, St Louis, 1998, Mosby.
3. Smith MC, Dunn MJ: Role of kidney in blood pressure regulation. In Jacobson HR and others, editors: *The principles and practice of nephrology,* Philadelphia, 1993, BC Decker.
4. Beck LH: Changes in renal function with aging, *Clin Geriatr Med* 14:199, 1998.
5. Ouslander JG: Aging and the lower urinary tract, *Am J Med Sci* 314:214, 1997.
6. Samsioe G: Urogenital aging—a hidden problem, *Am J Obstet Gynecol* 178:S245, 1998.
7. Bernier F, Jenkins P: The role of vaginal estrogen in the treatment of urogenital dysfunction in postmenopausal women, *Urol Nurs* 17:92, 1997.
8. Reilly NJ: Cancer of the bladder. In Karlowicz KA, editor: *Urologic nursing—principles and practice,* Philadelphia, 1995, Saunders.
9. Goldstein ML, Whitman T, Renshaw AA: Significance of cell groups in voided urine, *Acta Cytol* 42:290, 1998.
10. Wiener HG and others: Can urine bound diagnostic tests replace cystoscopy in the management of bladder cancer? *J Urol* 159:1876, 1998.
11. Karlowicz KA, Meredith CE: Adult voiding dysfunction. In Karlowicz KA, editor: *Urologic nursing—principles and practice,* Philadelphia, 1995, Saunders.

Resources

Resources for this chapter are listed after Chapter 43 on p. 1298.

43 NURSING MANAGEMENT
Renal and Urologic Problems

Patricia Bates

www.mosby.com/MERLIN/medsurg_lewis

LEARNING OBJECTIVES

1. Describe the pathophysiology, clinical manifestations, collaborative care, and drug therapy of cystitis, urethritis, and pyelonephritis.
2. Explain the nursing management of urinary tract infections.
3. Describe the immunologic mechanisms involved in glomerulonephritis.
4. Explain the clinical manifestations and nursing and collaborative management of acute poststreptococcal glomerulonephritis, Goodpasture's syndrome, and chronic glomerulonephritis.
5. Describe the common causes, clinical manifestations, collaborative care, and nursing management of nephrotic syndrome.
6. Compare and contrast the etiology, clinical manifestations, collaborative care, and nursing management of various types of urinary calculi.
7. Explain the common causes and management of renal trauma, renal vascular problems, and hereditary renal problems.
8. Describe the mechanisms of renal involvement in metabolic and connective tissue disorders.
9. Describe the clinical manifestations and collaborative care of renal and bladder cancer.
10. Describe the common causes and management of bladder dysfunctions.
11. Differentiate among ureteral, suprapubic, nephrostomy, and urethral catheters with regard to indications for use and nursing responsibilities.
12. Explain the nursing management of the patient undergoing nephrectomy or urinary diversion surgery.

Renal and urologic disorders encompass a wide spectrum of clinical problems. The diverse causes of these disorders may involve infectious, immunologic, obstructive, metabolic, collagen-vascular, traumatic, congenital, neoplastic, and neurologic mechanisms. This chapter discusses specific disorders of the kidneys, ureters, bladder, and urethra. Acute and chronic renal failure are discussed in Chapter 44. Female reproductive problems are discussed in Chapter 51. Male genitourinary problems are discussed in Chapter 52.

INFECTIOUS AND INFLAMMATORY DISORDERS OF THE URINARY SYSTEM

Urinary tract infections (UTIs) are the second most common bacterial disease. More than 1 million people are hospitalized annually because of UTIs. Nosocomial urinary infections are responsible for 40% of all hospital-acquired infections, and the majority of these are related to catheterization.[1] More than 15% of patients who develop gram-negative bacteremia die, and one third of these are caused by bacterial infections originating in the urinary tract. UTIs are the most common source of bacteremia in older adults.[2]

Infections of the urinary tract may appear as a variety of disorders. The common factor is a microbial invasion of the tissues of the urinary tract, most often by *Escherichia coli* (Table 43-1). Bacterial counts of 10^5 organisms or more generally indicate a UTI. However, bacterial counts as low as 10^2 to 10^3 in a person with symptoms are indicative of UTI. Viral, fungal, and parasitic infections are not as common but are seen most frequently in the patient who is immunosuppressed, has diabetes mellitus, or has taken multiple courses of antibiotics.

Classification

Infections may be broadly classified as upper and lower UTIs (Fig. 43-1) based on the patient's symptoms. Terminology may specifically delineate the site of inflammation or infection. Examples of terms are *pyelonephritis* (involvement of kidney and kidney pelvis) and *cystitis* (involvement of bladder). However, it may be difficult to determine the specific location of a UTI. A patient may have a simultaneous infection in both the upper and lower urinary tract, an infection of adjacent organs causing urinary infection–like symptoms, or no symptoms at all.

Determining whether a UTI is complicated or uncomplicated is a significant factor in determining the treatment plan. Uncomplicated infections are those that occur in an otherwise normal urinary tract. First-time infections in young women are usually uncomplicated. Complicated infections include the coexisting presence of obstruction, stones, or catheters; when

Reviewed by Mikel Gray, RN, PhD, CUNP, CCCN, FAAN, Associate Professor, Department of Urology and School of Nursing, University of Virginia Medical Center, Charlottesville, Va.

Table 43-1	Common Microorganisms Causing Urinary Tract Infections
*Escherichia coli**	*Proteus*
Enterococci	*Pseudomonas*
Klebsiella	*Staphylococci*
Enterobacter	*Candida*
Serratia	

*Causes about 80% of cases in persons who do not have urinary tract structural abnormalities or calculi.

diabetes or neurologic diseases exist; or when an infection is a recurrent one. The individual with a complicated infection is at risk for renal damage.

Only about one fourth of individuals who develop an acute infection go on to develop a recurrent UTI.[3] Recurrent UTIs can be classified as *relapses* (recurrence with the same strain of bacteria from within the urinary tract that occurs within 1 to 2 weeks of stopping antibiotic therapy) or *reinfections* (recurrence with a new organism following successful treatment).

Relapse can be further defined as states of unresolved bacteriuria or true bacterial persistence. Unresolved bacteriuria occurs when bacteria are resistant to the antibiotic used to treat an infection or when the infection is undertreated. Some bacteria, although initially sensitive to a drug, can mutate during therapy. Insufficient antibiotic concentrations in the urinary system may be attributed to renal insufficiency or an inability of the antibiotic to infiltrate the tissues (such as the prostate or urethra). Often the patient feels better and stops medication before an adequate course is completed. Bacterial persistence occurs when the infection is successfully treated but a persistent source of infection remains. This may result from infected stones, chronic pyelonephritis, obstructive uropathies, or foreign bodies. Urine cultures may be negative immediately following antibiotic therapy but will show growth again when cultured about 1 week after treatment.

Etiology

Defense Mechanisms. The urinary tract above the urethra is normally sterile. Several physiologic and mechanical defense mechanisms assist in maintaining sterility and preventing UTIs. These defenses include normal voiding with complete emptying of the bladder, normal antibacterial ability of the bladder mucosa and urine, ureterovesical junction competence, and peristaltic activity that propels urine toward the bladder. An alteration in any of these defense mechanisms increases the risk of contracting a UTI. Table 43-2 lists predisposing factors to urinary tract infections.

Source of Urinary Tract Infections. The organisms that usually cause UTIs are introduced via the ascending route from the urethra. Less common routes are via the bloodstream or lymphatic system. Most infections are due to gram-negative aerobic bacilli normally found in the gastrointestinal (GI) tract, although gram-positive organisms such as streptococci, enterococci, and *Staphylococcus saprophyticus* also can cause urinary infections. A common factor contributing to ascending infection is urologic instrumentation (e.g., catheterization, cystoscopic examinations). Instrumentation allows bacteria that are normally present at the opening of the urethra to enter the urethra or bladder. Sexual intercourse promotes milking of bacteria from the vagina and perineum

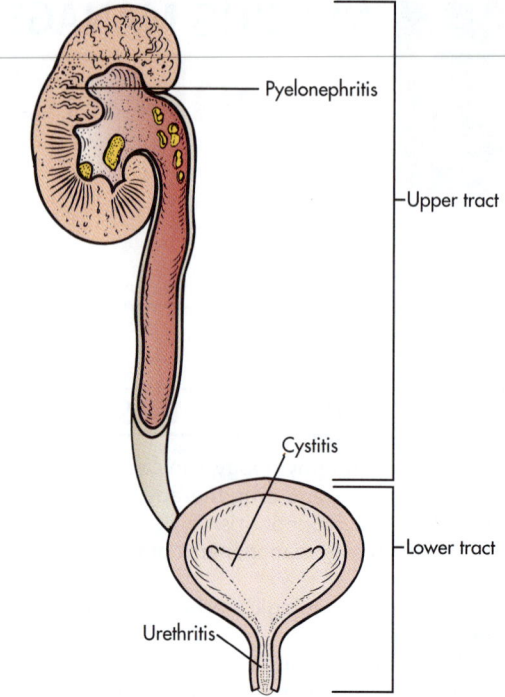

Fig. 43-1   Sites of infectious processes in the urinary tract.

Table 43-2	Predisposing Factors to Urinary Tract Infections

1. Renal scarring from previous UTI
2. Diminished ureteral peristalsis (e.g., pregnancy)
3. Compression of growing uterus against ureters (e.g., tumor, fibroids)
4. Urinary retention for any reason
5. Presence of a foreign body (e.g., urinary catheter)
6. Vesicoureteral reflux of urine in a retrograde direction from bladder toward the kidney
7. Humoral or cellular immunodeficiency in an otherwise normal urinary tract
8. Shorter urethra in females
9. Presence of urinary calculi
10. Neurogenic bladder
11. Congenital defects
12. Diabetes mellitus

and may cause minor urethral trauma that predisposes women to UTIs.

Rarely do UTIs result from a hematogenous route, where blood-borne bacteria secondarily invade the kidneys, ureters, or bladder from elsewhere in the body. For a kidney infection to occur from hematogenous transmission, there must be prior injury to the urinary tract, such as obstruction of the ureter, damage caused by stones, or renal scars.

An important source of UTIs is hospital-acquired, or nosocomial, infection. The cause of nosocomial infection is often *E. coli* and, less frequently, *Pseudomonas* organisms. Urologic instrumentation, particularly with an indwelling urinary catheter, is the most common predisposing factor.

The occurrence of UTIs is often related to the presence of abnormalities of the urinary tract, such as strictures and obstructions. An untreated UTI can lead to chronic pyelonephritis and a progressive decrease in renal function. If no abnormality exists, uncomplicated pyelonephritis rarely leads to progressive renal damage and renal failure.

CYSTITIS

Etiology and Pathophysiology

Although the majority of patients with cystitis are women, other groups with a high incidence are older men and young children (especially girls). These age and sex variations in the frequency of cystitis are related to anatomic differences or pathologic changes in the groups at risk. The adult female urethra is short, and its proximity to the rectum and vagina predisposes women to the risk of bladder contamination. Bacterial contamination of the bladder can be the result of poor personal hygiene practices and sexual intercourse.

In children and older men, UTIs are often associated with other preexisting problems. In children, vesicoureteral reflux is usually the preexisting abnormality. In men, the longer urethra (of which the proximal two thirds is normally sterile) and the antibacterial property of prostatic secretions provide protection from bacterial infections unless there are predisposing causes, such as benign prostatic hyperplasia.

Not all bacterial invasions of the bladder result in lower UTI or cause spread to the upper urinary tract (pyelonephritis). Once cystitis has occurred, it may remain localized in the urinary bladder for years without ascension to the kidneys or may be completely resolved after initial treatment. Although the bacterial infection may be self-limiting, the urinary tract should be evaluated if there is recurrence, even in the patient who has no symptoms. The risk of recurrent symptomatic infection is increased when there are urinary tract abnormalities.

Asymptomatic bacteriuria can occur and is not synonymous with UTI. It indicates that bacteria are present in the urine. Tissue invasion must occur for an infection to exist. Pyuria (the presence of white blood cells [WBCs] in the urine) usually signals this occurrence and is the characteristic laboratory finding in symptomatic UTI. Asymptomatic bacteriuria is more likely to occur in women over 65 years of age.[1] Asymptomatic bacteriuria may be important in a patient of any age if that person is at risk for complicated urinary infection and resultant renal damage.

Clinical Manifestations

The manifestations of cystitis are frequency and urgency of urination, suprapubic pain, dysuria, foul-smelling urine, and pyuria. Hematuria may or may not occur in symptomatic UTI.

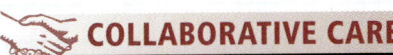

COLLABORATIVE CARE

Table 43-3 Cystitis

Diagnostic
Urinalysis
Urine for Gram's stain
Urine for culture and sensitivity (if indicated)
Evaluation of urinary tract (e.g., IVP, cystoscopy) (if indicated)

Collaborative Therapy
Uncomplicated
  Single-dose regimen
    Trimethoprim-sulfamethoxazole (Bactrim, Septra)
  1- to 3-day regimen
    Nitrofurantoin (Macrodantin, Furadantin)
    Cephalexin (Keflex)
    Ciprofloxacin (Cipro)
    Norfloxacin (Chibroxin, Noroxin)
    Ofloxacin (Floxin)
  Encouragement of high fluid intake

Recurring
  Continuous prophylaxis
    Trimethoprim-sulfamethoxazole (Bactrim, Septra)
    Nitrofurantoin (Macrodantin, Furadantin)
    Cephalexin (Keflex)
  Repeat of urine culture

IVP, intravenous pyelogram.

The presence of fever, nausea and vomiting, and flank tenderness usually indicates pyelonephritis. About one half of all persons with significant bacteriuria have no symptoms or may report nonspecific signs such as increased fatigue, anorexia, or changes in cognitive ability. The incidence of asymptomatic bacteriuria increases greatly with age.[4]

Diagnostic Studies

Examining the urine for the presence of WBCs by means of either a microscope or a urine dipstick is important in evaluating a person who complains of dysuria. The definitive diagnosis of cystitis is made on examination of a urine Gram's stain or by urine culture. Urine is usually cultured if the UTI is complicated or is unresponsive to therapy or if the diagnosis is questionable.[5] The best method for obtaining the urine culture is the midstream technique called *clean-catch urine.* (See Table 42-8 for an explanation of this technique.) If a satisfactory specimen cannot be obtained with this method, catheterization may be used.

The nurse should be aware that noninfectious agents also cause irritative bladder symptoms similar to UTI. The patient with a bladder tumor or the individual receiving intravesical chemotherapy or pelvic radiation often experiences urinary frequency, urgency, and dysuria. Nonbacterial inflammatory lesions such as interstitial cystitis also cause these symptoms.

Collaborative Care and Drug Therapy

Once cystitis has been diagnosed, appropriate antimicrobial therapy is initiated. The collaborative care and drug therapy of cystitis are summarized in Table 43-3. Uncomplicated cystitis

NURSING ASSESSMENT

Table 43-4 Urinary Tract Infection

Subjective Data

Important Health Information

Past health history: Previous urinary tract infections; urinary calculi, stasis, reflux, strictures, or retention; neurogenic bladder; pregnancy; prostatic hyperplasia; sexually transmitted disease; bladder cancer

Medications: Use of antibiotics, anticholinergics, antispasmodics

Surgery or other treatments: Recent urologic instrumentation (catheterization, cystoscopy, surgery)

Functional Health Patterns

Health perception–health management: Urinary hygiene practices; lassitude, malaise

Nutritional-metabolic: Nausea, vomiting, and anorexia; chills

Elimination: Urinary frequency, urgency, hesitancy; nocturia

Cognitive-perceptual: Suprapubic or low back pain, costovertebral tenderness; bladder spasms, dysuria, burning on urination

Objective Data

General

Fever

Urinary

Hematuria; cloudy, foul-smelling urine; tender, enlarged kidney

Possible Findings

Leukocytosis; urinalysis positive for bacteria, pyuria, RBCs, and WBCs; positive urine culture; IVP, CT scan, ultrasound, voiding cystourethrogram and cystoscopy demonstrating abnormalities of urinary tract

CT, computed tomography; *RBCs,* red blood cells; *UTI,* urinary tract infection; *WBCs,* white blood cells.

---

can be treated with short-term antibiotics, which consists of single-dose therapy or 1 to 3 days of therapy.[6]

Sulfamethoxazole combined with trimethoprim (Bactrim, Septra) has proved to be effective in treating UTIs. When these drugs are combined, resistance seems to develop less rapidly. Systemic antibiotics such as cephalexin (Keflex), nitrofurantoin (Macrodantin, Furadantin), and fluoroquinolones (ciprofloxacin [Cipro], norfloxacin [Chibroxin, Noroxin], enoxacin [Penetrex], levofloxacin [Levaquin], ofloxacin [Floxin]) can also be used.

High single-dose therapy has been effective when the infection is localized to the bladder and the organism is sensitive to antibiotics. Single-dose therapy results in lowered cost, increased compliance, and decreased potential for resistant organisms. Fosfomycin (Monurol) is a single-dose medication indicated exclusively for treatment of UTI. It has antibacterial activity for up to 3 to 5 days. However, if there is involvement of the kidney or if the patient is an older adult or has diabetes, single-dose therapy is not appropriate.

Phenazopyridine (Pyridium) may be used in cystitis to provide an analgesic effect on the urinary mucosa. This drug should relieve the burning sensation. The azo dye in the drug stains the urine reddish orange. It is important to tell the patient about the color change so that she or he does not think it is related to the infection. Phenazopyridine stain is also fairly permanent on underclothing.

Other drugs that may be used are methenamine mandelate (Mandelamine), methenamine hippurate (Hiprex), hyoscyamine sulfate (Cystospaz), and flavoxate (Urispas). Methenamine achieves its desired effect by decomposing to formaldehyde and ammonia. The urinary pH should be less than 6 for methenamine to be effective, so urinary pH should be tested to ensure the activity of the drug. Hyoscyamine and flavoxate help decrease bladder muscle irritability and spasm.

Many clinicians are now treating uncomplicated lower UTI with a 1 to 3 day course of antibiotics. As with single-dose ther-

apy, the candidate for 1 to 3 day therapy must be chosen to exclude the patient with UTI associated with fever or flank or back pain.

Patients with chronic UTIs require longer periods of treatment, sometimes several months. Initial treatment dosages are usually followed by smaller dosages of the same drug or a different drug to prevent reinfection or relapse (suppression therapy).

Antibiotic therapy is not usually recommended for asymptomatic bacteriuria unless symptoms develop or there is evidence of obstructive uropathy in the symptom-free patient. The risk of developing bacterial resistance and the inability to treat the patient when symptoms do occur is great. In general, asymptomatic bacteriuria in the older adult should not be treated. Prophylactic antibiotics may be ordered when a patient with asymptomatic bacteriuria undergoes surgery or genitourinary instrumentation.

Prophylactic antibiotic therapy is given to prevent recurrence after treatment of UTI. Women who have had more than three episodes of cystitis per year are considered candidates for prophylaxis. The three most common antibiotics used for prophylaxis are trimethoprim-sulfamethoxazole, nitrofurantoin, and cephalexin. In postmenopausal women, estrogen replacement therapy, particularly vaginally applied creams or estrogen rings, may also reduce the rate of recurrent UTI.[7]

NURSING MANAGEMENT: CYSTITIS

■ Nursing Assessment

Subjective and objective data that should be obtained from a patient with cystitis are presented in Table 43-4.

■ Nursing Diagnoses

Nursing diagnoses for the patient with cystitis may include, but are not limited to, those presented in NCP 43-1.

43-1   NURSING CARE PLAN   PATIENT WITH A URINARY TRACT INFECTION

Expected Patient Outcomes	Nursing Interventions and *Rationales*

NURSING DIAGNOSIS   **Hyperthermia** *related to* infection *as manifested by* elevation in temperature, tachycardia, tachypnea, chills, malaise.

- Normal body temperature.
- No chills.

- Assess vital signs q2-4hr *to plan appropriate intervention.*
- Administer antipyretics and antibiotics as ordered *to control fever and infection and promote comfort.*
- Ensure adequate hydration via oral or IV route *because fever increases fluid loss through insensible perspiration.*
- Monitor intake and output *to ensure adequate hydration and monitor renal function.*
- Cover patient lightly and keep patient dry *to prevent chilling and promote comfort.*
- Provide cooling sponge baths or compresses *to assist in temperature reduction by evaporation of moisture on skin.*

NURSING DIAGNOSIS   **Pain** *related to* inflammation of mucosal tissue of urinary tract *as manifested by* pain on urination, flank pain, suprapubic pain, lower back pain, bladder spasms.

- Satisfaction with pain control.
- No pain.

- Assess pain for location and severity *to plan appropriate interventions.*
- Position patient *for comfort.*
- Administer analgesics, antispasmodics, and phenazopyridine (Pyridium) as ordered *to promote comfort,* and note their effectiveness.
- Alert patient that phenazopyridine will color urine orange *to prevent concern over unusual appearance of urine.*
- Apply heating pad to painful area *because heat relieves pain associated with UTI.*

NURSING DIAGNOSIS   **Altered urinary elimination** *related to* UTI *as manifested by* urgency, frequency, nocturia, incontinence, or hematuria; verbalization of concern over altered elimination pattern.

- Normal urination pattern.

- Assess for changes in usual voiding pattern *to determine presence of UTI.*
- Instruct patient regarding reason for symptoms *to promote understanding and cooperation.*
- Encourage high fluid intake or administer IV fluids as ordered *to maintain a dilute, nonirritating urine and decrease bacterial concentration.*
- Obtain urine for culture and sensitivity *to determine cause of UTI or monitor effectiveness of treatment.*
- Administer antimicrobial medication as ordered *to eliminate symptoms by inhibiting bacterial growth.*
- Instruct patient about good perineal care and cleansing after each bowel movement *to prevent reintroducing infection.*
- Observe urine for color, odor, amount, and frequency *to evaluate effectiveness of treatment plan.*

NURSING DIAGNOSIS   **Risk for reinfection** *related to* lack of knowledge regarding measures to prevent recurrence (see Table 43-5).

■ Planning

The overall goals are that the patient with cystitis will have (1) relief from dysuria, (2) no upper urinary tract complications, and (3) no recurrent episodes of UTI.

■ Nursing Implementation

Health Promotion. Health promotion measures include recognizing the groups with a higher than normal incidence of UTIs. Especially for these individuals, health pro-

motion activities can help decrease the frequency of infections and promote early detection of infection. These activities include teaching preventive measures, such as emptying the bladder regularly and completely, evacuating the bowel regularly, wiping the perineal area from front to back after urination and defecation, and drinking an adequate amount of liquid each day. The standard adult requirement for daily liquid intake is approximately 15 ml per pound of body weight.[8] For example, a 135-pound person would require a minimum 2025 ml or more than eight 8-ounce glasses of liquids each day. Fluids such as coffee or colas containing caffeine, alcohol, and citrus juices may irritate the bladder and should be limited. In addition, it is important to teach the patient to seek early treatment once symptoms are identified.

The nurse can play a major role in the prevention of nosocomial infections. Debilitated persons, older adults, patients with severe underlying disease (cancer, cirrhosis, diabetes), and patients treated with immunosuppressive drugs, long-term corticosteroid therapy, or radiation are at high risk for UTIs. The patient undergoing instrumentation of the urinary tract is also at risk for developing nosocomial infections, and aseptic technique should always be followed for these procedures. Washing hands before and after contact with each patient and wearing gloves for care involving the urinary system are especially important. In general, catheterization of the bladder should be avoided if possible.

For the patient at risk for a nosocomial UTI, it is important to provide good perineal hygiene, especially after a bedpan is used. Incontinence should be avoided by answering the call light quickly or offering the bedpan or urinal at frequent intervals to the bedridden patient. If a catheter has been inserted, special catheter care measures must be employed as explained in the section on urethral catheterization (see p. 1289).

Acute Intervention. Acute intervention for a patient with cystitis includes an adequate fluid intake if this is not contraindicated. This means drinking more than the standard daily requirement. It is sometimes difficult to get the patient to maintain an adequate fluid intake because the person may think it will increase a feeling of urgency. Explain to the patient that fluids will increase frequency at first but will also dilute the urine, making the bladder less irritable. Fluids will help flush out bacteria before they have a chance to colonize in the bladder. Caffeine, alcohol, citrus juices, chocolate, and highly spiced foods or beverages should be avoided because they are potential bladder irritants. A heating pad or sitz bath may also help reduce discomfort. Treatment of cystitis does not usually require hospitalization.

The patient should be instructed about the prescribed drug therapy. Common side effects of the drugs should be explained, and the patient should be told to notify the health care provider if they occur. It is important for the patient to take the full course of antibiotics. Often patients stop antibiotic therapy once symptoms disappear. This practice can lead to inadequate treatment and recurrence of infection or to bacterial resistance to antibiotics. Sometimes a second medication or a reduced dose of medication is ordered after the initial course to suppress bacterial growth in certain patients susceptible to recurrent UTI.

The urine should be examined for gross or microscopic hematuria, presence of WBCs, malodor, and sediment. The patient should be instructed to watch for any changes in the color or consistency of the urine and a decrease in or cessation of symptoms as a sign of the effectiveness of therapy.

Ambulatory and Home Care. Home care for the patient with a UTI should emphasize the patient's compliance with the medication regimen. It is the nurse's responsibility to educate the patient about the need for ongoing care (Table 43-5). This includes taking antimicrobial medication as

---

🖊️ PATIENT TEACHING GUIDE

Table 43-5 | Urinary Tract Infection

The following are important to teach to the patient with a UTI to prevent recurrence:

1. Explain importance of taking all antibiotics as prescribed. Symptoms will improve after 1-2 days of therapy, but organisms may still be present.
2. Instruct the patient on appropriate hygiene, including
   - careful cleansing of perineal region
   - wiping from front to back after urinating
   - cleansing with soap and water after each bowel movement
3. Explain the importance of emptying the bladder before and after intercourse.
4. Instruct the patient to urinate when the urge occurs or at least every 2-4 hr during the day.
5. Instruct the patient about the need to maintain high fluid intake (seven to eight 8-ounce glasses of water per day).
6. Instruct the patient to avoid harsh soaps, bubble baths, powders, and sprays in the perineal area.
7. Instruct the patient to avoid tight-fitting pants and clothing on lower part of body.
8. Have the patient report symptoms or signs of recurrent urinary tract infection (e.g., cloudy urine, pain on urination, urgency, frequency).

---

ordered, maintaining more than an adequate daily fluid intake, emptying the bladder when the urge to urinate occurs or at least every 2 to 4 hours, urinating after intercourse, and discontinuing use of a diaphragm (if used).

The patient must understand the need for follow-up care with urine culture to determine that the infection has been adequately treated. Relapse with bacteria of the same species usually occurs within 1 to 2 weeks after completion of therapy. If the patient has been compliant, relapse suggests possible renal involvement or other uropathology in the infectious process. For the individual who has more than three episodes of cystitis in 1 year, the use of prophylactic antibiotic therapy may be ordered.

■ Evaluation

The expected outcomes for the patient with a urinary tract infection are presented in NCP 43-1.

ACUTE PYELONEPHRITIS
Etiology and Pathophysiology

Pyelonephritis is an acute or chronic inflammatory process of the renal pelvis and parenchyma of the kidney. Generally the inflammatory process is caused by bacterial invasion. Most infections are caused by the normal inhabitants of the intestinal tract (e.g., *E. coli, Proteus, Klebsiella, Enterobacter*).

Pyelonephritis usually ascends from the lower urinary tract. A preexisting factor is often present. In children it is usually associated with vesicoureteral reflux or other urinary tract abnormalities. In adults common preexisting factors are bladder tumors, prostatic hyperplasia, strictures, urinary stones, and pregnancy. Repeated attacks of acute pyelonephritis, especially in the presence of these abnormalities, can result in chronic pyelonephritis. The infection commonly starts in the renal medulla and spreads to the adjacent cortex. The infected portion of the kidney heals, resulting in fibrosis and scarring.

Clinical Manifestations

The clinical manifestations of acute pyelonephritis vary from mild lassitude to the sudden onset of chills, fever, vomiting, malaise, flank pain, dysuria, and frequent urination. Symptoms of cystitis may or may not be present. Costovertebral tenderness will be present on the affected side. The clinical manifestations usually subside within a few days, even without specific therapy. However, bacteriuria or pyuria may persist.

The results of a CBC show leukocytosis and a shift to the left with an increase in banded neutrophils. Urinalysis shows pyuria, bacteriuria, and varying degrees of hematuria. White cell casts may be found in the urine.

Bacteremia (presence of bacteria in blood) can occur secondary to a UTI ascending to the kidney and can result in sepsis. Some patients develop septic shock as a result of endotoxins produced by gram-negative bacteria that are released in the blood. (Septic shock is discussed in Chapter 61.) If bacteremia is a possibility, close observation and vital sign monitoring are essential. Prompt recognition and treatment of septic shock may prevent irreversible damage.

Collaborative Care and Drug Therapy

The diagnostic tests and collaborative therapy of acute pyelonephritis are summarized in Table 43-6. Severe infections or complicating factors require hospital admission. Urine cultures should always be obtained when pyelonephritis is suspected. In patients with more severe illness who are hospitalized, blood cultures should also be obtained. Intravenous pyelograms (IVPs) or excretory urograms are usually not obtained in the early stages of pyelonephritis to prevent the possible spread of infection.

An essential principle of management is to consider factors that may be contributing to the infection, such as an obstruction or a urinary tract anomaly. In addition to an IVP, other diagnostic procedures such as a cystourethrogram and cystoscopy may be used to evaluate any uropathies. It is essential to obtain follow-up urine cultures to determine the effectiveness of therapy.

The patient with mild symptoms may be treated as an outpatient with antibiotics for 14 to 21 days (see Table 43-6). IV antibiotics are often given initially in the hospital to achieve quick, high serum and urinary drug levels. If this treatment appears to be successful, the patient may be discharged on oral antibiotics for 14 to 21 days. Symptoms and signs typically improve or resolve within 48 to 72 hours after starting therapy.

Relapses may be treated with a 6-week course of antibiotics. Reinfections may be treated as individual episodes of disease or managed with long-term antibiotic therapy. Antibiotic prophylaxis may also be used for recurrent infections. The effectiveness of therapy is evaluated in accordance with the presence or absence of bacterial growth on urine culture.

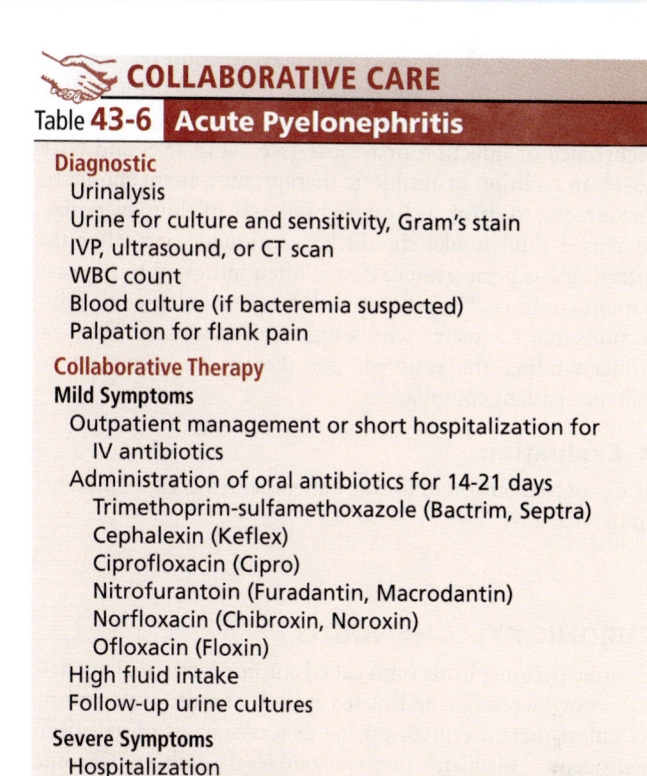

COLLABORATIVE CARE

Table 43-6 **Acute Pyelonephritis**

Diagnostic
Urinalysis
Urine for culture and sensitivity, Gram's stain
IVP, ultrasound, or CT scan
WBC count
Blood culture (if bacteremia suspected)
Palpation for flank pain

Collaborative Therapy

Mild Symptoms
Outpatient management or short hospitalization for IV antibiotics
Administration of oral antibiotics for 14-21 days
  Trimethoprim-sulfamethoxazole (Bactrim, Septra)
  Cephalexin (Keflex)
  Ciprofloxacin (Cipro)
  Nitrofurantoin (Furadantin, Macrodantin)
  Norfloxacin (Chibroxin, Noroxin)
  Ofloxacin (Floxin)
High fluid intake
Follow-up urine cultures

Severe Symptoms
Hospitalization
Parenteral antibiotics
  Ampicillin and aminoglycoside (e.g., gentamicin)
  Ciprofloxacin (Cipro)
  Ofloxacin (Floxin)
  Trimethoprim-sulfamethoxazole (Bactrim, Septra)
High fluid intake
Follow-up urine cultures

NURSING MANAGEMENT: PYELONEPHRITIS

■ Nursing Assessment

Subjective and objective data that should be obtained from a patient with a UTI are presented in Table 43-4.

■ Nursing Diagnoses

Nursing diagnoses for the patient with a UTI include, but are not limited to, those presented in NCP 43-1.

■ Planning

The overall goals are that the patient with pyelonephritis will have (1) relief of pain, (2) normal body temperature, (3) no complications, and (4) no recurrence of symptoms.

■ Nursing Implementation

Health Promotion. Health promotion and maintenance measures are similar to those for cystitis (see Health Promotion under Cystitis, p. 1265). In addition, it is important that the patient receive early treatment for cystitis to prevent ascending infections. Because the patient with structural abnormalities of the urinary tract is at high risk for infection, the need for regular medical care should be stressed.

Acute Intervention and Home Care. Nursing interventions vary depending on the severity of symptoms. These interventions include teaching the patient about the disease process with emphasis on (1) the need to continue medications as prescribed, (2) the need for a follow-up urine culture to ensure proper management, and (3) identification of recurrence of infection or relapse (see Table 43-5 and NCP 43-1). In addition to antibiotic therapy, the patient should be encouraged to drink at least eight glasses of fluid every day. Increased fluid intake should be continued, even after the infection has been treated. Rest is often indicated to increase patient comfort. The patient with frequent relapses or reinfections may be treated with long-term, low-dose antibiotics. Understanding the rationale for therapy is important to enhance patient compliance.

■ Evaluation

The expected outcomes for the patient with a UTI are presented in NCP 43-1.

CHRONIC PYELONEPHRITIS

Chronic pyelonephritis (also called chronic interstitial nephritis) is not the result of an isolated episode of acute pyelonephritis unless there are predisposing factors such as obstruction, neurogenic bladder, or vesicoureteral reflux. Chronic pyelonephritis is usually the end result of long-standing UTIs with relapses and reinfections.

The pathologic changes indicate that there have been repeated episodes of chronic inflammation and scarring. Grossly, both kidneys are irregularly and asymmetrically scarred. The renal pelvis and calyces are deformed, blunted, and dilated.

Clinical features of chronic pyelonephritis include a history of recurrent acute infections leading to progressive destruction of functioning nephrons resulting in chronic renal insufficiency. During active infection, urine cultures are positive and leukocyte casts are found on urinalysis. End-stage chronic pyelonephritis is not easily distinguished from other causes of chronic renal failure. IVP, renal biopsy, renal ultrasound, or computed tomography (CT) scan may be useful in delineating the severity of renal involvement after the infection has been resolved.

The level of renal function can vary in chronic pyelonephritis. The patient may have improvement in function after an acute exacerbation. Chronic pyelonephritis may progress to chronic renal failure. (Nursing and collaborative management of the patient with chronic renal failure is discussed in Chapter 44.)

URETHRITIS

Urethritis (inflammation of the urethra) is often difficult to diagnose, but the clinical manifestations are the same as those for cystitis. The female urethra may be extremely tender, or there may be a discharge, especially in men. Inflammatory changes may make recovery of bacteria difficult because they become entrapped in urethral tissue and do not appear in the urine. Urethritis may coexist with cystitis. Cultures on split urine collections (taken at beginning of urine flow and then midstream) or any urethral discharge may confirm a diagnosis of urethral infection. Causes of urethritis include a bacterial or viral infection, *Trichomonas* and monilial infection (especially

in women), *Chlamydia,* and gonorrhea (especially in men). (Gonococcal urethritis is discussed in Chapter 50.)

Detection of chlamydial organisms requires tissue culture or immunologic testing for chlamydial antigen in urethral or cervical specimens. Chlamydial infection is less likely to cause hematuria and suprapubic pain than bacterial infection.

Treatment is based on identifying and treating the cause and providing symptomatic relief. Sulfamethoxazole with trimethoprim or nitrofurantoin are examples of medications used for bacterial infections. Metronidazole (Flagyl) and clotrimazole (Mycelex) may be used for treating *Trichomonas.* Medications such as nystatin (Mycostatin) or fluconazole (Diflucan) may be prescribed for monilial infections. In chlamydial infections, doxycycline may be used. Women with negative urine cultures and no pyuria do not usually respond to antibiotics. Hot sitz baths without perfumed bath oil or bath salts may relieve the symptoms. The patient should be instructed to avoid the use of vaginal deodorant sprays, to properly cleanse the perineal area after bowel movements and urination, and to avoid intercourse until symptoms subside.

URETHRAL SYNDROME

Symptoms of dysuria, urgency, and frequency unaccompanied by significant bacteriuria (i.e., less than 10^2 to 10^3 per ml of urine) have been termed *acute urethral syndrome.* Clinically these patients cannot be readily distinguished from those with cystitis. When present, bacteria are usually *E. coli,* enterococci, or staphylococci. If few or no bacteria are detected, *Chlamydia trachomatis* or *Neisseria gonorrhoeae* (both sexually transmitted pathogens) may be the cause.

Vaginitis must be ruled out. If vaginitis is the cause, the symptoms may have a more gradual onset, and pruritis or vaginal discharge may be present.

Treatment depends on the causative agent. If bacteria are involved, the treatment is similar to that for cystitis. This patient responds well to single-dose therapy. Simultaneous treatment of the individual's sexual partner may be recommended. Heat or sitz baths may help alleviate symptoms. Acute symptoms of urethral syndrome tend to recur. The patient needs a great deal of reassurance.

INTERSTITIAL CYSTITIS

Interstitial cystitis is a chronic, painful inflammatory disease of the bladder that most commonly occurs in women. The etiology is unknown. Once thought to be psychologic in etiology, interstitial cystitis is now considered a physiologic syndrome with multifactorial etiologies.[9] The disease is characterized by severe bladder and pelvic pain, urinary frequency, and urgency. The inflammation can lead to scarring and stiffening of the bladder, decreased bladder capacity, bleeding, and ulcers of the bladder lining. Pyuria is usually not present. Hematuria is sometimes present. (The presence of hematuria more commonly suggests a lower urinary tract infection or tumor.) Urine cultures are negative.

The diagnosis is made following cystoscopy with the characteristic findings of reduced bladder capacity and the presence of superficial, often stellate, ulcers. In the earlier stages of the disease, only multiple petechiae-like hemorrhages may be found and the bladder capacity may be normal. A bladder biopsy may be done to rule out carcinoma in situ.

Specific treatments do not help all patients, but they are based on theories of physiologic causes and directed toward symptom relief. Hydraulic distention of the bladder under anesthesia, intravesical instillation of dimethyl sulfoxide (DMSO) and other medications, electrostimulation, and oral medications such as tricyclic antidepressants (which have anticholinergic, antihistamine effects on the bladder), antispasmodics, bladder anesthetics, and nonsteroidal anti-inflammatory drugs are often used as initial treatments. Pentosan polysulfate (Elmiron) is a newer oral medication that acts as a bladder protectant and brings symptom relief to many patients. This drug has a mild anticoagulant effect, and any bleeding (e.g., epistaxis, gum hemorrhage) should be noted. Dietary and activity changes, biofeedback, application of heat, diversional activities, and involvement in interstitial cystitis support groups are also helpful approaches for decreasing symptoms and managing the disease.

Cystectomy with urinary diversion is an approach occasionally used when other measures fail to control severe pain and when the patient is willing to risk the consequences and potential complications of this surgery. Even after surgery, some individuals continue to have pain.[10] No matter what treatment course is chosen, nurses caring for patients with interstitial cystitis must offer a great deal of support, empathy, and education about managing symptoms.

RENAL TUBERCULOSIS

Renal tuberculosis (TB) is rarely a primary lesion. It is usually secondary to TB of the lung. In a small percentage of patients with pulmonary TB, the tubercle bacilli reach the kidneys via the bloodstream. Onset occurs 5 to 8 years after the primary infection. The patient is often asymptomatic when the kidney is initially infiltrated with bacilli. Sometimes the patient complains of fatigue and develops a low-grade fever. As the lesions ulcerate, infection descends to the bladder, and the patient experiences frequent urination, burning on voiding, and epididymitis (in men). Symptoms of cystitis are the first sign in the majority of patients with renal TB. Renal lesions may calcify as they heal. Infrequently, renal colic, lumbar and iliac pain, and hematuria may be present. A diagnosis is based on localization of tubercle bacilli in the urine and on IVP findings.

Long-term complications of renal TB depend on the duration of the disease before treatment. Scarring of the renal parenchyma and the development of ureteral strictures occur. The earlier treatment is initiated, the less likely renal failure will develop. Reduced bladder volume may be irreversible in advanced disease. The patient may require long-term urologic follow-up. (Nursing and collaborative management for the patient with TB is discussed in Chapter 26.)

IMMUNOLOGIC DISORDERS OF THE KIDNEY

GLOMERULONEPHRITIS

Immunologic processes involving the urinary tract predominantly affect the renal glomerulus. The disease process results in glomerulonephritis (inflammation of the glomeruli), which affects both kidneys equally. Although the glomerulus is the primary site of inflammation, tubular, interstitial, and vascular changes also occur. Glomerulonephritis is divided into a number of classifications, which may describe (1) the extent of damage (diffuse or focal), (2) the initial cause of the disorder (systemic lupus erythematosus, scleroderma, streptococcal infection), or (3) the extent of changes (minimal or widespread).

Etiology and Pathophysiology

Two types of antibody-induced injury can initiate glomerular damage. In the first type, the antibodies have specificity for antigens within the glomerular basement membrane (GBM). These are termed *anti-GBM antibodies.* Immunoglobulins and complement are deposited along the basement membrane. The mechanism that causes a person to develop antibodies against its GBM is not known. Production of autoantibodies (antibodies to one's own tissue) may be stimulated by a structural alteration in the GBM or by a reaction of the basement membrane with an exogenous agent (e.g., hydrocarbon, viruses).

In the second type of immune process, the antibodies react with circulating nonglomerular antigens and are randomly deposited as immune complexes along the GBM. On electron microscopy of renal tissue sections, the deposits appear "lumpy-bumpy." In this immune complex process, the antigens do not come from the glomeruli but from either endogenous circulating native deoxyribonucleic acid (DNA) or exogenous sources (e.g., bacteria, viruses, chemicals, drugs). Bacterial products appear to be important in poststreptococcal glomerulonephritis. Viral agents have been recognized in certain cases of glomerulonephritis that develop after hepatitis A, B, or C and rubella (measles).

All forms of immune complex disease are characterized by an accumulation of antigen, antibody, and complement in the glomeruli, which can result in tissue injury. The immune complexes activate complement (see Chapter 12). Complement activation results in the release of chemotactic factors that attract polymorphonuclear leukocytes and causes the release of histamine and other vasoactive amines. The intrinsic clotting pathway may also be activated. The end result of these processes is glomerular injury as a result of inflammation.

Clinical Manifestations

There are many clinical manifestations of glomerulonephritis. They may include varying degrees of hematuria (ranging from microscopic to gross) and urinary excretion of various formed elements, including red blood cells (RBCs), WBCs, and some granular casts. Proteinuria and elevated blood urea nitrogen (BUN) and serum creatinine levels are other manifestations. In most cases, recovery from the acute illness is complete. However, if progressive involvement occurs, the result is destruction of renal tissue and marked renal insufficiency.

The patient's history provides important information related to glomerulonephritis. It is necessary to assess exposure to drugs, immunizations, microbial infections, and viral infections such as hepatitis. It is also important to evaluate the patient for more generalized conditions involving immune disorders, such as systemic lupus erythematosus and systemic progressive sclerosis (scleroderma).

ACUTE POSTSTREPTOCOCCAL GLOMERULONEPHRITIS

Acute poststreptococcal glomerulonephritis (APSGN) is most common in children and young adults, but all age-groups can be affected. APSGN develops 5 to 21 days after an infection of

COLLABORATIVE CARE

Table 43-7 | Acute Glomerulonephritis

Diagnostic
- History and physical examination
- Urinalysis
- CBC
- BUN, serum creatinine and albumin
- Complement levels and ASO titer
- Renal biopsy (if indicated)

Collaborative Therapy
- Rest
- Sodium and fluid restriction
- Diuretics
- Antihypertensive therapy
- Adjustment of dietary protein intake to level of proteinuria and uremia

ASO, antistreptolysin; *BUN,* blood urea nitrogen; *CBC,* complete blood count.

the pharynx or skin (e.g., streptococcal sore throat, impetigo) by certain nephrotoxic strains of group A β-hemolytic streptococci. The person produces antibodies to the streptococcal antigen. Although the specific mechanism is not known with certainty, the antigen-antibody complexes are deposited in the glomeruli and activate complement. Complement activation causes an inflammatory reaction to the injury. The response to the injury is also a decrease in the filtration of metabolic waste products from the blood and an increase in the permeability of the glomerulus to larger protein molecules.

Clinical Manifestations and Complications

The clinical manifestations of APSGN appear as a variety of signs and symptoms, which may include generalized body edema, hypertension, oliguria, hematuria with a smoky or rusty appearance, and proteinuria. Fluid retention occurs as a result of decreased glomerular filtration. The edema appears initially in low-pressure tissues, such as around the eyes (periorbital edema), but later progresses to involve the total body as ascites or peripheral edema in the legs. Smoky urine is indicative of bleeding in the upper urinary tract. The degree of proteinuria varies with the severity of the glomerulonephropathy. Hypertension primarily results from increased extracellular fluid volume.

The patient with APSGN may have abdominal or flank pain. At times the patient has no symptoms, with the problem found on routine urinalysis.

More than 95% of patients with APSGN recover completely or improve rapidly with conservative management. The prognosis for adults is less favorable than for children. Chronic glomerulonephritis develops in 5% to 15% of the affected persons, and irreversible renal failure occurs in less than 1% of patients.

Diagnostic Studies

The diagnosis of APSGN is based on a complete history and physical examination and laboratory studies (Table 43-7) to determine the presence or history of a group A β-hemolytic streptococcus in a throat or skin lesion. An immune response to

the streptococcus is often demonstrated by assessment of anti-streptolysin O (ASO) titers. The finding of decreased complement components (especially C3 and CH50) is indicative of an immune-mediated response. A renal biopsy may be performed to confirm the presence of the disease.

Dipstick and urine sediment microscopy will reveal the presence of erythrocytes in significant numbers. Erythrocyte casts are highly suggestive of acute glomerulonephritis. Proteinuria may range from mild to severe. Screening blood tests include BUN and serum creatinine to assess the extent of renal impairment.

NURSING AND COLLABORATIVE MANAGEMENT: ACUTE POSTSTREPTOCOCCAL GLOMERULONEPHRITIS

The management of APSGN focuses on symptomatic relief (see Table 43-7). Rest is recommended until the signs of glomerular inflammation (proteinuria, hematuria) and hypertension subside. Edema is treated by restricting sodium and fluid intake and by administrating diuretics. Severe hypertension is treated with antihypertensive drugs. Dietary protein intake may be restricted if there is evidence of an increase in nitrogenous wastes (e.g., elevated BUN value). The restriction varies with the degree of proteinuria. (Low-protein, low-sodium, fluid-restricted diets are discussed in Chapter 44.)

Antibiotics should be given only if the streptococcal infection is still present. Corticosteroids and cytotoxic drugs have not been shown to be of value.

One of the most important ways to prevent the development of APSGN is to encourage early diagnosis and treatment of sore throats and skin lesions. If streptococci are found in the culture, treatment with appropriate antibiotic therapy (usually penicillin) is essential. The patient must be encouraged to take the full course of antibiotics to ensure that the bacteria have been eradicated. Good personal hygiene is an important factor in preventing the spread of cutaneous streptococcal infections.

GOODPASTURE'S SYNDROME

Goodpasture's syndrome, an example of cytotoxic (type II) autoimmune disease, is characterized by the presence of circulating antibodies against GBM and alveolar basement membrane.[11] Although the primary target organ is the kidney, the lungs are also involved. The pathologic nature of the syndrome results when binding of the antibody causes an inflammatory reaction mediated by complement fixation and activation (see Chapter 12). The causative factors for development of autoantibody production are unknown, although type A influenza viruses, hydrocarbons, penicillamine, and unknown genetic factors may be involved.

Goodpasture's syndrome is a rare disease that is seen mostly in young male smokers. The clinical manifestations include hemoptysis, pulmonary insufficiency, crackles, rhonchi, renal involvement with hematuria and renal failure, weakness, pallor, and anemia. Pulmonary hemorrhage usually occurs and may precede glomerular abnormalities by weeks or months. Abnormal diagnostic findings include low hematocrit and hemoglobin levels, elevated BUN and serum creatinine levels, hematuria, and proteinuria. Circulating serum anti-GBM antibodies parallel the activity of the renal disease and are diagnostic of this syndrome.

NURSING AND COLLABORATIVE MANAGEMENT: GOODPASTURE'S SYNDROME

Until recently, the prognosis for the patient with Goodpasture's syndrome was poor. Management consists of corticosteroids, immunosuppressive drugs (e.g., cyclophosphamide [Cytoxan], azathioprine [Imuran]), plasmapheresis (see Chapter 12), and dialysis. Plasmapheresis removes the circulating anti-GBM antibody, and immunosuppressive therapy inhibits further antibody production. Renal transplantation can be attempted once the circulating anti-GBM antibody titer decreases. Although recurrences may develop, the disease is not a contraindication to transplantation. In selected patients with severe pulmonary hemorrhage, bilateral nephrectomy has been helpful. The exact mechanism for improvement has not been determined.

Nursing management appropriate for a critically ill patient who is experiencing symptoms of acute renal failure and respiratory distress is instituted. Death is often secondary to hemorrhage in the lungs and respiratory failure. (Nursing interventions for a patient in acute renal failure are discussed in Chapter 44, and nursing interventions for a patient with respiratory failure are discussed in Chapter 62.) Because this syndrome is rare and primarily affects previously healthy young men, support and understanding of the patient and family are of major importance. The patient and family need instructions concerning current therapy, medications, and complications of the disease process.

RAPIDLY PROGRESSIVE GLOMERULONEPHRITIS

Rapidly progressive glomerulonephritis (RPGN) is glomerular disease associated with rapid, progressive loss of renal function over days to weeks. Renal failure may occur within weeks to months in contrast to chronic glomerulonephritis, which develops insidiously and progresses over many years. The manifestations of RPGN are hypertension, edema, proteinuria, hematuria, and RBC casts.

RPGN can occur in a variety of situations: (1) as a complication of inflammatory or infectious disease (e.g., APSGN), (2) as a complication of a multisystemic disease (e.g., systemic lupus erythematosus, Goodpasture's syndrome), (3) as an idiopathic disease, or (4) in association with the use of certain drugs (e.g., penicillamine).

Treatment is directed toward correction of fluid overload, hypertension, uremia, and inflammatory injury to the kidney. Treatment includes corticosteroids, cytotoxic agents, and plasmapheresis. Dialysis therapy and transplantation are used to maintain the patient with RPGN. Following renal transplantation, RPGN may recur.

CHRONIC GLOMERULONEPHRITIS

Chronic glomerulonephritis is a syndrome that reflects the end stage of glomerular inflammatory disease. Most types of glomerulonephritis and nephrotic syndrome can eventually lead to chronic glomerulonephritis.

Table **43-8**	Causes of Nephrotic Syndrome

Primary Glomerular Disease
  Membranous proliferative glomerulonephritis
  Primary nephrotic syndrome
  Focal glomerulonephritis
  Inherited nephrotic disease

Extrarenal Causes
Multisystem Disease
  Systemic lupus erythematosus
  Diabetes mellitus
  Amyloidosis

Infections
  Bacterial (streptococcal, syphilis)
  Viral (hepatitis, human immunodeficiency virus
    infection)
  Protozoal (malaria)

Neoplasms
  Hodgkin's disease
  Solid tumors of lungs, colon, stomach, breast
  Leukemias

Allergens (e.g., Bee Sting, Pollen)
  Drugs
  Penicillamine
  Nonsteroidal antiinflammatory drugs
  Captopril (Capoten)
  Heroin

The syndrome is characterized by proteinuria, hematuria, and the slow development of uremic syndrome (see Chapter 44) as a result of decreasing renal function. Chronic glomerulonephritis does not usually follow an acute course. It progresses insidiously toward renal failure over a few to as many as 30 years.

Chronic glomerulonephritis is often found coincidentally when an abnormality on a urinalysis or elevated blood pressure is detected. It is common to find that the patient has no recollection or history of acute nephritis or any renal problems. A renal biopsy may be performed to determine the exact cause and nature of the glomerulonephritis. However, many institutions now prefer to use ultrasound and CT scanning as diagnostic measures.

Treatment is supportive and symptomatic. Hypertension and urinary tract infections should be treated vigorously. Protein and phosphate restrictions may slow the rate of progression of renal failure. (Management of chronic renal failure is discussed in Chapter 44.)

NEPHROTIC SYNDROME
Etiology and Clinical Manifestations

The term *nephrotic syndrome* describes a clinical course that can be associated with a number of disease conditions. Some of the more common causes of nephrotic syndrome are listed in Table 43-8. In adults about one third of patients with nephrotic syndrome will have a systemic disease such as diabetes or systemic lupus erythematosus. The remainder will be categorized as having idiopathic nephrotic syndrome.[12]

The characteristic manifestations include peripheral edema, massive proteinuria, hyperlipidemia, and hypoalbuminemia.

Characteristic blood chemistries include decreased serum albumin, decreased total serum protein, and elevated serum cholesterol. The increased glomerular membrane permeability found in nephrotic syndrome is responsible for the massive excretion of protein in the urine. This results in decreased serum protein and subsequent edema formation. Ascites and anasarca develop if there is severe hypoalbuminemia.

The diminished plasma oncotic pressure from the decreased serum proteins stimulates hepatic lipoprotein synthesis, which results in hyperlipidemia. Initially, cholesterol and low-density lipoproteins are elevated. Later the triglyceride level is also increased. Fat bodies (fatty casts) commonly appear in the urine.

Immune responses, both humoral and cellular, are altered in nephrotic syndrome. As a result, infection is an important cause of morbidity and mortality. Calcium and skeletal abnormalities may occur, including hypocalcemia, blunted calcemic response to parathyroid hormone, hyperparathyroidism, and osteomalacia.

With nephrotic proteinuria, loss of clotting factors can result in a relative hypercoagulable state. Hypercoagulability with thromboembolism is potentially the most serious complication of nephrotic syndrome. The renal vein is the site most commonly involved for thrombus formation. Pulmonary emboli occur in about 40% of nephrotic patients with thrombosis.

Collaborative Care

Treatment of nephrotic syndrome is symptomatic. The goals are to relieve edema and cure or control the primary disease. Management of the edema includes the cautious use of angiotensin-converting enzyme (ACE) inhibitors, nonsteroidal antiinflammatory drugs, and a low-sodium (2 to 3 g per day), low- to moderate-protein diet (0.5 to 0.6 kg per day). Dietary salt restrictions are a key to managing edema. In some individuals thiazide or loop diuretics may be needed. If urine protein loss exceeds 10 g/24 hr, additional dietary protein may be needed.

The treatment of hyperlipidemia is frequently unsuccessful. However, treatment with lipid-lowering agents, such as colestipol (Colestid), probucol (Lorelco), and lovastatin (Mevacor), may result in moderate decreases in serum cholesterol levels. If thrombosis is detected, anticoagulant therapy may be necessary for up to 6 months.

Corticosteroids and cyclophosphamide (Cytoxan) may be used for the treatment of severe cases of nephrotic syndrome. Prednisone has been effective to varying degrees in persons with lipoid nephrosis, membranous glomerulonephritis, proliferative glomerulonephritis, and lupus nephritis. Management of diabetes and treatment of edema are the only measures used for nephrotic syndrome related to diabetes.

NURSING MANAGEMENT: NEPHROTIC SYNDROME

A major nursing intervention for a patient with nephrotic syndrome is related to edema. It is important to assess the edema by weighing the patient daily, accurately recording intake and output, and measuring abdominal girth or extremity size. Comparing this information daily provides the nurse with a tool for assessing the effectiveness of treatment. The edematous

skin needs careful cleaning. Trauma should be avoided, and the effectiveness of diuretic therapy must be monitored.

The patient has the potential to become malnourished from the excessive loss of protein in the urine. Maintaining a low- to moderate-protein diet that is also low in sodium is not always easy. The patient is usually anorexic. Serving small, frequent meals in a pleasant setting may encourage better dietary intake.

Because the patient is susceptible to infection, measures should be taken to avoid exposure to persons with known infections. The person with nephrotic syndrome is often ashamed of an edematous appearance and needs support in dealing with an altered body image.

RENAL DISEASE AND ACQUIRED IMMUNODEFICIENCY SYNDROME

The patient with human immunodeficiency virus (HIV) infection can have a variety of renal manifestations, ranging from mild fluid and electrolyte abnormalities to progressive renal impairment resulting in end-stage renal disease.[13] The incidence of renal disease associated with HIV infection is about 10% and is highest among IV drug users.

HIV-associated renal syndromes include the following:

1. *Proteinuria and nephrotic syndrome,* which occurs in about 10% of patients with HIV infection. It may be the initial sign of HIV infection in some persons.
2. *HIV-associated nephropathy* (HIVAN), which is characterized by proteinuria, progressive azotemia, absence of hypertension, large kidney size on renal imaging studies, and unusually rapid progression to end-stage renal disease.
3. *Acute renal failure,* which is most commonly seen in the patient with acquired immunodeficiency syndrome (AIDS) who is critically ill with HIV-related infection or malignancy. Both oliguric and nonoliguric forms of renal failure can occur. The natural cause of acute renal failure secondary to AIDS is similar to acute renal failure associated with other acute illnesses (see Chapter 44). Survival and recovery usually depend on the treatment of the primary cause of renal failure and support of renal function by dialysis. (HIV infection is discussed in Chapter 13.)

OBSTRUCTIVE UROPATHIES

Obstruction of the urinary system may occur at any point from the kidney to the urethral meatus (Fig. 43-2). It may be congenital or acquired. Obstruction may be due to intrinsic causes such as anomalies, diverticuli, tumors, or benign growth within the urinary tract; extrinsic causes such as tumors, adhesions, retroperitoneal fibrosis, or prolapsed adjacent organs; or functional causes as a result of neurologic or psychogenic factors. Some common intrinsic obstructions are narrowing of the ureteropelvic junction, bladder neck contracture, benign prostatic hyperplasia, urethral stricture, and meatal stenosis. Common extrinsic causes include pelvic and abdominal tumors or a prolapsed uterus. Examples of functional causes are vesicosphincter dyssynergia after spinal cord injury and neurogenic bladder secondary to diabetes.

Damaging effects from urinary tract obstruction affect the system above the level of the obstruction. The severity of these

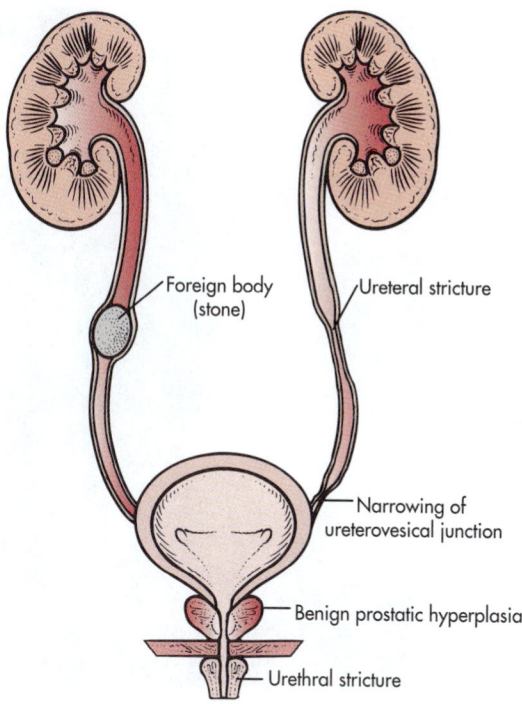

Fig. 43-2   Common causes of urinary tract obstruction.

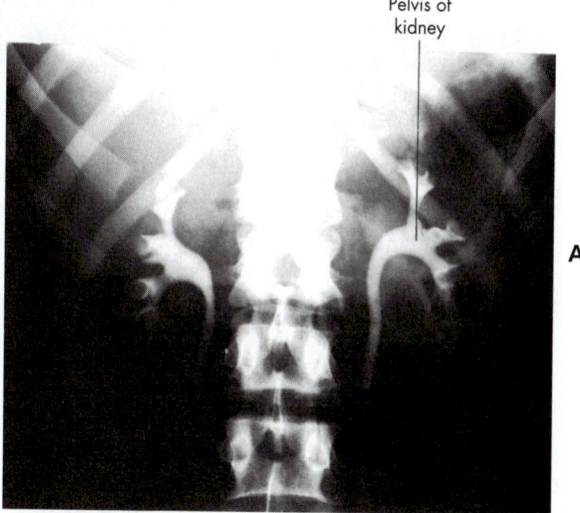

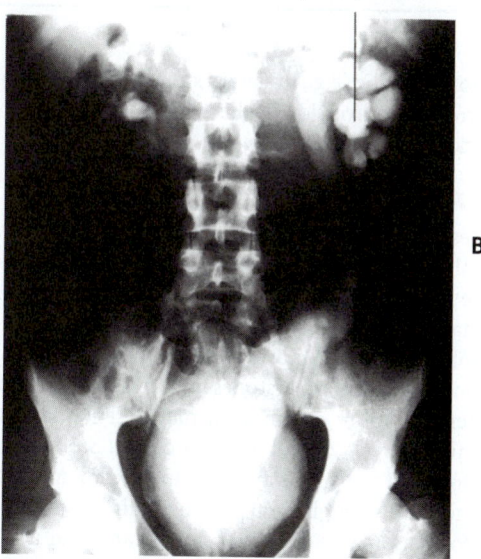

Fig. 43-3   **A,** Normal intravenous pyelogram (IVP). **B,** IVP showing hydronephrosis and hydroureter.

effects depends on the location, duration of obstruction, amount of pressure or dilation, presence of urinary stasis, and whether infection is present. Infection increases the risk of irreversible consequences.

Although obstruction distal to the prostate in men or the bladder neck in women causes mucosal scarring and a slower stream, it rarely results in major obstructive uropathy because the urethral wall pressure is less than that of the bladder neck and bladder. Urethral obstruction may contribute to outlet resistance and cause lower or upper urinary tract damage when other obstructive or dysfunctional factors are also present. For example, there is an increased risk of compromised renal function in the patient with a spinal cord injury with vesicosphincter dyssynergia.

When obstruction occurs at the level of the bladder neck or prostate, significant bladder changes can occur. Detrusor muscle fibers hypertrophy (increase in size) in order to contract harder to push urine out a narrower pathway. Over a long period of time, the detrusor loses its ability to compensate for this resistance. Muscle bundles separate and become less compliant. This separation is termed *trabeculation*. Trabeculaton is caused by the deposition of collagen in the bladder wall that separates the smooth muscle fascicles. Trabeculation may hasten the decompensation of the detrusor. The areas between these muscle bundles are called *cellules*. Because these areas have no muscle support, the bladder mucosa can herniate between detrusor muscle bundles, forming sacs that drain poorly, called *diverticuli*. Residual urine can be very high in a noncompensating bladder.

Pressure increases during bladder filling or storage and can be transmitted to the ureter when bladder outlet obstruction is present. This pressure overcomes the normal peristaltic pressure and leads to reflux (a backflow of urine); ureteral dilation, kinking, and tortuosity; hydroureter (dilation of the renal pelvis); and hydronephrosis (dilation of the calyces) and consequent chronic pyelonephritis and renal atrophy (Fig. 43-3). If

only one kidney is obstructed, the other kidney may try to compensate by hypertrophy, but the ureter will not be dilated on this contralateral side.

Partial obstruction may occur in the ureter or at the ureterovesical junction (UVJ). If the pressure remains low or moderate, the kidney may continue to dilate with no noticeable loss of function. There is an increased risk of pyelonephritis because of urinary stasis and reflux. If only one kidney is involved and the other kidney is functioning, the patient may be free of symptoms. If both kidneys or only one functioning kidney is involved (e.g., if the patient has only one kidney), alterations in renal function (e.g., increased BUN or serum creatinine levels) are found. If the obstruction progresses, oliguria or anuria develops. Often episodes of oliguria are followed by polyuria if the obstruction is a stone that becomes dislodged. Treatment requires locating and relieving the blockage. This can include

Table **43-9**	Risk Factors for the Development of Urinary Tract Calculi

Metabolic
  Abnormalities that result in increased urine levels of calcium, oxaluric acid, uric acid, or citric acid

Climate
  Warm climates that cause increased fluid loss, low urine volume, and increased solute concentration in urine

Diet
  Large intake of dietary proteins that increases uric acid excretion
  Excessive amounts of tea or fruit juices that elevate urinary oxalate level
  Large intake of calcium and oxalate
  Low fluid intake that increases urinary concentration

Genetic Factors
  Family history of stone formation, cystinuria, gout, or renal acidosis

Lifestyle
  Sedentary occupation, immobility

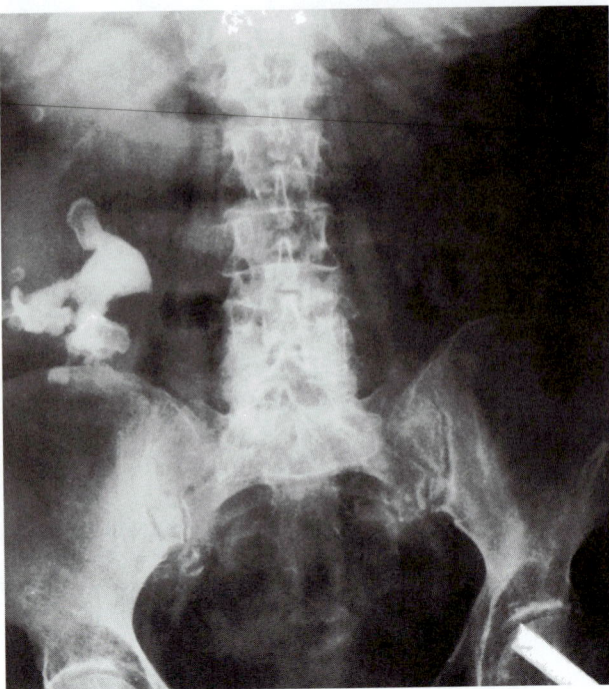

Fig. 43-4 X-ray of a staghorn calculus.

insertion of a tube (e.g., ureteral), surgical correction of the disease process, or diversion of the urinary stream above the level of blockage.

URINARY TRACT CALCULI

Each year an estimated 500,000 people in the United States have nephrolithiasis (kidney stone disease).[14] Many of these people require hospitalization. In the United States the incidence of urinary stone disease is highest in the Southeast and Southwest, followed by the Midwest. Except for struvite (magnesium-ammonium-phosphate) stones associated with UTI, stone disorders are more common in men.[15] The majority of patients are between 20 and 55 years of age. Stone formation is more frequent in Caucasians than in African-Americans. The incidence is also higher in persons with a family history of stone formation. Recurrence of stones can occur in up to 50% of patients.[14] There is seasonal variation, with stone formation occurring more often in the summer months, thus supporting the role of dehydration in this process. Stone formation in the kidney also seems to increase in incidence as countries become more industrialized, whereas the incidence of bladder stones decreases.

Etiology and Pathophysiology

Many factors are involved in the incidence and type of stone formation, including metabolic, dietary, genetic, climatic, lifestyle, and occupational influences (Table 43-9). Many theories have been proposed to explain the formation of stones in the urinary tract. No single theory can account for stone formation in all cases. Crystals, when in a supersaturated concentration, can precipitate and unite to form a stone. Keeping urine dilute and free-flowing reduces the risk of recurrent stone formation in many individuals. It is known that a mucoprotein (the matrix for the stone) is formed in the kidneys that form stones. Urinary pH, solute load, and inhibitors in the urine affect the formation of stones. The higher the pH, the less soluble are calcium and phosphate. The lower the pH, the less soluble are uric acid and cystine.

Other important factors in the development of stones include obstruction with urinary stasis and urinary infection with urea-splitting bacteria (e.g., *Proteus, Klebsiella, Pseudomonas,* and some species of staphylococci). These bacteria cause the urine to become alkaline and contribute to the formation of calcium-magnesium-ammonium phosphate stones (struvite or triple phosphate stones).[15] Infected stones, when they are entrapped in the kidney, may assume a staghorn configuration as they enlarge (Fig. 43-4). Infected stones are frequent in the patient with an external urinary diversion, long-term indwelling catheter, neurogenic bladder, or urinary retention. Genetic factors may also contribute to urine stone formation. Cystinuria is an autosomal recessive disorder. In this disorder there is greatly increased excretion of cystine.

Types

The term *calculus* refers to the stone and *lithiasis* refers to stone formation. There are five major categories of stones: (1) calcium phosphate, (2) calcium oxalate, (3) uric acid, (4) cystine, and (5) struvite (magnesium-ammonium phosphate) (Table 43-10). Stone composition may be mixed, although calcium stones are the most common. Calculi can be found in various locations in the urinary tract (Fig. 43-5).

Clinical Manifestations

Urinary stones cause clinical manifestations when they cause obstruction to urinary flow. Common sites of complete obstruction are at the ureteropelvic junction (UPJ), in the ureter at the point it crosses the iliac vessels, and at the uretero-vesical junction (UVJ). Symptoms include abdominal or flank pain (usually severe), hematuria, and renal colic. The pain may be associated with nausea and vomiting. The type of pain is determined by the location of the stone (see Fig. 43-5). If the stone is nonobstructing, pain may be absent. If it produces obstruction in a calyx or at the UPJ, the patient may experience

| Table **43-10** | | **Types of Urinary Tract Calculi** | | |

Urinary Stone	Incidence (%)	Characteristics	Predisposing Factors	Therapeutic Measures
Calcium oxalate*	35-40	Small, often possible to get trapped in ureter; more frequent in men than in women	Idiopathic hypercalcuria, hyperoxaluria, independent of urinary pH, family history	Increase hydration. Reduce dietary oxalate.[‡] Give thiazide diuretics. Give cellulose phosphate to chelate calcium and prevent GI absorption. Give potassium citrate to maintain alkaline urine. Give cholestyramine to bind oxalate. Give calcium lactate to precipitate oxalate in GI tract.
Calcium phosphate	8-10	Mixed stones (typically), with struvite or oxalate stones	Alkaline urine, primary hyperparathyroidism	Treat underlying causes and other stones.
Struvite (MgNH$_4$PO$_4$)	10-15	Three to four times as common in women than men, always in association with urinary tract infections, large staghorn type (usually)[†]	Urinary tract infections (usually *Proteus* organisms)	Administer antimicrobial agents, acetohydroxamic acid. Use surgical intervention to remove stone. Take measures to acidify urine.
Uric acid	5-8	Predominant in men, high incidence in Jewish men	Gout, acid urine, inherited condition	Reduce urinary concentration of uric acid. Alkalinize urine with potassium citrate. Administer allopurinol. Reduce dietary purines.[‡]
Cystine	1-2	Genetic autosomal recessive defect, defective absorption of cystine in GI tract and kidney, excess concentrations causing stone formation	Acid urine	Increase hydration. Give α-penicillamine and tiopronin to prevent cystine crystallization. Give potassium citrate to maintain alkaline urine.

*Calcium stones can exist as calcium oxalate, calcium phosphate, or a mixture of both. Calcium stones account for the majority of all stones.
†See Fig. 43-4.
‡See Table 43-11.

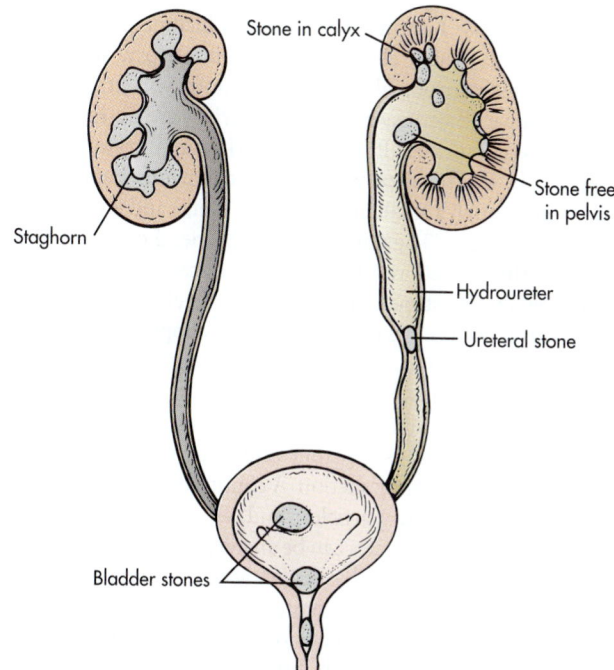

Fig. 43-5 Location of calculi in the urinary tract.

dull costovertebral flank pain or even colic. Pain resulting from the passage of a calculus down the ureter is intense and colicky. The patient may be in mild shock with cool, moist skin. As a stone nears the UVJ, pain will be felt in the lateral flank and sometimes down into the testicles, labia, or groin. Other clinical manifestations include the presence of urinary infection accompanied by fever, vomiting, nausea, and chills.

Diagnostic Studies

Diagnostic studies useful in the evaluation and management of renal lithiasis include urinalysis, urine culture, IVP, retrograde pyelogram, ultrasound, and cystoscopy. A plain film of the abdomen and renal ultrasound will usually diagnose most stones. An IVP or retrograde pyelogram can further localize the degree and site of obstruction and confirm the presence of nonradiopaque stones (uric acid, cystine). CT scans may be used to differentiate a nonopaque stone from a tumor.

Measurement of the urine and serum levels of various substances involved in stone formation (e.g., calcium, phosphate, oxalate, uric acid) is often done after a stone is discovered to determine possible metabolic causes and preventive management strategies. BUN and serum creatinine are determined to assess renal function. A careful history, including previous stone formation, prescribed and over-the-counter medications and dietary supplements, and familial stone formation, is useful.

Measurement of urine pH is useful in the diagnosis of struvite stones and renal tubular acidosis (tendency to alkaline pH) and uric acid stones (tendency to acidic pH). Retrieval and analysis of the stones are important in the diagnosis of the underlying problem contributing to stone formation. Chemical and crystallographic analyses are done.

Collaborative Care

Evaluation and management of a patient with renal lithiasis consist of two concurrent approaches. The first approach is directed toward management of the acute attack. This involves treating the symptoms of pain, infection, or obstruction as indicated for the individual patient. At frequent intervals, narcotics are typically required for relief of renal colic pain. Many stones pass spontaneously. However, stones larger than 4 mm are unlikely to pass through the ureter.

The second approach is directed toward evaluation of the etiology of the stone formation and the prevention of further development of stones. Information to be obtained from the patient includes family history of stone formation, geographic residence, nutritional assessment including the intake of vitamins A and D, activity pattern (active or sedentary), history of periods of prolonged illness with immobilization or dehydration, and any history of disease or surgery involving the GI or genitourinary (GU) tract.

Proper therapy for active stone formers requires a concerted management approach, with primary emphasis on teaching and on developing a therapeutic regimen with which the patient can reasonably comply (see Table 43-10). Adequate hydration, dietary sodium restrictions, dietary changes (Table 43-11), and the use of medications minimize urinary stone formation. Various medications are prescribed, depending on the specific problem underlying stone formation (see Table 43-10). These medications prevent stone formation in various ways, including altering urine pH, preventing excessive urinary excretion of a substance, or correcting a primary disease (e.g. hyperparathyroidism).

Treatment of struvite stones requires control of infection. This may be difficult if the stone remains in place. In addition to antibiotics, acetohydroxamic acid may be used in the treatment of kidney infections that result in the continual formation of struvite stones. Acetohydroxamic acid, an inhibitor of the chemical action caused by the persistent bacteria, can be used effectively to retard struvite stone formation. If the infection cannot be controlled, the stone may have to be removed surgically.

Indications for endourologic, lithotripsy, or open surgical stone removal include the following:

1. Stones too large for spontaneous passage
2. Stones associated with bacteriuria or symptomatic infection
3. Stones causing impaired renal function
4. Stones causing persistent pain, nausea, or ileus
5. Inability of patient to be treated medically
6. Patient with one kidney

Endourologic Procedures. If the stone is located in the bladder, a cystoscopy is done to remove small stones. For large stones a cystolitholapaxy is done. In this procedure large stones can be broken up with an instrument called a lithotrite (stone crusher). The bladder is then irrigated and the crushed stones washed out. A cystoscopic lithotripsy uses an ultrasonic lithotrite to pulverize stones. Complications associated with these cystoscopic procedures include hemorrhage, retained stone fragments, and infection.

Flexible ureteroscopes, inserted via a cystoscope, can be used to remove stones from the renal pelvis and upper urinary tract. Ultrasonic, laser, or electrohydraulic lithotripsy can be used in conjunction with the ureteroscope to pulverize and break the stone into fragments.[16]

In percutaneous nephrolithotomy (PNL) a nephroscope is inserted through a sinus tract from the skin into the kidney pelvis.[17] Stones can be fragmented using ultrasound, electrohydraulic, or laser lithotripsy. The stone fragments are removed and the pelvis irrigated. A percutaneous nephrostomy tube is usually left in place to ensure that the ureter is not obstructed. Complications include bleeding, injury to adjacent structures, and infection.

Lithotripsy. Lithotripsy techniques include percutaneous ultrasonic lithotripsy, electrohydraulic lithotripsy, laser lithotripsy, and extracorporeal shock-wave lithotripsy. Extracorporeal shock-wave lithotripsy and laser lithotripsy are the most common. In percutaneous ultrasonic lithotripsy an ultrasonic probe is placed in the renal pelvis via a percutaneous nephroscope (inserted through a small incision in the flank) and is positioned against the stone. (The patient is given general or spinal anesthesia for this procedure.) The probe produces ultrasonic waves, which break the stone into sandlike particles. Percutaneous lithotripsy is not used as much as a primary approach to renal or upper ureteral stones unless the stone is large and other lithotripsy procedures have failed.

The electrohydraulic lithotripsy probe is also placed directly on a stone, but it breaks the stone into small fragments that are removed by forceps or by suction. A continuous saline irrigation flushes out the stone particles, and all outflow drainage is strained so that the particles can be analyzed. The calculi can also be removed by forceps or basket extraction. Complications are rare but include hemorrhage, sepsis, and abscess. Postoperatively, the patient usually complains of moderate to severe colicky pain. The first few voidings are bright red; as the bleeding subsides, the urine becomes dark red or turns a smoky color. Antibiotics are usually given for 2 weeks to reduce the risk of infection.

🍊 NUTRITIONAL THERAPY

Table **43-11** **Urinary Tract Calculi**

The following is a list of foods high in purine, calcium, or oxalate content

Purine
High: Sardines, herring, mussels, liver, kidney, goose, venison, meat soups, sweetbreads
Moderate: Chicken, salmon, crab, veal, mutton, bacon, pork, beef, ham

Calcium
Milk, cheese, ice cream, yogurt, sauces containing milk; all beans (except green beans), lentils; fish with fine bones (e.g., sardines, kippers, herring, salmon); dried fruits, nuts; chocolate, cocoa, Ovaltine

Oxalate
Spinach, rhubarb, asparagus, cabbage, tomatoes, beets, nuts, celery, parsley, runner beans; chocolate, cocoa, instant coffee, Ovaltine, tea; Worcestershire sauce

Laser lithotripsy probes are used to fragment lower ureteral and large bladder stones. The medium used, a coumarin-based pulsed dye, works on a wavelength that fragments stones but does not injure the surrounding tissue.

In extracorporeal shock-wave lithotripsy, a noninvasive procedure, the patient is anesthetized (spinal or general) and placed in a water bath. Anesthesia is necessary to keep the patient very still during the procedure. Some of the newer-generation lithotripters do not require submersion and use other means of initiating shock waves. The lithotripters are categorized as electrohydraulic, electromagnetic, and piezoelectric. The second-generation lithotripters use less power to fragment stones. Lower power reduces a patient's pain, but usually some sedation or analgesia is necessary.

Fluoroscopy or ultrasound is used to focus the lithotripter on the affected kidney, and a high-voltage spark generator produces high-energy acoustic shock waves that shatter the stone without damaging the surrounding tissues. The stone is broken into fine sand, which is excreted into the patient's urine within a few days after the procedure.

Hematuria is common after lithotripsy procedures. A self-retaining ureteral stent is often placed after the procedure to promote passage of this sand and to prevent obstruction caused by *Steinstrasse* (a buildup of sand in the ureter). The stent is removed 1 to 2 weeks after lithotripsy. A primary advantage of these techniques compared with open surgery is the decrease in the length of hospitalization and the patient's earlier return to normal activities. Retreatment may be necessary, especially if a stone is large and in the mid or distal ureter.

Surgical Therapy. There are a small group of select patients who need open surgical procedures, such as the very obese patient or the individual with complex abnormalities in the calyces or at the UPJ. The type of open surgery needed depends on the location of the stone. A nephrolithotomy is an incision into the kidney to remove a stone. A pyelolithotomy is an incision into the renal pelvis to remove a stone. If the stone is located in the ureter, a ureterolithotomy is performed. A cystotomy may be indicated for bladder calculi. For open surgery on the kidney or ureter, a flank incision directly below the diaphragm and across the side is usually the preferred surgical approach. Complications related to hemorrhage are the most common following these surgical procedures.

Nutritional Therapy. A high fluid intake (at least 3000 ml per day) is recommended after an episode of urolithiasis to produce a urine output of at least 2 L per day. High urine output prevents supersaturation of minerals (i.e., dilutes the concentration) and flushes them out before the minerals have a chance to precipitate. Increasing the fluid intake is especially important for the patient who is active in sports, lives in a dry climate, performs physical exercise, has a family history of stone formation, or works in an occupation that requires outdoor work or a great deal of physical activity that can lead to dehydration.

Dietary intervention may be important in the management of urolithiasis. In the past, calcium restriction was routinely implemented for the patient with kidney stones. Recent research suggests that a high dietary calcium intake, which was previously thought to contribute to kidney stones, may actually lower the risk by reducing the urinary excretion of oxalate, a common factor in many stones. Initial nutritional management should include limiting oxalate-rich foods and thereby reducing oxalate excretion. Foods high in calcium, oxalate, and purines are presented in Table 43-11.

NURSING MANAGEMENT: RENAL CALCULI
■ Nursing Assessment
Subjective and objective data that should be obtained from a patient with urinary tract lithiasis are presented in Table 43-12.

■ Nursing Diagnoses
Nursing diagnoses for the patient with urinary tract lithiasis include, but are not limited to, those presented in NCP 43-2.

NURSING ASSESSMENT

Table **43-12** | **Urinary Tract Calculi**

Subjective Data	Objective Data
Important Health Information	**General**
Past health history: Recent or chronic UTI; bed rest; immobilization; previous urinary tract stones, obstruction, or kidney disease with urinary stasis; gout; prostatic hyperplasia; hyperparathyroidism	Guarding, fever
Medications: Prior use of medication for prevention of stones or treatment of UTI; allopurinol, analgesics	**Integumentary**
Surgery or other treatments: External urinary diversion, long-term indwelling urinary catheter	Warm, flushed skin or pallor with cool, moist skin (mild shock)
Functional Health Patterns	**Gastrointestinal**
Health perception–health management: Family history of renal calculi; sedentary lifestyle	Abdominal distention, absence of bowel sounds
Nutritional-metabolic: Nausea, vomiting: dietary intake of purines, calcium, oxalates, phosphates; low fluid intake; chills	**Urinary**
Elimination: Decreased urinary output, urinary urgency, frequency, feeling of bladder fullness	Oliguria, hematuria, tenderness on palpation of renal areas, passage of stone or stones
Cognitive-perceptual: Acute, severe, colicky pain in flank, back, abdomen, groin, or genitalia; burning on urination, dysuria, anxiety	**Possible Findings**
	Elevated BUN and serum creatinine levels; RBCs, WBCs, pyuria, crystals, casts, minerals, bacteria on urinalysis; elevated creatinine, uric acid, calcium, phosphorus, oxalate, or cystine values on 24 hr urine sample; calculi or anatomic changes on IVP or KUB x-ray; direct visualization of obstruction on cystoureteroscopy

BUN, blood urea nitrogen; *KUB,* kidneys, ureters, bladder; *UTI,* urinary tract infection.

43-2 NURSING CARE PLAN PATIENT WITH ACUTE RENAL LITHIASIS

Expected Patient Outcomes | **Nursing Interventions and *Rationales***

NURSING DIAGNOSIS **Pain** *related to* irritation of stone and inadequate pain control or comfort measures *as manifested by* complaints of pain, facial grimacing, restlessness.

- Minimal or no pain.
- Decrease in pain and satisfaction with pain control.

- Assess for pain location and severity *to plan appropriate interventions.*
- Encourage high fluid intake unless contraindicated *to promote passage of stone, dilute the urine, and reduce risk of additional stone formation.*
- Administer pain medication as ordered *to promote comfort.*
- Apply moist heat to flank area as needed *because heat reduces inflammation and reflex muscle spasm and promotes comfort.*

NURSING DIAGNOSIS **Anxiety** *related to* uncertain outcome and lack of knowledge regarding possible surgery *as manifested by* expressions of concern about future treatments.

- Relief of anxiety.
- Expression of confidence in treatment plan.

- Assess cause and level of anxiety *to plan appropriate interventions.*
- Explain surgical or nonsurgical procedure (include insertion of ureteral catheters) *because accurate information often decreases anxiety and fosters control.*
- Encourage patient to express feelings of anxiety, fear of surgery *to validate feelings and provide support.*

NURSING DIAGNOSIS **Ineffective management of therapeutic regimen** *related to* lack of knowledge about prevention of recurrence, diet, fluid requirements, and symptoms of recurrence *as manifested by* questions that indicate inadequate knowledge of disorder.

- Verbalization of correct self-care measures.
- Able to list symptoms of recurrence.

- Instruct patient during initial hospital stay regarding increasing fluids unless contraindicated and diet restrictions and rationale *to prepare for home self-care.*
- Inform patient about rationale, dose, frequency, and side effects of medication *to foster adherence to medication regimen.*
- Tell patient to strain all urine through a urine strainer or piece of gauze (if necessary) *to determine if stones are passed,* and to bring stone to physician for analysis.
- Educate patient about symptoms of recurrence (e.g., hematuria, flank pain) *to ensure early reporting and initiation of treatment.*

NURSING DIAGNOSIS **Altered urinary elimination** *related to* trauma or blockage of ureters or urethra *as manifested by* decrease in urinary output, bloody urine.

- Free flow of urine.
- Minimal to no hematuria.

- Monitor urine amount and character *to ensure patency in urinary system and that hematuria is not excessive.*
- Encourage increased fluid intake *because increased hydration flushes bacteria and blood and may facilitate passage of stone fragments.*

NURSING DIAGNOSIS **Risk for infection** *related to* introduction of bacteria following manipulations of the urinary tract.

- No urinary tract infections.

- Assess for elevation in temperature; chills; cloudy, foul-smelling urine *as indicators of potential infection.*
- Monitor vital signs and observe for fever *because abnormalities may indicate infection.*
- Report any fever or chills to physician *so prompt treatment can be initiated.*
- Administer antipyretics and antibiotics as ordered *to reduce fever and treat infection.*
- Encourage high fluid intake unless contraindicated *because stones form more rapidly in concentrated urine and increased fluids help the stone fragments pass down urinary tract.*

Continued

43-2 NURSING CARE PLAN   PATIENT WITH ACUTE RENAL LITHIASIS—continued

Expected Patient Outcomes	Nursing Interventions and *Rationales*

COLLABORATIVE PROBLEMS

Nursing Goals	Nursing Interventions and *Rationales*
POTENTIAL COMPLICATION ■ Monitor for signs of urinary obstruction and report occurrence. ■ Carry out medical and nursing interventions.	**Urinary obstruction** *related to* presence of stone in path of urine flow. ■ Assess patient for signs of urinary obstruction such as complaints of persistent pain, urgency along with inability to void and bladder distention *to ensure early identification of the problem.* ■ Monitor urine output and fluid intake *because decreased output relative to intake can suggest urinary obstruction.* ■ Notify physician of oliguria *so treatment can be started promptly.* ■ Strain all urine *to determine if stones are passed.* ■ Save stones *so they can be sent for analysis to determine chemical composition.*

■ Planning

The overall goals are that the patient with urinary tract calculi will have (1) relief of pain, (2) no urinary tract obstruction, and (3) an understanding of measures to prevent further recurrence of stones.

■ Nursing Implementation

Preventive measures relate to the person who is on bed rest or is relatively immobile for a prolonged time. It is important to maintain a high fluid intake and to prevent urinary stasis by turning the patient every 2 hours and helping the patient to sit or stand if possible. In the acute phase it is important to retrieve the stone if passed. All urine voided by the patient should be strained through gauze or a special urine strainer in an effort to detect the stone. Increased intake of fluids and ambulation help the stone pass down the urinary tract. The patient should not walk if pain is present during an attack of renal colic. Narcotics will be required for renal colic because the pain is excruciating. Pain management and patient comfort are primary nursing responsibilities (see NCP 43-2).

Stone formation can be prevented, and the recurrence rate can be greatly reduced. After the acute phase, it is important for the nurse to teach the patient ways to prevent recurrence. Dietary restriction of oxalate is important for the patient who has calcium oxalate stones. Diets that restrict purines may be helpful to the patient at risk for developing uric acid stones. Follow-up care includes monitoring the patient's compliance with fluid, dietary, and medication recommendations. Periodic urine cultures may be indicated. Testing the pH of the urine is important, especially to assess the effectiveness of acidifying or alkalinizing agents. It is important to emphasize the need to avoid inadvertent dehydration from excessive exercise and to increase fluid needs during illness and hot weather.

■ Evaluation

The expected outcomes for the patient with urinary calculi are presented in NCP 43-2.

STRICTURES

A *stricture* is a narrowing of the lumen and is sometimes congenital but is usually acquired. Strictures may occur in the bladder neck, urethra, or ureters. Strictures of the bladder neck may be congenital or may result from chronic prostatitis in men or cystitis in women. Causes of urethral strictures include trauma from accidents (e.g., those resulting in fractured pelvis), gonorrheal infections, and urethral instrumentation. The membranous urethra is a common site of stricture caused by instrumentation because of its location (the urethral curve just below the prostatic urethra) and because the surrounding rhabdosphincter muscles prevent easy distention. Meatal stenosis, a narrowing of the urethral opening, is also common. Ureteral strictures may be caused by severe or chronic infection, radiation therapy, and retroperitoneal abscess formation from inflammatory bowel disease and perforation.

Strictures can sometimes be avoided by the proper management of inflammatory processes or traumatic injuries. Treatment of existing strictures includes dilation, use of a catheter for temporary or permanent drainage for ureteral or urethral strictures, and surgery. Some patients are taught to dilate the urethra themselves between office visits to keep strictured areas open. Nursing interventions include informing the patient about the procedure; preparing the patient for the procedure; and assessing the patient's need for management, education, and follow-up care.

RENAL TRAUMA

A continual increase in the incidence of traumatic renal injuries is related to an increase in the mechanization and speed of transportation and to the increase in violent crimes and injuries. The majority of incidents occur in men younger than 30 years of age. Blunt trauma is the most frequent cause. Injury to the kidney should be considered in multiple or sports injuries, traffic accidents, and falls. It is especially likely when the patient injures the abdomen, flank, or back. Penetrating injuries may result from violent encounters (e.g., gunshot or stabbing incidents) or from surgical errors.

Clinical findings include a history of trauma to the area of the kidneys. Gross or microscopic hematuria may be present. Diagnostic studies include urinalysis, IVP with cystography, ultrasound, CT, or MRI evaluation. Renal arteriography may also be used. Both the injured kidney and the noninvolved kidney should be evaluated to provide information for further management.

The severity of renal trauma depends on the extent of the injury. Treatments range from bed rest, fluids, and analgesia to surgical exploration and repair or nephrectomy.

Nursing interventions vary with the type and extent of associated injuries. Specific interventions related to renal trauma include ensuring increased fluid intake, providing comfort measures, monitoring intake and output, observing for hematuria, determining the presence of myoglobinuria, assessing the cardiovascular status, and monitoring potentially nephrotoxic antibiotics.

RENAL VASCULAR PROBLEMS

Vascular problems involving the kidney include (1) nephrosclerosis, (2) renal artery stenosis, and (3) renal vein thrombosis.

NEPHROSCLEROSIS

Nephrosclerosis consists of sclerosis of the small arteries and arterioles of the kidney. There is decreased blood flow, which results in patchy necrosis of the renal parenchyma. Ischemic necrosis and destruction of glomeruli with subsequent fibrosis also occur.

Benign nephrosclerosis usually occurs in adults 30 to 50 years of age. It is caused by vascular changes resulting from hypertension and from the arteriosclerotic process. Arteriosclerotic vascular changes account for most of the loss of renal function associated with aging. There is a direct relation between the degree of nephrosclerosis and the severity of hypertension. The patient with benign nephrosclerosis may have normal renal function in the early stages. The only detectable abnormality may be hypertension.

Accelerated nephrosclerosis, or malignant nephrosclerosis, is associated with malignant hypertension, a complication of hypertension characterized by a sharp increase in blood pressure with a diastolic pressure greater than 130 mm Hg. The patient is usually a young adult, with a male-to-female predominance of 2:1. Renal insufficiency progresses rapidly.

Treatment of benign nephrosclerosis is the same as that of essential hypertension (see Chapter 31). Malignant nephrosclerosis is treated with aggressive antihypertensive therapy (see Chapter 31). The availability and use of antihypertensives have improved the prognosis for the patient with benign nephrosclerosis. Renal dysfunction and renal failure (in some persons) constitute two of the major complications of hypertension. The prognosis for the patient with malignant hypertension is poor, with the major cause of death related to renal failure.

RENAL ARTERY STENOSIS

Renal artery stenosis is a partial occlusion of one or both renal arteries and their major branches. It can be due to atherosclerotic narrowing or fibromuscular hyperplasia. Renal artery stenosis accounts for 1% to 2% of all cases of hypertension.

Renal artery stenosis is considered a major cause of hypertension when it develops abruptly, especially in the patient under 30 or over 50 years of age and in the patient with no familial history of hypertension. This contrasts with the age distribution for essential hypertension, which is 30 to 50 years of age. A renal arteriogram is the best diagnostic tool for identifying renal artery stenosis.

The goals of therapy are control of blood pressure and restoration of perfusion to the kidney. Surgical revascularization of the kidney is indicated when blood flow is decreased enough to cause renal ischemia or when evidence indicates that renovascular hypertension is present and surgical intervention may result in the patient becoming normotensive. The surgical procedure usually involves anastomoses between the kidney and another major artery, usually the splenic artery or aorta. Percutaneous transluminal angioplasty may be used as an alternative to surgery, especially in older patients who are poor surgical risks. In selected cases of unilateral renal involvement with high renin production, unilateral nephrectomy may be indicated.

RENAL VEIN THROMBOSIS

Renal vein thrombosis may occur unilaterally or bilaterally. Trauma, extrinsic compression (e.g., tumor, aortic aneurysm), renal cell carcinoma, pregnancy, contraceptive use, and nephrotic syndrome are associated with renal vein thrombosis.

The patient has symptoms of flank pain, hematuria, or fever or has nephrotic syndrome. Anticoagulation is important in treatment because there is a high incidence of pulmonary emboli. Corticosteroids may be used in the patient with nephrosis. Surgical thrombectomy may be performed instead of or along with anticoagulation.

HEREDITARY RENAL DISEASES

Hereditary renal diseases involve developmental abnormalities of the renal parenchyma. These abnormalities are either isolated or part of more complex malformation syndromes. The majority of inherited structural abnormalities are cystic. However, cysts may also develop as a result of obstructive uropathies, metabolic derangements, or neurologic diseases. Cysts may be evaluated to rule out any tumor content.

POLYCYSTIC RENAL DISEASE

Polycystic renal disease is one of the most common genetic diseases in humans and affects 600,000 people in the United States.[18] There are two forms of hereditary polycystic renal disease. It may be manifested in childhood or adulthood. The childhood form of polycystic disease is a rare autosomal recessive disorder that is often rapidly progressive.

The adult form of polycystic disease is an autosomal dominant disorder. It is latent for many years and is usually manifested between 30 and 40 years of age. It involves both kidneys and occurs in both men and women. The cortex and the medulla are filled with thin-walled cysts that are several millimeters to several centimeters in diameter (Fig. 43-6). The cysts enlarge and destroy surrounding tissue by compression. They are filled with fluid and may contain blood or pus.

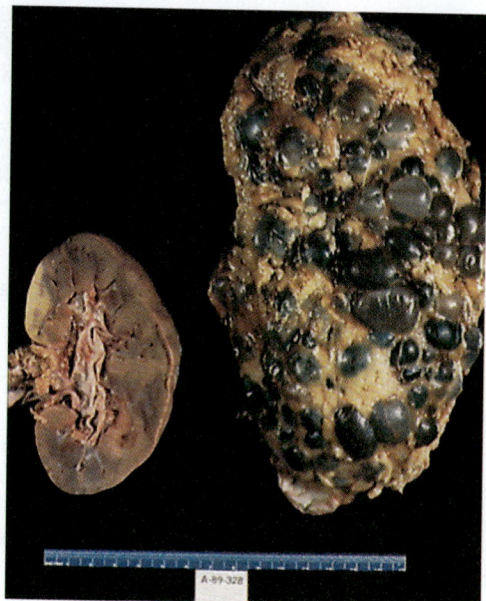

Fig. 43-6 Comparison of polycystic kidney with normal kidney.

Clinical Manifestations

In the patient with polycystic disease, symptoms appear when the cysts begin to enlarge. A common early symptom of adult cystic disease is abdominal or flank pain, which is either steady and dull or abrupt in onset, as well as episodic and colicky. This pain is often caused by bleeding into the cysts. On physical examination, palpable bilateral enlarged kidneys are often found. Other clinical manifestations include hematuria (from rupture of cysts), UTI, and hypertension. Diagnosis is based on clinical manifestations, family history, IVP, ultrasound, or CT scan. Usually the disease progresses to chronic renal failure, although some individuals have relatively mild disease and die from unrelated problems. Loss of kidney function to the point of end-stage renal disease occurs by age 60 in 50% of patients.[18]

Collaborative Care

There is no specific treatment for polycystic kidney disease. A major aim of treatment is to prevent infections of the urinary tract or to treat them with appropriate antibiotics if they occur. Nephrectomy may be necessary if pain, bleeding, or infection becomes a chronic, serious problem.

When the patient begins to experience progressive renal failure, the interventions are determined by the remaining renal function. Nursing measures are those used for management of end-stage renal disease (see Chapter 44). They include diet modification, fluid restriction, medications (e.g., antihypertensives), assisting the patient to accept the chronic disease process, and assisting the patient and family to deal with financial concerns and other issues related to the hereditary nature of the disease.

The patient who has adult polycystic disease often has children by the time the disease is diagnosed. Each child of a parent with polycystic kidney disease has a 50% chance of having the disease. The patient will need appropriate counseling regarding plans for having more children. In addition, genetic counseling resources should be provided for the children.

MEDULLARY CYSTIC DISEASE

Medullary cystic disease is a hereditary disorder that occurs in two forms. The recessive form is associated with renal failure before age 20; the dominant form is associated with renal failure after age 20. Most cysts are located in the medulla. The kidneys are asymmetric in shape and are significantly scarred. There are defects in the concentration ability of the kidneys. Polyuria, progressive renal failure, severe anemia, metabolic acidosis, and poor sodium conservation are common. Hypertension can be a terminal event. Genetic counseling may be helpful in family planning. Treatment measures are those related to end-stage renal disease (see Chapter 44).

ALPORT'S SYNDROME

Alport's syndrome is also known as chronic hereditary nephritis. Two forms of the disease exist: (1) classic Alport's syndrome, which is inherited as a sex-linked disorder with hematuria, sensorineural deafness, and deformities of the anterior surface of the lens; and (2) nonclassical Alport's syndrome, which is inherited as an autosomal trait that causes hematuria but not deafness or lens deformities. Men are affected earlier and more severely than women. The disease is frequently diagnosed in the first decade of life. The basic defect is altered synthesis of the glomerular basement membrane (GBM). The patient most commonly has hematuria and progressive uremia. Treatment is supportive. Corticosteroids and cytotoxic drugs are not effective. The disease does not recur after kidney transplantation.

RENAL INVOLVEMENT IN METABOLIC AND CONNECTIVE TISSUE DISEASES

Various metabolic and connective tissue disease processes may have an effect on renal function. The pathophysiologic effects on the renal parenchyma are not always specific to each process. The clinical course of renal involvement is that of chronic progressive nephropathy, which can result in uremia and death. Management includes treatment of the primary disorder along with symptomatic relief of renal involvement. If renal involvement progresses to chronic renal failure, management includes dialysis or transplantation (see Chapter 44). Nursing interventions include teaching the patient about the primary disease process, the renal involvement, and the resulting need to comply with dietary and fluid restrictions and medication.

Diabetic nephropathy is the major cause of end-stage renal failure in the United States. Diabetes mellitus may affect the kidneys in several ways. Microangiopathic changes in diabetes consist of diffuse glomerulosclerosis, involving thickening of the GBM and nodular glomerulosclerosis (Kimmelstiel-Wilson syndrome), which is characterized by nodular lesions. Nodular glomerulosclerosis is reasonably specific for type 1 diabetes mellitus. The diabetic patient prone to glomerulonephropathy (e.g., the presence of trace proteinuria or retinopathy) requires careful monitoring of glucose levels and insulin requirements.

Diabetic nephropathy can result in chronic renal failure. The patient with diabetes is especially susceptible to UTIs. Primary nursing interventions include teaching the patient about the increased risk of UTIs, the appropriate preventive measures, and when to seek additional medical care. (Diabetes mellitus is discussed in Chapter 46.)

Gout is a syndrome of acute attacks of arthritis caused by hyperuricemia (see Chapter 60). Monosodium urate crystals deposited in joints are responsible for the syndrome. Renal disease may develop as a result of damage caused by deposition of uric acid crystals in the renal interstitium and tubules.

Amyloidosis is a group of disorders manifested by impaired organ function from the infiltration of tissues with a hyaline substance (amyloid). The hyaline consists largely of protein. Kidney involvement is common in amyloidosis. Proteinuria is often the first clinical manifestation.

Systemic lupus erythematosus (SLE) is a connective tissue disorder characterized by the involvement of several tissues and organs, particularly the joints, skin, and kidneys (SLE is discussed in Chapter 60). Clinical manifestations of lupus nephritis are similar to those of other forms of glomerulonephritis. Most frequently found are microscopic hematuria and significant proteinuria. Renal failure frequently occurs in systemic lupus erythematosus and has a poor prognosis. The long-term course of the disorder is extremely variable. Corticosteroids are effective for the patient with severe renal disease. Recently, plasmapheresis therapy has been used.

Scleroderma (progressive systemic sclerosis) is a disease of unknown etiology characterized by widespread alterations of connective tissue and by vascular lesions in many organs (see Chapter 60). In the kidney, vascular lesions are associated with fibrosis. An immune complex mechanism has been postulated as a possible etiologic factor. The severity of renal involvement varies. The patient who develops severe renal lesions has a poor prognosis. Once uremia develops, about 70% die within 3 years.

NEOPLASTIC DISORDERS OF THE URINARY TRACT

RENAL TUMORS

Tumors of the kidney are responsible for approximately 12,000 deaths per year, and 30,000 new cases are diagnosed each year.[19] Renal tumors arise from the cortex or pelvis (and calyces). Tumors arising from both areas may be benign or malignant. However, malignant tumors are more frequent. Renal cell carcinoma (adenocarcinoma) is the most common type. Adenocarcinoma is twice as frequent in men as in women and is typically discovered when the person is 50 to 70 years old. Cigarette smoking is the most significant risk factor for the development of renal cell carcinoma. Other risk factors are the use of phenacetin-containing analgesics and exposure to asbestos, cadmium, and gasoline.

There are no characteristic early symptoms. Generalized symptoms of weight loss, weakness, and anemia are the earliest manifestations. The classic manifestations of gross hematuria, flank pain, and a palpable mass are those of advanced disease.[20] The most common sites of metastases include the

Table **43-13**	Robson's System of Staging Renal Carcinoma
Stage	Description
I	Limitation to renal capsule
II	Spreading to perirenal fat, but confined within fascia; includes metastasis to adrenal gland
III	Regional lymph node involvement, tumor thrombus in renal vein or vena cava, involvement of lymph nodes and renal vein or vena cava
IV	Presence of distant metastases

lungs, liver, and long bones. Local extension of renal cancer into the renal vein and vena cava is common. Renal cystic disease and renal-associated carcinomas may develop in the patient with end-stage renal disease on maintenance renal dialysis (see Chapter 44).

Several studies are used to diagnose adenocarcinoma of the kidney. IVP with nephrotomography is the primary examination by which most masses are detected and evaluated. Ultrasounds have improved the ability to differentiate between a tumor and a cyst. Angiography, percutaneous needle aspiration, CT, and magnetic resonance imaging (MRI) are also used in the diagnosis of renal tumors. Small renal tumors are found earlier because of the increased use of CT scans and MRI. Radionuclide isotope scanning is used to detect metastases.

Robson's system of staging renal carcinoma is presented in Table 43-13. Tumor, node, metastases (TNM) classification is also used for renal cancer staging. The treatment of choice is a radical nephrectomy. Radical nephrectomy is the removal of the kidney, adrenal gland, surrounding fascia, part of the ureter, and draining lymph nodes. Radiation therapy is used palliatively in inoperable cases and when there are metastases to bone or lungs. No effective chemotherapy is available for metastatic renal cell carcinoma. Biologic therapy, including α-interferon and interleukin-2 (IL-2), are most promising in the treatment of metastatic disease.[21] Side effects of IL-2 include capillary leakage syndrome, fever, chills, fatigue, and hypotension.

WILMS' TUMOR

Wilms' tumor is a common renal tumor of infants and children. Of these tumors, 40% are hereditary, with an autosomal dominant mode of transmission. The most common clinical manifestation is abdominal swelling or distention. This distention is often noticed by the parents or is found on a routine examination. Other symptoms include pain, fever, hematuria, and hypertension. Diagnostic studies for Wilms' tumor include ultrasound and renal arteriography.

These tumors respond well to multimodality therapy. Therapeutic treatment includes surgical removal of the involved kidney and radiation therapy. Radiation therapy is used postoperatively and for inoperable tumors, bilateral tumors, and

Table 43-14 Tumor–Node–Metastasis (TNM) Staging System for Bladder Cancer

Primary Tumor (T)

TX: Primary tumor cannot be assessed
T0: No evidence of primary tumor
Ta: Noninvasive papillary carcinoma
Tis: Carcinoma in situ ("flat tumor")
T1: Tumor invades subepithelial connective tissue
T2: Tumor invades superficial muscle (inner half)
T3: Tumor invades deep muscle or perivesical fat
T3a: Tumor invades deep muscle (outer half)
T3b: Tumor invades perivesical fat
T4: Tumor invades any of the following: prostate, uterus, vagina, pelvic wall, or abdominal wall
T4a: Tumor invades the prostate, uterus, or vagina
T4b: Tumor invades the pelvic wall or abdominal wall

Nodal Involvement (N)

Regional lymph nodes are those within the true pelvis; all others are distant nodes.

NX: Regional lymph nodes cannot be assessed
N0: No regional lymph node metastasis
N1: Metastasis in a single lymph node, 2.0 cm or less in greatest dimension
N2: Metastasis in a single lymph node, more than 2.0 cm but not more than 5.0 cm in greatest dimension; or multiple lymph nodes, none more than 5.0 cm in greatest dimension
N3: Metastasis in a lymph node more than 5.0 cm in greatest dimension

Distant Metastasis (M)

MX: Presence of distant metastasis cannot be assessed
M0: No distant metastasis
M1: Distant metastasis

American Joint Committee on Cancer Stage Groupings of Bladder Cancer

Stage 0a
  Ta, N0, M0
Stage 0is
  Tis, N0, M0
Stage I
  T1, N0, M0
Stage II
  T2, N0, M0
  T3a, N0, M0
Stage III
  T3b, N0, M0
  T4a, N0, M0
Stage IV
  T4b, N0, M0
  Any T, N1, M0
  Any T, N2, M0
  Any T, N3, M0
  Any T, any N, M1

metastases. Chemotherapy with actinomycin D and vincristine (Oncovin) is also frequently used.

BLADDER CANCER

In 1998 there were an estimated 54,400 new cases of bladder cancer and 12,500 deaths related to bladder cancer. Bladder cancer accounts for nearly 1 in every 20 cancers diagnosed in the United States.[19] The most frequent malignant tumor of the urinary tract is transitional cell carcinoma of the bladder. Most bladder tumors are papillomatous growths within the bladder. Cancer of the bladder is most common between the ages of 60 and 70 years and is at least three times as common in men as in women. Risk factors for bladder cancer include cigarette smoking, exposure to dyes used in the rubber and cable industries, and chronic abuse of phenacetin-containing analgesics. Women treated with radiation for cervical cancer and patients receiving cyclophosphamide (Cytoxan) also have increased risk, but the reason is unknown.[22]

Individuals with chronic, recurrent stones (often bladder) and chronic lower urinary infections have an increased risk of squamous cell cancer of the bladder. Patients who have indwelling catheters for long periods of time can develop these chronic conditions.

Clinical Manifestations and Diagnostic Studies

Gross, painless hematuria (chronic or intermittent) is the most common clinical finding and the first in 85% to 90% of patients. Bladder irritability with dysuria, frequency, and urgency may also occur. When cancer is suspected, urine specimens for cytology can be obtained to determine the presence of neoplastic or atypical cells. Exfoliated cells from the epithelial surface of the bladder can readily be detected in voided specimens. Other recent urine tests assess for specific factors associated with bladder cancer, such as bladder tumor antigens. Bladder cancers can be detected using IVP, ultrasound, CT, or MRI. However, the presence of cancer is confirmed by cytoscopy and biopsy.

The clinical staging of carcinoma of the bladder is determined by the depth of invasion of the bladder wall and surrounding tissue (Table 43-14). The Jewett-Strong-Marshall classification system broadly classifies bladder cancer as superficial (CIS, O, A), invasive (B1, B2, C), or metastatic (D1–D4) disease. Pathologic grading systems are also used to classify the malignant potential of tumor cells, indicating a scale from well-differentiated to anaplastic categories. Low-stage, low-grade bladder cancers are the most responsive to treatment and are more easily cured.

NURSING AND COLLABORATIVE MANAGEMENT: BLADDER CANCER

Collaborative care of bladder cancer is outlined in Table 43-15.

■ Surgical Therapy

Surgical therapies include a variety of procedures. Transurethral resection (TUR) with fulguration (electrocautery) is used for

COLLABORATIVE CARE

Table 43-15   Bladder Cancer

Diagnostic
  Urinalysis
  Intravenous pyelogram
  Cystoscopy with biopsy
  Cytology studies
  Ultrasound
  CT scan

Collaborative Therapy
  Surgical treatment
    Transurethral resection with fulguration
    Laser photocoagulation
    Open loop resection or fulguration
    Segmental cystectomy
    Radical cystectomy
  Radiation
  Intravesical immunotherapy
    Bacille Calmette-Guérin (BCG)
  Intravesical chemotherapy
    Thiotepa
    Mitomycin (Mutamycin)
    Doxorubicin (Adriamycin)
  Systemic chemotherapy

the diagnosis and treatment of superficial lesions with a low recurrence rate. This procedure is also used to control bleeding in the patient who is a poor operative risk or who has advanced tumors. With this technique the tumor mass is excised by means of a blade inserted through the cystoscope. The remaining portions of the tumor are cauterized.

A second technique, laser photocoagulation, is also used to treat superficial bladder cancers. This procedure can be repeated a number of times for recurrence. The advantages of laser include bloodless destruction of the lesion, minimal risk of perforation, and lack of need for a urinary catheter. Because laser destroys tumor tissue, pathologic evaluation cannot be done after this procedure.

A third technique used is open loop resection (snaring of polyp types of lesion) with fulguration. It is used for the control of bleeding, for large superficial tumors, and for multiple lesions. Treatment of large lesions entails a segmental resection of the bladder (segmental cystectomy).

Postoperative management of the patient who has had any of these surgical procedures includes instructions to drink large amounts of fluid each day, measurement of intake and output, avoidance of alcoholic beverages, use of analgesics and stool softeners (if necessary), and sitz baths to promote muscle relaxation and reduce urinary retention. The nurse should also help the patient and family cope with fears about cancer, surgery, and sexuality and should emphasize the importance of regular follow-up care. Frequent routine cystoscopies are required.

When the tumor is invasive or involves the trigone (the area where the ureters insert into the bladder) and the patient oth-erwise has a good life expectancy and has demonstrated no metastases beyond the pelvic area, a radical cystectomy with urinary diversion is the treatment of choice (see the following section on urinary diversion). A radical cystectomy involves the removal of bladder, prostate, seminal vesicles (in men) and uterus, cervix, urethra, and usually ovaries (in women).

■ Radiation Therapy and Chemotherapy

Radiation therapy is used with cystectomy or as the primary therapy when the cancer is inoperable or when surgery is refused. Increasingly radiation therapy is being combined with systemic chemotherapy. Sometimes combination systemic chemotherapy is used for bladder cancer, usually preoperatively or before radiation therapy, or is used to treat distant metastases.[23] Chemotherapy drugs used in treating invasive bladder cancer include cisplatin (Platinol), vinblastine (Velban), doxorubicin (Adriamycin), and methotrexate.

■ Intravesical therapy

Chemotherapy with local instillation of chemotherapeutic or immune-stimulating agents can be delivered directly into the bladder by a urethral catheter. Protocols vary, but intravesical therapy is usually initiated at weekly intervals for 6 to 12 weeks. They are instilled directly into the patient's bladder and retained for about 2 hours. The patient's position may be changed every 15 minutes for maximum contact in all areas of the bladder, especially if the tumor occurred on the bladder dome. The use of maintenance therapy after the initial induction regimen may be beneficial.

Bacille Calmette-Guérin (BCG), a weakened strain of *Mycobacterium bovis*, is the treatment of choice. It differs from other agents in that BCG stimulates the immune system rather than acting directly on cancer cells in the bladder. Thiotepa is an alkylating agent that is pharmacologically related to nitrogen mustard. Thiotepa may be used if BCG fails and a patient's bladder cancer returns.

Most patients have irritative voiding symptoms and hemorrhagic cystitis following intravesical therapy. Thiotepa can significantly reduce WBC and platelet counts in some individuals. BCG may cause flulike symptoms, hematuria, or systemic infection. Systemic side effects usually associated with chemotherapy, such as nausea, vomiting, and hair loss, are not experienced with intravesical chemotherapy.

Nursing responsibilities include encouraging the patient to increase the daily fluid intake and to quit smoking, assessing the patient for secondary urinary tract infection, and stressing the need for routine urologic follow-up. The patient may have fears or concerns about sexual activity or bladder function that will need to be addressed.

URINARY INCONTINENCE AND RETENTION

An estimated 13 million people (of which 11 million are women) in the United States suffer from urinary incontinence, or the unintentional loss of urine that is sufficient to be a problem.[24] Although about half of older people have episodes of incontinence, bladder problems are not a natural consequence of aging, and they are not exclusively a problem of older adults.[25]

Incontinence exacts physical (infection, pressure sores, perineal rashes), psychosocial (embarrassment, isolation, depression), and economic costs. However minor the problem, incontinence can cause severe psychologic distress. Incontinence is not an inevitable consequence of aging; in most cases among older adults, it can be significantly improved or corrected. *Retention* is the inability to urinate in spite of the presence of urine in the bladder. Both incontinence and retention may occur in the same person.

NORMAL BLADDER FUNCTION

Storage of urine in the bladder is mediated by relaxation of the detrusor muscle (which provides the propulsive force for emptying the bladder) and closure of the sphincters. The detrusor muscle is controlled by the parasympathetic nervous system through the pelvic nerves from sacral spinal cord segments S2, S3, or S4. These spinal segments are modulated by the pons (brainstem) and cortical centers in the brain. The smooth muscle of the trigonal portion of the bladder between the ureteral orifices and the posterior area of the bladder outlet is innervated by the sympathetic nervous system, in which α-receptors predominate. This layer of muscle acts as an involuntary internal sphincter. The external urethral sphincter and perineal muscles are under voluntary control.

The sensation of bladder fullness is transmitted via sensory nerves to the sacral cord. If not suppressed by cortical control, the sacral cord discharges motor impulses by reflex that cause powerful sustained detrusor contraction. Urination can be prevented by means of cortical suppression of the reflex arc or voluntary contraction of the external sphincter and perineal muscles. Urination occurs when detrusor contraction is coordinated with sphincter relaxation.

CAUSES OF URINARY INCONTINENCE AND RETENTION

Anything that interferes with bladder or urethral sphincter control can result in urinary incontinence. Causes may be transient (e.g., caused by confusion or depression, infection, medications, restricted mobility, or stool impaction). Congenital disorders that produce incontinence include exstrophy of the bladder, epispadias, spina bifida with myelomeningocele, and ectopic ureteral orifice. Acquired disorders are described in Table 43-16. Patients may have more than one type of incontinence.

Neurogenic Bladder

Neurogenic bladder is a general term referring to any bladder dysfunction resulting from a central nervous system (CNS) neurologic disorder. There are numerous causes of this condition, including such problems as CNS tumors, cerebrovascular accidents, multiple sclerosis, diabetic neuropathy, and spinal cord injury. A person with a neurogenic bladder may have problems with urgency, frequency, incontinence, inability to urinate, and obstruction-like symptoms. Long-term problems include formation of calculi, urinary tract infection, and progressive deterioration in renal function.

A simple way to classify neurogenic dysfunction is to identify whether there is a failure to store, failure to empty, or both problems and whether the dysfunction is of the bladder or urethra. Either or both problems lead to urinary tract damage if not treated. The type of dysfunction usually depends on where the problem affects the brain or spinal cord (e.g., cerebral centers, suprasacral spinal cord, sacral cord area). Lesions in the brain or upper spinal cord usually cause hyperreflexic symptoms, whereas lesions in the sacral cord cause arreflexia. Detrusor sphincter dyssynergia (the bladder and sphincter contract at the same time) is often associated with lesions in the suprasacral spinal cord. (A more detailed description of neurogenic bladder is found in Chapter 57.)

Urinary Retention

Retention can be found in association with incontinence but can also be independent of incontinence. Drugs that may cause retention include (1) antihypertensives (methyldopa [Aldomet], hydralazine [Apresoline]), (2) antiparkinsonian drugs (levodopa), (3) antihistamines, (4) anticholinergics (e.g., atropine, belladonna), (5) antispasmodics, (6) sedatives, and (7) anesthesia (especially spinal anesthesia).

Postoperative urinary retention is not uncommon and is related to preoperative medication (atropine and sedatives are frequently used), anesthesia, supine position after surgery, and low fluid intake. Postoperative retention may also be related to the effects of surgical manipulation of the bladder nerves.

Another cause of retention is urethral obstruction, which may be caused by congenital urethral stenosis, prostate cancer, benign prostatic hyperplasia, fecal impaction, or tumors (involving bladder outlet or large, displaced uterine myomas). Psychologic problems may also contribute to urinary retention. Psychogenic urinary retention is found more commonly in women than in men.

Diagnostic Studies

A complete history and physical examination (with particular attention to the GU system) are essential to obtain information on the patient's past and current urination patterns, current physical health, and underlying reasons for incontinence or retention. A drug history, including both prescription and over-the-counter drugs, should be obtained. It is advisable to ask the patient to keep a bladder diary that logs the times and precipitating factors for incontinence.

Diagnostic tests of urologic dysfunction are important in the evaluation of the function and structure of the urinary tract, especially the bladder. A urinalysis is essential. These tests may include IVP, cystoscopy (including urethroscopy), urodynamic studies (to assess sphincter, perineal, and muscle activity), and catheterization or ultrasound for residual urine.

Collaborative Care

An estimated 80% of incontinence can be improved.[25] Treatment should correct the factors responsible for incontinence or retention, if possible (see Table 43-16). Treatment includes

Table 43-16 **Acquired Disorders Causing Urinary Incontinence**

Type	Description	Causes	Treatment
■ Stress incontinence*	Sudden increase in intraabdominal pressure causes involuntary passage of urine. It can occur during coughing, heavy lifting, straining, or laughing.	Condition is found most commonly in women with relaxed pelvic musculature (frequently from obstetric complications or multiple pregnancies). Structures of the female urethra atrophy when estrogen decreases. Condition is found in men after prostate surgery for benign prostatic hyperplasia or prostatic carcinoma.	Perineal muscle exercises (e.g., Kegel exercises), weight loss if patient is obese, insertion of vaginal pessary, estrogen vaginal creams, condom catheters or penile clamp, surgery Urethral inserts, patches, or bladder neck support devices to correct underlying problem
■ Urge incontinence*	Condition occurs randomly when involuntary urination is preceded by warning of few seconds to few minutes. Leakage is periodic but frequent. Nocturnal frequency and incontinence are common. Condition may appear with varying severity during psychologic stress.	Condition is caused by uncontrolled contraction or overactivity of detrusor muscle. Bladder escapes central inhibition and contracts reflexively. Conditions include central nervous system disorders (e.g., cerebrovascular disease, Alzheimer's disease, brain tumor, Parkinson's disease), bladder disorders (e.g., carcinoma in situ, radiation effects, interstitial cystitis), interference with spinal inhibitory pathways (e.g., malignant growth in spinal cord, spondylosis), and bladder outlet obstruction, as well as conditions of unknown etiology.	Treatment of underlying cause, instruction to have patient urinate more frequently or on time schedule, anticholinergic drugs (e.g., propantheline), imipramine at bedtime, calcium channel blockers, condom catheters, vaginal estrogen creams
■ Overflow (paradoxic) incontinence	Condition occurs when the pressure of urine in overfull bladder overcomes sphincter control. Leakage of small amounts of urine is frequent throughout the day and night. Urination may also occur frequently in small amounts. Bladder remains distended and is usually palpable.	Disorder is caused by outlet obstruction (prostatic hyperplasia, bladder neck obstruction, urethral stricture) or by underactive detrusor muscle caused by myogenic or neurogenic factors (e.g., herniated disk, diabetic neuropathy). It may also occur after anesthesia and surgery (especially procedures such as hemorrhoidectomy, herniorrhaphy, cystoscopy). Neurogenic bladder (flaccid type) is another cause.	Urinary catheterization to decompress bladder, implementation of Credé's or Valsalva's maneuver, α-adrenergic blocker (e.g., prazosin) to decrease outlet resistance, bethanechol to enhance bladder contractions, intermittent catheterization, surgery to correct underlying problem
■ Reflex incontinence	Condition occurs when no warning or stress precedes periodic involuntary urination. Urination is frequent, is moderate in volume, and occurs equally during the day and night.	Spinal cord lesion above S2 interferes with central nervous system inhibition. Disorder results in detrusor hyperreflexia and interferes with pathways coordinating detrusor contraction and sphincter relaxation.	Treatment of underlying cause, bladder decompression to prevent ureteral reflux and hydronephrosis, intermittent self-catheterization, α-adrenergic blocker (e.g., prazosin) to relax internal sphincter, diazepam or baclofen to relax external sphincter, prophylactic antibiotics, surgical sphincterotomy
■ Incontinence after trauma or surgery	Vesicovaginal or urethrovaginal fistula may occur in women. Alteration in continence control in men involves proximal urethral sphincter (bladder neck and prostatic urethra) and distal urethral sphincter (external striated muscle).	Fistulas may occur during pregnancy, after delivery of baby, as a result of hysterectomy or invasive cancer of cervix, or after radiation therapy. Incontinence is found as postoperative complication after transurethral, perineal, or retropubic prostatectomy.	Surgery to correct fistula, urinary diversion surgery to bypass urethra and bladder, external condom catheter, penile clamp, placement of artificial implantable sphincter
■ Functional incontinence	Loss of urine due to problems of patient mobility or environmental factors	Elderly often have problems that affect balance and mobility	Modifications of environment or care plan that facilitate regular, easy access to toilet and promote patient safety (e.g., better lighting, ambulatory assistance equipment, clothing alterations, timed voiding, different toileting equipment)

*Patients can have combination of stress and urge incontinence that is referred to as mixed incontinence.

DRUG THERAPY

DRUG THERAPY

Table 43-17 Urinary Incontinence*

Muscarinic receptor antagonists and anticholinergics
  Oxybutynin (Ditropan)
  Tolterodine (Detrol)
  Propantheline (Pro-Banthine)
α-Adrenergic blockers
  Prazosin (Minipress)
  Phenoxybenzamine (Dibenzyline)
α-Adrenergic agonists
  Phenylpropanolamine
Tricyclic antidepressants
  Imipramine (Tofranil)
  Desipramine (Norpramin)
  Nortriptyline (Aventyl)
Calcium channel blockers
  Nifedipine (Adalat)
  Diltiazem (Cardizem)
  Verapamil (Calan, Isoptin)
Hormone replacement therapy

*The type of drug therapy depends on the type of incontinence.

behavioral techniques, electrostimulation, surgery, and medications.

Behavioral therapies help people regain control of their bladder. Bladder training teaches people to resist the urge to void and gradually expand the intervals between voiding. (Bladder training programs are described in Chapter 57.)

Pelvic floor electrical stimulation uses mild electrical pulses to stimulate muscle contractions. Electrical stimulation should be performed in conjunction with Kegel exercises (explained in next column).

Surgical approaches vary, depending on the underlying problem. For example, a transurethral resection of the prostate is used to treat benign prostatic hyperplasia. Urethral strictures are dilated. Several surgical procedures help correct anatomic malposition of the bladder neck and urethra that causes female stress incontinence. The Marshall-Marchetti procedure involves suspending the urethra and bladder neck by suturing the anterior vaginal wall on each side to the periosteum of the pubic bones and lower rectum through an abdominal incision. The Pereyra procedure and subsequent modifications involve suspending the tissues adjacent to the bladder neck to the abdominal fascia, mainly through a transvaginal approach.

Injection of urethral bulking agents, such as Teflon or collagen, and implantation of a prosthetic urethral sphincter are also done for stress incontinence in selected cases. There is risk of Teflon particles migrating to lungs; consequently, alternatives are more favorable. Augmentation enterocystoplasty (enlarging the bladder with a segment of bowel or stomach) may be attempted for severe urge incontinence when the disorder does not respond to other treatment measures and when kidney function may be compromised as a result of reflux.

Drug Therapy (Table 43-17)

Muscarinic receptor antagonists. This group of drugs is used to treat hyperreflexic bladders by suppressing the unwanted contractions that occur when the bladder has only a small volume of urine. Oxybutynin (Ditropan), which has both anti-

cholinergic and direct smooth-muscle relaxing properties, has been the gold standard of drug therapy for many years.[24] Oxybutynin is a nonselective muscarinic receptor antagonist that tends to produce significant anticholinergic effects such as drying of the mouth and eyes. Tolterodine (Detrol), a selective antimuscarinic agent, has recently been approved for use for treatment of overactive bladder. Propantheline (Pro-Banthine), an anticholinergic, inhibits the action of acetylcholine.

Other drug therapy. α-Adrenergic blockers such as prazosin (Minipress) and phenoxybenzamine (Dibenzyline) can be used to relax spastic bladder necks and prostatic smooth muscle. α-Adrenergic agonists, such as phenylpropanolamine, also increase urethral resistance. Imipramine and calcium channel blockers (see Table 43-17) reduce detrusor contractions and improve continence. Vaginal or oral estrogen replacement is often prescribed for postmenopausal women to restore urethral suppleness.

NURSING MANAGEMENT: URINARY INCONTINENCE

The nurse must recognize both the physical and the emotional problems that accompany incontinence. The patient's dignity, privacy, and feelings of self-worth must be maintained or enhanced. Most persons suffering from incontinence can be helped with proper diagnosis and modern therapeutic approaches.

A patient with stress incontinence can be taught to do pelvic floor (perineal) muscle exercises (Kegel exercises). The patient should contract the pelvic muscles, as though trying to stop the flow of urine, while relaxing the abdomen, thighs, and buttocks. Each contraction is held for a few seconds and followed by relaxation for the same period of time. Contraction and relaxation times are gradually increased. These exercises should be repeated in sets of 10 or more contractions and done four to five times each day over several weeks. Consistency and persistence are necessary for success, and exercise regimens have to be individualized. Vaginal weights (cones) or biofeedback may help patients gain awareness and control of their pelvic muscles. Vaginal weight training involves holding small weights within the vagina by tightening the vaginal muscles. These exercises should be performed for 15 minutes, twice daily, for 4 to 6 weeks.

The nurse has a major responsibility to help the patient with incontinence problems in a variety of settings. In the hospital, nursing measures aimed at maintaining urinary continence include identifying transient causes and assessing the patient for signs of bladder infection, fecal impaction, or bladder distention. The nurse should offer the urinal or bedpan or help the patient to the bathroom every 2 hours or at scheduled times.

Assuming the usual position for urination (standing for the man and sitting and leaning forward for the woman) or using relaxation techniques often help a patient urinate successfully, particularly in unfamiliar settings. Applying pressure over the bladder area (Credé's maneuver) may be helpful when bladder outlet obstruction is not a problem. The nurse should be sure the patient has privacy and is not rushed when trying to urinate. Techniques to stimulate urination include running water in the sink, placing hands in water, and pouring warm water over the perineum. Fluid intake patterns can be monitored and fluids encouraged.

The patient should be taught that incontinence is not a normal part of aging and that it can be eliminated or controlled in most cases. Local medical supply resources and suggestions for improving urinary control, including having the problem further evaluated, are helpful in discharge planning. The patient may feel more comfortable talking about incontinence when given this kind of permission to talk about a problem that is embarrassing to most people.

Fluid restriction, incontinence pads, and keeping a urinal in place at all times are only temporary measures to reduce the occurrence or effects of incontinence. Long-term use of these measures discourages continence and can lead to dehydration and skin problems.

If bladder retraining cannot be achieved, external appliances or intermittent self-catheterization may be indicated. Several external appliances that prevent soiling, decrease odor, and improve body image are available for men. External appliances for women are not useful in most situations. However, newly developed inserts, patches, pessaries, and bladder neck support devices are useful for some women with stress urinary incontinence.[26,27] Intermittent self-catheterization using a clean technique can be taught to selected patients. Keeping the skin clean and dry is essential to prevent skin irritation and breakdown. (Intermittent-catheterization is discussed on p. 1290)

INSTRUMENTATION

A catheter is a tubular instrument made of rubber, plastic, metal, or other material used to drain or inject gases or fluids through a body passage. The process of inserting the catheter into a body cavity or passage is termed *catheterization.* Indwelling catheters often have self-retaining balloons to keep the catheter in place. Nursing responsibility includes understanding the reason for catheterization, the scientific principles involved, aseptic technique, and the appropriate care of the patient after catheterization.

Table **43-18**	**Indications for Urinary Catheterization**

1. Relief of urinary retention caused by lower urinary tract obstruction, paralysis, or inability to void
2. Bladder decompression preoperatively and operatively for lower abdominal or pelvic surgery
3. Facilitation of surgical repair of urethra and surrounding structures
4. Splinting of ureters or urethra to facilitate healing after surgery or other trauma in area
5. Instillation of medications into bladder
6. Accurate measurement of urinary output in critically ill patient
7. Measurement of residual urine after urination
8. Study of anatomic structures of urinary system
9. Urodynamic testing
10. Collection of sterile urine sample in selected situations

The reasons for urinary catheterization are listed in Table 43-18. Two reasons that are *not* indications for catheterization are (1) routine acquisition of a sterile specimen for laboratory analysis and (2) convenience of the nursing staff or the patient's family. The risks of nosocomial infection are too high to allow catheterization of a patient for the convenience of hospital personnel or family members. Catheterization for sterile urine specimens may occasionally be indicated when patients have complicated urinary infection histories. These specimens have to be as free of contaminants as possible. A catheter should be the final means of providing the patient with a dry environment for prevention of skin breakdown and protection of dressings or skin lesions.

Urinary catheterization is commonly used in the management of the hospitalized patient. However, it is not without serious risks. The urinary tract is the most common site of nosocomial infections. Urinary catheterization is a major cause of UTIs. Scrupulous aseptic technique is mandatory when a urinary catheter is inserted. After insertion, maintenance and protection of the closed drainage system are major nursing responsibilities. Irrigation of the catheter should *not* be routinely performed.

While the patient has a catheter in place, nursing actions should include maintaining patency of the catheter, managing fluid intake, providing for the comfort and safety of the patient, and preventing infection. Attention should be given to the psychologic implications of urinary drainage. Concerns of the patient can include embarrassment related to exposure of the body, an altered body image, and fear concerning the care of the catheter that results in increased dependency.

Catheters vary in construction materials, tip shape (Fig. 43-7), and size of the lumen. Catheters are sized according to

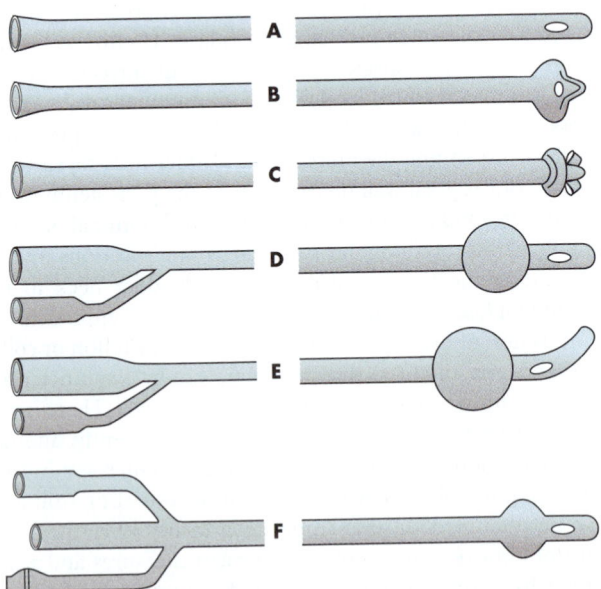

Fig. 43-7 Different types of commonly used catheters. **A,** Simple urethral catheter. **B,** Mushroom or dePezzar (can be used for suprapublic catheterization). **C,** Winged-tip or Malecot. **D,** Indwelling with inflated balloon. **E,** Indwelling with Coudé tip or Tiemann. **F,** Three-way indwelling (the third lumen is used for irrigation of the bladder).

the French scale. Each French unit equals 0.33 mm of diameter. The diameter measured is the internal diameter of the catheter. The size used varies with the size of the individual and the purpose for catheterization. In women, urethral catheter sizes 14F to 16F are the most common; in men, sizes 16F to 18F are used. Problems resulting from too small a catheter include possible obstruction of the urinary flow by blood clots, mineral sediment, or mucous plugs and difficulty in passing the catheter if resistance is met in the urethra. The primary problem resulting from too large a catheter is tissue erosion secondary to excessive pressure on the meatus or urethra. Four routes are used for urinary tract catheterization: urethral, ureteral, suprapubic, and via a nephrostomy tube.

URETHRAL CATHETERIZATION

The most common route of catheterization is insertion of the catheter through the external meatus into the urethra, past the internal sphincter, and into the bladder. Principles that should be considered in the management of the patient with a urethral catheter include the following:

1. The indwelling urinary catheter should be used *only* when absolutely necessary and never solely for the convenience of the caregivers. Its use should be discontinued as early as possible.
2. The catheterized patient, particularly the person who is ambulatory, should receive appropriate instruction regarding catheter care.
3. A sterile, closed drainage system should always be used in short-term catheterization. The distal urinary catheter and the proximal drainage tube should not be disconnected except for necessary catheter irrigation. Unobstructed downhill flow must be maintained. The collecting bag should be emptied regularly and kept below the level of the bladder. A poorly functioning catheter should be replaced. The leg bag should not be used for the short-term patient in the hospital setting because the risk of bacterial infection is great when the catheter is disconnected and the drainage bags are exchanged.
4. Perineal care (one to two times per day and when necessary) should include cleaning of the meatus-catheter junction with soap and water. Following this, an antimicrobial ointment may be applied. Lotion or powder should not be used near the catheter. The catheter should be properly secured to the leg to prevent movement and urethral traction.
5. Sterile technique must be used whenever the collecting system is opened. Catheter irrigation is performed only when obstruction or blood clots are suspected or, in the case of long-term catheterization, to reduce sediment buildup. If frequent irrigations are necessary in short-term catheterization for catheter patency, a triple-lumen catheter may be preferable, permitting continuous irrigations within a closed system. Small volumes of urine for culture can be aspirated from the distal catheter by means of a sterile syringe and a 21-gauge needle after the drainage tubing is clamped. The puncture site must first be prepared with a tincture of iodine or alcohol solution. Many drainage systems are now equipped with a sampling port. Silicone or plastic catheters do not self-seal. Urine for chemical analysis (e.g., electrolytes) can be obtained from the drainage bag.
6. When the patient is catheterized for less than 2 weeks, routine catheter change is not necessary. For long-term use of an indwelling catheter, replacement is necessary when concretions can be palpated in the catheter or when the catheter malfunctions. With long-term use of a catheter, the leg bag may be used. If the collection bag is reused, it should be washed in soap and water and rinsed thoroughly. When not reused immediately, it should be filled with $1/2$ cup of vinegar and drained. The vinegar is effective against *Pseudomonas* and other organisms and eliminates odors.

URETERAL CATHETERS

The ureteral catheter is placed through the ureters into the renal pelvis. The catheter is inserted either (1) by being threaded up the urethra and bladder to the ureters under cystoscopic observation or (2) by surgical insertion through the abdominal wall into the ureters. The ureteral catheter is used after surgery to splint the ureters and to prevent them from being obstructed by edema. The urine volume from the ureteral catheter should be recorded separately from other urinary catheters. The patient is usually kept on bed rest while a ureteral catheter is in place until specific orders indicate that ambulation is permissible. The self-retaining ureteral catheter is often inserted after a lithotripsy procedure or when ureteral obstruction from adjacent tumors or fibrosis threatens renal function. The double-J ureteral catheter is often used and allows the patient to ambulate. One end coils up in the kidney pelvis, while the other coils in the bladder.

The placement of the ureteral catheter should be checked frequently, and tension on the catheter should be avoided. The catheter drains urine from the renal pelvis, which has a capacity of 3 to 5 ml. If the volume of urine in the renal pelvis increases, tissue damage to the pelvis will result from pressure. Therefore the ureteral catheter should not be clamped. If the physician orders irrigation of the ureteral catheter, strict aseptic technique is required. If output is decreased, the physician should be notified immediately. Drainage should be checked often (at least every 1 to 2 hours). It is normal for some urine to drain around the ureteral catheter into the bladder. Accurate recording of urine output from both the ureters and the urethral catheter is essential. Sometimes a ureteral catheter may be used as a stent and is not expected to drain. It is important to check with the physician as to the type of catheter and what to expect.

SUPRAPUBIC CATHETERS

Suprapubic catheterization is the simplest and oldest method of urinary diversion. The two methods of insertion of a suprapubic catheter into the bladder are (1) through a small incision in the abdominal wall and (2) by the use of a trocar. A suprapubic catheter is placed while the patient is under general anesthesia for another surgical procedure or at the bedside with a local anesthetic. The catheter may be sutured into place, but a Foley catheter is usually used. The nursing responsibility includes taping the catheter to prevent dislodgment. The care of the tube and catheter is similar to that of the urethral catheter. A pectin-base skin barrier (e.g., Stomahesive) is effective around the insertion site in protecting the skin from breakdown.

The suprapubic catheter is used in temporary situations such as bladder, vesical neck, prostate, and urethral surgery. Suprapubic catheterization may be used instead of urethral catheterization, especially in the young or infant boy and when a urethral catheter cannot be inserted. The suprapubic catheter is also used long-term in selected patients (e.g., male quadriplegic patient who tends to form penoscrotal fistulas).

A suprapubic catheter is prone to poor drainage because of mechanical obstruction of the catheter tip by the bladder wall, sediment, and clots. Nursing interventions to ensure patency of the tube include (1) preventing tube kinking by coiling the excess tubing and maintaining gravity drainage, (2) having the patient turn from side to side, and (3) milking the tube. If these measures are not effective, the catheter is irrigated with sterile technique after a physician's order has been obtained.

If the patient experiences bladder spasms that are difficult to control, urinary leakage may result. Oxybutynin (Ditropan) or other oral antispasmodics or belladonna and opium (B & O) suppositories may be prescribed to decrease bladder spasms.

NEPHROSTOMY TUBES

The nephrostomy tube (catheter) is inserted on a temporary basis to preserve renal function when a complete obstruction of the ureter is present. It is inserted directly into the pelvis of the kidney and attached to connecting tubing for closed drainage. The principle is the same as with the ureteral catheter; that is, the catheter should never be kinked, laid or leaned on, or clamped. If the patient complains of excessive pain in the area or if there is excessive drainage around the tube, the catheter should be checked for patency. If irrigation is ordered, strict aseptic technique is required. No more than 5 ml of sterile saline solution is gently instilled at one time to prevent overdistention of the kidney pelvis and renal damage. Infection and secondary stone formation are complications associated with the insertion of a nephrostomy tube.

INTERMITTENT CATHETERIZATION

An alternative approach to a long-term indwelling catheter is intermittent catheterization.[28] It is being used with increasing frequency in conditions characterized by neurogenic bladder (e.g., spinal cord injuries, chronic neurologic diseases) or bladder outlet obstruction in men. This type of catheterization may also be used in the oliguric and anuric phases of acute renal failure to reduce the possibility of infection from an indwelling catheter. Intermittent catheterization is also used postoperatively, often after a surgical procedure for female incontinence or radioactive seed implantation into the prostate for cancer. The main goal of intermittent catheterization is to prevent urinary retention, stasis, and compromised blood supply to the bladder caused by prolonged pressure.

The technique consists of inserting a urethral catheter into the bladder every 3 to 5 hours. Some patients do intermittent catheterization only once or twice a day to measure residual urine and to ensure an empty bladder. Patients should be instructed to wash and rinse the catheter and their hands with soap and water before and after catheterization. Lubricant is necessary for men and may make catheterization more com-

fortable for women. The catheter may be inserted by the patient or the care provider. The bladder is emptied and the catheter is removed. The catheter can be dried and placed in a carrying pouch, purse, or folded in a paper towel until it is next needed. The same catheter can be used for weeks at a time. In general, patients should change the catheter every 2 to 4 weeks.

In the hospital, sterile technique is used. For home care, a clean technique that includes good hand washing with soap and water is used. There has been no significant increase in infection with the use of an appropriate clean technique as compared with sterile technique.[28] The patient is taught to observe for signs of UTI so that treatment can be instituted early. If indicated, some patients are placed on a regimen of prophylactic antibiotics.

SURGERY OF THE URINARY TRACT

RENAL AND URETERAL SURGERY

The most common indications for nephrectomy are a renal tumor, polycystic kidneys that are bleeding or severely infected, massive traumatic injury to the kidney, and the elective removal of a kidney from a donor. Surgery involving the ureters and kidneys is most commonly performed to remove calculi that become obstructive, correct congenital anomalies, and divert urine when necessary.

Preoperative Management

The basic needs of the patient undergoing renal and ureteral surgery are similar to those of any patient who experiences surgery (see Chapters 16 through 18). In addition, it is especially important preoperatively to ensure adequate fluid intake and a normal electrolyte balance. The patient should be told that there will probably be a flank incision on the affected side and that surgery will require a hyperextended, side-lying position. This position frequently causes the patient to experience muscle aches after surgery. If a nephrectomy is planned, the patient must be assured that one working kidney is sufficient to maintain normal renal function.

Postoperative Management

Specific postoperative needs of a patient are related to urine output, respiratory status, and abdominal distention.

Urine Output. In the immediate postoperative period, urine output should be determined at least every 1 to 2 hours. Drainage from various catheters should be recorded separately. The catheter or tube should not be clamped or irrigated without a specific order. The total urine output should be at least 30 to 50 ml per hour. It is also important to assess for urine drainage on the dressing and to estimate the amount. Daily weighing of the patient is important. The same scale should be used, properly balanced, and the patient should wear similar clothing and dressings each time.

It is important to observe and monitor the color and consistency of urine. Urine with increased amounts of mucus, blood, or sediment may occlude the drainage tubing or catheter.

Respiratory Status. Renal surgery is frequently performed through a flank incision just below the diaphragm and frequently involves removal of the twelfth rib. Postoperatively, it is important to ensure adequate ventilation. The patient is often reluctant to turn, cough, and deep breathe

Table **43-19**	Types of Urinary Diversion Surgery Requiring Collection Devices			
Type	Description	Advantages	Disadvantages	Special Considerations
▪ Ileal conduit	Ureters are implanted into part of ileum or colon that has been resected from intestinal tract. Abdominal stoma is created.	Relatively good urine flow with few physiologic alterations	External appliance necessary to continually collect urine	Surgical procedure is more complex. Postoperative complications may be increased. Reabsorption of urea by ileum occurs. Meticulous attention is necessary to care for stoma and collecting device.
▪ Cutaneous ureterostomy	Ureters are excised from bladder and brought through abdominal wall, and stoma is created. Ureteral stomas may be created from both ureters, or ureters may be brought together and one stoma created.	No need for major surgery as required with ileal conduit	External appliance necessary because of continuous urine drainage; possibility of stricture or stenosis of small stoma	Periodic catheterizations may be required to dilate stomas to maintain patency.
▪ Nephrostomy	Catheter is inserted into pelvis of kidney. Procedure may be done to one or both kidneys and may be temporary or permanent. It is most frequently done in advanced disease as palliative procedure.	No need for major surgery	High risk of renal infection; predisposition to calculus formation from catheter	Nephrostomy tube may have to be changed every month. Catheter must never be clamped.

because of the incisional pain. Adequate pain medication should be given to ensure the patient's comfort and ability to perform coughing and deep-breathing exercises. Frequently, additional respiratory devices such as an incentive spirometer are used every 2 hours while the patient is awake. In addition, early and frequent ambulation assists in maintaining adequate respiratory function.

Abdominal Distention. Abdominal distention is present to some degree in most patients who have had surgery on their kidneys or ureters. It is most commonly due to paralytic ileus caused by manipulation and compression of the bowel during surgery. Oral intake is restricted until bowel sounds are present (usually 24 to 48 hours after surgery). IV fluids are given until the patient can take oral fluids. Progression to a regular diet follows.

Laparoscopic Nephrectomy

Laparoscopic nephrectomy can be performed in selected situations to remove a diseased kidney. Laparoscopic nephrectomy can also be used to obtain a kidney from a living related donor to be transplanted into a person with end-stage renal disease. In contrast to the open incision of about 7 in (18 cm) required in a conventional nephrectomy, a laparoscopic nephrectomy is performed using five puncture sites of less than 0.5 inches (12 mm). One incision is to view the kidney and the other is to dissect it. The laparoscope contains a miniature camera so the surgeons can watch what they are doing on a video monitor. Once dissected, the kidney is maneuvered into a nylon impermeable

sack, and its contents can then be safely removed from the patient. As compared with a conventional nephrectomy, the laparoscopic approach is less painful and requires no sutures or staples, a shorter hospital stay, and a much faster recovery.

URINARY DIVERSION

Urinary diversion may be performed with and without cystectomy. Urinary diversion procedures are performed to treat cancer of the bladder, neurogenic bladder, congenital anomalies, strictures, trauma to the bladder, and chronic infections with deterioration of renal function. Numerous urinary diversion techniques and bladder substitutes are possible, including an incontinent urinary diversion, continent urinary diversion catheterized by patient, or an orthotopic bladder so the patient voids urethrally.[29] Types of these surgical procedures are presented in Table 43-19 and Fig. 43-8.

Incontinent Urinary Diversion

Incontinent urinary diversion is diversion to the skin, requiring an appliance. The simplest form is the cutaneous ureterostomy, but scarring and strictures led to the use of ileal or colonic conduits. The most commonly performed incontinent urinary diversion procedure is the ileal conduit (ileal loop). In this procedure a 6- to 8-inch (15 to 20 cm) segment of the ileum is converted into a conduit for urinary drainage. The colon (colon conduit) can be used instead of the ileum. The ureters are anastomosed into one end of the conduit, and the other end of the bowel is brought out through the abdominal

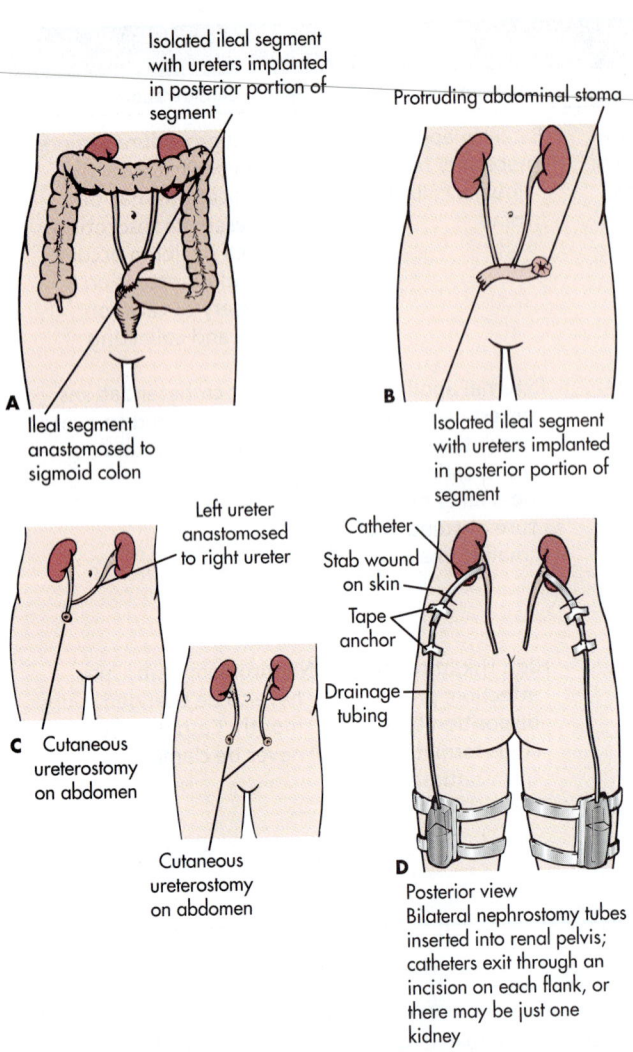

Fig. 43-8   Methods of urinary diversion. **A,** Ureteroileosigmo-idostomy. **B,** Ileal loop (or ileal conduit). **C,** Ureterostomy (transcutaneous ureterostomy and bilateral cutaneous ureterostomies). **D,** Nephrostomy.

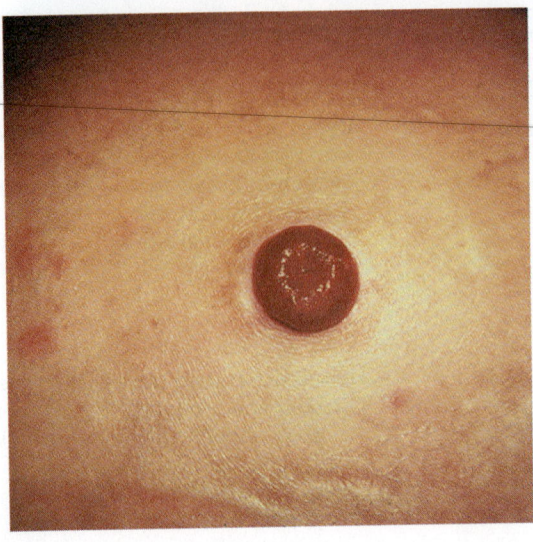

Fig. 43-9   Ideal urinary stoma. It is symmetric, has no skin breakdown, and protrudes about 1.5 cm; the mucosa is a healthy red and the configuration is flat when the patient is upright and supine.

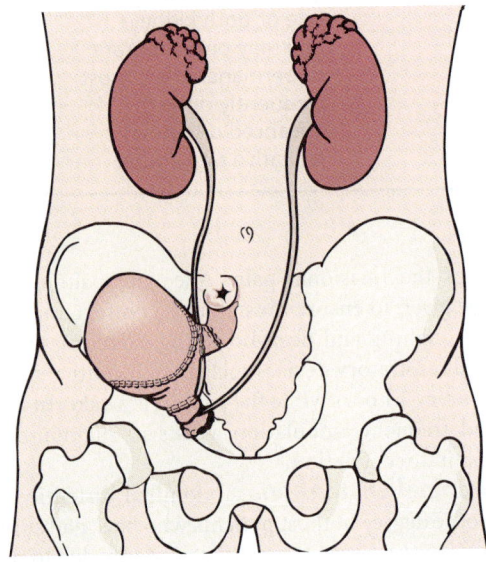

Fig. 43-10   Creation of a Kock pouch with implantation of ureters into one intussuscepted portion of the pouch and creation of a stoma with the other intussuscepted portion.

wall to form a stoma (Fig. 43-9). Although the segment of bowel remains supported by the mesentery, it is completely isolated from the intestinal tract. The bowel is anastomosed and continues to function normally. Because there is no valve and no voluntary control over the stoma, drops of urine flow from the stoma every few seconds, requiring the use of a permanent external collecting device. The visible stoma and the need for external collection devices are obvious disadvantages of this procedure. The lifelong care and dealing with the stoma and collection devices may be psychologically difficult. These problems have stimulated the increasing use of continent diversions and orthotopic bladder substitutes.

Continent Urinary Diversions

A *continent urinary diversion* is an intraabdominal urinary reservoir that is catheterizable or with an outlet controlled by the anal sphincter. Continent diversions are internal pouches created similarly to the ileal conduit. Reservoirs have been constructed from the ileum, ileocecal segment, or colon. Large segments of bowel are altered to prevent peristaltic action. A continence mechanism is formed between this large, low-pressure reservoir and the stoma by intussuscepting a portion of bowel. In this way, a patient does not leak involuntarily. The patient with a continent reservoir needs to self-catheterize every 4 to 6 hours but does not need to wear external attachments. Examples of continent diversions are the Kock (Fig. 43-10), Mainz, Indiana, and Florida pouches. A main difference between the various diversions is the segment of bowel used. For example, the Indiana pouch uses the right colon as

RESEARCH
IMPLICATIONS FOR NURSING PRACTICE

Quality of Life with Continent Urinary Diversion

Citation Sullivan LD and others: An evaluation of quality of life in patients with continent urinary diversions after cystectomy, *Br J Urol* 81:699, 1998.

Purpose To determine the long-term results and assess the quality of life in patients with continent urinary diversions after cystectomy.

Methods Eighty-six patients who received a continent urinary diversion were evaluated. The evaluation comprised a review of their hospital charts and clinic visits at 3 months and then yearly. Quality of life issues were assessed using a questionnaire pertaining to the patient's urinary symptoms, activity level, and overall well-being while living with a continent urinary diversion.

Results and Conclusions There was an acceptable rate of complications, with stone formation and urinary tract infection as the most common. Continence was rated as good in most patients, with no patient reporting complete incontinence. Undesirable urinary symptoms occurred less often than 20% of the time in most patients. Although there was a significant effect on sex life, the overall quality of life appeared to be very good, as 70% of the patients had no limitations to their activities.

Implications for Nursing Practice Bladder removal and urinary diversion result in significant physiologic and psychoemotional issues. Continent urinary diversions provide both a functional and a psychologic advantage to patients who have undergone a cystectomy. Patient counseling, education, and follow-up care and support can contribute to facilitating a positive outcome for patients.

a reservoir and has become a popular form of continent urinary diversion.

Orthotopic Bladder Substitution

Orthotopic bladder substitutes can be derived from various segments of the intestines. An isolated segment of the distal ileum is often preferred. Various procedures include the hemi-Kock pouch, Studer pouch, and the ileal W-neobladder. In these procedures the bowel is surgically reshaped to become a neobladder. The ureters and urethra are sutured into the neobladder. Orthotopic bladder substitution has been more commonly done in men because in women the urethra is usually removed when the bladder is resected.[30] The advantage of orthotopic bladder substitution is that it allows for natural micturition. Incontinence is a possible problem with this technique, and intermittent catheterization may need to be used.

NURSING MANAGEMENT: URINARY DIVERSION

■ Preoperative Management

The patient awaiting cystectomy and urinary diversion must be given a great deal of information. The nurse must assess ability and readiness to learn before initiating a teaching program. If the patient is not ready to learn, the teaching plan should be adjusted. The patient's anxiety and fear may be decreased by the information. However, the anxiety and fear may also interfere with learning. The patient's family should be involved in the teaching process. A discussion of the social aspects of living with a stoma (including clothing, changes in body image and sexuality, exercise, and odor) provides the patient with facts that may allay some fears. The patient who will have a continent diversion must be taught to catheterize and irrigate the pouch and be able to adhere to a strict catheterization schedule. The patient with an orthotopic neobladder may have problems with incontinence. Concerns about the effect on sexual activities should be discussed. The enterostomal therapy nurse should be involved in the preoperative phase of the patient's care. A visit from an ostomate or enterostomal therapy nurse can be helpful. Additional interventions are presented in NCP 43-3.

■ Postoperative Management

Nursing interventions during the postoperative period (see NCP 43-1 for care after an ileal conduit) should be planned to prevent surgical complications such as postoperative atelectasis and shock (see Chapter 18). After pelvic surgery, there is an increased incidence of thrombophlebitis. With removal of part of the bowel, there is an increased incidence of paralytic ileus and small bowel obstruction, the patient is NPO, and a nasogastric tube is necessary for 3 to 5 days.

Specific attention should be given to preventing injury to the stoma and maintaining urine output. Mucus is present in the urine because it is secreted by the intestines as a result of the irritating effect of the urine. The patient should be told that this is a normal occurrence. A high fluid intake is encouraged to "flush" the ileal conduit or continent diversion.

When an ileal conduit is created, the skin around the stoma requires meticulous care. Alkaline encrustations with dermatitis may occur when alkaline urine comes in contact with exposed skin (Fig. 43-11). Other common peristomal skin problems include yeast infections, product allergies, and shearing effect excoriations. Changing appliances (pouches) is discussed in Table 43-20. A properly fitting appliance is essential to prevent skin problems. The appliance should be about 0.1 inch (0.2 cm) larger than the stoma. It is normal for the stoma to shrink within the first few weeks after surgery. The urine is kept acidic to prevent alkaline encrustations.

Acceptance of the surgery and of alterations in body image is needed to ensure the patient's best adjustment. Concerns of the patient include fear that the stoma will be offensive to others and will interfere with sexual, personal, professional, and recreational activities. The patient should know that few activities, if any, will be restricted as a result of the urinary diversion.

43-3   NURSING CARE PLAN   PATIENT WITH AN ILEAL CONDUIT

Expected Patient Outcomes	Nursing Interventions and *Rationales*

NURSING DIAGNOSIS   **Anxiety** *related to* effects of ileal conduit on lifestyle and relationships; lack of knowledge regarding surgical procedure, appliance (pouch), and its use *as manifested by* frequent questions about surgical procedure; drawn facies; pallor, restlessness, inability to sleep.

- Knowledgeable about preoperative, operative, and postoperative procedures, including both stoma and appliance.

- Instruct patient in preoperative, operative, and postoperative procedures including diet, medications, nasogastric tubes, IVs, NPO status, pain management, turning, deep breathing, and leg exercises *to reduce anxiety and facilitate patient's progress through postoperative recovery.*
- Demonstrate how to apply appliance and use equipment *because knowledge before surgery reduces patient's postoperative concerns.*
- Answer questions honestly and provide emotional support *to reduce fear of the unknown and convey a caring attitude.*
- Arrange for visit with person with an ileal conduit or with enterostomal therapist *to provide patient with significant information related to ostomy care.*

NURSING DIAGNOSIS   **Risk for UTI** *related to* surgical procedure, ureteral obstruction, chronic use of external appliance, and incorrect or inadequate stoma care.

- No urinary tract infection.

- Assess patient for elevation in body temperature, pain in back or abdomen, bloody or cloudy urine, decrease in urinary output *to ensure early detection of UTI.*
- Empty appliance q2-3hr or when one-third full of urine *to reduce risk of urinary reflux.*
- Use bedside drainage bag at night *to prevent reflux of urine into conduit.*
- Instruct patient about symptoms to be reported *as indicators of possible infection.*
- Encourage high fluid intake *to maintain adequate urine flow.*

NURSING DIAGNOSIS   **Body image disturbance** *related to* effects of change in body function on lifestyle or relationships *as manifested by* negative feelings about self, refusal to look at or touch stoma or participate in self-care, expression of concern about effect on family and lifestyle.

- Acceptance of changes in body image and function.

- Encourage patient to share feelings *to provide opportunity to assist with issues and misconceptions and plan appropriate interventions.*
- Demonstrate willingness to listen and answer questions *to convey interest in the patient's concerns and to provide needed information.*
- Provide information about surgery and expected effects *to reduce anxiety associated with the unknown and altered body function.*
- Determine the need for additional support (e.g., psychiatric support, visit by an ostomate) *because these persons may provide new information and suggestions for ways to modify lifestyle.*
- Encourage gradual involvement in self-care *because independence in self-care helps improve self-esteem.*

NURSING DIAGNOSIS   **Ineffective management of therapeutic regimen** *related to* lack of knowledge regarding stoma and appliance care *as manifested by* expression of concern about how to manage ileal conduit, frequent questions or inaccurate responses regarding stoma care.

- Able to change stoma bag and cleanse stoma.
- Able to maintain permanent appliance.

- Demonstrate proper method of changing stoma bag and have patient give return demonstration *to teach correct care and evaluate learning.*
- Teach measures such as high fluid intake, regular activity, and urine acidification *to prevent urinary calculi and infection.*
- Teach practices such as proper stoma and pouch care; empty or change pouch when one-third to one-half full; avoid odor-producing foods such as onions, fish, eggs, cheese; drink cranberry juice or use a liquid appliance deodorant *to enable satisfactory self-care.*

Continued

43-3 NURSING CARE PLAN PATIENT WITH AN ILEAL CONDUIT—continued

Expected Patient Outcomes	Nursing Interventions and *Rationales*

NURSING DIAGNOSIS Risk for impaired skin integrity *related to* ill-fitting appliance, inadequate hygiene, and lack of knowledge regarding stoma care.

- Intact, viable stoma.
- Clean and intact skin surrounding stoma.

- Assess for improperly fitted appliance, reddened and irritated skin around stoma *to ensure prompt identification of the problem.*
- Check appliance position *to prevent leakage of caustic drainage onto skin.*
- Observe stoma for any bleeding or eroded areas *for early identification and treatment of complications.*
- Cleanse stoma as ordered *to reduce encrustations and bacterial contact with the stoma and surrounding skin.*
- Allow no tight clothing or binders over stoma *to enable unobstructed circulation of blood and flow of urine.*

NURSING DIAGNOSIS Risk for altered sexuality patterns *related to* perceived or actual effects of surgery on sexual activity.

- Satisfaction with sexual practices.

- Assess patient's concerns related to sexuality such as future sexual functioning and lack of understanding by significant other *to determine presence or extent of problem.*
- Provide accurate information related to sexual activity *so patient will know the effect of this surgery on sexual activities/practices.*
- Inform female patient about water-based vaginal lubricant for intercourse *to reduce dyspareunia related to inadequate vaginal lubrication;* teach Kegel exercises *to promote control of the pubococcygeal muscles around the vagina to ease dyspareunia.*

COLLABORATIVE PROBLEMS

Nursing Goals	Nursing Interventions and *Rationales*

POTENTIAL COMPLICATION Thrombophlebitis *related to* surgery involving pelvic manipulation.

- Monitor for signs of thrombophlebitis.
- Report deviations from acceptable parameters.
- Initiate appropriate medical and nursing interventions.

- Assess for signs of thrombophlebitis such as swelling, warmth, and pain in legs *to ensure early identification and treatment.*
- Teach patient method to do range-of-motion exercises for legs while in bed and instruct patient to keep legs uncrossed *to improve circulation in legs and reduce venous stasis.*
- Turn patient q2hr while in bed *to improve circulation to all body systems.*
- Increase activity level gradually and have patient ambulate as soon as possible *to improve circulation, especially in lower extremities.*
- Provide elastic compression stockings for legs as ordered *to provide support around veins and improve venous return of blood.*
- Administer anticoagulants if ordered *to reduce risk of thrombophlebitis by increasing clotting time.*

POTENTIAL COMPLICATION Paralytic ileus *related to* surgical manipulation of bowel.

- Monitor for signs of paralytic ileus.
- Report deviations from acceptable parameters.
- Initiate appropriate medical and nursing interventions.

- Assess patient for signs of paralytic ileus such as absence of bowel sounds, abdominal distention, cramping pain, nausea and vomiting *to enable early identification and treatment.*
- Maintain patency of nasogastric tube *to prevent accumulation and ensure removal of gastric secretions.*
- Encourage early ambulation *to promote peristalsis.*
- Administer IV fluids as ordered *to maintain fluid and electrolyte balance.*
- Monitor fluid and electrolyte levels *to identify imbalance and enable prompt treatment.*
- Assess for presence of bowel sounds, flatus, and bowel movements *as indicators of peristalsis.*

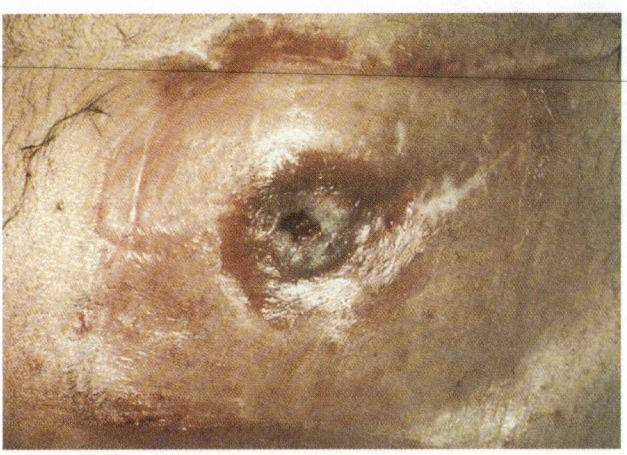

Fig. 43-11   Ammonia salt encrustation secondary to alkaline urine.

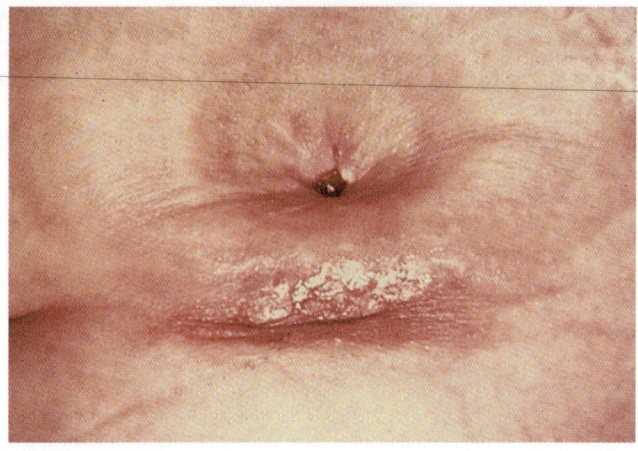

Fig. 43-12   Retracted urinary stoma with pressure sore from faceplate above stoma.

PATIENT & FAMILY TEACHING GUIDE
Table 43-20   Changing Ileal Conduit Appliances

Temporary Appliance	Permanent Appliance*
1. Cut hole in pouch to fit over stoma (pouch 3.2 mm [⅛ in] larger than stoma).	1. Keep appliance in place for 2-14 days.
2. Remove old pouch.	2. Change appliance when fluid intake has been restricted for several hours.
3. Clean area gently and remove old adhesive.	3. Have patient sit or stand in front of mirror.
4. Wash area with warm water.	4. Moisten edge of faceplate with adhesive solvent and gently remove.
5. Place wick (rolled-up 4 × 4 in pad) over stoma to keep area dry during rest of procedure.	5. Clean skin with adhesive solvent.
6. Dry skin around stoma.	6. Wash skin with warm water. (Patient may shower.)
7. Apply tincture of benzoin or other skin protectant around stoma to area where pouch will be placed.	7. Dry skin and inspect.
8. Apply pouch by first smoothing its edges toward side and lower portion of body.	8. Place wick (rolled up 4 × 4 in pad) over stoma to keep skin free of urine.
9. Remove wick and complete application of bag.	9. Apply skin cement to faceplate and skin.
10. If patient is usually in bed, apply bag so that it lies toward side of body.	10. Place appliance over stoma.
11. If patient is ambulatory, apply bag so that it lies vertically.	11. Wash removed appliance with soap and lukewarm water; soak in distilled vinegar; rinse with lukewarm water and air dry.
12. Connect drainage tubing to pouch.	
13. Keep drainage pouch on same side of bed as stoma.	

*Many disposable appliances with self-adhesive backing are used as permanent appliances.

Discharge planning after an ileal conduit includes teaching the patient symptoms of obstruction or infection and care of the ostomy. The patient with an ileal conduit is fitted for a permanent appliance 7 to 10 days after surgery and may need to be refitted at a later time, depending on the degree of stoma shrinkage. Appliances are made of a variety of products, including natural and synthetic rubbers, plastics, and metals. Most appliances have a faceplate that adheres to the skin, a collecting pouch, and an opening to drain the pouch. The faceplate may be secured to the skin with glues, adhesives, or adhering synthetic wafers. Some appliances do not require adhesives, but their design relies on pressure to keep the pouch in place. If improperly fitted or applied, the faceplate may cause skin problems (Fig. 43-12). The patient needs information on where to purchase supplies, emergency telephone numbers, location of ostomy clubs, and follow-up visits with an enterostomal therapist. Physician follow-up is imperative to monitor and correct homeostatic abnormalities and to prevent complications and renal function deterioration.

CRITICAL THINKING EXERCISES

CASE STUDY

Urinary Tract Infection

Patient Profile

Sue, a 28-year-old woman, was seen in the nurse practitioner's office for a history of painful, frequent urination.

Subjective Data

- Has had a history of painful, frequent urination with passage of small volumes of urine for 3 days
- Has had intermittent fever, chills, and back pain during these 3 days
- Was frightened when she saw blood in her urine
- Is anxious because her father died of kidney cancer

Objective Data

Physical Examination

- Complains of bilateral flank pain and abdominal tenderness to palpation
- Temperature is 100.4° F (38° C)

Diagnostic Study

- Urinalysis : pyuria and hematuria

Critical Thinking Questions

1. What are the most common organisms that cause UTIs?
2. What factors predispose a patient to a UTI?
3. What is the difference between upper and lower UTIs?
4. What nursing interventions will help Sue cope with her symptoms?
5. What can the nurse do to help Sue prevent another UTI?
6. Based on the data presented, write one or more appropriate nursing diagnoses. Are there any collaborative problems?

NURSING RESEARCH ISSUES

1. In the patient with UTI, what are the most effective methods to ensure compliance with therapy and follow-up care?
2. What therapeutic measures are most effective in treating stress incontinence?
3. What are the differences in quality of life of the patient with an ileal conduit as compared with the patient with a continent urinary diversion?
4. What are the most effective ways to manage pain following lithotripsy?
5. Does biofeedback improve the effectiveness of pelvic muscle exercises?

REVIEW QUESTIONS

The number of the question corresponds to the same-numbered objective at the beginning of the chapter.

1. In teaching a patient with pyelonephritis about the disorder, the nurse informs the patient that the organisms that cause pyelonephritis most commonly reach the kidneys through
   a. the bloodstream.
   b. the lymphatic system.
   c. a descending infection.
   d. an ascending infection.
2. The nurse teaches the female patient who has frequent urinary tract infections that she should
   a. urinate after sexual intercourse.
   b. take tub baths with bubble bath.
   c. take prophylactic sulfonamides for the rest of her life.
   d. restrict fluid intake to prevent the need for frequent voiding.
3. The immunologic mechanisms involved in glomerulonephritis include
   a. tubular blocking by precipitates of bacteria and antibody reactions.
   b. deposition of immune complexes and complement along the GBM.
   c. thickening of the GBM from autoimmune microangiopathic changes.
   d. destruction of glomeruli by proteolytic enzymes contained in the GBM.
4. One of the most important roles of the nurse in relation to acute poststreptococcal glomerulonephritis is to
   a. promote early diagnosis and treatment of sore throats and skin lesions.
   b. encourage patients to request antibiotic therapy for all upper respiratory infections.

   c. teach patients with APSGN that long-term prophylactic antibiotic therapy is necessary to prevent recurrence.
   d. monitor patients for respiratory symptoms that indicate that the disease is affecting the alveolar basement membrane.
5. The edema that occurs in nephrotic syndrome is due to
   a. decreased aldosterone secretion from adrenal insufficiency.
   b. increased hydrostatic pressure caused by sodium retention.
   c. increased fluid retention caused by decreased glomerular filtration.
   d. decreased colloidal osmotic pressure caused by loss of serum albumin.
6. A patient is admitted to the hospital with severe renal colic caused by renal lithiasis. The nurse's first priority in management of the patient is to
   a. administer narcotics as prescribed.
   b. obtain supplies for straining all urine.
   c. encourage fluid intake of 3 to 4 liters per day.
   d. keep the patient NPO in preparation for surgery.
7. The nurse recommends genetic counseling for the children of a patient with
   a. nephrotic syndrome.
   b. chronic pyelonephritis.
   c. malignant nephrosclerosis.
   d. adult-onset polycystic renal disease.
8. The nurse encourages strict diabetic control in the patient prone to diabetic nephropathy knowing that the renal tissue changes that may occur in this condition include
   a. uric acid calculi and nephrolithiasis.
   b. renal sugar-crystal calculi and cysts.
   c. lipid deposits in the glomeruli and nephrons.
   d. thickening of the GBM and glomerulosclerosis.

9. The nurse identifies a risk factor for kidney and bladder cancer in a patient who relates a history of
   a. aspirin use.
   b. tobacco use.
   c. chronic alcohol abuse.
   d. use of artificial sweeteners.

10. In planning nursing interventions to increase bladder control in the patient with urinary incontinence the nurse includes
    a. restricting fluid intake after dinner in the evening.
    b. using incontinence pads to prevent patient embarrassment.
    c. clamping and releasing a catheter to increase bladder tone.
    d. teaching the patient biofeedback mechanisms to suppress the urge to void.

11. A patient with a ureterolithotomy returns from surgery with a nephrostomy tube in place. Postoperative nursing care of the patient includes
    a. encouraging the patient to drink fruit juices and milk.
    b. forcing fluids of at least 2 to 3 L per day after nausea has subsided.
    c. notifying the physician if nephrostomy tube drainage is more than 30 ml/hr.
    d. irrigating the nephrostomy tube with 10 ml of normal saline solution as needed.

12. A patient has had a cystectomy and ileal conduit diversion performed. Four days postoperatively, mucous shreds are seen in the drainage bag. The nurse should
    a. notify the physician.
    b. notify the charge nurse.
    c. irrigate the drainage tube.
    d. chart it as a normal observation.

References

1. Marchiondo K: A new look at urinary tract infection, *AJN* 98:34, 1998.
2. Barnett BJ, Stephens DS: Urinary tract infection: an overview, *Am J Med Sci* 314:245, 1997.
3. Schaeffer AJ: Infections of the urinary tract. In Walsh PC and others, editors: *Campbell's urology,* ed 7, Philadelphia, 1998, Saunders.
4. Nicolle LE: Asymptomatic bacteriuria in the elderly, *Infect Dis Clin North Am* 11:647, 1997.
5. Hooton TM, Stamm WE: Diagnosis and treatment of uncomplicated urinary tract infection, *Infect Dis Clin North Am* 11:551, 1997.
6. Karlowicz KA: Pharmacologic therapy for acute cystitis in adults: a review of treatment options, *Urol Nurs* 17:106, 1997.
7. Stapleton A, Stamm WE: Prevention of urinary tract infection, *Infect Dis Clin North Am* 11:719, 1997.
8. Pearson BD: Liquidate a myth: reducing liquid intake is not advisable for elderly with urine control problems, *Urol Nurs* 13:86, 1993.
9. Kaufman MW and others: Caring for the patient with interstitial cystitis, *Medsurg Nurs* 6:203, 1997.
10. Irwin P, Galloway N: Surgical management of interstitial cystitis, *Urol Clin North Am* 21:145, 1994.
11. Wiseman KC: New insights on Goodpasture's syndrome, *ANNA J* 20:17, 1993.
12. Orth SR, Ritz E: The nephrotic syndrome, *N Engl J Med* 338:1202, 1998.
13. Humphreys MH: Human immunodeficiency virus–associated glomerulosclerosis, *Kidney Int* 48:311, 1995.
14. Kupin WL: A practical approach to nephrolithiasis, *Hosp Pract* 30:57, 1995.
15. Sosa RE, Martin TV: Critical challenges of renal calculi in women, *Medscape Women's Health* 1:8, 1996.
16. Wolf JS, Clayman RV: Percutaneous nephrostolithotomy. What is its role in 1997? *Urol Clin North Am* 24:43, 1997.
17. Nakada SY: The surgical management of renal stones: selecting what is best, *Infect Urol* 10:42, 1997.
18. Miller-Hjelle MA and others: Polycystic kidney disease: an unrecognized emerging infectious disease? *Emerg Infect Dis* 3:113, 1997.
19. American Cancer Society: *Cancer facts and figures,* Atlanta, 1998.
20. Lerner L, Heaney J: Incidentally detected renal tumors, *Hosp Pract* 32:53, 1997.
21. Bukowski RM, Novick AC: Clinical practice guidelines: renal cell carcinoma, *Cleve Clin J Med* 64(suppl 1):S1, 1997.
22. Cohen SM: Urinary bladder carcinogenesis, *Toxicol Pathol* 26:121, 1998.
23. McCaffrey JA, Bajorin DF, Scher HI, Bosl GJ: Combined-modality therapy for bladder cancer, *Oncology* 11(suppl 9):18, 1997.
24. Fourcroy JL: Urogynecology update: incontinence, *Hosp Pract* 33:63, 1998.
25. Urinary Incontinence Guideline Panel: *Urinary incontinence in adults: clinical practice guideline,* AHCPR pub no 92-0038, Rockville, Md, 1996, Agency for Health Care Policy and Research, Public Health Service, US Department of Health and Human Services.
26. Bernier F, Harris L: Treating stress incontinence with the bladder neck support device, *Urol Nurs* 15:5, 1995.
27. Gallo ML and others: Quality of life improvement and the reliance urinary control insert, *Urol Nurs* 17:146, 1997.
28. Hollander JB, Biokno AC: Clean intermittent catheterization: an update, *Infect Urol* 9:118, 1996.
29. Turner WH, Studer UE: Cystectomy and urinary diversion, *Semin Surg Oncol* 13:350, 1997.
30. Montie JE, Park JM: Orthotopic diversion in women, *Semin Urol Oncol* 15:184, 1997.

Resources

American Urological Association
1120 North Charles Street
Baltimore, MD 21201
410-727-1100
Fax: 410-223-4370
http://www.auanet.org/

Bladder Health Council
American Foundation for Urologic Disease
300 West Pratt Street, Suite 401
Baltimore, MD 21201
410-727-2908
800-242-2383

National Association for Continence (NAFC)
PO Box 8310
Spartanburg, SC 29305
864-579-7900
800-BLADDER (252-3337)
http://www.medhelp.org/agsg/agsg1172.htm

Simon Foundation for Continence
PO Box 835
Wilmette, IL 60091
800-23-SIMON (237-4666)
708-864-3913
http://www.simonfoundation.org/html/

Society of Urological Nurses and Associates
East Holly Avenue, Box 56
Pitman, NJ 08071-0056
East Holly Avenue
888-827-7862
Fax: 609-589-7463

United Ostomy Association
19772 MacArthur Boulevard, Suite 200
Irvine, CA 92612-2405
800-826-0826
http://www.uoa.org/

Also see Resources for Chapter 44 on p. 1341.

For additional Internet resources, see the website for this book at www.mosby.com/MERLIN/medsurg_lewis

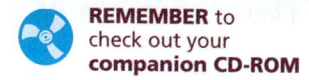

44

NURSING MANAGEMENT
Acute and Chronic Renal Failure

Gillian Brunier & Marilyn Bartucci

www.mosby.com/MERLIN/medsurg_lewis

LEARNING OBJECTIVES

1. Differentiate between acute and chronic renal failure.
2. Differentiate among the causes of prerenal, intrarenal, and postrenal acute renal failure.
3. Describe the clinical course of reversible acute renal failure.
4. Explain the collaborative care and nursing management of a patient in the oliguric and diuretic phases of acute renal failure.
5. Describe the systemic effects of chronic renal failure.
6. Explain the conservative collaborative care and the related nursing management of the patient with chronic renal failure.
7. Differentiate between peritoneal dialysis and hemodialysis in terms of purpose, indications for use, advantages and disadvantages, and nursing responsibilities.
8. Compare common vascular access sites used for hemodialysis.
9. Compare dialysis and renal transplantation as methods of treatment for end-stage renal disease.
10. Describe the nursing management of patients in the preoperative, intraoperative, and postoperative stages of kidney transplantation.
11. Explain the long-term problems of the patient with a kidney transplant.

Renal failure is severe impairment or total lack of kidney function. In renal failure there is an inability to excrete metabolic waste products and water, as well as functional disturbances of all body systems. Renal failure is classified as acute or chronic. Acute renal failure most commonly has a rapid onset. Although acute renal failure is potentially reversible, the mortality rate remains distressingly high in spite of advances in treatment.

Chronic renal failure usually develops insidiously over time and necessitates the initiation of dialysis or transplantation for long-term survival. The focus in chronic renal failure has changed from treating a terminally ill patient to dealing with a person who has a manageable chronic disease that requires long-term care. In dialysis, the change in focus is a result of technical advances. In renal transplant, the change in focus is a result of improved surgical techniques and immunosuppressive therapy.

ACUTE RENAL FAILURE

Acute renal failure is a clinical syndrome characterized by a rapid decline in renal function with progressive azotemia (an accumulation of nitrogenous waste products such as blood urea nitrogen [BUN]) and increasing levels of serum creatinine. *Uremia* is the condition in which azotemia progresses to a symptomatic state. Acute renal failure is usually associated with

a decrease in urinary output to less than 400 ml per day, although it is possible to have normal or increased urinary output. There is no correlation between the amount of urine produced and the severity of the renal failure.

Acute renal failure usually develops over hours or days with progressive elevations of BUN, creatinine, and potassium with or without oliguria. Most commonly, acute renal failure follows severe, prolonged hypotension or hypovolemia or contact with a nephrotoxic agent.

Etiology and Pathophysiology

The etiologies of acute renal failure are multiple and complex. They are categorized according to similar pathogenesis into prerenal, intrarenal (or renal parenchymal), and postrenal causes (Table 44-1).

Prerenal causes consist of factors outside the kidneys that reduce renal blood flow and lead to decreased glomerular perfusion and filtration. Hypovolemia can lead to decreased renal perfusion, as can cardiac failure, which decreases the effective circulating volume of the blood. Drugs that may start or complicate prerenal azotemia include nonsteroidal antiinflammatory drugs (NSAIDs), which block synthesis of vasodilating prostaglandins, and angiotensin-converting enzyme (ACE) inhibitors, which block synthesis of angiotensin II. Prerenal disease can lead to intrarenal disease (tubular necrosis) if renal ischemia is prolonged. Prerenal causes are the most common cause of acute renal failure, accounting for approximately 70% of all cases.[1]

Reviewed by Mary Jo Holechek, MS, CRNP, CS, CNN, Transplant Nurse Coordinator, Johns Hopkins Hospital, Baltimore, Md.

Table **44-1**	Common Causes of Acute Renal Failure		
Prerenal	**Intrarenal**		**Postrenal**

Prerenal	Intrarenal	Postrenal

■ Hypovolemia
   Hemorrhage
   Burns
   Dehydration
   Prolonged diarrhea or
     vomiting
■ Decreased cardiac output
   Myocardial infarction
   Cardiac arrhythmias
   Congestive heart failure
   Cardiogenic shock
   Pericardial tamponade
   Surgery (e.g., open heart)
■ Decreased peripheral
  vascular resistance
   Septic shock
   Anaphylaxis
   Neurologic injury
■ Renal vascular obstruction
   Thrombosis of renal arteries
   Bilateral renal vein
    thrombosis
   Embolism
	■ Nephrotoxic injury
	   Drugs (aminoglycosides [gentamicin, tobramycin,
	    amikacin], amphotericin B, cisplatin)
	   Radiographic contrast agents
	   Hemolytic blood transfusion reaction
	    (hemoglobin blocks tubules)
	   Severe crushing injury (myoglobin released from
	    muscles blocks tubules)
	   Chemicals (ethylene glycol, mercuric chloride,
	    carbon tetrachloride, lead, arsenic)
	■ Acute glomerulonephritis
	■ Acute pyelonephritis
	■ Toxemia of pregnancy
	■ Malignant hypertension
	■ Systemic lupus erythematosus
	■ Interstitial nephritis
	   Allergic (antibiotics [sulfonamides, rifampin],
	    nonsteroidal antiinflammatory drugs, ACE
	    inhibitors)
	   Infection (bacterial [e.g., acute pyelonephritis],
	    viral [e.g., CMV], fungal [e.g., candidiasis])
		■ Calculi formation
		■ Benign prostatic hyperplasia
		■ Prostate cancer
		■ Bladder cancer
		■ Trauma (to back, pelvis, or
		  perineum)
		■ Strictures
		■ Spinal cord disease

ACE, angiotensin-converting enzyme; *CMV,* cytomegalovirus.

Intrarenal causes include conditions that cause direct damage to the renal tissue (parenchyma) resulting in malfunctioning of nephrons. Intrarenal causes account for approximately 25% of all cases of acute renal failure.[1] Primary renal diseases such as acute glomerulonephritis and acute pyelonephritis may lead to acute renal failure. More commonly, acute tubular necrosis (ATN) is the predisposing insult. ATN may be caused by ischemia, nephrotoxins (e.g., antibiotics), hemoglobin released from hemolyzed red blood cells (RBCs), or myoglobin released from necrotic muscle cells. Nephrotoxic chemicals and drugs can cause obstruction of intrarenal structures by crystallization or actual damage to the epithelial cells of the tubules. The most common drugs that cause nephrotoxic injury are aminoglycoside antibiotics and radiocontrast agents. Hemoglobin and myoglobin block the tubules and cause renal vasoconstriction.

Postrenal causes involve mechanical obstruction of urinary outflow. As the flow of urine is blocked, urine backs up into the renal pelvis, ultimately resulting in renal failure. The most common causes are benign prostatic hyperplasia, calculi, trauma, prostate cancer, and tumors. Postrenal causes of acute renal failure account for less than 5% of cases, with a higher incidence among the elderly.[1] These causes are almost always treatable if identified before permanent kidney damage occurs.

The two major mechanisms that lead to acute renal failure are renal ischemia and nephrotoxic injury (Fig. 44-1). Acute renal failure that results from these two causes is usually referred to as ATN. Severe renal ischemia causes a disruption in the basement membrane and patchy destruction of the tubular epithelium. Nephrotoxic agents cause necrosis of tubular epithelial cells, which slough off and plug the tubules. Nephrotoxic injury usually leaves the basement membrane intact. ATN is potentially reversible if the basement membrane is not destroyed and if the necrotic tubular epithelium regenerates.

Possible pathologic processes involved in acute renal failure include the following:

1. *Renal vasoconstriction.* Hypovolemia and decreased renal blood flow stimulate renin release, which activates the angiotensin-aldosterone system (see Fig. 42-6) and results in constriction of the peripheral arteries and the renal afferent arterioles. With decreased renal blood flow, there is decreased glomerular capillary pressure and glomerular filtration rate (GFR), as well as tubular dysfunction and, ultimately, oliguria.

2. *Cellular edema.* Ischemia causes anoxia, which leads to endothelial cell edema. Cellular edema raises tissue pressures above capillary flow pressure; consequently, blood flow through the arterioles may still be altered after treatment of the underlying condition. Inadequate renal blood flow further depresses the GFR.

3. *Decreased glomerular capillary permeability.* Ischemia alters glomerular epithelial cells and thus decreases glomerular capillary permeability. This in turn reduces the GFR, which significantly reduces blood flow and leads to tubular dysfunction.

4. *Intratubular obstruction.* When tubules are damaged, interstitial edema occurs, and necrotic epithelial cells accumulate in the tubules. This accumulated debris also lowers the GFR by obstructing the tubules and increasing intratubular pressure.

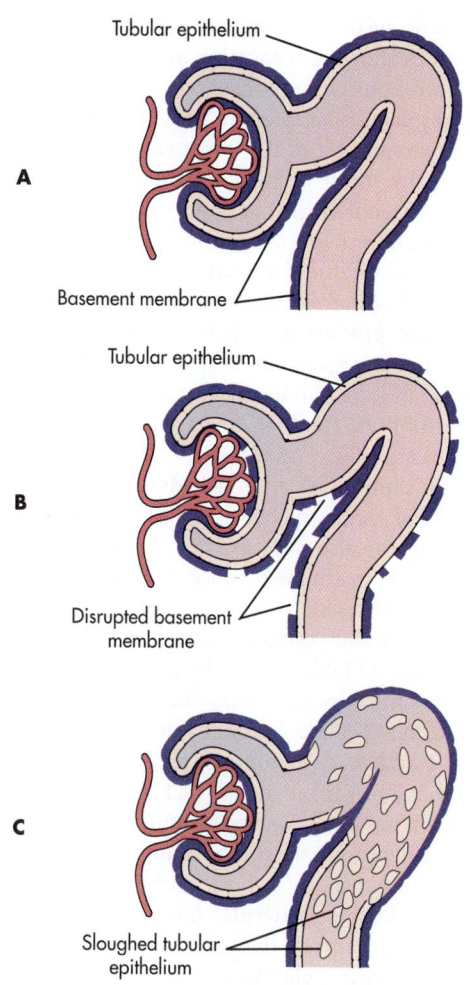

Fig. 44-1 Nephron destruction in acute renal failure. **A,** Normal nephron. **B,** Damage from renal ischemia results in disrupted basement membrane. **C,** Nephrotoxic agents can cause tubular injury.

5. *Leakage of glomerular filtrate.* Glomerular filtrate leaks back into plasma through holes in the damaged tubular membranes, which decreases intratubular fluid flow.

Clinical Course

Clinically acute renal failure may progress through the phases of oliguria, diuresis, and recovery. In some situations the patient does not recover from acute renal failure, and chronic renal failure results.

Oliguric Phase. The most common initial manifestation of acute renal failure is oliguria caused by a reduction in the GFR. The oliguria usually occurs within 1 to 7 days of the causative event. If the cause is ischemia, oliguria may occur within 24 hours, but when nephrotoxic drugs are involved, the onset may be delayed for as long as a week. Initially, the presence of anuria (≤400 ml urine output per 24 hours) is rare unless the precipitating cause is a urinary obstructive disorder. (Acute nonoliguric renal failure may also occur. In this situation, the onset may be less obvious with hypervolemia or an elevated BUN as the first presenting abnormality.) The du-

ration of the oliguric phase may range from a few days to several weeks. Some cases have lasted for several months. The average duration is about 10 to 14 days, but it rarely exceeds 4 weeks. The longer the oliguric phase lasts, the poorer the prognosis for recovery of renal function.

It is important to distinguish prerenal oliguria from oliguria of acute intrarenal failure. In prerenal oliguria there is no damage to the renal tissue. The oliguria is caused by a decrease in circulating blood volume (e.g., as a result of shock, burns, severe dehydration, decreased cardiac output) and is usually reversible. (Many causes of intrarenal failure are also potentially reversible.) With a decrease in circulating blood volume, autoregulatory mechanisms such as increases in angiotensin II, norepinephrine, and antidiuretic hormone (ADH) attempt to preserve blood flow to essential organs. Vasoconstriction occurs with sodium and water retention. Therefore prerenal oliguria is characterized by urine with a high specific gravity and a low sodium concentration.

In contrast, oliguria of intrarenal failure is characterized by urine with a normal specific gravity and a high sodium concentration, indicating that the injured tubules cannot respond to autoregulatory mechanisms. In addition, oliguria of intrarenal failure caused by ATN due to ischemia or toxins is characterized by the presence of granular or epithelial cell casts in the urine. The casts are formed from mucoprotein impressions of the necrotic renal tubular epithelial cells, which detach or slough into the tubules.

The manifestations of the oliguric phase are changes in urinary output, fluid and electrolyte abnormalities, and uremia. The nurse must be alert for the signs and symptoms of these changes.

Urinary changes. Urinary output decreases to less than 400 ml per 24 hours. The urine may be bloody but is usually not. A urinalysis may show casts, RBCs, white blood cells (WBCs), a specific gravity fixed at around 1.010, and urine osmolality at about 300 mOsm/kg (300 mmol/kg). This is the same specific gravity and osmolality as for plasma, reflecting tubular damage with a loss of concentrating ability by the kidney. Proteinuria may be present if the renal failure is related to glomerular membrane dysfunction.

Fluid volume excess. When urinary output decreases, fluid retention occurs. The severity of the symptoms depend on the extent of the fluid overload. The neck veins may become distended, the pulse may become more bounding, and peripheral and central edema and hypertension may develop. Fluid overload can eventually lead to congestive heart failure, pulmonary edema, and pericardial and pleural effusions.

Metabolic acidosis. In renal failure the kidneys cannot synthesize ammonia, which is needed for H^+ excretion, or excrete acid metabolites. The serum bicarbonate level decreases because bicarbonate is used up in buffering hydrogen ions. In addition, defective reabsorption and regeneration of bicarbonate occur. The patient may develop Kussmaul's respirations (rapid, deep respirations) to increase the excretion of carbon dioxide.

Sodium balance. Damaged tubules cannot conserve sodium. Consequently, the urinary excretion of sodium may increase, resulting in normal or below normal levels of serum sodium. Elevated sodium levels may be masked by hypervolemia (dilutional hyponatremia). However, excessive intake of sodium should be avoided because it can lead to volume expansion, hypertension, and congestive heart failure.

Potassium excess. The serum potassium levels increase, since the normal ability of the kidneys to excrete 80% to 90% of

Table **44-2**	Clinical Manifestations of Acute Renal Failure
Body System	**Clinical Manifestations**
Urinary	↓ Urinary output
	Proteinuria
	Casts
	↓ Specific gravity
	↓ Osmolality
	↑ Urinary sodium
Cardiovascular	Volume overload
	Congestive heart failure
	Hypotension (early)
	Hypertension (after development of fluid overload)
	Pericarditis
	Pericardial effusion
	Arrhythmias
Respiratory	Pulmonary edema
	Kussmaul's respirations
	Pleural effusions
Gastrointestinal	Nausea and vomiting
	Anorexia
	Stomatitis
	Bleeding
	Diarrhea
	Constipation
Hematologic	Anemia (development within 48 hr)
	Leukocytosis
	Defect in platelet functioning
Neurologic	Lethargy
	Convulsions
	Asterixis
	Memory impairment
Others	↑ Susceptibility to infection
	↑ BUN
	↑ Creatinine
	↑ Potassium
	↓ pH
	↓ Bicarbonate
	↓ Calcium
	↑ Phosphate

BUN, blood urea nitrogen.

the body's potassium is impaired. If the acute renal failure was caused by massive tissue trauma, the damaged cells release additional potassium to the extracellular fluid. Thus the patient with tissue injury may have an even higher serum potassium level. In addition, acidosis enhances the movement of potassium from intracellular to extracellular fluid.

When potassium levels exceed 6 mEq/L (6 mmol/L), treatment must be initiated immediately to prevent cardiac arrhythmias. Before clinical signs of hyperkalemia are apparent, the electrocardiogram (ECG) will show tall, peaked T waves, widening of the QRS complex, and ST depression. Progressive changes in the ECG, which are related to increasing potassium levels, are depicted in Fig. 15-13. The cardiac muscle is very intolerant of acute increases in potassium.

Calcium deficit and phosphate excess. A low serum calcium level results from decreased gastrointestinal (GI) absorption of calcium. To absorb calcium from the GI tract, activated vitamin D must be present. Only functioning kidneys can activate vitamin D, allowing absorption to occur. When calcium is removed from bones in response to parathyroid hormone secretion, phosphate is released as well. Elevated serum phosphate levels are a result of its decreased excretion by the kidneys. Normally most plasma calcium is found ionized (physiologically active form) or bound to protein. In renal failure it is unusual for hypocalcemia to be symptomatic because acidosis keeps more calcium in an ionized form. Sometimes a low serum level of ionized calcium can lead to tetany.

Nitrogenous product accumulation. The kidneys are the primary excretory organs for urea, an end product of protein metabolism, and creatinine, an end product of endogenous muscle metabolism. The BUN and serum creatinine levels are elevated in renal failure. An elevated BUN level must be interpreted with caution because dehydration and catabolism, caused by other factors such as infections, fever, severe injury, or GI bleeding, can also elevate BUN. The best serum indicator of renal failure is creatinine because it is not usually altered by other factors as is the BUN.

Eventually all body systems become involved in the acute uremic syndrome (Table 44-2). The extrarenal manifestations are generally similar to those found in the patient with chronic uremia (see Fig. 44-3 later in the chapter).

Diuretic Phase. The diuretic phase begins with a gradual increase in daily urine output of 1 to 3 L per day but may reach 3 to 5 L per day or more. Although urine output is increasing, the nephrons are still not fully functional. The high urine volume is caused by osmotic diuresis from the high urea concentration in the glomerular filtrate and the inability of the tubules to concentrate the urine. In this phase the kidneys have recovered their ability to excrete wastes but not to concentrate the urine. In this phase hypovolemia and hypotension can occur from massive fluid losses.

At this stage the uremia may still be severe, as reflected by low creatinine clearances and elevated serum creatinine and BUN levels. Because of the large losses of fluid and electrolytes, the patient must be monitored for hyponatremia, hypokalemia, and dehydration. The diuretic phase may last 1 to 3 weeks. Near the end of this phase the patient's acid-base, electrolyte, and waste product parameters begin to normalize.

Recovery Phase. The recovery phase begins when the GFR increases so that BUN and serum creatinine levels start to stabilize and then decrease. Although the major improvements occur in the first 1 to 2 weeks of this phase, renal function can continue to improve for up to 12 months after acute renal failure.

The outcome of acute renal failure is influenced by the patient's overall health, the severity of renal failure, and the number and type of complications. The mortality rate from acute renal failure varies from 30% to 60%, depending on the cause. Patients with ATN and oliguria have a 50% risk of mortality, especially when there is an underlying disease.[1] Many deaths are related to the underlying disease. However, the most common cause of death is infection. Infection occurs in 30% to 70% of individuals who develop acute renal failure. The incidence of infection is highest in the individual in whom surgery or traumatic injury contributed to renal failure.

Some individuals do not recover and progress to chronic renal failure. The older adult patient is less likely to recover normal renal function than the younger patient. Among the individuals who recover, the vast majority achieve clinically normal renal function with no complications (e.g., hypertension).

Diagnostic Studies

The most important tool for distinguishing prerenal, intrarenal, and postrenal causes is the history, including a thorough review of recent clinical events and drug therapy. Prerenal causes should be suspected when there is a history of heart disease or extracellular fluid volume loss or depletion. Intrarenal causes may be suspected if the patient has been taking potentially nephrotoxic medication or has a history of systemic disorders such as systemic lupus erythematosus. Postrenal causes are suggested by a history of changes in urinary stream, hematuria or pyuria, or cancer of the bladder or prostate.

Urinalysis is an important diagnostic test. Urine sediment containing abundant cells, casts, or proteins suggests intrarenal disorders. ATN is associated with abundant urinary casts. Normal urine sediment is possible in both prerenal and postrenal causes. Hematuria, pyuria, and crystals may be associated with postrenal causes.

If the cause of acute renal failure is difficult to determine from the history and physical examination, further testing may be necessary, such as a renal ultrasound, renal scan, retrograde pyelogram, computed tomography (CT) scan, or magnetic resonance imaging (MRI).

Collaborative Care

Because acute renal failure is potentially reversible, the primary goal of treatment is to maintain the patient in as normal a state as possible while the kidneys are repairing themselves (Table 44-3). The precipitating cause is determined and corrected if possible. Management is focused on controlling the patient's symptoms and preventing complications.

The first step is to determine if there is adequate intravascular volume and cardiac output to ensure adequate perfusion of the kidneys. Diuretic therapy is often administered along with volume expanders to prevent volume overload. Diuretic therapy includes loop diuretics (furosemide [Lasix], ethacrynic acid [Edecrin], bumetanide [Bumex]) or an osmotic diuretic (mannitol). If acute renal failure is already established, forcing fluids and diuresis is not effective and may in fact be harmful. Conservative therapy may be all that is necessary until renal function resumes. However, the general trend is to initiate early and frequent dialysis to minimize symptoms and prevent complications.

Fluid intake must be closely monitored during the oliguric phase. The common rule for calculating fluid replacement is to consider all losses for the previous 24 hours (e.g., urine, diarrhea, vomitus, blood) plus 500 to 600 ml for insensible losses (e.g., respirations, diaphoresis). For example, if a patient excreted 300 ml of urine on Tuesday with no other losses, fluid replacement on Wednesday would be 800 to 900 ml.

Hyperkalemia is one of the most dangerous complications in acute renal failure because it can cause life-threatening cardiac arrhythmias. The various therapies used to decrease potassium levels are listed in Table 44-4. Sodium polystyrene sulfonate (Kayexalate) should never be given to a patient with paralytic ileus.

COLLABORATIVE CARE

Table 44-3   Acute Renal Failure

Diagnostic
History and physical examination
Identification of precipitating cause
Serum creatinine and BUN levels
Serum electrolytes
Urinalysis
Renal ultrasound
Retrograde pyelogram (as indicated)
Renal scan (as indicated)
CT scan or MRI (as indicated)

Collaborative Therapy
Treatment of precipitating cause
Fluid restriction (500-600 ml plus previous 24 hr fluid loss)
Nutritional therapy
  Adequate protein provision (1.0-1.5 g/kg/day)
  Potassium restriction
  Phosphate restriction
  Sodium restriction
Measures to lower potassium (if elevated)*
Calcium supplements or phosphate-binding agents
Total parenteral nutrition (if indicated)†
Enteral nutrition (if indicated)†
Initiation of dialysis (if necessary)
Continuous renal replacement therapy (if necessary)

*See Table 44-4.
†Renal formulations of these two forms of nutrition are available.

Table 44-4   Therapies to Lower Serum Potassium Levels

1. **Regular Insulin Administration IV**
   Potassium moves into cells when insulin is given. Glucose is given concurrently to prevent hypoglycemia. When effects of insulin diminish, potassium shifts back out of cells.

2. **Sodium Bicarbonate**
   Therapy can correct acidosis and causes shift of potassium into cells.

3. **Calcium Gluconate IV**
   Therapy is given IV and generally used in advanced cardiac toxicity. Calcium raises the threshold for excitation resulting in arrhythmias.

4. **Dialysis**
   Hemodialysis can bring potassium levels to normal within 30 min to 2 hr. Peritoneal dialysis takes longer.

5. **Sodium Polystyrene Sulfonate (Kayexalate)**
   Cation-exchange resin is administered by mouth or retention enema. When resin is in the bowel, potassium is exchanged for sodium. Therapy removes 1 mEq of potassium per gram of drug. It is mixed in water with sorbitol to produce osmotic diarrhea, allowing for evacuation of potassium-rich stool from body.

6. **Dietary Restrictions**
   Daily potassium intake is limited to 40-50 mEq.

IV, intravenous.

The most common indications for the use of dialysis in acute renal failure include (1) volume overload resulting in congestive heart failure and pulmonary edema; (2) potassium level greater than 6 mEq/L (6 mmol/L) with ECG changes; (3) metabolic acidosis (serum bicarbonate level less than 15 mEq/L [15 mmol/L]); (4) BUN level greater than 120 mg/dl (43 mmol/L); (5) significant change in mental status; and (6) pericarditis, pericardial effusion, or cardiac tamponade. Laboratory values are only rough parameters, and clinical assessment is the most important guide in determining the need for dialysis.

If dialysis is required, there are two options available—hemodialysis (HD) and peritoneal dialysis (PD). HD has the advantage of efficiency and shorter duration compared with PD. However, it is technically more complicated because specialized equipment and vascular access is required and may require anticoagulation therapy to prevent blood clotting in the dialysis blood circuit. Rapid biochemical changes on HD may induce side effects such as hypotension. In most situations, HD is preferred to PD for treatment of acute renal failure because it is efficient and metabolic problems can be corrected safely and quickly. PD is simpler than HD but carries the risk of peritonitis, is less efficient in the catabolic patient, and takes longer. PD may be preferred for the individual with intracranial bleeding or cardiovascular instability. HD is preferred for the hypercatabolic patient and for the individual who has had abdominal or thoracic trauma or surgery. (HD and PD are discussed later in this chapter.)

Continuous renal replacement therapy (CRRT) may also be used in the treatment of acute renal failure.[2] (CRRT is discussed later in this chapter.) In the hemodynamically unstable patient, CRRT provides gradual removal of excess fluid and solutes. It is technically similar to HD and requires extracorporeal blood circulation via cannulation of an artery and vein or two veins. Blood removed from the artery or vein passes through a hemofilter where solutes and water are removed, and then the blood is returned to the patient. CRRT is used continuously and requires at least 12 to 24 hours to accomplish what can be done with 3 to 4 hours of HD. Larger amounts of fluid may be removed than with intermittent HD. It is the preferred treatment in the hemodynamically unstable patient with mild to moderate acute renal failure or fluid overload.

Nutritional Therapy. In the past, the regimen of fluid restriction and nutritional therapy was designed so that body weight would decrease by 0.25 to 0.5 kg per day from the loss of body tissue catabolized on the low-protein diet. Today, these severe restrictions are usually not necessary except during the interval between the diagnosis of oliguria and the establishment of dialysis and a nutritional regimen. However, a stable weight or a weight gain during this interval usually indicates hypervolemia.

If the patient does not receive adequate nutrition, catabolism of body protein will occur.[3] This process causes increased urea, phosphate, and potassium levels. The major goal of nutritional therapy is to decrease catabolism of the body's protein. Adequate energy must be provided from carbohydrate and fat sources to prevent ketosis from fat breakdown and gluconeogenesis from protein breakdown.[4] Nonprotein calories (35 to 55 kcal/kg body weight) should be provided daily. Protein intake is generally 1.0 to 1.5 g/kg. Essential amino acid supplements (e.g., Amin-Aid) may be given for amino acid and caloric supplementation, either orally or through tube feedings.

Potassium and sodium are regulated in accordance with plasma levels. Sodium is restricted as needed to prevent edema, hypertension, and congestive heart failure. Dietary fat intake is increased so that the patient receives at least 30% to 40% of total calories from fat. Intralipid (fat emulsions) infusions can also be given as a nutritional supplement, and it provides a good source of nonprotein calories (see Chapter 38). If a patient cannot obtain an adequate oral intake, enteral nutrition is the preferred route for nutritional support (see Chapter 38). When the GI tract is not functional, total parenteral nutrition (TPN) is necessary for the provision of adequate nutrition. TPN is most commonly used in the patient who has had extensive surgical procedures or multiple trauma. The patient treated with TPN may need daily HD or CRRT to remove the excess fluid. However, concentrated TPN formulas are available to minimize fluid volume.[4]

NURSING MANAGEMENT: ACUTE RENAL FAILURE

■ Nursing Assessment

An assessment of the patient in acute renal failure includes the specific areas presented in Table 44-2. It is important to monitor the blood pressure, pulse, respiratory rate and pattern, and temperature. The patient's general appearance should be assessed, including skin color, peripheral edema, neck vein distention, and bruises.

If HD is used for treating acute renal failure, the vascular access site should be observed for signs of inflammation. The patient's mental status and level of consciousness should also be determined. The oral mucosa should be examined for dryness and presence of inflammation. The lungs should be auscultated for the presence of crackles and rhonchi. Heart sounds should be monitored for the presence of S_3 sounds and murmurs. If a pulmonary artery catheter is inserted, the pulmonary artery pressures should be obtained. ECG readings should be obtained to assess for the presence of arrhythmias. Any urine output should be assessed, including volume, color, specific gravity, and the presence of blood, glucose, sediment, or protein.

■ Nursing Diagnoses

Nursing diagnoses for the patient with acute renal failure include, but are not limited to, the following:

- Fluid volume excess *related to* renal failure and fluid retention
- Risk for infection *related to* invasive lines, uremic toxins, and altered immune responses secondary to renal failure
- Altered nutrition: less than body requirements *related to* altered metabolic state and dietary restrictions
- Sensory-perceptual alterations *related to* uremic toxins and fluid and electrolyte and acid-base imbalances
- Altered thought processes *related to* effects of uremic toxins on central nervous system (CNS)
- Impaired skin integrity *related to* sites for vascular access or peritoneal dialysis and renal failure
- Fatigue *related to* anemia and uremic toxins
- Anxiety *related to* disease process, therapeutic interventions, and uncertainty of prognosis

- Potential complication: hyperkalemia *related to* decreased renal excretion of potassium
- Potential complication: arrhythmias *related to* electrolyte imbalances

Planning

The overall goals are that the patient with acute renal failure will (1) completely recover with no residual loss of kidney function, (2) be maintained in normal fluid and electrolyte balance, (3) have decreased anxiety, and (4) comply with and understand the need for careful follow-up care.

Nursing Implementation

Health Promotion. Prevention of acute renal failure is essential because of the high mortality rate and is primarily directed toward identifying and monitoring high risk populations, controlling industrial chemicals and nephrotoxic drugs, and preventing prolonged episodes of hypotension and hypovolemia. In the hospital the patient at greatest risk for developing acute renal failure is the person who has experienced massive trauma, major surgical procedures, extensive burns, cardiac failure, sepsis, or obstetric complications or the individual who has a baseline renal insufficiency as a result of chronic diseases such as hypertension, diabetes mellitus, or systemic lupus erythematosus. This patient must be monitored carefully for intake and output, fluid and electrolyte balance, and possible blood transfusion reactions. Extrarenal losses of fluid from vomitus, diarrhea, hemorrhage, and increased insensible losses must be assessed and recorded. Prompt replacement of lost extracellular fluids will help prevent ischemic tubular damage associated with trauma, burns, and extensive surgery. Intake and output records and the patient's weight provide valuable indicators of fluid volume status. Aggressive diuretic therapy for the patient with fluid overload as a result of any cause can lead to inadequate renal vascular perfusion.

Streptococcal infections must be identified and treated with antibiotics. Compliance with the antibiotic regimen is critical to eliminate the source of infection. Complications of streptococcal infections include acute poststreptococcal glomerulonephritis and rheumatic heart disease.

The older adult patient and the individual with diabetes who is undergoing multiple diagnostic studies, especially those requiring IV dye injection, need special attention to prevent the patient from sustaining a nephrotoxic injury secondary to the dye. Adequate hydration is critical. The individual with urinary tract infections needs prompt treatment and careful follow-up care. Other persons who are considered at risk are those taking chemotherapeutic drugs that cause hyperuricemia.

Industrial and agricultural chemicals and products (organic solvents, insecticides, cleaning agents) must be monitored regularly regarding their safety for both the employee and the general population. The individual who is taking drugs that are potentially nephrotoxic (see Table 42-3) must have renal function monitored with serum creatinine and BUN determinations. Nephrotoxic medications should be used sparingly in the high risk patient. When they must be used, nephrotoxic medications should be given in the smallest effective doses for the shortest possible periods. The patient should be cautioned about the abuse of over-the-counter analgesics (especially NSAIDs), since

some of these may precipitate renal failure in the patient with borderline renal insufficiency.

Acute Intervention. The patient with acute renal failure is critically ill and suffers not only from the effects of a renal disease but often from those effects of the nonrenal disease or condition (e.g., trauma, cardiac disease) that contributed to the renal failure. The nursing staff may become overly concerned with the patient's urinary output and forget to focus on the patient as a total person with many physical and emotional needs. Usually the changes caused by renal failure come on suddenly. Both the patient and the family need assistance in understanding that the functioning of the whole body can be disrupted by renal failure. However, these changes are potentially reversible.

The nursing role in managing fluid and electrolyte balance is important during the oliguric and diuretic phases. Observing and recording the accurate intake and output of fluids cannot be overemphasized. Daily weights measured with the same scale at the same time each day are essential in evaluating and detecting excessive gains or losses of body fluid (1 kg is equivalent to 1000 ml of fluid). The nurse must be knowledgeable about the common signs and symptoms that result from hypervolemia (in the oliguric phase) or hypovolemia (in the diuretic phase), hypernatremia or hyponatremia, hyperkalemia or hypokalemia, and other electrolyte imbalances that may occur in acute renal failure (see Chapter 15). Hyperkalemia is a leading biochemical cause of death in the oliguric phase of acute renal failure. Most typically, hyperkalemia is manifested by impairment of neuromuscular function and arrhythmias. Muscle weakness, abdominal cramps, flaccid paralysis, and absence of deep tendon reflexes are signs of neuromuscular impairment. Cardiac conduction abnormalities to watch for include a prolonged PR interval, prolonged QRS interval, peaked T wave, and depressed ST segment.

Because infection is the leading cause of death in acute renal failure, meticulous aseptic technique is critical. The patient should be protected from other individuals with infectious diseases. The nurse should be alert for local manifestations of infection (e.g., swelling, redness, pain) and systemic manifestations (e.g., anorexia, malaise, leukocytosis) because an elevated temperature may not be present in the patient with renal failure. (Patients with renal failure are usually hypothermic relative to healthy individuals.) If antibiotics are used to treat an infection, the type and dosage must be carefully considered because the kidneys are the route of excretion for many antibiotics.

Respiratory complications, especially pneumonitis, can be prevented. Humidified oxygen, intermittent positive-pressure breathing, turning, deep breathing, and ambulation are measures the nurse can use to help the patient maintain adequate respiratory ventilation.

Skin care and measures to prevent pressure ulcers should be performed, since the patient usually develops edema, as well as decreased muscle tone. Mouth care is important to prevent stomatitis, which develops when ammonia (produced by bacterial breakdown of urea) in saliva irritates the mucous membranes.

Ambulatory and Home Care. Recovery from acute renal failure is highly variable and depends on the underlying illness, the general condition and age of the patient, the length of the oliguric phase, and the management of the patient. The rest of the body, as well as the kidneys, has experienced a major insult. Good nutrition, rest, and limited activity are necessary to restore patients to their previous level of functioning. The diet should be high in calories, and protein and potassium intake should be regulated in accordance with renal function. Follow-up care and regular evaluation of renal function are necessary. The patient should be taught the signs and symptoms of recurrent renal disease, especially manifestations of fluid and electrolyte imbalances. Measures to prevent the recurrence of acute renal failure must be emphasized.

The long-term convalescence of 3 to 12 months may cause social and financial hardships for the family, and appropriate counseling and referrals should be done. Occasionally, renal function deteriorates, and manifestations of chronic renal failure develop. If the kidneys do not recover, the patient progresses to chronic renal failure.

■ Evaluation

The expected outcomes are that the patient with acute renal failure will

- regain and maintain normal fluid and electrolyte balance
- comply with treatment regimen
- experience no infectious complications
- have complete recovery

GERONTOLOGIC CONSIDERATIONS

Acute Renal Failure

The older adult is more susceptible than the younger adult to acute renal failure. Although decreased renal reserve function in advancing age is the primary risk factor, age itself and impaired function of other organ systems are independent risk factors. The aging kidney is less able to compensate for changes in fluid volume, solute load, and cardiac output. Common causes of acute renal failure in the older adult include dehydration, hypotension, diuretic therapy, aminoglycoside therapy, obstructive disorders (e.g., prostatic hyperplasia), surgery, infection, and radiocontrast agents. The prognosis after acute renal failure is generally worse in the older adult than in the younger person. The mortality rate after acute renal failure is 5% to 25% higher in the older adult than in the younger person, and death is usually caused by infection, GI hemorrhage, or myocardial infarction.[4]

CHRONIC RENAL FAILURE

Chronic renal failure involves progressive, irreversible destruction of the nephrons in both kidneys. The disease process progresses until most nephrons are destroyed and replaced by nonfunctional scar tissue. Although there are many different causes of chronic renal failure (Fig. 44-2), the end result is a systemic disease involving every body organ. (The specific disease processes are discussed in Chapter 43.)

The kidneys have remarkable functional reserve. Up to 80% of the GFR (reflected in creatinine clearance measurements) may be lost with few overt changes in the functioning of the body. A person is born with 2 million nephrons and can survive (albeit with difficulty) with as few as 20,000. In the vast majority of cases the individual passes through the early stages of

chronic renal failure without recognizing the disease state because the remaining nephrons hypertrophy to compensate. The prognosis and course of chronic renal failure are highly variable. Some individuals live normal, active lives with compensated renal failure, whereas others may rapidly progress to end-stage renal failure. When the creatinine clearance falls below 10 ml per minute (from the norm of 85 to 135 ml per minute for the average adult), some form of dialysis or transplantation is required for survival.

Although there are no distinct stages in chronic renal failure, the disease progression may be divided into three stages:

1. *Diminished renal reserve.* This stage is characterized by normal BUN and serum creatinine levels and an absence of symptoms.
2. *Renal insufficiency.* This stage occurs when the GFR is about 25% of normal. BUN and serum creatinine levels are increased. Easy fatigue and weakness are common symptoms. As the renal failure progresses, headaches, nausea, and pruritus may occur. Nocturia and polyuria occur as a result of the kidneys' loss of ability to concentrate urine.
3. *End-stage renal disease (ESRD) or uremia.* The last stage occurs when the GFR is less than 5% to 10% of normal or when creatinine clearances are less than 5 to 10 ml/min. It is at this stage that most patients have great difficulty carrying out basic activities of daily living (ADLs) because of the cumulative effect and extent of the symptoms.

Significance

In the United States over 290,000 individuals with ESRD are being treated with dialysis or have kidney transplants. This number could double in the next 7 years if current trends continue. Each year over 30,000 people die from various diseases of the kidneys.[5] During the 1970s, dramatic changes in the focus of treatment of chronic renal disease occurred. In July 1973 the federal government enacted a law that provided financial assistance through Medicare for all eligible persons who had ESRD and required treatment. (Medicare pays 80% of the cost of health care for ESRD patients.)

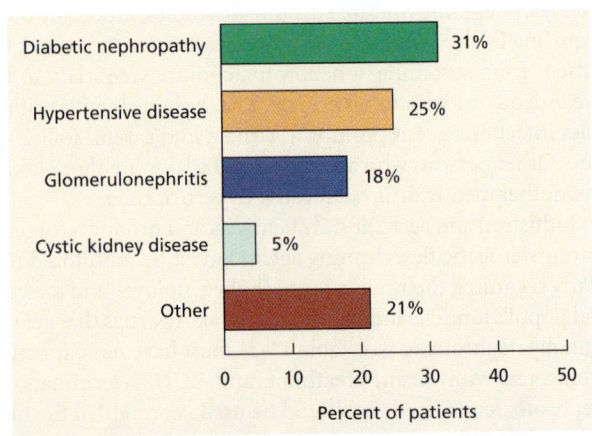

Fig. 44-2 Primary renal disease leading to end-stage renal failure.

Since 1973 many deaths have been prevented through the use of maintenance dialysis and renal transplantation. The majority of patients are treated with dialysis because (1) there is a lack of donated organs, (2) many patients do not want transplants, or (3) patients are medically unsuitable for the transplantation procedure. With the advancement of medical science each year, an increasing percentage of older individuals and patients with systemic disease (diabetics and patients with stable cancer) are being maintained on dialysis.

Every patient with ESRD, regardless of age, should be offered dialysis unless it is medically contraindicated or the patient refuses treatment. The Medicare program covers the cost of dialysis for most patients. For those not covered by Medicare, a variety of state and private programs are available. The incidence of patients being treated for ESRD is rising by an average of 9% per year. Older patients remain the fastest growing group entering the Medicare Renal Disease Program, with 34% of patients now over age 65.[5]

The increasing number of older adults with ESRD has changed the data related to the most common causes of chronic renal failure. Before the mid 1970s, glomerulonephritis and interstitial nephritis were the most common causes. Currently, diabetes and hypertension are the leading causes of chronic renal failure in the United States (see Fig. 44-2). In Canada the leading causes of ESRD are diabetes and glomerulonephritis.

Clinical Manifestations

As renal function progressively deteriorates, every body system becomes involved. The clinical manifestations are a result of retained substances, including urea, creatinine, phenols, hormones, electrolytes, water, and many other substances. Uremia is a syndrome that incorporates all the disturbances seen in the various systems throughout the body in chronic renal failure (Fig. 44-3). It is important to recognize that the manifestations of uremia vary among patients, according to the etiology of the renal failure, comorbid conditions, age, and degree of compliance with the prescribed medical regimen.

Urinary System. In the stage of renal insufficiency, the most noticeable sign is polyuria that is caused by the inability of the kidneys to concentrate urine. The patient will notice this most frequently at night when she or he must arise several times to urinate (nocturia). Because of the decrease in renal concentrating ability, the specific gravity of urine gradually becomes fixed at around 1.010 (the osmolar concentration of plasma). As renal failure progresses, oliguria develops, and later, anuria may develop. If the patient is still producing urine, common findings are proteinuria with casts, pyuria, and hematuria.

Metabolic Disturbances

Waste product accumulation. As the GFR decreases, the BUN and serum creatinine levels increase. The BUN influenced

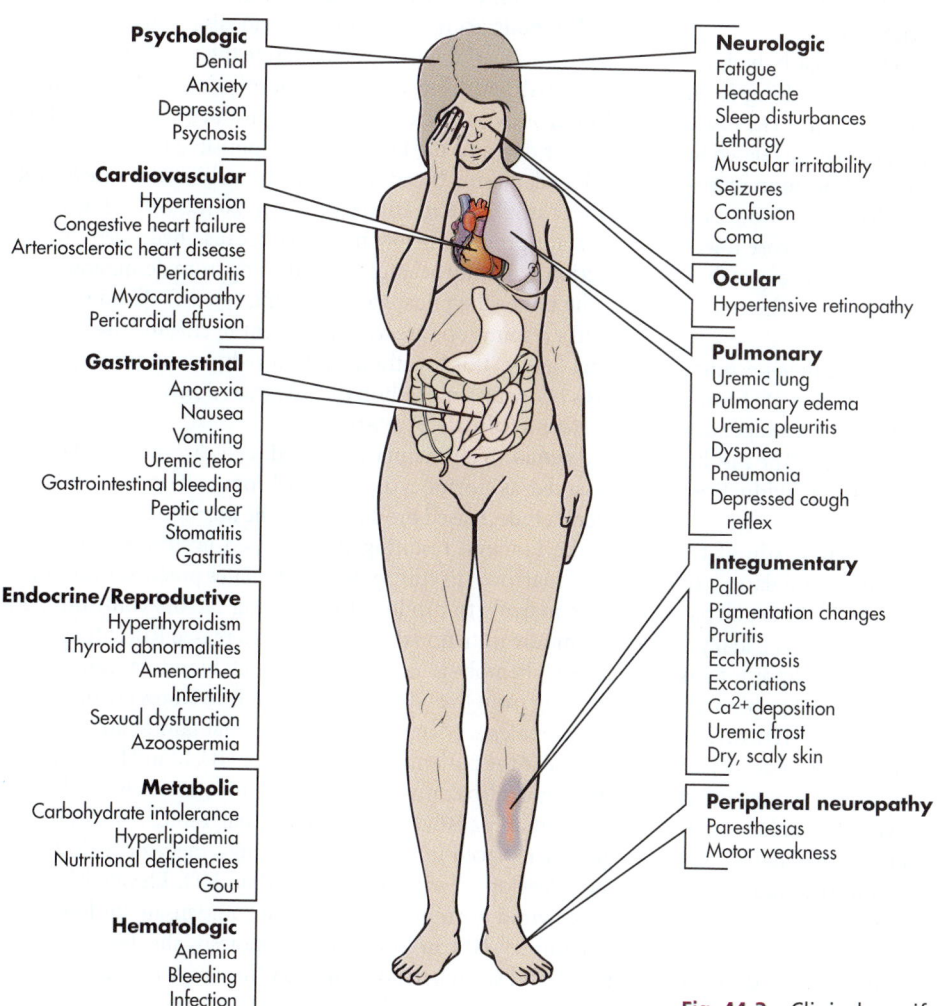

Fig. 44-3 Clinical manifestations of chronic uremia.

not only by renal failure but by protein intake, fever, and catabolic rate. For this reason serum creatinine and creatinine clearance determinations are considered more accurate indicators of renal function than BUN. As the BUN increases, nausea, vomiting, lethargy, fatigue, impaired thought processes, and headaches become common complaints.

The serum creatinine level in an older adult patient with ESRD is lower than the level expected in a younger person with the same degree of renal dysfunction. Decreased muscle mass and decreased muscle activity account for this finding because creatinine is an end product of muscle metabolism.

Altered carbohydrate metabolism. Defective carbohydrate metabolism is caused by impaired glucose use resulting from cellular insensitivity to the normal action of insulin. The exact nature of this insulin resistance is unclear but may be related to circulating insulin antagonists, alterations in hormone receptors, or abnormalities of transport mechanisms. Moderate hyperglycemia, hyperinsulinemia, and abnormal glucose tolerance tests are common findings. Insulin and glucose metabolism may improve (but not to normal values) after the initiation of dialysis.

The individual who has diabetes mellitus and then becomes uremic may require less insulin than before the onset of chronic renal failure. This is because both exogenous and endogenous insulin remain in circulation longer in renal failure. The insulin doses of insulin-dependent diabetics must be individualized and monitored carefully.

Elevated triglycerides. The hyperinsulinemia stimulates hepatic production of triglycerides, and the assimilation of triglycerides by peripheral tissues is diminished. Almost all patients with uremia develop hyperlipidemia, which is usually a type IV profile with elevated very-low-density lipoproteins (VLDLs), normal or decreased low-density lipoproteins (LDLs), and lowered high-density lipoproteins (HDLs). The reason for the altered lipid metabolism is related to decreased levels of the enzyme lipoprotein lipase, which is important in the breakdown of lipoproteins. Type IV hyperlipidemia is a definite risk factor for accelerated atherosclerosis (see Chapter 32). This dysfunction compounds the problem in the diabetic patient with renal disease who already has increased atherosclerotic changes.

The serum level of triglycerides does not usually decrease after dialysis is started. In the patient who is on chronic peritoneal dialysis, the level frequently becomes higher as a result of the increased amounts of glucose absorbed from the peritoneal dialysate fluid.

Electrolyte and Acid-Base Imbalances

Potassium. Hyperkalemia is the most serious electrolyte problem associated with renal failure. Fatal arrhythmias can occur when the serum potassium level reaches 7 to 8 mEq/L (7 to 8 mmol/L). Hyperkalemia results from the failure of the excretory ability of the kidneys, the breakdown of cellular protein with the subsequent release of potassium, and acidosis, which contributes to the shift of potassium from intracellular to extracellular spaces. Potassium can come from the diet, dietary supplements, medications, and intravenous infusions.

Calcium and phosphate. Calcium and phosphate alterations are discussed in the section on acute renal failure (p. 1302) and in the section on the musculoskeletal system (p. 1309).

Magnesium. Magnesium is primarily excreted by the kidneys. Hypermagnesemia is generally not a problem unless the patient is taking magnesium (e.g., milk of magnesia, magnesium citrate, antacids containing magnesium).

Sodium. Sodium levels can range from low to normal. Hypernatremia is unusual because whenever sodium is retained, so is water, resulting in a dilutional hyponatremia. Sodium retention can contribute to edema, hypertension, and congestive heart failure. Sodium intake must be individually determined but is generally restricted in all patients.

Metabolic acidosis. Metabolic acidosis results from the impaired ability of the kidneys to excrete the acid load (primarily ammonia) and from defective reabsorption and regeneration of bicarbonate. The average adult produces 80 to 90 mEq of acid per day, and the kidneys are responsible for excreting this acid load. Plasma bicarbonate usually stabilizes at a new steady state at around 16 to 20 mEq/L (16 to 20 mmol/L). It generally does not progress below this level because hydrogen ion production is usually balanced by buffering from demineralization of the bone (the phosphate buffering system). Although Kussmaul's respirations are less prominent in chronic than in acute renal failure, this breathing pattern reduces the severity of acidosis by increasing carbon dioxide excretion.

Hematologic System

Anemia. The anemia associated with chronic renal failure is classified as normocytic, normochromic. The main cause of anemia is decreased production of the hormone erythropoietin by the kidneys, resulting in decreased erythropoiesis by the bone marrow.[6] Erythropoietin stimulates precursor cells in the bone marrow to produce RBCs. Other factors contributing to anemia are nutritional deficiencies, decreased RBC life span, increased hemolysis of RBCs, frequent blood samplings, and bleeding from the GI tract. Sufficient iron stores are needed for erythropoiesis. Many patients with renal failure are iron deficient. For the patient on maintenance HD, blood loss in the dialyzer may also contribute to the anemic state. Folic acid, which is essential for RBC maturation, is dialyzable. If it is not adequately replaced in the diet or by drugs, megaloblastic anemia may develop in a patient on chronic HD. Elevated levels of parathyroid hormone (produced to compensate for low serum calcium levels) can inhibit erythropoiesis, shorten survival of RBCs, and stimulate bone marrow fibrosis, which can result in decreased numbers of hematopoietic cells.

Bleeding tendencies. The most common cause of bleeding in uremia is a qualitative defect in platelet function. This dysfunction is caused by impaired platelet aggregation and impaired release of platelet factor 3. The altered platelet function, hemorrhagic tendencies, and GI bleeding are usually reversible by HD or PD. In addition, there are alterations in the coagulation system with increased concentrations of both factor VIII and fibrinogen found in the serum of these patients.

Infection. Infectious complications are caused by changes in leukocyte function and altered immune response and function. A diminished inflammatory response occurs as a result of an altered chemotactic response by both neutrophils and monocytes. This impairment significantly decreases the accumulation of WBCs at the site of injury or infection. Both cellular and humoral immune responses are also suppressed. Characteristic clinical findings include lymphopenia, lymphoid atrophy (especially of the thymus), decreased antibody production, and suppression of the delayed hypersensitivity response. Other factors contributing to the increased risk of infection include protein malnutrition, hyperglycemia, and external trauma (e.g., catheters, needle insertions into vascular access sites).

Increased incidence of cancer. There is a significant increase in the incidence of neoplasms in the patient with renal failure who has not had transplants as compared with the general population. Lung, breast, uterus, colon, prostate, and skin malignancies are most commonly found.

Cardiovascular System. The most common cardiovascular abnormality is hypertension, which is usually caused by sodium retention and increased extracellular fluid volume. In some individuals, increased renin production contributes to the problem (see Fig. 42-6). Hypertension accelerates atherosclerotic vascular disease, produces intrarenal arterial spasm, and eventually leads to left ventricular hypertrophy and congestive heart failure.[7] Hypertension also causes retinopathy and encephalopathy.

Congestive heart failure from left ventricular hypertrophy can lead to pulmonary edema. Peripheral edema is also commonly present. Cardiac arrhythmias may result from hyperkalemia, hypocalcemia, and decreased coronary artery perfusion.

Uremic pericarditis develops and occasionally progresses to pericardial effusion and cardiac tamponade. Pericarditis is manifested by a friction rub, chest pain, and low-grade fever.

The vascular changes from long-standing hypertension and the accelerated atherosclerosis from elevated triglyceride levels are responsible for many of the cardiovascular complications (e.g., myocardial infarction, cerebrovascular accident), which are the leading causes of death for patients on chronic dialysis. Diabetes mellitus is also a major risk factor for the development of vascular problems.

Respiratory System. Respiratory changes include Kussmaul's respirations, dyspnea from congestive heart failure, pulmonary edema, uremic pleuritis (pleurisy), pleural effusion, and a predisposition to respiratory infections, which may be related to decreased pulmonary macrophage activity. The sputum is thick and tenacious. The cough reflex is depressed. "Uremic lung," or uremic pneumonitis, is typically found in chronic renal failure and shows up as an interstitial edema on chest x-ray. This condition usually responds to vigorous fluid removal during dialysis treatments.

Gastrointestinal System. Every part of the GI system is affected as a result of inflammation of the mucosa caused by excessive urea. Mucosal ulcerations, found throughout the GI tract, are caused by the increased ammonia produced by bacterial breakdown of urea. Stomatitis with exudates and ulcerations, a metallic taste in the mouth, and uremic fetor (a urinous odor of the breath) are commonly found. Anorexia, nausea, and vomiting caused by irritation of the GI tract by waste products contribute to weight loss. Diarrhea may occur because of hyperkalemia and altered calcium metabolism. Constipation or diarrhea may be a complication of taking iron salts, which are taken as part of anemia therapy, or a complication of taking calcium-containing phosphate binders, which are taken to facilitate phosphate excretion.

Neurologic System. Neurologic changes are expected as renal failure progresses. The exact cause of these changes is unknown, but they may be partially attributed to increased nitrogenous waste products, electrolyte imbalances, and axonal atrophy and demyelination of nerve fibers.[8] High levels of uremic toxins have been implicated in axonal damage.

In renal failure a general depression of the CNS results in lethargy, apathy, decreased ability to concentrate, fatigue, and altered mental ability. Seizures and coma may result from a rapidly increasing BUN and hypertensive encephalopathy.

Dialysis encephalopathy (dialysis dementia), a progressive neurologic impairment, is characterized by speech disturbances, dementia, lack of muscle coordination, and myoclonic seizures. A frequent cause of this problem is aluminum toxicity, which may result from ingestion of aluminum-containing antacids and a decreased ability of the kidneys to excrete aluminum. Phosphate-binding antacids (e.g., calcium acetate, calcium carbonate) that are not aluminum based are usually administered.

Peripheral neuropathy is initially manifested by a slowing of nerve conduction to the extremities. The patient complains of a restless leg syndrome and may describe it as "bugs crawling inside the leg." Paresthesias, especially of both feet and legs, may be described by the patient as a burning sensation. Eventually, motor involvement may lead to bilateral footdrop, muscular weakness and atrophy, and loss of deep tendon reflexes. Muscle twitching, jerking, asterixis (hand-flapping tremor), and nocturnal leg cramps also occur.

The treatment for neurologic problems is dialysis and, ultimately, transplantation. Altered mental status is often the signal that dialysis must be initiated. Dialysis should improve the general CNS symptoms and may halt the progression of neuropathies, but not necessarily. Motor neuropathy may not be reversible. The problem of uremic neuropathy is compounded in the diabetic patient who has diabetic neuropathy as well.

Musculoskeletal System. Renal osteodystrophy is a syndrome of skeletal changes found in chronic renal failure.[9] This syndrome is a result of alterations in calcium and phosphate metabolism (Fig. 44-4). Normally the calcium/phosphate ratio maintains the electrolytes in a soluble state. As the GFR decreases, phosphate cannot be excreted by the kidneys, thus increasing the serum phosphate.

Normally the kidneys metabolize vitamin D (formed in the skin or ingested) to its active form. The active form of vitamin D is needed for calcium absorption from the GI tract. In renal failure the kidneys fail to activate vitamin D, and calcium

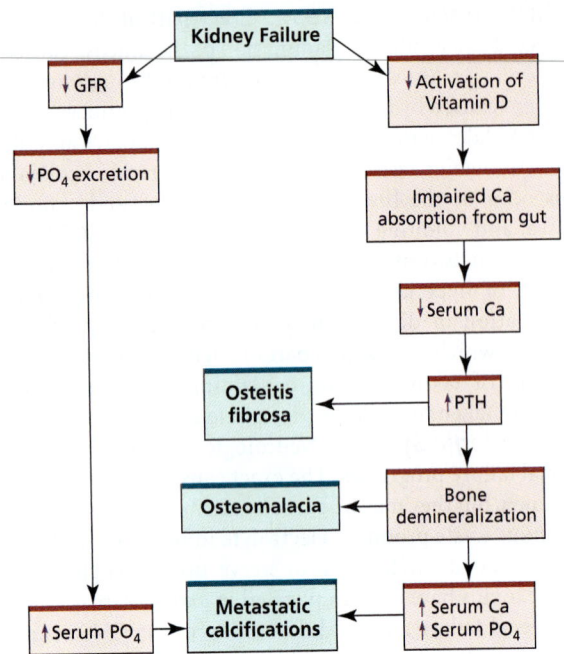

Fig. 44-4 Mechanisms of renal osteodystrophy.

absorption is impaired, thus lowering serum calcium. Low serum calcium stimulates the release of parathyroid hormone (PTH), which causes resorption of calcium and phosphate from the bone. This release increases serum calcium, as well as serum phosphate. When the phosphate level is high, it complexes with calcium, leading to the formation of metastatic calcifications that are deposited throughout the body.

The changes resulting from increased phosphate retention, bone resorption of calcium, inadequate calcium absorption, and elevated PTH levels lead to the following conditions:

1. *Osteomalacia.* This condition results from lack of mineralization of newly formed bone. It can be a result of hypocalcemia. It can also be caused by aluminum accumulation, since the primary route for aluminum excretion is through the kidneys. The primary source of aluminum is aluminum-based phosphate binders. Over the past decade, there has been a decreased use of aluminum-based phosphate binders and a concomitant decrease in the incidence of osteomalacia.

2. *Osteitis fibrosa.* This condition results from calcium resorption from the bone and replacement with fibrous tissue. Osteitis fibrosa is primarily a result of markedly elevated levels of PTH that cause bone resorption.[9]

3. *Metastatic calcification (soft-tissue calcification).* This condition results from calcium-phosphate deposits in soft tissues of the body. Common sites are the blood vessels, joints, lungs, muscles, myocardium, and eyes. "Uremic red eye" is caused by the irritation of the deposits in the eye. Metastatic calcifications in the arteries of the fingers and toes may cause gangrene. Intracardiac calcifications can disrupt the conduction system and cause cardiac arrest.

Integumentary System. The most noticeable change in the integumentary system is a yellowish discoloration of the skin. This change is a result of the absorption and retention of urinary chromogens that normally give the characteristic color to urine. The skin also appears pale as a result of anemia and is dry and scaly because of a decrease in oil and sweat gland activity. Decreased perspiration results from a decrease in the size of the sweat glands.

Pruritus most commonly results from a combination of the dry skin, calcium-phosphate deposition in the skin, and sensory neuropathy. The itching may be so intense that it can lead to bleeding or infection secondary to scratching. Uremic frost is a condition in which urea crystallizes on the skin and is usually seen only when BUN levels are extremely high. This is almost never seen unless the patient refuses dialysis or is withdrawn from dialysis.

The hair is dry and brittle and may fall out. The nails are thin, brittle, and ridged. Petechiae and ecchymoses may be present and are caused by clotting abnormalities.

Reproductive System. Both sexes characteristically experience infertility and a decreased libido. Women usually have decreased levels of estrogen, progesterone, and luteinizing hormone, causing anovulation and menstrual changes (usually amenorrhea). Menses and ovulation may return after dialysis is started. Men experience loss of testicular consistency, decreased testosterone levels, and low sperm counts. Sexual dysfunction in both sexes may also be caused by anemia, which causes fatigue and decreased libido. In addition, peripheral neuropathy can cause impotence in men and anorgasmy in women. Additional factors that may cause changes in sexual function are psychologic problems (e.g., anxiety, depression), physical stress, and side effects of medication.

Sexual function may improve with maintenance dialysis and may return to normal with successful transplantation. In rare cases pregnant dialysis patients have been able to carry a fetus to term, but there is significant risk to the mother and infant. Pregnancy in transplant patients is more common, but in this situation there is also a risk to both the mother and fetus.

Endocrine System. Many patients with chronic renal failure exhibit some clinical manifestations of hypothyroidism. Tests of thyroid function may yield low to low-normal levels for serum triiodothyronine (T_3) and thyroxine (T_4) levels. Neither the clinical significance nor the exact reason for these findings is known.

Psychologic Changes. Personality and behavior changes, emotional lability, withdrawal, and depression are commonly observed. Fatigue and lethargy contribute to the patient's feeling of sickness. The changes in body image caused by edema, integumentary disturbances, and access devices (e.g., fistulas, catheters) lead to further anxiety and depression. Decreased ability to concentrate and lessened mental activity can make the patient appear dull and disinterested in the environment. The patient is faced with significant changes in lifestyle, occupation, family responsibilities, and financial status. The patient's future depends on medications, dietary restrictions, dialysis, and possibly transplantation of another person's kidney. The patient will grieve the loss of renal function. This can be a prolonged process for some individuals.

Collaborative Conservative Care

When a patient is diagnosed as having chronic renal insufficiency, conservative therapy is attempted before maintenance

COLLABORATIVE CARE

Table **44-5** Chronic Renal Failure

Diagnostic
Identification of reversible renal disease
Renal ultrasound
Renal scan (if indicated)
CT scan (if indicated)
Hematocrit and hemoglobin level
BUN, serum creatinine, and creatinine clearance levels
Serum electrolytes
Urinalysis and urine culture

Collaborative Therapy
Correction of extracellular fluid volume overload or deficit
Nutritional therapy*
Erythropoietin therapy
Calcium supplementation, phosphate binders, or both
Antihypertensive therapy
Measures to lower potassium[†]
Adjustment of drug dosages to degree of renal function

*See Tables 44-6, 44-7, and 44-8.
[†]See Table 44-4.
BUN, blood urea nitrogen.

dialysis begins (Table 44-5). Every effort is made to detect and treat potentially reversible causes of renal failure (e.g., cardiac failure, dehydration, pyelonephritis, nephrotoxins, urinary tract obstruction, renal artery stenosis). Conservative therapy is directed toward preserving existing renal function, treating the symptoms, preventing complications, and providing for the patient's comfort.[10] Conservative therapy primarily consists of drug and nutritional therapy and supportive care. Patients with chronic renal insufficiency should be cautioned to avoid NSAIDs, since NSAIDs may block synthesis of prostaglandins in the kidney that promote vasodilation and thus may induce renal hypoperfusion.

Drug Therapy

Hyperkalemia. Acute hyperkalemia is usually treated with intravenous (IV) glucose and insulin or IV 10% calcium gluconate (see Table 44-4). Dietary restriction of foods high in potassium is needed. (Foods high in protein content are usually high in potassium.) Sodium polystyrene sulfonate (Kayexalate), a cation-exchange resin, is commonly used to lower potassium levels. The exchange resin, administered orally or rectally, exchanges 1 mEq of sodium for 1 mEq of potassium. The potassium is bound to the resin, which is excreted in the stool. To ensure excretion of potassium, a bulk laxative (usually sorbitol) is mixed with Kayexalate. The patient should be told to expect some diarrhea. Kayexalate should never be given to a patient with hypoactive bowels because fluid shifts could lead to bowel necrosis. As Kayexalate exchanges sodium for potassium the patient should be observed for sodium and water retention.

Hypertension. The progression of chronic renal failure can be delayed by controlling hypertension.[10] Treatment of hypertension initially consists of sodium and fluid restriction and the administration of antihypertensives. The antihypertensive drugs most commonly used are calcium channel blockers (e.g., nifedipine [Procardia], nicardipine [Cardene]) and ACE in-

hibitors (e.g., captopril [Capoten], enalapril [Vasotec]) (see Chapter 31). Calcium channel blockers have renoprotective properties. In addition to their antihypertensive action, ACE inhibitors decrease proteinuria and delay the progression of renal failure. ACE inhibitors should be used cautiously when ESRD occurs because they can further decrease GFR and increase serum potassium levels. The blood pressure should be measured in supine, sitting, and standing positions to effectively monitor the antihypertensive drugs. Treatment that is too vigorous can cause a hypotensive reaction in a patient who has compensated for long-standing hypertension. A significant decrease in blood pressure can lead to further renal problems because kidneys may be dependent on high blood pressure to be perfused via atherosclerotic blood vessels. Blood pressure control is essential to slow atherosclerotic changes that could further impair renal function.

Renal osteodystrophy. Phosphate intake is generally restricted to less than 1000 mg/day. Calcium-based phosphate binders such as calcium carbonate (e.g., Tums) and calcium acetate (e.g., PhosLo) are used frequently to bind the phosphate, which is then excreted in the stool. Giving a calcium-based binder when the phosphate levels are still high (6 mg/dl [1.98 mmol/L]) may cause the formation of calcium-phosphate deposits.

Because of dementia and bone disease (osteomalacia) associated with excessive absorption of aluminum, aluminum hydroxide gels or antacids (e.g., Alu-Cap, Amphojel, Basaljel, and Alternagel) are used less frequently to bind the phosphate. Magnesium-containing antacids (Maalox, Mylanta) should not be given because magnesium is dependent on the kidneys for excretion. Phosphate binders should be administered with each meal to be effective because most phosphate is absorbed within 1 hour after eating. Hypercalcemia may occur with calcium binders. Constipation is a frequent side effect of phosphate binders and may necessitate the use of stool softeners.

Hypocalcemia is often a problem because of the inability of the GI tract to absorb calcium in the absence of vitamin D. If hypocalcemia occurs in the setting of controlled serum phosphate levels and supplemental calcium, the active form of vitamin D should be given. It is commercially available in oral preparations such as calcitriol (Rocaltrol) and in IV form as calcitriol (Calcijex). Paricalcitol (Zemplar), a synthetically manufactured vitamin D analog, is also used to prevent and treat secondary hyperparathyroidism associated with renal failure. It is important to lower the phosphate level before administering calcium or vitamin D because these drugs may contribute to soft-tissue calcification if both calcium and phosphate levels are elevated.

If renal osteodystrophy remains severe, a subtotal parathyroidectomy may be performed to decrease the synthesis and secretion of PTH. In some situations a total parathyroidectomy is performed and some parathyroid tissue is transplanted into the forearm. The transplanted cells produce PTH as needed. If production of PTH becomes excessive, some of the cells can be removed using local anesthesia.

The most common methods for evaluating the status of the bone disease are skeletal x-ray, bone scans, bone biopsy, and bone densitometry. PTH and alkaline phosphatase levels should also be measured. The enzyme alkaline phosphatase is elevated when there is demineralization of the bone.

NUTRITIONAL THERAPY

Table 44-6 Daily Requirements for the Patient with Chronic Renal Failure

	Conservative Management	Hemodialysis	Peritoneal Dialysis
Fluid allowance	Urine output plus 500-600 ml	Urine output plus 1000 ml	Frequently no restriction
Protein*	0.6-0.8 g/kg body weight	1.0-1.5 g/kg IBW	1.2-2.0 g/kg IBW
Calories	35-40 kcal/kg EDW	35-40 kcal/kg EDW[†]	35-40 kcal/kg IBW[†]
Fat	Determined by caloric requirement	Determined by caloric requirement	Determined by caloric requirement
Carbohydrate	Unlimited intake of sugars and starches; bread and cereal products limited because of protein limit	Same as for conservative management	Dependent on individual patient needs
Iron	No supplementation	900 mg supplement	500-900 mg supplement
Potassium	2-3 g	2-3 g	3-4 g, no restrictions
Sodium	1-3 g	2 g	2-4 g
Phosphorus	700-1200 mg	700-1200 mg	700-1200 mg
Calcium	1000-2000 mg	1000-1500 mg	1000-1500 mg
Folic acid	1.0 mg supplement	1.0 mg supplement	1.0 mg supplement

*At least 70% of protein intake should be of high biologic value (e.g., coming from eggs, milk, and meat).
[†]Includes dialysate calories.
EDW, estimated dry weight; *IBW*, ideal body weight.

Anemia. The most important cause of renal anemia is a decreased production of erythropoietin. With the use of recombinant deoxyribonucleic acid (DNA) technology (see Chapter 12), human erythropoietin can now be made in large amounts and is available for the treatment of anemia.[6] It can be administered IV at the end of HD or subcutaneously for the PD patient. Erythropoietin has been effective in treating anemia. Clinically, a significant increase in hematocrit is usually not seen for 2 to 3 weeks. The patient who is receiving erythropoietin has an improved cardiac performance and exercise tolerance and an enhanced quality of life.

A common adverse effect of exogenous erythropoietin is the development or aggravation of hypertension. The underlying mechanism is related to the hemodynamic changes (e.g., increased whole blood viscosity) that occur as the patient's anemia is corrected. Another side effect of erythropoietin therapy is the development of functional iron deficiency as a result of the increased demand for iron to support erythropoiesis. Most patients receive oral iron supplements; however, the GI side effects of iron supplements may lead to patients not taking the medication. Parenteral iron is used if iron deficiencies persist in spite of oral iron intake. Orally administered iron should not be taken at the same time as phosphate binders because the aluminum and calcium bind the iron. Supplemental folic acid (1 mg or more daily) is usually given because it is needed for RBC formation and is usually deficient in these patients.

Blood transfusions should be avoided in treating anemia unless the patient experiences an acute blood loss or has symptomatic anemia (i.e., dyspnea, excess fatigue, tachycardia, palpitations, chest pain). Undesirable effects of transfusions are the suppression of erythropoiesis as a result of a decrease in the hypoxic stimulus, the possible transmission of hepatitis or human immunodeficiency virus (HIV), and the possibility of iron overload because each unit of blood contains about 250 mg of iron.

Complications of drug therapy. Most drugs are excreted partially or totally by the kidneys. Drug dosages must be adapted to the degree of renal failure. Drug toxicity is a serious problem in the patient with uremia. Delayed and decreased elimination leads to an accumulation of drugs in the body. Increased sensitivity to the drug may result as drug levels increase in the blood and tissues. Drugs of particular concern include digitalis preparations, antibiotics, and pain medication.

Digitalis preparations are excreted largely by the kidneys. Loading doses may not have to be changed, but maintenance dosages may have to be adjusted. Dialysis does not affect body levels of digoxin, but it does affect potassium levels, which can potentiate the action of digitalis.

Aminoglycosides (gentamicin, kanamycin, tobramycin [Nebcin]), penicillin in high doses, and tetracyclines are potentially nephrotoxic. The frequency of doses or the dose of many antibiotics, such as vancomycin (Vancocin) and gentamicin, must be decreased because they are dependent on the kidney for excretion. These drugs can accumulate to toxic levels if appropriate precautions are not taken.

Meperidine should never be administered to a patient with chronic renal failure because the liver metabolizes it to normeperidine, which is dependent on the kidneys for excretion. If normeperidine accumulates, seizures can result. Other pain medications are appropriate, but they may need to be given less frequently and in smaller doses.

Nutritional Therapy

Protein restriction. Before the use of maintenance dialysis, Giovannetti and Giordano designed a 20 g, high-quality protein diet to prevent the accumulation of nitrogenous waste products. This diet provided the essential amino acids from eggs and milk. No meat was allowed. In addition to eggs and milk, low-protein vegetables, noodles, butter balls, and high-carbohydrate foods were included. Patient acceptance of this dietary regimen was poor, and patients were malnourished and vitamin deficient.

The current diet is designed to be as normal as possible to maintain good nutrition (Table 44-6). For the patient who is not undergoing dialysis, one guide is to restrict protein intake

NUTRITIONAL THERAPY

Table 44-7 | Chronic Renal Failure*

General Principles
1. Protein, sodium, potassium, phosphorus, and fluids are controlled to meet each patient's needs.
2. Protein sources should be of high biologic value.
3. High-sodium and high-potassium foods should be avoided.
4. Sufficient calories and nutrients are provided to meet daily requirements.

Meal	Exchanges	Sample Menu 1	Sample Menu 2	Sample Menu 3
Breakfast	1 fruit	60 ml grape juice	60 ml apple juice	Applesauce
	1 bread	Toast or corn flakes	Tortilla	Grits
	1 meat	Scrambled egg	Fried egg	Poached egg
	3 fats	2 tsp margarine or butter	2 tsp butter	2 tsp butter
		30 ml cream	30 ml cream	30 ml cream
		Jelly	Jam	Jam
	Beverage	250 ml decaf coffee	250 ml decaf coffee	250 ml decaf coffee
	Dairy	120 ml milk	120 ml milk	120 ml milk
Lunch	1 meat	Salt-free tuna (¼ cup)	2 enchiladas (using ¼ cup ground beef, 2 corn tortillas, and shredded lettuce)	Fried chicken leg
	2 breads	2 slices bread		Cornbread
				½ cup rice
	Vegetable	Lettuce and cucumber	Chili sauce	Zucchini
	Fruit	Canned plums	Canned pears	Canned peaches
	2 fats	2 tbs salt-free mayonnaise	2 tbs oil for cooking	1 tsp butter
		Hard candy	Jelly beans	1 tbs oil for cooking
				Hard candy
	Beverage	250 ml carbonated beverage	250 ml carbonated beverage	250 ml carbonated beverage
Dinner	1 meat	1 oz fried fresh fish	1 oz chicken	1 oz pork
	1 bread	½ cup mashed potatoes (using presoaked potatoes)	1 salt-free corn or flour tortilla to make chicken taco	Salt-free corn on the cob
	Vegetable	Salt-free green peas	Tossed salad	Salt-free green beans
	Fruit	Fruit cocktail	Canned pineapple	Grapes
	3 fats	30 ml cream	30 ml cream	2 tsp butter
		1 tbs fat for cooking	2 tbs salt-free dressing	
		1 tsp butter		
	Beverage	250 ml fruit punch	250 ml fruit punch	250 ml fruit punch
		250 ml decaf coffee	250 ml decaf coffee	250 ml decaf coffee
Snack		120 ml gelatin dessert with whipped topping	180 ml Popsicle	Butter balls
		140 ml carbonated beverage†	80 ml carbonated beverage	320 ml carbonated beverage

*Each diet plan contains 40 g protein, 40 mEq potassium, 2 g sodium, and 1500 ml fluid. To increase the protein to 60 g, the dietician can add 3 oz meat; 1 egg and 2 oz meat; 120 ml milk, 1 egg, and 1½ oz meat; or 120 ml milk and 2½ oz meat. With the increase in protein, the potassium level also increases to 60 mEq.
†Coke is an acceptable beverage.

to 0.6 to 0.8 g/kg of ideal body weight (IBW) per day when the creatinine clearance is less than 25 ml per minute.[10] Some treatment centers use a routine 40 g protein diet (Table 44-7). Because this diet is deficient in vitamins, multivitamins are prescribed.

Protein restriction may reduce the decline of renal function in the patient with chronic renal insufficiency. A low-protein (0.6 to 0.8 g/kg body weight per day), low-phosphorus diet supplemented with amino acids and their ketoanalogues can slow the progression of renal failure.[11] Keto acids of essential amino acids are a dietary supplement. The rationale for using this treatment is that in the body, nonessential amino acids transfer amine groups to the essential keto acids synthesizing essential amino acids. Thus the nitrogen present in nonessential amino acids is used, and the total nitrogen intake is kept to an absolute minimum. Keto acid supplements are available in liquid preparations. Modest protein restriction (0.6 to 0.8 g/kg per day) appears to be a relatively safe therapeutic option for patients with moderate renal insufficiency. For patients with more severe renal insufficiency, low-protein diets should be used with caution, since these patients are at risk for developing malnutrition.

Once the patient is started on dialysis, protein intake can be increased to 1.0 to 1.5 g/kg of IBW per day. Dietary protein guidelines for the patient on PD differ from those for the patient on HD. Because excessive amounts of protein are lost in the dialysate during peritoneal dialysis, the protein intake must be high enough to compensate for the losses so that the nitrogen balance is maintained. The recommended protein intake is 1.2 to 2.0 g/kg of IBW per day, depending on the individual needs of the patient. For all patients with renal failure, at least 70% of protein intake should come from eggs, milk, poultry, and meat; these foods are considered to have high biologic value because they contain all of the essential amino acids.

Sufficient calories from carbohydrates and fat are needed to minimize catabolism of body protein and to maintain body weight. Therefore 100 g of carbohydrates and an appropriate amount of fat are prescribed to maintain an intake of 2000 to 2500 calories per day (35 kcal/kg body weight per day). See Table 44-6 for specific guidelines.

Lowering the protein intake decreases the metabolic end products of urea, potassium, phosphate, and hydrogen. As the BUN level decreases, the symptoms of nausea, vomiting, fatigue, and headache become less troublesome. However, dietary protein restriction should not be prescribed for chronic renal failure patients who are malnourished, and the ongoing assessments of a skilled dietician are necessary. A patient experiences increased anorexia from the progression of chronic renal failure and may spontaneously decrease protein intake to a low level in spite of nutritional counseling. Dialysis for this type of patient may need to be started early to prevent severe malnutrition and increased risk of morbidity and mortality.

Commercially prepared products that are high in calories and low in protein, sodium, and potassium are available. Liquid and powder preparations include Nepro, Microlipid, SumaCal, Suplena, and Polycose. Products containing only the essential amino acids (Amin-Aid) can also be used as dietary supplements.

Water restriction. Water intake depends on the daily urine output. Generally, 500 to 600 ml (from insensible loss) plus an amount equal to the urine output is allowed for a patient with chronic renal failure who is not on dialysis. This amount of fluid is in addition to the fluid found in food. Foods that are liquid at room temperature (e.g., Jell-O and ice cream) should be counted as fluid intake. The fluid allotment should be spaced throughout the day so that the patient does not become uncomfortable from thirst. During chronic HD, fluid intake is adjusted so that ideally the patient gains no more than 1.0 to 1.5 kg between dialyses.

NUTRITIONAL THERAPY

Table 44-8 High-Potassium Foods

100-250 mg K+	250-350 mg K+	>350 mg K+
Fruits		
1 medium tangerine	½ cup prune juice	⅒ honey dew melon
½ cup fresh pineapple	3 apricots	1 medium banana
1 medium orange	1 fresh peach	10 dried prunes
1 dried fig	½ fresh papaya	10 dates
½ grapefruit	¼ cantaloupe	½ cup raisins
1 fresh pear		½ avocado
½ cup grapefruit juice		1 nectarine
½ cup orange juice		
½ cup pineapple juice		
½ cup apricot nectar		
Cooked Vegetables		
½ cup broccoli	½ cup tomato juice	½ cup parsnips
½ cup rutabagas	½ cup vegetable juice	Artichokes
½ cup pared and boiled potatoes	½ cup rhubarb	1 baked potato
½ cup yams	½ cup pumpkin	
2½-in diameter tomato	½ cup winter squash	
½ cup brussels sprouts		
½ cup pinto beans		
Miscellaneous		
2 tbs wheat germ	1 oz chocolate	1 cup milk
2 slices whole grain bread		1 tbs dark molasses
2 ounces meat		
2 tbs cocoa		
1 cup bran cereal		
20 pecans		
10 peanuts		
10 walnuts		
1 tbs light molasses		

Sodium and potassium restriction. The amount of sodium and potassium restriction depends on the ability of the kidneys to excrete these electrolytes. Sodium-restricted diets may vary from 1000 to 4000 mg (1 mEq = 23 mg of sodium), depending on the degree of edema and hypertension. (The average daily intake of sodium is 3 g to 7 g.) Sodium and salt should not be equated because the sodium content in 1 g of sodium chloride is equivalent to 400 mg of sodium. The patient should be instructed to avoid foods known to be high in sodium such as cured meats, pickled foods, canned soups and stews, frankfurters, cold cuts, soy sauce, and salad dressings (see Table 33-11). Most salt substitutes should not be used because they contain potassium chloride.

Controlled dietary restrictions of potassium range from 1500 to 4000 mg (1 mEq = 39 mg of potassium). Some PD patients do not need potassium restrictions. For every 20 g increase in dietary protein, the potassium intake is increased by 500 mg. This makes it virtually impossible to restrict potassium to 40 mEq (1.6 g) in an 80 g protein diet because most foods that are high in protein are also high in potassium. Foods with high potassium levels that should be avoided are dried fruits, legumes, oranges, bananas, melons, deep green and deep yellow vegetables, beans, and peas (Table 44-8).

NURSING MANAGEMENT: CONSERVATIVE THERAPY OF CHRONIC RENAL FAILURE
Nursing Assessment

The nurse should obtain a complete history of any existing renal disease or family history of renal disease because many renal disorders have a hereditary basis. Information on long-term health problems such as hypertension, diabetes, recurrent urinary tract infections, and systemic lupus erythematosus must be obtained. Because many medications are potentially nephrotoxic, both current and past use of prescription and over-the-counter medications must be determined.

The nurse should assess the patient's dietary habits and discuss any problems. Accurate height and weight assessment and information about recent weight gain or loss must be obtained.

Clinical manifestations of chronic renal failure are related to alterations in multiple body systems (see Fig. 44-3). The nurse must be aware of the wide diversity of problems in the patient. Fatigue, lethargy, and pruritus are often the early symptoms of chronic renal failure; hypertension and changes in urine characteristics are often the first signs.

Family and other support systems should be assessed. The chronicity of renal disease and the long-term nature of treatment modalities affect every area of a person's life, including family relationships, social and work activities, and self-image. The choice of treatment modality may be related to support systems available to the patient.

■ Nursing Diagnoses

Nursing diagnoses for chronic renal failure may include, but are not limited to, those presented in NCP 44-1.

■ Planning

The overall goals are that a patient with chronic renal failure will (1) demonstrate knowledge and ability to comply with the therapeutic regimen, (2) participate in decision making for the plan of care and future treatment modality, (3) demonstrate effective coping strategies, and (4) continue with activities of daily living within physiologic limitations.

■ Nursing Implementation

Health Promotion. Individuals must be instructed on the importance of maintaining an adequate fluid intake each day (at least 2 L). They should be advised that any changes in urine appearance (color, odor), frequency, or volume must be reported to the health care provider.

If a patient has a history of renal disease, hypertension, or diabetes mellitus or a family history of renal disease, regular checkups including serum creatinine, BUN, and urinalysis are essential. If a patient must be prescribed a potentially nephrotoxic drug, it is important to monitor renal function with serum creatinine and BUN determinations.

Acute Intervention. The specific nursing management related to various problems is included in NCP 44-1. In addition, it is important to educate the patient and family because diet, medications, and follow-up medical care are the responsibilities of the patient (Table 44-9). The patient should obtain a daily weight, learn to take daily blood pressures, and be able to identify signs and symptoms of edema, hyperkalemia, and other electrolyte imbalances. The patient and family must understand the importance of strict dietary adherence. The dietician and the nurse should meet with the patient and family on a continuing basis to assist in diet planning. A diet history and consideration of cultural variations make diet planning and adherence more easily achieved goals.

The patient needs a complete understanding of the drugs, the dosages, and the common side effects. It may be helpful to make a list of the medications and the times of administration that can be posted in the home in a convenient location. The patient must be instructed to avoid certain over-the-counter drugs such as laxatives and antacids that contain magnesium.

It is important that the patient be motivated to assume the primary role in the management of the disease. The period of conservative management provides a good opportunity to evaluate each patient's ability to manage the disease. This is a critical factor in considering each patient as a candidate for home dialysis or transplantation.

Ambulatory and Home Care. The length of time a patient can be maintained on conservative therapy is highly variable and depends on the progression of renal failure. When conservative therapy is no longer effective, hemodialysis, peritoneal dialysis, and transplantation are the available treatment options.

While the patient is being maintained on conservative therapy, the decision regarding future therapies, if any, should be made. This should be done before complications such as mental status changes, bleeding, progressive neuropathies, and persistent congestive heart failure occur.

The patient and family need a clear explanation of what is involved in dialysis and transplantation. If alternative treatments

44-1 NURSING CARE PLAN PATIENT WITH CHRONIC RENAL FAILURE

| Expected Patient Outcomes | Nursing Interventions and *Rationales* |

NURSING DIAGNOSIS **Fluid volume excess** *related to* inability of kidneys to excrete fluid, inadequate dialysis, and excessive fluid intake *as manifested by* edema, hypertension, bounding pulse, weight gain, shortness of breath, pulmonary edema.

- No edema.
- No evidence of dyspnea.
- Dry weight remaining within 2 lb (1 kg) of patient's dry weight.
- Blood pressure within limits for patient.

- Monitor for increase in blood pressure, periorbital sacral and peripheral edema, dyspnea, and pericardial friction rub, *which are indicators of fluid excess.*
- Auscultate lungs for crackles *to identify fluid in the lungs.*
- Teach patient how to maintain a low-sodium diet *to help control edema and hypertension.*
- Teach patient fluid control measures and importance of daily weights *to help monitor and control fluid overload and related hypertension.*
- Teach patient on hemodialysis or peritoneal dialysis what the individual goal weight or dry weight is and how this may change *to help maintain better fluid balance.*
- Provide skin care with special emphasis on edematous areas *because these areas are prone to breakdown.*

NURSING DIAGNOSIS **Impaired skin integrity** *related to* decrease in oil and sweat gland activity, deposition of calcium-phosphate precipitates, capillary fragility, excess fluid, and neuropathy *as manifested by* itching, bruising, dry skin, edema, excoriation.

- No itching or skin dryness.
- Intact, clean skin.

- Assess skin for changes in color, texture, turgor, and vascularity *to provide direction for appropriate interventions.*
- Inspect patient for bruises, purpura, and signs of infection *to detect early signs of problems.*
- Provide skin care with tepid water, xipamide (Aquaphor), or bath oils *to relieve itching and moisturize dry, cracked skin.*
- Apply ointments or creams (lanolin, Aquaphor) following bath or shower *to relieve itching and promote comfort.*
- Administer antihistamines and antipruritics as prescribed *to relieve itching.*
- Trim patient's nails short and keep them clean *to reduce tissue damage from scratching and prevent infection.*
- Monitor serum calcium and phosphate levels *since elevated blood levels may lead to calcium-phosphate precipitation in the skin.*

NURSING DIAGNOSIS **Risk for injury: fracture** *related to* alterations in the absorption of calcium and excretion of phosphate, altered vitamin D metabolism.

- Slowing of bone disease.
- Serum calcium levels >8 mg/dl (2.0 mmol/L) and phosphate levels <5.5 mg/dl (1.8 mmol/L).
- No bone fractures.

- Assess for hypocalcemia, elevated serum phosphate levels, muscle pain, and limited mobility of joints *to detect potential risks for injury.*
- Observe for manifestations of bone pain *as a possible indicator of bone injury.*
- Provide range-of-motion exercises and encourage ambulation *to foster osteoblast activity and decrease bone resorption.*
- Provide safe environment *to reduce the risk of injury.*
- Administer calcium supplements, vitamin D, and phosphate binders as ordered *to prevent or treat the bone demineralization.*
- Give calcium supplements or phosphate binders with meals *to increase their effectiveness by binding dietary phosphorus to form insoluble calcium phosphate or aluminum phosphate, which is excreted in feces.*
- Instruct patient in the importance of taking these drugs with meals *to facilitate compliance with therapeutic regimen.*
- Ensure that patient understands and follows dietary restrictions of phosphate.
- Observe for hypocalcemia when using calcium supplements.
- Explain to patient the potential for fracture *to reduce the risk of unsafe practices that might result in a traumatic or pathologic fracture.*

Continued

44-1 NURSING CARE PLAN PATIENT WITH CHRONIC RENAL FAILURE
—continued

| Expected Patient Outcomes | Nursing Interventions and *Rationales* |

NURSING DIAGNOSIS Activity intolerance *related to* anemia secondary to uremia and blood loss during dialysis *as manifested by* fatigability, shortness of breath, pallor, dyspnea, tachycardia.

- Hematocrit in acceptable range.
- Able to perform activities of daily living without undue fatigue.

- Monitor hematocrit and hemoglobin levels *as an indicator of the patient's oxygen-carrying capacity.*
- Administer iron between meals and erythropoietin as ordered *to maintain normal erythropoiesis and stimulate production of RBCs.*
- Do not administer folic acid before or during hemodialysis *because folic acid is dialyzable and would be lost in the dialysate.*
- Provide adequate periods of rest *to enable patient to recuperate from past activities and participate in future activity.*
- Teach patient to plan activities *to avoid fatigue.*
- Minimize blood loss during dialysis and watch for any bleeding sites *because bleeding reduces RBCs and can result in decreased O_2 at cellular level.*
- Assess patient's response to activity *to make appropriate adjustments in plan of care.*

NURSING DIAGNOSIS Altered nutrition: less than body requirements *related to* restricted level of nutrients (especially protein), nausea, vomiting, anorexia, stomatitis, and altered metabolism of nutrients *as manifested by* loss of appetite, loss of weight, alterations in electrolyte balance.

- Maintenance of ideal body weight.
- Albumin and total protein within acceptable limits.

- Monitor weight, BUN, serum creatinine, albumin, total protein, and serum electrolytes *as indicators of effectiveness of dialysis, nutritional status, and response to treatment.*
- Provide frequent mouth care *to prevent stomatitis, remove foul tastes, and increase patient's comfort.*
- Provide small, frequent meals *because smaller, more frequent feedings reduce nausea and vomiting.*
- Allow patient freedom in choosing food and fluid intake within limitations *to increase the patient's sense of control.*
- Provide at least 2000-2500 kcal/day with a high-carbohydrate intake *to minimize catabolism of body protein and maintain body weight.*
- Restrict protein and phosphate to prescribed amount *to decrease the metabolic end products of urea, potassium, phosphate, and hydrogen.*
- Provide hard candy, gum, and lollipops *to improve taste and increase carbohydrate intake if patient is not a diabetic.*

NURSING DIAGNOSIS Constipation *related to* decreased mobility, antacid intake, fluid restrictions, dietary modification, or electrolyte imbalances *as manifested by* lack of usual bowel elimination.

- Usual bowel elimination pattern.

- Administer stool softeners as prescribed *to prevent constipation by maintaining soft stools.*
- Teach patient to avoid over-the-counter laxatives that contain magnesium *since hypermagnesemia could develop.*
- Encourage ambulation to patient's ability *to increase bowel peristalsis.*

NURSING DIAGNOSIS Diarrhea *related to* GI inflammation secondary to urea or as side effect of sorbitol-Kayexalate treatment *as manifested by* frequent, loose-to-watery stools.

- Usual bowel elimination pattern.

- Record and measure stool *to monitor fluid and electrolyte losses.*
- Monitor serum electrolytes (especially potassium, calcium, and bicarbonate levels) when patient has persistent diarrhea *because altered levels can result in significant problems.*
- Encourage oral intake of fluids containing electrolytes *to replace losses.*
- Clean perianal area gently and apply lotions *to maintain perianal skin integrity.*
- Increase oral fluid intake to prescribed maximum and return to normal diet as tolerated *to promote return to normal bowel functioning.*

Continued

44-1 **NURSING CARE PLAN** **PATIENT WITH CHRONIC RENAL FAILURE**
—continued

Expected Patient Outcomes	Nursing Interventions and *Rationales*

NURSING DIAGNOSIS **Anticipatory grieving** *related to* loss of kidney function *as manifested by* expression of feelings of sadness, anger, inadequacy, hopelessness.

- Acceptance of chronic disease.

- Listen to concerns of patient *to convey a caring attitude and foster the nurse-patient relationship and to determine how patient is handling the situation.*
- Allow patient time to mourn loss of body function *so patient can deal with feelings and identify ways of coping with losses more effectively.*
- Include family members in discussions of patient's concerns *to enable them to assist the patient and foster their support and understanding.*

NURSING DIAGNOSIS **Self-esteem disturbance** *related to* enforced lifestyle changes, dependency on dialysis, chronic fatigue, body image changes, occupational problems, and role maintenance *as manifested by* expression of feelings of inadequacy and unworthiness, concerns about family finances and functioning.

- Positive feelings about self.
- Participation in treatment regimen.
- Adaptation of lifestyle to changing health status.

- Provide opportunity for patient to discuss concerns *to determine how patient is dealing with the changes in her or his life.*
- Refer patient to social worker and for counseling if indicated *to provide additional assistance for management of chronic illness.*
- Assure patient of self-worth *to raise self-esteem by reinforcing positive attributes.*
- Encourage patient and significant others to share feelings *because verbalization helps clarify feelings and may provide insight into solutions.*
- Arrange for patient to talk with other patients in similar circumstances *to provide support and understanding.*

NURSING DIAGNOSIS **Sensory-perceptual alterations** *related to* CNS changes induced by uremic toxins *as manifested by* confusion, slowing of thought processes, decreased attention and memory span, disorientation, changes in sensorium (e.g., somnolence, stupor), changes in mood (e.g., irritability, depression), changes in behavior (e.g., withdrawal).

- Mental alertness and appropriate interaction with environment.

- Provide explanation to patient and family of effects of uremia on nervous system *to reduce anxiety over changes in mentation.*
- Assess patient's level of consciousness and mental status at regular intervals *because minor confusion and irritability can progress and indicate a worsening of condition.*
- Discuss significant material for brief rather than long time periods *to reduce confusion and increase possibility that information will be understood and retained.*
- Provide calm, nonstimulating environment *to prevent increasing patient's confusion and agitation.*

NURSING DIAGNOSIS **Risk for sexual dysfunction** *related to* effects of uremia on reproductive and endocrine systems and the psychosocial impact of renal failure and its treatment.

- Satisfaction with sexual relationship by patient and significant other.

- Assess female patients for amenorrhea and decreased libido; assess male patients for impotence, atrophy of testicles, and gynecomastia *to determine presence and extent of risk factors for sexual dysfunction and plan appropriate interventions.*
- Discuss meaning of sexuality with patient and significant other *to determine significance of problem.*
- Encourage patient and partner to discuss feelings openly and to use other means of sexual expression besides intercourse; explore new patterns of sexual activity if previous patterns lead to anxiety *to ensure continued expression of sexual feelings.*

Continued

44-1   NURSING CARE PLAN   PATIENT WITH CHRONIC RENAL FAILURE
—continued

Expected Patient Outcomes	Nursing Interventions and *Rationales*

NURSING DIAGNOSIS   **Risk for infection** *related to* suppressed immune system, access sites, and malnutrition secondary to dialysis and uremia.

- No infections.
- WBC count within normal range.

- Assess for chills, fever, tachycardia; redness, swelling, or drainage in area of break in skin *to detect signs of possible infection.*
- Provide frequent oral and personal hygiene *to reduce risk of self-contamination.*
- Instruct patient to avoid exposure to people with infections *because the patient has an altered immune response and therefore has an increased risk of infection.*
- Watch for local and systemic manifestations of infection *to promote early identification and treatment.*
- Maintain aseptic technique when performing dialysis *to prevent the introduction of organisms.*
- Avoid invasive procedures such as catheterization *to avoid introduction of organisms.*

COLLABORATIVE PROBLEMS

Nursing Goals	Nursing Interventions and *Rationales*

POTENTIAL COMPLICATION   **Hypertension** *related to* sodium and water retention and alterations of renin-angiotensin system.

- Monitor for hypertension.
- Report deviations from acceptable parameters.
- Carry out appropriate medical and nursing interventions.

- Assess patient for elevated blood pressure, headache, dizziness, shortness of breath, chest pain, edema *to identify the presence and effects of hypertension.*
- Take vital signs q4hr *to provide a database for ongoing analysis of patient's response to treatment.*
- Administer antihypertensive medications as ordered.
- Observe for orthostatic hypotension and other side effects of medication *because overtreatment may cause problems.*
- Instruct patient to change positions slowly *to minimize dizziness caused by orthostatic hypotension.*
- Explain the actions and side effects of drugs and risks of uncontrolled hypertension (e.g., stroke) *to foster adherence to medication regimen.*

POTENTIAL COMPLICATION   **Hyperkalemia** *related to* decreased renal function, increased tissue catabolism, and shift of potassium into extracellular fluid *related to* metabolic acidosis.

- Monitor for signs of hyperkalemia.
- Report deviations from acceptable parameters.
- Carry out appropriate medical and nursing interventions.

- Assess for signs of hyperkalemia such as serum potassium >5.5 mEq/L (5.5 mmol/L), muscle weakness, arrhythmias, paresthesias, intestinal colic and diarrhea, peaked T waves on ECG *to ensure early identification and treatment.*
- Discuss importance of following prescribed diet and avoiding foods high in potassium *to prevent complications of hyperkalemia.*
- Monitor serum potassium and notify physician of elevated levels and ECG results *because elevated potassium can cause life-threatening cardiac arrhythmias.*
- Be prepared to administer treatment for hyperkalemia *because this is a medical emergency requiring prompt treatment.*

POTENTIAL COMPLICATION   **Peripheral neuropathy** *related to* effects of uremia on peripheral nerves.

- Monitor for peripheral neuropathies.
- Report deviations from acceptable parameters.
- Carry out appropriate medical and nursing interventions.

- Assess patient for decreased sensation, numbness, burning of feet, muscle cramps, restlessness of legs, loss of muscle strength, footdrop *to identify presence of peripheral neuropathy.*
- Explain to patient reason for neuropathy *to increase understanding and decrease anxiety.*
- Prevent trauma and excess stimulation to extremities *because areas with diminished sensation are extremely prone to injury.*
- Instruct patient to avoid tight clothing and restricting bed linens *to prevent inadvertent injury since the affected areas have decreased sensation.*
- Teach patient to examine areas of decreased sensation *to observe for injury.*
- In collaboration with physical therapy department, develop exercise regimen *to maintain prescribed level of activity.*
- Assess adequacy of dialysis therapy *because dialysis may reduce the symptoms and halt the progress of neuropathies.*

Table **44-9**   **Chronic Renal Failure**

1. Explain dietary (protein, sodium, potassium, phosphate) and fluid restrictions.
2. Encourage discussion of difficulties in modifying diet and fluid intake.
3. Explain signs and symptoms of electrolyte imbalance, especially high potassium.
4. Teach alternative ways of reducing thirst, such as sucking on ice cubes, lemon, or hard candy.
5. Explain the rationale for prescribed medications and common side effects. Examples:
    - Calcium supplements or phosphate binders should be taken with meals.
    - Iron supplements should be taken between meals.
6. Explain the importance of reporting any of the following:
    - Weight gain greater than 2 lb (1 kg)
    - Increasing blood pressure
    - Shortness of breath
    - Edema
    - Increasing fatigue or weakness
    - Confusion or lethargy
7. Encourage patient and family to share concerns about lifestyle changes, living with a chronic illness, decisions about type of dialysis or transplantation.

are presented early in the course of therapy, the patient will have an opportunity to carefully consider choices. The patient will feel more control over her or his life and health care when educated about treatment and treatment options and when active in the decision-making process. The patient should be informed that if dialysis is chosen, the option of transplantation still remains. It should be emphasized that if a transplanted organ fails, the patient can return to dialysis. Some individuals with chronic renal failure have received more than one kidney transplant.

■ **Evaluation**

The expected outcomes for the patient with chronic renal failure are presented in NCP 44-1.

DIALYSIS

Dialysis is the movement of fluid and molecules across a semipermeable membrane from one compartment to another. Clinically, dialysis is a technique in which substances move from the blood through a semipermeable membrane and into a dialysis solution (dialysate). Dialysis is used to correct fluid and electrolyte imbalances and to remove waste products in renal failure. Dialysis can also be used to treat drug overdoses. The two methods of dialysis are peritoneal dialysis (PD) and hemodialysis (HD) (Table 44-10). In PD the peritoneal membrane is used as the semipermeable membrane. In HD an artificial membrane (usually made of cellulose-based or synthetic materials) is used as the semipermeable membrane that is in contact with the patient's blood.

Dialysis is begun when the patient's uremic state can no longer be adequately managed conservatively. A general guideline is to start dialysis when the GFR (or creatinine clearance) is less than 5 to 10 ml per minute. However, this criterion varies widely in different clinical situations, and the physician determines when to start dialysis based on the patient's clinical status. Certain uremic complications, including encephalopathy, neuropathies, uncontrollable hyperkalemia, pericarditis, and accelerated hypertension, indicate a need for immediate dialysis.

GENERAL PRINCIPLES

Solutes and water move across the membrane from the blood to the dialysate or from the dialysate to the blood in accordance with concentration gradients. The principles of diffusion, osmosis, and ultrafiltration are involved in dialysis (Fig. 44-5). *Diffusion* is the movement of solutes from an area of greater concentration to an area of lesser concentration. In renal failure, urea, creatinine, uric acid, and electrolytes (potassium, phosphate) move from the blood to the dialysate with the net effect of lowering their concentration in the blood. RBCs, WBCs, and large plasma proteins are too large to diffuse through the pores of the membrane.

Osmosis is the movement of fluid from an area of lesser to an area of greater concentration of solutes. Glucose is added to the dialysate bath and creates an osmotic gradient across the membrane to remove excess fluid from the blood.

Ultrafiltration (water and fluid removal) results when a pressure gradient across the dialyzer membrane is created by an increased pressure in the blood compartment (positive pressure) or a decreased pressure in the dialysate compartment (negative pressure). Extracellular fluid moves into the dialysate because of the pressure gradient. In peritoneal dialysis, excess fluid is removed by increasing the osmolality of the dialysate with the addition of glucose. In HD, excess fluid is removed by creating a pressure differential between the blood and the dialysate solution with a combination of positive pressure in the blood compartment or a negative pressure in the dialysate compartment.

PERITONEAL DIALYSIS

Although PD was first used in 1923, it did not come into widespread use for chronic treatment until the 1970s with the development of soft, pliable peritoneal solution bags and the introduction of the concept of continuous PD. In the United States, approximately 15% of patients receiving dialysis treatments are on peritoneal dialysis.[5] In Canada, approximately 36% of patients are on PD because of the decreased availability of HD. In recent years the use of PD to treat chronic renal failure has increased considerably. The large surface area of the peritoneum makes it a good semipermeable membrane for performing clinical dialysis.

Table **44-10** **Comparison of Peritoneal Dialysis and Hemodialysis**

| Peritoneal Dialysis | | Hemodialysis | |
Advantages	Disadvantages	Advantages	Disadvantages
Immediate initiation in almost any hospital Less complicated than hemodialysis Portable system with CAPD Fewer dietary restrictions Relatively short training time Usable in the patient with vascular access problems Less cardiovascular stress Home dialysis possible Preferable for the diabetic patient	Bacterial or chemical peritonitis Protein loss into dialysate Exit-site and tunnel infections Self-image problems with catheter placement Hyperglycemia Aggravated hyperlipidemia Surgery for catheter placement Contraindication in the patient with multiple abdominal surgery or trauma Specially trained personnel needed	Rapid fluid removal Rapid removal of urea and creatinine Effective potassium removal Less protein loss Lowering of serum triglycerides Home dialysis possible Temporary access can be placed at bedside	Vascular access problems Dietary and fluid restrictions Heparinization may be necessary Extensive equipment necessary Hypotension during dialysis Added blood loss that contributes to anemia Specially trained personnel necessary

CAPD, continuous ambulatory peritoneal dialysis.

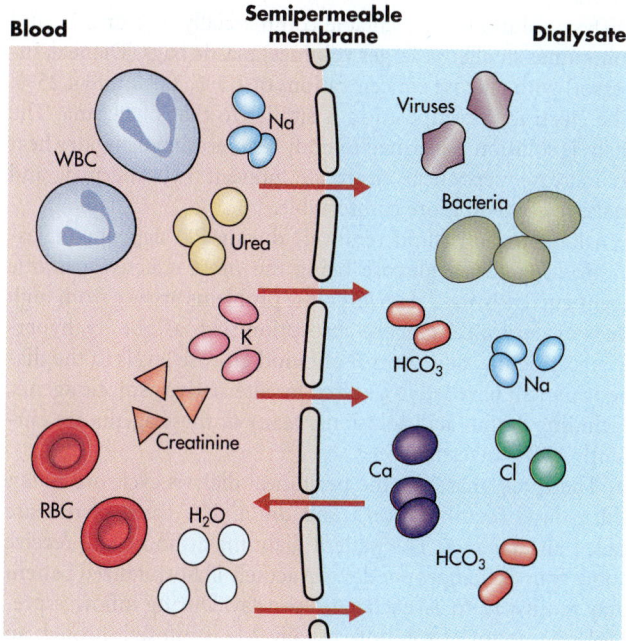

Fig. 44-5 Osmosis and diffusion across a semipermeable membrane.

Catheter Placement

Peritoneal access is obtained by inserting a catheter through the anterior abdominal wall (Fig. 44-6). The prototype of the catheter that is used was developed by Tenckhoff in 1968 and is made of silicone rubber tubing (see Fig. 44-6). The current version of this catheter is about 25 cm long and has one or two Dacron cuffs at the subcutaneous and peritoneal ends of the catheter that anchor it securely and prevent the migration of microorganisms down the shaft from the skin. Within a few

weeks, fibrous tissue grows into the Dacron cuff, anchors the catheter in place, and prevents bacterial penetration into the peritoneal cavity. The tip of the catheter rests in the peritoneal cavity and has many perforations spaced throughout the distal end of the tubing to allow fluid to flow in and out of the catheter. Other types of catheters for chronic PD are variations of the Tenckhoff catheter, including the Toronto-Western, Purdue-Column Disc, and Gore-Tex catheters (Fig. 44-7).

The technique for catheter placement varies. Although it is possible to place a permanent catheter in the peritoneal cavity with a trocar, it is usually done via surgery so that its placement can be directly visualized, thus minimizing potential complications. Preparation of the patient for catheter insertion includes emptying the bladder and bowel, weighing the patient, and obtaining a signed consent form. In the nonsurgical approach, an area approximately 2 cm below the umbilicus is anesthetized with a local anesthetic, and the abdomen is distended with dialysis solution. A trocar, with the catheter threaded through or over it, is inserted into the peritoneal cavity. When the patient feels pressure in the rectal area and has the urge to defecate, the trocar is withdrawn, and the catheter is in place.

In the surgical approach a midline umbilical incision is made, and a small puncture is made to one side and below this incision. The distal end of the catheter is placed in the peritoneum and it is tunneled under the skin to the puncture site. After the catheter is inserted, the skin is cleaned with an antiseptic solution, and a sterile dressing is applied. Complications of catheter insertion include perforation of the bladder, the bowel, or a blood vessel and the introduction of bacteria.

The catheter is connected to a sterile tubing system and anchored to the abdomen with tape. The catheter is irrigated immediately with heparinized dialysate (usually 500 ml) to clear blood and fibrin from it. The irrigations may continue for 12 to 24 hours using small volumes of dialysate. This procedure helps prevent the catheter from clogging, resulting in poor drainage

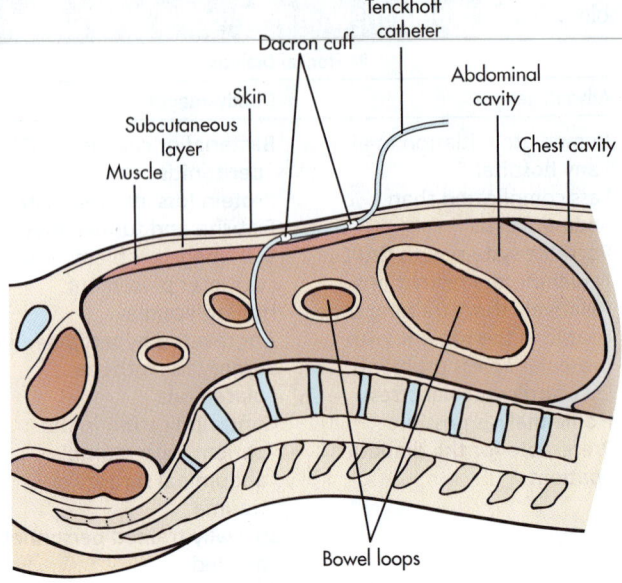

Fig. 44-6 Tenckhoff catheter used in peritoneal dialysis.

Dialysis Solutions and Cycle

Dialysis solutions are available commercially in 1 or 2 L (and sometimes smaller or larger volumes) plastic bags (Dianeal, Inpersol) with glucose concentrations of 1.5%, 2.5%, and 4.25%. The electrolyte composition is similar to that of plasma. The dialysis solution is warmed to body temperature using dry heat to increase peritoneal clearance, prevent hypothermia, and make the patient more comfortable.

Ultrafiltration (fluid removal) during PD depends on osmotic forces with glucose being the most effective osmotic agent currently used. However, the problems arising from high rates of peritoneal glucose absorption such as obesity, hypertriglyceridemia, and control of blood glucose levels in the diabetic patient have led to a search for alternative osmotic agents, including amino acid solutions. Many of these agents are currently under investigation.

The three phases of the peritoneal dialysis cycle are *inflow* (fill), *dwell* (equilibration), and *drain*. The three phases are called an *exchange*. The patient dialyzing at home will receive about four exchanges per day. An acutely ill hospitalized patient may receive 12 to 24 exchanges per day. During inflow, a prescribed amount of solution, usually 2 L, is infused through an established catheter over about 10 minutes. The flow rate may be decreased if the patient becomes uncomfortable. After the solution has been infused, the inflow clamp is closed before air enters the tubing.

The next part of the cycle is the dwell phase, or equilibration, during which diffusion and osmosis occur between the patient's blood and the peritoneal cavity. The duration of the dwell time can last 20 to 30 minutes to 8 or more hours, depending on the method of PD. Drain time takes 15 to 30 minutes and may be facilitated by gently massaging the abdomen or changing the patient's position. The cycle starts again with the infusion of another 2 L of solution. For manual PD, a period of about 30 to 50 minutes is required to complete an exchange.

and inflow. More frequently today, this procedure is carried out as day surgery and the patient is discharged home with a sterile dressing covering the PD catheter. The patient then needs explicit instructions on keeping the dressing dry and an appointment to visit the dialysis clinic in a few days.

Before the start of PD, it is preferable to allow a waiting period of 7 to 14 days for proper sealing of the catheter and for tissue ingrowth into the cuffs. However, some centers start dialysis 5 to 7 days after catheter insertion. About 2 to 4 weeks after catheter implantation, the exit site should be clean, dry, and free of redness and tenderness (Fig. 44-8). Once the catheter incision site is healed, the patient may shower and then pat the catheter and exit site dry. Daily catheter care includes the application of an antiseptic solution and a clean dressing, as well as examination of the catheter site for signs of infection.

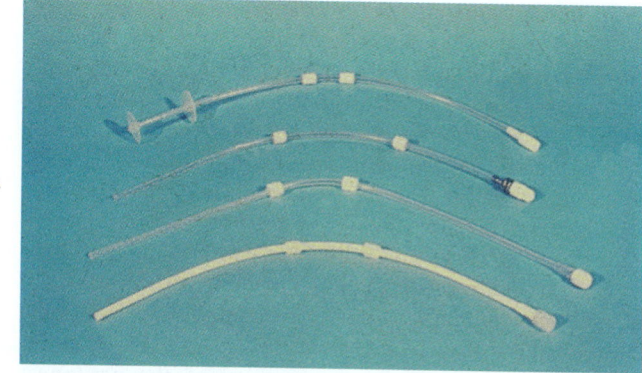

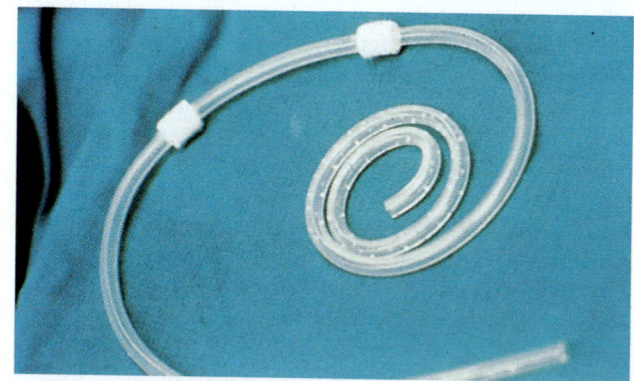

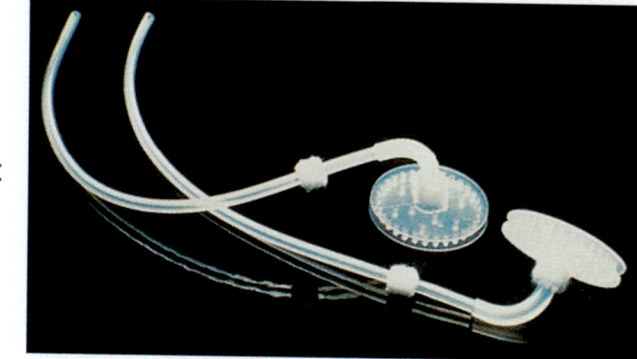

Fig. 44-7   A, Peritoneal catheters used for peritoneal dialysis. **B,** Bent neck curl catheters. **C,** Disk catheters.

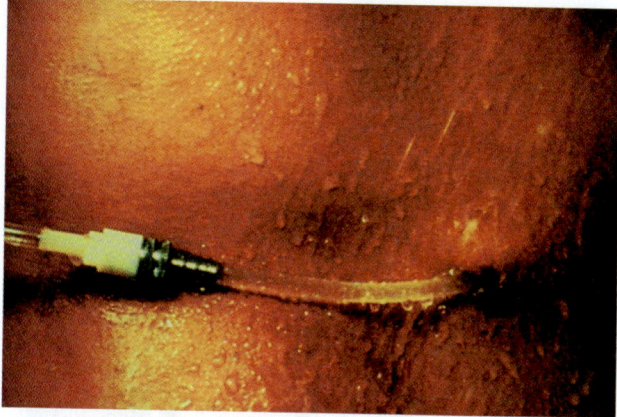

Fig. 44-8   Placement of peritoneal catheter.

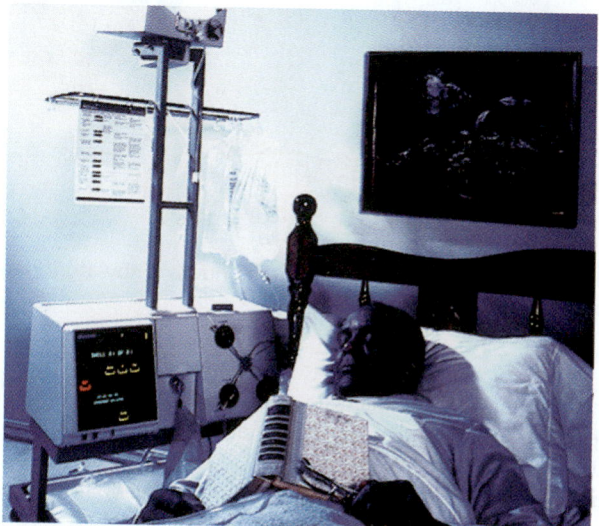

Fig. 44-9   Automated peritoneal dialysis cycler that can be used while the patient is sleeping or for hospitalized patients who require frequent exchanges.

Peritoneal Dialysis Systems

Two types of PD currently being used are automated peritoneal dialysis (APD) and continuous ambulatory peritoneal dialysis (CAPD).

Automated Peritoneal Dialysis. An automated device called a *cycler* is used to deliver the dialysate for APD (Fig. 44-9). The automated cycler times and controls the fill, dwell, and drain phases. The machine cycles four to eight exchanges per night with 1 to 2 hours per exchange. Alarms and monitors are built into the system to make it safe for the patient to dialyze while sleeping. It may be easier to teach the patient and family to use the PD machine at home compared with the HD equipment. APD includes the following variations: continuous cyclic peritoneal dialysis (CCPD), intermittent peritoneal dialysis (IPD), and nightly peritoneal dialysis (NPD). In CCPD the dialysis solution can be left in the peritoneal cavity during the day between nightly cycling, or the peritoneal cavity can be left "dry" during the day. With IPD and NPD, cycling is performed five to seven nights per week, and the abdomen is left empty between dialysis.

Continuous Ambulatory Peritoneal Dialysis. CAPD is carried out manually by exchanging 1.5 to 3 L (usually 2 L) of peritoneal dialysate usually four times daily with dwell times of 4 to 10 hours. One schedule, for example, starts the exchanges at 7 AM, 12 noon, 5 PM, and 10 PM. In this procedure the person instills 2 L of dialysate from a collapsible plastic bag into the peritoneal cavity through a disposable plastic tube.

Technical advances in CAPD systems, including Y sets and twin bag systems, allow the bag and line to be disconnected after the instillation of the fluid and decrease the risk of peritonitis. After the equilibration period the line is reconnected to

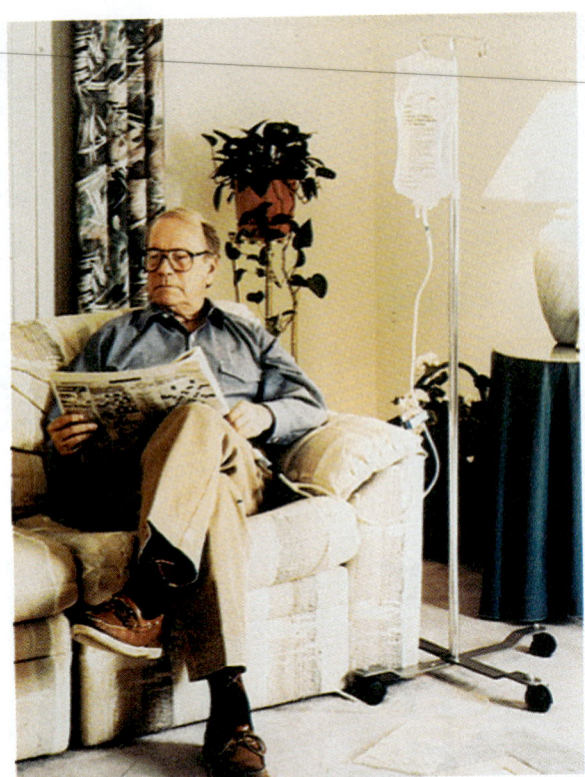

Fig. 44-10 Infusion period for a continuous ambulatory peritoneal dialysis patient.

the catheter, and the dialysate (effluent) is drained from the peritoneal cavity, and a new 2 L bag of dialysate solution is infused (Fig. 44-10). It is critical in PD to maintain aseptic technique to avoid peritonitis. Several tubing connections and devices are commercially available to help maintain an aseptic system.

Contraindications for PD include the following:

1. History of multiple abdominal surgical procedures or severe abdominal pathology (e.g., severe pancreatitis, diverticulitis)
2. Recurrent abdominal wall or inguinal hernias
3. Excessive obesity with large abdominal wall and fat deposits
4. Preexisting vertebral disease (e.g., chronic back problems)
5. Severe obstructive pulmonary disease

Complications of Peritoneal Dialysis

Exit Site Infection. Infection of the peritoneal catheter exit site is most commonly caused by *Staphylococcus aureus* or *S. epidermidis* (from skin flora). Superficial exit-site infections caused by these organisms are generally resolved with antibiotic therapy. Clinical manifestations of an exit site infection include redness at site, tenderness, and drainage. If not treated immediately, subcutaneous tunnel infections usually result in abscess formation and may cause peritonitis and necessitate catheter removal.

Peritonitis. Peritonitis results from contamination of the dialysate or tubing or from progression of exit site or tunnel infections. Less commonly peritonitis results from bacte-

ria in the intestine crossing over into the peritoneal cavity. Peritonitis is usually caused by *S. aureus* or *S. epidermidis.*[12] The primary clinical manifestation of peritonitis is a cloudy peritoneal effluent that has a WBC count of over 100 cells per microliter (particularly neutrophils). GI manifestations may also be present, including diffuse abdominal pain, diarrhea, vomiting, abdominal distention, and hyperactive bowel sounds. Fever may or may not be present. Cultures, Gram's stain, and a cell count and a differential of peritoneal effluent are used to confirm the diagnosis of peritonitis. Antibiotics are given by mouth, IV, or, most commonly, intraperitoneally. The patient is usually treated on an outpatient basis. Repeated infections may necessitate the removal of the peritoneal catheter and termination of peritoneal dialysis. The formation of adhesions in the peritoneum can result from repeated infections and can interfere with the peritoneal membrane's ability as a dialyzing surface.

Abdominal Pain. Although not severe, pain is a common complication caused by the low pH of the dialysate solution, peritonitis, intraperitoneal irritation (which usually subsides in 1 to 2 weeks), and placement of the catheter. Pain can also occur when the tip of the catheter touches the bladder, bowel, or peritoneum. A change in the position of the catheter should correct this problem. Accidental infusion of air or infusing the dialysate too rapidly may cause referred pain in the shoulder. If the infusion rate is decreased, the pain usually subsides.

Outflow Problems. When outflow is less than 80% of inflow immediately after catheter placement, it may be caused by a kink in the tunnel segment of the catheter, omentum wrapped around the catheter, or migration of the catheter out of the pelvic region. Persistent outflow problems may require radiologic or surgical manipulation of the catheter. Outflow problems after the catheter has settled into place are often a result of a full colon; bowel evacuation frequently relieves the problem.

Hernias. Because of increased intraabdominal pressures secondary to the dialysate infusion, hernias can develop in predisposed individuals such as multiparous women and older men. However, in most situations after hernia repair, peritoneal dialysis can be restarted after several days using small dialysate volumes and keeping the patient supine.

Lower Back Problems. Increased intraabdominal pressure can cause or aggravate lower back pain. The lumbosacral curvature is increased by intraperitoneal infusion of dialysate. Orthopedic binders and a regular exercise program for the back muscles have been beneficial for some patients.

Bleeding. Effluent drained after the first few exchanges may be pink or slightly bloody because of the trauma of catheter insertion. Bloody effluent over several days or the new appearance of blood in the effluent can indicate active intraperitoneal bleeding. If this occurs, the blood pressure and hematocrit should be checked. Blood may also be present in the effluent of women who are menstruating or ovulating, but this requires no intervention.

Pulmonary Complications. Atelectasis, pneumonia, and bronchitis may occur from repeated upward displacement of the diaphragm, resulting in decreased lung expansion. The longer the dwell time, the greater the likelihood of pulmonary complications. Frequent repositioning and deep-breathing exercises can help alleviate pulmonary complications. When lying in bed, elevation of the head of the bed may prevent these problems.

Protein Loss. The peritoneal membrane is permeable to plasma proteins, amino acids, and polypeptides. Therefore these substances are lost in the dialysate fluid. The amount of loss may be as much as 9 to 12 g per day. This protein loss may be increased up to 40 g per day during episodes of peritonitis as the membrane becomes more permeable. The patient can maintain a positive nitrogen balance with satisfactory protein intake.

Carbohydrate and Lipid Abnormalities. Dialysate glucose is absorbed via the peritoneum and may amount to as much as 100 to 150 g per day. Continuous absorption of glucose results in increased insulin secretion and increased plasma insulin levels. The hyperinsulinemia stimulates hepatic production of triglycerides (see p. 1308).

Encapsulating Sclerosing Peritonitis and Loss of Ultrafiltration. *Encapsulating sclerosing peritonitis* is a term applied to the development of a thick fibrous membrane that surrounds and compresses the bowel. Intestinal obstruction and strangulation are common complications. This condition generally necessitates changing the patient to HD because of the loss of ultrafiltration. It can also occur as a result of unknown reasons or accidental infusion of disinfecting agents. Loss of ultrafiltration is associated with rapid glucose absorption.

Effectiveness of and Adaptation to Chronic Peritoneal Dialysis

The use and popularity of chronic PD is increasing. The technique is associated with a short training program, independence, and ease of traveling. Clinically, the patient on PD does at least as well as the patient on HD and sometimes better. There are fewer dietary restrictions, and greater mobility is possible than with conventional HD. The major disadvantage is the possibility of developing peritonitis. As further improvements in techniques are made (e.g., improved connecting and sterilizing devices, in-line filters, improved catheters), the incidence of peritonitis should decrease.

PD is especially indicated for the individual who has vascular access problems and responds poorly to the hemodynamic stresses of HD (e.g., the older adult patient with diabetes and cardiovascular disease). The diabetic patient with ESRD does better on PD than on HD. The advantages of PD for the diabetic patient include better blood pressure control, stable cardiovascular status without rapid fluid shifts, better control of blood glucose by intraperitoneal insulin (which can often eliminate the need for subcutaneous insulin), and avoidance of the risk of retinal hemorrhage from heparin use during HD.

HEMODIALYSIS

In 1943 Willem Kolff in the Netherlands performed the first successful dialysis on a human being with the use of a rotating-drum dialyzer. He initiated dialysis treatment in the United States in the 1950s.

Vascular Access Sites

Vascular access is one of the major problems with HD. To carry out HD, a high blood flow is required. Before 1960, HD re-

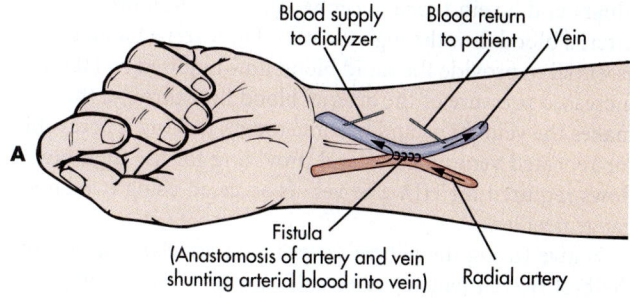
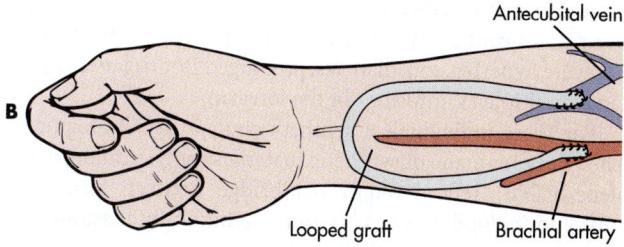
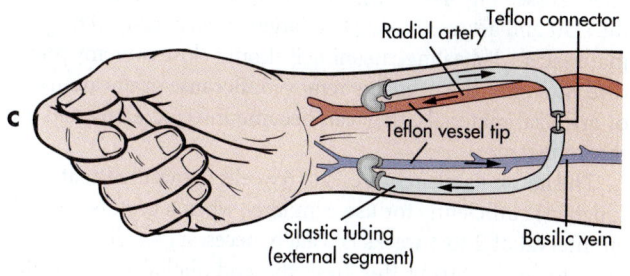

Fig. 44-11 Methods of vascular access for hemodialysis. **A,** Internal arteriovenous fistula. **B,** Looped graft in forearm. **C,** External cannula or shunt.

quired the insertion of needles into arteries and veins for each dialysis. Chronic dialysis was not possible with this technique.

Shunts. In 1960 Scribner developed a Teflon silicone rubber cannula that could be inserted into the radial artery and into an adjacent forearm vein (Fig. 44-11, *C*). The cannula is implanted subcutaneously in both the artery and vein and is connected to a silicone rubber tubing that exits from the skin. The two ends are connected by a U-shaped shunt that has a connector at its midpoint. The U portion of the shunt is external. This connection can be opened after clamping on both sides to attach the patient to the dialysis machine. The external access cannula is commonly referred to as an *external shunt* and can be used immediately. The external shunt is associated with many complications, including infection and bleeding. Because of these complications and the availability of other access alternatives, it is very rarely used for chronic dialysis. Although not commonly used, it can be used as a temporary access for continuous renal replacement therapy (see p. 1329).

Internal Arteriovenous Fistulas and Grafts. In 1966 the use of the subcutaneous internal arteriovenous native fistula (see Fig. 44-11, *A*) was introduced by Cimino and Brescia. An arteriovenous (AV) fistula is created most commonly in the forearm by a side-to-side, end-to-side, or end-to-end anastomosis between an artery (usually radial or ulnar) and a vein (usually cephalic). The fistula provides for arterial blood flow through the vein. The arterial blood flow is essential to provide the rapid blood flow required by HD. The increased pressure of the arterial blood flow through the vein makes the vein dilate and become tough, making it accessible for repeated venipuncture and providing for the high blood flows required for HD. The vein is accessed using two large-gauge needles.

Native (using the person's own blood vessels) fistulas have the best overall patency rates and least number of complications of all vascular accesses; however, they are suitable only for the patient with relatively healthy blood vessels.[13] Therefore native fistulas cannot always be created in patients with a history of severe hypertension, diabetes, prolonged IV drug use, or previous multiple IV infusions in the forearm.

For these individuals a synthetic graft is usually required. The grafts are made of synthetic materials (polytetrafluoroethylene [PTFE], Teflon) and form a "bridge" between the arterial and venous blood supplies.[13] Grafts are surgically anastomosed between an artery (usually brachial) and a vein (usually antecubital) (see Fig. 44-11, *B*). The graft, like the fistula, is under the skin and accessed using two large-gauge needles. The graft material is self-healing, meaning it should close over any puncture sites after the needle is removed. Because grafts are made of artificial materials, they can become infected easily and are thrombogenic.

The native fistula requires 4 to 6 weeks to mature (dilate and toughen) sufficiently for use. Similarly, when a graft is created, an interval of 2 to 4 weeks is usually necessary to allow for the graft to heal. During this time the endothelial cells are deposited on the inside of the graft, and these cells help seal the needle puncture site after the dialysis needle is removed. Some dialysis centers use the graft earlier.

Two 14- to 16-gauge needles are inserted into the fistula or graft (local anesthesia may be used) to obtain vascular access. One needle is placed to pull blood from the circulation to the HD machine, and the other needle is used to return the dialyzed blood to the patient. The needles are attached via tubing to dialysis lines. Normally, a thrill can be felt by palpating the area of anastomosis, and a bruit can be heard with a stethoscope. The bruit and thrill are created by arterial blood rushing into the vein. Blood pressures, IV insertion, and venipuncture should not be performed on the affected extremity. This prevents infection and potential sources of clotting of the vascular access. Vascular access can be difficult to obtain in patients with ESRD. Protection of the vascular access site is of paramount importance.

The subcutaneous AV fistula is much less likely to clot and become infected than a graft. Native fistulas seem to get better as the years go by. Thrombosis in grafts is common. Grafts can lead to the development of distal ischemia (steal syndrome) because arterial blood is being shunted. This is usually seen soon after surgery and may require surgical correction. Another complication is the development of an aneurysm at the fistula site. When a graft becomes infected, it is a serious problem that is frequently associated with bacteremia and may require the removal of the graft.

Temporary Vascular Access. In some situations when temporary vascular access is required quickly, percutaneous cannulation of the subclavian, internal jugular, or femoral vein is used. A flexible Teflon, silicone rubber, or polyurethane catheter is inserted into one of these large veins and provides easy immediate access to circulation without the need for the patient to have surgery or to sacrifice a peripheral artery or vein. The catheters usually have a double lumen with an internal septum separating the two segments (Fig. 44-12). One lumen is used for blood removal and the other for blood return. The procedure for percutaneous cannulation is similar to the method of insertion of a pulmonary artery catheter (see Chapter 63).

Percutaneous cannulas in the subclavian or jugular veins can be left in place for 1 to 3 weeks. Femoral-vein cannulas can remain in place for up to 1 week.

Technical complications of subclavian vein catheterization include brachial plexus problems, hemothorax, and pneumothorax. A moderate risk of infection also exists. While the catheter is in place, the patient is usually comfortable and can be ambulatory. No medications should be administered or blood withdrawn from this catheter by nondialysis staff. Trained dialysis staff may inject heparin into the lumen of the catheter at the end of dialysis and remove the heparin before starting dialysis. Subclavian vein thrombosis and stenosis is a complication of subclavian cannulation.

Although jugular vein cannulation is associated with a low incidence of thrombosis, short-term jugular vein access with stiff catheters is often unacceptable to the patient since the catheter is in the patient's neck and can cause discomfort and restrict movement.

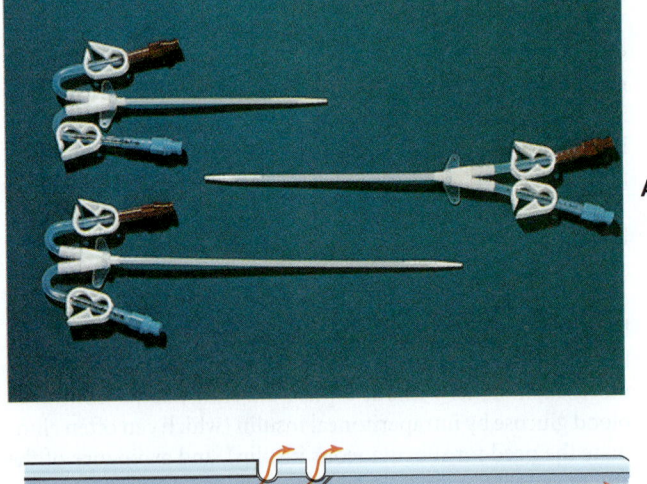

Fig. 44-12   Temporary double-lumen, single-needle vascular access catheter for acute hemodialysis. **A,** The soft, flexible dual-lumen polyurethane tube is attached to a Y hub. **B,** Blood is withdrawn continuously through the outer lumen upstream and returned through the inner lumen downstream, thus reducing recirculation.

Disadvantages of femoral-vessel cannulization include the following: (1) the catheter can remain in place only a short time, (2) the location encourages catheter kinking, and (3) the groin is not a clean site. Complications of femoral catheterization consist of femoral vein thrombosis with pulmonary emboli (especially if the treatment is prolonged), infections, immobility, and inadvertent blood vessel punctures with hematoma formation.

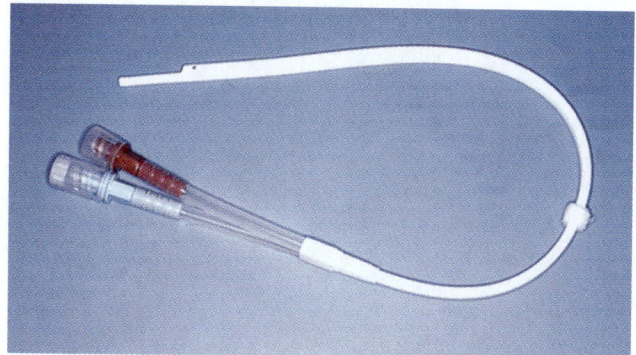

Fig. 44-13 Silastic permanent catheter used for permanent or temporary access.

A permanent, soft, flexible Silastic double-lumen catheter is being used more commonly (Fig. 44-13). It exits on the upper chest wall and is tunneled subcutaneously to the internal or external jugular vein. It has two Dacron cuffs, which reside subcutaneously to prevent infection and anchor the catheter, thus eliminating the need for sutures. The catheter must be placed radiologically. It is used as a temporary access while awaiting fistula placement and development or long-term access when other forms of vascular access have failed.

When dialysis is indicated, a permanent access is created, and a temporary access is used until the permanent access is ready to use. A subcutaneous AV fistula is created or a graft inserted, and the patient is hemodialyzed via a subclavian or jugular catheter until the AV fistula or graft is ready. Preferably the AV fistula or graft will be surgically created while the patient is being maintained on conservative therapy, well in advance of ESRD.

Dialyzers

The coil dialyzer was the first type of dialyzer used in which blood flowed through a series of cellophane tubes. Historically, this was later replaced by a flat plate dialyzer (Kiil) in which blood flowed between sheets of membrane outside of which the dialysate passed. Today the dialyzer is a long plastic cartridge that contains thousands of parallel hollow tubes or fibers (Fig. 44-14).

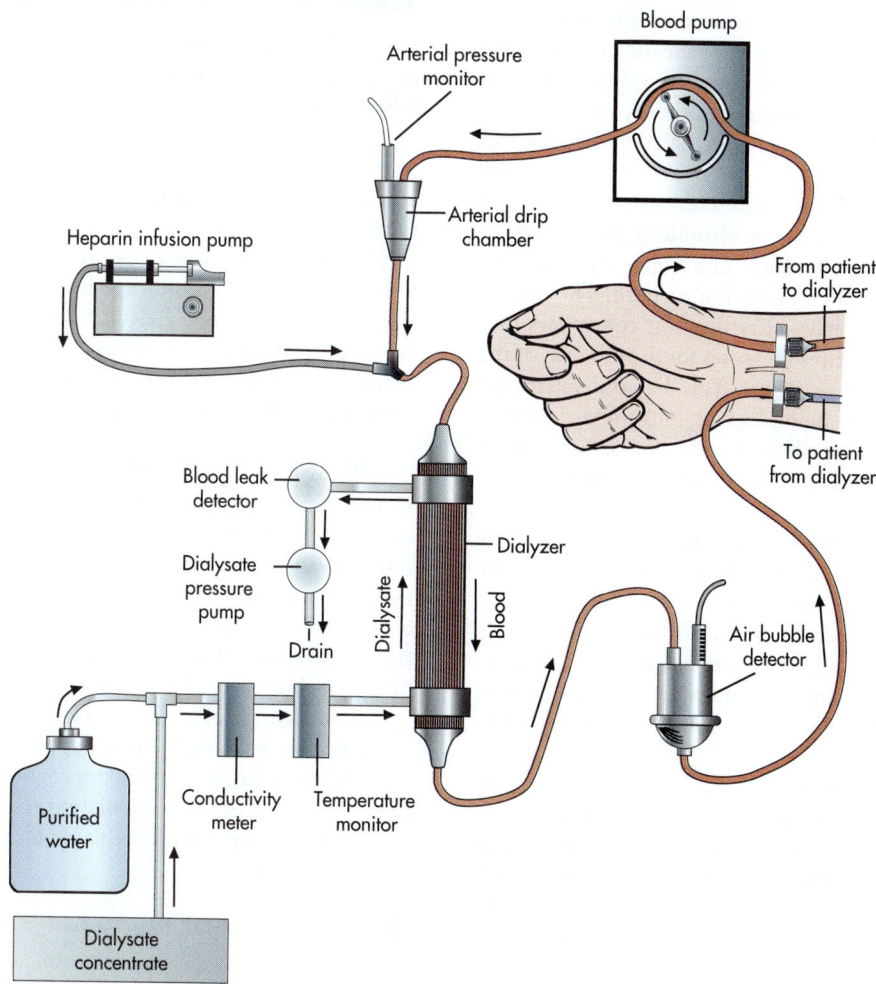

Fig. 44-14   Components of a hemodialysis system.

The fibers are the semipermeable membrane made of cellulose-based or other synthetic materials. The blood is pumped into the top of the cartridge and is dispersed to all of the fibers. Dialysis fluid (dialysate) is pumped into the cartridge and bathes the outside of the fibers with dialysis fluid. Ultrafiltration, diffusion, and osmosis occur across the pores of this semipermeable membrane. When the dialyzed blood reaches the end of the thousands of semipermeable fibers, it converges into a single tubing that returns it to the patient. Various dialyzers differ in regard to surface area, membrane composition and thickness, clearance of waste products, and removal of fluid.

Procedure

To initiate chronic dialysis, two needles are placed in the fistula or graft. The needle closest to the fistula is used to obtain "arterial" blood from the patient and send it to the dialyzer with the assistance of a blood pump. The dialyzer and blood lines are usually primed with up to 1000 ml of saline solution so no air is in the system. On initiation of hemodialysis, the saline solution is discarded as blood fills the dialyzer circuit. Heparin is added to the blood as it flows into the dialyzer because any time blood contacts a foreign substance it has a tendency to clot. Once the blood enters the extracorporeal circuit, it is propelled through the top of the dialyzer by a blood pump at a flow rate of 200 to 500 ml/min, while the dialysate (warmed to body temperature) circulates in the opposite direction at a rate of 300 to 900 ml/min. Blood is returned from the dialyzer to the patient via the "venous" line through the second needle.

In addition to the dialyzer, there is a dialysate delivery and monitoring system (Fig. 44-15). This system pumps the dialysate through the dialyzer, countercurrent to the blood flow. Adjustments can be made for ultrafiltration by creating a positive pressure in the blood side or a negative pressure on the dialysate side or by a combination of both. The newest dialysis delivery systems have ultrafiltration controllers that equalize negative and positive pressures for the removal of the precise amount of fluid per hour. The dialysis system has alarm systems to warn of blood leaking into the dialysate or air leaking into the blood; alterations in dialysate temperature, concentration, or pressure; and extremes in blood pressure readings.

Dialysis is terminated by flushing the dialyzer with saline solution to return all blood to the patient's fistula or graft. The needles are then removed from the patient, and firm pressure is applied to the venipuncture sites until the bleeding stops. On occasion the access site can begin to bleed again. If this occurs, pressure should be applied, but not so firmly that flow through the access is occluded because this could result in clotting.

Before beginning treatment, the nurse must complete an assessment that includes fluid status (weight, blood pressure, peripheral edema, lung and heart sounds), condition of vascular access, temperature, and general condition of the skin. The difference between the last postdialysis weight and the present predialysis weight determines the ultrafiltration or the amount of weight to be removed. Ideally, no more than 1.0 to 1.5 kg should be gained between treatments to avoid causing hypotension associated with the removal of larger volumes of fluid. While the patient is on dialysis, vital signs should be taken

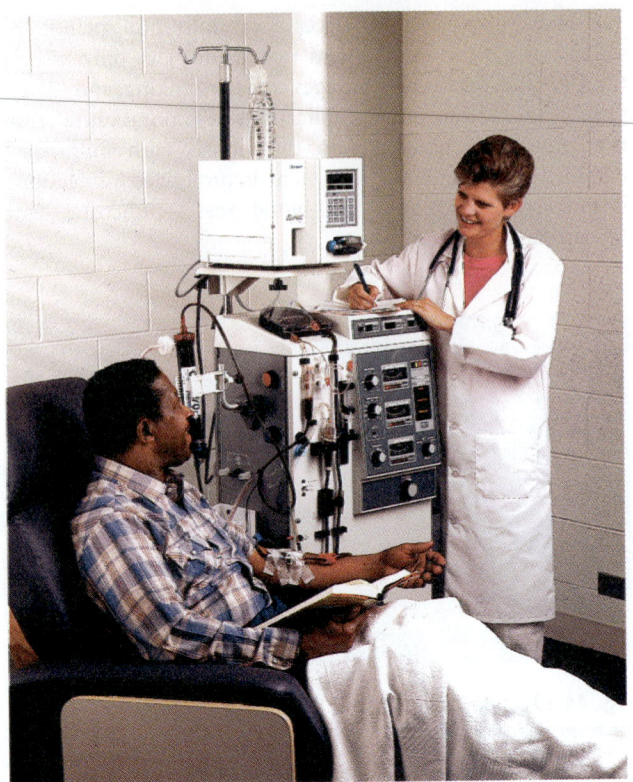

Fig. 44-15   The Baxter ISSO™ Hemodialysis Instrument is used to perform in-center hemodialysis treatments on renal failure patients.

at least every 30 to 60 minutes, since rapid changes may occur in the blood pressure.

Most maintenance dialysis units use reclining chairs in an attempt to create a nonhospital environment. Most people sleep, read, talk, or watch television during dialysis. HD usually lasts 3 to 4 hours and occurs three times per week. While patients are attached to dialysis machines, they can engage in meaningful interaction with the staff.

Settings for Hemodialysis

HD can be done in an inpatient (hospital) or outpatient (clinic or hospital) setting. Inpatient dialysis is used for treating seriously ill patients. In outpatient dialysis the patient comes to the hospital or a satellite unit for treatment. The patient may choose self-care in either setting with backup support from trained personnel if needed. The patient who chooses self-care often puts in the needles and sets up the machine.

Another choice of setting for HD is the home. In 1963 home HD training was started. Today less than 2% of patients on HD use it.[5] One of the main advantages of home HD is that it allows greater freedom in choosing dialysis times. Today home PD is the treatment choice for more patients because it is less technically demanding.

Complications of Hemodialysis

Hypotension.   Hypotension that occurs during HD primarily results from rapid removal of vascular volume (hypovolemia), decreased cardiac output, and decreased systemic vascular resistance. The drop in blood pressure during dialysis may precipitate light-headedness, nausea, vomiting, seizures, vision changes, and coronary ischemia. The usual treatment for hypotension includes decreasing the volume of fluid being removed and infusion of 0.9% saline solution (100 to 300 ml). If a patient experiences recurrent hypotensive episodes, a reassessment may have to be done of dry weight and blood pressure medications. Blood pressure medications should be held before dialysis if there is hypotension during dialysis.

Muscle Cramps. Muscle cramps are a common problem in the patient on dialysis and are associated with significant discomfort and pain. They result from too rapid removal of sodium and water or from neuromuscular hypersensitivity. Treatment includes reducing the ultrafiltration rate and administering a hypertonic solution or normal saline bolus.

Loss of Blood. Blood loss may result from residual blood not being rinsed from the dialyzer, from accidental separation of blood tubing or dialysis membrane rupture, or from bleeding after the removal of needles at the end of dialysis. In a patient who has received too much heparin or has clotting problems, there can be significant postdialysis bleeding. It is essential to rinse back all blood, to closely monitor heparinization to avoid excess anticoagulation, and to hold pressure on access sites until the risk of bleeding has passed.

Hepatitis. The cause of hepatitis in the patient on dialysis is related to blood transfusions, IV drug abuse, or the lack of adherence to precautions used to prevent the spread of infection. Although the patient is frequently free of symptoms if he or she develops hepatitis B as a result of the immunocompromised state, the patient can become a carrier of hepatitis B. The incidence of hepatitis B has decreased with frequent testing for hepatitis B surface antigen (HBsAg) in patients, isolation of dialysis patients who are positive for hepatitis B, the use of disposable equipment, and the use of infection control precautions. All patients and personnel in dialysis units should receive hepatitis B vaccine.

Currently hepatitis C is responsible for the majority of cases of hepatitis in dialysis patients. (Hepatitis is discussed in more detail in Chapter 41.) Currently the Centers for Disease Control and Prevention (CDC) does not recommend isolation of the HD patient positive for hepatitis C antibody. Infection control precautions are mandated in the care of the patient with hepatitis C to protect the patient and staff. (Infection control precautions are discussed in Chapter 11.) There is currently no vaccine for hepatitis C.

Sepsis. Sepsis is most often related to infections of vascular access sites. Bacteria can also be introduced during the dialysis treatment as a result of poor technique or interruption of blood tubings or dialyzer membranes. Bacterial endocarditis can occur because of the frequent and prolonged access to the vascular system. Aseptic technique is essential to prevent this problem. Nurses must monitor patients for signs and symptoms of sepsis HD such as fever accompanied by decreasing blood pressure.

Disequilibrium Syndrome. Disequilibrium syndrome develops as a result of rapid changes in the composition of the extracellular fluid. Urea, sodium, and other solutes are removed more rapidly from the blood than from the cerebrospinal fluid and the brain. This creates a high osmotic gradient in the brain resulting in the shift of fluid into the brain,

causing cerebral edema. Manifestations include nausea, vomiting, confusion, restlessness, headaches, twitching and jerking, and seizures. In addition, the rapid changes in osmolality may cause muscle cramps and contribute to hypotension. Treatment consists of slowing or stopping dialysis and infusing hypertonic saline solution, albumin, or mannitol to draw fluid from the brain cells back into circulation. It is more commonly observed in the initial treatment of the patient when the BUN level is high. First dialyses are purposely short and inefficient to limit total solute removal.

Effectiveness of and Adaptation to Hemodialysis

HD is still an imperfect technique in treating ESRD. It cannot fully replace the metabolic and hormonal functions of the kidneys. HD can relieve most of the symptoms of chronic renal failure and, if started early, can prevent certain complications. However, it does not alter the accelerated atherosclerosis.

The yearly death rate of patients on maintenance dialysis has increased from about 10% to almost 20%.[5] The major reason for this is the increased proportion of older adult patients who are now receiving dialysis as maintenance therapy. The majority of deaths are caused by cardiovascular-related disease (cerebrovascular accident or myocardial infarction). Infectious complications are the second leading cause of death. Many of the complications associated with chronic renal failure continue after the transplantation period and can affect the success of a kidney transplant.

Individual adaptation to maintenance HD varies considerably. Initially many patients feel positive about the machine because it makes them feel better. Some people come to hospitals or satellite units for dialysis because they know that if they are not treated, they will become sicker and die. Dependence on a machine is a reality. Many patients have dreams about being tied to the machine. Depression and suicidal tendencies may be manifested in noncompliance with diet or drug therapy or in a large weight gain. A primary nursing goal is to help the patient regain or maintain positive self-esteem and continue to be productive in society.

CONTINUOUS RENAL REPLACEMENT THERAPY

CRRT is an alternative or adjunctive method for treating acute renal failure.[14] CRRT provides a means by which solutes and fluids can be removed slowly and continuously in the hemodynamically unstable patient. CRRT is especially useful in the individual with fluid overload regardless of the cause of the overload (e.g., acute renal failure with or without hemodynamic instability, pulmonary edema).[15] If a patient with acute renal failure has life-threatening manifestations of uremia (e.g., hyperkalemia, pericarditis), HD is indicated for therapy rather than any of the continuous renal replacement therapies. However, CRRT can be used in conjunction with HD for continuous fluid removal.

There are several technical variations of CRRT. Both fluid and solute removal can be achieved with continuous therapies. There are two types of CRRT differentiated by whether arterial or venous access is required (Table 44-11). The continuous arteriovenous therapies (CAVTs) require arterial access because arterial pressure is needed to pump blood through the circuit. Vascular access is achieved by means of an

Table **44-11**	Types of Continuous Renal Replacement Therapies
Term	**Description**
SCUF	Slow continuous ultrafiltration
CAVH	Continuous arteriovenous hemofiltration
CVVH	Continuous venovenous hemofiltration
CAVHD	Continuous arteriovenous hemodialysis
CVVHD	Continuous venovenous hemodialysis
CAVHDF	Continuous arteriovenous hemodiafiltration
CVVHDF	Continuous venovenous hemodiafiltration

AV Scribner external shunt (rarely used) or cannulation of the femoral artery and vein or a subclavian vein. The CAVTs include slow continous ultrafiltration (SCUF), continuous arteriovenous hemofiltration (CAVH), and continuous arteriovenous hemodialysis (CAVHD). Continuous venovenous therapies (CVVT) achieve the same goals as CAVT but use venous access necessitating the use of a blood pump to propel the blood through the circuit. In many clinical situations CVVT is preferred because it is difficult to obtain and maintain arterial access for long periods of time.

In CRRT a highly permeable hollow fiber hemofilter removes plasma water and nonprotein solutes, which are collectively termed *ultrafiltrate*. When the hydrostatic pressure exceeds the oncotic pressure, water and nonprotein solutes pass out of the filter into the extracapillary space and drain through the ultrafiltrate port into a collection device (Fig. 44-16). The remaining fluid continues through the filter and returns to the patient through the venous access site. While the ultrafiltrate pours out of the hemofilter, fluid and electrolyte replacements can be infused into the venous port. This fluid is designed to replace volume and solutes such as sodium, chloride, bicarbonate, and glucose and is free of unwanted solutes such as creatinine, urea, potassium, and phosphates. The infusion rate of replacement fluids is determined in accordance with the ultrafiltration rate to control weight reduction and fluid and electrolyte elimination. Replacement fluid may also be infused into the arterial port. This method of fluid replacement allows for greater clearance of urea and can decrease filter clotting. Like HD, CRRT provides for the removal of fluid, electrolytes, and solutes. However, several of its features differ from HD, including the following:

1. It is continuous rather than intermittent.
2. Solute removal occurs by means of convection rather than by osmosis and diffusion (no dialysate required).
3. It has fewer or no effects on cardiovascular stability (e.g., hypotension).
4. It does not require the specialized skills of an HD nurse.
5. It does not require complicated HD equipment.

CRRT can be continued as long as 30 to 40 days, but the hemofilter is changed about every 24 to 48 hours because of loss of filtration efficiency or clotting. The ultrafiltrate should be clear yellow, and specimens may be obtained for evaluation of serum chemistries. If the ultrafiltrate becomes bloody or blood tinged, a possible rupture in the filter membrane should be sus-

pected, and treatment should be suspended immediately to prevent blood loss and infection.[16]

During CRRT the nurse must monitor fluid and electrolyte balance. Hourly intake and output measurements and daily weights must be recorded. Vital signs and hemodynamic status should be monitored hourly. Although reductions in central venous pressure and pulmonary artery pressure are expected, there should be little change in mean arterial pressure or cardiac output. Assessment and care of the vascular access sites are important.

An alternative to CAVH is CAVHD. During CAVHD a bag of PD solution is connected to the end of the hemofilter opposite the ultrafiltration port and infused, creating a diffusion gradient. The advantage of CAVHD is that urea and creatinine clearances are greater than during CAVH. The increased rate of solute removal can reduce the incidence of uremia, acidosis, and electrolyte imbalances. High ultrafiltration rates can be achieved by changing the glucose concentration of the dialysis solution to create a greater osmotic gradient.

KIDNEY TRANSPLANTATION

Major advances have been made in the art and science of organ transplantation since the first kidney transplant was performed in 1954 in Boston between identical twins. The advances made in organ procurement and preservation, surgical techniques, tissue typing and matching, understanding the immune system, immunosuppressant therapy, and preventing and treating rejection have dramatically increased the demand for organs for transplantation.

The supply and demand discrepancy is most severe in kidney transplantation because almost 210,000 patients are on dialysis. Kidney transplantation is extremely successful, with 1-year graft survival rates at almost 90% for cadaver-donated kidneys and 90% to 95% for recipients of live donor kidneys. At the end of 1997 nearly 35,000 patients were awaiting cadaveric kidney transplants, but less than 8600 cadaveric kidney transplants were performed during the same year.[17] Transplantation from a cadaver donor usually requires a prolonged waiting period, averaging close to 2 years. In 1997 there were approximately 3100 living related and 650 living unrelated (spousal and biologically unrelated) kidney transplants.[5]

The advantages of kidney transplantation as compared with dialysis include the reversal of many of the pathophysiologic changes associated with renal failure as normal kidney function is restored. It also eliminates the dependence on dialysis and the accompanying dietary restrictions, provides the opportunity to return to normal life activities (including work), and is less expensive than dialysis after the first year.

RECIPIENT SELECTION

Appropriate recipient selection is important for a successful outcome. Candidacy is determined by a variety of medical and psychosocial factors that vary among transplant centers. A careful evaluation is completed in an attempt to identify and minimize potential complications after transplantation. Certain patients, particularly those with cardiovascular disease and those with diabetes mellitus, are considered high risk. However, with a careful evaluation and monitoring, these high-risk patients can achieve the same success rates as other patients.[18] Some patients who are approaching ESRD may undergo transplant

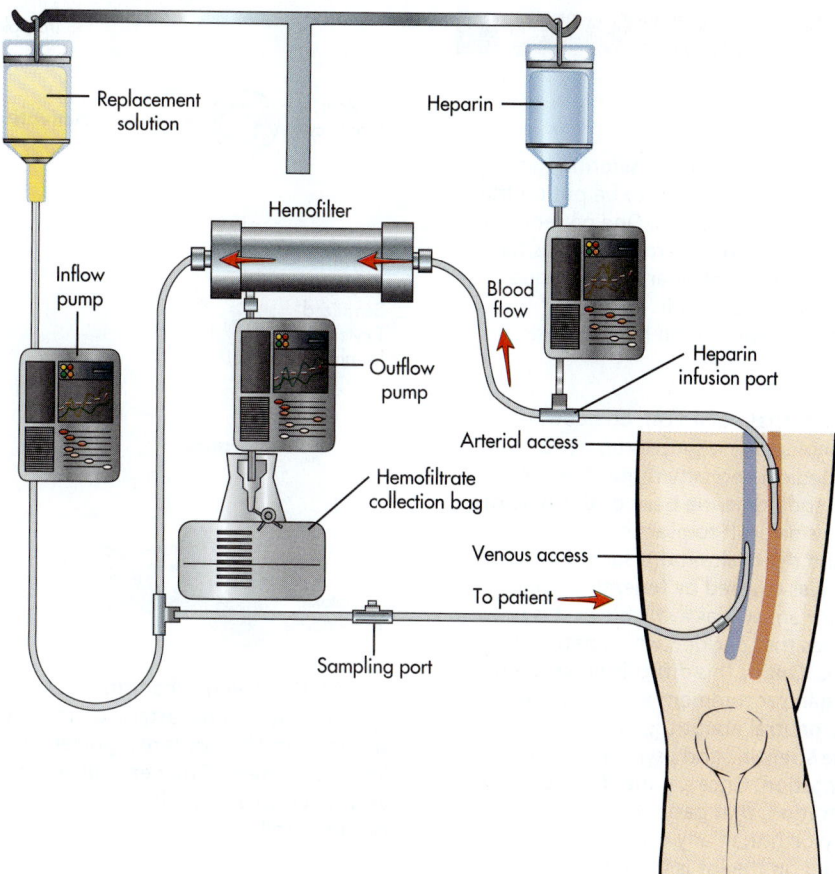

Fig. 44-16 Continuous arteriovenous hemofiltration.

surgery before they require dialysis. This approach is most advantageous for patients with diabetes, who have a much higher mortality rate on dialysis than nondiabetics.

Contraindications to transplantation include disseminated malignancies, refractory cardiac failure, chronic respiratory failure, extensive vascular disease, chronic infection (including HIV), and unresolved psychosocial disorders (e.g., noncompliance with medical regimens, alcoholism, drug addiction). Having hepatitis B or C is not an absolute contraindication to transplantation.

Surgical procedures may be required before transplantation based on the results of the recipient evaluation. For example, a bilateral nephrectomy may be considered in a patient with (1) intractable hypertension secondary to renin activity in the person's own kidneys, (2) any problem causing repeated urinary tract or kidney infections, and (3) polycystic kidney disease with grossly enlarged kidneys or repeated infection or bleeding in the cysts. However, pretransplant nephrectomies are rarely performed. Some patients may undergo coronary artery bypass graft surgery for advanced coronary artery disease in preparation for kidney transplantation.

Histocompatibility Studies

ABO blood group antigens must be compatible (see Table 28-8). Histocompatibility testing is performed to determine the degree of genetic similarity between the donor and recipient. Human leukocyte antigens (HLAs), which identify the individual's genetic makeup, are determined to assess histocompatibil-

ity (see Chapter 12). All recipients and donors express HLA antigens on all nucleated cells. The recognition of non-self HLA antigens by the recipient's immune system initiates the attack against the transplanted organ (Fig. 44-17).

The HLA antigens are located on chromosome 6. Major HLA loci that have been identified in this region include A, B, C, D, and D-related (DR) (see Fig. 12-10). Each locus may have multiple alleles (antigens). Each person has two antigens at each locus, one inherited from each parent. Because the genes that code for HLA are closely linked, they are inherited as a group or haplotype. One haplotype is inherited from each parent (see Fig. 12-10).

The purpose of histocompatibility testing is to identify the two antigens at each locus for both donors and potential recipients. A serologic test is used to type for the antigens at all five loci (A, B, C, D, and DR) with lymphocytes taken from peripheral blood. Currently only the A, B, and DR antigens are thought to be clinically significant for renal transplantation. Because there are two antigens at each of the loci, a total of six antigens are identified. The total time required for HLA typing is about 4 to 6 hours.

In cadaveric transplantation an attempt is made to match as many antigens as possible between the HLA-A, HLA-B, and HLA-DR loci. Antigen matches of five and six antigens and certain four-antigen matches have been found to have better outcomes. A good match is less important if a donor is available because limited "cold times" (i.e., the time from when the kidney is removed from the donor and revascularized in the recipient) allow for better outcomes.

ETHICAL DILEMMAS

Allocation of Resources

SITUATION

The nurse on the transplant team is considering her feelings about two patients who want to be put on the waiting list for kidney transplantation. One patient is a 40-year-old school teacher who is married and has two children. The other patient is a 58-year-old alcoholic who has spent most of his adult life in and out of prison. Currently both patients are on hemodialysis.

DISCUSSION

It is tempting to believe that nurses can be neutral, basing our allocation of scarce resources on need rather than worth. Medical necessity rather than societal contribution should be the basis of this type of decision. However, it is difficult to practice patient-neutral care in life and death situations such as this. Before renal dialysis was covered by federal funding and before the equipment was as available as it is now, there were committees that decided which patients would receive dialysis. Out of this difficult process has grown a national organ procurement system which is, in itself, set up to be neutral about the patient in all respects except those scientific and psychologic areas relevant to transplantation. Once a patient is placed on the list for transplantation, that patient is deemed of no greater or lesser worth than any other patient. However, being placed on the list is itself a value laden process, not just a neutral medical assessment. In kidney transplantation, there is no option but to transplant the organ into the best matched patient, regardless of the person's position on the list or the health professional's opinion of the patient's worth.

ETHICAL AND LEGAL ISSUES

- Blaming the patient for his disease and his lifestyle choices does not contribute to the appropriate professional detachment owed to all patients. Unless past medical history or current compliance will affect treatment decisions, they are best left out of consideration for allocation of scarce resources.
- Organ transplantation systems are based on medical necessity, prognosis, and need. If two patients of equal medical standing are on the list for organ transplantation, the first one on the list has priority unless the patient's tissue type does not appropriately match that of the donor kidney.
- Any attempt to bring moral judgments about the worth of patients into the selection process for allocation of scarce resources raises the questions of criteria and authority.
- Since organ donation is voluntary and altruistic in the United States, any concerns that the system of procurement and transplantation is not fair may negatively affect the pool of available organs.

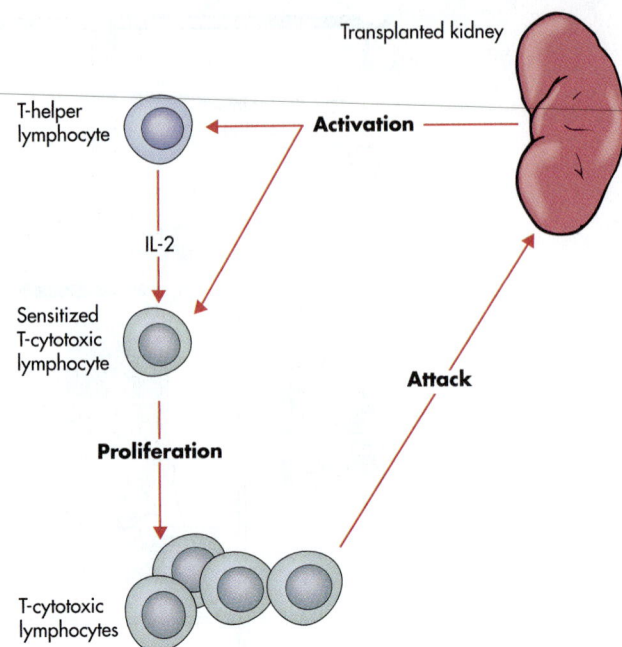

Fig. 44-17 The mechanism of action of T-cytotoxic lymphocyte activation and attack of renal transplanted tissue. The transplanted kidney is recognized as foreign and activates the immune system. T-helper cells are activated to produce IL-2, and T-cytotoxic lymphocytes are sensitized. After these T-cytotoxic cells proliferate, they attack the transplanted kidney.

kidney. A positive crossmatch indicates that the recipient has cytotoxic antibodies to the donor and is an absolute contraindication to transplantation. The potential recipient may have been exposed to antigens similar to those of the donor by means of previous blood transfusions, pregnancy, or a previous kidney transplant. If transplanted, the kidney would undergo hyperacute rejection. This procedure takes about 3 to 5 hours. A negative crossmatch indicates that no preformed antibodies are present and it is safe to proceed with transplantation.

Crossmatching is also performed to detect preformed cytotoxic antibodies in the recipient serum to HLA antigens on lymphocytes from random donors. In this situation, rather than using specific donor lymphocytes, the recipient serum is mixed with a randomly selected panel of donor lymphocytes to determine reactivity. This is called the panel of reactive antibodies (PRA) and indicates the recipient's sensitivity to various HLA antigens. The results are calculated in percentages. A high PRA indicates that the person has a large number of cytotoxic antibodies, which means that there is a poor chance of finding a crossmatch-negative donor. In patients awaiting transplantation a PRA panel is usually done on a monthly basis.

All patients wishing to be transplanted must have these tests done. If a patient is awaiting a cadaveric kidney, the information related to HLA will be entered into the national transplant database.

Donor Sources

Kidneys for transplantation may be obtained from blood type–compatible cadavers, blood relatives, or emotionally related individuals, such as spouses, adoptive parents or children, and, less commonly, friends. In 1997 about 25% of the total

Another test done is termed a *crossmatch*. This is done at the time a living donor is being evaluated and just before surgery for live and cadaver donors. A crossmatch uses serum from the recipient mixed with donor lymphocytes to test for any preformed cytotoxic (anti-HLA) antibodies to the potential donor

number of kidney transplants performed involved living related donors, and about 5% were from living unrelated donors.[5]

Live Donors. Advantages of a live donor include the following:

1. Patient and graft survival rates are improved, even with unrelated donors who may have no HLA antigens in common with the recipient.
2. The kidney is immediately available (no 2- to 3-year wait).
3. It is elective surgery with the recipient in the best possible medical condition.
4. The kidney usually functions immediately because there is minimal cold time.

Live donors must undergo extensive evaluation to be certain that they are in good general health and have no history of diseases that would place them at risk for developing kidney or other significant diseases later on, such as diabetes, hypertension, or cystic kidney disease. In addition to a compatible blood type, the recipient must have a negative crossmatch with the donor indicating there are no preformed antibodies to the donor's HLA.

Crossmatches for live donors are done at the time of evaluation and 1 day before the transplant. The second crossmatch ensures that no new antibodies have developed in the interval. Once donor and recipient compatibility are confirmed, the donor is scheduled to see the nephrologist for a complete history and physical examination and laboratory studies. Laboratory studies include a 24-hour urine study for creatinine clearance and total protein, complete blood count (CBC), and chemistry and electrolyte profile. Blood tests to rule out the presence of infectious diseases that could be transmitted from the donor to the recipient are also obtained. These include hepatitis B and C, HIV, and cytomegalovirus (CMV). An ECG and chest x-ray are also done. The next phase of the evaluation involves a renal ultrasound and a renal arteriogram to ensure that the blood vessels supplying each kidney are normal. An arteriogram is done to determine which kidney will be removed for transplantation and to ensure that there are no anatomic abnormalities that would preclude transplantation.

The donor must also be evaluated by a transplant psychologist or social worker who will determine if the individual is emotionally stable and can deal with the issues related to organ donation. All donors must be informed regarding the risks and benefits of donation, the potential short- and long-term complications, what the evaluation entails, and what can be expected during the hospitalization and recovery phases. Although the cost of the evaluation and surgery are covered by the recipient's insurance, there is no compensation available for lost wages during the posthospitalization recovery period, which can be as long as 6 weeks for jobs requiring heavy manual labor. Most transplant centers have an interdisciplinary team comprising transplant surgeons, nephrologists, nurse coordinators, psychologists, and social workers who participate in the donor evaluation and selection process.

Cadaver Donors. Cadaver kidney donors are previously healthy individuals who have suffered an irreversible brain injury. The most common causes of injury are cerebral trauma from motor vehicle accidents or gunshot wounds, intracerebral or subarachnoid hemorrhage, and anoxic brain damage resulting from a cardiac arrest. The brain-dead donor must have effective cardiovascular function and must be supported on a ventilator to preserve organ viability. The age range of most suitable kidney donors is 2 to 70 years of age. The age of the donor is generally less important than the quality of kidney function. The donor must be free of IV drug abuse, malignancies, sepsis, chronic diseases that result in renal damage (e.g., diabetes mellitus, hypertension, systemic lupus erythematosus), and communicable diseases, including HIV, hepatitis, syphilis, and tuberculosis. Permission from the donor's legal next-of-kin is required after brain death is determined even if the donor carried a signed donor card.

The kidneys are removed attached to the aorta and vena cava and flushed with a sterile, cold preservation solution and either preserved in the iced solution or on a pulsatile perfusion machine that continuously pumps the preservation solution through the kidneys. Kidneys can be preserved for up to 72 hours, but most transplant surgeons prefer to transplant kidneys before the cold time reaches 24 hours. Experience has shown that longer cold time increases the likelihood that the kidney will not function immediately, and the transplant recipient will require dialysis until the acute tubular necrosis (ATN) caused by the prolonged cold time resolves.

Kidneys are distributed by the United Network for Organ Sharing (UNOS) using an objective computerized point system. All kidney transplant candidates' ABO and HLA typing are entered into the national computer at the time they are listed. When a donor becomes available, the donor's HLA, ABO, and other key information are compared through the computer with the ABO and HLA typing of all patients awaiting transplantation in the local area where the donor is hospitalized. ABO compatibility between donor and recipient is mandatory. A national search is also conducted. If a six HLA-antigen match is identified nationally, one of the donor kidneys must be sent to that recipient's transplant center. If there is no six HLA-antigen match, the potential recipient with the best HLA match in the local area receives the most points. Additional points are given for waiting time compared with other recipients in the same locale. Potential recipients who have a high PRA ($> 80\%$) also receive extra points because the presence of these antibodies severely limits the number of kidneys for which they would be eligible. Once the patient with the most points is identified, she or he is called in for the transplant. The transplant is not done until the final crossmatch comes back negative.

SURGICAL PROCEDURE
Live Donor

The donor nephrectomy is usually performed by a urologist or transplant surgeon at the same time that the recipient is being surgically prepared for the kidney transplant in an adjoining operating room. After routine operative preparation and induction of general anesthesia for a conventional nephrectomy, the donor is placed in a lateral decubitus position on the operating table so the flank is presented laterally. An incision is made at the level of the eleventh rib. The rib is often removed to provide adequate visualization of the kidney. The kidney is carefully dissected free with its renal artery and vein. The ureter is also dissected with great care to preserve the periureteral vascular supply. The renal artery and vein are clamped and divided. The kidney is removed; flushed with a chilled, sterile electrolyte solution; and prepared for transplant into the recip-

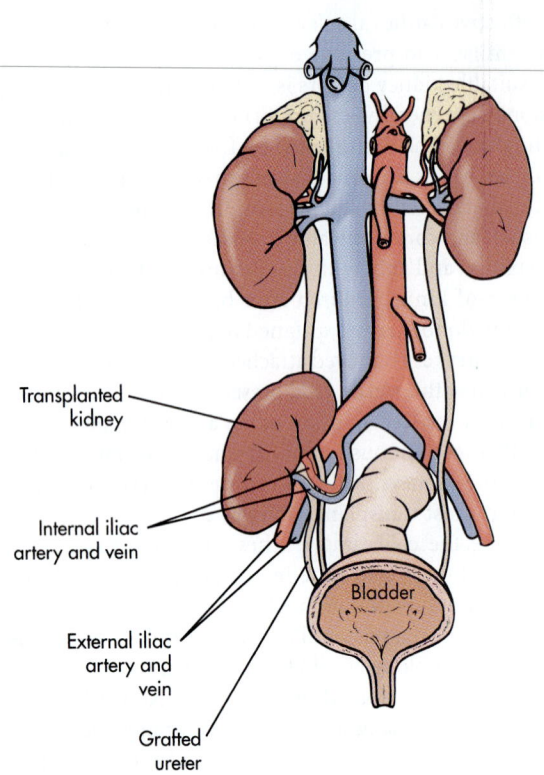

Fig. 44-18 Surgical placement of transplanted kidney.

ient. The whole procedure takes about 2 hours. Immediately after removal the organ is carried to the recipient's operating room for placement. This very limited cold time is a key reason for the success of living donor transplants.

Laparoscopic donor nephrectomy is an alternative to a conventional nephrectomy. (Laparoscopic nephrectomy is discussed in Chapter 43.) The laparoscopic approach significantly decreases the hospital stay, pain, debilitation, and length of time off work. For this reason it has increased the number of people willing to donate a kidney.

Kidney Transplant

The transplanted kidney is placed extraperitoneally in the iliac fossa. Intraperitoneal placement may be indicated in certain circumstances, such as in a small person for whom the transplanted kidney is too large to fit in the extraperitoneal space or in individuals who have received previous transplants or have inadequate extraperitoneal vascular access.[19]

Before any incisions are made, a urinary catheter is placed into the bladder. An antibiotic solution is instilled to distend the bladder and decrease the risk of infection. An incision is made extending from the iliac crest to the symphysis pubis. The peritoneum is left intact and retracted upward while the common iliac, external iliac, and hypogastric arteries and common and external iliac veins are dissected free.

Efficient revascularization is critical to prevent ischemic injury to the kidney. In the live donor kidney transplant, an end-to-side anastomosis between the donor renal artery and the recipient hypogastric artery or internal iliac artery is made. In the cadaver transplant, the donor renal artery is anastomosed to the side of the recipient hypogastric artery or internal iliac artery (Fig. 44-18).

The kidney is positioned in the iliac fossa, and the iliac vein is clamped until the donor renal vein is anastomosed to the recipient iliac vein. When the clamp is released and blood flow to the kidney is reestablished, the kidney becomes firm and pink. Urine may begin to flow from the ureter immediately. Mannitol or furosemide (Lasix) may be administered intravenously to promote diuresis.

The donor ureter in most cases is tunneled through the bladder submucosa before entering the bladder cavity and sutured in place. This is termed *ureteroneocystostomy*. This allows the bladder to clamp down on the ureter as it contracts for micturition, thereby preventing reflux of urine up the ureter into the transplanted kidney. On closing, a drain is inserted adjacent to the incision to facilitate removal of excess blood and serum from the operative site. The transplant surgery takes approximately 3 to 4 hours.

NURSING MANAGEMENT: KIDNEY TRANSPLANT RECIPIENT

Nursing care of the kidney transplant recipient is challenging, complex, and rewarding. The successful recovery and rehabilitation of the recipient is made possible with careful nursing assessment, diagnosis, intervention, and evaluation of all body systems. With a hospital length of stay averaging 7 days, time and attention must be paid to discharge planning and teaching needs early in the hospital course.

■ Preoperative Care

Nursing care of the patient in the preoperative phase includes emotional and physical preparation for surgery. Since the patient and family may have been waiting 2 to 3 years for the kidney transplant, a review of the operative procedure and what can be expected in the immediate postoperative recovery period is necessary. It is important to stress that there is a 20% chance the kidney will not function immediately and dialysis may be required for the first few weeks. In addition, the need for immunosuppressive medications and the importance of preventing infection after surgery must be stressed.

To ensure the patient is in optimal physical condition for surgery, an ECG, chest x-ray, and laboratory studies are ordered. Dialysis may be required before surgery to achieve optimal fluid, electrolyte, and acid-base balance, as well as remove excess nitrogenous wastes. A patient on peritoneal dialysis must empty the peritoneal cavity of all dialysate solution before going to surgery. Because dialysis may be required after transplant, the patency of the vascular access must be maintained. Before surgery, the extremity containing the vascular access should be lightly wrapped with Kerlix and labeled "dialysis access." This identification will remind all health care professionals to avoid using the affected extremity for blood pressure measurement, blood drawing, or IV infusions.

■ Postoperative Care

Live Donor. The usual postoperative care is similar to that after a conventional or laparoscopic nephrectomy (see Chapter 43). Often the donor is the forgotten person because most of the attention is focused on the kidney recipient. The pain of a conventional nephrectomy is greater than that of the iliac fossa incision used for the recipient. Most donors are ready to be discharged from the hospital in 3 to 5 days and can usually return to work in 4 to 6 weeks. Patients with laparoscopic nephrectomy have much less pain than with conventional nephrectomy, are able to be discharged from the hospital in 2 to 3 days, and return to work in 2 to 3 weeks. Renal function studies and a complete blood count are performed before discharge. The donor is seen by the surgeon within 2 weeks after discharge.

The majority of kidney donors feel good about donation because of the improved health of their close family member or friend. If the kidney does not function immediately or is rejected, the donor may feel disappointed, angry, or guilty. The donor is a healthy individual who donated a kidney and took a leave from work and family to do so. Nurses caring for live donors need to acknowledge the precious gift they have given.

Recipient. The first priority of care during this period is maintenance of fluid and electrolyte balance. In many centers, kidney transplant recipients spend the first 24 hours in the intensive care unit because of the close monitoring required. Renal function with rapid diuresis may begin soon after the blood supply to the transplanted kidney is reestablished. This diuresis is due to (1) the new kidney's ability to filter blood urea nitrogen, which acts as an osmotic diuretic; (2) the abundance of fluids administered intravenously during the operation; and (3) the renal tubular dysfunction, which inhibits the kidney from concentrating urine normally. Urine output during this phase may be as high as 1 L per hour, slowing down as the BUN and serum creatinine levels return toward normal. For every ml of urine output, IV fluid is administered hourly for the first 12 to 24 hours. Central venous pressure readings are essential for monitoring postoperative fluid status. Dehydration must be avoided to prevent subsequent renal hypoperfusion and renal tubular damage. Electrolyte monitoring to assess for hypokalemia often associated with rapid diuresis and for hyponatremia resulting from the inability of the kidney tubules to concentrate urine is critical. Treatment with potassium supplements or 0.9% normal saline solution infusion may be indicated. Intravenous sodium bicarbonate may also be required.

As mentioned earlier, 20% of patients receiving cadaver kidneys preserved for longer than 24 hours experience delayed graft function. The ischemic damage from prolonged preservation results in ATN. The period of ATN can last anywhere from several days to weeks, with gradually improving kidney function. Most of these patients will be discharged from the hospital on dialysis. This is extremely discouraging for the patient, who needs reassurance that renal function usually improves. Dialysis will be discontinued when urine output increases and serum creatinine and urea nitrogen begin to normalize. Some patients have high-output ATN; that is, they are able to excrete the fluid but unable to excrete metabolic wastes and control electrolytes. Other patients have oliguric or anuric ATN. These patients are at risk for fluid overload in the immediate postoperative period.

A sudden decrease in urine output in the early postoperative period warrants concern. It may be caused by dehydration, rejection, a technical complication, or an obstruction that impedes urine flow. A common cause of early obstruction is a blood clot in the urinary catheter. Because the catheter remains in the bladder for 3 to 5 days to allow the bladder anastomosis

to heal, patency must be maintained. If blood clots are suspected, careful sterile catheter irrigation can dislodge the occluding clots. This should not be attempted without an order from the physician.

Most patients undergo ultrasonography within 24 hours of transplantation to assess vascular supply and to look for any fluid collections such as hematoma, lymphocele, or urine leak. Hydronephrosis, with or without a dilated ureter, may indicate obstruction. A radionucleotide renal scan is performed to assess blood supply to the kidney, as well as the kidney's ability to concentrate and then excrete the radioisotope iodohippurate sodium iodine 131 (Hippuran[131]). Hippuran[131] is injected through a peripheral vein and timed scanning is performed over the kidney, ureter, and bladder. Abnormal results can include minimal isotope filtering into the kidney, indicating an inadequate blood supply; isotope slowly filtering through the kidney into the ureter, demonstrating ATN; isotope being filtered only to a certain point in the urinary tract, suggesting obstruction; or isotope filtering outside the urinary tract, demonstrating urine leakage or extravasation.

Once the patient has sufficiently recovered from the operative procedure, nursing care involves ongoing assessment, diagnosis, intervention, and evaluation of the patient's response to the transplant. These include the prevention and treatment of rejection, infection, complications of surgery, and complications of immunosuppression. Patient education to ensure a smooth transition from hospital to home is an integral part of the nursing care.

IMMUNOSUPPRESSIVE THERAPY

The goal of immunosuppression is to adequately suppress the immune response to prevent rejection of the transplanted kidney while maintaining sufficient immunity to prevent overwhelming infection. Many of the medications used to achieve immunosuppression have adverse effects. By using a combination of medications that work in different phases of the immune response, lower doses of each drug produce effective immunosuppression while minimizing side effects.[20] Immunosuppressive protocols are highly variable among transplant centers, with different combinations of medications used. Most kidney transplant patients are initially on triple therapy consisting of combination of drugs that suppress the immune system in different ways. Doses of maintenance drugs may be decreased over time, and some patients can be weaned off corticosteroids (prednisone) after 1 to 2 years.

The major groups of immunosuppressive agents are (1) cyclosporine (Sandimmune, Neoral), tacrolimus (Prograf/FK506), or sirolimus (Rapamune); (2) mycophenolate mofetil (CellCept), azathioprine (Imuran), or cylophosphamide (Cytoxan); and (3) corticosteroids. Antithymocyte globulin (ATG), antilymphocyte globulin (ALG), and muromonab-CD3 are IV medications used for short periods to prevent or reverse acute rejection. The drugs, route of administration, mechanism of action, and adverse side effects are presented in Table 44-12.

Cyclosporine and Similar Drugs

Cyclosporine (Sandimmune), first used in Europe in 1978, is now being used in most kidney transplant centers in the United

DRUG THERAPY

Table 44-12   Immunosuppressive Therapy for Renal Transplant Recipients

Agent	Route of Administration	Mechanism of Action	Adverse Side Effects
Azathioprine (Imuran)	IV, PO	Antimetabolite that suppresses proliferation of rapidly dividing cells, including sensitized T and B lymphocytes	Bone marrow suppression (leukopenia, anemia, thrombocytopenia), drug-induced hepatitis, oral lesions, increased susceptibility to infection, alopecia, malignancies, pancreatitis
Corticosteroids Prednisone, Deltasone Methylprednisolone (Solu-Medrol)	 PO IV	Suppresses inflammatory response; prevents proliferation of T-cytotoxic lymphocytes; inhibits cytokine production	Cushingoid syndrome (peptic ulcer, hypertension, GI bleeding, aseptic necrosis, sodium and water retention, acne, muscle weakness, fat dystrophy, capillary fragility, delayed healing, hyperglycemia, mood alterations); bacterial, fungal, and viral infections
Cyclophosphamide (Cytoxan)	PO	Alkylating agent that interferes with DNA, RNA, and protein synthesis	Alopecia, leukopenia, hemorrhagic cystitis
ATG, ALG	IV	Polyclonal antibody directed against lymphocytes, reduces circulating lymphocytes, decreases lymphocyte proliferation	Serum sickness (fever, chills, malaise, joint and muscle pain), leukopenia, anaphylactic shock, rash, local phlebitis, thrombocytopenia, infection, lymphoma
Cyclosporine (Sandimmune)	PO, IV	Prevents production and release of interleukin 2 (IL-2) and gamma interferon; inhibits maturation of T-cytotoxic lymphocyte precursors	Hepatotoxicity, nephrotoxicity, lymphomas, infections, hirsutism, hypertension, tremors, gingival hyperplasia, hypermagnesemia, seizures
Cyclosporine (Neoral)	PO	Microemulsion available in capsules or oral solution with more consistent absorption than Sandimmune	Same as above
Tacrolimus (Prograf, FK506)	PO	Prevents production and release of IL-2 and gamma interferon; inhibits maturation of T-cytotoxic lymphocyte precursors	Hepatotoxicity, nephrotoxicity, neurotoxicity, hyperglycemia, gastrointestinal toxicity, alopecia, seizures, hypertension, lymphoma
Mycophenolate mofetil (CellCept)	PO	Antimetabolite that inhibits purine synthesis; suppresses proliferation of T and B cells	Gastrointestinal toxicity (diarrhea, nausea, vomiting), leukopenia, thrombocytopenia
Sirolimus (Rapamune)	PO	Suppresses lymphocyte proliferation; inhibits B cells from synthesizing antibodies	Gastrointestinal toxicity (diarrhea, nausea, vomiting)
Muromonab-CD3 (Orthoclone OKT3)	IV	Monoclonal antibody that binds to CD3 receptors on lymphocytes and lyses cells	Fever, tachycardia, infections, headache, vomiting, chills, joint and muscle pain, diarrhea, hypertension, hypotension, bronchospasm, infection, aseptic meningitis, malignancies
Daclizumab (Zenapax)	IV	Monoclonal antibody (hybrid of human and mouse) that acts as an IL-2 receptor antagonist by inhibiting the binding of IL-2; inhibits T cell activation and proliferation	Gastrointestinal toxicity (nausea, diarrhea, constipation, abdominal pain)
Basiliximab (Simulect)	IV	Same as above	Same as above

ALG, antilymphocytic globulin; *ATG,* antithymocytic globulin; *DNA,* deoxyribonucleic acid; *HLA,* human leukocyte antigen; *PO,* oral; *RNA,* ribonucleic acid.

States. The mechanism of action of this fungus extract is to prevent the production and release of interleukin-2 (IL-2) from T-helper lymphocytes (see Fig. 44-17). Since the proliferation and maturation of T-cytotoxic lymphocytes is mediated by IL-2, cyclosporine alters the cell-mediated immune attack against the transplanted kidney. This drug does not cause bone marrow depression or alter the normal inflammatory response. Cyclosporine is used in conjunction with corticosteroids or with a combination of corticosteroids and mycophenolate mofetil. Many of the side effects of cyclosporine are dose related. Cyclosporine is nephrotoxic, and absorption is incomplete and inconsistent from dose to dose. For this reason, drug levels are followed closely to prevent toxicity. Neoral, a microemulsion of cyclosporine, is replacing Sandimmune because of better and more consistent absorption.[24] Neoral and Sandimmune are not biocompatible and should never be given in exchange for the other.

Like cyclosporine, tacrolimus (Prograf, FK506) inhibits cytokine production (including IL-2), inhibits expression of IL-2 receptors, and blocks cell division. It is 100 times more potent than cyclosporine. It is never used in combination with cyclosporine because of the nephrotoxicity of both drugs. Tacrolimus does not cause hirsutism or gingival hyperplasia and is often selected over cyclosporine for women and adolescents because of these body image effects.

Sirolimus (Rapamune, rapamycin) is a new immunosuppressive agent with structural similarities to tacrolimus. Sirolimus suppresses lymphocyte proliferation and inhibits B cells from synthesizing antibodies. In relatively low doses it has a synergistic effect with cyclosporine, corticosteroids, or both.

Mycophenolate Mofetil

Mycophenolate mofetil (CellCept) is a lymphocyte-specific inhibitor of purine synthesis with antiproliferative effects on both T and B lymphocytes.[22] This drug appears to be most effective when used in combination with the immunosuppressant agents cyclosporine, tacrolimus, or sirolimus. Its effects are additive because it acts later in the lymphocyte activation pathway by an entirely different mechanism. Mycophenolate mofetil is being used in place of azathioprine (Imuran) at many transplant centers in the immunosuppressive regimen because of its greater lymphocyte-specific effects.

Antithymocyte Globulin and Antilymphocyte Globulin

ALG and ATG are also used as immunosuppressive therapy in many transplant centers. These agents are prepared by immunizing horses, rabbits, or goats with human lymphoblasts (for ALG) or thymocytes (for ATG). The antibody made against human lymphocytes is then purified and administered intravenously. The actual mechanism of action of ATG and ALG is not known. These polyclonal antibody preparations, which are directed against lymphocytes, induce lymphopenia and decrease the proliferative response of T lymphocytes, possibly as a result of the generation of T-suppressor lymphocytes. ATG and ALG are used for induction to prevent rejection immediately after transplantation or less commonly to treat an acute rejection episode.

Allergic reactions to the foreign proteins, manifested by fever, arthralgias, and tachycardia, are common but usually not severe enough to preclude use. These reactions can be attenuated by administering the preparation slowly, over 4 to 6 hours, and premedicating patients with acetaminophen (Tylenol), diphenhydramine HCl (Benadryl), or methylprednisolone (Solu-Medrol). Patients may develop antibodies against the antisera, limiting the drugs' effectiveness during subsequent courses of treatment. The main toxicities of these antisera are lymphopenia and thrombocytopenia caused by antibody contaminants that are not completely removed during preparation of the antisera.

Monoclonal Antibodies

Monoclonal antibodies are used for preventing and treating acute rejection episodes. (Monoclonal antibodies are discussed in Chapter 12.) Muromonab-CD3 was the first of these monoclonal antibodies to be used in clinical transplantation. It is a mouse monoclonal antibody that reacts with the CD3 antigen found on the surface of human thymocytes and mature T cells. Therefore muromonab-CD3 is an anti–antigen-receptor antibody that interferes with the function of the T lymphocyte, the pivotal cell in the response to graft rejection. This agent reverses 95% of acute rejection episodes. Muromonab-CD3 is administered via IV push daily for 10 to 14 days.

Unfortunately all T cells are affected rather than just the subset active in graft rejection. Within minutes after the initial infusion of muromonab-CD3, circulating T cells become essentially undetectable.

A flulike syndrome occurs that lasts through the first few days of treatment. Side effects include fever, rigors, headache, myalgias, and various gastrointestinal disturbances. To reduce the expected side effects of CD3, patients should receive acetaminophen, diphenhydramine, and corticosteroids at the time of IV infusion. Newer-generation monoclonal antibodies include daclizumab (Zenapax) and basiliximab (Simulect). These monoclonal antibodies are a hybrid of mouse and human antibodies and have fewer side effects than muromonab-CD3.

COMPLICATIONS OF TRANSPLANTATION
Rejection

Rejection is one of the major problems following kidney transplantation. Rejection can be hyperacute, acute, or chronic.

Hyperacute Rejection. Hyperacute (antibody-mediated) rejection occurs minutes to hours after transplantation. Preformed cytotoxic antibodies from pregnancy, blood transfusions, or previous transplants bind to donor antigens in the kidney. Renal vessels thrombose and the kidney dies. There is no treatment and the transplanted kidney is removed. Hyperacute rejection can usually be prevented by avoiding the transplantation of a kidney with HLA antigens to which the recipient has been sensitized. However, on occasion the final crossmatch does not detect these preformed antibodies.

Acute Rejection. Acute rejection most commonly occurs 4 days to 4 months after transplantation. This type of rejection is mediated by the recipient's T-cytotoxic cells, which attack the foreign kidney. It is not uncommon to have at least one rejection episode, especially with cadaver kidneys. These episodes are usually reversible with additional immunosuppressive therapy, which consists of increased doses of corticosteroids, muromonab-CD3, ALG, or ATG. Signs of rejection include increasing serum creatinine, elevated BUN, fever, weight gain, decreased urine output, increasing blood pressure, and tenderness over the transplanted kidney. It is sometimes difficult to distinguish between acute rejection and nephrotoxicity from cyclosporine or tacrolimus.

Chronic Rejection. Chronic rejection is a process that occurs over months or years and is irreversible. The kidney is infiltrated with large numbers of T and B cells characteristic of an ongoing, low-grade immunologically mediated injury. Chronic rejection is associated with a gradual occlusion of the renal blood vessels. Signs include proteinuria, hypertension, and increasing serum creatinine levels. There is no definitive therapy for this type of rejection. Switching immunosuppressive therapy has brought some improvement for some patients. Treatment is mainly supportive. This type of rejection is difficult to manage and is not associated with the optimistic prognosis of acute rejection. Patients with chronic rejection should be put on the transplant list in the hope that they can be retransplanted before dialysis is required.

Infection

Infection remains a major cause of morbidity and mortality after transplantation.[23] The transplant recipient is at risk for infection because of alteration of the body's normal defense mechanisms by surgery, immunosuppressive medications, and the effects of ESRD. Any underlying systemic illness such as diabetes mellitus, systemic lupus erythematosus, malnutrition, and older age further compounds the effects on the immune response. The signs and symptoms of infection can be subtle. Nurses caring for transplant recipients must be astute in their observation and assessment because prompt diagnosis and treatment of infectious disease can improve patient outcomes.

The most common infections observed in the first month after transplantation are similar to those acquired by any postoperative patient, such as pneumonia, wound infections, IV line and drain infections, and urinary tract infections.[24] In addition, fungal and viral infections are prevalent secondary to the patient's immunosuppressed state. Fungal infections from *Candida, Cryptococcus, Pneumocystis carinii,* and other fungi are difficult to treat.

Viral infections, especially the herpesvirus group—CMV, Epstein-Barr virus (EBV), herpes simplex virus (HSV), and varicella-zoster virus (VZV)—may be primary or reactivated.[25] Primary infections occur as new infections after transplantation from an exogenous source such as the donated organ or blood transfusion. Reactivation occurs when a virus exists in a patient and becomes reactivated after transplantation because of immunosuppression.

Because of the donor shortage and high frequency of CMV in donors, it is not practical to match CMV status between the donor and recipient. If a CMV-negative recipient receives a CMV-positive organ, he or she is given CMV immune globulin that contains CMV antibodies. This therapy will prevent the disease from occurring or at least decrease the severity of the disease. If primary CMV is diagnosed or there is symptomatic reactivation of CMV, ganciclovir (Cytovene) will be given along with immune globulin.

Hypertension

Hypertension is a well-known complication of kidney failure that unfortunately is rarely cured by kidney transplant. In fact, hypertension occurs in approximately 70% of kidney transplant recipients. In kidney transplant recipients, hypertension has been attributed to acute or chronic rejection episodes, the effects of antirejection drugs (corticosteroids, cyclosporine, and tacrolimus), the presence of diseased native kidneys, and weight gain following the transplant. Less common factors include blockage of the artery perfusing the transplanted kidney (renal artery stenosis) and recurrence of the original kidney disease in the transplanted kidney.

Malignancies

The incidence of malignancies (approximately 5% of patients) in kidney transplant recipients is 100 times greater than that in the general population. In general, the primary reason for this increased incidence is related to an altered immune system secondary to immunosuppressive therapy. The malignancies include cancer of the skin and lips, lymphomas, and cervical cancer.

Recurrence of Renal Disease

Recurrence of the same type of renal disease that destroyed the original kidney takes place in some kidney transplant recipients. It is most common with certain types of glomerulonephritis and can result in the loss of a functioning kidney transplant. Patients must be advised before transplant if they have a disease known to recur.

Vascular Disease

Patients who receive transplants have an increased incidence of atherosclerotic vascular disease. Coronary artery disease is a leading cause of death after renal transplantation. Atherosclerotic vascular disease is a problem because of an inability to alter the process that started with renal failure, and because hypertension and hyperlipidemia are present and enhanced by immunosuppression with corticosteroids, cyclosporine, and tacrolimus.

ETHICAL DILEMMAS

Withdrawing Treatment

SITUATION

A 70-year-old patient with diabetes mellitus and chronic renal failure who has been on dialysis for 10 years tells the nurse he wants to discontinue his dialysis. His quality of life has diminished during the past 2 years since his wife died. He is not a prospective transplant patient. How should the nurse respond to the patient's request?

DISCUSSION

The first concern about a patient's wish to discontinue life support treatment should be his or her mental state. Is the patient clinically depressed, mentally affected by the progress of the disease or condition, or affected by the medication or treatment? If a psychiatric consultation finds that the patient is not impaired, then a competent adult patient has expressed a legally valid treatment directive. The nurse should explain the consequences of withdrawing treatment to the patient and the family, and offer a referral to hospice care. The physician should be contacted to confer with the patient and his family, and should offer palliative support.

ETHICAL AND LEGAL ISSUES

- There is no ethical responsibility to continue or finish a treatment once it has begun, especially if the patient no longer consents to it or it is no longer having the intended outcome.
- Dialysis therapy may treat renal failure, but it cannot cure it. The goal of technologic intervention is to relieve the patient's pain and suffering. But once the patient perceives that the burden of the treatment itself outweighs the benefits, a competent adult patient may decide to request the withdrawal of treatment.
- Competent adults have the legal right to have any form of treatment withheld or withdrawn, including life-sustaining treatment.

Aseptic Bone Necrosis

Aseptic necrosis of the hips, knees, and other joints can occur in kidney transplant recipients. This problem is primarily the result of chronic corticosteroid therapy and may be potentiated by altered calcium metabolism. The incidence of aseptic necrosis has decreased in the last 10 years because of lower corticosteroid doses with the discovery of cyclosporine and tacrolimus. Some patients have been successfully withdrawn from corticosteroids 1 to 2 years after transplantation and eliminated the risk of this complication.[26]

GERONTOLOGIC CONSIDERATIONS

Chronic Renal Failure

The incidence of ESRD in the United States and Canada is increasing most rapidly in older patients. Currently the average age of patients on dialysis is 60.2 years. In 1986 the average age of patients on dialysis was 56.[5] The most common diseases leading to renal failure in the older adult are hypertension and diabetes.

The health problems of the older ESRD patient differ significantly from the younger patient. For example, the incidence of other chronic illnesses increases with advancing age. Physiologic changes of clinical importance in the older ESRD patient include diminished cardiopulmonary function, bone loss, immunodeficiency, altered protein synthesis, and altered drug metabolism. Malnutrition is common in the older ESRD patient for a variety of reasons, including lack of mobility, lack of understanding of basic nutritional requirements, social isolation, physical disability, impaired cognitive function, and malabsorption problems.[27]

The older patient and the family need to consider what is the best form of dialysis. Home peritoneal dialysis allows the patient to be more mobile and to enjoy an increased sense of control over the illness. Peritoneal dialysis is not as hemodynamically stressful as HD. On the other hand, PD requires self-care or assistance from a family member. The older adult may not want to burden the family to get involved in the medical care. Establishing vascular access for HD may be difficult in an older patient.

Withdrawal from dialysis accounts for 9% of deaths in ESRD patients in the United States and Canada. For patients over 70 years old, voluntary withdrawal is the most common cause of death in U.S. dialysis patients.[5] If a patient decides to withdraw from dialysis, it is crucial to support the patient, family, and dialysis staff. In the early years of the ESRD program, the older adult was not placed on dialysis. The availability of chronic PD changed this situation. The increasing number of elderly, debilitated ESRD patients on dialysis has raised a number of ethical concerns about the appropriateness of using scarce technical resources in a population with limited life expectancy.

On the other hand, substantial evidence exists showing success of dialysis (especially PD) in the elderly. Quality of life has also been reported to be good to excellent in many older ESRD patients. There appears to be no justification for excluding the older adult from dialysis programs. Rationing dialysis on the basis of age alone is not supported based on currently available outcome and quality of life data.

CRITICAL THINKING EXERCISES

CASE STUDY

Chronic Renal Failure

Patient Profile

Sue, a 46-year-old school teacher, has been treated for type 1 diabetes mellitus since the age of 15. She has been followed by her nephrologist for the past several years for manifestations of increasing chronic renal failure. Eight weeks ago she had an AV fistula created in day surgery in preparation of needing hemodialysis. Over the past week she has experienced anorexia, nausea, vomiting, and headaches.

Subjective Data

- Complains of swelling in her feet and hands
- Has gained 10 pounds (4.5 kg) in the past 2 weeks
- Complains of dyspnea and weakness when walking

Objective Data

Laboratory Data

- Creatinine clearance 8.2 ml/min
- Serum creatinine 12.8 mg/dl (1132 μmol/L)
- BUN 125 mg/dl (45 mmol/L)
- Potassium 6 mEq/L (6 mmol/L)
- Hematocrit 20%

Chest X-ray

- Pulmonary edema and cardiomegaly

Critical Thinking Questions

1. Explain the basic pathologic changes that resulted in the development of diabetic nephropathy.
2. What are the indications for dialysis in this patient?
3. Identify the abnormal diagnostic study results and why each would occur.
4. Explain why Sue developed each of her clinical manifestations.
5. What are important nursing interventions for Sue and her family?
6. Based on the assessment data provided, write one or more nursing diagnoses. Are there any collaborative problems?

NURSING RESEARCH ISSUES

1. What is the psychosocial impact of home peritoneal dialysis on the spouse and family?
2. What nursing strategies promote compliance in the dialysis patient?
3. Are the stressors for older (>65 years) dialysis patients different from those of younger patients?
4. What is the impact of kidney transplantation on rehabilitation and functional capacity?
5. What is the quality of life for a living-related donor following surgery?
6. What are the needs of the family when a patient chooses to withdraw from dialysis treatment?

REVIEW QUESTIONS

The number of the question corresponds to the same-numbered objective at the beginning of the chapter.

1. A patient is admitted to the hospital in chronic renal failure. The nurse understands that this condition is characterized by
   a. a rapid decrease in urinary output with azotemia.
   b. progressive irreversible destruction of the kidneys.
   c. an increasing creatinine clearance with a decrease in urinary output.
   d. prostration, somnolence, and confusion with coma and imminent death.

2. Prerenal causes of acute renal failure include
   a. hypovolemia and cardiogenic shock.
   b. prostate cancer and calculi formation.
   c. acute glomerulonephritis and neoplasms.
   d. septic shock and nephrotoxic injury from drugs.

3. During the oliguric phase of acute renal failure the nurse monitors the patient for
   a. hypernatremia and CNS depression.
   b. Kussmaul's respirations and hypotension.
   c. pulmonary edema and electrical changes in cardiac activity.
   d. urine with high specific gravity and low sodium concentration.

4. If a patient is in the diuretic phase of acute renal failure, the nurse must monitor for which serum electrolyte imbalances?
   a. Hyperkalemia and hyponatremia
   b. Hyperkalemia and hypernatremia
   c. Hypokalemia and hyponatremia
   d. Hypokalemia and hypernatremia

5. A systemic effect of chronic renal failure that is usually reversed by the initiation of dialysis is
   a. anemia.
   b. hyperlipidemia.
   c. psychologic changes.
   d. nausea and vomiting.

6. Measures indicated in the conservative therapy of chronic renal failure include
   a. decreased fluid intake, carbohydrate intake, and protein intake.
   b. increased fluid intake, decreased carbohydrate intake and protein intake.
   c. decreased fluid intake and protein intake, increased carbohydrate intake.
   d. decreased fluid intake and carbohydrate intake, increased protein intake.

7. One of the major disadvantages of peritoneal dialysis is that
   a. hypotension is a constant problem because of continuous fluid removal.
   b. blood loss can be extensive because of the use of heparin to keep the catheter patent.
   c. solutes are removed more rapidly from the blood than from the CNS, causing disequilibrium syndrome.
   d. high glucose concentrations of the dialysate necessary for ultrafiltration cause carbohydrate and lipid abnormalities.

8. To assess the patency of a newly placed arteriovenous graft for dialysis the nurse should
   a. irrigate the graft daily with low-dose heparin.
   b. monitor for any increase in blood pressure in the affected arm.
   c. listen with a stethoscope over the graft for the presence of a bruit.
   d. frequently monitor the pulses and neurovascular status distal to the graft.

9. A patient in end-stage renal disease on hemodialysis is considering asking a relative to donate a kidney for transplant. In assisting the patient to make a decision about his treatment, the nurse informs the patient that
   a. successful transplantation usually provides better quality of life than that offered by dialysis.
   b. if rejection of the transplanted kidney occurs, no further treatment for the renal failure is available.
   c. the immunosuppressive therapy that is required following transplantation causes fatal malignancies in many patients.
   d. hemodialysis replaces the normal functions of the kidneys and patients do not have to live with the continual fear of rejection.

10. Following a kidney transplant the nurse teaches the patient that signs of rejection include
    a. fever, weight loss, increased urinary output, increased blood pressure.
    b. fever, weight gain, increased urinary output, increased blood pressure.
    c. fever, weight loss, increased urinary output, decreased blood pressure.
    d. fever, weight gain, decreased urinary output, increased blood pressure.

11. Most of the long-term problems that occur in the patient with a kidney transplant are a result of
    a. chronic rejection.
    b. immunosuppressive therapy.
    c. recurrence of the original renal disease.
    d. failure of the patient to follow the prescribed regimen.

References

1. Biology of acute renal failure: therapeutic implications, *Kidney Int* 52:1102, 1997.
2. Stark J: Dialysis choices: turning the tide in acute renal failure, *Nursing* 27:41, 1997.
3. Franz M, Horl WH: Protein catabolism in acute renal failure, *Miner Electrolyte Metab* 23:189, 1997.
4. Ikizler TA, Himmelfarb J: Nutrition in acute renal failure patients, *Advances in Renal Replacement Therapy* 4:54, 1997.
5. *United States Renal Data System,* Washington, DC, 1998, Department of Health and Human Services.
6. Henry DH, Spivak JL: Clinical use of erythropoietin, *Curr Opin Hematol* 2:118, 1995.
7. Calkins ME: Pathophysiology of congestive heart failure in ESRD, *ANNA J* 23:457, 1996.
8. Pirzada NA, Morgenlander JC: Peripheral neuropathy in patients with chronic renal failure. A treatable source of discomfort and disability, *Postgrad Med* 102:249, 1997.
9. Headley CM: Osteitis fibrosa: treatment trends, *ANNA J* 25:21, 1998.
10. Kobrin S, Aradhye S: Preventing progression and complications of renal disease, *Hosp Med* 33:11, 1997.
11. Levey AS and others: Effects of dietary protein restriction on the progression of advanced renal disease in the modification of diet in renal disease study, *Am J Kidney Dis* 27:652, 1996.
12. Brunier G: Peritonitis in patients on peritoneal dialysis: a review of pathophysiology and treatment, *ANNA J* 22:575, 1995.
13. Berkoben M, Schwab SJ: Maintenance of permanent hemodialysis vascular access patency, *ANNA J* 22:17, 1995.
14. Gretz N, Quintel M, Kranzlin B: Extracorporeal therapies in acute renal failure: different therapeutic options, *Kidney Int* 64(suppl):S57, 1998.

15. Giuliano KK, Pysznik EE: Renal replacement therapy in critical care: implementation of a unit-based continuous venovenous hemodialysis program, *Crit Care Nurse* 18:40, 1998.

16. Joy MS and others: A primer on continuous renal replacement therapy for critically ill patients, *Ann Pharmacother* 32:362, 1998.

17. United Network for Organ Sharing (UNOS) Scientific Registry, 1998.

18. Cecka M: Clinical outcome of renal transplantation. Factors influencing patient and graft survival, *Surg Clin North Am* 78:133, 1998.

19. Odland MD: Surgical technique/post-transplant surgical complications, *Surg Clin North Am* 78:55, Richmond, VA, 1998.

20. First MR: Clinical application of immunosuppressive agents in renal transplantation, *Surg Clin North Am* 78:61, 1998.

21. Corbett J, Ross K: Neoral: the new cyclosporine, *ANNA J* 25:71, 1998.

22. Hoffmann RL, Reeder SJ: Mycophenolate mofetil (CellCept): the newest immunosuppressant, *Crit Care Nurse* 18:50, 1998.

23. Sia IG, Paya CV: Infectious complications following renal transplantation, *Surg Clin North Am* 78:95, 1998.

24. Schlatter S, McNatt GE: Risk of community infections in transplant patients: a literature review, *ANNA J* 22:590, 1995.

25. Lott S: Cytomegalovirus prophylaxis in kidney transplant recipients, *ANNA J* 22:599, 1995.

26. Is corticosteroid withdrawal after kidney transplantation a good idea? *Drugs and Therapy Perspectives* 11:13, 1998.

27. Winchester JF, Rakowski TA: End-stage renal disease and its management in older adults, *Clin Geriatr Med* 14:255, 1998.

Resources

American Council on Transplantation
700 N. Fairfax Street, Suite 505
Alexandria, VA 22314

American Kidney Fund
7315 Wisconsin Avenue
Bethesda, MD 20814-3266
800-638-8299
http://www.arbon.com/kidney/info.htm

American Nephrology Nurses' Association
ANNA National Office
East Holly Avenue, Box 56
Pitman, NJ 08071-0056
800-203-5561
Fax: 609-589-7463
http://www.inurse.com/~anna/

American Society for Artificial Internal Organs
P.O. Box C
Boca Raton, FL 33429-0468
561-391-8589
Fax: 561-368-9153
http://www.asaio.com

American Society of Transplant Physicians
6900 Grove Road
Thorofare, NJ 08086-9447
609-848-6205
Fax: 609-848-4016
http://www.astp.org/

American Society of Transplant Surgeons
P.O. Box 510
Thorofare, NJ 08086-0510
609-384-8256
Fax: 609-251-0278
http://www.asts.org

International Society for Peritoneal Dialysis
c/o Georgetown University Hospital
3800 Reservoir Road NW, PHC-6003
Washington, DC 20007
202-784-3662
Fax: 202-687-2808
http://www.ispd.org

International Society of Nephrology
http://www.med.ualberta.ca/isn/

National Association for Patients on Hemodialysis and Transplantation (NAPHT)
211 East 43rd Street, Suite 301
New York, NY 10017
212-867-4486

National Kidney Foundation
30 East 33rd St.
New York, NY 10016
212-889-2210
800-622-9010
http://www.kidney.org/

National Kidney and Urologic Diseases Information Clearinghouse (NKUDIC)
9000 Rockville Pike
Bethesda, MD 20892
301-468-6345
http://www.niddk.nih.gov/health/kidney/nkudic.htm

Nephroworld
http://www.nephroworld.com

Renalnet
http://www.renalnet.org/renalnet/renalnet.cfm

For additional Internet resources, see the website for this book at **www.mosby.com/MERLIN/medsurg_lewis**

PROBLEMS RELATED TO REGULATORY MECHANISMS

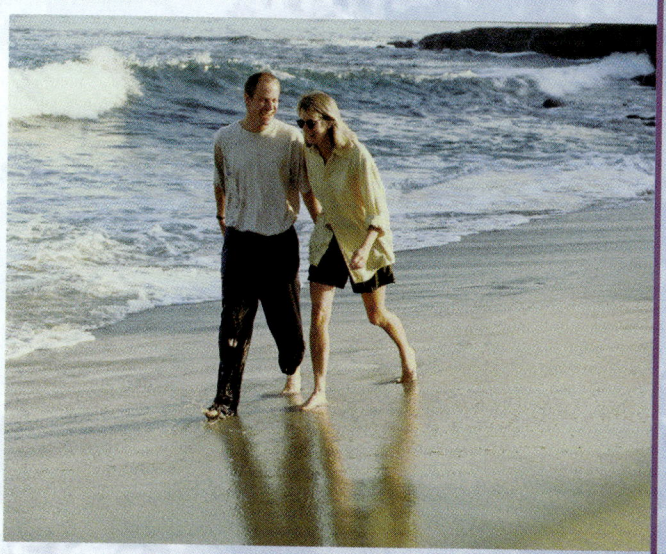

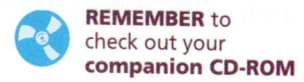
45 NURSING ASSESSMENT
Endocrine System

Linda B. Haas

LEARNING OBJECTIVES

1. Identify the common characteristics and functions of hormones.
2. Identify the locations of the endocrine glands.
3. Describe the functions of hormones secreted by the pituitary, thyroid, parathyroid, and adrenal glands and the pancreas.
4. Describe the locations and roles of hormone receptors.
5. Identify the significant subjective and objective assessment data related to the endocrine system that should be obtained from a patient.
6. Describe the appropriate technique used in the physical assessment of the thyroid gland.
7. Describe age-related changes in the endocrine system and differences in assessment findings.
8. Differentiate normal from common abnormal findings in the assessment of the endocrine system.
9. Describe the purpose, significance of results, and nursing responsibilities related to diagnostic studies of the endocrine system.

The endocrine system is an integrated chemical communication and coordination system that enables reproduction, growth and development, and regulation of energy. With the nervous and immune systems, the endocrine system maintains the internal homeostasis of the body and coordinates responses to external and internal environmental changes. The endocrine system is composed of glands or glandular tissues that synthesize, store, and secrete chemical messengers (hormones) that travel through the blood to specific target cells throughout the body. The specificity of this system is determined by the affinity of receptors on the target organs and tissues for a particular hormone, the "lock-and-key" mechanism (Fig. 45-1).

The endocrine glands include the hypothalamus, pituitary, thyroid, parathyroids, adrenals, pancreas, ovaries, testes, pineal, and thymus[1] (Fig. 45-2). The pineal gland, which secretes melatonin (a hormone that is secreted in response to light/dark cycles) is not discussed, because the significance of this gland in humans is not well understood.[2,3] The thymus gland, which secretes hormones (e.g., thymosin), is important in the function of the immune system and is discussed in Chapter 12. In addition to the glands mentioned above, other organs of the body secrete hormones. For example, the kidneys secrete erythropoietin, the heart secretes atrial natriuretic factor, and the gastrointestinal tract secretes numerous peptide hormones (e.g., gastrin). These hormones are discussed in the respective assessment chapters.

STRUCTURES AND FUNCTIONS OF THE ENDOCRINE SYSTEM

Glands

Endocrine organs (glands and cells) are ductless but highly vascularized. They synthesize hormones and secrete them into blood, where they eventually affect specific target tissues. For instance, the thyroid (gland) synthesizes thyroxine (the hormone), which influences all body tissues (target tissue).

Hormones

Characteristics. A *hormone* is a chemical substance synthesized and secreted by a specific organ or tissue. Hormones are carried by the blood to other sites in the body where their actions are exerted. Most hormones have common characteristics, including (1) secretion in minute but effective amounts at variable but predictable rates, (2) circulation through the blood, and (3) binding to specific cellular receptors either in the cell membrane or within the cell.

Many hormones (e.g., somatostatin, vasoactive intestinal peptide) are synthesized and secreted by several tissues and stimulate different physiologic responses depending on the source and target tissue. For example, somatostatin is found in several areas of the brain, including the part of the hypothalamus that controls the anterior pituitary. In this instance, somatostatin inhibits growth hormone and thyroid-stimulating hormone (TSH) release. Somatostatin is also synthesized and secreted by the delta cells of the pancreas where it inhibits insulin and glucagon release.

Structure. Structurally the major hormones are amines, peptides (proteins), and steroids. Amine hormones are derived from the amino acid tyrosine. For example, catecholamines released from the adrenal medulla are derived

Reviewed by Susan Harrington, RN, MN, ARNP, Family Nurse Practitioner, University of Washington, Seattle, Wash.

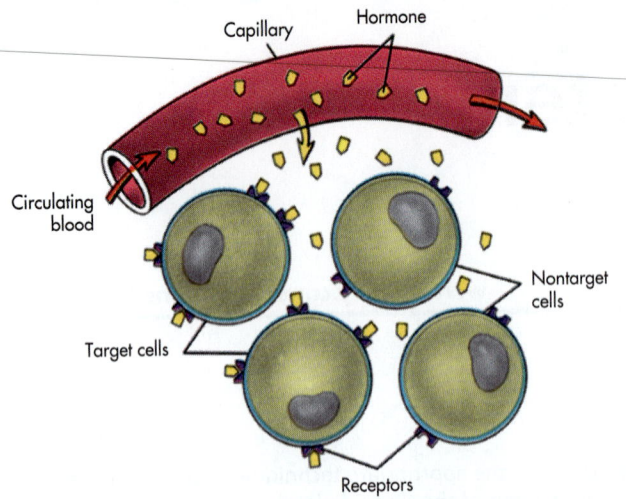

Fig. 45-1   The target cell concept. A hormone acts only on cells that have receptors specific to that hormone, because the shape of the receptor determines which hormone can react with it. This is an example of the lock-and-key model of biochemical reactions.

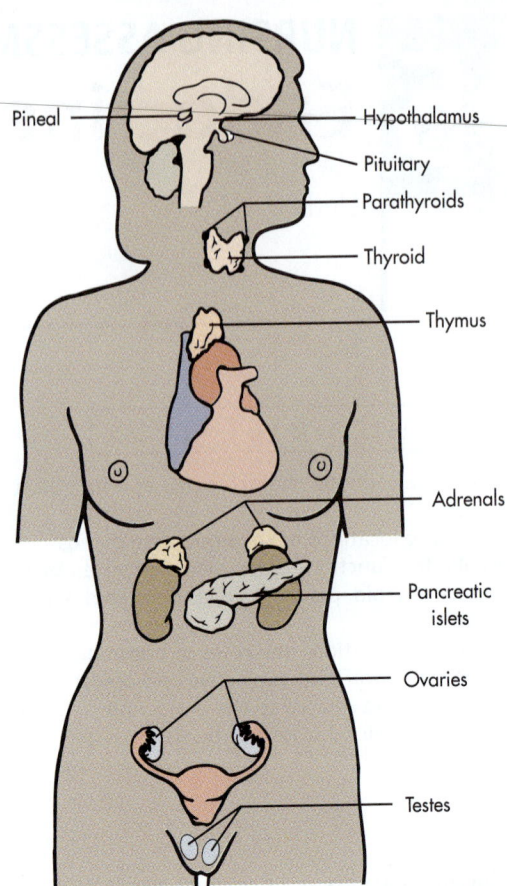

Fig. 45-2   Location of the major endocrine glands. The parathyroid glands actually lie on the posterior surface of the thyroid.

from the amino acid tyrosine. Catecholamines produce their effects by binding to receptors located on cell membranes. Thyroid hormones are also derived from the amino acid tyrosine. However, thyroid hormones bind to receptors in the cell nucleus.

Peptide hormones, which are strings of amino acids in various configurations, are unable to penetrate cell membranes because of their large size and lipid insolubility. Therefore they bind to cell membrane receptors. Some protein hormones are initially synthesized as part of larger structures (prohormones) and are not active until they have been cleaved from the prohormone. For example, proinsulin has little biologic activity, and insulin cannot exert its action until it is cleaved from proinsulin.

Steroid hormones, which have 17 carbon atoms arranged in three or four rings, are secreted by the adrenal cortices and gonads. Steroid hormones are synthesized from cholesterol, are lipid soluble, and are able to diffuse into cells and bind with cytoplasmic receptors. This hormone-receptor complex translocates to the cell nucleus to produce changes.

Transport.   Steroid and thyroid hormones are not water soluble. Therefore the majority of these hormones are bound to plasma proteins for transport in the blood. When the hormones are bound to transport proteins, they can travel in the blood and not be degraded by the liver. The hormone/transport complex also acts as a reservoir. Although hormones are inactive when bound to plasma proteins, they can be released when appropriate and immediately exert their action at the target tissue. Peptide hormones and catecholamines are water soluble. Thus they do not need to be bound to proteins and circulate freely in the blood.

Functions.   Hormones modulate or control a number of physiologic activities. Important hormonal functions are related to reproduction, responses to stress and injury, electrolyte balance, energy metabolism, growth, maturation, and aging. For examples, the thyroid hormone triiodothyronine regulates cellular metabolic rates, and insulin activates intra-

cellular glucose transport proteins, which in turn enable glucose to enter cells. Table 45-1 summarizes the major hormones, glands or tissues from which they are synthesized, target organs or tissues, and functions.

Mechanism of Action.   Hormones can produce their effects in several different ways, including the activation of second messengers such as cyclic adenosine monophosphate (cAMP), the synthesis of protein via increases in messenger ribonucleic acid (mRNA) levels, and directly within the cell. Hormones initiate these effects via the binding with a receptor.

Hormone Receptors

Specificity.   The specificity of hormone–target cell interaction is determined by receptors. *Receptors,* or *hormone-binding sites,* are glycoprotein macromolecules of the target cell that interact with a hormone in the first step of the hormone's action. The receptor allows the hormone to recognize the cell. Steroid hormone receptors are in the cytoplasm of the target cell, thyroid and some steroid hormone receptors are in the nucleus, and receptors for other hormones are in the cell membrane.[1]

Intracellular hormone-receptor complexes, such as those seen in steroid hormone action, translocate to the cell nucleus where they bind to specific sites on DNA to stimulate or inhibit the synthesis of mRNA. When new mRNA is synthesized, it migrates to the cytoplasm, where it stimulates the synthesis of new protein. These new proteins produce specific effects in the target cell (Fig. 45-3).[4] This process requires minutes to days. In

Table **45-1**   **Major Endocrine Glands and Hormones**

Hormones	Target Tissue	Functions
Anterior Pituitary (adenohypophysis)		
Growth hormone (GH) or somatotropin	All body cells	Promotes protein anabolism (growth, tissue repair) and lipid mobilization and catabolism
Thyroid-stimulating hormone (TSH) or thyrotropin	Thyroid gland	Stimulates synthesis and release of thyroid hormones, growth and function of thyroid
Adrenocorticotropic hormone (ACTH) or corticotropin	Adrenal cortex	Fosters growth of adrenal cortex; stimulates secretion of glucocorticoids
Gonadotropic hormones	Reproductive organs	Stimulates sex hormone secretion, reproductive organ growth, reproductive processes
■ Follicle-stimulating hormone (FSH)		
■ Luteinizing hormone (LH)		
Melanocyte-stimulating hormone (MSH)	Melanocytes in skin	Increases melanin production in melanocytes to make skin darker in color
Prolactin	Ovary and mammary glands in females	Stimulates milk production in lactating women; increases response of follicles to LH and FSH; has unclear function in men
Posterior Pituitary (neurohypophysis)		
Oxytocin	Uterus; mammary glands	Stimulates milk secretion, uterine motility
Antidiuretic hormone (ADH) or vasopressin	Renal tubules, vascular smooth muscle	Promotes reabsorption of water
Thyroid		
Thyroxine (T_4)	All body tissues	Precursor to T_3
Triiodothyronine (T_3)	All body tissues	Regulates metabolic rate of all cells and processes of cell growth and tissue differentiation
Calcitonin (CT)	Bone tissue	Regulates calcium and phosphorus blood levels, lowering of blood Ca^{2+} levels
Parathyroids		
Parathyroid hormone (PTH) or parathormone	Bone, intestine, kidneys	Regulates calcium and phosphorus blood levels (bone demineralization and increased intestinal absorption)
Adrenal Medulla		
Epinephrine (adrenalin)	Sympathetic effectors	Enhances and prolongs effects of sympathetic nervous system
Norepinephrine	Sympathetic effectors	Response to stress; enhances and prolongs effects of sympathetic nervous system
Adrenal Cortex		
Corticosteroids (e.g., cortisol, hydrocortisone)	All body tissues	Promotes metabolism, response to stress
Androgens (e.g., testosterone and androsterone) and estrogen	Sex organs	Promotes masculinization in men, growth and sexual activity in women
Mineralocorticoids (e.g., aldosterone)	Kidney	Regulates sodium and potassium balance and thus water balance
Pancreas		
Islets of Langerhans		
Insulin (from beta cells)	General	Promotes movement of glucose out of blood and into cells
Glucagon (from alpha cells)	General	Promotes movement of glucose from storage and into blood
Somatostatin	Pancreas	Inhibits insulin and glucagon secretion
Gonads		
Women: Ovaries		
Estrogen	Reproductive system, breasts	Stimulates development of secondary sex characteristics, preparation of uterus for fertilization and fetal development; stimulates bone growth
Progesterone	Reproductive system	Maintains lining of uterus necessary for successful pregnancy
Men: Testes		
Testosterone	Reproductive system	Stimulates development of secondary sex characteristics, spermatogenesis

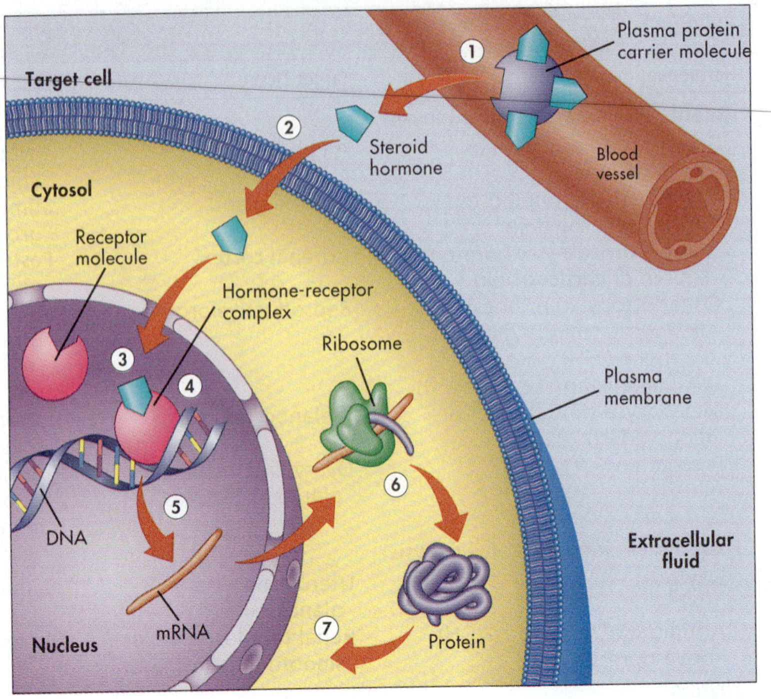

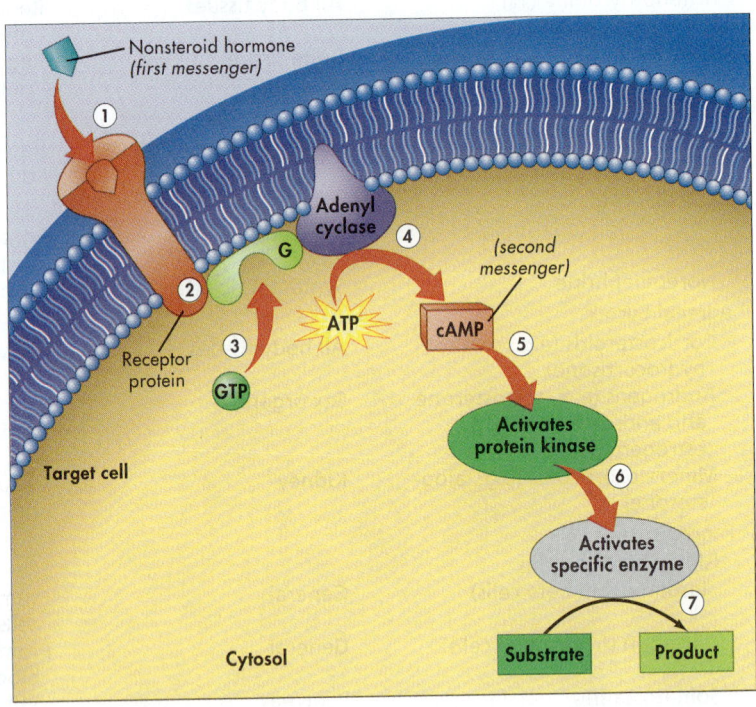

Fig. 45-3 Steroid hormone mechanism. According to the mobile-receptor hypothesis, lipid-soluble hormone molecules detach from a carrier protein *(1)* and pass through the plasma membrane *(2)*. The hormone molecules then pass into the nucleus where they bind with a mobile receptor to form a hormone-receptor complex *(3)*. This complex then binds to a specific site on a DNA molecule *(4)*, triggering transcription of the genetic information encoded there *(5)*. The resulting mRNA molecule moves to the cytosol, where it associates with a ribosome, initiating synthesis of a new protein *(6)*. This new protein—usually an enzyme or channel protein—produces specific effects in the target cell *(7)*.

Fig. 45-4 Example of a second-messenger mechanism. A nonsteroid hormone (first messenger) binds to a fixed receptor in the plasma membrane of the target cell *(1)*. The hormone-receptor complex activates the G protein *(2)*. The activated G protein reacts with guanosine triphosphate (GTP), which in turn activates the membrane-bound enzyme adenyl cyclase *(3)*. Adenyl cyclase removes phosphates from ATP, converting it to cAMP (second messenger) *(4)*. cAMP activates protein kinases *(5)*. Protein kinases activate specific intracellular enzymes *(6)*. These activated enzymes then influence specific cellular reactions, thus producing the target cell's response to the hormone *(7)*.

contrast, thyroid hormones bind to receptors in the cell nucleus.[5] Thyroid hormone promotes synthesis of structural and functional cellular components.

Peptide (protein) and amine hormone receptors are located in the cell membrane. The hormone-receptor complex is then linked to effector molecules via coupling by G proteins.[6] The effector molecules can stimulate or inhibit secondary messengers within the cell, which in turn alter the cell's metabolism or gene expression. These intracellular effector molecules activate secondary messengers such as cAMP and nitric oxide (NO). cAMP exerts its action by activating kinases to regulate intracellular activity (Fig. 45-4). NO activates cyclic guanosine monophos-

phate (cGMP) and is a major regulator of peripheral blood flow. NO is also an important messenger in the brain.

Regulation of Hormonal Secretion. The regulation of endocrine activity is controlled by specific mechanisms of varying levels of complexity. These mechanisms stimulate or inhibit hormone synthesis and secretion. One such mechanism, simple feedback, which may be negative or positive, is based on the blood level of a particular substance. This substance may be a hormone or other chemical compound regulated by, or responsive to, a hormone.

Negative feedback. In negative feedback, high levels of the substance inhibit hormone synthesis and secretion, and low

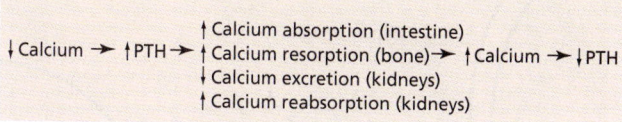

Fig. 45-5 Simple negative feedback: calcium and parathyroid hormone (PTH).

Table **45-2**	Factors Influencing Insulin Secretion	
Stimulate Secretion	**Inhibit Secretion**	
↑ Glucose levels	↓ Glucose levels	
↑ Amino acid levels	↓ Amino acid levels	
↑ Gastrointestinal hormone levels	↓ Potassium levels	
↑ Vagal stimulation	↑ Steroid hormone levels	
↑ Fats	↑ Catecholamine levels	
	↑ Somatostatin levels	
	↑ Glucagon levels (usually)	
	↑ Insulin levels	

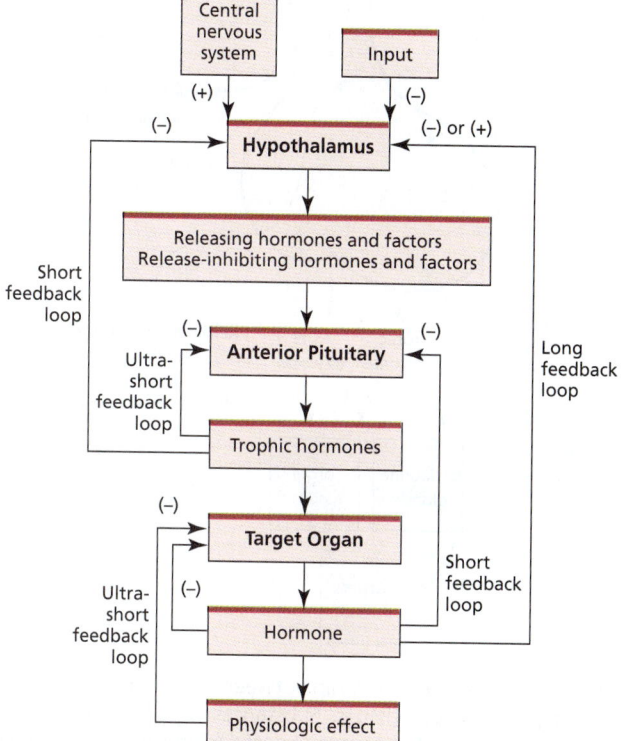

Fig. 45-6 General model for control and negative feedback to hypothalamus-pituitary target organ systems. Negative feedback regulation is possible at three levels: target organ (ultrashort feedback), anterior pituitary (short feedback), and hypothalamus (long feedback).

levels stimulate hormone synthesis and secretion. Negative feedback is similar to the functioning of a thermostat in which cold air in a room activates the thermostat to release heat, and hot air turns off the thermostat to prevent more warm air from entering the room. A physiologic example of this is the relationship between calcium and parathyroid hormone (PTH). Low blood calcium levels stimulate the parathyroid glands to release PTH, which acts on bone, the intestine, and the kidneys to increase blood calcium levels. The increased blood calcium levels then inhibit further PTH release (Fig. 45-5).

Positive feedback. In positive feedback, high levels of a substance stimulate hormone synthesis and secretion, and low levels inhibit hormone synthesis and secretion. An example of positive feedback is the stimulatory effect of increased luteinizing hormone (LH) levels on ovarian estradiol secretion during the menstrual cycle.

Complex feedback system. Another level of complexity exists in feedback systems. An example of this is regulation of thyroid hormones (Fig. 45-6). The synthesis and release of TSH or thyrotropin from the anterior pituitary is stimulated by

thyrotropin-releasing hormone (TRH), which is secreted by the hypothalamus. The thyroid hormones, T_3 and T_4, have an inhibitory effect on the secretion of both TRH from the hypothalamus and TSH from the anterior pituitary.

Another example of a complex feedback system is insulin regulation (Table 45-2). High levels of circulating glucose, amino acids, and fats (as seen after a meal) stimulate insulin secretion. In addition, gastrointestinal or enteric hormones such as gastrin and gastric inhibitory polypeptide enhance insulin release after a meal, as does vagal stimulation. After a high-protein meal, the secretion of both glucagon and insulin increases. Glucagon increases gluconeogenesis and insulin has an anabolic effect on protein synthesis. Insulin secretion is inhibited by low circulating levels of glucose and amino acids, high circulating levels of steroids and catecholamines (as seen in stress), hypokalemia, and other pancreatic hormones such as glucagon and somatostatin.

Nervous system control. In addition to chemical regulation, some endocrine glands are directly affected by the activity of the nervous system. Pain, emotion, sexual excitement, and stress can stimulate the nervous system to modulate hormone secretion. Neural involvement is initiated by the central nervous system (CNS) and implemented by the autonomic nervous system (ANS). For example, stress is sensed by the CNS and the ANS secretes catecholamines to inhibit insulin secretion so that the liver can produce glucose to enable the individual to physiologically deal with stress.

Rhythms. Another regulatory mechanism affecting many hormonal secretions involves the rhythms of secretions. These rhythms originate in brain structures. A common physiologic rhythm is the diurnal (circadian) rhythm, in which a hormone level fluctuates predictably during a 24-hour period. These rhythms may be related to sleep-wake or dark-light cycles. For example, cortisol rises early in the day, declines toward evening, and rises again toward the end of sleep to peak by morning (Fig. 45-7). Growth hormone (GH) and prolactin secretion peak during sleep. TSH secretion is also maximal during sleep and ebbs 3 hours after a person awakens in the morning. The menstrual cycle is an example of a body rhythm that is longer than 24 hours (infradian). These rhythms must be considered when interpreting hormone levels on laboratory results. (See diagnostic studies section in this chapter and Chapter 48.)

Neuroendocrine System

The ANS and endocrine system are interrelated and interdependent, and together integrate stimuli to allow a coordinated response to internal or external environmental changes. The ANS controls endocrine gland blood flow and hormone

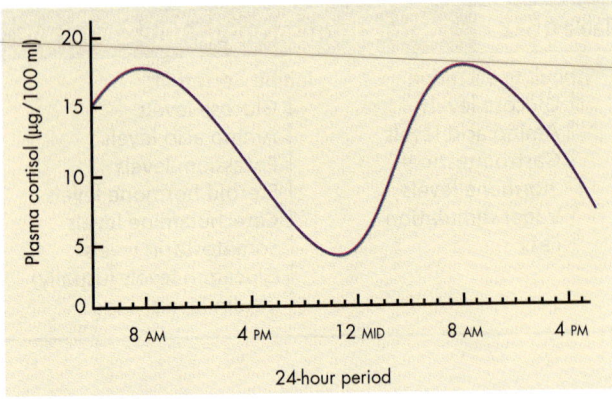

Fig. 45-7 Circadian rhythm of cortisol secretion.

Table **45-3**	Hormones of the Hypothalamus

Releasing Hormones
 Corticotropin-releasing hormone (CRH)
 Thyrotropin-releasing hormone (TRH)
 Growth hormone–releasing factor or somatotropin-
  releasing hormone
 Gonadotropin-releasing hormone
 Prolactin-releasing hormone

Inhibiting Hormones
 Somatostatin (inhibits growth hormone release)
 Prolactin-inhibiting hormone

secretion, and hormones have a regulatory effect on nervous tissue. For example, testosterone and estrogen affect the hypothalamic neuronal synthesis and release of gonadotropin-releasing hormone (GnRH), which in turn affects the release of follicle-stimulating hormone (FSH) and LH. Hormones can also influence behavior.[7] For example, excess growth hormone, cortisol, and PTH can cause mood swings. Depression has been associated with adrenal insufficiency.

Substances can be hormones in one instance and neurotransmitters or modulators in another. For example, catecholamines are hormones when they are secreted by the adrenal medulla and neurotransmitters when they are secreted by nerve cells in the brain and peripheral sympathetic nervous system. The differentiating factor is the mode of transport. When epinephrine travels through the blood, it is a hormone and affects a number of organs and tissues. When it travels across synaptic junctions, it acts as a neurotransmitter producing a specific effect on the effector tissue.

Hypothalamus. The hypothalamus is the most central part of the diencephalon area of the brain. The hypothalamus and the pituitary gland integrate communication between the nervous and endocrine systems.[8] CNS input is mediated by hypothalamic hormones and neurotransmitters (norepinephrine, dopamine, serotonin, and acetylcholine), which helps regulate pituitary hormone secretion. Hypothalamic hormones can stimulate or inhibit the synthesis and release of anterior pituitary hormones (Table 45-3). Two major hormones synthesized in the hypothalamus are antidiuretic hormone (ADH, vasopressin) and oxytocin.

The hypothalamus and pituitary gland communicate via veins called the median eminence portal system (Fig. 45-8).

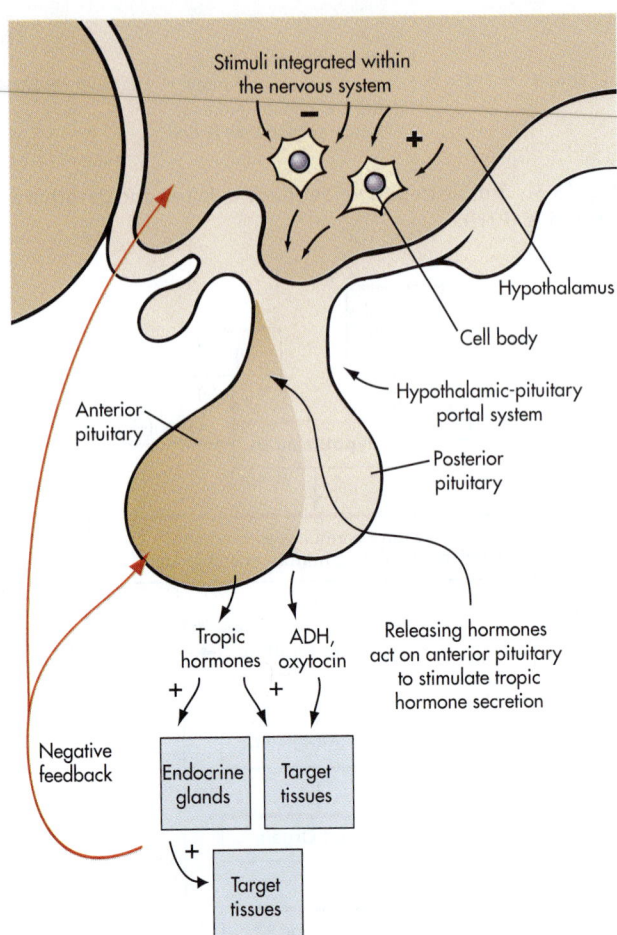

Fig. 45-8 General relationship between the hypothalamus, the pituitary, and target tissues. Substances called releasing hormones or releasing factors are secreted from the hypothalamic neurons as a result of certain stimuli. They pass through the hypothalamic-pituitary portal system to the anterior pituitary. The releasing hormones either stimulate or inhibit the secretion of anterior pituitary hormones. Secreted hormones from cells within the anterior pituitary pass through the blood and influence the activity of their target tissues. In response to stimulation of hypothalamic neurosecretory cells, action potentials pass along the axons of the neurosecretory cells to the posterior pituitary. The action potentials cause the release of neurohormones from the posterior pituitary and pass through the blood to target tissues. *ADH,* antidiuretic hormone.

ADH and oxytocin are secreted into the portal vessels and travel to the posterior pituitary, where they are stored until needed. A major function of the hypothalamus is the secretion of releasing and inhibiting hormones that travel through this portal system to the anterior pituitary. There they interact with specific receptors and rapidly stimulate or inhibit the synthesis and release of anterior pituitary hormones (see Table 45-3).

The hypothalamus also contains neurons, which receive data from the brainstem and limbic system. These neurons also influence the limbic system, the brainstem, and spinal cord. This creates a circuit to facilitate the coordination of the endocrine system, ANS, and expression of complex behavioral responses, such as anger and feelings of fear and pleasure, to ensure homeostasis. The hypothalamus may also have a role in libido.[8]

Pituitary Gland

The pituitary gland (hypophysis) weighs approximately 0.6 g and is located in the sella turcica at the base of the brain above the sphenoid bone. It is connected to the hypothalamus by the infundibular (hypophyseal) stalk. The pituitary consists of two parts, the anterior (adenohypophysis) and the posterior (neurohypophysis) lobes, which are derived from different embryonic tissue.

Anterior Pituitary. The anterior lobe accounts for 80% of the gland by weight. Anterior pituitary function is regulated by the integrated effects of hypothalamic releasing and inhibiting hormones and feedback effects from circulating hormones. Hormones secreted by the anterior pituitary include GH, TSH, adrenocorticotropic hormone (ACTH), prolactin, gonadotropic hormones (e.g., FSH, LH), and β-lipotropin (see Table 45-1).

Posterior Pituitary. The posterior pituitary is an extension of the hypothalamus. The cell bodies of neurons that carry posterior pituitary hormones are in the hypothalamus, and the axons terminate in the posterior pituitary or neurohypophysis. The posterior pituitary lies behind the anterior pituitary and consists of unmyelinated nerve fibers and the terminals of axons. The hormones of the posterior pituitary, ADH or vasopressin and oxytocin, are produced in the hypothalamus as prohormones, travel down the nerve fibers, and are stored in the posterior pituitary near capillaries. The hormones are released into the general circulation after appropriate stimulation.

Antidiuretic hormone. The major physiologic role of ADH is regulation of fluid volume by stimulating reabsorption of water in the renal tubules. ADH, also called vasopressin, can be a potent vasoconstrictor. The most important stimulus to ADH secretion is increased osmotic pressure of body fluid as reflected by increased plasma osmolality (a measure of solute concentration of circulating blood). Plasma osmolality is increased by decreased extracellular fluid or increased sodium concentration. The increased plasma osmolality activates osmoreceptors, which are extremely sensitive, specialized neurons near the supraorbital nucleus of the hypothalamus. These activated osmoreceptors then stimulate ADH release. Therefore when body fluids become highly concentrated, osmoreceptors stimulate ADH release. In the absence of ADH, dilute urine is excreted.

Nonosmotic stimuli to ADH secretion include decreased blood volume, orthostatic changes in blood pressure, hypotension, pain, nausea, vomiting, hypoglycemia, and many pharmacologic agents (e.g., epinephrine, general anesthesia, lithium, narcotics, nicotine, tricyclic antidepressants). ADH release is inhibited by an increase in fluid volume, hypothermia, β-adrenergic agonists, and alcohol.[9]

Oxytocin. Oxytocin stimulates ejection of milk into mammary ducts and contraction of uterine smooth muscle. Oxytocin secretion is increased by stimulation of touch receptors in the nipples of lactating women. Oxytocin secretion is inhibited by endorphins and alcohol.[9]

Thyroid Gland

The thyroid gland is located in the anterior portion of the neck in front of the trachea. It consists of two encapsulated lateral lobes connected by a narrow isthmus (Fig. 45-9). The thyroid is

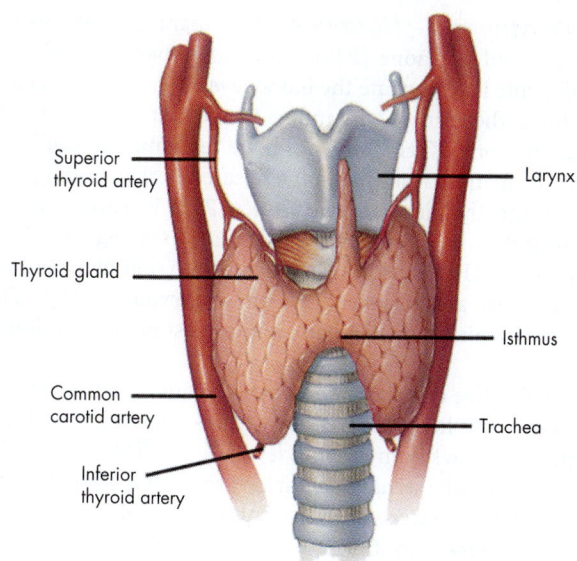

Fig. 45-9   Frontal view of thyroid gland.

a highly vascular organ and is regulated by TSH from the anterior pituitary.

Thyroxine (T₄) and Triiodothyronine (T₃). The major function of the thyroid gland is the production, storage, and release of the thyroid hormones, T_4 (thyroxine) and T_3 (triiodothyronine). T_4 is the precursor for T_3, which is the more active hormone. About 10% of circulating T_3 is secreted directly by the thyroid gland, and the remainder is obtained by peripheral conversion of T_4. Iodine is necessary for the synthesis of thyroid hormones. T_4 and T_3 affect metabolic rate, caloric requirements, oxygen consumption, carbohydrate and lipid metabolism, growth and development, brain functions, and nervous system activity. More than 99% of thyroid hormones are bound to plasma proteins, especially thyroxine-binding globulin synthesized by the liver. Only the unbound "free" hormones are biologically active.

Thyroid hormone production and release is stimulated by TSH from the anterior pituitary gland. Low circulating levels of thyroid hormone stimulate the release of TRH by the hypothalamus and TSH by the anterior pituitary. High circulating thyroid hormone levels have an inhibitory effect on the secretion of both TRH from the hypothalamus and TSH from the adenohypophysis.

Calcitonin. Calcitonin is a hormone produced by C cells (parafollicular cells) of the thyroid gland in response to high circulating calcium levels. Secretion is inhibited by somatostatin. In pharmacologic doses, calcitonin inhibits calcium resorption from bone, increases calcium storage in bone, and increases renal excretion of calcium and phosphorus, thereby lowering serum calcium levels.[10]

Parathyroid Glands

The parathyroid glands are small, oval structures arranged in pairs behind each thyroid lobe. Occasionally they are found in the chest. There are usually four glands. The major cell type of the glands is epithelial, and the gland is richly supplied with blood by fenestrated capillaries from the inferior and superior thyroid arteries.

Parathyroid Hormone. The parathyroids secrete parathyroid hormone (PTH), also called parathormone. Its major role is to regulate the blood level of calcium. PTH acts on bone, the kidneys, and indirectly the gastrointestinal (GI) tract. In bone, PTH stimulates bone resorption and inhibits bone formation, resulting in the release of calcium and phosphate into the blood. In the kidney, PTH increases calcium reabsorption and phosphate excretion (see Fig. 45-5). In addition, PTH stimulates the renal conversion of vitamin D to its most active form (1,25-dihydroxyvitamin D_3). This active vitamin D then enhances the intestinal absorption of calcium.

PTH is free of pituitary and hypothalamic control. The secretion of this hormone is directly regulated by a feedback system. When the serum calcium level is low, PTH secretion increases; when the serum calcium level rises, PTH secretion falls. In addition, high levels of active vitamin D inhibit PTH and low levels of magnesium stimulate PTH secretion.

Adrenal Glands

The adrenal glands are small, paired, highly vascularized glands located near the upper poles of each kidney and lateral to the lower thoracic and upper lumbar vertebrae. Each gland weighs about 4 g and consists of two parts, the inner medulla and the outer cortex. Each has distinct functions.

Adrenal Medulla. The adrenal medulla constitutes 10% to 20% of the gland and consists of sympathetic postganglionic neurons. The medulla secretes the catecholamines epinephrine (the major hormone [75%]), norepinephrine (25%), and dopamine. Catecholamines, usually considered neurotransmitters, are hormones when secreted by the adrenal medulla, because they are released into the circulation and transported to their target organs. Catecholamines exert their effects after binding to adrenergic receptors on cells, and they have widespread effects on all body systems.

Adrenal Cortex. The adrenal cortex, the outer part of the adrenal gland, constitutes 80% to 90% of the gland. It secretes more than 50 steroid hormones, which are classified as glucocorticoids, mineralocorticoids, and androgens. Cholesterol is a precursor for steroid hormone synthesis. Glucocorticoids (e.g., cortisol) are named for their effects on glucose metabolism. Mineralocorticoids are essential for the maintenance of fluid and electrolyte balance. Adrenal androgens and estrogens (sex steroids) are produced and secreted in small but significant amounts.

Cortisol, the most abundant and potent glucocorticoid, is necessary to maintain life. Approximately 75% to 80% of circulating cortisol is bound to transcortin (corticosteroid-binding globulin) and about 15% to albumin. The free cortisol (5% to 10% of total) binds with receptors in the cytoplasm and nucleus of a target cell.[11] The hormone-receptor complex exerts cortisol's effects within the nucleus of the target tissue. Cortisol is secreted in a diurnal pattern (see Fig. 45-7). Major functions of cortisol are to facilitate hepatic gluconeogenesis by facilitating conversion of protein to glucose and inhibiting protein synthesis and to decrease peripheral glucose use in the fasting state. In addition, cortisol contributes to lipid and nucleic acid metabolism and physiologic responses to many hormones. Cortisol is also critical in the body's response to stress. Glucocorticoids stimulate lipolysis in adipose tissue, thereby mobilizing glycerol and free fatty acids.[12]

Other effects of glucocorticoids include their antiinflammatory action and supportive actions in stressful situations. Cortisol decreases the inflammatory response by stabilizing the membranes of cellular lysosomes and preventing increased capillary permeability. The lysosomal stabilization reduces the release of proteolytic enzymes and thereby their destructive effects on surrounding tissue. Cortisol can also inhibit production of prostaglandins, thromboxanes, and leukotrienes and alter the cell-mediated immune response. Cortisol helps maintain vascular integrity and responsiveness and fluid volume, and it has mineralocorticoid effects because it can bind to mineralocorticoid receptors. A marked increase in the rate of cortisol secretion by the adrenal cortex can aid the body in coping more effectively with stressful situations (see Chapter 7).

The major control of cortisol is by means of a negative feedback mechanism that involves the secretion of corticotropin-releasing hormone (CRH) from the hypothalamus. CRH stimulates the secretion of ACTH by the anterior pituitary. Cortisol levels are also increased by surgical stress, burns, infection, fever, psychoses, acute anxiety, and hypoglycemia.

Aldosterone, a potent mineralocorticoid, maintains extracellular fluid volume. It acts at the renal tubule to promote renal reabsorption of sodium and excretion of potassium and hydrogen ions. Aldosterone synthesis and secretion are stimulated by angiotensin II (see Fig. 42-6), hyponatremia, and hyperkalemia and inhibited by atrial natriuretic factor and hypokalemia.

Adrenal androgens are the third class of steroids synthesized and secreted by the adrenal cortex. The normal adrenal cortex secretes small amounts of androgens. Adrenal androgens stimulate pubic and axillary hair growth and sex drive in females. In the female, androgens are converted to estrogen in the peripheral tissues. In postmenopausal women the adrenal cortex is the major source of endogenous estrogen (see Chapters 48 and 49). Adrenal androgen effects in men are negligible in comparison with testosterone secreted by the testes.

Pancreas

The pancreas is a long, tapered, lobular, soft gland that weighs between 60 and 90 g. It lies behind the stomach and anterior to the first and second lumbar vertebrae. The pancreas performs exocrine and endocrine functions (see Chapter 37). The islets of Langerhans are the areas of endocrine activity; they release their secretions into the portal circulation. However, the secretions are also paracrine. (Paracrine secretions diffuse to neighboring cells to exert their action, rather than traveling to their target tissues through the blood like endocrine secretions.) The islets account for less than 2% of the gland and consist of alpha, beta, and delta cells. Glucagon is synthesized by the alpha cells, insulin by the beta cells, and gastrin and somatostatin by the delta cells.

Glucagon. Glucagon is synthesized and released from pancreatic alpha cells in response to low levels of blood glucose, protein ingestion, and exercise. Glucagon stimulates hepatic glycogenolysis and gluconeogenesis and ketogenesis. Usually, glucagon and insulin function in a reciprocal manner to maintain normal blood glucose levels (euglycemia). The exception is after ingestion of a high-protein carbohydrate-free diet, in which case both hormones are secreted. In this instance, glucagon counteracts the inhibitory effect of insulin on gluconeogenesis, and euglycemia is maintained.[13]

Insulin. Insulin is the principal regulator of the metabolism and storage of ingested carbohydrates, fats, and proteins.[14] Insulin facilitates glucose transport across cell membranes in most tissues. However, the brain, nerves, the lens of the eye, hepatocytes, erythrocytes, and cells in the intestinal mucosa and kidney tubules are not dependent on insulin for glucose uptake. An increased blood glucose level is the major stimulus for insulin synthesis and secretion. Other stimuli to insulin secretion are increased amino acid levels; specific GI hormones, which enhance the response to glucose; and vagal stimulation. Insulin secretion is usually inhibited by low blood glucose levels, glucagon, somatostatin, hypokalemia, and catecholamines (see Table 45-2).

A major effect of insulin on glucose metabolism occurs in the liver, where the hormone enhances glucose incorporation into glycogen and triglyceride by altering enzymatic activity and inhibiting gluconeogenesis. Another major effect occurs in peripheral tissues where insulin facilitates glucose transport into cells, transport of amino acids across muscle membranes and their synthesis into protein, and transport of triglyceride into adipose tissue. Thus insulin is a storage, or anabolic, hormone.

The endocrine system is concerned with the regulation of body processes and the maintenance of internal homeostasis despite vastly changing substrates, as is seen in glucose homeostasis after food ingestion. After a meal, insulin is responsible for the storage of nutrients (anabolism). In the fasting state (during which ingested glucose is not readily available), hormones such as catecholamines, cortisol, epinephrine, and glucagon break down stored complex fuels (catabolism) to provide simple glucose as fuel for energy.

Heart

Atrial Natriuretic Factor. Naturietic hormones are a family of peptides; the most abundant is atrial natriuretic factor (ANF). ANF is produced by right atrial myocytes; it helps maintain fluid homeostasis. Its release is stimulated by an increase in the stretch of the atrial wall caused by an abnormally high blood volume or blood pressure. These receptors in the atrial myocytes are also stimulated by high serum sodium levels. ANF acts on the kidneys to inhibit the reabsorption of sodium ions. When sodium is lost, water follows, resulting in a decrease in blood volume and a decrease in blood pressure. ANF also inhibits renin, ADH, and the action of angiotensin II on the adrenal glands, thereby suppressing aldosterone secretion. ANF also causes vasodilation.[15]

GERONTOLOGIC CONSIDERATIONS

Effects of Aging on the Endocrine System

Normal aging has many effects on the endocrine system (Table 45-4). General changes include increased connective tissue in the glands, decreased blood supply, and decreased metabolism resulting in an increased half-life. This can be manifested by events such as changes in a hormone's basal level, response to stimuli, transport of the hormone, target organ responsiveness,

and catabolism. Often one change such as decreased response to stimuli is offset by another such as decreased metabolic clearance rate so that the net effect is normal hormone levels. Because radioimmunoassays of hormone levels have become widely available, problems previously attributed to age-related endocrine changes have been found to be the effects of specific illnesses, health problems, or nutritional deficits affecting the endocrine system.

Assessment of the effects of aging on the endocrine system is difficult because the subtle changes of aging often mimic symptoms of endocrine disorders. However, there are endocrine changes with clinical significance. Aging is associated with altered hypothalamic neurotransmitters, and the hypothalamus is less sensitive to feedback inhibition. In addition, increased PTH secretion is often seen and may be related to the bone changes seen in older adults. In addition to endocrine changes related to aging, the nurse must be aware that endocrine problems may occur differently in an older adult than in a younger person.[16] Altered PTH secretion usually manifests as hyperparathyroidism. Because of altered PTH secretion the older adult often has altered mental status, fatigue, and generalized weakness rather than the kidney stones and peptic ulcers seen in a younger person.

Some symptoms of hypothyroidism in the older adult are similar to those in a younger person but are more likely to be overlooked because the symptoms, such as fatigue, mental impairment, sluggishness, and constipation, are often attributed solely to aging.[17] The older person with hypothyroidism has symptoms unique to the age set, including more disturbances of the CNS, such as syncope, convulsions, dementia, and coma. There is often pitting edema and deafness. The older patient with hyperthyroidism frequently has manifestations related only to the cardiovascular system, such as palpitations, angina, atrial fibrillation, and breathlessness. The older adult may also have depression, anorexia, and constipation (apathetic hyperthyroidism). Thus signs and symptoms often attributed to "old age" may actually indicate an endocrine problem.

ASSESSMENT OF THE ENDOCRINE SYSTEM

Hormones affect every body tissue and system, causing great diversity in the signs and symptoms of endocrine dysfunction.[7] Therefore assessment of the endocrine system is often difficult and requires keen clinical skills to detect manifestations of disorders (Table 45-5). Endocrine dysfunction may result from deficient or excessive hormone secretion, transport abnormalities, an inability of the target tissue to respond to a hormone, or inappropriate stimulation of the target-tissue receptor. If the patient has a specific problem, an appropriate health history should be taken and the system involved should be assessed. For instance, a chief complaint of tachycardia indicates the need for a cardiovascular assessment and for information related to stress, diet, exercise, and sleep. The nurse must also remember the possibility of endocrine dysfunction and assess for hyperthyroidism.

Endocrine disorders may have nonspecific or specific manifestations. For example, weight loss may be a sign of panhypopituitarism, hyperthyroidism, occasionally hypothyroidism, Addison's disease, pheochromocytoma, relative or absolute insulin deficiency, or hyperparathyroidism. Alternatively, it may

Table **45-4** **Effects of Aging on the Endocrine System**

Hormone	Basal Level	Secretion	MCR	Target Organ Response	Clinical Significance
Posterior Pituitary					
ADH	↑	↑	—	↓ (renal)	Sodium imbalance, syndrome of inappropriate ADH, hyponatremia
Anterior Pituitary					
GH	↓	↓	—	—	Unknown significance
TSH	—	—	—	—	
ACTH	—	—	—	—	
Prolactin	—	—	?	?	
LH and FSH	↑	↑	?	↓	
Thyroid					
T₄	—	↓	↓	↓	Atypical presentation of hyperthyroidism
T₃	—	—	↓	↓	Increased hypothyroidism
Parathyroids					
PTH	↑	↑	?	↓ (renal)	Hypercalcemia, hypercalciuria, increased bone resorption
Adrenal Cortex					
Cortisol	—	↓	↓	↓	
Androgens	↓	↓	?	?	
Aldosterone	↓	↓	↓	?	Decreased response to sodium restriction and upright posture
Adrenal Medulla					
Epinephrine	—	—	—	↓	Decreased response to β-blockers (e.g., less of a decrease in heart rate and cardiac output)
Norepinephrine	↑	↑	↑	↓	Increased sympathetic nervous system activity, possible increase in hypertension
Pancreas					
Insulin	↑	↓	—	↓	Impaired glucose tolerance
Gonads					
Estrogen	↓	↓	—	?	Increased hot flashes, decreased vaginal secretions, increased risk for atherosclerosis, osteoporosis
Testosterone	↓	↓	?	?	Decreased ejaculatory force
Kidneys					
Renin	↓	↓	?	?	Decreased response to sodium restriction, upright posture
Vitamin D	↓	N/A	?	↓	Decreased intestinal absorption of calcium

↑, increased; ↓, decreased; —, no change; ?, no data or conflicting data.
ACTH, adrenocorticotropic hormone; *ADH,* antidiuretic hormone; *FSH,* follicle-stimulating hormone; *GH,* growth hormone, *LH,* luteinizing hormone; *MCR,* metabolic clearance rate; *N/A,* not applicable; *TSH,* thyroid stimulating hormone.

be due to malignancy, GI or emotional problems, or a well-planned weight reduction program. A careful health history will yield data to help sort out possible causes. Some signs of endocrine dysfunction are specific, such as the classic "polys" (polyuria, polydipsia, and polyphagia) in diabetes mellitus and exophthalmos in hyperthyroidism. Specific signs make the assessment easier; nonspecific signs and symptoms such as tachycardia and fatigue are more problematic. The lack of clear-cut manifestations of endocrine problems requires a conscientious and detailed health history.

Certain guidelines should be used in the assessment of endocrine dysfunction. Nonspecific changes should alert the clinician to the possibility of an endocrine disorder. The most common nonspecific symptoms are fatigue and depression, often accompanied by other manifestations. The latter includes changes in energy level, alertness, sleep patterns, mood, affect,

weight, skin, hair, personal appearance, and sexual function (Table 45-6).

Subjective Data

Important Health Information

Past health history. During an assessment, the patient should be questioned about the general state of health and if there have been any changes. In addition, the patient or significant other should be specifically questioned about previous or concurrent endocrine abnormalities. The presence of delay or acceleration in growth and development and abnormal secondary sex characteristics (e.g., facial hair in a woman or decreased need for shaving in a man) should also be documented.

Medications. The patient should be questioned as to whether any hormone replacements are being taken, and the reasons for these hormones. This is particularly important if

HEALTH HISTORY

Table 45-5 | Endocrine System

Health Perception–Health Management
- What is your usual day like?
- Have you noticed any changes in your ability to perform your usual activities compared with last year, 5 years ago?*

Nutritional-Metabolic
- What is your weight and height?
- How much do you want to weigh?
- Have there been any changes in your appetite or weight?*
- Have you noticed any changes in the distribution of the hair anywhere on your body?*
- Have you noticed any changes in the color of your skin, particularly on your face, neck, hands, or body creases?*
- Has the texture of your skin changed? For example, does it seem thicker and drier than it used to?*
- Have you noticed any difficulty swallowing, or are your shirts more difficult to button?*
- Do you feel more nervous than you used to? Do you notice your heart pounding, or that you sweat when you do not think you should be sweating?
- Do you have difficulty holding things because of shakiness of your hands?*
- Do you feel that most rooms are too hot or too cold? Do you frequently have to put on a sweater, or feel as though you need to open windows when others in the room seem comfortable?*

Elimination
- Do you have to get up at night to urinate? If so, how many times? Do you keep water by your bed at night?
- Have you ever had a kidney stone?*
- Describe your usual bowel pattern. Have you noted any bowel changes?*
- Do you use anything, such as laxatives, to help you move your bowels?*

Activity-Exercise
- What is your usual activity pattern during a typical day?
- Do you have a planned exercise program? If yes, what is it and have you had to make any changes in this routine lately? If so, why and what kinds of changes?
- Do you experience fatigue with or without activity?*

Sleep-Rest
- How many hours do you sleep at night? Do you feel rested on awakening?
- Are you ever awakened by sweating during the night?*
- Do you have nightmares?*
- Does anyone in your family complain about your snoring?*

Cognitive-Perceptual
- How is your memory? Have you noticed any changes?
- How long can you concentrate on any one thing? Has this changed lately?
- Have you experienced any blurring or double visions?*
- When was your last eye examination?

Self-Perception–Self-Concept
- Have you noticed any changes in your physical appearance or size?*
- Are you concerned about your weight?*
- Do you feel you are able to do what you think you should be capable of doing? If not, why not?
- Does your health problem affect how you feel about yourself?*

Role-Relationship
- Are you married? Do you have any children? Do you think you are able to take care of your family, home? If no, why not?
- Have there been any changes in your ability to function at work, at school?*

Sexuality-Reproductive
Women
- When did you start to menstruate? Was this earlier or later than other women in your family? Do you have scant, heavy, or irregular menstrual flows?
- How many children have you had? How much did they weigh at birth? Were you told you had diabetes during any pregnancy?*
- Were you able to nurse your children if you wanted to?
- Are you attempting to get pregnant but cannot?*
Men
- Have you noticed any changes in your ability to have an erection?*
- Are you trying to have children but cannot?*

Coping–Stress Tolerance
- Where do you work? What kind of work do you do? Are you able to do what is expected of you and what you expect of yourself?
- What kind of stressors do you have at work (school)?
- If retired, what do you do with your time? What did you do before you retired?
- If unemployed, are you looking for work?
- Is your income adequate for your needs?
- How do you deal with stress or problems?
- What is your support system? Whom do you turn to when you have a problem?

Value-Belief
- Do you think medicine should still be taken even though you feel OK?
- Does your health plan cause any conflict in your value-belief system?*

*If yes, describe.

Table 45-6 Nonspecific Manifestations of Hormone Dysfunction

Manifestations	Panhypopituitary Hormone — Hypo	ADH — Hyper	ADH — Hypo	Thyroid Hormone — Hyper	Thyroid Hormone — Hypo	Cortisol — Hyper	Cortisol — Hypo	Mineralocorticoids — Hyper	Mineralocorticoids — Hypo	Insulin — Hyper	Insulin — Hypo	PTH — Hyper	PTH — Hypo
Nutrition and elimination													
Weight	↓↓	↑	↓	↓↑	↓↑	↑↑+	↓↓++			↑↓	↓↓++	↓↓	+
Appetite	↓			+	++	+	++			←	++	↑↑←	
Growth abnormality (children)	+			↓	+								
Abdominal pain	↓		↓	↓	+		+					←	
Stool output				←	+	←	+	←		←	←		
Urine output		↓	↓		→		←	+					
Cardiovascular system													
Blood pressure		←		←	→	+	←	←	+	→		+	
Pulse				+	+	+	+			+		+	
Anemia	+												
Neurologic system													
Temperature			←	←	→	+	←			↑		←	+
Sleep disturbances	+			+	+	+	+			++		+	
Seizures	+	+	+		+		+			+		+	
Mood													
Depression or apathy	+	+	+		+	+	+			+		+	+
Skin													
Body hair	↓↓		→	→→	→	→→	→					→→	
Pigmentation													
Reproductive or sexual system													
Male dysfunction	++			++	++	++	++		+	++		+	+
Female dysfunction	++			++	++	++	++		+	++		+	+

↑, increased; +, present; ↓, decreased.

the patient is taking large doses of glucocorticoids because abrupt discontinuance of these medications may cause an Addisonian crisis. In addition, regular long-term glucocorticoid therapy can result in potentially serious side effects and complications (see Table 47-19).

Insulin replacement should be identified in terms of type, amount, and timing of replacement. In addition, some medications may adversely affect endocrine function. Corticosteroids may cause glucose intolerance in the susceptible patient by increasing glycogenolysis and insulin resistance. There is a greater glucose-lowering effect of sulfonylureas and insulin when taken with large doses (>4 g per day) of aspirin. Dicumarol can cause adrenal hemorrhage and resultant adrenal insufficiency. Lithium carbonate has many adverse effects on the endocrine system, including diffuse nontoxic goiter, hypercalcemia, hyperparathyroidism, transient hyperglycemia, and impotence or sexual dysfunction. Many medications affect blood glucose levels (see Table 47-10).

Surgery or other treatments. The nurse should inquire about previous hospitalizations, surgeries, chemotherapies, and radiation treatments (especially of the neck). A history of a severe blow to the head could indicate pituitary or hypothalamic trauma.

Functional Health Patterns

Health perception–health management pattern. The nurse should ask about energy levels, particularly as compared with the patient's past energy level. Fatigue and hyperactivity are two common problems associated with endocrine problems. Inquiry should also be made about the patient's general health care and health care behaviors. Such an inquiry might result in the identification of vague, nonspecific symptoms that could suggest an endocrine problem.

Heredity and general health can play a major role in the occurrence of endocrine problems. The patient should be questioned about the following conditions in family members: diabetes mellitus or insipidus; hyperthyroidism or hypothyroidism, goiter; hypertension or hypotension; obesity; infertility; growth problems; pheochromocytoma (neoplastic tumor of the adrenal medulla or sympathetic ganglia); autoimmune diseases (e.g., Addison's disease); and adrenal hyperplasia. Further information may be elicited by asking additional questions such as the following: Are there any other members of your family who have, or have had, a similar problem? This frequently uncovers evidence of a familial tendency that cannot be found in any other way.

Nutritional-metabolic pattern. Because a major function of the endocrine system is regulating metabolism and maintenance of homeostasis, the patient with endocrine dysfunction will often experience alterations in nutritional-metabolic patterns. Changes in appetite and weight can indicate endocrine dysfunction. Weight loss with increased appetite may indicate hyperthyroidism or diabetes mellitus, particularly type 1. Weight loss with decreased appetite may indicate hypopituitarism, hypocortisolism, or gastroparesis from diabetes mellitus. Weight gain may indicate hypothyroidism and, if the weight gain is concentrated in the truncal area, hypercortisolism. In addition, weight gain in a genetically susceptible patient may increase the risk for type 2 diabetes mellitus.

Assessment of the endocrine system includes growth and development patterns, weight distribution and changes, and comparisons of these factors with normal findings. Height should be measured in all patients. The charts used should be race specific because significant racial differences exist in normal children. For example, Caucasian children usually are smaller than African-American children but larger than Asian children. Familial patterns should always be assessed. A helpful guide in growth assessment is that approximate normal growth rates are 3 inches (7.5 cm) per year from ages 1 to 7 and 2 inches (5 cm) per year from ages 8 to 15. Heights more than 3 standard deviations below the mean should be investigated.[18] Approximate average heights for children and young teenagers can be estimated on the basis of age using the following formula:

$$\text{Height (inches)} = 2.5 \times \text{Age (years)} + 30$$

In adults, weight changes may indicate endocrine dysfunction. Body mass index (BMI) is a common way to assess obesity (see Table 38-7). This estimation takes height into account. It is derived by dividing the weight (in kilograms) by the height (in meters squared): BMI = Weight (kg)/Height (m^2). A BMI of 25 is the upper limit of normal; 25 to 29.9 indicates that a patient is overweight; and 30 or above indicates obesity. A weight increase of more than 1 kg per day usually indicates fluid retention.

Changes in hair distribution and skin and hair color and texture can all indicate endocrine dysfunction. Hair loss can indicate hypopituitarism, hypothyroidism, hypoparathyroidism, or increased testosterone and other androgens. Increased body hair may indicate hypercortisolism. Decreased skin pigmentation can occur in hypopituitarism, hypothyroidism, and hypoparathyroidism, whereas increased skin pigmentation, particularly in sun-exposed areas, can indicate hypocortisolism. A patient with hypothyroidism or excess growth hormone may complain of coarse, leathery skin. A patient with hyperthyroidism may comment about fine, silky hair. A history of hypertension may indicate excess ADH, aldosterone, or cortisol.

Difficulty swallowing or a change in neck size may indicate thyroid hyperplasia or inflammation. Questions related to increased sympathetic nervous system activity (e.g., nervousness, palpitations, sweating, tremors) may assist the nurse in identifying a thyroid disorder or pheochromocytoma. Heat or cold intolerance may indicate hyperthyroidism or hypothyroidism, respectively. The patient should be questioned about dietary intake. This record should be examined for the presence of foods that contain thyroid-inhibiting substances (goitrogens) (see Table 47-7).

Elimination pattern. Because maintenance of fluid balance is a major role of the endocrine system, questions related to elimination patterns may uncover endocrine dysfunction. For instance, increased thirst and urination can indicate diabetes mellitus or insipidus. A history of nephrolithiasis (kidney stones) may indicate excess PTH. The patient should be asked about the frequency and consistency of bowel movements. Hyperdefecation may indicate hyperthyroidism. Large-volume, watery stools or fecal incontinence may indicate autonomic gastroenteropathy of diabetes mellitus. Constipation is also seen in the gastroenteropathy of diabetes mellitus, as well as in hypothyroidism, hypoparathyroidism, and hypopituitarism.

Activity-exercise pattern. The major effect of endocrine dysfunction on activity-exercise pattern will be an inability to maintain previous activity levels. Although a patient with hyperthyroidism may seem to have excess energy, fatigue is common. A patient with an endocrine dysfunction will almost always manifest apathy and frequently depression. This indicates the need for the nurse to specifically question the patient or significant other to describe current activity in relation to previous activity patterns. In addition, in diabetes mellitus, the patient's activity-exercise patterns will help determine diabetes management, including insulin therapy.

Sleep-rest pattern. It is important that the nurse obtain a detailed sleep history. Sleep disturbances are frequently seen in endocrine dysfunction. The patient with diabetes mellitus or insipidus will complain of nocturia, which can severely disrupt normal sleep patterns. The patient with tightly controlled type 1 diabetes mellitus who complains of sweating or nightmares may be experiencing hypoglycemia. The hyperthyroid patient may complain of inability to sleep, as may one with hypercortisolism. The patient with hypothyroidism, hypocortisolism, or hypopituitarism may tell the nurse of sleeping all the time, yet still being fatigued. The significant other of a patient with excess growth hormone may tell the nurse of an inability to sleep because of the patient's snoring.

Cognitive-perceptual pattern. The nurse can question both the patient and significant other to determine if any cognitive changes are present. Memory deficits, inability to concentrate, and decreased energy levels are common in endocrine disorders. As mentioned, depression and apathy are frequent in endocrine disorders. Visual changes can also occur. A patient with hyperglycemia may complain of blurred vision. Diplopia may indicate pressure from a pituitary tumor. Exophthalmos secondary to hyperthyroidism can cause corneal drying and other visual disturbances.

Self-perception–self-concept pattern. Endocrine disorders may affect the patient's self-perception because of associated physical changes. Changes in weight, size, and level of fatigue should be determined. Weight changes often occur, and both increases and decreases can affect self-perception. Increases in the size of the head, hands, or feet in the adult (e.g., change in ring, glove, or shoe size) may indicate excess growth hormone. In addition, the fatigue so often experienced by a patient with an endocrine disorder often affects feelings about self.

The chronicity of many endocrine disorders and need for continued therapy can affect the patient's self-perception. The patient can be asked to describe the effects of the present illness on self-perception.

Role-relationship pattern. The nurse should ask whether there have been any changes in the patient's ability to maintain roles at home, at work, or in the community. Often the patient with an endocrine disorder will be unable to sustain life's roles. However, in most cases the patient can be advised that, with adequate management, previous roles can be resumed. This can be very reassuring for the patient and family.

Sexuality-reproductive pattern. Problems with menstruation and pregnancy in a woman may indicate an endocrine disorder. Consequently, a detailed history of menstruation and pregnancy should be obtained. Menstrual irregularities are seen in disorders of the ovaries, pituitary, thyroid, and adrenal glands. A female patient with a history of large babies may have had undiagnosed gestational diabetes, which may put her at a higher risk to develop type 2 diabetes mellitus. A history of inability to lactate may indicate a pituitary disorder.

Male sexual dysfunction is also frequently seen in endocrine disorders. It usually takes the form of impotence, although retrograde ejaculation can occur in diabetes mellitus. Infertility in either sex warrants a full reproductive and endocrine workup.

Coping–stress tolerance pattern. Stressors of all kinds affect the endocrine system. Areas that can cause a great deal of stress should be investigated. The patient should be asked about place of employment, kind of work, ability to meet job requirements, and the amount of stress involved. The nurse should ask whether the job provides an adequate income to identify financial stressors. Usual coping patterns are also discussed. The nurse then determines whether previous coping patterns are still successful. It is often useful to ask family members or a significant other about the patient's coping strategies and reaction to stress.

Value-belief pattern. When dealing with a patient with a chronic condition, identification of the patient's value-belief patterns can assist the health care team to identify appropriate regimens. This is particularly important in a condition such as diabetes mellitus, which may require major lifestyle changes for successful management. Other endocrine disorders, such as hypothyroidism or hypocortisolism, can be easily managed with oral medication taken faithfully. Identification of a patient's ability to make lifestyle changes or take daily medication (and increase this medication as indicated) is an important nursing function.

Objective Data
Physical Examination
Mental-emotional status. Throughout the examination the patient's orientation, alertness, memory, affect, personality, anxiety, and speech pattern should be objectively assessed. Endocrine disorders commonly cause changes in mental status and level of consciousness.

General appearance

Inspection. The nurse should observe the patient's general appearance, including physical growth and development, level of consciousness and orientation, and appearance and appropriateness of dress for ambient temperature. Endocrine dysfunction can subtly or markedly affect the size, shape, color, and maturation of the body. Assessment should include the following:

1. *Body size:* height and weight compared with a table of standards or estimation of normality; size of head and extremities, proportionality and posture; facial features
2. *Integumentary system:* skin color, pigmentation, texture, coarseness, leathery texture, excessive thinness, size of sweat glands, diaphoresis, acne, striae, ecchymosis, vitiligo (patchy loss of pigmentation)
3. *Hair:* texture, distribution, brittleness, alopecia (patchy baldness)
4. *Face:* color; erythema, especially on cheeks (plethora); pained, anxious expression
5. *Eyes:* eyebrows, hair distribution; visual acuity, lens opacity; shape, position, movement of eyelids; lid lag; visual fields; extraocular movements; edema
6. *Nose:* mucosa, noisy breathing
7. *Mouth:* buccal mucosa, condition of teeth, malocclusion and mottling, tongue size and fasciculations (local-

ized, uncoordinated, uncontrollable twitching of a single muscle group), size and shape of jaw

8. *Voice:* huskiness or hoarseness, volume, pitch, slurring
9. *Neck:* symmetry, alignment; forceful carotid pulsations; unusual bulging of the thyroid lobes behind the sternocleidomastoid muscles; trachea in midline; dullness, thickening, flabbiness of vocal chords; polyps; gray-brown hyperpigmentation on posterior neck and axillae (acanthosis nigricans); when inspecting the thyroid gland, observation should be made first in the normal position, preferably with side lighting, then in slight extension, and then as the patient swallows some water
10. *Extremities:* size, shape, symmetry, proportionality (distance from symphysis pubis to foot: approximately half of total height), edema
    a. *Hands:* tremors (a piece of paper is placed on outstretched fingers, palm down, to assess fine tremors); muscle strength, grip, thenar (ball of the thumb) wasting, Dupuytren's contracture, clubbing, muscle wasting
    b. *Legs:* muscle weakness (assessed by having the seated patient extend one leg to a horizontal position; ability to hold this position for 2 minutes usually indicates normal muscle strength), bowing, color and amount of hair, size of feet, corns, calluses, pedal pulses
    c. *Toes:* maceration, fissures, deformities, toenails with fungal infection
11. *Reflexes:* particularly deep tendon reflexes, relaxation time
12. *Pulses:* rate and force
13. *Thorax:* gynecomastia in men
14. *Abdomen:* increased pigmentation of scars, purplish striae, pain on light palpation
15. *Genitalia:* decreased hair distribution (diamond pattern in women may indicate virilizing adrenal tumor), size of testes, clitoral enlargement

Palpation. The thyroid is the only palpable endocrine gland. Thyroid palpation requires considerable practice, as well as validation by an experienced examiner. Palpation can cause the release of thyroid hormone into the circulation, increasing the patient's symptoms and potentially causing a thyroid storm. (Hyperthyroidism is discussed in Chapter 47.) In the patient with a visibly enlarged thyroid, palpation of the thyroid should be deferred if a more experienced clinician will be examining the patient.

To palpate the thyroid, the nurse identifies other midline neck structures (see Fig. 45-9). The thyroid can be palpated anteriorly and posteriorly. Water should always be available for the patient to swallow as part of this examination.

For anterior palpation the nurse stands in front of the patient, with the patient's neck flexed. The nurse places the thumb horizontally with the upper edge along the lower border of the cricoid cartilage. The thumb is then moved over the isthmus as the patient swallows water. The fingers are then placed laterally to the anterior border of the sternocleidomastoid muscle, and each lateral lobe is palpated before and while the patient swallows water.

For posterior palpation the examiner stands behind the patient. With the thumbs of both hands resting on the nape of the patient's neck, the nurse uses the index and middle fingers of both hands to feel for the thyroid isthmus and for the anterior

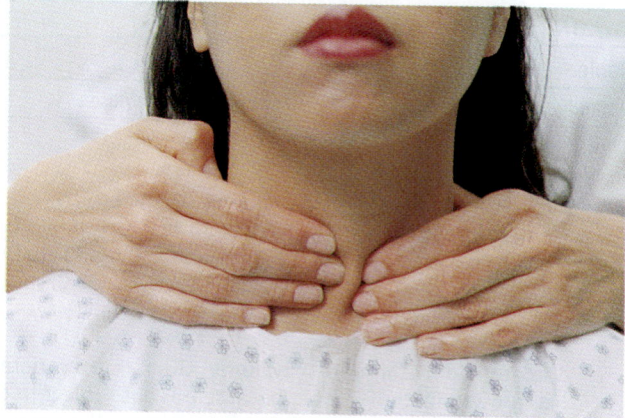

Fig. 45-10   Posterior palpation of the thyroid gland.

surfaces of the lateral lobes. To facilitate the examination of each lobe and to relax the neck muscles, the nurse asks the patient to flex the neck slightly forward and to the right. The thyroid cartilage is displaced to the right by the left hand and fingers. The nurse palpates with the right hand after placing the thumb deep and behind the sternocleidomastoid muscle with the index and middle fingers in front of it; the area is palpated with the right hand (Fig. 45-10). While this is done, the patient is asked to swallow water. This procedure is then repeated on the left side. The thyroid is palpated for its size, shape, symmetry, tenderness, and for any nodules. In the average person the thyroid is often not palpable. If palpable, it usually feels smooth with a firm consistency and is not tender with gentle pressure. Nodules, enlargement, asymmetry, or hardness is abnormal, and the patient should be referred for further evaluation.

Other assessment skills.   Percussion and auscultation are not normally part of an endocrine assessment. When an enlarged thyroid has been noted, however, the lateral lobes should be auscultated with the stethoscope bell to determine the presence of a bruit.

Assessment of vital signs should include the following:

1. Temperature: Hyperthermia or hypothermia
2. Pulse: Rate and rhythm
3. Respirations: Change in rate or rhythm
4. Blood pressure: Widening of the pulse pressure, hypotension, hypertension, or orthostatic hypotension (see Chapter 31)
5. Heart sounds: Systolic murmur at apex or pulmonic area (possible indication of increased blood flow as a result of hyperthyroidism)

DIAGNOSTIC STUDIES OF THE ENDOCRINE SYSTEM

Diagnostic studies common to the endocrine system are presented in Table 45-7. Accurately performed laboratory tests aid and confirm diagnoses of problems of the endocrine system.[19]

Hormone Assays

These tests can measure absolute hormone levels and estimate the production, transport, and catabolism of hormones.

Text continues on p. 1365

DIAGNOSTIC STUDIES

Table **45-7**   **Endocrine System**

Study	Description and Purpose	Nursing Responsibility
Pituitary Studies **Serum Studies**		
■ Growth hormone (GH) (somatotropin)	Evaluates GH hypersecretion. After an overnight fast, GH should be <5 ng/ml (5.0) in men and <10 ng/ml (10.0) in women. Values >50 ng/ml (50.0) suggest acromegaly.	Inform patient that blood sample will be drawn. Make sure that patient takes nothing by mouth after midnight and does not smoke. Send samples to laboratory immediately. Observe venipuncture site for bleeding or hematoma formation. Observe venipuncture site for bleeding or hematoma formation.
■ Somatomedin C (insulin-like growth factor I [IGF-I], growth factor I)	Evaluates GH; it is less variable than GH because it is not subject to circadian rhythm and fluctuations. *Normal values* are 135-250 ng/ml; low levels indicate GH deficiency, and high levels indicate GH excess. Values increase during puberty and pregnancy.	
■ GH release after exercise	Evaluates GH reserve in suspected hypopituitarism. Exercise stimulates GH secretion. Patient exercises vigorously for ½ hour before blood sample drawn. GH values should rise above 20 ng/ml after exercise.	Have patient fast for 12 hours. Explain procedure. Monitor pulse rate before and after exercise. May be contraindicated in patient with coronary artery insufficiency or exercise-induced asthma. Send sample to laboratory immediately.
■ Insulin-induced hypoglycemia	Used in examination of patients with suspected hypopituitarism. IV injection of regular insulin is given, based on body weight (usually 0.1 U/kg). Basal samples of GH, cortisol, and glucose are drawn. Blood samples are drawn at 30, 45, 60, and 90 minutes after injection. If test is terminated because of hypoglycemia (glucose level less than 40 mg/dl [40 ng/L]), samples are drawn for GH and cortisol levels 30 minutes after IV dextrose. GH level should rise twofold to threefold over baseline levels. Response is subnormal or absent in GH deficiency.	Ensure that patient fasted overnight (water is allowed) and that bed rest was prescribed. Have 5% cortisone, 20 ml of 50% dextrose, and IV solution of 5% glucose at bedside for use if severe hypoglycemia occurs and test will continue. Weigh patient. Continually assess patient's mental status because seizures, cardiac arrhythmias, and coma can result from hypoglycemia (test is contraindicated in patients with seizure disorders, cardiac disease, hypocortisolism, and hypothyroidism.) Assess capillary glucose levels immediately with BGM. Note on laboratory slips times that blood is drawn. Provide 25 g glucose and breakfast after last sample.
■ Prolactin level	Evaluates prolactin levels. Decreased levels in postpartum women attempting to nurse may be associated with Sheehan's syndrome. *Normal values* <20 ng/ml (<20 µg/L) (nonlactating); levels greater than 200 ng/ml (200 µg/L) indicate pituitary tumors.	Have patient fast. Inform patient that blood sample will be drawn. Draw blood within 3-4 hours after patient awakens. Observe venipuncture site for bleeding or hematoma formation.
■ Gonadotropin levels Follicle-stimulating hormone (FSH) Luteinizing hormone (LH)	Useful in distinguishing primary gonadal problems from pituitary insufficiency. Normal levels vary according to age and sex. In women, there are marked differences during menstrual cycle and in postmenopausal period. Levels are low in pituitary insufficiency and high in primary gonadal failure. In women, values for FSH are basal rate—2-15 mIU/ml (2-15 IU/L); ovulatory surge—8-40 mIU/ml (8-40 IU/L); and postmenopausal level—greater than 50 mIU/ml (40 IU/L). In women, values for LH are basal rate—2-20 mIU/ml (2-20 IU/L); ovulatory surge—30-140 mIU/ml (30-140 IU/L); and postmenopausal level—greater than 50 mIU/ml (50 IU/L). In men, values for FSH are 2-15 mIU/ml (2-15 IU/L) and LH 3-25 mIU/ml (3-25 IU/L).	Ensure that patient has fasted. Inform patient that three blood samples may be drawn 30 minutes apart for FSH. For women, note on laboratory slip time of menstrual cycle or whether she is postmenopausal.

Continued

DIAGNOSTIC STUDIES

Table **45-7**   **Endocrine System—cont'd**

Study	Description and Purpose	Nursing Responsibility
Serum Studies—cont'd		
■ Water deprivation test	Used to differentiate causes of polyuria, including pituitary diabetes insipidus (DI), nephrogenic DI, syndrome of inappropriate ADH, and psychogenic polydipsia. ADH or vasopressin diluted in saline solution are administered intravenously over a 2-hour period. With normal patients and with patients with psychogenic DI, urine osmolality is >600 mOsm/kg and plasma osmolality <300 mOsm/kg after ADH administration. With pituitary DI, plasma osmolality is >300 mOsm/kg; with dilute urine, it is <270 mOsm/kg. With nephrogenic DI, there is little or no response to ADH.	Have patient discontinue tea, coffee, alcohol, and smoking after midnight. Obtain baseline weight and urine and plasma osmolality. Ensure that fluid is withheld. Weigh patient and take three postural BP measurements (lying and standing BP measurements separated by 2 minutes) hourly. Assess urine hourly for volume and specific gravity. Send hourly samples for urine osmolality. Draw sample for plasma osmolality when (1) urine samples are collected and (2) orthostatic hypotension and postural tachycardia appear. Assess weight at 4, 6, 7, and 8 hours. Patients must be very closely supervised during this test.
Radiologic Studies		
■ Skull x-ray, CT scan, MRI	Useful in evaluating sella turcica for volume, enlargement, or erosion when disease of hypothalamic-pituitary axis is suspected. Compare with normal measurement of sella turcica in relation to patient's height.	Inform patient of the need to lie as still as possible during test; explain that tests are painless and noninvasive. Explain procedure.
Thyroid Studies		
Serum Studies		
■ T_4	Measures total serum level of T_4. Useful in evaluating thyroid function and monitoring thyroid therapy. *Normal values* are 5-12 µg/dl (51-142 nmol/L).	Inform patient that fasting is not necessary. Inform patient that blood samples will be drawn. Observe venipuncture site for bleeding or hematoma formation.
■ T_3	Measures serum levels of T_3. It is helpful in diagnosing hyperthyroidism if T_4 levels are normal. *Normal values* are 65-195 ng/dl (1.0-3.0 nmol/L).	Same as above.
■ T_3 resin uptake (T_3RU)	This study indirectly measures binding capacity of thyroid-binding globulin. *Normal values* are 25-35% (0.25-0.35).	Same as above.
■ Free T_4	Measures active component of total T_4. *Normal values* are 1.0-3.5 ng/dl (12.9-45.0 pmol/L).	Same as above.
■ Free T_3	Measures active component of total T_3. *Normal values* are 0.26-0.65 ng/dl.	Same as above.
■ Thyroid ^{131}I uptake (radioactive iodine uptake)	Provides direct measure of thyroid activity. Useful for evaluation of functional activity of solitary thyroid nodules. Small tracer dose of ^{131}I is given orally or intravenously. Serum uptake measurements are drawn at 2 to 4 and at 24 hours. *Normal serum values* for 2-4 hours are 3-10%; for 24 hours, they are 5-30%. Values are affected by drugs, seafood, certain radiographic contrast media, and antiseptics containing iodine.	Instruct patient to discontinue thyroid medication and to start T_3 (Cytomel) 2-3 times/day for 4 weeks. Tell patient to report for further testing in 10-14 days. Collect 24-hour urine specimen.
■ Thyroid-stimulating hormone (TSH)	This test measures level of TSH, which is markedly elevated in primary hypothyroidism. *Normal values* are 0.3-5.4 µU/ml (0.3-5.4 mU/L).	Inform patient that fasting is not necessary. Inform patient that blood sample will be drawn. Observe venipuncture site for bleeding or hematoma formation.
■ Calcitonin	High calcitonin level with normal serum calcium level is associated with medullary thyroid carcinoma. *Normal values* are ≤155 pg/ml (155 ng/L) for men and 105 pg/ml (105 ng/L) for women.	Ensure that patient has fasted. Inform patient that blood sample will be drawn. Observe venipuncture site for bleeding or hematoma formation.

Continued

DIAGNOSTIC STUDIES

Table 45-7 Endocrine System—cont'd

Study	Description and Purpose	Nursing Responsibility
Thyroid Studies—cont'd **Radiologic Studies**		
• Thyroid scan	Used to evaluate nodules of the thyroid. Tracer dose of technetium is given intravenously. Scanner passes over thyroid and makes graphic record of radiation emitted. Normal thyroid scan reveals homogeneous pattern with symmetric lobes.	Determine whether other tests requiring iodine preparation (IV pyelogram, saturated solution of potassium iodine, or barium enema) have been done within 30 days (can invalidate test). Explain procedure to patient.
Parathyroid Studies **Serum Studies**		
• Parathyroid hormone (PTH)	Measures PTH level in serum. Normal range depends on assay used (check with laboratory). This study must be interpreted in terms of concomitantly drawn serum calcium level.	Fasting specimen preferred. Inform patient that blood sample will be drawn. Sample must be kept on ice. Observe venipuncture site for bleeding or hematoma formation.
• Total serum calcium	Measures total serum calcium to help detect bone and parathyroid disorders. Hypercalcemia can indicate primary hyperparathyroidism, and hypocalcemia can indicate hypoparathyroidism. *Normal values are 9.0-11.0 mg/dl or 4.5-5.5 mEq/L (2.25-2.74 mmol/L).*	Fasting specimen preferred. Inform patient that blood sample will be drawn. Observe venipuncture site for bleeding or hematoma formation. Ensure that prolonged tourniquet application does not cause falsely elevated values. Adjust total calcium for albumin levels. Using following formula: Total serum calcium (mg/dl) − Albumin (g/dl) + 4.0 = Adjusted total serum calcium.
• Phosphorus	Measures inorganic phosphorus. Hyperphosphatemia indicates primary hypoparathyroidism or secondary causes (e.g., renal failure); hypophosphatemia indicates hyperparathyroidism. Phosphorus and calcium levels are inversely related. *Normal values are 2.8-4.5 mg/dl (0.90-1.45 mmol/L).*	Need for fasting varies with lab. Determine fasting requirement. Inform patient that blood sample will be drawn. Observe venipuncture site for bleeding or hematoma formation.
• 1,25-Dihydroxyvitamin D_3	This test is used to evaluate calcium and phosphorus levels and bone disease. *Normal values are 15-60 pg/ml.*	Inform patient that blood sample will be drawn. Observe venipuncture site for bleeding or hematoma formation.
Radiologic Studies		
• Skeletal x-ray, CT scans	Used to determine bone disease and osteoporosis. Fractures or deformities can be caused by the demineralization produced by excessive PTH.	Monitor patient's exposure to x-rays. Inform patient that tests are painless and noninvasive and that no special preparation is required for x-ray studies. For CT scan, give patient radiolabeled agent 4 hours before scan.
Adrenal Studies **Serum Studies**		
• Cortisol	Measures amount of cortisol in serum and evaluates status of adrenocortical function. *Normal values are 5-25 μg/dl (0.14-0.69 μmol/L) at 8 AM, <10 μg/dl (<0.28 μmol/L) at 8 PM.*	Inform patient that blood sample will be taken. Observe venipuncture site for bleeding and hematoma formation. Ensure collection of properly timed blood sample. Draw specimen early in morning when cortisol levels are highest. Mark time on laboratory slip. Minimize stress to avoid raising level.
• Aldosterone	Normal values are 5-20 ng/dl (140-556 pmol/L) (upright posture) and 8.5 ng/dl (237 pmol/L) supine position.	Increases with low-salt diet (less than 2 g/day), stress, an upright posture, and diuretics; decreases with a high-salt diet, ACE inhibitors such as captopril, and lying in supine position. Determine which maneuvers will be done and advise patient.

Continued

DIAGNOSTIC STUDIES

Table **45-7**	**Endocrine System—cont'd**	
Study	**Description and Purpose**	**Nursing Responsibility**

Adrenal Studies—cont'd
Serum Studies—cont'd

■ ACTH stimulation	Used to evaluate adrenal function. After baseline samples are drawn, 250 µg synthetic ACTH is given as IV or IM bolus; samples are drawn 30 and 50 minutes after bolus. Baseline ACTH sample is often drawn in case results are abnormal. Plasma cortisol at 60 minutes should be (1) greater than baseline and (2) greater than 20 µg/dl.	Inject ACTH with a plastic syringe and collect samples for ACTH in plastic, heparinized tubes. Administer test with continuous-infusion method. Monitor site and rate of IV infusion. Ensure sample collection at appropriate times.
■ Dexamethasone suppression (overnight)	Assesses adrenal function and is especially helpful if hyperactivity is suspected. Useful in evaluation of Cushing's syndrome. Dexamethasone (Decadron) 2 mg is given at 11 PM to suppress secretion of corticotropin-releasing hormone. Plasma cortisol sample is drawn at 8 AM. Cortisol level less than 5 µg/dl (138 nmol/L) indicates normal adrenal response (50% decrease in cortisol production).	Ensure that patient has fasted. Inform patient that blood sample will be taken. Observe venipuncture site for bleeding and hematoma formation. Do not test acutely ill patients; those under stress are not tested. ACTH may override suppression. Screen patient for drugs such as estrogen and glucocorticoids, which may give false-positive results. Ensure accurate timing of medication and sample collection.
■ Metyrapone suppression	Used to evaluate feedback response of hypothalamus and pituitary and adrenal glands and to differentiate causes of endogenous glucocorticoid overproduction. Metyrapone (30 mg/kg) is given at midnight. Sample is drawn at 8 AM for plasma 11-deoxycortisol (Compound S), cortisol, and ACTH. Normal response is 11-deoxycortisol: 7-232 µg/dl (202-6696 nmol/L) and ACTH >250 pg/ml (55.1 pmol/L). To validate blockage by metyrapone, cortisol must be (1) less than 8 µg/dl (220 nmol/L) and (2) less than 45% of Compound S level.	Weigh patient. Administer metyrapone with milk and snack at midnight. (Note that metyrapone can cause gastrointestinal distress and confusion.) Draw ACTH into heparinized plastic tube with plastic syringe. Ensure that patient has not ingested estrogens, phenytoin, and phenobarbital because these substances invalidate test.

Urine Studies

■ 17-Ketosteroids	Measures androgen metabolites in urine and evaluates adrenal cortical and gonadal function. *Normal values* are 10-22 mg/day (35-76 µmol/day) for men and 6-16 mg/day (21-55 µmol/day) for women.	Instruct patient regarding 24-hour urine collection. Tell patient that specimen must be kept refrigerated or iced during collection. Determine whether preservative is required for method used.
■ Aldosterone	Measures urinary aldosterone level to evaluate adrenal function. Useful in determining therapy for hypertension. *Normal values* are 2-26 µg/24 hours (5.5-72 nmol/day).	Ensure that patient is on unrestricted diet with normal salt intake and no medication for 3 weeks before collection. Instruct patient regarding 24-hour urine collection.
■ Free cortisol	Preferred test to evaluate hypercortisolism. Can also be used to screen for endogenous glucocorticoids. *Normal values* are less than 100 mg/24 hours.	Instruct patient regarding 24-hour urine collection and avoidance of stressful situations and excessive physical exercise. Tell patient that some drugs (e.g., reserpine, diuretics, phenothiazines, and amphetamines) may elevate levels. Ensure that patient is on low-sodium diet.
■ Vanillylmandelic acid	Measures urinary excretion of catecholamine metabolite and is helpful in diagnosing pheochromocytoma. *Normal values* are less than 8 mg/14 hours (40 µmol/day); pheochromocytoma is indicated with values of 10-250 mg/24 hours (51-126 µmol/day).	Keep 24-hour urine collection at pH of less than 3.0 with hydrochloric acid as preservative. Know that newer methods are not affected by dietary intake. Consult with laboratory or physician about patient discontinuing any drugs 3 days before urine collection.

Continued

DIAGNOSTIC STUDIES

Table **45-7**   Endocrine System—cont'd

Study	Description and Purpose	Nursing Responsibility
Pancreatic Studies		
Serum Studies		
▪ Fasting blood sugar (FBS) levels	Measures circulating glucose level. *Normal serum values* for adults are 70-110 mg/dl (3.9-6.7 mmol/L); for pregnant women they are 60-90 mg/dl (3.3-5 mmol/L).	Ensure that patient has fasted at least 4 hours. Inform patient that blood sample will be drawn. Observe venipuncture site for bleeding or hematoma formation.
▪ Oral glucose tolerance	A. This 2-hour test is used to diagnose diabetes mellitus if FBS is equivocal. Patient drinks 75 g of glucose; samples for glucose are drawn immediately and at 30, 60, and 120 minutes. *Normal values* are <200 mg/dl (11.1 mmol/L) at 30, 60, and 90 minutes and <140 mg/dl (7.8 mmol/L) at 120 minutes.	Ensure that tests are not done on patients who are malnourished, confined to bed for over 3 days, or severely stressed. Instruct patient to refrain from smoking and caffeine and to fast for 12 hours before test. Ensure that patient's diet 3 days before test included 150-300 g of carbohydrate with intake of at least 1500 calories per day. Screen for estrogens, phenytoin, and corticosteroids, and check for hypokalemia, which may impair glucose tolerance.
	B. This 5-hour test is used to evaluate hypoglycemia. Patient drinks 100 g of glucose; samples of glucose are drawn immediately and at 30, 60, 90, 120, 180, 240, and 300 minutes. Baseline cortisol level test is done if patient becomes symptomatic. Patients with reactive hypoglycemia have adrenergic symptoms and glucose less than 60 mg/dl (3.3 mmol/L) between 30 minutes and 5 hr after glucose ingestion.	Simultaneously monitor glucoses with capillary BGM.
▪ Capillary glucose monitoring	Used to give immediate glucose values with glucose oxidase or electrochemical methods. Capillary values (whole blood) are usually 10-15% less than serum values.	Obtain large drop of blood from clean finger, touch strip to drop of blood (not finger), time accurately, and compare colors in good lighting, if using visual method. Use digital readout if available. Use automatic finger-puncture device if available. Be sure to change section of device that touches patients' fingers between patients.
▪ Glycosylated hemoglobin	Measures degree of glucose control during previous 3 months (life span of hemoglobin molecule). *Normal values* are 4-6% (values vary widely, check with laboratory.)	Inform patient that fasting is not necessary and that blood sample will be drawn. Observe venipuncture site for bleeding or hematoma formation.
Urine Studies		
▪ Glucose (Clinistix, Labstix, Multistix, Clinitest)	Estimates amount of glucose in urine by using reducing substance. Results have wide range from negative (no glucose) to 2% (large amount of glucose).	Use freshly voided urine specimen collected at appropriate time. Know that many different drugs alter glucose readings and that errors are great if directions for timing are not followed exactly. Follow package directions.
▪ Ketone (Acetest, Ketostix, Labstix, Multistix)	Measures amount of acetone excreted in urine as result of incomplete fat metabolism. Positive result can indicate lack of insulin and diabetic acidosis.	Use freshly voided urine specimen. Test is often done with glucose test. Directions must be followed exactly. Certain drugs can produce false-positive and false-negative results.
▪ Glucose and acetone (Ketodiastix)	Measures glucose and acetone levels.	Know that large amounts of urinary acetone may depress glucose measurement.

ACE, angiotensin-converting enzyme; *BGM*, blood glucose monitoring.

Hormones with fairly constant basal levels (e.g., T$_4$) require only a single measurement. Hormones with pulsatile secretion (e.g., LH) may require multiple samples with a measurement taken from pooled aliquots. Notation of sample time on the laboratory slip and sample is important for hormones with circadian or sleep-related secretion (e.g., cortisol, GH).

On occasion, multiple blood sampling is indicated, such as in suppression tests (e.g., dexamethasone suppression) and stimulation tests (e.g., glucose tolerance). To decrease patient discomfort and minimize the effects of stress hormones, the nurse initiates an intravenous infusion of normal saline solution with a stopcock between the extension and the infusion tubing. After insertion of the infusion, 15 to 30 minutes should be allowed for stress hormones to normalize. Baseline samples are then drawn, the appropriate medication is given through the stopcock, and samples are withdrawn through the stopcock at the appropriate times. A heparin lock may be used in place of the saline infusion. It is necessary to draw and discard 1.5 to 3 ml of blood from the patient before drawing the sample for measurement. This prevents saline or heparin dilution.

In general, tests of endocrine function require patient fasting and the elimination of as many environmental stimuli as possible. This necessitates inactivity throughout the test; such inactivity can be achieved with bed rest with the head of the bed elevated or through the use of a recliner chair. The patient should refrain from smoking or taking food or fluids by mouth. A thorough explanation of the test and the reasons for reducing environmental stimuli reassures patients and helps them cooperate. The patient should be monitored frequently during the test and not just when samples are being taken.

During endocrine testing there are instances in which simultaneous blood and urine samples or special preservatives are needed for samples. The nurse ensures thorough patient instruction, as well as correct and complete sample collection. When a patient is having multiple endocrine testing, such as with suspected pituitary disease, a fluid volume deficit may occur. Nursing interventions in this instance include recording the amount of blood and urine taken per test, assessing for dehydration, and promptly notifying the physician if blood loss through sample collection is excessive or the patient becomes dehydrated. Using the saline infusion method helps offset fluid volume deficit.

Types of Laboratory Tests.
Several types of laboratory tests are used to determine endocrine status, including immunoassay, immunometric, receptor, chromatographic, and in vitro bioassays.[20] The immunoassay, a displacement assay, uses antibodies specific for a hormone or parts of a hormone and can measure very small amounts of circulating hormones. It is used for peptide, steroid, and thyroid hormones. Immunometric assays can measure minute hormone levels and are used for TSH measurements. Radioreceptor assays measure the ability of a hormone to bind to its receptor. Receptor measurements are useful in states of hormone resistance such as those seen with insulin, PTH, and vitamin D. Chromatographic assay allows measurement of several hormones in the same sample. In vitro bioassays can provide information about the transport, clearance rate, and enzymatic transformation of a substance before it binds to its receptor.

Specific diagnostic studies related to the endocrine system are summarized in Table 45-7. Because of the interrelatedness of the endocrine system, nursing interventions are focused on reducing the stress and anxiety often associated with diagnostic testing. Unless nursing measures related to patient instruction and expectations are initiated, the effect of stress hormones can produce inaccurate and misleading results.

Normal values and collection procedures vary among laboratories. It is therefore important to check with the laboratory doing the testing to determine the correct collection and transport procedures and normal values.

REVIEW QUESTIONS

The number of the question corresponds to the same-numbered objective at the beginning of the chapter.

1. A characteristic common to all hormones is that they
   a. circulate in the blood bound to plasma proteins.
   b. influence cellular activity of specific target tissues.
   c. accelerate the metabolic processes of all body cells.
   d. enter cells to alter the cell's metabolism or gene expression.

2. A patient is receiving radiation therapy for cancer of the kidney. The nurse monitors the patient for signs and symptoms of damage to the
   a. pancreas.
   b. thyroid gland.
   c. adrenal glands.
   d. posterior pituitary gland.

3. A patient has a serum sodium level of 152 mEq/L (152 mmol/L). The normal hormonal response to this situation is
   a. release of ADH.
   b. release of renin.
   c. secretion of aldosterone.
   d. secretion of corticotropin-releasing hormone.

4. All cells in the body are believed to have intracellular receptors for
   a. insulin.
   b. cortisone.
   c. growth hormone.
   d. thyroid hormones.

5. When obtaining subjective data from a patient during assessment of the endocrine system, the nurse asks specifically about
   a. energy level.
   b. intake of vitamin C.
   c. employment history.
   d. frequency of sexual intercourse.

6. An appropriate technique to use during physical assessment of the thyroid gland is
   a. asking the patient to hyperextend the neck during palpation.
   b. percussing the neck for dullness to define the size of the thyroid.
   c. having the patient swallow water during inspection and palpation of the gland.
   d. using deep palpation to determine the extent of a visibly enlarged thyroid gland.

7. The older adult with hypothyroidism is more likely than a younger person to have disturbances of
   a. bone metabolism.
   b. cardiovascular function.
   c. gastrointestinal function.
   d. central nervous system function.

8. An abnormal finding by the nurse during an endocrine assessment would include
   a. joint pain.
   b. blood pressure of 100/70.
   c. decreased skin pigmentation.
   d. soft, formed stool every other day.

9. A patient has a serum cortisol level of 3 µg/dl at 8 AM. If this finding reflects a primary dysfunction of the adrenal glands, the nurse would expect further diagnostic testing to reveal
   a. increased serum ACTH.
   b. decreased urinary aldosterone.
   c. increased urine 17-ketosteroids.
   d. serum cortisol level less than 5 µg with dexamethasone suppression.

References

1. Baxter JD, Frohman L, Felig P: Introduction to the endocrine system. In Felig P, Baxter JD, Frohman L, editors: *Endocrinology and metabolism,* ed 3, New York, 1995, McGraw-Hill.
2. Hagan RM, Oakley NR: Melatonin comes of age? *Trends Pharmacol Sci* 16:50, 1995.
3. Reppert SM, Weaver RR: Melatonin madness, *Cell* 83:1059, 1995.
4. Gill GN: Biosynthesis, secretion, and metabolism of hormones. In Felig P, Baxter JD, Frohman LC, editors: *Endocrinology and metabolism,* ed 3, New York, 1995, McGraw-Hill.
5. Oppenheimer JH, Schwartz HL, Strait KA: The molecular basis of thyroid hormone action. In Braverman LE, Utiger RD, editors: *Werner and Ingbar's the thyroid, a fundamental and clinical text,* ed 7, Philadelphia, 1996, Lippincott.
6. Catt KJ: Molecular mechanisms of hormone action: control of target cell function by peptide and catecholamine hormones. In Felig P, Baxter JD, Frohman LA, editors: *Endocrinology and metabolism,* ed 3, New York, 1995, McGraw-Hill.
7. Loriaux TC: Endocrine assessment: red flags for those on the front lines, *Nurs Clin North Am* 31:695, 1996.
8. Cooper PF, Martin JB: Physiology and pathophysiology of the endocrine brain and hypothalamus. In Becker KL, editor: *Principles and practices of endocrinology and metabolism,* ed 2, Philadelphia, 1995, Lippincott.
9. Robertson GL: Posterior pituitary. In Felig P, Baxter JD, Frohman LA, editors: *Endocrinology and metabolism,* ed 3, New York, 1995, McGraw-Hill.
10. Baran DT: The skeletal system in thyrotoxicosis. In Braverman LE, Utiger RD, editors: *Werner and Ingbar's the thyroid: a fundamental and clinical text,* ed 7, Philadelphia, 1996, Lippincott.
11. Carlstedt-Duke J and others: Molecular mechanisms of hormone action: regulation of target cell function by the steroid hormone receptor supergene family. In Felig P, Baxter JD, Frohman LA, editors: *Endocrinology and metabolism,* ed 3, New York, 1995, McGraw-Hill.
12. Miller WL, Tyrell JB: The adrenal cortex. In Felig P, Baxter JD, Frohman LA, editors: *Endocrinology and metabolism,* ed 3, New York, 1995, McGraw-Hill.
13. Felig P, Bergman M: The endocrine pancreas: diabetes mellitus. In Felig P, Baxter JD, Frohman LC, editors: *Endocrinology and metabolism,* ed 3, New York, 1995, McGraw-Hill.
14. Scheen AJ, Lefebvre PJ: Insulin action in man, *Diabetes Metab* 22:105, 1996.
15. Seely EW, Williams GH: The endocrine heart. In Becker KL, editor: *Principles and practice of endocrinology and metabolism,* ed 2, Philadelphia, 1995, Lippincott.
16. Winger JM, Hornick T: Age-associated changes in the endocrine system, *Nurs Clin North Am* 31:827, 1996.
17. Grunewald DA, Matsumoto AM: Aging and endocrinology. In Becker KL, editor: *Principles and practice of endocrinology and metabolism,* ed 2, Philadelphia, 1995, Lippincott.
18. Aceto TJ and others: Short stature and slow growth in the infant and child. In Becker KL, editor: *Principles and practice of endocrinology and metabolism,* ed 2, Philadelphia, 1995, Lippincott.
19. Rusterholtz A: Interpretation of diagnostic laboratory tests in selected endocrine disorders, *Nurs Clin North Am* 31:715, 1996.
20. Pekary AE, Hershman JM: Hormone assays. In Felig P, Baxter JD, Frohman LC, editors: *Endocrinology and metabolism,* ed 3, New York, 1995, McGraw-Hill.

Resources

Resources for this chapter are listed after Chapter 47 on p. 1448.

46 NURSING MANAGEMENT
Patient with Diabetes Mellitus

Virginia Valentine

www.mosby.com/MERLIN/medsurg_lewis

DIABETES MELLITUS

Diabetes mellitus is a serious health problem throughout the world. An estimated 15.7 million people have diabetes mellitus in the United States alone. It is estimated that, counting both diagnosed and undiagnosed diabetes, as many as 5.9% of the United States population has diabetes mellitus.[1] Diabetes mellitus contributed to more than 162,000 deaths in 1996. Diabetes is the seventh leading cause of death listed on U.S. death certificates, but diabetes is believed to be underreported on death certificates, both as a condition and as cause of death.[1] Diabetes is the leading cause of new cases of blindness. African-Americans are 1.7 times more likely than Caucasians to have diabetes.[1] It increases the risk of coronary artery disease twofold or more. More than 60% to 65% of people with diabetes mellitus have hypertension.[1] The staggering cost from both direct and indirect medical expenditures attributable to diabetes in 1997 was estimated at $98 billion. Hospitalization costs accounted for the greatest proportion of direct medical costs (62%).[2] These dollar amounts do not reflect the impact that the diagnosis of diabetes has on the lives of patients and their families.

Etiology and Pathophysiology

Diabetes mellitus is not a single disease. Rather, it is a group of genetically and clinically heterogeneous disorders characterized by abnormalities in glucose homeostasis resulting in hyperglycemia. The hyperglycemia of diabetes is caused by a decrease in the secretion or activity of insulin. These insulin alterations result in disordered metabolism of carbohydrate, fat, and protein. In time, structural abnormalities in a variety of organs and organ systems, especially the heart, kidneys, and eyes, develop. The complications arise primarily from microangiopathy, macroangiopathy, and neuropathy. Chronic hyperglycemia is generally recognized as contributing to the development of these complications. In addition, diabetes mellitus is associated with complications in pregnancy.

Diabetes mellitus is a heterogeneous syndrome for which several theories of etiology have been proposed. Current theories link the causes of diabetes, singly or in combination, to genetic, autoimmune, viral, and environmental factors such as obesity and stress. There are primarily two types of diabetes mellitus: type 1, in which insulin production by the β-cells is reduced or completely absent and for which the management requires insulin replacement; and type 2, which is the more prevalent type of diabetes mellitus (approximately 90% of patients). Table 46-1 depicts the distinguishing characteristics of type 1 and type 2 diabetes mellitus.

Normal Insulin Metabolism. Insulin is a hormone produced by the β-cells in the islets of Langerhans of the pancreas. Under normal conditions, insulin is continuously released into the bloodstream in small pulsatile increments (a basal rate), with increased release (bolus) when food is ingested (Fig. 46-1). The activity of released insulin lowers blood glucose and facilitates a stable, normal glucose range of approximately 70 to 110 mg/dl (3.9 to 6.0 mmol/L). The average amount of insulin secreted daily by an adult is approximately 40 to 50 U or 0.6 U/kg of body weight. Other hormones (glucagon, epinephrine, growth hormone, cortisol, and somatostatin) work to counter the effects of insulin and are often referred to as counterregulatory hormones because they stimulate glycogen release and breakdown or antagonize the effect of insulin and thereby increase blood glucose levels. Insulin and these counterregulatory substances provide a sustained but regulated release of glucose for energy during

Reviewed by Carol Blainey, RN, MN, Associate Professor, Biobehavioral Nursing and Health Systems, University of Washington School of Nursing, Seattle, Wash.

Table **46-1**	Characteristics of Type 1 and Type 2 Diabetes Mellitus	
Factor	**Type 1 Diabetes Mellitus**	**Type 2 Diabetes Mellitus**
■ Age at onset	Usually in young person but possible at any age	Usually age 35 yr or older but possible at any age
■ Type of onset	Signs and symptoms abrupt, but disease process may be present for several years	Insidious
■ Genetic susceptibility	HLA-DR3, HLA-DR4, and others	Frequent genetic tendency, no relation to HLA
■ Environmental factors	Virus, toxins	Obesity, lack of exercise
■ Islet cell antibodies	Often present at onset	Absent
■ Endogenous insulin	Minimal or absent	Possibly excessive; adequate but delayed secretion or reduced but not absent secretion
■ Nutritional status	Thin, catabolic state	Obese or possibly normal
■ Symptoms	Thirst, polyuria, polyphagia, fatigue	Frequently none or mild
■ Ketosis	Prone at onset or during insulin deficiency	Resistant except during infection or stress
■ Dietary management	Essential	Essential, possibly sufficient for glycemic control
■ Insulin	Required for all	Required for 30-40%
■ Oral agents	Not beneficial	Usually beneficial
■ Vascular and neurologic complications	In majority of patients after ≥5 yr	Frequent

HLA, human leukocyte antigen.

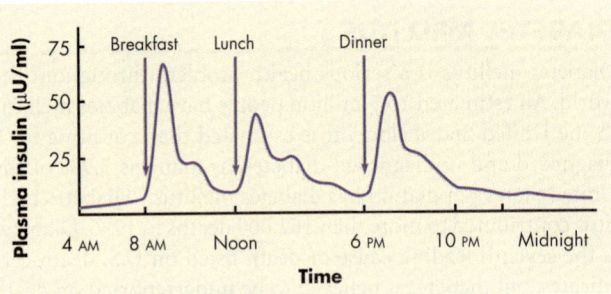

Fig. 46-1 Normal endogenous insulin secretion. In the first hour or two after meals, insulin concentrations rise rapidly in blood and peak at about 1 hour. After meals, insulin concentrations promptly decline toward preprandial values as carbohydrate absorption from the gastrointestinal tract declines. After carbohydrate absorption from the gastrointestinal tract is complete and during the night, insulin concentrations are low and fairly constant, with a slight increase at dawn.

food intake and periods of fasting and usually maintain blood glucose levels within the normal range. Abnormal production of any or all of these hormones may be present in diabetes.

Once insulin is released into the bloodstream from the β-cells as proinsulin, it is routed through the liver. Within the liver, approximately 50% to 70% of received insulin is extracted from the blood. Insulin is formed from proinsulin after cleavage of the C-peptide chain.[3] The presence of C peptide in serum and urine is a useful indicator of β-cell function. The remaining insulin (now active A- and B-peptide chains) functions to promote glucose transport from the bloodstream across the cell membrane to the cytoplasm of the cell. The rise in plasma insulin after a meal stimulates storage of glucose as glycogen in liver and muscle, enhances fat deposition in adipose tissue, inhibits protein degradation, and accelerates the processes of amino acid transport into cells and protein synthesis. The fall in insulin level during normal overnight fasting facilitates the release of stored glucose from the liver, protein from muscle, and fat from adipose tissue.[4] For this reason insulin is known as the storage hormone.

Skeletal muscle and adipose tissue have specific receptors for insulin and are considered to be insulin-dependent tissues. Other tissues (e.g., brain, liver, and blood cells) do not directly depend on insulin for glucose transport but require an adequate glucose supply.

Classification of Diabetes Mellitus

The diagnostic label of diabetes mellitus carries many psychologic and socioeconomic ramifications and therapeutic requirements. Therefore accurate classification of the degree of glucose intolerance and the type of diabetes is important. In 1997 an expert committee supported by the American Diabetes Association (ADA), the National Institute of Diabetes and Digestive and Kidney Diseases at the National Institutes of Health, and the Division of Diabetes Translation at the Centers

Table 46-2	Types of Diabetes Mellitus and Other Categories of Glucose Intolerance
Types	**Characteristics**
■ Type 1	May be of any age, is usually thin, and usually has abrupt onset of signs and symptoms with insulinopenia before age 30. Patient often has strongly positive urine ketone tests in conjunction with hyperglycemia and depends on insulin therapy to prevent ketoacidosis and to sustain life.
■ Type 2	Is usually older than 30 yr at diagnosis, often obese, and has relatively few classic symptoms. Patient is not prone to ketoacidosis except during periods of stress. Although not dependent on exogenous insulin for survival, patient may require it for adequate control of hyperglycemia. Primarily insulin resistant.
■ Impaired glucose tolerance	Has plasma glucose levels that are higher than normal but not diagnostic for diabetes mellitus. In response to glucose challenge, 2 hr plasma glucose ≥140 mg/dl (7.8 mmol/L) and <200 mg/dl (11.1 mmol/L).
■ Impaired fasting glucose	Fasting plasma glucose ≥110 mg/dl (6.1 mmol/L) and <126 mg/dl (7.0 mmol/L).
■ Gestational diabetes mellitus	Has onset or discovery of glucose intolerance during pregnancy.

for Disease Control and Prevention revised the classification system and diagnostic criteria for diabetes, marking the first changes since 1979.[5] The classification system is based not on the treatment of the disease but on the presence and degree of hyperglycemia and the presenting history and symptoms (Table 46-2). The classification scheme also includes the person who has had or who is having glucose intolerance without overt signs of diabetes mellitus. Recognition of this difference allows a person at risk for diabetes to be followed up without being misclassified or mismanaged.

According to the new criteria, the diagnosis of diabetes mellitus is made when the fasting plasma glucose level equals or exceeds 126 mg/dl (7.0 mmol/L), when a random plasma glucose measurement equals or exceeds 200 mg/dl (11.1 mmol/L), or when plasma glucose 2 hours after a glucose challenge is equal or greater than 200 mg/dl (11.1 mmol/L). When the fasting blood glucose level is greater than 110 mg/dl (6.1 mmol/L) but less than 126 mg/dl (7.0 mmol/L), the individual is considered to have impaired fasting glucose. *Impaired glucose tolerance* is classified as a 2 hour plasma glucose level higher than normal but lower than that considered diagnostic for diabetes mellitus (≥140 mg/dl [7.8 mmol/L] and less than 200 mg/dl [11.1 mmol/L]).

As shown in Fig. 46-2 there are altered mechanisms in type 1 and type 2 diabetes in different tissue sites. The development of hyperglycemia arises from different causes. Type 1 diabetes results from progressive destruction of β-cell function as a result of an autoimmune process in a susceptible individual. Islet cell antibodies and insulin autoantibodies cause a reduction in β-cells of 80% to 90% of normal before hyperglycemia and symptoms occur. Type 2 diabetes is a combination of genetically determined defects in skeletal muscle, fat, and liver receptors for insulin and β-cell secretory exhaustion. Excessive hepatic glucose production eventually adds to the fasting and postprandial hyperglycemia.[4] Because of these possibilities for malfunctioning, diabetes mellitus must be considered a heterogeneous disease that cannot be managed by only one treatment regimen.

Type 1 Diabetes Mellitus. Type 1 diabetes is characterized by autoimmune β-cell destruction, which is attributed to a genetic predisposition coupled with one or more viral agents and possibly chemical agents. It is not known conclusively that these are the only factors involved.

The complexity may be better appreciated in relationship to information about human leukocyte antigens (HLAs), which are proteins on the cell surface controlled by genes on chromosome 6. (See Chapter 12 for a discussion of HLAs and disease associations.) Five groups of these antigens have been recognized (A, B, C, D, and DR), and these groups can appear in many variations. Results of family studies confirm that susceptibility to type 1 diabetes is strongly linked to the HLA-DR3 and DR4 loci.[6,7] The individual at highest risk for type 1 diabetes has one or more of the following HLA types: B8, DR3, B15, DR4.[6,7] Theoretically, when an individual with these genetic characteristics is exposed to viral infections, the β-cells are destroyed directly, or an autoimmune process is triggered, which in turn destroys the β-cells. A combination of both processes may occur. Current research continues to seek genetic markers to identify a person at risk for type 1 diabetes who is free of symptoms and to study immunologic parameters that may be manipulated to prevent or cure type 1 diabetes.

Genetic counseling for parents is based on statistical risk. If one child has type 1 diabetes, other siblings have a 5% to 10% chance of type 1 diabetes developing (up to 45% if the sibling is an identical twin). The offspring of a father with type 1 diabetes has a risk of 4% to 6%, double that of offspring of type 1 diabetic mothers (2% to 3%).[7]

The onset and progression of hyperglycemic symptoms are usually more rapid and acute in type 1 diabetes as compared with type 2, and successful treatment depends on insulin replacement. If the disease process is allowed to progress without treatment, diabetic ketoacidosis with nausea and vomiting, electrolyte imbalance, weight loss, and muscle wasting may develop. Without treatment (i.e., insulin) ketoacidosis can progress to coma and death.

Once treatment is initiated, the patient with type 1 diabetes may go into a remission (often called the "honeymoon" period). During this time, the patient needs very little insulin to control blood glucose. The honeymoon period occurs because, even as insulin islet cell antibodies destroy β-cells, β-cells continue to produce insulin. Eventually, blood glucose levels climb, more insulin is needed, and the honeymoon period ends. The honeymoon period may last up to a year, depending on the patient.

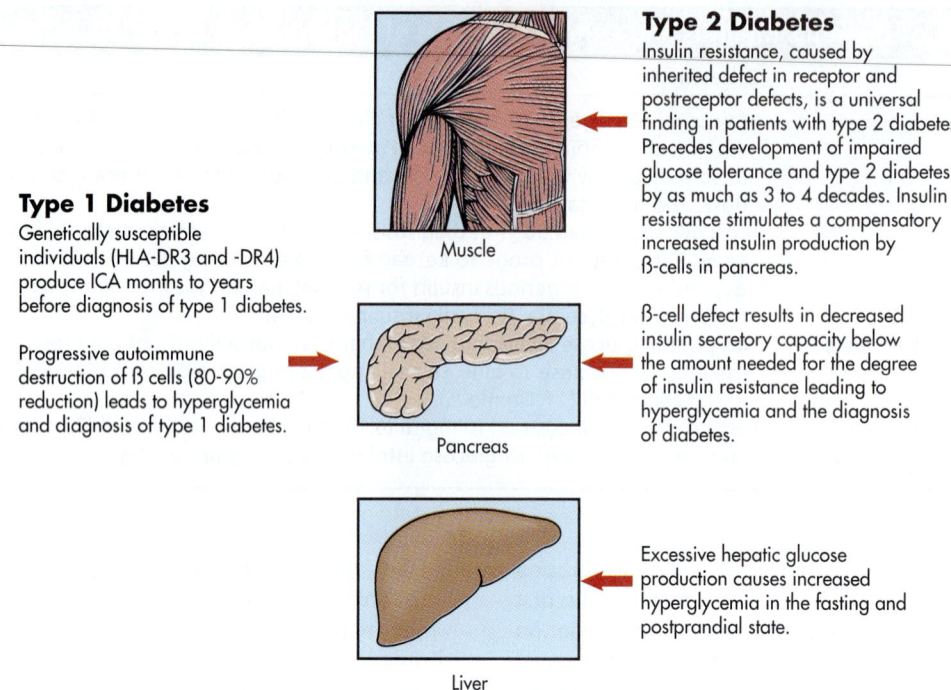

Type 2 Diabetes

Insulin resistance, caused by inherited defect in receptor and postreceptor defects, is a universal finding in patients with type 2 diabetes. Precedes development of impaired glucose tolerance and type 2 diabetes by as much as 3 to 4 decades. Insulin resistance stimulates a compensatory increased insulin production by ß-cells in pancreas.

Type 1 Diabetes

Genetically susceptible individuals (HLA-DR3 and -DR4) produce ICA months to years before diagnosis of type 1 diabetes.

Progressive autoimmune destruction of ß cells (80-90% reduction) leads to hyperglycemia and diagnosis of type 1 diabetes.

Muscle

ß-cell defect results in decreased insulin secretory capacity below the amount needed for the degree of insulin resistance leading to hyperglycemia and the diagnosis of diabetes.

Pancreas

Excessive hepatic glucose production causes increased hyperglycemia in the fasting and postprandial state.

Liver

Fig. 46-2   Altered mechanisms in type 1 and type 2 diabetes. *ICA,* islet cell antibodies.

Type 2 Diabetes Mellitus.   Approximately 90% of people with diabetes mellitus have type 2. Type 2 diabetes has a strong genetic influence (almost 100% concordance in monozygotic twins), but no correlation with HLA type has been found.

Genetic counseling for the type 2 group is based on a known higher familial risk. The siblings of a person with type 2 diabetes have a 7% to 14% risk for type 2 diabetes developing. The offspring of parents who both have type 2 diabetes have a 15% to 45% chance of the disease developing. Children and young adults with type 2 diabetes have a 50% chance of transmitting the disease to their children.[7]

Prevalence of diabetes increases with age, with about half of cases in people older than age 55. It was formerly called non–insulin-dependent diabetes mellitus or maturity-onset diabetes. These names are no longer used because they do not accurately characterize the treatment or the pathophysiology. Prevalence of type 2 varies by race and is highest among Native-Americans such as the Pima tribe (one out of two adults has type 2 diabetes mellitus). Hispanic populations are two times as likely to develop diabetes as non-Hispanic whites. Overall, the prevalence of diagnosed and undiagnosed diabetes in adults is about 30% higher in African-Americans than in Caucasians.[1] Obesity appears to play a major role in type 2 diabetes.

In addition to older age at onset, type 2 diabetes mellitus is distinguished by an endogenous insulin supply sufficient to inhibit the development of diabetic ketoacidosis (DKA), which occurs when endogenous insulin is markedly reduced or absent. The pathophysiologic factors that have been identified in type 2 diabetes include (1) decreased tissue (e.g., fat, muscle) responsiveness to insulin as a result of receptor or postreceptor defects; (2) overproduction of insulin early in the disease, but eventual decreased secretion of insulin from β-cell exhaustion; and (3) abnormal hepatic glucose regulation. These factors result in what is often referred to as peripheral insulin resis-

tance. This resistance stimulates increased insulin production as a compensatory response, which may also predispose the patient to weight gain. A reduced-calorie diet for the obese patient with type 2 diabetes tends to reverse this phenomenon.[4] The patient with type 2 diabetes may benefit from oral antidiabetic agents, which have been found to be physiologically effective in several ways, including increasing insulin production, improving cell receptor binding, and regulating hepatic glucose production.

In type 2 diabetes mellitus the onset of hyperglycemic symptoms may occur over a long period. The person may "adjust" to the persistent feelings of fatigue, thirst, polyuria, and blurred vision without realizing that the diabetic disease process is producing the symptoms.[8] If the patient with type 2 diabetes has marked hyperglycemia (e.g., 500 to 1000 mg/dl; 27.6 to 55.1 mmol/L), a sufficient endogenous insulin supply may prevent DKA from occurring, but fluid and electrolyte loss may become severe and lead to hyperosmolar coma. (See Fig. 46-13 for the sequence of events associated with hyperosmolar hyperglycemia.) During precipitating and acute situations (such as acute illness), the patient with type 2 diabetes may briefly require insulin administration. It is also possible for the type 2 patient to have DKA if a precipitating stress event is severe and strains the available endogenous insulin supply. The fact that some persons with type 2 diabetes may require insulin during times of stress or for treatment of hyperosmolar nonketotic hyperglycemia does not mean that these persons are "insulin dependent" or will require long-term insulin treatment.[9]

Clinical Manifestations

Normally, insulin and its counterregulatory hormones maintain blood glucose within a range of 70 to 110 mg/dl (3.9 to 6.0 mmol/L). Elevated blood glucose levels produce symptoms related to the degree of actual or relative insulin deficiency. When an absolute insulin deficiency or decreased insulin activ-

COLLABORATIVE CARE

Table **46-3** **Diabetes Mellitus**

Diagnostic

Complete history and physical examination
Blood tests, including fasting blood glucose,
postprandial blood glucose, glycosylated hemoglobin,
cholesterol and triglyceride levels, blood urea nitrogen
and serum creatinine, electrolytes
Urine for complete urinalysis, microalbuminuria,
culture and sensitivity, glucose and acetone
Funduscopic examination—dilated eye examination
Neurologic examination
Blood pressure
Monitoring of weight
Doppler scan

Collaborative Therapy

Calculated food plan
Exercise plan
Insulin or oral hypoglycemia agent (if indicated)
Dental examination
Podiatric examination
Specific teaching and follow-up programs

ity occurs, glucose is not used properly. Glucose remains in the bloodstream and produces an osmotic effect on intracellular and interstitial fluid. This shift in fluid balance results in clinical symptoms of frequent urination (polyuria) and thirst (polydipsia). Without sufficient insulin the patient may experience hunger (polyphagia) as the body turns to other energy sources besides glucose: first fat and then protein. Varying degrees of polyuria, polydipsia, and polyphagia are the hallmark symptoms of diabetes mellitus. Acute and chronic complications from hyperglycemia are closely associated with the type of diabetes mellitus and the circumstances in which it occurs.

Diagnostic Studies

The classification of diabetes depends on appropriate and accurate diagnostic studies (Table 46-3). Urine tests are not sufficient for diagnosing diabetes mellitus because variables such as age, medications, and a normally low renal threshold for glucose may show glycosuria without the presence of diabetes or glucose intolerance.

When overt symptoms of hyperglycemia (polyuria, polydipsia, and polyphagia), together with fasting blood glucose levels of 126 mg/dl (7.0 mmol/L) or greater are present, further glucose tolerance tests are usually not warranted. However, when oral glucose tolerance tests are used, the accuracy of test results depends on adequate patient preparation and attention to the many factors that may influence the outcome of such tests. For example, factors that can cause falsely elevated values include recent severe restrictions of dietary carbohydrate, acute illness, medications such as contraceptives and glucocorticoids, and restricted activity such as bed rest. A patient with impaired gastrointestinal (GI) absorption may also have false-negative test results.

Because diabetes is a multisystem, multiproblem disease, all laboratory studies must be correlated with clinical findings. The most common finding in overt diabetes mellitus is an elevated blood glucose level (≥126 mg/dl [7.0 mmol/L]). Glucose

values differ depending on the source of the sample and the site from which the blood is taken, the timing in relation to meals, and the time of day. Arterial blood values tend to be higher than venous blood samplings. Postprandial (after meals) and late afternoon values also tend to be higher.

In the presence of abnormal insulin use, fat metabolism is altered. This results in elevations of lipid, cholesterol, and triglyceride levels that are associated with the vascular disorders of diabetes.

The results of urine tests for glucose and acetone depend on age, severity of diabetes, and renal function. Blood glucose is a better measurement of glycemic status because glycosuria may not be evident when hyperglycemia is present. The presence of ketonuria and elevated serum ketones accompanied by marked hyperglycemia is the heralding sign of DKA. When a person without diabetes fasts, ketonuria also develops as a result of fat breakdown but without accompanying hyperglycemia.

Glycosylated hemoglobin is a measurement that is useful in determining glycemic levels over time. The hemoglobin of red blood cells (RBCs) attracts a certain amount of glucose (approximately 4% to 6% in the nondiabetic person). When blood glucose is elevated over time, or when the person has frequent wide fluctuations in glycemic levels, the amount of glucose attached to the hemoglobin molecule increases. The glucose remains attached to the RBC for the life of the cell (120 days). Therefore a glycosylated hemoglobin test indicates the overall glucose control for the past 120 days. Laboratory methods may differ in this assay because some methods measure the entire glycosylated hemoglobin molecule, whereas other methods measure only a specific glycosylated hemoglobin, hemoglobin A1, or hemoglobin A1c. The ideal goal range for glycosylated hemoglobin is a value that is less than 1% to 2% above the laboratory normal. Diseases affecting RBCs (e.g., sickle cell anemia) also affect the glycosylated hemoglobin results and should be taken into consideration in the interpretation of this test result. The glycosylated albumin (fructosamine), a glycosylated serum protein test, reflects blood glucose control over the preceding 7 to 10 days. The reliability and clinical applicability of these tests is under evaluation.[10]

Proteinuria is a sign of early nephropathy. Analysis for microalbuminuria may show early nephropathy long before routine urinalysis displays proteinuria.[11] Microalbuminuria tests are now the recommended method for early detection of nephropathy. The presence of protein in the urine as detected by microalbuminuria urinalysis should be followed with a 24-hour urine collection for determination of creatinine clearance and serum creatinine. It is important to monitor renal function because the patient with diabetes in the later stages of renal disease may require a reduction in insulin dose as a result of both a decrease in caloric intake and an alteration in insulin function and metabolism in chronic renal failure[11] (see Chapter 44).

The Doppler instrument is used to diagnose the presence or degree of peripheral vascular disease. It is a device similar to an electronic stethoscope that amplifies sound. The procedure is noninvasive and can measure blood pressure in the lower extremities and blood flow velocity. It can indicate areas of stenosis or occlusion and is useful as an indicator of the need for additional vascular tests.

Collaborative Care

Management of diabetes mellitus is primarily aimed at achieving a balance of diet, activity, and medications together with

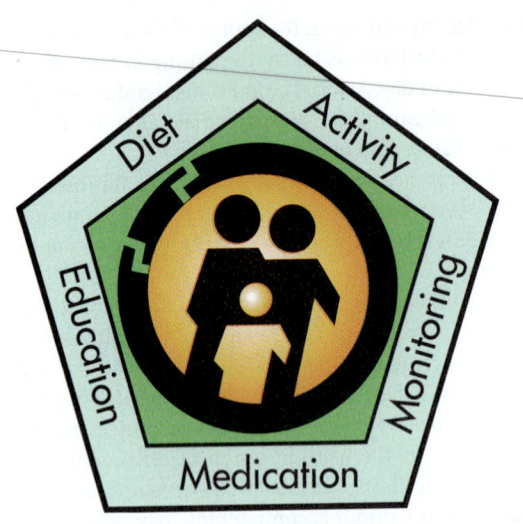

Fig. 46-3   The five aspects of diabetes management make up the complete program for good control.

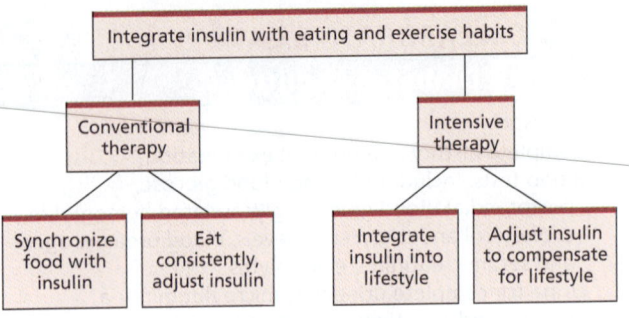

Fig. 46-4   Nutritional therapy for type 1 diabetes.

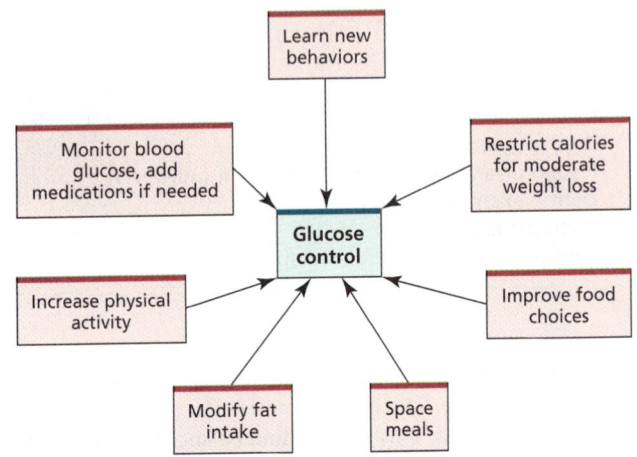

Fig. 46-5   Nutritional therapy for type 2 diabetes.

appropriate monitoring and patient and family education (Table 46-3 and Fig. 46-3). These components are equally necessary for effective control of diabetes.

Nutritional Therapy.   Nutritional therapy is the cornerstone of care for the person with diabetes. Achieving nutritional goals requires a coordinated team effort that includes the person with diabetes. Today there is no one "diabetic" or "ADA" diet. In an institutional setting, the prescribed diet is often labeled "ADA," indicating that the meal plan follows the American Diabetes Association's current nutritional recommendations.

The recommended diet can only be defined as a dietary prescription based on nutritional assessment and goals. Because of the complexity of nutritional issues, it is recommended that a registered dietician, with expertise in diabetes management, be a member of the treatment team. Effective self-management training requires an individualized approach that is appropriate for the personal lifestyle and diabetes management goals of the patient. Monitoring of glucose and glycosylated hemoglobin, lipids, and renal status is essential to evaluate nutrition-related outcomes. Nutritional assessment is used to determine what the individual with diabetes is able and willing to do. Sensitivity to cultural, ethnic, and financial considerations is important when developing individual meal planning approaches.

Goals of nutritional therapy.   The overall goal is to assist people with diabetes in making changes in nutrition and exercise habits leading to improved metabolic control. Additional specific goals include the following:

1. Maintenance of as near-normal blood glucose levels as possible by balancing food intake with insulin (either endogenous or exogenous) or oral glucose-lowering medications and activity levels.
2. Achievement of optimal serum lipid levels.
3. Provision of adequate calories for maintaining or attaining reasonable weights for adults, normal growth and development rates in children and adolescents, increased metabolic needs during pregnancy and lactation, or recovery from catabolic illnesses. *Reasonable weight* is defined as the weight an individual and health care

provider acknowledge as achievable and maintainable, both short-term and long-term. This may not be the same as the usually defined desirable or ideal body weight.

4. Prevention and treatment of acute complications, such as hypoglycemia, and long-term complications, such as renal disease, neuropathy, hypertension, and cardiovascular disease.
5. Improvement of overall health through optimal nutrition. The food guide pyramid summarize and illustrate nutritional guidelines and nutrient needs for all healthy Americans and can be used by the patient with diabetes (see Chapter 38).

Type 1 diabetes.   Meal planning should be based on the individual's usual food intake with insulin therapy integrated into the usual eating and exercise patterns. It is recommended that the individual using insulin therapy eat meals at consistent times synchronized with the action time of the insulin preparation used. Additionally, the individual must monitor blood glucose levels and adjust insulin doses for the amount of food eaten. Intensified insulin therapy, such as multiple daily injections or use of an insulin pump, allows considerable flexibility in food selection and can be adjusted for deviations from usual eating and exercise habits (Fig. 46-4).

Type 2 diabetes.   The emphasis for nutritional therapy in type 2 diabetes should be placed on achieving glucose, lipid, and blood pressure goals. Weight loss and hypocaloric diets usually improve short-term glycemic levels and have the potential to increase long-term metabolic control. However, traditional dietary strategies and even very-low-calorie diets have usually

NUTRITIONAL THERAPY
Table 46-4   Diabetes Mellitus

Factor	Type 1 Diabetes Mellitus	Type 2 Diabetes Mellitus
■ Total calories	Increase in caloric intake possibly necessary to achieve desirable body weight and restore body tissues	Reduction in caloric intake desirable for the obese patient
■ Effect of diet	Diet and insulin necessary for glucose control	Diet alone possibly sufficient for glucose control
■ Distribution of calories	Equal distribution of carbohydrates through meals or adjustment of carbohydrates for insulin activity	Equal distribution not essential; low-fat desirable; consistency of carbohydrate intake at meals desirable
■ Consistency in daily intake	Necessary for glucose control	Desirable for weight reduction
■ Uniform timing of meals	Crucial for NPH/Lente insulin programs; flexibility with multidose rapid-acting insulin	Desirable but not essential
■ Intermeal and bedtime snacks	Frequently necessary	Not recommended
■ Nutritional supplement for exercise programs	Carbohydrates 20 g/hr for moderate physical activities	Necessary if patient controlled on sulfonylurea or insulin

not been effective in achieving long-term weight loss, and the focus is more rationally placed on glucose and lipid goals.

Although weight loss is desirable, and some individuals are able to lose weight and maintain weight loss, several strategies can be implemented to improve metabolic control. No one proven strategy or method can be uniformly recommended. A nutritionally adequate meal plan with a reduction of total fat, especially saturated fats, can be employed. Spacing meals is another strategy that can be adopted to spread nutrient intake throughout the day. A weight loss of 11 to 22 lb (5 to 10 kg) has been shown to improve diabetes control, even if desirable body weight is not achieved. Weight loss is best attempted by a moderate decrease in calories and an increase in caloric expenditure. Regular exercise and learning new behaviors and attitudes can help facilitate long-term lifestyle changes. Monitoring of blood glucose levels, glycosylated hemoglobin, lipids, and blood pressure is essential (Fig. 46-5). Table 46-4 describes dietary strategies for type 1 and type 2 diabetes. General guidelines for patient teaching are shown in Table 46-5.

Food composition. Distribution of nutrients is based on guidelines for all adults. There are limited data on which to establish firm nutritional recommendations for protein. Dietary protein derived from both animal and vegetable sources should make up about 10% to 20% of calories. The remaining 80% to 90% of calories should be distributed between dietary fat and carbohydrates. Less than 10% of these calories should be from saturated fats. The distribution of calories from fat and carbohydrates can vary and can be individualized based on the nutritional assessment and treatment goals. Consideration of the individual's usual eating habits, lifestyle, body weight, and quality of life is essential for successful meal planning.

Another topic to consider is the glycemic index, which refers to the ranking of foods by comparing the glycemic effect on blood glucose in reference to white bread. This type of information is useful in considering ways to select and prepare foods for more predictable glycemic control. It has been concluded that starches and sucrose do not act differently in the context of

a mixed meal when it comes to glycemic effect. It is important for patients to understand the principles underlying the glycemic index, or how foods of different composition affect blood glucose. Mixed meal, method of food preparation, and fiber content also play an important role.[12]

Scientific research has not supported the belief that simple sugars should be avoided and replaced with complex carbohydrates. Fruits and milks have been shown to have a lower glycemic response than most starches, and sucrose produces a glycemic response similar to that of bread, rice, and potatoes. Even though various starches do have different glycemic responses, from a clinical perspective, priority should be given to the total amount of carbohydrate consumed rather than the source of carbohydrate. The American Diabetes Association advises that the use of sucrose as a part of the meal plan does not impair blood glucose control in individuals with type 1 or type 2 diabetes. Sucrose and sucrose-containing foods must be substituted for other carbohydrates and not simply added to the meal plan. In making such substitutions, the nutrient content of concentrated sweets and sucrose-containing foods, as well as the presence of other nutrients frequently ingested with sucrose such as fat, must be considered.[12]

Diet teaching. Most often the dietician initially teaches the principles of the dietary prescription. However, the nurse should be knowledgeable about diabetes dietary principles to answer questions and to help the patient make appropriate selections and decisions. The nurse should include the family of the patient when teaching the diet plan. Particular attention and teaching efforts are effectively directed to the person who will be cooking. It is important, however, that the responsibility for maintaining a diabetic diet not fall to someone other than the patient with diabetes. Reliance on another person to make health decisions fosters dependence and should be avoided except in special situations.

Areas of concern

Alcohol. Alcohol is high in calories, has no nutritive value, and promotes hypertriglyceridemia. In addition, it has detrimental effects on the liver (see Chapter 41). The

Table **46-5** **Diet Guidelines**

Principles that both the nurse and dietician should teach and reinforce include the following:

1. **Eat according to the prescribed meal plan.** A dietary prescription is individualized to reflect the dietary needs related to a specific patient's body weight, occupation, age, activities, and type of diabetes. Individual responses to a dietary prescription should be monitored, and appropriate adjustments should be made when necessary.

2. **Never skip meals.** This is particularly important for the patient taking insulin or oral agents (OAs). The body requires food at regularly spaced intervals throughout the day. Insulin and OAs are prescribed to fit this schedule. Omission or delay of meals can result in hypoglycemia.

3. **Learn to recognize appropriate food portions.** Practice can result in accurate portion allotments.

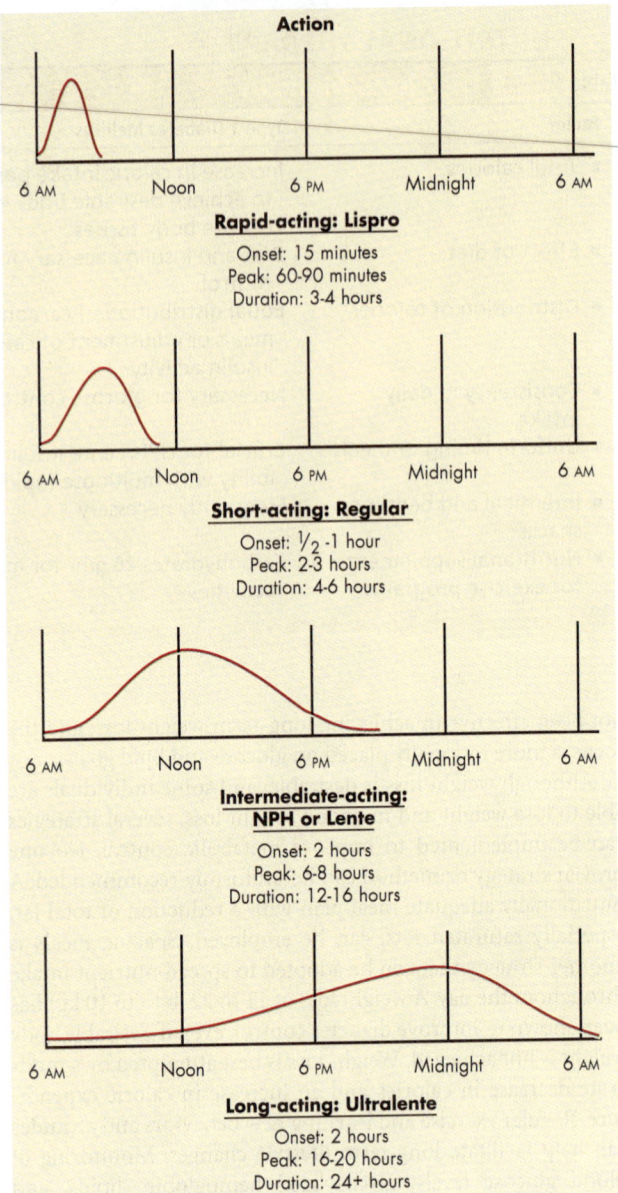

Fig. 46-6 Commercially available insulin preparations showing onset, peak, and duration.

inhibitory effect of alcohol on gluconeogenesis can cause severe hypoglycemia in patients on glucose-lowering agents. A patient can reduce this risk by eating carbohydrates when drinking alcohol. Alcohol may produce a disulfiram (Antabuse) effect (nausea and vomiting, flushing, respiratory distress, chest pain) proportional to the amount ingested with certain oral agents.

However, if the patient chooses, a drink can be included in the meal plan. One drink has approximately 135 calories. The patient with diabetes should drink alcohol with food, use sugar-free mixes, and drink dry, light wines.

Dietetic foods. The word *dietetic* is confusing because it does not always refer to a lack of calories. The caloric value of dietetic foods should be considered if weight loss is a dietary goal. Dietetic foods are expensive and, although convenient, are not necessary. The patient can be taught to make intelligent decisions regarding the use of nondietetic foods by reading labels. The increasing availability of foods prepared with artificial sweeteners allows greater freedom in the diet. Recipes that use artificial sweeteners are also available.

Drug Therapy: Insulin. The two types of glucose-lowering agents (GLAs) used in the treatment of diabetes are insulin and oral antidiabetes agents (OAs).

Indications for use. Exogenous insulin is needed when a patient has inadequate insulin to meet specific metabolic needs, and the combination of nutritional therapy, exercise, and OAs cannot maintain a satisfactory blood glucose level. Exogenous insulin is required for the management of type 1 diabetes. Exogenous insulin may be prescribed for the patient with type 2 diabetes during periods of severe stress, such as illness or surgery, or when attempts at glycemic control by means of diet, exercise, or OAs fail.

Types of insulin. Exogenous insulin has commonly been obtained from the pancreases of pigs and cows. These two forms of insulin are similar to human insulin protein chains, with pork insulin being more similar to human insulin. However, these sources have become expensive to obtain. Also, although the purification process for extracting the insulin islets has improved to where only minuscule amounts of for-

eign protein are present, these substances can initiate insulin allergies. Insulins marked "purified" have had nearly all extraneous pancreatic proteins removed.

Today, biosynthetic insulin is used almost exclusively. Human insulin is produced by genetically altering common bacteria or yeast using recombinant deoxyribonucleic acid (DNA) technology (see Fig. 12-12). This insulin exhibits chemical and biologic properties identical to human insulin produced by human β-cells. The advantage of these new insulins is a reduced allergic response and a more predictable insulin activity. The purified and human insulins are the preferred type of drug.

In addition to origin and purity, insulins differ in regard to onset, peak action, and duration (Fig. 46-6). The specific properties of each type of insulin are matched with the patient's diet and activity. Not all patients respond to insulin exactly as shown in Table 46-6. The action times are listed as approximate guidelines. Human insulin may have slightly less activity time.

Table **46-6** Insulin Regimens

Regimen	Type of Insulin Used	Time Administered and Expected Time-Action Curve*	Advantages	Disadvantages
Single dose	Intermediate insulin (I)		One injection should cover noon and PM meal. Hypoglycemia during sleep is not a problem.	No fasting, breakfast, or nighttime coverage of hyperglycemia is available.
Split-mixed dose (70/30 premix)	Intermediate and regular or Humalog insulin (I + R or I + H)		Two injections provide coverage for 24 hr.	Two injections are required. Patient must adhere to a set meal pattern.
Split-mixed dose	Intermediate and regular or Humalog insulin (I + R or I + H)		Three injections provide coverage for 24 hr, particularly during early AM hours. Potential is reduced for 2-3 AM hypoglycemia.	Three injections are required.
Multiple dose	Intermediate and regular or Humalog insulin (I + R or I + H)		More flexibility is allowed at mealtimes and for amount of food intake.	Four injections are required. Premeal blood glucose checks, establishing and following individualized algorithm are necessary. Patients with type 1 will require basal insulin (I or LA) during the day.
Multiple dose† (split dose long-acting insulin [Ultra Lente])	Regular or Humalog and long acting insulin (R + LA or H + LA)		Insulin delivery pattern more closely simulates normal endogenous insulin pattern. Some flexibility is allowed in food intake pattern. Regimen gives a basal insulin coverage and regular or Humalog insulin covers meal blood glucose excursions.	Required three or four injections and blood glucose check premeal and on retiring. Establishing and following individualized algorithm are necessary.

*H = lispro (Humalog) or rapid-acting insulin (R) = ——
I = intermediate insulin = ——
LA = long-acting insulin = ——
R = regular insulin = ——
†Insulin delivery through a pump is similar to this regimen.

By adding zinc, acetate buffers, and protamine to insulin in various ways, the onset of activity, peak, and duration times can be manipulated.[13] A new class of insulins, synthetic analogs, were introduced in 1996 with the advent of lispro insulin (Humalog). Lispro is a synthetic product made by exchanging the amino acids proline and lysine at positions 28 and 29 on the beta chain of the insulin molecule.[14] This change in structure results in a change in time of action. Regular human insulin self-associates into hexameric structures that require 30 minutes to 1 hour to break apart in subcutaneous deposits. This is the cause of the 30- to 60-minute delay in onset of action for regular insulin. Lispro's structure permits rapid dissociation and therefore an onset of action of approximately 15 minutes. This rapid-acting insulin has a peak of 30 to 90 minutes and duration of 4 hours or less. This time action profile makes lispro a preferred meal coverage insulin. Lispro can be used wherever regular insulin is used, but because of its limited duration of action, a basal background insulin must be used in conjunction with the meal coverage when lispro is used for patients with type 1 diabetes.[14] Different combinations of insulins can be used to tailor treatment to the patient's specific pattern of blood glucose levels. Formulas are classified as rapid acting (e.g., lispro insulin [Humalog]), short acting (e.g., regular insulin [Humulin]), intermediate acting (e.g., NPH insulin [Humulin L]), and long acting (Ultralente insulin [Humulin U]). In the future the same technology used to make lispro insulin will be used to create new insulins with different times of action.

All insulin preparations start with regular insulin as a base; zinc is added to make Lente insulin, and zinc and protamine are added to make NPH to prolong the action of insulin. These binding agents can cause an allergic reaction at the injection site. Lispro or regular insulin is prescribed when a rapid onset of glucose-lowering action is needed, such as before meals and during periods of acute illness, surgery, or stress. Both regular and lispro insulin can be administered IV; however, regular is used in emergencies because there is no difference between lispro and regular in half-life (9 minutes).

Insulins are commonly used in combination to mimic the normal endogenous insulin secretion (see Fig. 46-1). The timing of insulin administration in relation to meals is important. Regular insulin should be taken 30 to 45 minutes before meals to ensure the onset of action in conjunction with meal absorption. Examples of insulin combination regimens, onset, peak, and descriptions of the advantages and disadvantages of each regimen are presented in Table 46-6. Ideally, regimens should be mutually selected by the patient and the health care provider. The criteria for selection are based on the type of diabetes and the required, desired, and feasible levels of glycemic control.

Because a single injection of a modified insulin rarely provides adequate glycemic control for most insulin-dependent patients, lispro or regular insulin is mixed with the modified insulin in the same syringe to avoid unnecessary injections. On the basis of current insulin formulations and use, the effect of NPH and lispro or regular insulin mixed in any proportion is the same as if the two were injected separately. The commercially available 70/30 or 50/50 mixtures of NPH and regular insulin appear to have the same activity as their component insulins given at separate injection sites. Stable mixtures with lispro and intermediate-acting insulin will probably be on the market in the near future.

✎ **PATIENT TEACHING GUIDE**

Table **46-7** | **Insulin Therapy**

1. Wash hands thoroughly.
2. Roll intermediate or long-acting insulin bottle between palms of hands to mix insulin. *Note:* Always inspect insulin bottle before using it for first time. Make sure that it is of proper type and concentration, expiration date has not passed, and top of bottle is in perfect condition.
3. Prepare insulin injection in same manner as for any injection.
4. Select proper injection site and inject following procedure for any SC injection.* In sites where SC tissue is adequate, inject commercial insulin needles at 90-degree angle. For sites with minimal SC tissue, pinch up skin and insert needle at 45-degree angle.
5. If blood appears in syringe after needle is inserted, select new site for injection. Aspiration is not necessary.
6. After injecting insulin, apply some pressure with dry cotton ball (or 2 × 2) at site when withdrawing needle.
7. Hold ball in place for a few seconds but do not massage.
8. Destroy and dispose of single-use syringe safely. *Note:* When instructing patient to self-inject insulin, use the following guidelines (if appropriate):
   - Aspiration does not need to be done before injection.
   - Disposable syringes can be reused for several injections.

*See Fig. 46-8.
SC, subcutaneous.

Mixing human regular and lente insulins results in blunting of the usual peak action of the regular insulin, but not lispro, presumably because the excess zinc in the Lente insulin binds regular insulin. A patient is sometimes given the option to mix regular and Lente or Ultralente and should be instructed to give the injection immediately after mixing if combining a Lente insulin and regular in the same syringe. Lispro can be mixed with the Lente insulins with no change in effect.

As a protein, insulin requires special storage considerations. Heat and freezing alter the insulin molecule. Insulin in use may be left at room temperature for up to 4 weeks unless the room temperature is higher than 70° F (21° C) or below freezing. Extra insulin may be stored in the refrigerator. The same principles apply for a patient with diabetes who is traveling. Insulin can be stored in a thermos or cooler to keep it cool (not frozen) if the patient is traveling in hot climates.

Administration of insulin

Injection. Because insulin is inactivated by gastric juices, it must be administered by injection. Daily administration of insulin is most commonly done by means of subcutaneous (SC) injection, although intramuscular (IM) or IV administration of regular insulin can be done when immediate onset of action is desired. The half-life of regular insulin in the circulation is 9 minutes, necessitating a continuous IV infusion for administration rather than a bolus IV injection. The steps in administering an SC insulin injection are outlined in Table 46-7. The tech-

1. Wash hands.
2. Gently rotate NPH insulin bottle.
3. Wipe off tops of insulin vials with alcohol sponge.
4. Draw back amount of air into the syringe that equals total dose.

5. Inject air equal to NPH dose into NPH vial. Remove syringe from vial.

6. Inject air equal to regular dose into regular vial.

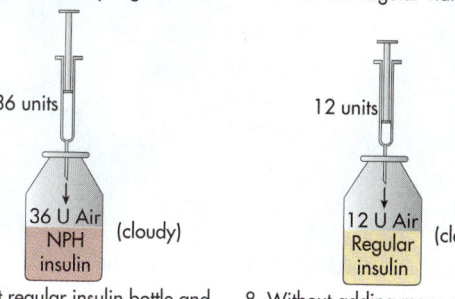
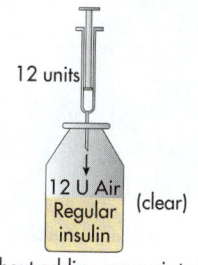

7. Invert regular insulin bottle and withdraw regular insulin dose.

8. Without adding more air to NPH vial, carefully withdraw NPH dose.

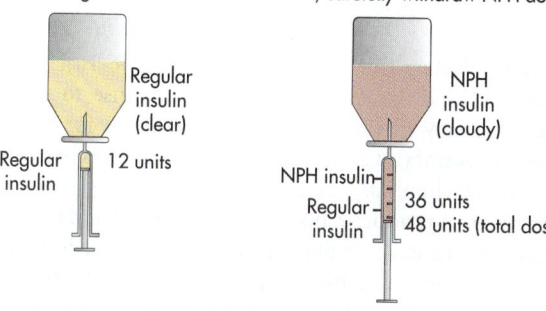

Fig. 46-7 Mixing insulins. This step-order process avoids the problem of contaminating regular insulin with intermediate-acting insulin.

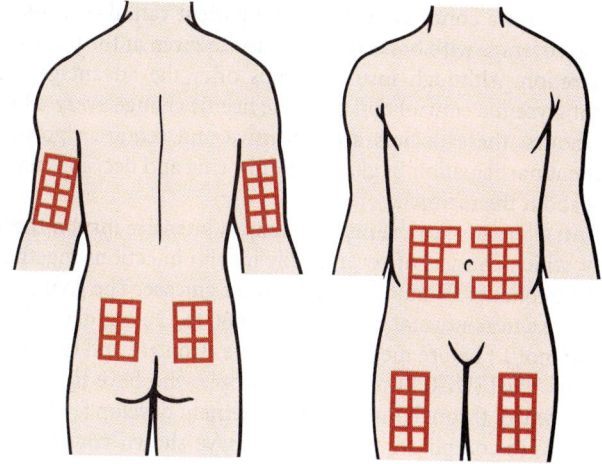

Fig. 46-8 Injection sites for insulin.

nique should be taught to new insulin users and reviewed periodically with long-term users. It should never be assumed that because insulin is being used, the patient knows and practices the correct insulin injection technique. Inaccurate preparation is often caused by poor eyesight. Air bubbles in the syringe may not be seen, or the scale on the syringe may be read improperly. Administration systems, such as the insulin "pen," or "prefilled syringe," are available for patient convenience and are sometimes useful for visually or manually impaired persons.

The patient receiving mixed insulins (e.g., regular and an intermediate-acting insulin) must learn the proper technique for combining both in the same syringe if commercially prepared premixed insulins are not used (Fig. 46-7). Insulins should not be mixed if they differ in purity or species of origin.

Recommended sites for insulin injection are noted in Fig. 46-8. The speed with which peak serum concentrations are reached varies with the anatomic site for injection. The fastest absorption is from the abdomen, then the arm, thigh, and buttock. Because of the variability in absorption and the decreased frequency of lipoatrophy in a patient treated with human or purified pork insulins, rotation of injection sites is no longer the recommended injection technique when these types of insulin are used. The patient should rotate the injection sites within a particular area, such as the abdomen, for a period, and then, if rotation to the thigh is desired, the patient can adjust the regimen to the new peak and action times for the new site.

The patient should also be cautioned about injecting into a site that is to be exercised. For example, the patient should not inject insulin into the thigh and then go jogging. Exercise of the area containing the injection site together with the increased body heat generated by the exercise may increase the rate of absorption and speed the onset of insulin action.

Insulin administration also requires the appropriate syringe. Most commercial insulin is available as U100, indicating that each milliliter contains 100 U of insulin. U100 insulin must be used with an U100-marked syringe. For a user taking smaller doses of insulin, insulin syringes with larger black lines are marked for 25, 30, or 50 U and are available for use with U100 insulin. One important distinction regarding the different-size syringes is that the 100 U syringe is marked in 2 U increments, whereas the 50 U and 30 U syringes are marked in 1 U increments. To avoid serious dosing errors, the patient must use the correct syringe and not switch back and forth between different-size syringes. Before the development of U100 insulin, insulin was available in concentrations of U40 and U80. U500 insulin is available for patients requiring very large doses of insulin.

Some patients may prefer to use their syringe more than once. Insulin preparations have bacteriostatic additives that inhibit growth of bacteria commonly found on the skin. Many studies have shown that it is both safe and practical for the syringe to be reused if the patient desires. The syringe should be discarded when the needle becomes dull, has been bent, or has come in contact with any surface other than the skin. If reuse is planned, the needle must be recapped after each use.[15]

Another change in the insulin injection routine relates to the use of the alcohol swab on the skin before injection. When instructing a patient on the technique of insulin injection, the use of the alcohol wipe is optional. Routine hygiene such as washing with soap and rinsing with water is adequate.[16]

Alternative delivery methods. Continuous SC insulin infusion is currently being accomplished through insulin pumps. The pump devices are able to deliver insulin continuously in titrated amounts through tubing attached to a small pump device on one end and to a needle on the other end, which is placed subcutaneously in the skin. The pump delivers a preprogrammed dose of insulin that is designed to match the patient's basal profile to achieve a nearly normal insulin delivery on a continuous basis. The patient can also regulate meal coverage with bolus doses of insulin given at the patient's discretion. Although insulin pumps offer the advantages of tight glycemic control and only one needle change every 48 to 72 hours, these devices are expensive and require vigorous patient participation in glucose monitoring and decision making about the regimen.

An alternative to the insulin pump is intensive insulin therapy, which consists of several daily insulin injections together with frequent self-monitoring of blood glucose. The goal is to achieve a near-normal glucose level of 80 to 120 mg/dl (4.45 to 6.7 mmol/L) before meals. The Diabetes Control and Complications Trial (DCCT) proved that people who have tight glucose control through intensive management develop fewer and less severe complications.[17] Studies have shown comparable control outcomes in patients receiving intensive therapy and patients with an insulin pump. Because the required patient participation is similar, intensive therapy may be instituted before the initiation of pump use.[17] Because of the specialized nature of these insulin delivery systems and devices, expert guidance from a physician and a nurse educator is essential.

Intensive insulin therapy is not for everyone. Children are already at increased risk for low blood glucose (hypoglycemia), which can impair normal brain development. This risk is increased with intensive insulin therapy. In the elderly, intensive insulin therapy increases the risk of hypoglycemia, which could result in heart attacks or strokes during periods of low blood glucose in older adults with atherosclerosis.[18]

Another insulin administration technique under investigation is aerosol inhalation. In a small study, aerosol insulin, inhaled in 5 to 10 times the amount of insulin found in normal injections, effectively controlled blood glucose levels.[19] No adverse respiratory tract or hypoglycemic symptoms were reported. If further studies of aerosol insulin prove the effectiveness of this method, persons with diabetes may have a more convenient method to control their blood glucose levels.

Problems with insulin therapy. Hypoglycemia, allergic reactions, lipodystrophy, and the Somogyi effect are the problems associated with insulin therapy. Hypoglycemia is discussed in detail later in this chapter.

Allergic reactions. There are three types of allergic reactions to insulin. Local reactions may occur as itching, erythema, and burning around the injection site. Local reactions may be self-limiting within 1 to 3 months or may improve with a low dose of antihistamine.

A "true" insulin allergy is a systemic response with urticaria and possibly anaphylactic shock generally resulting from the use of animal insulins. Fortunately, this type of allergy is rare, particularly since human insulin has become available.

Lipodystrophy. Lipodystrophies (hypertrophy or atrophy of SC tissue; lipoatrophy) may occur if the same injection sites are used frequently (Fig. 46-9). Hypertrophy, a thickening of the SC tissue, eventually regresses if the patient does not use the site for at least 6 months. The use of hypertrophied sites may result in erratic insulin absorption. Lipoatrophies have been most commonly associated with beef or beef and pork insulin and rarely with human insulin. Site rotation on a daily or weekly basis is not necessary with human insulin.

Somogyi effect and dawn phenomenon. The Somogyi effect is characterized by wide differences in early morning

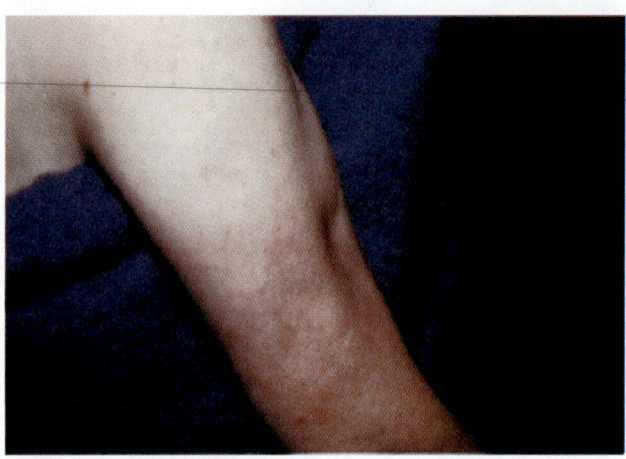

Fig. 46-9   Lipodystrophy of the arm.

(low) and fasting (high) glucose levels (Fig. 46-10). The blood glucose level drops below normal in response to too much insulin usually in the night (see Table 46-20 for the causes of hypoglycemia). Counterregulatory hormones are released, stimulating lipolysis, gluconeogenesis, and glycogenolysis, which in turn produce rebound hyperglycemia and ketosis. The danger of this effect is that, when blood glucose is measured, the patient (or the health care professional) may assess the situation as hyperglycemia and increase the insulin dose. The Somogyi effect is associated with the occurrence of undetected hypoglycemia during sleep, although it can happen at any time. The patient may report headaches on awakening and may recall night sweats or nightmares. When the Somogyi effect occurs at night, the patient's blood glucose is elevated on awakening in the morning.

With the dawn phenomenon, hyperglycemia is also present on awakening in the morning and ketonuria may be present. The cause is theorized to be a dawn release of endogenous growth hormone or cortisol, diurnal variation of insulin clearance, and insulin sensitivity. Both growth hormone and cortisol are counterregulatory hormones to insulin and raise the blood glucose level. The dawn phenomenon affects the majority of diabetics and tends to be most severe when growth hormone is at its peak in adolescence and young adulthood.

Careful assessment is required to document each phenomenon because the treatment for each differs. The treatment for the Somogyi effect is less insulin. The treatment for the dawn phenomenon is an adjustment in the timing of insulin administration or an increase in insulin. The assessment must include insulin dose, injection sites, and variability in the time of meals or insulin administration. In addition, the patient is asked to measure and document bedtime, between 2 and 4 AM, and morning fasting blood glucose levels on several occasions. If the predawn levels are below 60 mg/dl (3.3 mmol/L) and signs and symptoms of hypoglycemia are present, the insulin dosage should be reduced. If the 2 to 4 AM blood glucose is high, the insulin dosage should be increased.[20] In addition, the patient should be counseled on appropriate bedtime snacks.

Drug Therapy: Oral Agents. Currently, four classes of medications are available to improve diabetes control for patients with type 2 diabetes. Oral agents are listed in Table 46-8.

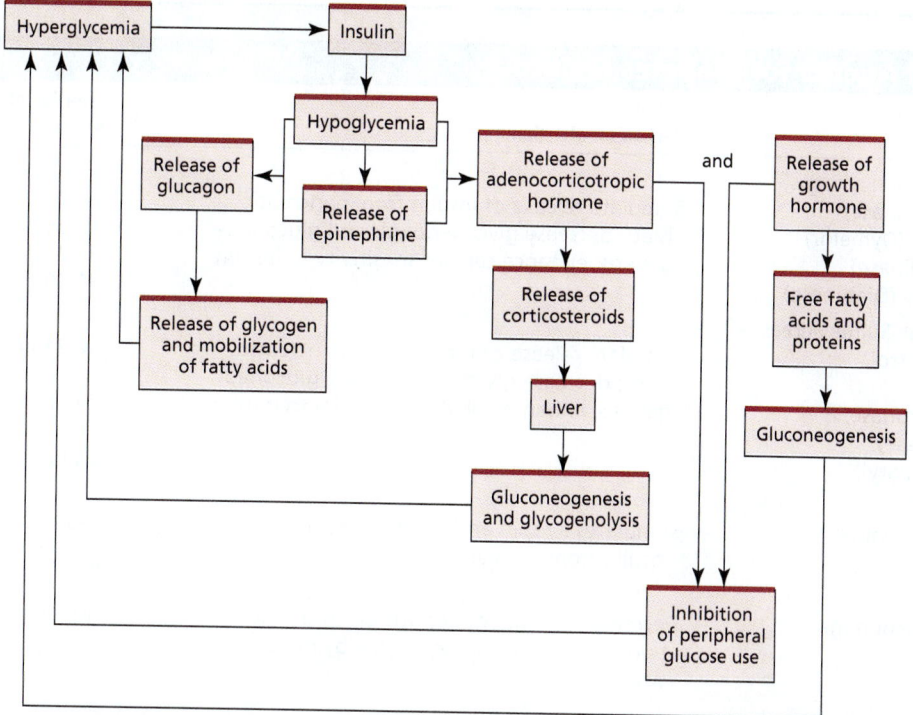

Fig. 46-10   The Somogyi effect.

Sulfonylureas. Sulfonylureas were found to have blood glucose–lowering effects during research on their antibiotic properties in the 1940s. They are called first generation or second generation depending on when they were introduced into clinical use in the United States. The first generation of these drugs used in the treatment of diabetes mellitus included tolbutamide (Orinase), acetohexamide (Dymelor), tolazamide (Tolinase), and chlorpropamide (Diabinese). A second generation of sulfonylureas, approved for use in the United States more recently, includes glipizide (Glucotrol and Glucotrol XL), glyburide (Micronase, DiaBeta, Glynase), and glimepiride (Amaryl).

Second-generation drugs have fewer adverse effects, are about 100 times more potent by weight, and have more predictable action times and half-lives.[21] Their drug interaction potential is lower because they bind to circulating proteins differently. The main disadvantage of second-generation drugs is their increased expense.

Meglitinides. Repaglinide (Prandin), classified as a meglitinide, stimulates the pancreas to secrete insulin, which is an action similar to that of the sulfonylureas. However, it has a more rapid onset and shorter duration of action. It is most effectively used before meals.

Biguanides. Metformin (Glucophage) is a biguanide glucose-lowering agent. Worldwide, metformin is widely used as a monotherapy and in combination with a sulfonylurea. Unlike sulfonylureas, metformin is not bound to plasma proteins, is not metabolized, and is eliminated rapidly by the kidney. The glucose-lowering effect occurs without stimulation of insulin secretion and results mainly by decreasing the rate of hepatic glucose production (gluconeogenesis). The presence of insulin is required for metformin to be effective. Metformin may also act by augmenting glucose uptake by muscle tissues. Because metformin does not cause clinical hypoglycemia, it is actually an antihyperglycemic drug. It does not cause weight gain and helps combat hypertriglyceridemia.[20] Side effects include GI problems such as nausea, diarrhea, and flatulence. Lactic acidosis is also a potential side effect for which the patient and nurse should monitor. Metformin is contraindicated in patients with renal insufficiency (serum creatinine >1.5 mg/dl for men and >1.4 mg/dl for women), congestive heart failure, or alcohol abuse.[22]

Alpha glucosidase inhibitors. Carbohydrate absorption inhibitors is another class of oral antidiabetes agents that work in the small intestine. Alpha glucosidase inhibitors, such as acarbose (Precose) and miglitol (Glyset), slow the breakdown of disaccharides and polysaccharides and other complex sugars into monosaccharides on the brush border of the small intestine. The enzymatic generation and subsequent absorption of glucose is delayed, and the postprandial blood glucose, which is usually high after a meal high in carbohydrates, is improved. The most common side effects of these medications include flatulence and mild abdominal pain. Many of the symptoms are dose related and transient, occurring with the highest frequency during the first few weeks of therapy. Titration of acarbose up from 25 mg with the first bite of a meal to 50 to 100 mg with each meal will help minimize the GI side effects. Dosages at different meals can be determined and adjusted by postprandial monitoring of blood glucose, usually 1 to 2 hours after meals. This drug can be used as a monotherapy or in combination with other oral agents or insulin.

Thiazolidinediones. Thiazolidinediones are a new class of agents that improve peripheral insulin resistance in skeletal muscle without stimulating insulin secretion. These agents work

DRUG THERAPY

Table 46-8 Oral Agents for Diabetes Mellitus*

Type	Mechanism of Action	Duration of Action
First-Generation Sulfonylureas		
Tolbutamide (Orinase)	Stimulate release of insulin from pancreatic islets; decrease glycogenolysis and gluconeogenesis; enhance cellular sensitivity to insulin	6-12 hr
Acetohexamide (Dymelor)		12-24 hr
Tolazamide (Tolinase)		12-24 hr
Chlorpropamide (Diabinese)		36-60 hr
Second-Generation Sulfonylureas		
Glipizide (Glucotrol, Glucotrol XL)	Stimulate release of insulin from pancreatic islets; decrease glycogenolysis and gluconeogenesis; enhance cellular sensitivity to insulin	10-24 hr
Glyburide (Micronase, DiaBeta, Glynase)		24 hr
Glimepiride (Amaryl)		24 hr
Meglitinides		
Repaglinide (Prandin)	Stimulates a rapid and short-lived release of insulin from the pancreas	2-3 hr
Biguanide		
Metformin (Glucophage)	Decreases the rate of hepatic glucose production; augments glucose uptake by muscle tissues	12-24 hr
Alpha-Glucosidase Inhibitors		
Acarbose (Precose)	Works on the brush border of the small intestine to slow the breakdown of disaccharides and polysaccharides into monosaccharides; delays subsequent absorption of glucose	Affects postprandial absorption of carbohydrates
Miglitol (Glyset)		
Thiazolidinediones		
Rosiglitazone (Avandia)	Decreases peripheral insulin resistance in skeletal muscle without stimulating insulin secretion	>24 hr
Pioglitazone (Actos)		

*Side effects can be minimized if OA choice is matched appropriately to patient's needs. OAs are not appropriate for ketosis-prone patients and pregnant patients and should be used cautiously if at all in patients with renal or hepatic dysfunction.

using a novel action that stimulates glucose transport in muscle and, to a lesser degree, hepatic tissues. Fasting and glucose-stimulated insulin levels are reduced while glucose disposal is increased in obese, insulin-resistant patients. Thus these agents reduce insulin resistance and improve glycemia both as monotherapy and in combination with sulphonylureas or metformin. Troglitzone (Rezulin), the first thiazolidinedione, was approved in 1997. However, because of reported cases of hepatic failure, this agent was removed from the market in 1999. Newer thiazolidinediones include rosiglitazone (Avandia) and pioglitazone (Actos). There are still potential liver problems with these agents. Liver function tests are required at baseline, then every 2 months for the first year and periodically thereafter.

Indication for use. OAs are not oral insulin or a substitute for insulin. The patient must have some functioning endogenous insulin for OAs to be effective. They may be used in combinations of oral agents or with insulin to achieve goal-range control. Guidelines for assessing patients receiving OAs are shown in Table 46-9.

In the patient with newly diagnosed diabetes, therapy with OAs may not be started until the patient has been given an opportunity to try dietary control. Even if OA therapy is initially successful, the patient may eventually fail to maintain control and insulin therapy may have to be initiated.

The hypoglycemic action of OAs can be enhanced and prolonged by means of the concurrent administration of drugs such as anticoagulants, salicylates, alcohol, and propranolol. Drugs that can oppose OA action include thyroid preparations, corticosteroids, and thiazide diuretics.

Other Drugs Affecting Blood Glucose Levels. The patient with diabetes may be concurrently taking other medications. Both the patient and the health care provider must be aware of drug interactions that can potentiate hypoglycemic and hyperglycemic effects. For example, beta-adrenergic drugs block the hepatic glycogenolytic response that occurs in response to hypoglycemia. Thiazide diuretics can also potentiate hyperglycemia by inducing potassium loss. A list of medications that may influence glycemic control is pre-

Table **46-9**   **Assessing the Patient Treated with Glucose-Lowering Agents**

For patient with newly diagnosed diabetes or for reevaluation of GLA regimen	
Cognitive	Is patient or responsible other able to understand why insulin or OAs are being used as part of diabetes management? Is patient or responsible other able to understand concepts of asepsis, combining insulins, insulin-OA actions, and side effects? Is patient able to remember to take >1 dose/day? Does patient take medications at right times in relation to meals?
Psychomotor	Is patient or responsible other physically able to prepare and administer accurate doses of GLA?
Affective	What emotions and attitudes are patient and responsible others displaying in regard to diagnosis of diabetes and insulin or OA treatment?
For follow-up of GLA-treated patient	
Effectiveness of therapy	Is patient having symptoms of hyperglycemia? Does blood glucose and urine record show good or poor control? Is glycosylated hemoglobin consistent with glucose records?
Side effects of GLA therapy	Is atrophy or hypertrophy present at injection sites? Has patient had hypoglycemic episodes? If so, how often? What time of day? Are there complaints of nightmares, night sweats, or early morning headaches? Has patient had skin rash or GI upset since taking OA?
Self-management behaviors	If patient is having hypoglycemic episodes, how are those episodes managed? How much insulin or OA is patient taking and at what times of day? Is patient adjusting insulin or OA dose? Under what circumstances and by how much? Has exercise pattern changed? Is patient adhering to number of prescribed calories? Are meals taken at times corresponding to peak insulin action?

GLA, glucose lowering agent.

DRUG THERAPY

Table **46-10**   **Blood Glucose Level Effects**

Glucose-Lowering Effect

Acetaminophen	Clofibrate	Potassium salts
Alcohol	Dicumarol	Probenecid
Allopurinol (Zyloprim)	Fenfluramine	Salicyclates in large doses
α-Glucosidase inhibitors	Histamine antagonists	Sulfonylureas
Anabolic steroids	Insulin	Thiazolidinediones (rosiglitazone)
β-Adrenergic blockers	Monoamine oxidase inhibitors	Tricyclic antidepressants
Biguanides	Phenylbutazone	Urinary acidifiers
Chloramphenicol		

Glucose-Raising Effect

Acetazolamide (Diamox)	Ethacrynic acid (Edecrin)	Marijuana
Asparaginase (Elspar)	Morphine	Nicotine
Caffeine in large doses	Epinephrine	Nifedipine (Procardia)
Arginine HCl	Furosemide (Lasix)	Phenobarbital
Barbiturates	Glucagon	Phenothiazines
β-Adrenergic blockers	Glucose	Phenytoin (Dilantin)
Birth control pills	Glycerin	Rifampin
Cholestyramine (Questran)	Glycerol	Thiazide diuretics
Corticosteroids	Levodopa	Urinary alkalizing agents
Calcitonin	Lithium	

sented in Table 46-10. Medications may have to be changed or dosages adjusted if the patient is also taking GLAs.

Exercise

Regular, consistent exercise is considered an essential part of diabetic management. Exercise contributes to weight loss, reduces triglycerides and cholesterol, increases muscle tone, and improves circulation. In type 1 diabetes, exercise may increase insulin sensitivity, thereby allowing a lowering of the insulin dose. In type 2 diabetes, exercise contributes to weight loss and improves insulin binding on cell receptors. However, the patient should be aware that exercise is perceived by the body as a stress, and that counterregulatory hormones are increased to ensure that adequate glucose is readily available.

PATIENT TEACHING GUIDE

Table 46-11   Exercise

1. Exercise does not have to be vigorous to be effective. The blood glucose–reducing effects of exercise can be attained with mild exercise such as brisk walking. The exercises selected should be enjoyable to foster regularity.
2. Exercise is best done after meals, when the blood glucose level is rising.
3. Exercise plans should be individualized for each patient and monitored by the health care provider.
4. It is important to self-monitor blood glucose levels before, during, and after exercise to determine the effect exercise has on blood glucose level at particular times of the day.
5. Be alert to the possibility of delayed exercise-induced hypoglycemia, which may occur several hours after the completion of exercise.
6. Taking a GLA does not mean that planned or spontaneous exercise cannot occur. It is important to compensate for extensive planned and spontaneous activity by monitoring blood glucose level to make adjustments in the insulin dose (if taken) and food intake.

Table 46-12   Activities That Affect Caloric Expenditure

Light Activity (100-200 cal/hr)	Moderate Activity (200-350 cal/hr)	Vigorous Activity (400-900 cal/hr)
Driving a car	Active housework	Aerobic exercise
Fishing	Bicycling	Bicycling
Light housework	Bowling	Hard labor
Secretarial work	Brisk walking	Ice skating
Teaching	Dancing	Outdoor sports
Walking casually	Gardening	Running
	Golf	Soccer
	Roller skating	Tennis
		Wood chopping

As a result, hyperglycemia may occur in situations of poorly controlled diabetes or in insulin-dependent patients who exercise at a time of day when insufficient insulin is available. Additional information about exercise and diabetes that is important for both the patient and the health care provider is provided in Table 46-11.

Hypoglycemia is likely to occur if the insulin-dependent patient exercises at a time when the GLA action is peaking or if exercise is strenuous and prolonged and carbohydrate is not replaced. This can also occur if a normally sedentary patient with diabetes has an unusually active day. Exercise can be scheduled about 1 hour after a meal, or a 10 to 15 g carbohydrate snack can be eaten before exercising to avoid hypoglycemia. For every 45 minutes to 1 hour of strenuous exercise such as tennis, the patient should repeat the 10 to 15 g carbohydrate snack. (See Table 46-12 for guidelines on calories burned per hour for different activities.)

Hyperglycemia may occur if exercise is scheduled at a time when insulin action is waning. When the insulin dose is insufficient to cover the amount of exercise, the increase in blood glucose created by the counterregulatory hormones may not be curtailed. Again, the patient can guard against this situation by scheduling exercise when sufficient insulin is available. Some patients may have to inject a small bolus of regular insulin if the blood glucose level is elevated before exercising to prevent progressive hyperglycemia.[24]

Monitoring Blood Glucose

Glucose levels must be determined daily to monitor the interactions and effect of diet, exercise, and medication on an individual diabetic regimen. Detection of extreme or episodic hyperglycemia is necessary to avoid DKA and hyperglycemic hyperosmolar nonketosis (HHNK). Traditionally, monitoring has been accomplished by checking for the presence and degree of glycosuria. This technique provides only gross, semiquantitative information. Many factors affect urine test results, such as age, medications, disease, and the individual renal threshold. Urine testing also cannot measure the presence or degree of hypoglycemia. Urine testing for ketonuria, however, is a valuable aid in determining the advent of DKA and is recommended for every patient with type 1 diabetes when the patient is experiencing hyperglycemia or acute illness. Second-voided specimens, which were previously recommended for the patient using urine testing, have been shown to constitute an unnecessary step.

Self-Monitoring. Self-monitoring of blood glucose using capillary blood glucose monitoring (CBGM) technology is a more reliable technique for measuring blood glucose. Commercially available glucose-testing products, including disposable lancets and lancet holders, are widely available. A small drop of capillary blood (usually from a finger stick) is dropped onto a reagent strip. After a specified time, the strip is read either visually or by a machine. The machines are either reflectance meters or sensors. Reflectance meters work by measuring the amount of light reflected onto a strip that has reacted with a color change in response to the reaction of glucose with the reagent strip. Sensors use the measurement of conductivity of electricity as it is affected by the glucose in the blood. The technology of CBGM is a rapidly changing field with newer and more convenient systems being introduced every year. Blood glucose monitoring technology uses a noninvasive spectroscopy, or the use of laser light on a skin surface. Implantable sensors for continuous glucose monitoring are also being considered in research trials.[25] A diabetes educator should be consulted to learn the latest in monitoring technology.

Many meters are computerized and are becoming increasingly sophisticated. Some models are capable of storing results of previous blood glucose tests. These tests can be retrieved to provide a more complete picture of blood glucose fluctuations over time and to guide adjustment to the regimen.

The blood glucose level reported by a laboratory is often higher than the patient's home glucose monitor or the hospital's portable meter. This is because a finger stick is based on a capillary whole blood sample rather than a plasma sample, so it may be approximately 10% to 15% lower. Plasma or serum gives a higher glucose reading.[3] To further complicate this

PATIENT TEACHING GUIDE

Table 46-13 | Capillary Blood Glucose Monitoring

1. Hands are washed in warm water. Cleaning the site with alcohol is not necessary and may even interfere with test results.
2. If it is difficult to obtain an adequate drop of blood for testing, the patient should warm the hands in warm water or let the arms hang dependently for a few minutes before the finger puncture is made.
3. The puncture is made on the side of the finger pad rather than near the center. Fewer nerve endings are along the side of the finger pad.
4. The puncture should be only deep enough to obtain a sufficiently large drop of blood. Unnecessarily deep punctures may cause pain and bruising.

process, some monitors are calibrated to give whole blood results while other meters are calibrated to give values equivalent to plasma concentrations. This must be determined by reading the literature accompanying the particular monitor and strips being used by the patient. Finally, home monitoring equipment must be cleaned and calibrated regularly to maintain its accuracy.

The technique for using a blood glucose–monitoring product accompanies each product. Because errors in monitoring technique can cause errors in clinical management strategies that may be based on erroneous CBGM information, patient training should be emphasized not only at the initial session but at follow-up visits with any member of the health care team. Patient technique should be reassessed at 30 to 180 days after initial training and yearly thereafter.[26] The major source of variability in results obtained with CBGM devices is attributable to the user.[27] Table 46-13 lists the steps that the patient performing CBGM should be taught.

The advantages of CBGM are that it ensures immediate information about blood glucose levels and produces accurate records with daily glucose fluctuations and trends.[28] CBGM is the preferred glucose-monitoring method for the patient with type 1 diabetes. The type 2 diabetic patient may also benefit from CBGM by seeing the correlation between dietary choices and blood glucose levels. As weight is lost and blood glucose levels are lowered, the obese type 2 patient may also gain reinforcement from CBGM.

The frequency of monitoring depends on the glycemic goals the patient and health care provider set and the intensity of the treatment regimen. The patient receiving two or more injections per day may want to test before meals every day. If the glycemic control is relatively stable, the patient may elect to test two or more times a day on certain days of the week. Testing is most often done before meals but can be done any time the patient needs to know the way a factor, such as exercise or stress, is affecting the blood glucose level. The frequency of recording CBGM results to guide therapy decisions should be mutually determined by the health care provider and the patient.

Ideally, a patient should be motivated to learn not only CBGM technique but also how to interpret the results. Most patients find that CBGM brings about physiologic and emotional benefits, as well as a willingness to be an active partner in

the treatment. Achieving the desired level of patient participation also requires time and effort from the health care professional. The nurse involved in this aspect of management should anticipate a close working relationship with the patient for a period of 3 to 6 months as the patient learns refinements of the technique and appropriate decision making regarding changes in diet, medication, and exercise. A patient who is visually impaired, color blind, or limited in manual dexterity needs careful evaluation of the glucose-monitoring method most appropriate for that patient's needs. Glucose monitors are now commercially available for the visually impaired.

NURSING MANAGEMENT: DIABETES MELLITUS

■ Nursing Assessment

Initial subjective and objective data that should be obtained from a person with diabetes mellitus are presented in Table 46-14. After the initial assessment, periodic patient assessments should be done on a schedule as outlined in Table 46-15.

■ Nursing Diagnoses

Nursing diagnoses for the patient with diabetes mellitus may include, but are not limited to, those found in NCP 46-1.

■ Planning

The overall goals are that the patient with diabetes mellitus will (1) be an active participant in the management of the diabetes regimen; (2) experience minimal or no episodes of DKA, HHNK, or hypoglycemia; (3) prevent or delay the occurrence of chronic complications of diabetes; and (4) adjust lifestyle to accommodate diabetes regimen with a minimum of stress.

■ Nursing Implementation

Health Promotion. The role of the nurse in health promotion and maintenance relates to the identification, monitoring, and education of the patient at risk for the development of diabetes mellitus. The American Diabetes Association now recommends routine screening for diabetes for all adults over age 45, and if normal, it should be repeated at 3-year intervals. This screening should include a fasting plasma glucose, although a screening may be done by capillary glucose in some instances. Testing should be considered at a younger age or be carried out more frequently in individuals who meet the criteria listed in Table 46-16.[5]

A person with impaired glucose tolerance with plasma levels of glucose that are higher than normal is also at increased risk for diabetes. In addition, the presence of pancreatic or endocrine disease or the use of certain medications such as corticosteroids also alerts the nurse to evaluate this person for diabetes.

Acute Intervention. The nurse is involved with the care of a patient with diabetes in many acute situations, such as DKA, hypoglycemia, and HHNK. Nursing management for hypoglycemia, DKA, and HHNK are discussed starting on p. 1396. Other areas of acute intervention relate to management during stress, such as during acute illness and surgery.

Stress of acute illness and surgery. Both emotional and physical stress can increase the blood glucose level and result in hyperglycemia. However, it is impossible to avoid stress totally

NURSING ASSESSMENT

Table 46-14 | Diabetes Mellitus

Subjective Data

Important Health Information

Past health history: Mumps, rubella, coxsackievirus or other viral infections; recent trauma, infection, or stress; pregnancy, gave birth to infant >9 lb; chronic pancreatitis; Cushing's syndrome, acromegaly

Family history: History of type 1 or type 2 diabetes mellitus

Medications: Use of and compliance with insulin or OAs; use of glucocorticoids, diuretics, phenytoin (Dilantin)

Surgery and other treatments: Any recent surgery

Functional Health Patterns

Health perception–health management: Positive family history; malaise

Nutritional-metabolic: Obesity; weight loss (type 1), weight gain (type 2): thirst, hunger; nausea and vomiting; poor healing especially involving the feet, compliance with diet in patients with previously diagnosed diabetes

Elimination: Constipation or diarrhea; frequent urination, nocturia, incontinence; skin infections

Activity-exercise: Muscle weakness, fatigue

Cognitive-perceptual: Abdominal pain, headache; blurred vision; numbness or tingling of extremities; pruritus

Sexuality-reproductive: Impotence; frequent vaginal infections; decreased libido

Coping–stress tolerance: Depression, irritability, apathy

Value-belief: Commitment to lifestyle changes involving diet, medication, and activity patterns

Objective Data

Eyes

Soft, sunken eyeballs; vitreal hemorrhages, cataracts

Integumentary

Dry, warm, inelastic skin; pigmented lesions (on legs); ulcers (especially on feet), loss of hair on toes

Respiratory

Rapid, deep respirations (Kussmaul respirations)

Cardiovascular

Hypotension; weak, rapid pulse

Gastrointestinal

Dry mouth, vomiting, fruity breath

Neurologic

Altered reflexes, restlessness, confusion, stupor, coma

Musculoskeletal

Muscle wasting

Possible Findings

Serum electrolyte abnormalities; fasting blood glucose level ≥126 mg/dl (7.0 mmol/L); glucose tolerance test ≥200 mg/dl (11.1 mmol/L); leukocytosis; elevated blood urea nitrogen, creatinine, triglycerides, cholesterol, LDL, VLDL; glycosylated hemoglobin ≥6%; glycosuria; ketonuria; albuminuria; acidosis

LDL, low density lipoproteins; *VLDL,* very low density lipoproteins.

in life situations such as deaths in the family, job interviews, and final examinations. These situations may require extra insulin to avoid hyperglycemia.

Common stress-evoking situations include acute illness and the controlled stress of surgery. The patient with diabetes who has a minor illness such as a cold or the flu should continue drug therapy and food intake. A carbohydrate liquid substitution such as regular soft drinks, gelatin dessert, or beverages such as Gatorade may be necessary. The patient should understand that food intake is important during this time because the body requires extra energy to deal with the stress of the illness. Extra insulin may be necessary to meet this demand without DKA concurrently developing.

Blood glucose monitoring should be done every 1 to 2 hours by either the patient or a person who can assume responsibility for care during the illness. Urine output and the presence and degree of ketonuria should be monitored, particularly when fever is present. Fluid intake should be increased to prevent dehydration, with a minimum of 4 oz per hour for an adult.

The patient should be instructed to contact the health care provider when a blood glucose level more than 250 mg/dl (13.9 mmol/L), fever, ketonuria, and nausea and vomiting occur. The health care provider should supervise the necessary adjustments in the treatment regimen during times of stress. Eventually, the well-informed patient will be able to make most adjustments independently on the basis of past successful experiences.

Surgery is controlled stress, and adjustments in the diabetes regimen can be planned to ensure glycemic control. The patient is given IV fluids and insulin immediately before, during, and after surgery when there is no oral intake. The type 2 diabetic patient receiving OAs usually has the OAs discontinued 48 hours before surgery and is treated with insulin during the surgical period. The patient should understand that this is a temporary measure and is not to be interpreted as a worsening of diabetes.

The nurse caring for an unconscious surgical patient receiving insulin must be alert for hypoglycemic signs such as sweating, tachycardia, and tremors. The nurse should be aware that blood glucose monitoring must also be done frequently.

Ambulatory and Home Care. The nurse may be involved in any or all aspects of management, but the focus of nursing care has two aims: to care for the patient during acute episodes and to assist the patient in learning to live with diabetes every day. Both aims require the nurse to be thoroughly familiar with diabetes and its management and to educate the patient with diabetes about all aspects of the disease.

Patients are often treated in outpatient diabetes clinics. Frequently these clinics are staffed by diabetes nurse specialists. These specialists have preparation beyond the baccalaureate degree in diabetes and work collaboratively with physicians to manage patients with diabetes. The diabetes nurse specialist is also often available to the nursing staff for consultation in the acute care setting.

Table **46-15**	Standards of Medical Care for a Patient with Diabetes Mellitus		
Item	Initial Visit	Every 3 Mo	Every 12 Mo
Assessment of Glycemic Control			
Symptoms of hypoglycemia	X	X	
Symptoms of hyperglycemia	X	X	
Record of blood tests	X	X	
Glycosylated hemoglobin	X	X	
Assessment for Complications			
Postural blood pressure and pulse (BP goal <130/85)	X	X	
Weight	X	X	
Funduscopic—dilated eye examination	X	X	
Ophthalmologist or optometrist			X
Cardiac examination	X		X
Neurologic examination			X
Sensory: monofilament foot examination	X		X
Motor: ankle reflexes, muscle bulk and tone	X		X
Pelvic examination as indicated for vaginal discharge		As needed	X
Extremities			
Feet: calluses, toenails, ulcers	X	X	
Peripheral pulses			
Dorsalis pedis	X		
Posterior tibial	X		X
Popliteal	X		X
Femoral	X		X
Assessment of Educational Needs			
Diet	X	X	
Medication management	X	X	
Monitoring skills	X	X	
Diagnostic Studies			
Blood glucose level	X	X	
Blood urea nitrogen and creatinine level	X		
Urinalysis for microalbuminuria	X		X
Electrocardiogram	X*		X
Lipid profile	X		X
Fasting triglyceride level	X		X

*If appropriate to age and history.

The nurse may request consultation with a diabetes educator who is certified by the National Certification Board for Diabetes Educators. Certified diabetes educators (CDEs) have met stringent preparation and experience criteria and have demonstrated expertise in the field of diabetes education. Nurses, dieticians, pharmacists, physicians, and other health care professionals who make up the diabetes management team are eligible to apply for the CDE credential. The certified diabetes educator is designated with the initials CDE after the name.

The effect of the diagnosis of diabetes cannot be overestimated. An assessment of the patient's perception of what it means to have diabetes must be carefully assessed before patient education is designed and implemented. The nurse should foster a positive attitude about the prescribed regimen and assist the patient in developing an individualized management plan. Learning goals should be mutually determined by the patient and the nurse on the basis of individual needs and therapeutic requirements. The nurse should assess the patient's feelings and facilitate acceptance of diabetes mellitus and its treatment over time.

A clinical pathway for home care of the patient with diabetes mellitus is provided on p. 1389.

Insulin therapy. Nursing responsibilities for the patient receiving insulin include proper administration, assessment of the patient's use of and response to insulin therapy, and education of the patient regarding administration, adjustment to, and side effects of insulin (see Table 46-6). Table 46-9 lists guidelines for the nurse assessing a patient using glucose-lowering agents, including insulin and OAs.

The patient with newly diagnosed diabetes should be assessed for the ability to understand the purpose of insulin therapy; the interaction of insulin, diet, and activity; and the ways side effects may be manifested. The patient or significant other also has to be able to prepare and inject the insulin. If the patient or family lacks the psychomotor skills to prepare insulin, the nurse may have to find additional resources to assist the patient.

Some patients find it difficult to inject themselves. This may be due to fear of the needle or anger and lack of acceptance of the disease. The nurse should determine the emotions and attitude of the patient and family regarding insulin therapy.

46-1 NURSING CARE PLAN PATIENT WITH DIABETES MELLITUS*

| Expected Patient Outcomes | Nursing Interventions and *Rationales* |

Ambulatory and Home Care

NURSING DIAGNOSIS **Ineffective management of therapeutic regimen** *related to* inadequate knowledge of adequate exercise program, diet and weight control, administration and potential side effects of glucose-lowering agents (GLAs), glucose monitoring, and care during acute minor illness *as manifested by* frequent questioning regarding diabetic management, inaccurate responses to questions about diabetic management.

- Participation in exercise program.
- Appropriate dietary preparation and intake.
- Safe, effective administration of GLA.
- Demonstration of proper blood glucose testing and recording of measurements.
- Plan of action for self in event of illness and symptoms lasting >24 hr.

- Plan individualized exercise program with patient *because exercise is an integral part of diabetic management.*
- Review steps to prevent hyperglycemia and hypoglycemia *because activity changes can cause changes in insulin needs.*
- Review diet and problem areas with patient *to provide appropriate teaching.*
- Counsel on weight loss if appropriate *because excess weight complicates diabetic management.*
- Refer to dietician *because dietary management of diabetes can be complex and requires ongoing monitoring.*
- Review GLA administration; have patient give return demonstration of insulin injection *to ensure proper technique.*
- Assess injection sites *to determine need for changing sites or initiating treatment to problematic areas.*
- Review symptoms and treatment of hypoglycemia *so early treatment can be initiated.*
- Demonstrate glucose testing; have patient give return demonstration *to ensure proper technique.*
- Review glucose records with patient and explain how to identify trends *to improve glucose control.*
- Remind patient to call physician if blood glucose is >250 mg/dl (13.9 mmol/L) and ketonuria is present *so appropriate adjustments can be made to prevent development of diabetic ketoacidosis (DKA).*
- Review effect of stress on glycemic control *so patient is aware that stress can increase glucose level.*
- Review sick-day care *so patient can make appropriate adjustments in diabetic management.*
- Assist patient in devising a sick-day plan, including foods to have on hand and family member or friend who can be with patient during illness episode, *to be ready to properly manage diabetes when illness occurs.*
- Review symptoms needing attention of physician, including blood glucose level >250 mg/dl (13.9 mmol/L), ketonuria, fever, nausea, and vomiting *so patient can contact physician when necessary to prevent occurrence of DKA and hyperglycemic hyperosmolar nonketosis (HHNK).*

NURSING DIAGNOSIS **Risk for infection** *related to* depressed immune system, inadequate circulation, and environmental pathogens.

- Verbalization of steps to prevent infection (skin care, foot care, regular dental care).
- Recognition of signs of infection and need for intervention.

- Assess for signs of infection such as fever, redness, swelling, or pus at trauma or pressure site; fever *to ensure early recognition and treatment.*
- Assess oral cavity, skin, pulses, particularly lower extremities and pedal pulses, *to detect areas of infection or poor circulation.*
- Review skin and foot care; have patient give return demonstration of foot care *to ensure patient understanding.*
- Review signs of infection, including redness, swelling, pus, and when to contact health care provider *to ensure patient recognizes infection and notifies health care provider if indicated so treatment can be initiated.*

Continued

46-1   NURSING CARE PLAN   PATIENT WITH DIABETES MELLITUS*—continued

Expected Patient Outcomes	Nursing Interventions and *Rationales*

NURSING DIAGNOSIS   **Self-esteem disturbance** *related to* lifestyle changes imposed by diabetes and its treatment and frustration at progression of disease *as manifested by* negative feelings about self, resistance to incorporating treatment regimen into lifestyle.

- Verbalization of positive attitude about self and ability to manage disease.
- Plan for continued contact with health care provider for health monitoring.

- Encourage patient to discuss diagnosis and its implications *so appropriate counseling and interventions can be planned.*
- Suggest individualized diabetes education and support group *to increase patient's knowledge base and meet other people with diabetes.*
- Suggest creative approaches to problems with patient *because patient may be overwhelmed initially by complexity of disease management.*
- Assure patient of continued value and self-worth *to minimize impact of diabetes on patient's self-esteem.*

COLLABORATIVE PROBLEMS

Nursing Goals	Nursing Interventions and *Rationales*

Acute Management

POTENTIAL COMPLICATION   **DKA and HHNK** *related to* inadequate insulin and excess blood glucose secondary to increased caloric intake, physical or emotional stress, or undiagnosed diabetes.

- Monitor for signs of DKA and HHNK.
- Report deviations from acceptable parameters.
- Carry out appropriate medical and nursing interventions.

- Assess for signs of DKA such as increase in urination; vomiting; somnolence; dehydration; dry, loose skin; hypotension with weak, rapid pulse; coma; hyperglycemia >250 mg/dl (13.9 mmol/L); presence of urine ketones; pH <7.3 *to ensure early recognition and intervention.*
- Assess for signs of HHNK such as hyperglycemia >500 mg/dl (27.8 mmol/L), serum osmolality >300 mOsm/kg (300 mmol/kg), absence of ketonuria *to detect signs of HHNK.*
- Administer insulin per physician order *to stabilize blood glucose level.*
- Administer fluid and electrolyte replacement as ordered *to correct dehydration.*
- Monitor input and output and vital signs *to detect signs and symptoms of inadequate tissue perfusion.*
- Assess for precipitating factors *to prevent recurrence and identify teaching needs.*

POTENTIAL COMPLICATION   **Hypoglycemia** *related to* low blood glucose secondary to too much insulin.

- Monitor for signs of hypoglycemia.
- Report deviations from acceptable parameters.
- Carry out appropriate medical and nursing interventions.

- Assess for signs of hypoglycemia such as cold sweats; weakness; trembling; nervousness; irritability; pallor; increase in heart rate; confusion; fatigue; abnormal behavior *to ensure prompt identification and treatment.*
- Check blood glucose if time permits (e.g., when symptoms are mild) *to provide an indicator for treatment.*
- Provide quick-acting carbohydrate source such as 6-8 oz orange juice, 1 cup milk, or 6-8 oz soft drink *to quickly reverse hypoglycemia;* give orally only if patient is alert enough to swallow *to prevent aspiration.*
- Repeat oral dose in 10-15 min if no improvement. If no improvement or patient is comatose, administer 1 mg glucagon subcutaneously or 30-50 ml of 50% IV dextrose per physician order *to stimulate hepatic response to convert glycogen to glucose.*
- When patient improves and is alert, provide long-acting carbohydrate or next scheduled meal *to keep blood glucose level within acceptable range.*
- Assess for precipitating factors such as history of too much insulin, too little food, unusual amounts of exercise, or delayed eating *to prevent recurrence and identify precipitating factors.*

*This care plan is intended to be used for persons with newly diagnosed diabetes.

Table 46-16 Criteria for Testing in Asymptomatic, Undiagnosed Individuals

Type 1 diabetes: Testing presumably healthy individuals for the presence of any immune markers, outside of a clinical trials setting, is not recommended.

Type 2 diabetes: In asymptomatic, undiagnosed individuals, testing for diabetes should be considered in all individuals at age 45 years and above; if normal, it should be repeated at 3-year intervals.

Testing* should be considered at a younger age, or be carried out more frequently, in individuals who

- are obese (≥120% desirable body weight or a body mass index ≥27 kg/m^2)
- have a first-degree relative with diabetes
- are members of a high risk ethnic population (African-American, Hispanic, Native-American, Asian)
- delivered a baby weighing >9 lb or were diagnosed with gestational diabetes mellitus
- are hypertensive (≥140/90 mm Hg)
- have an HDL cholesterol level ≤35 mg/dl (9.1 mmol/L) or a triglyceride level ≥250 mg/dl (2.82 mmol/L)
- on previous testing had impaired glucose tolerance or impaired fasting glucose

Adapted from American Diabetes Association Clinical Practice Recommendations.
*The fasting plasma glucose is the preferred diagnostic test because of its ease of administration, convenience, acceptability to patients, and lower cost.

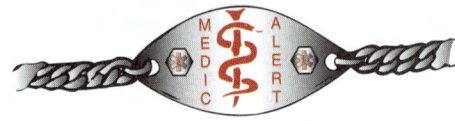

Name				Phone		
Address						
Physician				Phone		
Address				ORAL		
INSULIN	DOSAGE	TIME		MEDICATION	DOSAGE	TIME
Regular				Orinase		
PZI				Diabinese		
Globin				Dymelor		
NPH				Tolinase		
Lente				DBI		
Semilente				DBI TD		
Ultralente						
				Date		

I am a DIABETIC

If unconscious or behaving abnormally, I may be having a reaction associated with diabetes or its treatment.

If I can swallow give me sugar, candy, or a sweet drink. If I do not recover promptly, call a physician or send me to the hospital.

If I am unconscious or cannot swallow, do not attempt to give me anything by mouth, but call a physician or send me to the hospital immediately.

Fig. 46-11 Medical alerts. A patient with diabetes should carry a card and wear a bracelet or necklace that indicates diabetes. If the patient with diabetes is unconscious, these measures will ensure prompt and appropriate attention.

Follow-up assessment of the patient who has been using insulin therapy also includes an inspection of injection sites for allergic reactions, a review of insulin preparation and injection technique, a history pertaining to the occurrence of hypoglycemic episodes, and the patient's method for handling hypoglycemic episodes. A review of the patient's record of urine and blood glucose tests is also important in assessing overall glycemic control.

Oral agents. Nursing responsibilities for the patient taking OAs are similar to those for the patient taking insulin. Proper administration, assessment of the patient's use of and response to the OA, and education of the patient and the family about OAs are all part of the nurse's function. Table 46-9 lists guidelines for the nurse assessing a patient starting therapy with OAs and the follow-up assessment. The assessment done by the nurse can be invaluable in determining the most appropriate oral agent for a patient. The assessment includes the patient's mental status, eating habits, home environment, attitude toward diabetes, and use of oral agents. For example, if the patient is older, lives alone, or has difficulty remembering to follow a medication and diet schedule, a shorter-acting OA may be preferable. Some patients may assume that their diabetes is not a serious condition if they are taking only a pill for glycemic control. The patient needs to understand the importance of diet and not skipping meals. The patient should not take extra pills if overeating has occurred. The patient also needs to know that if on sulfonylureas, hypoglycemic reactions may be severe and prolonged and that health care provider supervision may be necessary, particularly for the older patient.

The patient should also be instructed to contact a physician if periods of illness or extreme stress occur. During such a period, insulin therapy may be required to prevent or treat hyperglycemic symptoms and HHNK.

Personal hygiene. The potential chronic complications of infections, neuropathy, and microangiopathy require the patient with diabetes to participate in effective hygiene practices related to skin and dental care. Because of susceptibility to periodontal disease and pyorrhea, daily brushing and flossing should be encouraged. When dental work must be done, the dentist should be informed that the patient has diabetes.

Daily baths should be part of routine care, with particular emphasis given to foot care. (See Table 46-25 for patient teaching guide.) If cuts, scrapes, or burns occur, they should be treated promptly. The area should be washed, and a nonabrasive or nonirritating antiseptic ointment must be applied. The area should be covered with a dry, sterile pad. If the injury does not begin to heal within 24 hours or if signs of infection develop, the health care provider should be notified immediately.

Medical identification and travel. The patient should be instructed to carry medical identification at all times indicating diabetes. An identification card (Fig. 46-11) can supply valuable information, such as the name of the health care provider and the type and dose of insulin or OA. A Medic Alert bracelet or necklace should be worn by every person with diabetes. Police, paramedics, and many private citizens are aware of the need to look for this identification when working with sick or unconscious persons.

Travel for a patient with diabetes requires planning in advance. The patient should have all supplies in carry-on luggage and keep them at hand at all times. This includes insulin, syringes, quick-acting carbohydrate, and glucagon. Extra insulin should be available in case a bottle breaks or gets lost. If

CLINICAL PATHWAY Home Care of Diabetes Mellitus

ICD-9 Code(s) 250.9, 250.91, 250.11, 250.70

Patient Name _____ Pt. ID No. _____ SOC Date _____ Discharge Date _____

Date Noted	Expected Outcomes	Achieved			Variance Codes	Date Noted	Nursing Diagnoses	Date Closed
		Y	N	Date				
	1. Stable endocrine status by visit no. ___ as noted by blood glucose in range of ___ to ___.						Cardiac output, decreased Outcome(s) no. ____ :	
	2. Patient/caregiver demonstrates compliance with treatment regimen to include dietary and exercise requirements, as well as general health issues by visit no.___						Coping, ineffective family/patient Outcome(s) no. ____ :	
	3. Patient/caregiver demonstrates understanding and compliance with blood glucose testing, insulin administration, and medication regimens as evidenced by return demonstration by visit no. ___						Denial, ineffective Outcome(s) no. ____ :	
							Knowledge deficit: medication and therapeutic regimen Outcome(s) no. ____ :	
	4. Patient/caregiver demonstrates understanding of home safety, general emergency measures related to disease condition, infection control, and proper disposal of contaminated wastes by visit no. ___.						Management of therapeutic regimen, ineffective Outcome(s) no. ____ :	
							Nutrition, altered: risk for more than body requirements Outcome(s) no. ____ :	
	5. Other:						Tissue perfusion, altered: peripheral, renal Outcome(s) no. ____ :	
	6. Other:						Noncompliance (specify) Outcome(s) no. ____ :	
	7. Other:						Other: Outcome(s) no. ____ :	

Adapted from Marrelli TM, Hilliard LS: *Home care and clinical paths: effective care across the continuum,* St Louis, 1996, Mosby.   *Continued*

the patient is planning a trip out of the country, it is wise to have a letter from the physician explaining that the patient has diabetes and requires all the materials, particularly syringes, for ongoing health care.

Some travel involves time changes such as traveling coast to coast or across the international date line. The patient should contact the health care provider to plan an appropriate insulin schedule. Many patients find it easier and more predictable to take only regular insulin every 4 to 6 hours to cover insulin needs while on long airplane trips instead of trying to anticipate the peak of intermediate insulin and the availability of meals. During travel, most patients find it helpful to keep watches set to the time of the city of origin until they reach their destination. The key to travel when taking insulin is to know the type of insulin being taken, its onset of action, and the anticipated peak time. Meals or carry-along food can then be planned around this schedule.

Patient Teaching. The major educational objective is to match the level of self-management to the ability of the individual patient. Ideally, the patient should be taught about the disease and encouraged to achieve self-management with guidance only from the health care provider. The more in control the patient with diabetes can feel, the more likely the patient is to accept and adhere to the management program. The basis of self-management is a sound educational program related to diabetes. A knowledgeable patient

CLINICAL PATHWAY   Home Care of Diabetes Mellitus—continued

Assessments/Instructions/Interventions	VS No. _	VS No. _	VS No. _	VS No. _	VS No. _	VS No. _	VS No. _	VS No. _	VS No. _
Explain patient rights and responsibilities.									
Assess for home safety management.									
Assess vital signs.									
Assess endocrine status.									
Assess hydration and nutrition status.									
Assess weight.									
Assess coping skills of patient/family/caregiver.									
Assess patient/caregiver's strengths/weaknesses related to therapeutic regimen.									
Assess patient/caregiver's willingness and ability to provide home therapeutic regimen.									
Assess patient/caregiver's understanding of disease process and compliance with therapeutic regimen.									
Refer to dietician for nutritional needs.									
Instruct on home safety.									
Instruct on medication regimen and compliance issues.									
Instruct patient/caregiver on signs of hypoglycemia and hyperglycemia and emergency measures related to those conditions.									
Instruct patient/caregiver on blood glucose testing.									
Instruct patient/caregiver on self/caregiver administration of insulin.									
Instruct patient/caregiver on home maintenance program (including exercise and correct nutritional intake). _____ on visit no. ____.									
Venipuncture for ordered laboratory tests.									
Other:									

Medical Supplies/Home Medical Equipment Needs
1. Blood glucose meter
2. Insulin syringes/insulin
3. Other _____

Variance codes

Case manager name_____

1. Patient related   Team member signature _____ Initials _____
2. Situation related   Team member signature _____ Initials _____   _____
3. Systems related   Team member signature _____ Initials _____   Patient signature
                                                                                           (involved in care planning)

---

should be able to make minor adjustments in insulin dosage and diet prescription to compensate for special circumstances, such as illness or increased exercise.

Not all patients with diabetes are capable of self-management. If the patient is not able to manage the disease, a family member may be able to assume this role. If the patient or the family cannot make decisions related to diabetes management, the nurse may identify appropriate resources outside the family. These resources can assist the patient and the family in outlining a feasible treatment program that meets their capabilities. Patient and health care provider resources are listed at the end of this chapter.

The American Diabetes Association offers pamphlets, booklets, and a bimonthly magazine called Diabetes Forecast for patients of all ages. Affiliates of the American Diabetes Association are located in all states, and most can be reached by dialing 800-DIABETES. The American Diabetes Associa-

tion also publishes materials and sponsors conferences for health care professionals concerned with diabetes education, research, and management of patients. It gives recognition to education programs that meet the national standards of diabetes education and can provide a list of these programs. Drug companies manufacturing diabetes-related products also have free educational material for patients and health care providers.

Treatment programs take time to learn. The theory and textbook information are only the beginning. The information must then be incorporated into the patient's lifestyle. The health care provider who educates the patient and family understands that the education process initially takes weeks to months and provides periodic reassessment after the basics have been learned and integrated.

Another useful strategy is to divide the teaching content into the level that must be learned right away and the level

Table **46-17**	Levels of Diabetes Education

Level 1

Educational Guidelines for Initial Management of Diabetes

Provide content required at time of diagnosis and represent basic or survival needs. Level is based on limitations of patient and family to accept and assimilate all there is to know about diabetes at time of diagnosis and limitations of some settings to provide additional education.

Example

Capillary blood glucose monitoring and insulin administration and hypoglycemia prevention and management.

Level 2

Educational Guidelines for Home Management of Diabetes

Place emphasis on increasing knowledge and flexibility as some experience is gained in living with diabetes. This is perceived as essential for every patient but must be tailored to individual needs and capacity. This type of educational experience is preferably offered in a nonhospital environment as close to home as possible.

Example

Goals for control, diabetes diet management, and sick-day guidelines.

Level 3

Education Guidelines for Improvement of Lifestyle

Present form of advanced learning viewed as enriching patient's life with flexibility, insight, and self-determination. Most patients are forced to discover this information by trial and error through experience. Although no educational program can or should entirely replace personal experience, the process need not be experienced by each person.

Example

Exercise, adjusting insulin and lifestyle, stress management.

RESEARCH
IMPLICATIONS FOR NURSING PRACTICE

Diabetes Self-Care

Citation Coates VE, Boore JR: The influence of psychological factors on the self-management of insulin-dependent diabetes mellitus, *J Adv Nurs* 17:528, 1998.

Purpose To determine the influence that perceived health beliefs, perceived control of diabetes, and knowledge have on the practice and outcomes of diabetes self-management.

Methods A mailed survey was completed by 263 patients (ages 18 to 35) with type 1 diabetes mellitus who were treated in a diabetes clinic. The questionnaires included items related to health beliefs, perceived control, and knowledge of diabetes. Glycosylated hemoglobin levels and clinic attendance as obtained from the medical records were used as indicators of self-care practice.

Results and Conclusions Most patients shared the belief that the consequences of diabetes were serious, and most had a sense of internal control and a high level of knowledge about diabetes. However, neither perceptions of control nor health belief had a demonstrable effect on either of the outcome measures (glycosylated hemoglobin or clinic attendance). Only 22% attended the clinic on all six appointment days.

Implications for Nursing Practice Although assessment of knowledge and beliefs is useful to planning care, it may not be predictive of how well patients followed through with prescribed therapy. Additional markers of patient compliance or outcomes are also needed. These results support the notion that care for diabetic patients must be tailored to meet their individual needs.

---

that can be scheduled for another time. Levels of diabetes education include survival, home management, and improvement of lifestyle. These levels are outlined in Table 46-17. The levels provide the diabetes educator with some structure for patient education and relieve the expectation that the patient will have to be taught everything in a short time.

In 1984 the National Diabetes Advisory Board established a set of standards to be used for ensuring the quality of diabetes patient education programs. The American Diabetes Association then developed a set of review criteria that specify the conditions under which each standard is to be met for a diabetes education program to be "recognized." It is believed that meeting the national standards and obtaining recognition will result in improvement in the overall quality of diabetes patient education programs.[29]

After the initial diagnosis of diabetes has been made, the lifelong process of patient education begins. The nurse's understanding of diabetes mellitus is central to a successful teaching program. An assessment of the patient's knowledge of diabetes and lifestyle preferences is useful in planning the teaching program. Table 46-18 is an example of a diabetes patient education record that can provide the nurse with a framework related to the patient's learning needs. Based on the information obtained from the record, an educational plan can be developed to meet the patient's individual needs. Table 46-19 is a summary of educational needs that can be used to track the progress of the patient's educational program. The nurse should assess the patient's knowledge base frequently so that gaps in knowledge or incorrect or inaccurate ideas can be quickly corrected. The record can be reviewed with the patient to outline and contract for additional educational information. The record can also provide an efficient way for other health care providers to be aware of what the patient knows or needs to learn.

Follow-up Nursing Management.   Although the educational emphasis is on self-care, the patient should be encouraged to also be a partner in care with the health care provider. In addition to carrying out the daily management routines, maintaining a schedule of regular follow-up to assess the progress of the disease and additional education are necessary. Table 46-15 outlines a suggested follow-up schedule to aid in the long-term care of a patient with diabetes and to meet American Diabetes Association Standards of Care.

Table **46-18**   **Diabetes Patient Education Record**

1. **Demographic information**   Date: _____
   Name: _____   Age: _____
   Race: _____ Sex (circle): M F Participant status (circle): Inpatient Outpatient
   Level of education: _____ Occupation: _____
   Physician's name: _____ Marital status (circle): Single Married Widowed Divorced

2. **General medical condition**
   Height: _____ Weight: _____ %Ideal weight: _____ Blood pressure: _____
   Hb$_{A1c}$: _____ Total cholesterol level: _____ HDL: _____ Triglyceride level: _____
   Allergies: _____
   Other medications: _____
   Other medical problems: _____
   Present health status: _____
   _____

3. **Diabetes history**
   Types of diabetes: _____ Duration of diabetes: _____
   Treatment plan (check): _____ Insulin _____ OAs _____ Diet alone
   Monitoring system: Type: _____ Test times: _____ Product: _____ Usual AM glucose level: _____
   Attach monitoring log, if appropriate.
   Name and type of insulin or OA: Dose   Times taken
   _____
   _____
   Describe any side effects of OAs/insulin: _____
   Complications (check):
   ____ Retinopathy ____ Neuropathy ____ Renal ____ Foot ____ Macrovascular ____ Other (specify) _____
   Describe: _____
   Incidences of DKA, hypoglycemia, hyperglycemia (date, etc.): _____

4. **Dietary habits**
   If prescribed, daily caloric intake: _____ Food or foods to avoid: _____
   Indicate times of Breakfast _____ Lunch _____ Dinner _____
   Attach dietary recall data or nutrition workup, if appropriate.

5. **Physical activity habits**
   Does patient have regular exercise program (20 min, 3 days/wk)? Yes _____ No _____
   If yes, indicate:
   Type   Duration   Intensity (Circle)
   _____   _____   Light   Medium   Heavy
   _____   _____   Light   Medium   Heavy
   _____   _____   Light   Medium   Heavy

6. **Diabetes education history**
   Prior diabetes education? Patient/NP _____ Yes _____ No   Significant other _____ Yes _____ No
   Prior education: _____
   Special educational needs: _____
   Will significant other participate in program? Yes _____ No _____ Relationship: _____
7. **Source of referral (check one)**
   _____ Physician/NP _____ Self-referred _____ Facility staff _____ Community agency _____ Other (specify): _____
8. **Social history**
   Cigarettes/day: _____ Alcoholic drinks/wk: _____
   No. in household: _____ Relationship: _____
   Types of health/medical insurance: _____
   _____

Modified from *Meeting the standards: a manual for completing the ADA application for recognition*, ed 5, American Diabetes Association, 1998.

COMPLICATIONS OF DIABETES

With the discovery and initial administration of insulin, it was believed that a cure for diabetes had been found. However, 70 years of insulin therapy has proved that insulin is not the total answer in the treatment of diabetes. Hyperglycemia-related problems do not cause death as often as they did before insulin was discovered. Other chronic complications of long-term disease are responsible for more than 75% of all diabetic deaths.

The acute problems of diabetes are associated with severe, untreated hyperglycemia (e.g., DKA, HHNK) or the hypoglycemic side effects of treatment with GLAs. Chronic problems are primarily those of end organ disease from microangiopathy, macroangiopathy, and neuropathy. Hyperglycemia plays a significant role in these complications as shown by the DCCT. Hyperglycemia may damage cells and tissue in at least two ways:

1. Metabolic dysfunction in the breakdown of glucose may lead to accumulation of damaging by-products (e.g., sorbitol).
2. Glucose becomes abnormally bound to protein structures of the body and produces deleterious effects in nerves and blood vessels over time.

In June 1993 the National Institute of Diabetes and Digestive and Kidney Diseases announced the results of a landmark medical study that began in 1983. Called the Diabetes Control

| Table **46-19** | **Summary of Educational Needs Assessment and Progress Form** |

Content Area	Preprogram*		Taught†	Postprogram‡	
Patient			Date/initial/method		
1. Understands general facts of diabetes	Y	N		Y	N
2. Is well adjusted psychologically in relation to diabetes	Y	N		Y	N
3. Adequately or appropriately involves family in diabetes care	Y	N		Y	N
4. Understands and practices effective nutritional management	Y	N		Y	N
5. Understands benefits of and engages in appropriate exercise	Y	N		Y	N
6. Monitors blood or urine glucose levels appropriately	Y	N		Y	N
7. Properly uses insulin or OAs	Y	N		Y	N
8. Knows relationship among nutrition, exercise, and medication	Y	N		Y	N
9. Recognizes and responds appropriately to symptoms of hypoglycemia and hyperglycemia	Y	N		Y	N
10. Understands effects of illness on diabetes management and responds appropriately	Y	N		Y	N
11. Practices proper hygiene (skin care, foot care, dental care) to prevent complications of diabetes	Y	N		Y	N
12. Cooperates in therapeutic management and rehabilitation of diabetes complications	Y	N		Y	N
13. Understands benefits and responsibilities of self-management in diabetes	Y	N		Y	N
14. Effectively uses available health care systems	Y	N		Y	N
15. Makes appropriate use of community resources	Y	N		Y	N

Modified from *Meeting the standards: a manual for completing the ADA application for recognition,* ed 5, American Diabetes Association, 1998.
*Preprogram: Did patient know content before education?
†Taught: Was content taught? Put date, initials (instructor's name must accompany initials at least once); method of instruction (L, lecture; D, demonstration; R, return demonstration; V, video; X, other); and format (1/1, one to one; CL, classroom; G, group; SI, self-instruction module).
‡Postprogram: Did patient know content after education?

and Complications Trial (DCCT), it compared different forms of diabetes treatment in preventing or slowing the complications of diabetes. The trial included more than 1400 people with insulin-dependent diabetes at 29 medical centers in the United States and Canada, half with no retinopathy at baseline (the primary prevention cohort) and the other half with mild retinopathy (the secondary intervention cohort). Patients were randomly assigned to one of two groups: intensive or standard treatment. The intensive treatment group took three or more insulin injections a day or used an insulin pump. The patients in the standard treatment group took one to two injections a day and tested their blood glucose once or twice a day. The intensive group was distinguished from the standard treatment group in terms of glycosylated hemoglobin levels and capillary blood glucose values throughout the study (average glycosylated hemoglobin in the intensive treatment group was about 7.2% and the standard treatment group was about 9% on a normal range of 4.0% to 6.05%).

The results found that in the primary prevention cohort, intensive therapy reduced the adjusted mean risk for the development of retinopathy by 76%, as compared with conventional therapy. In the secondary intervention cohort, intensive therapy slowed the progression of retinopathy by 54%. In the two cohorts combined, intensive therapy reduced the occurrence of microalbuminuria by 39% and of albuminuria (urinary albumin excretion of 300 μg per 24 hours) by 54%, and that of clinical neuropathy by 60%. The chief adverse event associated with intensive therapy was a twofold to threefold increase in severe hypoglycemia.[30]

The American Diabetes Association issued a position statement regarding the DCCT:

A primary treatment goal should be blood glucose control at least equal to that achieved in the intensively treated cohort. This goal may not apply to all patients with diabetes and must be based on clinical judgment. Of importance, intensively treated patients had a threefold greater risk of hypoglycemia than did patients in the control group. Because serious hypoglycemia is dangerous, "tight" control goals may have to be sacrificed in people in whom frequent or severe hypoglycemia cannot be avoided by treatment modification.[31]

ACUTE METABOLIC COMPLICATIONS

The acute problems of DKA and HHNK coma arise from events associated with hyperglycemia and insufficient insulin. A problem that may arise from too much insulin or an excessive dose of an OA is hypoglycemia (also referred to as insulin reaction or low blood glucose), which occurs when the level of available blood glucose falls. It is important for the health care provider to be able to distinguish between hyperglycemia and hypoglycemia because hypoglycemia can constitute a serious threat and requires immediate attention. Table 46-20 compares the manifestations, causes, management, and prevention of hyperglycemia and hypoglycemia.

Diabetic Ketoacidosis

DKA, also referred to as diabetic acidosis and diabetic coma, may develop quickly or over several days or weeks. It can be caused by too little insulin accompanied by increased caloric intake, physical or emotional stress, or undiagnosed diabetes. DKA is most likely to occur in type 1 diabetes but may be seen in type 2 in conditions of severe illness or stress when extra demand for insulin cannot be met by the pancreas.

Table 46-20   Comparison of Hyperglycemia and Hypoglycemia

Hyperglycemia	Hypoglycemia	Hyperglycemia	Hypoglycemia
Manifestations*	Blood glucose <50 mg/dl (2.8 mmol/L)	**Treatment**	Immediate ingestion of 5-20 g of simple carbohydrates
Elevated blood glucose†	Cold, clammy skin	Physician's attention	Ingestion of another 5-20 g of simple carbohydrates in 15 min if no relief obtained
Increase in urination	Numbness of fingers, toes, mouth	Continuance of diabetes medication as ordered	Contacting of physician if no relief obtained
Increase in appetite followed by lack of appetite	Rapid heartbeat	Frequent checking of blood and urine specimens and recording of results	Discussion with physician about medication dosage
Weakness, fatigue	Emotional changes	Hourly drinking of fluids	
Blurred vision	Headache		
Headache	Nervousness, tremors	**Preventive Measures**	
Glycosuria	Faintness, dizziness	Taking of prescribed dose of medication at proper time	Taking of prescribed dose of medication at proper time
Nausea and vomiting	Unsteady gait, slurred speech	Accurate administration of insulin/OA	Accurate administration of insulin/OA
Abdominal cramps	Hunger	Maintenance of diet	Ingestion of all ordered diet foods at proper time
Progression to DKA or HHNK	Changes in vision	Maintenance of good personal hygiene	Provision of compensation for exercise
	Seizures, coma	Adherence to sick-day rules when ill	Ability to recognize and know symptoms and treat them immediately
Causes		Checking of blood for glucose as ordered	Carrying of simple carbohydrates
Too much food	Alcohol intake with food	Contacting of physician regarding ketonuria	Education of friends, family, fellow employees about symptoms and treatment
Too little or no diabetes medication	Too little food—delayed, omitted, inadequate intake	Wearing of diabetic identification	Checking blood glucose as ordered
Inactivity	Too much diabetic medication		
Emotional, physical stress	Too much exercise without compensation		
Poor absorption of insulin	Diabetes medication or food taken at wrong time		
	Loss of weight with change in medication		
	Use of β-blockers interfering with recognition of symptoms		

*There is usually a gradual onset of symptoms in hyperglycemia and a rapid onset in hypoglycemia.
†Specific clinical manifestations related to elevated levels of blood glucose vary according to the patient.

When the insulin supply is insufficient, glucose cannot be properly used for cellular energy. In response to cellular starvation, the body releases and breaks down stored fats and protein to provide the needed energy. Free fatty acids from stored triglycerides are released and metabolized in the liver in such large quantities that ketones are formed (ketonemia). Excess ketones alter the pH balance, and acidosis develops. More water is lost as ketones are excreted (ketonuria) in an attempt to balance the pH (Fig. 46-12).

Gluconeogenesis from protein is the last resource used by the body as a compensatory response to provide a cellular energy source. The result is an increase in blood glucose and nitrogen. However, because of the prevailing insulin deficiency, this glucose resource cannot be used and the blood glucose level rises further, adding to the osmotic diuresis. Dehydration and loss of electrolytes, particularly potassium, ensue. The patient's skin becomes dry and loose, and the eyeballs become soft and sunken. Hypotension with a weak, rapid pulse may develop.

Vomiting caused by the acidosis results in more fluid and electrolyte losses. The continual bicarbonate loss adds to the acidosis. Finally, Kussmaul's respirations (rapid, deep breathing associated with dyspnea) begin to remove carbonic acid through the exhalation of carbon dioxide. Acetone is noted on the breath as a sweet, fruity odor.

Renal failure may eventually occur from hypovolemic shock. This failure causes the retention of ketones and glucose, and the acidosis progresses. The patient becomes comatose as a result of the neurologic stressors of dehydration, electrolyte imbalance, and acidosis. If the condition is not treated, death is inevitable.

Collaborative Care

Before the advent of self-monitoring of blood glucose, patients with DKA required hospitalization for treatment. Today, hospitalization may not be required. In instances where fluid and electrolyte imbalance is not severe and self-monitoring of blood glucose can be done by the patient or someone in the household, less severe forms of DKA may be managed on an outpatient basis. However, other factors, such as the presence of fever, nausea and vomiting, or diarrhea; altered mental status; nature of the cause of the ketoacidosis; and availability of frequent communication with the physician (every few hours), must also be considered in this decision.

Regardless of the setting in which it occurs, DKA is a serious condition that proceeds rapidly and must be treated promptly. (See Table 46-21 for the emergency management of a patient with DKA.) Treatment is aimed at immediate administration of insulin, replacement of fluid to correct hypovolemia, and replacement of electrolytes to correct imbalances.

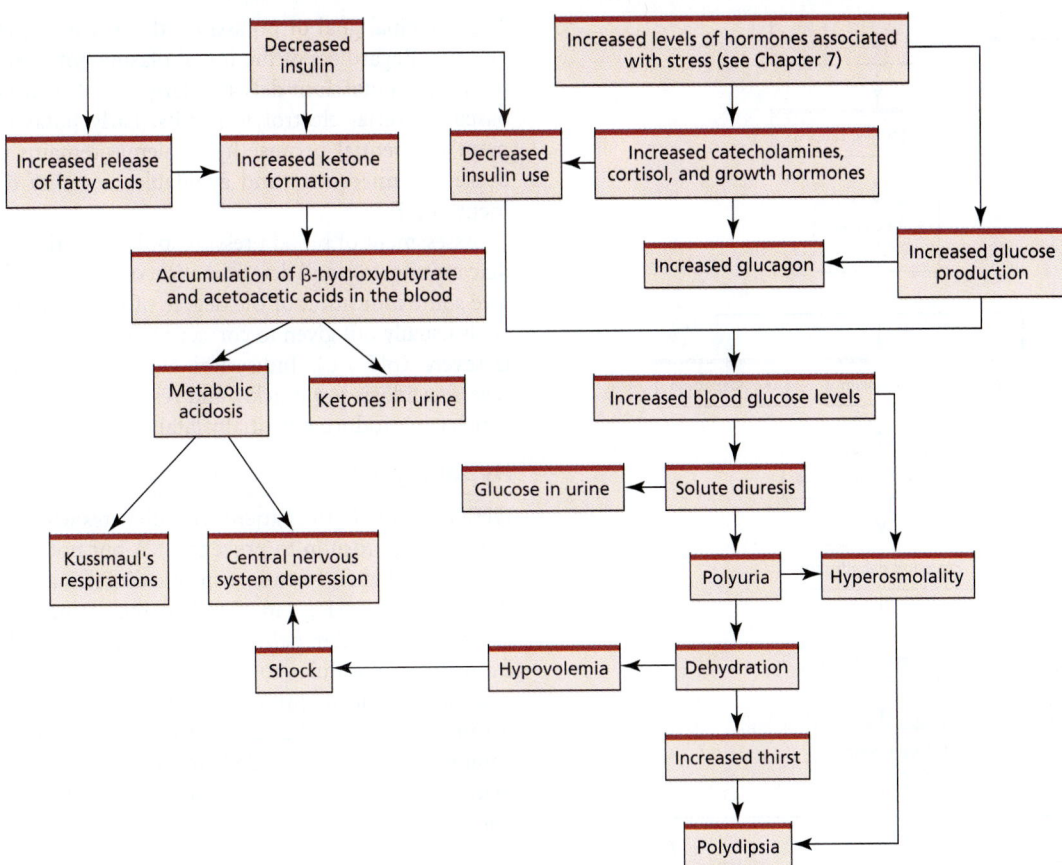

Fig. 46-12   Diabetic ketoacidosis.

✚ **EMERGENCY MANAGEMENT**

Table **46-21**	**Diabetic Ketoacidosis**	
Etiology	**Assessment Findings**	**Interventions**
Undiagnosed diabetes mellitus Inadequate treatment of existing diabetes mellitus Insulin not taken as prescribed Infection Change in diet, insulin, or exercise regimen	▪ Dry mouth ▪ Thirst ▪ Abdominal pain ▪ Nausea and vomiting ▪ Gradually increasing restlessness, confusion, lethargy ▪ Flushed, dry skin ▪ Eyes appear sunken ▪ Breath odor of ketones ▪ Rapid, weak pulse ▪ Labored breathing (Kussmaul's respirations) ▪ Fever ▪ Urinary frequency ▪ Serum glucose >300 mg/dl (16.7 mmol/L) ▪ Glucosuria and ketonuria	**Initial** ▪ Ensure patient airway. ▪ Administer oxygen via nasal cannula or non-rebreather mask. ▪ Establish IV access with large-bore catheter. ▪ Begin fluid resuscitation with normal saline solution 1 L/hr until BP stabilized and urine output 60 ml/hr. ▪ Begin continuous IV insulin (0.1 U/kg/hr). ▪ Identify history of diabetes, time of last food, and time/amount of last insulin injection. **Ongoing Monitoring** ▪ Monitor vital signs, level of consciousness, cardiac rhythm, oxygen saturation, and urine output. ▪ Assess breath sounds for fluid overload. ▪ Monitor serum glucose and serum potassium. ▪ Anticipate possible administration of sodium bicarbonate with severe acidosis (pH <7.0).

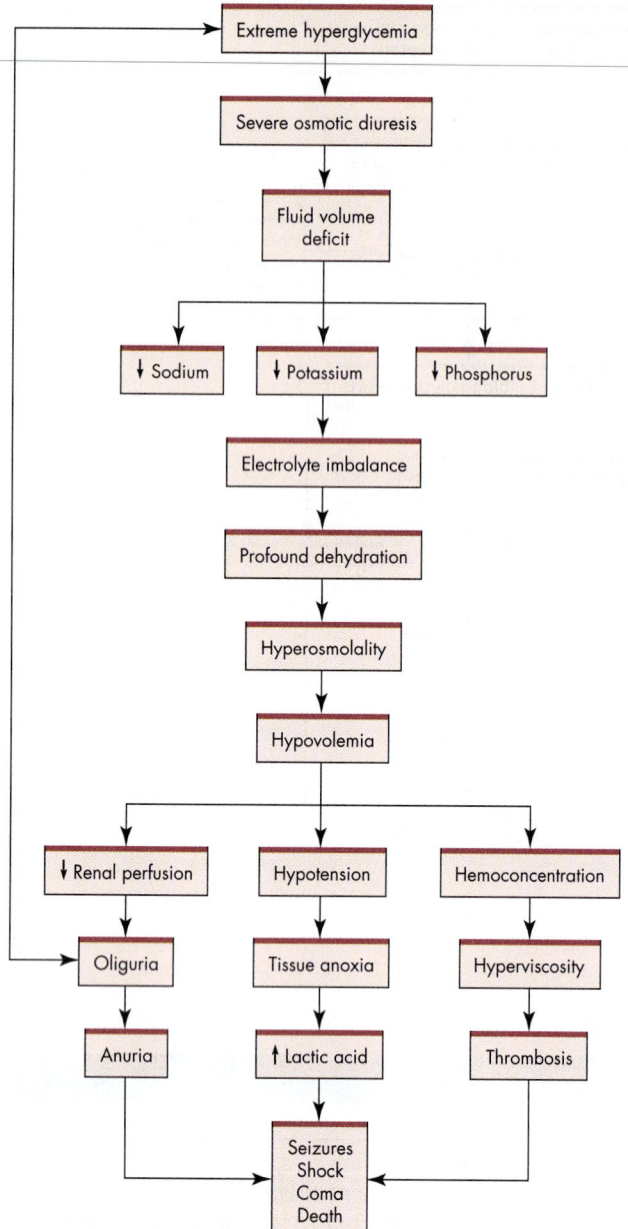

Fig. 46-13 Pathophysiology of hyperglycemic hyperosmolar nonketosis (HHNK).

The preferred treatment for DKA is the low-dose insulin IV infusion method. In this method 5 to 10 U of insulin per hour in normal saline solution is administered until ketoacidosis is reversed.[32] This insulin therapy is continued until a blood glucose level of 250 mg/dl (13.9 mmol/L) is reached. When the blood glucose level reaches 250 mg/dl (13.9 mmol/L), a solution containing 5% to 10% glucose (e.g., 5% dextrose in saline solution) is given to prevent hypoglycemia along with IV or SC insulin as needed to maintain blood glucose control.

Fluid and electrolyte therapy is aimed at replacing extracellular and intracellular water and deficits of sodium, chloride, bicarbonate, potassium, phosphate, magnesium, and nitrogen.

The principal goal of potassium therapy is to prevent hypokalemia. Regardless of the initial plasma potassium value, the total body potassium deficit is large. Treatment decisions are based on serial electrolyte results. Early potassium replacement is essential because hypokalemia remains a significant cause of unnecessary and avoidable mortality during treatment of DKA.

Assessment of blood pressure, pulse, and tissue turgor; cardiac monitoring; and determination of central venous pressure give some indication of the degree of hypovolemia. Bicarbonate is usually not given to correct acidosis unless the condition is severe (pH 7.0). Indiscriminate use of bicarbonate may reverse acidosis too quickly and result in severe hypokalemia, which can produce potentially fatal cardiac arrhythmias.

Hyperglycemic Hyperosmolar Nonketosis

HHNK occurs in the patient with diabetes who is able to produce enough insulin to prevent DKA but not enough to prevent severe hyperglycemia, osmotic diuresis, and extracellular fluid depletion (Fig. 46-13). The increasing hyperglycemia causes intracellular dehydration because of a shift of fluid from the intracellular to the extracellular space. This causes neurologic abnormalities such as somnolence, coma, seizures, hemiparesis, and aphasia. HHNK often occurs in the older adult patient with type 2 diabetes. There is usually a history of inadequate fluid intake, increasing mental depression, and polyuria.

Collaborative Care

HHNK constitutes a medical emergency. This acute complication has a mortality rate greater than 50%.[33] The immediate therapy to reverse this hyperosmolar state consists of the rapid administration of IV solutions. From 6 to 20 L of fluid may have to be given during the first 24 to 48 hours. Depending on the degree of dehydration, either 0.9% or 0.45% sodium chloride is used. Regular insulin is given IV to aid in reducing the hyperglycemia. When blood glucose levels fall to 250 mg/dl (13.9 mmol/L), IV fluids containing glucose should be administered. Electrolytes are monitored and replaced as needed. Vital signs, intake and output, tissue turgor, and cardiac monitoring are assessed to monitor fluid and electrolyte replacement.

The management for both DKA and HHNK is similar except that HHNK requires greater fluid replacement (Table 46-22). Once the patient is stabilized, attempts to detect and correct the underlying precipitating cause should be initiated.

NURSING MANAGEMENT: DIABETIC KETOACIDOSIS AND HYPERGLYCEMIC HYPEROSMOLAR NONKETOSIS

When hospitalized, the patient is closely monitored with appropriate blood and urine tests. The nurse is responsible for monitoring blood glucose and urine for output and ketones, as well as using laboratory data to direct care.

Areas that need monitoring are administration of IV fluids to correct dehydration, administration of insulin therapy to reduce blood glucose and serum acetone, administration of

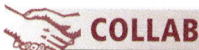

COLLABORATIVE CARE

Table 46-22	**Diabetic Ketoacidosis and Hyperglycemic Hyperosmolar Nonketosis**

Diagnostic
 Blood work, including immediate blood glucose, complete blood count, ketones, pH, electrolytes, blood urea nitrogen, arterial blood gases
 Urinalysis, including specific gravity, pH, sugar, acetone

Collaborative Therapy
 Administration of rapid-acting insulin IV
 Administration of IV fluids
 Electrolyte replacement
 Assessment of mental status
 Recording of intake and output
 Central venous pressure monitoring (if indicated)
 Assessment of blood glucose level
 Assessment of blood and urine for ketones
 Electrocardiogram monitoring

electrolytes to correct electrolyte imbalance, assessment of renal status, assessment of the cardiopulmonary status related to hydration and electrolyte levels, and monitoring of the level of consciousness.

The nurse must also monitor the signs of potassium imbalance resulting from hypoinsulinemia and osmotic diuresis (see Chapter 15). When treatment for hyperglycemia is begun with insulin, potassium loss may initially be increased. As insulin is replaced, potassium moves back into the cell. This movement of potassium into and out of extracellular fluid influences cardiac functioning. For this reason, cardiac monitoring is a useful aid in detecting hyperkalemia and hypokalemia because characteristic changes indicating potassium excess or deficit are observable on electrocardiographic readings. Vital signs should be assessed often to determine the presence of fever, hypo-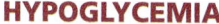volemic shock, tachycardia, and Kussmaul's breathing.

HYPOGLYCEMIA

Hypoglycemia, or low blood glucose, occurs when proportionately too much insulin is in the blood for the available glucose. This causes the blood glucose level to drop to less than 50 mg/dl (2.8 mmol/L). This type of hypoglycemia is different from the condition commonly termed *reactive hypoglycemia* (see p. 1402).

Hypoglycemic symptoms may also occur when a very high blood glucose level falls too rapidly (e.g., a blood glucose level of 300 mg/dl [16.7 mmol/L] falling quickly to 180 mg/dl [10 mmol/L]). Although the blood glucose level is above normal by definition and measurement, the sudden metabolic shift can evoke hypoglycemic symptoms. This type of situation can be induced by too vigorous management of hyperglycemia with insulin.

The balance between blood glucose and insulin can be disrupted by the administration of too much insulin, the ingestion

of too little food, unusual amounts of exercise, and delayed eating. Insulin reactions can occur at any time, but most reactions occur when the GLA is at its peak of action or when the patient's daily routine is disrupted without adequate adjustments in diet, medications, and activity. Although hypoglycemia is more common with insulin therapy, it can occur with OAs and may be severe and persist for an extended time as a result of the longer half-lives of active metabolites of some OAs.

A decrease in available blood glucose can result in sympathetic nervous system activation with the release of epinephrine. This results in manifestations of cold sweats, weakness, trembling, nervousness, irritability, pallor, and increased heart rate. The clinical manifestations of hypoglycemia vary with each patient. The brain depends on a constant supply of glucose because it is unable to store glucose or glycogen. If that supply is inadequate, the patient will experience confusion, fatigue, and abnormal behavior that can resemble alcohol intoxication.

In recent years the physiology of glucose recovery has been shown to depend on glucagon and epinephrine. In type 1 diabetes, secretion and use of one or both of these substances may be impaired. As a result, some type 1 patients do not have the early warning symptoms produced by epinephrine. Rather, they have neuroglycopenia, that is, the more advanced symptoms of cerebral glucose deficit. The symptoms of this condition are irritability, irrational behavior, dizziness, tremors, and loss of consciousness. This may result from the development of autonomic neuropathy or from treatment with beta-adrenergic blocking agents. These patients must be managed with intensive education and instruction in the prevention of hypoglycemia.

NURSING AND COLLABORATIVE MANAGEMENT: HYPOGLYCEMIA

The preferred treatment of hypoglycemia is prevention. However, if hypoglycemia occurs, the patient should be able to reverse the situation before medical assistance is required. The patient's ability to do this depends on the state of alertness and ability to swallow and the availability of a quick-acting carbohydrate source.

At the first sign of hypoglycemia the patient should ingest 5 to 20 g of a simple (fast-acting) carbohydrate, such as 120 to 180 ml of orange juice, 180 to 240 ml of regular soft drink, two packets of sugar, or five or six hard candies. Overtreatment with large quantities of quick-acting carbohydrates such as a whole candy bar should be avoided.

If the symptoms are still present after 10 to 15 minutes, ingestion of 5 to 20 g of carbohydrate should be repeated.[34] Once the symptoms have improved, the patient should eat a longer-lasting carbohydrate such as bread or milk to prevent symptoms from recurring. Commercial products such as gels or tablets containing specific amounts of quick-acting carbohydrate are convenient for carrying in a purse or pocket to be used in such situations. High-fat foods and high-protein foods should not be used initially to correct hypoglycemia. These

COLLABORATIVE CARE

Table 46-23 Hypoglycemia

Diagnostic
Stat blood glucose
History (if possible)

Collaborative Therapy
Determination of cause of hypoglycemia (after correction of condition)

Conscious Patient
Administration of 5-20 g of quick-acting CHO
(e.g., 6-8 oz of regular soda, 1 tbs syrup or honey, 4 tsp jelly, 4-6 oz orange juice, 8 oz milk, 2½ tsp sugar, commercial dextrose products [per label instructions])
Repetition of treatment in 15 min (if no improvement)
Administration of additional food of longer-acting CHO (e.g., slice of bread, crackers) after subsiding of symptoms
Immediate notification of health care provider or emergency service (if patient outside hospital) if symptoms not subsiding after 2 to 3 administrations of quick-acting CHO

Worsening Symptoms or Unconscious Patient
SC or IM injection of 1 mg glucagon
Administration of 50 ml 50% IV glucose

CHO, carbohydrate.

Table 46-24 Mechanisms of Macrovascular Disease in Diabetes

Cellular Mechanisms
Arterial endothelial cell injury (sorbitol accumulation, hypoxia, hypertension, immune complexes)
Foam cell activation (smooth muscle cell migration, monocyte/macrophage activation)

Hemostatic Mechanisms
Platelet dysfunction (aggregation, thromboxane production, growth factor release)
Clotting factor abnormalities (raised fibrinogen, factor VII, factor VIII, reduced fibrinolysis)
Cell-cell forces (RBC rigidity)

Lipoprotein Abnormalities
Hypertriglyceridemia (increased VLDL, remnant particles, reduced lipoprotein lipase activity, reduced HDL in type 2 diabetes mellitus)
Hypercholesterolemia (increased LDL in type 2 diabetes mellitus)
Apolipoprotein abnormalities (e.g., glycosylation)

Other Mechanisms
Chronic renal disease secondary to diabetes (raised VLDL, LDL; lowered HDL; hypertension)
Increased arterial wall proteoglycans (trapping of lipoproteins, local cell activation)
Abnormalities of collagen, fibronectin (synthesis, glycosylation)
Insulin-induced lipogenesis, esterification
Intramural coronary vascular (macro and micro) disease

HDL, high density lipoproteins; *LDL*, low density lipoproteins; *VLDL*, very low density lipoproteins.

food sources are metabolized too slowly to be effective as immediate treatment.

If there is little discernible improvement in the patient's condition after two to three doses of 5 to 20 g of simple carbohydrate within 30 minutes or if the patient is not alert enough to swallow, 1 mg of glucagon may be administered with the same technique used for an insulin injection, although an IM injection in a site such as the deltoid will result in a quicker response. Glucagon stimulates a strong hepatic response to convert glycogen to glucose and therefore make glucose rapidly available. Once the patient is receiving medical care, a concentrated glucose solution may also be administered slowly IV until the patient regains consciousness. Blood glucose level must be carefully monitored during the treatment. (See Table 46-23 for a summary of collaborative care of hypoglycemia.)

With effective treatment, hypoglycemia can be quickly reversed. Once the acute hypoglycemia has been reversed, the nurse should explore with the patient the reasons why the situation developed. This assessment may indicate the need for additional education of the patient and the family to avoid future episodes of hypoglycemia. The danger of hypoglycemic reactions must be stressed because memory and learning impairment can result from repeated episodes of severe hypoglycemia.

DKA, HHNK, and hypoglycemia constitute potentially life-threatening situations and may be frightening to the patient and the family. The nurse should attempt to keep the family members informed about the patient's progress to relieve their anxiety. The nurse's calm, competent manner in caring for the patient can provide assurance to the acutely ill patient and the family.

CHRONIC COMPLICATIONS
Angiopathy

Angiopathy, or blood vessel disease, is estimated to account for the majority of deaths among patients with diabetes. Many factors, including genetics, diet, and lipid metabolism, are being investigated for their role in the development of angiopathy. These chronic blood vessel dysfunctions are divided into two categories: macroangiopathy and microangiopathy.

Macroangiopathy. Macroangiopathy, or disease of large and medium-sized blood vessels, is essentially atherosclerosis and arteriosclerotic vascular disease characterized by a higher frequency and earlier onset than in the nondiabetic population. The degree of vascular damage appears to be related to the duration of the diabetes and not to its severity. Although atherosclerotic plaque formation is believed to have a genetic origin, its development seems to be promoted by the altered lipid metabolism common to diabetes (Table 46-24). Tight glucose control may help delay the atherosclerotic process.[30]

The complications resulting from macroangiopathy are cerebrovascular, cardiovascular, and peripheral vascular disease. Although genetic makeup cannot be altered, a patient with diabetes can diminish other risk factors associated with macroangiopathy, such as obesity, smoking, hypertension, high fat intake, and low activity level.

In addition to the association of type 1 and type 2 diabetes with ischemic heart disease, some have suggested that insulin resistance may be implicated in the pathogenesis of essential

PATIENT TEACHING GUIDE

Table 46-25   Foot Care

1. Wash feet daily with a mild soap and *warm* water. Test water temperature with hands first.
2. Pat feet dry gently, especially between toes.
3. Examine feet daily for cuts, blisters, swelling, and red, tender areas. Do not depend on feeling sores. If eyesight is poor, have others inspect feet.
4. Use lanolin on feet to prevent skin from drying and cracking. Do not apply between toes.
5. Use mild foot powder on sweaty feet. Powder feet only, not shoes.
6. Do not use commercial remedies to remove calluses or corns.
7. Cleanse cuts with *warm* water and mild soap, covering with clean dressing. Do not use iodine, rubbing alcohol, or strong adhesives.
8. Report skin infections or nonhealing sores to health care provider immediately.
9. Cut toenails even with rounded contour of toes. Do not cut down corners. Soak nails before cutting.
10. Separate overlapping toes with cotton or lamb's wool.
11. Break in new shoes slowly. Avoid open-toe, open-heel, and high-heel shoes. Leather shoes are preferred to plastic ones. Wear slippers with soles. Do not go barefoot. Shake out shoes before use.
12. Wear clean, absorbent (cotton or wool) socks or stockings that have not been mended. Colored socks must be colorfast.
13. Do not wear clothing that leaves impressions, hindering circulation.
14. Do not use hot water bottles or heating pads to warm feet. Wear socks for warmth.
15. Guard against frostbite.
16. Exercise feet daily either by walking or by flexing and extending feet in suspended position. Avoid prolonged sitting, standing, and crossing of legs.

Table 46-26   Types of Diabetic Retinopathy

Type	Pathologic Alteration
Background	Microvasculature of retina of eye is damaged. Capillaries become damaged, resulting in development of microaneurysms (seen as tiny red dots on retina).
Preproliferative	Possible progression from background retinopathy represents further destruction of retinal capillaries and development of capillary dropout.
Proliferative	Abnormal blood vessels (neovascularization) grow on surface of retina. Vessels can grow into chamber of vitreous surface and can hemorrhage, filling vitreous chamber with blood.

Modified from Peragallo V: *A core curriculum for diabetes education,* Chicago, 1993, American Association of Diabetes Educators.

hypertension and dyslipidemia. The term *syndrome X* is applied to the clinical association of insulin resistance, hypertension, and increased very-low-density lipoprotein (VLDL) and decreased high-density lipoprotein (HDL) cholesterol concentrations. The role of insulin resistance in the pathogenesis of cardiovascular disease is not well understood; in the United States, insulin resistance probably combines with dyslipidemia in contributing to greater risk of cardiovascular disease in patients with diabetes mellitus.[35]

Microangiopathy. Microangiopathy, or disease of the small blood vessels, is different from macroangiopathy in that it is specific to diabetes. Microangiopathy is the result of thickening of the basement membranes in the capillaries and arterioles, a highly characteristic concomitant of long-term diabetes mellitus. Although microangiopathy can be found throughout the body, the areas most noticeably affected are the eyes (retinopathy), the kidneys (nephropathy), and the skin (dermopathy). Thickening of the basement membrane has been found in some persons with diabetes before or at the time of diagnosis or before the onset of symptoms of diabetes mellitus. However, clinical manifestations usually do not appear until 15 to 20 years after the onset of diabetes.[36] However, Native-Americans with diabetes mellitus have an earlier onset of microangiopathy relative to other groups.

Peripheral Vascular Disease

Peripheral vascular disease (PVD) is a combination of microangiopathy and macroangiopathy, as well as clotting abnormalities. The legs and feet are most often affected in diabetes mellitus, and associated problems account for 20% of hospitalizations of patients with diabetes. The sequelae of PVD can lead to infection, gangrene, and amputation. Signs of PVD include intermittent claudication, pain at rest, cold feet, loss of hair, delayed capillary filling, and dependent rubor. The disease is diagnosed by history, Doppler findings, and angiography. Management centers on control or reduction of risk factors, particularly smoking, high cholesterol intake, and hypertension. Antibiotics are necessary when infection is present. If the infection cannot be reversed with antibiotic therapy, amputation may be necessary. Proper care of the feet is crucial for the patient with PVD; guidelines for patient teaching regarding foot care are listed in Table 46-25. Approximately 6% of the U.S. diabetic population (14 million) experience lower-extremity amputation because of diabetic foot ulcers.[37]

Diabetic Retinopathy

The term *retinopathy* literally means disease of the retina; however, diabetic retinopathy refers to the microangiopathic process seen in a patient with diabetes. After 10 years with diabetes mellitus, 50% of patients demonstrate diabetic retinopathy; after 15 years, approximately 80% of patients have some retinal disease.

The primary problems in diabetic retinopathy are microvascular damage and occlusion of retinal capillaries. Retinopathy can be classified as background retinopathy, preproliferative retinopathy, and proliferative retinopathy. The types are outlined in Table 46-26. In background retinopathy, the most common form, partial occlusion of the small blood vessels in the retina causes the development of microaneurysms in the capillary walls. These microaneurysms are so weak that capillary fluid leaks out, causing retinal edema and eventually hard exudates or intraretinal hemorrhages. Vision may be affected if the macula is involved. Preproliferative retinopathy is distinct from background retinopathy and indicates further destruction of retinal capillaries.

Proliferative retinopathy, the most severe form, involves the retina and the vitreous. When retinal capillaries become occluded, new blood vessels are formed (neovascularization) to supply the retina with blood. These new vessels hemorrhage easily and may produce vitreous contraction. The vessels are torn and bleed into the vitreous cavity, preventing light from reaching the retina. The patient sees black or red spots or lines. If these new blood vessels pull the retina while the vitreous contracts, causing a tear, partial or complete retinal detachment will occur. If the macula is involved, vision is lost. Without treatment, more than half of patients with proliferative diabetic retinopathy will be blind.[38]

The earliest and most treatable stages of diabetic retinopathy often produce no visual symptoms. Because of this, the patient with diabetes must have regular examinations by an ophthalmologist for early detection and appropriate treatment. Careful ophthalmoscopic and slit lamp microscopic retinal examinations are the most important diagnostic tools to identify diabetic fundus changes. Fluorescein angiography demonstrates dye leakage from abnormal retinal and subretinal vessels and identifies retinal areas amenable to focal laser treatment. If the vitreous humor is opaque in advanced disease, ultrasonography may be useful to identify retinal detachments.

The two most common forms of treatment of diabetic retinopathy are early photocoagulation of the retina and vitrectomy. Photocoagulation by laser converts light energy into heat and coagulates the tissue in the area where the light is directed. It is particularly useful with neovascularization because the laser obliterates new vessels, stopping the hemorrhage. Panretinal photocoagulation (PRP) is a scatter technique in which thousands of laser burns are placed in the retinal periphery. PRP is generally recommended when there is moderate to severe neovascularization. PRP destroys the hypoxic retina, reducing its oxygen requirement and reducing the stimulus for new blood vessel growth.

Topical anesthetic is generally adequate for laser treatment. Pain is usually transient but occasionally requires retrobulbar anesthesia. The patient may experience some loss of peripheral or central vision, and the dark adaptation may be affected.

Photocoagulation is not possible when there is significant vitreous or retinal hemorrhage. In these cases, vitrectomy is useful. *Vitrectomy* is the aspiration of blood, membrane, and fibers from the inside of the eye through a small incision just behind the cornea. Vitrectomy is indicated when there is vitreal hemorrhage that does not clear or when the hemorrhage is obscuring the retina in the patient who needs photocoagulation. This type of surgery is also helpful in patients with traction retinal detachments. Vitrectomy is an intraocular procedure, and possible complications include the risk of further vitreous hemorrhage, cataract formation, glaucoma, and infec-

tion. Despite the risks, vitrectomy has been an important development in treating the ocular complications of diabetes mellitus.

Persons with diabetes are also prone to other visual problems. Glaucoma occurs as a result of the occlusion of the outflow channels secondary to neovascularization. This type of glaucoma is difficult to treat and often results in blindness. Cataracts occur with increasing frequency in the patient with diabetes. Although the process is similar to that of senile cataracts, it occurs at an earlier age in the patient with diabetes. Diabetic retinopathy may occur concurrently with nephropathy and parallel its progression. Although the vast majority of diabetic patients have some degree of retinopathy, nephropathy develops in only 35% to 45% of patients with type 1 diabetes.[36]

Nephropathy

Diabetic nephropathy is now the leading cause of end-stage renal disease (ESRD) in the United States.[38] Mild proteinuria develops in 70% of persons with diabetes mellitus and may progress to more serious involvement and ESRD. This occurs as a result of microvascular abnormalities associated with diabetes mellitus, but these processes are not clearly understood.

Microangiopathy in the kidneys causes diffuse and nodular glomerulosclerosis. Diffuse glomerulosclerosis affects the basement membranes of all glomerular capillaries, usually in both kidneys. The basement membranes become thickened and leaky. Sclerosis of glomerular vascular tufts leads to progressive renal failure. In nodular glomerulosclerosis (Kimmelstiel-Wilson lesions), nodules develop in the glomeruli. In advanced cases most glomeruli are involved. In more than 70% of patients, the course of diabetic nephropathy is complicated by the presence of hypertension. The monitoring and treatment of hypertension are important parts of diabetes management and are believed to be significant factors in controlling the progression of nephropathy. (See Chapter 31 for a discussion of hypertension and Chapter 44 for a discussion of acute and chronic renal failure.) The majority of type 1 diabetes patients with diabetic nephropathy die of cardiovascular disease. The risk of cardiovascular disease is 30 to 40 times higher in patients with nephropathy than in those diabetics who did not develop renal diseases.[38]

ESRD requires treatment by either dialysis or kidney transplantation. A patient in the later stages of nephropathy may require an adjustment in insulin and OAs because of a loss of the insulin-degradative function of the kidneys and an abnormal peripheral insulin response.

Neuropathy

Neuropathy is probably one of the most common complications of diabetes in adults. However, its cause is unclear. Mononeuropathic conditions (i.e., single nerve branch involvement) are theorized to develop from microangiopathy, whereas the more diffuse neuropathic conditions are attributed to metabolic defects and the accumulation of by-products in the nerve tissue. The result is reduced nerve conduction and demyelinization. Neuropathy can precede, accompany, or follow the diagnosis of diabetes.

The two major categories of diabetic neuropathy are neuropathic conditions of the peripheral nervous system, includ-

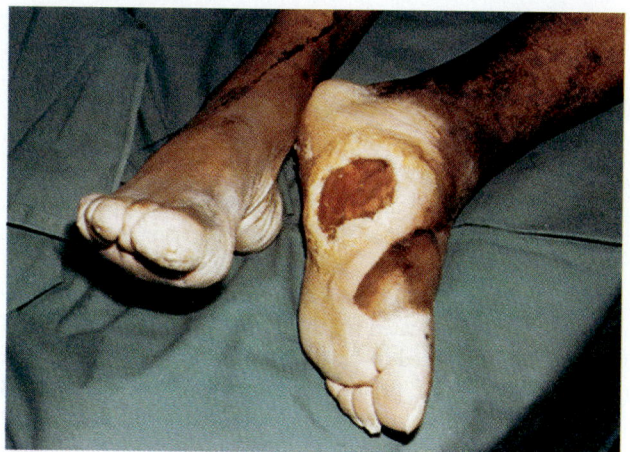

Fig. 46-14   Neuropathy: neurotrophic ulceration.

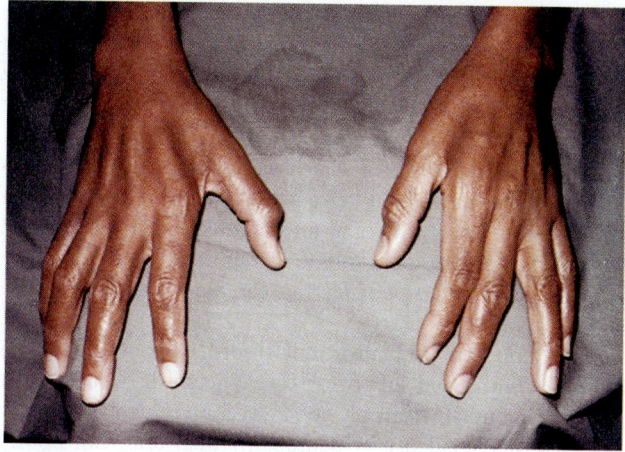

Fig. 46-15   Diabetic neuropathy: muscle atrophy.

ing symmetric peripheral polyneuropathy, mononeuropathic disorders, and diabetic amyotrophy; and autonomic neuropathic conditions, including cardiovascular abnormalities, GI abnormalities, urinary bladder abnormalities, and sexual dysfunction. Symmetric peripheral polyneuropathy affects all the extremities but most often affects the legs. Symmetric peripheral polyneuropathy is usually bilateral and symmetric and is thought to be due to both metabolic and vascular mechanisms. The patient has pain and paresthesias. The pain, described as burning, cramping, crushing, or tearing, is usually worse at night and may occur only at that time. It may be relieved by walking.

The paresthesias are associated with tingling, burning, and itching sensations. Complete or partial loss of sensitivity to touch and temperature is common. Foot injury and ulcerations can occur without the patient ever having pain (Fig. 46-14). The patient may report a feeling of walking on pillows or numb feet. At times the skin becomes so sensitive (hyperesthesia) that even light pressure from bed sheets cannot be tolerated. Neuropathy in the hands causes atrophy of the small muscles, limiting fine movement (Fig. 46-15).

Mononeuropathic conditions tend to occur unilaterally and are characterized by a sudden onset of pain with weakness or paralysis. Although the extremities are most often affected, cranial nerves III, IV, and VI may be involved.

No direct treatment for neuropathy is known. Treatment is aimed at relief of symptoms, particularly pain. Medications commonly used include tricyclic antidepressants (e.g., amitriptyline [Elavil]) and topical creams (e.g., capsaicin [Zostrix]). Better glucose control may also aid in the reduction of symptoms. As nerve conduction improves, the pain may initially increase before relief is noted.

Neuropathy affecting the autonomic nervous system may produce nocturnal diarrhea, postural hypotension, impotence, and neurogenic bladder. Nocturnal diarrhea is not associated with abdominal cramping. It affects few persons with diabetes and does not disturb diabetic control. *Gastroparesis diabeticorum* is delayed gastric emptying that can produce anorexia, nausea, vomiting, and persistent feelings of fullness. Gastroparesis can trigger hypoglycemia by delaying food absorption. Metoclopramide (Reglan), a dopamine

receptor antagonist and serotonin antagonist, stimulates esophageal and gastric emptying and has been used in the treatment of gastroparesis. Other drugs that are sometimes useful to increase intestinal motility are domperidone (Motillium) and cisapride (Propulsid).

The cardiovascular abnormalities associated with autonomic neuropathy are postural hypotension, resting tachycardia, and painless myocardial infarction. A patient with postural hypotension should be instructed to change from a lying or sitting position slowly.

Reports of the prevalence of erectile dysfunction (ED) among men with diabetes vary from 30% to 60%. ED associated with diabetes mellitus is believed to result from damage to the sacral parasympathetic nerves. Determining whether ED is of organic or psychologic origin is an important part of the assessment. Organic ED usually develops insidiously, whereas psychologic ED is often acute in onset. Measuring nocturnal penile tumescence (extent and duration of penile erection) during rapid eye movement phases of sleep is one assessment method to establish the presence of organic disease. Nonsurgical devices and surgical prosthetic implantations have been developed that make vaginal penetration possible. Decreased libido is a problem with some women with diabetes. Monilial and nonspecific vaginitis are also common. Organic ED or sexual dysfunctioning in either the male or the female patient requires sensitive therapeutic counseling for both the patient and the patient's partner. (See Chapter 52 for a further discussion of erectile dysfunction.)

A neurogenic bladder develops as sensation in the inner bladder wall decreases, causing urinary retention. A patient with retention has infrequent voiding, difficulty in voiding, and a weak stream of urine. Emptying the bladder every 3 hours in a sitting position helps prevent stasis and subsequent infection. Tightening the abdominal muscles during voiding and using the Credé maneuver (mild massage downward over the lower abdomen and bladder) may also help with complete bladder emptying. Cholinergic drugs such as bethanechol (Urecholine) may be used. The patient may also have to learn self-catheterization (see Chapter 43).

Neuropathic arthropathy, or Charcot's joints, results in ankle and foot changes that ultimately lead to joint dysfunction and footdrop. These changes occur gradually and promote an abnormal distribution of weight over the foot. New pressure points emerge, and neuropathic ulcers often develop. The ulcers resemble a "BB-shot" or "punched-out" wound and are initially painless when peripheral polyneuropathy is present. Infection is a danger and may penetrate to underlying bone tissue, necessitating the long-term use of antibiotics and weeks of avoidance of weight bearing on the affected limb. The ideal treatment is prevention. Table 46-25 outlines rules for foot care that can reduce the patient's risk for infection and possible amputation.

The treatment of neuropathic disorders involves effective diabetic control and supportive care. There is no known cure. The patient under relatively good glycemic control appears to have a lower incidence of neuropathy than one with poorly controlled disease. However, neuropathy can occur despite good control.

Skin Changes

Skin disorders such as diabetic dermopathy and *necrobiosis lipoidica diabeticorum* are attributed to microangiopathy. Shin spots are brown spots located on the anterior surfaces of the lower extremities. They are harmless and painless and initially measure less than 1 cm in diameter. Necrobiosis lipoidica diabeticorum, which is believed to be the result of trauma, consists of lesions similar to those of diabetic dermopathy but is more likely to be associated with ulcerations and necrosis. The lesions are reddish yellow and atrophic. Skin grafts are sometimes required because of the slow healing of the lesions. Necrobiosis lipoidica diabeticorum is present most often in women with type 1 diabetes and may precede the onset of overt diabetes.

Infection

A patient with diabetes is more susceptible to infections than other patients. The mechanisms for this phenomenon include a defect in the mobilization of inflammatory cells and an impairment of white blood cells in the process of phagocytosis. Recurring or persistent infections such as *Candida albicans,* as well as boils and furuncles in the undiagnosed patient, often lead the health care provider to suspect diabetes. Loss of sensation (neuropathy) may delay the detection of an infection.

Persistent glycosuria may encourage bladder infections, especially in a neurogenic bladder. Decreased circulation as a result of angiopathy can prevent or delay the healing process. Protein waste during hyperglycemia and DKA is also responsible for poor healing. Antibiotic therapy has prevented infection from being a major cause of death in diabetic patients. The treatment of infections must be prompt and vigorous.

■ GERONTOLOGIC CONSIDERATIONS ■

Diabetes Mellitus

The prevalence of diabetes is about 18% in persons between age 65 and 74. The increased blood glucose levels and decreased glucose tolerance make diabetes more difficult to diagnose in the older adult. Aging is also associated with an increase in the prevalence of other factors that tend to impair carbohydrate metabolism and are more likely to be treated with medications that impair insulin action (e.g., corticosteroids, antihypertensives, phenothiazines). The clinical manifestations of renal, retinal, and neurologic complications of diabetes generally take 10 to 20 years to develop. Attempts to normalize glucose are associated with an increased frequency of hypoglycemia. Therefore in the older patient there is less reason for treatment of hyperglycemia based on the prevention of these specific diabetic complications. Whereas it is generally agreed that treatment is usually indicated for this patient, the goals for control probably do not need to be as near normoglycemia as in the younger population. Because of the physiologic changes that occur with aging, the therapeutic outcome for the older adult with diabetes who receives OAs may be altered. The second-generation OAs such as glyburide and glipizide have increased potency but appear to have fewer side effects and fewer drug interaction problems when compared with the first-generation agents. Insulin therapy may be instituted if OAs fail. However, for accurate insulin administration, it is important to recognize the limitations among some individuals related to manual dexterity and visual acuity.

The patient education issues for the older patient that should be addressed are self-care in terms of vision, mobility, mental status, functional ability, and finances; the effect of multiple medications; eating habits; undetected hypoglycemia; and quality of life issues.

Patient teaching should be based on the individual's needs, using a slower pace with simple printed or audio materials. It is important to include family or a support person in the teaching.

REACTIVE HYPOGLYCEMIA

Many people claim to have reactive hypoglycemia. However, reactive hypoglycemia occurs infrequently in persons other than those with diabetes treated with insulin or sulfonylureas. Reactive hypoglycemia results from an uncompensated reduction in blood glucose level. The symptoms are similar to those of the hypoglycemia of diabetes: sudden onset of hunger, diaphoresis, tremulousness, weakness, nervousness (adrenergic) and headache, confusion, slurred speech, behavioral aberrations, focal neurologic signs, and coma (neuroglycopenic). These symptoms mimic the effects of anxiety and stress and are often misinterpreted.

Idiopathic hypoglycemia (i.e., hypoglycemia of no known cause) is particularly difficult to document. Various physiologic disturbances have been suggested, but subtle abnormalities of insulin response to food (particularly excessive or delayed secretion) seem the most likely possibilities. A definite diagnosis can be made only if the plasma glucose concentration is less than 50 mg/dl (2.8 mmol/L) accompanied by symptoms of hypoglycemia and relieved by eating. The usual treatment is a diet balanced in protein and carbohydrate with frequent small meals.

If a patient claims to have reactive hypoglycemia, it should be determined whether this has been medically diagnosed or self-diagnosed. Because of the similarity to symptoms of anxiety reaction, careful assessment of the symptoms and the treatment is important.

CRITICAL THINKING EXERCISES

CASE STUDY

Diabetic Ketoacidosis

Patient Profile

John, a 34-year-old man, was admitted to the emergency department after he was found comatose in his apartment by his wife.

Subjective Data (provided by wife)

- Was diagnosed with diabetes mellitus 12 months ago
- Was taking 48 U of insulin daily: 12 U of regular insulin plus 20 U of NPH before breakfast, 8 U of regular insulin before dinner, and 8 U of NPH at bedtime
- Has history of flu for 1 week with vomiting and anorexia
- Stopped taking insulin 2 days ago when he was unable to eat

Objective Data

Physical Examination
- Breathing is deep and rapid
- Acetone smell on breath
- Skin flushed and dry

Diagnostic Studies
- Blood glucose level of 730 mg/dl (40.5 mmol/L)
- Urine acetone of 3+ with Acetest tablets
- Blood pH of 7.26

Critical Thinking Questions

1. Briefly explain the pathophysiology of the development of diabetic ketoacidosis (DKA) in this patient.
2. What clinical manifestations of DKA does this patient exhibit?
3. What factors precipitated this patient's DKA?
4. What distinguishes this case history from one of hyperglycemic hyperosmolar nonketosis or hypoglycemia?
5. What educational needs must be met before the patient's discharge?
6. What role does John's wife play in the management of his diabetes?
7. Based on the assessment data presented, write one or more appropriate nursing diagnoses. Are there any collaborative problems?

NURSING RESEARCH ISSUES

1. What degree of pain does the patient associate with capillary blood glucose monitoring?
2. How often does the patient make phone contact with a diabetes patient educator when this service is available free as compared with when there is a charge?
3. Is the patient willing to maintain tight glycemic control in the present to prevent chronic complications from diabetes in the future?
4. Does the frequency of review of major diabetes education issues affect the frequency of occurrence of acute complications of diabetes?

REVIEW QUESTIONS

The number of the question corresponds to the same-numbered objective at the beginning of the chapter.

1. The polydipsia and polyuria related to diabetes are caused primarily by
   a. the release of ketones from cells during fat metabolism.
   b. fluid shifts resulting from the osmotic effect of hyperglycemia.
   c. damage to the kidneys from exposure to high levels of glucose.
   d. changes in RBCs resulting from attachment of excessive glucose to hemoglobin.

2. In planning care for a patient with type 2 diabetes admitted to the hospital with pneumonia, the nurse recognizes that the patient
   a. must receive insulin therapy to prevent the development of ketoacidosis.
   b. has islet cell antibodies that have destroyed the ability of the pancreas to produce insulin.
   c. has minimal or absent endogenous insulin secretion and requires daily insulin injections.
   d. may have sufficient endogenous insulin to prevent ketosis but is at risk for development of hyperosmolar coma.

3. A diabetic patient has a serum glucose level of 824 mg/dl (45.7 mmol/L) and is somnolent and unresponsive. Following assessment of the patient the nurse suspects diabetic ketoacidosis rather than hyperglycemic hyperosmolar nonketosis based on the finding of
   a. polyuria.
   b. severe dehydration.
   c. rapid, deep respirations.
   d. decreased serum potassium.

4. A diabetic patient takes a combination of regular and NPH insulin twice a day for glucose control. The nurse teaches the patient to be alert for hypoglycemia
   a. immediately after breakfast and dinner.
   b. immediately after lunch and dinner.
   c. in the late afternoon and at bedtime.
   d. immediately after dinner and at bedtime.

5. The nurse assists the patient with dietary management of diabetes with the knowledge that a diabetic diet is designed
   a. to be used only for type 1 diabetes.
   b. for use during periods of high stress.
   c. to normalize blood glucose by elimination of sugar.
   d. to help normalize blood glucose through a balanced diet.

6. In teaching a newly diagnosed type 1 diabetic "survival skills," the nurse includes information about
   a. weight-loss measures.
   b. elimination of sugar from diet.
   c. need to reduce physical activity.
   d. capillary blood glucose monitoring.

7. An appropriate instruction for the patient with diabetes related to care of the feet is
   a. use heat to increase blood supply.
   b. avoid softening lotions and creams.
   c. inspect all surfaces of the feet daily.
   d. use iodine to disinfect cuts and abrasions.

References

1. Centers for Disease Control and Prevention: *National diabetes fact sheet—1998*, Atlanta, Ga, 1998.
2. Report from the American Diabetes Association: Economic consequences of diabetes mellitus in the US in 1997, *Diabetes Care* 21:246, 1998.
3. Davidson MB: *Diabetes mellitus: diagnosis and treatment*, ed 4, Philadelphia, 1998, Saunders.
4. DeFronzo R: Pathogenesis of type 2 diabetes: metabolic and molecular implications for identifying diabetes genes, *Diabetes Rev* 5:177, 1997.
5. Report of the expert committee on the diagnosis and classification of diabetes mellitus, *Diabetes Care* 21(suppl 1):55, 1998.
6. Peakman M and others: Persistant activation on CD8+ T-cells characterizes prediabetic twins, *Diabetes Care* 19:1177, 1996.
7. Dorman JS and others: *Risk factors for insulin dependent diabetes, diabetes in America*, NIH pub no 95-1468, 1995, National Diabetes Data Group, Bethesda, MD.
8. Leahy JL: Impaired beta-cell function with chronic hyperglycemia "overworked beta-cell" hypothesis, *Diabetes Rev* 4:298, 1996.
9. Kelley DB, editor: *American Diabetes Association complete guide to diabetes*, Alexandria, 1997, American Diabetes Association.
10. Goldstein DE: How much do you know about glycated hemoglobin testing? *Clinical Diabetes* 13:60, 1995.
11. Mahnensmith RL: Diabetic nephropathy: a comprehensive approach, *Hosp Pract* 28:129, 1993.
12. American Diabetes Association position statement: nutritional recommendations and principles for people with diabetes mellitus, *Diabetes Care* 21(suppl 1):32, 1998.
13. Kestel F: Are you up to date on diabetes medications? *AJN* 94:48, 1994.
14. Herter CD: Insulin lispro: the next step, *Clinical Diabetes* 15:51, 1997.
15. Position statement on insulin administration by the American Diabetes Association, *Diabetes Care* 21(suppl 1):72, 1998.
16. McCarthy JA, Covarrubias B, Sink P: Is the traditional alcohol wipe necessary before an insulin injection? Dogma disputed, *Diabetes Care* 16:402, 1993.
17. Farkas-Hirsch R, editor: *Intensive diabetes management*, Alexandria, 1995, American Diabetes Association.
18. American Diabetes Association position statement: implications of the Diabetes Control and Complication Trial, *Diabetes Care* 21(suppl 1):88, 1998.
19. Valensi P and others: Effect of insulin concentration on bioavailability during nasal spray administration, *Pathol Biol* 44:235, 1996.
20. Ahern JA: Steps to reduce the risks of severe hypoglycemia, *Diabetes Spectrum* 10:39, 1997.
21. Edelman SV: Prescribing oral antidiabetic agents: general considerations, *Clinical Diabetes* 16:37, 1998.
22. Bihm B, Wilson BA: Metformin (Glucophage): new treatment for NIDDM, *Medsurg Nurs* 4:236, 1995.
23. Bressler R, Johnson DG: Pharmacologic regulation of blood glucose levels in non–insulin dependent diabetes mellitus, *Arch Intern Med* 157:836, 1997.
24. Jakicic JM, Leermakers EA: Commit to get fit: exercise for life, *Diabetes Spectrum* 9:202, 1996.
25. Shichiri M and others: Enhanced, simplified glucose sensors: long-term clinical application of wearable artificial endocrine pancreas, *Artif Organs* 22:32, 1998.
26. The National Steering Committee for Quality Assurance in Capillary Blood Glucose Monitoring: Proposed strategies for reducing user error in capillary blood glucose monitoring, *Diabetes Care* 16:493, 1993.
27. American Diabetes Association technical review: tests of glycemia in diabetes, *Diabetes Care* 18:1896, 1995.
28. Position statement of the American Diabetes Association: tests of glycemia in diabetes, *Diabetes Care* 21(suppl 1):69, 1998.
29. American Diabetes Association national standards for diabetes self-management education programs and American Diabetes Association review criteria, *Diabetes Care* 21(suppl 1):95, 1998.
30. The Diabetes Control and Complications Trial Research Group: The effect of intensive treatment of diabetes on the development and progression of long-term complications in insulin-dependent diabetes mellitus, *N Engl J Med* 329:977, 1993.
31. American Diabetes Association position statement: implications of the Diabetes Control and Complications Trial, *Diabetes Care* 21(suppl 1):88, 1998.
32. Genuth S: Diabetic ketoacidosis and hyperosmolar hyperglycemic nonketotic syndrome in adults. In Lebovitz HE, editor: *Therapy for diabetes mellitus and related disorders*, ed 2, Alexandria, 1994, American Diabetes Association.
33. Foster DW: Diabetes mellitus. In Isselbacher KJ and others, editors: *Harrison's principles of internal medicine*, ed 14, New York, 1998, McGraw-Hill.
34. Reising DL: Acute hypoglycemia, *Nursing* 25:41, 1995.
35. American Diabetes Association Consensus Development Conference on Insulin Resistance, *Diabetes Care* 21:310, 1998.
36. Nathan DM: Long-term complications of diabetes mellitus, *N Engl J Med* 328:1676, 1993.
37. Kaufman MW, Bowsher JE: Preventing diabetic foot ulcers, *Medsurg Nurs* 3:204, 1994.
38. Seaquist ER: Microvascular complications of diabetes. Strategies for managing retinopathy, nephropathy, and neuropathy, *Postgrad Med* 103:61, 1998.

Resources

Academy for the Advancement of Diabetes Research and Treatment
http://drinet.med.miami.edu

American Association of Clinical Endocrinologists
1000 Riverside Ave., Suite 205
Jacksonville, FL 32204
http://www.aace.com

American Association of Diabetes Educators (AADE)
100 W Monroe, 4th floor
Chicago, IL 60603
312-424-2426
800-338-3633
http://www.diabetesnet.com/aade.html

American Diabetes Association—National Service Center
1660 Duke Street
Alexandria, VA 22314
800-232-3472
http://www.diabetes.org/default.htm

Canadian Diabetes Association
15 Toronto Street, Suite #800
Toronto, Ontario M5C 2E3
CANADA
416-363-3373
800-226-8464
http://www.diabetes.ca

Diabetes Mall on the Net
http://www.diabetesnet.com/

Diabetes Resources on the Internet
http://vigora.com/resources/

Endocrine Society
4350 East West Highway
Bethesda, MD 20814-4410
301-941-0252
Fax: 301-941-0259
http://www.endo-society.org/

Joslin Diabetes Center DNA Core Facility
Room 616
One Joslin Place
Boston, MA 02215
617-735-1932
Fax: 617-735-1915
http://dnacore.joslab.harvard.edu/core/home.html

Juvenile Diabetes Foundation International—The Diabetes Research
    Foundation
120 Wall Street
New York, NY 10005-4001
800-JDF-CURE
212-785-9500
Fax: 212-785-9595
http://www.jdfcure.org

National Diabetes Information Clearinghouse
1 Information Way
Bethesda, MD 20892-3570
301-654-3327
Fax: 301-907-8906
http://www.niddk.nih.gov/health/diabetes/ndic.htm

National Institute of Diabetes, and Digestive and Kidney Diseases
Building 31, Room 9A-52
Bethesda, MD 20892
301-496-5877
http://www.niddk.nih.gov

Pituitary Tumor Network Association
P.O. Box 1958
Thousand Oaks, CA 91358
805-499-2262
Fax: 805-499-1523
http://www.pituitary.com

Thyroid Foundation of Canada
96 Mack Street
Kingston, Ontario K7L 1N9
CANADA
613-544-8364
800-267-8822
Fax: 613-544-9731
http://home.ican.net/~thyroid/Canada.html

For additional Internet resources, see the website for this book at
www.mosby.com/MERLIN/medsurg_lewis

47

NURSING MANAGEMENT
Endocrine Problems

Linda B. Haas

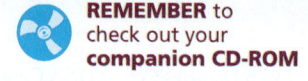

REMEMBER to check out your **companion CD-ROM**

www.mosby.com/MERLIN/medsurg_lewis

LEARNING OBJECTIVES

1. Describe the pathophysiology, clinical manifestations, collaborative care, and nursing management of the patient with an imbalance of hormones produced by the anterior pituitary gland.
2. Describe the pathophysiology, clinical manifestations, collaborative care, and nursing management of the patient with an imbalance of hormones produced by the posterior pituitary gland.
3. Describe the pathophysiology, clinical manifestations, collaborative care, and nursing management of the patient with thyroid enlargement or dysfunction.
4. Describe the pathophysiology, clinical manifestations, collaborative care, and nursing management of the patient with an imbalance of the hormone produced by the parathyroid glands.
5. Describe the pathophysiology, clinical manifestations, collaborative care, and nursing management of the

patient with an imbalance of hormones produced by the adrenal cortices.
6. Describe the pathophysiology, clinical manifestations, collaborative care, and nursing management of the patient with an excess of hormones produced by the adrenal medullae.
7. Name the endocrine disorders characterized by excesses and deficits in fluid volume, and describe the appropriate nursing interventions.
8. Describe the systemic effects of replacement and pharmacologic use of corticosteroid therapy.
9. List the nursing assessments, interventions, rationales, and expected outcomes related to patient education for chronic management of endocrine problems.

DISORDERS OF THE ANTERIOR PITUITARY GLAND

GROWTH HORMONE EXCESS
Etiology and Pathophysiology

Growth hormone (GH), an anabolic hormone, promotes protein synthesis and mobilizes glucose and free fatty acids. Overproduction of GH, which is usually caused by a benign pituitary adenoma (tumor), causes gigantism or acromegaly characterized by soft tissue and boney overgrowth.

Gigantism results when the onset occurs before closure of the epiphyses, while the long bones are still capable of longitudinal growth. The onset usually occurs in early childhood but may occur at puberty. The excessive growth is usually proportional. These children may grow as tall as 8 feet (240 cm) and weigh more than 300 lb (136 kg).[1]

Acromegaly, with a prevalence of approximately 60 cases per million and an incidence of 1000 cases per million per year in the United States, is rare, but it is more common than gigantism.[1]

Clinical Manifestations

Symptoms of acromegaly begin insidiously in the third and fourth decades of life, and both genders are affected equally. When the problem develops after epiphyseal closure, bones increase in thickness and width. Physical features include enlargement of the hands, feet, and paranasal and frontal sinuses and deformities of the spine and mandible (Fig. 47-1). In addition, enlargement of soft tissue (e.g., tongue, skin, abdominal organs) causes manifestations such as speech difficulties and hoarseness, coarsening of facial features, abdominal distention, and sleep apnea. The sleep apnea may be related to upper airway narrowing or may be central in origin.[2] Persons with acromegaly may have hypertension, cardiomegaly, left ventricular hypertrophy, diaphoresis, oily skin, peripheral neuropathy, proximal muscle weakness, and joint pain. Women exhibit menstrual disturbances.[1]

The enlarged pituitary gland can exert pressure on surrounding structures, leading to visual disturbances and headaches. Because GH mobilizes stored fat for energy, it increases free fatty acids levels in the blood and predisposes the patient to atherosclerosis. The hormone also antagonizes the action of insulin and can cause hyperglycemia. Prolonged secretion of GH is diabetogenic (see Chapter 46).

Diagnostic Studies

In addition to the history and physical examination, diagnosis of GH excess requires evaluation of plasma GH and somatomedin

---

Reviewed by Susan Harrington, RN, MN, ARNP, Family Nurse Practitioner, University of Washington, Seattle, Wash.

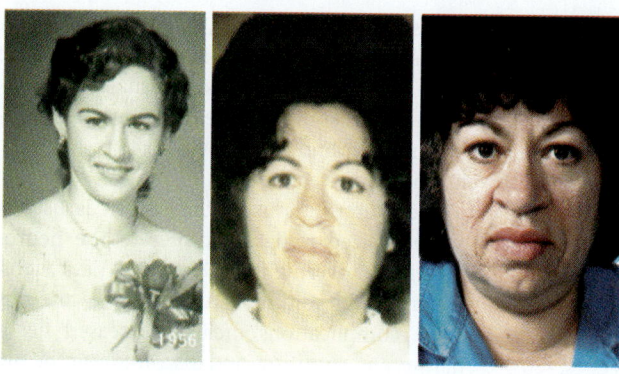

Fig. 47-1 Progressive development of facial features of acromegaly.

C (insulin-like growth factor 1 [IGF-1]) levels, IGF binding protein 3 (IGFBP-3) levels, and GH response to an oral glucose challenge.[2] Magnetic resonance imaging (MRI), used for further evaluation and tumor localization, is a sensitive method for identification, localization, and determination of extension of the tumor into surrounding tissue.[3] High-resolution computed tomography (CT) scanning with contrast media may also be used to localize the tumor. The patient with macroadenoma (10 mm) will require a complete ophthalmologic examination, including visual fields, because of potential pressure of the tumor on the optic chiasm or nerve.

Collaborative Care

The therapeutic goal in gigantism and acromegaly is to return GH levels to normal. This is accomplished by surgery, radiation, drug therapy, or a combination of these three. The prognosis depends on age at onset, age when treatment is initiated, and tumor size. Usually bone growth can be arrested, and soft tissue hypertrophy can be reversed. However, sleep apnea and diabetic and cardiac complications may persist in spite of treatment.

Surgical Therapy. Surgery is the usual treatment and offers the best hope for a cure, especially for microadenomas (<10 mm). Surgery is most commonly accomplished with the transsphenoidal approach, in which an incision is made in the inner aspect of the upper lip and gingiva. The sella turcica is entered through the floor of the nose and sphenoid sinuses (Fig. 47-2). The goal of transsphenoidal microsurgery is to remove only the GH-secreting adenoma. However, the pituitary gland may be destroyed or removed in some instances. Removal of the entire gland results in permanent deficiencies of hormones of the anterior pituitary. Rather than replacing the tropic hormones, which requires parenteral administration, the essential hormones produced by target organs (glucocorticoids, thyroid hormone, and certain sex hormones) can be given orally. Testosterone can be administered to men via a transdermal patch or self-administered intramuscularly (IM) every 2 weeks. Hormone replacement must be continued throughout life.

Radiation Therapy. External radiation normalizes GH levels in 30% to 70% of patients treated in this manner, although it may be months to years before GH levels normalize.[4] If a tumor is large or has a great deal of supersellar extension, surgery may be followed by radiation. Depending on the amount of radiation and the patient's susceptibility, the patient may experience local skin changes, alopecia, or oral

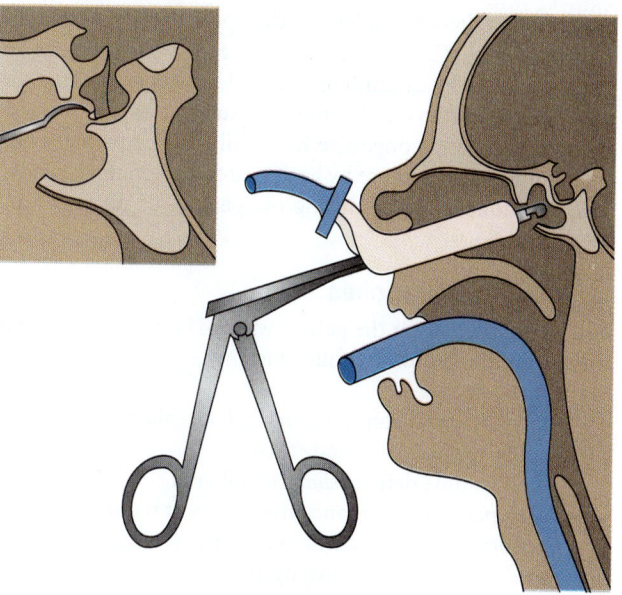

Fig. 47-2 Surgery on the pituitary gland is most commonly performed with the transsphenoidal approach. An incision is made in the inner aspect of the upper lip and gingiva. The sella turcica is entered through the floor of the nose and sphenoid sinuses.

complications. Hypopituitarism is a common sequela that often requires hormone replacement therapy.

Stereotactic radiosurgery (gamma surgery) may be applied to small, surgically inaccessible pituitary tumors. This procedure consists of radiation delivered to a single site from multiple angles and can be used to occlude blood vessels feeding the tumor, thereby starving it. The radiation source is arranged on a helmet device on the patient's head and focused on the tumor.[5]

Drug therapy may include the use of bromocriptine (Parlodel), a dopamine agonist, or octreotide (Sandostatin), a somatostatin analog that reduces GH levels to within the normal range in many patients. The GH-lowering effects of these drugs are seldom complete or permanent, and they are often used as adjuncts to other therapies or to reduce tumor size before surgery.[6]

NURSING MANAGEMENT: GROWTH HORMONE EXCESS

■ Nursing Assessment

The nurse assesses for signs and symptoms of abnormal tissue growth and evaluates the physical size of each patient. Assessment of children includes evaluation of growth and development with the use of growth charts (see Chapter 45). Accelerated growth, especially if greater than 5 to 6 inches (12 to 15 cm) per year and if inconsistent with familial patterns, constitutes cause for medical referral. The adult should be questioned about increases in hat, ring, glove, and shoe sizes. The patient can be questioned about changes in appearance noted in serial photographs.

When first seen, the patient usually has experienced undesirable changes in appearance and may have substantial alterations in self-image. The individual also commonly exhibits symptoms of diabetes mellitus such as polydipsia, polyuria, and blurred vision. Cardiovascular disease may be present. The patient should be carefully monitored for hyperglycemia and cardiovascular signs and symptoms such as angina pectoris, hypertension, and congestive heart failure. The patient needs unconditional acceptance by health care workers and considerable emotional support during the periods of diagnosis and treatment.

■ Nursing Diagnoses

Nursing diagnoses for the patient with GH excess may include, but are not limited to, the following:

- Body image disturbance *related to* enlargement of the hands, feet, jaw, soft body tissue
- Fluid volume deficit *related to* polyuria
- Sleep pattern disturbance *related to* soft tissue swelling
- Sensory-perceptual alteration *related to* visual defect *secondary to* enlarged pituitary gland

■ Planning

The overall goals are that the patient with GH excess will (1) accept and cope effectively with altered body image, (2) maintain adequate fluid volume, (3) experience restful sleep patterns, (4) develop no complications, and (5) state and accept the need for long-term follow-up.

■ Nursing Implementation

Health Promotion. At this time there are no known preventive measures for GH excess. Efforts are directed at early detection of the GH excess and treatment of the underlying cause.

Acute Intervention

Surgical care. The individual treated surgically needs skilled neurosurgical nursing care and must be prepared before surgery for postoperative care. Nursing interventions include preoperative installation of bacitracin nose drops,[5] discussion of mouth breathing, mouth care, ambulation, pain control, activity, and hormone replacement. The patient should be instructed to avoid vigorous coughing, sneezing, and straining at stool (Valsalva's maneuver) to prevent cerebrospinal fluid leakage from the point at which the sella turcica was entered.[5]

After surgery in which a transsphenoidal approach has been used, the head of the patient's bed should be elevated at a 30-degree angle at all times. This elevation avoids pressure on the sella turcica and decreases headaches, a frequent postoperative problem. Mild analgesia is given for headaches. The nurse should perform mouth care every 4 hours to keep the surgical area clean and free of debris and to promote patient comfort. Tooth brushing should be avoided for at least 10 days to prevent disrupting the suture line and to avoid discomfort.

Any clear nasal drainage should be sent to the laboratory to be tested for glucose. A level greater than 30 mg/dl (1.67 mmol/L) indicates cerebrospinal fluid leakage from an open connection to the brain, which places the patient at an increased risk for meningitis. Complaints of persistent and severe generalized or supraorbital headache may indicate cerebrospinal fluid leakage into the sinuses. A cerebrospinal fluid leak usually resolves within 72 hours when treated with head elevation and bed rest. If the leak persists, daily spinal taps may be done to reduce pressure to below normal levels and allow the fossa to heal. Intravenous (IV) antibiotics are usually administered when there is a cerebrospinal fluid leak to prevent meningitis. If the leak does not respond to treatment in 48 to 72 hours, surgical intervention may be required.

If stereotactic radiosurgery is used, the patient is usually moved from the specialized radiation center to the neurosurgical nursing unit for overnight observation. Vital signs, neurologic status, and fluid volume status must be carefully monitored. Possible complications include increased headaches, seizures, nausea and vomiting, and discomfort at the pin sites. All staff members should know how to remove a stereotactic frame in case of an emergency. The patient with a history of seizures is at increased risk for seizures for 24 hours after the procedure. The anterior and posterior pin sites should be cleaned with hydrogen peroxide and covered with clean dressings. Family members can be instructed in pin-site care if the patient is discharged the day after the procedure.[7]

A common postoperative occurrence is transient diabetes insipidus (DI).[5] The signs of DI are discussed in more detail later in this chapter. To assess for DI, serum sodium and fluid balance must be closely monitored. The DI may occur because of the loss of antidiuretic hormone (ADH), which is stored in the posterior lobe of the pituitary gland or cerebral edema related to manipulation of the pituitary stalk during surgery. If DI develops and ingestion of free water and nonsalty fluids does not allow the patient to keep up with urinary water losses, IV fluids are indicated. Vasopressin (Pitressin) is given IM, subcutaneously (SC), or intranasally as needed if the urine output exceeds 800 to 900 ml over 2 hours or if the urine specific gravity is less than 1.005. When vasopressin is used in a patient with known cardiovascular disease, the patient should be closely monitored because this drug may lead to vasoconstriction and angina.

Ambulatory and Home Care. If a hypophysectomy (removal of pituitary gland) is performed or the pituitary is damaged, hormone replacement will be necessary.[4] Permanent ADH, cortisol, and thyroid hormone replacement will be needed. Because these medications must be taken for life, careful patient education is necessary when replacement of these hormones is necessary.

Hypopituitarism causes infertility because of deficient sex hormones secondary to loss of gonadotropins. In addition, gamete (ova and sperm) production ceases because of a lack of stimulation from the gonadotropins, follicle-stimulating hormone (FSH), and luteinizing hormone (LH). However, if an individual with deficient FSH and LH wishes to have children, these hormones can be replaced with intermittent SC injections with possible restoration of fertility.

Because surgery may result in pituitary destruction with permanent hormone deficiencies and possible altered fertility, the patient needs assistance in working through the grieving process associated with these losses. It is important that the patient be aware of the disease progression if surgery is not done so that an informed decision can be made. The need for continued drug therapy reduces the patient's perception of independence and requires considerable emotional adjustment. The nurse must consider the emotional impact of a hypophysectomy when counseling the patient and planning the educational program related to hormone replacement. Referral to the Acromegaly Network Association (619-431-2625) may be helpful.

■ Evaluation

The expected outcomes are that the patient

- is adequately prepared for all collaborative care therapies
- experiences a complication-free postoperative course
- maintains adequate fluid and electrolyte balance
- is able to cope with altered body image
- knows how and when to take hormone replacement (if indicated)
- states the importance of long-term follow-up and has a follow-up medical appointment

EXCESSES OF OTHER TROPIC HORMONES

Excesses of other tropic hormones and overproduction of a single anterior pituitary hormone usually produce syndromes related to hormone excess from the target organ. If adrenocorticotropic hormone (ACTH) is involved, Cushing's disease (hypercortisolism) results; if thyroid-stimulating hormone (TSH) levels are excessive, hyperthyroidism develops.

In some instances, excess secretion of a pituitary hormone may be appropriate, such as when there are alterations in the negative feedback system. (See Chapter 45 for a discussion of negative feedback.) In the adult, hypersecretion of FSH and LH occurs in primary gonadal failure. The resultant low levels of sex hormones cause oversecretion of gonadotropins by the pituitary gland and are not indicative of intracranial disease. Thus excess FSH and LH may indicate a pathologic gonadal process such as orchitis (testicular inflammation resulting in decreased testosterone), or the excess may be a normal consequence of aging such as menopause. Sex hormone replacement therapy normalizes gonadotropin activity but does have side effects (see Chapters 48 and 51).

Sometimes symptoms of excess gonadotropins signify pituitary disease and require prompt referral for a definitive diagnosis. This is true of inappropriate lactation in either gender and precocious puberty in children.

Prolactin-secreting adenomas (prolactinomas) are the most frequently occurring pituitary tumor. The affected patient may experience headaches and visual problems. The visual problems are secondary to pressure on the optic chiasm. Women may have galactorrhea, menstrual abnormalities, or infertility. In men, impotence and decreased libido and sperm density may result. Treatment is achieved with surgery, radiation, or drug therapy using bromocriptine (Parlodel) or cabergoline (Doxtinex).[8]

HYPOFUNCTION OF THE PITUITARY GLAND

Hypopituitarism is a rare disorder that involves a decrease in one or more of the anterior pituitary hormones.

Etiology and Pathophysiology

Primary hypofunction may be a result of developmental or autoimmune disorders, infections, tumors, vascular diseases, or destruction of the gland. The most common cause of pituitary hypofunction is a tumor, but destruction of the pituitary can also result from trauma, radiation, and surgical procedures. Cranial radiation used in the treatment of other conditions may cause hypothalamic dysfunction, which often results in pituitary dysfunction. Failure to secrete GH and gonadotropins is the most common abnormality, followed by deficiencies of TSH, ACTH, and prolactin.[9] The manifestations of hypopituitarism depend on the specific pituitary hormones that are lacking. Infertility may be caused by primary gonadal failure or may be the first indication of pituitary hypofunction. In the latter case the gonads lack tropic hormone stimulation.

Clinical Manifestations

Clinical findings associated with pituitary hypofunction vary with the degree and speed of onset of pituitary dysfunction and are related to hyposecretion of the target glands. The symptoms are often nonspecific and commonly include weakness, fatigue, headache, sexual dysfunction, fasting hypoglycemia, dry and sallow skin, diminished tolerance for stress, and poor resistance to infection. In the adult, premature, fine wrinkling around the eyes and mouth is common. Psychiatric symptoms include apathy, mental slowness, and delusions. Orthostatic hypotension may also occur. If a pituitary tumor exerts pressure on the optic chiasm, there may be asymmetric visual field changes. If the tumor is large, blindness in one or both eyes may occur.

Hyposecretion of GH during childhood results in growth retardation. Growth may be normal for the first 1 or 2 years but then slows progressively. Intelligence is usually normal. Adults with GH deficiency have an increased cardiovascular mortality rate. In addition, they have decreased muscle strength, defective renal function and thermoregulation, altered thyroid metabolism, and reduced basal metabolic rate. These adults are also easily fatigued and have truncal obesity and altered body image.[10,11]

Anorexia and bulimia (see Chapter 38) are associated with decreased pituitary hormone secretion. These conditions usually affect young women with distorted body images. The patient decreases caloric intake and may increase exercise levels to the point where body weight and body fat percentage fall below a critical level for normal hypothalamic-pituitary-gonadotropin function, leading to amenorrhea. Decreased circulating thyroid hormone with inadequate TSH response and glucocorticoid and androgen abnormalities can also occur.

In women, hypofunction can follow a postpartum hemorrhage. This is called *postpartum pituitary necrosis*, or *Sheehan's syndrome*. Sheehan's syndrome should be suspected when failure to lactate and amenorrhea occur in a patient with a history of postpartum hemorrhage. The vascularity of the pituitary gland increases during pregnancy, making it vulnerable to hemorrhage. If hemorrhagic shock occurs during childbirth, the pituitary gland can become hypoxic, causing a slow degeneration and necrosis of the gland.[12] Panhypopituitarism may develop over a span of 10 to 15 years. The patient does not lactate secondary to postpartum hemorrhage after childbirth and is subsequently infertile because of prolactin, FSH, and LH deficiencies. Later, hypothyroidism develops and is followed by corticosteroid deficiency. Mental disorders are common, and because lethargy and apathy are characteristic of thyroid and corticosteroid hormone deficiencies, affected women rarely seek treatment. Many women with Sheehan's syndrome are diagnosed only after an acute Addisonian crisis (discussed later in this chapter). Some are never diagnosed or treated and succumb to this life-threatening condition.

When pituitary hypofunction affects FSH and LH, sexual development is impaired and features remain childlike. FSH and LH deficiencies in the adult woman are first manifested as menstrual irregularities, diminished libido, and changes in secondary sex characteristics (e.g., decreased breast size). If the cause is Sheehan's syndrome, lactation fails and infertility occurs. Men with FSH and LH deficiencies experience testicular atrophy, diminished spermatogenesis, loss of libido, impotence, and decreased facial hair and muscle mass.

If hypopituitarism is not detected and treated, the patient eventually develops deficiencies of thyroid hormone and the adrenal corticosteroids. The latter deficiency causes a tendency toward shock and may result in an episode of acute adrenal insufficiency (refractory and life-threatening shock from sodium and water depletion).

Collaborative Care

For GH deficiency, replacement therapy with recombinant GH is available. Prepubertal children, whose bones are undergoing more rapid growth spurts, respond better than postpubertal children do. GH therapy is costly, but it is recommended for children with growth retardation caused by GH deficiency and children with chronic renal failure before renal transplantation, and it may be useful in Turner's syndrome.[13] Adults with GH deficiency respond well to GH replacement and experience increased energy and lean body mass and improved body image. The major side effect of GH replacement is fluid retention.[10,11]

Treatment of hypopituitarism consists of surgery or radiation for tumor removal, permanent target gland hormone replacement, and a nutritious dietary plan. Replacement therapy is carried out with corticosteroids, thyroid hormone, and sex hormones. Gonadotropins can sometimes restore fertility.

NURSING MANAGEMENT: HYPOFUNCTION OF THE PITUITARY GLAND

A primary nursing role in anterior pituitary insufficiency is assessment and recognition of subtle signs and symptoms. The patient with hypopituitarism may first exhibit symptoms in stressful situations such as trauma or surgery. In addition, hypopituitarism may be detected in the patient with symptoms of failure to grow, infertility, or amenorrhea. Failure to grow may indicate pituitary dwarfism, and infertility and amenorrhea can be signs of Sheehan's syndrome or a pituitary adenoma.

Children affected by pituitary dwarfism exhibit slow but proportional growth. Except for their small size, they may appear completely normal. When the age of puberty is reached, however, sexual maturation may not occur. If it does occur, the epiphyses will close, ending the possibility of further longitudinal bone growth despite hormone replacement. For this reason and because normal stature and psychosocial development are more likely to be achieved with early initiation of treatment, these children must be identified and treated early. (See a pediatric text for a complete discussion of pituitary dwarfism.)

The nurse should be alert for the possibility of Sheehan's syndrome and refer any woman with the following characteristics for diagnosis and treatment:

1. History of hemorrhage or other hypoxic episode during the birth of youngest child
2. Failure to lactate after birth—this is usually the preeminent clue
3. Scanty, irregular, or absent menses
4. Decrease in secondary sex characteristics (or complaints of being "less womanly" than before)
5. Signs and symptoms of hypothyroidism
6. Signs and symptoms of glucocorticoid insufficiency without the "bronzing" of the skin associated with the condition

Although Sheehan's syndrome has been considered a relatively rare condition, there is evidence that it has been seriously underdiagnosed. The disease is devastating to affected women but is largely reversible with hormone replacement.[12] If the disease is not detected and treated early, the woman is likely to need considerable help in rebuilding her life. Marital, vocational, or psychologic counseling may be needed, and appropriate referrals should be made. The nature of the physiologic problem should be explained to significant others, and their help should be enlisted in the rehabilitative process.

DISORDERS OF THE POSTERIOR PITUITARY GLAND

The hormones secreted by the posterior pituitary are antidiuretic (ADH), also called arginine vasopressin (AVP), and oxytocin. These hormones are formed in the hypothalamus and stored in the posterior pituitary. ADH contributes to fluid balance by controlling renal reabsorption of free water (Fig. 47-3). It also has potent vasoconstrictive properties. Oxytocin controls lactation and uterine contractions. Oxytocin excess is not recognized as a clinical problem. This hormone is administered pharmacologically in the management of labor.

SYNDROME OF INAPPROPRIATE ANTIDIURETIC HORMONE

Etiology and Pathophysiology

Syndrome of inappropriate antidiuretic hormone (SIADH), also called Schwartz-Bartter syndrome, occurs when ADH is released in amounts far in excess of those indicated by the plasma osmotic pressure (Fig. 47-4). This syndrome is associated with diseases that affect osmoreceptors in the hypothalamus and is more common in the elderly.[14] SIADH is characterized by fluid retention, serum hypoosmolality, dilutional hyponatremia, hypochloremia, concentrated urine in the presence of normal or increased intravascular volume, and normal renal function.

SIADH has various causes (Table 47-1). Although ectopic ADH production by carcinomas is not a primary pituitary disorder, it has similar clinical manifestations and nursing management. The most common ADH-secreting tumor is bronchogenic carcinoma. Other pulmonary conditions, such as pneumonia, tuberculosis, lung abscess, and positive-pressure

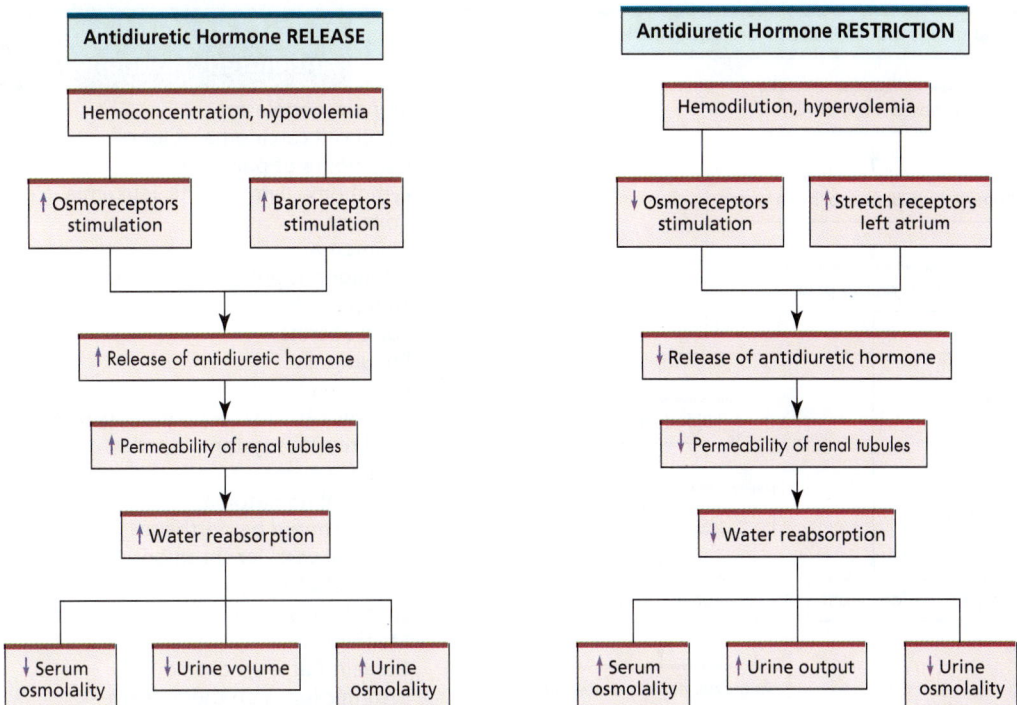

Fig. 47-3   Physiology of the release and restriction of antidiuretic hormone.

breathing, have been associated with SIADH. The syndrome is also associated with such diverse conditions as trauma (all types but most frequently head trauma), meningitis, subarachnoid hemorrhage, acquired immunodeficiency syndrome (AIDS), peripheral neuropathy, delirium tremens, Addison's disease, psychoses, vomiting, stress, and many medications.[15]

SIADH tends to be self-limiting when caused by head trauma or drugs but chronic in nature when associated with tumors or metabolic diseases. Treatment of the underlying cause or discontinuing the causal medication is indicated to improve the clinical course.

Clinical Manifestations

The excess ADH increases renal tubular permeability and reabsorption of water into the circulation. Consequently, extracellular fluid (ECF) volume expands, plasma osmolality declines, the glomerular filtration rate rises, and sodium levels decline (dilutional hyponatremia). This hyponatremia causes muscle cramps and weakness. The patient with SIADH will experience low urinary output and increased body weight without edema. As plasma osmolality and serum sodium levels continue to decline, cerebral edema may occur, leading to lethargy, anorexia, confusion, headache, seizures, and coma.

Diagnostic Studies

The diagnosis of SIADH is made by simultaneous measurements of urine and serum osmolality. The dilutional hyponatremia is indicated by serum sodium less than 134 mEq/L, serum osmolality less than 280 mOsm/kg (280 mmol/kg), and urine specific gravity greater than 1.005.[16] A serum osmolality much lower than the urine osmolality indicates the inappropri-

ate excretion of concentrated urine in the presence of very dilute serum. Associated manifestations correlate with the serum sodium level. Initially, thirst, dyspnea on exertion, fatigue, and dulled sensorium may be evident. As the serum sodium level falls (usually below 120 mEq/L [120 mmol/L]), symptoms become more severe and include vomiting, abdominal cramps, muscle twitching, and seizures.[15] Other laboratory findings are a decreased blood urea nitrogen (BUN), creatinine clearance, hemoglobin, and hematocrit.[16]

Collaborative Care

The treatment goal is to restore normal fluid volume and osmolality. If symptoms are mild and serum sodium is greater than 125 mEq/L (125 mmol/L), the only treatment may be restriction of fluids to 800 to 1000 ml per day. This restriction should result in gradual, daily reductions in weight, a progressive rise in serum sodium concentration and osmolality, and symptomatic improvement. If fluid restriction alone does not improve the symptoms, 3% to 5% (hypertonic) saline solution may be administered IV. A diuretic such as furosemide (Lasix) may be used to promote diuresis if the serum sodium is less than 105 mEq/L (105 mmol/L) or cardiac symptoms or seizures develop. Because furosemide increases potassium excretion, potassium supplements may be needed.

In chronic SIADH, water restriction of 800 to 1000 ml/day is recommended. Regardless of the etiology, demeclocycline (Declomycin), a tetracycline that causes nephrogenic diabetes insipidus, is useful. This drug blocks the action of ADH at the level of the distal and collecting tubules, regardless of the ADH source.

Syndrome of Inappropriate Antidiuretic Hormone (SIADH)

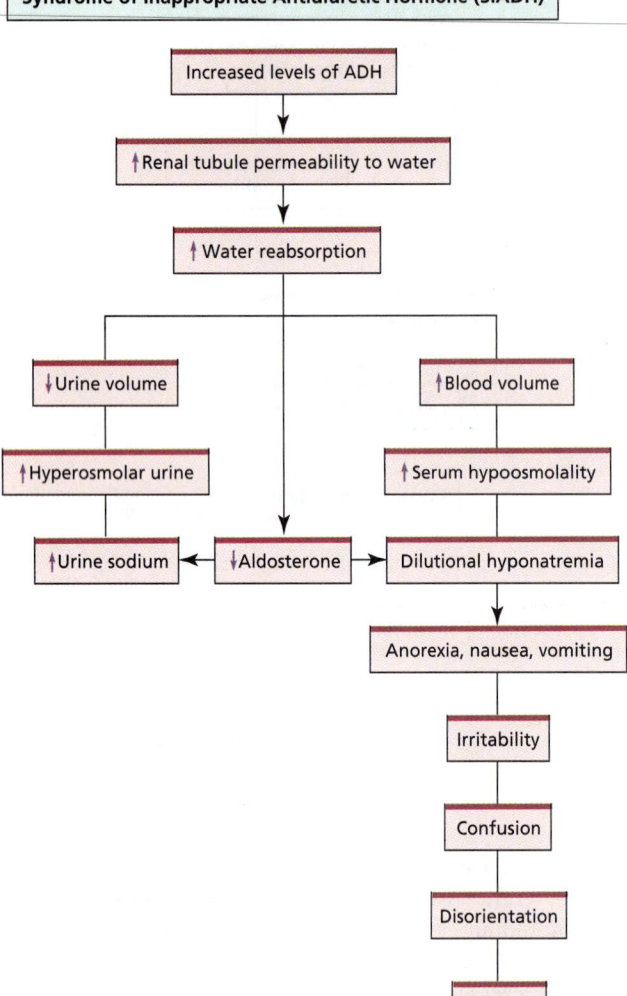

Fig. 47-4 Pathophysiology of syndrome of inappropriate antidiuretic hormone (SIADH).

Table 47-1   Causes of Syndrome of Inappropriate Antidiuretic Hormone

- Malignant neoplasms
  - Small-cell carcinoma of lung
  - Carcinoma of pancreas
  - Lymphoma, lymphocytic leukemia, Hodgkin's disease
  - Thymoma
- Nonmalignant pulmonary diseases
  - Tuberculosis
  - Lung abscess
  - Pneumonia
  - Empyema
  - Chronic obstructive pulmonary disease
- Central nervous system disorders
  - Skull fracture
  - Subdural hematoma
  - Subarachnoid hemorrhage
  - Cerebral vascular thrombosis
  - Cerebral atrophy
  - Encephalitis
  - Meningitis
  - Guillain-Barré syndrome
  - Systemic lupus erythematosus
- Drugs
  - Chlorpropramide
  - Vincristine
  - Vinblastine
  - Cyclophosphamide
  - Carbamazepine
  - Oxytocin
  - General anesthesia
  - Narcotics
  - Tricyclic antidepressants
- Miscellaneous causes
  - Hypothyroidism
  - Positive pressure mechanical ventilation

From Moses A, Streeten D: Disorders of the neurohypophysis. In Isselbacher K and others, editors: *Harrison's principles of internal medicine,* ed 14, New York, 1998, McGraw-Hill.

NURSING MANAGEMENT: SYNDROME OF INAPPROPRIATE ANTIDIURETIC HORMONE

■ Nursing Assessment

Careful nursing assessment of the patient who has had surgery or is susceptible to the syndrome (Table 47-2) can help in the early detection of SIADH. The nurse should be alert for low urinary output with a high specific gravity, a sudden weight gain, or a serum sodium decline.

■ Nursing Diagnoses

Nursing diagnoses for the patient with SIADH may include, but are not limited to, the following:

- Altered urinary elimination *related to* excess ADH levels
- Fluid volume excess *related to* excess ADH

■ Planning

The overall goals are that the patient with SIADH will (1) maintain fluid and electrolyte balance and (2) adhere to fluid restriction and drug therapy.

■ Nursing Implementation

Health Promotion. At this time there are no known preventive measures for SIADH. Health promotion is focused on early identification of those at risk and appropriate interventions. Patients at risk include those who have had intracranial trauma or surgery and those who have tumors or infections (e.g., meningitis).

Acute Intervention. If a patient has SIADH, nursing measures include the assessments and interventions presented in Table 47-2.

Ambulatory and Home Care. When SIADH is chronic, the patient must learn to self manage treatment regimens. Fluids are restricted to 800 to 1000 ml per day. Sucking on hard candy or ice chips can help decrease thirst. If drinking liquids is an aspect of socialization, the patient should be assisted in planning fluid intake so liquid allowances are saved for social occasions. The patient may be treated with a diuretic to remove excess fluid volume. The diet should be supplemented with sodium and potassium, especially if diuretics are

Table **47-2**	Syndrome of Inappropriate Antidiuretic Hormone

Assessment*
- Accurate hourly intake (oral and parenteral) and output
- Hourly measurement of urine specific gravity
- Daily weights
- Level of consciousness
- Observation for signs of hyponatremia every 2 hr (decreased neurologic function, seizures, nausea and vomiting, muscle cramping)
- Monitoring of heart and lung sounds and blood pressure

Interventions
- Restriction of total fluid intake to no more than 1000 ml/day (including that taken with medications); restriction of oral intake to 700 ml < urine output until normalization of serum sodium (if appropriate)
- Positioning head of bed flat or with no more than 10° of elevation to enhance venous return to heart and increase left atrial filling pressure, reducing antidiuretic hormone release
- Positioning side rails up because of potential alterations in mental status
- Turning of patient every 2 hr, proper positioning, range-of-motion exercise, massage (if patient bedridden)
- Use of seizure precautions such as padded side rails and dim lighting
- Assistance with ambulation
- Provision of frequent oral hygiene

*Use a flow sheet for assessment documentation.

prescribed. Solutions of these electrolytes must be well diluted to prevent gastrointestinal (GI) irritation or damage. They are best taken at mealtime to allow mixing with and dilution by food. The patient should be taught the symptoms of fluid and electrolyte imbalances, especially those involving sodium and potassium, so that responses to treatment can be monitored (see Chapter 15). If a patient is to be treated with demeclocycline (Declomysin) the need for close follow-up care should be stressed because of the nephrotoxic side effects and the potential for fungal infections associated with this drug.

■ Evaluation

The expected outcomes are that the patient with SIADH

- has an adequate fluid and electrolyte balance
- understands the need for, and has a plan for, adhering to the meal plan and drug regimen

DIABETES INSIPIDUS
Etiology and Pathophysiology

Central DI occurs when any organic lesion of the hypothalamus, infundibular stem, or posterior pituitary interferes with ADH synthesis, transport, or release. Brain tumors, pituitary or other cranial surgery, closed head trauma, granulomatous dis-

ease, central nervous system (CNS) infections, and vascular disorders may cause DI. Central DI may also be caused by osmoreceptor destruction or have no apparent cause (idiopathic).[17]

Clinical Manifestations

DI is characterized by increased thirst (polydipsia) and increased urination (polyuria) (Fig. 47-5). The primary characteristic of DI is the excretion of large quantities of urine (5 to 20 L per day) with a very low specific gravity (less than 1.003) and urine osmolality of <100 mOsm/kg (<100 mmol/kg). Serum osmolality is usually greater than 295 mOsm/kg (295 mmol/kg). In the milder form, urinary output may be lower (2 to 4 L per day). Most patients compensate for fluid loss by drinking large amounts of water so that serum osmolality is normal or only moderately elevated. The patient with central DI particularly favors cold or iced drinks. The patient is usually fatigued from nocturia and may experience generalized weakness.

Central DI usually occurs suddenly. After intracranial surgery, central DI usually has a triphasic pattern: the acute phase, with abrupt onset of polyuria; an interphase, where urine volume apparently normalizes; and a third phase, where central DI is permanent. The third phase is usually apparent within 10 to 14 days postoperatively. Neurogenic DI that results from head trauma is usually self-limiting and improves with treatment of the underlying problem. DI following cranial surgery is more likely to be permanent.

If oral fluid intake cannot keep up with urinary losses, severe fluid volume deficit results. This deficit is manifested by weight loss, poor tissue turgor, hypotension, tachycardia, constipation, and shock. In addition, the patient shows CNS manifestations, ranging from irritability and mental dullness to coma. These symptoms are related to rising serum osmolality and hypernatremia. Because of the polyuria, severe dehydration and hypovolemic shock may occur.

Diagnostic Studies

Because DI may be pituitary (central, neurogenic), renal (nephrogenic), or psychologic (psychogenic) in origin, identification of the cause of the DI is the initial step. A complete history and physical is done. An attempt is made to rule out psychogenic DI related to emotional disturbances. Psychogenic DI is associated with overhydration and hypervolemia rather than with dehydration and hypovolemia seen in other forms of DI. A water deprivation test is usually done to confirm the diagnosis of central DI (see Table 45-7).

Collaborative Care

The therapeutic goal is maintenance of fluid and electrolyte balance. This goal may be accomplished by IV administration of fluid (saline and glucose) and by hormone replacement, with ADH (vasopressin) administered either SC, IM, or IV. In acute DI, fluids should be administered at a rate that decreases the serum sodium by about 1 mEq/L every 2 hours.[16] Clofibrate (Atromid), carbamazepine (Tegretol), and thiazide diuretics may also be prescribed for symptomatic DI. For long-term therapy, desmopressin acetate (DDAVP), an analog of ADH that is administered as a nasal preparation and does not have the vasoconstrictive effect, is the preferred therapy.

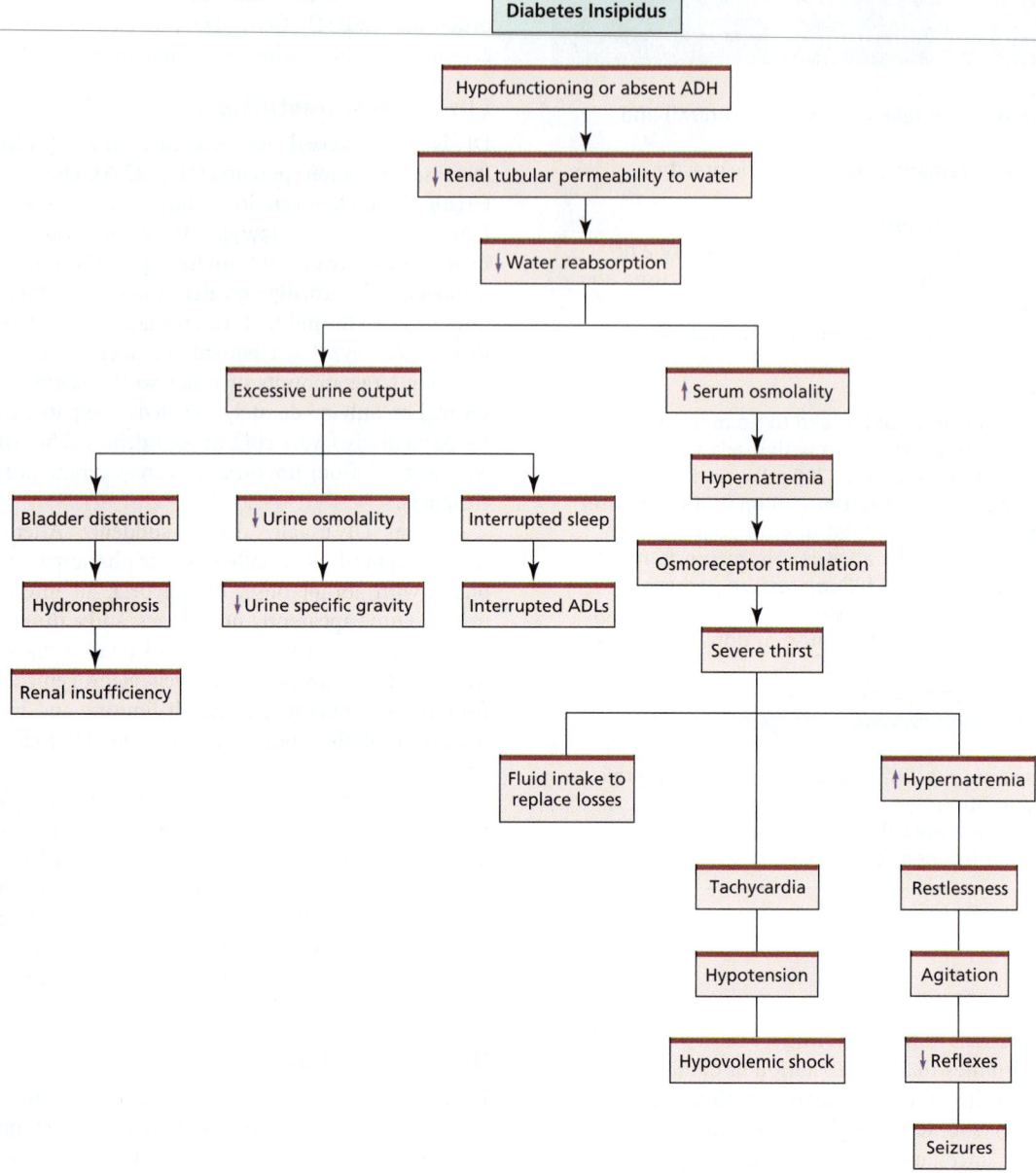

Fig. 47-5   Pathophysiology of diabetes insipidus (DI). *ADH,* antidiuretic hormone; *ADLs,* activities of daily living.

NURSING MANAGEMENT: DIABETES INSIPIDUS

■ Nursing Assessment

Nursing care of the patient with DI is based on the clinical symptoms. Fluid volume deficit manifested by hypotension, tachycardia, and rapid, shallow respirations can be detected early by frequent assessment. Polyuria and nocturia can cause disturbances in rest and sleep patterns.

■ Nursing Diagnoses

The nursing diagnoses for the patient with DI may include, but are not limited, to the following:

- Altered urinary elimination *related to* inadequate secretion of, or renal sensitivity to, ADH
- Sleep pattern disturbance *related to* nocturia

■ Planning

The overall goals are that the patient with DI will (1) maintain fluid and electrolyte balance, (2) have normal sleep patterns, and (3) comply with drug therapy.

■ Nursing Implementation

Health Promotion. At this time there are no known preventive measures for DI. Health promotion is focused on early identification of those at risk and appropriate interventions. Patients at risk include those who have had intracranial trauma or surgery, brain tumors, infections, and vascular diseases.

Acute Intervention. Fluids must be replaced orally or intravenously, depending on the patient's condition and ability to drink copious amounts of fluids. Adequate fluids should be kept at the bedside. If IV glucose is used, urine should be assessed for glucose. If positive, the physician should be notified, because glucosuria causes an osmotic diuresis, which increases the fluid volume deficit. Accurate records of intake and output, urine specific gravity, and daily weights are mandatory in the assessment of fluid volume status. The patient is often listless, tired, and discouraged. Support and reassurance that the sleep disturbances are temporary may be helpful. Perineal care should be done at least twice daily for the bedridden female patient to cleanse urine from the perineum.

If a water deprivation test is done, the patient's baseline weight, heart rate, urine and plasma osmolalities, urine specific gravity, and blood pressure are obtained. All fluids are withheld for 8 to 16 hours. The patient may be anxious and should be reassured that the test will be stopped if fluid volume deficit becomes severe. The patient should be observed throughout the test because of the craving to drink. During the test, the patient's blood pressure, weight, and urine osmolality are assessed hourly. The test continues until urine osmolalities stabilize (hourly increase less than 30 mOsm/kg [30 mmol/kg] in 2 consecutive hours) or body weight declines by 5%, or orthostatic hypotension develops.[18] Aqueous vasopressin is then given IV, and urine osmolality is measured 1 hour later. In central DI, the rise in urinary osmolality after vasopressin exceeds 9%.[17]

When the patient affected by DI is hospitalized, often for emergency treatment of hypertonic encephalopathy, the therapeutic goal is to restore fluid balance. Desmopressin acetate is administered as a nasal or subcutaneous preparation. Overmedication can precipitate volume excess. The patient should be assessed for weight gain, headache, restlessness, and chest pain. The adequacy of treatment is assessed by monitoring fluid intake and output and by urine specific gravity. Increased urine volume with lower specific gravity is related to an inadequate pharmacologic effect, and the physician should be notified immediately.

Ambulatory and Home Care. The patient who requires long-term ADH replacement needs instruction in self-management. Desmopressin acetate is usually taken intranasally twice daily. Nasal irritation, headache, and nausea may indicate overdosage, whereas failure to improve may indicate underdosage. The patient should be instructed to report any of these symptoms. The need for close follow-up should be stressed.

DISORDERS OF THE THYROID GLAND

Thyroid hormones, thyroxine (T_4) and triiodothyronine (T_3), which is the more active form, regulate energy metabolism and growth and development. Thyroid disorders are manifested as hyperfunction (thyrotoxicosis), hypofunction, inflammation, or enlargement (goiter). A goiter may interfere with surrounding structures and can be associated with increased, normal, or decreased hormone production.

HYPERTHYROIDISM

Hyperthyroidism is defined as sustained increased synthesis and release of thyroid hormones by the thyroid gland. *Thyrotoxicosis* is hypermetabolism that results from excess circulating levels of T_4, T_3, or both. Hyperthyroidism and thyro-

toxicosis usually occur together as in Graves' disease. However, in some forms of thyroiditis, thyrotoxicosis may occur without hyperthyroidism.[19]

Hyperthyroidism is second only to diabetes mellitus among noniatrogenic-occurring endocrine diseases. The incidence of hyperthyroidism is 4 to 10 times greater in women, and the highest frequency is in the 30- to 50-year-old age-group. Iodine deficiency is believed to predispose the patient to thyrotoxicosis and other thyroid diseases with a greater incidence in iodine-poor geographic locations. The most common form of thyrotoxicosis is Graves' disease, followed by multinodular goiter, thyroiditis, and exogenous thyroid administration.[20]

Etiology and Pathophysiology

Graves' Disease. *Graves' disease* (diffuse toxic goiter) is a multisystem autoimmune disease of unknown etiology marked by diffuse thyroid enlargement, increased production of thyroid hormone, and usually ophthalmopathy. The patient who is genetically susceptible becomes sensitized to and develops antibodies against various antigens within the thyroid gland and often to other tissues as well. The hyperthyroidism and diffuse thyroid hyperplasia are caused by antibodies that attack thyroid tissue and thus stimulate hyperplasia. These antibodies are found in the serum of the individual with Graves' disease and are known collectively as thyroid-stimulating antibodies (TSAbs). TSAbs stimulate the TSH receptor on the thyroid and by acting like TSH, inappropriately activate the production of thyroid hormones.

Graves' disease occurs more frequently in women in their fourth to sixth decades. A concordance rate of 50% in identical twins indicates genetic and environmental components in the expression of the disease. The disease is characterized by remissions and exacerbations, with or without treatment. It may progress to destruction of thyroid tissue, causing hypothyroidism. Precipitating factors such as insufficient iodine supply, infections, and stressful life events may interact with genetic factors that control immunology and metabolic abnormalities to cause Graves' disease.[20]

Nodular Goiters. Nodular goiters are characterized by small, discrete, autonomously functioning (not TSH dependent) nodules that secrete thyroid hormone. If associated with signs of hyperthyroidism, a nodule is termed *toxic*. There may be multiple nodules (multinodular goiter) or a single nodule (uninodular goiter, thyroid adenoma).

The frequency of toxic multinodular goiter is highest in women in the sixth and seventh decades of life, and it is more common in iodine-deficient areas. There is usually a history of preexisting simple goiter for years before the onset of demonstrable thyrotoxicosis. The manifestations are slower to develop and usually less severe than in Graves' disease. Multinodular goiter is usually not associated with exophthalmos (eyeball protrusion from the orbit). These nodules may be benign or malignant. Uninodular goiter is characterized by a single nodule. These single adenomas are usually larger than 3 cm in diameter, and although encapsulated and benign, they are considered true tumors.[21]

Clinical Manifestations

The clinical manifestations of hyperthyroidism are related to the effects of excess thyroid hormones in two ways. The first is

Table **47-3** **Clinical Manifestations: Thyroid Hormone Dysfunction**

Hypofunction	Hyperfunction	Hypofunction	Hyperfunction
Cardiovascular System		**Musculoskeletal System**	
Increased capillary fragility	Systolic hypertension	Fatigue	Fatigue
Decreased pulse rate	Increased rate and force of cardiac contractions	Weakness	Muscle weakness (especially proximal)
Varied changes in blood pressure	Bounding, rapid pulse	Muscular aches and pains	Proximal muscle wasting
Cardiac hypertrophy, weak contractility	Increased cardiac output	Slow movements	Pretibial myxedema
Distant heart sounds	Cardiac hypertrophy	Arthralgia	Dependent edema
Anemia	Systolic murmurs		Osteoporosis
Tendency to develop congestive heart failure, angina, myocardial infarction	Arrhythmias	**Nervous System**	
	Palpitations	Apathy	Difficulty in focusing eyes
	Atrial fibrillation (more common in the older adult)	Lethargy	Nervousness
	Angina	Forgetfulness	Fine tremor (of fingers and tongue)
Respiratory System		Slowed mental processes	Insomnia
Dyspnea	Increased respiratory rate	Hoarseness	Lability of mood, delirium
Decreased breathing capacity	Dyspnea on mild exertion	Slow, slurred speech	Restlessness
		Prolonged relaxation of deep tendon muscles	Personality changes of irritability, agitation
Gastrointestinal System		Stupor, coma	Exhaustion
Decreased appetite	Increased appetite, thirst	Paresthesias	Hyperreflexia of tendon reflexes
Nausea and vomiting	Weight loss	Anxiety, depression	Depression, fatigue, apathy (in the older adult)
Weight gain	Increased peristalsis	Polyneuropathy	Lack of ability to concentrate
Constipation	Diarrhea, frequent defecation		Stupor, coma
Distended abdomen	Increased bowel sounds		
Enlarged, scaly tongue	Splenomegaly	**Reproductive System**	
	Hepatomegaly	Prolonged menstrual periods or amenorrhea	Menstrual irregularities
		Decreased libido	Amenorrhea
Integumentary System		Infertility	Decreased libido
Dry, thick, inelastic, cold skin	Warm, smooth, moist skin		Impotence in men
Thick, brittle nails	Thin, brittle nails detached from nail bed (onydrolysis)		Gynecomastia
Dry, sparse, coarse hair	Hair loss (may be patchy)		Decreased fertility
Poor turgor of mucosa	Acropachy (clubbing)	**Other**	
Generalized interstitial edema	Palmar erythema	Increased susceptibility to infection	Intolerance to heat
Puffy face	Fine silky hair	Increased sensitivity to narcotics, barbiturates, anesthesia	Increased sensitivity to stimulant drugs
Decreased sweating	Premature graying (in men)	Intolerance to cold	Elevated basal temperature
Pallor	Diaphoresis	Decreased hearing	Lid lag, stare
	Vitiligo	Sleepiness	Eyelid retraction
		Goiter	Exophthalmos
			Goiter
			Rapid speech

their direct effect of increasing metabolism. The second is an increased tissue sensitivity to stimulation by the sympathetic division of the autonomic nervous system. Thyroid hormones increase the number of β-adrenergic receptors, thereby increasing sensitivity to the activity of catecholamines (epinephrine and norepinephrine), although the absolute levels of these hormones are not elevated.[20] (The manifestations of thyroid hyperfunction are summarized in Table 47-3.) A patient with advanced disease may exhibit many of the symptoms, whereas a patient in the early stages of hyperthyroidism may exhibit only weight loss and increased nervousness. In the elderly patient with this disorder the only symptoms may be those

related to cardiovascular function (apathetic hyperthyroidism).[22] Table 47-4 compares features of hyperthyroidism in young and older adult patients.

Ophthalmopathy. Ophthalmopathy may be infiltrative or noninfiltrative.[20] In infiltrative ophthalmopathy, the eyeballs protrude from the orbits (exophthalmos, proptosis). This exophthalmos is due to impaired venous drainage from the orbit, which causes increased fat deposits and fluid (edema) in the retroorbital tissues (Fig. 47-6). Because of increased pressure, the eyeballs are forced outward and protrude. This sign, which is seen in 20% to 40% of patients with Graves' disease, is autoimmune in nature. It is usually bilateral

Table 47-4	Comparison of Hyperthyroidism in Younger and Older Patients	
	Young Adult	**Older Adult**
■ Common causes	Graves' disease in >90% of cases	Graves' disease or toxic nodular goiter
■ Syndrome	Nervousness, irritability, weight loss, palpitations, heat intolerance, and warm, fine skin	Cardiac (angina, arrhythmia, congestive heart failure) Weight loss Myopathy
■ Goiter	In >90% of cases	In about 50% of cases
■ Eye signs	Endocrine exophthalmos reflects autoimmune pathogenesis of Graves' disease	Eye signs less frequent
■ Cardiac features	Tachycardia without heart disease	Underlying cardiac disease common
■ Thyroxine (T_4)	Elevated in >90% of cases	Elevated somewhat less often
■ Triiodothyronine (T_3)	Elevated	Elevated
■ Thyroid-stimulating hormone	Low	Low

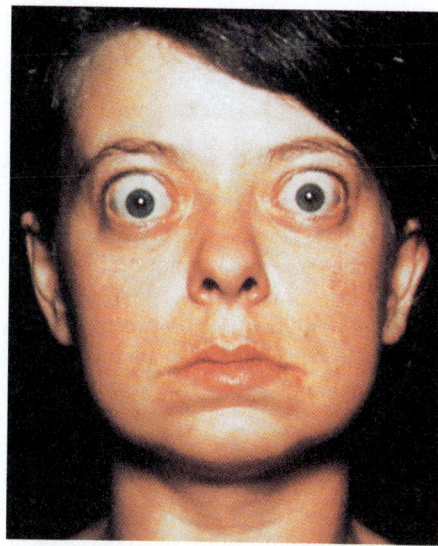

Fig. 47-6   Exophthalmos secondary to Graves' disease.

but can be unilateral or asymmetric. In noninfiltrative ophthalmopathy, the upper lids are usually retracted and elevated, with the sclera above the iris visible. When the eyelids do not close completely, the exposed corneal surfaces become dry and irritated. Serious consequences, such as corneal ulcers and eventual loss of vision, can occur.

Complications

Thyrotoxic crisis (thyroid storm) is an acute but rare condition in which all hyperthyroid manifestations are heightened. It is potentially fatal, but death is rare when treatment is vigorous and initiated early. The cause is presumed to be stressors such as infection, trauma, or surgery in a patient with preexisting hyperthyroidism, either diagnosed or undiagnosed. The physiologic factor or factors that initiate thyrotoxic crisis are unknown.

Manifestations include severe tachycardia, heart failure, shock, hyperthermia (up to 105.3° F [40.7° C]), restlessness,

agitation, abdominal pain, nausea, vomiting, diarrhea, delirium, and coma. Measures must be taken to prevent death. Treatment is aimed at reducing circulating thyroid hormone levels and the clinical manifestations of this disorder by appropriate drug therapy. Therapy is directed at fever reduction, fluid replacement, and elimination or management of the initiating stressor(s).[23]

Diagnostic Studies

Serum T_4 and T_3 can be measured with radioimmunoassay techniques (see Table 45-7) and will be elevated. TSH levels, the most sensitive marker, are low in hyperthyroidism. T_3 resin uptake (T_3RU) is also elevated. T_3RU varies inversely with the amount of thyroid hormone that is protein bound and therefore inactive; that is, a high T_3RU indicates that more hormone than normal is biologically active. Free T_4 and T_3 are usually elevated in thyrotoxicosis. The electrocardiogram (ECG) may show tachycardia, atrial fibrillation, and alterations in P and T waves.

In the nonpregnant, nonlactating patient, a 6- or 24-hour radioactive iodine uptake (RAIU) may be done. This test is contraindicated for pregnant or lactating women because radioactive iodine can cross the placenta and destroy the fetal thyroid or enter breast milk and destroy the infant's thyroid. This test can differentiate Graves' disease from other forms of thyroiditis. The patient with Graves' disease will show a diffuse, homogeneous uptake of 35% to 95%, whereas the patient with thyroiditis will show an uptake of less than 2%. The person with nodular goiter will show an uptake in the high normal range.[24,25]

Collaborative Care

The therapeutic goals are to block the adverse effects of thyroid hormones and stop their oversecretion. The diagnostic studies and collaborative care measures are summarized in Table 47-5. Therapy involves drug therapy with antithyroid medications and β-adrenergic receptor blockers, thyroid ablation with radioactive iodine, and subtotal thyroidectomy after adequate preparation. The choice of treatment is influenced by the patient's age, severity of the disorder, complicating features

COLLABORATIVE CARE

Table 47-5   Hyperthyroidism

Diagnostic Studies
History and physical examination
Ophthalmologic examination
ECG
Laboratory tests
  Serum T_3RU, T_4, free T_3, TSH levels
  TRH stimulation test
Nuclear medicine—thyroid scan

Collaborative Therapy
Graves' Disease
Antithyroid drugs
  Propylthiouracil
  Methimazole (Tapazole)
β-Adrenergic blockers such as propranolol (Inderal)
Ablation of thyroid tissue
  Radioactive iodine (^{131}I)
  Subtotal thyroidectomy
High-caloric diet

Multinodular Goiter
Antithyroid drugs
  Propylthiouracil
  Methimazole (Tapazole)
Ablation of thyroid tissue by radioactive iodine

ECG, electrocardiogram; *TRH*, thyrotropin-releasing hormone; *T_3RU*, T_3 resin uptake; *TSH*, thyroid-stimulating hormone.

(including pregnancy), and patient's preferences. If surgery is to be performed, the patient is usually given antithyroid drugs to produce a euthyroid state and possibly iodine and β-adrenergic blockers to relieve symptoms preoperatively.

Surgical Therapy. Preoperatively, any other associated disorders, such as cardiac disease or diabetes mellitus, must be controlled before surgery. For thyroidectomy to be effective, approximately 90% of thyroid tissue must be removed. If too much tissue is taken, the gland will not regenerate after surgery and hypothyroidism will develop. Occasionally the recurrent laryngeal nerve or parathyroid glands may be damaged during surgery.

Drug Therapy

Thioamides. The most commonly used antithyroid drugs are classified as thioamides. Propylthiouracil (PTU) and methimazole (Tapazole) are clinically the most commonly used drugs. These drugs inhibit the synthesis of thyroid hormones. PTU also blocks peripheral conversion of T_4 to T_3. Although there is considerable individual variation, improvement usually begins 1 to 2 weeks after the initiation of therapy, and good results are seen within 4 to 8 weeks. Therapy is usually continued for 6 months to 2 years to allow for spontaneous remission. The major disadvantages of antithyroid drugs are patient noncompliance and a high rate of recurrence of hyperthyroidism when the drugs are discontinued. In addition, agranulocytosis may occur in rare situations. Indications for use of antithyroid drugs include Graves' disease in the young patient, hyperthyroidism during pregnancy, and the need to make a patient euthyroid before surgery or radiation.

Iodine. Iodine (e.g., Lugol's solution, potassium iodide) in large doses inhibits synthesis of active thyroid hormones T_3 and T_4 and blocks the release of these hormones into circulation. Its maximal effect is usually seen within 1 to 2 weeks. After that time, a reduction in the therapeutic effect may be seen, and long-term iodine therapy is not effective in controlling hyperthyroidism. Usually one drop of a saturated solution of potassium iodide is administered three times daily before surgery. Iodine decreases the size and vascularity of the thyroid, making resection safer and easier. Administration of PTU, with iodine therapy added 10 days before surgery, is a common method for surgical preparation of a patient with hyperthyroidism.

β-Adrenergic blockers. Propranolol (Inderal) is the most frequently used β-adrenergic blocker. It relieves the symptoms of thyrotoxicosis that result from increased β-adrenergic receptors caused by excess thyroid hormones. These symptoms include heat intolerance, palpitations, nervousness, tremor, and muscle weakness. Propranolol is used with other antithyroid treatment and rapidly relieves the symptoms that cause such discomfort to the patient with hyperthyroidism. Propranolol is not used in the patient with asthma or heart disease. Atenolol (Tenormin) may be used instead.

Radioactive iodine. Radioactive iodine (radioiodine) limits thyroid hormone secretion by damaging or destroying thyroid tissue. Between 8 and 12 mCi (296 and 444 MBq) is administered orally. This treatment is effective but often results in hypothyroidism.[25] Radioactive iodine has a delayed response, and maximum effects may not be seen for 2 to 3 months. However, it is effective and inexpensive and can be administered on an outpatient basis. The patient is treated with PTU or propranolol before and during the first 3 months after the initiation of radioactive iodine therapy and for relief of hypermetabolic symptoms until the effects of irradiation become apparent. Thyroid ablation with ^{131}I is not indicated in pregnant women because radioactive iodine crosses the placenta and destroys the fetal thyroid.

Nutritional Therapy. The potential for nutritional deficits is high when an increased metabolic rate is present. A high-caloric diet (4000 to 5000 kcal/day) may be ordered to satisfy hunger and prevent tissue breakdown. This is accomplished with six full meals a day and snacks high in protein, carbohydrates, minerals, and vitamins, particularly vitamin A, thiamin, vitamin B_6, and ascorbic acid. The protein allowance should be 1 to 2 g/kg of ideal body weight. Increased carbohydrates should compensate for disturbed metabolism, provide energy, and spare protein. A registered dietician should be consulted for guidance in meeting the nutritional needs of a patient with hyperthyroidism.

Highly seasoned and high-fiber foods should be avoided because they stimulate the already hyperactive gastrointestinal tract. Substitutes should be provided for caffeine-containing liquids such as coffee, tea, and cola because the stimulating effects of these fluids increase the restlessness and sleep disturbances. Milk is an excellent food source that provides calcium and protein.

NURSING ASSESSMENT

Table 47-6 Hyperthyroidism

Subjective Data

Important Health Information

Past health history: Preexisting goiter; recent infection or trauma, immigration from iodine-deficient area, autoimmune disease

Medications: Use of thyroid hormones

Functional Health Patterns

Health perception–health management: Positive family history of thyroid or autoimmune disorders

Nutritional-metabolic: Insufficient iodine intake; weight loss; increased appetite, thirst; nausea

Elimination: Diarrhea; polyuria; sweating

Activity-exercise: Dyspnea on exertion; palpitations; muscle weakness, fatigue

Sleep-rest: Insomnia

Cognitive-perceptual: Chest pain; nervousness; heat intolerance, pruritis

Sexuality-reproductive: Decreased libido; impotence; gynecomastia (in men); amenorrhea (in women)

Coping–stress tolerance: Emotional lability, irritability, restlessness, personality changes, delirium

Objective Data

General

Agitation, rapid speech and body movements; hyperthermia, enlarged or nodular thyroid gland

Eyes

Exophthalmos, eyelid retraction; infrequent blinking

Integumentary

Warm, diaphoretic, velvety skin; thin, loose nails; fine, silky hair and hair loss; palmar erythema; clubbing; white pigmentation of skin (vitiligo), diffuse edema of legs and feet

Respiratory

Tachypnea

Cardiovascular

Tachycardia, bounding pulse, systolic murmurs, arrhythmias, hypertension

Gastrointestinal

Increased bowel sounds; hepatosplenomegaly

Neurologic

Hyperreflexia, diplopia, fine tremors of hands, tongue, eyelids; stupor, coma

Musculoskeletal

Muscle wasting

Reproductive

Menstrual irregularities, infertility; decreased libido; impotence, gynecomastia in men

Possible Findings

Elevated serum T_3, T_4, and T_3 resin uptake; decreased serum TSH; chest x-ray showing cardiac hypertrophy

NURSING MANAGEMENT: HYPERTHYROIDISM

■ Nursing Assessment

Subjective and objective data that should be obtained from an individual with hyperthyroidism are presented in Table 47-6.

■ Nursing Diagnoses

Nursing diagnoses for the patient with hyperthyroidism may include, but are not limited to, those presented in NCP 47-1.

■ Planning

The overall goals are that the patient with hyperthyroidism will (1) experience relief of symptoms, (2) have no serious complications related to the disease or treatment, and (3) cooperate with the therapeutic plan.

■ Nursing Implementation

Health Promotion. There are currently no preventive measures for hyperthyroidism. Health promotion is focused on preventing relapse in patients who have been treated for hyperthyroidism. Thyrotoxicosis may recur after a period of time, requiring further treatment. Factors that may precipitate relapse include exposure to dietary sources of iodine. Iodine is widespread and can be found in red food dye, preser-vatives such as iodates in flour, some public drinking systems, health food products such as kelp tablets, and milk from cows treated with iodine or iodophors used to clean milk vats.[26]

Acute Intervention. A restful, calm, quiet room should be provided because increased metabolism causes sleep disturbances. Provision of adequate rest may be a challenge because of the patient's irritability and restlessness. Interventions may include (1) placing the patient in a cool room, away from very ill patients and noisy, high-traffic areas; (2) using light bed coverings and changing the linen frequently if the patient is diaphoretic; (3) encouraging and assisting with exercise involving large muscle groups (tremors can interfere with small-muscle coordination) to allow the release of nervous tension and restlessness; (4) restricting visitors who upset the patient; and (5) establishing a supportive, trusting relationship to help the patient cope with aggravating events and lessen anxiety.

If exophthalmos is present there is a potential for corneal injury related to irritation and dryness. The patient may also have orbital pain. Nursing interventions to relieve eye discomfort and prevent corneal ulceration include applying artificial tears to soothe and moisten conjunctival membranes. Salt restriction may help reduce periorbital edema. Elevation of the patient's head promotes fluid drainage from the periorbital

47-1 NURSING CARE PLAN PATIENT WITH HYPERTHYROIDISM

| Expected Patient Outcomes | Nursing Interventions and *Rationales* |

NURSING DIAGNOSIS **Activity intolerance** *related to* fatigue, exhaustion, and heat intolerance secondary to hypermetabolism *as manifested by* complaints of weakness, inability to perform usual activities, short attention span, memory lapses, dyspnea, tachycardia, irritability.

- Decreased perception of weakness and fatigue.

- Assess for signs of activity intolerance *because hyperthyroidism results in protein catabolism, overactivity, and increased metabolism leading to exhaustion.*
- Monitor vital signs q4hr and before and after activities *because tachycardia and BP elevations can indicate excessive activity.*
- Assist patient with self-care as needed *to make certain patient's daily needs are met.*
- Limit ambulation to short walks *to avoid fatiguing patient.*
- Schedule activities of daily living and treatments *to promote adequate rest periods.*

NURSING DIAGNOSIS **Risk for injury: corneal ulceration** *related to* decreased blinking or inability to close eyelids secondary to exophthalmos.

- No evidence of corneal damage.

- Assess patient for complaints of eye pain, feeling of grittiness or "sand" in eyes, proptosis, inability to close eyelids completely, lid lag, lid retraction, visible sclera above iris, and "stare" *to determine if risk factors are present and initiate appropriate interventions.*
- Restrict patient's salt intake *to reduce periorbital edema.*
- Raise head of bed at night *to promote fluid drainage.*
- Teach patient to exercise extraocular muscles daily *to maintain flexibility.*
- Cover patient's eyes with mask or tape shut if eyes will not close if exophthalmos is severe *to prevent corneal drying and, at night, to promote sleep.*
- Apply methylcellulose eyedrops (artificial tears) *to soothe and moisten conjunctival membranes.*

NURSING DIAGNOSIS **Risk for injury** *related to* fine muscle tremors, fatigue, inattentiveness, incoordination.

- No accidental injury.

- Assess for complaints of inability to perform tasks requiring small muscles; restlessness, fatigue; fine muscle tremors; uncoordinated movements; pretibial myxedema *to determine risk for injury and plan appropriate interventions.*
- Assist patient as necessary with tasks requiring fine motor skill; reduce environmental hazards *to reduce exposure to high-risk activities.*
- Assist patient with ambulation *to prevent injury from falling or bumping into items.*
- Teach patient safety practices *to reduce possibility of injury and increase patient's sense of control.*
- Avoid use of caffeine *because it stimulates catecholamines, which can increase fine muscle tremors.*

NURSING DIAGNOSIS **Altered nutrition: less than body requirements** *related to* hypermetabolism and inadequate diet *as manifested by* complaints of weight loss; body weight 20% less than ideal.

- Maintenance of weight (or gain weight).
- Alleviation (or prevention) of nutritional deficiency.

- Assess patient's eating habits and weight pattern *to determine extent of the problem and plan appropriate interventions.*
- Teach and provide high-calorie, high-vitamin, high-mineral diet that includes between meal and bedtime snacks *because hyperthyroidism increases metabolic rate with resulting need to prevent muscle breakdown and weight loss.*
- Weigh patient daily *to evaluate effectiveness of nutritional plan.*
- Monitor BUN and albumin levels *to evaluate protein levels to determine extent of protein malnutrition.*

Continued

area; the patient should sit upright as much as possible. Dark glasses reduce glare and prevent irritation from smoke, air currents, dust, and dirt. If the eyelids cannot be closed, they should be lightly taped shut for sleep. To maintain flexibility, the patient should be taught to exercise the intraocular mus-

cles several times a day, by turning the eyes in the complete range of motion. Good grooming can be helpful in reducing the loss of self-esteem that can result from an altered body image. If the exophthalmos is severe, treatment may involve suturing the eyelids together, administering corticosteroids,

47-1 NURSING CARE PLAN PATIENT WITH HYPERTHYROIDISM—continued

Expected Patient Outcomes   Nursing Interventions and *Rationales*

NURSING DIAGNOSIS **Anxiety** *related to* lack of knowledge about management and course of disease, hypermetabolism, and presence of hypertension *as manifested by* inability to verbalize information regarding medication, verbalization of inability to cope with stress.

- Verbalization of knowledge of management and course of disease.
- Verbalization of decrease in anxiety.

- Teach patient about disease management, including medication regimen, potential for hypertension, chronic nature of disease, and dietary implications, *because knowledge decreases anxiety and increases a sense of control.*
- Assist patient to develop strategies for behavior change *to incorporate medication regimen into lifestyle.*
- Promote rest and relaxation *because anxiety often causes difficulty with rest and sleep.*
- Teach patient strategies for coping with stress *to prevent increasing anxiety.*
- Administer medications as ordered *because decrease in disease activity will decrease anxiety.*

NURSING DIAGNOSIS **Hyperthermia** *related to* impaired temperature adaptation, hypermetabolism; and altered perception of ambient temperature *as manifested by* verbalization of feelings of excess warmth; elevated temperature; diaphoresis.

- Decrease in perspiration.
- Increase in comfort.

- Assess for elevated temperature, diaphoresis, and heat intolerance *to determine extent of problem and plan interventions.*
- Maintain cool environmental temperature; provide light, loose clothing; bathe patient and change linen frequently *to promote patient comfort.*
- Encourage fluids to 3 L/day *to replace fluid loss.*

COLLABORATIVE PROBLEMS

Nursing Goals   Nursing Interventions and *Rationales*

POTENTIAL COMPLICATION **Congestive heart failure** *related to* cardiac hypertrophy, hypertension, arrhythmias.

- Monitor for signs of congestive heart failure.
- Report deviations from acceptable parameters.
- Carry out appropriate medical and nursing interventions.

- Assess for complaints of dyspnea, fatigue, chest pain; edema; cardiac enlargement; atrial fibrillation; diaphoresis *to determine presence of congestive heart failure.*
- Reduce environmental stressors; promote rest and relaxation *to reduce cardiac workload.*
- Assess tolerance to activity *so appropriate assistance can be provided.*
- Discourage physical activity that is not well tolerated *to prevent stressing heart beyond its limit to respond.*
- Administer cardiotonics (e.g., digoxin [Lanoxin]) as ordered *to stabilize cardiac status.*
- Monitor vital signs and cardiac status frequently *to evaluate effectiveness of plan.*

---

radiation of retroorbital tissues, orbital decompression, or corrective lid or muscle surgery.

Thyroid surgery. When subtotal thyroidectomy is the treatment of choice, the patient must be adequately prepared to avoid postoperative complications. The signs and symptoms of thyrotoxicosis must be alleviated as much as possible, and cardiac problems must be controlled before surgery. If iodine is used to relieve hyperthyroid symptoms, it should be mixed with water or juice, sipped through a straw, and administered after meals. The patient must be assessed for signs of iodine toxicity such as swelling of buccal mucosa and other mucous membranes, excessive salivation, nausea and vomiting, and skin reactions. If toxicity occurs, iodine administration should be discontinued and the physician notified.

Preoperative teaching should include comfort and safety measures in which the patient can participate. Coughing, deep breathing, and leg exercises should be practiced and their

importance explained. The patient should be taught how to support the head manually while turning in bed, because this maneuver minimizes stress on the suture line after surgery. Range-of-motion exercises of the neck should be practiced. The nurse should explain routine postoperative care such as IV infusions. The patient should be told that talking is likely to be difficult for a short time after surgery.

The hospital room must be prepared before the patient's return from surgery. Oxygen, suction equipment, and a tracheostomy tray should be readily available. A tracheostomy tray is required in case airway obstruction occurs. Although this rarely happens, it is an emergency situation. Recurrent laryngeal nerve damage leads to vocal cord paralysis. If there is paralysis of both cords, spastic airway obstruction will occur, requiring an immediate tracheostomy.

Respiration may also become difficult because of excess swelling of the neck tissues, hemorrhage, hematoma formation,

RESEARCH
IMPLICATIONS FOR NURSING PRACTICE

Patients with Thyroid Cancer

Citation Dow KH, Ferrell BR, Anello C: Balancing demands of cancer surveillance among survivors of thyroid cancer, *Cancer Practice* 5:289, 1997.

Purpose To explore and describe the demands of long-term cancer surveillance among survivors of thyroid cancer and how these perceived demands influenced their quality of life.

Methods The sample included 34 patients with a history of thyroid cancer on thyroid hormone replacement therapy. The mean age of the patients was 40 years. Patients participated in the study at the time they were undergoing thyroid hormone withdrawal for the purpose of body scanning for detection of cancer recurrence or metastatic disease. In addition to completing a demographic data collection tool, the participants were asked three open-ended questions about their quality of life during the thyroid hormone withdrawal period.

Results and Conclusions The patients experienced profound changes in quality of life during the withdrawal phase. Patients reported changes in physical, psychologic, and social well-being related to the thyroid hormone withdrawal (hypothyroidism). Regardless of the prognosis, patients expressed concerns about the possibility of disease recurrence.

Implications for Nursing Practice Symptoms related to thyroid hormone withdrawal (which is necessary for diagnostic testing) can produce profound and debilitating symptoms in hypothyroid patients. Because thyroid cancer tends to affect young to middle-aged adults, the withdrawal of thyroid hormone can greatly affect work and life schedules. These withdrawal effects occur at the same time the patient is coping with the stress of additional testing.

and laryngeal stridor. Laryngeal stridor (harsh, vibratory sound) may occur during respiration as a result of tetany, which occurs if the parathyroid glands are removed or damaged during surgery. To treat tetany, calcium salts such as calcium gluconate and calcium chloride should be readily available for IV administration.

After a thyroidectomy the nurse should do the following:

- Assess the patient every 2 hours for 24 hours for signs of hemorrhage or tracheal compression such as irregular breathing, neck swelling, frequent swallowing, sensations of fullness at the incision site, choking, and blood on the anterior or posterior dressings.
- Place the patient in a semi-Fowler's position and support the head with pillows, avoiding flexion of the neck and any tension on the suture lines.
- Monitor vital signs. Complete the initial assessment by checking for signs of tetany secondary to hypoparathyroidism (e.g., tingling in toes, fingers, or around the

mouth; muscular twitching; apprehension) and by evaluating difficulty in speaking and hoarseness. Trousseau's sign and Chvostek's sign should be monitored for 72 hours (see Fig. 15-14). Some hoarseness is to be expected for 3 to 4 days after surgery because of edema.

- Control postoperative pain by giving medication.[27]

The neck incision should be supported and range-of-motion exercises should be carried out three or four times daily to promote comfort and the return of full range of motion. The patient should be taught to avoid movements that cause flexion, extension, rotation, and lateral bending of the neck. The appearance of the incision may be distressing. The patient can be reassured that the scar will fade in color and eventually look like a normal neck wrinkle. A scarf, jewelry, high collar, or other covering can effectively camouflage a fresh scar.

If postoperative recovery is uneventful, the patient is ambulated the first day, takes fluid as soon as tolerated, and eats a soft diet by the second day after surgery. Recommended foods should be kept readily available.

Ambulatory and Home Care. Nursing interventions with the patient's significant others include assisting them to perform the nursing interventions. In addition, the nurse should instruct them about the nature of the patient's illness to enable them to understand the physical and emotional manifestations that the patient experiences. Exploring or suggesting ways they can help reduce stressful situations and providing a nonjudgmental atmosphere for them to express difficulties in accepting and dealing with the patient's demands and behavior can be helpful.

Follow-up care is important for the patient who has undergone thyroid surgery. Hormone balance should be monitored periodically to ensure that normal function has returned. Most patients experience a period of relative hypothyroidism soon after surgery because of the substantial reduction in the size of the thyroid. However, the remaining tissue usually hypertrophies, recovering the capacity to produce the hormone needed by the body; but this takes time. The administration of thyroid hormone is avoided because exogenous hormone inhibits pituitary production of TSH and delays or prevents the restoration of normal gland function and thyroid tissue regeneration.

The patient can do a great deal to prevent complications and promote a return to normal function during the hypothyroid period after surgery. Caloric intake must be reduced substantially below the amount that was required before surgery to prevent weight gain. The surgeon may suggest avoiding foods that contain thyroid-inhibiting substances (goitrogens) (Table 47-7). Adequate iodine is necessary to promote thyroid function, but excesses inhibit the thyroid. Seafood once or twice a week or normal use of iodized salt should provide sufficient intake. Regular exercise helps stimulate the thyroid and should be encouraged. Exposure to alternating extremes of temperature, such as hot and cold showers, also promotes thyroid hyperplasia but is not acceptable to many individuals because of cold intolerance. High environmental temperature should be avoided because it inhibits thyroid regeneration.

Regular follow-up care is necessary. The patient should be seen biweekly for a month and then at least semiannually to assess for the development of hypothyroidism. If a complete

Table **47-7**	**Common Exogenous Goitrogens**

Foods
  Potent goitrogens
    Turnips
    Rutabagas
    Soybeans (especially when fed to infants in formula)
    Skins of peanuts
    Milk from kale-fed cattle
  Less potent goitrogens
    Seafood
    Green leafy vegetables
    Peanuts
    Peaches
    Peas
    Strawberries
    Carrots
    Cabbage
    Mustard seed
    Radishes

Drugs
  Thyroid inhibitors
    Propylthiouracil
    Methimazole
    Carbimazole
    Iodine in large doses
  Others
    Sulfonamides
    Salicylates
    p-Aminosalicylic acid
    Phenylbutazone
    Lithium
    Amiodarone

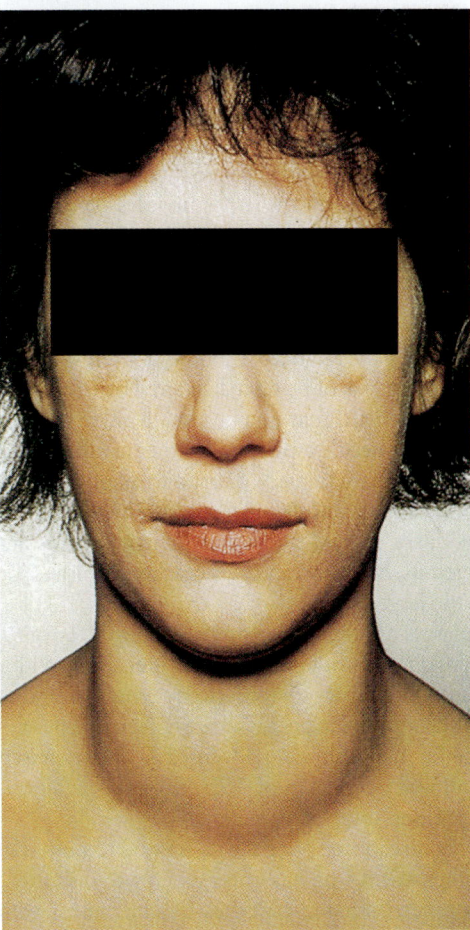

Fig. 47-7   Simple goiter.

thyroidectomy has been performed, the patient needs instruction in lifelong pharmacologic thyroid replacement. Failure of thyroid function is considered by some authorities to be the normal end stage of Graves' disease. The patient should be taught the signs and symptoms of progressive thyroid failure and instructed to seek medical care if these develop. Hypothyroidism is relatively easy to control with oral administration of thyroid preparations.

Radioactive iodine therapy. Radioactive iodine therapy (ablation) is usually administered on an outpatient basis and is the therapy of choice for the adult beyond childbearing years. Because the usual therapeutic dose of radioactive iodine is only 7 to 10 mCi, no radiation safety precautions are necessary. The patient should be instructed that radiation thyroiditis and parotiditis are possible and may cause dryness and irritation of the mouth and throat. Relief may be obtained with frequent sips of water, ice chips, or the use of a salt and soda gargle three to four times per day. This gargle is made by dissolving 1 teaspoon of salt and 1 teaspoon of baking soda in 2 cups of warm water. The discomfort should subside in 3 to 4 days. If dryness and irritation persist, the patient should contact a clinician. Because of the high frequency of hypothyroidism after radioactive iodine therapy, the patient and significant others should be taught the symptoms of hypothyroidism and instructed to seek medical help if these symptoms occur.

■ Evaluation

The expected outcomes are that the patient with hyperthyroidism

- experiences relief of symptoms
- has no serious complications related to the disease or treatment
- cooperates with the therapeutic plan

THYROID ENLARGEMENT

Enlargement of the thyroid gland is called *goiter* (Fig. 47-7). Goiter may result from hypertrophy caused by excess TSH stimulation, which in turn can be caused by inadequate circulating thyroid hormones. Goiter may also be caused by growth-stimulating immunoglobulins and other growth factors. Goitrogens (see Table 47-7), which inhibit synthesis of thyroid hormone, can cause goiter but usually only in the individual who lives in an iodine-deficient area (endemic goiter).

TSH and T_4 are measured to determine whether a goiter is associated with hyperthyroidism, hypothyroidism, or normal thyroid function. Thyroid antibodies are measured to assess for thyroiditis. Treatment with thyroid hormone may prevent further thyroid enlargement. Surgery to remove large goiters may be necessary.

THYROID NODULES

A thyroid nodule, a palpable deformity of the thyroid gland, may be benign or malignant. Malignant tumors of the thyroid gland are rare. Both single and multinodular thyroids carry a risk of cancer. The major sign of thyroid cancer is the appearance of a hard, painless nodule in an enlarged thyroid.

A thyroid scan shows whether nodules on the thyroid are "hot" or "cold." When a person is given tracer doses of ^{131}I, thyroid tumors on the thyroid may or may not take up the radioactive iodine. Tumors that take up the radioactive iodine are termed *hot nodules* and are nearly always benign. If the nodule does not take up the radioactive iodine, it is termed a *cold nodule* and has a higher risk of being malignant. High-resolution ultrasonography and MRI may also be used to aid in diagnosis. Needle biopsy (fine-needle aspiration) of the nodule is usually done to identify malignant tissue.[28] Measurement of serum calcitonin is also helpful in diagnosis, since increased levels are associated with medullary thyroid carcinoma. Benign nodules are usually not dangerous, but they can cause tracheal compression if they become too large.

Neoplasms are treated by surgical removal. Surgical procedures may range from unilateral total lobectomy with removal of the isthmus to total thyroidectomy with bilateral neck dissection. Many thyroid cancers are TSH dependent, and thyroid hormone in hyperphysiologic doses is often prescribed to inhibit pituitary secretion of TSH. External radiation may be used to prolong survival.

Nursing care for the patient with thyroid tumors is similar to care for the patient who has undergone thyroidectomy and also includes general nursing measures for the patient with cancer (see Chapter 14).

THYROIDITIS

Thyroiditis is an inflammatory process in the thyroid and can have several causes. Subacute granulomatous thyroiditis (de Quervain's thyroiditis), which causes thyrotoxicosis, is thought to be caused by a viral infection. Acute thyroiditis is due to bacterial or fungal infection. Subacute and acute forms of thyroiditis have abrupt onsets and the thyroid is painful. Chronic autoimmune thyroiditis (Hashimoto's thyroiditis), leading to hypothyroidism, is insidious in onset. Hashimoto's thyroiditis is a chronic autoimmune disease in which thyroid tissue is replaced by lymphocytes and fibrous tissue. It is the most common cause of goiterous hypothyroidism in the United States. Silent thyroiditis, a form of lymphocytic thyroiditis, has a variable onset. This condition may occur in the postpartal period. It is believed to be an autoimmune disease and may be early Hashimoto's thyroiditis.

T_4 and T_3 are initially elevated in subacute, acute, and silent thyroiditis but may become depressed with time. TSH levels are low and then elevated. Thyroid hormone levels are usually low in chronic Hashimoto's thyroiditis, and TSH is high. Suppression of RAIU is seen in subacute and silent thyroiditis. Antithyroid antibodies are present in Hashimoto's thyroiditis.

NURSING AND COLLABORATIVE MANAGEMENT: THYROIDITIS

Recovery from thyroiditis may be complete in weeks or months without treatment. If the condition is bacterial in origin, treatment may include specific antibiotics or surgical drainage. In subacute and acute forms, salicylates and nonsteroidal anti-inflammatory drugs (NSAIDs) are used. If there is no response to these drugs in 48 hours, corticosteroids are given. Propranolol or atenolol may be used for the cardiovascular symptoms of a hyperthyroid condition. Thyroid hormone is used if the patient is hypothyroid.

Nursing care of the patient with thyroiditis includes education regarding normal thyroid function and what is happening in the patient's specific instance. Other nursing interventions depend in part on the therapeutic management. Nursing interventions include reassurance, support, and assistance during the recovery period. The patient should be instructed to remain under close health supervision so that progress can be monitored and to report any change in symptoms to the health care provider.

The patient with thyroiditis of autoimmune origin may be susceptible to other autoimmune diseases such as Addison's disease, pernicious anemia, or premature gonadal failure or Graves' disease. The patient should be taught the signs and symptoms of these disorders, particularly Addison's disease. Because stress may aggravate these autoimmune diseases, stress management is an important part of patient education (see Chapter 7). The patient should also be given a list of common goitrogens (see Table 47-7) and encouraged to avoid them as much as possible.

A patient receiving thyroid hormone replacement or corticosteroids must be taught the expected side effects of these drugs and measures to manage them. The patient should also be instructed in unexpected side effects and told when and to whom these should be reported. Toxic symptoms should be clearly defined, and the patient should be instructed to report them. Table 47-3 lists signs of hyperthyroidism that are the same as toxic symptoms of thyroid hormone replacement. Patient handouts written in understandable language should accompany verbal instruction. The handouts should be reviewed with the patient to assess understanding, and information should be clarified when necessary. The patient treated surgically needs care similar to that given to the person undergoing thyroidectomy.

HYPOTHYROIDISM
Etiology and Pathophysiology

Hypothyroidism usually results from insufficient circulating thyroid hormone as a result of a variety of abnormalities. Hypothyroidism can be primary, related to destruction of thyroid tissue or defective hormone synthesis, or secondary, related to pituitary disease with decreased TSH secretion or to hypothalamic problems with decreased TRH secretion. It may also be transient, related to a thyroiditis or discontinuance of thyroid hormone therapy.[29] All hypothyroid states have certain features in common, regardless of the cause. Some differences depend on the patient's age at onset of the deficiency.

Hypothyroidism may occur in infancy (cretinism), childhood, or adulthood. Cretinism is caused by thyroid hormone deficiencies during fetal or early neonatal life. It can be caused by maternal iodine deprivation or congenital thyroid abnormalities. Cretinism occurs in 1 of 3700 births in the United States and is more frequent in females.[30] Juvenile hypothyroidism has causes similar to those seen in the adult and requires prompt diagnosis and treatment to prevent developmental retardation.

ETHICAL DILEMMAS

Alternative Healers

SITUATION

Although thyroid replacement therapy is the planned treatment, the patient's cultural healer tells her not to take the medication and that she should begin an herbal regimen instead. Should the nurse intervene?

DISCUSSION

Knowledge of a patient's cultural background and setting is important to a successful treatment plan. If the nurse can learn about the healing practices and come to know the healers in the community, a partnership can develop between traditional and allopathic (Western) medicine. Education can be conducted in both directions, and the cultural healer's methods can be used in conjunction with the prescribed treatment. However, if the nurse reacts negatively and denigrates or condemns traditional healing, the patient may be forced to choose between what is culturally appropriate, acceptable, and known, and that which is required by the Western medical establishment. Hostility between Western medical professionals and traditional healing does not benefit the patient and may, in fact, dissuade the community from seeking medical attention. It is always in the patient's best interests for providers to be knowledgeable of the cultures of the people they serve and to develop relationships with traditional healers.

ETHICAL AND LEGAL PRINCIPLES

- Patient autonomy (the right of a patient to decide for himself or herself) should be upheld.
- Planning appropriate and effective health care should take into consideration a patient's religious and cultural values and beliefs.
- In some situations, Western (allopathic) medicine can no longer provide definitive care (e.g., terminally ill cancer patient), and alternative medicine may provide the patient with hope and support.

In areas where iodine intake is adequate, such as the United States, the most common cause of primary hypothyroidism in the adult is atrophy of the thyroid gland. This atrophy is the end result of both Hashimoto's thyroiditis and Graves' disease. These autoimmune diseases destroy the thyroid gland. Thyroid deficiency also occurs when pituitary TSH production is inadequate. Iatrogenic causes of hypothyroidism include surgical removal of the thyroid, destruction of the thyroid gland by radiation, and surgical removal of the pituitary gland. Occasionally, hypothyroidism develops as a result of the ingestion of excessive amounts of goitrogens (see Table 47-7). The person with underlying autoimmune disease is particularly susceptible to goitrogens.

Although the typical patient with hypothyroidism is a woman over age 50, the disease can occur at any age and in either sex. An increased incidence has been correlated with the previous therapeutic use of radioactive iodine. Hypothyroidism is more common in iodine-deficient areas of the world, such as Zaire and Nepal, and iodine deficiency is the most common cause of hypothyroidism worldwide.[30]

Clinical Manifestations

The major manifestations of cretinism are defective physical development and mental retardation. Although affected infants usually appear normal at birth, cretinism should be suspected when there is a long gestational period and a large infant who fails to thrive. Affected infants may exhibit a large posterior fontanel, squinting, excessive sleeping, thickened skin and lips, enlarged tongue, abdominal distention with vomiting, a hoarse cry, dull facial expression, feeding and respiratory difficulty, peripheral cyanosis, supraclavicular and periorbital edema, umbilical hernia, and hypothermia.

Hypothyroidism in childhood is usually due to autoimmune thyroiditis. Intellectual development is normal, but the child may seem mentally sluggish. Physical and sexual development are altered. Although there is generalized muscle hypertrophy, the face remains childlike, and eruption of permanent teeth, linear growth, and sexual maturation are delayed. In addition, there is a high frequency of other autoimmune diseases.[30,33]

Hypothyroidism in the adult is characterized by an insidious and nonspecific slowing of body processes. The adult with hypothyroidism often is fatigued and lethargic and may experience personality changes. The mental changes seen in hypothyroidism include impaired memory, slowed speech, decreased initiative, and somnolence. In addition, cold intolerance, hair loss, dry and coarse skin, brittle nails, hoarseness, muscle weakness and swelling, overall weakness, constipation, weight gain, and menorrhagia are common.

Unless hypothyroidism occurs after thyroidectomy or thyroid ablation, or during treatment with antithyroid drugs, the onset of symptoms may occur over months to years. The symptoms are so insidious that medical attention is seldom sought. The patient's family and friends are often unaware of the changes. The severity of the symptoms depends on the degree of thyroid hormone deficiency and results from the long-term physiologic effects of thyroid hormone deficiency. They may involve any body system but are more pronounced in cardiovascular, GI, reproductive, and hematopoietic systems.

Hypothyroid heart disease includes cardiomyopathy, pericardial effusion, and coronary atherosclerosis. Bradycardia and weakened cardiac contractility lead to decreased cardiac output. Pericardial effusion, however, seldom results in hemodynamic compromise. Increased serum cholesterol and triglyceride levels and the accumulation of mucopolysaccharides in the intima of small blood vessels can result in coronary atherosclerosis. This accumulation is seldom symptomatic (i.e., characterized by angina) because of the decreased myocardial oxygen consumption that has been observed in hypothyroidism.

The brain is affected by diminished cerebral blood flow related to decreased cardiac output. This is manifested by mental sluggishness, inattentiveness, memory loss, lethargy, and changes in affect. Although some individuals with hypothyroidism exhibit a jocular air regarding their condition, others appear depressed. They express distress and describe an impaired self-image in regard to their disabilities and altered appearance. Although the patient with hypothyroidism sleeps long hours, stage 3 and stage 4 sleep are reduced.

GI motility is decreased in hypothyroidism, and achlorhydria (absence of hydrochloric acid) is common. Constipation, which is a common complaint, may progress to obstipation and, rarely, to intestinal obstruction. The underlying metabolic disease makes the individual a high-risk candidate for intestinal surgery.

Women with hypothyroidism frequently complain of menorrhagia. Some affected individuals have been treated for menorrhagia for years and may have undergone hysterectomy before the hypothyroidism was diagnosed. In addition, anovulatory cycles with subsequent infertility may occur.

Anemia is a common feature of hypothyroidism. Erythropoietin levels may be low or normal. Oxygen demand is decreased in the periphery, and there is hypocellular bone marrow. The result is a low hematocrit. Other hematopoietic problems are cobalamin, iron, and folate deficiencies and a predisposition to bruising.

The term *myxedema* is often used synonymously with hypothyroidism but actually connotes severe, long-standing hypothyroidism. Myxedema is the accumulation of hydrophilic mucopolysaccharides in the dermis and other tissues. This mucinous edema causes the characteristic facies of hypothyroidism and puffiness, periorbital edema, and masklike affect.

Complications

The mental sluggishness, drowsiness, and lethargy of hypothyroidism may progress gradually or suddenly to a notable impairment of consciousness or coma. This situation, termed *myxedema coma,* constitutes a medical emergency. Myxedema coma can be precipitated by infection, drugs (especially narcotics, tranquilizers, and barbiturates), exposure to cold, and trauma. It is characterized by subnormal temperature, hypotension, and hypoventilation. For the patient to live, vital functions must be supported, and IV thyroid hormone must be administered.

Diagnostic Studies

T_4, T_3, and T_3RU levels are usually low in hypothyroidism. These values, correlated with symptoms gathered from the history and physical examination, confirm the diagnosis. Serum TSH levels help determine the cause of hypothyroidism. Serum TSH is high when the defect is in the thyroid and low when it is in the pituitary or hypothalamus. An increase in TSH after TRH injection suggests hypothalamic dysfunction, whereas no change suggests anterior pituitary dysfunction (Table 47-8). In the well elderly, T_3, T_4, and TSH levels are unchanged.

Clinical diagnosis of hypothyroidism in the elderly adult can be difficult. The typical manifestations of hypothyroidism, which are often considered normal changes of aging, include fatigue; cold, dry skin; hoarseness; hair loss; constipation; and cold intolerance.

Collaborative Care

The therapeutic objective in hypothyroidism is restoration of a euthyroid state as safely and rapidly as possible with hormone replacement therapy. In the adult a low-calorie diet is indicated to promote weight loss.

Synthetic oral thyroxine (Synthroid, Levothroid, Noroxine) is the drug of choice to treat hypothyroidism. In the young, otherwise healthy patient, the maintenance replacement dose can be started at once.[25] In the older adult patient and the person with compromised cardiac status, a small initial dose is recommended because the usual dose may increase myocardial oxygen consumption.[34] The resultant oxygen demand may cause angina and cardiac arrhythmias. Any chest pain experienced by a patient starting thyroid replacement should be reported

DIAGNOSTIC STUDIES

Table 47-8 Hypothyroidism

Study	Finding
Serum T_3RU	Low
Serum T_3	Low
Serum T_4	Low
Serum cholesterol	Increased
ECG	Bradycardia, low voltage
Serum TSH	High (if thyroid diseased), low (if pituitary diseased)
TRH stimulation test	Increase in TSH if hypothalamus diseased, no change in TSH if pituitary diseased

immediately, and ECG and serum cardiac enzyme tests must be performed. The dose is increased at 1- to 4-week intervals. It is important that the patient take replacement medication regularly. Lifelong thyroid replacement therapy is usually required for both adults and children.

NURSING MANAGEMENT: HYPOTHYROIDISM

■ Nursing Assessment

Assessment of the patient who is suspected of having hypothyroidism should include questions about weight gain, mental changes, fatigue, slowed and slurred speech, cold intolerance, skin changes such as increased dryness or thickening, constipation, and dyspnea. In addition, the nurse should assess for recent introduction of iodine-containing medications or ingestion of large amounts of goitrogens.[31,35] The patient should be assessed for bradycardia; distended abdomen; dry, thick, cold skin; thick, brittle nails; paresthesias; and muscular aches and pains.

■ Nursing Diagnoses

Nursing diagnoses for the patient with hypothyroidism may include, but are not limited to, those presented in NCP 47-2.

■ Planning

The overall goals are that the patient with hypothyroidism will (1) experience relief of symptoms, (2) maintain a euthyroid state, (3) maintain a positive self-image, and (4) comply with lifelong thyroid replacement therapy.

■ Nursing Implementation

Health Promotion. The nurse plays an important role in the detection of hypothyroidism. Careful assessment may reveal the early and subtle changes that indicate dysfunction, particularly when caring for the patient with a condition, such as family history, that may predispose him or her to endocrine dysfunction. Promotion and maintenance of thyroid function requires an adequate dietary intake of iodine for hormone production. The importance of adequate nutrition is illustrated by

47-2 NURSING CARE PLAN PATIENT WITH HYPOTHYROIDISM

Expected Patient Outcomes	Nursing Interventions and *Rationales*

NURSING DIAGNOSIS Hypothermia *related to* cold intolerance *as manifested by* complaints of feeling cold, shivering.

- Satisfaction with temperature of environment.
- Personal comfort.

- Provide extra clothing, blankets, warm environment *to increase patient's comfort.*
- Explain to patient and significant others that decreased heat production causes discomfort *to increase understanding of and empathy for patient's condition.*

NURSING DIAGNOSIS Altered nutrition: more than body requirements *related to* hypometabolism *as manifested by* weight gain greater than 10% more than ideal body weight.

- Maintenance of weight in usual range.

- Provide low-calorie, high-protein diet; include foods high in cobalamin, folic acid, iron, and vitamin C *to reduce tendency for weight gain while preventing muscle wasting and anemia.*
- Explain the need for fewer calories *so patient will be more agreeable to dietary restrictions.*
- Assist patient to develop method of monitoring weight and caloric intake *so excess weight gain can be avoided.*
- Encourage small, frequent meals *because early satiety and decreased gastrointestinal motility can cause gas and discomfort.*

NURSING DIAGNOSIS Constipation *related to* gastrointestinal hypomotility *as manifested by* irregular, hard stools.

- Daily soft formed stool.

- Assess bowel pattern and characteristics *to plan appropriate interventions.*
- Provide 2-3 L of fluids per day *to maintain soft stool.*
- Encourage activity *to stimulate peristalsis.*
- Administer laxatives or stool softeners if necessary *to stimulate GI motility.*
- Offer foods high in bulk and roughage *to increase fecal mass.*

NURSING DIAGNOSIS Activity intolerance *related to* decreased metabolic rate and mucin deposits in joints and interstitial spaces *as manifested by* generalized weakness and muscle and joint stiffness.

- Able to participate in self-care activities with minimal discomfort and fatigue.

- Assess ability to participate in self-care activities *to determine extent of problem and plan appropriate interventions.*
- Monitor vital signs and comfort level *to determine effect of activities and plan activity increases.*
- Administer thyroid hormone as ordered *to correct hypometabolic state.*
- Plan frequent rest periods *to improve patient's tolerance and comfort level.*
- Apply splints and hot packs if appropriate *to relieve joint stiffness and pain by immobilization.*
- Pace activities to match patient's abilities *to allow maximum participation.*

NURSING DIAGNOSIS Altered thought processes *related to* diminished cerebral blood flow secondary to decreased cardiac output *as manifested by* forgetfulness, memory loss, and personality changes.

- Maintenance of orientation to reality at highest level possible.

- Assess thinking processes such as memory; attention span; orientation to time, person, and place *to enable appropriate planning.*
- Repeat information to patient *because this person requires more time to comprehend.*
- Explain cause of symptoms to patient and family *to reduce anxiety and frustration.*
- Provide clock and calendar *to maintain orientation to time and day.*
- Provide written handouts with all instructions *to help patient remember and thereby enhance adherence to regimen.*

the thyroid enlargement and marginal hypothyroidism that can develop in the individual with iodine deficiencies (endemic goiter). Thyroid hormone production also requires an adequate intake of protein.

Acute Intervention. If the patient has myxedema coma, mechanical respiratory support will be necessary, as well as cardiac monitoring. The nurse will be administering all medications IV since the paralytic ileus associated with myxedema coma causes unreliable absorption of oral medications. If the patient is hyponatremic, hypertonic saline may be administered until the serum sodium reaches 130 mEq/L (130 mmol/L). The nurse should monitor core temperature because the patient with myxedema coma is often extremely hypothermic.[36]

For assessment of the patient's progress, vital signs, body weight, fluid intake and output, and visible edema should be monitored. Cardiac assessment is especially important because the cardiovascular response to the hormone determines the medication regimen. Energy level and mental alertness should be noted. These should increase within 2 to 14 days and continue to rise steadily to normal levels.

Ambulatory and Home Care. Repeated patient education is imperative (Table 47-9). Initially the hypothyroid patient needs more time than usual to comprehend all of the necessary information. It is important to provide written instructions, repeat the information often, and assess the patient's comprehension level regularly. The need for lifelong drug therapy must be stressed. The signs and symptoms of hypothyroidism or hyperthyroidism that indicate hormone imbalance should be included in the teaching plan. It is sometimes difficult for the patient to recognize signs of overdosage or underdosage; therefore a family member or friend should be included in the instruction process. Forgetfulness is an early indication of thyroid deficiency.

The patient must be taught to contact a clinician immediately if signs of overdose such as orthopnea, dyspnea, rapid pulse, palpitations, nervousness, or insomnia appear. The patient with diabetes mellitus should test his or her capillary blood glucose at least daily because return to the euthyroid state frequently increases insulin requirements. In addition, thyroid preparations potentiate the effects of other common drug groups, such as anticoagulants, antidepressants, and digitalis compounds. Thus the patient should be taught the toxic signs and symptoms of these medications and should remain under close medical observation until stable.

With treatment, striking transformations occur in both appearance and mental function. Most adults return to a normal state. Cardiovascular conditions and (occasionally) psychosis may persist despite corrections of the hormonal imbalance. Relapses occur if treatment is interrupted.

■ Evaluation

The expected outcomes are that the patient with hypothyroidism will

- have relief from symptoms
- maintain a euthyroid state as evidenced by normal thyroid hormone and TSH levels
- state the need for and a plan to adhere to lifelong therapy

---

✎ PATIENT TEACHING GUIDE

Table **47-9** **Hypothyroidism**

1. Provide a comfortable, warm environment because of intolerance to cold.
2. Take measures to prevent skin breakdown. Use soap sparingly, and apply an emollient or lotion. An alternating-pressure mattress may be helpful.
3. Avoid using sedatives. If they must be used, use the lowest possible dose, and family members should closely monitor mental status, level of consciousness, and respirations.
4. Prevent constipation by a gradual increase in exercise, increased fiber in diet, stool softeners as advised, and maintenance of a regular bowel elimination time (usually in the morning). Avoid enemas because they produce vagal stimulation, which can be hazardous if cardiac disease is present.
5. Understand the nature of the thyroid hormone deficiency and the self-care practices necessary to prevent complications.

DISORDERS OF THE PARATHYROID GLANDS

HYPERPARATHYROIDISM
Etiology and Pathophysiology

Hyperparathyroidism is a condition involving increased secretion of parathyroid hormone (PTH). PTH helps regulate calcium and phosphate levels by stimulating bone resorption, renal tubular reabsorption of calcium, and activation of vitamin D. Until recently, this dysfunction was considered rare. However, with the increased use of routine evaluation of serum calcium levels the prevalence in the general population is estimated to be 0.04%, and the annual incidence in persons over 40 years of age ranges between 0.1% and 0.5%.[37,38]

Hyperparathyroidism is classified as primary, secondary, or tertiary. Primary hyperparathyroidism is due to an increased secretion of PTH leading to disorders of calcium, phosphate, and bone metabolism. The excessive concentration of circulating PTH usually leads to hypercalcemia and hypophosphatemia. The most common cause is a benign neoplasm or a single adenoma (80% of cases) in the parathyroid gland. Secondary hyperparathyroidism appears to be a compensatory response to states that induce or cause hypocalcemia, the main stimulus of PTH secretion. Disease conditions associated with secondary hyperparathyroidism include vitamin D deficiencies, malabsorption, chronic renal failure, and hyperphosphatemia. Tertiary hyperparathyroidism occurs when there is hyperplasia of the parathyroid glands and a loss of negative feedback from circulating calcium levels. Thus there is autonomous secretion of PTH, even with normal calcium levels. It is observed in the patient who has had a kidney transplant after a long period of dialysis treatment for chronic renal failure (see Chapter 44).

Primary hyperparathyroidism is more common in women and usually occurs between 30 and 70 years of age. The peak incidence is in the fifth and sixth decades of life. Previous head and neck radiation may predispose a patient to the

Table **47-10**	Clinical Manifestations: Parathyroid Dysfunction	
System	Hypofunction	Hyperfunction
Cardiovascular	Decreased contractility of heart muscle Decreased cardiac output Prolongation of QT and ST intervals on ECG Arrhythmias	Arrhythmias Shortened QT interval on ECG Hypertension
Gastrointestinal	Abdominal cramps Urinary and fecal incontinence (in older adult)	Vague abdominal pain Anorexia Nausea and vomiting Constipation Pancreatitis Peptic ulcer disease Cholelithiasis Weight loss
Integumentary	Dry, scaly skin Hair loss on scalp and body Brittle nails, transverse ridging Changes in developing teeth, lack of tooth enamel	Skin necrosis Moist skin
Musculoskeletal	Fatigue Weakness Painful muscle cramps Skeletal x-ray changes, osteosclerosis Soft-tissue calcification Difficulty in walking	Skeletal pain Backache Weakness, fatigue Pain on weight bearing Osteoporosis Pathologic fractures of long bones Compression fractures of spine Decreased muscle tone
Neurologic	Personality changes Psychiatric manifestations of depression, anxiety Irritability Memory impairment Headache Seizures Positive Chvostek's sign or Trousseau's phenomenon Tremor Paresthesias of perioral area, hands, feet Hyperactive deep-tendon reflexes Disorientation, confusion (in older adult)	Personality disturbances Emotional irritability Memory impairment Psychosis Delirium, confusion, coma Incoordination Hyperactive deep-tendon reflexes Abnormalities of gait Psychomotor retardation Headache
Renal	Urinary frequency	Hypercalciuria Kidney stones (nephrolithiasis) Urinary tract infections Polyuria
Other	Eye changes, including lenticular opacities, cataracts, papilledema	Corneal calcification on slit-lamp examination

development of parathyroid adenoma in a small group of patients.[38] Increased PTH has a multisystem effect (Table 47-10). In the bones, subperiosteal bone resorption, decreased bone density, cyst formation, and general weakness can occur as a result of the effect of PTH on osteoclastic (bone resorbers) and osteoblastic (bone formers) activity.

In the kidneys the excess calcium cannot be reabsorbed, leading to increased levels of calcium in the urine (hypercalciuria). This urinary calcium, along with a large amount of urinary phosphate, can lead to calculi formation. In addition, in the kidneys, PTH stimulates the synthesis of a biologically active form of vitamin D, a potent stimulator of calcium transport in the intestine. In this way, PTH indirectly increases GI absorption of calcium, contributing further to the high serum calcium levels.

Clinical Manifestations and Complications

Hyperparathyroidism has varying symptoms (see Table 47-10). The major symptoms include weakness, loss of appetite, constipation, increased need for sleep, emotional disorders, and shortened attention span. Major signs include loss of calcium from bones (osteoporosis), broken bones, and kidney stones (nephrolithiasis). Neuromuscular abnormalities are characterized by muscle weakness, particularly in the proximal muscles of the lower extremities. Asymptomatic cases are being identified with increasing frequency with routine calcium screening.

Serious complications of hyperparathyroidism are renal failure, pancreatitis, collapse of vertebral bodies, cardiac changes, and long bone and rib fractures.

Diagnostic Studies

PTH, as measured by radioimmunoassay, will be elevated. Serum calcium levels usually exceed 10 mg/dl (2.50 mmol/L). Because of its inverse relation with calcium, the serum phosphorus level is usually below 3 mg/dl (0.1 mmol/L). Elevations in other laboratory tests include urine calcium, serum chloride, uric acid, creatinine, amylase (if pancreatitis is present), and alkaline phosphatase (if bone disease has begun). If bone changes are present, radiologic studies may reveal subperiosteal resorption. Imaging such as MRI, CT scanning, and ultrasound may be used for localization of the adenoma.[39]

Collaborative Care

The treatment objectives are to relieve symptoms and prevent complications caused by excess PTH. The choice of therapy depends on the urgency of the clinical situation, the degree of hypercalcemia, the underlying disorder, the status of renal and hepatic function, the clinical presentation of the patient, and the particular advantages and disadvantages of the different therapeutic modalities.

If the symptoms are mild or if the patient is elderly or at increased surgical risk from other health problems, a conservative management approach is used. This includes an annual examination with tests for serum PTH, calcium, phosphorus, and alkaline phosphatase levels and renal function, x-rays to assess for metabolic bone disease, and measurement of urinary calcium excretion. Continued ambulation and the avoidance of immobility are critical aspects of management.

Parathyroid tumors should be removed surgically. The parathyroid glands occasionally lie in ectopic sites such as the mediastinum. This situation requires a highly skilled surgeon to open the chest and explore the area behind the sternum. Generally, a single gland is removed if an adenoma is the cause of the hyperparathyroidism. When cancer is the cause, all the parathyroid glands are removed. With a total parathyroidectomy, the patient will need to take calcium supplements for life.

Specific management measures include maintenance of a high fluid intake and a moderate calcium intake. The diet should contain 8 to 10 g of sodium per day to replace losses from increased urine output. Phosphorus is usually supplemented, unless contraindicated by an increased risk for urinary calculi formation.

Drug Therapy. Plicamycin (Mithracin), an antihypercalcemic agent, lowers serum calcium within 48 hours. However, because of toxic side effects, its use is limited to the patient with metastatic parathyroid carcinoma and severe bone disease. Biphosphonates such as pamidronate (Aredia) may be used. They inhibit osteoclastic bone resorption and rapidly normalize serum calcium levels. Estrogen or progestin therapy can reduce serum and urinary calcium levels in the postmenopausal woman and may retard demineralization of the skeleton.[39] Oral phosphate may be used to inhibit the calcium-absorbing effects of vitamin D in the intestine. Phosphates should be used only if a patient has normal renal function and low serum phosphate levels. Diuretics may be given to increase the urinary excretion of calcium.

In severe hyperparathyroidism, normal saline is given IV to correct fluid volume deficit and promote calcium excretion. Furosemide (Lasix) is given orally or IV to promote sodium loss and decrease renal tubular reabsorption of calcium. Plicamycin (Mithracin) may be administered IV to inhibit osteoclastic bone resorption.[40]

NURSING MANAGEMENT: HYPERPARATHYROIDISM

■ Nursing Assessment

Subjective and objective data that should be obtained from an individual with hyperparathyroidism are presented in Table 47-11.

■ Nursing Diagnoses

Nursing diagnoses for the patient with hyperparathyroidism may include, but are not limited to, those presented in NCP 47-3.

■ Planning

The overall goals are that the patient with hyperparathyroidism will (1) maintain satisfactory activity level, (2) keep a consistently high fluid intake, (3) not experience any serious complications related to the disease or its treatment, (4) maintain a positive self-image, and (5) accept and comply with the long-term nature of the problem.

■ Nursing Implementation

If surgery is performed, close monitoring of the patient's vital signs is required. Other aspects of care are similar to that after thyroidectomy. The major postoperative complications are tetany and fluid and electrolyte disturbances. Tetany is usually apparent early in the postoperative period but may develop over several days. Mild tetany, characterized by unpleasant tingling of the hands and around the mouth, may be present but should abate without problems. If tetany becomes more severe (e.g., muscular spasms or laryngospasms develop), IV calcium may be given. Strict monitoring of intake and output is necessary to evaluate fluid status. Calcium, potassium, phosphate, and magnesium levels are assessed frequently, as well as Chvostek's and Trousseau's signs (see Fig. 15-14). Mobility is encouraged to promote bone calcification.

If surgery is not performed, treatment to relieve symptoms and prevent complications is carried out. The nurse can assist the patient with hyperparathyroidism to adapt the meal plan to her or his lifestyle. A referral to a dietician may be useful. Since immobility can aggravate the bone loss, the nurse can assist the patient to implement an exercise prescription and identify resources, such as shopping malls and YMCAs or YWCAs, as places to exercise safely. The patient should be encouraged to keep the annual appointments, and the tests being performed should be explained. The patient should also be instructed in the symptoms of hypocalcemia and hypercalcemia and to report these should they occur. Hypocalcemia and hypercalcemia are discussed in Chapter 15.

■ Evaluation

Expected outcomes for the patient with hyperparathyroidism are addressed in NCP 47-3.

NURSING ASSESSMENT
Table 47-11 Hyperparathyroidism

Subjective Data

Important Health Information
Past health history: Vitamin D deficiency; malabsorption, malnutrition; chronic renal failure
Medications: Compliance with renal failure medication (e.g., phosphate binders, calcium supplements)
Surgery or other treatments: Previous head or neck radiation

Functional Health Patterns
Health perception–health management: Malaise
Nutritional-metabolic: Anorexia, nausea, vomiting, weight loss
Elimination: Polyuria, dysuria, constipation
Activity-exercise: Weakness, fatigue
Sleep: Increase in sleeping
Cognitive-perceptual: Irritability, depression; generalized skeletal pain with pain on weight bearing, headache, abdominal and back pain, arthralgias; renal colic
Coping–stress tolerance: Irritability, memory impairment, personality changes

Objective Data

General
Apathy

Integumentary
Moist skin, skin necrosis

Cardiovascular
Hypertension, arrhythmias (especially bradycardias)

Neurologic
Drowsiness, slow mentation, confusion, delirium, poor coordination, hyperactive deep tendon reflexes

Musculoskeletal
Fractures, decreased muscle tone, abnormal gait

Possible Findings
Elevated serum calcium (>10 mg/dl), parathyroid hormone, chloride, alkaline phosphatase, uric acid, creatinine; decreased serum phosphate (<3 mg/dl); hypercalciuria; guaiac-positive stool and emesis (peptic ulcer); subperiosteal bone resorption and demineralization on x-ray examination; enlarged parathyroids on ultrasonography

HYPOPARATHYROIDISM
Etiology and Pathophysiology

Hypoparathyroidism, or inadequate circulating PTH, is uncommon. It is characterized by hypocalcemia resulting from a lack of PTH to maintain serum calcium levels. PTH resistance at the cellular level may also occur (pseudohypoparathyroidism). This is caused by a genetic defect resulting in hypocalcemia in spite of normal or high PTH levels and is often associated with hypothyroidism and hypogonadism.

The most common cause of hypoparathyroidism is iatrogenic, that is, accidental removal of the parathyroids or damage to the vascular supply of the glands during neck surgery (e.g., thyroidectomy, radical neck surgery). Idiopathic hypoparathyroidism resulting from the absence, fatty replacement, or atrophy of the glands is a rare disease that usually occurs early in life and may be associated with other endocrine disorders. Affected patients may have antiparathyroid antibodies. Hypomagnesemia is increasingly being recognized as a cause of hypoparathyroidism. Hypomagnesemia, as seen in alcoholism or malabsorption, impairs PTH secretion and its action on bone and kidneys.[37]

Clinical Manifestations

The clinical features of acute hypoparathyroidism are due to a low serum calcium level (see Table 47-10). Sudden decreases in calcium concentration give rise to a syndrome called *tetany.* This state is characterized by tingling of the lips, fingertips, and occasionally feet and increased muscle tension leading to paresthesias and stiffness. Painful tonic spasms of smooth and skeletal muscles (particularly of the extremities and face), dysphagia, a constricted feeling in the throat, and laryngospasms are also present. Chvostek's sign (facial muscle spasm when the face is tapped below the temple) and Trousseau's sign (carpopedal spasm when arterial circulation is interrupted by applying a blood pressure cuff for 3 minutes; see Fig. 15-14) are usually positive. Respiratory function may be severely compromised by accessory muscle spasm and laryngeal spasm–induced airway obstruction. Patients are usually anxious and apprehensive. Abnormal laboratory findings include decreased serum calcium and PTH levels and increased serum phosphate levels. Other causes of chronic hypocalcemia include chronic renal failure, vitamin D deficiency, and hypomagnesemia.

Collaborative Care

The main objectives of treatment are to treat tetany when present and prevent long-term complications by maintaining normal serum calcium levels (eucalcemia).

Tetany is treated with IV infusion or slow push of calcium salts. Long-term therapy consists of the administration of vitamin D and possibly supplemental calcium and oral phosphate binders.[41]

Emergency treatment of tetany requires the administration of IV calcium. Generally, in adults, 10 to 20 ml of a 10% solution of calcium gluconate is infused over 10 minutes. Calcium salts can cause hypotension and cardiac arrest; thus a slow IV push is required.[41] In addition, these salts can cause venous irritation and inflammation if leakage occurs into extravascular tissues. For long-term management, oral calcium supplements may be prescribed. Calcium carbonate, an antacid, is readily available but may alter acid-base balance. It also stimulates secretion of hydrochloric acid, which could be a problem for the patient with an ulcer. Calcium gluconate, which is available in tablet form, should be chewed into fine particles before swallowing. Acid aids in the gastrointestinal absorption of calcium

47-3 NURSING CARE PLAN PATIENT WITH HYPERPARATHYROIDISM

Expected Patient Outcomes	Nursing Interventions and *Rationales*

NURSING DIAGNOSIS **Activity intolerance** *related to* muscle weakness and fatigue *as manifested by* complaints of weakness and fatigue, pain on weight bearing.

- Decreased fatigue and weakness.
- Activities of daily living needs met by self or others.

- Assist with ambulation and limit ambulation to short walks *to demonstrate a caring attitude and prevent fatigue.*
- Assist patient with self-care as needed *to ensure activities of daily living needs are met and to conserve energy.*
- Plan activities of daily living and treatment *to allow for adequate rest periods.*
- Provide patient with walker or cane as necessary *as aids to safe ambulation and to keep patient ambulatory.*

NURSING DIAGNOSIS **Altered urinary elimination** *related to* renal involvement secondary to hypercalcemia *as manifested by* hypercalciuria, renal stones.

- No renal stones.
- Prompt detection and early treatment of renal stones.

- Instruct patient about symptoms of renal stones such as flank pain and hematuria *to ensure early reporting of symptoms.*
- Strain urine *to detect stones.*
- Keep fluids within easy reach and offer frequently; encourage fluid intake to point of moderate overhydration (4000 ml or more fluid output per day) *to keep fluid level high so kidneys are flushed and stone formation is less likely.*

NURSING DIAGNOSIS **Altered nutrition: less than body requirements** *related to* anorexia and nausea *as manifested by* loss of weight and complaints of loss of appetite and nausea.

- Maintenance of adequate food and fluid intake.
- Maintenance of stable weight.

- Administer mouth care frequently with use of flavored mouthwash or toothpaste *to keep mouth fresh.*
- Eliminate noxious odors from environment *to prevent this potential cause of a decreased appetite.*
- Reduce milk products *to reduce nausea.*
- Teach calorie counting *so that caloric intake is sufficient to maintain weight.*
- Serve small amounts of food frequently *to prevent bloating and a premature sense of fullness.*

NURSING DIAGNOSIS **Constipation** *related to* dehydration and inactivity *as manifested by* complaints of rectal fullness and pressure, pain on defecation, hard stools, <3 stools per week.

- Regular evacuation (preferably daily) of soft or formed stools.
- Prompt detection of constipation or impaction.

- Encourage fluid intake to 3000 ml per day *to increase fluid content of fecal mass.*
- Administer prune juice daily *because it contains dihydroxyphenyl isatin, which acts as a laxative.*
- Maintain diet high in bulk *to increase fecal mass.*
- Request order for stool softener from physician.
- Encourage frequent, short walks *to promote increased peristalsis and movement of fecal mass.*
- Promote maintenance of regular habit of defecation consistent with preadmission pattern *to foster bowel regularity.*

NURSING DIAGNOSIS **Risk for injury: fractures and joint contractures** *related to* decreased bone density, weakness, improper body alignment, and immobility.

- No occurrence of deformity or accidental injury.

- Monitor for complaints of bone and joint pain, weakness, backache, impaired mobility, unsteady gait *to detect potential for injury.*
- Assist patient with ambulation, reduce safety hazards in environment, and maintain bed in low position *to reduce potential for injury.*
- Alert other hospital departments about handling and positioning patient during tests *to avoid accidental injury caused by lack of knowledge of patient's musculoskeletal fragility.*

Continued

47-3　NURSING CARE PLAN　PATIENT WITH HYPERPARATHYROIDISM
—continued

Expected Patient Outcomes	Nursing Interventions and *Rationales*

NURSING DIAGNOSIS **Body image disturbance** *related to* weight loss, weakness, fatigue, and mental status changes *as manifested by* verbalization of negative feelings about self; expression of feelings of hopelessness; hostile, angry behavior; self-isolation.

■ Statements and actions indicative of improved self-image. ■ More positive mental outlook.	■ Encourage patient to ventilate feelings about physical and emotional changes *because venting of feelings helps clarify issues.* ■ Compliment patient when appropriate *to promote a positive body image.* ■ Reassure patient that fatigability and depression will improve when hormone imbalance is corrected *to foster hope and a positive attitude.* ■ Encourage short walks to social areas *to prevent isolation.* ■ Ascertain which activities the patient has enjoyed in past; encourage continued involvement in those activities that are appropriate to setting and patient's condition.

NURSING DIAGNOSIS **Altered thought processes** *related to* slowed mentation, depression, and drowsiness *as manifested by* disorientation, inappropriate behavior or response, difficulty in concentrating.

■ Maintenance of reality-based orientation. ■ Appropriate actions and reactions.	■ Assess sensory-perceptual status *to plan appropriate interventions.* ■ Orient patient as indicated *to assist with reality orientation.* ■ Provide calm, restful environment *to minimize confusion and foster rest.* ■ Explain actions in simple language *to avoid increasing patient's confusion.* ■ Monitor and record level of consciousness and orientation every shift *to evaluate effectiveness of plan and alter as appropriate.*

COLLABORATIVE PROBLEMS

Nursing Goals	Nursing Interventions and *Rationales*

POTENTIAL COMPLICATION **Tetany** *related to* hypocalcemia secondary to low serum calcium following parathyroidectomy.

■ Monitor for signs of tetany, including neuromuscular irritability, Chvostek's sign, and Trousseau's sign. ■ Report deviations from acceptable parameters. ■ Carry out appropriate nursing and medical interventions.	■ Assess the patient for circumoral and hand paresthesias that do not subside *as a precursor to tetany.* ■ Be prepared to administer calcium gluconate intravenously if ordered *to treat hypocalcemia.*

gluconate, so it should be taken at the end of a meal. Oral calcium supplements are given four times a day.

Specific hormone replacement of PTH is not used to treat hypoparathyroidism because of expense and the need for parenteral administration. Vitamin D is used in chronic and resistant hypocalcemia to enhance intestinal calcium absorption and bone resorption. The preferred preparations are dihydrotachysterol (Hytakerol) and calcitriol (1,25-dihydroxycholecalciferol [Rocaltrol]). These drugs are more potent, raise calcium levels rapidly, and are quickly metabolized. Rapid metabolism is desired because vitamin D is a fat-soluble vitamin and toxicity can cause irreversible renal impairment. Oral vitamin D (ergocalciferol) may also be prescribed.

NURSING MANAGEMENT: HYPOPARATHYROIDISM

■ Nursing Assessment

Nursing care of a patient with hypoparathyroidism requires close assessment for signs of tetany. The patient should be observed closely for carpopedal spasm (Trousseau's phenomenon) while blood pressures are being taken because this is an early sign of tetany. Periodic assessment for Chvostek's sign is advisable. Tingling in the fingertips and around the mouth, irritability, anxiety, apprehension, muscular hypertonicity, and cramps may precede acute tetany. It is important to note any allergy to iodine because it may be used in associated diagnostic testing, such as an intravenous pyelogram (IVP).

■ Nursing Diagnoses

Nursing diagnoses for the patient with hypoparathyroidism may include, but are not limited to, the following:

- Impaired skin integrity *related to* dry, scaly skin
- Activity intolerance *related to* fatigue, weakness, and painful muscle cramps
- Altered thought processes *related to* personality and psychiatric changes and memory impairment
- Ineffective management of therapeutic regimen *related to* lack of knowledge regarding signs and symptoms of calcium deficiency, calcium-rich foods and supplements, and chronic nature of the problem
- Potential complication: arrhythmia
- Potential complication: tetany

■ Planning

The overall goals are that the patient with hypoparathyroidism will (1) develop no complications such as tetany or arrhythmias, (2) recognize signs and symptoms of hypoparathyroidism and hyperparathyroidism, and (3) comply with periodic assessment of calcium level.

■ Nursing Implementation

Health Promotion. Health promotion is directed at identifying patients at risk. This includes patients who have undergone thyroid removal (thyroidectomy).

Acute Intervention. If tetany or generalized muscle cramps develop, rebreathing may partially alleviate the symptoms. The patient who can cooperate should be instructed to breathe in and out of a paper bag or breathing mask. This reduces carbon dioxide excretion from the lungs, increases carbonic acid levels in the blood, and lowers body pH. Because an acidic environment enhances both solubility and the degree of ionization of calcium, the proportion of total body calcium available in physiologically active form (i.e., ionized calcium) is increased, temporarily relieving the functional hypocalcemia.

IV calcium salts should be available at the bedside for treatment of acute tetany. Calcium salts must be infused slowly because high blood levels can cause serious cardiac arrhythmias or cardiac arrest. The patient who has been digitalized is particularly vulnerable. Because calcium-induced ventricular standstill occurs in systole, this type of arrest is less likely than other types to respond to resuscitation. ECG monitoring is indicated. Side rails should be padded as a seizure precaution. The patient should be kept in a nonstimulating environment, assisted with hygienic needs, and given support and encouragement until free of symptoms.

Ambulatory and Home Care. The patient with hypoparathyroidism needs instruction in the management of long-term nutrition and drug therapy. A high-calcium meal plan includes foods such as dark green vegetables, soy beans, and tofu. The patient should be told that foods containing oxalic acid (e.g., spinach and rhubarb), phytic acid (e.g., bran and whole grains), and phosphorus reduce calcium absorption. Calcium supplements of at least 1 g per day for the patient under 40 years of age and 2 g per day for the patient more than 40 years of age are usually prescribed. These supplements are best administered 2 to 3 hours after meals. Although calcium carbonate often leads to constipation and flatulence, bran and whole grain foods should not be used for treatment. Alternative nursing interventions include providing stool softeners, adequate fluids, and fresh fruits.

The patient should be instructed with written handouts about the signs and symptoms of hypocalcemia and hypercalcemia and to report these to a clinician as soon as possible if they occur. If manifestations of hypocalcemia occur, calcium supplementation should be increased. The need for lifelong treatment and health supervision should be stressed. The patient's calcium levels should be monitored three to four times a year. Treatment modification is often necessary because hypercalcemia can develop without apparent cause. Thorough patient instruction and frequent serum calcium assessment should allow a normal life expectancy. The patient needs support and encouragement to continue with the regimen. The patient may dislike taking so many pills.

■ Evaluation

The expected outcomes are that the patient with hypoparathyroidism

- experiences no complications of the disease
- states the signs and symptoms of hypoparathyroidism
- has a follow-up appointment and states the importance of periodic assessment of calcium levels

DISORDERS OF THE ADRENAL CORTEX

There are three main classifications of adrenal steroid hormones. Glucocorticoids regulate metabolism, increase blood glucose levels, and are critical in the physiologic stress response. In humans the primary glucocorticoid is cortisol. Mineralocorticoids regulate sodium and potassium balance. The primary mineralocorticoid is aldosterone. Androgens contribute to growth and development in both genders and to sexual activity in adult women. The term *corticosteroid* refers to any one of these three types of hormones produced by the adrenal cortex.

CUSHING'S SYNDROME
Etiology and Pathophysiology

Cushing's syndrome is a spectrum of clinical abnormalities caused by excess corticosteroids, particularly glucocorticoids. Several conditions can cause Cushing's syndrome (Table 47-12). The most common cause is iatrogenic administration of exogenous cortisol. Approximately 85% of endogenous Cushing's syndrome is due to an ACTH-secreting pituitary tumor (Cushing's disease). Other causes include adrenal tumors and ectopic ACTH production by tumors outside the hypothalamic-pituitary-adrenal axis (usually of the lung or pancreas). Cushing's disease and primary adrenal tumors are more common in women 20 to 40 years of age (Fig. 47-8), whereas ectopic ACTH production is more common in men.[42]

Clinical Manifestations

The clinical manifestations of Cushing's syndrome can be seen in most body systems and are related to excess levels of corti-

Table **47-12**	**Causes of Cushing's Syndrome**

Prolonged administration of high doses of corticosteroids
ACTH-secreting pituitary tumor (Cushing's disease)
Cortisol-secreting neoplasm within the adrenal cortex that can be either carcinoma or adenoma
Excess secretion of ACTH from carcinoma of lung or other malignant growth outside pituitary or adrenals

ACTH, adrenocorticotropic hormone.

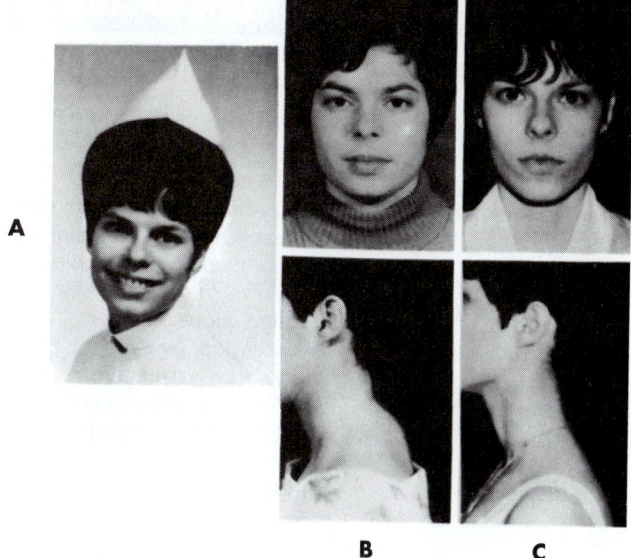

Fig. 47-8　A woman with Cushing's syndrome resulting from right adrenal cortical adenoma. **A,** Patient at age 18, 2 years before surgery. **B,** Patient at age 20, 1 month before surgery. **C,** Patient at age 21, 1 year after surgery. (From Williams GH, Dluhy RG: Diseases of the adrenal cortex. In Isselbacher K and others, eds: *Harrison's principles of internal medicine,* ed 14, New York, 1998, McGraw-Hill.)

costeroids (Table 47-13). Although manifestations of glucocorticoid excess usually predominate, symptoms of mineralocorticoid and androgen excess may also be seen.

Glucocorticoid excess causes pronounced changes in personal appearance (Fig. 47-9). These signs and symptoms logically flow from the known actions of glucocorticoids. Weight gain, the most common feature, results from the accumulation of adipose tissue in the trunk, face, and cervical area. Transient weight gain from sodium and water retention may be present because of the mineralocorticoid effects of cortisol. Glucose intolerance occurs because of cortisol-induced insulin resistance and increased gluconeogenesis by the liver.

Protein wasting is caused by the catabolic effects of cortisol on peripheral tissue. Muscle wasting leads to muscle weakness, especially in the extremities. Loss of protein matrix in bone leads to osteoporosis with subsequent pathologic fractures, vertebral compression fractures, and bone and back pain. Loss of collagen makes the skin weaker and thinner; therefore it bruises easier. Catabolic processes predominate, and wound healing is delayed. Mood disturbances (irritability, anxiety, euphoria), insomnia, irrationality, and occasionally psychosis may occur. The skin and mucous membranes may take on a bronze or brownish color because of the melanotropic activity of ACTH.

Mineralocorticoid excess may cause hypertension, whereas adrenal androgen excess may cause pronounced acne, virilization in women, and feminization in men. Menstrual disorders and hirsutism in women and gynecomastia and impotence in men are seen more commonly in adrenal carcinomas.

The clinical presentation, as revealed by the history and physical examination, is the first indication of Cushing's syndrome. Of particular importance are (1) centripedal (truncal) obesity or generalized obesity; (2) "moon facies" (fullness of the face) with facial plethora; (3) purplish-red striae, which are usually depressed below the skin surface, on the abdomen, breast, or buttocks; (4) hirsutism; (5) menstrual disorders; (6) hypertension; and (7) unexplained hypokalemia.

Diagnostic Studies

Abnormal findings include granulocytosis, lymphocytopenia, eosinopenia, hyperglycemia, glycosuria, hypercalciuria, and osteoporosis (as observed on x-rays). Hypokalemia and alkalosis are seen in ectopic ACTH syndrome and adrenal carcinoma. Plasma ACTH may be low, normal, or elevated depending on the underlying problem. High or normal levels indicate ACTH-dependent Cushing's syndrome, whereas low or undetectable levels indicate an adrenal or exogenous etiology. When Cushing's syndrome is suspected, a 24-hour urine collection for free

cortisol and a low-dose dexamethasone suppression test (see Chapter 45) are done. If these results are borderline, a high-dose dexamethasone suppression test is done.[43] False-positive results can occur in depressed patients, those under acute stress, and those who are active alcoholics. Plasma cortisol (the primary glucocorticoid) levels may be elevated, with loss of diurnal variation. CT scanning and MRI may be used for tumor localization.

Collaborative Care

The treatment of choice for Cushing's disease is transsphenoidal surgical removal of the pituitary adenoma (hypophysectomy) (see earlier in this chapter). Adrenalectomy is indicated for adrenal tumors or hyperplasia. Currently transperitoneal or retroperitoneal laparoscopic surgery is performed to remove adrenal tumors less than 5 cm in size. Occasionally, bilateral adrenalectomy is necessary (Table 47-14). Patients with ectopic ACTH-secreting tumors are managed with treatment of the neoplasm.

If surgery is anticipated, the patient should be brought to optimal physical condition. Hypertension and hyperglycemia must be controlled, and hypokalemia is corrected with diet and potassium supplements. A high-protein meal plan helps correct the protein depletion. Vitamin A supplementation may be given to counteract the problem of delayed wound healing.[43]

Drug Therapy.　In inoperable cases or in cases in which residual disease remains, treatment with mitotane (Lysodren) may be used. This drug suppresses cortisol production, alters peripheral metabolism of cortisol, and decreases plasma and urine corticosteroid levels. The action of this drug results in a "medical adrenalectomy." Metyrapone, ketoconazole (Nizoral),

| Table **47-13** | **Clinical Manifestations: Adrenal Cortical Hormone Dysfunction** |

System	Hypofunction	Hyperfunction
Glucocorticoids		
General appearance	Weight loss	Truncal (centripedal) obesity, thin extremities, rounding of face (moon face), fat deposits on back of neck and on shoulders ("buffalo hump")
Integumentary	Bronzed or smoky hyperpigmentation of face, neck, hands (especially creases), buccal membranes, nipples, genitalia, and scars (if pituitary function normal); vitiligo, alopecia	Thin, fragile skin; purplish-red striae; petechial hemorrhages; bruises; florid cheeks (plethora); acne; poor wound healing
Cardiovascular	Hypotension, tendency to develop refractory shock, vasodilation	Hypervolemia, hypertension, edema of lower extremities
Gastrointestinal	Anorexia, nausea and vomiting, cramping abdominal pain, diarrhea	Increase in secretion of pepsin and hydrochloric acid, anorexia
Urinary		Glycosuria, hypercalciuria, kidney stones
Musculoskeletal	Fatigability	Muscle wasting in extremities, proximal muscle weakness, fatigue, osteoporosis, awkward gait, back and joint pain, weakness, growth retardation (in children)
Immune	Propensity toward autoimmune diseases	Inhibition of immune response, suppression of allergic response, inhibition of inflammation
Hematologic	Anemia, lymphocytosis	Leukocytosis, lymphopenia, polycythemia, increased coagulability
Fluids and electrolytes	Hyponatremia, hypovolemia, dehydration, hyperkalemia	Sodium and water retention, edema, hypokalemia
Metabolic	Hypoglycemia, insulin sensitivity, fever	Hyperglycemia, negative nitrogen balance, dyslipidemia
Emotional	Neurasthenia, depression, exhaustion or irritability, confusion, delusions	Psychic stimulation, euphoria, irritability, hypomania to depression, emotional lability
Mineralocorticoids		
Fluid and electrolytes	Sodium loss, decreased volume of extracellular fluid, hyperkalemia, salt craving	Marked sodium and water retention, tendency toward edema, marked hypokalemia
Cardiovascular	Hypovolemia, tendency toward shock, decreased cardiac output, decreased heart size	Hypertension, hypervolemia
Androgens		
Integumentary	Decreased axillary and pubic hair (in women)	Hirsutism, acne
Reproductive	No effect in men, decreased libido in women	Menstrual irregularities and enlargement of clitoris (in females); gynecomastia and testicular atrophy (in males)
Musculoskeletal	Decrease in muscle size and tone	Increase in muscle development

and aminoglutethimide (Cytadren) may be used to inhibit cortisol synthesis. The relatively common side effects of these agents include anorexia, nausea and vomiting, GI bleeding, depression, vertigo, skin rashes, and diplopia. The GI side effects may be minimized by administering mitotane (Lysodren) with meals and with a bedtime snack. Ketoconazole, which inhibits synthesis of gonadal and adrenal corticosteroids, may also be used. The side effects from this medication are fewer than those of other adrenal suppressants.

If Cushing's syndrome has developed during the course of prolonged administration of glucocorticoids (e.g., cortisol), one or more of the following alternatives may be tried: (1) gradual discontinuance of glucocorticoid therapy, (2) reduction of the glucocorticoid dose, and (3) conversion to an alternate-day regimen. Gradual tapering of the glucocorticoids is necessary to avoid

potentially life-threatening adrenal insufficiency. An alternate-day regimen is one in which twice the daily dosage of a shorter-acting glucocorticoid is given every other morning to minimize hypothalamic-pituitary-adrenal suppression, growth suppression, and altered appearance. This regimen is not used when the corticosteroids (i.e., cortisol and aldosterone mimicking drugs) are given as physiologic replacements.

NURSING MANAGEMENT: CUSHING'S SYNDROME

■ Nursing Assessment

Subjective and objective data that should be obtained from a patient with Cushing's syndrome are presented in Table 47-15.

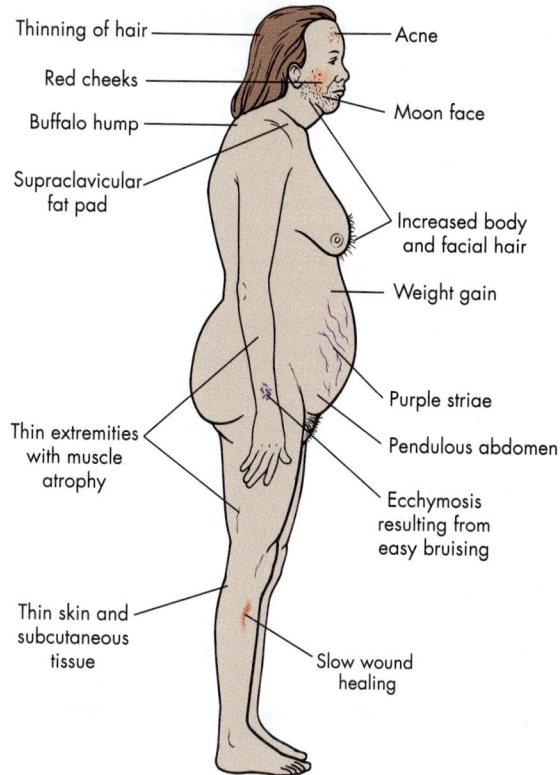

Fig. 47-9 Common characteristics of Cushing's syndrome.

Labels: Thinning of hair — Acne — Red cheeks — Moon face — Buffalo hump — Supraclavicular fat pad — Increased body and facial hair — Weight gain — Thin extremities with muscle atrophy — Purple striae — Pendulous abdomen — Ecchymosis resulting from easy bruising — Thin skin and subcutaneous tissue — Slow wound healing

COLLABORATIVE CARE
Table 47-14 Cushing's Syndrome

Diagnostic
- History and physical examination
- Mental status examination
- Plasma cortisol levels for diurnal variations
- Plasma ACTH level
- Complete blood count
- Blood chemistries for sodium, potassium, glucose
- Dexamethasone suppression test
- 24-hour urine for free cortisol
- Examination of visual fields
- CT scan, MRI

Collaborative Therapy
- Adrenal cortical adenoma, carcinoma, or hyperplasia
  - Surgical adrenalectomy
    - Laparoscopic adrenalectomy
  - Medical adrenalectomy
- Pituitary corticotropin (ACTH) hypersecretion
  - Transsphenoidal resection of microadenoma
  - Radiation
  - Treatment with hypothalamic serotonin antagonist (cyproheptadine)
- Surgical removal of nonendocrine ACTH-producing tumors, adrenalectomy (if pituitary tumor inoperable)
- Discontinuance of or alteration in administration of exogenous corticosteroids

NURSING ASSESSMENT
Table 47-15 Cushing's Syndrome

Subjective Data

Important Health Information
Past health history: Pituitary tumor (Cushing's disease); adrenal, pancreatic, or pulmonary neoplasms; GI bleeding; frequent infections
Medications: Use of corticosteroids

Functional Health Patterns
Health perception–health management: Malaise
Nutritional-metabolic: Weight gain, anorexia
Elimination: Polyuria; prolonged wound healing, easy bruising
Activity-exercise: Weakness, fatigue
Sleep: Insomnia, poor sleep quality
Cognitive-perceptual: Headache; back, joint, bone, and rib pain; poor concentration and memory
Self-perception–self-concept: Negative feelings regarding changes in personal appearance
Sexuality-reproductive: Amenorrhea, impotence, decreased libido
Coping–stress tolerance: Anxiety, mood disturbances, emotional lability, psychosis

Objective Data

General
Truncal obesity, supraclavicular fat pads, buffalo hump, moon facies

Integumentary
Plethora; hirsutism of body and face, thinning of head hair; thin, friable skin; acne; petechiae; purpura; hyperpigmentation; purplish-red striae on breasts, buttocks, and abdomen; edema of lower extremities

Cardiovascular
Hypertension

Musculoskeletal
Muscle wasting, thin extremities, awkward gait

Reproductive
Gynecomastia, testicular atrophy (in men), enlarged clitoris (in women)

Possible Findings
Hypokalemia, hyperglycemia, dyslipidemia; polycythemia, granulocytosis, lymphocytopenia, eosinopenia; elevated plasma cortisol; high, low, or normal ACTH levels; abnormal dexamethasone suppression test; elevated urine free cortisol, 17-ketosteroids; glycosuria, hypercalciuria; osteoporosis on x-ray

47-4   NURSING CARE PLAN   PATIENT WITH CUSHING'S SYNDROME

| Expected Patient Outcomes | Nursing Interventions and *Rationales* |

NURSING DIAGNOSIS   **Risk for infection** *related to* lowered resistance to stress and suppression of immune system.

- No infection.
- Early detection and treatment of any infectious process.

- Assess for inadequate protein stores, proteinuria, muscle wasting, poor wound healing *as indicators of risk for infection.*
- Assess potential infection sites such as urinary and respiratory tracts, skin, and IV lines *so infection can be detected early and treatment initiated promptly.*
- Note pain, loss of function, and purulent drainage *because other signs and symptoms of infection may be minimal or absent.*
- Provide private room, if possible; maintain meticulous asepsis and prevent contact with contagious individuals *to reduce the risk of cross-contamination because patient has an increased susceptibility to infection.*
- Instruct patient in self-care practices *to avoid infection (e.g., hand washing).*
- Refer patient to dietician for high-protein diet instruction *to help correct the protein depletion caused by excess glucocorticoids.*
- Instruct patient and family to be alert for slight changes in signs and symptoms of infection *since the usual immune and inflammatory responses are suppressed* and to report these to clinician immediately *so treatment can be initiated promptly.*

NURSING DIAGNOSIS   **Risk for injury: fracture** *related to* decreased muscle strength, fatigue, osteoporosis, and increased protein catabolism.

- No accidental injury.

- Assess for complaints of weakness, fatigue, back and rib pain; difficulty in ambulating, impairment in mobility; impairment in judgment; drowsiness; hypocalcemia *to detect injury risk factors.*
- Provide cane or walker as necessary *to provide patient with stabilizing device.*
- Keep side rails up if patient's judgment is impaired *to reduce possibility of falls.*
- Instruct patient in high-calcium diet *to replace lost calcium and prevent increasing the severity of osteoporosis.*
- Reinforce dietary instructions. Instruct patient and family in provisions of a safe environment (e.g., nonskid surfaces in wet areas, use of railings, good lighting).

NURSING DIAGNOSIS   **Altered nutrition: more than body requirements** *related to* increased appetite, high caloric content of foods, and inactivity *as manifested by* statement of increased appetite; weight greater than 10% optimum for height.

- Maintenance of body weight if appropriate or no more than 1-2 lb loss per week.

- Obtain dietary consult for instruction in low-caloric, high-nutrition diet (including protein and calcium) *because excess glucocorticoids produce weight gain and calcium and protein loss.*
- Assist with appropriate menu choices *to reinforce dietary instructions.*
- Provide low-calorie, high-vitamin snacks.

NURSING DIAGNOSIS   **Self-esteem disturbance** *related to* altered body image, emotional lability, and diminished physical capabilities *as manifested by* verbalization of negative feelings regarding personal appearance and inability to perform usual activities.

- Verbalization of acceptance of appearance by patient and family.
- Self-care methods to improve appearance.

- Explain to patient and family that physical and emotional changes are related to hormone imbalance and that most will disappear when hormone imbalance is corrected *to increase their understanding and assist with coping.*
- Accept and respect patient as a person *to maintain patient's self-worth.*
- Encourage good grooming and use of attractive attire *to improve patient's appearance and self-esteem.*
- Compliment patient when appropriate *to boost morale by providing positive feedback.*

Continued

47-4 NURSING CARE PLAN PATIENT WITH CUSHING'S SYNDROME—continued

Expected Patient Outcomes	Nursing Interventions and *Rationales*

NURSING DIAGNOSIS | **Impaired skin integrity** *related to* excess corticosteroids, immobility, and altered skin fragility *as manifested by* edema; thin, fragile skin; impaired healing.

- Intact skin.
  - Assess skin *for early detection of trauma.*
  - Protect patient from bumping and bruising *to prevent injury to easily traumatized tissue.*
  - Change patient's position frequently *to minimize pressure over bony prominences and improve circulation in edematous tissue.*
  - Provide good skin care, particularly to edematous areas and areas over bony prominences *because these areas have decreased circulation.*

Nursing Diagnoses

Nursing diagnoses for the patient with Cushing's syndrome may include, but are not limited to, those presented in the NCP 47-4.

Planning

The overall goals are that the patient with Cushing's syndrome will (1) experience relief of symptoms, (2) experience no serious complications, (3) maintain a positive self-image, and (4) actively participate in the therapeutic plan.

Nursing Implementation

Health Promotion. Health promotion is focused on identifying patients at risk for Cushing's syndrome. Patients receiving long-term, exogenous cortisol for a variety of diseases are at risk. Careful patient teaching related to the medication usage and monitoring of side effects are important preventive measures.

Acute Intervention. The patient with Cushing's syndrome is seriously ill. Because the therapeutic interventions have many side effects, the focus of daily assessment is on signs and symptoms of hormone and drug toxicity and complicating conditions such as cardiovascular disease, diabetes mellitus, infection, nephrolithiasis, and pathologic fractures. Daily nursing assessment includes the following:

1. Vital signs every 4 hours, particularly blood pressure
2. Daily weights (gain possibly indicates volume excess)
3. Signs and symptoms of infection, especially pain, loss of function, and purulent drainage, because other signs and symptoms of inflammation such as fever and redness may be minimal or absent
4. Location, time, and duration of abdominal pain
5. Signs and symptoms of abnormal thromboembolic phenomena, such as sudden chest pain, dyspnea, or tachypnea
6. Capillary blood glucose monitoring
7. Bone pain or limitations of range of motion, especially in the lower back
8. Changes in mental status, particularly depression

The patient needs a great deal of emotional support. Changes in appearance such as centripedal obesity, multiple bruises, hirsutism in women, and gynecomastia in men can be distressing. The patient may feel unattractive, repulsive, or unwanted. A survey of patients with Cushing's syndrome showed that 71% reported that their lives had been very adversely affected by this condition.[44] The nurse can help by remaining sensitive to patients' feelings and offering respect and unconditional acceptance.[45] The patient can be reassured that the physical changes and much of the emotional lability are related to side effects of drug therapy and will resolve when hormone levels return to normal.

If treatment involves surgical removal of a pituitary adenoma, an adrenal tumor, or one or both adrenal glands, nursing care will have an additional focus on preoperative and postoperative care. Before surgery the patient should be brought to optimal physical condition. Hypertension and hyperglycemia must be controlled, and hypokalemia is corrected with diet and potassium supplements. A high-protein meal plan helps correct the protein depletion. Surgery on glandular structures poses risks beyond those of other types of operations. Because glands are highly vascular, the risk of hemorrhage is increased. Manipulation of glandular tissue during surgery may release large amounts of hormone into the circulation, producing marked fluctuations in the metabolic processes affected by these hormones.

Preoperative teaching for an adrenalectomy should include information that intermittent pneumatic leg compression may be used to prevent venous thrombosis.[43] In addition, teaching should include that IV infusion and nasogastric suctioning are likely after surgery. Information and instruction about exercises, coughing, and deep breathing are particularly important because patients are prone to thrombosis and infection. If an open surgical approach is used, an upper abdominal incision will be made, increasing the difficulty of coughing and deep breathing. Except for the patient with adrenal cancer or a tumor larger than 5 cm, a laparoscopic adrenalectomy may be performed. This procedure is done via a transperitoneal or retroperitoneal approach. Because this procedure is associated with a faster and less complicated recovery, its use is increasing.[46]

Postoperatively, blood pressure, fluid balance, and electrolyte levels tend to be unstable because of hormone fluctuations. High doses of glucocorticoids (e.g., cortisone) are administered IV during surgery and for several days afterward to ensure adequate responses to the stress of the procedure. If large amounts of endogenous hormone have been released into the systemic circulation during surgery, the patient is likely to develop hypertension, increasing the risk of hemorrhage. High levels of glucocorticoids also increase susceptibility to infection and delay healing.

Any rapid or significant changes in blood pressure, respirations, or heart rate should be reported. Fluid intake and output should be monitored carefully and assessed for potential imbalance. The critical period for circulatory instability ranges from 24 to 48 hours after surgery. IV glucocorticoids are given, and the dose and rate of flow are adjusted to the patient's clinical manifestations and fluid and electrolyte balance. Oral doses are given as tolerated. The IV line may be kept in place after IV glucocorticoids are withdrawn to keep a line open for quick administration of glucocorticoids or vasopressors. Morning urine levels of cortisol (obtained at the same time each morning) are measured to evaluate the effectiveness of the surgery.

If glucocorticoid dosage is tapered too rapidly after surgery, acute adrenal insufficiency may develop. Vomiting after the nasogastric tube is removed, increased weakness, dehydration, and hypotension may indicate hypocortisolism. In addition, the patient may complain of painful joints, pruritus, or peeling skin and may experience severe emotional disturbances. These signs and symptoms should be reported so that drug doses can be adjusted. The nurse must constantly be alert for signs of glucocorticoid imbalance. After surgery the patient is usually maintained on bed rest until the blood pressure stabilizes. The nurse must be alert for subtle signs of postoperative infections because the usual immune and inflammatory responses are suppressed. Meticulous care must be used when changing the dressing and during any other procedures that necessitate access to body cavities, circulation, or areas under the skin so that infection is prevented.

Ambulatory and Home Care. The discharge instructions are based on the patient's lack of endogenous corticosteroids and resulting inability to react to stressors physiologically. Patients should wear Medic Alert bracelets at all times and carry medical identification and instructions in a wallet or purse. Exposure to extremes of temperature, infections, and emotional disturbances should be avoided as much as possible. Stress may produce or precipitate acute adrenal insufficiency because the remaining adrenal tissue cannot meet an increased hormonal demand. Many patients can be taught to adjust their corticosteroid replacement therapy in accordance with their stress levels. The nurse should consult with each patient's physician to determine the parameters for dosage changes if this plan is feasible. If the patient cannot adjust his or her own medication or if weakness, fainting, fever, or nausea and vomiting occur, the patient should contact the clinician for a possible adjustment in corticosteroid dosage. Lifetime replacement therapy is required by many patients, but it may take several months to adjust the hormone dose satisfactorily, and patients should be prepared for this.

■ Evaluation

Expected outcomes for the patient with Cushing's syndrome are addressed in NCP 47-4.

ADRENOCORTICAL INSUFFICIENCY/ADDISON'S DISEASE

Etiology and Pathophysiology

Adrenocortical insufficiency (hypofunction of the adrenal cortex) may be primary (Addison's disease) or secondary, from a lack of pituitary ACTH. In Addison's disease, all three classes of adrenal corticosteroids (glucocorticoids, mineralocorticoids, and androgens) are reduced. In secondary adrenocortical insufficiency, corticosteroids and androgens are deficient but mineralocorticoids rarely are. ACTH deficiency may be caused by pituitary disease or suppression of the hypothalamic-pituitary axis as a result of the administration of exogenous glucocorticoids.[47]

In the United States, the most common cause of primary Addison's disease (which is a rare condition) is autoimmune. Adrenal tissue is destroyed by antibodies against the patient's own adrenal cortex. Often, other endocrine conditions are present and Addison's disease is considered a component of polyendocrine deficiency syndrome. Tuberculosis can cause Addison's disease, but this is now rare in areas in which tuberculosis is controlled. Less common causes include infarction, fungal infections (e.g., histoplasmosis), AIDS, and metastatic cancer. Iatrogenic Addison's disease may be due to adrenal hemorrhage, often related to anticoagulant therapy, antineoplastic chemotherapy, ketoconazole (Nizoral) therapy for AIDS, or bilateral adrenalectomy.

Clinical Manifestations

Progressive weakness, fatigue, weight loss, and anorexia are primary features. Skin hyperpigmentation, a striking feature, is seen primarily in sun-exposed areas of the body, at pressure points, over joints, and in creases, especially palmar creases. It is most likely due to increased secretion of melanocyte stimulating hormone and ACTH. These tropic hormones are increased because of low glucocorticoid levels. Other frequent manifestations are hypotension, hyponatremia, hyperkalemia, nausea and vomiting, and diarrhea. The most dangerous feature of Addison's disease is hypotension, which may cause shock, especially during stress. Circulatory collapse from this cause is unresponsive to the usual treatment (vasopressors and fluid replacement) and requires glucocorticoid administration to reverse the hypotension.

Patients with secondary adrenocortical hypofunction may have many signs and symptoms in common with patients with Addison's disease but are characteristically not hyperpigmented because ACTH and related peptide levels are low. When severe dehydration, hyponatremia, and hyperkalemia are present, a diagnosis of primary adrenocortical insufficiency is favored because of the severe mineralocorticoid insufficiency associated with this disorder.

Complications

Patients with adrenocortical insufficiency are at risk for acute adrenal insufficiency (Addisonian crisis), which is a life-threatening emergency caused by insufficient adrenocortical hormones or a sudden sharp decrease in these hormones. It may occur during stress (e.g., from infection, surgery, trauma, hemorrhage, or psychologic distress); following sudden withdrawal of corticosteroid hormone replacement therapy (which

COLLABORATIVE CARE

Table **47-16** Addison's Disease

Diagnostic
History and physical examination
Plasma cortisol levels
Serum electrolytes
ACTH-stimulation test
Tuberculin test
CT scan, MRI

Collaborative Therapy
Daily glucocorticoid replacement (two thirds on awakening in morning, one third in late afternoon)*
Daily mineralocorticoid in morning*
Salt additives for excess heat or humidity

*For conditions of normal daily stress in individuals with usual daytime activity.

PATIENT TEACHING GUIDE

Table **47-17** Addison's Disease

1. Names and dosages of drugs
2. Actions of drugs
3. Symptoms of overdosage and underdosage
4. Conditions requiring increased medication (e.g., trauma, infection, surgery, emotional crisis)
5. Course of action to take relative to changes in medication
   - Increase in dose of corticosteroid
   - Administration of large dose of corticosteroid IM—including demonstration and return demonstration
   - Consultation with clinician
6. Prevention of infection and need for prompt and vigorous treatment of existing infections
7. Need for lifelong replacement therapy
8. Need for lifelong medical supervision
9. Need for medical identification device

is often done by a patient who lacks knowledge of the importance of replacement therapy); after adrenal surgery; or following sudden pituitary gland destruction (pituitary apoplexy).

Severe manifestations of glucocorticoid and mineralocorticoid deficiencies are exhibited, including hypotension (particularly postural), tachycardia, dehydration, hyponatremia, hyperkalemia, hypoglycemia, fever, weakness, and confusion. GI manifestations include nausea, vomiting, diarrhea, and vague abdominal pain.

Diagnostic Studies

In addition to clinical features, a diagnosis of Addison's disease can be made when cortisol levels are subnormal or fail to rise over basal levels with an ACTH stimulation test. Other abnormal laboratory findings include hyperkalemia, hypochloremia, hyponatremia, hypoglycemia, anemia, and increased blood urea nitrogen levels. Urine levels of free cortisol are low. A failure of cortisol levels to rise in response to ACTH stimulation indicates primary adrenal disease. A positive response to ACTH stimulation indicates a functioning adrenal gland and points to probable pituitary disease (see Chapter 45). An ECG may show low voltage and a vertical QRS axis. In addition, peaked T waves caused by hypokalemia may be evident.[42] CT scans and MRI are used to localize tumors or identify adrenal calcifications or enlargement (Table 47-16).

Collaborative Care

Treatment of adrenocortical insufficiency is focused on management of the underlying cause when possible. The mainstay of treatment for adrenocortical insufficiency is replacement therapy with glucocorticoids and mineralocorticoids. Hydrocortisone, the most commonly used form of replacement therapy, also has mineralocorticoid properties (Table 47-17). Management of Addisonian crisis requires immediate glucocorticoid replacement therapy. Treatment must be vigorous and directed toward shock management. IV hydrocortisone 100 mg every 6 hours, sodium, fluids, and dextrose (for hypoglycemia) are necessary for 24 hours or until blood pressure returns to normal.[48]

NURSING MANAGEMENT: ADDISON'S DISEASE

■ Nursing Assessment

Nursing assessment related to the patient with Addison's disease includes assessment of subjective data such as weight loss, hyperpigmentation, loss of body hair, anorexia, salt craving, nausea and vomiting, cramping abdominal pain, and diarrhea. Patients may also complain of exhaustion, profound weakness, inability to perform usual activities, muscle aches, light-headedness, lack of interest in usual activities and relationships, confusion, inability to tolerate any stress, decreased libido, and amenorrhea.

Objective data noted during the physical examination include emaciation, pale skin (but bronzed in sun-exposed areas, scars, buccal mucosa, and genitalia), and sparse body hair (particularly axillary and genital). Irritability, confusion, disorientation, or depression may also be noted. Skin tenting (delayed return of skin to flat position after pinching) may be observed with poor skin turgor. Hypotension (particularly postural), decreased cardiac output and heart size, muscle wasting, and weakness may also be present. Laboratory values may indicate hyponatremia, hyperkalemia, hypoglycemia, low serum cortisol, increased serum ACTH, decreased 24-hour urine free cortisol, and lack of response to an ACTH stimulation test (see Table 45-7).

■ Nursing Diagnoses

Nursing diagnoses for the patient with Addison's disease may include, but are not limited to, the following:

- Activity intolerance *related to* weakness and hypotension
- Self-care deficits *related to* weakness, lack of interest, and depression
- Altered nutrition: less than body requirements *related to* weakness, anorexia, and nausea and vomiting
- Self-esteem disturbance *related to* inability to perform usual activities, loss of hair, skin hyperpigmentation, and diagnosis of chronic illness

- Altered health maintenance *related to* lack of knowledge of management of lifelong hormone replacement therapy
- Decreased cardiac output *related to* hypotension and volume depletion
- Altered sexuality patterns *related to* weakness, malaise, depression, and changing self-concept
- Potential complication: hypotension

■ Planning

The overall goals are that the patient with Addison's disease will (1) manage self-care activities, (2) experience relief of symptoms, (3) learn to adjust medication dosage to life situations, (4) avoid acute adrenocortical insufficiency, and (5) actively participate in long-term therapeutic plan.

■ Nursing Implementation

Acute Intervention. When the patient with Addison's disease is hospitalized, whether for diagnosis, an acute crisis, or some other health problem, frequent nursing assessment is necessary. Vital signs and signs of fluid volume deficit and electrolyte imbalance should be assessed every 30 minutes to 4 hours for the first 24 hours depending on the patient's instability. In addition, the following nursing assessments and orders should be included: daily weights, diligent corticosteroid administration, protection against exposure to infection (reverse isolation), and complete assistance with daily hygiene. The patient should be protected from noise, light, and environmental temperature extremes. The patient cannot cope with these stresses because she or he cannot produce corticosteroids, in particular glucocorticoids.

If the hospitalization was due to adrenal crises, the patient usually responds by the second day and can start oral corticosteroid replacement. Because discharge frequently occurs before the usual maintenance dose of corticosteroids is reached, the patient should be instructed on the importance of keeping scheduled follow-up appointments.

Ambulatory and Home Care. The nurse has an important role in the long-term management of Addison's disease. Because of the serious nature of the disease and the need for lifelong replacement therapy, a well-organized and carefully presented teaching plan is vital to the health of the patient. Table 47-18 outlines the major areas that must be included in the teaching plan.

Glucocorticoids are usually given in divided doses, two thirds in the morning and one third in the afternoon. Mineralocorticoids are given once daily, usually in the morning. This dosage schedule reflects normal circadian rhythm in endogenous hormone secretion and decreases the side effects associated with steroid replacement therapy. A hormone-deficit patient receiving glucocorticoid replacement is less apt to exhibit harmful symptoms from the medication than a patient receiving pharmacologic doses of these drugs. Because the aim of replacement therapy is to return to normal hormone levels, nursing care is designed to help the patient maintain hormone balance and manage the medication regimen. Glucocorticoids are stimulating to the CNS and thus may cause insomnia if taken late in the evening.

Because the patient with Addison's disease is unable to tolerate physical or emotional stress, without additional exogenous corticosteroids, long-term care revolves around recognizing the

---

DRUG THERAPY

Table **47-18** Use of Corticosteroids

Hormone Replacement
Adrenal insufficiency
Congenital adrenal hyperplasia

Therapeutic Effect
- Allergic reactions
  Anaphylaxis
  Bee stings
  Contact dermatitis
  Drug reactions
  Serum sickness
  Urticaria
- Collagen diseases
  Giant cell arteritis
  Mixed connective tissue disorders
  Polymyositis
  Polyarteritis nodosa
  Systemic lupus erythematosus
- Eye disease
  Inflammation
- Gastrointestinal diseases
  Inflammatory bowel disease
  Nontropical sprue
- Hypercalcemia
  Thyroid storm
- Endocrine diseases
  Hypercalcemia
  Hashimoto's thyroiditis
  Thyroid storm
- Immunosuppression (after organ transplantation)
- Liver diseases
  Alcoholic hepatitis
  Autoimmune hepatitis
- Nephrotic syndrome
- Neurologic disease
  Prevention of cerebral edema and increased intracranial pressure
  Malignancies, leukemia, lymphoma
  Head trauma
- Pulmonary diseases
  Aspiration pneumonia
  Asthma
  Chronic obstructive pulmonary disease
- Rheumatoid arthritis
- Skin diseases

---

need for extra medication and techniques for stress management. The need for glucocorticoid hormone is proportional to stress levels. A patient who cannot produce endogenous hormone must adjust the dose of exogenous hormone to the stress level. Examples of situations requiring glucocorticoid adjustment are fever, influenza, extraction of teeth, and rigorous physical activity, such as playing tennis on a hot day or running a marathon. Doses are usually doubled when minor stress occurs (e.g., a respiratory infection or dental work) and tripled when major stress occurs. When in doubt, it is better to err on the side of overreplacement. If vomiting or diarrhea occurs, as may happen with influenza, the clinician must be notified immediately because electrolyte replacement may be necessary. In addition, these symptoms may be early indicators of crisis. Overall, however, patients who take their medications consistently can anticipate a normal life expectancy.

Patients must be taught the signs and symptoms of glucocorticoid deficiency and excess and to report to their clinicians so that dosages can be adjusted to each patient's need. It is critical that the patient wear an identification bracelet and carry a wallet card stating that the patient has Addison's disease so that appropriate therapy can be initiated in case of an unexpected trauma, accident, or crisis. The patient should be instructed in and given handouts related to other medications that cause a need to increase glucocorticoid dosage (e.g., phenytoin [Dilantin], barbiturates, rifampin [Rifadin], and antacids).[43] Estrogen inhibits steroid metabolism. Patients using mineralocorticoid therapy should be instructed how to take their blood pressure and given parameters to report to their clinicians, because untoward changes may indicate a need for dosage adjustment.

The patient should carry an emergency kit at all times. The kit should consist of 100 mg of IM hydrocortisone, syringes, and instructions for use. The patient and significant others should be instructed in how to give an IM injection in case the replacement therapy cannot be taken orally. The patient should verbalize instructions, practice IM injections with saline, and have written instructions as to when to alter the dose.[49]

■ Evaluation

The expected outcomes are that the patient with adrenal insufficiency

- is able to manage self-care activities
- experiences relief of symptoms
- states and demonstrates how to adjust medication doses for potential stressors
- states how to avoid acute adrenal insufficiency
- states the importance of lifelong follow-up medical care and has an appointment for follow-up

CORTICOSTEROID THERAPY

Cortisol and related glucocorticoids are used to relieve the signs and symptoms associated with many diseases (see Table 47-18). The long-term administration of glucocorticoids in therapeutic doses often leads to serious complications and side effects (Table 47-19). Therefore glucocorticoid therapy is not recommended for minor chronic conditions. Rather, therapy should be reserved for diseases in which there is a risk of death or permanent loss of function and conditions in which short-term therapy is likely to produce remission or recovery. The potential benefits of treatment must always be weighed against the risks.

Effects of Corticosteroid Therapy

The therapeutic actions of glucocorticoids include the following:

1. *Antiinflammatory action.* Glucocorticoids decrease the number of circulating lymphocytes, monocytes and macrophages, and eosinophils. They enhance the release of polymorphonuclear leukocytes from bone marrow, in-

---

DRUG THERAPY

Table **47-19** Side Effects of Corticosteroids

- Susceptibility to infection is increased. Infection develops more rapidly and spreads more widely in the cushingoid individual.
- Blood pressure is increased because of excess blood volume and potentiation of vasoconstrictor effects. Hypertension in turn predisposes patient to cardiac failure.
- Glucose intolerance affects more than 90% of individuals with cushingoid patterns.
- Protein depletion decreases bone formation, density, and strength and predisposes patient to pathologic fractures, especially compression fractures of the vertebrae (osteoporosis).
- Hypocalcemia related to anti–vitamin D effect may occur.
- Decreased mucus production predisposes patient to stomach and duodenal ulceration (peptic ulcer).
- Patients undergoing surgery are at increased risk for dehiscence and evisceration. Healing is delayed.
- Hypokalemia may develop, and potassium supplements may be indicated.
- Skeletal muscle atrophy occurs, and muscle weakness predisposes patient to accidental injury.
- Suppression of pituitary ACTH synthesis occurs. Glucocorticoid deficiency is likely if hormones are withdrawn abruptly.
- Mood and behavior changes (feelings of invulnerability and depression) may be observed.
- Fat from extremities is redistributed to trunk and face.

---

hibit the accumulation of leukocytes at the site of inflammation, and inhibit the release of substances involved in the inflammatory response (e.g., kinins, prostaglandins, and histamine) from the leukocytes. Therefore manifestations of inflammation, including redness, tenderness, heat, swelling, and local edema, are suppressed.

2. *Immunosuppression.* Glucocorticoids cause atrophy of lymphoid tissue, suppress cell-mediated immune responses, and decrease production of antibodies.

3. *Maintenance of normal blood pressure.* Glucocorticoids potentiate the vasoconstrictor effect of norepinephrine and act on the renal tubules to increase sodium reabsorption and enhance potassium and hydrogen excretion. Retention of sodium (and subsequently water) increases blood volume and helps maintain blood pressure. Mineralocorticoids have a direct effect on sodium reabsorption in the distal tubule of the kidney and as a result increase sodium and water retention.

4. *Carbohydrate and protein metabolic effects.* Glucocorticoids antagonize the effects of insulin and can induce glucose intolerance by increasing hepatic glycogenolysis and insulin resistance. They also stimulate the breakdown of protein for gluconeogenesis, which can lead to skeletal muscle wasting. Although glucocorticoids mobilize free fatty acids and redistribute fat in cushingoid patterns, the mechanism for this process is unknown. Glucocorticoids also decrease the conversion of T_4 to T_3.[50]

Complications of Corticosteroid Therapy

Beneficial and harmful effects of the corticosteroids relate to their physiologic actions. A beneficial effect in one situation may be a harmful one in another. For example, the vasopressive effect of the hormone is critical in enabling the organism to function in stressful situations but can produce hypertension when the substance is used for drug therapy. Inhibition of cell division is therapeutic and sometimes curative in the treatment of malignancies, but it slows healing after trauma or surgery. Suppression of inflammation and the immune response may help save the life of the victim of anaphylaxis and the transplant recipient, but it causes reactivation of latent tuberculosis and greatly reduces resistance to other infections. In addition, glucocorticoids inhibit the antibody response to vaccines. Specific side effects related to corticosteroid therapy are listed in Table 47-19.

NURSING AND COLLABORATIVE MANAGEMENT: CORTICOSTEROID THERAPY

Many patients receive corticosteroid therapy, in particular glucocorticoid therapy, for nonendocrine reasons (see Table 47-18), and thorough instruction is necessary to ensure patient cooperation. Corticosteroids are taken once daily or once every other day. They should be taken early in the morning with food to decrease gastric irritation. Because exogenous corticosteroid administration may suppress endogenous ACTH and therefore endogenous cortisol (suppression is time and dose dependent), the danger of abrupt cessation of corticosteroid therapy must be emphasized to patients and significant others.

Because patients often receive corticosteroid treatment for prolonged periods of time (more than 3 months), glucocorticoid-induced osteoporosis is an important concern. Therapies to reduce the resorption of bone may include increased calcium intake, vitamin D supplementation, biphosphonates, and institution of a low-impact exercise program. Further instruction and interventions to minimize the side effects and complications of corticosteroid therapy are shown in Table 47-20.

PRIMARY HYPERALDOSTERONISM
Etiology and Pathophysiology

Primary hyperaldosteronism (aldosteronism, Conn's syndrome) is characterized by excessive aldosterone secretion caused by an adenoma of the adrenal zona glomerulosa or bilateral adrenal hyperplasia. This disorder is seen in approximately 2.0% of patients with hypertension.[51] It is more common in women, and the usual age of diagnosis is between 20 and 40 years.[47] The main effects of aldosterone are sodium retention and potassium and hydrogen ion excretion. Thus the hallmark of this disease is hypertension with hypokalemic alkalosis.

Clinical Manifestations

The sodium retention leads to hypernatremia, hypertension, and headache. Edema does not usually occur because the rate of sodium excretion is reset, which prevents more severe sodium retention. However, there is an increased loss of potassium. The potassium wasting leads to hypokalemia, which causes generalized muscle weakness, tiredness, cardiac arrhythmias, glucose intolerance, and metabolic alkalosis that may lead to tetany.[51]

PATIENT TEACHING GUIDE
Table 47-20 Corticosteroid Therapy

1. Provide a diet plan high in protein, calcium (at least 1500 mg per day), and potassium but low in fat and concentrated simple carbohydrates such as sugar, honey, syrups, and candy.
2. Identify measures to ensure adequate rest and sleep, such as daily naps and avoidance of caffeine late in the day.
3. Develop and maintain an exercise program to help maintain bone integrity.
4. Instruct on how to recognize edema and ways to restrict sodium intake to less than 2000 mg per day if edema occurs.
5. Monitor glucose levels, symptoms and signs of hyperglycemia (e.g., polydipsia, polyuria, blurred vision), and glycosuria (glucose in the urine). Need to report hyperglycemic symptoms or capillary glucose levels greater than 180 mg/dl (10 mmol/L) or urine positive for glucose.
6. Notify a clinician if experiencing postprandial heartburn or epigastric pain that is not relieved by antacids.
7. See an eye specialist yearly to assess for possible cataracts.
8. Get up slowly from bed or a chair, and use good lighting to avoid accidental injury.
9. Maintain good hygiene practices. Avoid contact with persons with colds or other contagious illnesses to avoid infection.

Diagnostic Studies

The diagnosis of hyperaldosteronism should be suspected in all patients with hypokalemia and hypertension who are not being treated with diuretics. Diagnostic tests show increased plasma aldosterone and serum sodium levels and decreased serum potassium levels. An IV saline infusion test is often performed. In this test, 2 L of normal saline is infused over 4 hours, with plasma aldosterone levels measured at the beginning and end of the infusion. If aldosterone fails to suppress (i.e., is <10 ng/dl [277 pmol/L]), the patient probably has hyperaldosteronism. Adenomas are localized by means of a CT scan. If a tumor is not found, plasma 18-hydroxycorticosterone is measured after overnight bed rest. A level greater than 50 ng/dl (1387 pmol/L) indicates an adenoma.

NURSING AND COLLABORATIVE MANAGEMENT: PRIMARY HYPERALDOSTERONISM

The treatment for adenoma is unilateral adrenalectomy. Before surgery, patients should be treated with a low-sodium diet, potassium-sparing diuretics, and antihypertensive agents to control serum potassium levels and blood pressure. Spironolactone (Aldactone) binds to the mineralocorticoid receptor in the terminal distal tubules and collecting ducts of the kidney and increases excretion of sodium and water and retention of potassium.[52] Oral potassium supplements and sodium restrictions are also necessary. Potassium supplementation and a potassium-sparing diuretic should not be started simultaneously because of the danger of hyperkalemia. Patients with bilateral hyperplasia are treated with spironolactone (Aldactone); amiloride (Midamor), another potassium-sparing diuretic; or aminoglutethimide (Cytadren), which blocks aldosterone synthesis. Calcium channel blockers may also be used.[51]

Nursing care includes careful assessment for signs of hypokalemia, tetany (Chvostek's sign, Trousseau's sign), fluid and electrolyte balance, and cardiovascular status. Blood pressure should be monitored frequently before and after surgery because unilateral adrenalectomy is successful in controlling hypertension in only 50% of patients with adenoma.

Patients receiving maintenance therapy with spironolactone (Aldactone) or amiloride need instruction about the possible side effects of gynecomastia, impotence, and menstrual disorders, as well as knowledge about the signs and symptoms of hypokalemia and hyperkalemia. Patients should be taught how to monitor their own blood pressure and the need for frequent monitoring. The need for continued health supervision should be stressed.

SECONDARY HYPERALDOSTERONISM

Secondary hyperaldosteronism occurs in response to an extra-adrenal stimulus (often angiotensin), renal artery stenosis, or juxtaglomerular cell tumors. If treatment of the primary disorder is not possible, angiotensin-converting enzyme inhibitors are useful in inhibiting the powerful mineralocorticoid.

CONGENITAL ADRENAL HYPERPLASIA SYNDROMES

The adrenal glands normally produce small amounts of androgens. Overproduction of these hormones can be caused by adrenogenital syndromes. Causes of these syndromes are congenital enzymatic deficiencies leading to hypocortisolism. The hypocortisolism causes increased ACTH secretion, which overstimulates the adrenals and causes hypertrophy and excess androgen production. The onset of symptoms may occur from birth to early adult life and depends on the enzymes affected. In some deficiencies, males show precocious sexual development, whereas in others, sexual development may fail to occur. Females can show signs of masculinization and menstrual irregularities.

DISORDERS OF THE ADRENAL MEDULLA

PHEOCHROMOCYTOMA
Etiology and Pathophysiology

Disorders of the adrenal medulla are uncommon. Defects in norepinephrine release in autonomic nervous system failure may be associated with orthostatic hypotension, and defective adrenal epinephrine secretion and pancreatic glucagon secretion may affect the recovery from hypoglycemia in persons with diabetes mellitus.[53] However, the most common of these rare disorders of the adrenal medulla is pheochromocytoma, a neoplasm that produces excessive catecholamines. Most of these tumors (95%) are benign and encapsulated. Pheochromocytoma can occur at any age and in either gender, but it is found most commonly in patients between 30 and 50 years of age.[54]

Clinical Manifestations

The most striking clinical features of pheochromocytoma are severe, episodic hypertension accompanied by the classic triad of severe, pounding headache, tachycardia, and profuse sweating. Attacks of episodic hypertension are due to sympathetic nervous system stimulation usually from norepinephrine and are often accompanied by anxiety and palpitations. Attacks may be provoked by many medications, including antihypertensives, opiates, radiographic contrast media, and tricyclic antidepressants.[54] The duration of the attacks may vary from a few minutes to several hours. Untreated, pheochromocytoma may lead to diabetes mellitus, cadiomyopathy, and manifestations of uncontrolled hypertension and death.

Diagnostic Studies

Measurement of urinary metanephrines (catecholamine metabolites) is the simplest and most reliable test. Values are elevated in at least 90% of persons with pheochromocytoma. Vanillylmandelic acid (VMA) may also be measured in a 24-hour urine sample. However, this test has more false-negative results than urine metanephrines.[53] Plasma catecholamines are also elevated. It is preferable to measure catecholamines during an attack. CT scans and MRI are used for tumor localization.

Collaborative Care

Treatment consists of surgical removal of the tumor. Surgery may be done via laparoscopic adrenalectomy or by open abdominal incision. Regardless of the approach, this is one of the few conditions in which dangerously high blood pressure may be corrected surgically. Before surgery the patient is hospitalized for treatment to correct hypovolemia and cardiovascular complications to decrease the risk of surgery. Complete removal of the tumor cures the hypertension in the majority of individuals. In the others, hypertension persists or returns but is usually well controlled by standard therapy.

Preoperatively, sympathetic blocking agents (e.g., phenoxybenzamine [Dibenzyline], prazosin [Minipress], terazosin [Hytrin], or doxazosin [Cardura]) are administered to reduce the blood pressure and alleviate other symptoms of catecholamine excess. Because this management may result in orthostatic hypotension, the patient must be advised to make postural changes cautiously. Calcium channel blockers may be used to treat the hypertension and avoid the orthostatic hypotension in patients with cardiovascular disease. If surgery is not an option, metyrosine (Demser) is used to diminish catecholamine production by the tumor and simplify chronic management.

NURSING MANAGEMENT: PHEOCHROMOCYTOMA
■ Nursing Assessment

Case finding is an important nursing function. Any patient with hypertension accompanied by symptoms of sympathoadrenal discharge should be referred to a physician for definitive diagnosis. An important part of the nursing assessment is observation of the patient for the classic triad of symptoms of pheochromocytoma; severe, pounding headache; tachycardia; and profuse sweating. Blood pressure should be monitored immediately if the patient is experiencing an attack. The nurse should be prepared to check blood pressure when any of the drugs that might precipitate an attack are given.

■ Nursing Diagnoses

Nursing diagnosis for the patient with pheochromocytoma may include, but are not limited to, the following:

- Decreased cardiac output *related to* variations in blood pressure
- Sleep pattern disturbance *related to* interrupted sleep
- Body image disturbance *related to* anxiety caused by catecholamine surges.

■ Planning

The goals are that the patient with pheochromocytoma will (1) experience relief of symptoms, (2) experience no serious complications, and (3) maintain a positive self-image.

■ Nursing Implementation

The nurse should attempt to make the patient with pheochromocytoma as comfortable as possible. All diagnostic samples should be collected appropriately. Capillary blood glucose levels should be monitored to assess for diabetes mellitus. Patients should be monitored closely if any medications are used that may precipitate an attack. Patients need rest, nourishing food, and emotional support during this period. Preoperative and postoperative care is similar to that for any patient undergoing adrenalectomy except that blood pressure fluctuations from catecholamine imbalances tend to be severe and must be carefully monitored. In addition, blood may be transfused preoperatively to reduce postoperative hypotension.[55]

Since the hypertension may persist, even when the tumor is removed, the nurse should stress the importance of follow-up care and routine blood pressure monitoring. If metyrosine is being used, the patient should be instructed to rise slowly and hold onto a secure object, because this medication can cause orthostatic hypotension.

■ Evaluation

The expected outcomes are that the patient with pheochromocytoma

- experiences relief of symptoms
- does not experience any complications
- maintains a positive self-image

CRITICAL THINKING EXERCISES

CASE STUDY

Graves' Disease

Patient Profile
Sally C., a 43-year-old woman, was admitted to the hospital with a high fever. Following an endocrine workup, she was diagnosed as having Graves' disease.

Subjective Data
- Reports recent job loss because of inability to cope with job stress
- Reports symptoms that include fatigue, unintentional weight loss, insomnia, palpitations, and heat intolerance

Objective Data
Physical Examination
- Has a fever of 105° F (40.6° C)
- Has blood pressure of 150/78, pulse of 118, and respiratory rate of 24
- Has hot, moist skin
- Has fine tremors of the hands
- Has 4+ deep tendon reflexes and muscle strength of 1 to 2

Collaborative Care
- Subtotal thyroidectomy planned for 2 months later
- Started on propylthiouracil and propranolol

Critical Thinking Questions

1. What is the etiology of the patient's symptoms?
2. What diagnostic studies were probably ordered? What would the results have been to establish the diagnosis of Graves' disease?
3. Why was surgery delayed?
4. What was the purpose of the pharmacologic intervention?
5. What are the patient's immediate learning needs and her learning needs preoperatively and postoperatively?
6. What are the nursing interventions for successful long-term management of this patient after the subtotal thyroidectomy?
7. Based on the assessment data presented, write one or more appropriate nursing diagnoses pertinent to this patient while hospitalized. Are there any collaborative problems?

NURSING RESEARCH ISSUES

1. Is sucking on hard candy or ice chips more effective in decreasing the subjective sensation of thirst in patients with SIADH?
2. Do patients with hyperthyroidism sleep better in a private hospital room than in a hospital room shared with another patient?
3. What is the difference in the mental status of hypothyroid patients before and after thyroid replacement therapy?
4. What are the presenting symptoms of infection in patients with Cushing's syndrome?
5. Is a nurse-directed dosage adjustment more effective in preventing symptoms in the patient lacking endogenous cortisol who is exposed to stress than a patient-directed dosage adjustment?
6. Does regular exercise prevent bone loss in patients receiving glucocorticoid therapy?

REVIEW QUESTIONS

The number of the question corresponds to the same-numbered objective at the beginning of the chapter.

1. Following a hypophysectomy for treatment of acromegaly a patient develops hypopituitarism. The nurse teaches the patient that
   a. hormone replacement with ACTH, TSH, FSH, and LH will be necessary.
   b. permanent ADH replacement will be needed if the postoperative diabetes insipidus does not reverse.
   c. frequent monitoring of blood and urine glucose is needed to identify the development of diabetes mellitus.
   d. the elimination of the source of excess growth hormone will reverse the physiologic effects of acromegaly.

2. A patient with a head injury develops SIADH. Symptoms the nurse would expect to find include
   a. edema.
   b. weight gain.
   c. serum sodium of 140 mEq/L (140 mmol/L).
   d. urine specific gravity of 1.004.

3. The physician prescribes levothyroxin for a patient with myxedema. Following teaching regarding this therapy the nurse determines that further instruction is needed when the patient says,
   a. "I can expect to return to normal function with the use of this drug."
   b. "I can expect the medication dose to be increased every several weeks."
   c. "I will only need to take this medication until my symptoms are improved."
   d. "I will report any chest pain or difficulty breathing to the doctor right away."

4. Following thyroid surgery the nurse suspects damage or removal of the parathyroid glands when the patient develops
   a. laryngeal stridor.
   b. muscle weakness.
   c. hoarseness and difficulty swallowing.
   d. hyperthermia and severe tachycardia.

5. An important nursing intervention when caring for a patient with Cushing's syndrome is to
   a. restrict protein intake.
   b. observe for signs of hypotension.
   c. administer corticosteroids in equal doses.
   d. protect the patient from exposure to infection.

6. After an adrenalectomy for pheochromocytoma, the patient is most likely to experience
   a. hypokalemia.
   b. hyperglycemia.
   c. marked sodium and water retention.
   d. marked fluctuations in blood pressure.

7. Before surgery a patient with hyperaldosteronism is being treated with spironolactone (Aldactone). The nurse evaluates a successful response to this therapy when the
   a. blood pressure increases.
   b. urine output decreases.
   c. urine sodium decreases.
   d. serum potassium increases.

8. To control the side effects of pharmacologic corticosteroid therapy the nurse teaches the patient to
   a. increase calcium intake to 1500 mg per day.
   b. perform glucose monitoring for hypoglycemia.
   c. carry an emergency kit of hydrocortisone in case of severe stress.
   d. avoid abrupt position changes because of orthostatic hypotension.

9. The nurse teaches the patient that the best time to take cortisone for replacement purposes is
   a. once a day at bedtime.
   b. every other day on awakening.
   c. on arising and in the late afternoon.
   d. at consistent intervals every 6 to 8 hours.

References

1. Melmed S: Acromegaly. In Melmed S, editor: *The pituitary*, Cambridge, Mass, 1995, Blackwell Science.
2. Melmed S and others: Recent advances in pathogenesis, diagnosis, and management of acromegaly, *J Clin Endocrinol Metab* 80:3395, 1995.
3. Mohammed-Zadeh L: MR imaging of macroadenomas, *Radiol Technol* 67:29, 1995.
4. O'Halloran DJ, Shalet SM: Radiotherapy for pituitary adenomas: an endocrinologist's perspective, *Clin Oncol* 8:79, 1996.
5. Counsell C: Management of the patient with a pituitary tumor resection, *DCCN* 15:75, 1996.
6. Sherman RG, Lasseter DH: Pharmacologic management of patients with the diseases of the endocrine system, *Dent Clin North Am* 40:727, 1996.
7. Krause EA: Radiosurgery: a nursing perspective, *J Neurosci Nurs* 23:24, 1991.
8. Vance ML: New directions in the treatment of hyperprolactinemia, *Endocrinologist* 7:153, 1997.
9. Dexter RN: Hypopituitarism. In Becker KL, editor: *Principles and practice of endocrinology and metabolism*, ed 6, Philadelphia, 1995, Lippincott.
10. Jorgenson JOL and others: Adult growth hormone deficiency, *Horm Res* 42:235, 1994.
11. Wallymahmed M: Growth hormone deficiency in adults, *Nurs Times* 9:50, 1997.
12. Carlson HE: The pituitary gland in pregnancy and the puerperium. In Melmed S, editor: *The pituitary*, Cambridge, Mass, 1995, Blackwell Science.
13. Furlanetto RW and others: Guidelines for the use of growth hormone in children with short stature. A report by the Drug and Therapeutics Committee of the Lawson Wilkins Pediatric Endocrine Society, *J Pediatr* 127:857, 1995.
14. Winger JM, Hornick T: Age-associated changes in the endocrine system, *Nurs Clin North Am* 31:827, 1996.
15. Miller M: Inappropriate antidiuretic hormone secretion. In Bardin CW, editor: *Current therapy in endocrinology and metabolism*, ed 6, St Louis, 1997, Mosby.
16. Parobek V, Alaimo I: Fluid and electrolyte management in the neurologically-impaired patient, *J Neurosci Nurs* 28:322, 1996.
17. Robertson GL: Posterior pituitary. In Felig P, Baxter JD, Frohman LA, editors: *Endocrinology and metabolism*, ed 3, New York, 1995, McGraw-Hill.
18. Chernecky CC, Berger BJ: *Laboratory tests and diagnostic procedures*, Philadelphia, 1997, Saunders.
19. Braverman LE, Utiger RD: Introduction to thyrotoxicosis. In Braverman LE, Utiger RD, editors: *Werner and Ingbar's the thyroid: a fundamental and clinical text*, ed 7, Philadelphia, 1996, Lippincott-Raven.
20. Utiger RD: The thyroid: physiology, thyrotoxicosis, hypothyroidism, and the painful thyroid. In Felig P, Baxter JD, Frohman LA, editors: *Endocrinology and metabolism*, ed 3, New York, 1995, McGraw-Hill.
21. Hay ID, Morris JC: Toxic adenoma and toxic multinodular goiter. In Braverman LE, Utiger RD, editors: *Werner and Ingbar's the thyroid: a fundamental and clinical text*, ed 7, Philadelphia, 1996, Lippincott-Raven.
22. Mariotti S and others: The aging thyroid, *Endocr Rev* 16:686, 1995.
23. Dillman WH: Thyroid storm. In Bardin CW, editor: *Current therapy in endocrinology and metabolism*, ed 7, St Louis, 1997, Mosby.
24. Ladenson PW: Diagnosis of thyrotoxicosis. In Braverman LE, Utiger RD, editors: *Werner and Ingbar's the thyroid: a fundamental and clinical text*, ed 7, Philadelphia, 1996, Lippincott-Raven.
25. Streff MM, Pachucki-Hyde LC: Management of the patient with thyroid disease, *Nurs Clin North Am* 31:779, 1996.
26. Wartofsky L: Treatment options for hyperthyroidism, *Hosp Pract* 31:69, 1996.

27. McKennis A, Waddington C: Nursing interventions for potential complications after thyroidectomy, *ORL Head Neck Nurs* 15:27, 1997.

28. Gharib H: Management of thyroid nodules: another look, *Thyroid Today* 20: 1, 1997.

29. Bravermann LE, Utiger RD: Introduction to hypothyroidism. In Braverman LE, Utiger RD, editors: *Werner and Ingbar's the thyroid: a fundamental and clinical text,* ed 7, Philadelphia, 1996, Lippincott-Raven.

30. Moltz KC, Postellon DC: Congenital hypothyroidism and mental development, *Compr Ther* 20:342, 1994.

31. Braverman LE, Roti E: Effects of iodine on thyroid function, *Acta Med Austriaca* 23:4, 1996.

32. Aceto TJ and others: Short stature and slow growth in the infant and child. In Becker KL, editor: *Principles and practice of endocrinology and metabolism,* ed 2, Philadelphia, 1995, Lippincott.

33. MacGillivray MH: Disorders of growth and development. In Felig P, Baxter JD, Frohman LC, editors: *Endocrinology and metabolism,* ed 3, New York, 1996, McGraw-Hill.

34. Finucane P, Anderson C: Thyroid disease in older patients. Diagnosis and treatment, *Drugs Aging* 6:268, 1996.

35. Wartofsky L: The scope and impact of thyroid disease, *Clin Chem* 42:121, 1996.

36. Pittman CS, Zayed AA: Myxedema coma. In Bardin CW, editor: *Current therapy in endocrinology and metabolism,* ed 6, St Louis, 1997, Mosby.

37. Strewler GJ, Rosenblatt M: Mineral metabolism. In Felig P, Baxter JD, Frohman LC, editors: *Endocrinology and metabolism,* ed 3, New York, 1995, McGraw-Hill.

38. Silverberg SJ, Fitzpatrick LA, Bilezikian JP: Primary hyperthyroidism. In Becker KL, editor: *Principles and practice of endocrinology and metabolism,* ed 2, Philadelphia, 1995, Lippincott.

39. Horowitz M and others: Primary hyperparathyroidism, *Clin Geriatr Med* 10:757, 1994.

40. Attie JN: Primary hyperparathyroidism. In Bardin CW, editor: *Current therapy in endocrinology and metabolism,* ed 6, St Louis, 1997, Mosby.

41. Zeiger MA: Hypoparathyroidism, pseudohypoparathyroidism, and pseudopseudohypoparathyroidism. In Clark OH, Duh QY, editors: *Textbook of endocrine surgery,* Philadelphia, 1997, Saunders.

42. Miller WL, Tyrell JB: The adrenal cortex. In Felig P, Baxter JD, Frohman LA, editors: *Endocrinology and metabolism,* New York, 1995, McGraw-Hill.

43. Prinz RA, Falimirski ME: Operative approaches to the adrenal gland. In Clark OH, Duh QY, editors: *Textbook of endocrine surgery,* Philadelphia, 1997, Saunders.

44. Gotch P: Cushing's syndrome from the patient's perspective, *Endocrinol Metab Clin North Am* 23:607, 1994.

45. Davis-Martin S: Disorders of the adrenal glands, *J Am Acad Nurse Pract* 8:323, 1996.

46. Gagner M: Laparoscopic adrenalectomy. In Clark OH, Duh QY, editors: *Textbook of endocrine surgery,* Philadelphia, 1997, Saunders.

47. Gumowski J, Loughran M: Diseases of the adrenal gland, *Nurs Clin North Am* 31:747, 1996.

48. Malcoff CD, Carey RM: Adrenal insufficiency. In Bardin CW, editor: *Current therapy in endocrinology and metabolism,* St Louis, 1997, Mosby.

49. Braatvedt GD, Newrick PG, Corrall RJM: Patient's self administration of hydrocortisone, *BMJ* 301:1312, 1990.

50. Magiakou MA, Chrousos GP: Corticosteroid therapy, nonendocrine disease, and corticosteroid withdrawal. In Bardin CW, editor: *Current therapy in endocrinology and metabolism,* ed 6, St Louis, 1997, Mosby.

51. Gill JR: Hyperaldosteronism. In Becker KL, editor: *Principles and practice of endocrinology and metabolism,* ed 2, Philadelphia, 1995, Lippincott.

52. Obara T, Ito Y, Fujimoto Y: Hyperaldosteronism. In Clark OH, Duh QY, editors: *Textbook of endocrine surgery,* Philadelphia, 1997, Saunders.

53. Cryer PE: Disease of the sympathochromaffin system. In Felig P, Baxter JD, Frohman LC, editors: *Endocrinology and metabolism,* ed 3, New York, 1995, McGraw-Hill.

54. Keiser HR: Pheochromocytoma and other diseases of the sympathetic nervous system. In Becker KL, editor: *Principles and practice of endocrinology and metabolism,* ed 2, Philadelphia, 1995, Lippincott.

55. Bravo EL: Pheochromocytoma. In Bardin CW, editor: *Current therapy in endocrinology and metabolism,* ed 6, St Louis, 1997, Mosby.

Resources

Addison's Disease, National Institute of Diabetes and Digestive and Kidney Diseases
2 Information Way
Bethesda, MD 20892-3570
http://www.niddk.nih.gov

American Association of Clinical Endocrinologists
1000 Riverside Avenue, Suite 205
Jacksonville, FL 32204
http://www.aace.com

American Society for Bone and Mineral Research
1200—19th Street NW, Suite 300
Washington, DC 20036-2401
202-857-1161
Fax: 202-223-4579
http://www.asbmr.org/

American Thyroid Association
Montefiore Medical Center
111 East 210th Street
Bronx, NY 10467
Fax: 718-882-6085
http://www.thyroid.org

Endocrine Nurses Society
2258 SE Darline Avenue
Gresham, OR 97080
503-215-1082
http://www.endo-nurses.org/

Endocrine Society
4350 East West Highway
Bethesda, MD 20814-4410
301-941-0252
Fax: 301-941-0259
http://www.endo-society.org/

Pituitary Tumor Network Association
http://www.pituitary.com/

Thyroid Foundation of Canada
96 Mack Street, Kingston, Ontario K7L 1N9
613-544-8364
800-267-8822
Fax: 613-544-9731
http://home.ican.net/~thyroid/Canada.html

For additional Internet resources, see the website for this book at www.mosby.com/MERLIN/medsurg_lewis

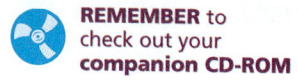

48

NURSING ASSESSMENT
Reproductive System

Nancy MacMullen & Laura Dulski

www.mosby.com/MERLIN/medsurg_lewis

LEARNING OBJECTIVES

1. Describe the structures and functions of the male and female reproductive systems.
2. Explain the functions of the major hormones essential for the structure and function of the reproductive systems.
3. Describe the physiologic and psychologic changes of a man and of a woman during the stages of sexual response.
4. Describe age-related changes in the reproductive systems and differences in assessment findings.
5. Identify significant subjective and objective data related to the reproductive systems and information about sexual function that should be obtained from a patient.
6. Describe noninvasive techniques used in the physical assessment of the reproductive systems.
7. Differentiate normal from abnormal findings obtained from a physical assessment of the reproductive systems.
8. Describe the purpose, significance of results, and nursing responsibilities related to diagnostic studies of the reproductive systems.

STRUCTURES AND FUNCTIONS OF THE MALE AND FEMALE REPRODUCTIVE SYSTEMS

The reproductive system is interrelated with other systems, including the neurologic, endocrine, and urinary systems, and also with general physiologic function. For example, estrogen (produced primarily in a woman's ovaries) influences bone density and testosterone (produced primarily in a man's testes) influences muscle mass. The reproductive system is responsible for the perpetuation of the species through fertilization, implantation, maintenance of pregnancy, and birth of a baby. The reproductive system is also directly related to sexual function and is therefore intricately interwoven into the complex, sensitive, and frequently stress-laden area of psychosocial mores and cultural values regarding sex.

Male Reproductive System

The male reproductive system consists of the external structures—the penis and the scrotum—and the internal structures, including the prostate gland, the seminal vesicles, and several ducts (Fig. 48-1). The scrotum lies within the scrotal sac, which is a thin, loose outer layer of skin over a more muscular internal layer. The scrotum consists of two halves divided by a septum; each half contains a testis, an epididymis, and a spermatic cord. The testis is an ovoid, smooth, firm organ measuring 3.5 to 5.5 cm deep and 2 to 3 cm wide.[1] Within the testes are the seminiferous tubules, where spermatozoa (immature sperm) are formed at a rate of 10 to 30 billion per month. The tubules

lead into a system of small ducts that conduct sperm to the epididymis.

The epididymis is a soft, cordlike structure that measures almost 2½ inches (530 cm) in length if stretched out. It lies in the anterior plane and along the posterolateral surface of each testis. This organ may be considered to be a large duct. It stores the sperm as they mature and until they are released by ejaculation or until they disintegrate and are reabsorbed by the body. The ductus deferens (vas deferens) begins in the epididymis within the scrotal sac, goes up, goes through the scrotum and continues proximally through the inguinal ring, and then posteriorly above the bladder and down again behind the bladder, where it is joined by ducts from the seminal vesicles. It then continues down through the prostate gland, connecting with the urethra (Fig. 48-2). The duct system emerging from each testis conveys sperm into the urethra.

The spermatic cord is composed of the ductus deferens and the arteries, veins, and lymph vessels supplying the testes and the epididymis. All of these structures are enclosed by the cremaster muscle and by layers of fascia. The spermatic cord extends from the scrotum up to the external inguinal ring. The cord ends there, and its components, primarily the ductus deferens, continue along a backward course toward the scrotum.

The prostate gland, the seminal vesicles, and Cowper's (bulbourethral) glands are the accessory glands of the male reproductive system. These glands produce and secrete seminal fluid, which surrounds the sperm and forms the ejaculate. The prostate gland lies underneath the bladder. Its posterior surface approximates the rectal wall. The normal prostate measures 2 cm wide and 3 cm long and is divided into the right and left lateral lobes and an anteroposterior median lobe. As the ejaculate passes through the urethra, it receives an alkaline secretion

Reviewed by Linda Monfore Fluke, RN, MN, ARNP, Adult and Geriatric Nurse Practitioner, State of Washington, Seattle, Wash.

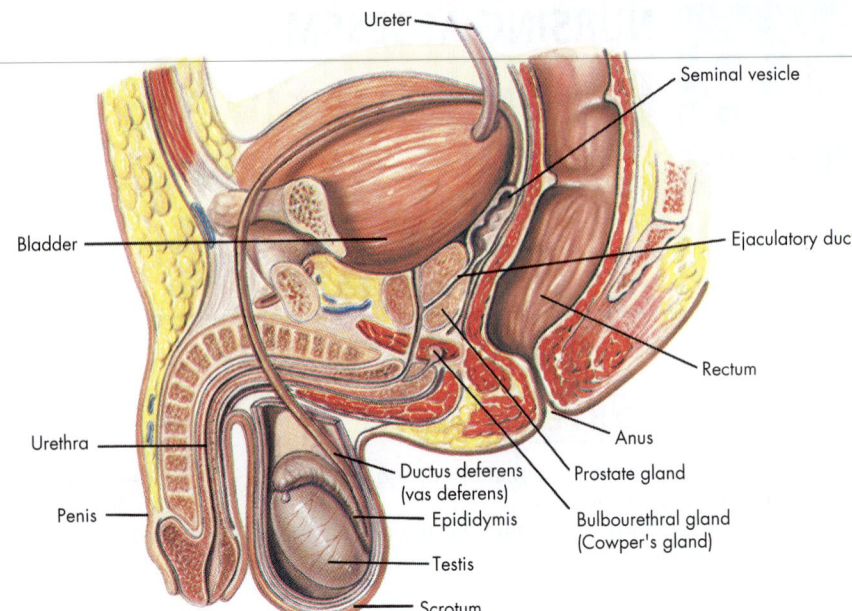

Fig. 48-1 External and internal male sex organs.

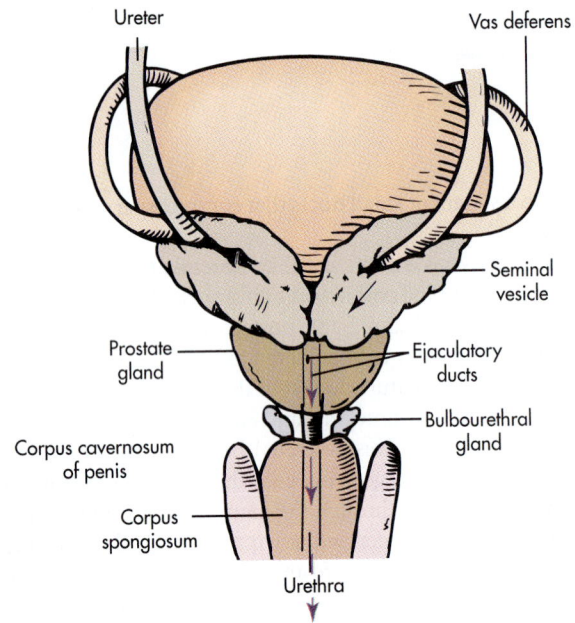

Fig. 48-2 Formation of the ejaculatory ducts by union of the seminal vesicles with the ductus deferens just before entrance into the prostate gland. The ejaculatory ducts open into the prostatic portion of the urethra.

from the prostate gland. The seminal vesicles lie just behind the bladder and between the rectum and the bladder. The ducts of the seminal vesicles fuse with the ductus deferens to form the ejaculatory ducts that enter the prostate gland. Cowper's glands lie on each side of the urethra and slightly posterior to it, just below the prostate. The ducts of these glands enter directly into the urethra. The secretion from the prostate makes up most of the fluid in the ejaculate. By comparison, the seminal vesicles and Cowper's glands contribute a minimum amount of fluid to the ejaculate. These various secretions serve as a medium for the transport of sperm and create an alkaline, nutritious environment that promotes sperm motility and survival.

The urethra extends from the bladder, through the prostate, and ends in a slitlike opening (the meatus) on the ventral side of the glans, the end of the penis. The glans is covered by a fold of skin, the prepuce (or foreskin), which forms at the junction of the glans and the shaft of the penis. In circumcised men the prepuce has been removed. The broadened segment of the glans at the junction is the corona. The shaft of the penis consists of erectile tissue composed of the corpus cavernosum and corpus spongiosum, the fibrous sheath that encases the erectile tissue, and the urethra. The skin covering the penis is thin, loose, and essentially hairless.

Female Reproductive System

The female reproductive system consists of the breasts, the uterus, the ovaries, the fallopian tubes, the vagina, and the external genitalia (the vulva), as well as ligaments and pelvic bones.

Breasts. The breasts are a secondary sex characteristic that develops during puberty in response to estrogen and progesterone. Cyclic hormonal changes lead to regular changes in breast tissue to prepare it for lactation when fertilization and pregnancy occur. The breasts are also considered a major organ of sexual stimulation and response among some cultures.

The breasts extend from the second to the sixth ribs, with the tail reaching the axilla (Fig. 48-3). The fully mature breast is dome shaped and contains a pigmented center termed the *areola*. The areolar region contains Montgomery's tubercles, which are similar to sebaceous glands and assist in moistening the nipple. During lactation, the alveoli or acini secrete milk. The milk then flows into a ductal system and is transported to the lactiferous sinuses. The nipple contains 15 to 20 tiny openings through which the milk flows during breastfeeding. The breast's rich lymphatic network drains primarily into the axillary, the infraclavicular, and the supraclavicular channels. This system is often responsible for the metastasis of a malignant tumor from the breast to other parts of the body (Fig. 48-4). The fibrous and fatty tissue that supports and separates the channels of the mammary duct system is primarily responsible for the varying sizes and shapes of the breasts in different individuals.

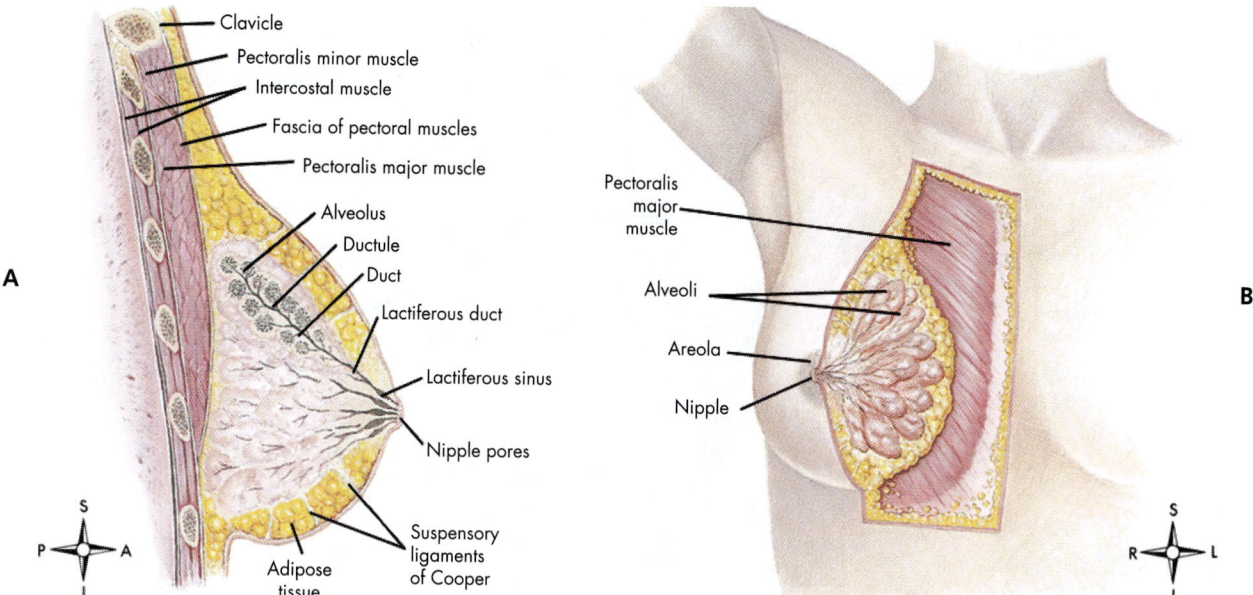

Fig. 48-3 The female breast. **A,** Sagittal section of a lactating breast. Notice how the glandular structures are anchored to the overlying skin and to the pectoral muscles by suspensory ligaments of Cooper. Each lobule of glandular tissue is drained by a lactiferous duct that eventually opens through the nipple. **B,** Anterior view of a lactating breast. In nonlactating breasts the glandular tissue is much less prominent, with adipose tissue comprising most of each breast.

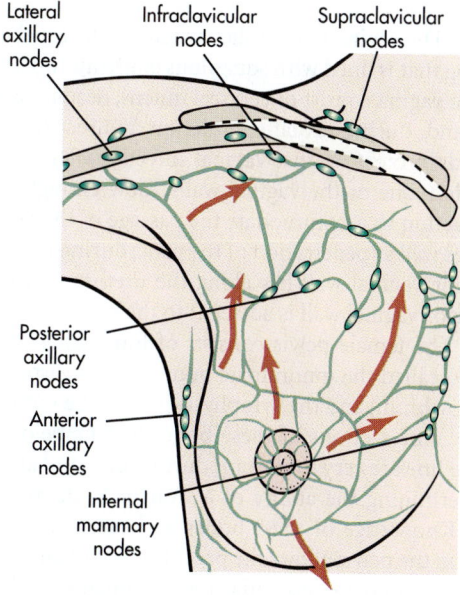

Fig. 48-4 Lymphatic drainage of the breast. *Arrows* indicate direction of drainage.

Pelvic Organs

Ovaries. The ovaries are usually located on either side of the uterus, just behind and below the fallopian (uterine) tubes (Fig. 48-5). The ovaries are firm and solid, averaging 1.5 cm wide, 3 cm long, and 2 cm deep. Their functions include ovulation, as well as secretion of the two major reproductive hormones, estrogen and progesterone. The outer zone of the ovary contains follicles with germ cells, or oocytes. Each follicle contains a primordial (immature) oocyte surrounded by granulosa and theca cells. These two layers protect and nourish the oocyte until the follicle reaches maturity and ovulation occurs. However, not all follicles reach maturity. In a process termed *atresia*, most of the primordial follicles become smaller and are reabsorbed by the body; thus the number of follicles declines from 2 to 4 million at birth to approximately 300,000 to 400,000 at menarche. This number continues to decrease throughout a woman's reproductive years.[2] The vast majority of oocytes are destroyed by atresia. Fewer than 500 are actually released by ovulation during the reproductive years of the normal healthy woman.

Fallopian tubes. Normally, each month during a woman's reproductive years, one ovarian follicle reaches maturity, and the ovum is ovulated, or expelled, from the ovary through the stimulus of the gonadotropic hormones, follicle-stimulating hormone (FSH) and luteinizing hormone (LH). The ovum then travels up a fallopian tube where fertilization by a sperm may occur, assuming that sperm are present. An ovum can be fertilized up to 72 hours after its release. Sperm are viable for 24 to 48 hours.[3]

The distal ends of the fallopian tubes consist of fingerlike projections called *fimbriae* that "massage" the ovaries at ovulation to help extract the mature ovum. The tubes, which average 4.8 inches (12 cm) in length, extend from the fimbriae to the superior lateral borders of the uterus. Fertilization usually takes place within the outer one third of the tubes.

Uterus. The uterus is a pear-shaped, hollow, muscular organ (see Fig. 48-5). It is located between the bladder and the rectum. In the mature nulliparous (never pregnant) female the uterus is approximately 6 cm long and 4 cm wide. The uterine walls consist of an outer serosal layer, the perimetrium, a middle muscular layer, the myometrium, and an inner mucosal layer, the endometrium.

The uterus consists of the fundus, the body (or the corpus), and the cervix. The body makes up about 80% of the uterus and connects with the cervix at the isthmus, or the neck. The cervix

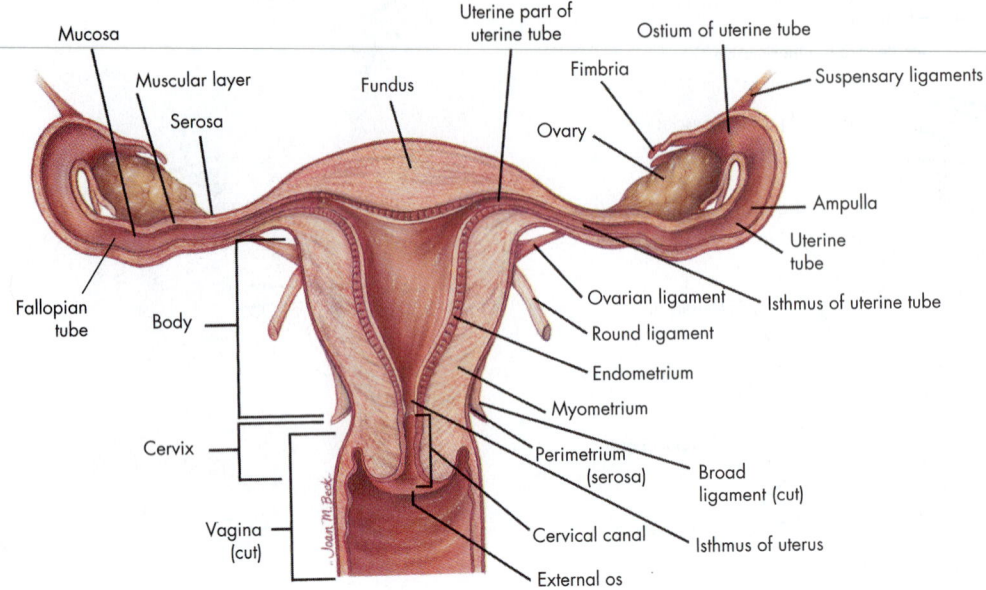

Fig. 48-5 Anatomy of the female reproductive tract.

is the lower portion that invaginates (projects) into the anterior wall of the vaginal canal. It makes up about 15% to 20% of the uterus in the nulliparous female. The cervix consists of the ectocervix, the outer portion that protrudes into the vagina, and the endocervix, the canal in the opening of the cervix. The ectocervix is covered with squamous epithelial cells, which give it a smooth, pinkish appearance. The endocervix contains a lining of columnar epithelial cells, which give it a rough, reddened appearance. The junction at which the two types of epithelial cells meet is termed the *squamocolumnar junction* and contains the optimal types of cells needed for an accurate Papanicolaou (Pap) smear to screen for malignancies. The presence of endocervical cells in the sample taken for a Pap smear ensures that the squamocolumnar junction, or the transformation zone, has been sampled. Cells taken from the vagina provide a less accurate diagnosis and therefore are not included in the routine Pap smear.[2] The cervical canal is 2 to 4 cm long and is relatively tightly closed. The cervix, however, allows sperm to enter the uterus and also allows menses to be expelled. The columnar epithelium, under hormonal influence, provides enough elasticity at labor for the cervix to stretch so that a fetus can pass. The entrance of sperm into the uterus is facilitated by mucus produced by the cervix under the influence of estrogen. Under normal conditions, the cervical mucus becomes watery and more abundant at ovulation. This mucus can stretch several inches (spinnbarkeit) and allows for the easy entrance of sperm into the uterus. The postovulatory cervical mucus, under the influence of progesterone, is thick and inhibits sperm passage. Knowledge of these physiologic changes is used in natural approaches to family planning.

The anterior and posterior peritoneal covering of the uterus is called the *broad ligament.* It separates the uterus from the bladder and the rectum but does not provide support for the uterus or the adnexa (ovaries and tubes). The cardinal ligaments, which extend from the isthmus of the uterus to the pelvic wall, also offer only minimal support. The round ligament, which extends anteriorly to the labia majora, provides some support but is easily weakened by pregnancy. The firmest support for the uterus is provided by the uterine sacral ligaments, which pull the uterus back and away from the vaginal orifice.

Vagina. The vagina is a tubular structure 3 to 4 inches (8 to 10 cm) long that is lined with squamous epithelium. The secretions of the vagina consist of cervical mucus, desquamated epithelium, and, during sexual stimulation, a direct transudate. These fluids protect against vaginal infection. The muscular and erectile tissue of the vaginal walls allow enough dilation and contraction to accommodate the passage of the fetus during labor, as well as penetration of the penis during intercourse. The anterior vaginal wall lies along the urethra and bladder. The posterior vaginal wall is adjacent to the rectum.

Pelvis. The female pelvis consists of four bones: two hipbones (also called the innominate bones and consisting of the ilium, the ischium, and the symphysis pubis), the sacrum, and the coccyx. The sections of these bones that lie below the iliopectineal line are very important during birth and are often a factor determining the ability of a woman to deliver a child vaginally. Knowledge of these bones and the landmarks that they form in the pelvis allows the practitioner to estimate pelvic measurements and the potential for a woman's pelvis to accommodate the birth of a full-term fetus. Specialty references discuss the specific techniques of clinical pelvimetry.

The pelvis is also divided into the true pelvis and the false pelvis. The true pelvis encompasses the brim, the cavity, and the outlet and is the bony passageway through which the fetus passes during birth. The false pelvis consists of the superior portion of the iliac bones, above the brim or the iliopectineal line.[2]

External Genitalia. The external portion of the female reproductive system (Fig. 48-6), commonly called the *vulva,* consists of the mons pubis, the labia majora, the labia minora, the clitoris, the urethral meatus, the ducts of Skene's glands, the vaginal orifice, and the Bartholin's glands.

The mons pubis is a fatty layer lying over the pubic bone. It contains coarse hair that lies in an upside-down triangular pat-

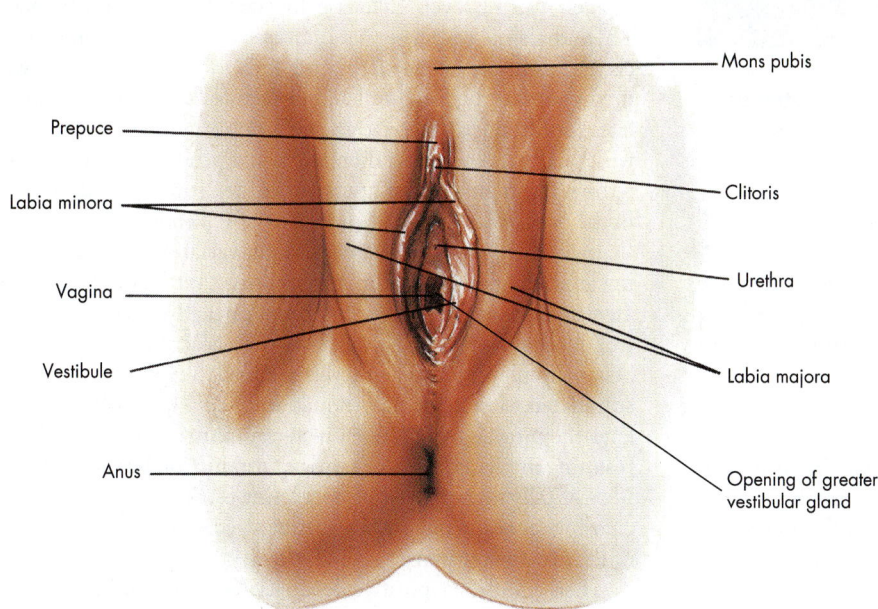

Fig. 48-6   External female genitalia.

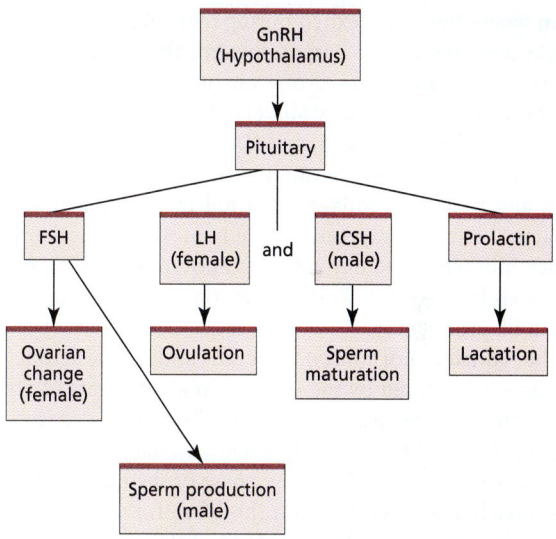

Fig. 48-7   The hypothalamic-pituitary-gonadal axis. Only the major pituitary hormone actions are depicted. *FSH,* follicle-stimulating hormone; *GnRH,* gonadotropin-releasing hormone; *ICSH,* interstitial cell–stimulating hormone; *LH,* luteinizing hormone.

tern. (The male hair pattern is diamond shaped.) The labia majora are folds of adipose tissue that form the outer borders of the vulva. These hair-covered folds contain sweat glands and sebaceous glands. The hairless labia minora form the borders of the vaginal orifice and extend anteriorly to enclose the clitoris. The vestibule is a boat-shaped fossa between the labia minora, extending from the clitoris at the anterior end to the vaginal opening at the posterior end. The perineum is the area between the vagina and the anus.

In a virgin the vaginal orifice usually but not always contains a thin membrane called the *hymen,* which varies the size of the vaginal orifice in individuals from that of a pinhole to an opening large enough to allow two fingers to enter. Frequently, the hymen is torn during first sexual intercourse, and only tags remain. In many societies, the bleeding that occurs with this tearing has been used to validate virginity. However, not all hymens are torn by the first intercourse. Some are already well stretched or are torn because of childhood activity, tampon usage, or accidents.

The clitoris is homologous (similar) to the male penis; it is the erectile tissue that becomes engorged during sexual excitation. It lies anterior to the urethral meatus and the vaginal orifice and is usually covered by the prepuce or hood. Clitoral stimulation is an important part of sexual activity for many women.

Skene's glands and ducts lie alongside the urethral meatus and have no known function. They are homologous to the male prostate. Bartholin's glands, which are at the posterior and lateral aspects of the vaginal orifice, secrete a thin, mucoid material believed to contribute slightly to lubrication during sexual intercourse. These glands are not usually palpable unless sebaceous-like cysts form or an infection, especially a sexually transmitted disease, arises.

Neuroendocrine Regulation

The hypothalamus and pituitary gland (see Chapter 45) and the gonads (organs of reproduction) secrete numerous hormones (Fig. 48-7). These hormones regulate the processes of

ovulation, spermatogenesis (formation of sperm), and fertilization, as well as the formation and function of the secondary sex characteristics. The cyclic changes in the amounts of these hormones secreted by the anterior pituitary gland cause cyclic changes in the ovaries. The hypothalamus secretes gonadotropin-releasing hormones (GnRHs), which stimulate the pituitary gland to secrete its hormones, including FSH and LH. LH in males is sometimes called interstitial cell–stimulating hormone (ICSH). The gonadal hormones are estrogen, progesterone, and testosterone.

In women, FSH production by the pituitary stimulates the growth and maturity of the ovarian follicles to cause ovulation.

Table 48-1 Gonadal Feedback Mechanisms

Negative Feedback

↓ Estrogen → ↑ GnRH → ↑ FSH → ↑ Estrogen
(hypothalamus) (pituitary) (ovaries)

Positive Feedback

↑ Estrogen → ↑ GnRH → ↑ LH
(hypothalamus) (pituitary)

Testes (Negative Feedback)

↓ Testosterone → ↑ GnRH → ↑ FSH and ICSH → ↑ Testosterone
(hypothalamus) (pituitary) (testes)

FSH, follicle-stimulating hormone; *GnRH,* gonadotropin-releasing hormone; *ICSH,* interstitial cell–stimulating hormone; *LH,* luteinizing hormone.

The mature follicle produces estrogen, which in turn suppresses the release of FSH. Another hormone, inhibin, is also secreted by the ovarian follicle and inhibits both GnRH and FSH secretion. In men, FSH stimulates the seminiferous tubules to produce sperm.

LH contributes to the ovulatory process because it causes follicles to complete maturation and undergo ovulation. It also causes the development of a ruptured follicle, or the area on the ovum where the ovum exited during ovulation. The ruptured follicle develops into a corpus luteum, from which progesterone is secreted. Progesterone maintains the rich vascular state of the uterus (secretory phase) in preparation for fertilization and implantation. In men, LH or ICSH is responsible for the production of testosterone by the interstitial cells of the testes and thus is essential for the full maturation of sperm. Prolactin has no known function in men but, with other hormones, stimulates the development and growth of the mammary glands in women. During lactation, it initiates and maintains milk production.

The gonadal hormones, estrogen and progesterone, in women are produced by the ovaries. Small amounts of an estrogen precursor are also produced in the adrenal cortices. Estrogen is essential to the development and maintenance of the secondary sex characteristics, the phase of the menstrual cycle immediately after menstruation (proliferative phase), and the uterine changes essential to pregnancy. Estrogen has also been found in the urine of men, although its role and importance are not well understood. In men, this hormone is produced predominantly in the adrenal cortex.

Progesterone plays a major role in the menstrual cycle but most specifically in the secretory phase. Like estrogen, progesterone is involved in the bodily changes associated with pregnancy. Adequate progesterone is necessary to maintain an implanted egg.

The major gonadal hormone of men, testosterone, is produced by the testes. Testosterone is responsible for the development and maintenance of secondary sex characteristics, as well as for adequate spermatogenesis. Androgens are produced in females by the adrenal glands and ovaries, though in small amounts.

The circulating levels of gonadal hormones are controlled primarily by a negative feedback process. Receptors within the hypothalamus and pituitary are sensitive to the circulating blood levels of the hormones (Table 48-1). Increased levels of hormones stimulate a hypothalamic response to decrease the high circulating levels. Likewise, low circulating levels provoke a hypothalamic response that increases the low circulating levels. For example, if the circulating level of testosterone is low, the hypothalamus is stimulated to secrete GnRH. This stimulates the pituitary to secrete greater amounts of FSH and ICSH, which in turn causes an increase in the production of testosterone. The high levels of testosterone then stimulate a decrease in the production of GnRH and thus of FSH and ICSH.

In women, however, there is a slight variation. The circulating levels are controlled through a combination of both a negative and a positive feedback system. A negative feedback control mechanism exists, similar to that described previously. When circulating estrogen levels are low, the hypothalamus is stimulated to increase its production of GnRH. GnRH stimulates the pituitary to secrete greater amounts of FSH and LH, resulting in higher levels of estrogen production by the ovaries. Reciprocally higher levels of circulating estrogen result in a decreasing secretion of GnRH and thus a decrease in the secretion of FSH by the pituitary.

There is also a positive feedback control mechanism in women. Thus, with increasing levels of circulating estrogen, a greater level of GnRH is produced, resulting in an increased level of LH from the pituitary. Likewise, lowered levels of estrogen result in a lowered level of LH.

Menarche

Menarche is the first episode of menstrual bleeding, indicating a female has reached puberty. This usually occurs around 13 years of age, although there is individual variation according to race, nutrition, health, and heredity.

As puberty approaches, there are changes associated with the elevated rate of estrogen and progesterone secretion by the ovaries. These changes include the development of breast buds, the development of pubic hair, and later the development of axillary hair. During this time, there is a decrease in the sensitivity of the hypothalamic-pituitary axis that allows for increased secretion of FSH and LH and a resultant increase in estrogen. It is during this time that the adult pattern of gonadotropin secretion occurs, resulting in the menstrual cycle. Menstrual cycles are often irregular during the first few years of menarche because of anovulation.

Menstrual Cycle

The major functions of the ovaries are ovulation and the secretion of hormones. These functions are accomplished during the normal menstrual cycle, a monthly process mediated by the hormonal activity of the hypothalamus, the pituitary gland, and the ovaries. Menstruation occurs during each month in which an egg is not fertilized (Fig. 48-8). The endometrial cycle is divided into three phases labeled in relation to uterine and ovarian changes: (1) the proliferative or follicular phase, (2) the secretory or luteal phase, and (3) the menstrual or ischemic phase. The length of the menstrual cycle ranges from 20 to 40 days, the average being 28 days.

The menstrual cycle begins on the first day of menstruation, which usually lasts 3 to 5 days. During this time, estrogen and progesterone levels are low, but FSH levels begin to increase. During the follicular phase, a single follicle matures fully under the stimulation of FSH. (The mechanism that ensures that usually only one follicle reaches maturity is not known.) The ma-

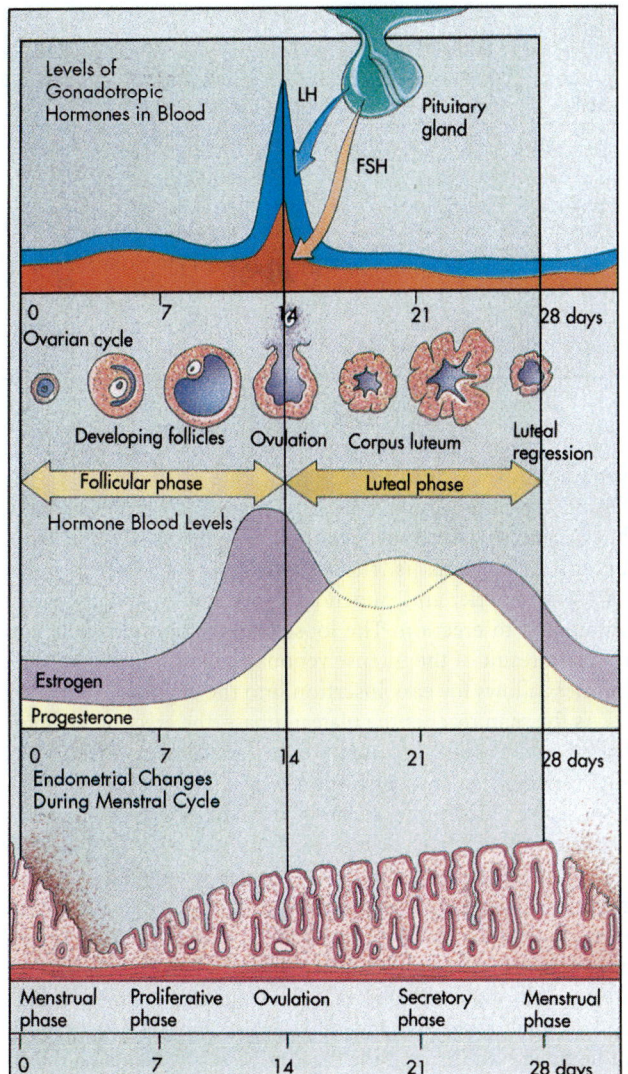

Fig. 48-8 Events of the menstrual cycle. The various lines depict the changes in blood hormone levels, the development of the follicles, and the changes in the endometrium during the cycle. *FSH,* follicle-stimulating hormone; *LH,* luteinizing hormone.

Table **48-2**	Common Manifestations During the Climacteric	
Premenopausal	**Postmenopausal**	
Irregular menses	Atrophic vaginitis	
Vasomotor instability (hot flashes)	Occasional vasomotor symptoms	
Nervousness	Atrophy of genitourinary tissue with decreased support	
Perimenopausal	Osteoporosis	
Cessation of menses		
Frequent vasomotor symptoms		
Atrophy of genitourinary tissue (e.g., vaginal epithelium)		
Stress and urge incontinence		

During the follicular phase, the endometrial lining of the uterus also undergoes change. As larger amounts of estrogen are produced, the endometrial lining undergoes proliferative changes, and there is an increase in cellular growth, including an increase in the length of blood vessels and glandular tissue.

With ovulation and the resulting increased levels of progesterone, the luteal, or secretory, phase begins. In this phase, the blood vessels begin to coil, increasing the surface area of the vascular supply. The glandular tissues mature and secrete a glycogen-rich substance, and the glandular ducts dilate. If the corpus luteum regresses (when fertilization does not occur) and estrogen and progesterone levels fall, the endometrial lining can no longer be supported. As a result, the blood vessels contract, and tissue begins to slough (fall away). This sloughing results in the menses and the start of the menstrual phase.

Menopause

Menopause is the cessation of the menses for the remainder of a woman's lifetime. It is usually considered complete after 1 year of amenorrhea (absence of menstruation). The average age at which menopause occurs is 52 years, but this can vary.[4] The climacteric, also commonly known as the perimenopause, is the period during which symptoms of approaching menopause begin, menopause actually occurs, and equilibrium after menopause is established (Table 48-2). Ovulation decreases over a period of years. In a way, the factors that result in menopause are established during fetal life. Approximately 2 to 4 million oocytes are present by the 20th week of gestation, after which time the number begins to decline. The average woman ovulates 400 to 500 times during a lifetime. Most follicles undergo atresia and are then called atretic follicles.[2] In 40 to 50 years after birth the full store of oocytes is greatly depleted. Because the number of oocytes decreases during the climacteric, the amount of estrogen produced also begins to decrease.

The decreasing level of estrogen causes a gradual increase in FSH and LH as a result of the negative feedback process. By the time menopause occurs, there is a tenfold to twentyfold increase in FSH. These elevated FSH levels may take several years to return to premenopausal levels. The reduced estrogen level

ture follicle stimulates estrogen production, causing a negative feedback with resulting decreased FSH secretion.

Although the initial stage of follicular maturation is stimulated by FSH, complete maturation and ovulation occur only with the presence of LH. When estrogen levels peak on about the twelfth day of the cycle, there is a surge of LH, which triggers ovulation a day or two later. After ovulation (maturation and release of an ovum), LH promotes the development of the corpus luteum.

The fully developed corpus luteum continues to secrete estrogen and initiates progesterone secretion. If fertilization occurs, high levels of estrogen and progesterone continue to be secreted as a result of the continued activity of the corpus luteum from stimulation by human chorionic gonadotropin (hCG). If fertilization does not take place, menstruation occurs because of a decrease in estrogen production and progesterone withdrawal.

also causes a decrease in the frequency of ovulation and results in atrophy of the secondary sex characteristics.

The reason for "hot flashes" or vasomotor instability is not clearly understood. It has been theorized that temperature regulators in the brain are in proximity to the area where GnRH is released. However, lowered estrogen levels are correlated with dilation of cutaneous blood vessels, resulting in "hot flashes" and increased sweating. The more sudden the withdrawal of estrogen (e.g., surgical removal of the ovaries), the more likely the symptoms will be severe if no replacement is provided. These symptoms subside over time, with or without hormone replacement therapy. Autonomic nervous system instability may also be related to emotional irritability during the climacteric, but this "symptom" has been greatly exaggerated in literature and myth. Atrophy of the vaginal epithelium often causes vaginal dryness that is responsible for mild to moderate dyspareunia (painful intercourse). This can lead to unnecessary and premature cessation of sexual activity. Dryness is a problem that can be easily corrected with water-soluble lubricants or, if needed, with hormonal creams or systemic hormone replacement therapy. In general, the extent and severity of the symptoms of the climacteric vary and are not easily predicted, even with a detailed history of family patterns.

Osteoporosis, a condition in which the bone mass is decreased because of increased bone resorption, is prevalent in menopausal women. This condition puts women at a much greater risk for sustaining fractures of the spine, vertebrae, wrists, and hips. Such fractures can be life threatening in older women. Although the exact mechanism is not known, cessation of estrogen production is associated with accelerated bone loss. Hormone replacement therapy in the postmenopausal period can help protect women from osteoporosis and cardiovascular disease. Combined estrogen and progesterone therapy reduces the risk of endometrial cancer associated with the use of estrogen alone. Research on hormonal replacement therapy and breast cancer is underway; past study results have been equivocal.[5]

The changes of menopause and particularly the risk of osteoporosis create a dilemma in the care of menopausal women. The use of estrogen replacement therapy often reduces the risk of such symptoms but can create other potentially serious side effects. Adequate calcium intake and exercise both before and after menopause are also important factors in the prevention of osteoporosis (see Chapter 59).

Phases of the Sexual Response

It is helpful to look at the structural homologues in the male and female reproductive systems to understand the sexual response (Table 48-3). Masters and Johnson described the sexual response in terms of the excitement, plateau, orgasmic, and resolution phases.[6] These phases are discussed for the male and the female as the sexual response.

Orgasm does not occur in every sexual encounter. In addition, orgasm does not depend on anatomic features such as the size of the penis or of the vaginal canal. The sexual response is a complex interplay of psychologic and physiologic phenomena and is therefore influenced by daily stress, as well as by illness and crisis.

Male Sexual Response.   The penis and the urethra are essential to the transport of sperm into the vagina and the cervix during intercourse. This transport is facilitated by penile erection in response to sexual stimulation during the ex-

Table **48-3**	Structural Homologues of the Male and Female Reproductive Systems
Male	**Female**
Penis	Clitoris
Scrotal ridge	Labia minora
Scrotum	Labia majora
Testes	Ovaries
Cowper's glands	Bartholin's glands
Prostate gland	Skene's ducts
Prostatic utricle (blind pouch of urethra)	Vagina

citement phase. Erection results from the filling of the large venous sinuses within the erectile tissue of the penis. In the flaccid state the sinuses hold only a small amount of blood, but during the erection stage they are congested with blood. Because the penis is richly endowed with sympathetic, parasympathetic, and pudendal nerve endings, it is readily stimulated to erection. The loose skin of the penis becomes taut as a result of the intense venous congestion. This erectile tautness allows for easy insertion into the vagina.

As the man reaches the plateau phase, the erection is maintained, and a small increase in diameter occurs as a result of a slight increase in vasocongestion. There is also an increase in testicle size. Sometimes a change in color occurs in the glans penis, which becomes more reddish-purple.

The subsequent contraction of the penile and urethral musculature during the orgasmic phase propels the sperm outward through the meatus. In this process, termed *ejaculation,* sperm are released into the ductus deferens during contractions. They advance through the urethra, where fluids from the prostate and seminal vesicles are added to the ejaculate. The sperm continue their path through the urethra, receiving a small amount of fluid from the Cowper's glands, and are finally ejaculated through the urinary meatus. Orgasm is characterized by the rapid release of the vasocongestion and myotonia that have developed. The rapid release of muscular tension (through rhythmic contractions) occurs primarily in the penis, the prostate gland, and the seminal vesicles.

After ejaculation, a man enters the resolution phase. During this phase the penis undergoes involution, gradually returning to its unstimulated, flaccid state.

Female Sexual Response.   The changes that occur in a woman during sexual excitation are similar to those in a man. In response to stimulation the clitoris swells (becomes congested, as does the penis in a man), and vaginal lubrication increases from secretions from the cervix and Bartholin's glands and sweating of the vaginal walls. This initial response is the excitation phase.

As excitation is maintained in the plateau phase, the vagina expands and the uterus is elevated (in the man, correspondingly, there is an increase in testicular size). In the orgasmic phase, contractions occur in the uterus from the fundus to the lower uterine segment. There is a slight relaxation of the cervical os, which helps the entrance of the sperm, and rhythmic contractions of the vagina. Muscular tension is rapidly released through rhythmic contractions in the clitoris, the vagina, and the uterus. This phase is followed by a resolution phase in which these organs return to their preexcitation state. However,

Table 48-4   Reproductive System

Changes	Differences in Assessment Findings
Male	
Penis	
Decreased subcutaneous fat, decreased skin turgor	Easily retractable foreskin (if uncircumcised), decrease in size, fewer sustained erections
Testes	
Decreased testosterone production	Decrease in size, change in position (lower), increase in firmness
Prostate	
Benign hyperplasia	Enlargement
Breasts	
Enlargement	Gynecomastia (abnormal enlargement)
Female	
Breasts	
Decreased subcutaneous fat, increased fibrous tissue, decreased skin turgor	Less resilient, looser, more pendulous tissue, decreased size, duct around nipple may feel like stringy strand
Vulva	
Decreased skin turgor	Atrophy, decreased amount of pubic hair, decreased size of clitoris, decreased size of labia
Vagina	
Atrophy of tissue, decreased muscle tone	Pale mucosa, dryness of mucosa, less intense sexual response, relaxation of outlets, mucosa thins, vagina narrower and shorter
Urethra	
Decreased muscle tone	Cystocele (protrusion of bladder through vaginal wall)
Uterus	
Decreased thickness of myometrium	Decrease in size, uterine prolapse
Ovaries	
Decreased ovarian function	Nonpalpable ovaries, decreased size

Table 48-5   Sexual Function

Male
Increased stimulation necessary for erection
Decreased need to ejaculate
Decreased ability to attain erection
Possible decreased response to sexual stimuli

Female
Decreased vaginal lubrication
Possible decreased response to sexual stimuli

women do not have to go through the resolution (refractory) recovery state before they can be orgasmic again. They can be multiorgasmic without resolution between orgasms.

GERONTOLOGIC CONSIDERATIONS

Effects of Aging on the Reproductive Systems and the Sexual Response

With advancing age, changes occur in the male and female reproductive systems. In women, many of these changes are related to the altered estrogen production that is associated with menopause. Age-related changes in the reproductive systems and differences in assessment findings are presented in Table 48-4.

Gradual changes resulting from advancing age occur in the sexual responses of men and women (Table 48-5). These changes occur at different rates and to varying degrees. The cumulative effects of these changes, as well as the negative social attitude toward sexuality in older adults, can affect the sexual practices of people in this age-group. Nurses have an important role in providing accurate and unbiased information about sexuality and age. Nurses should emphasize the normalcy of sexual activity in older adults. Counseling may be necessary to help older patients accommodate to these normal physiologic changes.[7]

ASSESSMENT OF THE MALE AND FEMALE REPRODUCTIVE SYSTEMS

Subjective Data

Important Health Information. Problems in other systems are often interrelated with problems and stresses within the reproductive system. The nurse must elicit general information, as well as information specifically relating to the reproductive system. Reproduction and sexual issues are often considered extremely personal and private. The nurse must develop trust to elicit such information. A professional demeanor is important when taking a reproductive or sexual history.

Past health history. Every woman who enters the health care system should have a complete obstetric and gynecologic history taken (Table 48-6). The gynecologic history provides information related to such problems as pelvic pain, exposure to sexually transmitted diseases, vaginal infections, and the presence of symptoms such as vaginal discharge and dyspareunia that need treatment. An obstetric history provides important information related to family planning and fertility counseling most relevant to the individual.

In addition, the nurse should obtain data related to in utero exposure to diethylstilbestrol (DES). DES was frequently administered to women to prevent spontaneous abortions during the 1940s and 1950s, with a national decline in use during the 1960s. It is associated with cervical adenosis and cervical and vaginal adenocarcinoma in women who were exposed to it in utero. Male offspring of mothers given DES experience congenital anomalies such as structural defects of the genitourinary tract and decreased sperm levels, as well as an increase in the incidence of penile cancer.

Table 48-6 | Gynecologic and Obstetric History Format

General Gynecologic Information

External genitalia
_____ Pain
_____ Rashes
_____ Lesions
_____ Other
_____ Vaginal discharge
Amount _____
Color _____
Consistency _____
Odor _____
Past history of vaginal infection _____ Yes _____ No
If yes, type _____
_____ Pain during intercourse
_____ Bleeding after intercourse

Sexually transmitted diseases (STDs)
_____ Chlamydia   _____ Syphilis
_____ Genital herpes   _____ Yeast infection
_____ Gonorrhea   _(Candida albicans)_
_____ HIV
_____ Other (specify) _____

Gynecologic history
Last Pap Smear _____ Abnormal _____ (Yes or No)
_____ Uterine fibroids Treatment if any _____
_____ Endometriosis   Treatment if any _____
_____ Ovarian cyst _____
Did your mother take hormones when she was pregnant
    with you? (Yes, No, or Not Sure)
Any difficulties in getting pregnant? (Yes, No, or
    Has not attempted)
Gynecologic surgery (e.g., D&C, cryosurgery)
    Type _____
    Reason _____
    Year _____

Obstetric Information
_____ Number of pregnancies
_____ Number of full-term births
_____ Number of preterm births
_____ Number of live births
_____ Number of spontaneous abortions (miscarriages)
_____ Number of therapeutic abortions
_____ Number of ectopic (tubal) pregnancies
_____ Number of cesarean sections
Problems during pregnancy, if any _____
_____
_____
_____

Menstrual Information
Age at onset _____
Last menstrual period _____
Cycle (frequency) _____ Irregular periods _____ Length _____
Duration of each menses _____
Number of pads or tampons used on heaviest days _____
Clots _____ Spotting (other than during menses) _____
Dysmenorrhea (describe) _____
Treatment _____
    Change in flow or amount (yes or no)
    Explain _____
Menopause _____ Menopausal symptoms _____
Hormonal replacement _____ (yes or no)
    What _____ Dose _____
If menopausal, have you noticed any vaginal
    bleeding? _____
Birth control method (if applicable) _____
    Length _____ Previous methods _____

Breast Information
_____ Monthly breast self-exam (yes or no)
Breast lumps (location) _____
Treatment, if any _____
_____ Mammogram (date) _____
_____ Breast pain
    Onset _____
    Severity _____
    Previous occurrence _____
_____ Breast discharge
    Onset _____
    Amount _____
    Color _____
    Odor and consistency _____
    Breastfeeding _____ (yes or no)
Where are you in your menstrual cycle (in case any
    breast abnormality is found)? _____
_____

D&C, dilation and curettage.

Common pediatric illnesses that affect reproductive function are mumps and rubella. The occurrence of mumps in young men has been associated with an increase in sterility because of bilateral testicular atrophy secondary to orchitis. In the health history, the nurse should elicit whether male patients have had mumps, been immunized, or had any indications of sterility.

Rubella is of primary concern to women of childbearing age. If rubella occurs during the first 3 months of pregnancy, the possibility of congenital anomalies is increased. For this reason, nurses should encourage immunization for all women of childbearing age who have not been immunized for rubella or have not already had the disease. However, women should not be immunized if they are already pregnant. Women are also advised not to conceive for at least 3 months after immunization.

The presence of a chronic disease such as diabetes mellitus that can affect the functioning of the reproductive system must be determined. Men who have diabetes mellitus frequently experience impotency problems because of associated neuropathies. Impotence and retrograde ejaculation are additional manifestations of diabetes mellitus in men. In women with uncontrolled diabetes mellitus, pregnancy and the use of oral contraceptives may constitute significant risks to health. Likewise, in women, a history of cardiovascular disease, including hypertension, thrombophlebitis, and angina, causes a higher incidence of morbidity and mortality with pregnancy or oral con-

Table 48-7	Surgeries of the Reproductive System
Surgery	**Definition**
Men	
Herniorrhaphy	Repair of hernia
Orchiectomy	Removal of a testis
Prostatectomy	Removal of prostate gland
Repair of testicular torsion	Correction of axial rotation of spermatic cord, which cuts off blood supply to the testicle, epididymis, and other structures
Varicocelectomy	Repair of varicose vein of scrotum
Vasectomy	Removal of part of vas deferens, can be an elective procedure for sterilization or contraception
Women	
Cryosurgery	Use of subfreezing temperature to destroy tissue, especially in treatment of abnormal cells
Dilation and curettage	Dilation of uterus and scraping of endometrium, performed to diagnose disease of uterus, correct heavy or prolonged vaginal bleeding, or empty uterus of products of conception; also used in the treatment of infertility to correlate state of endometrium and time of cycle
Hysterectomy	Removal of uterus
Oophorectomy	Removal of one or both ovaries
Repair of cystocele	Correction of protrusion of urinary bladder through vaginal wall
Repair of rectocele	Correction of protrusion of rectum and posterior vaginal wall into vagina
Salpingectomy	Removal of one or both fallopian tubes
Tubal sterilization	Ligation of fallopian tubes

traceptive use. Anemia is also relevant to women's reproductive health. Anemia can result from or be aggravated by menstrual flow. Fear of painful intercourse can occur in women because of the physiologic changes of vaginal atrophy and decreased vaginal lubrication.

A history of a stroke (cerebrovascular accident [CVA]) should be determined. In men, strokes may cause physiologic or psychologic impotence. Men who have suffered heart attacks frequently experience impotence. This impotence is often caused by the fear of precipitating another heart attack as a result of the increased heart rate associated with sexual activity. This same concern is shared by the woman both as a partner and as the person recovering from a heart attack. The interviewer must be sensitive to this concern. Questions asked about the original cardiac event may elicit fear and thus indicate a need for counseling and support regarding safe sexual practices related to cardiac health.

Questions relating to endocrine disorders, particularly hypothyroidism and hyperthyroidism, must also be asked because these disorders directly interfere with women's menstrual cycles and with sexual performance in men. Finally, men and women should be assessed for kidney and urinary tract disorders because sexual functioning and reproductive capacity can be affected by genitourinary problems. When taking a sexual or reproductive history, it is helpful to begin with the least sensitive information (e.g., menstrual history) before asking questions regarding more sensitive issues such as sexual practices or sexually transmitted diseases.

Medications. A pharmacologic profile of prescribed and over-the-counter drugs is necessary for all patients. Particularly relevant in assessment of the reproductive system is the use of diuretics (sometimes prescribed for premenstrual edema), psychotropic agents (which may interfere with sexual performance), and antihypertensives (some of which have been implicated in impotence). Thus patients who use drugs such as methyldopa (Aldomet), clonidine (Catapres), guanethidine (Ismelin), and hydralazine (Apresoline) must be closely assessed for these problems. All drugs taken by female patients should be evaluated for possible teratogenic effects in women of childbearing age.

In women, the use of oral contraceptives or other hormones should be noted. The use of estrogen replacement therapy is relevant for women because of its effect on the prevention of osteoporosis and coronary artery disease. Recent data suggest that estrogen may also have beneficial effects on memory and cognitive function in older women.[8] In women with a uterus, the concurrent use of a progestational agent should be documented. The use of estrogen alone has been shown to increase the incidence of endometrial cancer. The nurse must also note the use of drugs such as alcohol, marijuana, barbiturates, amphetamines, and phencyclidine hydrochloride (PCP), or "angel dust," which can have serious behavioral or physiologic effects on the functioning of the reproductive system.

Oral contraceptive use can aggravate the symptoms of certain neurologic dysfunctions, such as seizures or migraine headaches. However, the use of lower doses in current contraceptives makes these side effects less problematic. A history of cholecystitis and hepatitis is important information because these conditions may be contraindications for oral contraceptives; cholecystitis is often aggravated by oral contraceptives, and chronic active inflammation of the liver generally precludes the use of estrogen products because they are metabolized by the liver. Other contraindications to oral contraceptive use may be chronic obstructive pulmonary disease because progesterone thickens respiratory secretions.

Surgery or other treatments. Any hospitalizations or surgeries should be noted in the health history. In particular, certain types of surgeries should be noted (Table 48-7). Therapeutic or spontaneous pregnancy interruptions are also documented at this time.

HEALTH HISTORY

Table 48-8   **Reproductive System**

Health Perception–Health Management
- Have you had or been immunized for rubella?
- Are you currently attempting to become pregnant?
- Explain how you examine your breasts (testes).
- When was your last mammogram? Pap smear? Rectal exam? What were the results?
- Do you have any chronic illnesses such as diabetes?
- Do you have any vaginal or urethral discharge?
- What is "safe sex"?
- Do you protect yourself from unwanted pregnancy, HIV, and sexually transmitted diseases? How?

Nutritional-Metabolic
- Have you ever been told you were anemic?
- Do you think you get enough calcium in your diet? What calcium-rich foods do you eat regularly? Do you take a calcium supplement?
- What is your average daily caloric intake? (For pregnant, lactating, obese, or underweight patients)
- How do you feel about your weight? Would you like to be thinner/heavier? Are you on a diet currently?

Elimination
- Do you have any problems with urination? Bowel movements?
- Have you ever had a bladder infection? If so, when? How often does this problem occur? Does anything make it better?
- Do you use laxatives? How often? Have you ever made yourself vomit after eating?

Activity-Exercise
- Tell me what activities you typically do each day.
- Can you dress yourself? Feed yourself? Walk without help?

Cognitive-Perceptual
- Do you have any problems with your balance?
- Are you having any pain in your private parts?
- Do you have pain during sexual activity or intercourse?
- Are you forgetful at times?

Self-Perception–Self-Concept
- Has the problem in your reproductive system affected how you feel about yourself as a woman/man?
- Tell me how your problem has affected your sex life.

Role-Relationship
- What effect has your reproductive problem/pregnancy had on your work, family, or social life?
- Are you experiencing any role-associated problems in your family?*

Sexuality-Reproductive
- Are you satisfied with your present means of sexual expression? If no, explain.
- Have you had any recent changes in your sexual practices?
- Does your problem of your reproductive system affect your ability to have a satisfactory sex life?

Coping–Stress Tolerance
- What is stressful in your life right now?
- How do you handle your health problem(s)?
- Whom do you go to for support? Does this help?

Value-Belief
- What do you believe about your health problem(s)?
- Does your medical treatment contradict your personal beliefs?
- Do you use home remedies? What are they?
- Have you been seen by a homeopath, naturopath, or chiropractor?

Note: Some questions apply only to a woman or a man.
*If yes, describe.
HIV, human immunodeficiency virus

Functional Health Patterns. The key questions to ask a patient with a reproductive problem are presented in Table 48-8.

Health perception–health management pattern. The patient's sexual and contraceptive practices are important aspects of health management (Table 48-9). The patient's knowledge of safe sexual practices should be determined. Exposure to environmental toxins and sexually transmitted diseases can adversely affect fertility and reproductive health. Monthly breast self-examination (BSE), mammography according to age-specific guidelines, and routine Pap smears are integral to a woman's health. Testicular self-examination (TSE) should be practiced by all men, starting in adolescence. Prostate examination should be done annually by a health care professional for all men over age 40.

Initial questions asked of the female patient usually refer to the breast. The nurse asks the patient whether she performs a monthly BSE (see Chapter 49). If a lump is present, its onset, size, and consistency should be noted. The nurse also asks whether there has been an increase or a decrease in the size and shape of the lump since its onset or discovery. The patient is also questioned about breast pain or tenderness. She should describe the degree and severity of pain; breast pain or tenderness is not usually present with a malignant mass, particularly in the early stages.

The nurse should also inquire about a history of breast cancer in a woman's mother, maternal aunt, or sister because such a history increases the patient's risk of developing breast cancer. A family history of cancer, particularly cancer of the reproduc-

Table 48-9   Sexual History Format

How long have you been sexually active?
How frequently do you have penile-vaginal intercourse?
How frequently do you masturbate?
How many sexual partners do you have?
What is your sexual preference?
How frequently do you have oral sex?
How frequently do you have rectal intercourse?
Have you ever had an STD? If yes, what?
Are you using a contraceptive method? If yes, what kind? How often? Is it satisfactory?
Do you consider your sex life satisfactory?
How often have you experienced impotence or difficulty with vaginal lubrication or pain with intercourse?
Has your sex life changed? If yes, how?
Would you like to see your sex life change? If yes, how?
How would your partner rate your sex life?

STD, sexually transmitted disease.

tive organs, is important information related to health counseling. Determination of a familial tendency for diabetes mellitus, hypothyroidism, hyperthyroidism, hypertension, stroke, angina, myocardial infarction, endocrine disorders, or anemia is also important.

The nurse must determine if the patient is allergic to sulfonamides, penicillin, rubber, or latex. Sulfonamides and penicillin are used frequently in the treatment of reproductive and genitourinary problems such as vaginitis and gonorrhea. Rubber or latex are commonly used in diaphragms and condoms. An allergy to these substances precludes their use as contraceptive methods.

Assessment of the reproductive system is incomplete without a knowledge of the patient's lifestyle choices. The nurse should know whether a woman uses cigarettes, alcohol, caffeine, or other drugs because these substances can be detrimental to both mother and fetus. Cigarette smoking may delay conception. Maternal smoking during pregnancy may result in an infant of low birth weight and increases the risk of spontaneous abortion, fetal death, neonatal death, and sudden infant death syndrome (SIDS). Cigarette smoking can increase the risk of morbidity in women using contraceptives and is associated with early menopause. These substances may also adversely affect the sperm count in men and cause impotence or decreased libido.

Nutritional-metabolic pattern. Anemia is a common problem in women in their reproductive years, particularly during pregnancy and the postpartum period. The adequacy of the diet should be evaluated with this problem in mind. Women should be encouraged to gain adequate but not excessive weight during pregnancy. The nurse should determine whether specific dietary recommendations from the health care provider are being followed throughout pregnancy.

A thorough nutritional and psychologic history should be taken to assess for the presence of an eating disorder. Anorexia can cause amenorrhea and the subsequent problems, such as osteoporosis, that are related to estrogen cessation. The nurse has the opportunity to help prevent the debilitating condition of osteoporosis. From early adolescence, women can be coun-

seled regarding adequate calcium intake and the role of calcium in the prevention of osteoporosis. The patient's daily calcium intake should be estimated to determine whether there is a need for supplementation. Folic acid intake for women in their reproductive years should be evaluated because a deficiency can result in spina bifida and other neural tube defects in the fetus.[9,10]

Elimination pattern. Many gynecologic problems can result in genitourinary problems. Stress and urge incontinence are common in older women because of relaxation of the pelvic musculature caused by multiple births or advancing age. Vaginal infections predispose patients to chronic or recurrent urinary tract infections. The proximity of the reproductive organs and the genitourinary tract make metastasis of malignant tumors to this site a possibility to be considered. Benign prostatic hyperplasia is a common problem of aging in men. It can impede normal urination, causing retention and difficulty in initiating the stream.

Activity-exercise pattern. Weight-bearing exercise decreases the risk of osteoporosis in women. The amount, type, and intensity of exercise should be documented. Lack of stress on bones, secondary to lack of exercise, is an important factor in the development of osteoporosis. Anemia, secondary to menorrhagia, can result in fatigue and activity intolerance and can interfere with satisfactory performance of the activities of daily living. Exercise should be encouraged during pregnancy, following guidelines regarding the type of exercise, the intensity, and the frequency of workouts.

Sleep-rest pattern. Sleep disturbances occur during pregnancy because of nocturia and the woman's inability to find a comfortable sleeping position. Sleep patterns may be affected during the postpartum period and also while raising young children. The hot flashes and sweating often present during the perimenopause can cause serious sleep interruption when the woman is awakened in a drenching sweat. The need to change her nightgown and bedding further disrupts her sleep. Insomnia is also a common complaint of perimenopausal women. Daytime fatigue often results from such nighttime awakenings.

Cognitive-perceptual pattern. Changes in balance and sensory perception accompany normal pregnancy. Aches and pains during gestation are caused by stretching of muscles and ligaments to accommodate the growing fetus. Pelvic pain is associated with various gynecologic disorders such as pelvic inflammatory disease, ovarian cysts, and endometriosis.

Reproduction and sexual issues are often considered highly personal and private and are not easily discussed by many patients. The nurse must strive to develop trust and must maintain a professional demeanor when eliciting a reproductive history.

Dyspareunia (painful intercourse) can be particularly problematic for a woman. The pain associated with intercourse can make her reluctant to participate in sexual activity and strain her relationship with her sexual partner. The woman should be referred to her health care provider if dyspareunia is present.

Self-perception–self-concept pattern. For both men and women, there may be body image changes associated with developmental changes. Menarche and puberty herald the appearance of secondary sexual characteristics, which may result in either pride or embarrassment. Adolescent problems related to body image include acne, myopia, obesity, anorexia nervosa, bulimia, and scoliosis.

Pregnancy may affect a woman's body image in a negative way as her size increases and her functional abilities decrease. Changes in body shape become more threatening to the woman as the pregnancy progresses.

The reproductive changes of aging such as pendulous breasts and vaginal dryness in women and decreased size of the penis in men may lead to emotional distress. The subtle changes associated with sexuality and advancing age may challenge the self-concept of many persons.

Role-relationship pattern. The addition of a new baby into the family may change family dynamics. Indeed, one maternal task is to integrate the new member of the household into the family.

The changes occurring during adolescence and the need to challenge parental authority may lead to stress among family members. Conflicts that arise during the adolescent's quest for identity can add further tension. Risk-taking behaviors, such as smoking and substance abuse on the part of the adolescent, are often symptomatic of the problem.

As the years go by, role relationship patterns change as children begin their careers and move away from home. This again rearranges the family configuration.

The nurse seeks information about the type of family to which the patient belongs. Questions regarding recent changes or family conflicts should be asked. It is important to ascertain the patient's role in the family as a starting point in determining family dynamics.

A thorough health history also includes information about the patient's occupation and potential hazards associated with it. For example, exposure to toxic chemicals can affect sexual functioning and reproductive capacity.

Sexuality-reproductive pattern. The extent and depth of the interview about a patient's sexuality depend primarily on the expertise of the interviewer and on the needs and the willingness of the patient. Before taking a sexual history, interviewers should assess their comfort with their own sexuality, because any discomfort in questioning becomes obvious to the patient. Interviews must be carried out in an environment that provides reassurance, confidentiality, and a nonjudgmental attitude. It is best to begin with the least sensitive areas and then move to more sensitive areas. For this reason, sexual histories are frequently initiated during the review of the genitourinary and gynecologic systems. Early questioning can relate to menstruation, the onset of puberty, and the presence or absence of symptoms of genitourinary problems. These questions thus serve as an introduction for both the care provider and the patient before they move into more sensitive areas. Questions about sexuality should always be asked in a straightforward and nonjudgmental manner. Table 48-9 outlines questions appropriate for an initial assessment or annual examination. Both men and women should be asked about their general satisfaction with sexuality. Indications of sexual dysfunction may require referral or consultation with a sex counselor. A thorough genitourinary history must also be collected for the assessment of the reproductive system to be complete.

Problems of the reproductive system can cause physiologic or psychologic problems that can lead to painful intercourse, impotence, sexual dysfunction, or infertility. Both the cause and the effect of such problems should be determined.

The patient should be questioned about sexual beliefs and practices and whether orgasm is achieved. The patient's satisfaction with the opportunities for sexual gratification is important information that should be elicited. Any unexplained change in sexual practices or performance should be explored. This is an appropriate time to discuss methods of birth control and safe sex.

Menstrual history data are used in the detection of pregnancy, infertility, and numerous other gynecologic concerns. Changes in the usual menstrual pattern must be explicitly described to determine whether the change is transient and unimportant or connected with a more serious gynecologic problem. Metrorrhagia (spotting or bleeding between menstruations), menorrhagia (excessive menstrual bleeding), amenorrhea (lack of menstruation), and postcoital bleeding are examples of such problems. Changes in menstrual patterns associated with the use of contraceptive pills, intrauterine devices (IUDs), subdermal estrogen-only implant (Norplant), or medroxyprogesterone (Depo-Provera) injections must be identified. Contraceptive pills usually decrease the amount and duration of flow, whereas IUDs may cause an increase in the amount and duration. IUDs also frequently increase the severity of dysmenorrhea.

Patterns of sexual relationships also provide important information. A history of multiple sex partners increases the risk of contracting a sexually transmitted disease. For a woman, this can increase the risk of pelvic inflammatory disease, which can compromise her ability to become pregnant.

Coping–stress tolerance pattern. The stress related to situational or maturational crises such as pregnancy, menopause, or the climacteric may cause an increased dependence on support systems. It is essential for the nurse to ascertain who the support people are in the patient's life. The diagnosis of a sexually transmitted disease can cause stress to the patient and the partner. Means to manage such stress should be explored.

Value-belief pattern. Sexual and reproductive functioning is closely related to cultural, religious, moral, and ethical values. The nurse should be aware of his or her own beliefs in these areas and should recognize and sensitively react to the patient's personal beliefs associated with reproductive issues.

Objective Data

Physical Examination. The examination of the external genitalia uses inspection and palpation.

Male genitalia. An examination may be performed with the patient lying or standing. The standing position is generally preferred. The examiner should be seated in front of the standing patient. Gloves should be used during examination of the male genitalia.

Pubes. The nurse observes the diamond-shaped pattern of hair distribution. The absence of hair is not normal. The skin is also evaluated.

Penis. The nurse notes the size and skin texture of the penis and any lesions, scars, or swelling. The location of the urethral meatus, as well as the presence or absence of a foreskin, should be noted. If present, the foreskin should be retracted to note cleanliness and replaced over the glans after observation. The glans are compressed to note any discharge and its amount, color, and odor if present. The nurse also palpates the penile shaft for tenderness or masses and observes the ventral and dorsal aspects.

Scrotum and testes. The nurse performs a complete skin examination by lifting each testis to inspect all sides of the scrotal sac. Palpation of the scrotum is done to note changes in consistency or the presence of masses. It is important to note if the testes are descended. The left testis usually hangs lower than the right. Undescended testis is a major risk factor for testicular cancer, as well as a potential cause of male infertility. The patient should also be taught TSE (see Chapter 52).

Inguinal region and spermatic cord. The examiner inspects the inguinal regions for rashes, lesions, or lymphadenopathy, which may suggest pelvic organ infection. The nurse has the patient cough or bear down and notes any conspicuous bulging in the inguinal canals. The nurse also palpates the area for any bulging as the patient again coughs or bears down. The nurse palpates the inguinal and femoral pulses and the local lymph nodes.

The spermatic cord is located posteriorly in the scrotal sac. The nurse follows the cord on each side. The inguinal region is gently palpated using the forefinger or small finger and by pushing up through the loose scrotal skin to the abdominal wall along the inguinal region. The internal inguinal ring meets and impedes the finger. At this point, the patient again bears down and coughs. The nurse determines whether the strain produces a bulging of the intestines through the ring, indicating the presence of a hernia, a condition that requires follow-up.

Anus and prostate. The anal sphincter and perineal regions are inspected for lesions, masses, and hemorrhoids. A digital examination is required for all patients who have symptoms of prostate trouble, such as difficulty in initiating the flow and the urge to void frequently; this examination should be performed annually for all men over 40 years of age.

Female breasts and external genitalia. Physical examination of women often begins with inspection and palpation of the breasts and then proceeds to the abdomen. Examination of the abdomen provides an opportunity to detect pain or any masses that may involve the genitourinary system.

Breasts. Breasts are examined first by visual inspection. The nurse, with the patient seated, observes the breasts for symmetry, size, shape, skin color and texture, vascular patterns, and the presence of unusual lesions. The patient is asked to put her arms at her sides, arms overhead, lean forward, and press hands on hips. The nurse observes for any abnormalities during these maneuvers. The axillae and the clavicular areas are then palpated for enlarged lymph nodes.

After the patient assumes a supine position, a pillow is placed under the back on the side to be examined. The patient is asked to put the arm above and behind the head. These maneuvers flatten breast tissue and make palpation easier. The breast is then palpated in a systematic fashion using a vertical line, a clockwise, or a spoke approach. The nurse should use the distal finger pads for palpation. The tail of Spence should be included in the examination because this area and the upper outer quadrant are the areas where most breast malignancies develop.

Finally, the nurse should palpate the area around the areolae for masses. The nipple should be compressed to determine the presence of discharge or any masses. The color, consistency, and odor of any discharge should be documented.

External genitalia. The nurse uses gloves for examination of the external genitalia. The mons pubis, the labia majora, the labia minora, the perineum, and the anal region are inspected for characteristics of skin, hair distribution, and contour. Lesions, swelling, and discharge are noted.

The nurse separates the labia to fully inspect the clitoris, the urethral meatus, the vaginal orifice, the hymen, the perineum, and the anal region. Any inflammation or cysts on Bartholin's glands or Skene's glands are noted.

Internal pelvic examination. During the speculum examination, the nurse observes the walls of the vagina and the cervix for inflammation, discharge, polyps, and suspicious growths. During this examination, it is possible to take a Pap smear and collect secretions for culture and study under the microscope (i.e., wet smears).

After the speculum examination, a bimanual examination is performed to allow assessment of the size, shape, and consistency of the uterus, ovaries, and tubes. The tubes are not normally palpable. Details of the pelvic and bimanual examinations are described in physical assessment textbooks. Because these skills are not usually within the scope of the nurse generalist, they are not described here.

Table 48-10 illustrates a recording format for the physical assessment findings of the male and female reproductive

Table **48-10** Recording the Normal Physical Assessment of the Reproductive System	
Male	**Female**
Penis and Scrotum	**Breasts**
Diamond-shaped hair distribution	Symmetric or slightly asymmetric
Testes	Nipples everted
Descended bilaterally	No nipple discharge
3 cm wide, 4.5 cm long	No dimpling or retraction
Smooth, firm	No masses, lesions, or tenderness
Skin	No axillary nodes
No lesions, redness, swelling, masses, or inflammation	Appropriate for age and parity
Circumcised penis	**Vulva**
Meatus patent, no discharge	Triangular hair distribution
No masses, slight tenderness	No lesions, redness, swelling, masses, or inflammation
No inguinal hernias	Patent vaginal orifice, no discharge
Epididymis	Nonpalpable Skene's ducts and Bartholin's glands, no tenderness
Nontender	Intact clitoris and urethral meatus
No masses	
Rectum	
No hemorrhoids	

COMMON ASSESSMENT ABNORMALITIES

Table **48-11** Breast

Finding	Description	Possible Etiology and Significance
■ Nipple inversion or retraction	Recent onset, erythematous, pain, unilateral	Abscess, inflammation, cancer
	Recent onset (usually within past year), unilateral presentation, lack of tenderness	Neoplasm
■ Nipple secretions Galactorrhea (female)	Milky, no relationship to lactation, unilateral or bilateral or intermittent or consistent presentation	Drug therapy, particularly phenothiazines, tricyclic antidepressants, methyldopa; hypofunction or hyperfunction of thyroid or adrenal glands; tumors of hypothalamus or pituitary gland; excessive estrogen; prolonged suckling or breast foreplay
Galactorrhea (male)	Milky, bilateral presentation	Chorioepithelioma of testes
Purulent	Gray-green or yellow color; frequent unilateral presentation; association with pain, erythema, induration, nipple inversion	Puerperal (after birth) mastitis (inflammatory condition of breast) or abscess
	Same as above but usually without nipple inversion	Infected sebaceous cyst
Serous discharge	Clear appearance, unilateral or bilateral or intermittent or consistent presentation	Intraductal papilloma
Dark green or multicolored discharge	Thick, sticky, and frequently bilateral	Mammary duct ectasia (dilation of mammary ducts)
Serosanguineous or bloody drainage	Unilateral presentation	Papillomatosis (widespread development of nipplelike growths), intraductal papilloma, carcinoma (male and female)
■ Scaling or irritation of nipple	Unilateral or bilateral presentation, crusting, possible ulceration	Paget's disease, eczema, infection
■ Nodules, lumps, or masses	Multiple, bilateral, well-delineated, soft or firm, mobile cysts; pain; premenstrual occurrence	Fibrocystic changes
	Rubbery consistency, fluid-filled interior, pain	Mammary duct ectasia
	Soft, mobile, well-delineated cyst, absence of pain	Lipoma, fibroadenoma
	Erythema, tenderness, induration	Infected sebaceous cysts, abscesses
	Usually singular, hard irregularly shaped, poorly delineated, nonmobile	Neoplasm

systems. Tables 48-11 through 48-13 summarize common assessment abnormalities of the breasts, the female reproductive system, and the male reproductive system, respectively.

DIAGNOSTIC STUDIES OF THE REPRODUCTIVE SYSTEM

Many diagnostic tests that are performed to assess problems occurring in other body systems also provide valuable data on the condition of the reproductive system. Table 48-14 summarizes the most commonly used diagnostic studies in the assessment of the reproductive system and the nurse's responsibility regarding these diagnostic tests.[11,12]

To understand many of the diagnostic studies of the reproductive system, it is important to understand the concepts of sensitivity and specificity. *Sensitivity* addresses the issue of how

well a test identifies people with a particular disease. The goal of sensitivity testing is to avoid the occurrence of false-negative results, that is, to avoid saying that someone does not have a particular health problem when, in fact, the disease is present. It is considered a screening test. *Specificity* testing answers the question of how well a test eliminates those individuals without the disease. The goal of sensitivity testing is to avoid false-positive results. It is the nurse's responsibility to ensure that the patient understands the purpose of any test being performed.

Urine Studies

Pregnancy Testing. Occurrence of pregnancy is generally validated by measuring the output of human chorionic gonadotropin (hCG) in the urine by means of an immunologic test. A solution containing monoclonal antibodies specific for

COMMON ASSESSMENT ABNORMALITIES

Table 48-12   Female Reproductive System

Finding	Description	Possible Etiology and Significance
■ Vulvar discharge	Plaquelike consistency, frequent itching and inflammation, lack of odor	Candidiasis (Candida or yeast infection), vaginitis
	Grayish color, copious flow, frothy appearance, vulvar irritation	Bacterial vaginosis infection
	Purulent odor, grayish-green or yellow color	Trichomonas vaginalis
	Bloody color	Chlamydia trachomatis or Neisseria gonorrhoeae infection, menstruation, trauma, cancer
■ Vulvar erythema	Bright or beefy red color, itching	Candida albicans, allergy, chemical vaginitis
	Reddened base, painful vesicles or ulcerations	Genital herpes
	Macules or papules, itching	Chancroid (STD), contact dermatitis, scabies, pediculosis
■ Vulvar growths	Soft, fleshy growth; nontender	Condyloma acuminatum
	Flat and warty appearance, nontender	Condyloma latum
	Same as either of above, possible pain	Neoplasm
	Reddened base, vesicles, and small erosions; pain	Lymphogranuloma venereum, genital herpes, chancroid
	Indurated, firm ulcers; lack of pain	Chancre (syphilis), granuloma inguinale
■ Abdominal pain or tenderness	Intermittent or consistent tenderness in right or left lower quadrant	Salpingitis (infection of fallopian tube), ectopic pregnancy, ruptured ovarian cyst, PID, tubal or ovarian abscess
	Periumbilical location, consistent occurrence	Cystitis, endometritis (inflammation of endometrium), ectopic pregnancy

PID, pelvic inflammatory disease.

hCG is mixed with a small amount of urine. The presence of hCG causes a change in color of the tested urine. To reduce cross-reactivity with LH and other pituitary hormones, the beta subunit of hCG is measured.

Home pregnancy test kits use the same assay principle described in the preceding paragraph. Positive results are based on the presence of hCG in urine. Some tests can detect pregnancy as early as the first day after the expected period. These tests are 97% accurate, but a negative test should be repeated in 2 weeks to achieve the greatest accuracy.[13] Serum pregnancy tests have also been developed, and they are almost 100% accurate.

Hormone Studies. Although estrogen studies are performed on urine, the results are frequently inaccurate because of variable estrogen levels during the normal cycle and the difficulty in estimating the day of the cycle in women with irregular menses. Adrenal androgens are precursors of estrogens and can be measured in the urine of both men and women. FSH can be measured in a 24-hour urine specimen. Increased and decreased FSH levels can indicate gonad failure resulting from pituitary dysfunction.

Blood Studies

Recently, serum pregnancy tests using radioimmunoassays have been developed. One test, a radioimmunoassay for the beta subunit of hCG, is so sensitive that a pregnancy can be detected before a woman misses her menstrual period.

The prolactin assay is used primarily in the workup of a patient with amenorrhea. High levels of prolactin are normally associated with low levels of estrogen, such as those that occur during lactation. However, the same finding can occur with pituitary adenomas, especially with otherwise unexplained galactorrhea.

Serum progesterone and estradiol are sometimes tested in ovarian function assessment, particularly for amenorrhea. In addition, hormonal blood studies are essential components of a thorough fertility workup.

Biologic tumor markers are often secreted by germinal cell cancers of the testis. The two most common markers are alpha-fetoprotein (AFP) and hCG. Measurement of these markers is useful in monitoring therapy (marker levels rise as disease progresses and fall with disease regression) because marker levels may rise months before new disease or metastasis is evident.

Syphilis Studies

The types of tests performed to diagnose syphilis can be classified as nontreponemal or treponemal. Nontreponemal tests such as the Venereal Disease Research Laboratory (VDRL) test and the rapid plasma reagin (RPR) test are inexpensive and reliable but have high levels of false-positive results (i.e., good sensitivity but poor specificity). These tests detect the presence of antibodies in the serum of infected patients. Nonspecific antibodies can be produced during many pathologic processes, especially some types of autoimmune diseases, and can yield false-positive test results.

Treponemal tests such as the fluorescent treponemal antibody absorption (FTAAbs) test are highly reliable and should be used after a positive nontreponemal test, even if it is weakly positive or questionable. This test measures specific antibodies to *Treponema pallidum*. The FTAAbs test does not assess the

COMMON ASSESSMENT ABNORMALITIES

Table 48-13 Male Reproductive System

Finding	Description	Possible Etiology and Significance
▪ Penile growths or masses	Indurated, smooth, disklike appearance; absence of pain; singular presentation	Chancre
	Papular to irregularly shaped ulceration with pus, lack of induration	Chancroid
	Ulceration with induration and nodularity	Cancer
	Flat, wartlike nodule	Condyloma latum
	Elevated, fleshy, moist, elongated projections with single or multiple projections	Condyloma acuminatum
	Localized swelling with retracted, tight foreskin	Paraphimosis (inability to replace foreskin to its normal position after retraction), trauma
▪ Vesicles, erosions, or ulcers	Painful, erythematous base; vesicular or small erosions	Genital herpes, balanitis (inflammation of glans penis), chancroid
	Painless, singular, small erosion with eventual lymphadenopathy	Lymphogranuloma venereum, cancer
▪ Scrotal masses	Localized swelling with tenderness, unilateral or bilateral presentation	Epididymitis (inflammation of epididymis), testicular torsion, orchitis (mumps)
	Swelling, tenderness	Incarcerated hernia
	Unilateral or bilateral presentation; swelling without pain; translucent, cordlike or wormlike appearance	Hydrocele (accumulation of fluid in outer covering of testes), spermatocele (firm, sperm-containing cyst of epididymis), varicocele (dilation of veins that drain testes), hematocele (accumulation of blood within scrotum)
	Firm, nodular testes or epididymis; frequent unilateral presentation	Tuberculosis, cancer
▪ Penile discharge	Clear to purulent color, minimal to copious flow	Urethritis or gonorrhea, *Chlamydia trachomatis* infection, trauma
▪ Penile or scrotal erythema	Macules and papules	Scabies, pediculosis
▪ Inguinal masses	Bulging, unilateral presentation during straining	Inguinal hernia
	Shotty, 1-3 cm nodules	Lymphadenopathy

adequacy of treatment of syphilis; the test remains reactive even after treatment. Antibody titers obtained with a VDRL test are used to measure the adequacy of therapy.

The most specific and direct examination for syphilis is dark-field microscopy of a specimen obtained from a potential syphilitic lesion (chancre). Unfortunately, the chancre is frequently gone by the time other symptoms occur, so the test cannot be performed. Other miscellaneous tests of secretions involve wet mounts, cultures, and stains to detect specific reproductive problems (see Table 48-14).

Cytologic Studies

The Pap smear is a screening test to detect abnormal cells obtained from the cervix, vagina, or nipple. It is performed by obtaining cells from the cervical canal, preferably the endocervix, as well as from the vagina, and placing these cells in a fixative for examination by a cytologist for cellular abnormalities. Pap smears are more accurate if performed at midcycle or during the secretory phase of the menstrual cycle because there is a greater likelihood that abnormal cells will be detected during these times. A Pap smear should be performed annually or more frequently in women with a history of dysplasia or exposure to DES. Pap smears are necessary in women who have had a hysterectomy because abnormal vaginal cells can sometimes be detected.

Although a Pap smear is highly accurate in detecting cervical cancer, a negative Pap test does not rule out endometrial cancer. Specific tests are available to obtain a smear directly from the endometrium. Uterine aspiration and cannulation into the uterine cavity make it possible to obtain endometrial tissue. Cytologic studies are also performed on any nipple discharge.

Radiologic Studies

Mammography has become one of the most frequently used diagnostic tools in reproductive system assessment (see Chapter 49). Unfortunately, its frequent use has been highly criticized because of the potential risks of radiation. However, increased awareness of the risks from radiographic studies has resulted in valuable improvements in the technique of mammography, particularly in lowering the exposure per examination. The American Cancer Society recommends that a screening mammogram be performed every 1 to 2 years for women between the ages of 40 and 49 and yearly after age 50.[14]

DIAGNOSTIC STUDIES

Table 48-14 Male and Female Reproductive Systems

Study	Description and Purpose	Nursing Responsibility
Urine Studies		
▪ Pregnancy testing	hCG is detected in urine to ascertain whether a woman is pregnant. Hydatidiform mole and chorioepithelioma (in men and women) may also be detected.	Obtain thorough menstrual history from patient, including birth control methods. Determine presence or absence of presumptive signs of pregnancy (e.g., breast changes or increased whitish vaginal discharge).
▪ Hormone testing Testosterone levels	Tumors and developmental anomalies of the testes can be detected.	Instruct patient to collect 24-hr urine specimen. Keep it refrigerated.

Follicle-stimulating hormone (FSH) assay	Test indicates gonadal failure because of pituitary dysfunction.
	Female:
	  Follicular phrase: 2-5 IU/24 hr
	  Midcycle: 8-40 IU/24 hr
	  Luteal phase: 2-10 IU/24 hr
	  Menopause: 35-100 IU/24 hr
	Male:
	  2-15 IU/24 hr
		Instruct patient to collect 24-hr urine specimen. Indicate phase of menstrual cycle, if menopausal, and if on oral contraceptives or hormones.

Blood Studies		
▪ Prolactin assay	This test detects pituitary dysfunction that can cause amenorrhea.	Observe venipuncture site for bleeding or hematoma formation.
▪ Serum hCG assay	hCG is detected in serum to ascertain whether a woman is pregnant (see entry on pregnancy testing).	Instruct patient to have blood drawn in laboratory. Elicit where she is in her menstrual cycle, whether she has missed menses, and if so, how late she is.
▪ Serum androstenedione and testosterone levels	These tests ascertain whether elevated androgens are due to adrenal or ovarian dysfunction. Serum testosterone is also drawn to assess cause of amenorrhea.	Collect health history to eliminate potential sources of interference with accuracy of results (e.g., use of steroids or barbiturates or presence of hypothyroidism or hyperthyroidism).
▪ Serum progesterone	This test is frequently used to detect functioning corpus luteum cyst.	Observe venipuncture site for bleeding or hematoma formation. Include last menstrual period and trimester of pregnancy since progesterone levels vary with gestation.
▪ Serum estradiol	This test measures ovarian function. It is particularly useful in assessing estrogen-secreting tumors and states of precocious female puberty. Normal values depend on laboratory that performs test and should be obtained from that laboratory. May be used to confirm perimenopausal time. Increased serum estradiol levels in men may be indicative of testicular tumors.	Observe venipuncture site for bleeding or hematoma formation.

▪ Serum FSH	This test indicates gonadal failure due to pituitary dysfunction; used to validate menopause.
	Female:
	  Follicular phase: 4-30 mIU/ml
	  Midcycle: 10-90 mIU/ml
	  Luteal phase: 4-30 mIU/ml
	  Menopause: 40-250 mIU/ml
	Male:
	  4-25 mIU/ml
		No food or fluid restrictions required. State phase of menstrual cycle, if menopausal, or if on oral contraceptive or hormones

Continued

DIAGNOSTIC STUDIES

Table 48-14   Male and Female Reproductive Systems—cont'd

Study	Description and Purpose	Nursing Responsibility
Syphilis Studies		
■ Nontreponemal serologic tests: Wassermann (complement fixation) Venereal Disease Research Laboratory (VDRL) (flocculation) Rapid plasma reagin (RPR) (agglutination)	These tests are nonspecific antibody tests used to screen for syphilis. Positive readings can be made within 1-2 wk after appearance of primary lesion (chancre) or 4-15 wk after initial infection.	Tell the patient that fasting is unnecessary. Inform patient that blood sample will be drawn. Observe venipuncture site for bleeding or hematoma formation. Obtain data to determine presence or absence of problems such as hepatitis, pregnancy, and autoimmune diseases that may interfere with the accuracy of results.
■ Treponemal test Fluorescent treponemal antibody absorption (FTAAbs)	This test detects syphilis antibodies. It also detects early syphilis with great accuracy. It is usually performed if results of nontreponemal testing are questionable.	Tell the patient that fasting is unnecessary. Inform patient that blood sample will be drawn. Observe venipuncture site for bleeding or hematoma formation.
Miscellaneous Studies		
■ Dark-field microscopy	Direct examination of specimen obtained from potential syphilitic lesion (chancre) is performed to detect treponema.	Avoid direct skin contact with open lesion.
■ Wet mounts	Direct microscopic examination of specimen of vaginal discharge is performed immediately after collection. This determines presence or absence and number of *Trichomonas* organisms, bacteria, white and red blood cells, and candidal buds or hyphae. Other clues or causes of inflammation or infection may be determined.	Explain procedure and purpose to patient. Instruct patient not to douche before examination. Prepare for collection of specimens (glass slide, 10-20% potassium hydroxide [KOH] solution, sodium chloride [NaCl] solution, and cotton-tipped applicators).
■ Cultures	Culture of specimens of vaginal, urethral, or cervical discharge are taken and used to assess presence of gonorrhea or chlamydia. Rectal and throat cultures may also be taken, depending on data obtained from sexual history.	Obtain specific contact and sexual history inclusive of oral and rectal intercourse. Instruct against douching before examination. Obtain urethral specimen from men before they void. Instruct women who are sexually active with multiple partners to have at least a yearly culture for gonorrhea and chlamydia. Instruct sexually active men to have any discharge evaluated immediately to rule out gonorrhea strains that do not cause classic symptoms of dysuria.
■ Gram's stain	This presumptive test is used for rapid detection of gonorrhea. Presence of gram-negative intracellular diplococci generally warrants initiation of treatment. Not highly accurate for women.	Same as above.
Cytologic Studies		
■ Pap smear	Microscopic study of exfoliated cells via special staining and fixation technique detects abnormal cells. Cells most commonly studied are those obtained directly from endocervix, cervix, vaginal pool, and endometrial lining of uterine cavity.	Instruct women who are sexually active and who are over age 18 to have Pap smears according to American Cancer Society guidelines. Arrange for smear at midcycle time. Instruct patients not to douche for at least 24 hr before examination. Collect careful menstrual and gynecologic history.
■ Nipple discharge test	Cytologic study of nipple discharge is performed.	Indicate whether hormonal preparations or other drugs are being taken, breastfeeding, or history of amenorrhea. Instruct patient during demonstration of breast self-examination or examination of breasts that nipple discharge should always be evaluated.

Continued

DIAGNOSTIC STUDIES

Table **48-14**	Male and Female Reproductive Systems—cont'd	
Study	**Description and Purpose**	**Nursing Responsibility**
Radiologic Studies		
▪ Soft tissue mammography	Low-dose x-ray image of breast tissue on photographic film is used to assess breast masses, recent breast enlargement, and nipple discharge to detect malignancy. It is usually an outpatient procedure.	Instruct patient about risks (radiation) and advantages of the examination. Instruct regarding American Cancer Society recommendations.
▪ Contrast mammography	This test is used to evaluate abnormal nipple discharge. It is particularly effective in detecting nonpalpable intraductal papillomas. Test consists of injection of radiopaque dye in breast duct.	Determine actual or possible allergy to contrast medium.
▪ Ultrasound	This test measures and records high-frequency sound waves as they pass through tissues of variable density. It is very useful in detecting masses greater than 3 cm, such as ectopic pregnancies, IUDs, ovarian cysts, and hydatidiform moles.	Instruct patient that a full bladder may be required depending on the reason for the study.
Invasive Procedures		
▪ Breast biopsy	Histologic examination of excised breast tissue is performed, either by needle-aspiration or excisional biopsy.	Before surgery, instruct patient about operative procedures and sedation. After surgery, perform wound care and instruct patient about breast self-examination.
▪ Hysterosalpingogram	This test involves instillation of radioscopic dye through cervix into uterine cavity and subsequently through and out fallopian tubes. Spot x-ray images are taken to detect abnormalities of uterus and its adnexa (ovaries and tubes) as dye progresses through them. Test may be most useful in diagnostic assessment of fertility (e.g., to detect adhesions near ovary, an abnormal uterine shape, or blockage of tubal pathways).	Inform patient about procedure and that it may be fairly uncomfortable, especially shoulder pain. Determine possibility of dye allergy.
▪ Colposcopy	Direct visualization of cervix with binocular microscope that allows magnification and study of cellular dysplasia and vascular and tissue abnormalities of cervix. This test is used as a follow-up study for abnormal Pap smears and for examination of women exposed to DES in utero. Biopsy of cervix may be taken during colposcopic examination. This test is valuable in decreasing number of false-negative cervical biopsies.	Instruct patient about this outpatient procedure. Inform patient that this examination is similar to speculum examination. Explain purpose of procedure and prepare patient for it.
▪ Conization	Cone-shaped sample of squamocolumnar tissue of cervix is removed for direct study.	Explain purpose and method of procedure and that it requires use of surgical facilities and anesthesia. Instruct patient to rest for at least 3 days after procedure. Also discuss necessity for 3-wk follow-up check.
▪ Loop electrosurgical excision of transformation zone (LEETZ)	Excision of cervical tissue via an electrosurgical instrument.	Explain purpose and method of procedure and that it may be done in the physician's office for further diagnostic testing.
▪ Loop electrosurgical excision procedure (LEEP)	Same as above.	Same as above.

Continued

DIAGNOSTIC STUDIES

Table 48-14   Male and Female Reproductive Systems—cont'd

Study	Description and Purpose	Nursing Responsibility
Operative Procedures—cont'd		
■ Culdotomy, culdoscopy, and culdocentesis	Culdotomy is an incision made through posterior fornix of cul-de-sac and allows visualization of peritoneal cavity (i.e., uterus, tubes, and ovaries). Culdoscope can then be used to study these structures closely. This technique is valuable in fertility evaluations. Withdrawal of fluid (culdocentesis) allows examination of fluid characteristics.	Explain purpose and method of procedure. Prepare patient for vaginal operation with preoperative instruction and sedation. Perform assessment of bleeding and discomfort after surgery.
■ Laparoscopy (peritoneoscopy)	This method of entry into the abdomen allows visualization of pelvic structures via fiberoptic scopes inserted through small abdominal incisions. Instillation of carbon dioxide into cavity improves visualization. This technique is used in diagnostic assessment of uterus, tubes, and ovaries. Can be used in conjunction with tubal sterilization.	Explain purpose and method of procedure. Before surgery, instruct patient about procedure, prepare abdomen, and reassure patient about sedation. Tell patient to rest for 1-3 days after surgery. Inform patient of probability of shoulder pain because of air in the abdomen.
■ Dilation and curettage	The operative procedure dilates cervix and allows curetting of endometrial lining. This test is used in assessment of abnormal bleeding patterns and cytologic evaluation of lining.	Before surgery, instruct patient about procedure and sedation. Tell patient that overnight hospitalization is occasionally required. Perform postoperative assessment of degree of bleeding (frequent pad check during first 24 hr).
Fertility Studies		
■ Semen analysis	Semen is assessed for volume (2-5 ml), viscosity, sperm count (>20 million/ml), sperm motility (60% motile), and percent of abnormal sperm (60% with normal structure).	Instruct patient to bring in fresh specimen within 2 hr after ejaculation.
■ Basal body temperature assessment	This measurement indicates indirectly whether ovulation has occurred. (Temperature rises at ovulation and remains elevated during secretory phase of normal menstrual cycle.)	Instruct woman to take her temperature using special basal temperature thermometer (calibrated in tenths of degrees) every morning before getting out of bed. Tell woman to record temperature on graph.
■ Huhner test or Sims-Huhner	Mucus sample of cervix is examined within 2-8 hr after intercourse. Total number of sperm is assessed in relation to number of live sperm. This test is performed to determine whether cervical mucus is "hostile" to passage of sperm from vagina into uterus.	Instruct couples to have intercourse at estimated time of ovulation and be present for test within 2-8 hr after intercourse.
■ Endometrial biopsy	In this outpatient procedure, small curette is used to obtain piece of endometrial lining to assess endometrial changes common to progesterone secretion after ovulation.	Tell patient that test must be performed postovulation. Explain that procedure should cause only short period of uterine cramping.
■ Hysterosalpingogram	Same as operative procedures.	Same as operative procedures.
■ Serum progesterone	Same as blood studies.	Same as blood studies.

DES, diethylstilbestrol; *hCG*, human chorionic gonadotropin; *IUDs*, intrauterine device

REVIEW QUESTIONS

The number of the question corresponds to the same-numbered objective at the beginning of the chapter.

1. A normal reproductive function that may be altered in a patient who undergoes a prostatectomy is
   a. sperm production.
   b. production of testosterone.
   c. production of seminal fluid.
   d. release of sperm from the epididymis.

2. Estrogen production by the mature ovarian follicle causes
   a. decreased secretion of FSH and LH.
   b. increased production of GnRH and FSH.
   c. release of GnRH and increased secretion of LH.
   d. decreased release of FSH and decreased progesterone production.

3. Female orgasm is the result of
   a. clitoral swelling and increased vaginal lubrication.
   b. vaginal enlargement and secretion with penile insertion.

    c. clitoral swelling, vaginal lubrication, and uterine elevation.

    d. rapid release of vasocongestion and myotonia in the reproductive structures.

4. An age-related finding noted by the nurse during assessment of the older woman's reproductive system would include

    a. gynecomastia.

    b. presence of a cystocele.

    c. soft, nontender, fleshy vulvar lesions.

    d. soft, mobile, well-delineated cysts in the breast.

5. Significant data collection regarding past health history during assessment of male and female reproductive systems should include

    a. extent of sexual activity.

    b. general satisfaction with sexuality.

    c. self-image and relationships with others.

    d. in utero exposure to diethylstilbestrol (DES).

6. After age 40 every man should have an annual examination involving palpation of the

    a. testes.

    b. prostate.

    c. spermatic cord.

    d. inguinal canals.

7. An abnormal finding noted during physical assessment of the male reproductive system is

    a. slight clear urethral discharge.

    b. the glans covered with prepuce.

    c. rubbery feeling of the testes on palpation.

    d. urethral meatus on the ventral side of the glans.

8. The American Cancer Society's criteria for mammography include

    a. a baseline mammogram for all women at age 50.

    b. a yearly mammogram for women over age 50.

    c. mammography only when a discernible mass is found.

    d. a mammogram every 1 to 2 years for women over age 40 only if they are at high risk for breast cancer.

References

1. Bates B, Bickley LS, Hoekelman RA: *A guide to physical examination and history taking*, ed 6, Philadelphia, 1995, Lippincott.
2. Seeley R, Stephens T, Tate P: *Anatomy and physiology*, ed 3, St Louis, 1995, McGraw-Hill.
3. Scanlon VC, Saunders T: *Understanding human structure and function*, Philadelphia, 1997, Davis.
4. Benson R, Pernoll M: *Handbook of obstetrics and gynecology*, ed 9, New York, 1994, McGraw-Hill.
5. Allen KM, Phillips JM: *Women's health across the lifespan: a comprehensive perspective*, Philadelphia, 1997, Lippincott.
6. Masters WH, Johnson E: *Human sexual response*, Boston, 1966, Little, Brown.
7. Bolten A and others: Love and sex after 60: how physical changes affect intimate expression, *Geriatrics* 49:21, 1994.
8. Henderson VW: Estrogen, cognition, and a woman's risk of Alzheimer's disease, *Am J Med* 103:11S, 1997.
9. Butterworth CE, Bendich A: Folic acid and the prevention of birth defects, *Annu Rev Nutr* 16:73, 1996.
10. Jorde LB, Carey JC, White RL: *Medical genetics*, ed 2, St Louis, 1998, Mosby.
11. Tilkian SM, Conover MB, Tilkian AG: *Clinical and nursing implications of laboratory tests*, St Louis, 1996, Mosby.
12. Corbett JV: *Laboratory tests and diagnostic procedures with nursing diagnoses*, East Norwalk, Conn, 1996, Appleton & Lange.
13. Munroe W: Home diagnostic kits, *Am Pharm* 34:50, 1994.
14. Youngkin EQ, Davis MS: *Women's health: a primary care clinical guide*, East Norwalk, Conn, 1994, Appleton & Lange.

Resources

Resources for this chapter are listed after Chapter 51 on p. 1552.

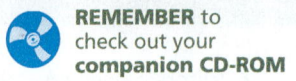
NURSING MANAGEMENT

49 Breast Disorders

Shannon Ruff Dirksen & Sharon Mantik Lewis

LEARNING OBJECTIVES

1. Assess breast tissue by inspection and palpation using appropriate examination techniques.
2. Teach breast health awareness and breast self-examination, including rationale, technique, and reasons for referral.
3. Describe the types, causes, clinical manifestations, and appropriate nursing and collaborative management of common benign breast disorders.
4. Identify the known risk factors for breast cancer.
5. Describe the pathophysiology, clinical manifestations, and collaborative care of breast cancer.
6. Identify the types of, indications for, and complications of surgical interventions for breast cancer.
7. Explain the physical and psychologic preoperative and postoperative aspects of nursing management for the patient undergoing a mastectomy.
8. Describe the indications for reconstructive breast surgery; types, potential risks, and complications of reconstructive breast surgery; and nursing management after reconstructive breast surgery.

Breast disorders are a significant health concern to women. In a woman's lifetime, there is a one in eight chance that she will be diagnosed with breast cancer. An estimated 178,700 new cases of breast cancer were diagnosed in women in the United States in 1998.[1] About 1000 new cases were diagnosed in men. Whether benign or malignant, intense feelings of shock, fear, and denial often accompany the initial discovery of a lump or change in the breast. These feelings are associated both with the fear of survival and with the possible loss of a breast. Throughout history, the female breast has been regarded as a symbol of beauty, sexuality, and motherhood. The potential loss of a breast, or part of a breast, may be devastating for many women because of the significant psychologic, social, sexual, and body image implications associated with it.

HEALTH PROMOTION

Early Detection

Health promotion practices apply to all women, regardless of their age or menstrual status. It is critical that breast disorders be detected early, diagnosed accurately, and treated promptly. A variety of factors influence the potential for cure, the length of a disease-free period, and the overall length of survival after a diagnosis of breast cancer. Research indicates that 97% of patients diagnosed with localized breast cancer with little or no

Reviewed by Rebecca Crane, RN, PhD, AOCN, Oncology Clinical Nurse Specialist, John Wayne Cancer Institute, Saint John's Health Center, Santa Monica, Calif; and Marci Lovett, RN, MN, FNP, CS, Project Manager, Iris Cantor Center for Breast Imaging, UCLA Medical Center, Los Angeles, Calif.

axillary node involvement will be alive in 5 years. Conversely, only 21% of patients diagnosed with advanced-stage breast cancer with metastases to distant sites will survive 5 years.[2] The essential factors in the early detection of breast cancer and other breast-related problems are the regular performance of routine mammography, regular clinical breast examination (CBE), and breast self-examination (BSE). The frequency of these examinations is determined by the woman's age, the presence of significant risk factors, and her past medical history (Table 49-1). Current guidelines established in the United States by the American Cancer Society and the National Cancer Institute regarding breast surveillance practices include the following:

1. Annual screening mammography for asymptomatic women beginning at age 40 every 1 to 2 years and an annual mammogram for women 50 years of age or older[3]
2. Physical examination of the breasts by a trained health professional (CBE) every 3 years between ages 20 and 40 and every year thereafter
3. Monthly BSE over age 18

The benefits of early detection of breast cancer are well established. The use of a screening mammography has significantly improved early and accurate detection of breast malignancies. Mammography can identify breast abnormalities that may be cancer before physical symptoms appear.[2] Women at high risk for disease, such as those with a family history of breast cancer, should consult their physician about having mammograms earlier and more frequently. Women who have regular mammograms starting when they are 40 to 49 years old have 17% fewer breast cancer deaths.[3] Despite the promise of reduced mortality rates, only 31% of all women follow mammography guidelines.

Table **49-1** Risk Factors for Breast Cancer	
Increased Risk	**Comments**
Female	Women account for 99% of breast cancer cases.
Age 50 or over	Nearly two thirds of breast cancers are found in postmenopausal women.
Family history	Breast cancer in a maternal first-degree relative, particularly when premenopausal or bilateral, increases risk; 85-90% of women with breast cancer have no family history. Gene mutations (BRCA-1 or 2) play a role in 5-10% of breast cancer cases.
Personal history of breast cancer, colon cancer, endometrial cancer	Personal history significantly increases risk of breast cancer, risk of cancer in other breast, and recurrence.
Onset of menarche at age 12 yr or younger; onset of menopause at age 55 years or older	Active menstruation for 40 yr or more results in twice the breast cancer risk.
First full-term pregnancy after age 30; nulliparity	Prolonged exposure to unopposed estrogen increases risk for breast cancer.
Benign breast disease with atypical epithelial hyperplasia	Atypical changes in breast biopsy increase the risk of breast cancer fivefold.
Obesity	Fat cells store estrogen.
Exposure to ionizing radiation	Radiation damages DNA.

Improved imaging techniques have reduced the radiation exposure that accompanies mammography to insignificant levels. Therefore the benefits of mammography outweigh the risks from radiation exposure. Ultrasound (echogram, sonogram) is another diagnostic procedure that can be used to differentiate a benign cyst (fluid filled) from a malignant mass (solid). An ultrasound will not detect microcalcifications, which are often the only indicators of very small tumors. Thermography is not currently recommended as a screening method for a breast mass because the results are inconclusive. (See Table 48-14 for a more detailed discussion of diagnostic studies of the breast.)

Education and encouraging women to perform BSE are recommended to decrease mortality rates from breast cancer. In recent years there has been some controversy regarding the value of BSE and its role in reducing mortality rates from breast cancer in women.[4] Until the issue is resolved, BSE should be used as a supplement rather than a substitute for screening by mammography and CBE.

Although the reasons that women report for failing to practice regular BSE have changed somewhat over the years, many women still do not regularly examine their breasts. Some reasons cited by women for not practicing BSE are embarrassment, lack of confidence in ability to do BSE, inadequate knowledge of the procedure, and not remembering to do BSE. Factors that increase BSE compliance include a reminder system, confidence in BSE skill, encouragement from health care providers and significant others, and BSE instruction that involves the woman's active participation.[5,6]

The nurse who is teaching BSE must emphasize that early detection and treatment enhance survival rates. Efforts must be directed toward teaching women the importance of BSE, how to perform it, and what to do if a problem is detected. BSE teaching techniques should include allowing time for the woman to ask questions about the procedure and to perform a return demonstration. The technique for BSE has been established by the American Cancer Society and the National Cancer Institute (Fig. 49-1). BSE should be done monthly at a regular time when the breasts are not tender. In premenopausal women, the best time is 7 days after the start of menstruation. At this time, hormonal stimulation of the breasts is at its lowest point. In most women, nodularity and tenderness will be minimal. For women on oral contraceptives (about 20% to 25% of women ages 15 to 45) the first day of a new package may be a helpful reminder. Postmenopausal women and women who have had hysterectomies should set a regular date for monthly BSE. The monthly date of a birthday or the first day of the month are common choices for many women.

BSE should be done in good light and should include inspection before a mirror and careful, systematic palpation. The entire breast, axilla, and clavicle should be examined. The woman should be taught the BSE procedure by a health care provider using the woman's own hand on her breast. A gentle circular motion over wet, soapy skin is particularly useful if she is in the shower. The woman should be told what to look for, such as a lump, nipple discharge, nipple retraction, redness, pain or tenderness, dimpling of the skin, or edema. Some teaching techniques involve using silicone breast models that simulate normal and abnormal breast tissue to help women learn to identify problems. The woman should be shown the normal variations in her own breasts so that she will be able to detect changes. Finally, she should be reminded that most breast problems are not related to malignancy.

Follow-up Care

If a problem is suspected, the woman should see her primary care provider or contact a comprehensive breast center as soon as possible so that additional diagnostic studies can be promptly initiated. If the problem is not serious, the woman's anxiety can be quickly relieved. If a serious problem is suspected or diagnosed, definitive treatment should not be delayed. Even when the woman faithfully practices BSE, she should have an annual breast examination by a qualified health care provider and a mammogram if age appropriate. The care and attention to detail shown by the clinician in performing BSE reinforces the practice of BSE by the patient.

ASSESSMENT OF BREAST DISORDERS

The most frequently encountered breast disorders in women are fibrocystic changes, carcinoma, fibroadenoma, intraductal papilloma, and ductal ectasia including dilated ducts

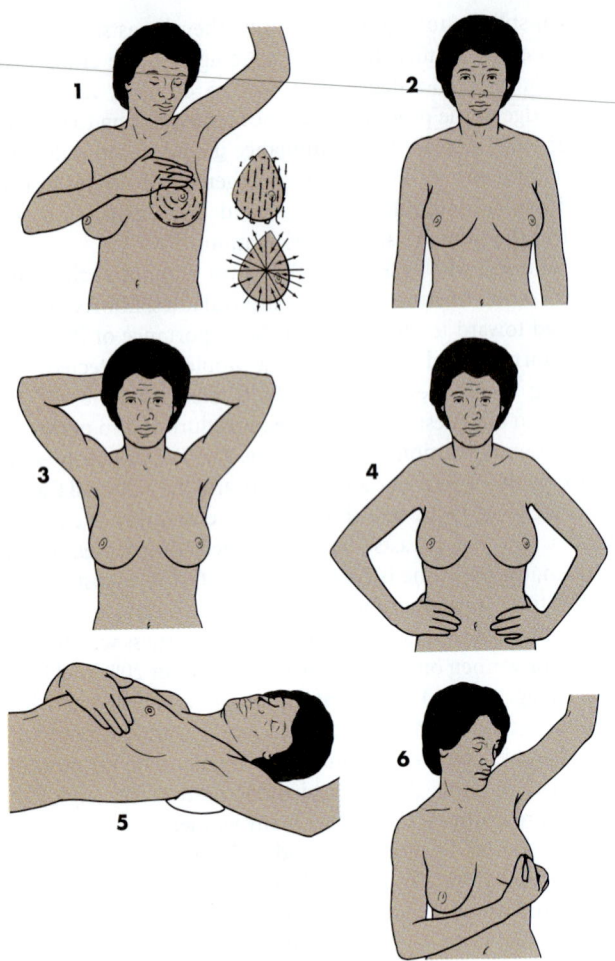

Fig. 49-1 Breast self-examination and patient instruction. *(1)* While in the shower or bath, when the skin is slippery with soap and water, examine your breasts. Use the pads of your second, third, and fourth fingers to firmly press every part of the breast. (While examining your left breast, use your right hand, and use your left hand to examine your right breast.) Check for any lump, hard knot, or thickening of the tissue. *(2)* Look at your breasts in a mirror. Stand with your arms at your side. *(3)* Raise your arms overhead and check for any changes in the shape of your breasts, dimpling of the skin, or any changes in the nipple. *(4)* Next, place your hands on your hips and press down firmly, tightening the pectoral muscles. Observe for asymmetry or changes, keeping in mind that your breasts probably do not exactly match. *(5)* Feel your breasts while lying down. When examining your right breast, place a folded towel under your right shoulder and put your right hand behind your head. Using the pads of the fingers on your left hand, examine the entire breast using small circular motions in a spiral or in an up-and-down motion so that the entire breast area is examined. Repeat the procedure using your right hand to examine your left breast. Repeat pattern of palpation under the arm. *(6)* Finally, gently squeeze the nipple of each breast between your thumb and index finger to check for any discharge.

(Table 49-2). In men, gynecomastia is overwhelmingly the most frequently observed breast disorder.

Many factors must be considered when the nurse is assessing a breast problem. Gender and age are important variables. Only 1% of breast carcinomas occur in males. Benign lesions

occur more frequently in premenopausal women. Breast cancer is predominantly found in postmenopausal women, and the incidence increases with age. Family history is also a significant risk factor. Although it is not as common, premenopausal breast cancer tends to be more aggressive.

The history of the breast disorder assists in establishing the diagnosis. The presence of nipple discharge, pain, rate of growth of the lump, and correlation with the menstrual cycle should all be investigated (see Table 49-2).

The size and location of the lump or lumps should be carefully documented, and the physical characteristics of the lesion, such as consistency, mobility, and shape, should be assessed. If nipple discharge is present, the color and consistency should be noted, as well as whether it occurs from single or multiple ducts or from one or both breasts.

Diagnostic Studies

Several techniques can be used to screen for breast disease or provide a diagnosis of a suspicious physical finding. Mammography is a method used to visualize the internal structure of the breast using low-dose x-rays (Fig. 49-2). This simple, safe procedure can detect tumors and cysts that cannot be felt by palpation. The minimum size detectable by physical examination is 1 cm. It may take 10 years or longer to grow a tumor this size. Mammography can detect masses of 0.5 cm.

Calcifications are the most easily recognized mammogram abnormality. These deposits of calcium crystals form in the breast for many reasons, such as inflammation, trauma, and aging. Although most calcifications are benign, they also may be associated with preinvasive cancer.[7]

A comparison of current and prior mammograms may show early cancer tissue changes. Because some tumors metastasize late in the preclinical course, early detection by mammography allows for early treatment and the prevention of metastasis of these smaller lesions. In younger women mammography is less sensitive because of the greater density of breast tissue, resulting in more false-negative results.[8] From 10% to 15% of breast cancers cannot be seen on mammography and are detected only by palpation. Suspicious masses should be biopsied even if mammogram findings are unremarkable.

Definitive diagnosis of a mass can be made only by means of histologic examination of biopsied tissue. Biopsy techniques include fine-needle aspiration (FNA) biopsy, stereotactic core biopsy, or open surgical biopsy.

FNA biopsy is performed by inserting a needle into the lesion and aspirating tissue into a syringe. Three or four passes are usually made. FNA and cytologic evaluation may be helpful in making a diagnosis and planning treatment. It should be done only if an experienced cytologist is available and all suspicious lesions read as negative are followed with a more definitive biopsy procedure. If the aspirated specimen is positive for malignancy, the patient can be given this information at the same visit and begin learning about the treatment options.

Stereotactic core biopsy is a reliable diagnostic technique for obtaining a biopsy. In this procedure mammography is used to locate the lesion. The skin is anesthetized, and a small skin incision is made to allow the entrance of a biopsy gun device. The gun is fired and removes a core sample of the lesion. This is repeated several times, and the core samples are sent for pathologic analysis. This technique has several advantages over an

Table 49-2	Differential Diagnosis of Selected Breast Masses	
Condition	**Risk Factors**	**Clinical Picture**
■ Breast cancer	Genetic predisposition Radiation Advanced age or over age 50 Menarche/menopausal ages Proliferative breast disease (atypia) Alcohol intake	Breast mass (movable or fixed) Abnormal breast findings may also accompany mass, such as increase in breast size, dimpling, nipple inversion, or bloody discharge
■ Puerperal mastitis	Lactating woman Occurs spontaneously in approximately 2% of all postpartum lactating mothers (both primipara and multipara), usually 2-4 weeks after birth	Warm to touch Indurated Usually unilateral Most common etiology is *Staphylococcus aureus*
■ Nonpuerperal mastitis	Rare condition Usually women in late adolescence or midyears	Palpable mass Usually an obscure organism Should rule out syphilis or tuberculosis
■ Ductal ectasia (plasma cell mastitis or comedomastitis)	Perimenopausal woman—most common in women in their 50s Previous lactation Inverted nipples	Fixation of nipple Usually accompanied by nipple discharge of thick gray material Often associated with breast pain
■ Physiologic nodularity (fibrocystic breast changes)	Most common between ages 35 and 50	Not usually discrete masses, nodularity instead; usually accompanied by cyclic pain and tenderness; mass(es) usually cyclic in occurrence
■ Cysts	Most common between ages 30 and 50	Palpable mass; may have multiple microcysts
■ Fibroadenoma	Peak age range between ages 21 and 25 Most occur before age 30 Most common among African-American women	Often bilateral Most common size at diagnosis is 2-3 cm Rapid growth Accounts for 2-3% of all breast masses
■ Fat necrosis	50% report previous history of trauma to breast	Usually a hard, tender, mobile, indurated mass with irregular borders
■ Intraductal papilloma (benign lesion of lactiferous duct)	Peak age at 40	Usually associated with serous, serosanguineous, or bloody nipple discharge on affected side

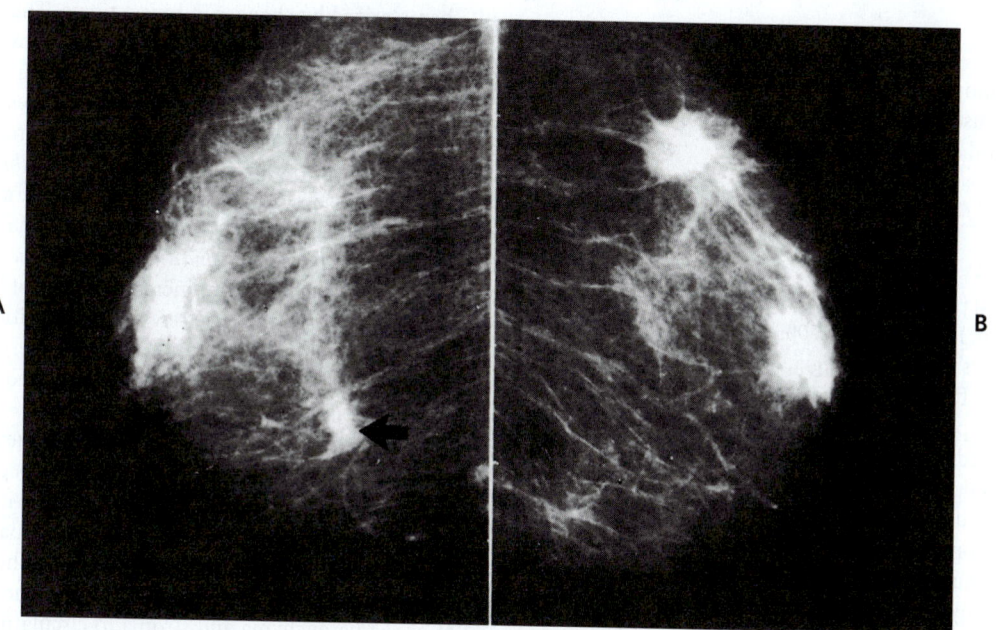

Fig. 49-2 Mammogram showing bilateral invasive ductal carcinoma. **A,** The larger left mass was palpable. **B,** The smaller right mass was clinically occult.

RESEARCH
IMPLICATIONS FOR NURSING PRACTICE

Experience of Women Attending Breast Cancer Screening

Citation Bakker D and others: The experience and satisfaction of women attending breast cancer screening, *Oncol Nurs Forum* 25:115, 1998.

Purpose To determine women's satisfaction and experience with breast cancer screening and associated factors.

Methods Asymptomatic women (*n* = 315), age 50 years or older, with no previous history of breast malignancy participated in the study. Data were collected from the entire sample immediately after screening using a self-report questionnaire and from a subgroup of 256 women by telephone interview 3 weeks after screening.

Results and Conclusions Women reported a high level of satisfaction with their screening experience, including respect for privacy, encouragement to ask questions, and provision of information. Two areas of concern that participants identified were mammogram discomfort and fear about radiation risks. Since the degree of satisfaction that participants in health services report has been shown to influence attendance patterns, assessing breast screening programs from the perspective of attendees is necessary.

Implications for Nursing Practice As health educators, nurses play an important role in providing breast cancer screening information to women. As well as being knowledgeable about screening guidelines and the benefits of screening, nurses also must recognize women's concerns about radiation risks and pain or discomfort with the procedure and be prepared to provide teaching and support for these women.

open surgical biopsy, including decreased length of time for procedure, the use of local anesthesia, outpatient procedure, reduced cost, and decreased recovery time.[9]

BENIGN BREAST PROBLEMS

MASTALGIA

Mastalgia (breast pain) is the most common breast-related complaint in women. It affects up to 70% of all women.[10] The most common form is cyclic mastalgia, which coincides with the menstrual cycle. It is described as diffuse breast tenderness or heaviness. Breast pain may last 2 to 3 days or most of the month. The pain is related to hormonal sensitivity. Noncyclic mastalgia has no relationship to the menstrual cycle. It may be constant or intermittent throughout the month. Symptoms include a burning, aching, or soreness in the breast. The etiology of the pain may be due to trauma, fat necrosis, or duct ectasia.

Mammography is frequently done to exclude cancer and provide information on the etiology of mastalgia. Some relief may occur with caffeine and dietary fat reduction and the continual wearing of a support bra. Hormonal therapy may be recommended, including oral contraceptives, gamma-linolenic acid (evening primrose oil), tamoxifen (Nolvadex), and danazol (Danocrine).[11]

BREAST INFECTIONS
Mastitis

Mastitis is an inflammatory condition that occurs most frequently in lactating women. Lactational mastitis manifests as a localized area that is erythematous, painful, and tender to palpation. Fever is usually present. The infection develops when organisms, usually staphylococci, gain access to the breast through a cracked nipple. In its early stages, mastitis can be cured with antibiotics. Breastfeeding should continue unless an abscess is forming or a purulent drainage is noted. The mother may wish to use a nipple shield or to hand-express milk from the involved breast until the pain subsides. The woman should see her health care provider promptly to begin a course of antibiotic therapy. Any breast that remains red, tender and not responsive to antibiotics needs follow-up care for inflammatory breast cancer.

Lactational Breast Abscess

If lactational mastitis persists after several days of antibiotic therapy, a lactational breast abscess may have developed. In this condition the skin may become red and edematous over the involved breast, often with a corresponding palpable mass, and the patient may have an elevated temperature. Antibiotics alone constitute insufficient treatment for a breast abscess. Surgical incision and drainage is necessary. The drainage is cultured, sensitivities are obtained, and therapy with an appropriate antibiotic is begun. Often the woman will find it necessary to express and discard milk from the affected breast until the abscess is resolved.

FIBROCYSTIC CHANGES

Fibrocystic changes in the breast constitute a benign condition characterized by changes in breast tissue. The changes include the development of excess fibrous tissue, hyperplasia of the epithelial lining of the mammary ducts, proliferation of mammary ducts, and cyst formation. These changes produce pain by nerve irritation from connective tissue edema and by fibrosis from nerve pinching. The use of the term *fibrocystic disease* is incorrect because the cluster of problems is actually an exaggerated response to hormonal influence. It has been suggested that the term *fibrocystic condition* or *fibrocystic complex* be used. Fibrocystic changes do not increase the risk of breast cancer for the majority of patients. Masses or nodularities can appear in both breasts and are often found in the upper, outer quadrants and usually occur bilaterally. It is the most frequently occurring breast disorder.

Fibrocystic changes occur most frequently in women between 35 and 50 years of age but often begin in women as young as 20 years of age. Pain and nodularity often increase over time but tend to subside after menopause unless high doses of estrogen replacement are used. The cause of these fibrocystic changes is thought to be heightened responsiveness of breast parenchyma and stroma to circulating estrogens and progesterones. Predominantly affected are women with premenstrual abnormalities, nulliparous women, women with a history of spontaneous abortion, nonusers of oral contraceptives, and women with early menarche and late menopause. Fibrocystic changes often exacerbate in the premenstrual phase and subside after menstruation.

Manifestations of fibrocystic breast changes include one or more palpable lumps that are usually round, well delineated, and freely movable within the breast. Some lumps are fibrous and do not contain cysts. There may be accompanying discomfort ranging from tenderness to pain. The lump is usually observed to increase in size and perhaps in tenderness before menstruation. Cysts may enlarge or shrink rapidly. Nipple discharge associated with fibrocystic breasts is often milky, watery-milky, yellow, or green.

Mammography may be helpful in distinguishing fibrocystic changes from breast cancer. However, in some women the breast tissue is so dense that it is difficult to obtain a worthwhile mammogram study. In these situations, ultrasound may be more useful in differentiating a cystic mass from a solid mass.

NURSING AND COLLABORATIVE MANAGEMENT: FIBROCYSTIC CHANGES

With the initial discovery of a discrete mass in the breast by a woman or her health care provider, aspiration or surgical biopsy may be indicated. A wait of 7 to 10 days may be planned if the nodularity is recurrent to note changes as the menstrual cycle changes. With large or frequent cysts, surgical removal may be favored over repeated aspiration. An excisional biopsy should be done if no fluid is found on aspiration, if the fluid that is found is hemorrhagic, or if a residual mass remains. This surgery is performed in an office or day surgery unit with the patient under local anesthesia.

Biopsies in women with fibrocystic disease may be indicated for women with an increased risk for breast cancer (see Table 49-1). Hyperplastic changes approximating the histologic appearance of carcinoma in situ (atypical hyperplasia) and a family history of breast cancer increase the probability of developing breast cancer.

The woman with cystic changes should be encouraged to return regularly for follow-up examinations throughout life. She should also be taught BSE to self-monitor the problem. Severe fibrocystic changes may make palpation of the breast more difficult. Any new lumps or changes in the breasts should be evaluated, and changes in symptoms should be reported and investigated.

Many types of treatment have been suggested for a fibrocystic condition. These include the use of a good support bra, dietary therapy (low-salt diet, restriction of methylxanthines such as coffee and chocolate), vitamin E therapy, analgesics, danazol (Danocrine), diuretics, hormone therapy, antiestrogen therapy, and surgical therapy (subcutaneous mastectomy).[12] Although many of these treatments have not been scientifically proven to be beneficial, many women report less discomfort with these measures. Danazol has been used for patients with severe pain. It decreases follicle-stimulating hormone (FSH) and luteinizing hormone (LH), resulting in reduced estrogen production and subsequent decreased pain and nodularity. The androgenic side effects of danazol (acne,

edema, hirsutism) often make this therapy intolerable for many women.

Because stress can be a contributing factor in breast discomfort, efforts should be directed toward the reduction of stress. Many of these approaches are considered experimental. The large number of possible interventions indicates the uncertainty surrounding the causes and treatment of fibrocystic conditions.

The role of the nurse in the care of the patient with fibrocystic breast changes is primarily one of teaching. A woman with fibrocystic breasts should be told that she may expect recurrence of the cysts in one or both breasts until menopause and that cysts may enlarge or become painful just before menstruation. Additionally, she should be reassured that cysts do not "turn into" cancer. Any new lump that does not respond in a cyclic manner over 1 to 2 weeks should be examined promptly. The woman should be carefully instructed in BSE, using her own breasts. Teaching breast models can also be helpful.

FIBROADENOMA

Fibroadenoma is a common cause of discrete benign breast lumps in young women. It generally occurs in women between 15 and 25 years of age and is the most frequent cause of breast tumors in women under 25 years of age. Fibroadenomas tend to develop more frequently and at a younger age in African-American women.[13] The possible cause of fibroadenoma may be increased estrogen sensitivity in a localized area of the breast. Fibroadenomas are usually small, painless, round, well delineated, and very mobile. They may be soft but are usually solid, firm, and rubbery in consistency. There is no accompanying retraction or nipple discharge. The lump is often painless. The fibroadenoma may appear as a single unilateral mass, although multiple bilateral fibroadenomas have been reported. Growth is slow and often ceases when size reaches 2 to 3 cm. Size is not affected by menstruation. However, pregnancy can stimulate dramatic growth. Fibroadenomas are rarely associated with cancer.

NURSING AND COLLABORATIVE MANAGEMENT: FIBROADENOMA

Fibroadenomas are easily detected by physical examination and are often visible on mammography. Definitive diagnosis, however, requires biopsy and tissue examination by a pathologist. Treatment is by excision, which is not urgent in women under 25 years of age. In women over 35 years of age all new lesions should be examined using an excisional biopsy. Fibroadenomas are not reduced by radiation and are not affected by hormone therapy. The nurse frequently has the opportunity to counsel a young woman with fibroadenomas. During this contact the benign nature of the lesion should be stressed and follow-up examinations and BSE should be encouraged.

NIPPLE DISCHARGE

Nipple discharge may occur spontaneously or as a result of nipple manipulation. A milky secretion is due to inappropriate lactation (galactorrhea) as a result of such problems as drug therapy, endocrine problems, and neural disorders. It may also be idiopathic.

Secretions can also be serous, grossly bloody, or brown to green. These may be caused by either benign or malignant disease. A slide can be made of the secretion to detect specific disease. Diseases associated with nipple discharge include malignancies, cystic disease, intraductal papilloma, and ductal ectasia. Treatment depends on identification of the cause. In most cases, nipple discharge is not related to malignancy. If galactorrhea is accompanied by amenorrhea, various gynecologic endocrinopathies should be explored.

Intraductal Papilloma

Intraductal papillomas are benign, wartlike growths found in the mammary ducts, usually near the nipple. Typically, there is an associated bloody nipple discharge, a mass, or both. Intraductal papillomas usually affect women 40 to 60 years of age. A single duct or several ducts may be involved. Treatment includes excision of the papilloma and the involved duct or duct system.

Ductal Ectasia

Ductal ectasia is a benign breast disease of perimenopausal and postmenopausal women involving the ducts in the subareolar area. It usually involves several bilateral ducts. Nipple discharge is the primary symptom. This discharge is multicolored and sticky. Ductal ectasia is initially painless but may progress to burning, itching, and pain around the nipple, as well as swelling in the areolar area. Inflammatory signs are often present, the nipple may retract, and the discharge may become bloody in more advanced disease. Ductal ectasia is not associated with malignancy. If an abscess develops, warm compresses and antibiotics are usually effective treatments. Therapy consists of close follow-up examinations or surgical excision of the involved ducts.

GYNECOMASTIA IN MEN

Gynecomastia, a transient enlargement of one or both breasts, is the most common breast problem in men. The condition is usually temporary and benign. Gynecomastia in itself is not an established risk factor for breast cancer. The most common cause of gynecomastia is a disturbance of the normal ratio of active androgen to estrogen in plasma or within the breast itself. Other causes include tumor of the testes or pituitary, medication with estrogen or steroidal compounds, or failure of the liver to inactivate circulating estrogen, as in liver failure (e.g., cirrhosis).[14]

Gynecomastia may also be a symptom of other problems. It is seen accompanying developmental abnormalities of the male reproductive organs. It may also accompany organic diseases, including testicular tumors, cancer of the adrenal cortex, pituitary adenomas, hyperthyroidism, and liver disease. Gynecomastia may occur as a side effect of drug therapy, particularly with administration of estrogens and androgens, digitalis, isoniazid (INH), ranitidine (Zantac), and spironolactone (Aldactone). Use of heroin and marijuana can also cause gynecomastia.

Pubertal Gynecomastia

Pubertal gynecomastia caused by increased estrogen production is seen most often in boys between the ages of 13 and 17. It is usually limited, although occasionally the localized hyperplasia may measure 2 to 3 cm in size. Pubertal gynecomastia is almost always self-limiting, and disappears within 4 to 6 months of onset. Parents and the affected boy should be reassured that in almost all cases this is a normal physiologic phenomenon that will disappear spontaneously and will require no treatment. Rarely, unilateral gynecomastia in the young male may be marked and fail to regress. This is the only indication for surgical intervention.

Senescent Gynecomastia

Senescent gynecomastia occurs in 40% of older men. A probable cause is the elevation in plasma estrogen in older adult men as the result of an increase in the peripheral conversion of androgens to estrogens with age. Although initially unilateral, the tender, firm, centrally located enlargement may become bilateral. When gynecomastia is characterized by a discrete, circumscribed mass, it must be diagnosed to differentiate it from the rarer breast cancer in males. Senescent hyperplasia requires no treatment and generally regresses within 6 to 12 months.

■─── **GERONTOLOGIC CONSIDERATIONS** ───■

Age-Related Breast Changes

Loss of subcutaneous fat and structural support and atrophy of mammary glands often result in pendulous breasts in the postmenopausal woman. The nurse should encourage older women to wear a well-fitting bra. Adequate support can improve physical appearance and reduce pain in the back, shoulders, and neck. It can also prevent intertrigo (dermatitis caused by friction between opposing surfaces of skin). Surgical lifting of sagging breasts is possible and may be desirable when reconstruction after a mastectomy is performed.

The decrease in glandular tissue in older women makes a breast mass easier to palpate. This decreased density is probably age related and occurs even with women on hormone replacement therapy. Rib margins may be palpable in the older adult woman and can be confused with a mass. As a woman becomes more familiar with her own breasts and is reassured about her findings, the anxiety about this finding should decrease. The nurse should encourage the older woman to continue BSE and to have annual mammograms and clinical examinations because the incidence of breast cancer increases with age.

BREAST CANCER

Breast cancer is the most common malignancy in American women. It is second only to lung cancer as the leading cause of death from cancer in women. The number of deaths of women from breast cancer appears to be leveling off.[1] Each year in the United States, approximately 184,000 cases of breast cancer occur in women and about 46,000 women die of the disease. At the present time the American Cancer Society predicts that one of every eight American women will develop breast cancer during her lifetime.[2]

Although the vast majority of breast problems occur in women, men can also have breast cancer. Therefore it is critical that men know the importance of reporting any change in their breasts. One out of every 100 cases of breast cancer occurs in men. Predisposing risk factors include states of hyperestrogenism, a family history of breast cancer, and radiation exposure. A thorough examination of the male breast should be a routine part of a physical examination.

Etiology and Risk Factors

Although the etiology is not completely understood, a number of factors are thought to relate to the cause of breast cancer.

Table 49-3	Types of Breast Cancer
Type	**Frequency of Occurrence**
Infiltrating ductal carcinoma (not otherwise specified)	80%
Medullary	5-8%
Colloid (mucinous)	2-4%
Tubular	1-2%
Papillary	1-2%
Infiltrating lobular carcinoma	10-15%
Noninvasive	4-6%
Ductal carcinoma in situ	2-3%
Lobular carcinoma in situ	2-3%

Heredity or genetically related susceptibility is considered to play a role. Hormonal regulation of the breast is related to the development of breast cancer, but the mechanisms are poorly understood. Sex hormones may act as tumor promoters if initiating agents have induced malignant changes. Additional factors under study include physical inactivity, dietary fat intake, obesity, and alcohol intake.[2] Environmental factors such as chemical and pesticide exposure and radiation may also play a role.

Some factors that place a woman at higher risk for breast cancer have been identified (see Table 49-1). Women are at far greater risk than men because 99% of breast cancers occur in women. Increasing age also increases the risk of developing breast cancer. The incidence of breast cancer in women under 25 years of age is very low and increases gradually until age 60. After age 60 the incidence increases dramatically.[9] Positive family history is an important risk factor, especially if the involved member with breast cancer was premenopausal, had bilateral disease, and is a first-degree relative (i.e., mother, sister, daughter). Having any first-degree relative with breast cancer increases a woman's risk of breast cancer 1.5 to 3 times, depending on age.[11] Controversy exists as to whether hormone replacement therapy (HRT), primarily estrogen, in postmenopausal women increases breast cancer risk. Some studies suggest that risk increases only with prolonged HRT use.[15] Other studies suggest that adding progesterone to the estrogen decreases risk.[16] The Nurses' Health Study has linked long-term oral contraceptive use to an increased risk of breast cancer.[17] Given that estrogen protects against heart disease and hip fractures, each woman and her health care provider must weigh the risk of these problems against the risk of developing breast cancer.

Risk factors appear to be cumulative. Therefore the presence of other risk factors may greatly increase the overall risk, especially for those with a positive family history. Identification of risk factors indicates an increased need for careful clinical surveillance of the patient and participation in cancer screening measures. However, about 60% of women who develop breast cancer have none of the identifiable risk factors.[18]

As many as 5% to 10% of all breast cancer patients may have inherited a specific genetic abnormality contributing to the development of their breast cancer.[19] The first genetic alteration to be identified was in the tumor suppressor gene, p53. The BRCA-1 gene, located on chromosome 17, is a tumor suppressor gene which inhibits tumor development when functioning normally. Women who have BRCA-1 mutations have an 85% to 90% lifetime chance of developing breast cancer. The BRCA-2

gene, located on chromosome 11, is another tumor suppressor gene.[20] Mutations in the two known BRCA genes may cause 90% of all inherited breast cancers. As many as 1 in 200 to 400 women in the United States may be carriers. Women with a strong family history of breast cancer may wish to consider testing in a program that includes pre- and post-test counseling. Routine screening for genetic abnormalities in women without evidence of a strong family history of breast cancer is not warranted. Genetic screening is expensive and often not covered by insurance.

Pathophysiology

Various types of breast cancer have been identified based on their histologic characteristics and growth pattern of the tumor (Table 49-3). The main components of the breast are lobules (milk-producing glands) and ducts (milk passages that connect the lobules and the nipple). In general breast cancer arises from the epithelial lining of the ducts (ductal carcinoma) or from the epithelium of the lobules (lobular carcinoma). Breast cancers may be invasive or in situ. Most breast cancers arise from the ducts and are invasive. Subtypes of invasive ductal cancer with unusual growth patterns include medullary, colloid, tubular, and papillary. Lobular carcinomas may be either infiltrating or in situ.

The natural history of breast cancer varies considerably from patient to patient. Cancer growth can range from slow to rapid. Factors that affect cancer prognosis are size, axillary node involvement (the more nodes involved, the worse the prognosis), tumor differentiation, DNA content (characteristics of malignant cells), and estrogen and progesterone receptor status. The histologic type of breast cancer seems to have little prognostic significance once the tumors are truly invasive.

Noninvasive Breast Cancer. The increased use of screening mammography has led to more women being diagnosed with noninvasive breast cancer. These intraductal cancers include ductal carcinoma in situ (DCIS) and lobular carcinoma in situ (LCIS). While DCIS behaves as an early malignancy, LCIS would be better called lobular neoplasia. DCIS tends to be unilateral and most likely would progress to invasive cancer if left untreated. LCIS appears to be more of a risk factor for breast cancer, and women with this condition have a higher risk of developing an invasive breast cancer in the same or opposite breast.

Although the management of these two disorders is controversial, patients with DCIS and LCIS have historically been treated with mastectomy. Once diagnosed, all treatment options should be discussed with the patient, including prophylactic bilateral mastectomy with breast reconstruction, breast-conserving treatment (lumpectomy), and radiation therapy.

Paget's Disease. Paget's disease is a breast malignancy characterized by a persistent lesion of the nipple and areola with or without a palpable mass. Itching, burning, bloody nipple discharge with superficial erosion, and ulceration may be present. Diagnosis of Paget's disease is confirmed by pathologic examination of the erosion. Nipple changes are often diagnosed as an infection or dermatitis, which can lead to treatment delays. (This is different from Paget's disease of the bone that is discussed in Chapter 59.) The treatment of Paget's disease is a simple or modified radical mastectomy. Prognosis is good when the cancer remains in the nipple only. The nursing care for the patient with Paget's disease is the same as the care for a patient with any breast carcinoma.

Inflammatory Breast Cancer. Inflammatory breast cancer, the most malignant form of all breast cancers, is rare. It is an aggressive and fast-growing cancer. The skin of the breast looks red, feels warm, and has a thickened appearance that is often described as resembling an orange peel. Sometimes the breast develops ridges and small bumps that look like hives. The inflammatory changes, often mistaken for an infection, are caused by cancer cells blocking lymph channels. Metastases occurs early and widely. Radiation, chemotherapy, and hormone therapy are more likely to be used for treatment than surgery.

Clinical Manifestations

Breast cancer is detected as a single lump or mammographic abnormality in the breast. It occurs most often in the upper, outer quadrant of the breast because most of the glandular tissue is there (Fig. 49-3). The rate at which the lesion grows varies considerably. Slow-growing lesions are often associated with a lower mortality rate. If palpable, breast cancer is characteristically hard, irregularly shaped, poorly delineated, nonmobile, and nontender.

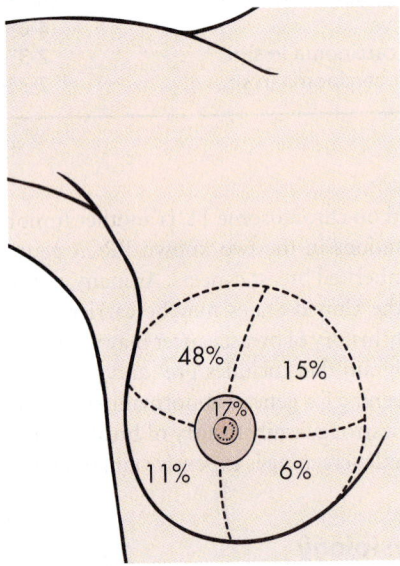

Fig. 49-3   Distribution of carcinomas in different areas of the breast.

Table **49-4**	**Common Sites of Breast Cancer Recurrence and Metastasis**
Site	**Clinical Presentation**
Local Recurrence	
Skin	Firm, discrete nodules; occasionally pruritic, usually painless
Regional Recurrence	
Lymph nodes	Enlarged nodes in axilla or supraclavicular area, usually nontender, superior vena caval obstruction from enlarged supraclavicular nodes (oncologic emergency), pain in shoulder and arm of affected side
Distant Metastases	
Skeletal metastasis	Localized pain of gradually increasing intensity, percussion tenderness at involved sites, pathologic fracture caused by involvement of bone cortex, hypercalcemia from skeletal metastasis or endocrine therapy
Spinal cord metastasis	Progressive back pain, localized and radicular; muscular weakness, usually in lower extremities; paresthesias in one or more extremities; bowel or bladder sphincter dysfunction; paralysis from epidural spinal cord compression
Brain metastasis	Headache, unilateral sensory loss, focal muscular weakness, hemiparesis, incoordination (ataxia), visual defects, speech disorder (dysphasia), impaired cognition, behavioral or mental changes, loss of sphincter control, papilledema, persistent nausea and vomiting, seizure activity, progressive decrease in level of consciousness
Pulmonary metastasis (including lung nodules and pleural effusions)	Dependent on sites and extent of pulmonary metastases; chest pain, dyspnea on exertion, shortness of breath, tachypnea, nonproductive cough (not present in all patients); adventitious breath sounds, dullness to percussion, restricted chest-wall expansion on affected side with pleural effusion
Liver metastasis	Abdominal distention; right lower quadrant abdominal pain sometimes with radiation to scapular area; nausea and vomiting, anorexia, weight loss; weakness and fatigue; hepatomegaly, ascites, jaundice; peripheral edema; elevated liver enzymes
Bone marrow metastasis	Anemia; infection; increased bleeding, bruising, petechiae; weakness and fatigue; mild confusion, light-headedness; dyspnea

A small percentage of breast cancers cause nipple discharge. The discharge is usually unilateral and may be clear or bloody. Nipple retraction may occur. Plugging of the dermal lymphatics can cause skin thickening and exaggeration of the usual skin markings, giving the skin the appearance of an orange peel (peau d'orange). In large cancers, infiltration, induration, and dimpling (pulling in) of the overlying skin may occur.

Complications

The main complication of breast cancer is recurrence (Table 49-4). Recurrence may be local or regional (skin or soft tissue near the mastectomy site, axillary or internal mammary lymph nodes) or distant (most commonly bone, lung, brain, and liver). However, metastatic disease can be found in any distant site.

About 50% to 75% of patients with node-positive disease have recurrences, compared with about 25% to 33% of those with negative nodes. Seventy percent of all recurrences occur during the 3 to 4 years following diagnosis.

Widely disseminated or metastatic disease involves the growth of colonies of cancerous breast cells in parts of the body distant from the breast. Metastases primarily occur through the lymphatic chains, principally those of the axilla (see Fig. 48-4). However, the cancer can spread to other parts of the body without invading the axillary nodes even when the primary breast tumor is small. Even in node-negative breast cancer, there is a possibility of distant metastasis. Prognosis is directly related to the number of nodes involved and other factors discussed in the section on diagnostic studies.

Chemotherapy is the usual treatment for recurrent disease. Hormonal therapy or radiation therapy may be used alone or in combination with chemotherapy when recurrent disease occurs.

Diagnostic Studies

In addition to tissue studies used to diagnose breast cancer, other tests done on breast tissue are useful in predicting the risk of recurrence or metastatic breast disease. These tests include axillary lymph node status, tumor size and histologic characteristics, estrogen and progesterone receptor status, DNA content analysis (ploidy status), and cell proliferative indices (Table 49-5).

Axillary lymph node involvement is one of the most important prognostic factors in early-stage breast cancer.[21] The presence of metastasis in axillary nodes can be determined by pathologic examination of as few as 6 to 10 nodes. The more nodes involved, the greater the risk of relapse. Nodal status is often grouped into three subsets: negative nodes (30% to 35% recurrence at 10 years), one to three positive nodes (55% to 65% recurrence at 10 years), and four or more positive nodes (80% to 90% recurrence at 10 years).

New studies are addressing better methods to identify key lymph nodes for removal. A new technique called *lymphatic mapping* and *sentinel lymph node biopsy* helps the surgeon identify the lymph node(s) that drain first from the tumor site (sentinel node).[22] A radioisotope with blue dye is injected into the tumor site, and with the aid of a gamma probe, it is determined in which node(s) the radioisotope is located. A local incision is made and the surgeon dissects the blue-stained sentinel node, which is then subsequently analyzed by pathologic studies.

Tumor size is a valuable prognostic variable: the larger the tumor, the greater the risk of relapse. The wide variety of histo-

logic types of breast cancer explains the heterogeneity of the disease. In general, the more well differentiated the tumor, the less aggressive it is. Poorly differentiated tumors appear morphologically disorganized and aggressive.

Another diagnostic test useful both for treatment decisions and prediction of prognosis is estrogen and progesterone receptor status. Receptor-positive tumors commonly (1) show histologic evidence of being well differentiated, (2) frequently have a diploid DNA content and low proliferative indices, (3) have a low propensity for visceral recurrence, and (4) are frequently hormone dependent and responsive to hormonal therapy. Receptor-negative tumors (1) are frequently poorly differentiated histologically, (2) have a high incidence of aneuploidy (abnormally high or low DNA content) and higher proliferative indices, (3) frequently recur at visceral sites, and (4) are usually unresponsive to hormonal therapy.

Flow cytometry can be used to measure DNA content (ploidy status) and cell proliferation. The technique uses a flow cytometer to measure certain characteristics of malignant cells that are difficult to measure by microscopy. This test quantifies

---

COLLABORATIVE CARE
Table 49-5 | Breast Cancer

Diagnostic
History including risk factors
Physical examination of breast and lymphatics
Mammography
Ultrasound
Biopsy
Estrogen-progesterone receptor assays
Other molecular studies (DNA ploidy, S phase, p53, HER-2/neu)

Staging Workup
Complete blood count, platelet count
Calcium and phosphate levels
Liver function tests
Sentinel lymph node biopsy
Chest x-ray
Bone scan
CT scan of chest, abdomen, pelvis
MRI (if indicated)

Collaborative Therapy
Surgery
   Breast-conserving (lumpectomy) with or without axillary node sampling or dissection
   Modified radical mastectomy (may include reconstruction)
Radiation therapy
   Primary radiotherapy
   Adjuvant radiotherapy
   Palliative radiotherapy
Chemotherapy
   Adjuvant chemotherapy
   Chemotherapy of recurrent disease
Hormonal therapy
   Hormones (e.g., tamoxifen [Nolvadex])
Surgical hormonal therapy

CT, computed tomography; *DNA,* deoxyribonucleic acid; *MRI,* magnetic resonance imaging.

cellular DNA content and determines if a tumor is diploid (DNA content equal to that in normal cells) or aneuploid (abnormally high or low DNA content). Ploidy correlates with tumor aggressiveness. Diploid tumors have been shown to have a significantly lower risk of relapse than aneuploid tumors.

Cell-proliferative indices indirectly measure the rate of tumor cell proliferation. The percent of tumor cells in the S phase of the cell cycle (see Fig. 14-1) is another important prognostic indicator. Patients with cells that have high S-phase fractions have a higher risk for recurrence and earlier cancer death.

Another prognostic indicator is the genetic marker HER-2/neu (also called c-erb-B2 or neu). Amplification and overexpression of this gene have been associated with a poor prognosis in breast cancer, advanced-stage ovarian cancer, and endometrial cancer.[23] People with this gene have tumors that are routinely resistant to some forms of chemotherapy and more responsive to others.

Collaborative Care

Historically, radical ablative surgery was the standard of care. Presently there is a wide range of treatment options available to both the patient and the care providers attempting to make critical decisions about what treatment to select (see Table 49-5). Many prognostic factors are considered when treatment decisions are made about a specific breast cancer. These factors include lymph node status, tumor size, histologic classification, and the identification of special histologic subtypes. All of these factors enter into the staging of breast cancer. The most widely accepted staging method is the American Joint Committee on Cancer's (AJCC's) TNM system (Table 49-6).[24] This system uses tumor size (T), nodal involvement (N), and presence of metastasis (M) to determine the stage of disease. The stages range from I to IV, with stage I being very small tumors (less than 2 cm) with no lymph node involvement and no metastasis. Classification within these stages depends on the size of the tumor and the number of lymph nodes involved. Stage IV indicates the presence of metastatic spread, regardless of tumor size or lymph node involvement. The therapeutic regimen is often dictated by the clinical stage classification of the cancer. (Side effects and appropriate nursing management of general treatment modalities for cancer are discussed in Chapter 14.)

In spite of the advent of new prognostic indicators such as flow-cytometric determination of DNA content and analysis of cell-cycle phases, the single most powerful prognostic factor related to local recurrence or metastasis after primary therapy is still the presence or absence of malignant cells in axillary lymph nodes.

Surgical Therapy. Breast conservation surgery with radiation therapy and modified radical mastectomy with or without reconstruction are currently the most common options for resectable breast cancer.[25] Most women diagnosed with early-stage breast cancer (tumors smaller than 4 to 5 cm) are candidates for either treatment choice. Ten-year overall survival with lumpectomy and radiation is about the same as that with modified radical mastectomy.[21]

Axillary node dissection. Axillary lymph node dissection is often performed regardless of the treatment option selected. Examination of nodes provides the most powerful prognostic data currently available. Knowing the status of the lymph nodes helps determine further treatment (chemotherapy, hormone

Table **49-6**	**TNM Classification of Breast Cancer**		
Primary Tumor (T)			
T0	No evidence of primary tumor		
Tis	Carcinoma in situ		
T1	Tumor ≤2 cm		
T2	Tumor >2 cm but ≤5 cm		
T3	Tumor >5 cm		
T4	Extension to chest wall, inflammation		
Regional Lymph Nodes (N)			
N0	No tumor in regional lymph nodes		
N1	Metastasis to movable ipsilateral nodes		
N2	Metastasis to matted or fixed ipsilateral nodes		
N3	Metastasis to ipsilateral internal mammary nodes		
Distant Metastasis (M)			
M0	No distant metastasis		
M1	Distant metastasis (includes spread to ipsilateral supraclavicular nodes)		
Stage Grouping			
Stage 0	TIS	N0	M0
Stage I	T1	N0	M0
Stage IIA	T0	N1	M0
	T1	N1	M0
	T2	N0	M0
Stage IIB	T2	N1	M0
	T3	N0	M0
Stage IIIA	T0	N2	M0
	T1	N2	M0
	T2	N2	M0
	T3	N1, N2	M0
Stage IIIB	T4	Any N	M0
	Any T	N3	M0
Stage IV	Any T	Any N	M1

therapy, or both). For all cases of invasive breast cancer, a typical lymph node dissection has always involved the removal of 10 to 15 lymph nodes. However, this technique may not be necessary or appropriate for some women with very small invasive breast cancers or with noninvasive (in situ) cancers.

Sentinel lymph node biopsy shows promise for reducing unnecessary lymph node dissection. If the sentinel node does not show any signs of cancer, no further lymph nodes are removed. Because this technique is still under study, ongoing research will reveal which patients are most appropriate for lymph node preservation.

Lymphedema (accumulation of lymph in soft tissue) can occur as a result of the excision or radiation of lymph nodes.[26] When the axillary nodes cannot return lymph fluid to the central circulation, the fluid accumulates in the arm, causing obstructive pressure on the veins and venous return. The patient may experience heaviness, pain, impaired motor function in the arm, and numbness and paresthesia of the fingers as a result of lymphedema. Cellulitis and progressive fibrosis can result from lymphedema.

Although lymphedema is not always preventable, it can be controlled somewhat after surgery or radiation. Frequent and sustained elevation of the arm, exercises, regular use of a custom-fitted pressure sleeve, and treatment with an inflatable sleeve (pneumomassage) are all helpful in preventing or reducing lymphedema.[18]

Breast conservation surgery. Breast conservation surgery (lumpectomy) involves the removal of the entire tumor along with a margin of normal tissue. Following surgery, radiation therapy is delivered to the entire breast, ending with a boost to the tumor bed. This treatment method is an option when the tumor is less than 4 cm and can be totally removed. If there is evidence of systemic disease, chemotherapy may be given before radiation therapy. Contraindications to breast conservation surgery include breast size too small to yield an acceptable cosmetic result, tumor exceeding 4 cm, masses and calcifications that are multifocal (within the same breast quadrant), masses that are multicentric (in more than one quadrant), or diffuse calcifications in more than one quadrant.

One of the main advantages of breast conservation surgery and radiation is that it preserves the breast, including the nipple. The goal of the combined surgery and radiation is to maximize the benefits of both cancer treatment and cosmetic outcome while minimizing risks. Disadvantages of this surgery include the increased cost of the surgery plus radiation over surgery alone and the possible side effects of radiation. Table 49-7 describes treatment options, side effects, complications, and patient issues related to the most common surgical procedures currently used to treat breast cancer.

Modified radical mastectomy. The modified radical mastectomy includes removal of the breast and axillary lymph nodes, but it preserves the pectoralis major muscle. This surgery would be selected over breast conservation therapy if the tumor is too large to excise with good margins and attain a reasonable cosmetic result. Some patients may select this surgical procedure over lumpectomy when presented with the choice of either procedure.

When a modified radical mastectomy is performed, the patient has the option of breast reconstruction. If the patient chooses to have reconstructive surgery, it can be performed immediately following the mastectomy or it can be delayed until postoperative recovery is complete (about 6 months).

Follow-up care. After surgery, the woman must be followed up for the rest of her life at regular intervals. Most women have professional examinations every 3 months for 2 years, every 6 months for the next 3 years, and then annually thereafter. In addition, the woman must continue to practice a monthly BSE on both breasts or the remaining breast and the mastectomy site. The most common sites of recurrence of breast cancer are at the surgical site and in the opposite breast. The woman should also have yearly mammography of the remaining breast or breast tissue.

Adjuvant Therapy. The decision to recommend adjuvant (additional) therapy after surgery depends on the number of involved nodes, menstrual status, age, cell type, size and extent of the cancer, presence or absence of estrogen receptors, and other preexisting health problems that can complicate treatment. Adjuvant therapies include radiation therapy and systemic therapies such as chemotherapy, hormonal manipulation, and biologic therapy. Adjuvant therapy for men with breast cancer is the same as adjuvant therapy for women.[27]

Radiation therapy. The three situations in which radiation therapy may be used for breast cancer are (1) as the primary treatment to destroy the tumor or as a companion to surgery to prevent local recurrence, (2) to shrink a large tumor to operable size, and (3) as the palliative treatment for pain caused by local recurrence and metastases. Lumpectomy is almost always followed by radiation.

Primary radiation therapy. When radiation therapy is the primary treatment, it is usually performed after local excision of the breast mass. The breast (and the regional lymph nodes in some cases) are radiated daily over the course of approximately 5 to 6 weeks. An external beam of radiation is used to deliver an approximate total dose of 4500 to 5000 cGy (4500 to 5000 rads; 1 rad = 1 cGy). A "boost" treatment to the full breast may also be given, either before or after therapy has been completed. The boost is a dose of radiation delivered to the area in which the original tumor was located. It can be given by external beam and usually adds 10 treatments to the total number given. Esophagitis, tracheitis, fatigue, skin changes, and breast edema may be temporary side effects of external beam radiation therapy. Radiation of the axilla is also effective in decreasing the incidence of axillary recurrence. Chemotherapy may be used systemically to enhance the local effects of radiation. (Nursing management of the patient receiving radiation therapy is discussed in Chapter 14.)

Radiation therapy as adjunct to surgery. Although an uncommon treatment mode, preoperative radiation therapy can be used to reduce the size of a large tumor mass to operable proportions by destroying the cancer cells. Additionally, because the malignant cells are partially or completely destroyed, the rate of local recurrence decreases. The disadvantages of potential delayed wound healing and increased lymphedema do not seem to outweigh the advantages of preoperative radiation in cases in which the cancer is locally advanced.

The decision to use radiation therapy after mastectomy is based on the probability of the presence of local residual cancer cells. Radiating the area will not prevent the appearance of distant metastasis at a later date. The site of radiation therapy (lymph nodes, chest wall, or both) depends on the degree of possible spread of the cancer.

Palliative radiation therapy. In addition to reducing the primary tumor mass with a resultant decrease in pain, radiation therapy is also used to stabilize symptomatic metastatic lesions in such sites as bone, soft-tissue organs, the brain, and the chest. Radiation therapy relieves pain and is often successful in controlling recurrent or metastatic disease for long periods.

Systemic therapy. The goal of systemic therapy is to destroy or control tumor cells that have spread to distant sites. The vast majority of women with breast cancer have no evidence of metastatic disease at the time of diagnosis. However, micrometastases have probably occurred even in stage I disease and especially in stage II disease, making breast cancer a systemic disease at the time of diagnosis. Because of the high risk for recurrent disease, nearly all women with evidence of node involvement, particularly those who are hormone-receptor negative, will have some type of systemic therapy. Certain women, particularly those who are premenopausal, are known to be at higher risk for recurrent or metastatic disease. These women are often recommended for systemic therapy even when no evidence of node involvement is found. Weighing the different risk factors to determine the need for adjuvant therapy in a node-negative patient is a complex process.[27]

Systemic therapy as an adjuvant to primary local treatment, in the absence of demonstrable metastases, significantly decreases

Table 49-7 Breast Cancer: Treatment Options, Side Effects, Complications, and Patient Issues

Procedure	Description	Hospitalization	Side Effects	Potential Complications		Patient Issues
				Short Term	**Long Term**	
Modified radical mastectomy	Removal of breast, preservation of pectoralis muscle, axillary node dissection	Hospital stay is 1-2 days	Chest wall tightness Phantom breast sensations Arm swelling Sensory changes	Skin flap necrosis Seroma Hematoma Infection	Muscle atrophy Muscle weakness Lymphedema	Loss of breast Incision Body image Need for prosthesis Impaired arm mobility
Breast conservation surgery (lumpectomy) with radiation therapy	Wide excision of tumor, axillary node dissection, radiation therapy	Hospital stay is 1-2 days Radiation 5-6 weeks	Breast soreness Breast edema Skin reactions Arm swelling Sensory changes in breast and arm Fatigue	Moist desquamation* Hematoma Seroma Infection	Fibrosis Rib fractures* Lymphedema Myositis Pneumonitis*	Prolonged treatment* Impaired arm mobility Change in texture and sensitivity of breast
Tissue expansion and breast implants	Expander used to slowly stretch tissue; saline gradually injected into reservoir over weeks to months Insertion of implant under musculofascial layer of chest wall	Outpatient or overnight hospital stay	Discomfort	Skin flap necrosis Wound separation Seroma Hematoma Infection	Capsular contractions	Body image Prolonged physician visits (expander implants)
Musculocutaneous flap procedures	A musculocutaneous flap (muscle, skin, blood supply) is transposed from latissimus dorsi or transverse rectus abdominis to chest wall	Hospital stay is 3-5 days	Pain related to two surgical sites and extensive surgery	Delayed wound healing Cellulitis Skin flap necrosis Abdominal hernia		Prolonged postoperative recovery New breast tissue Similar to normal breast

Sources: Bostwick J, Carlson GW: Reconstruction of the breast, *Surg Oncol Clin North Am* 6:71, 1997; and Knobf MT: Treatment options for early stage breast cancer, *Medsurg Nurs* 3:249, 1994.
*Specific to radiation therapy.

cancer recurrence rates and increases survival. Current types of systemic therapy available for breast cancer treatment include chemotherapy, hormonal manipulation, and biologic therapy.

Chemotherapy. Chemotherapy refers to the use of cytotoxic drugs to destroy cancer cells. The greatest benefits from chemotherapy have been achieved among premenopausal women with node findings that are positive for malignancy. Some studies indicate improved outcomes for postmenopausal women as well.

In some instances chemotherapy is being used preoperatively. Preoperative chemotherapy may be more convenient than postoperative administration and can decrease the size of the primary tumor, possibly permitting less extensive surgery. Also, it has been shown that preoperative chemotherapy suppresses tumor growth and prolongs survival.

Breast cancer is one of the solid tumors that is most responsive to chemotherapy. The use of combinations of drugs is clearly superior to the use of a single drug. The benefit of combination treatment results from the use of drugs that have different actions on cell growth and division. Two common combination-therapy protocols are cyclophosphamide (Cytoxan), methotrexate, 5-fluorouracil (5-FU), vincristine (Oncovin), and prednisone (CMFVP); and cyclophosphamide, doxorubicin (Adriamycin), and 5-FU (CAF). Paclitaxel (Taxol) and docetaxel (Taxotere) show promise for treating metastatic breast cancer.[28] Capecitabine (Xeloda), used to treat metastatic breast cancer, is administered orally and causes minimal hair loss and limited bone marrow depression. Vinorelbine (Navelbine), a relatively new chemotherapeutic drug for treating metastatic breast cancer, is well tolerated with fewer and milder side effects than other chemotherapy drugs.

Because healthy cells are also affected by chemotherapy, a variety of side effects accompany this treatment modality. The incidence and severity of predictable and commonly observed side effects will be influenced by the specific drug combination, drug schedule, and dose intensity of the drug or drugs. Usually body organs with rapidly growing cells are the most strongly affected. The most common side effects involve the gastrointestinal (GI) tract, bone marrow, and hair follicles, resulting in nausea, anorexia, weight loss, bone marrow suppression and subsequent fatigue, and alopecia (hair loss). When prednisone is added to the chemotherapy regimen, the side effects related to myelosuppression and GI toxicity are reduced.

Herceptin is an antibody to HER-2/neu, an antigen that often appears on the surface of breast cancer cells. After the antibody attaches to the antigen, it is taken into the cells and eventually kills them. It can be used in combination with standard therapy to treat patients with metastatic breast cancer.

Hormonal therapy. Estrogen can promote growth of breast cancer cells if the cells are estrogen-receptor positive. If the source of estrogen is removed, tumor regression may occur. The source of estrogen (especially estradiol) can be greatly reduced by surgical ablation (e.g., oophorectomy, adrenalectomy, hypophysectomy) or with additive hormonal therapy.[18] Hormonal therapy is widely used to treat recurrent or metastatic cancer but may occasionally be used as an adjuvant to primary treatment.

Two advances have increased the use of hormone therapy. First, hormone receptor assays, which are reliable tests, have been developed to identify women who are likely to respond to hormone therapy. Both estrogen and progesterone receptor status of the tumor can be determined. The importance of these assays is their ability to predict whether hormone manipulation is a treatment option for women with breast cancer, either at the time of initial therapy or if the cancer recurs. Second, drugs have been developed that can inactivate the hormone-secreting glands as effectively as surgery or radiation, without the side effects of these therapies or the need to supplement other hormones no longer secreted by the ablated gland.

Not all breast malignancies are estrogen dependent. Although normal breast tissue contains receptor sites for hormones, malignant cell transformation alters these receptor sites in some cells. If a malignant cell retains hormone receptor sites, it continues to depend on estrogen for cell division. The receptor sites that are altered as a result of malignant transformation are no longer controlled by hormones. Premenopausal and perimenopausal women are more likely to have tumors that are not hormone dependent, whereas women who are postmenopausal are more likely to have hormone-dependent tumors. Chances of tumor regression observed with hormone manipulation are minimal in women whose tumors are lacking estrogen and progesterone receptors. Receptor status probably has no relation to response to chemotherapy. Receptor status may change following hormonal therapy, radiotherapy, or chemotherapy.

Tamoxifen citrate (Nolvadex) is the usual first choice of treatment in postmenopausal, estrogen receptor–positive women with or without nodal involvement. Tamoxifen, an antiestrogen drug, blocks the estrogen receptor sites of malignant cells and thus inhibits the growth-stimulating effects of estrogen. It is commonly used to prevent or treat recurrent breast cancer. Side effects of tamoxifen are minimal but include hot flashes, nausea, vomiting, dry skin, vaginal bleeding, menstrual irregularities, and other effects commonly associated with decreased estrogen.

Women with breast cancer have an increased risk of a second primary breast tumor. Tamoxifen reduces not only the risk of recurrent breast cancer but also that of new primary tumors. Although originally prescribed for 1 to 2 years, it is often used now for longer periods of time.[27] The risk for endometrial cancer increases following tamoxifen therapy for invasive breast cancer. However, it is generally agreed that the net benefit greatly outweighs the risk. Endometrial cancers occurring after tamoxifen therapy do not appear to be of a different type than endometrial cancers in non–tamoxifen-treated patients.

Initial results from clinical trials have shown that tamoxifen may significantly prevent breast cancer in high risk individuals.[29] Women who took tamoxifen in these trials had a rate of breast cancer half as high as women taking a placebo. Side effects from tamoxifen in postmenopausal women include blood clots and increased risk for endometrial cancer. Current trials are examining the effect of taking tamoxifen for 2 years versus 3 to 5 years to prevent cancer relapse. Raloxifene (Evista), a drug used to prevent bone loss, may also reduce the risk of breast cancer without stimulating endometrial growth. Raloxifene acts as an estrogen antagonist at hormone-sensitive breast cancer tissue. (Raloxifene is discussed in the section on osteoporosis in Chapter 59.)

Toremifene citrate (Fareston), an antiestrogen agent similar to tamoxifen, is indicated as first-line treatment for

NURSING ASSESSMENT

Table **49-8** Breast Cancer

Subjective Data	Objective Data
Important Health Information	**General**
Past health history: Benign breast disease with atypical changes; previous unilateral breast cancer; menstrual history (early menarche with late menopause); pregnancy history (nulliparity or first full-term pregnancy after age 30); previous endometrial, ovarian, or colon cancer; hyperestrogenism and testicular atrophy (in men)	Axillary and supraclavicular lymphadenopathy
	Integumentary
	Firm, discrete nodules at mastectomy site (possible indicator of local recurrence); peripheral edema (possible indicator of metastasis)
Medications: Use of estrogens, especially as postmenopausal hormone replacement therapy and in oral contraceptives	**Respiratory**
Surgery and other treatments: Exposure to excessive radiation	Pleural effusions (possible indicator of metastasis)
	Gastrointestinal
Functional Health Patterns	Hepatomegaly, jaundice; ascites (possible indicators of liver metastasis)
Health perception–health management: Positive family history (especially mother or sister); alcohol use; mammography history; palpable change found on BSE	**Reproductive**
Nutritional-metabolic: Obesity; anorexia (possible indicator of metastasis)	Hard, irregular, nonmobile breast lump most often in upper, outer sector, possibly fixated to fascia or chest wall; nipple inversion or retraction, erosion; edema ("orange peel"), erythema, induration, infiltration, or dimpling (in later stages)
Cognitive-perceptual: Headache, back, arm, or bone pain (possible indicators of metastasis)	**Possible Findings**
Sexuality-reproductive: Unilateral nipple discharge (clear, milky, or bloody); change in breast contour, size, or symmetry	Finding of mass or change in tissue on breast examination; positive results of mammography or ultrasonography; positive results of FNA or surgical biopsy or similar results with a needle biopsy
Coping–stress tolerance: Chronic psychologic stress	
Self-perception–self-concept: Anxiety regarding threat to self-esteem	

FNA, fine needle aspiration.

metastatic breast cancer in postmenopausal women with estrogen receptor–positive or estrogen receptor–unknown tumors. Aromatase inhibitor drugs, which block the synthesis of estrogen from precursor molecules, are used in the treatment of advanced breast cancer in postmenopausal women with disease progression. These drugs include aminoglutethimide (Cytadren), anastrozole (Arimidex), and letrozole (Femara).

Additional drugs that may be used to suppress hormone-dependent breast tumors include megestrol (Megace), diethylstilbestrol (DES), and fluoxymesterone (Halotestin). Less common hormone-deprivation strategies include bilateral oophorectomy, adrenalectomy, and hypophysectomy.

Biologic Therapy. The use of biologic therapy represents an attempt to stimulate the body's natural defenses to recognize and attack cancer cells. (The use of these therapies is discussed in Chapter 14.)

Bone Marrow and Stem Cell Transplantation. Autologous bone marrow or stem cell transplantation combined with high-dose chemotherapy has been used to treat patients with advanced metastatic breast cancer. In this technique patients donate their own bone marrow or peripheral blood from which stem cells are harvested. Then they receive high doses of chemotherapy, which causes bone marrow suppression. The patient subsequently undergoes autologous bone marrow or stem cell transplantation. (Bone marrow and stem cell transplantation are discussed in Chapter 14.)

NURSING MANAGEMENT: BREAST CANCER

■ Nursing Assessment

Subjective and objective data that should be obtained from an individual suspected of having or diagnosed as having breast cancer are presented in Table 49-8.

■ Nursing Diagnoses

Nursing diagnoses related to the care of a patient diagnosed with breast cancer vary. Following diagnosis and before a treatment plan has been selected, the following diagnoses would apply:

- Decisional conflict *related to* lack of knowledge about treatment options and their effects
- Fear *related to* diagnosis of breast cancer
- Body image disturbance *related to* anticipated physical and emotional effects of treatment modalities

If a mastectomy is planned, the nursing diagnoses may include, but are not limited to, those presented in NCP 49-1. Nursing diagnoses for the patient receiving radiation therapy or chemotherapy are presented in NCP 14-1.

■ Planning

The overall goals are that the patient with breast cancer will (1) actively participate in the decision-making process related to treatment options, (2) fully comply with the therapeutic plan, (3) manage the side effects of adjuvant therapy, and (4) be

49-1 NURSING CARE PLAN PATIENT AFTER A MODIFIED RADICAL MASTECTOMY*

Expected Patient Outcomes	Nursing Interventions and *Rationales*

NURSING DIAGNOSIS **Pain** *related to* surgical incision and manipulation of tissue *as manifested by* verbalization regarding presence and degree of pain at operative area.*

- Absence of or tolerable level of pain.
- Satisfaction with pain control.

- Administer analgesics as prescribed *to relieve pain.*
- Position arm *to prevent tension on suture line and provide support.*
- Encourage use of noninvasive pain management strategies such as distraction, guided imagery, and relaxation *to complement analgesics and decrease need for analgesia.*

NURSING DIAGNOSIS **Fear** *related to* diagnosis of cancer *as manifested by* questioning, insomnia, reduced attention span, crying.*

- Verbalization of fear.
- Support of significant others.
- Confidence in ability to cope.

- Encourage woman to talk about feelings and diagnosis of cancer *to promote successful resolution of fear and establish effective coping mechanisms.*
- Provide accurate information *to promote understanding, clarify information, and reduce anxiety.*
- Provide opportunity for significant others to discuss situation and learn about support groups *because their fear about the diagnosis and outcome can decrease their effectiveness as a support system.*

NURSING DIAGNOSIS **Body image disturbance** *related to* loss of body part *as manifested by* verbalization of concern about appearance and feelings of loss of femininity, refusal to view incision, fear of intimacy.

- Verbalization of feelings about surgery and change in body image.
- Indication of beginning of resolution of negative feelings toward self.
- Acceptance of altered body image.

- Assess degree of self-esteem disturbance *so appropriate interventions can be initiated.*
- Arrange for Reach for Recovery visitor or similar community resource *to serve as a role model and provide hope for recovery and a normal future.*
- Provide information regarding prosthesis fitting and breast reconstruction (if patient is interested) *so patient can make informed decisions regarding options.*
- Assist patient to verbalize feelings and encourage open communication with significant others *to promote grief work and maintain support from family/friends.*
- Share information regarding community resources (e.g., support groups, information services) *to enable patient to find a place to exchange concerns and feelings about the experience.*

NURSING DIAGNOSIS **Ineffective management of therapeutic regimen** *related to* lack of knowledge regarding BSE and signs and symptoms to report to health care provider *as manifested by* lack of knowledge of or confidence in performing BSE; lack of information about plans for follow-up care, signs and symptoms of recurrent or metastatic disease.*

- Practice of monthly BSE.
- Early recognition of recurrent or metastatic disease.

- Teach or evaluate BSE performance *to ensure that patient is performing correctly.*
- Reinforce importance of annual mammogram *because it is a recommended screening technique for identification of local recurrence after mastectomy and for assessing other breast.*
- Provide information about signs and symptoms to report to health care provider (e.g., new and persistent problems such as skin changes at surgical site, new changes in breast or chest wall).

NURSING DIAGNOSIS **Impaired physical mobility** *related to* pain *as manifested by* limitation in movement or upper extremity on surgical side.

- Return to usual arm and shoulder function.

- Assess degree of mobility impairment *to provide baseline data and to plan appropriate interventions.*
- Treat pain *to promote participation in exercise plan.*
- Flex and extend fingers in postoperative period *to maintain range of motion and promote arm circulation.*
- Carry out postmastectomy exercises *to prevent contractures and muscle shortening, maintain muscle tone, and improve lymph and blood circulation.*
- Assist woman to resume activities of daily living as tolerated or as directed by physician *to reduce dependent behaviors, raise self-esteem, and maintain mobility of affected arm.*
- Emphasize bilateral activity of upper extremities *to prevent guarding of operative side and loss of function.*

Continued

49-1 **NURSING CARE PLAN** **PATIENT AFTER A MODIFIED RADICAL MASTECTOMY*—continued**

| Expected Patient Outcomes | Nursing Interventions and *Rationales* |

COLLABORATIVE PROBLEMS

| Nursing Goals | Nursing Interventions and *Rationales* |

POTENTIAL COMPLICATION

Lymphedema *related to* impaired lymphatic drainage and lack of knowledge of preventive measures.

- Monitor for signs of lymphedema.
- Report deviations from acceptable parameters.
- Carry out appropriate medical and nursing interventions.

- Assess woman for signs of lymphedema such as edema in hand or arm on operative side, heaviness, or localized pain *to enable early diagnosis and intervention to prevent and treat the complication.*
- Instruct patient about self-care strategies and precautions to reduce risk of lymphedema *so patient will be an active, informed participant in self-care.*
- Do not perform venipunctures or take BP measurements on affected arm *to reduce risk of constriction, infection, and lymphedema in affected arm.*
- Avoid dependent arm position *to allow proper wound healing and decrease stress to incision site.*
- Elevate arm and hand on pillow *to use gravity to assist with drainage of fluid.*
- Perform hand and wrist movements, elbow flexion, and extension hourly or as indicated *to maintain circulation and range of motion of affected arm.*
- Encourage participation in activities of daily living and self-care as much as possible *to promote patient's independence and maintain use of affected arm.*
- Use elastic sleeve if ordered *to apply mechanical pressure to reduce fluid collection in affected arm and promote venous return.*

*Nursing diagnoses with an asterisk also apply to the patient following breast conservation therapy.

satisfied with the support provided by significant others and health care providers.

■ Nursing Implementation

Acute Intervention. The time between the diagnosis of breast cancer and the selection of a treatment plan is a difficult period for the woman and her family. Although the primary care provider has discussed treatment options, the woman often relies on the nurse to clarify and expand on these options. During this time, the woman may be very self-focused, verbalizing her conflict and indecision frequently. Appropriate nursing interventions during this period include exploring the woman's usual decision-making patterns, helping the woman accurately evaluate the advantages and disadvantages of the options, providing information relevant to the decision, and supporting the patient once the decision is made.

During this period the woman may exhibit signs of distress or tension, such as tachycardia, increased muscle tension, and restlessness, whenever she focuses on the decision to be made. The nurse should assess the woman's body language, motor activity, and affect during periods of high stress and indecision so appropriate interventions can be carried out.

Regardless of the surgery planned, the patient must be provided with sufficient information to ensure informed consent. Some patients need extensive, detailed information. For others, this only increases anxiety. Sensitivity to individual needs is essential. Preoperative diagnostic studies must be completed. Teaching in the preoperative phase includes instruction in turning, coughing and deep breathing, a review of postoperative exercises, and an explanation of the recovery period from the time of surgery until discharge.

The woman who has breast conservation surgery usually has an uneventful postoperative course with only a moderate amount of pain. If an axillary lymph node dissection has occurred or if a woman has had a modified radical mastectomy, specific interventions will be needed.

Restoring arm function on the affected side after mastectomy and axillary lymph node dissection is one of the most important goals of nursing activities. The woman should be placed in a semi-Fowler's position with the arm on the affected side elevated on a pillow. Flexing and extending the fingers should begin in the recovery room with progressive increases in activity encouraged. (Information pertaining to arm exercises and care also apply to women who have had an axillary node dissection after lumpectomy or total mastectomy.) Postoperative mastectomy exercises are instituted gradually at the surgeon's direction (Fig. 49-4). These exercises are designed to prevent contractures and muscle shortening, maintain muscle tone, and improve lymph and blood circulation. The difficulty and pain encountered by the woman in performing the previously simple tasks included in the exercise program may cause

ETHICAL DILEMMAS

Passive Euthanasia and Suffering

SITUATION

A terminally ill 50-year-old woman with metastatic breast cancer resistant to chemotherapy and radiation has developed severe bone pain that is not being managed adequately by her present dose of IV morphine. This is exhibited by moaning at rest and verbalizing severe pain from any movement to reposition her. Even though she appears to sleep at intervals, she requests pain medicine frequently, and her family is demanding additional pain medicine for her. At the team conference the nurses have discussed concerns that additional pain medicine could hasten her death.

DISCUSSION

A medical intervention for the purpose of causing death in order to reduce a patient's suffering is *active euthanasia* and is not legal in the United States. The *intent* in active euthanasia is that the patient die. In *passive euthanasia*, the intent is to reduce pain and suffering and to allow the disease to take its course; the *consequence* may be a hastened death. Although most cancer pain can be managed by health care professionals trained in pain management, a specific patient's suffering may not be helped significantly. Relieving this patient's pain may cause her death to come earlier, but alleviation of pain and suffering is the goal.

ETHICAL AND LEGAL PRINCIPLES

- Euthanasia (good death) can be classified as active or passive. Active euthanasia involves the intentional act to cause the death of another. Passive euthanasia results from the omission of treatment that would sustain life or from the provision of pain medication at a dose that could hasten death. The difference is ambiguous and is often thought to be irrelevant.
- In the theory of double effect it is permissible to provide high levels of medication to provide pain relief even if the secondary effect of that medication is to hasten death.
- The principles of beneficence and nonmaleficence may be considered to conflict in this case. Providing pain relief is beneficent, but hastening a death by an increased dosage could be viewed as harmful. Refusing to give adequate pain relief is harmful to the patient, but not hastening the patient's death is beneficent.

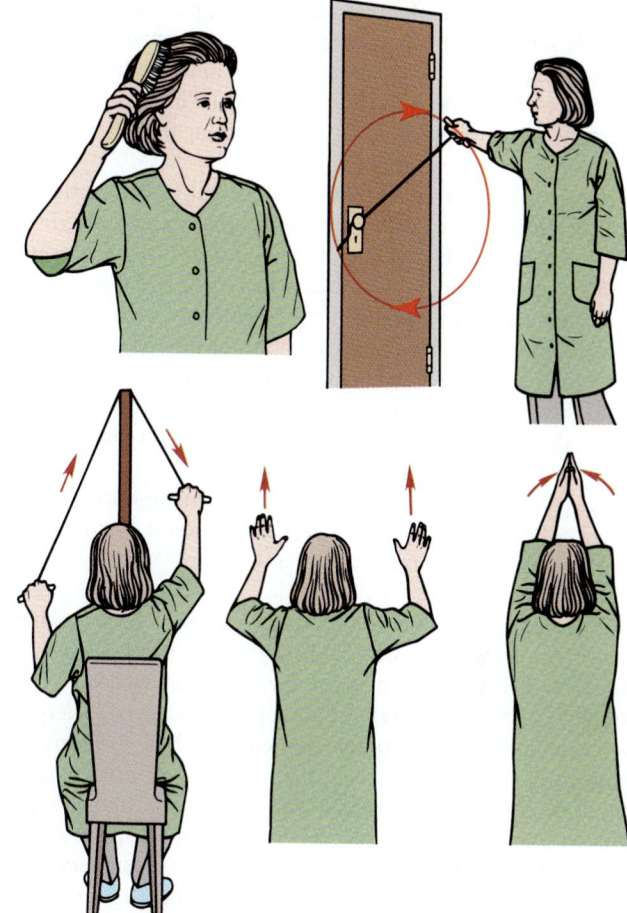

Fig. 49-4 Postoperative mastectomy exercises.

frustration and depression. The goal of all exercise is a return to full range of motion gradually within 4 to 6 weeks.

Postoperative discomfort can be minimized by administering analgesics about 30 minutes before initiating exercises. When showering is appropriate, the flow of warm water over the involved shoulder often has a soothing effect and reduces joint stiffness. Whenever possible, the same nurse should work with the woman so that progress can be monitored and problems can be identified.

Measures to prevent or reduce lymphedema must be used by the nurse and taught to the woman. The affected arm should never be dependent, even while the person is sleeping. Blood pressure readings, venipunctures, and injections should not be done on the affected arm. Elastic bandages should not be used in the early postoperative period because they inhibit collateral lymph drainage. The woman must be instructed to protect the arm on the operative side from even minor trauma such as a pinprick or sunburn. If trauma to the arm occurs, the area should be washed thoroughly with soap and water. A topical antibiotic ointment and a bandage or other sterile dressing should be applied. The surgeon must be advised of the trauma, and the site of injury must be observed closely for evidence of inflammation. The patient must know and understand that she is at risk of developing lymphedema for the rest of her life.[26]

When lymphedema is acute, an intermittent pneumatic compression sleeve may be prescribed. This device applies mechanical massage to the arm. Manual massage is also effective in mobilizing subcutaneous accumulations of fluid. Elevation of the arm so that it is level with the heart, diuretics, and isometric exercises may be recommended to reduce the fluid volume in the arm. The patient may need to wear a fitted elastic pressure-gradient sleeve during waking hours to maintain maximum volume reduction.

Psychologic care. Throughout interactions with a woman with breast cancer, the nurse must keep in mind the extensive psychologic impact of the disease. All aspects of care must include sensitivity to the woman's efforts to cope with a life-threatening disease. An open relationship in which the woman can express her fears and feelings is essential. The nurse can help meet the woman's psychologic needs by doing the following:

1. Assisting her to develop a positive but realistic attitude
2. Helping her identify sources of support and strength to her, such as her partner, family, and spiritual practices
3. Encouraging her to verbalize her anger and fears about her diagnosis and the impact it will have on her life
4. Promoting open communication of thoughts and feelings between the patient and her family
5. Providing accurate and complete answers to questions about her disease, treatment options, and reproductive or lactation issues (if appropriate)
6. Offering information about community resources, such as Reach to Recovery, Y-Me, CanSurmount, Encore, and local support organizations and groups

The nurse can promote the woman's recovery by arranging a visit from a woman who had similar treatment, such as a Reach to Recovery volunteer, if the service is available. The Reach to Recovery program of the American Cancer Society is a rehabilitation program for women who have had breast surgery. It is designed to help them meet their psychologic, physical, and cosmetic needs. The volunteers, who are all women who have had breast cancer, can answer questions about what to expect at home, how to tell people about the surgery, and what prosthetic devices are available. If a Reach to Recovery volunteer is not available, it is the nurse's responsibility to be knowledgeable about the needs of the woman after breast surgery. The American Cancer Society and the National Cancer Institute can provide excellent materials to assist the nurse in meeting the special needs of women with breast cancer.

The professional staff must never underestimate the tremendous psychologic impact that a diagnosis of cancer and subsequent breast surgery can have on a woman. Emotional complications are common. The nurse's accepting, concerned attitude can do a great deal to relieve the feelings of anger and depression experienced by many patients.

Ambulatory and Home Care. The nurse should explain the follow-up routine to the patient and emphasize the importance of beginning and continuing BSE and annual mammography. Immediately after surgery, symptoms that should be reported to the clinician include fever, inflammation at surgical site, erythema, and unusual swelling. Other changes to report are new back pain, weakness, constipation, shortness of breath, and confusion. If adjuvant therapy is to be used, the woman should have specific instructions about appointment times and treatment locations and management of side effects.

For women who have had a mastectomy, the nurse should stress the importance of wearing a well-fitting prosthesis. A variety of products are available to meet the specific needs of the individual woman. A well-trained salesperson can help the woman select a suitable prosthesis. There are both physical and psychologic advantages to the use of a prosthesis; the return of a normal external appearance is especially important to most women.

The implications of the loss of a breast on the sexual identity and relationships of the woman vary. A preoperative sexual assessment provides helpful baseline data that the nurse

can use to plan postoperative interventions. Often the husband, sexual partner, or family members may need assistance in dealing with their emotional reactions to the diagnosis and surgery for them to act as effective means of support for the patient.[30] There are no physical reasons for a mastectomy to prevent sexual satisfaction. The woman taking tamoxifen may have a decreased sexual drive or vaginal dryness. She may need to use lubrication to prevent discomfort during intercourse. If difficulty in adjustment or other problems develop, counseling may be necessary to deal with the emotional component of a mastectomy and the diagnosis of cancer.

Depression may occur with the continued stress and uncertainty of a cancer diagnosis. A woman's self-esteem and identity may also be threatened. Special nursing interventions are necessary in terms of both psychologic support and self-care teaching, if a recurrence of cancer is found. The support of family and friends and participation in a cancer support group are important aspects of care that are helpful in improving quality of life and have been found to have a clinically significant impact on survival.[31]

■ Evaluation

The expected outcomes for the patient after a modified radical mastectomy are presented in NCP 49-1.

MAMMOPLASTY

Mammoplasty is the surgical change in the size or shape of the breast. It may be done electively for cosmetic purposes to either enlarge or reduce the size of the breasts. It may also be done to reconstruct the breast after a mastectomy.

Health care providers should remain nonjudgmental toward women who desire mammoplasty. The desire to alter the appearance of the breasts has special significance for each woman as she attempts to alter or re-create her body image. It is important for the nurse to be aware of the cultural value placed on the breast by the woman. It is important that the woman have a realistic idea about what mammoplasty can accomplish and about possible complications, such as hematoma formation, hemorrhage, and infection. If an implant is involved, capsular contracture and loss of the implant are possible.

Breast Augmentation

In augmentation mammoplasty (the procedure to enlarge the breasts), an implant is placed in a surgically created pocket between the capsule of the breast and the pectoral fascia. Most implants are silicone envelopes filled with a fluid such as dextran, saline, or silicone. Because of their resemblance to the human breast, implants filled with silicone were the most widely used. In 1992 the Food and Drug Administration suspended the routine use of silicone implants in response to potential hazards related to silicone leakage. Allegations of associated immune-related diseases caused or exacerbated by the presence of silicone gel implants have caused considerable controversy and litigation. Their use is approved only when medically prescribed in clinical trials.

In the United States saline-filled implants are usually used. Saline-filled implants are silicone shells filled with normal saline. Soybean implants are an alternative form of implant. This implant has an outer shell of silicone and is filled with highly refined soybean oil. A major advantage of soybean implants is that it is easier for x-rays to penetrate the implant, so better visualization of breast tissue is possible with mammography.

Breast Reduction

For some women, large breasts can be a source of pain and embarrassment. They can interfere with normal daily activities such as walking, typing, and driving a car. Overly large breasts can interfere with self-esteem and self-image and can lead to back, shoulder, and neck problems. They may make stylish dressing more difficult. Reduction in the size of the breasts can have positive effects on both the psychologic and the physical health of the patient. Reduction mammoplasty is performed by resecting wedges of tissue from the upper and lower quadrants of the breast. The excess skin is removed, and the areola and nipple are relocated on the breast. Lactation can usually be accomplished if massive amounts of tissue are not removed and the nipples are left connected during surgery.

NURSING MANAGEMENT: BREAST AUGMENTATION AND REDUCTION

Breast augmentation and breast reduction may be done in the outpatient surgical area, or it may involve overnight hospitalization. General anesthesia is used. Drains are generally placed in the surgical site to prevent hematoma formation and then removed 2 to 3 days after surgery or when drainage is under 20 ml per day. The drainage must be examined for color and odor to detect postoperative infection or hemorrhage. The woman's temperature should also be monitored. Dressings should be changed as necessary and prescribed using sterile technique. After surgery the woman should be assured that the appearance of the breast will improve when healing is completed. Depending on physician instructions, the patient may be instructed to wear a bra that provides good support continuously for 2 to 3 days after breast reduction or augmentation. Depending on the extent of the operation, most women can resume normal activities within 2 to 3 weeks. Strenuous exercise may not be appropriate until several weeks later.

Breast Reconstruction

Breast reconstruction can be done at the time of mastectomy or any time after mastectomy. Recent advances in techniques have made breast reconstruction a satisfactory alternative for many women. The possibility of breast reconstruction may encourage women to seek professional help if a breast lump is detected. Women are demanding more information about and participation in treatment decisions, and breast reconstruction is becoming more common and accepted.

Indications. The main indication for breast reconstruction is to improve the woman's self-image and regain a sense of normality.[32] Present techniques cannot restore lactation, nipple sensation, or erectility. Therefore the erotic functions of the breast are not present. Although the breast will not fully resemble its premastectomy appearance, the reconstructed appearance usually represents an improvement over the mastectomy scar (Fig. 49-5). The contour of the breast is restored without the use of an external prosthesis.

Timing of Reconstruction. Reconstructive surgery may be done simultaneously with a mastectomy or some time

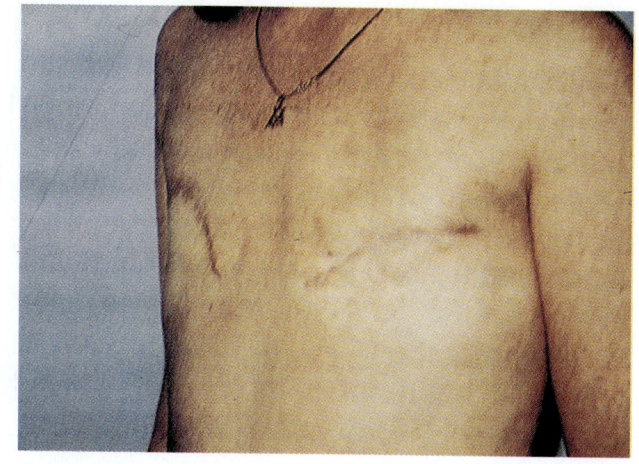

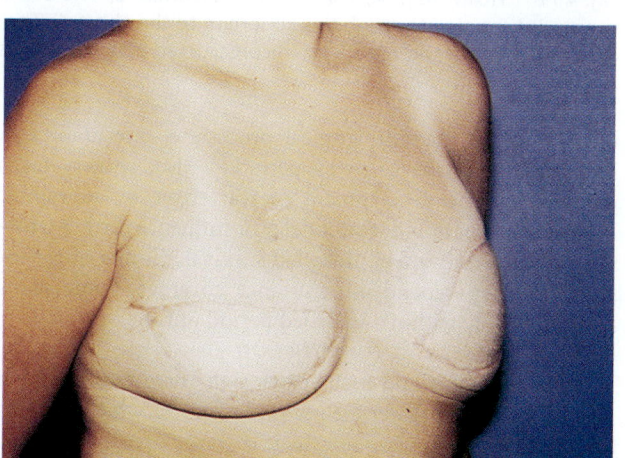

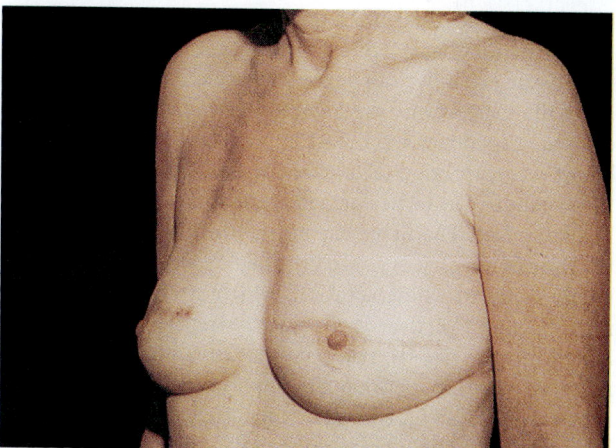

Fig. 49-5   **A,** Appearance of chest following bilateral mastectomy. Postoperative breast reconstruction before, **B,** and after, **C,** nipple-areolar reconstruction.

afterward to achieve symmetry and to restore or preserve body image. The timing of reconstruction surgery should be individualized, based on the psychologic needs of the patient. The timing of reconstruction ranges from during the initial mastectomy surgery to many years after surgery. Immediate breast reconstruction after mastectomy is being performed with increasing frequency.[33] The advantages to immediate

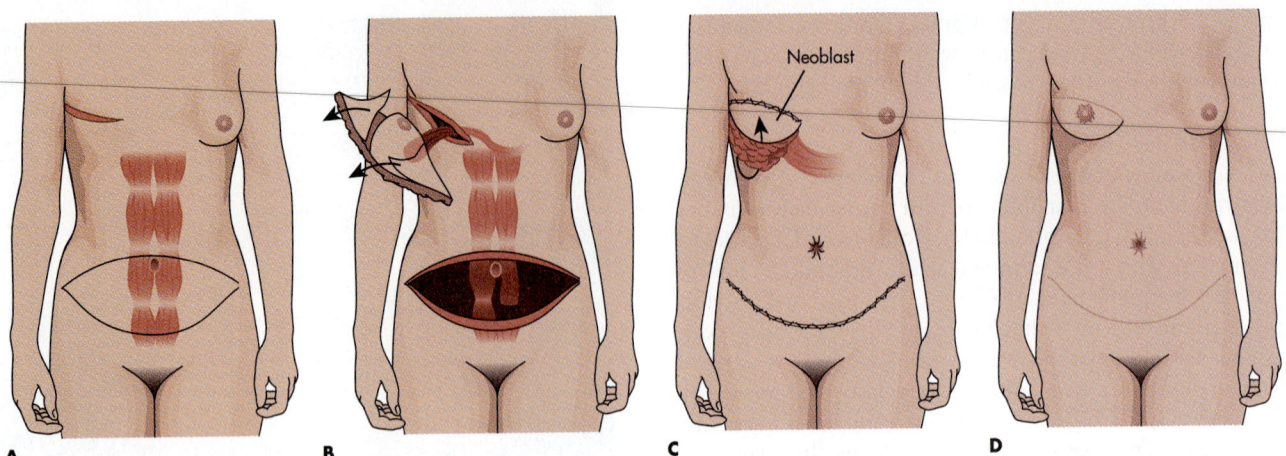

Fig. 49-6   TRAM flap. **A,** TRAM flap is planned. **B,** The abdominal tissue, while attached to the rectus muscle, nerve, and blood supply, is tunneled through the abdomen to the chest. **C,** The flap is trimmed to shape the breast. The lower abdominal incision is closed. **D,** Nipple and areola are reconstructed after the breast is healed.

reconstruction are one surgical procedure, one anesthesia induction, and one recovery period.[33] Also, surgery takes place before the development of scar tissue or adhesions. Early reconstruction does not delay or influence further treatment or adversely affect predicted survival. Timing of reconstruction may depend on insurance coverage. Some plans reimburse only within a specified period of time.

Techniques of Reconstruction

Breast implants and tissue expansion. Breast implants are placed in a pocket under the pectoralis muscle, which protects the implant and provides soft tissue coverage over the implant. Implants can be placed either at the time of mastectomy or later. Because many mastectomy patients have insufficient tissue, simple placement of an implant may lead to small breast reconstruction that is tight or firm.

A tissue expander can be used to stretch the skin and muscle at the mastectomy site before inserting implants. The use of tissue expanders and breast implants is the most common breast reconstruction technique currently used. Placement of the expander can be performed at the time of mastectomy or at a later date. The tissue expander, which is fully deflated at the time of surgery, is gradually filled by weekly injections of sterile water or saline solution, which stretch the skin and muscle. Once the tissue is adequately stretched and the anticipated breast size is reached, the expander is surgically removed and a permanent implant is inserted. Some expanders are designed to remain in place and become the implant, eliminating the need for a second surgical procedure. Tissue expansion does not work well in individuals with extensive scarred tissue from surgery or radiation therapy.

The body's natural response to the presence of a foreign substance is the formation of a fibrous capsule around the implant. If excessive capsular formation occurs as a result of infection, hematoma, trauma, or reaction to a foreign body, a contracture can develop, resulting in a deformed breast. Surgeons differ in their approaches to the prevention of contracture formation, although gentle manual massage around the implant is routine. Prevention of the problems that cause excessive capsule formation is critical. Other postoperative complications include skin ulceration, hypertrophic scar formation, intercostal neuralgia, and wound infection.

Musculocutaneous flap techniques. If insufficient muscle is left after mastectomy or if the chest wall has been radiated, the person's own musculocutaneous flaps may be used to repair the soft-tissue defects. Current restrictions on the use of silicone implants have resulted in an increased use of autologous tissue reconstruction.[33] Flaps are most often taken from the back (latissimus dorsi muscle) or the abdomen (transverse rectus abdominis muscle). In the latissimus dorsi musculocutaneous flap a block of skin and muscle from the patient's back is used to replace tissue removed during mastectomy. A small implant may be needed beneath the flap to gain reasonable breast shape and size. A disadvantage of this technique is an additional scar on the back.

The transverse rectus abdominis musculocutaneous (TRAM) flap is the most frequently used flap operation.[33] The rectus abdominis muscles are paired flat muscles running from the rib cage down to the pubic bone. Arteries running inside the muscle provide branches at many levels, and these branches supply the fat and skin across a large expanse of the abdomen. With this technique the surgeon elevates a large block of tissue from the lower abdominal area, but leaves it attached to the rectus muscle (Fig. 49-6). This tissue is then tunneled under the skin up to the area where the breast will be reconstructed. Then it is molded and fashioned to form a breast. The abdominal incision is closed, giving the patient a result that is similar to having an abdominoplasty. This surgical procedure can last 2 to 4 hours, with recovery taking 4 to 6 weeks. Complications include bleeding, hernia, and infection. An implant may be used in addition to the flap if the flap does not provide the desired cosmetic result alone.

Nipple-areolar reconstruction. The majority of patients who have breast reconstruction also have nipple-areolar reconstruction. Nipple reconstruction gives the reconstructed breast a much more natural appearance. Nipple-areolar reconstruction is usually done a few months after breast reconstruction. Tissue to construct a nipple may be taken from the opposite breast or from a small flap of tissue on the reconstructed breast mound. The areola may be grafted from the labia, skin in area of the groin, or lower abdominal skin, or it may be tattooed with a permanent pigmented dye. In some patients a small implant may be placed under the completed nipple areolar reconstruction to add additional projection.

CRITICAL THINKING EXERCISES

CASE STUDY

Breast Cancer

Patient Profile

Karen G., a 46-year-old woman, discovered a large lump in the upper outer quadrant of her left breast while showering.

Subjective Data

- Has family history of breast cancer—mother diagnosed at age 48
- Had onset of menarche at age 11
- Has two daughters, first birth at age 33
- Has no previous history of breast cancer
- States she is afraid she has cancer

Objective Data

- Palpable 1.5 cm mass in upper outer quadrant of left breast
- Left breast mass confirmed by mammogram
- Otherwise normal physical examination
- Fine-needle aspiration biopsy of mass indicates diagnosis of cancer

Collaborative Care

- Scheduled for lumpectomy and axillary lymph node dissection

Critical Thinking Questions

1. What characteristics of malignancy could be determined by palpation of Karen's breast mass?
2. What information would the nurse provide to Karen about her planned therapy?
3. What information about breast cancer risks is important to provide to Karen and her daughters? What early detection measures are important for them to know?
4. What are the possible complications the patient may face after a lumpectomy?
5. What are common postoperative exercises that Karen will need to practice?
6. What community resources are available to help Karen and her family adjust to the change in her body and to cope with the diagnosis of cancer? How can the nurse access these resources?
7. Based on the assessment data presented, write one or more appropriate nursing diagnoses. Are there any collaborative problems?

NURSING RESEARCH ISSUES

1. What are the major concerns of women who are diagnosed with breast cancer?
2. Does attendance at a cancer support group decrease anxiety in women who elect to have breast conservation surgery and radiation?
3. What are the informational and support needs of family members of the woman with cancer?
4. Do elderly women experience more or less sensory changes after breast surgery than young women?
5. Does perceived susceptibility to breast cancer increase a woman's motivation to participate in breast cancer screening?
6. What effect does dietary intake of caffeine have on a woman's perception of the severity of fibrocystic changes in the breast?
7. What influence does immediate versus delayed reconstruction have on the psychosocial adjustment of a woman after a mastectomy?
8. What is the influence of individualized teaching by a health professional on the frequency of breast self-examination practice in women?

REVIEW QUESTIONS

The number of the question corresponds to the same-numbered objective at the beginning of the chapter.

1. The nurse teaches a patient that BSE involves both the palpation of the breast tissue and
   a. hard squeezing of the breast tissue.
   b. palpation of cervical lymph nodes.
   c. a mammogram to evaluate breast tissue.
   d. inspection of the breasts for any changes.
2. An occupational health nurse is planning a program on BSE for women in the company. To best promote learning and compliance of the participants the nurse includes
   a. a movie that demonstrates the procedure of BSE.
   b. distribution of detailed written instructions for use at home.
   c. explanations emphasizing the value of early detection of breast cancer.
   d. an opportunity to practice BSE on themselves with individual guidance from the nurse.
3. In teaching a patient with painful fibrocystic breast changes about the condition, the nurse explains that
   a. all discrete breast lumps must be biopsied to rule out malignant changes.
   b. the lumps will become progressively larger and more painful, eventually necessitating surgical removal.
   c. the symptoms will probably subside following menopause unless hormone replacement is used.
   d. restrictions of coffee and chocolate and supplements of vitamin E are effective treatments for most postmenopausal patients.
4. While discussing risk factors for breast cancer with a group of women, the nurse stresses that the greatest risk factor for breast cancer is
   a. being a female over the age of 50.
   b. experiencing menstruation for 40 years or more.
   c. using estrogen replacement therapy during menopause.
   d. having a paternal grandmother with postmenopausal breast cancer.
5. A patient has an excisional biopsy of a breast nodule that is positive for cancer. The nurse explains that of the other tests done to determine the risk for cancer recurrence or spread, the result that supports the most favorable prognosis is
   a. cells with low S-phase fractions.
   b. absence of an HER-2/neu genetic marker.
   c. absence of axillary lymph node involvement.
   d. estrogen and progesterone receptor–positive tumors.

6. A patient diagnosed with breast cancer has been offered the treatment choice of breast conservation surgery with radiation or a modified radical mastectomy. When questioned by the patient about these options, the nurse informs the patient that the lumpectomy with radiation
   a. preserves the normal appearance and sensitivity of the breast.
   b. provides a shorter treatment period with fewer long-term complications.
   c. has about the same 10-year survival rate as the modified radical mastectomy.
   d. reduces the fear and anxiety that accompany the diagnosis and treatment of cancer.

7. Postoperatively the nurse teaches the patient with a modified radical mastectomy to prevent lymphedema by
   a. using a sling to keep the arm flexed at the side.
   b. exposing the arm to sunlight to increase circulation.
   c. wrapping the arm with elastic bandages during the night.
   d. avoiding unnecessary trauma (e.g., venipuncture, BP) to the arm on the operative side.

8. To prevent capsular formation following breast reconstruction with implants, the nurse teaches the patient to
   a. bind the breasts tightly with elastic bandages.
   b. gently massage the area around the implant.
   c. avoid strenuous exercise until implant healing has occurred.
   d. exercise the arm on the affected side to promote drainage.

References

1. Landis SH and others: Cancer statistics 1998, *CA Cancer J Clin* 48:1, 1998.
2. American Cancer Society: *Cancer facts and figures 1998: selected cancers,* Atlanta, 1998, American Cancer Society.
3. National Institutes of Health Consensus Development Panel: National Institutes of Health Consensus Development Conference Statement: breast cancer screening for women ages 40–49, *J Natl Cancer Inst* 89:1, 1998.
4. National Cancer Institute: PDQ: detection and prevention, *http://www.icic.nci.nih.gov/clinpdg/screening/breastcancer-physician.html#1.*
5. Champion V, Menon U: Predicting mammography and breast self-examination in African-American women, *Cancer Nurs* 20:315, 1997.
6. Womeodu RJ, Bailey JE: Barriers to cancer screening, *Med Clin North Am* 80:115, 1996.
7. Harvard Women's Health Watch: *Benign breast conditions 5:4,* Boston, 1998, Harvard Women's Health.
8. Weber E: Questions and answers about breast cancer diagnosis, *AJN* 97:34, 1997.
9. Witmer DR, Dickson-Witmer D, Teixido R: Initial 100 consecutive stereotactic core breast biopsies in a private breast center setting, *Del Med J* 69:297, 1997.
10. Adner D, Shriver C: Cyclical mastalgia: prevalence and impact in an outpatient breast clinic sample, *Am Coll Surg* 185:466, 1997.
11. Perna W: Mastalgia: diagnosis and treatment, *J Am Acad Nurse Pract* 8:579, 1996.
12. Cady B and others: Evaluation of common breast problems: guidance for primary care providers, *CA Cancer J Clin* 48:49, 1998.
13. Robinson K, McCance K: Alterations of the reproductive systems. In McCance K, Huether S, editors: *Pathophysiology—biologic basis for disease in adults and children,* ed 3, St Louis, 1998, Mosby.
14. Thompson J, Wilson S: *Health assessment for nursing practice,* St Louis, 1996, Mosby.
15. Colditz G: The benefits of hormone replacement therapy do not outweigh the increased risk of breast cancer, *J NIH Research* 8:41, 1996.
16. Stanford J: The benefits of hormone replacement therapy outweigh the breast cancer risks for some women, *J NIH Research* 8:40, 1996.
17. Nurses Health Study: Risks and benefits of oral contraceptives and postmenopausal hormones, *Nurses' Health Study Newsletter* 5:6, 1998.
18. Dow K: Breast cancer. In Varrichio C and others, editors: *A cancer source book for nurses,* ed 7, Atlanta, 1997, American Cancer Society.
19. Lessick M, Wickham R, Rehwaldt M: Breast and ovarian cancer: genetic update and implications for nursing, *Medsurg Nurs* 6:341, 1997.
20. Calzone K: Issues in breast cancer susceptibility testing, *Innovations in Breast Cancer Care* 2:66, 1997.
21. Moore M, Kinne D: The surgical management of primary invasive breast cancer, *CA Cancer J Clin* 45:279, 1995.
22. Harvard Women's Health Watch: Sentinel node biopsy, 5:7 Boston, 1998, Harvard Women's Health.
23. Cirisano F, Karlan B: The role of HER-2/neu oncogene in gynecologic cancers, *J Soc Gynecol Investig* 3:99, 1996.
24. American Joint Committee on Cancer: *Manual for staging of cancer,* ed 4, Philadelphia, 1992, Lippincott.
25. Gross R: Current issues in the surgical treatment of early stage breast cancer, *Clin J Oncol* 2:55, 1998.
26. Price J, Purtell J: Prevention and treatment of lymphedema after breast cancer, *AJN* 97:34, 1997.
27. Hortobaggi G, Buxdar A: Current status of adjuvant systemic therapy for breast cancer: progress and controversy, *CA Cancer J Clin* 45:199, 1995.
28. Marty M and others: Prospects with docetaxel in the treatment of patients with breast cancer, *Eur J Cancer* 33(suppl 7):526, 1997.
29. Early Breast Cancer Trialists: Tamoxifen for early breast cancer: an overview of the randomized trials, *Lancet* 351:9114, 1998.
30. Pelushi J: The lived experience of surviving breast cancer, *Oncol Nurs Forum* 24:1343, 1997.
31. Ferrell B and others: Quality of life in breast cancer survivors: implications for developing support services, *Oncol Nurs Forum* 25:887, 1998.
32. Neil K, Armstrong N, Burnett C: Choosing reconstruction after mastectomy: a qualitative analysis, *Oncol Nurs Forum* 25:743, 1998.
33. Bostwick J, Carlson GW: Reconstruction of the breast, *Surg Oncol Clin North Am* 6:71, 1997.

Resources

American Cancer Society—Reach to Recovery
1599 Clifton Road NE
Atlanta, GA 30329
404-320-3333
http://www.cancer.org

Breast Cancer Information Center
http://breast-cancer.sciweb.com/index.html

Breast Cancer Information Clearinghouse (BCIC)
http://nysernet.org/bcic/

National Alliance of Breast Cancer Organizations
9 East 37th Street, 10th Floor
New York, NY 10016
212-719-0154
800-719-9154
Fax: 212-689-1213
http://www.nabco.org

National Breast Cancer Coalition
1707 L Street, NW, Suite 1060
Washington, DC 20036
202-296-7477
Fax: 202-265-6854
http://www.natlbcc.org/

National Lymphedema Network
2211 Post Street, Suite 404
San Francisco, CA 94115-3427
415-921-1306
800-541-3259
Fax: 415-921-4284
http://www.wenet.net/~lymphnet/

OncoLink (cancer information site)
http://www.oncolink.upenn.edu

For additional Internet resources, see the website for this book at **www.mosby.com/MERLIN/medsurg_lewis**

NURSING MANAGEMENT

50 Sexually Transmitted Diseases

Janis Luft

www.mosby.com/MERLIN/medsurg_lewis

LEARNING OBJECTIVES

1. Identify the factors contributing to the high incidence of sexually transmitted diseases.
2. Explain the etiology, clinical manifestations, complications, and diagnostic abnormalities of gonorrhea, syphilis, genital herpes, chlamydial infections, and condylomata acuminata.
3. Compare primary genital herpes with recurrent genital herpes.
4. Explain the collaborative care and drug therapy of gonorrhea, syphilis, genital herpes, chlamydial infections, and condylomata acuminata.
5. Identify nursing assessment and nursing diagnoses for patients who have a sexually transmitted disease.
6. Describe the nursing role in the prevention and control of sexually transmitted diseases.
7. Describe the nursing management of patients with sexually transmitted diseases.

SEXUALLY TRANSMITTED DISEASES

Sexually transmitted diseases (STDs) are infectious diseases usually associated with intimate sexual contact. Historically they have been referred to as venereal diseases. Many diseases can be sexually transmitted (Table 50-1). Some STDs, such as chancroid and granuloma inguinale, are more common in tropical and semitropical areas. However, with the mobility of modern society, their occurrence in other areas of the world is increasing. Diseases that are associated with sexual transmission can also be contracted by other routes such as through blood, blood products, and accidental inoculation. Common STDs are discussed in this chapter. Human immunodeficiency virus (HIV) infection and related problems are discussed in Chapter 13. Hepatitis B and hepatitis C infection and related problems are discussed in Chapter 41.

Significance

In the United States all cases of gonorrhea and syphilis must be reported to the state or local health officer. In spite of this requirement, there are many unreported and undiagnosed cases. Often, various STDs coexist; for instance, if a person has gonorrhea, chlamydial infection may also be present. In 1994 and again in 1996, reported cases of chlamydia exceeded those of gonorrhea in the United States. The incidence of gonorrhea steadily increased after 1966 but began to decline in 1975. This trend continued throughout the past two decades, possibly influenced by more focused control activities, changes in surveillance and reporting procedures, and changes in host factors. There were 325,883 cases of gonorrhea reported in the United States in 1996. This was a 17% decrease from 1995.[1]

Resistant strains of gonorrhea accounted for almost 30% of all cases.[1] In 1996 29% of isolates collected by the Gonococcal Isolate Surveillance Project (GISP) were resistant to penicillin, tetracycline, or both. Between 1991 and 1996, the percentage of GISP isolates that were penicillinase-producing *Neisseria gonorrhoeae* (PPNG) declined from 13.1% to 5.8%.[1] In contrast, isolates with chromosomally mediated resistance to penicillin increased from 6.4% in 1991 to 9.1% in 1996. The prevalence of chromosomally mediated tetracycline resistance, 14.3% in 1996, has been relatively stable since 1992. The proportion of GISP isolates demonstrating decreased susceptibility to ciprofloxacin (Cipro), one of the currently recommended treatments for gonorrhea, has decreased from a high of 1.3% in 1994 to 0.5% in 1996.[1] Teenagers and young adults account for 25% to 40% of all gonorrhea cases reported. Most states have enacted laws that permit examination and treatment of minors without parental consent.

The incidence of primary and secondary syphilis has changed since 1941 (Fig. 50-1), mainly because of the availability of penicillin. In 1996 11,387 cases of primary and secondary syphilis were reported to the Centers for Disease Control and Prevention (CDC), the lowest rate of infection since 1960.[1] The reasons for this decline are unclear, but the recognition of the epidemic rise of syphilis and a renewed priority in screening, treating, and educating high risk populations by health care providers may have been factors. Still this disease remains an important health problem. Syphilis is an ulcerative disease, and as such facilitates transmission of HIV infection during sexual

Reviewed by Stephine Heitkemper, RN, ARNP, Nurse Practitioner, Women's Health Care Specialist, Washington State Health Department, Olympia, Wash.

Table **50-1**	Microorganisms Responsible for Diseases Transmitted by Sexual Activity	
Organism	**Disease**	
Chlamydia trachomatis	Nongonococcal urethritis (NGU); cervicitis; lymphogranuloma venereum	
Cytomegalovirus (CMV)	Multiple diseases	
Hepatitis B virus	Hepatitis B	
Herpes simplex virus (HSV)	Genital herpes	
Human immuno-deficiency virus (HIV)	HIV infection, acquired immuno-deficiency syndrome (AIDS)	
Human papillomavirus	Genital and anal warts	
Molluscum conta-giosum virus	Molluscum contagiosum	
Neisseria gonorrhoeae	Gonorrhea	
Treponema pallidum	Syphilis	

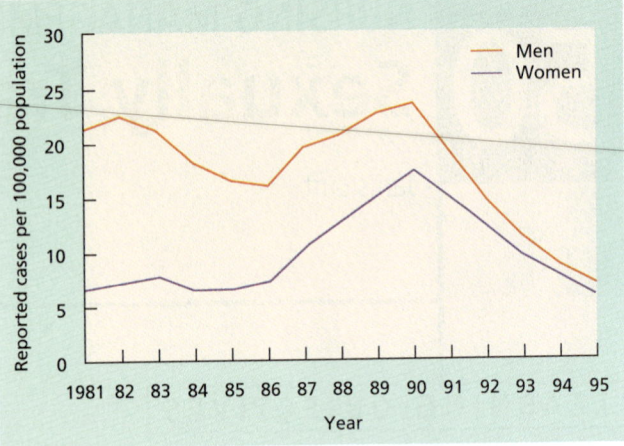

Fig. 50-1 Syphilis. Reported by sex: United States, 1981 to 1995.

contact. If untreated in early pregnancy, syphilis can lead to fetal infection or perinatal death.

Because genital herpes and condylomata acuminata (genital warts) are not reportable diseases in most states, their true incidence is difficult to determine. It is estimated that more than 45 million people in the United States are infected with genital herpes. Since the early 1970s, the prevalence of herpes simplex virus type 2 (HSV-2) has risen by 30%.[2]

Infections caused by bacterium *Chlamydia trachomatis* are the most prevalent bacterial STDs in the United States today. In 1996 490,000 cases of chlamydia were reported to the CDC.[1] Chlamydial infections are a major contributor to pelvic inflammatory disease (PID), ectopic pregnancy, and infertility among women and nongonococcal urethritis in men, and perinatal transmission of the organism can cause neonatal conjunctivitis and pneumonia.[3] Genital warts, the primary clinical manifestation of human papillomavirus (HPV), have become increasingly common with an estimated annual incidence of 500,000 to 1 million cases.

Factors Affecting Incidence of Sexually Transmitted Diseases

There are contributing factors to the increased incidence of STDs. Earlier reproductive maturity and increased longevity have resulted in a longer sexual life span. The increase in the total population has resulted in an increase in the number of susceptible hosts. Other factors include greater sexual freedom, changing roles of women, changes in the institutions of marriage and the family, decreased social control by religious institutions, and an increased emphasis on sexuality on the part of the media. In many studies, the incidence of drug abuse is closely correlated with increasing numbers of cases of STDs.[4] In addition, increased leisure time, inexpensive travel, and urbanization have brought together people of varying cultural backgrounds and value systems.

Changes in the methods of contraception are also reflected in the incidence of STDs. The condom is considered to be the only contraceptive device that is prophylactic in regard to STDs. Although condom use is increasing in selected populations, it is not used frequently in the general population.[5,6] Commonly used oral contraceptives cause the secretions of the cervix and the vagina to become more alkaline. This change produces a more favorable environment for the growth of organisms that cause STDs at these sites. Women who take oral contraceptives have a lower risk of PID as a result of the ability of the cervical mucus to act as a barrier against bacteria. However, the proliferation of chlamydia, the leading cause of nongonococcal PID, may be enhanced by oral contraceptive use. Whether or not intrauterine device (IUD) users are at increased risk of PID is controversial,[7,8] but it is clear that IUDs confer no protection against STDs. Long-acting contraceptives such as levonorgestrel (Norplant) and medroxyprogesterone (Depo-Provera) have been shown to lower concurrent use of condoms, even among women with risk factors for STDs.[4] Both Norplant and Depo-Provera confer no protection against STDs. Lack of awareness of this fact may be a factor leading to STDs in persons using these products.

GONORRHEA

Etiology and Pathophysiology

Gonorrhea is caused by *Neisseria gonorrhoeae*, a gram-negative diplococcus. Mucosa with columnar epithelium is susceptible to gonococcal infection. This tissue is present in the genitalia (the urethra in men, the cervix in women), the rectum, and the oropharynx. The disease is spread by direct physical contact with an infected host, usually during sexual activity. Neonates can develop a gonococcal infection after passage through an infected birth canal. The delicate gonococcus is easily killed by drying, heating, or washing with an antiseptic solution. Consequently, indirect transmission by instruments or linens is rare. The incubation period is 3 to 4 days. The disease confers no immunity to subsequent reinfection. Gonococcal infection elicits an inflammatory response, which, if left untreated, leads to the formation of fibrous tissue and adhesions. This fibrous scarring is subsequently responsible for many complications such as strictures and tubal abnormalities, which can lead to tubal pregnancy, chronic pelvic pain, and infertility.

Clinical Manifestations

Men. The initial site of infection in heterosexual men is usually the urethra. Symptoms of urethritis consist of dysuria and profuse, purulent urethral discharge developing 2 to 5 days after infection. Men generally seek medical assistance early in the disease because their symptoms are usually obvious and distressing. It is very unusual for men with gonorrhea to be asymptomatic.

Women. Most women who contract gonorrhea are asymptomatic or have minor symptoms that are often overlooked, making it possible for them to remain a source of infection. A few women may complain of vaginal discharge, dysuria, or frequency of urination. Changes in menstruation may be a symptom, but these changes are often disregarded by the woman. After the incubation period, redness and swelling occur at the site of contact, which is usually the cervix or urethra. A purulent exudate often develops with a potential for abscess formation. The disease may remain local or can spread by direct tissue extension to the uterus, fallopian tubes, and ovaries. Although the vulva and vagina are uncommon sites for a gonorrheal infection, they may become involved when little or no estrogen is present, as is the case in prepubertal girls and postmenopausal women. Because the vagina acts as a natural reservoir for infectious secretions, transmission is often more efficient from men to women than it is from women to men.

General. Anorectal gonorrhea may be present, particularly in homosexual men, and is usually caused by anal intercourse. Gonococcal proctitis in women probably results from rectal coitus, as well as contamination from infected vaginal secretions. Most patients with rectal infections have no significant symptoms. A small percentage of individuals develop gonococcal pharyngitis resulting from orogenital sexual contact. When the gonococcus can be demonstrated by culture, individuals of either gender are infectious to their sexual partners.

Complications

Because men often seek treatment early in the course of the disease, they are less likely to develop complications. The complications that do occur in men are prostatitis, urethral strictures, and sterility from orchitis or epididymitis. Because women who are free of symptoms seldom seek treatment, complications are more common and usually constitute the reason for seeking medical attention. PID, Bartholin abscess, ectopic pregnancy, and infertility are the main complications of gonorrhea in women. A small percentage of infected persons, mainly women, may develop a disseminated gonococcal infection (DGI). In disseminated infection the appearance of skin lesions, fever, arthralgia, or arthritis usually causes the patient to seek medical help.

Eye Infections in Newborns. Almost all states have a health department regulation or law requiring the instillation of a prophylactic drug such as erythromycin (0.5%) or silver nitrate into the eyes of all newborns.[9] The incidence of gonorrheal eye infections in newborns (ophthalmia neonatorum)

is therefore relatively rare today. Untreated infected infants develop permanent blindness.

Diagnostic Studies

The most reliable way to confirm gonococcal infection is to isolate the organism in culture. The immediate identification of *N. gonorrhoeae* is usually made with a Gram's stain of smears made from the exudate. The slides should be interpreted by an experienced technician so that a correct diagnosis is made initially, since some patients fail to return for follow-up care. Cultures of the discharge or secretion can provide a definitive diagnosis after incubation for 24 to 48 hours. For culture, a specific medium (Thayer-Martin), which encourages the growth of the gonococcus, is used. If laboratory facilities are not readily accessible, special holding media are available.

Newer nonculture techniques, including DNA probe techniques and polymerase chain reaction (PCR), do not involve bacterial culture and are useful in situations where culture facilities are unavailable. The new tests are rapidly approaching the specificity and sensitivity of culture methods. The use of DNA amplification techniques (PCR) holds promise for noninvasive testing of genital secretions or urine in the near future. These techniques offer a quicker approach to detecting infection with high rates of sensitivity and specificity.[10,11]

For men, a presumptive diagnosis of gonorrhea is made if there is a history of sexual contact with an infected individual followed within a few days by a urethral discharge. Typical clinical manifestations, combined with a positive finding in a gram-stained smear of the purulent discharge from the penis, gives an almost certain diagnosis. Culture of the discharge is indicated for men whose smears are negative in the presence of strong clinical evidence.

Making a diagnosis of gonorrhea in women on the basis of symptoms is difficult because most women are symptom free or have complaints that may be confused with other conditions. Smears and purulent discharge do not establish a diagnosis of gonorrhea because the female genitourinary tract normally harbors a large number of organisms that resemble *N. gonorrhoeae*. A culture must be performed to confirm the diagnosis. Although the cervix is the most common site of sampling, specimens may also be taken from the urethra, anus, or oropharynx to confirm the diagnosis. The CDC recommends that all women treated for gonorrhea have a rectal culture done.

Collaborative Care

Drug Therapy. A history of sexual contact with a partner known to have gonorrhea is considered good evidence for the presence of gonorrhea. Because of a short incubation period and high infectivity, treatment is instituted without awaiting culture results, even in the absence of any signs or symptoms. The treatment of gonorrhea in the early stage is curative. Traditionally, the drug of choice for gonorrheal therapy had been penicillin, but changes have been made because of resistant strains of *N. gonorrhoeae* and the presence of coexisting chlamydial infection (Table 50-2).

Recently, a rapid increase in the number of cases of gonorrhea caused by resistant strains of *N. gonorrhoeae* has been identified

(Fig. 50-2). Antibiotic resistance can occur as a result of the bacteria producing penicillinase (these strains first appeared in 1976), as well as chromosomally mediated resistance to penicillin (strains displaying this mechanism first appeared in 1983). The recent increase in the rate of chromosomally mediated penicillin-resistant strains of *N. gonorrhoeae* is a worrisome trend. Resistance to ciprofloxacin (Cipro) was first reported in certain strains in 1991, and although still somewhat rare is a cause for concern.

There is no clinical distinction between infections caused by drug-resistant or drug-sensitive strains of *N. gonorrhoeae*. It was therefore anticipated that there would be increased numbers of disease-related complications (e.g., PID, DGI), extended periods of infectiveness resulting in increased numbers of sex partners becoming infected, and increased cost of treatment. As a result, ceftriaxone (Rocephin), a penicillinase-resistant cephalosporin, became part of the treatment plan. Cefixine (Suprax) given orally one time is also effective. The high frequency (up to 45%) of coexisting chlamydial and gonococcal infections has led to the addition of doxycycline (Vibramycin) to the treatment regimen. The expense of diagnosing chlamydial infection and the sequelae of chlamydial infection make this strategy cost-effective. Patients with coexisting syphilis are likely to be cured by the same drugs.

All sexual contacts of patients with gonorrhea must be treated to prevent reinfection after resumption of sexual relations. The "ping-pong" effect of reexposure, treatment, and reinfection can cease only when infected partners are treated simultaneously. Additionally, the patient should be counseled to abstain from sexual intercourse and alcohol during treatment. Sexual intercourse allows the infection to spread and can retard complete healing as a result of vascular congestion. Alcohol has an irritant effect on the healing urethral walls. Men should be cautioned against squeezing the penis to look for further discharge. Follow-up examination and reculture should be done at least once after treatment, usually in 4 to 7 days. Relapse, reinfection, and complications should be treated appropriately.

SYPHILIS

Etiology and Pathophysiology

The causative organism of syphilis is *Treponema pallidum*, a spirochete. It is extremely fragile and easily destroyed by drying, heating, or washing. The organism is thought to enter the body through very small breaks in the skin or mucous membranes. Its entry is facilitated by the minor abrasions that often occur during intercourse. Not all people who are exposed to syphilis acquire the disease; about one third become infected after intercourse with an infected person. In addition to sexual contact, syphilis may be spread through contact with infectious lesions and sharing of needles among drug addicts. Congenital syphilis is transmitted from an infected mother to the fetus in utero. The incubation period for syphilis ranges from 10 to 90 days but is usually considered to be 3 weeks.

Data from the CDC show the number of reported syphilis cases in 1996 to be the lowest since 1959.[1] However, the disease remains a significant problem among African-Americans (Fig. 50-3). More so than for gonorrhea, persons with untreated syphilis tend to be young persons of a low educational and socioeconomic level, a group that also has high rates of prostitution and drug abuse. This group of people has been extremely hard to reach for education and case finding.

Syphilis is a disease of the blood vessels. The tissue reaction to the presence of *T. pallidum* multiplying in the lymphatics and the perivascular spaces is characterized by dilation and

---

🤝 COLLABORATIVE CARE

Table 50-2 Gonorrhea

Diagnostic
History and physical examination
Gram-stained smears of urethral or endocervical exudate
Cultures for *N. gonorrhea*
Testing for other STDs (syphilis, HIV, chlamydia)

Collaborative Therapy
Uncomplicated gonorrhea: cefixine (Suprax) 400 mg orally in a single dose or ceftriaxone (Rocephin) 125 mg IM in a single dose or ciprofloxacin (Cipro) 500 mg orally in a single dose PLUS azithromycin (Zithromax) 1 gm orally in a single dose or doxycycline (Vibramycin) 100 mg orally twice a day for 7 days
Follow-up cultures after completion of treatment (usually 7 days)
Case finding
Treatment of contacts
Instruction on abstinence from sexual intercourse and alcohol
Reexamination if symptoms persist or recur after completion of treatment
Repeat of serologic test for syphilis at 1 month

Modified from Centers for Disease Control: STD treatment guidelines, *MMWR* 47(RR-1):1, 1998.
IM, intramuscular.

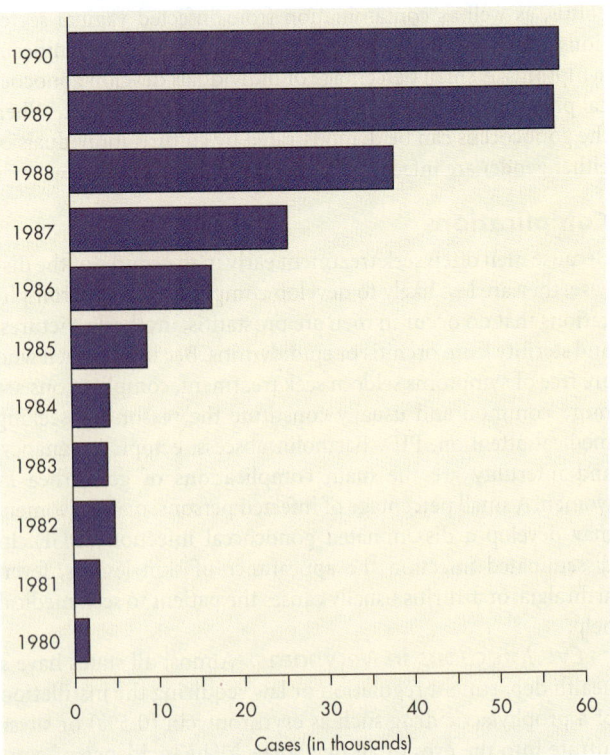

Fig. 50-2 Antibiotic-resistant gonorrhea. Reported cases: United States, 1980 to 1990.

swelling of the capillaries and proliferation of the endothelium and a perivascular infiltration of lymphocytes, giant cells, and fibroblasts, with the formation of new blood vessels. Scar tissue formation is the method of healing in syphilis. The severity and extent of the damage vary.

There is an association between syphilis and HIV infection. Persons at high risk for acquiring syphilis are also at an increased risk for acquiring HIV. Often, both infections are present in the same person. The presence of syphilitic lesions on the genitals enhances HIV transmission. HIV-infected patients with syphilis appear to be at greatest risk for clinically significant central nervous system (CNS) involvement and may require more intensive treatment with penicillin than do other patients with syphilis. Therefore the evaluation of all patients with syphilis should also include testing for HIV antibodies with the patient's consent.

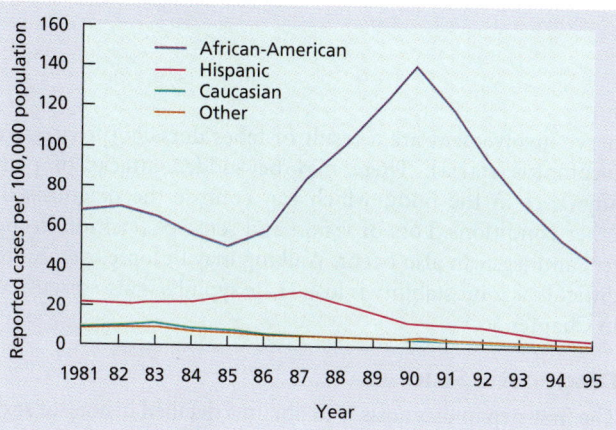

Fig. 50-3 Rate of primary and secondary syphilis in men and women in the United States, by ethnic origin, 1981 to 1995.

Clinical Manifestations

Syphilis has a variety of signs and symptoms that can mimic a number of less serious diseases. Consequently, compared with other venereal diseases, it is more difficult to recognize syphilis. If it is not treated, specific clinical stages are characteristic of the progression of the disease (Table 50-3). Chancres, which are painless indurated lesions found on the penis, vulva, and lips and in the mouth, vagina, and rectum, are seen in the primary stage at the site of bacterial invasion (Fig. 50-4). There, *T. pallidum* multiples in the epithelium, producing a granulomatous tissue reaction (chancre). Some of these microorganisms drain with the lymph into adjacent lymph nodes.

Secondary syphilis is systemic. During this stage bloodborne bacteria spread to all major organ systems. Manifestations characteristic of the secondary stage include cutaneous eruptions, alopecia (hair loss), and generalized adenopathy. The cutaneous eruptions include a bilateral, symmetric rash usually involving the palms and soles; mucous patches in the mouth, tongue, or cervix; and condylomata (moist papules) in the anal and genital area (Fig. 50-5). Latent syphilis follows the secondary stage and is a period during which the immune system is able to suppress the infection. There are no signs or symptoms of syphilis during this time. The diagnosis is established by the finding of a positive specific treponemal antibody test for syphilis together with a normal cerebrospinal fluid (CSF) examination and the absence of clinical manifestations of syphilis on physical examination and chest radiograms. About 70% of untreated patients with latent syphilis never develop clinically evident late syphilis, but the occurrence of a spontaneous cure is in doubt.[12]

Late syphilis (also called tertiary syphilis) is the most severe stage of the disease. Because antibiotics can cure syphilis, manifestations of late syphilis are rare. However, when it does occur, it is responsible for significant morbidity and mortality. The

Table **50-3**	Stages of Syphilis		
Clinical Stage	**Characteristic Findings**	**Communicability**	**Duration of Stage**
Primary	Chancre	Exudate from chancre highly infectious; blood is infectious	3-8 wk
Secondary	Cutaneous eruptions, alopecia, systemic symptoms (malaise, arthralgia, headache, occasionally liver and kidney dysfunction), regional adenopathy 6-12 wk after chancre	Exudate from skin and mucous membrane lesions highly infectious	1-2 yr
Latent	Absence of signs or symptoms	Noninfectious after 4 yr, possible placental transmission	Throughout life or progression to late stage
Late*	Appearance 3-20 yr after initial infection	Noninfectious	Chronic (without treatment), possibly fatal
Benign	Gummas (chronic, destructive lesions affecting any organ of body, especially skin, bone, liver, mucous membranes)	Spinal fluid possibly containing organism	
Cardiovascular	Aortic valve insufficiency or saccular aneurysm of thoracic aorta, aortitis		
Neurosyphilis	General paresis (personality changes from minor to psychotic, tremors, physical and mental deterioration)		
	Tabes dorsalis (ataxia, areflexia, paresthesias, lightning pains, damaged joints [Charcot's joints])		

*Several forms such as cardiovascular and neurosyphilis occur together in approximately 25% of untreated cases.

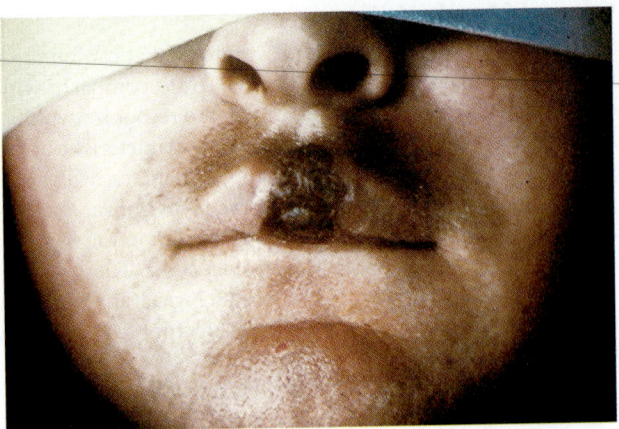

Fig. 50-4   Primary syphilis chancre on upper lip.

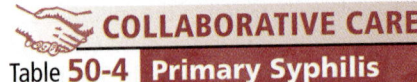

COLLABORATIVE CARE

Table **50-4**   **Primary Syphilis**

Diagnostic
History and physical examination
Dark-field microscopy
Nontreponemal or treponemal serologic testing
Testing for other STDs (HIV, gonorrhea, chlamydia)

Collaborative Therapy
Appropriate drug therapy (See Table 50-5)
Confidential counseling and testing for HIV infection
Case finding
Surveillance
   Repeat of quantitative nontreponemal tests at 3, 6, and 12 mo
   Examination of cerebrospinal fluid at 1 year if treatment involves alternative antibiotics

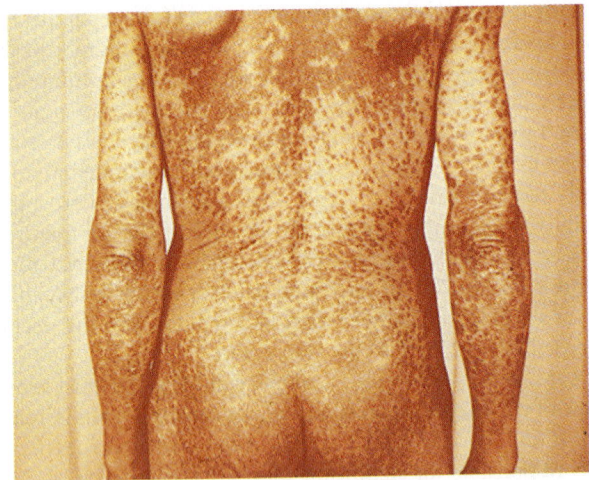

Fig. 50-5   Generalized posterior cutaneous eruptions in secondary syphilis. Distribution of lesions is bilateral and symmetric.

pathogenesis of the manifestations of this stage is unclear. Gummas (destructive skin, bone, and soft-tissue lesions associated with late syphilis) are probably caused by a severe hypersensitivity reaction to the microorganism. Within the cardiovascular system late syphilis may cause aneurysms, heart valve insufficiency, and heart failure. Within the CNS the presence of *T. pallidum* in CSF may cause manifestations of neurosyphilis (see Table 50-3).

Complications

Complications of the disease occur chiefly in late syphilis. The gummas of benign late syphilis may produce irreparable damage to bone, liver, or skin but seldom result in death. In cardiovascular syphilis, the resulting aneurysm may press on the structures such as intercostal nerves, causing pain. The possibility of rupture exists as the aneurysm increases in size. Scarring of the aortic valve results in aortic valve insufficiency and eventually heart failure.

Neurosyphilis (general paresis) is responsible for degeneration of the brain with mental deterioration. Evidence of other neurologic deficits may be present. Problems related to sensory nerve involvement are a result of tabes dorsalis (progressive locomotor ataxia). There may be sudden attacks of pain anywhere in the body, which can confuse the diagnosis of other conditions. Loss of vision and sense of position in the feet and legs can also occur. Walking may become even more difficult as joint stability is lost. (Late syphilis is also discussed in Chapter 56.)

Diagnostic Studies

The first step in diagnosis is to obtain a detailed history of sexual behavior. A physical examination should be done to identify any suspicious lesions, as well as to note other significant signs and symptoms.

The presence of spirochetes on dark-field microscopy of tissue scrapings from primary or secondary lesions can confirm a clinical diagnosis of syphilis. However, syphilis is more commonly diagnosed by a serologic test. Tests for syphilis may be classified as those performed for screening and those performed for confirmation of a positive screening test. Nonspecific antitreponemal antibodies can be detected by tests such as the Venereal Disease Research Laboratory (VDRL) test and the rapid plasma reagin (RPR) test. These nontreponemal tests are suitable for screening purposes and usually become positive 10 to 14 days after the appearance of a chancre. The fluorescent treponemal antibody absorption (FTAAbs) test and the microhemagglutination (MHA) test detect specific antitreponemal antibodies and are suitable for confirming the diagnosis.

False-negative and false-positive test results do occur with the nontreponemal tests (VDRL, RPR). A false-negative result may be obtained during primary syphilis if the test is done before the individual has had time to produce antibody. A false-positive finding may occur with other diseases or conditions such as hepatitis, infectious mononucleosis, after smallpox vaccination, collagen diseases (systemic lupus erythematosus), narcotic addiction, pregnancy, or aging. Positive nontreponemal test results should be confirmed by more specific treponemal tests to rule out other causes. In the CSF, changes such as increased white blood cell count, increased total protein, and a positive treponemal antibody test are diagnostic of asymptomatic neurosyphilis.

DRUG THERAPY

Table 50-5 Syphilis

Stage	Benzathine Penicillin G (IM)	Aqueous Crystalline Penicillin (IV)	Other Antibiotics*
Early syphilis (primary, secondary, and early latent)	At single visit		Doxycycline, tetracycline, erythromycin
Syphilis lasting >1 year Symptomatic neurosyphilis	Three weekly injections	Daily for 14 days followed by penicillin G benzathine weekly for 3 doses	Doxycycline, tetracycline, erythromycin

Modified from Centers for Disease Control: *STD treatment guidelines of USPHS,* Atlanta, 1998, Centers for Disease Control and Prevention.
*Given when penicillin is contraindicated.

If a patient is treated with antibiotics early in the course of the disease on the basis of the history and the symptoms, the serologic testing may not indicate the presence of syphilis. Once a person has positive serologic findings for syphilis, indicating the presence of antibodies, these findings may remain positive for an indefinite period in spite of successful treatment.

Collaborative Care

Drug Therapy. Management of syphilis is aimed at eradication of all syphilitic organisms (Table 50-4). However, treatment cannot reverse damage that is already present in the late stage of the disease. Parenteral penicillin remains the treatment of choice for all stages of syphilis. To date, there is no evidence to suggest a decrease in the effectiveness of penicillin against *T. pallidum.* Table 50-5 describes therapy for the various stages of syphilis and is in accordance with U.S. Public Health Service recommendations. All stages of syphilis should be treated.

Appropriate antibiotic treatment of maternal syphilis before the eighteenth week of pregnancy prevents infection of the fetus. Appropriate treatment after 18 weeks of pregnancy cures both mother and fetus because the antibiotics can cross the placental barrier. Treatment administered in the second half of pregnancy may pose a risk of premature labor. Some authorities recommend hospitalization and fetal monitoring of women at 20 weeks of gestation or greater.[13] All patients with neurosyphilis must be carefully monitored, with periodic serologic testing, clinical evaluation at 6-month intervals, and repeat CSF examinations for at least 3 years. Specific management is based on the presenting symptoms.

GENITAL HERPES

Etiology and Pathophysiology

There are two different strains of herpes simplex virus (HSV) that cause infection—type 1 and type 2. In general, HSV type 1 (HSV-1) causes infection above the waist, involving the gingivae, the dermis, the upper respiratory tract, and the CNS. HSV type 2 (HSV-2) most frequently infects the genital tract and the perineum (i.e., locations below the waist). However, either strain can cause disease on the mouth or the genitals. HSV-1 can be transmitted from mouth to genitals, and HSV-2 can be transmitted from genitals to mouth through oral-genital contact.

In the course of the primary infection, HSV is established in the sensory nerve ganglion innervating the primary site. The virus remains dormant within sensory and autonomic nerve ganglia and can cause recurrence of the disease. Upon activation, the virus travels down the nerve axon to the skin or to the mucous membrane. Additional sexual contact is therefore not necessary for a recurrence of HSV infection. The recurrent infection produces a syndrome similar to but less intense than the primary infection.

Because HSV is readily inactivated at room temperature and by drying, airborne and fomitic spread have not been documented as significant means of transmission. The virus enters through the mucous membrane or through breaks in the skin during contact with an infected person. When a person is infected with HSV, the virus usually persists within the individual for life. Approximately 500,000 people a year contract genital herpes. The incubation period ranges from 1 to 45 days with an average of 6 days. Viral shedding even in the absence of an identifiable lesion is a well-established phenomenon. It is estimated that up to 80% of those infected with HSV are asymptomatic or unaware of their infection.[14]

Clinical Manifestations

A patient with primary HSV-2 infections may initially complain of burning or tingling at the site of inoculation. Vesicular lesions, which may occur on the penis, scrotum, vulva, perineum, perianal region, vagina, or cervix, contain large quantities of infectious viral particles (Fig. 50-6). The lesions rupture and form shallow, moist ulcerations. Finally, crusting and epithelialization of the erosions occur. Primary infections tend to be associated with local inflammation and pain, accompanied by systemic manifestations of fever, headache, malaise, myalgia, and regional lymphadenopathy.

Urination may be painful from urine touching active lesions. Retention may occur as a result of HSV urethritis or cystitis. A purulent vaginal discharge may develop with HSV cervicitis. The duration of symptoms is longer and the frequency of complications is greater in women. Many HSV-2 infections, both primary and secondary, are asymptomatic; the exact percentage is unknown. Transmission of genital herpes therefore can occur by sexual contact with an excretor of virus who is free of symptoms. Primary lesions are generally present for 17 to 20 days, but new lesions sometimes continue to develop for 6 weeks.

After the first infection, HSV-2 establishes latency in the sacral ganglia and may be reactivated periodically. Recurrent attacks occur in about 50% to 80% of individuals during the

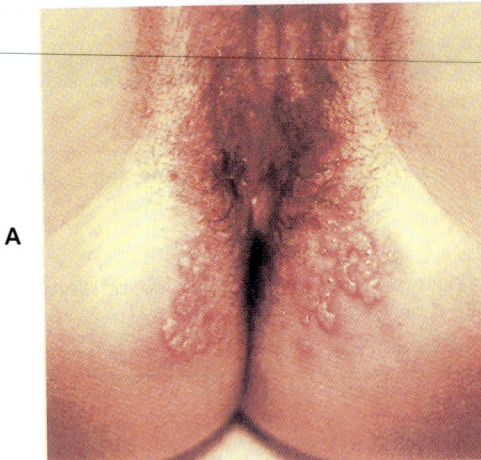

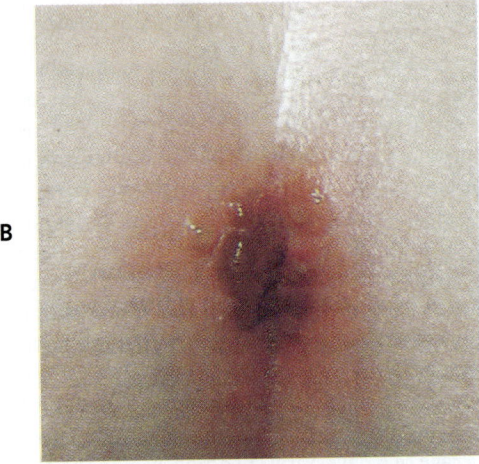

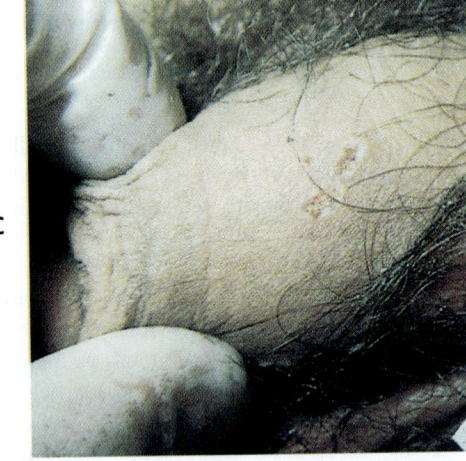

Fig. 50-6   Unruptured vesicles of herpes simplex virus type 2. **A,** Vulvar and **B,** perianal area. **C,** Penile herpes simplex, ulcerative stage.

year following the primary episode. Stress, sexual activity, sunburn, and fever tend to trigger recurrence. Many patients can predict a recurrence by noticing early symptoms of tingling, burning, and itching at the site where lesions eventually arise. The symptoms of recurrent episodes are less severe, and the unilateral lesions heal within 8 to 12 days. With time the recurrent lesions generally occur less frequently.

Although viral transmission is easier when overt genital lesions are present, there does not appear to be any predictability as to when viral transmission is possible once the primary HSV-2 infection has occurred. It has been shown that women with recurrent symptomatic genital herpes shed the virus up to 1% of the time even when no visible lesions are present. The person with HSV is capable of transmitting the virus at any time, even when he or she is asymptomatic. Suppressive therapy with antiviral agents can reduce but not eradicate asymptomatic shedding. Barrier forms of contraception, especially condoms, used during asymptomatic periods decrease transmission of the disease. When lesions are present, the patient should avoid sexual activity altogether because even barrier protection is not satisfactory in eliminating disease transmission.

Complications

Although most infections are of a relatively benign nature, complications of genital herpes may involve the CNS, causing aseptic meningitis and lower motor neuron damage.[15] Neuron damage may result in atonic bladder, impotence, and constipation. The most common complication is autoinoculation of the virus to extragenital sites such as fingers (whitlow), lips, and breasts.

Herpes Simplex Virus Infection in Pregnancy. Studies indicate no difference in the length or severity of symptoms in pregnant or nonpregnant women.[16] Some studies have suggested that HSV increases the incidence of spontaneous abortion. However, a recent large prospective study of high risk pregnant women showed that while 2% or more of susceptible women become infected during pregnancy, acquisition of new disease before labor does not seem to adversely affect pregnancy outcome. New infections near the time of labor increase the risk of neonatal herpes and perinatal morbidity.[17] Although women with recurrent HSV infections are not at higher risk for transmitting the virus to their infants, an active genital lesion at the time of delivery is usually an indication for cesarean section delivery, since most infections to neonates occur during passage through an infected birth canal.

Diagnostic Studies

Diagnosis of genital herpes is usually based on the patient's symptoms and history. The diagnosis can be confirmed through isolation of the virus from active lesions by means of tissue culture. Tzanck- or Pap-stained smears from lesions may show the cellular characteristics of viral infection, including multinucleated giant cells and intranuclear inclusions. Rapid testing using anti-HSV antibodies in direct immunofluorescence tests or in an enzyme-linked immunosorbent assay (ELISA), and DNA hybridization is now available with sensitivity ranging from 75% to 90%. Herpes antibody tests are unreliable for distinguishing between HSV-1 and HSV-2 antibodies. Highly accurate serologic methods have been developed, based on identification of specific antibody to the glycoprotein G component of the outer membrane of the virus. The Western blot technique is becoming more available but remains very expensive. Thus these tests have limited availability.

Collaborative Care

Drug Therapy. The skin lesions of genital herpes heal spontaneously unless secondary infection occurs. Symptomatic

COLLABORATIVE CARE

Table 50-6   Genital Herpes

Diagnostic
History and physical examination
Viral isolation by tissue culture
Cytologic examination of vesicular exudate for
multinucleated giant cells

Collaborative Therapy
Primary Infection
Acyclovir (Zovirax) 400 mg orally three times a day for
7-10 days OR acyclovir 200 mg orally five times a day
for 7-10 days OR famciclovir (Famvir) 250 mg orally
three times a day for 7-10 days OR valcyclovir (Valtrex)
1 gm orally twice a day for 7-10 days.

Recurrent Infection
Acyclovir 400 mg orally three times a day for
5 days OR acyclovir 200 mg orally five times a day for
5 days OR famciclovir 125 mg orally twice a day for 5
days OR valcyclovir 500 mg orally twice a day for 5 days
Attempt to identify trigger mechanisms
Yearly Pap smear
Abstinence from sexual contact while lesions are
present; however, may shed virus without lesions
Provision of symptomatic interventions
Confidential counseling and testing for HIV

Daily Suppressive Therapy for Frequent Recurrence
Acyclovir 400 mg orally twice a day OR famciclovir 250
mg orally twice a day OR valcyclovir 250 mg twice a day

Severe Infection
Acyclovir (Zovirax) 5-10 mg/kg IV for 5-7 days

Modified from Centers for Disease Control: STD treatment guidelines, *MMWR*
47(RR-1): 1, 1998.
*When treatment is started during the prodrome or within 1 day after onset of
lesions, many patients who have recurrent disease benefit from episodic therapy.

Table 50-7   Comparison of Gonorrhea and Chlamydia

Site of Infection	N. gonorrhoeae	C. trachomatis
Men		
Urethra	Urethritis	Nongonococcal urethritis; post-gonococcal urethritis
Epididymis	Epididymitis	Epididymitis
Rectum	Proctitis	Proctitis
Conjunctiva	Conjunctivitis	Conjunctivitis
Systemic	Disseminated gonococcal infection	Reiter syndrome
Women		
Urethra	Acute urethral syndrome	Acute urethral syndrome
Bartholin's gland	Bartholinitis	Bartholinitis
Cervix	Cervicitis	Cervicitis; atypical cervical cells
Fallopian tube	Salpingitis	Salpingitis
Conjunctiva	Conjunctivitis	Conjunctivitis
Liver capsule	Perihepatitis	Perihepatitis
Systemic	Disseminated gonococcal infection	Arthritis-dermatitis syndrome

From McCance KL, Huether SE: *Pathophysiology: the biologic basis for disease in adults and children,* ed 3, St Louis, 1998, Mosby.

treatment such as good genital hygiene and the wearing of loose-fitting cotton undergarments should be encouraged (Table 50-6). The lesions should be kept clean and dry. To ensure complete drying of the perineal area, women may use a hair dryer set on a cool setting. Frequent sitz baths may soothe the area and reduce inflammation. Techniques to reduce pain on urination include pouring a pitcher of water onto the perineal area while voiding to dilute the urine and voiding in a warm tub of water. Pain may require a local anesthetic such as lidocaine (Xylocaine) or systemic analgesics such as codeine and aspirin. Patients are advised to abstain from sexual contact while lesions are present. However, sexual transmission of HSV has been documented even in the absence of clinical lesions, and the use of condoms should be encouraged.

Three antiviral agents are available for the treatment of HSV: acyclovir (Zovirax), valacyclovir (Valtrex), and famciclovir (Famvir). These purine analogues inhibit herpetic viral replication and are prescribed for primary and recurrent infections. Acyclovir, valacyclovir, and famciclovir are also used to suppress frequent recurrences (more than six episodes per year). Although not a cure, these drugs shorten the duration of viral shedding and the healing time of genital lesions and suppress 75% of recurrences with daily use. Continued use of oral acyclovir for up to 5 years is safe and effective, but it should be interrupted after 1 year to assess the patient's rate of recurrent

episodes. Adverse reactions are mild and include headache, occasional nausea and vomiting, and diarrhea. The safety of these drugs for treatment of pregnant women has not been established. Acyclovir ointment appears to be of no clinical benefit in the treatment of recurrent lesions, either in speed of healing or in resolution of pain, and is not commonly recommended. IV acyclovir is reserved for severe or life-threatening infections in which hospitalization is required for treatment of disseminated infections, CNS (meningitis), or pneumonitis. With high-dose IV use nephrotoxicity has been observed.

CHLAMYDIAL INFECTIONS

Urogenital Infections

Chlamydia trachomatis, a gram-negative bacterium, is recognized as a genital pathogen that is responsible for an increasing variety of clinical illnesses. Numerous different serotypes, or strains, of *C. trachomatis* cause urogenital infection (e.g., nongonococcal urethritis [NGU] in men and cervicitis in women), ocular trachoma, and lymphogranuloma venereum. Between 1987 and 1996 reported rates of genital chlamydia soared from 47.8 cases per 100,000 to 194.5 cases per 100,000.[1]

Chlamydia trachomatis is now a reportable disease in all states except Alaska and the District of Columbia. It is the most prevalent bacterial STD in the United States.[1] Symptoms, however, may be absent or minor in most infected women and in many men.

Because chlamydial infections are closely associated with gonococcal infections, clinical differentiation may be difficult (Table 50-7). Both infections are therefore usually treated

Table **50-8**	Risk Factors for Chlamydial Infection

Age <25 years
Multiple sex partners
Sex partners who have had multiple partners
History of STDs
Use of nonbarrier contraception
Bleeding inducible by swabbing of cervical mucosa

concurrently even without diagnostic evidence. The incubation period of 1 to 3 weeks for chlamydial infection is longer than that for gonorrhea, and the symptoms are often milder. The high incidence of recurrence may be because of failure to treat the sexual partners of infected persons. Table 50-8 lists the risk factors for chlamydial infection. Because of the high prevalence of asymptomatic infections, screening of high risk populations is needed to identify those infected.

Clinical Manifestations and Complications

As with gonorrhea, chlamydial infections result in a superficial mucosal infection that can become more invasive. Infections and associated signs and symptoms in men include urethritis (dysuria, urethral discharge), epididymitis (unilateral scrotal pain, swelling, tenderness, fever), and proctitis (rectal discharge and pain during defecation). Infections and associated signs and symptoms in women include cervicitis (mucopurulent discharge and hypertrophic ectopy [area that is edematous and bleeds easily]), urethritis (dysuria, frequent urination, and pyuria), bartholinitis (purulent exudate), pelvic inflammatory disease (abdominal pain, nausea, vomiting, fever, malaise, abnormal vaginal bleeding, and menstrual abnormalities), and perihepatitis (fever, nausea, vomiting, and right upper quadrant pain).[18] A large number of women with chlamydial cervicitis have been found to have a male partner with NGU.

Complications often develop from poorly managed, inaccurately diagnosed, or undiagnosed chlamydial infections. Infection in men may result in epididymitis, with possible infertility and Reiter's disease (a systemic condition characterized by urethritis, conjunctivitis, arthritis, and mucocutaneous lesions). Complications from chlamydial infections in men are rare; in women, infection with *C. trachomatis* is a major cause of PID and ectopic pregnancy. For this reason, in 1993 the CDC issued a recommendation that all females younger than 20 years of age be routinely screened for chlamydia at their annual gynecologic examination. They further advised annual screening of all sexually active women older than 20 years of age with one or more risk factors for disease (e.g., new sexual partner in the past 3 months, multiple sexual partners, lack of barrier contraception.) Chlamydial infection can also be transmitted from a mother to the newborn, causing neonatal inclusion conjunctivitis or pneumonia.

Diagnostic Studies and Collaborative Care

Chlamydial infections in men can be diagnosed by excluding gonorrhea. If no gram-negative intracellular diplococci are found on the gram-stained smear of male urethral discharge or the sediment of first-catch urine specimen, a culture is done. If both are negative and signs of inflammation are present (e.g.,

polymorphonuclear leukocytes [PMNs] on the gram-stained smear), a diagnosis of NGU *Chlamydia* infection can be made. The availability of nonculture tests has made the screening of both men and women more effective. Direct fluorescent antibody (DFA) tests, enzyme immunoassay (EIA), and DNA hybridization tests (using specific DNA probes) do not require special handling of specimens, are less expensive, and are easier to perform than are cell cultures. New techniques using nucleic acid amplification including PCR and ligase chain reaction promise to surpass culture as the gold standard of chlamydial testing. Tests being developed are highly sensitive and specific and may not require pelvic examination for obtaining appropriate sample material.[10,19]

Drug Therapy. Chlamydial infections respond to treatment with doxycycline (Vibramycin), azithromycin (Zithromax), or ofloxacin (Floxin). For doxycycline, the dosage is 100 mg two times a day. The dosage of ofloxacin is 300 mg twice a day. Both drugs are taken for 7 days. Azithromycin (1 g in a single dose) offers the advantage of ease of administration, but the safety and efficacy in patients under 15 years of age has not been established. Both of these medications are contraindicated in pregnancy. Erythromycin or amoxicillin is the drug of choice for use in pregnant patients. Follow-up care should include advising the patient to return if symptoms persist or recur, treatment of sex partners, and encouraging the use of condoms during all sexual contacts.

Lymphogranuloma Venereum

Lymphogranuloma venereum (LGV) is a chronic sexually transmitted disease caused by specific strains of *C. trachomatis*. LGV is rare in the United States. LGV is endemic in other areas of the world, including Africa, India, Southeast Asia, South America, and the Caribbean.

The strain of *C. trachomatis* that causes LGV probably enters the skin and mucous membranes through tiny abrasions. LGV begins as a skin lesion and spreads via the regional lymphatics. It may also spread systemically through the bloodstream and enter the CNS. Penile, vulvar, and anal infection can lead to inguinal and femoral lymphadenopathy. Marked inflammation occurs, resulting in necrosis, buboes (greatly enlarged, inflamed lymph nodes), abscesses of inguinal lymph nodes, and infection of surrounding tissue. Healing occurs by fibrosis after several weeks or months and results in scarring, which damages the lymph nodes and disrupts nodal function.

Constitutional symptoms that occur during the stage of regional lymphadenopathy include fever, chills, headache, meningismus (meningitis-like symptoms), anorexia, myalgia, and arthralgia. Complications of untreated anorectal infection include perirectal abscess; fistula in ano; and rectovaginal, rectovesical, and ischiorectal fistulas. LGV is treated with a 2-week course of tetracycline. Sex partners should also be treated.

CONDYLOMATA ACUMINATA

Condylomata acuminata (genital warts) is caused by human papilloma virus (HPV) and is a highly contagious STD seen frequently in young, sexually active adults. It is often found in conjunction with other STDs. Accurate incidence data are not available because it is not a reportable condition. The genitalia and anorectal region, as well as the urethra, bladder, and oral mucosa, may be affected. The incubation period of the virus is generally 1 to 6 months, but may be longer. Prevention is hampered by a high proportion of asymptomatic infections and lack of curative treatment.

Minor trauma during intercourse can cause abrasions that allow HPV to enter the body. The epithelial cells infected with HPV undergo transformation, proliferate, and form a warty growth. Immunosuppressed persons, pregnant women, and diabetics are the individuals most susceptible to HPV.

Clinical Manifestations and Complications

Condylomata acuminata lesions are discrete single or multiple papillary growths that are white to gray. The warts may grow and coalesce to form large, cauliflower-like masses. In men, the warts may occur on the penis and scrotum, around the anus, or in the urethra. In women, the warts may be located on the vulva, the vagina, and the cervix and in the perianal area (Fig. 50-7).

During pregnancy, genital warts tend to grow rapidly. An infected mother may transmit the condition to her newborn. Cesarean delivery is not routinely indicated unless the birth canal becomes blocked by massive warts. Bleeding on defecation may occur with anal warts.

Subclinical Human Papillomavirus Infections.
Research has linked HPV infection with cervical and vulvar cancer in women and with anorectal and squamous cell carcinoma of the penis in men. To date more than 60 types of HPV have been identified, at least 15 of which invade the genital tract. Some of these types appear to be harmless and self-limiting (e.g., types 6 and 11 commonly found in genital warts), while others seem to have oncogenic (cancer-causing) potential (e.g., types 16, 18, and 31).[20] Up to two thirds of the early lesions caused by these viruses are undetectable by visual examination. Flat subclinical lesions are commonly found on the cervix, introitus, and perianal and intraanal mucosa of women and on the penis, perianal, and anal mucosa of men[21,22] and are strongly associated with the development of dysplasia and neoplasia at these sites.

Diagnostic Studies and Collaborative Care

Diagnosis of condylomata can be made on the basis of the gross appearance of the lesions. However, the warts may be confused with condylomata lata of secondary syphilis, carcinoma, or benign neoplasms. Serologic and cytologic testing should be done to rule out these conditions. If dysplasia is confirmed by the Pap smear, a colposcopic examination and directed biopsies should be performed. Virapap, a test that uses DNA hybridization techniques, can be used to determine some molecular types of HPV present in a lesion. Currently, HPV cannot be confirmed by culture.

The primary goal when treating visible genital warts is the removal of symptomatic warts. The removal may or may not decrease infectivity. Genital warts are difficult to treat and often require multiple office visits with a variety of treatment modalities. One common treatment is the use of 80% to 90% trichloroacetic acid (TCA) applied directly to the wart surface. Petroleum jelly is applied to the surrounding normal skin to minimize irritation before a small amount of TCA is applied to the wart with a cotton swab. A sharp stinging pain is often felt with initial acid contact, but this quickly subsides. TCA is not washed off after treatment. It can be used in pregnant women.

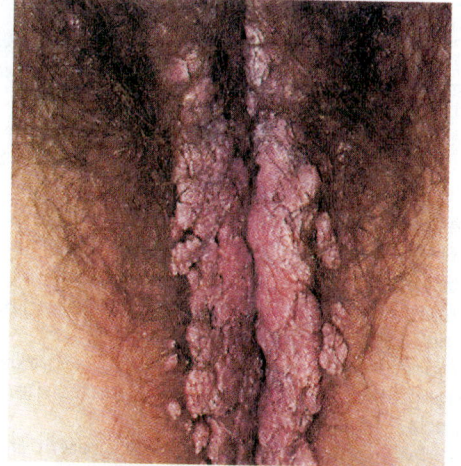

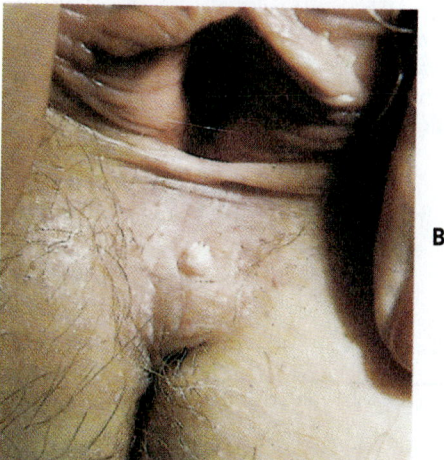

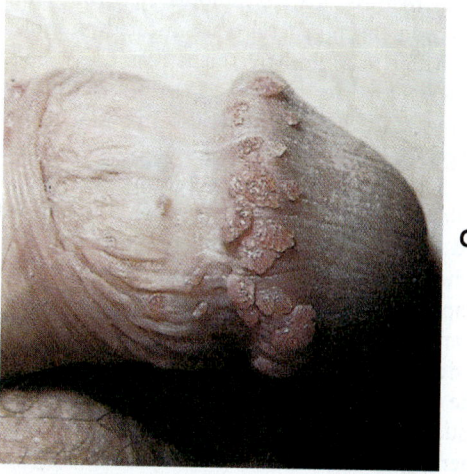

Fig. 50-7   Condyloma. **A,** Severe vulvular condyloma; **B,** perineal wart; **C,** multiple genital warts (condylomata acuminata) of the glans penis.

Podophyllin (10% to 25%), a cytotoxic agent, is recommended therapy for small external genital warts. When podophyllin is used, it is applied carefully to each wart, with normal tissue being avoided, and is then thoroughly washed off in 1 to 4 hours. This substance encourages the sloughing off of skin containing viral particles. Podophyllin has local (e.g., pain, burning) and systemic (e.g., nausea, dizziness, leukopenia,

NURSING ASSESSMENT

Table 50-9　Sexually Transmitted Disease

Subjective Data	Objective Data
Important Health Information	**General**
Past health history: Contact with individuals with STDs, multiple sexual partners, pregnancy	Fever, lymphadenopathy (generalized or inguinal)
Medications: Use of oral contraceptives; allergy to any antibiotics, especially penicillin	**Integumentary**
	Syphilis: Primary: painless, indurated genital, oral, or perianal lesions; secondary: bilateral, symmetric rash on palms, soles, or entire body, mucous patches on mouth or tongue, alopecia
Functional Health Patterns	*Genital herpes:* Painful genital or anal vesicular lesions
Health perception–health management: Shared needles during IV drug use; malaise	*Condylomata:* Single or multiple gray or white genital or anal warts (possibly becoming massive)
Nutritional-metabolic: Nausea, vomiting, anorexia; pharyngitis, oral lesions, itching at infected site; chills; alopecia	**Gastrointestinal**
Elimination: Dysuria, urinary frequency, retention; urethral discharge; tenesmus, proctitis	Purulent rectal discharge (indicator of gonorrhea), rectal lesions, proctitis
Cognitive-perceptual: Arthralgia; headache; painful, burning lesions	**Urinary**
Sexuality-reproductive: Dyspareunia; vaginal discharge, menstrual abnormalities; presence of genital or perianal lesions	Urethral discharge, erythema
	Reproductive
	Cervical discharge, lesions, inflamed Bartholin's glands
	Possible Findings
	Gonorrhea: Positive Gram's stain, smears, and cultures for *N. gonorrhoeae*
	Syphilis: Positive findings on VDRL and RPR, spirochetes on dark-field microscopy
	Genital herpes: Positive tissue culture for HSV-2, anti–HSV-2 antibody assay
	Chlamydia: Positive culture for *Chlamydia* organism

HSV-2, herpes simplex virus type 2; *RPR,* rapid plasma reagin; *STD,* sexually transmitted disease; *VDRL,* venereal disease research laboratory.

respiratory distress) toxic symptoms. It is contraindicated in pregnant women. In general, warts located on moist surfaces respond better to topical treatment (e.g., TCA, podophyllin) than do warts on drier surfaces.

Patient-managed treatment is also an option. Podofilox liquid and gel are available by prescription (Condylox and Condylox Gel). The patient applies the solution or gel for 3 successive days followed by 4 days of no treatment. Treatment can be repeated up to 4 weeks or until resolution of the lesions. Imiquimod cream (Aldara) is an immune response modifier that is applied every other day for up to 16 weeks or until the lesions are resolved. None of these treatments is recommended for use during pregnancy or lactation.

If the warts do not regress with any of these therapies, treatments such as cryotherapy with liquid nitrogen, electrocautery, laser therapy, 5-fluorouracil (5% cream), and surgical excision may be indicated. Because treatment does not destroy the virus, merely the infected tissue, recurrences and reinfection are possible, and careful long-term follow-up is advised.

NURSING MANAGEMENT: SEXUALLY TRANSMITTED DISEASES

■ Nursing Assessment

Subjective and objective data that should be obtained from a person with a sexually transmitted disease are presented in Table 50-9.

■ Nursing Diagnoses

Nursing diagnoses for the patient with a sexually transmitted disease include, but are not limited to, the following:

- Risk for infection *related to* lack of knowledge about mode of transmission, inadequate personal and genital hygiene, and failure to practice precautionary measures
- Anxiety *related to* impact of condition on relationships, disease outcome, and lack of knowledge of disease
- Altered health maintenance *related to* lack of knowledge about disease process, appropriate follow-up measures, and possibility of reinfection

■ Planning

The overall goals are that the patient with a sexually transmitted disease will (1) demonstrate understanding of the mode of transmission of STDs and the the risk posed by STDs, (2) complete treatment and return for appropriate follow-up, (3) notify or assist in notification of contacts about their need for testing and treatment, (4) abstain from intercourse until infection is resolved, and (5) demonstrate knowledge of safer sex practices.

■ Nursing Implementation

Health Promotion. Many approaches to curtailing the spread of STDs have been advocated and have met with varying degrees of success. Nurses should be prepared to discuss

PATIENT TEACHING GUIDE

Table 50-10   Sexually Transmitted Disease

1. Instruct patient in hygienic measures, such as washing and urinating after intercourse to destroy many causative organisms.
2. Explain the importance of taking all antibiotics as prescribed. Symptoms will improve after 1-2 days of therapy, but organisms may still be present.
3. Teach patient about the need for treatment of sexual partners with antibiotics to prevent transmission of disease.
4. Instruct patient to abstain from sexual intercourse during treatment and to use condoms when sexual activity is resumed to prevent spread of infection and prevent reinfection.
5. Explain the importance of follow-up examination and reculture at least once after treatment if appropriate to confirm complete cure and prevent relapse.
6. Allow patient and partner to verbalize concerns to clarify areas that need explanation.
7. Instruct patient about symptoms of complications and need to report problems to ensure proper follow-up and early treatment of reinfection.
8. Explain precautions to take, such as being monogamous; asking potential partners about sexual history; avoiding sex with partners who use IV drugs or who have visible oral, inguinal, genital, perineal, or anal lesions; using condoms; voiding and washing genitalia after coitus to reduce the occurrence of reinfection.
9. Inform patient regarding state of infectivity to prevent a false sense of security, which might result in careless sexual practices and poor personal hygiene.

practices with all patients, not only those who are perceived to be at risk. These "safe" sex practices include abstinence, monogamy with an uninfected partner, avoidance of certain high risk sexual practices, and use of condoms and other barriers to limit contact with potentially infectious body fluids or lesions. Sexual abstinence is a certain method of avoiding all STD's, but few adults consider this a feasible alternative to sexual expression. Limiting sexual intimacies outside of a well-established monogamous relationship can reduce the risk of contracting a STD. A patient teaching guide related to the patient with an STD is presented in Table 50-10.

All sexually active women should be screened for cervical cancer. Women with a history of STDs are at greater risk for cervical cancer than those women without this history. Pap smears are discussed in Chapter 51.

Measures to prevent infection. An inspection of the sexual partner's genitals before coitus is recommended. The presence of discharge, sores, blisters, or rash should be viewed with concern. A patient who is aware of specific signs and symptoms of infection can intelligently make the decision to continue the sexual interaction with modifications or elect not to have sexual relations. The patient should remember that, when engaging in sex, there is exposure to the infections of everyone with whom the partner has ever had sex. Men should be told that some protection is provided if they void immediately following intercourse and wash their genitalia and the adjacent areas with soap and water. Women may also benefit from postcoital voiding and washing. However, it should not be assumed that this provides adequate protection against STDs after exposure to infection. Although spermicidal jellies and creams have a mild detergent effect that may reduce the risk of contracting STDs, this has not been proven. These same barriers can serve as supplementary lubrication, thereby decreasing irritation and friction and chances for development of a minor laceration that could serve as an entry point for the organism.

Proper use of a latex condom provides a highly effective mechanical barrier to infection. The condom should be undamaged and correctly in place throughout all phases of sexual activity. The use of a spermicide such as nonoxynol-9 (which inactivates most STD organisms) in the vagina and concurrent use of a condom may further reduce the risk of disease.[22] Some studies have shown that condoms are less likely to be used by couples using a nonbarrier method of birth control (such as oral contraceptives, contraceptive injections or implants, IUD, or sterilization.)[4,6] The patient should be strongly cautioned that although these methods are highly effective in preventing pregnancy, they do not protect against STDs. Another deterrent to condom usage is alcohol and drug use. In one survey by the CDC, one fourth of high school students questioned reported that they had used drugs or alcohol with previous sexual intercourse.[4] Use of barrier contraceptives requires planning and motivation, both of which are impaired with alcohol or drug ingestion. The patient should be given specific verbal and written instructions on the proper use of condoms (see Chapter 13). The objections to condom usage, such as interference with spontaneity and the presence of a barrier, should be discussed by the partners. Information about the mechanics of sexual arousal and incorporating a condom into lovemaking can help in overcoming patient or partner resistance to its use. The Reality female condom is a lubricated polyurethane sheath with a ring at each end designed for vaginal wear (see Chapter 13). Laboratory studies indicate that it is an effective barrier to microorganisms, including viruses, but clinical trials are currently lacking for STDs.[23]

Sexual contact with persons known or suspected to have HIV infection should be avoided (see Chapter 13). Among couples with one infected partner, consistent and scrupulous condom use can reduce transmission to the uninfected partner. A sexually active homosexual man can reduce risk by minimizing the number of sexual contacts. Unprotected anal intercourse and other high-risk behaviors should be eliminated, and condoms should be used if sexual contact continues. Interpersonal skills necessary for this interview include respect, compassion, and a nonjudgmental attitude. Counseling should be tailored to the individual patient.

The nurse can initiate an interview to establish the patient's risk for contracting an STD. Questions to ask include number of partners, type of birth control used, use of condoms, use of IV drugs, and sexual preference. Patient education can be planned based on the response to these questions.

Screening programs. Screening programs that are used to detect infected patients can also help prevent certain STDs. For

ETHICAL DILEMMAS

Confidentiality

SITUATION

A nurse in a clinic gives the positive results of a test for *Chlamydia* to a patient and advises her to tell her sexual partners that she has this disease. The patient refuses to tell her boyfriend because he will know that she has had sex with another partner. Should the nurse contact the boyfriend?

DISCUSSION

A patient has the right to confidential diagnosis and treatment. However, if the boyfriend is not treated and continues to have sex with this (treated) patient, she will be reinfected. If he has additional partners, he could transmit the disease to them which, if left untreated, could lead to irreversible damage to the reproductive tract. While this disease could potentially endanger others, it is not life threatening. Education, not violation of confidentiality or coercion, is the key issue. The patient should be educated about reinfection and the long-term effects on others that this disease may have. The nurse should discuss the potential for reinfection if the boyfriend is not treated and encourage the patient to inform her partners of her diagnosis.

ETHICAL AND LEGAL PRINCIPLES

- Providers of health care have a legal obligation to maintain their patients' confidentiality unless required by law to report those who pose a risk to the health or life of innocent parties.
- Health care professionals have an ethical obligation to do no harm.
- Health care professionals have a primary responsibility to their patients. If trust cannot be maintained between health care professionals and their patients, patients may choose not to seek medical attention.

---

many years, there have been various screening programs to find cases of syphilis. With the decline of infection rates across the United States, many states have eliminated laws requiring premarital testing for syphilis. Many institutions offer voluntary prenatal HIV testing and counseling for pregnant women.

Screening programs have been developed and implemented for detection of gonorrhea and chlamydia. These programs are targeted to women because women are more likely to have asymptomatic gonorrhea and thereby serve as sources of infection. Routine gonorrheal and chlamydial testing during pelvic examinations and prenatal visits are being performed as a major part of these programs. Their effectiveness is well documented.[24] Mass application of screening programs for genital chlamydial infections, genital herpes, and HPV infections (warts) may also be possible with the advent of rapid, cost-effective tests.

Case finding. Interviewing and case finding are other processes used to control venereal disease. These activities are directed toward locating and examining all contacts of each known patient with an STD as soon after sexual exposure as possible, so that effective treatment can be initiated. Trained interviewers may often find cases even if they are supplied with only limited information. The caseworkers, who are often nurses, are aware of the social implications of these diseases and the need for discretion. Sexual contacts are often not informed about the origin of the information naming them as a contact so that greater cooperation and privacy is ensured.

Educational and research programs. Nurses can actively encourage their communities to provide better education about STDs for their citizens. Teenagers, who are known to have a high incidence of infection, should be a prime target for such educational programs. Hot-line services, school nurses, nurse practitioners, nurse midwives, and outreach programs sponsored by the CDC in the United States and Canada's Health Protection Branch are effective. The National Gay Task Force and the Herpes Resource Center were established to provide education and support where needed. Knowledge and understanding of the disease can decrease the STD epidemic. Currently, efforts are being made to develop immunizing agents for syphilis, gonorrhea, genital herpes, HPV, and HIV. The development of effective vaccines is viewed by many clinicians as a prerequisite for eradication of sexually transmitted diseases.

Acute Intervention

Psychologic support. The diagnosis of an STD may be met with a variety of emotions, such as shame, guilt, anger, and a desire for vengeance. The nurse should provide counseling and try to help the patient verbalize feelings. Couples in marital or committed relationships are confronted with an added problem when an STD is diagnosed. The implication of sexual activity by one of the partners with a person outside the relationship must be faced. Other concerns relative to their relationship are present, and the acute problem may serve as an incentive for further problem solving. Support and counseling for the couple are needed. A referral for professional counseling to explore the ramifications of an STD in their relationship may be indicated.

A patient who has contracted genital herpes is faced with the fact that repeated infections can occur and that no cure is available. This can be frustrating and disruptive to the patient's physical, emotional, social, and sexual lives. Helping the patient identify and avoid any factors that may precipitate the condition is indicated. Informing the patient that the incidence and severity of recurrences will decrease over time may provide some support.

HPV infections involve a prolonged course of treatment. The patient can become frustrated and distressed because of frequent office visits, associated costs, potential for unpleasant side effects as a result of treatment, and effects of the infection on future health and sexual relationships. Tremendous support and a willingness to listen to the patient's concerns are needed.

Compliance and follow-up. A nurse working in public health facilities, clinics, or other outpatient settings may care for a patient with an STD more often than a nurse in a hospital. This nurse is in a position to explain and interpret treatment measures such as the purpose and possible side effects of prescribed drugs and the need for follow-up care.

Frequently, single-dose treatment for gonorrhea, chlamydial infection, and syphilis helps prevent the problems associated with noncompliance with drug therapy. The patient requiring multiple-dose therapy should be given special instructions in completing the prescribed regimen and should be informed about problems resulting from noncompliance. All patients should return to the treatment center for a repeat culture from the infected sites or for serologic testing at designated times to determine the effectiveness of the treatment. Informing the patient that cures are not always obtained on the first treatment can reinforce the need for a follow-up visit. The patient should also be advised to inform sexual partners of the need for testing and treatment, regardless of whether they are free of symptoms or experiencing symptoms.

Hygiene measures. The patient with an STD should have certain hygiene measures emphasized. An important measure is frequent hand washing and bathing; this results in the destruction of many of the causative organisms of STDs. Bathing and cleaning of the involved areas can provide local comfort and prevent secondary infection. Douching may spread the infection or undermine local immune responses and is therefore contraindicated. The synthetic materials used in most undergarments frequently increase or exacerbate local irritations by trapping moisture. Cotton undergarments provide better absorption and are cooler and more comfortable for the patient with an STD.

Sexual activity. Sexual abstinence is indicated during the communicable phase of the disease. If sexual activity occurs before treatment of the patient has been completed, the use of condoms may prevent the spread of infection and reinfection. Condom usage after treatment should be encouraged to prevent future exposure to infection. The patient can also choose to relate to a partner in an intimate way that avoids both coitus and oral-genital contact. It is important to note that even single-dose treatments can take up to 1 week to be effective and thus the patient is infective during this period.

Ambulatory and Home Care. Because many STDs are cured with a single dose or short course of antibiotic therapy, many persons are casual about the outcome of these diseases. The consequences of this attitude can include delays in treatment, noncompliance with instructions, and subsequent development of complications. The complications are serious and costly; they can result in disfigurement and destruction of important tissues and organs.

Surgery and prolonged therapy are indicated for many patients with disease-related complications. Major surgical procedures such as resection of an aneurysm or aortic valve replacement may be necessary to treat cardiovascular problems caused by syphilis. Pelvic surgery and procedures to correct fertility problems secondary to an STD may include lysis of adhesions, dilation of strictures, reconstructive tuboplasty, and in vitro fertilization.

■ Evaluation

Expected outcomes for the patient with an STD are that the patient

- describes modes of transmission
- uses appropriate hygienic measures
- experiences no reinfection
- demonstrates compliance with follow-up protocol

CRITICAL THINKING EXERCISES

CASE STUDY

Chlamydia

Patient Profile

Sara M. is a 17-year-old female who visits the outpatient Teen Clinic seeking birth control pills.

Subjective Data

- Had first-time intercourse with boyfriend 2 weeks ago
- Did not use condom or spermicide
- Has not asked boyfriend about his sexual practices
- Denies any symptoms

Objective Data

- Has hypertrophic ectopy noted during Pap test
- Tests positive for chlamydia
- Crying and very upset when informed of positive test result

Collaborative Care

- Doxycycline 100 mg bid for 7 days

Critical Thinking Questions

1. What were Sara's risk factors for acquiring chlamydial infection?
2. What complications could have occurred if Sara's infection had not been detected?
3. What impact is her diagnosis likely to have on Sara's self-image? On her relationship with her boyfriend?
4. What instructions should Sara receive to ensure successful treatment? To prevent reinfection? To prevent further transmission of the infection?
5. What does she need to know about other STDs? What other testing would you recommend?
6. Based on the assessment data presented, write one or more nursing diagnoses. Are there any collaborative problems?

NURSING RESEARCH ISSUES

1. What are the best strategies for encouraging safer sex practices and condom use among high risk populations?
2. What is the level of teens' knowledge of risk, transmission, and impact of STDs? How can teaching about STDs best be adapted to their developmental level?
3. Does education about safer sex practices increase preventive behaviors?

REVIEW QUESTIONS

The number of the question corresponds to the same-numbered objective at the beginning of the chapter.

1. The individual with the lowest risk for sexually transmitted pelvic inflammatory disease is a woman who
   a. uses oral contraceptives.
   b. uses an intrauterine device for contraception.
   c. uses barrier methods of contraception.
   d. uses a Norplant implant or injectible Depo-Provera for contraception.

2. While obtaining subjective assessment data from a woman reported as a sexual contact of a man with chlamydia, the nurse understands that symptoms of chlamydial infections in women
   a. are frequently absent.
   b. mimic those of genital herpes.
   c. include a macular palmar rash in later stages.
   d. may involve chancres hidden inside the vagina.

3. A primary HSV infection differs from recurrent episodes in that
   a. it is of shorter duration than recurrent episodes.
   b. only primary infections are sexually transmissible.
   c. systemic manifestations such as fever and myalgia are more common.
   d. transmission of the virus to a fetus is less likely during primary infection.

4. The nurse explains to a patient with gonorrhea that treatment will include both ceftriaxone and a tetracycline agent because
   a. most patients do not respond to ceftriaxone alone.
   b. coverage with more than one antibiotic prevents reinfection.
   c. no single agent successfully eradicates all strains of gonorrhea.
   d. the high rate of coexisting chlamydia and gonorrhea indicates dual coverage.

5. The patient with an STD who is most likely to have a nursing diagnosis of body image disturbance that hinders future sexual relationships is the patient with
   a. gonorrhea.
   b. primary syphilis.
   c. chlamydial infection.
   d. condylomata acuminata.

6. Teaching by the nurse to prevent infection and transmission of STDs includes explanations of
   a. the appropriate use of birth control pills.
   b. sexual positions used to avoid infection.
   c. sexual practices that are considered high risk.
   d. the necessity of annual Pap smears for patients with HPV.

7. An appropriate nursing intervention to provide emotional support to a patient with an STD is to
   a. use concerned listening when the patient expresses negative feelings.
   b. offer many alternatives that the patient can use to change sexual relationships.
   c. reassure the patient that the disease is curable with appropriate treatment.
   d. help the patient who is an innocent sexual partner forgive the infecting partner.

References

1. US Department of Health and Human Services, Division of STD Prevention: *Sexually transmitted disease surveillance, 1996:* Atlanta, 1997, Centers for Disease Control.
2. Fleming DT and others: Herpes simplex virus type 2 in the United States, 1976 to 1994, *N Engl J Med* 337:16, 1997.
3. Centers for Disease Control: *Chlamydia trachomatis* genital infections—United States, 1995, *MMWR* 46:9, 1997.
4. Centers for Disease Control: Youth risk behaviour surveillance—United States, 1995, *MMWR* 44:SS-4, 1996.
5. Centers for Disease Control: Update: barrier protection against HIV infection and other sexually transmitted diseases, *MMWR* 42:30, 1993.
*6. Rannie K, Craig DM: Adolescent females' attitudes, subjective norms, perceived behavioral control, and intention to use latex condoms, *Public Health Nursing* 14:1, 1997.
7. Sarma SP, Garafalo K, Graves WL: Use of intrauterine device by inner city women, *Arch Fam Med* 7:130, 1998.
8. Pasquale S: Clinical experience with today's IUDs, *Obstet Gynecol Surv* 51(12 suppl):S25, 1996.
9. Finelli L and others: Early syphilis: relationship to sex, drugs, and changes in high-risk behavior from 1987–1990, *Sex Transm Dis* 20:2, 1993.
10. Wagar EA: Direct hybridization and amplification application for the diagnosis of infectious diseases, *J Clin Lab Anal* 10:6, 1996.
11. Young H and others: Non-cultural detection of rectal and pharyngeal gonorrhoeae by the Gen-Probe PACE 2 assay, *Genitourin Med* 73:1, 1997.
12. Lukehart SA, Holmes KK: Syphilis. In Fauci AS and others, editors: *Harrison's principles of internal medicine,* ed 14, New York, 1998, McGraw-Hill.
13. Brunham RC and others: Sexually transmitted diseases in pregnancy. In Holmes KK, editor: *Sexually transmitted diseases,* ed 2, New York, 1990, McGraw-Hill.
*14. Andrist LC: Genital herpes: overcoming barriers to diagnosis and treatment, *AJN* 97:10, 1997.
15. Catotti DN and others: Herpes revisited, *Sex Transm Dis* 20:2, 1993.
16. Corey L: Genital herpes. In Holmes KK, editor: *Sexually transmitted diseases,* ed 2, New York, 1990, McGraw-Hill.
17. Brown ZA and others: The acquisition of herpes simplex virus during pregnancy, *N Engl J Med* 337:8, 1997.
*18. Erickson MF: Chlamydial infections: combating the silent threat, *AJN* 94:16B, 1994.
19. LeBar WD: Keeping up with new technology: new approaches to diagnosis of *Chlamydia* infection, *Clin Chem* 42:5, 1996.
*20. Carson S.: Human papillomatous virus infection update: impact on women's health, *Nurs Pract* 22:4, 1997.
21. Beutner KR: Human papilloma virus infection of the vulva, *Semin Dermatol* 15:1, 1996.
22. Mayman R and others: Penile condyloma: a gynecological epidemic disease. A review of the current approach and management aspects, *Obstet Gynecol Surv* 49:11, 1994.
23. US Department of Health and Human Services, Public Health Service: *1998 sexually transmitted diseases treatment guidelines,* Atlanta, 1998, Centers for Disease Control.
24. US Department of Health and Human Services, Public Health Service: *Recommendations for the prevention and management of* Chlamydia trachomatis *infections, 1998,* Atlanta, 1998, Centers for Disease Control.

*Nursing research-based articles.

Resources

American Venereal Disease Association
Box 385
University of Virginia Hospital
Charlottesville, VA 22908

National Herpes Hotline
Herpes Resource Center
13827 Research Triangle Park
Raleigh, NC 27709
800-230-6039
http://www.ashastd.org/herpes/hrc.html

Sex Information and Education Council of the United States
130 West 42nd Street, Suite 350
New York, NY 10036-7802
212-819-9770
Fax: 212-819-9776
http://www.siecus.org

For additional Internet resources, see the website for this book at www.mosby.com/MERLIN/medsurg_lewis

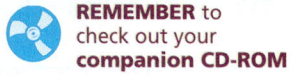
51 NURSING MANAGEMENT
Female Reproductive Problems

Susan Flagler & Kathryn Patterson

www.mosby.com/MERLIN/medsurg_lewis

LEARNING OBJECTIVES

1. Describe the advantages and disadvantages of common contraceptive methods.
2. Identify causative factors and the strategies to diagnose and treat infertility.
3. Discuss the nursing management of women who miscarry or terminate a pregnancy.
4. Describe the etiology, clinical manifestations, and collaborative and nursing management of menstrual problems and irregular vaginal bleeding.
5. Identify the risk factors for and symptoms of ectopic pregnancy.
6. Discuss the changes that accompany perimenopause and postmenopause and their collaborative and nursing management.
7. Identify the clinical manifestations of rape and the appropriate collaborative and nursing management.
8. Differentiate among the common problems that affect the vulva, vagina, and cervix and the related collaborative care and nursing management.

9. Describe the assessment and collaborative care and nursing management of women with pelvic inflammatory disease.
10. Describe the clinical manifestations, complications, collaborative care, and nursing management of endometriosis.
11. Describe the manifestations and collaborative care of benign tumors of the female reproductive system.
12. Identify the clinical manifestations, diagnostic studies, collaborative care, and surgical interventions of malignancies of the uterus, ovaries, and vulva.
13. Describe the preoperative and postoperative nursing management for the patient requiring major surgery of the female reproductive system.
14. Identify the nursing responsibilities in caring for women receiving radiation therapy for cancers of the reproductive system.
15. Describe common problems with cystoceles, rectoceles, and fistulas and the related collaborative care.

CONTRACEPTIVE METHODS

Although contraceptive methods are not reproductive problems, they have an important influence on the health of women in their reproductive years. Pregnancy and childbirth carry a higher risk, although extremely small, of death to a woman than either the use of oral contraceptives or the early termination of pregnancy.[1] Nearly half of the pregnancies occurring in the United States are unintended ones, even with the availability of safe and effective birth control methods. An unintended pregnancy is more likely than an intended pregnancy to compromise a woman's health and socioeconomic status.[2] Most unintended pregnancies occur when a method of birth control is not used or not used correctly. By providing accurate contraceptive information, nurses in all settings can positively influence women's health. Women's knowledge and ability to use contraceptive methods correctly can result in planned pregnancies at desired intervals.

Several contraceptives have health benefits beyond preventing pregnancy. These are referred to as the noncontraceptive benefits. Barrier methods such as condoms and diaphragms

reduce the spread of sexually transmitted diseases (STDs). Decreased vaginal and cervical infections reduce the risk of developing more serious conditions such as pelvic inflammatory disease or cervical cancer. Oral contraceptives can improve women's health by decreasing their risk for endometrial and ovarian cancer. In women over 35 years of age, oral contraceptives can have a positive effect on bone calcium content.[3] In addition, women on oral contraceptives report fewer problems with dysmenorrhea (painful uterine cramping) and have lighter menstrual flow resulting in decreased potential for anemia.[4]

Selection of Contraceptive Method

An ideal contraceptive is one that is safe, simple to use, inexpensive, reversible, and does not interfere with sexual activity. No current single method meets all of these criteria. Thus the selection of a method involves the careful consideration of the risks and benefits of the various methods. Each woman's active involvement in selecting the method is essential.[1] Most women use several methods over time. Temporary methods are used to delay or space childbearing. Permanent methods such as voluntary surgical contraception or sterilization (i.e., tubal ligation) are used by women who have completed their childbearing or do not wish to have any children.

Reviewed by Katherine A. Howe, RN, MSN, MEd, Women's Health Nurse Practitioner, Center for Women's Health, The Toledo Hospital, Toledo, Ohio.

Table **51-1**	Methods of Birth Control		
Description	**Side Effects and Complications**	**Patient Education**

Temporary

Combined Estrogen-Progesterone

Combination pill contains both estrogen and progesterone (standard and low-dose) taken usually on fifth through twenty-fifth day of each cycle. Prevents ovulation, causes changes in endometrium, alterations in cervical mucus, and tubal transport. Simple and unobtrusive in use, 99% effective. Failure from irregular or incorrect use.	Side effects of nausea, spotting and breakthrough bleeding, postpill amenorrhea, breast tenderness, headache, irritability, nervousness, depression, and decreased libido; complications are benign liver tumors, gallstones, myocardial infarction, thromboembolism, stroke (smokers over age 35 yr at higher risk); contraindications are history of cardiovascular disease, breast or pelvic cancer, and caution with diabetes mellitus, sickle cell disease. Provides no protection against HIV transmission.	Instruct patient in correct use of pills. Tell patient to take pill same time each day; if forgotten one day, take two next day. Review side effects, contraindications. Explain that patient should report cramps or swelling of legs, chest pain. Discuss need for periodic (every 12 mo) checkup that involves weight, BP, Pap smear, hematocrit. Review danger signs of drug. Take drug history, asking about use of phenytoin (Dilantin), phenobarbital, antibiotic (e.g., ampicillin, rifampin [Rifamale]), which decrease contraceptive action. Inform patient that method is usually not recommended for persons over age 35 yr who smoke. Discourage smoking.
Morning-after pill (Ovral) ethinyl estradiol 50 μg and norgestrel 0.5 mg. Another use of combined hormonal contraception. 98.4% effective. Creates hostile uterine lining and alters tubal transport.	Nausea for 1 or 2 days. Would not prevent an ectopic pregnancy.	Take two Ovral within 72 hr of coitus. Repeat if vomiting occurs. Take second dose 12 hr later. Menses should begin within 2-3 wk. Start an ongoing method of contraception immediately after menses.

Progestin Only

Progestin-only pills (Minipills) are taken daily, with no pill-free days. Preferred for women who are breast feeding. Does not suppress lactation. Inhibits ovulation. Thickens cervical mucus. Alters uterine lining. Lower cardiovascular risk than combined pills.	Menstrual changes; breakthrough bleeding, prolonged cycles or amenorrhea. Increase in functional cysts of the ovary. Increase in ectopic pregnancy.	Use alternate contraception when starting progestin-only pills or if pill is missed. Take pill at same time every day. Keep record of menses and get pregnancy test if 2 wk late.
Depo-Provera (DMPA) is a progestin-only drug given by injection every 3 mo. A private, convenient, and highly effective method.	May cause amenorrhea, headaches, bloating, and weight gain. Return of fertility may be delayed for several months. May cause bone mineral loss.	Return every 3 mo for injection. Discontinue method for several months before planning to conceive.
Norplant is a progestin-only subdermal implant. Six silicone capsules provide protection for 5 yr. Continuous, long-term contraception. Failure rate is extremely low. Does not suppress lactation.	Surgical removal of capsules after 5 yr. Menstrual irregularities, especially during the first year. Later may cause amenorrhea. May cause abdominal pain, headaches, weight gain, acne, and bone mineral loss.	Is effective after 24 hr. Keep arm dry for 48 hr after insertion. Report arm pain. Implants are soft and flexible and cannot break. Expect some irregular bleeding. Report any other changes. Remove implants in 5 yr. Continue to protect against STDs.

Barrier Method

Cervical cap

Rubber thimble-shaped shield covering cervix held in place only by suction. Spermicide in inner surface provides mechanical barrier to sperm. Fitting by trained professional. Effectiveness similar to diaphragm; failure from dislodgement and improper fit.	Allergy to latex, rubber, or spermicide, possible cervical irritation or erosion from suction.	Provide sufficient time for practice with insertion and removal (more time than for diaphragm). Give instruction for cleaning, storing, and inspecting for damage. Inform patient that it can be used with abnormalities of vaginal canal but not with cervical inconsistencies, genital infections or cervical malignancy.

Continued

Table **51-1**	Methods of Birth Control—cont'd	
Description	**Side Effects and Complications**	**Patient Education**
Barrier Method—cont'd		
Condom		
Male: thin rubber, latex, or animal membrane sheath fitting over erect penis and providing mechanical barrier to sperm. Simple method to use, no prescription necessary. 85% effective; failure from tearing or slipping during coitus. Used with spermicide. Affords some protection against STDs and HIV transmission.	Possible allergy to latex, rubber, possible decrease in sensation and interference with foreplay.	Advise patient to roll sheath along entire penis, leaving slack at end to receive semen. Inform patient that sharp object (e.g., fingernails) may tear condom. Tell patient to hold sheath in place when penis is withdrawn to prevent emptying of sperm in or near vagina.
Female: double ring system fitted into vagina up to 8 hr before intercourse. No prescription necessary; 88% effective. Affords protection against HIV, cytomegalovirus, and hepatitis B.	No significant side effects; generally acceptable to couple.	Discuss insertion, lubrication, method of removal. More expensive than male condom.
Diaphragm		
Dome-shaped latex cup with flexible metal ring (varies in size) covering cervix. Inner surface coated with spermicide before insertion. Provides mechanical barrier to sperm. Prescription method; fitting by professional; recurrent motivation to use necessary. 87% effective; failure from improper fitting or placement of device.	Allergy to latex, spermicide.	Demonstrate how to hold, insert, and remove device, using model. Allow for insertion and removal practice sessions. Advise patient that insertion may be any time up to 6 hr before coitus, but removal should be 6-8 hr after coitus. Tell patient that bowel and bladder should be emptied before insertion. Give instructions for cleansing and storing, checking for holes or deterioration. Advise patient that diaphragm must be refitted following pregnancy, weight loss, or weight gain. Advise patient that it is not suitable if severe pelvic relaxation is present.
Foam, creams, jellies and suppositories		
Available without prescription. Contain nonoxynol 9 or octoxynol 9; viricidal and bactericidal activity.	Allergy to spermicide. Alteration of normal vaginal flora.	Discuss how to use. Advise patient to void after coitus. Most effective when used in combination with other barrier methods.
Other Methods		
IUD		
Insertion into uterus of flexible objects made of plastic containing fine copper wire or progesterone with string that protrudes into vagina. The method of action is not fully clear. After insertion, no additional equipment necessary; 97-99% effective; failure mainly from undetected expulsion. Most common type used today is Copper T380, effective for 10 years.	Increased menstrual flow and cramping, especially during early months of use; possible complications of ectopic pregnancy, pelvic infection. Undetected expulsion of IUD resulting in pregnancy.	Discuss techniques and experience of insertion and removal. Inform women that the IUD is not advised if future pregnancies are wanted, and about any risk for STDs. Instruct patient to check for string in vagina after each period; report to provider if unable to locate. Discuss need for annual pelvic examination and Pap smear.

Continued

Selecting the method most suitable for her current circumstances should be accomplished when the woman has a full understanding of the benefits, risks, and drawbacks involved with each of the available methods. Benefits might include effectiveness in preventing pregnancy and infection. Drawbacks might include side effects, cost, or messiness of the method. Primary care providers are responsible for ensuring that medical contraindications do not exist for any prescribed contraceptive methods. Table 51-1 presents a description of common contraceptive methods, their side effects, and related patient education. Figure 51-1 shows various temporary contraceptive methods.

Table 51-1	Methods of Birth Control—cont'd	
Description	**Side Effects and Complications**	**Patient Education**
Other Methods—cont'd		
Natural family planning		
Periodic abstinence during fertile portion of menstrual cycle. Requires strong motivation, self-control; complies with all religious doctrines; 60-65% effective; failure from difficulty in determining precise day of ovulation, irregularity of menses.	Inaccurate or incomplete knowledge of menstrual cycle.	Discuss methods to establish baseline menstrual patterns and identify ovulation. Give instructions in use of calendar, cervical mucus, or basal body temperature method to determine ovulation and fertile period.
Permanent		
Tubal		
Variety of abdominal and vaginal surgical procedures (laparotomy, laparoscopy, culdoscopy) that permanently prevent sperm and ovum from meeting. Crushing, ligating, clipping, or plugging of fallopian tubes (potentially reversible procedure); 99.96% effective; failure due to recanalization of fallopian tubes, erroneous ligation.	Bowel injury, hemorrhage, or infection.	Determine whether temporary contraceptives were used and reason for patient's dissatisfaction. Counsel regarding effects of procedure on physiology and sexual performance. Assist in obtaining written informed consent for procedure. Inform patient that procedure requires short-term hospitalization or can be done on outpatient basis.
Vasectomy		
Bilateral surgical ligation or occlusion of the vas deferens, nearly 100% effective.	Hematoma, swelling, psychologic adjustment.	Inform patient that procedure is usually done as outpatient procedure and takes 15-30 min. Tell patient that alternative form of contraception is needed until no sperm is seen on examination. Explain that procedure does not affect masculinity.

BP, blood pressure; *DES*, diethylstilbestrol; *HIV*, human immunodeficiency virus; *IUD*, intrauterine device; *STD*, sexually transmitted disease.

Hormonal Contraceptive Methods

Oral Contraceptives. Oral contraceptives containing a combination of estrogen and progesterone are the most widely used reversible method of contraception in the United States and Canada. So called "low-dose" pills containing 35 μg or less of estrogen, and new synthetic progesterones provide the same high level of effectiveness as earlier pills while producing fewer side effects. Primary care providers may prescribe progestin-only or minipills for women with cardiovascular problems or who have other contraindications for taking estrogen. Progestin-only pills must be taken at the same time daily and continuously without a break. This differs from combination estrogen-progesterone pills that are taken every day for 3 weeks followed by 1 week of placebo pills. During this week withdrawal bleeding occurs.

Injectable and Subdermal Methods. Progestin-only injectable methods such as medroxyprogesterone acetate (Depo-Provera) and subdermal implants such as levonorgestrel (Norplant) have effectiveness rates greater than the combined oral contraceptives. Depo-Provera injections are prescribed to be given every 3 months in a deep muscle such as the gluteus maximus. Crystals form from the injected solution and create the "deposit" that releases small amounts of progesterone over time. The site should not be massaged after the injection as this could interfere with the crystal formation. Norplant prevents pregnancy for 5 years, but it must be both placed and removed surgically. Progestin-only methods are associated with irregular vaginal bleeding, which is the major reason women discontinue these methods. In addition, progestin-only methods are associated with weight gain, amenorrhea, headaches, and bone mineral loss.[5] Fully informed consent is important for all contraceptives. Failure to fully inform women about what to expect has greater consequences with longer-acting methods. No counterinjection can be given to neutralize Depo-Provera, and surgical removal is necessary to stop the effects of Norplant.

Intrauterine Devices

Intrauterine devices (IUDs) are effective contraceptives that provide long-term pregnancy prevention without unwanted metabolic effects. The mechanism by which IUDs prevent conception is not completely understood. IUDs are thought to prevent fertilization by immobilizing sperm and preventing them from migrating from the vagina to the fallopian tubes and by speeding the transit of the ovum through the fallopian tube. The most often used IUD, the Copper-T 380, is approved for 10 years and has a typical failure rate of less than 1% in the first year of use.[1]

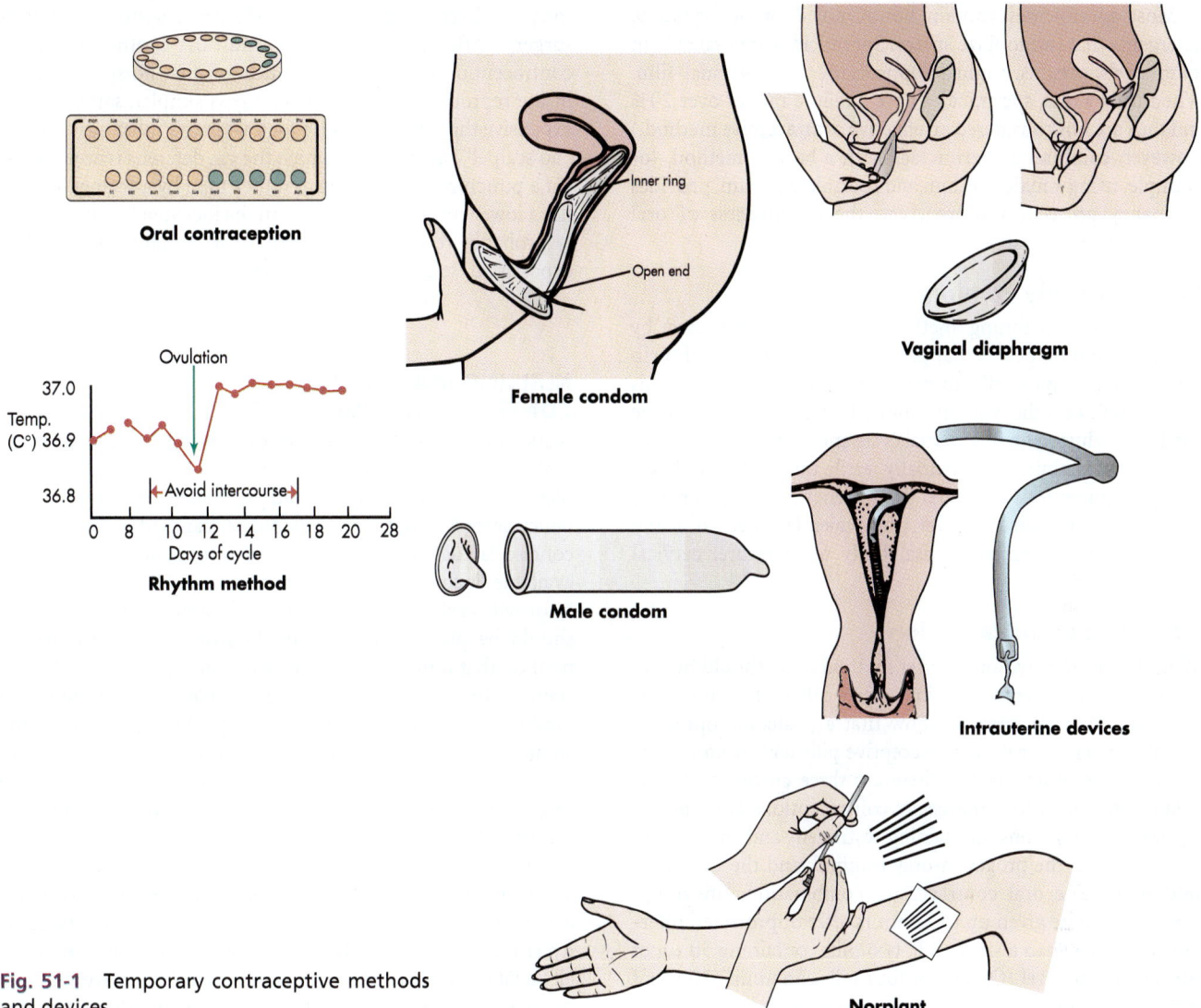

Oral contraception

Rhythm method

Female condom

Male condom

Vaginal diaphragm

Intrauterine devices

Norplant

Fig. 51-1 Temporary contraceptive methods and devices.

Two potential problems for IUD users are pelvic infection and ectopic pregnancy. In the past, certain models of IUDs were implicated in causing pelvic infections and subsequent infertility. Now it is clear that the risk of pelvic infection is increased only during the first 3 weeks following IUD insertion. Prophylactic antibiotics may be prescribed at the time of IUD insertion.[4] To reduce the risk of postinsertion infection, women desiring an IUD must be carefully screened and treated for genital tract infections before insertion. Three weeks after insertion, women with IUDs have the same relative risk of pelvic inflammatory disease as other women. The few women who become pregnant with their IUDs in place (typically 2 or less out of 100) have a 25% to 50% chance of losing the pregnancy by spontaneous abortion and approximately 5% chance of having an ectopic pregnancy. Since an ectopic pregnancy can be life threatening, women with IUDs must understand the importance of contacting a primary care provider if their menstrual periods are late or if they experience irregular spotting or bleeding.

Since the IUD offers no protection against STDs, women in long-term, mutually monogamous relationships are the best candidates. Many primary care providers discourage IUDs for women who consider having children in the future. Other providers view the IUD as an option for women who have not completed their childbearing, as long as the risks have been fully discussed. The IUD is not a good choice for women who are at risk for STDs or who have an impaired response to infection (e.g., individuals with diabetes mellitus or who are taking corticosteroids or HIV patients) because of their greater risk for developing a pelvic infection.

Barrier Methods and Spermicides

With typical use, barrier methods are less effective in preventing pregnancy than are hormonal methods. However, condoms are highly effective in preventing the transmission of HIV and other STDs. Hormonal methods provide little or no protection against infection. Male condoms are readily available, inexpensive, and should be used, even during pregnancy, whenever the possibility of an STD exists. Female condoms are more expensive than male condoms but provide another option for women wanting protection from pregnancy and STDs.

Most spermicides contain nonoxynol 9 or octoxynol 9, detergents that immobilize sperm. Spermicides are available in foams, gels, creams, vaginal suppositories, and vaginal film. When used alone, spermicides have a failure rate of over 20% and thus are not considered an effective contraceptive method.[1] However, combining spermicides with a barrier method, for example, using a male condom and spermicidal foam, provides pregnancy protection approaching the effectiveness of oral contraceptives.

Natural Family Planning

Natural family planning methods are most often used by women who have beliefs that preclude other methods of birth control. The typical effectiveness varies widely because this method relies on the woman's ability to accurately predict the fertile time during her menstrual cycle and on partner and self-control in abstaining at potentially fertile times. Natural family planning methods are based on the length and regularity of the woman's menstrual cycles (the "calendar method") and tracking the variations of basal body temperature, cervical mucus, or both.

Emergency Contraception

All oral contraceptive and barrier method users should be told about emergency contraception, often called the "morning-after pill." Women need to know that a postcoital option is available when their oral contraceptive pills have been forgotten or the condom breaks. There are three currently recommended methods for emergency contraception: oral contraceptive combinations containing estrogen and norgestrel/levonorgestrel, the progestin-only minipill, and the Copper-T 380A IUD. The oral contraceptive combination, "morning-after pill," can be given up to 72 hours after unprotected intercourse. Rather than a single pill, two pills containing 50 μg of estrogen (norgestrel [Ovral]) or four pills containing 30 μg of estrogen are prescribed to be taken at once and repeated 12 hours later.[6] The major side effects are nausea and vomiting. This contraceptive combination prevents pregnancy by blocking ovulation.

Recently the progestin minipill has been shown to be more effective than combination contraceptives and produces fewer side effects.[6] Due to the small amount of progestin in each minipill, 20 pills are needed for each dose. Again, therapy must be started within 72 hours of unprotected sex.

Insertion of a copper IUD within 5 to 7 days after unprotected intercourse is also a highly effective postcoital method. It is not clear how the device works but is thought to interfere with sperm transport or implantation.[6] Better utilization of emergency contraceptive methods could significantly reduce unintended pregnancies and, hence, the termination of pregnancies.

Permanent Methods of Contraception

Increasing numbers of men and women are choosing voluntary surgical contraception or sterilization to provide themselves with permanent contraception. Close to 100% effective, the first year failure rate for bilateral tubal ligation is 0.4% and for males with vasectomies only 0.15%.[1] Women who were unknowingly pregnant at the time of surgery and surgical error account for the majority of failures. For males having vasectomies, the failure rate is due to spontaneous recanalization of the vas deferens or the occlusion of the wrong structure during surgery.[1] After a vasectomy, men must use another method of contraception until clinical verification that no sperm remain in the reproductive tract. Vasectomy is simpler, safer, and less expensive than the procedure for a woman's tubal ligation. The "no scalpel" vasectomy in which the vas deferens is approached via a puncture in the scrotum rather than by a scalpel incision has a lower complication rate than the incisional method.[7] This is probably related to reduced tissue handling required to expose and isolate the vas deferens.[8]

NURSING MANAGEMENT: CONTRACEPTIVE METHODS

Nurses in many settings have the opportunity to provide information about contraceptive methods to individuals and couples who currently want to avoid pregnancy or to space a pregnancy according to their needs. Nurses can best assist by giving concise, factual, unbiased information about all of the methods available, including the benefits and risks. When feasible, this information should also be supplied in written form. Emphasis should be placed on the individual or couple selecting the method that is most compatible with current personal circumstances. Individuals considering permanent sterilization or long-term methods, for example, Depo-Provera or Norplant, should be counseled regarding discomfort and possible complications of surgery, as well as the consequences of the choice (e.g., sterilization is not reversible; Depo-Provera may delay return to fertility for 9 months).

Contraceptive needs typically change over a woman's lifetime. The woman's personal considerations such as the importance of avoiding pregnancy at a given time, cost, pattern of sexual activity, risk of exposure to STDs, and access to medical care should all be taken into account. Factors important to one woman may not match what is important to another woman nor match what the nurse thinks is most important. However, the best method is the one the woman will use consistently and safely. Women selecting a hormonal method, diaphragm, IUD, or surgical sterilization should see their primary care providers. Nurses should know the available resources for contraceptive referral within their communities. These resources may include Planned Parenthood, health departments, and community clinics.

Nurses should teach women how to use the method selected. If the method is tied to the act of intercourse (e.g., spermicides, condoms, diaphragms), women must know how and when it should be placed or inserted and how and when it should be removed. Women selecting oral contraceptives should know what to do if a pill is missed and when using a back-up method is indicated. Women taking oral contraceptives should be advised to keep an additional method on hand, such as foam and condoms, so it is readily available when needed. Both barrier and oral contraceptives method users should be told about the availability of emergency contraception.

Nurses can assist women to use their methods safely by giving accurate information. Foremost is educating women about the specific danger signs. This should be done both verbally and in writing. While serious complications are rare, women should know the possible danger signs and what should be done when a danger sign is recognized. For example, women selecting "the pill" may be taught the danger signs using the acronym *ACHES*. ACHES stands for the following signs: *A,* abdominal pain; *C,* chest pain, cough, shortness of breath; *H,* headache, dizziness, weakness, or numbness; *E,* eye problems, speech problems; and *S,* severe leg pain. If any of these danger signs are present, the woman should contact her primary care provider promptly.

Nurses should also educate women that discomforts, such as nausea or breast tenderness, when first starting oral contraceptives are not danger signs. Teaching women what can be done to minimize discomfort is important so they feel better and are less likely to discontinue the method. Also any misconceptions a woman may have about the method should be corrected. For example, some women have the misconception that after several years on oral contraceptives the pills should be discontinued to give the body a break from taking hormones. This is not true. On the contrary, continuing oral contraceptives increases the noncontraceptive benefits, such as reducing the risks for endometrial and ovarian cancer, with no detrimental effects on future fertility.

The woman's safety may also depend on protection from STDs. Women using nonbarrier methods who may be at risk for STDs should be encouraged to use condoms before any penetration with every act of intercourse. Many women are not aware that genital herpes and human papillomavirus (HPV) can be transmitted when their partners are unaware of being infected or have no evidence of disease.

INFERTILITY

Infertility is the inability to achieve a pregnancy after at least 1 year of regular intercourse without contraception.[9] Approximately 15% of couples in North America are involuntarily infertile. Evaluation and therapeutic measures can be invasive, expensive, and take a year or more, with only 50% eventually conceiving.[10] Understandably, infertility can constitute a physical and emotional life crisis.

Etiology

Infertility may be caused by either female factors or male factors. Conditions that cause male infertility are discussed in Chapter 52. In up to 20% of the couples evaluated, the cause of infertility may remain unexplained.[9] The most frequent female causes of infertility include ovulation factors such as anovulation or inadequate corpus luteum, tubal obstruction or dysfunction such as endometriosis or damage from pelvic infection, and uterine or cervical factors such as leiomyoma or structural anomalies.[9] Risk factors for infertility include increasing age, tobacco and illicit drug use, extremes of exercise activity, severe dietary restrictions, and specific occupational and environmental exposures.[9] The infertility risk for women aged 35 to 44 years is double the risk for women 30 to 34 years old.[11] One third of women older than 35 years who desire pregnancy experience infertility.

Diagnostic Studies

Evaluation of infertility is generally conducted over a series of visits (Table 51-2). A detailed history and general physical examination of the woman and her partner provide the basis for selecting diagnostic studies. The possibility of medical or gynecologic diseases is explored before tests are performed to

Table **51-2**	**Evaluation of the Infertile Couple**

Initial Visit
Clinical
  History/physical for both partners
  Extensive review of menstrual pattern
Laboratory
  Testing to assess specific medical findings
  Assess for sexually transmitted diseases
  Papanicolaou smear
  Semen analysis
Education
  Health maintenance (breast and scrotal
    self-examinations)
  Discussion of possible future testing options and cost
Ovulation Monitoring
  Instruction for at-home ovulation testing using basal
    body temperature, cervical mucus evaluation, and uri-
    nary LH test kit
Second Visit (scheduled in midcycle, periovulatory phase)
Clinical
  Postcoital test
Laboratory
  Schedule for midluteal progesterone/prolactin level
  Sperm penetration assay
Education
  Review ovulation monitoring data and techniques
  Review laboratory findings from last visit
Third Visit (at postovulatory part of cycle)
Clinical
  Endometrial biopsy
Laboratory
  Draw blood for midluteal progesterone/prolactin levels
Education
  Discuss need to assess tubal/uterine integrity (hystero-
    salpingogram vs. laparoscopy)
Fourth Visit (conclusion of initial work-up)
Education
  Outline biochemical/physiologic bases of couple's
    infertility
  Outline management plans with time and cost for each
  Discuss referral for possible assisted reproductive
    technologies (ART)

Modified from Stenchever MA: *Office gynecology,* ed 2, St Louis, 1997, Mosby. *LH,* luteinizing hormone.

evaluate whether the cause is female infertility. These tests include ovulatory studies, tubal patency studies, and postcoital studies.[11]

Ovulatory Studies. A basal body temperature record is kept to determine whether there is regular ovulation (Fig. 51-2). The woman is instructed to take and graph her temperature on awakening before any activity. The same site (e.g., oral) for taking the temperature should be used each time. Any cause for variation, such as sleeplessness or illness, should be noted. As ovulation approaches, the production of estrogen increases and may cause a drop in temperature. When ovulation occurs, progesterone is produced, causing a rise in temperature. The temperature graph thus helps to detect ovulation and suggest the timing of intercourse if pregnancy is

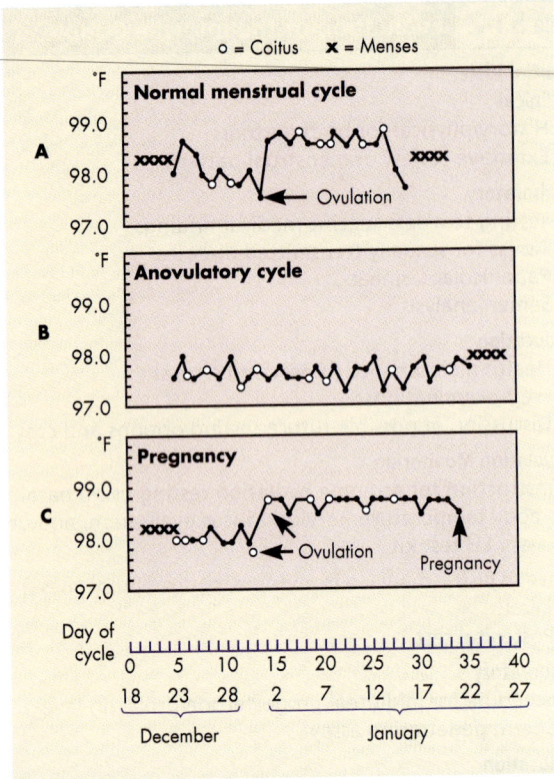

Fig. 51-2 Basal body temperature chart. **A,** Typical biphasic temperature curve indicative of ovulation and normal progesterone effect. **B,** Irregular monophasic curve characteristic of anovulatory cycles. **C,** Ovulatory curve with sustained temperature elevation following conception and the first missed period.

desired. Rigid adherence to a schedule can produce psychologic stress sufficient to inhibit sexual relations.

Simple rapid ovulation prediction kits are now available for use by women at home. These kits are generally used daily to measure luteinizing hormone (LH) levels in urine samples. Ovulation occurs about 28 to 36 hours after the first rise of LH, so intercourse can be timed accordingly. Other tests for ovulation include cervical and vaginal smears, endometrial biopsy, and plasma progesterone levels.

Tubal Patency Studies. Tubal factors (occlusion or deformity) are assessed most commonly by means of hysterosalpingogram. This procedure consists of the radiographic visualization of the uterus and tubes by injecting a radiopaque dye through the cervix. Tubal patency, shape, position, and any distortions of the endometrial cavity can be determined. Laparoscopy may be used when hysterosalpingogram is contraindicated or a pelvic cause appears likely.

Postcoital Studies. Examination of the cervical mucus can reveal whether it undergoes favorable changes at ovulation, enabling penetration, survival, and normal motility of the sperm. A postcoital examination can determine whether the cervical environment is favorable for the sperm. The couple is asked to have intercourse about the time ovulation is expected and 2 to 12 hours before the office visit. Douching or bathing should be avoided before the test. The cervical and vaginal secretions are aspirated and examined for the number and motility of sperm present.

NURSING AND COLLABORATIVE MANAGEMENT: INFERTILITY

The management of infertility problems depends on the cause. If infertility is secondary to an alteration in ovarian function, supplemental hormone therapy to restore and maintain ovulation may be attempted. Drugs used to induce ovulation include clomiphene citrate (Clomid), human menopausal gonadotropin (Pergonal), and bromocriptine (Parlodel). When a tubal blockage exists, the woman should be referred to a specialist to discuss whether surgical correction or in vitro fertilization is more appropriate.[9] Chronic cervicitis and inadequate estrogenic stimulation are cervical factors causing infertility. Antibiotic therapy is indicated for cervicitis. Inadequate estrogenic stimulation is treated by the administration of estrogens.

When a couple has not succeeded in conceiving while under infertility management, an option is intrauterine insemination with the husband's or donor's sperm. If this technique does not succeed, in vitro fertilization (IVF) may be used. IVF is the removal of mature oocytes from the woman's ovarian follicle via laparoscopy, followed by fertilization of the ova with the partner's sperm in a Petri dish. When fertilization and cleavage have occurred, the resulting embryos are transferred into the woman's uterus. The procedure requires 2 to 3 days to complete and is used in cases of fallopian tube obstruction, oligospermia, and unexplained infertility. IVF is costly and emotionally stressful, but it has become a recognized and accepted method of therapy for infertile couples.

Assisted reproductive technologies (ART) continue to develop rapidly since the first IVF baby was born in 1978. ARTs include IVF, gamete intrafallopian transfer (GIFT), zygote intrafallopian transfer (ZIFT), donor gametes, and embryo cryopreservation. With the increasing sophistication of embryo cryopreservation, assisted hatching, and intracytoplasmic sperm injection, couples will have an increased potential for pregnancy. The use of ART poses many ethical, legal, and social concerns.

Nurses can assist women experiencing infertility by providing information about the reproductive process and infertility evaluation and addressing the psychologic and social distress that can accompany infertility. Removing or reducing psychologic stress can improve the emotional climate, making it more conducive to achieving a pregnancy.

The nurse has a major responsibility for teaching and providing emotional support throughout the infertility testing and treatment period. Feelings of anger, frustration, grief, and helplessness may heighten as more and more diagnostic tests are performed. Infertility can generate great tension in a marriage as the couple exhausts their financial and emotional resources. Few insurance carriers cover the high cost of infertility testing or the therapeutic measures associated with infertility. Recognizing and taking steps to deal with the psychologic factors that surface can assist the couple to better cope with the situation. Couples should be encouraged to participate in a support group for infertile couples as well as individual therapy.

ABORTION

An *abortion* is the loss or termination of a pregnancy before 20 weeks or a fetal weight of less than 500 g. Abortions are classified as spontaneous (occurring naturally) or induced (occur-

Table 51-3 **Induced Abortion**

Method	Length of Pregnancy	Procedure	Advantages	Disadvantages
Early Abortion				
▪ Menstrual extraction	Usually up to 2 wk after first missed period	Catheter is inserted through cervix into uterus, and suction is applied. Endometrium and contents of uterus are aspirated.	Low cost, simple, done at outpatient facility without anesthesia or cervical dilatation, minimally traumatic	Continuation of pregnancy possible, potential for uterine injury and bleeding
▪ Suction curettage	Up to 14 wk	Cervix is usually dilated, uterine aspirator is introduced, and suction is applied, removing endometrial tissue and implanted pregnancy.	Outpatient procedure, most often involving local anesthesia, 1- to 2-day recovery period	Infection, uterine perforation possible
▪ Dilation and evacuation (D & E)	10-16 wk (approximate)	Cervix is dilated, and products of conception are removed by vacuum cannula and the use of other instruments as needed.	Safe and effective procedure for more advanced pregnancy, outpatient procedure with general anesthesia, 2-day recovery period	More psychologic trauma, more expensive, greater risk with general anesthesia and more invasive procedure
Late Abortion				
▪ Instillation of drugs				
Hypertonic saline solution	After 16 wk	About 200 ml of amniotic fluid is withdrawn, and a similar amount of 20% normal saline solution is injected. Uterus is apparently irritated and begins to contract within 12-36 hr. Contractions may be assisted with IV oxytocin.	Inexpensive, readily available, feticidal	Hypernatremia, infection, hemorrhage, disseminated intravascular coagulation, more emotional trauma because of time required
Prostaglandins	After 16 wk	Amniocentesis is done, and 8 ml of prostaglandin is inserted into amniotic sac, resulting in stimulation of smooth muscle of uterus. Expulsion of uterine contents occurs within 24 hr.	Fast induction, no need for surgery	Nausea and vomiting, abdominal cramps, cervical laceration, possible delivery of live fetus, high cost
▪ Hysterotomy	16-20 wk	Miniature cesarean section is performed. Incision is made into uterus and contents are removed.	Concurrent sterilization procedure possible	More difficult and expensive in time and money, surgical incision with possible complications

ring as a result of mechanical or medicinal interruption). Miscarriage is the common term indicating the unintended loss of a pregnancy. Habitual abortion is defined by a history of three or more previous abortions.

Spontaneous Abortion

Approximately 70% of all conceptions never achieve fetal viability with nearly 50% being lost before the first missed menses.[9] Spontaneous abortion is the loss of pregnancy before 20 weeks of gestation that had been clinically recognized by ultrasound or a reliable pregnancy test. Fetal chromosomal anomalies account for 60% of miscarriages before 8 weeks of gestation. Other causes of spontaneous abortions include endocrine abnormalities, maternal infection, acquired anatomic abnormalities (such as uterine fibroids or endometriosis), immunologic factors, and environmental factors.[9]

Uterine cramping in the presence of vaginal bleeding is an indication of a spontaneous abortion. Cramping is usually absent in vaginal bleeding caused by other conditions, such as polyps. Serial serum beta-human chorionic gonadotropin hormone (β-hCG) and vaginal ultrasound examination of the pelvis are the most reliable indicators of an early abortion. The gestational sac can be visualized using ultrasound as early as 6 weeks of gestation.

Treatment for a possible spontaneous abortion is limited. Although bed rest and abstention from sexual activity are often recommended, there is no evidence that these measures or any active medical management improves the outcome. The woman is advised to report any bleeding to her primary care provider. An estimated 80% of patients proceed to abortion regardless of management. If the products of conception do not pass on their own or bleeding becomes excessive, a dilation and curettage (D&C) is generally performed. A D&C procedure involves dilating the uterine cervix and scraping the endometrium of the uterus to empty the uterus of the products of conception.

NURSING MANAGEMENT: SPONTANEOUS ABORTION

Women who are threatening to abort (bleeding and cramping) may be admitted to the hospital. Nurses must attend to both the physical and emotional needs of patients. Vital signs and estimated blood loss are monitored. Any tissue or clots that might contain tissue are saved to be examined for traces of the fetus and placenta. Women may be very distressed and experience both physical and emotional pain. Nurses should use comfort measures to provide the needed physical and mental rest. Arranging for someone significant to the patient to stay with the patient provides important emotional support. The nurse should offer other resources for support of the grieving process that may result from this loss.

Induced Abortion

Pregnancy termination or an abortion that is induced for medical and personal reasons is one of the most commonly performed surgical procedures. In Europe, pharmacologic methods (e.g., RU-486) of abortion induction are available and soon will be approved in the United States. A woman's right to seek safe pregnancy termination and in what circumstances that termination may occur continue to be matters of debate and controversy. Early pregnancy termination involves fewer health risks to a woman than carrying a pregnancy to term.[1]

Techniques. The decision about which technique to use to terminate a pregnancy depends on the length of the pregnancy and the woman's condition. Early abortion methods include menstrual extraction, suction curettage, and dilation and evacuation (D&E). Table 51-3 lists current surgical techniques for abortion.

Suction curettage may be performed up to 14 weeks of gestation and accounts for more than 90% of abortion procedures.[11] Late or second-trimester abortions are most often used to terminate pregnancies when a fetal anomaly has been detected. Late termination procedures involve intrauterine instillation of prostaglandins or hypertonic saline that precipitate uterine contractions and the eventual expulsion of the fetus.

NURSING MANAGEMENT: INDUCED ABORTIONS

Pregnancy terminations are usually sought because women have decided that an abortion is better than any other option. Women seeking abortions experience less distress afterwards if the decision has been freely made after the consideration of the options

of keeping the pregnancy and the child as well as keeping the pregnancy and relinquishing the child. Once the decision has been made, the woman and her significant others need support and acceptance. The patient should be prepared in advance for what to expect both emotionally and physically. Grief and sadness are normal postabortion feelings and should not be misconstrued as otherwise. As with any surgical procedure, the patient needs to understand the instructions to be carried out

PATIENT TEACHING GUIDE

Table 51-4 Characteristics of the Menstrual Cycle

Characteristic	Patient Education
Menarche Occurs between ages of 9 and 16 yr; average age at onset is 12 or 13 yr	See physician regarding possible endocrine or developmental abnormality when delayed.
Interval Usually is 21-35 days, but regular cycles as short as 17 or as long as 45 days are considered normal if pattern is consistent for individual	Keep written record to identify own pattern of menstrual cycle. Expect some irregularity in premenopausal period. Be aware that drugs (phenothiazines, narcotics, contraceptives) and stressful life events can result in missed periods.
Duration Menstrual flow generally lasts 2-8 days	Realize that pattern is fairly constant but that wide variations do exist.
Amount Menstrual flow varies from 20-80 ml per menses; average is 30 ml; amount varies among women and in the same woman at different times; it is usually heaviest first 2 days	Count pads or tampons used per day. The average tampon or pad completely saturated absorbs 20-30 ml. Very heavy flow is indicated by complete soaking of 2 pads in 1-2 hr. Know that flow increases and then gradually decreases in premenopausal period. IUD or drugs such as anticoagulants and thiazides can produce heavy menses.
Composition Menstrual discharge is mixture of endometrium, blood, mucus, and vaginal cells; it is dark red and less viscous than blood and usually does not clot	Realize that clots indicate heavy flow or vaginal pooling.

before and after the procedure. The nurse's compassionate care can be a positive factor in the patient's experience.

Follow-up care includes instructions on signs and symptoms of possible complications, including an increase in vaginal bleeding, severe abdominal cramping, and signs associated with infection, such as fever and foul drainage. The importance of avoiding intercourse, tampons, and douching until reexamination should be stressed. The patient needs to return for reexamination in 2 weeks. Contraception can be started the day of the procedure or during the patient's return visit in accordance with her needs and desires.

PROBLEMS RELATED TO MENSTRUATION

To better understand problems of menstruation, key aspects of normal menstrual cycles must be understood. Menstrual cycles are influenced by hormones from the hypothalamus (gonadotropin-releasing hormone) and anterior pituitary (follicle-stimulating hormone and luteinizing hormone).[12] These hormones influence the development of a dominant follicle and egg within one ovary and the resulting production of estrogen during the follicular phase of the cycle. The estrogen from the ovary causes the growth of the endometrial lining of the uterus. Following ovulation, the corpus luteum (site of ovulation) produces progesterone that further develops and stabilizes the endometrial lining, building a suitable lining to receive a fertilized egg. The progesterone dominant part of the menstrual cycle is called the luteal phase because of the essential part the corpus luteum plays. When a fertilized egg does not implant in the endometrial lining, the corpus luteum is not maintained and production of progesterone falls. In response to decreasing levels of progesterone, the endometrial lining is shed. This shedding is referred to as *menstruation* or the

woman's menses or her period. The first day of menses is considered the start or day 1 of the menstrual cycle.

Menses may be irregular during the first few years after menarche and the years preceding menopause. Once established, a woman's menstrual cycles usually have a predictable pattern. However, considerable normal variation exists among women in cycle length as well as in the duration, amount, and character of the menstrual flow (Table 51-4). Women's awareness of normal menstrual variation may reduce unfounded concerns.

PREMENSTRUAL SYNDROME

Premenstrual syndrome (PMS) constitutes a group of somatic, behavioral, cognitive, and mood symptoms distressing enough to impair interpersonal relationships or interfere with usual activities. Because there are many symptoms associated with PMS it is difficult to concisely define it. However, PMS symptoms always occur cyclically during the luteal phase before the onset of menstruation and are not present at other times of the month.[13]

Etiology and Pathophysiology

The etiology and pathophysiology of PMS are not well understood. PMS is thought to have a biologic trigger with compounding psychosocial factors. Women with PMS may have a genetically determined sensitivity to one or more of the neurotransmitter systems, such as serotonin. This sensitivity results in heightened responses to the normal cyclic fluctuations of ovarian hormones.[11] Other proposed causes of PMS include estrogen and progesterone imbalances and nutritional deficiencies of pyridoxine (vitamin B_6) or magnesium.[13]

Clinical Manifestations

PMS is extremely variable in its clinical manifestations. Variation is common between women and, for an individual

RESEARCH

IMPLICATIONS FOR NURSING PRACTICE

Relationship Between Stress, Hormones, and Premenstrual Symptoms

Citation Woods NF and others: Luteal phase ovarian steroids, stress arousal, premenses perceived stress, and premenstrual symptoms, *Res Nurs Health* 21:1269, 1998.

Purpose To examine the relationships among perceived stress, ovarian hormones (estradiol and pregnanediol), stress arousal indicators (urine levels of catecholamines and cortisol), and premenstrual symptoms, including sense of turmoil (e.g., anxiety, irritability, and depression) and fluid retention.

Methods Women (n=74) with low symptom severity, premenstrual syndrome (PMS), or premenstrual magnification of symptoms (PMM) kept a daily diary of symptoms and stress ratings as well as daily urine samples for one menstrual cycle. Multiple regression analyses were performed to test models of premenstrual symptoms in the different groups.

Results and Conclusions In the women with low symptoms and PMS, the premenses global stress rating was the single significant factor accounting for turmoil symptoms. Cortisol levels were also a significant factor in predicting symptoms in women with PMS. Epinephrine and norepinephrine were both associated with symptoms but in opposite directions. Epinephrine was positively related to turmoil ratings while norepinephrine was inversely related.

Implications for Nursing Practice The results support the importance of perceived stress, stress arousal hormones, and ovarian hormone patterns in accounting for two of the more distressing symptoms associated with PMS, which are fluid retention and turmoil. Strategies to reduce stress arousal, including relaxation, biofeedback, and guided imagery techniques, may be useful techniques for further study in this population. Such results also point to the physiologic basis for symptom experiences of PMS.

woman, from one cycle to another. Commonly occurring physical symptoms include breast discomfort, peripheral edema, abdominal bloating, episodes of binge eating, and headache. Abdominal bloating and breast swelling are apparently caused by local fluid shifts because total body weight does not generally change. Symptoms of autonomic nervous system arousal such as heart palpitations and dizziness have been reported by women with PMS. Anxiety, depression, irritability, and mood swings are some of the emotional symptoms women may experience.

Diagnostic Studies and Collaborative Care

PMS can be diagnosed only when other possible causes for the symptoms have been eliminated. A focused health history and physical examination are done to identify any underlying conditions, such as thyroid dysfunction, uterine fibroids, or depression, that may account for the symptoms. While laboratory work such as thyroid function tests can help determine whether the symptoms are attributed to another condition, no definitive diagnostic test is available for PMS.

When PMS is a possible diagnosis, women are given a symptom diary to record their symptoms prospectively for two or three menstrual cycles. Diagnosis is based on an evaluation of the woman's symptoms. Evaluation of at least two cycle records must show no or low symptoms in the follicular phase (first part of menstrual cycle) and presence of symptoms or magnified symptoms in the luteal phase for a diagnosis of PMS.[14]

Nonpharmacologic and pharmacologic strategies that aid in relieving some PMS symptoms are shown in Fig. 51-3. No simple treatment is available. The goal of treatment is to reduce the severity of symptoms and enhance the woman's sense of control and quality of life. The nonpharmacologic approaches include diet changes, exercise, stress management, education, and counseling.[14] To decrease autonomic nervous system arousal women should avoid caffeine, reduce refined carbohydrates, exercise on a regular basis, and practice relaxation techniques. Increasing calcium intake may also help to reduce symptoms associated with PMS. Techniques for stress reduction include yoga, meditation, imaging, and biofeedback training. Eating complex carbohydrates high in fiber, foods rich in vitamin B_6, and sources of tryptophan (dairy and poultry) are thought to promote serotonin production. Vitamin B_6 may be found in foods such as pork, milk, egg yolk, and legumes.

Exercise results in a release of endorphins, leading to mood elevation. Aerobic exercise can also have a relaxing effect. The patient's lifestyle and interests should be considered when an exercise program is being planned. Because fatigue tends to exaggerate the symptoms of PMS, adequate rest in the premenstrual period is a priority.

The patient should be informed about PMS and the current theories on its etiology and treatment. Explanations help the woman with PMS understand the complexity of PMS and ways she can regain a better sense of control. The patient needs to be assured that her symptoms are real, PMS exists, and she is not "crazy." Acknowledgment of her PMS can be therapeutic.[13] Educating the woman's partner about the nature of PMS assists the partner to better understand PMS and to provide support to the woman in making lifestyle changes to reduce her PMS.

Drug Therapy. Pharmacologic treatment strategies should be considered when symptoms persist. Presently, no single drug is being prescribed for the treatment of PMS symptoms. One therapy may be tried for a time and if no improvement is observed, another approach is tried. Some treatments are symptom specific. For fluid retention, diuretics such as spironolactone (Aldactone) are used. For reducing cramps, backache, and headache, prostaglandin inhibitors such as ibuprofen (Motrin, Advil) are used. To improve negative mood, vitamin B_6 supplementation (50 mg daily) may by used. For anxiety, buspirone (BuSpar) taken during the luteal phase or on an as needed basis has helped some women.

Other pharmacologic treatments are directed at PMS in general. Selective serotonin reuptake inhibitors (SSRIs) (sertra-

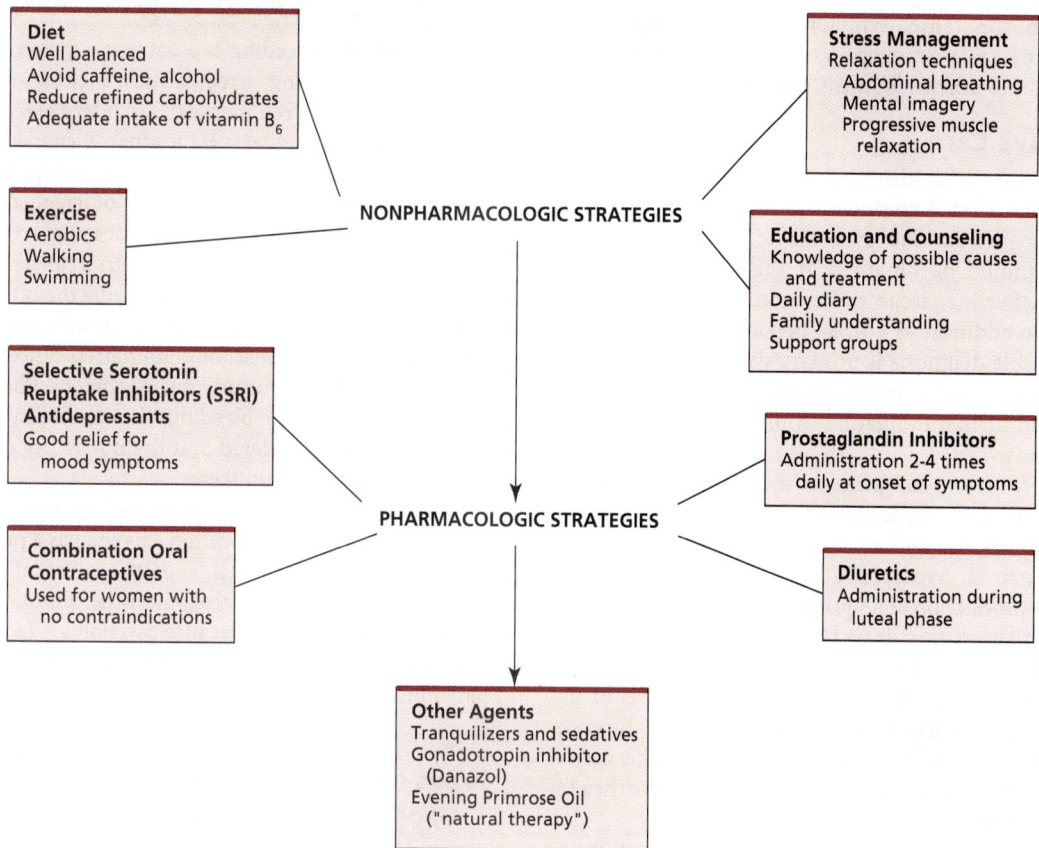

Fig. 51-3   Treatment strategies for premenstrual syndrome.

line [Zoloft]), a type of antidepressant, have provided significant relief to about 60% of women with severe PMS.[14] General treatments include combined oral contraceptives, tranquilizers such as alprazolam (Xanax), and gonadotropin inhibitors such as danazol (Danocrine). Although progesterone was previously used, it is not currently used. Evening Primrose Oil, a natural therapy, may help some women.

DYSMENORRHEA

Dysmenorrhea is defined as abdominal cramping pain or discomfort associated with menstrual flow. The degree of pain and discomfort varies with the individual. The two types of dysmenorrhea are primary (when no pathology exists) and secondary (when a pelvic disease or condition is the underlying cause). Dysmenorrhea is one of the most common gynecologic problems, affecting approximately 50% of all women.[11]

Etiology and Pathophysiology

Primary dysmenorrhea is not a disease. It is caused by either an excess of prostaglandin F_2 alpha (PGF_2 alpha) and/or an increased sensitivity to it. The sequential stimulation of the endometrium by estrogen followed by progesterone results in a dramatic increase in prostaglandin production by the endometrium. With the onset of menses, degeneration of the endometrium releases prostaglandins. Locally, prostaglandins increase myometrial contractions and constriction of small endometrial blood vessels with consequent tissue ischemia

and increased sensitization of the pain receptors resulting in menstrual pain. Prostaglandins absorbed into the circulatory system may be responsible for symptoms of headache, diarrhea, and vomiting, which are other manifestations of dysmenorrhea. Primary dysmenorrhea begins in the few years after menarche, typically with the onset of regular ovulatory cycles.

Secondary dysmenorrhea is usually acquired after adolescence, occurring most commonly in the 30s and 40s. Common pelvic conditions that cause secondary dysmenorrhea include endometriosis, chronic pelvic inflammatory disease, uterine leiomyomas, and adenomyosis. Because secondary dysmenorrhea is caused by multiple conditions, symptoms vary. However, a symptom shared in common is increasingly painful menses.[13]

Clinical Manifestations

Primary dysmenorrhea starts 12 to 24 hours before the onset of menses. The pain is most severe the first day of menses and rarely lasts more than 2 days.[11] Characteristic manifestations include lower abdominal pain that is colicky in nature, frequently radiating to the lower back and upper thighs. The abdominal pain is often accompanied by nausea, diarrhea or loose stools, fatigue, headache, and lightheadedness.

Secondary dysmenorrhea usually occurs after the woman has experienced problem-free periods for some time. The pain, which may be unilateral, is generally more constant in nature and usually continues longer than in primary dysmenorrhea.

Depending on the cause, symptoms such as dyspareunia (painful intercourse), painful defecation, or irregular bleeding, may occur at times other than menstruation.[13]

Collaborative Care

Evaluation begins with distinguishing primary from secondary dysmenorrhea. A complete health history with special attention to menstrual and gynecologic history and pelvic examination should be obtained. If the history reveals an onset shortly after menarche and symptoms only associated with menses in addition to normal pelvic examination findings, the probable diagnosis is primary dysmenorrhea. If any cause or etiology is evident, the diagnosis is secondary dysmenorrhea and further evaluation would be indicated by the possible diagnosis.

Nondrug treatment for primary dysmenorrhea includes heat applied to the lower abdomen or back and regular exercise. Regular exercise is thought to be beneficial because it may reduce endometrial hyperplasia and subsequently reduce prostaglandin production. The primary drug therapy is nonsteroidal antiinflammatory drugs (NSAIDs) such as ibuprofen. NSAIDs should be started at the first sign of menses and continued every 4 to 8 hours to maintain a sufficient level of the drug to inhibit prostaglandin synthesis for the usual duration of discomfort. Birth control pills provide another pharmacologic choice. Birth control pills can decrease dysmenorrhea by reducing the endometrial growth.

Acupuncture, exercise, and transcutaneous nerve stimulation provide varying degrees of relief. (See Chapter 8 for discussion of alternative therapies.) These methods may be used for women who obtain inadequate relief from medications or who prefer not to take medications. Patients who are unresponsive to these treatments should be evaluated for chronic pelvic pain.

Treatment of secondary dysmenorrhea depends on the cause. Some but not all individuals with secondary dysmenorrhea will be helped by the approaches used for primary dysmenorrhea. Additional drug or surgical intervention would relate to the underlying causes of dysmenorrhea.

NURSING MANAGEMENT: DYSMENORRHEA

Women often ask nurses what can be done for minor discomforts associated with menstrual cycles. They should be advised that during acute pain, relief may be obtained by lying down for short periods, drinking hot beverages, applying heat to the abdomen or back, and taking an antiinflammatory drug for mild analgesia. The nurse can also suggest noninvasive pain-relieving practices such as distraction and guided imagery.

Other health care measures can reduce the discomfort of dysmenorrhea. These include regular exercise, maintenance of proper nutritional habits, avoidance of constipation, maintenance of good body mechanics, and avoidance of stress and fatigue, particularly during the time preceding menstrual periods. Staying active and interested in activities may also help. Women should be taught why dysmenorrhea occurs as well as how to treat it. Education and supportive therapy can provide women with a foundation for coping with this common occurrence and increase feelings of control and self-reliance.

PROBLEMS RELATED TO VAGINAL BLEEDING

Irregular vaginal bleeding is a common gynecologic concern. Frequently occurring irregularities include *oligomenorrhea* (long intervals between menses), *secondary amenorrhea* (cessation of menses for at least 6 months), *menorrhagia* (excessive menstrual bleeding), and *metrorrhagia* (irregular bleeding or bleeding between menses). The cause of irregular bleeding may vary from anovulatory menstrual cycles to more serious causes such as ectopic pregnancy or endometrial cancer. The age of the woman provides direction for identifying the cause of bleeding. For example, a postmenopausal woman with irregular bleeding must always be evaluated for endometrial cancer but does not need to be evaluated for possible pregnancy. For a 20-year-old woman with irregular bleeding, the possibility of pregnancy must always be considered and the possibility of endometrial cancer would be very unlikely.

Irregular bleeding may be caused by dysfunction of the hypothalamic-pituitary-ovarian axis such as a pituitary adenoma. Changes in lifestyle such as marriage, recent moves, a death in the family, financial stress, and other emotional crises can cause such dysfunction. Because psychologic factors can influence endocrine function, they should be considered when the patient is evaluated.

Types of Irregular Bleeding

Oligomenorrhea and Secondary Amenorrhea. Anovulation is the most common cause for missing menses once pregnancy has been ruled out. Additional causes of amenorrhea are listed in Table 51-5. *Secondary amenorrhea* is cessation of menses after menses have occurred. *Primary amenorrhea* is not having menarche by age 16 years or by age 14 years if secondary sex characteristics are present.[13]

For several years following menarche and then before menopause, ovulation is often erratic. Thus oligomenorrhea resulting from anovulation is common for women at the beginning and end of menstruation. In anovulatory cycles, the corpus luteum that produces progesterone does not form. This may result in a situation referred to as unopposed estrogen. When estrogen is unopposed by progesterone, it can cause excessive build-up of the endometrium. Persistent overgrowth of the endometrium increases a woman's risk for endometrial cancer. To reduce this risk, progesterone or birth control pills are prescribed to ensure that the patient's endometrial lining is shed at least four to six times per year.

Menorrhagia. The excessive bleeding of menorrhagia may be increased duration (more than 7 days), increased amount (more than 80 ml), or both. Approximately 80% of menorrhagia is anovulatory uterine bleeding. Here, an unopposed estrogen state continues to build-up the endometrium until it becomes unstable, resulting in menorrhagia. For young women with excessive bleeding, clotting disorders should be considered. Uterine fibroids (leiomyomas) are a common cause of menorrhagia for women in their 30s and 40s.

Metrorrhagia. Metrorrhagia, also referred to as spotting or breakthrough bleeding, is bleeding between menstrual periods. For all reproductive age women, pregnancy complications such as spontaneous abortion or ectopic pregnancy must be considered as a possible cause. Other causes include

Table **51-5**	Causes of Amenorrhea

Hypothalamic-Pituitary Axis

Reversible CNS-mediated insults (e.g., emotional stress, anorexia nervosa or severe dieting, strenuous exercise, postpill syndrome, chronic or acute illness)

Prolactinoma and other causes of hyperprolactinemia (e.g., drugs)

Craniopharyngioma and other brainstem or parasellar tumors

Congenital conditions (e.g., isolated gonadotropin deficiency)*

Trauma (e.g., head injury with hypothalamic contusion)

Infiltrative processes (e.g., sarcoidosis)

Vascular disease (e.g., hypothalamic vasculitis)

Pituitary tumors

Sheehan's syndrome

Ovaries

Autoimmune disease (often involving thyroid, adrenal, and islet cells)

Premature menopause (idiopathic) or resistant-ovary syndrome

Polycystic ovary disease

Tumors

Congenital or genetic conditions (e.g., Turner's syndrome)*

Infection (e.g., mumps oophoritis)

Toxins (especially alkylating chemotherapeutic agents)

Radiation

Trauma, torsion (rare)

Uterovaginal Outflow Tract

Asherman's syndrome (postcurettage loss of endometrium)

Müllerian dysgenesis*

Hormonal Synthesis and Action

Male pseudohermaphroditism (e.g., testicular feminization)*

17-Hydroxylase deficiency*

*Usually presents as primary amenorrhea.
CNS, central nervous system.

cervical or endometrial polyps, infection, and carcinoma. Spotting is common during the first four cycles of birth control pills. If spotting continues past the woman's fourth cycle of pills, a different pill formulation can be prescribed when other causes of metrorrhagia have been ruled out. Spotting with long-acting progestin therapy is also common. For postmenopausal women, endometrial cancer must be considered whenever spotting is experienced. In postmenopausal women, exogenous estrogen administration during hormone replacement therapy is a common cause of metrorrhagia. *Menometrorrhagia* is excessive bleeding that occurs at irregular intervals. It may be caused by endometrial cancer or uterine fibroids.

Diagnostic Studies and Collaborative Care

Because irregular vaginal bleeding has multiple causes, diagnostic and collaborative care vary as well. A health history and physical examination directed at the most likely causes of vagi-

nal bleeding for the woman's age-group is the first step. These findings provide the basis for selecting the necessary laboratory tests and diagnostic procedures. Treatment depends on the nature of the problem (menorrhagia or amenorrhea), degree of threat to the patient's health, and whether children are desired in the future.

Birth control pills may be prescribed for a woman with amenorrhea to ensure regular shedding of endometrium if she also wants contraception. If she does not need birth control, progesterone may be prescribed to ensure a shedding of the endometrial lining four to six times per year. On the other hand, if she wants to become pregnant, a fertility drug may be prescribed.

The treatment goal for women with menorrhagia is to minimize further blood loss. If menorrhagia is the result of anovulatory cycles, the endometrium needs to be stabilized by a combination of oral estrogen and progesterone. This can usually be accomplished on an outpatient basis. With severe bleeding, hospitalization is indicated. All patients with menorrhagia should to be evaluated for anemia and treated as indicated.

Surgical Therapy. Surgery may be indicated depending on the underlying cause of the irregular vaginal bleeding. Dilation and curettage (D&C) was once a common therapy for excessive bleeding or for spotting in perimenopausal women. Now D&C is used only in extreme cases of bleeding or for older women when endometrial biopsy and ultrasonography have not provided the necessary diagnostic information.[11] Endometrial ablation done by laser or electrosurgical technique has been successful with 85% of patients with uncontrolled menorrhagia. If menorrhagia is caused by uterine fibroids, a hysterectomy may be performed or a *myomectomy,* removal of fibroids without removal of the uterus, may be performed if the patient wants to preserve her uterus.

NURSING MANAGEMENT:
IRREGULAR VAGINAL BLEEDING

For some women, infrequent or no menses might seem a desirable state. Educating women about characteristics of the menstrual cycle assists them to identify normal variations. Table 51-4 includes characteristics of the menstrual cycle and related patient education. This knowledge can help dispel apprehension and misconceptions. If the patient's menstrual cycle pattern does not fall within the range of normal, the nurse should urge her to visit her primary care provider. Myths concerning activities allowed during menstruation are common. The nurse should be prepared to clarify the facts. The patient should be assured that bathing and hair washing are safe. A daily warm tub bath may actually relieve some of the associated pelvic discomfort. Women can swim, exercise, have intercourse, and basically continue their usual daily activities.

Frequent changing of tampons or pads meets comfort and hygiene needs during menstruation. The selection of internal or external sanitary protection is a matter of personal preference. Tampons are convenient and make menstrual hygiene easier, whereas pads may provide better protection. Using a

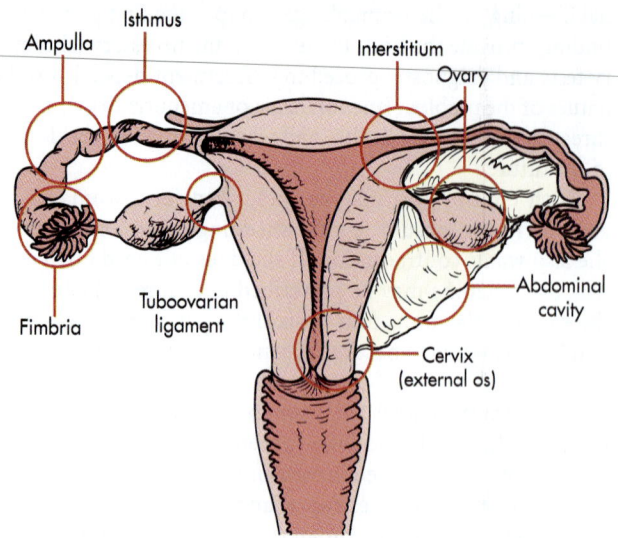

Fig. 51-4 Sites of implantation of ectopic pregnancies. Order of frequency of occurrence is ampulla, isthmus, interstitium, fimbria, tuboovarian ligament, ovary, abdominal cavity, and cervix (external os).

combination of tampons and pads and avoiding superabsorbent tampons may decrease the risk of *toxic shock syndrome* (TSS).[13] TSS is an acute condition caused by the toxin of *Staphylococcus aureus*. TSS causes high fever, vomiting, diarrhea, weakness, myalgia, and a sunburnlike rash.

Whenever excessive, the amount of the patient's vaginal bleeding should be assessed as accurately as possible. The number and size of pads or tampons used and the degree of saturation should be reported and recorded. The patient's fatigue level, along with variations in blood pressure and pulse, should be monitored because anemia and hypovolemia may be present. If a surgical procedure is indicated, the nurse should provide appropriate preoperative and postoperative care.

ECTOPIC PREGNANCY

An *ectopic pregnancy* is the implantation of the fertilized ovum anywhere outside the uterine cavity. Between 97% and 98% of ectopic pregnancies occur in the fallopian tube. The remaining 2% to 3% may be ovarian, abdominal, or cervical (Fig. 51-4). Ectopic pregnancy is a life-threatening condition. Earlier identification has contributed to a decrease in mortality. However, in the United States 40 to 50 deaths per year occur as a result of ectopic pregnancy, and ectopic pregnancy is the leading cause of maternal mortality among African-American women.[15] Any blockage of the tube or reduction of tubal peristalsis that impedes or delays the zygote passing to the uterine cavity can result in tubal implantation. Risk factors for ectopic pregnancy include a history of pelvic inflammatory disease, prior ectopic pregnancy, current progestin-releasing IUD, progestin-only birth control failure, and prior pelvic or tubal surgery.[15] Addi-

tional risk factors for ectopic pregnancy include procedures used in infertility treatment including in vitro fertilization procedures, embryo transfer, and ovulation induction. After implantation, the growth of the gestational sac expands the tubal wall until eventually the tube ruptures, causing acute peritoneal symptoms. Less acute symptoms usually begin by 6 to 8 weeks after the last normal menstrual period and weeks before rupture would occur.

Clinical Manifestations

The classic symptoms of ectopic pregnancy are abdominal or pelvic pain, missed menses, and irregular vaginal bleeding.[15] Pain is almost always present and caused by distention of the fallopian tube. It may start unilaterally and then spread to become bilateral. The character of the pain varies among women and can be colicky or vague. If tubal rupture occurs, the pain is intense and may be referred to the right shoulder because of irritation of the diaphragm by blood released into the abdominal cavity. With rupture, the risk of hemorrhage and hypovolemic shock is present. Suspected rupture is treated as an emergency.

More than 75% of women with an ectopic pregnancy realize they have missed their last menstrual period. Vaginal bleeding is most often spotting, but may be heavier and can be confused with menses. Irregular bleeding occurs in 75% of the women with ectopic pregnancy.

Diagnostic Studies

Because of the life-threatening nature of ectopic pregnancy, it should be considered whenever pregnancy is even remotely possible. Ectopic pregnancy can be a diagnostic challenge as a result of its similarity to other pelvic and abdominal disorders, such as salpingitis, spontaneous abortion, ruptured ovarian cyst, appendicitis, and peritonitis. A sensitive serum pregnancy test should be performed. If the test is negative, an ectopic pregnancy is highly unlikely. If ectopic pregnancy cannot be excluded by the pregnancy test, further evaluation is warranted. If the patient is in a stable condition, a combination of serial beta-human chorionic gonadotropin (β-hCG) and vaginal ultrasonography is used. In a normal pregnancy, β-hCG is expected to double about every 48 hours. If the β-hCG level fails to double, the patient may have an ectopic pregnancy. Ultrasound can be used to confirm the presence of an intrauterine pregnancy once the β-hCG level has reached 2000 mIU/ml.

Absence of a normal intrauterine pregnancy means that the diagnosis is very likely spontaneous abortion or ectopic pregnancy. With a spontaneous abortion, serial β-hCG levels decrease over time. Women with bleeding in pregnancy should have their Rh status determined with appropriate follow-up if Rh negative. A complete blood count is obtained when there is any concern regarding the amount of blood loss or if surgery is contemplated. A gradually decreasing hematocrit may indicate internal bleeding.

Collaborative Care

Surgery remains the primary approach for treating ectopic pregnancies and should be performed immediately. However, medical management with methotrexate is being used with increasing success with patients who are hemodynamically stable and have an adnexal mass less than 3 cm in size. The most conservative surgical approach is used to limit damage to the reproductive system as much as possible. Therefore removal of the pregnancy from the tube is preferred to removing the tube. Laparoscopy is preferable to laparotomy, since it decreases blood loss and the hospital stay.[15] If the patient is unstable, as may happen with tubal rupture, conservative surgical approaches may not be possible. Further, the patient may need a blood transfusion and supplemental IV fluid therapy to relieve shock and restore a satisfactory blood volume for safe anesthesia and surgery. The use of microsurgery techniques has resulted in fewer repeated ectopic pregnancies and a higher rate of future successful pregnancies.

NURSING MANAGEMENT: ECTOPIC PREGNANCY

Nursing care depends on the condition of the patient. Before the diagnosis has been confirmed the nurse should be alert to signs of increasing pain and vaginal bleeding, which may indicate that rupture of the tube has occurred. Vital signs are monitored closely, along with observation for signs of shock. Explanations and preparation for diagnostic procedures are given when appropriate. Preparation of the patient for abdominal surgery may follow rapidly. The patient's emotional status should be assessed. Reassurance and support for the surgery should be given to both the patient and her family. Postoperatively, the patient may express a fear of future ectopic pregnancies and have many questions about the impact of this experience on her future fertility.

PERIMENOPAUSE AND POSTMENOPAUSE

The *perimenopause* is a normal life transition that begins with the first signs of change in menstrual cycles and ends 6 to 12 months after menopause. *Menopause* is the single day that marks the last naturally occurring menstrual period. The date of the last menses is determined in retrospect, when a woman has not had a period for 12 months. The average age when natural menopause occurs is 50 years. However, wide variation exists, and menopause during a woman's fourth decade would not be considered premature.[13] *Artificial menopause* results from surgical removal of both ovaries or may occur as a side effect of radiation, chemotherapy, and certain drugs, particularly drugs that inhibit gonadotropin-releasing hormone (e.g., leuprolide [Lupron]). *Postmenopause* refers to any time after menopause.

Changes in the ovary start the cascade of events that finally result in menopause. The regression of the follicles within each ovary begins with puberty and accelerates after age 35 years. With age, fewer and fewer follicles remain that are responsive to follicle-stimulating hormone (FSH). FSH normally stimulates the dominant follicle to secrete estrogen. When the follicles can no longer respond to FSH, ovarian production of estrogen and progesterone decline. However, perimenopausal women can get pregnant until menopause has occurred.

Table 51-6	Signs and Symptoms of Estrogen Deficiency

Vasomotor
   Hot flashes
Genitourinary
   Atrophic vaginitis
   Dyspareunia secondary to poor lubrication
   Incontinence
Psychologic
   Emotional lability
   Change in sleep pattern
   Decreased REM sleep
Skeletal
   Increased fracture rate, particularly of vertebral bodies but also of humerus, distal radius, and upper femur
Cardiovascular
   Decreased high-density lipoproteins (HDL)
   Increased low-density lipoproteins (LDL)
Dermatologic
   Diminished collagen content of skin
   Breast tissue changes

REM, rapid eye movement.

Clinical Manifestations

The perimenopause is a time of erratic hormonal fluctuation. Thus irregular vaginal bleeding is common. With decreasing estrogen, hot flashes and other symptoms begin. The signs and symptoms of diminished estrogen are listed in Table 51-6. Postmenopause is associated with changes in bone density, lipid levels, and skin as discussed in Chapter 48. The loss of estrogen plays a significant role in the cause of age-related alterations. Changes most critical to a woman's well-being are the increased risks for coronary artery disease and osteoporosis secondary to bone density loss. Other changes include a redistribution of fat, a tendency to gain weight more easily, muscle and joint pain, loss of skin elasticity, changes in hair amount and distribution, and atrophy of external genitalia and breast tissue.

Hallmarks of the perimenopause are hot flashes and irregular menses. *Vasomotor* instability (hot flash) is described as a sensation of warmth in the upper part of the chest, neck, and face followed by profuse perspiration and sometimes chilling. These sensations last from several seconds to 5 minutes and occur most often at night, thereby disturbing sleep. Hot flashes can be triggered by situations that affect body temperature, such as eating a hot meal, hot weather, drinking an alcoholic beverage, stress, or warm clothing.

Atrophic vaginal changes secondary to decreased estrogen include thinning of the vaginal mucosa and disappearance of rugae. Vaginal secretions also decrease and become more alkaline. Because of these changes, the vagina is easily traumatized and susceptible to infection. Dyspareunia may also occur.

Atrophic changes in the lower urinary tract also occur with a decrease in estrogen. Bladder capacity decreases and the bladder and urethral tissue lose tone. These changes can cause symptoms that mimic a bladder infection (dysuria, urgency, frequency) when no infection is present.

Whether decreasing estrogen is responsible for the psychologic changes associated with perimenopause is not clear.[16] The attributed depression, irritability, and cognitive problems could result from life stressors or sleep deprivation from hot flashes. Studies conducted in both Canada and the United States have not found a statistically significant relationship between perimenopause and depression.[16] Other studies have found that women who are most likely to be depressed believe depression is related to menopause, are concerned about menopause and aging, or have a previous history of depression or unemployment.

Collaborative Care

Educating women about perimenopausal changes is essential. Women need to be told what to expect and options for symptom management. The advantages and risks of hormone therapy should be discussed thoroughly. This discussion needs to include the individual woman's risks and benefits based on her family and personal medical history. As long as no absolute contraindications exist for hormone therapy, it should be the woman's choice whether or not she takes hormone replacement therapy.

The diagnosis of perimenopause should be made only after careful consideration of other possible causes for the woman's symptoms. Depression, thyroid dysfunction, anemia, or anxiety reactions could be responsible for the same symptoms. Because of the erratic hormonal fluctuations before menopause, routine testing of the serum FSH level is not indicated. After age 50 years, postmenopause can be diagnosed by an FSH of 30 mIU/ml or greater if the woman is not on any hormonal medication.[13]

Nonhormonal Therapy. The frequency and severity of hot flashes can be reduced by avoiding things that increase heat production and by promoting heat loss. Keeping a cool environment as well as reducing caffeine and alcohol intake reduce heat production. Behavioral changes, such as slowing down and reducing tension with relaxation techniques, also help. To promote heat loss at night when hot flashes can disrupt sleep, increase air circulation in the room and avoid bedding that traps the heat such as heavy quilts. Loose fitting clothes do not retain body heat as well as clothes with tight necks and wrists. Cool cloths applied to flushed areas also aid heat loss. Daily Vitamin E in doses up to 600 IU is reported to reduce hot flashes.[17]

Skin and urogenital changes may be self managed by nonhormonal approaches. Dry skin can be improved by reducing the use of soap and the number of showers or baths and using body lotions. Stress incontinence can be decreased with the practice of Kegel exercises. Dyspareunia related to vaginal dryness can be managed with a water-soluble lubricant.

Symptoms of anxiety or depression can be reduced by improving nutrition, exercise, and sleep. For better sleep, alcohol and sleep-interfering drugs should be avoided and techniques employed to reduce hot flashes. Employing techniques to decrease stress also decreases depression and anxiety.

Hormonal Therapy. Significant beneficial effects are associated with postmenopausal hormonal therapy. Initially, the regimen involved estrogen alone, so it was called estrogen replacement therapy (ERT). Concern about the increased risk of endometrial cancer with unopposed estrogen led to development of replacement therapy with estrogen and progesterone. This regimen is referred to as hormone replacement therapy (HRT). Some HRT regimens include low-dose testosterone to increase libido.[18] Women using ERT or HRT have a decrease in heart disease, which is a reason to use HRT even when the woman does not have vasomotor instability. HRT also helps to retard bone loss and prevent osteoporosis. HRT also minimizes atrophic changes to the genitourinary tissues.[11] There is some evidence to suggest that estrogen replacement in women may reduce the risk of Alzheimer's disease.[19]

Whether women on ERT or HRT have an increased risk for breast cancer is still controversial.[11] Known or suspected breast cancer is a contraindication to estrogen use.[13] Long-term use of ERT increases the risk for endometrial cancer, but this increased risk is eliminated with 12 or more days of progesterone per month. The risk for endometrial cancer is present only in those women who still have a uterus. Some women have an increase in their hyperlipidemia with progesterone. However, this is not a contraindication to HRT. The lowest dose of progesterone should be used and serum lipid levels monitored. Women have increased cardiovascular benefit from estrogen replacement, and the addition of progesterone does not decrease the cardioprotective effects of estrogen.

In addition to known or suspected breast cancer, other absolute contraindications for HRT include abnormal vaginal bleeding, pregnancy, active thrombophlebitis or thromboembolic disorder, and current liver dysfunction.[13] Whether a personal history of breast cancer and/or a family history of breast cancer are contraindications for HRT remains controversial. HRT is not contraindicated for women who smoke cigarettes or who have diabetes mellitus.

HRT may be started before menopause to control hot flashes and changes related to decreased estrogen. In the absence of menopausal symptoms, HRT is initiated as soon as possible after menopause to achieve the maximum health benefits. Many different regimens of HRT are available, including continuous combined estrogen and progesterone therapy to various sequential and cyclic patterns. The choice of HRT regimen should be tailored to the individual woman. Factors for consideration include her concern about cancer, previously used regimens and side effects, tolerance of hormonal side effects, and presence of perimenopausal symptoms.

The side effects of estrogen include nausea, fluid retention, headache, and breast enlargement. Side effects of progesterone include increased appetite, weight gain, irritability, depression, spotting, and breast tenderness. To minimize these unwanted side effects, the lowest possible but still beneficial dose of each should be used.

Protective effects from estrogen are achieved by 0.625 mg of conjugated estrogen (Premarin) daily. For symptom relief, a higher dose may be needed. To receive a protective benefit of progesterone, 5 to 10 mg of medroxyprogesterone (Provera) is indicated for 12 days of each month on a cyclic regimen or 2.5 mg if a continuous regimen. If the estrogen needs to be increased for symptom relief, the progesterone should also be increased. Other forms of progesterone include norethindrone (Aygestin) and micronized progesterone (Prometrium).[13] Estrogen comes in a variety of forms: oral tablets, vaginal creams, dermal patches, rings placed around the cervix, and subcutaneous pellets. Vaginal creams are especially useful for urogenital symptoms. Transdermal (skin patches) estrogen has the advantage of bypassing the liver but the disadvantage of causing skin irritation.

A new class of drugs called SERMS (selective estrogen receptor modulators) are now available. These drugs have some of the positive benefits of estrogen, such as preventing bone loss, without the negative effects such as endometrial hyperplasia. Raloxifene (Evista) is a nonsteroidal drug that competes with estrogen for estrogen receptor sites and decreases bone loss and serum cholesterol but has minimal effects on breast and uterine tissue. These drugs are also discussed with respect to their potential role in the management of osteoporosis in Chapter 59.

Nutritional Therapy.   Good nutrition can decrease the risk of cardiovascular disease and osteoporosis in addition to assisting with vasomotor symptoms. A daily intake of about 30 kcal/kg body weight with maintenance of sound nutrition is recommended. A decrease in metabolic rate and careless eating habits rather than menopause itself can be the cause for weight gain and related fatigue. An adequate intake of calcium and vitamin D can help maintain healthy bones and thereby counteract the effect of decreased estrogen that makes bones become lighter and more fragile. Postmenopausal women should have a daily calcium intake of 1200 to 1500 mg. Calcium supplements are best absorbed when taken with meals. Either dietary calcium or calcium supplements may be used.

The diet should be high in complex carbohydrates and Vitamin B complex, especially B_6. Phytoestrogens from plant sources have been shown to be beneficial in some women.[20] Examples of foods containing phytoestrogens include soy, tofu, chickpeas, and sunflower seeds.

NURSING MANAGEMENT: PERIMENOPAUSE

Nurses can play a key role in helping women to understand perimenopausal changes and their options to minimize unwanted symptoms and decrease their risk for cardiovascular disease and osteoporosis. Nurses can foster a positive image of perimenopause as a time of vitality and attractiveness. Perimenopause can provide women with an incentive to enhance self-care.

Nurses should provide health education teaching and reassurance to perimenopausal women distraught by their symptoms. The woman should be taught that the symptoms are normal and only temporary. Nondrug approaches to managing symptoms should be taught. Any misconceptions about menopause and HRT should be clarified by the nurse to reduce unnecessary anxiety. The decision to use HRT is personal. The nurse should support a woman's decision not to take HRT by discussing alternative ways (e.g., diet and exercise) to manage symptoms related to decreasing estrogen.

A regular program of exercise and physical activity can improve circulation, maintain good muscle tone, and delay some aspects of aging for postmenopausal women. Exercising for 20 to 60 minutes at least three times a week stimulates osteoblastic activity, thereby stimulating calcium deposition into bone and delaying osteoporosis.

Sexual function can continue with little change in the vast majority of postmenopausal women. Cessation of menstrua-

tion and ability to bear children should not be equated with cessation of sexual capability. Femininity and libido do not disappear with menopause. Atrophic changes in vaginal epithelium associated with decreased estrogen may lead to dyspareunia (painful coitus). A water-soluble lubricant (e.g., Replens, Astroglide) is often effective in managing this problem. An active sex life helps increase lubrication and maintain the pliability of vaginal tissues. The patient should be given an opportunity to candidly discuss concerns related to sexual functioning.

The nurse should be alert to the risks, benefits, and possible side effects of the drugs that the patient is taking and should be able to explain them for the patient. Hormonal therapy may be continued indefinitely as part of a plan to prevent the development or worsening of osteoporosis.

RAPE

Rape is defined as any nonconsensual sexual act. Violence against women is a significant health and societal problem. Within the United States, one out of every eight adult women has been forcibly raped sometime in her life.[16] Because over 80% of adult women are raped by an acquaintance or intimate partner, rape is one of the most underreported crimes. Also, women may not report rape because they fear that they would not be able to withstand the stresses of prosecution or that they would be met with disbelief and humiliation from the police, the medical staff, or their peers.

Changes in residency and place of employment may occur as a consequence of the experience because of fear or inability to maintain previous relationships. Rape trauma dramatically disrupts the homemaking and parenting roles normally performed by the adult woman. The survivor's partner and family have a tremendous potential for both negative and positive influence. They can revictimize her and increase her burden in resolving the rape, or they can provide her with support and find support themselves in resolving a shared crisis.

Clinical Manifestations

Physical.   Of the rape survivors who seek help immediately after the assault, between one half and two thirds will not have any evidence of physical trauma.[16] Evidence of trauma may be limited because women do not resist for fear of physical danger and injury. When present, physical injuries may include bruising and lacerations to the perineum, hymen, vulva, vagina, cervix, and anus. In general, the more serious injuries involve nongenital areas, such as the face, neck, and extremities, and often occur after the rape. Fractures, subdural hematomas, cerebral concussions, and intraabdominal injuries have resulted in the need for hospitalization. Sexual assault also places women at risk for STDs and pregnancy.

Psychologic.   Immediately after the assault, women are often in a state of crisis. They may show shock, numbness, denial, or withdrawal. Some women may seem unnaturally calm; others may be crying or expressing anger.[16] Then feelings of humiliation, degradation, embarrassment, anger, self-blame, and fear of another assault are commonly expressed. These symptoms usually decrease after 2 weeks, and survivors may appear to have adjusted. Yet any time from 2 to 3 weeks

✚ EMERGENCY MANAGEMENT

Table 51-7 Sexual Assault

Etiology	Assessment Findings	Interventions
Sexual molestation Sodomy Assault involving genitalia (male or female) without consent	• Emotional or physical manifestations of shock • Hysteria • Crying • Anger • Silence • Decreased level of consciousness • Hyperventilation • Oral, vaginal, and rectal injuries • Extragenital injuries • Pain in genital area or extragenital area	**Initial** • Treat shock and other urgent medical problems, (e.g., head injury, hemorrhage, wounds, fractures). • Assess emotional state. • Contact support person (i.e., social worker, rape advocate, sexual assault nurse examiner). • Do *not* clean the patient until all evidence is collected. Make sure the patient does not wash, douche, urinate, brush teeth, or gargle. • Place sheet on floor. Then have patient stand on sheet to remove clothing. Place sheet with clothing in paper bag. • Obtain forensic evidence per local protocol (i.e., body hair, nail scrapings, tissue, dried semen, vaginal washing, blood samples). • Maintain chain of evidence for all legal specimens. Clearly label evidence and keep in locked cabinet until given to law enforcement agency. • Obtain baseline HIV, syphilis, and other STD screening. • Determine method of contraception, date of last menstrual period, and date of last tetanus immunization. • Consider tetanus prophylactis if lacerations contain soil/dirt. • Vaccinate against Hepatitis B. **Ongoing Monitoring** • Monitor vital signs and emotional status. • Provide clothing as needed. • Counsel patient regarding confidential HIV and STD testing.

to months after the assault, symptoms may return and become more severe. About 50% of women are clinically depressed. Many women experience psychologic effects for 2 years. Suicidal ideation may occur during this time.

Some rape survivors have long-term psychologic problems. The rape trauma syndrome is a classification of posttraumatic stress disorder. Flashbacks, intrusive recall, sleep disturbances, and numbing of feelings are common initial symptoms. Women feel embarrassment, self-blame, and powerlessness. Later symptoms include mood swings, irritability, and anger. Feelings of despair, shame, and hopelessness are often the cause of the anger.[16] These feelings may be internalized and expressed as depression.

Collaborative Care

In the acute care of a rape survivor, ensuring the woman's emotional and physical safety has the highest priority. Other care includes prevention of STDs and pregnancy, collecting evidence for possible prosecution, and arranging both initial and long-term follow-up.[11] The patient's immediate and long-term need for emotional support is given special consideration. Table 51-7 outlines the emergency management of the patient who has been sexually assaulted. Most emergency departments (ED) have identified personnel who have received special train-

ing in order to work with women who have been raped. Special procedures are followed in taking the history and conducting the examination in order to preserve all evidence in case of future prosecution.

When the survivor of a rape is admitted to the ED or clinic, a specific chain of events occurs (Table 51-8). A signed informed consent is obtained from the woman before any data are collected. All materials gathered are well documented, labeled, and given to the appropriate person, such as the pathologist or a police officer. The materials are handled by as few people as possible, and signatures of all responsible for keeping and handling the data are obtained. Many items can be used as evidence if the victim chooses to file a complaint. Consequently, the integrity of the material must be maintained. The nurse's involvement in the medicolegal process depends on the policies of the individual institution and state law.

A gynecologic and sexual history and an account of the assault (who, what, when, and where), as well as a general physical and pelvic examination, add further information about the rape incident. Laboratory tests are done primarily to determine the presence of sperm in the vagina and to identify any existing STDs or pregnancy. The woman's physical injuries are attended to and prophylaxis for STDs, tetanus, hepatitis B, and pregnancy are administered.

| Table **51-8** | **Checklist for Evaluation for Alleged Rape** |

1. Medicolegal
Valid written consent for examination, photographs, laboratory tests, release of information, and laboratory samples
Appropriate "chain of evidence" documentation

2. History
History of assault (who, what, when, where)
Penetration, ejaculation, extragenital acts
Activities since assault (e.g., changed clothes, bathed, douched)
Inquire about safety
Menstrual and contraceptive history
Medical history
Emotional status
Current symptoms

3. General Physical Examination
Vital signs and general appearance
Extragenital trauma—mouth, breasts, neck
Cuts, bruises, scratches (photograph taken)

4. Pelvic Examination
Vulvar trauma, erythema; hymen, anal, and rectal status
Matted hairs or free hairs
Vaginal examination with unlubricated speculum for discharge, blood, lacerations
Uterine size
Adnexa, especially hematomas

5. Laboratory Samples
Vaginal vault content sampling
Vaginal smears—microscope evaluation for trichomonads and semen
Oral or rectal swabs and smears, if indicated
Blood samples—VDRL serology, pregnancy test; serologic testing for HIV and hepatitis B infection
Freeze serum sample for later testing
Cultures—cervix and other areas (if indicated) for gonorrhea and chlamydia
Fingernail scrapings
Pubic hair scrapings
Clipping of matted pubic hairs

6. Treatment
Care of injuries and emotional trauma
Antibiotic prophylaxis for venereal disease, if appropriate; ceftriaxone 250 mg IM followed by doxycycline 100 mg PO bid for 7 days
Protection against pregnancy if any risk with Ovral 2 tabs PO within 72 hr of rape and 2 tabs PO 12 hr later
Protection of legal rights
Recommendation of continued follow-up and services of rape crisis center
Repetition of gonorrhea and chlamydial culture 14-21 days later; consider herpes culture
Repetition of serologic testing for HIV and hepatitis B 8-12 wk later
Pregnancy test if appropriate

VDRL, Venereal Disease Research Laboratory.

The health care provider cannot legally state that rape occurred. However, the provider can swear that the findings show that sexual intercourse took place and describe any injury that was inflicted. These findings, along with others such as the police report and examination of the rape scene, can form the foundation for the rapist's conviction.

Follow-up physical and psychologic care is essential. Women should return weekly for the first month following the rape. This includes the time period when women's psychologic reactions may be the most severe.[16] Providers should have the telephone numbers and names of contact persons for local resources for rape survivors, including rape crisis centers, legal and law enforcement authorities, and human services. Follow-up for physical concerns should include a pregnancy test in 2 to 3 weeks. Testing for HIV, syphilis, and hepatitis B may be done at 6 weeks. The HIV test and any other indicated tests should be repeated 3 to 6 months after the rape.

NURSING MANAGEMENT: RAPE

Nurses can assist all women in becoming aware of rape prevention tactics (Table 51-9). They should also be encouraged to learn some basic techniques of self-defense. Local high schools and the YWCA usually have self-defense classes in which formal

PATIENT TEACHING GUIDE

| Table **51-9** | **Rape Prevention** |

1. See that there are lights at all entrances to your home.
2. Keep your doors locked and do not open them to a stranger; ask for identification if a service person comes to the door.
3. Do not advertise that you live alone; list only your initials with your last name in the telephone directory or on the mailbox; never reveal to a caller that you are home alone.
4. Avoid walking alone in deserted areas; walk to the parking lot with a friend; be sure you see each other leave.
5. Have your keys ready as you approach your car or home.
6. Keep all doors locked and windows up when driving.
7. Never get on an elevator with a suspicious person; pretend you have forgotten something and get off.
8. Say what you mean in social situations; be sure your voice and body language reflect your response.
9. Carry a loud whistle and use it when you think you are in danger.
10. Yell "fire" if you are attacked and run toward a lighted area.

instruction is given. Practicing the various techniques with a friend builds a woman's confidence in her ability to fight back. Learning self-defense can make the woman less vulnerable and more self-reliant.

When a rape survivor is brought to the clinic or emergency room, she should be given the highest priority for care and treatment. A quiet, private area should be used for the initial assessment and the examinations that follow. The patient should not be left alone. Whenever possible, the same nurse should remain with her throughout her stay and provide needed emotional support. The patient's actions and words as she describes the rape incident may be inconsistent, confused, and inappropriate. The nurse should maintain a nonjudgmental attitude.

The patient usually has many feelings and thoughts about the rape and generally wants to talk about them to an interested listener. Talking may help the patient feel better and gain understanding of her reactions to the incident. When the nurse listens carefully, the patient feels that she is not alone and is better able to gain control over the situation.

The nurse should assess the patient's stress level before preparing her for the various procedures that follow. The patient's coping mechanisms are supported when she knows what to expect and what is expected of her, as well as why the particular procedure must be done. Because the pelvic examination may trigger a flashback of the rape, the nurse should answer all related questions before the examination and be a supportive presence during the examination.

Following the examinations, the patient's physical comfort needs should be considered. She may need safety pins or needle and thread for her torn clothing or a cool drink to relieve her thirst. Most women who have been raped feel dirty and would appreciate a place to wash as well as use of mouthwash, especially if oral sex was involved.

The nurse can also further emphasize and elaborate on any prescribed treatment. The patient's understanding of the possible side effects of the medications given should be assessed. The patient is urged to see her own primary care provider if care was given elsewhere. The importance of follow-up should be emphasized. Many rape survivors are unaware of the availability of financial compensation (a law in most states) and appreciate information about the application process. This compensation is to assist them in paying for emergency services and for emotional injuries that may temporarily interfere with their ability to work.

When the patient is discharged, the nurse should make certain the patient has transportation home. If friends or family members are not available, the hospital or clinic should make arrangements with an appropriate community resource. The patient should not be sent home alone.

Many communities today have rape crisis centers. These public service organizations have trained professional and nonprofessional volunteers who provide an emotional support system for rape survivors on request. Their programs provide advocacy to ensure dignified treatment throughout the medical and police procedures, short-term counseling for the woman and her family, and court assistance and public education on rape-related issues. The nurse should be able to give the patient the names and local telephone numbers of such organizations.

CONDITIONS OF THE VULVA, VAGINA, AND CERVIX

Etiology and Pathophysiology

Infection and inflammation of the vagina, cervix, and vulva tend to occur when the natural defenses of the acidic vaginal secretions (maintained by sufficient estrogen levels) and the presence of *Lactobacillus* are disrupted. The woman's resistance may also be decreased as a result of aging, poor nutrition, and the use of drugs that alter the mucosa. Organisms gain entrance to the areas through contaminated hands, clothing, and douche nozzles and during intercourse, surgery, and childbirth. Table 51-10 relates the specific etiologic factors, clinical manifestations and diagnostic methods, and collaborative care of common inflammations and infections.

Most lower genital tract infections are related to sexual intercourse. Intercourse can transmit organisms, injure tissues, and alter the acid-base balance of the vagina. All of these increase risk for inflammations or infections such as bacterial vaginosis or chlamydial cervicitis. Vulvar infections caused by viruses such as herpes and genital warts can be sexually transmitted when no lesions are apparent. Drugs such as oral contraceptives, antibiotics, and corticosteroids may produce changes in the vagina and trigger an overgrowth of the organisms present. For example, *Candida albicans* may be present in small numbers in the vagina. An overgrowth of this organism causes yeast vaginitis.

Clinical Manifestations

Abnormal vaginal discharge and vulvar lesions are the two main classifications of clinical manifestations. Cervicitis and vaginal problems may be accompanied by an abnormal vaginal discharge. In addition to a thick, white, curdy discharge, women with monilial vaginitis often experience intense itching and dysuria, which is the result of urine coming into contact with fissures and irritated areas on the vulva. The hallmark of bacterial vaginosis is the fishy odor of the discharge. Women with cervicitis may notice spotting after intercourse.

Common vulvar lesions include herpes infection and genital warts. Initial or primary herpes infections may be extremely painful and tender, or they may go unnoticed. Herpes begins as a small vesicle followed by superficial red ulcers. Most herpes lesions are painful. Dysuria is common when urine touches the lesion. Genital warts, caused by the human papillomavirus (HPV), vary in appearance. Irregularly shaped "cauliflower" type lesions are common. Genital warts are painless unless traumatized. (See Chapter 50 for discussion of STDs.)

Older women may develop vulvar dystrophies including lichen sclerosis and squamous cell hyperplasia.[11] These conditions are associated with intense itching. The lesions are white initially although scratching in response to itching produces changes in the appearance.

Collaborative Care

Genital problems are evaluated by performing a history and physical examination and obtaining the appropriate laboratory and diagnostic studies. Since many problems may be related to sexual activity, a sexual history is essential. The nature of the problem directs specific aspects of the evaluation. A herpes culture should be taken of any ulcerative lesions. A blood test for syphilis may be done when ulcerative lesions are present. Gen-

Table **51-10**   Infections of the Lower Genital Tract

Infection/Etiology	Clinical Manifestations and Diagnostic Methods	Drug Management

■ Monilial vaginitis
  Candida albicans
  (fungus)
	Commonly found in mouth, gastrointestinal tract, and vagina; pruritus, thick white curd-like discharge; KOH microscopic examination—pseudohyphae; pH 4.0-4.7.	Antifungal agents (e.g., Monistat, Gyne-Lotrimin, Mycelex [available over the counter]) available in cream or suppository.

■ Trichomoniasis
  Trichomonas vaginalis
  (protozoa)
	Sexually transmitted; pruritus, frothy greenish or gray discharge; hemorrhagic spots on cervix or vaginal walls; saline microscopic examination—swimming trichomonads; pH 5.0-7.0.	Metronidazole (Flagyl) orally in single dose for patient and partner.

■ Bacterial vaginosis
  Gardnerella vaginalis
  Corynebacterium vaginale
	Watery discharge with fishy odor; may or may not have other symptoms; saline microscopic examination—epithelial cells; pH 5.0-5.5.	Sexually transmitted; metronidazole (Flagyl) 500 mg orally or clindamycin (Cleocin) 300 mg orally bid for 7 days; examine and treat partner.

■ Cervicitis
  Chlamydia trachomatis
  Neisseria gonorrhoeae
  Staphylococcus aureus
	Sexually transmitted; mucopurulent discharge with postcoital spotting from cervical inflammation; culture for chlamydia and gonorrhea.	Azithromycin (Zithromax) PO single dose or Doxycycline PO bid for 7 days and Ciprofloxacin (Cipro) PO single dose or Cefriaxone (Rocephin) IM in single dose. Treat partners with same drugs.

■ Severe recurrent vaginitis
  Candida albicans
  (most often)
	May be indication of HIV infection; all women who are unresponsive to first-line treatment should be counseled and offered HIV testing.	Drug appropriate to opportunistic organism.

ital warts are usually identified by their clinical appearance. Vulva dystrophies may be examined using a colposcope and biopsies taken for diagnosis.

Problems involving vaginal discharge are evaluated by microscopy and cultures. The most common vaginal conditions (bacterial vaginosis, monilial vaginitis, and trichomoniasis) are diagnosed by a procedure called a wet mount. The findings characteristic of each condition are shown in Table 51-10. To assess for cervicitis, endocervical cultures are obtained for chlamydia and gonorrhea. If purulent discharge is observed coming from the cervix, a sample of endocervical cells may be taken to conduct a Gram stain. The gram-stained slide is examined on high power to identify white blood cells and any intracellular gram-negative diplococci (indicative of gonorrhea). STDs are discussed in Chapter 50.

Drug therapy is based on the diagnosis and is shown in Table 51-10.[21] Antibiotics taken as directed will cure bacterial infections. Antifungal preparations, usually creams, are indicated for monilial vaginitis. Women with vaginal conditions or cervical infection should abstain from intercourse for at least 1 week. Douching should be avoided. Douching disrupts the normal protective mechanisms within the vagina and may increase the number of pathogens and move them higher into the genital tract. Sexual partners must be evaluated and treated if the patient is diagnosed with trichomoniasis or cervicitis.

Viral infections such as herpes and genital warts cannot be cured. Systemic antiviral drugs may reduce the duration and severity of recurrent herpes outbreaks. Nondrug measures such as wearing loose fitting clothes and sitz baths may decrease discomfort. Many women with visible genital warts want them removed for cosmetic reasons. Application of liquid nitrogen is a common treatment. Women with genital warts or those who have partners with genital warts are advised to get annual Pap tests. The reason for this is that certain subtypes of the wart virus appear to cause cervical cancer.

Pharmacologic treatment of vulvar dystrophies is symptomatic because no cures are available. Treatment involves controlling the itching and hence the scratching. Interrupting the "itch-scratch cycle" prevents further secondary damage to the skin. Women should be monitored annually for squamous cell cancer, since it also presents as a vulvar lesion.

NURSING MANAGEMENT: CONDITIONS OF THE VULVA, VAGINA, AND CERVIX

Nurses have the opportunity to educate women about common genital conditions and about how they can reduce their risks. Understanding the symptoms that may indicate a problem helps women seek care in a timely manner. Matters involving genitals or sexual intercourse are frequently difficult for people to discuss. The nurse's nonjudgmental attitude in providing information allows women to feel more comfortable and ask the questions that may be especially worrisome.

When a woman is diagnosed with cervicitis or a vaginal or vulvar condition, nurses should ensure that the patient fully understands the directions for treatment. Taking the full course of medication is especially important to decrease the chance of relapse. Because genitals are such a private area, use of graphs and models is especially helpful for patient teaching. When a woman is using a vaginal medication such as an antifungal

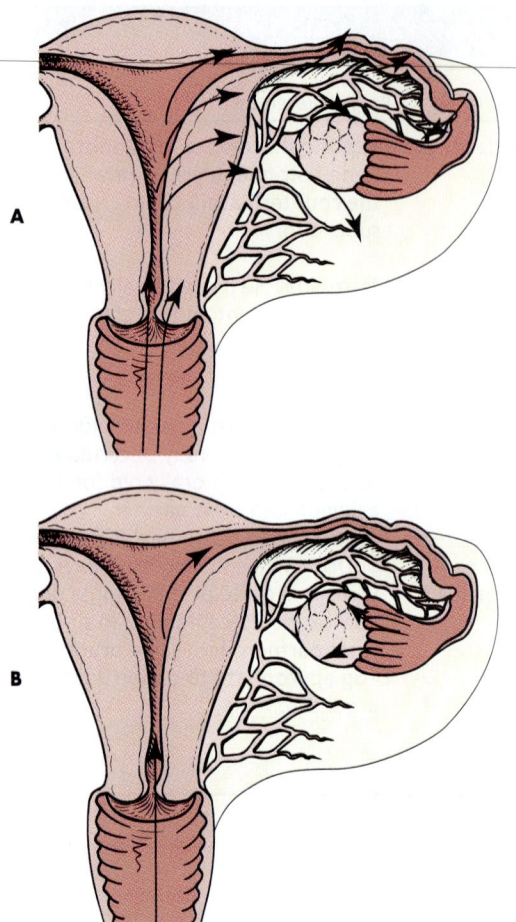

Fig. 51-5 Common routes of the spread of pelvic inflammatory disease. **A,** Direct spread of bacterial infection other than *Neisseria gonorrhoeae.* **B,** Direct spread of *Neisseria gonorrhoeae.*

cream for the first time, showing her the applicator and how to fill it is important. The woman should be taught where and how the applicator should be inserted using visual aids or models. Vaginal creams should be inserted before going to bed so that the medication remains in the vagina for a long period of time. Women using vaginal creams or suppositories may wish to use panty liners during the day, when the residual medication may drain out.

PELVIC INFLAMMATORY DISEASE

Pelvic inflammatory disease (PID) is an infectious condition of the pelvic cavity that may involve infection of the fallopian tubes (salpingitis), ovaries (oophoritis), and pelvic peritoneum (peritonitis). A tuboovarian abscess may also form. PID is referred to as "silent" when women do not perceive any symptoms. Other women with PID are in acute distress.

Etiology and Pathophysiology

PID is often the result of untreated cervicitis. The organism infecting the cervix ascends higher into the uterus, fallopian tubes, ovaries, and peritoneal cavity (Fig. 51-5). *Chlamydia trachomatis* or *Neisseria gonorrhoeae* are the most common

causative organisms of PID. These organisms, as well as mycoplasma, streptococci, and anaerobes, may gain entrance during sexual intercourse or after pregnancy termination, pelvic surgery, or childbirth. It is important to remember that not all PID is the result of STDs.

Women at increased risk for chlamydial infections (i.e., those women younger than 24 years of age and having multiple sex partners or a new sex partner) should be routinely tested for chlamydia. Chlamydial infections can be asymptomatic and so unknowingly transmitted during intercourse. Even silent PID can cause damage that cannot be reversed. PID remains a major cause of female infertility.

Clinical Manifestations

Women with PID usually go to a care provider because they are experiencing lower abdominal pain. The pain typically starts gradually and is constant. The intensity may vary from mild to severe, and movements such as walking can increase the pain. Pain increases during intercourse. Spotting after intercourse and abnormal vaginal discharge are common. Fever and chills may also be present. Women with less acute symptoms notice increased cramping pain with menses, irregular bleeding, and some pain with intercourse. Women who have mild symptoms may go untreated either because they did not seek care or the health care provider misdiagnosed the complaints.

PID is a clinical diagnosis based on the patient's signs and symptoms. The diagnosis of PID is based on data obtained during the bimanual portion of the pelvic examination.[21] Women with PID have lower abdominal tenderness, bilateral adnexal tenderness, and tenderness when the cervix is moved. Additional criteria useful for diagnosis include fever and abnormal vaginal or cervical discharge. Cultures for gonorrhea and chlamydia should be obtained from the endocervix. A pregnancy test should always be done. Drug therapy should begin when the minimal criteria are met and should not await culture results.

When the patient's pain or obesity compromise the pelvic examination and a tuboovarian abscess may be present, a vaginal ultrasound is indicated. Although the patient will already have met the minimal criteria for diagnosing and treating PID, if a tuboovarian abscess is present, hospitalization is necessary.

Complications

Immediate complications of PID include septic shock and *Fitz-Hugh-Curtis syndrome,* which occurs when PID spreads to the liver and causes acute perihepatitis. The patient will have symptoms of right upper quadrant pain, but liver function tests will be normal. Pelvic and tuboovarian abscesses may "leak" or rupture, resulting in pelvic or generalized peritonitis. As the general circulation is flooded with bacterial endotoxins from the infected areas, septic shock may result. Also, embolic episodes may occur as the result of thrombophlebitis of the pelvic veins.

Long-term complications include ectopic pregnancy, infertility, and chronic pelvic pain. PID can cause adhesions and strictures to develop in the fallopian tubes. Ectopic pregnancy may result when a tube is partially obstructed because the sperm can pass through the stricture but the fertilized ovum cannot reach the uterus. After one episode of PID, the risk of having an ectopic pregnancy increases tenfold. Further damage can result in closure of the fallopian tubes and cause infertility.

NURSING ASSESSMENT

Table 51-11   Pelvic Inflammatory Disease

Subjective Data

Important Health Information

Past health history: Use of IUD; previous PID, gonorrhea, or chlamydia; multiple sexual partners; exposure to partner with urethritis; infertility

Medications: Use of and allergy to any antibiotics

Surgery or other treatments: Recent abortion or pelvic surgery

Functional Health Patterns

Health perception–health management: Malaise

Nutritional-metabolic: Nausea, vomiting; chills

Elimination: Urinary frequency, urgency

Cognitive-perceptual: Lower abdominal and pelvic pain; low back pain; pain on fundal palpation and cervical motion; onset of pain just after a menstrual cycle; dysmenorrhea, dyspareunia, dysuria, vulvar pruritus

Sexuality-reproductive: Abnormal vaginal bleeding and menstrual irregularity; vaginal discharge

Objective Data

General

Fever

Reproductive

Mucopurulent cervicitis, vulval maceration, vaginal discharge (heavy and purulent to thin and mucoid), tenderness on motion of cervix and uterus; presence of inflammatory masses on palpation

Possible Findings

Leukocytosis: elevated erythrocyte sedimentation rate; positive culture of secretions or endocervical fluid; pelvic inflammation and positive endometrial biopsy on laparoscopic examination; abscess or inflammation on ultrasonography

PID, pelvic inflammatory disease.

Collaborative Care

PID is usually treated on an outpatient basis. The patient is given a combination of antibiotics such as cefoxitin (Mefoxin) and doxycycline (Vibramycin) to provide broad coverage against the causative organisms. The patient must have no intercourse for 3 weeks. Her partners must be examined and treated. An important part of care is physical rest and oral fluids. The patient's return to the clinic for reevaluation in 48 to 72 hours, even if symptoms are improving, is an essential part of outpatient care.

Some cases of PID require hospitalization. If outpatient treatment is not successful or if the patient is acutely ill or in severe pain, admission to the hospital is indicated. Maximum doses of parenteral antibiotics can be given in the hospital. Some providers believe the addition of corticosteroids to the antibiotic regimen reduces the inflammation, allowing for faster recovery and improvement in subsequent fertility. Application of heat to the lower abdomen or sitz baths may be used to improve circulation and decrease pain. Bed rest in the semi-Fowler's position promotes drainage of the pelvic cavity by gravity and may prevent the development of abscesses high in the abdomen. Analgesics to relieve pain and IV fluids to prevent dehydration are also prescribed.

An indication for surgery is the presence of abscesses that fail to resolve with IV antibiotics. The abscess may be drained by laparoscopy or laparotomy. At one time, a hysterectomy was the standard approach for tuboovarian abscess. Now this is only done in extreme cases. When surgery is necessary, the capacity for childbearing is preserved whenever possible.

NURSING MANAGEMENT: PELVIC INFLAMMATORY DISEASE

Subjective and objective data that should be obtained from the woman with PID are presented in Table 51-11.

Prevention, early recognition, and prompt treatment of vaginal and cervical infections can help prevent PID and its serious complications. Nurses can provide accurate information about factors, such as multiple sexual partners and intercourse without a condom, that place women at increased risk for PID. Nurses should urge women to seek medical attention for any unusual vaginal discharge or possible infection of their reproductive organs. Women should be helped to understand that all discharge is not indicative of infection, but early diagnosis and treatment of an infection, if present, can prevent serious complications. Women should be informed of the methods to decrease the risk of getting STDs and to recognize the signs of infection in their partners.

The patient may have guilt feelings about having PID, especially if it was associated with an STD. She may also be concerned about the complications associated with PID, such as adhesions and strictures of the fallopian tubes, infertility, and the increased incidence of ectopic pregnancy. Discussion with the patient regarding her feelings and concerns can assist her to cope more effectively with them. Nursing diagnoses related to PID may include, but are not limited to, those presented in NCP 51-1.

For patients requiring hospitalization, nurses have an important role in implementing drug therapy, monitoring the patient's health status, and providing symptom relief and patient education. Vital signs and the character, amount, color, and odor of the vaginal discharge should be recorded. Explanations about the need for limited activity, being in a semi-Fowler's position, and increased fluid intake should increase patient cooperation. Assessing the degree of abdominal pain provides information about the effectiveness of drug therapy.

The nurse can use interventions such as applying heat to the lower abdomen, giving sitz baths, and giving analgesics to reduce pain. Usually the pain is dull and constant in character. The location and intensity of the pain may vary. With effective antibiotics the pain should gradually subside. Subsequent use of barrier methods (e.g., condoms and diaphragm) of birth control with spermicide and avoidance of intercourse during menses may reduce the risk of reinfection.[4]

51-1   NURSING CARE PLAN   PATIENT WITH PELVIC INFLAMMATORY DISEASE

Expected Patient Outcomes	Nursing Interventions and *Rationales*

NURSING DIAGNOSIS   **Pain** *related to* infectious process *as manifested by* crampy, continuous, bilateral lower abdominal pain, guarding behavior, altered muscle tone.

- Satisfactory level of pain control.

- Assess degree of pain *to plan appropriate interventions.*
- Provide comfort measures (e.g., backrub, nonstimulating environment, heat to lower abdomen) *to increase patient comfort.*
- Administer analgesics (e.g., ibuprofen [Motrin]) as ordered *to relieve the pain.*
- Instruct patient to restrict movement *to avoid increasing pain.*

NURSING DIAGNOSIS   **Risk for infection transmission** *related to* vaginal discharge and lack of knowledge of proper hygiene and appropriate sexual practices.

- Knowledge and use of principles of medical asepsis.
- Avoidance of practices that could lead to transmission of disease.

- Assess for purulent vaginal discharge, inadequate hand washing, improper disposal of perineal pads, unsafe sexual practices *as possible sources of transmission of infection.*
- Use and teach strict medical asepsis when in contact with discharge (e.g., proper hand washing, careful handling and disposal of perineal pads); explain need for precautions related to vaginal discharge and encourage patient's participation in them; advise patient against sexual contact while infected *to prevent transmission of infection.*

NURSING DIAGNOSIS   **Anxiety** *related to* imposed activity restrictions, perceived loss of control, and lack of knowledge of outcome on reproductive status and course of disease *as manifested by* restlessness, frequent questioning about restricted activity and outcome, irritability, crying spells.

- Understanding of possible outcomes of disease process on reproductive status.

- Assess degree of anxiety and areas of questioning and concern *to plan appropriate interventions.*
- Maintain bed rest in semi-Fowler's position *to promote drainage of pelvic cavity by gravity and possibly prevent development of an abscess.*
- Explain need for limited activity *to improve patient's understanding and increase cooperation.*
- Discuss possible outcomes of disease process *to assist patient in considering a realistic outcome.*
- Provide counsel for patient and significant others *to demonstrate caring and understanding.*
- Clarify course of disease *so patient can prepare herself and be an informed partner in the plan of care.*

ENDOMETRIOSIS

Endometriosis is the presence of normal endometrial tissue in sites outside the endometrial cavity. The most frequent sites are in or near the ovaries, the uterosacral ligaments, and the uterovesical peritoneum (Fig. 51-6). However, endometrial tissues can be in many other locations such as the stomach, lungs, intestines, and spleen. The tissue responds to the hormones of the ovarian cycle and undergoes a mini–menstrual cycle similar to the uterine endometrium. About 7% to 10% of all women have endometriosis, so it is a common problem for women during their reproductive years.

Endometriosis occurs among all ethnic groups from early adolescence to the perimenopause. However, most typically, the patient with endometriosis is in her late 20s or early 30s, Caucasian, and has never had a full-term pregnancy. While not a life-threatening condition, endometriosis is responsible for considerable pain and loss of work time. Endometriosis is found in 30% to 60% of women who seek evaluation for infertility.[11]

Etiology and Pathophysiology

The etiology of endometriosis is not well understood and many theories about the cause of endometriosis have been proposed.

A widely held view is that retrograde menstrual flow passes through the fallopian tubes carrying viable endometrial tissues into the pelvis. Here the tissue attaches to various sites shown in Fig. 51-6. Another theory suggests that undifferentiated celomic cells (embryonic peritoneal cavity cells) remain dormant on the peritoneal surface until the ovaries produce sufficient hormones to stimulate their growth and cyclic changes.[11]

Clinical Manifestations

A wide range of symptoms and severity exist, and the magnitude of a woman's symptoms do not match the clinical extent of her endometriosis. The most common symptoms are secondary dysmenorrhea (50%), infertility (25% to 50%), pelvic pain and dyspareunia (20%), and irregular bleeding (12% to 14%).[11] Less common symptoms include backache, painful bowel movements, and dysuria. These symptoms may or may not correspond to the woman's menstrual cycles. With menopause, estrogen is no longer produced in the ovaries, which may lead to the disappearance of the symptoms.

When the ectopic endometrial implants "menstruate," the blood collects in cystlike nodules that have a characteristic bluish black look. Nodules in the ovaries are sometimes called

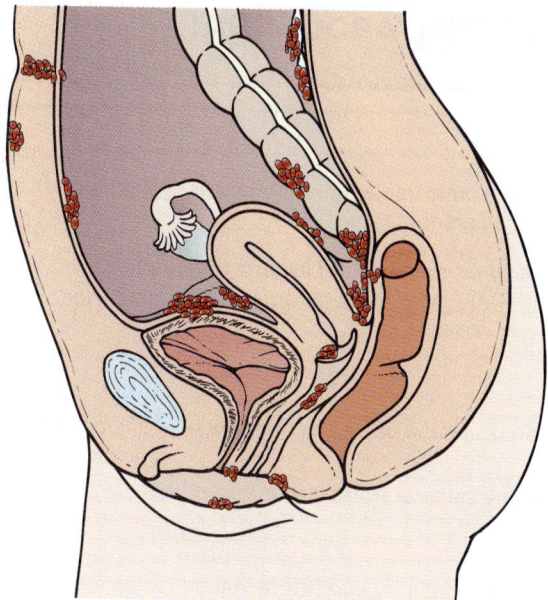

Fig. 51-6   Common sites of endometriosis.

chocolate cysts because of the thick, chocolate-colored material they contain. When a cyst ruptures, the pain may be acute and the resulting irritation promotes the formation of adhesions, which fix the affected area to another pelvic structure. The adhesions may become severe enough to cause a bowel obstruction or painful micturition. Adhesions involving the uterus, tubes, or ovaries may result in infertility.

Collaborative Care

Endometriosis may be suspected from a woman's history of the characteristic symptoms and the health care provider's palpation of firm nodular lumps in the adnexa on bimanual examination. However, laparoscopy is necessary for a definitive diagnosis. The treatment of endometriosis is influenced by the patient's age, desire to get pregnant, symptom severity, and the extent and location of the disease. When symptoms are not disruptive, a watch and wait approach is used. When endometriosis is identified as a possible cause of infertility, therapy will proceed more rapidly.

Surgical Therapy. The only cure for endometriosis is surgical removal of all the implants. Surgical therapy may be conservative or definitive. Conservative surgery is done to confirm the diagnosis or to remove implants. It involves removal or destruction of endometrial implants and lysing or excision of adhesions by means of laparoscopic laser surgery and laparotomy. Gonadotropin-releasing hormone agonist therapy (e.g., leuprolide acetate) can be administered for 4 to 6 months to reduce the size of the lesions before surgery. By reducing the extent of the surgery, this preoperative drug treatment helps reduce the development of adhesions that may further threaten fertility.

For women wishing to get pregnant, conservative surgical therapy is used to remove implants that may block the fallopian tube. Also, adhesions are removed from the tubes, ovaries, and pelvic structures. Efforts are made to conserve all tissues necessary to maintain fertility.

Definitive surgery involves removal of the uterus, tubes, ovaries, and as many endometrial implants as possible. The individual woman should be actively involved in making the decision about preserving part or all of her ovaries, if surgically possible. Her feelings about maintaining her cyclical ovarian function must be explored. The health care provider should assess the woman's risk for ovarian cancer and provide this information for her consideration.

Drug Therapy. Drug therapy is used to reduce symptoms. Drugs are selected to inhibit estrogen production by the ovary so that the endometrial tissue shrinks. The various drugs used imitate a state of pregnancy or menopause, since both natural conditions relieve symptoms. Continuous use (for 9 months) of combined progestin and estrogen causes regression of endometrial tissue. Ovulation is suppressed and pseudopregnancy (hyperhormonal amenorrhea) is produced. Another approach to hormonal treatment is danazol (Danocrine), a synthetic androgen that inhibits the anterior pituitary. When given in dosages of up to 800 mg/day for 6 to 9 months, the drug produces a pseudomenopause (ovarian suppression), with consequent atrophy of ectopic endometrial tissue. Subjective relief of symptoms is noted within 6 weeks of danazol use. Side effects include weight gain, acne, hot flashes, and hirsutism. These side effects and the expense of this drug restrict its use.

The newest and most expensive drug therapy is injectable gonadotropin-releasing hormone analog (leuprolide [Lupron]). It causes a hypoestrogenic state resulting in amenorrhea. The side effects reported by patients are usually the same as menopause (hot flashes, vaginal dryness, and emotional lability). Loss of bone density has also been reported in women who remain on the therapy longer than 6 months. Endometriosis is controlled but not cured by hormonal therapy. Persistent lesions give rise to subsequent recurrences once the menstrual cycle is reestablished.

NURSING MANAGEMENT: ENDOMETRIOSIS

Nurses should educate women about endometriosis with special attention to the common symptoms. Dysmenorrhea after years of relatively pain-free menses and the inability to achieve pregnancy may serve as clues to the presence of endometriosis. When women understand the symptoms that might suggest endometriosis, they are more likely to see their primary care providers sooner when symptoms develop.

Education of the patient and reassurance that a life-threatening situation does not exist may permit her to accept a conservative and progressive treatment. When the symptoms are less severe, teaching about nondrug comfort measures may be very helpful. Nurses often assist patients to fully understand the drugs that have been ordered to treat their condition. The action of the prescribed drug should be explained, as well as the possible side effects. Psychologic support may be needed for the women experiencing severe disabling pain, sexual difficulties secondary to dyspareunia, and infertility.

If conservative surgery is the treatment selected, the nursing care is similar to the general preoperative and postoperative care of a patient undergoing laparotomy. If definitive surgery is planned, the nursing care is similar to the patient undergoing an abdominal hysterectomy (see NCP 51-2 on p. 1538). The nurse must know the extent of the procedure so that appropriate postoperative teaching can be done.

51-2 NURSING CARE PLAN PATIENT WITH A TOTAL ABDOMINAL HYSTERECTOMY

| Expected Patient Outcomes | Nursing Interventions and *Rationales* |

NURSING DIAGNOSIS **Urinary retention** *related to* loss of bladder tone, uncomfortable urinating position, and pain *as manifested by* distention of bladder, voiding of small amounts.

- Able to urinate in suffi-cient quantities without difficulty.

- Measure intake and output *to determine if satisfactory fluid balance is maintained.*
- Encourage fluids orally within limitations of diet *to ensure adequate quantity of urine to stim-ulate urge to urinate.*
- Percuss bladder *to detect distention.*
- Catheterize as ordered.
- Report any complaints of backache and decreased output *as these are signs of a possible liga-tion of a ureter.*
- Provide routine catheter care if indwelling catheter is in place *to ensure catheter patency and free flow of urine.*

NURSING DIAGNOSIS **Body-image disturbance** *related to* perceived loss of femininity and future inability to conceive *as manifested by* crying, weeping, depression; verbalization of perceived loss of femininity and/or ability to conceive.

- Accurate statements of effects of hysterectomy.
- Verbalization of confi-dence in ability to adjust to postsurgical state.

- Assess depth of impact of surgery on body image *to determine need and plan for intervention.*
- Provide factual information regarding anticipated bodily changes *so patient will have accu-rate information.*
- Provide information on hormone replacement *so patient is informed about possible treatment of surgical menopause.*
- Encourage discussion with patient, significant others, and health professionals *to minimize emotional impact of hysterectomy through open discussion.*

NURSING DIAGNOSIS **Altered sexuality patterns** *related to* perceived lack of desirability and lack of knowledge regarding resumption of sexual activity *as manifested by* frequent questioning about future sexual response, lack of desire to resume presurgical sexual practices.

- Optimism that satisfac-tory sexual practices can be resumed when indi-cated by surgeon.

- Facilitate discussion of sexuality with significant other *to clarify areas of misunderstanding and foster mutual approach to any problems.*
- Reassure patient that energy and desire will return after a period of convalescence *to prevent discouragement and depression.*
- Explain psychologic and physiologic implications of hysterectomy related to a woman's sex-uality *to provide accurate facts and decrease fear of consequences of hysterectomy.*

NURSING DIAGNOSIS **Altered health maintenance** *related to* lack of knowledge regarding activity restrictions and hormone replacement therapy (HRT) *as manifested by* questioning about postdischarge plans.

- Ability to make appro-priate decisions related to occupational and leisure activity and HRT.

- Encourage expression of concerns *to clarify areas of concern.*
- Assess knowledge level.
- Provide information regarding HRT *so patient has accurate knowledge base to make decisions.*
- Provide timetable for gradual resumption of presurgery activity *so patient does not resume activities too soon or delay resumption of activities unnecessarily.*

NURSING DIAGNOSIS **Pain** *related to* incision and manipulation of internal organs *as manifested by* statements about pain, guarding of incision, reluctance to ambulate, facial grimacing.

- Verbalization of satis-factory level of pain control.

- Assess degree of pain *to plan appropriate interventions.*
- Provide comfort measures (e.g., backrub, heat to lower abdomen) *to increase patient comfort.*
- Administer analgesics as ordered *to relieve the pain.*
- Instruct patient on methods for moving and coughing while supporting abdominal incision.

Continued

51-2 NURSING CARE PLAN   PATIENT WITH A TOTAL ABDOMINAL HYSTERECTOMY—continued

Expected Patient Outcomes	Nursing Interventions and *Rationales*

COLLABORATIVE PROBLEMS

Nursing Goals	Nursing Interventions and *Rationales*

POTENTIAL COMPLICATION

- Monitor for signs of paralytic ileus and report if present.
- Carry out appropriate medical and nursing interventions.

Paralytic ileus *related to* surgical manipulation of bowel and immobility.

- Assess for distended abdomen, complaints of gas pains, decreased bowel sounds *to detect presence of paralytic ileus.*
- Encourage ambulation q4hr *to promote bowel peristalsis.*
- Insert rectal tube as ordered *to expel flatus and promote patient comfort.*
- Withhold food and fluids if paralytic ileus is present *to prevent nausea and vomiting.*

POTENTIAL COMPLICATION

- Monitor for signs of thromboembolism and report if present.
- Carry out appropriate medical and nursing interventions.

Thromboembolic phenomenon *related to* immobility and irritation of vessels of pelvis and upper thigh.

- Assess lower extremities for warmth, color, blanching, pain, and sensation q8hr *to detect impaired circulation.*
- Assess for signs of pulmonary embolism such as chest pain, tachycardia, and dyspnea.
- Report and record signs and symptoms of thrombophlebitis *so early treatment can be initiated.*
- Encourage foot-leg exercises while in bed; ambulate q4hr and avoid prolonged sitting *to promote good circulation and prevent stasis.*
- Reapply elastic compression gradient stockings every shift *to apply even pressure to veins to prevent venous stasis.*

BENIGN TUMORS OF THE FEMALE REPRODUCTIVE SYSTEM

LEIOMYOMAS

Etiology

Leiomyomas (fibroids, myomas, fibromyomas, fibromas) are the most common benign tumors of the female genital tract (Fig. 51-7). By 30 years of age, 10% of Caucasian women and 30% of African-American women have uterine leiomyomas. The cause of leiomyomas is unknown. They appear to depend on ovarian hormones because they grow slowly during the reproductive years and undergo atrophy after menopause. Leiomyomas consist of smooth muscle cells.

Clinical Manifestations

The majority of women with fibroids do not have any symptoms. Of the women with leiomyomas who develop symptoms, the most common is menorrhagia. Although rarely experienced with leiomyomas, pain is associated with infection or twisting of the pedicle from which the tumor is growing. Dysmenorrhea and dyspareunia may occasionally occur. Pressure on surrounding organs may result in rectal, bladder, and lower abdominal discomfort. Large tumors may cause a general enlargement of the lower abdomen. These tumors are sometimes associated with miscarriage and infertility.

Collaborative Care

Clinical diagnosis is based on the characteristic pelvic findings of an enlarged uterus distorted by nodular masses. Treatment

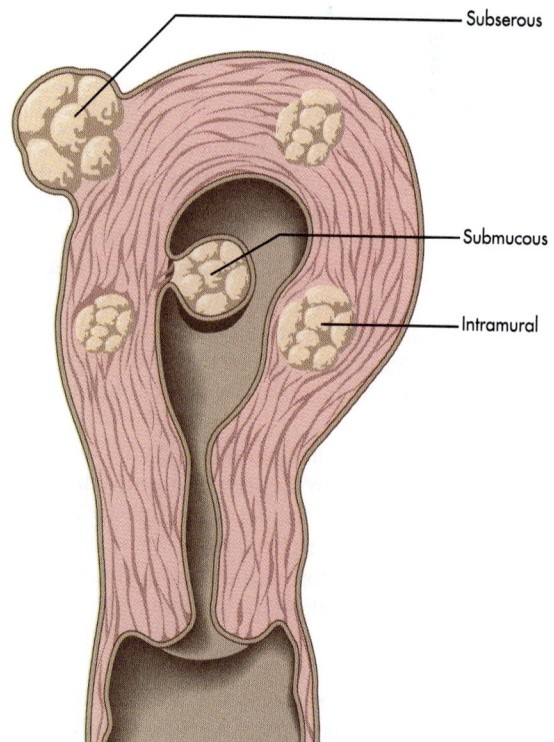

Fig. 51-7 Leiomyomas. Uterine section showing whorl-like appearance and locations of leiomyomas, which are also called uterine fibroids.

depends on the symptoms, the age of the patient, her desire to bear children, and the location and size of the tumor or tumors. If the symptoms are minor, the provider may elect to follow the patient closely for a time. If the woman is experiencing menorrhagia, the use of aspirin is discouraged because of its effect on platelets.

Persistent heavy menstrual bleeding causing anemia and large or rapidly growing fibroids are indications for surgery. The fibroids are removed by hysterectomy or myomectomy. A myomectomy is performed for women who wish to have children. In this case, only the fibroids are removed in order to preserve the uterus. Small fibroids may be removed using a hysteroscope and laser resection instruments.[4] In cases of large leiomyomas, a gonadotropin-releasing hormone agonist (e.g., leuprolide) may be used preoperatively to shrink the size of the leiomyomas. However, the risks and benefits of this drug should be fully discussed, including the potential for irreversible loss of bone mass.

CERVICAL POLYPS

Cervical polyps are benign pedunculated lesions that generally arise from the endocervical mucosa and are seen protruding through the cervical os during a speculum examination. Polyps are a characteristic bright cherry red and are soft and fragile in consistency. They are generally small, measuring less than 3 cm in length, and may be single or multiple. Their origin is unknown. Symptoms are usually not present, but metrorrhagia and bleeding after straining and coitus can occur. Polyps are prone to infection. When the polyp is small, it can be excised in an outpatient procedure. If the point of attachment of the polyp cannot be identified and is not accessible to cautery, a polypectomy is performed in an operating room. All tissue removed is sent for pathologic review because polyps occasionally undergo malignant changes.

BENIGN OVARIAN TUMORS

Benign tumors of the ovary are many and varied. The cause of most of them is unknown. For purposes of clarity, they are divided into cysts and neoplasms. Cysts are usually soft, surrounded by a thin capsule, and are seen mainly during the reproductive years (Fig. 51-8). Follicle and corpus luteum cysts are common ovarian cysts. Epithelial ovarian neoplasms are extremely varied. They may be cystic or solid, small or extremely large. Cystic teratomas or dermoids originate from germ cells and can contain bits of any type of body tissue, such as hair or teeth.

Ovarian masses are often asymptomatic until they are large enough to cause pressure in the pelvis. Constipation, menstrual irregularities, urinary frequency, a full feeling in the abdomen, anorexia, and peripheral edema may occur, depending on the size and location of the tumor. There may be an increase in abdominal girth. Pelvic pain may be present if the tumor is growing rapidly. Severe pain results when the cyst twists on its pedicle (twisted ovarian cyst).

Pelvic examination reveals a mass or an enlarged ovary that demands further investigation. If the mass is cystic and smaller than 8 cm, the patient is asked to return for reexamination in 4 to 6 weeks. If the mass is cystic and greater than 8 cm or is solid, laparoscopic surgery or laparotomy is performed. Immediate

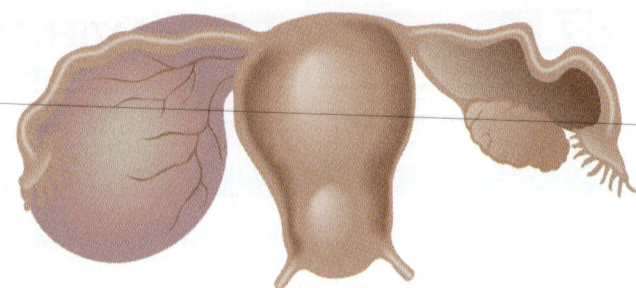

Fig. 51-8 Ovarian cysts can occur on both ovaries and have different sizes.

surgery is necessary if the ovarian mass causes the ovary to rotate, cutting off circulation. Surgical techniques are used to save as much of the ovary as possible.

MALIGNANT TUMORS OF THE FEMALE REPRODUCTIVE SYSTEM

CERVICAL CANCER

In 1998, there were approximately 13,700 cases of invasive cervical cancer diagnosed and approximately 4900 women in the United States died from cervical cancer. The mortality rate was twice as high for African-American women as compared with Caucasian women. The incidence is also higher among Hispanic women than Caucasian women. An increased risk of cervical cancer is associated with low economic status, early sexual activity (before 17 years of age), multiple sexual partners, infection with HPV, and smoking.[9]

The number of deaths from cervical cancer has fallen steadily over the past 40 years. This is attributable to better and earlier diagnosis with the widespread use of the Pap test. In addition to cancer, the Pap test detects precancerous changes called cervical intraepithelial neoplasia (CIN) or dysplasia. By treating dysplasia, progression to cervical cancer can be prevented. The American Cancer Society recommends annual Pap tests beginning with the onset of sexual activity. Following three negative Pap tests, less frequent tests may be recommended by the health care provider.

Etiology and Pathophysiology

The progression from normal cervical cells to dysplasia and on to cervical cancer appears to be related to repeated injuries to the cervix.[22] The progression occurs slowly over years rather than months. There is a relationship between certain subtypes of HPV and cervical cancer.[9] However, a cofactor such as smoking is thought to be needed in addition to the specific subtype of HPV. Women who smoke have a 50% higher risk for developing cervical cancer than nonsmokers. This risk is greatest in those with longer duration of smoking, increased number of cigarettes smoked, and use of unfiltered cigarettes.[11]

Clinical Manifestations

Precancerous changes are asymptomatic, highlighting the importance of routine screening. CIN occurs mainly in young women. The peak incidence of CIN is in women in their early

Table **51-12**	Classification of Cytologic Findings of Pap Tests			
Papanicolaou Class	**Dysplasia**	**CIN**	**Bethesda System**	
Class I Normal smear	Negative	Negative	Within normal limits	

Class II
  Atypical cells,
  no dysplasia
	Reactive atypia
	Koilocytosis or HPV
	Mild dysplasia
		Koilocytosis or HPV
		CIN 1
			Regeneration, repair
			Inflammation
			Low-grade squamous intraepithelial lesion	

Class III
  Abnormal cells consistent
  with dysplasia
	Moderate dysplasia	CIN 2		

Class IV
  Abnormal cells consistent
  with CIS
	Severe dysplasia, CIS	CIN 2
		CIN 3
			High-grade squamous intraepithelial lesion	

Class V
  Abnormal cells consistent
  with invasive or squamous
  cell origin
	Squamous cell
	carcinoma
		Squamous cell
		carcinoma
			Squamous cell carcinoma	

CIN, cervical intraepithelial neoplasia; *CIS*, carcinoma in situ; *HPV*, human papillomavirus.

CULTURAL & ETHNIC CONSIDERATIONS

Cancer of the Female Reproductive System

- Japanese women have a low incidence of ovarian cancer. However, second and third generation Japanese women in the United States have much higher rates, similar to Caucasian women born in the United States. Dietary practices may explain this difference.
- Five-year survival rate for endometrial cancer (all stages combined) is 80% for Caucasian women and 55% for African-American women.
- Cervical cancer has a higher incidence among Hispanic, African-American, and Native-American women than Caucasians.
- Mortality rates from cervical cancer are more than twice as high among African-American women as among Caucasian women.

30s. The average age for women with invasive cervical cancer is 50 years. Early cervical cancer is generally asymptomatic, but leukorrhea and intermenstrual bleeding eventually occur. The discharge is usually thin and watery but becomes dark and foul smelling as the disease advances, suggesting the presence of an infection. The vaginal bleeding is initially only spotting, but as the tumor enlarges, it becomes heavier and more frequent. Pain is a late symptom and is followed by weight loss, anemia, and cachexia.

Diagnostic Studies

A Pap test, the Schiller iodine test, colposcopy, and a biopsy may be used to diagnose cervical cancer. (These diagnostic tests are described in Chapter 48.) Various classification systems are used to interpret the cytologic findings. Examples are given in Table 51-12. The current trend is to use the Bethesda system because it improves accuracy and quality of diagnosis by standardizing diagnostic reports. Pap tests are less than 100% accurate. There are problems with both false-positive and false-negative reports. New techniques for cervical cancer screening are being explored.

Collaborative Care

The finding of an abnormal Pap smear indicates the need for follow-up. The type of follow-up depends on the Pap findings. Women with minor changes (Class II) may be followed with a repeated Pap test in 3 to 4 months. Up to 80% may revert to normal spontaneously. Women with more prominent changes (Class III or greater) receive additional procedures, such as colposcopy and biopsy, before a definitive diagnosis can be made. Colposcopy involves examination of the cervix with a binocular microscope with low levels of magnification (10× to 40×). The procedure helps in the identification of possible epithelial abnormalities and suggests areas for biopsy. Biopsies are sent to pathology for evaluation. Colposcopy and biopsy have improved diagnosis and allowed more focused treatments to be selected.

The type and extent of the biopsy vary with the abnormality seen. A punch biopsy may be done on an outpatient basis with special punch biopsy forceps. The excision of a cone-shaped section of the cervix may be used for both diagnosis and treatment. Conization is accomplished using one of several techniques. The choice of procedure is determined by the provider's experience and the availability of equipment. Cryotherapy (freezing) and laser cone vaporization destroy the tissue. Laser cone excision and loop electrosurgery excision procedure (LEEP) remove the identified tissue and allow for histologic examination to ensure that all microinvasive tissue has been removed. These procedures can be performed in the office with some mild analgesics or relaxants. Complications of these procedures include excessive bleeding and possible cervical stenosis with healing.

Table 51-13   International Classification of Clinical Stages of Carcinoma of the Cervix

Stage	Extent	Treatment
Stage 0	In situ, intraepithelial	Cervical conization, total hysterectomy, cryosurgery, laser surgery
Stage I	Strict confinement to cervix (no consideration of extension to corpus)	
Stage IA	Microinvasive (early stromal invasion)	Radiation or surgery
Stage IB	All other cases of stage I	Radiation, Wertheim's hysterectomy
Stage II	Extension beyond cervix but not to pelvic wall, involvement of vagina, but not as far as lower third	
Stage IIA	No obvious parametrial involvement	Radiation, Wertheim's hysterectomy
Stage IIB	Obvious parametrial involvement	Radiation; if this fails, pelvic exenteration may be required
Stage III	Extension to pelvic wall, no cancer-free space between tumor and pelvic wall on rectal examination, involvement of lower third of vagina, hydronephrosis or nonfunctioning kidney	Radiation
Stage IIIA	No extension to pelvic wall	
Stage IIIB	Extension to pelvic wall or hydronephrosis or nonfunctioning kidney	
Stage IV	Extension beyond true pelvis or clinical involvement of the mucosa of bladder or rectum, no stage IV classification with bullous edema alone	Radiation, surgery (e.g., exenteration)
Stage IVA	Spread to adjacent organs	
Stage IVB	Spread to distant organs	

Treatment of cancer of the cervix is guided by the stage of the tumor (Table 51-13) and the patient's age and general state of health. There are four procedures in which fertility can be preserved. Conization may be the only type of therapy needed for CIN if analysis of removed tissue demonstrates that a wide area of normal tissue surrounds the excised tissue. Laser treatments using a directed infrared beam is effective in the destruction of dysplasic tissue. Cautery and cryosurgery may also be used.

Invasive cancer of the cervix is treated with surgery, radiation, or a combination of the two are used to remove or destroy the involved areas and lymphatic drainage. Surgical procedures commonly carried out include hysterectomy, Wertheim or radical hysterectomy (involving adjacent structures), and rarely pelvic exenteration. Radiation may be external (e.g., cobalt) or internal (e.g., cesium or radium). Standard radiation treatment is 4 to 6 weeks of external radiation followed with one or two treatments with internal implants.[22] (Radiation therapy is discussed in Chapter 14.)

ENDOMETRIAL CANCER

Cancer of the endometrium is the most common gynecologic malignancy, accounting for nearly 50% of female genital tract neoplasms. In 1998 there were approximately 36,100 cases of endometrial cancer and 6300 deaths. Endometrial cancer has a relatively low mortality, with a survival rate of 94% if the cancer has not spread at the time of diagnosis.[22] About 25% of endometrial cancer is diagnosed before menopause. The average age at the time of diagnosis is 61 years.

Etiology and Pathophysiology

The major risk factor for endometrial cancer is estrogen, in particular unopposed estrogen. Additional risk factors include increasing age, nulliparity, obesity, hypertension, and diabetes mellitus. Obesity is a risk factor because adipose (fat) cells store estrogen, which increases endogenous estrogen and increases its availability. Pregnancy and birth control pills are protective factors.

Cancer arises from the lining of the endometrium. Most tumors are pure adenocarcinomas. The precursor may be a hyperplasic state that progresses to invasive carcinoma. Hyperplasia occurs when estrogen is not counteracted by progesterone. Direct extension develops into the cervix and through the uterine serosa. As invasion of the myometrium occurs, regional lymph nodes, including the paravaginal and paraaortic, become involved. Hematogenous metastases develop concurrently. The usual sites of metastases are lung, bone, liver, and eventually the brain. Malignant cells can be found in the peritoneal cavity, presumably by tubal transport, and their presence is included in staging. Prognostic factors include histologic differentiation, uterine size at time of diagnosis, myometrial invasion, peritoneal cytology, lymph node and adnexal metastases, and tumor size. Endometrial cancer grows slowly, metastasizes late, and is amenable to therapy if diagnosed early.

Clinical Manifestations

The first sign of endometrial cancer is abnormal uterine bleeding, usually in postmenopausal women. Because perimenopausal women have sporadic periods for a time, it is important that this sign not be ignored or automatically blamed on menopause. Pain occurs late in the disease process, and other symptoms that may arise are related to metastasis to other organs.

Collaborative Care

Endometrial biopsy has replaced a D&C as a diagnostic procedure for endometrial cancer. Endometrial biopsy, often an office procedure, involves obtaining endometrial tissue from the uterus. Any occurrence of spotting or unexpected bleeding in a postmenopausal woman mandates obtaining a tissue sample to exclude endometrial cancer. The American Cancer Society recommends an endometrial biopsy be performed at menopause and then periodically in women who are at risk. The Pap test is not a reliable diagnostic tool for endometrial cancer, but it can rule out cervical cancer.

Treatment of endometrial cancer is a total hysterectomy and bilateral salpingo-oophorectomy with selective node biopsies. Surgery may be followed by radiation, either to the pelvis or abdomen externally or intravaginally, to decrease local recurrence.[22] Treatment of advanced or recurrent disease is difficult. Hormonal therapy (e.g., progesterone) is the treatment of choice when the progesterone receptor status is positive and the tumor is well differentiated. Chemotherapy is considered when progesterone therapy is unsuccessful. The most common agents used are doxorubicin (Adriamycin) and cisplatin (Platinol).[22]

OVARIAN CANCER

Because most women with ovarian cancer have advanced disease at diagnosis, it causes more deaths than any other cancer of the female reproductive system. Ovarian cancer is responsible for 32% of all cancers of the female reproductive system, but carries a mortality rate over 50%.[11] It occurs most frequently in women between 55 and 65 years of age.[11] The median age of women with ovarian cancer is 60 years. Caucasian women of North American or European descent are also at greater risk for ovarian cancer as compared with African-American women.

Etiology and Pathophysiology

Risk factors include family history of ovarian cancer, increasing age, and high-fat diet. However, many women diagnosed with ovarian cancer have none of these risks. Women who have mutations of the BRCA-1 gene have increased susceptibility (60% higher risk) for ovarian cancer.[23] The BRCA genes are tumor suppressor genes. They inhibit tumor growth when functioning normally. When they mutate, they lose their tumor suppressor ability, and hence there is increased risk for women to develop cancer (ovarian and breast). Breast feeding, multiple pregnancies, oral contraceptive use (greater than 5 years), and early age at first birth seem to reduce the risk of ovarian cancer. It is thought that these factors have a protective effect because they reduce the number of ovulatory cycles the woman experiences.

Between 80% and 85% of ovarian cancers are epithelial carcinomas, that is, they arise from malignant transformation of the surface epithelial cells. Germ cell tumors account for another 10%. Histologic grading is an important prognostic determinant. Generally, tumors are divided into well differentiated (grade I), moderately well differentiated (grade II), and poorly differentiated (grade III). Grade III lesions carry a worse prognosis than the other grades.

Ovarian cancer has two patterns of metastasis: lymphatic and direct. Primary lymphatic drainage of the ovary is through the retroperitoneal nodes surrounding the renal hilum. Secondary drainage is through the iliac lymphatics. Tertiary drainage is through the inguinal lymphatics. Ovarian cancer also metastasizes directly to the abdominal cavity, the diaphragm, and the omentum.

Clinical Manifestations

In its early stages, ovarian cancer is usually asymptomatic. As the malignancy grows, a variety of symptoms, such as an increase in abdominal girth, bowel and bladder dysfunction, pain, menstrual irregularities, and ascites, can occur. An ovarian malignancy should be considered when abnormal uterine bleeding occurs.

Diagnostic Studies

Unlike the Pap test used to screen for cervical cancer, no screening test exists for ovarian cancer. For women at risk for ovarian cancer, a combination of serum CA-125 and ultrasound is recommended in addition to a yearly pelvic examination. CA-125 is positive in 80% of women with epithelial ovarian cancer and is used to monitor the course of disease.[22] However, values of CA-125 may be elevated with other nonovarian malignancies or with benign conditions such as fibroids or endometriosis.

Collaborative Care

Since early ovarian cancer is usually asymptomatic, yearly bimanual pelvic examinations should be performed to identify the presence of an ovarian mass. Postmenopausal women should not have palpable ovaries, so a mass of any size should be suspected as possible ovarian cancer. When a suspicious mass in the ovarian area is palpated, laparoscopy is performed to establish the diagnosis. Women identified as high risk based on family and health history may require additional surveillance and counseling regarding options such as prophylactic oophorectomy and birth control pills. It is important to note that while oophorectomy significantly reduces the risk of ovarian cancer it does not completely eliminate the possibility of disease.

If the mass is malignant, staging is critical for guiding treatment decisions. Because of the numerous metastatic pathways for ovarian cancer, accurate staging usually involves multiple biopsies. Stage I describes disease limited to the ovaries; stage II, disease limited to the true pelvis; stage III, disease limited to the abdominal cavity; and stage IV, distant metastatic disease.

The usual treatment for stage I malignancies is a total abdominal hysterectomy and bilateral salpingo-oophorectomy with removal of as much of the tumor as possible (i.e., tumor debulking). The remaining tissues in the abdomen and pelvis are carefully scrutinized. Ascitic fluid is submitted for cytologic study, and appropriate biopsies are performed to determine the stage of the disease.

The addition of chemotherapy or the instillation of intraperitoneal radioisotopes is usually suggested for stage I disease. The patient with stage II disease may receive external abdominal and pelvic radiation, intraperitoneal radiation, or systemic combined chemotherapy after tumor-reducing surgery. After completion of systemic chemotherapy, in the patient who is clinically free of symptoms, a "second-look" surgical procedure is often performed to determine whether there is any evidence of disease. This option does not necessarily improve the outcome. If no disease is found, the patient is monitored for recurrent disease.

Chemotherapy (e.g., cisplatin [Platinol] or carboplatin [Paraplatin]) is used for the treatment of stage III and stage IV diseases. Altretamine (Hexalen) is used for palliative treatment of persistent, recurrent ovarian cancer. Paclitaxel (Taxol) and topotecan (Hycamtin) are used to treat metastatic ovarian cancer. Surgical debulking is often done in conjunction with chemotherapy for advanced disease. Intraperitoneal chemotherapy, although associated with substantial side effects, is coming into wider use for the patient who has minimum residual disease after surgery. Unfortunately, the malignancy may have metastasized to the peritoneum, omentum, or bowel surface before discovery of the tumors. In these situations the prognosis is poor. Recurrent pleural effusion causing shortness of breath and discomfort may require frequent paracenteses, but the fluid accumulates again. Radiation and chemotherapy may be used to shrink the size of the tumor, relieving pressure and pain.

VAGINAL CANCER

Primary vaginal cancers are rare, representing less than 2% of genital cancers. The peak incidence is between 50 and 70 years of age. Vaginal tumors are usually secondary sites or metastases of other cancers such as cervical or endometrial cancer. The most common type of vaginal cancer is squamous cell carcinoma. Intrauterine exposure to diethylstilbestrol (DES) places a woman at risk for clear cell adenocarcinoma of the vagina. Treatment of vaginal cancer depends on the type of cells involved and the stage of the disease, the size of the tumor, and the location of the tumor. Squamous cell carcinomas can be treated with both surgery and radiation.

VULVAR CANCER

Cancer of the vulva is relatively rare, accounting for about 5% of cancers of the female reproductive system.[9] Similar to cervical cancer, preinvasive lesions referred to as vulvar intraepithelial neoplasia (VIN) precede invasive vulvar cancer. The invasive form occurs mainly in women over 60 years of age with the highest incidence being in the 70s.[22] Patients with vulvar neoplasia may have symptoms of vulvar itching or burning, pain, bleeding, or discharge. Women who are immunosuppressed, have diabetes mellitus, hypertension, and chronic vulvar dystrophies are at a higher risk for developing vulvar cancer.[9] Several subtypes of HPV have been identified in some but not all vulvar cancers.[4]

Diagnosis of vulvar cancer is based on the pathology report on the biopsy of the suspicious lesion. VIN is managed by eradicating the lesion medically with 5-fluorouracil (5-FU) or surgical excision. Larger lesions may require more extensive surgery and skin graft. The traditional treatment for vulvar cancer has been radical vulvectomy. However, the procedure results in extensive morbidity related to scarring and wound breakdown. For this reason, more conservative surgical techniques such as radical hemivulvectomy are being used. Cure rates are comparable between the radical vulvectomy and hemivulvectomy. Morbidity and loss of function has been significantly decreased with the hemivulvectomy.

SURGICAL PROCEDURES FOR FEMALE REPRODUCTIVE SYSTEM

A variety of surgical procedures (Table 51-14) are performed when benign or malignant tumors of the genital tract are found. A hysterectomy may be done either vaginally or abdominally. A vaginal route is often used when vaginal repair is to be done in addition to removal of the uterus. The abdominal route is used when large tumors are present and the pelvic cavity is to be explored or when the tubes and ovaries are to be removed at the same time (Fig. 51-9). The abdominal route can present more postoperative problems because it involves an incision and the opening of the abdominal cavity. In both vaginal and abdominal hysterectomies the ligaments that support the uterus are attached to the vaginal cuff so that normal depth of the vagina is maintained. Laparoscopy assisted vaginal hysterectomy is becoming more common as a means of decreasing morbidity associated with abdominal hysterectomy.[24,25]

Table **51-14**	Surgical Procedures on the Female Reproductive Tract
Type of Surgery	**Description**
Subtotal hysterectomy	Removal of uterus without cervix (rarely done today)
Total hysterectomy	Removal of uterus and cervix
Panhysterectomy (TAH-BSO)	Removal of uterus, cervix, fallopian tubes, and ovaries
Simple vulvectomy	Excision of vulva and wide margin of skin
Radical vulvectomy	Excision of tissue from anus to few cm above symphysis pubis (skin, labia majora and minora, and clitoris) with superficial and deep lymph node dissection
Vaginectomy	Removal of vagina
Radical hysterectomy (Wertheim)	Panhysterectomy, partial vaginectomy, and dissection of lymph nodes in pelvis
Pelvic exenteration	Radical hysterectomy, total vaginectomy, removal of bladder with diversion of urinary system and resection of bowel with colostomy
Anterior pelvic exenteration	Above operation without bowel resection
Posterior pelvic exenteration	Above operation without bladder removal

TAH-BSO, total abdominal hysterectomy and bilateral salpingo-oophorectomy.

RADIATION THERAPY FOR CANCERS OF THE FEMALE REPRODUCTIVE SYSTEM

Radiation is used to cure, control, or palliatively treat cancers of the female reproductive system either alone or in combination with other treatments. The goal of radiation therapy is to deliver a specific amount of high-energy (or ionizing) radiation to the cancer with minimal damage to the normal surrounding tissue.[22] Radiation therapy may be external or internal.

External Radiation Therapy

With external radiation therapy, a source outside of the body delivers electromagnetic radiation in the form of waves.[22] The waves are produced by highly specialized machines or from rays emitted from a radioactive source. Higher energy machines, such as the betatron, penetrate deeper with a more sharply

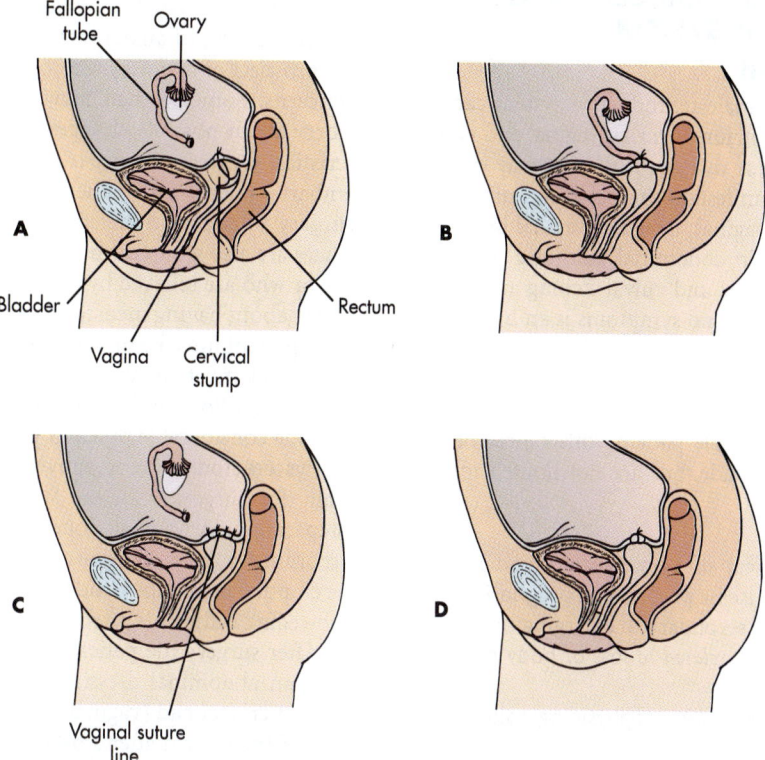

Fig. 51-9 **A,** Cross section of subtotal hysterectomy. Note that cervical stump, fallopian tubes, and ovaries remain. **B,** Cross section of total hysterectomy. Note that fallopian tubes and ovaries remain. **C,** Cross section of vaginal hysterectomy. Note that fallopian tubes and ovaries remain. **D,** Total hysterectomy, salpingectomy, and oophorectomy. Note that uterus, fallopian tubes, and ovaries are completely removed.

defined beam. This reduces the side effects that patients experience. The radiation treatment plan is based on a thorough evaluation of the patient. The plan includes the total amount of radiation to control the tumor, the daily dose, schedule, and arrangement of the radiation beams.[22] (External radiation therapy is discussed in Chapter 14.)

Internal Radiation Therapy

Use of internal radiation therapy allows the radiation to be placed near or into the tumor. This method can deliver a high dose of radiation directly to the tumor. The dose decreases sharply the farther away from the source, causing less damage to the surrounding normal tissue. A variety of forms are used to deliver internal radiation including wires, capsules, needles, tubes, and grains or seeds. Internal radiation is used in the management of cervical and endometrial cancer because of the accessibility of these body parts and the favorable results obtained. Radium and cesium are two commonly used isotopes. In preparation of the patient for the treatment, a cleansing enema is given to prevent straining at stool, which could cause displacement of the isotope. An indwelling catheter is inserted to prevent a distended bladder from coming into contact with the radioactive source.

A variety of applicators have been developed for intrauterine treatment. Applicators are inserted into the endometrial cavity and vagina of an anesthetized patient in the operating room. When the applicator contains the radioactive material, this is known as preloading.[22] In afterloading, the applicator is implanted in the operating room but is not loaded with the radioactive material until its correct placement is verified and the patient has been returned to her room. Radiation exposure to the patient is precisely controlled. The radiation exposure to the physician and other personnel involved in the implantation is reduced when the afterload technique is used. The applicator is secured with vaginal packing and is left in place for 24 to 72 hours. The radiation oncologist determines the exact amount of radioactive substance to be used and the length of time it will be left in place so that destruction of cancer cells can occur with minimal damage to normal cells.

During the treatment the patient is placed in a lead-lined private room and is on absolute bed rest. She may be turned from side to side. The presence of an intrauterine applicator produces uterine contractions that may require analgesics. The destruction of cells results in a foul-smelling vaginal discharge, and a deodorizer is helpful. Nausea, vomiting, diarrhea, and malaise may develop as a systemic reaction to the radiation.

At the end of the prescribed period of radiation, the radioactive material and the catheter are removed. The patient is allowed off bed rest and is discharged from the hospital when stable. Late complications that may arise after radiation of the uterus include fistulas (vesicovaginal, ureterovaginal), cystitis, phlebitis, hemorrhage, and fibrosis. If fibrosis occurs, the vaginal wall becomes smaller in diameter and shorter. Dilation of the vagina through intercourse or the use of a sequentially sized dilators may be indicated. The patient is urged to report any unusual symptoms or complaints to her physician. (Internal radiation and related nursing care are discussed in Chapter 14.)

NURSING MANAGEMENT: CANCERS OF THE FEMALE REPRODUCTIVE SYSTEM

■ Nursing Assessment

Malignant tumors of the female reproductive system can be found in the cervix, endometrium, ovaries, vagina, and vulva. The patient with any of these malignant tumors may experience a variety of clinical manifestations, including leukorrhea (white discharge from the vagina), irregular vaginal bleeding, vaginal discharge, increase in abdominal pain and pressure, bowel and bladder dysfunction, and vulvar itching and burning. Assessment for these signs and symptoms is an important nursing responsibility.

■ Nursing Diagnoses

Nursing diagnoses for the female patient with cancer of the reproductive system may include, but are not limited to, the following:

- Anxiety *related to* threat of a malignancy and lack of knowledge about the disease process and prognosis
- Pain *related to* pressure secondary to enlarging tumor
- Body image disturbance *related to* loss of body part and loss of good health
- Altered sexuality patterns *related to* physiologic alterations and fatigue
- Ineffective breathing pattern *related to* presence of ascites and effusions
- Anticipatory grieving *related to* poor prognosis of advanced disease

■ Planning

The overall goals are that the patient with a malignant tumor will (1) actively participate in treatment decisions, (2) achieve satisfactory pain and symptom management, (3) recognize and report problems promptly, (4) maintain preferred lifestyle as long as possible, and (5) continue to practice cancer detection strategies.

■ Nursing Implementation

Health Promotion. Through their contact with women in a variety of settings, nurses can teach women the importance of routine screening for cancers of the reproductive system. Cancer can be prevented from ever occurring when screening can reveal precancerous conditions of the vulva, cervix, or endometrium. Also, routine screening increases the chance that a cancer will be identified in its early stage. When cancer is identified earlier, treatment can be more conservative and the woman's prognosis is better. A yearly pelvic examination and Pap test allows the health care provider to detect lesions on the vulva or any uterine or ovarian irregularities and screen for cervical cancer. Nurses can assist women to view routine cancer screening as an important self-care activity.

Educating women about risk factors for cancers of the reproductive system is also very important. Limiting sexual activity during adolescence, using condoms, having fewer sexual partners, and not smoking reduce the risk of cervical cancer.[22] A high-fat diet increases risk for ovarian cancer. Therefore, when high risk behaviors are identified, nurses should assist women with behavior change.

Acute Intervention with Surgery. All patients experience a degree of anxiety when surgery is contemplated, but the prospect of major gynecologic surgery may heighten these concerns. Some women may fear a loss of femininity and worry about possible changes in their secondary sex characteristics. Others may experience feelings of guilt, anger, or embarrassment. Still others may focus on the effect the surgery will have on their reproductive and sexual functions. There are also women who view the whole process as annoying or who are relieved by the thought of no longer having to worry about having menstrual periods or becoming pregnant. Each patient must be understood in light of her fears and concerns and must be approached and evaluated individually. The nurse who exhibits interest and a willingness to listen can provide considerable psychologic support.

Hysterectomy. Preoperatively, the patient is prepared physically for surgery with the standard perineal or abdominal preparation. A vaginal douche and enemas may be given, according to the preference of the surgeon. The bladder should be emptied before the patient is sent to the operating room. An indwelling catheter is often inserted preoperatively.

After surgery the patient who has had a hysterectomy will have an abdominal dressing (abdominal hysterectomy) or a sterile perineal pad (vaginal hysterectomy). (See NCP 51-2 for care of the patient after a total abdominal hysterectomy.) The dressing should be observed frequently for any sign of bleeding during the first 8 hours after surgery. A moderate amount of serosanguineous drainage on the perineal pad is expected following a vaginal hysterectomy.

The patient may experience urinary retention postoperatively because of temporary bladder atony resulting from edema or nerve trauma. This problem is more acute when a radical hysterectomy has been performed. At times an indwelling catheter is used for 1 to 2 days postoperatively to maintain constant drainage of the bladder and prevent strain on the suture line. If an indwelling catheter is not used, catheterization may be necessary if the patient has not urinated for 8 hours postoperatively. If residual urine is suspected after the removal of an indwelling catheter, catheterization is done to prevent bladder infection caused by pooling of urine. Accidental ligation of a ureter is a serious surgical complication. Any complaint of backache or decreased urine output should be reported to the surgeon.

Abdominal distention may develop from the sudden release of pressure on the intestines when a large tumor is removed or from paralytic ileus secondary to anesthesia and pressure on the bowel. Food and fluids may be restricted if the patient is nauseated. A rectal tube may be prescribed to relieve abdominal flatus, and ambulation is encouraged. A Fleet enema or suppository is frequently given on the third postoperative day.

Special care must be taken to prevent the development of thrombophlebitis of the veins in the pelvis or legs. Frequent changes of position and the avoidance of high Fowler's position and pressure under the knees minimize stasis and pooling of blood. Special attention must be given to patients with varicosities. Leg exercises to promote circulation and the use of elastic gradient compression stockings or elastic bandages can be helpful.

The loss of the uterus may bring about grief responses similar to any great personal loss. The ability to bear children is central to society's image of being a female. Although not experienced by all women, grief over this loss is normal. Eliciting the woman's feelings and concerns about her surgery, will provide the needed information to give understanding care. When surgery removes the ovaries as well, women experience surgical menopause. Estrogen is no longer available from the ovaries, so symptoms of estrogen deficiency will arise. To counter this, hormone therapy may be initiated in the early postoperative period.

Discharge teaching should prepare the patient for what to expect following surgery (e.g., she will not menstruate). Teaching should include specific activity restrictions. Intercourse should be avoided until the wound is healed (about 4 to 6 weeks). However, intercourse is not contraindicated once healing is complete. Sutures at the top of the vagina can tear and produce considerable bleeding if genital sex is engaged in too early or too vigorously. Secondary sex characteristics are not affected unless the ovaries have been removed. If a vaginal hysterectomy is performed, the woman needs to know that there may be a temporary loss of vaginal sensation. She should be reassured that sensation will return in several months.

Physical restrictions are limited for a short time. Heavy lifting should be avoided for 2 months. Activities that may increase pelvic congestion, such as dancing and walking swiftly, should be avoided for several months, whereas activities such as swimming may be both physically and mentally helpful. Wearing a girdle is allowed and may provide comfort. Once the patient has been assured that healing is complete, all previous activity can be resumed.

Salpingectomy and oophorectomy. Postoperative care of the woman who has undergone removal of a fallopian tube (*salpingectomy*) or an ovary (*oophorectomy*) is similar to that for any patient having abdominal surgery. One exception is that if a large ovarian cyst is removed, there may be abdominal distention caused by the sudden release of pressure on the intestines. An abdominal binder may provide relief until the distention subsides.

When both ovaries are removed (bilateral oophorectomy), surgical menopause results. The symptoms are similar to those of regular menopause but may be more severe because of the sudden withdrawal of hormones. Attempts may be made to leave at least a portion of an ovary. Replacement therapy with estrogen is given to most patients to avoid symptoms of menopause and to prevent bone loss and the development of osteoporosis.

Vulvectomy. Although cancer of the vulva is relatively uncommon, it is important that the nurse recognize the extent of the vulvectomy and the significant effect it is likely to have on the patient's life. An honest, open attitude with the patient and her partner preoperatively can be most helpful in the postoperative period.

After a vulvectomy, the patient returns to the unit with a wound in the perineal area extending to the groin. The wounds may be covered or left exposed and frequently have drains attached to portable suction (e.g., Hemovac). A heavy pressure dressing is often in place for the first 24 to 48 hours.

The wounds are cleaned with normal saline solution or an antiseptic twice daily. Solutions can be applied with an aseptic bulb syringe or a WaterPik machine. A heat lamp or a hair dryer is then used to dry the area. Wound care must be meticulous to prevent infection, which results in delayed healing.

Special attention to bowel and bladder care is needed. A low-residue diet and fecal softeners prevent straining at stool and wound contamination. An indwelling catheter is used to provide urinary drainage. Great care is taken not to dislodge the catheter because the extensive edema in the area would make its reinsertion difficult. Heavy, taut sutures are often used to close the wounds, resulting in severe discomfort for the patient. In other instances the wound may be allowed to heal by granulation. Analgesics may be required frequently to control pain. Careful positioning of the patient through the use of strategically placed pillows provides comfort. Ambulation is usually begun on the second postoperative day, but this varies with the preference of the surgeon. Anticoagulant therapy to prevent vascular complications is common.

Because the surgery causes mutilation of the perineal area and the healing process is slow, the patient is likely to become discouraged. Opportunities for the patient to express her feelings and concerns about the operation should be provided. The patient needs specific instructions in self-care before she is discharged. She should be told to report any unusual odor, fresh bleeding, breakdown of incision, or perineal pain. Home care nursing can benefit the patient during her adjustment period. Sexual function is often retained. Whether clitoral sensation is retained may be critical to some women, particularly if it was a primary source of orgasmic satisfaction. A discussion of alternative methods of achieving sexual satisfaction may also be indicated.

Pelvic exenteration. When other forms of therapy are ineffective in checking the spread of cancer and no metastases have been found outside of the pelvis, pelvic exenteration may be performed. Although different types are done, this radical surgery usually involves removal of the uterus, ovaries, fallopian tubes, vagina, bladder, urethra, and pelvic lymph nodes (Fig. 51-10). In some situations, the descending colon, rectum, and anal canal may also be removed. Candidates for this procedure are selected on the basis of their likelihood of surviving the surgery and their ability to adjust to and accept the resulting limitations.

The postoperative care involves that of a patient who has had a radical hysterectomy, an abdominal perineal resection, an ileostomy or colostomy, a cystectomy, and urinary diversion surgery. The physical, emotional, and social adjustments to life on the part of the woman and her family are great. There are urinary or fecal diversions in the abdominal wall, a reconstructed vagina, and the onset of menopausal symptoms.

The patient's rehabilitative process should keep pace with her acceptance of the situation. Much understanding and support is needed from the nursing staff during a long hospital stay. The patient should be gently encouraged to regain her independence. She needs to verbalize her feelings about her altered body structure to an interested and concerned listener. Inclusion of the family in the plan of care is important.

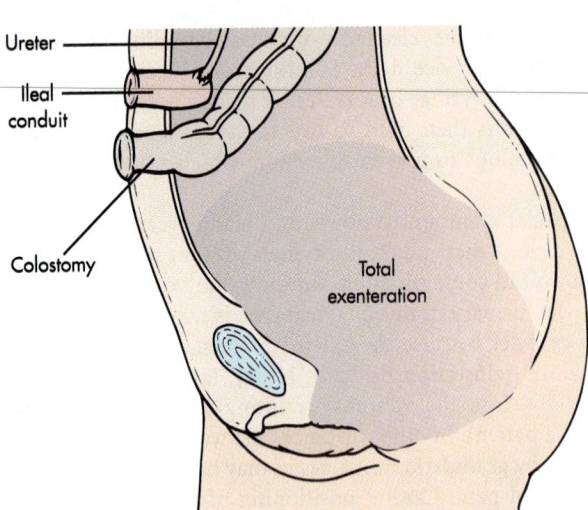

Fig. 51-10   Total exenteration is removal of all pelvic organs with creation of an ileal conduit and colostomy.

The patient needs to return to her physician at specified intervals. Early recurrence of the cancer may then be identified and treated. At this time the patient's physical and emotional adjustment to the changes in body image produced by the surgery and her ability to carry out any treatment measures can also be assessed. Additional teaching and counseling can then be provided.

Acute Intervention with Radiation Therapy. Nursing management of a patient receiving internal radiation therapy requires special considerations. The nurse should not stay in the immediate area any longer than is necessary to give proper care and attention. No individual nurse should attend the patient for more than 30 minutes per day. The nurse should stay at the foot of the bed or at the entrance to the room to minimize radiation exposure. Visitors should be told to stay 6 feet away from the bed and limit visits to less than 3 hours a day. Efficient organization of nursing care is essential so the nurse does not stay in the immediate area of the patient any longer than is necessary. The reasons for these precautions should be explained fully to the patient and her visitors. (A more detailed discussion of nursing care of the patient with an internal implant is given in Chapter 14.)

When the patient is to receive external radiation, she should be told to urinate immediately before the treatment to minimize radiation exposure to the bladder. She should be advised about the radiation side effects, including enteritis and cystitis, that may occur. These are natural reactions to radiotherapy and do not indicate an overdose. The patient should be fully informed of the possible side effects and measures to use to reduce their impact.

■ Evaluation

The expected outcomes are that the patient with a malignant tumor of the reproductive system will

- actively participate in treatment decisions
- achieve satisfactory pain and symptom management

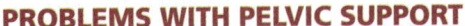

- recognize and report problems promptly
- maintain preferred lifestyle as long as possible
- continue to practice cancer detection strategies

PROBLEMS WITH PELVIC SUPPORT

The most common occurring problems with pelvic support are uterine prolapse, cystocele, and rectocele. Vaginal birth increases the risk for these problems, but women without any children can also have them. Obesity, chronic coughing, and straining during bowel movements can increase the likelihood of these problems. The decreased estrogen that normally accompanies the perimenopause also reduces some connective tissue support.

Uterine Prolapse

Uterine prolapse is the downward displacement of the uterus into the vaginal canal (Fig. 51-11). Prolapse is rated by degrees. In first-degree prolapse, the cervix rests in the lower part of the vagina. Second-degree prolapse means the cervix is at the vaginal opening. A third-degree prolapse means the uterus protrudes through the introitus. Symptoms vary with the degree of prolapse. The patient may describe a feeling of "something coming down." She may have dyspareunia, a dragging or heavy feeling in the pelvis, backache, and bowel or bladder problems if cystocele or rectocele are also present. Stress incontinence is a common and troubling problem. When third-degree uterine prolapse occurs, the protruding cervix and vaginal walls are subjected to constant irritation, and tissue changes may occur.

Therapy depends on the degree of prolapse and how much the woman's daily activities have been affected. Pelvic muscle strengthening exercises (Kegel exercises) may be effective for some women. If not, a pessary may be used. A *pessary* is a devise that is placed in the vagina to help to support the uterus. A wide variety of shapes exist including rings, arches, and balls. Most are made of plastic or wire coated with plastic. When a woman first receives a pessary, she also needs instructions for its cleaning and follow-up. Pessaries that are left in place for long periods are associated with erosion, fistulas, and an increased incidence of vaginal carcinoma. If more conservative measures are not successful, surgery is indicated. Surgery generally involves a vaginal hysterectomy with anterior and posterior repair of the vagina and underlying fascia.

Cystocele and Rectocele

Cystocele occurs when support between the vagina and bladder is weakened (Fig. 51-12). Similarly, a *rectocele* results from weakening between the vagina and rectum. These problems are common and asymptomatic in many women. With large cystoceles, complete emptying of the bladder can be difficult, predisposing women to bladder infections. A woman with a large rectocele may not be able to completely empty her rectum when defecating unless she helps to push the stool out by putting her fingers in her vagina.

As with uterine prolapse, Kegel exercises may be used to strengthen the weakened perineal muscles if the cystocele or rectocele is not too problematic. A pessary may be helpful for cystoceles. Surgery designed to tighten the vaginal wall is generally the method of treatment. A cystocele is corrected with a

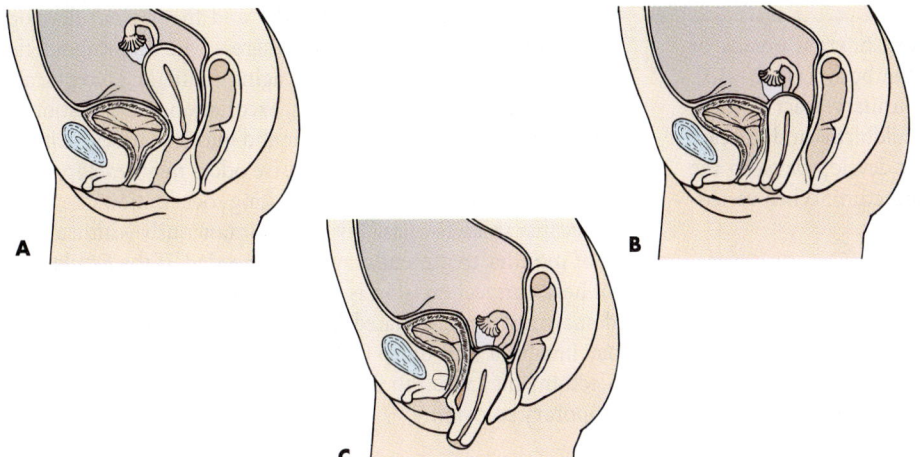

Fig. 51-11 Uterine prolapse. **A,** First-degree prolapse. **B,** Second-degree prolapse. **C,** Third-degree prolapse.

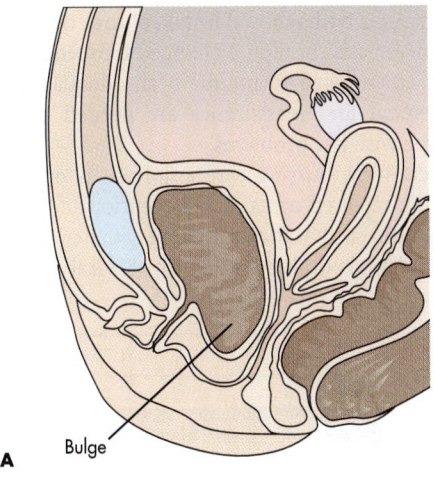

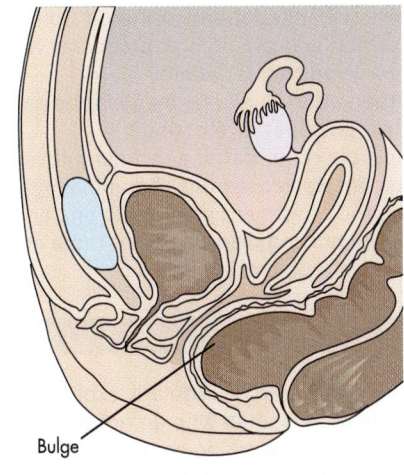

Fig. 51-12 **A,** Cystocele. **B,** Rectocele.

procedure called an anterior colporrhaphy, whereas a posterior colporrhaphy is done for a rectocele. If further surgery is needed to relieve stress incontinence, procedures to support the urethra and restore the proper angle between the urethra and the posterior bladder wall are used.

NURSING MANAGEMENT: PROBLEMS WITH PELVIC SUPPORT

Nurses can assist women to avoid or decrease problems with pelvic support by teaching them how to do Kegel exercises to strengthen their pelvic floor muscles. Women of all ages can benefit from these exercises. However, Kegel exercises are especially important following childbirth or whenever women begin to have incontinence. To instruct a patient in this exercise, she should be told to pull in or contract her muscles as if she were trying to stop the flow of urine. She should hold the contraction for several seconds and then relax. Sets of 5 to 10 contractions each should be done several times daily.

If vaginal surgery is necessary, the preoperative preparation usually includes a cleansing douche the morning of surgery. A cathartic and a cleansing enema are usually given when a rectocele repair is scheduled. A perineal shave is done.

In the postoperative period, the goals of care are to prevent wound infection and pressure on the vaginal suture line. This necessitates perineal care at least twice a day and after each urination or defecation. An ice pack applied locally may relieve the initial perineal discomfort and swelling. A disposable glove filled with ice and covered with a cloth works well in these instances. Later, sitz baths may be used. A heat lamp may be used to help dry the area and enhance the healing process.

After an anterior colporrhaphy, an indwelling catheter is usually left in the bladder for 4 days to allow the local edema to subside. The catheter keeps the bladder empty, thereby preventing strain on the sutures. Catheter care with an antiseptic is generally done twice daily. After posterior colporrhaphy, straining at stool is avoided by means of a low-residue diet and the prevention of constipation. A stool softener is usually given each night.

Discharge instructions should be reviewed before the patient leaves the hospital. They include the use of douches or mild laxatives as needed; restriction of heavy lifting and prolonged standing, walking, or sitting; and avoidance of intercourse until the physician gives permission. There may be a loss of vaginal sensation, which can last for several months. The patient needs to be reassured that this situation is temporary.

FISTULAS

A *fistula* is an abnormal opening between internal organs or between an organ and the exterior of the body (Fig. 51-13). Gynecologic procedures cause 75% of urinary tract fistulas. Other causes include injury during childbirth and disease processes such as carcinoma. Fistulas may develop between the vagina and the bladder, urethra, ureter, or rectum. When vesico-vaginal fistulas (between the bladder and the vagina) develop, some urine leaks into the vagina, whereas with rectovaginal fistulas (between the rectum and the vagina), flatus and feces escape into the vagina. In both instances, excoriation and irritation of the vaginal and vulvar tissues occur and may lead to severe infections. In addition to wetness, offensive odors may develop, causing embarrassment and severely limiting socialization.

Because small fistulas may heal spontaneously within a matter of months, treatment may not be needed. If the fistula does not heal, surgical excision is required. Inflammation and tissue edema must be eliminated before surgery is attempted. This may involve a wait of up to 6 months for the surgery. The fistulectomy may result in the patient's having an ileal conduit or temporary colostomy.

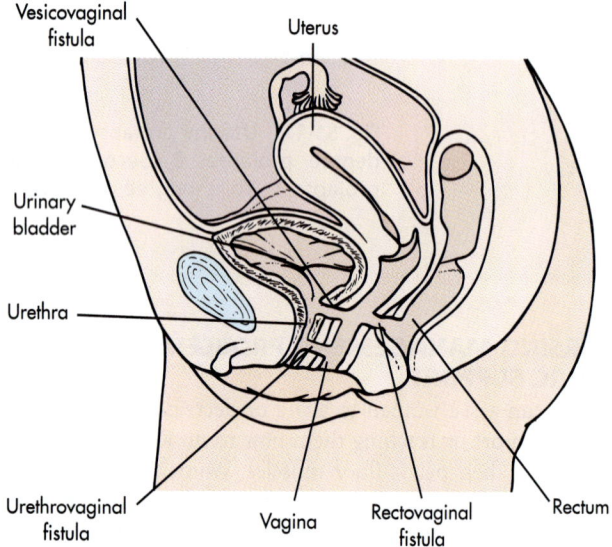

Fig. 51-13 Common fistulas involving the vagina.

NURSING MANAGEMENT: FISTULAS

Perineal hygiene is of great importance, both preoperatively and postoperatively. The perineum should be cleansed every 4 hours. Warm sitz baths should be taken three times daily if possible. Perineal pads should be changed frequently. The patient should be encouraged to maintain an adequate fluid intake. Encouragement and reassurance are needed in helping the patient cope with her problems.

Postoperatively, nursing care emphasis is on avoidance of stress on the repaired areas and prevention of infection. Care should be taken so that the indwelling catheter, usually in place for 7 to 10 days, is draining at all times. Oral fluids should be

CRITICAL THINKING EXERCISES

CASE STUDY

Total Abdominal Hysterectomy

Patient Profile

Marion P., a 40-year-old woman with two children, consulted her health care provider about experiencing menorrhagia and occasionally metrorrhagia for the past 5 months. She was diagnosed with leiomyomas, and a total abdominal hysterectomy was recommended.

Subjective Data

- Was initially reluctant about surgery
- States family is complete
- Concerned that she may actually have uterine cancer

Objective Data

Physical Examination
- Has several large, firm masses thought to be leiomyomas in body of uterus
- Had otherwise normal physical examination

Postoperative Status
- Returned to room with indwelling urinary catheter in place
- Legs wrapped in full-length elastic compression gradient stockings

Critical Thinking Questions

1. What are the common causes of menorrhagia and metrorrhagia?
2. What clinical manifestations may result from leiomyomas?
3. What physical and psychologic preoperative preparation should be given to this patient?
4. What observation should be made in the patient's immediate postoperative period?
5. What possible complications, including their basis for development, can arise after abdominal hysterectomy?
6. Based on the assessment data, write one or more appropriate nursing diagnoses. Are there any collaborative problems?

NURSING RESEARCH ISSUES

1. Do women who exercise regularly experience less dysmenorrhea than women who do not exercise regularly?
2. Do working or nonworking women experience more episodes of vasomotor instability during the perimenopausal period?
3. Are women who use a female condom satisfied with this form of birth control?
4. Does the emotional response of the nurse caring for a rape victim help or hinder effective intervention?
5. What parameters can a nurse use in deciding how much information to provide to a woman who is to have a pelvic exenteration?

urged to provide for internal catheter irrigation. Minimal pressure and strict asepsis are used if catheter irrigation becomes necessary. The first stool after bowel surgery may be purposely delayed to prevent contamination of the wound. Later, stool softeners or mild laxatives may be given. See Chapter 43 for care of a patient with an ileal conduit and Chapter 40 for care of a patient with a colostomy. Surgical repair of fistulas is not always effective, even in the best conditions. Therefore supportive nursing care for the patient and her significant others is especially important.

REVIEW QUESTIONS

The number of the question corresponds to the same-numbered objective at the beginning of the chapter.

1. In assisting a sexually active woman to choose a birth control method, the nurse advises the patient that taking oral contraceptives may cause
   a. later infertility.
   b. infection of the uterus.
   c. toxic shock syndrome.
   d. thromboembolic disorders.

2. In telling a patient with infertility what she and her partner can expect, the nurse explains that
   a. the cause should be diagnosed by the second visit.
   b. an hysterosalpingogram is a common diagnostic study.
   c. if postcoital studies are normal, infection tests will be done.
   d. the reason will remain unexplained for 50% of couples.

3. A patient with a spontaneous abortion is more likely than the patient with an induced abortion to have
   a. a D&C performed.
   b. feelings of loss and grief.
   c. emotional support from family and friends.
   d. physical complications such as infection.

4. An appropriate question to ask the patient with painful menstruation to differentiate primary dysmenorrhea from secondary dysmenorrhea is
   a. "Does your pain become worse with activity or overexertion?"
   b. "Have you had a recent personal crisis or change in your lifestyle?"
   c. "Is your pain relieved by nonsteroidal antiinflammatory medications?"
   d. "When in your menstrual history did the pain with your period begin?"

5. In caring for a patient after an ectopic pregnancy was surgically removed, the nurse advises the patient that
   a. most ectopic pregnancies attach to the ovary.
   b. she will not be able to get pregnant in the future.
   c. bed rest must be maintained for 24 hours to assist healing.
   d. having one ectopic pregnancy increases her risk for another.

6. To prevent or decrease age-related pathology that occurs after menopause in a patient who chooses not to take hormone therapy, the nurse teaches the patient that the most important self-care measure is
   a. maintaining usual sexual activity.
   b. increasing the intake of dietary calcium.
   c. performing regular aerobic, weight-bearing exercise.
   d. taking vitamin E and vitamin B-complex supplements.

7. The first nursing intervention for the patient who has been raped is to
   a. treat urgent medical problems.
   b. contact a support person for the patient.
   c. provide supplies for the patient to cleanse self.
   d. document bruises and lacerations of the perineum and cervix.

8. The patient's history indicating thick, white, curdlike vaginal discharge and vulvar pruritus is most consistent with
   a. bacterial vaginosis.
   b. chlamydial cervicitis.
   c. monilial vaginitis.
   d. trichomoniasis.

9. The nurse caring for a patient with pelvic inflammatory disease places her in semi-Fowler's position. The rationale for this measure is to
   a. relieve pain.
   b. prevent the complication of sterility.
   c. improve circulation and promote healing.
   d. promote drainage to prevent abscesses.

10. In planning care for the patient receiving medical management of endometriosis, the nurse includes teaching regarding the side effects of
    a. estrogen supplementation.
    b. large doses of vitamins A and E.
    c. hormonal suppression of ovulation.
    d. long-term use of NSAIDs.

11. A 31-year-old woman who wishes to have children is diagnosed with leiomyoma. The nurse plans care for the patient based on the knowledge that
    a. a hysterectomy will be necessary to treat the tumor.
    b. a myomectomy may be performed to maintain fertility.
    c. hormonal therapy to shrink the tumor and increase fertility can be used.
    d. aspirin and other NSAIDs used to control pain may cause fetal defects.

12. A 52-year-old woman who has not had a menstrual period for 18 months tells the nurse she has recently had some spotting. The nurse advises the patient that
    a. she should keep a menstrual calendar for the next 6 months.
    b. this problem should be further investigated by an endometrial biopsy.
    c. this is a common, but not serious, problem that can occur after menopause.
    d. warm douching is recommended to promote healing of fragile vaginal tissue.

13. The nurse plans early and frequent ambulation for the patient who has undergone an abdominal hysterectomy in order to
    a. prevent urinary retention.
    b. promote pelvic circulation.
    c. relieve abdominal distention.
    d. maintain a sense of normalcy.

14. Nursing responsibilities related to the patient receiving internal radiation for uterine cancer include
    a. maintaining absolute bed rest.
    b. allowing the patient bathroom privileges only.
    c. limiting an individual nurse's contact with the patient to 1 hour per day.
    d. allowing visitors to stay as long as desired if they stay 6 feet (2 meters) from the bed.

15. When instructing a woman how to do Kegel exercises, the nurse should advise her
    a. to tighten abdominal muscles and hold her breath.
    b. to tilt the pelvis forward keeping her back as straight as possible.
    c. to bear down like having a bowel movement and hold her breath.
    d. to tighten her perineal muscles as if trying to stop the flow of urine.

References

1. Hatcher RA and others: *Contraceptive technology*, ed 16, New York, 1994, Irvington.
2. Grimes DA: *Contraception Report* 9:4, 1998.
3. DeCherney A: Bone sparing properties of oral contraceptives, *Am J Obstet Gynecol* 174:15, 1996.
4. MacKay H, Trent MD: Gynecology. In Lawrence M: *Current medical diagnosis and treatment*, ed 37, Stamford, Conn, 1998, Appleton & Lange.
5. Kaunitz AM: Long-acting injectable contraception with depot medroxyprogesterone acetate, *Am J Obstet Gynecol* 170:1543, 1994.
6. Stewart F: Promoting emergency contraception, *Hosp Pract* 33:61, 1998.
7. Davis LE, Stockton MD: Office procedures: No scalpel vasectomy, *Prim Care* 24:433, 1997.
8. Holt BA, Higgins AF: Minimally invasive vasectomy, *Br J Urol* 77:585, 1996.
9. Carlson KJ, Eisenstat SA, editors: *Primary care of women*, St Louis, 1995, Mosby.
10. Schroeder CJ, Krysa LW: The comfort and discomfort of infertility, *JOGNN* 25:167, 1996.
11. Johnson CA and others: *Women's health care handbook*, Philadelphia, 1996, Hanley & Belfus/Mosby.
12. Speroff L, Glass RH, Kase NG: *Clinical gynecologic endocrinology and infertility*, ed 5, Baltimore, 1994, Williams & Wilkins.
13. Youngkin EQ, Davis MS: *Women's health*, ed 2, Stamford, Conn, 1998, Appleton & Lange.
14. Freeman EW and others: PMS: new treatments that really work, *Contemp OB/GYN* 41:25, 1996.
15. Leppart PC, Howard FM: *Primary care of women*, Philadelphia, 1997, Lippincott-Raven.
16. Rosenfeld JA: *Women's health in primary care*, Baltimore, 1997, Williams & Wilkins.
17. LeBoeuf, FJ, Carter SG: Discomforts of the perimenopause, *JOGNN* 25:173, 1996.
18. Gelfand MM: Women and androgen—HRT, *Women's Health Digest* 3:236, 1997.
19. Paganini-Hill A, Henderson VW: Estrogen replacement therapy and risk of Alzheimer's disease, *Arch Intern Med* 156:221, 1996.
20. Taylor M: Alternatives to conventional hormone replacement therapy, *Complement Ther* 23:514, 1997.
21. Center for Disease Control and Prevention: 1998 Guidelines for treatment of sexually transmitted diseases, *MMWR* 47, 1998.
22. Moore GJ: *Women and cancer*, Boston, 1997, Jones & Bartlett.
23. Schwartz PE: Prophylactic oophorectomy for the prevention of epithelial ovarian cancer revisited, *Eur Menopause J* 4:105, 1997.
24. Reisner JG, Miollis M: Laparoscopically assisted vaginal hysterectomy in a community hospital, *J Reprod Med* 42:542, 1997.
25. Riza ED: Laparoscopically assisted vaginal hysterectomy: report of 190 cases, *J Laparoendosc Adv Surg Techniques* 7:13, 1997.

Resources

Association of Women's Health, Obstetric, & Neonatal Nurses (AWHONN)
2000 L Street, Suite 740
Washington, D.C. 20036
800-673-8499 (U.S.)
800-245-0231 (Canada)
Fax: 202-737-0575
http://www.awhonn.org/

National Center for Education in Maternal and Child Health
2000 15th Street, North, Suite 701
Arlington, VA 22201-2617
703-524-7802
Fax: 703-524-9335
http://www.ncemch.georgetown.edu/

For additional Internet resources, see the website for this book at
www.mosby.com/MERLIN/medsurg_lewis

52 | NURSING MANAGEMENT
Male Genitourinary Problems

Cindy Meredith

www.mosby.com/MERLIN/medsurg_lewis

LEARNING OBJECTIVES

1. Describe the pathophysiology, clinical features, diagnostic studies, and collaborative care of benign prostatic hyperplasia.
2. Describe the nursing management of benign prostatic hyperplasia.
3. Describe the pathophysiology, clinical features, diagnostic studies, and collaborative care of cancer of the prostate.
4. Describe the nursing management of prostate cancer.
5. Describe the pathophysiology, clinical features, diagnostic studies, and collaborative and nursing management of problems of the penis, problems of the scrotum, and prostatitis.
6. Explain the nursing management of problems related to male sexual functioning.
7. Identify the psychologic and emotional implications of problems related to the male genitourinary organs.

Problems of the male genitourinary system can involve a variety of structures (Fig. 52-1) and create anxiety for both the patient and nurse providing care. Anxiety and fear may also cause the patient to delay seeking help for a problem or practicing health-promoting behaviors. Our society often does not encourage men to admit to or seek help for problems related to their sex organs. The nurse should be particularly sensitive to the possible embarrassment associated with a male genitourinary problem.

PROBLEMS OF THE PROSTATE GLAND

BENIGN PROSTATIC HYPERPLASIA

The most common problem of the adult male genitourinary system is *benign prostatic hyperplasia* (BPH), a term referring to an increase in the number of epithelial and especially stromal tissue within the prostate gland. The problem occurs in about 50% of men over 50 years of age and 75% of men over 70 years of age. BPH is most likely to develop in the innermost part of the prostate,[1] and cancer is most likely to develop in the outer part of the prostate gland (Fig. 52-2).[2] Prostatic hyperplasia does not predispose to the development of cancer of the prostate.

Etiology and Pathophysiology

BPH begins with enlargement of the glandular tissue. Although the cause is not completely understood, it is thought that the primary cause is an increased number of cells resulting from endocrine changes associated with the aging process. Excessive accumulation of dihydroxytestosterone (the principal intraprostatic androgen), stimulation of estrogen, and local growth hormone action are proposed causes.

Clinical Manifestations

The patient seeks assistance for relief of the symptoms related to urinary obstruction. Symptoms are usually gradual in onset and may not be noticed until prostatic enlargement has been present for some time. There is no direct relationship between the degree of obstruction and the size of the prostate. Mild hyperplasia can cause severe obstruction, whereas severe hyperplasia can result in few bladder symptoms. It is often the location of the enlargement rather than the size that causes the symptoms. Treatment is generally based on the degree to which the symptoms bother the patient rather than on the size of the prostate alone.

Early symptoms are usually minimal because the bladder can compensate for a small amount of resistance to urine flow.[3] With increasing blockage, obstructive symptoms of BPH develop. Symptoms include a decrease in the caliber and force of the urinary stream, hesitancy in initiating voiding, dribbling at the end of urination, and a feeling of incomplete bladder emptying because of urinary retention. Irritative symptoms include nocturia and urgency, which can develop from inflammatory, infectious, or neoplastic causes.

Self-assessment such as the one developed by the American Urological Association (AUA) (Table 52-1) and quality-of-life questionnaires have been developed to facilitate assessment of the symptom burden. Such tools are also used to facilitate decisions regarding treatment options.

Reviewed by Donna Berry, PhD, RN, AOCN, Research Assistant Professor, University of Washington, School of Nursing, Seattle, Wash.

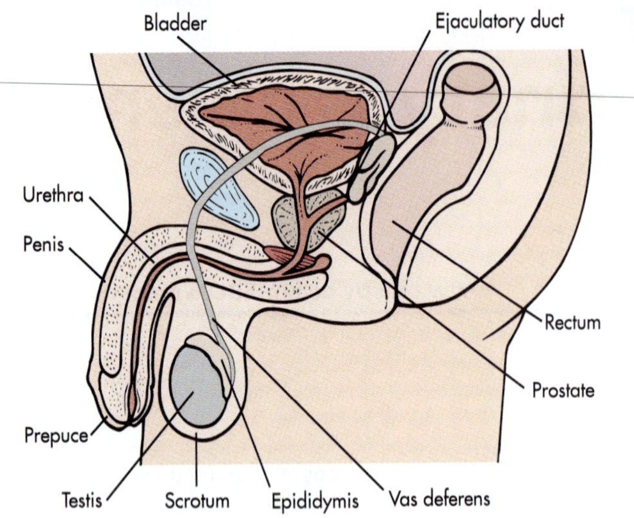

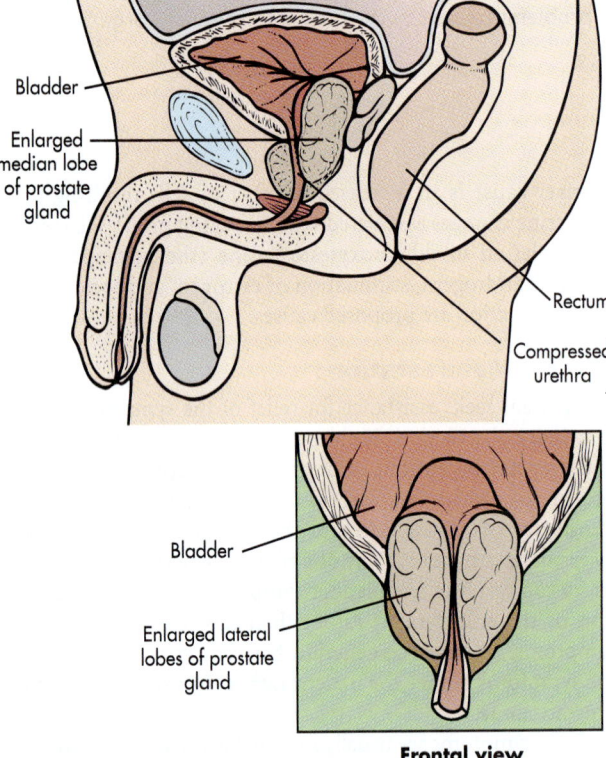

Fig. 52-1   Areas of the male reproductive system in which problems are likely to develop.

Fig. 52-2   Benign prostatic hyperplasia.

Complications

The patient with BPH is at increased risk for urinary tract infection. The bladder does not empty completely because of partial or complete obstruction of the proximal urethra. The residual urine provides a favorable environment for bacterial growth. Calculi may develop because of the alkalinization of the residual urine. Breakage of tiny overstretched blood vessels in the bladder may produce hematuria. Increased pressure in the bladder can cause wall thickening and the formation of diverticula.

More serious complications resulting from urinary retention are bladder dysfunction, abnormally distended ureters (hydroureters), destruction of the kidney's parenchyma from the back pressure of the urine (hydronephrosis), and infection (pyelonephritis). These complications can lead to renal failure.

Diagnostic Studies

The primary diagnostic test for BPH is a digital rectal examination (DRE) to palpate for enlargement and assess whether the gland is hard, nodular, or "boggy." In the early stages of BPH, the specific gravity of the urine may be unchanged or elevated because the patient may restrict fluid intake to decrease the need to void. If hydronephrosis with renal impairment has occurred, the specific gravity will be about 1.010, which is the specific gravity of plasma. The presence of bacteria, white blood cells, or microscopic hematuria found on urinalysis may indicate the presence of infection or inflammation. If BPH has been a long-standing problem, the blood urea nitrogen (BUN) and serum creatinine levels may be elevated because of renal involvement. The prostate-specific antigen (PSA) blood level is examined as a potential indicator of prostatic cancer.

Secondary diagnostic screening may include a transrectal ultrasound (TRUS) scan of the prostate, urodynamic flow studies, and cystoscopy. A TRUS scan is useful in locating specific areas of enlargement or tumors. A biopsy can be taken during the ultrasound procedure. Locating and possible staging of cancer growths provide important information in deciding whether surgery or another treatment option should be the first approach to care.

Urine flow studies are helpful in determining the extent of obstruction. Measuring the urinary flow rate helps gauge the extent of blockage and aid in determining the type of treatment needed. Cystourethroscopy may be done to evaluate bladder neck obstruction in patients scheduled for surgery. Diagnostic studies are outlined in Table 52-2.

Collaborative Care

The goal of collaborative management is to restore bladder drainage, relieve the patient's symptoms, and prevent or treat the complications of BPH.

Conservative Therapy

The primary treatment for BPH is now referred to as "watchful waiting." When there are no symptoms or only mild ones, a conservative, noninvasive wait-and-see approach is taken. If the patient begins to have signs or symptoms that indicate an increase in uretheral obstruction, further treatment is indicated. The numerous treatment options for BPH can be categorized as pharmacologic, nonsurgical invasive, and surgical invasive options.[4,5]

Drug Therapy. Hormone manipulation can be used to cause regression of hyperplastic tissue through suppression of androgens. Finasteride (Proscar) blocks the enzyme 5-α-reductase, which is necessary for the conversion of testosterone to dihydroxytestosterone, the principal intraprostatic androgen. Studies have shown a decrease in prostate size and an increase in urine flow. This medication must be taken on a continuous

Table **52-1**	American Urological Association Symptom Index to Determine Severity of Prostatic Problems

Questions to Be Answered	American Urological Association (AUA) Symptom Score* (Circle 1 number on each line)					
	Not At All	Less Than 1 Time in 5	Less Than Half the Time	About Half the Time	More Than Half the Time	Almost Always
Over the past month, 1. How often have you had a sensation of not emptying your bladder completely after you finished urinating?	0	1	2	3	4	5
2. How often have you had to urinate again, less than 2 hr after you finished urinating?	0	1	2	3	4	5
3. How often have you found you stopped and started again several times when you urinated?	0	1	2	3	4	5
4. How often have you found it difficult to postpone urination?	0	1	2	3	4	5
5. How often have you had a weak urinary stream?	0	1	2	3	4	5
6. How often have you had to push or strain to begin urination?	0	1	2	3	4	5
7. How many times did you most typically get up to urinate from the time you went to bed at night until the time you got up in the morning?	0 (None)	1 (1 Time)	2 (2 times)	3 (3 times)	4 (4 times)	5 (5 times or more)
Sum of circled numbers (AUA Symptom Score):*_____						

From Barry B and others: The American Urological Association symptom index for benign prostatic hyperplasia, *J Urol* 148:1547, 1992. Used with permission.
*Score is interpreted as: 0-7, mild; 8-19, moderate; and 20-35, severe.

COLLABORATIVE CARE

Table **52-2**	Benign Prostatic Hyperplasia

Diagnostic

Primary Screening
History including symptoms of voiding problems
Physical examination including digital rectal exam (DRE)
Urinalysis with culture
Serum creatinine and BUN
Prostate-specific antigen (PSA)

Secondary Screening
Urodynamic flow studies
Transrectal ultrasound
Cystoscopy (for surgical candidates)

Collaborative Therapy

"Watchful waiting" and patient education
Catheterization (intermittent or indwelling)
High fluid intake
Antibiotics
Finasteride (Proscar) therapy
Alpha-adrenergic receptor blockers
   Prazosin (Minipress)
   Terazosin (Hytrin)
   Tamsulosin (Flomax)
Coils and stents
Balloon dilation
Thermoregulatory procedures (TUMA)
Laser ablation
Transurethral incision of the prostate (TUIP)
Transurethral resection of the prostate (TURP)
Open prostatectomy (>60 g)
   Suprapubic
   Retropubic
   Perineal

BUN, blood urea nitrogen.

basis to achieve therapeutic results. The major side effects are erectile dysfunction, which develops in about 10% of patients, and decreased libido.[6]

α-Adrenergic receptor blockade is another drug treatment option in the treatment of BPH. This type of drug causes smooth muscle relaxation in the prostate and the bladder neck. This relaxation ultimately facilitates urinary flow through the prostatic urethra. Several alpha-adrenergic blockers, such as prazosin (Minipress), doxazosin (Cardura), terazosin (Hytrin), and tamsulosin (Flomax), are currently being used. Alpha-adrenergic blockers do not decrease the prostate hyperplasia. Side effects, including postural hypotension, dizziness, and fatigue, can be a problem, especially if the patient is also taking cardiac or antihypertensive medication.

Herbal medicines extracted from plants (phytotherapy) have been used in the management of BPH. In particular, phytotherapy involving plant extracts, such as saw palmetto have been used. Although some data suggest improvement of urinary symptoms based on patient self-report, additional studies are needed.[10]

Nonsurgical Invasive Care

Intermittent catheterization or an indwelling catheter can temporarily be used to reduce symptoms and bypass the obstruction. Long-term catheter use should be avoided because of the increased risk of infection. If BPH becomes symptomatic, other nonsurgical invasive options may be tried before surgery. These outpatient options include stents or coils, prostatic balloon dilation, heat, and experimental approaches such as transurethral needle ablation (TUNA)[7] or percutaneous radical cryosurgical ablation (PRCSA).

One nonsurgical therapeutic option is the placement of stents (stainless steel) or coils (titanium) in the prostatic urethra. These devices hold back the walls of the prostate to allow for the unobstructed flow of urine. In the majority of cases the stents become covered by epithelium, reducing the risk of

---

Table 52-3 | **Treatment Options for Benign Prostatic Hyperplasia**

Treatment Options	Advantages	Disadvantages
Nonsurgical Invasive		
▪ Stents and coils	Local anesthesia Minimal hemorrhage Short operative time Usually an outpatient procedure	Short-term incontinence
▪ Balloon dilation	Topical or local anesthesia Simple, short procedure Less expensive Outpatient procedure No impotence or retrograde ejaculation	Later treatment may be necessary Long-term effectiveness not known Tissue sample unavailable for histologic examination
▪ Heat (transurethral microwave antenna [TUMA])	Short procedure No retrograde ejaculation Decrease nocturia	Cell death in normal as well as benign and malignant tissue Potential for urinary retention
Surgical		
▪ Laser ablation (transurethral ultrasound-guided laser-induced prostatectomy [TULIP]; visual laser ablation of the prostate [VLAP])	Short procedure Little bleeding No fluid absorption Decreased incidence of retrograde ejaculation	Postoperative urinary retention Tissue sample unavailable for histologic examination
▪ Transurethral resection of the prostate (TURP)	No external incision Erectile dysfunction and long-term incontinence unlikely	Not all prostatic tissue removed Regular follow-up less likely
▪ Transurethral incision of the prostate (TUIP)	Maintenance of antegrade ejaculation Short operating time Minimal complications	Temporary solution Effective on small glands (< 30 g) Cancer can be missed Possible rectal injury
▪ Suprapubic prostate resection	Better exploration and visualization Choice for larger prostate	Increased risk of urinary tract infection, spasms, incontinence, hemorrhage Recovery longer than TURP Difficult in obese patient
▪ Retropubic prostate resection	Removal of large mass high in pelvic area Direct visualization of prostate possible Bladder not incised Voiding problems are rare	Difficult in obese patient High risk for hemorrhage Slight risk of erectile dysfunction
▪ Perineal prostate resection	Able to remove large mass low in pelvic area and lymph nodes Direct visualization of prostate and surrounding tissue	High risk of erectile dysfunction Possible urinary incontinence Higher risk of infection

encrustation and infection. The procedure is used most often for men who have medical contraindications to surgery because only local anesthesia is required for this procedure. The advantages and disadvantages of the various treatment options are compared in Table 52-3.

Another nonsurgical approach is prostatic balloon dilation, which uses a balloon device to dilate the urethra by stretching, fracturing, or compressing the gland to enlarge the passage and allow for free flow of urine. After dilation the balloon is removed, and the urethra is assessed for an increase in diameter. If the procedure is successful, an indwelling catheter is left in place for the first 24 hours to monitor urinary output and the extent of hematuria. The dilation procedure may be repeated if the first attempt is unsuccessful. The procedure is not a permanent solution to the problem of an enlarged prostate but does offer a nonsurgical, cost-saving option to appropriate patients, particularly those who are surgical risks. The balloon technique is contraindicated in patients with atonic bladder because dilation alone will not allow proper emptying of the bladder.

Microwave therapy involves the use of heat to reduce the prostatic tissue.[8,9] There are two basic types of microwave treatment. Hyperthermia involves either a transurethral or transrectal (rarely used today) heated probe. The transurethral probe raises the temperature in the prostate gland to between 107.6° and 111° F (42° and 44° C). The heat causes an inflammatory reaction but is not hot enough to result in tissue necrosis. After a series (between 3 and 20) of 1-hour treatments the obstruction is generally relieved.

In transurethral microwave thermal therapy (sometimes referred to as transurethral microwave antenna [TUMA] therapy, a one-time treatment), a microwave uretheral probe or catheter heats the prostatic tissue above 113° F (45° C) to produce tissue necrosis. A rectal temperature probe is often used during the procedure to be sure that the rectal temperature is kept below 110° F (43.5° C) to prevent rectal tissue damage. The patient is generally sent home with an indwelling catheter for 2 to 7 days to maintain urinary flow and to facilitate the passing of small clots or necrotic tissue. Prescriptions for an antibiotic, pain medication, and bladder antispasmodic medications are generally sent home with the patient. The procedure is not appropriate for men with rectal problems. Anticoagulant therapy should be stopped 10 days before treatment. Mild side effects include occasional problems of bladder spasm, hematuria, dysuria, and retention.

Surgical Therapy

Surgery is indicated when there is a decrease in urine flow sufficient to cause discomfort, persistent residual urine, acute urinary retention because of obstruction with no reversible precipitating cause, or hydronephrosis. Treatment of symptomatic BPH primarily involves resection of the prostate. The selection of a surgical approach to remove the tissue depends on the size and position of the prostatic enlargement (Fig. 52-3). No correlation has been found between symptoms and the size of the prostate.

It is the location of the enlargement rather than the amount that produces symptoms. The nurse can help the patient ask appropriate questions regarding the impact of a particular type of surgery.

Laser Ablation. A transurethral, ultrasound-guided, laser-induced prostatectomy (TULIP) is a specially designed laser used to decrease the obstructive tissue. A second approach is visual laser ablation of the prostate (VLAP), which uses a

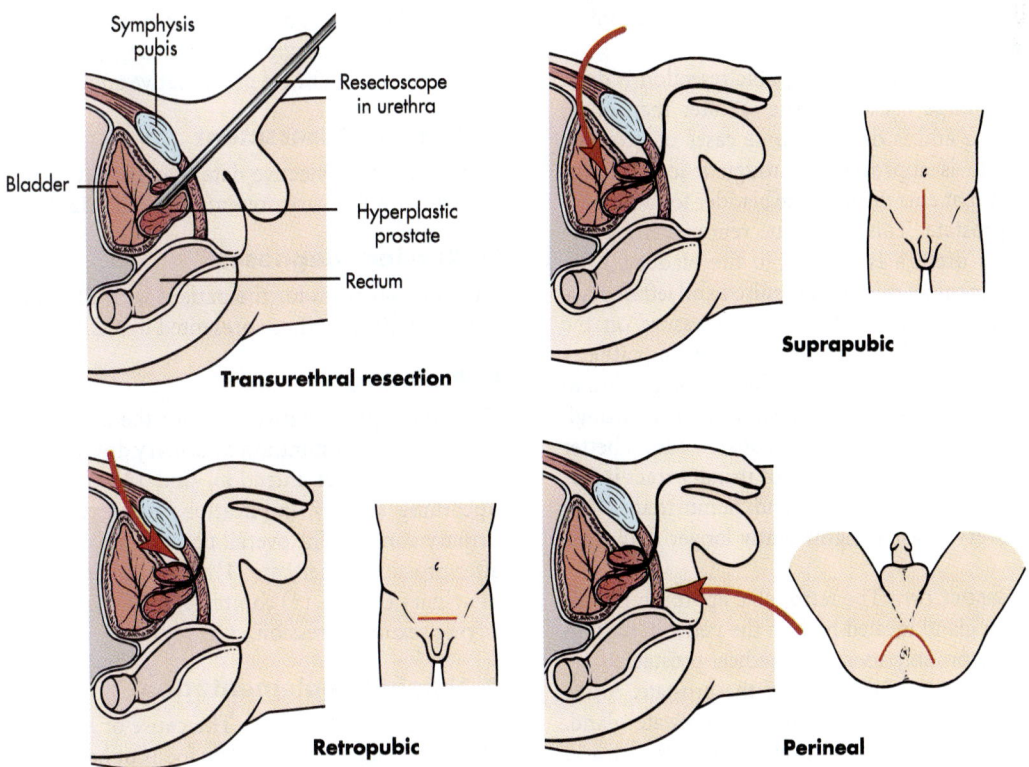

Fig. 52-3 Four types of prostatectomy.

standard cystoscope and allows direct visualization. Both approaches use the neodymium:yttrium-aluminum-garnet (Nd:YAG) laser, which produces coagulation necrosis and ultimately shrinkage of the prostate gland.

Transurethral Resection of the Prostate. Transurethral resection of the prostate (TURP) is the most common route for partial removal of the prostate. No external surgical incision is made because a resectoscope is passed through the urethra to excise and cauterize prostatic tissue. A large (no. 18 to no. 22) three-way indwelling catheter with a 30 ml balloon containing 30 to 60 ml of sterile water is usually inserted into the bladder after the procedure to provide hemostasis and facilitate urinary drainage. The bladder is irrigated, either continuously or intermittently, for approximately the first 24 hours to prevent obstruction from mucus threads and blood clots.

A TURP is often the surgery of choice for the debilitated patient or for the patient with moderate prostatic enlargement. The advantages of a TURP are that it does not involve an external incision and is less likely to result in erectile dysfunction or long-term urinary incontinence. A disadvantage is that it does not completely remove all prostatic tissue, leaving the potential for recurrence of hyperplasia, possible prostatic cancer, and sometimes the false impression that there is no need for yearly DREs.

Transurethral Incision of the Prostate. A transurethral incision of the prostate (TUIP) can be performed in high risk patients, those with mild obstruction, or younger patients. Transurethral slits or incisions are made into the prostatic tissue to relieve bladder neck obstruction. This method is usually used to treat intravesical obstruction related to BPH. The incision can be made unilaterally or bilaterally with a variety of instruments (including laser) at different locations around the bladder neck. The patient is discharged with an indwelling catheter for the first 24 hours to monitor urinary output and hematuria.

Suprapubic Resection. A suprapubic resection is done when an extremely large mass of tissue (greater than 60 g) obstructs the urethra and is done in some cases of prostatic cancer. The prostate is approached through a low midline abdominal incision that cuts through the bladder to the anterior or aspect of the prostate. This technique removes the gland completely, and the urethra is sutured to the bladder. After surgery, a suprapubic catheter is often required and left in place through the abdominal incision to prevent pressure on the suture line and to aid in bladder healing. An indwelling catheter with a 30 ml balloon is placed in the bladder via the urethra to avoid strictures. The bladder is irrigated continuously through the urethral catheter for 24 hours. This approach allows better exploration, but it has an increased risk of urinary tract infections, incontinence, bladder spasms, and hemorrhage. The postoperative recovery phase is significantly longer than after a TURP.

Retropubic Resection. The retropubic approach is used to remove a massive gland located high in the pelvic area. This approach is more commonly used for a radical prostatectomy with lymph node dissection for cancer of the prostate. A low midline abdominal incision is made into the prostate gland. After surgery, the patient has a large indwelling catheter with a 30 ml balloon placed in the bladder via the urethra. A surgical drain may be left at the site of the abdominal incision to aid in the removal of drainage from the area. Although the bladder is not incised in this approach, direct visualization of the prostate is possible. The risk of hemorrhage remains high. Both suprapubic and retropubic resections are difficult in the obese patient.

Perineal Resection. The perineal approach is used on rare occasions to remove a large mass located low in the pelvic area or for cancer of the prostate. The incision is made between the scrotum and the anus. Because of the possibility of inadvertently entering the rectum, the bowel is prepared with enemas, antibiotics, and a low-residue diet. After surgery, an indwelling catheter with a 30 ml balloon is left in the urethra. A surgical drain may be placed in the incision site to promote drainage of the area. Careful dressing changes and perineal care after each bowel movement are important for comfort and to prevent incisional infection. Although all open procedures carry some risk of erectile dysfunction, the perineal approach has the highest incidence. Urinary incontinence may also be a problem. This approach also has an increased risk of incisional infection because of the closeness of the anus.

Complications of Prostatic Surgery. The major postoperative complications of these types of surgery are hemorrhage, infection, bladder spasm, urinary incontinence, and erectile problems. The Campbell-Walsh procedure, a nerve-sparing surgical technique, greatly reduces the incidence of erectile dysfunction. Patients should be encouraged to talk with their physician or qualified nurse about postoperative management of urinary incontinence or erectile dysfunction.[13]

NURSING MANAGEMENT: BENIGN PROSTATIC HYPERPLASIA

Because the nurse is most directly involved with care of prostate patients having surgical interventions, the focus of nursing management will be on preoperative and postoperative care.[11]

■ Nursing Assessment

Subjective and objective data that should be obtained from a patient with BPH are presented in Table 52-4.

■ Nursing Diagnoses

Nursing diagnoses for the patient with BPH may include, but are not limited to, those presented in NCP 52-1.

■ Planning

The overall preoperative goals for the patient having prostatic surgery are (1) restoration of urinary drainage, (2) treatment of any urinary tract infection, and (3) understanding of the upcoming surgery, implications for sexual functioning, and urinary control. The overall postoperative goals for the patient after prostate surgery are (1) no complications, (2) restoration of urinary control, (3) complete bladder emptying, and (4) satisfying sexual expression.

■ Nursing Implementation

Health Promotion. The cause of BPH is largely attributed to the aging process. The focus of health promotion is on early detection and treatment. The American Cancer Society,

NURSING ASSESSMENT

Table 52-4   Benign Prostatic Hyperplasia

Subjective Data	Objective Data
Important Health Information	**General**
Medications: Estrogen or testosterone supplementation	Older adult male
Surgery or other treatments: Previous treatment for BPH	**Urinary**
Functional Health Patterns	Distended bladder on palpation; smooth, firm, elastic enlargement of prostate on rectal examination
Health perception–health management: Knowledge of the condition	**Possible Findings**
Nutritional-metabolic: Voluntary fluid restriction	Enlarged prostate on ultrasonography; vesicle neck obstruction on cystourethroscopy; residual urine with postvoiding catheterization; presence of white blood cells, bacteria, or microscopic hematuria with infection; elevated BUN and serum creatinine levels with renal involvement
Elimination: Urinary urgency, diminution in caliber and force of urinary stream; hesitancy in initiating voiding; postvoiding dribbling; urinary retention; incontinence	
Sleep: Nocturia	
Cognitive-perceptual: Dysuria, sensation of incomplete voiding; bladder discomfort	
Sexuality-reproductive: Anxiety about sexual dysfunction	

along with the AUA, recommends a yearly medical history and DRE for men over 40 years of age in an effort to provide early detection of prostate problems. After 50 years of age, and when symptoms of prostatic hyperplasia become evident, further diagnostic screening may be necessary (see Table 52-2).

Some men find that the ingestion of alcohol and caffeine tends to increase prostatic symptoms because the diuretic effect of these substances increases bladder distention. Compounds found in common cough and cold remedies such as pseudoephedrine (in Sudafed) and phenylephrine (in Allerest and Coricidin preparations) often worsen the symptoms of BPH. These drugs are alpha-adrenergic agonists that cause smooth muscle contraction. If this happens, the patient should avoid these drugs.

The patient with obstructive symptoms should be advised to urinate every 2 to 3 hours and when first feeling the urge so urinary stasis and acute urinary retention are minimized. Fluid intake should be maintained at a normal level to avoid dehydration or fluid overload. The patient may believe that if he restricts his fluid intake, symptoms will be less severe, but this only increases the chances of an infection. However, if the patient increases his intake too rapidly, bladder distention can develop because of the prostatic obstruction.

Acute Intervention

Preoperative care. Urinary drainage must be restored before surgery. Prostatic obstruction may have resulted in retention or inability to void. A urethral catheter such as a Coudé (curved-tip) catheter may be needed to restore drainage. If a sizable obstruction of the urethra exists, a filiform catheter with sufficient rigidity to pass the obstruction may be inserted by a urologist. Aseptic technique is important at all times to avoid introducing bacteria into the bladder.

Antibiotics are usually administered before any invasive surgical procedure. Any infection of the urinary tract must be treated before surgery. Restoring urine drainage and encouraging a high fluid intake (2 to 3 L/day, unless contraindicated) are also helpful in managing the infection.

The patient is often concerned about the impact of the impending surgery on his sexual functioning. Data gathered from the health history relating to sexual activities will identify possible problem areas. The nurse should provide an opportunity for the patient and partner to express their concerns. The patient needs to know how the surgery may affect sexual functioning. All types of prostatic surgery generally result in some degree of retrograde ejaculation. The patient should be informed that the ejaculate may be decreased in amount or totally absent. This may decrease orgasmic sensations felt during ejaculation. Retrograde ejaculation is not harmful because the semen is simply eliminated during the next urination.

Postoperative care. The main complications of prostatectomy are hemorrhage, bladder spasms, urinary incontinence, and infection. The plan of care should be adjusted to the type of surgery, the reasons for surgery, and the patient's response to surgery.

After prostatectomy the bladder may be continuously irrigated with sterile normal saline solution or another prescribed solution to remove clotted blood from the bladder and ensure drainage of urine. Some form of irrigation (continuous or intermittent) may be used for 24 hours or until no clots are noted draining from the bladder.

Blood clots are normal after a prostatectomy for the first 24 to 36 hours. However, large amounts of bright red blood in the urine can indicate hemorrhage. Postoperative hemorrhage may occur from displacement of the catheter, dislodging a large clot, or increases in abdominal pressure. Release or displacement of the catheter dislodges the balloon that provides counterpressure on the operative site. Traction on the catheter may be applied to provide counterpressure (tamponade) on the bleeding site in the prostate, decreasing bleeding. Such traction can result in local necrosis if pressure is applied for too long. Pressure should therefore be relieved on a scheduled basis by qualified personnel. Activities that increase abdominal pressure, such as sitting or walking for prolonged periods and straining to have a bowel movement (Valsalva's maneuver), should be avoided in the postoperative recovery period.

Bladder spasms are a distressing complication for the patient after transurethral and suprapubic prostatectomy. They occur as a result of irritation of the bladder mucosa from the

52-1 NURSING CARE PLAN PATIENT UNDERGOING TRANSURETHRAL RESECTION

Expected Patient Outcomes	Nursing Interventions and *Rationales*

Preoperative

NURSING DIAGNOSIS **Pain** *related to* bladder distention secondary to enlarged prostate *as manifested by* complaints of discomfort caused by inability to void, palpable bladder, no urine output, diaphoresis, restlessness.

- No complaints of pain.

- Assist with insertion of indwelling catheter (usually done by urologist) *to reduce pain by providing urinary drainage.*
- Monitor intake and output *to evaluate adequacy.*
- Percuss bladder for distention *to validate adequate emptying of the bladder.*
- Assess comfort status *to continue or revise plan as necessary.*
- Maintain patency of catheter *to ensure continuous flow of urine from the bladder.*

NURSING DIAGNOSIS **Risk for infection** *related to* indwelling catheter, environmental pathogens, and urinary stasis.

- No evidence of urinary tract infection.

- Assess for elevated temperature and cloudy, foul-smelling urine *to identify symptoms of infection and initiate appropriate interventions.*
- Do urinalysis for culture *to determine presence and cause of infection.*
- Give patient 8 oz of water or other noncitrus, noncaffeine fluids every waking hour *to prevent urinary stasis and dilute the urine.*
- Observe strict aseptic technique for catheter care *to minimize the risk of introducing an infectious organism.*

NURSING DIAGNOSIS **Fear** *related to* actual or potential sexual dysfunction, possible diagnosis of cancer, and lack of knowledge regarding surgical procedure and postoperative care *as manifested by* verbalization of fear about impact of surgery on sexuality; questioning or inaccurate comments about surgical course.

- Decreased fear about effect of surgery on sexuality and surgical course as shown by accurate knowledge base.
- Correct responses to questions.
- Calm demeanor.

- Perform preoperative teaching *to provide information regarding the preoperative and postoperative routines.*
- Assess patient's concerns related to sexual functioning and correct misconceptions and inaccuracies *to plan appropriate interventions that address unique concerns.*
- Provide opportunity for private conversation for patient to ask personal questions *because a private setting facilitates open discussion.*
- Inform patient about retrograde ejaculation *because this often occurs in prostatic surgery and is not harmful because the fluid is eliminated during the next urination.*

Postoperative

NURSING DIAGNOSIS **Pain** *related to* irrigations and clots, presence of catheter, and surgical procedure *as manifested by* expression of pain; nonverbal signs of pain such as moaning, crying, legs drawn to abdomen.

- Decreased or no pain.

- Maintain patency of catheter *because clots cause obstruction of urine flow resulting in bladder spasms.*
- Irrigate catheter if occluded with clots (according to aseptic technique and institution protocols) *so urine can flow freely.*
- Instruct patient to try not to urinate around catheter *because this increases the occurrence of spasm.*
- Give belladonna and opium suppository as needed; instruct patient in relaxation techniques such as deep breathing exercises and distraction therapy or visual imagery *to relieve pain and decrease spasm.*

Continued

| 52-1 | NURSING CARE PLAN | **PATIENT UNDERGOING TRANSURETHRAL RESECTION**—continued |

Expected Patient Outcomes   Nursing Interventions and *Rationales*

NURSING DIAGNOSIS | **Ineffective management of therapeutic regimen** *related to* lack of knowledge regarding need for follow-up care and activity restriction postoperatively *as manifested by* questioning or inaccurate comments about postoperative activity.

- No postoperative bleeding because of performing activities that increase intraabdominal pressure.

- Teach patient that some prostatic tissue is present that could become malignant *so patient understands need for annual prostatic examination.*
- Instruct patient to avoid heavy lifting (>10 lb [4.5 kg]), straining during defecation, prolonged periods of travel, stair climbing, driving, and sexual activity until surgeon approves such activity *to prevent increases in intraabdominal pressure and the possibility of bleeding.*
- Teach patient to increase fiber in diet, use of stool softeners, and to avoid straining during bowel movements *to prevent constipation and prevent increased intraabdominal pressure.*

NURSING DIAGNOSIS | **Urge incontinence** *related to* poor sphincter control *as manifested by* urinary urgency.

- Absence of or satisfactory control of dribbling.

- Teach patient Kegel exercises *to strengthen sphincter tone.*
- Advise patient about devices to control dribbling and absorbent materials *so patient is aware of various devices and can make an informed decision among alternatives.*

NURSING DIAGNOSIS | **Risk for infection** *related to* indwelling catheter, bladder irrigations, environmental pathogens, inadequate oral intake, and poor catheter care.

- No evidence of infection.

- Assess for fever, diaphoresis, self-restriction of fluid intake, cloudy urine *to determine if risk factors or signs and symptoms of infection are present.*
- Monitor temperature q4hr first 48 hr postoperatively *because fever is a good indicator of infection.*
- Give patient 8 oz of water hourly while awake *to maintain good urine flow and dilute the urine.*
- Observe strict aseptic technique for catheter care and bladder irrigations *to prevent introducing infectious organisms.*

COLLABORATIVE PROBLEMS

Nursing Goals   Nursing Interventions and *Rationales*

POTENTIAL COMPLICATION | Hemorrhage *related to* surgical procedure

- Monitor for and report signs of hemorrhage.
- Carry out appropriate medical and nursing interventions.

- Observe urinary drainage and report bright red bleeding in larger than expected quantities immediately *because this could indicate hemorrhage and the need for immediate intervention.*
- Monitor blood pressure, pulse, and respirations and report abnormalities *because increasing pulse and respirations and decreasing BP can indicate hemorrhage.*
- Maintain catheter drainage *to prevent obstruction and allow monitoring of bleeding and urine flow.*
- Do not perform rectal treatments such as enemas or rectal temperatures (except belladonna and opium suppositories for bladder spasms) *because bleeding could be initiated.*
- Teach patient not to strain during bowel movement; limit ambulation and chair sitting to 15 min tid *to decrease pressure on operative area.*

insertion of the resectoscope, the presence of a catheter, or clots leading to obstruction of the catheter. The patient should be instructed not to urinate around the catheter because this increases the likelihood of spasm. If bladder spasms develop, the catheter should be checked for clots. If present, the clots should be removed by irrigation so urine can flow freely. Bel-

ladonna and opium suppositories, or other antispasmodics (e.g., oxybutynin [Ditropan]) along with relaxation techniques, are used to relieve the pain and decrease spasm. The catheter is often removed 2 to 4 days after surgery. The patient should urinate within 6 hours after catheter removal. If he cannot, a catheter is reinserted for a day or two. If the problem continues, the nurse may need to instruct the patient in clean intermittent self-catheterization (see Chapter 43).

Sphincter tone may be poor immediately after catheter removal, resulting in urinary incontinence or dribbling. This is a common but distressing situation for the patient. Sphincter tone can be strengthened by having the patient practice Kegel exercises (pelvic floor muscle technique) 10 to 20 times per hour while awake. The patient should be encouraged to practice starting and stopping the stream several times during urination. This facilitates learning the pelvic floor exercises. It usually takes several weeks to achieve urinary continence. In some instances, control of urine may never be fully regained. Continence can improve for up to 12 months. If continence has not been achieved by that time, the patient may be referred to a continence clinic. A variety of methods, including biofeedback, have been used to achieve positive results. The patient can also be instructed to use a penile clamp, condom catheter, or incontinence pads or briefs to avoid embarrassment from dribbling. In severe cases, an occlusive cuff that serves as an artificial sphincter can be surgically implanted to restore continence. The nurse should assist the patient in finding ways to manage the problem that will allow him to continue socializing and interacting with others.

The patient should be observed for signs of postoperative infection. If an external wound is present, the area should be observed for redness, heat, swelling, and purulent drainage. Special care must be taken if a perineal incision is present because of the proximity of the anus. Rectal procedures, such as taking rectal temperatures and administering enemas, should be avoided. The insertion of well-lubricated belladonna and opium suppositories is acceptable.

Careful aseptic technique should be used when irrigating the bladder because bacteria can easily be introduced into the urinary tract. Proper care of the catheter is important. To prevent urethral irritation and minimize the risk of bladder infection, the catheter must be secured to the leg or abdomen with tape or catheter strap. The catheter should be connected to a closed-drainage system and should not be disconnected unless it is being removed, changed, or irrigated. The secretions that accumulate around the meatus can be cleansed daily with soap and water.

Dietary intervention and stool softeners are important in the postoperative period to prevent the patient from straining while having bowel movements. Straining increases the intraabdominal pressure, which can lead to bleeding at the operative site. A diet high in fiber facilitates the passage of stool.

Ambulatory and Home Care. Discharge planning and home care issues are important aspects of care after prostatectomy. Instructions include (1) caring for an indwelling catheter, if one is in place; (2) managing of urinary incontinence; (3) maintaining oral fluids between 2000 and 3000 ml per day; (4) observing for signs and symptoms of urinary tract and wound infection; (5) preventing constipation; (6) avoiding heavy lifting (more than 10 pounds [4.5 kg]); and (7) refraining from driving or intercourse for 6 weeks after surgery or as directed by the surgeon.

After prostatic surgery the patient may be concerned about erectile dysfunction. Physiologic erectile dysfunction may occur when nerves are cut or damaged during surgery. The patient often experiences anxiety over the loss of his sex role,

---

his self-esteem, and the quality of sexual interaction with his sexual partner. Sexual counseling and treatment options may be necessary if erectile dysfunction becomes a chronic or permanent problem. Patients may also require counseling regarding treatment options, which include drug therapy, vacuum or constriction devices, implants, and surgery.

Many men experience retrograde ejaculation after prostatectomy because of trauma to the internal sphincter. Semen is discharged into the bladder at orgasm and may produce cloudy urine when the patient urinates after orgasm. The nurse should discuss these changes with the patient and his partner and allow them to ask questions and express their concerns.

The bladder may take up to 2 months to return to its normal capacity. The patient should be instructed to drink at least 1 to 2 L of fluid per day and to urinate every 2 to 3 hours to flush the urinary tract. Bladder irritants such as caffeine products, citrus juices, and alcohol should be avoided or limited to small amounts. Because the patient may be experiencing incontinence or dribbling, he may incorrectly believe that decreasing fluid intake will relieve this problem. Urethral strictures may result from instrumentation or catheterization. Treatment ranges from teaching the patient intermittent clean catheterization to urethral dilation.

The patient must be advised that he should continue to have a yearly DRE if he has had any procedure other than complete removal of the prostate. Hyperplasia or cancer can occur in the remaining prostatic tissue.

■ Evaluation

Expected outcomes for the patient with BPH are addressed in NCP 52-1.

CANCER OF THE PROSTATE

Cancer of the prostate is the most common cancer in men. It is the second leading cause of cancer death in men, after lung cancer. Because of new screening procedures (e.g., prostate-specific antigen), subclinical prostate cancer is being diagnosed with increasing frequency. In 1998 an estimated 184,500 men in the

United States were diagnosed with prostate cancer. Continued increases in prostatic cancer are projected, primarily because of an aging population.

Etiology and Pathophysiology

Prostate cancer is an androgen-dependent adenocarcinoma. Factors such as sexual activity, socioeconomic class, and alcohol use have not been shown to be significant risk factors. In addition, patients with BPH are at no greater risk for prostate cancer. Researchers are now investigating high fat diets and environmental factors for possible links to prostate cancer. A family history of prostate cancer is a major risk factor. Approximately 9% of prostate cancers may be familial.[12]

A higher incidence exists in men 60 years of age or older, in African-American men, and in married men.[13] African-Americans have the highest incidence of prostate cancer, and tend to have more aggressive tumors at diagnosis and higher mortality rates.[14]

The tumor is slow growing and usually begins in the posterior or lateral portions of the prostate. It can spread by three routes: direct extension, via the lymphatics, and via the bloodstream. Direct extension is by continuity to the seminal vesicles, urethral mucosa, bladder wall, and external sphincter. The cancer later spreads through the perineural lymphatic system to the regional lymph nodes. The veins from the prostate seem to be the mode of spread to the pelvic bones, head of the femur, lower lumbar spine, liver, and lungs.

Clinical Manifestations and Complications

Prostate cancer is asymptomatic in the early stages. Eventually the patient may have symptoms similar to those of BPH, including dysuria, hesitancy, dribbling, frequency, urgency, hematuria, nocturia, and retention. The prostate feels hard, enlarged, and fixed on rectal examination. The enlargement is usually unilateral. Pain in the lumbosacral area, which radiates down to the hips or legs, when coupled with urinary symptoms may indicate metastasis.

Early recognition and treatment is required to control growth, prevent metastasis, and preserve quality of life. The tumor can spread to pelvic lymph nodes, bones, bladder, lungs, and liver. Once the tumor has spread to distant sites, the major problem becomes the management of pain. As the cancer spreads to the bones, pain can become severe, especially in the back and the legs because of compression of the spinal cord and osteoblastic lesions.

Diagnostic Studies

Improved diagnostic techniques have greatly enhanced the physician's ability to detect cancer of the prostate at an earlier stage. Primary screening for prostate cancer consists of palpation of the gland during DRE, a blood test for PSA (a glycoprotein that is detected only in the epithelial cells of the prostate), and TRUS. The American Cancer Society and the AUA recommend yearly DREs for all men over age 40. Current evidence strongly suggests that the combination of DRE and serum PSA level measurement increases the chances of early detection of prostate cancer. Ultrasonography of the prostate allows the physician to visualize the outer lobes of the prostate and pinpoint potential cancer sites. When a suspicious area is located, a special biopsy needle can be inserted and the specimen examined.

Elevated levels of PSA (normal level, 0 to 4 ng/ml [0 to 4 µg/L]) and the prostatic isoenzyme of acid phosphatase (prostatic acid phosphatase [PAP]) are both suggestive of cancer of the prostate. Elevated PSA levels indicate prostatic pathology, although not necessarily cancer of the prostate. Mild elevations in PSA may occur in BPH, acute or chronic prostatitis, urinary retention, or infarction of the prostate. In addition, cystoscopy, indwelling urethral catheters, and prostate biopsies may produce an elevation. An elevated PSA alerts the physician to the possibility of cancer of the prostate. In prostate cancer, serum PSA levels are a useful marker of tumor volume. For example, the higher the serum value the greater the tumor mass. Finasteride (Proscar), which is taken to reduce prostatic hyperplasia in men with BPH, may reduce the levels of PSA by almost 50%.[12] This should be considered when evaluating PSA blood levels.

PSA is also useful in following patients after treatment for localized disease. When treatment has been successful in removing all prostatic tissue, the PSA should fall to undetectable levels.

Elevated PAP is specifically indicative of cancer of the prostate. In advanced prostate cancer, serum alkaline phosphatase is increased as a result of bone metastasis. Investigation is now under way to locate a serum marker for prostate cancer similar to CA-125 in ovarian cancer.

When an elevated PSA level or a positive finding on digital rectal examination is noted, the prostate gland is biopsied. This is done through a transrectal needle biopsy. Six systematic samples of prostate tissue are taken for histologic examination. Other tests used to determine the location and extent of the spread of the cancer may include transrectal ultrasound, computed tomography (CT), and magnetic resonance imaging (MRI).

Collaborative Care

The collaborative care of cancer of the prostate depends on the stage of the cancer. Prostatic cancer is staged on the basis of tumor volume and spread (Table 52-5). The TNM staging system is also used to stage prostate cancer (see Chapter 14). Surgery is the most accurate method of staging the extent of the tumor growth and lymph node involvement. At all stages, there is more than one possible treatment option. The decision of which treatment course to pursue is made jointly by the patient and the physician based on a careful analysis of the facts and the patient's unique situation.[15] Table 52-6 summarizes the various treatment options available.

Surgical Therapy.   Surgery is often the first line of treatment, particularly in the earlier stages of the disease. In stage A or B a TURP or total prostatectomy may be the treatment depending on the location and symptoms. Patients who are asymptomatic may be observed carefully, with annual DRE and PSA testing. For patients in good health with stage C tumor, surgery is usually a radical prostatectomy involving resection of the prostate gland, seminal vesicles, and part of the ampulla of the vas deferens.[16] Surgery is usually not considered an option for stage D cancer except to relieve obstruction because metastasis has already occurred.

A nerve-sparing surgical technique is sometimes used to decrease the incidence of erectile dysfunction following a radical prostatectomy.[17,18] This surgery is useful only for patients

Table 52-5	Whitmore-Jewett Staging Classification of Prostate Cancer

Stage A: Clinically Unrecognized
| A1 | <5% of prostatic tissue neoplastic |
| A2 | >5% of prostatic tissue neoplastic, all high-grade tumors |

Stage B: Clinically Intracapsular
| B1 | Nodule <2 cm and surrounded by palpably normal tissue |
| B2 | Nodule >2 cm or multiple nodules |

Stage C: Clinically Extracapsular, Localized to Periprostatic Area
| C1 | Minimal extracapsular extension |
| C2 | Large tumors involving seminal vesicles, adjacent structures, or both |

Stage D: Metastatic Disease
| D1 | Pelvic lymph node metastases or ureteral obstruction causing hydronephrosis |
| D2 | Distant metastases to bone, viscera, or other soft-tissue structures |

COLLABORATIVE CARE

Table 52-6	Prostate Cancer

Diagnostic
Digital rectal examination (DRE)
Prostate specific antigen (PSA)
Prostatic acid phosphatase (PAP) in advanced stages
Transrectal ultrasound (TRUS)
Biopsy, needle aspiration, open biopsy
Bone scan
Grading and staging

Collaborative Therapy
Stage A
Continue medical follow-up, observation, TURP or total prostatectomy
Radiation therapy

Stage B
TURP
Total prostatectomy with or without lymphadenectomy
Radiation therapy

Stage C
Hormone manipulation (e.g., luteinizing hormone–releasing hormone analogues) or orchiectomy
Radical resection of prostate
Radiation therapy

Stage D
Hormone therapy
Radiation to metastatic bone areas
Chemotherapy

TURP, transurethral resection of prostate.

who are younger and have negative lymph nodes, no elevation of serum alkaline phosphatase levels, and no clinical evidence of extracapsular extension. Patients with extensive disease or older men may not benefit from the nerve-sparing operation. However, a patient with a localized nodule or with small-volume disease may benefit. Up to 70% of patients undergoing a nerve-sparing operation will retain erectile function postoperatively.

Radiation Therapy. External beam radiation therapy is commonly used in the management of prostate cancer, especially in men over age 70. As compared with surgery, there is a reduced risk of erectile dysfunction. Long-term outcomes of radiation therapy compared with prostatectomy show few differences. Potential side effects of radiation include diarrhea, cystitis, and erectile dysfunction. Sexual potency may not be affected when lower-dose, well-controlled radiation therapy is used.[19-21] Radiation therapy may also be combined with the antiandrogen agents such as goserelin (Zoladex).[22]

Interstitial radioactive seed implants (brachytherapy) have been used for the past 25 years to treat prostate cancer. Radioactive implants are placed in the prostate tissue through a transrectal approach. This therapy may be used in conjunction with external beam radiation therapy. Brachytherapy is discussed in Chapter 14.

Drug Therapy. A unique feature of prostate cancer is that cell growth initially depends on the presence of androgens. Hormone therapy is focused on reducing the levels of circulating androgens and is used in the management of extraprostatic (metastatic) disease. Hormone or antiandrogen therapy is rarely used alone in the treatment of prostate cancer.[12]

Current antiandrogen therapy involves agents such as leuprolide (Lupron) and goserelin (Zoladex) that are agonists of luteinizing hormone–releasing hormone (LHRH), a hypothalamic hormone that controls the release of luteinizing hormone (LH) and follicle-stimulating hormone (FSH) from the anterior pituitary. By binding the LHRH receptor sites there is a reduction in release of FSH and LH and as a result a decrease in testosterone levels. Antiandrogen medications are given by

monthly subcutaneous or intramuscular injections, require monitoring, and must be taken indefinitely. More recent developments include a suspension preparation that can be administered every 3 months.[12] Side effects include hot flashes, loss of libido, and erectile dysfunction.

Another classification of antiandrogens primarily used in combination with LHRH agonists are drugs that compete with circulating androgens at the receptor sites. Flutamide (Eulexin), nilutamide (Nilandron), and bicalutamide (Casodex) are nonsteroidal androgen receptor blockers. They can be used in combination with goserelin or leuprolide. The combination has been found to be safe and well tolerated as a potency-sparing, androgen-ablative therapy. These agents may also be used in combination with finesteride (Proscar) to reduce androgenic effects.[23,24] Adverse effects of antiandrogen drugs are similar to LHRH agonists and include loss of libido, erectile dysfunction, and hot flashes. The loss of libido and erections are not as great when antiandrogens are used alone as when combined with LHRH agonists. However, breast pain and gynecomastia may occur in men treated with antiandrogens.

Surgical removal of the prostate followed by orchiectomy (removal of the testes) removes the source of 90% of circulating androgens. Orchiectomy often provides rapid relief of bone pain. Orchiectomy alone may induce sufficient shrinkage of the prostate to relieve urinary obstruction in later stages of disease when surgery is not an option. While an orchiectomy can cause emotional distress, the physiologic side effects are less than when chemical androgen suppression is used. Men are often

NURSING ASSESSMENT

Table 52-7   Cancer of the Prostate

Subjective Data	Objective Data
Important Health Information *Medications:* Testosterone supplements; use of any medications affecting urinary tract such as morphine, anticholinergics, monoamine oxidase inhibitors, and tricyclic antidepressants **Functional Health Patterns** *Health perception–health management:* Positive family history; increasing fatigue and malaise *Nutritional-metabolic:* High-fat diet; anorexia, weight loss (possible indicators of metastasis) *Elimination:* Hesitancy or straining to start stream, urinary urgency, frequency, retention with dribbling, weak stream, hematuria *Sleep:* Nocturia *Cognitive-perceptual:* Dysuria; low back pain radiating to legs or pelvis, bone pain (possible indicators of metastasis) *Self-preception–self-concept:* Anxiety regarding self-concept	**General** Older adult male; pelvic lymphadenopathy (late sign) **Urinary** Distended bladder on palpation; unilaterally hard, enlarged, fixed prostate on rectal examination **Musculoskeletal** Pathologic fractures (metastasis) **Possible Findings** Elevated serum PSA; elevated serum acid phosphatase PAP (metastasis); nodular and irregular prostate on ultrasonography, positive biopsy results; anemia

PSA, prostate specific antigen.

able to continue having erections and orgasmic sensations, even though ejaculation is absent.

Estrogen (e.g., diethylstilbestrol) treatment may be substituted for orchiectomy. It causes regression of the size of the prostate and of metastatic bone lesions. The minimum dose that is capable of suppressing plasma testosterone to castration levels is used. Estrogen therapy often results in gynecomastia, mood swings, decreased libido, hot flashes, and total loss of erectile functioning. Estrogen treatment is declining in popularity because of more serious side effects such as heart attack, stroke, and pulmonary embolism.

Chemotherapy is occasionally used in late-stage disease with some success. It does appear to reduce pain associated with prostate cancer. However, it has not been shown to improve survival or quality of life.

Other Therapies. Prostatic cryosurgery is an experimental but promising approach to treating cancer of the prostate. The treatment takes about 2 hours under general or spinal anesthesia and does not involve a major abdominal incision. Liquid nitrogen is circulated in probes inserted into the prostate gland through tiny punctures in the perineum. Possible complications of prostatic cryosurgery include the development of a urethrorectal fistula (an opening between the urethra and the rectum) or a urethrocutaneous fistula (an opening between the urethra and the skin), tissue sloughing, erectile dysfunction, urinary incontinence, and hemorrhage.

NURSING MANAGEMENT: PROSTATIC CANCER
■ Nursing Assessment

Subjective and objective data that should be obtained from an individual with cancer of the prostate are presented in Table 52-7.

■ Nursing Diagnoses

Nursing diagnoses for the patient with cancer of the prostate depend on the stage of the cancer. General nursing diagnoses, which may or may not apply to every patient with cancer of the prostate, may include, but are not limited to, the following:

- Decisional conflict *related to* numerous alternative treatment options
- Pain *related to* surgery, prostatic enlargement, bone metastasis, and bladder spasms
- Urinary retention *related to* obstruction of urethra or bladder neck by the prostate, blood clots, and loss of bladder tone
- Altered urinary elimination *related to* bladder neck sphincter damage
- Constipation or diarrhea *related to* treatment interventions
- Sexual dysfunction *related to* effects of treatment
- Anxiety *related to* uncertain outcome of disease process on life and lifestyle and effect of treatment on sexual functioning

■ Planning

The overall goals are that the patient with cancer of the prostate will (1) be an active participant in the treatment plan, (2) have satisfactory pain control, (3) follow the therapeutic plan, (4) accept the effect of the therapeutic plan on sexual function, and (5) find a satisfactory way to manage the impact on bladder or bowel function.

■ Nursing Implementation

Health Promotion. One of the most important roles for nurses in relation to prostate cancer is to encourage patients to have an annual prostate examination to facilitate early detection of this malignant tumor. Because of their

RESEARCH
IMPLICATIONS FOR NURSING PRACTICE

Uncertainty and Prostate Cancer

Citation Germino BB and others: Uncertainty in prostate cancer: ethnic and family patterns, *Cancer Pract* 6:107, 1998.

Purpose To examine the relationship of sense of uncertainty with family coping, psychologic adjustment to illness, and spiritual factors. In addition, to determine whether these relationships were similar for white and African-American patient and family caregivers.

Method A sample of 403 white and African-American men and their family caregivers were interviewed either 1 week after postsurgical catheter removal or at the beginning of primary radiation treatment. All men were diagnosed with stage B prostate cancer. Tools included measures of uncertainty, adult role behavior, problem solving, social support, importance of God in one's life, family coping, psychologic adjustment to illness, and perceptions of health and illness.

Results and Conclusions In African-American and white family care providers, the more uncertainty experienced, the less positive they felt about treatment and the patient recovering from the illness. For white patients and family members higher levels of uncertainty were related to lower scores on adult role behavior (e.g., shopping), less active problem solving, and less perceived social support. Higher levels of uncertainty were related to poorer social environment for African-American patients and white family members.

Implications for Nursing Practice Uncertainty accompanying the diagnosis and treatment (surgery versus radiation) of prostate cancer is a common experience for both the patient and the family caregivers. This study demonstrates that there are differences between African-Americans and whites in the relationship of uncertainty to a number of coping variables. The results have implications for the assessment and management of psychosocial responses to cancer and cancer treatments. The nurse should consider the sociocultural perspective of the individual patient and his family members when planning care.

increased risk of prostate cancer, African-American men in particular should be encouraged to participate in prostate screening programs or to consult a clinician on an annual basis. All men should have an annual DRE beginning at 40 years of age.

Acute Intervention. Preoperative and postoperative phases of therapy are the same as for BPH. Nursing interventions for the patient who undergoes radiation therapy and chemotherapy are discussed in Chapter 14. An additional consideration is the psychologic response of the patient to a diagnosis of cancer. The nurse should provide sensitive, caring support for the patient and his family to help them cope with the diagnosis of cancer.[25,26] Prostate support groups are available for men and their families to encourage them to be active, informed participants in their own care.

Ambulatory and Home Care. If the patient is discharged with an indwelling catheter in place, the nurse must teach appropriate catheter care. The patient should be instructed to clean the urethral meatus with soap and water once a day; maintain a high fluid intake; keep the collecting bag lower than the bladder at all times; keep the catheter securely anchored to the inner thigh or abdomen; and report any signs of bladder infection, such as bladder spasms, fever, or hematuria. If urinary incontinence is a problem, patients should be encouraged to practice pelvic floor muscle exercises (Kegel exercises) at every urination and throughout the day. Continuous practice during the 4- to 6-week healing process improves the success rate. Products used for incontinence specifically designed for men are available through home care product catalogs and many retail stores.

Cancer of the prostate has a high cure rate if detected and treated early. However, prognosis for stage D prostate cancer is very unfavorable. Pain control is the primary nursing intervention for the terminally ill patient. Hospice care is often appropriate and most beneficial to the patient and family. (Hospice care is discussed in Chapter 2.)

■ Evaluation

The expected outcomes are that the patient with prostate cancer will

- be an active participant in the treatment plan
- have satisfactory pain control
- follow the therapeutic plan
- accept the effect of the treatment on sexual function
- find a satisfactory way to manage the impact on bladder or bowel function

PROSTATITIS
Etiology and Pathophysiology

A number of inflammatory conditions can affect the prostate gland after a male reaches puberty. The four most common forms of prostatitis are acute bacterial prostatitis, chronic bacterial prostatitis, nonbacterial prostatitis, and prostatodynia. Bacterial prostatitis generally results from organisms reaching the prostate gland by one of the following routes: ascending from the urethra, descending from the bladder, and invasion via the bloodstream or the lymphatic channels.

Bacterial prostatitis is frequently associated with urethritis or an infection of the lower urinary tract. It can also be associated with an indwelling urethral catheter, urethral instrumentation, or trauma. Common causative organisms are *Escherichia coli*, *Pseudomonas*, *Enterobacter*, *Proteus*, *Chlamydia trachomatis*, *Neisseria gonorrhoeae*, and group D streptococci. Chronic bacterial prostatitis should be considered in men with a history of recurrent bacteriuria.

Nonbacterial prostatitis may occur after a viral illness, or it may be associated with other sexually transmitted diseases (STDs), particularly in a younger adult. The etiology is not known, and a culture reveals no causative organisms. Prostatodynia has the same symptoms as prostatitis (irritation and pelvic pain on urination) but no evidence of inflammation. The condition is generally limited to younger men.

Clinical Manifestations and Complications

Acute bacterial prostatitis results in manifestations of fever; chills; dysuria; urethral discharge; increased urinary frequency and urgency; low back, rectal, pelvic, and perineal pain; and acute cystitis with cloudy, smelly urine. The prostate is extremely swollen, tender, firm, and warm to touch. The complications of prostatitis are epididymitis and cystitis. Sexual functioning may be affected as manifested by post-ejaculation pain, libido problems, and erectile dysfunction. Prostatic abscess is a rare complication.

The symptoms of chronic prostatitis may be absent or are generally milder than those of acute prostatitis.[27] These include backache, perineal pain, ejaculatory pain, mild dysuria, and increased frequency of urination.[28] Factors that may contribute to chronic prostatitis include urethral obstruction, persistent infections above the urethra, and prostatic pathologic conditions such as congestion, hyperplasia, and prostatic calculi. Chronic prostatitis can predispose the patient to recurrent urinary tract infections. The prostate feels irregularly enlarged, firm, and slightly tender on palpation.

Diagnostic Studies

A prostatitis symptom severity index and symptom frequency assessment questionnaire has been developed as a primary screening tool.[29] Complaints of lower abdominal, testicular, penile, and ejaculatory pain are found more often in prostatitis when compared with BPH. If a patient with prostatitis has a fever, the white blood cell (WBC) count may be elevated. An increased PSA level can be found in acute prostatitis, a moderate increase in chronic prostatitis, and a minimal increase in nonbacterial prostatitis.[30] The urine is often cloudy with a foul odor and may test positive for bacteria. The patient may be instructed to void into two or three separate containers for a split-specimen urinalysis. The first container shows many more WBCs and bacteria than subsequent containers. On palpation, the prostate gland may be normal or may appear enlarged and tender, and in long-standing cases, may reveal the presence of calculi. Cystoscopy, catheterizations, and prostatic massage are avoided during the acute phase to minimize the risk of introducing the organisms into the bladder and to avoid further pain. Prostatic massage may be used in chronic prostatitis to express secretions for culture and sensitivity. A transrectal ultrasound (TRUS) scan may be done before the massage to prevent unnecessary prolonged treatment.

NURSING AND COLLABORATIVE MANAGEMENT: PROSTATITIS

Collaborative care of acute bacterial prostatitis usually consists of administering an antibiotic for 3 to 6 weeks that concentrates in the prostatic tissue. Most antibiotics cannot penetrate the prostate because the low pH of the gland precludes solubility of the drugs. The specific antibiotics for acute bacterial prostatitis are ciprofloxacin (Cipro) and trimethoprim-sulfamethoxazole (Bactrim). Antispasmodics, analgesics, and stool softeners are often prescribed to provide relief from painful symptoms. Other interventions include increasing fluid intake, use of warm sitz baths, antiinflammatory agents, and rest.

Collaborative care of chronic prostatitis may consist of long-term (12 to 16 weeks) administration of antibiotics, antiinflammatory agents, frequent prostatic massage and ejaculations, sitz baths, and stool softeners. Antibiotics include ciprofloxacin, trimethoprim-sulfamethoxazole, carbenicillin, tetracycline, doxycycline, and erythromycin. If the infection is sexually transmitted, both the patient and partner need to be treated.

Nonbacterial prostatitis and prostatodynia are difficult to treat because no bacteria are found in the urine or prostatic fluid. Treatment generally consists of antiinflammatory agents, hot sitz baths, and sexual activities that result in ejaculation. TUMA therapy may be a treatment option when traditional therapy is unsuccessful.[31]

The patient with acute bacterial prostatitis experiences prostate pain when standing, when urinating, and during ejaculation. Nursing interventions are aimed at relief of pain and fever, bed rest, and the maintenance of adequate hydration. The patient with chronic prostatitis should be instructed regarding the long-term nature of the problem. Because the prostate can serve as a source of bacteria, fluid intake should be kept at a high level. Antibiotics may have to be taken for a number of months. Activities that drain the prostate, such as intercourse (use a condom to protect the partner from infection), masturbation, and prostatic massage, are often helpful in the long-term management of this problem. Chronic prostatitis may eventually lead to erectile dysfunction, for which the patient may need to seek treatment.

PROBLEMS OF THE PENIS

Health problems of the penis are rare if sexually transmitted infectious diseases are excluded (see Chapter 50). Problems of the penis may be classified as congenital, problems of the prepuce, problems with the erectile mechanism, and cancer.

CONGENITAL PROBLEMS

Hypospadias is a urologic abnormality in which the urethral meatus is located on the ventral surface of the penis anywhere from the corona to the perineum. Hormonal influences in utero, environmental factors, and genetic factors are possible causes. Surgical repair of hypospadias may be necessary if it is associated with chordee, or if it prevents intercourse or normal urination. Surgery may also be done for cosmetic reasons or emotional well-being.

Epispadias, an opening of the urethra on the dorsal surface of the penis, is a complex birth defect that is usually associated with other genitourinary tract defects. Corrective surgery to place the urethra in a normal position in the penis is usually done in early childhood.

PROBLEMS OF THE PREPUCE

Problems of the prepuce in the United States are rare because circumcision has been a routine procedure for most male infants for many years. The trend is now shifting away from routine circumcision to one of preference, which may result in an increased incidence of problems.

Circumcision, the surgical removal of the foreskin of the penis, may be done for religious, cultural, or hygienic reasons.

Parents are encouraged to make the final decision after consideration of all the advantages and disadvantages.

Phimosis is caused by edema or inflammation of the foreskin of an uncircumcised male. This results in the foreskin constricting around the head of the penis, making retraction difficult. It is generally caused by poor hygiene techniques that allow bacterial and yeast organisms to become trapped under the foreskin.

Paraphimosis is edema of the retracted uncircumcised foreskin, preventing normal return over the glans. This can occur when the foreskin is pulled back during bathing, use of urinary catheters, or intercourse and is not placed back in the forward position. Antibiotics, warm soaks, and sometimes circumcision or dorsal slit of the prepuce may be required. Careful cleaning followed by replacement of the foreskin generally prevents these problems.

PROBLEMS OF THE ERECTILE MECHANISM

Priapism is a painful erection lasting longer than 6 hours. Causes of priapism include thrombosis of the corpora cavernosal veins, leukemia, sickle cell anemia, diabetes mellitus, degenerative lesions of the spine, neoplasms of the brain or spinal cord, prolonged foreplay, injection of vasoactive medications into the corpus cavernosa, and cocaine use. Treatment may include sedatives, injection of smooth muscle relaxants directly into the penis, aspiration and irrigation of the corpora cavernosa with a large-bore needle, or the surgical creation of a shunt to drain the corpora. Prolonged priapism constitutes a medical emergency. Complications may include penile tissue necrosis caused by lack of blood flow or hydronephrosis from bladder distention. After an episode of priapism, the patient may be unable to achieve a normal erection.

Peyronie's disease, sometimes referred to as curved or crooked penis, is caused by plaque formation in one of the corpora cavernosa of the penis. The palpable, nontender, hard plaque formation is usually found on the posterior surface. It may result from trauma to the penile shaft or may occur spontaneously. The plaque prevents adequate blood flow into the spongy tissue, which results in a curvature during erection. The condition is not dangerous but can result in painful erections, erectile dysfunction, or embarrassment. If conservative measures do not correct the problem, surgery may be necessary.

CANCER OF PENIS

Cancer of the penis is rare apart from cancers associated with the STD human papillomavirus (HPV) and in men who were not circumcised as infants. The tumor may appear as a superficial ulceration or a pimple-like nodule. The nontender warty lesion may be mistaken for a venereal wart. The majority of malignancies (95%) are well-differentiated squamous cell carcinomas. Treatment in the early stages is laser removal of the growth. A radical resection of the penis may be done if the cancer has spread. Surgery, radiation, or chemotherapy may be tried depending on the extent of the disease, lymph node involvement, or metastasis.

PROBLEMS OF THE SCROTUM AND ITS CONTENTS

EXTERNAL PROBLEMS

The skin of the scrotum is susceptible to a number of common skin diseases. The most common conditions of the scrotal skin are fungal infections, dermatitis (neurodermatitis, contact dermatitis, and seborrheic dermatitis), and parasitic infections (scabies and lice). These conditions involve discomfort for the patient but are associated with few, if any, severe complications (see Chapter 22).

CONGENITAL PROBLEMS

Cryptorchidism (undescended testes) is failure of the testes to descend into the scrotal sack before birth. It is the most common congenital testicular condition. It may occur bilaterally or unilaterally and may be the cause of infertility if corrective surgery is not done by 2 years of age. The incidence of testicular cancer is also higher if the condition is not corrected before puberty. Surgery is performed to locate and suture the testis or testes to the scrotum.

Absence of the vas deferens is a rare condition associated most often with cystic fibrosis. With the advent of advanced techniques to treat infertility, this defect can be circumvented by aspirating the sperm directly from the testis.

"DES sons" are the male children of women who took diethylstilbestrol (DES) during pregnancy. Until recently it was thought that only females were affected in utero if their mothers took DES during pregnancy. The impact on males is now seen in the form of undescended or underdeveloped testes, a micropenis or small penis, varicocele, or epididymal cysts. These males also have an increased rate of infertility.[32]

ACQUIRED PROBLEMS

Problems that develop within the scrotum usually are first noticed as a mass or as scrotal edema. Some problems produce pain, whereas others do not. Acquired conditions affecting scrotal contents in the adult include epididymitis, hydrocele, spermatocele, varicocele, orchitis, torsion, and testicular cancer (Fig. 52-4).

Epididymitis

Epididymitis is an inflammatory process of the epididymis, usually secondary to an infectious process (sexually or nonsexually transmitted), trauma, or urinary reflux down the vas deferens. When the problem is associated with prostatitis it is usually painful. Swelling may progress to the point that the epididymis and testis are indistinguishable. In younger men, less than 35 years of age, the most common cause is through sexual transmission of either gonorrhea or chlamydia. The use of antibiotics is important for both partners if the transmission is through sexual contact. Patients should be encouraged to refrain from sexual intercourse during the acute phase. If they do engage in intercourse, a condom should be used. Conservative treatment consists of bed rest with elevation of the scrotum, use of ice packs, and analgesics. Ambulation places the scrotum in a dependent position and increases pain. Most tenderness subsides within 1 week, although swelling may last for weeks or months.

Hydrocele

A *hydrocele* is a nontender, fluid-filled mass that results from interference with lymphatic drainage of the scrotum and swelling of the tunica vaginalis that surrounds the testis. Diagnosis is fairly simple because the mass can be seen by shining a

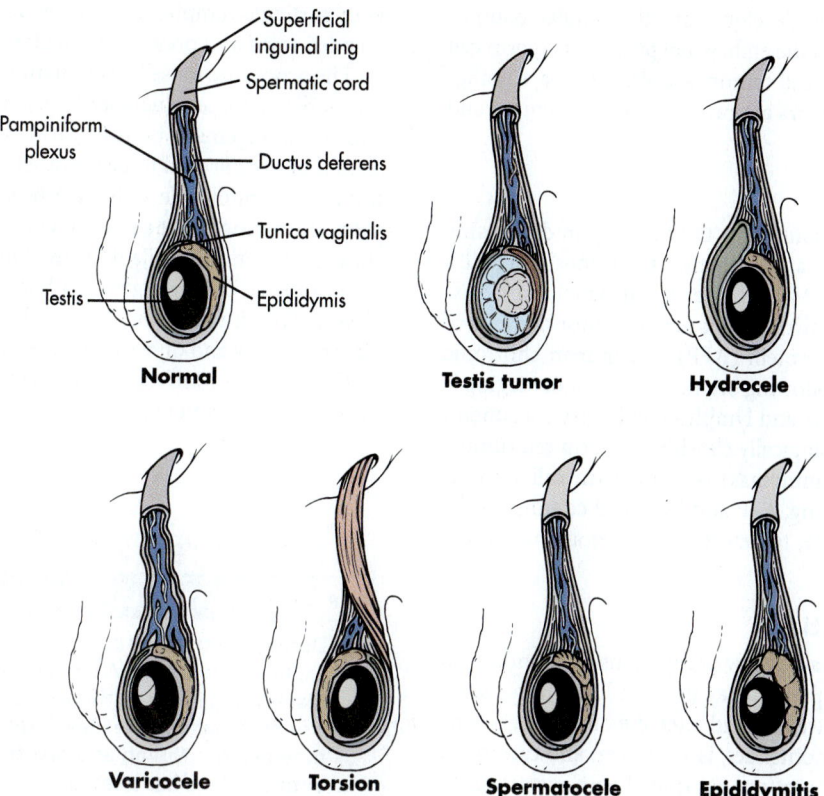

Fig. 52-4 Scrotal masses.

flashlight through the scrotum (transillumination). No treatment is indicated unless the swelling becomes very large and uncomfortable, in which case aspiration or surgical drainage of the mass is performed.

Spermatocele

A *spermatocele* is a firm, sperm-containing, painless cyst of the epididymis that may be visible with transillumination. The cause is unknown, and surgical removal is the treatment. It is important for the patient to see his doctor if he feels any lumps. He would be unable to distinguish this cyst from cancer when performing self-examination.

Varicocele

A *varicocele* is a dilation of the veins that drain the testes. The scrotum feels wormlike when palpated. The cause of the problem is unknown. The varicocele is usually located on the left side of the scrotum as a consequence of retrograde blood flow from the left renal vein. Surgery is indicated if the patient is infertile, since persistent varicoceles are associated with 40% to 50% of the causes of infertility. Repair of the varicocele may be through injection of a sclerosing agent or by surgical ligation of the spermatic vein.

Orchitis

In *orchitis* the testis is acutely inflamed, painful, tender, and swollen. It generally occurs after an episode of bacterial or viral infections such as mumps, pneumonia, tuberculosis, or syphilis. It can also be a side effect of epididymitis, prostatectomy, trauma, infectious mononucleosis, influenza, catheterization, or complicated urinary tract infection. Mumps orchitis is a condition contributing to infertility and could easily be decreased by childhood vaccination against mumps. Treatment involves the use of antibiotics (if the organism is known), pain medications, or bed rest with the scrotum elevated on an ice pack.

Torsion

Testicular torsion involves a twisting of the spermatic cord that supplies blood to the testes and epididymis. It is most commonly seen in young males under the age of 20. Torsion constitutes a surgical emergency. The patient experiences severe scrotal pain, tenderness, swelling, nausea, and vomiting. Urinary complaints, fever, and WBCs or bacteria in the urine are absent. The pain does not usually subside with rest or elevation of the scrotum. Unless it resolves spontaneously, surgery to untwist the cord and restore the blood supply must be performed quickly. The torsion causes ischemia to the testis, leading to necrosis and the possible need for removal.

Testicular Cancer

Etiology and Pathophysiology

Testicular tumors occur primarily in men between 20 and 40 years of age. Testicular tumors are more common in males who have had undescended testes (cryptorchidism) or a family history of testicular cancer or anomalies. Other predisposing factors include a history of mumps, orchitis, inguinal hernia in childhood, maternal exposure to DES, and testicular cancer in the contralateral testis.

Testicular tumors may develop from the cellular components of the testis or from the embryonal precursors (germ cell tumors). Testicular germ cell tumors are almost always malignant. Non–germ cell tumors are rare, are usually benign, and can occur at any age.

Diagnostic Studies

Palpation of the scrotal contents is the first step in diagnosing testicular cancer. Additional tests that aid in diagnosis include a testicular sonogram and MRI. If a testicular neoplasm is suspected, blood may be drawn to look for the tumor markers of glycoproteins alpha-fetoprotein (AFP) and human chorionic gonadotropin (hCG). Following orchiectomy, tumor staging is done on the testicle tissue and lymph node biopsy specimens. Testicular cancer is histologically classified as germ cell tumors (seminomas and nonseminomas) or non–germ cell tumors. After diagnosis and staging, AFP and hCG will continue to be monitored, if appropriate, to detect metastases and assess the response to therapy.

Clinical Manifestations

Germ cell tumors may have a slow or rapid onset depending on the type of tumor. The patient may notice a lump in his scrotum, as well as scrotal swelling and a feeling of heaviness. The scrotal mass usually is nontender, is very firm, and cannot be transilluminated. Manifestations associated with metastasis to other systems include back pain, cough, dyspnea, hemoptysis, dysphagia (difficulty swallowing), alterations in vision or mental status, papilledema, and seizures.

NURSING AND COLLABORATIVE MANAGEMENT: TESTICULAR CANCER

As with many forms of cancer, the survival of the patient is closely associated with early recognition of the tumor. The scrotum is easily examined, and beginning tumors are usually palpable. Every male between puberty and 40 years of age should be taught and encouraged to perform a monthly testicular self-examination for the purpose of detecting testicular tumors or other scrotal abnormalities such as varicoceles. The nurse should teach the patient how to do a self-examination

with particular emphasis on males with a history of an undescended testis or a previous testicular tumor.

The procedure for self-examination is not difficult. The male may indicate some reluctance to examine his own genitals, but with encouragement he can learn this simple procedure. He should be encouraged to perform self-examinations frequently until he is comfortable with the procedure. The scrotum should then be examined once a month. Videotapes and illustrations on shower hangers are available as teaching aids and ideally should be introduced during high school or college physical education classes. Free information is available through the American Cancer Society and on various Internet medical websites.

Guidelines for self-examination of the scrotum are presented in Table 52-8 and Fig. 52-5. The nurse should make this pro-

---

🖊 **PATIENT TEACHING GUIDE**

Table 52-8 **Testicular Self-Examination**

1. During a shower or bath is the easiest time to examine the testes. Warm temperatures make the testes hang lower in the scrotum (See Fig. 52-5).
2. Use both hands to feel each testis. Roll the testis between the thumb and first three fingers until the entire surface has been covered. Palpate each one separately.
3. Identify the structures. The testis should feel round and smooth, like a hard-boiled egg. Differentiate the testis from the epididymis. The epididymis is not as smooth as the egg-shaped testis. One testis may be larger than the other. Size is not as important as texture. Check for lumps, irregularities, pain in the testes, or a dragging sensation. Locate the spermatic cord, which is usually firm and smooth and goes up toward the groin.
4. Choose a consistent day of the month, such as a birth date, that is easy to remember to examine the testes. The examination can be performed more frequently if desired.
5. Notify the doctor at once if any abnormalities are found.

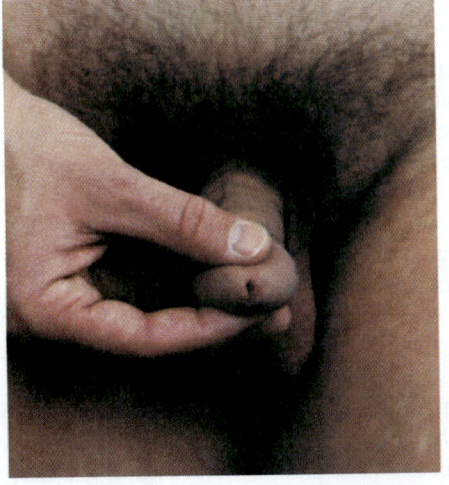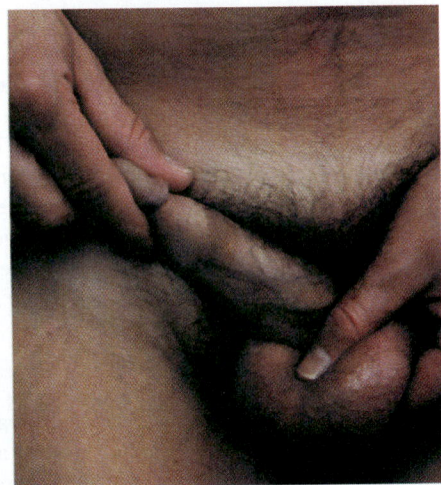

Fig. 52-5 Testicular self-examination.

cedure as simple and uncomplicated for the man as possible. The man should choose a technique that is comfortable and consistent for him. It may be his first step toward a lifetime of healthy living practices.

Collaborative management of testicular cancer generally involves a radical orchiectomy (surgical removal of the affected testis, spermatic cord, and regional lymph nodes). Radiation of the remaining lymph nodes may be used if the tumor is radiosensitive. Single or multiple chemotherapeutic agent regimens, including bleomycin (Blenoxane), vincristine (Oncovin), cisplatin (Platinol), vinblastine (Velban), and etoposide (VePesid), are also used before or after surgery, depending on the histologic conditions and disease stage.[33,34]

The prognosis for patients with testicular cancer has improved, and 75% of the patients obtain complete remission if the disease is detected in the early stages. All patients with testicular cancer, regardless of pathology or stage, require meticulous follow-up and regular physical examinations, chest radiography, CT scan, and assessment of hCG and AFP (if appropriate). The goal is to detect relapse when the tumor burden is minimal. Some studies have indicated a higher risk of second cancers in these men.[35] Secondary malignancies that occur as a result of chemotherapy and radiation are described in Chapter 14. The man with testicular cancer should have the opportunity to discuss fertility and sperm banking before any treatment. The nurse should be sensitive to any psychosocial problems this type of cancer can have on a man's feelings of maleness or self-worth.[36] Treatment has the potential to interfere with both erections and fertility.

SEXUAL FUNCTIONING

VASECTOMY

Vasectomy is the bilateral surgical ligation or resection of the vas deferens performed for the purpose of sterilization (Fig. 52-6). The procedure requires only 15 to 30 minutes and is usually performed with the patient under local anesthesia on an outpatient basis. Vasectomy is considered a permanent form of sterilization, although some successful reversals (vasovasotomy) have been reported.

After vasectomy, the patient should not notice any difference in the look or feel of the ejaculate, because its major component is seminal and prostatic fluid. The patient will need to use an alternative form of contraception until semen examination reveals no sperm. This usually requires at least 10 ejaculations or 6 weeks to evacuate sperm distal to the surgical site. Sperm cells continue to be produced by the testes but are absorbed by the body rather than being passed through the vas deferens. Occasionally postoperative hematoma and swelling of the scrotum occur.

Vasectomy does not affect the production of hormones, ability to ejaculate, or physiologic mechanisms related to erection or orgasm. Psychologic adjustment may be a problem after surgery. It may be very difficult for the patient to separate vasectomy from castration at a subconscious level. Some men may develop erectile dysfunction or may feel the need to become much more sexually active than they were in the past to prove their masculinity. Careful discussion of the procedure

and its outcome before the surgery can be helpful in detecting patients who may have problems with psychologic adjustment. Surgery should be delayed for these patients.

ERECTILE DYSFUNCTION

Over 20 million men in the United States experience erectile dysfunction.[37] The problem is increasing in all segments of the sexually active male population and impacts both the man and his partner. In younger men the increase is attributed to an increase in substance abuse, such as recreational drugs and alcohol. Middle-aged men are affected by modern medical technology, such as major organ transplants, bypass surgeries, and chemotherapeutic agents. The older population (men over 70 years of age) are living longer, fuller lives and expect to remain sexually active, regardless of any existing medical conditions. Stress factors associated with modern lifestyles are affecting men of all ages and contribute greatly to the overall causes of erectile failure.

Etiology and Pathophysiology

Erectile dysfunction is the inability to attain or maintain an erect penis that allows satisfactory sexual performance. This problem occurs at some time or other for almost all sexually active males. The problem can occur at any age, although it most often begins among males between 55 and 65 years of age. Erection is a parasympathetic reflex initiated mainly by certain tactile, visual, and mental stimuli. It consists of dilation of the arteries and arterioles of the penis, which in turn fills and distends spaces in its erectile tissue and compresses veins. When this occurs, more blood enters the penis through the dilated arteries than leaves it through the constricted veins. The penis then becomes larger and rigid, or, in other words, erection occurs. Problems occur when these spaces (corporeal bodies) fail to fill when desired or when they empty before orgasm.

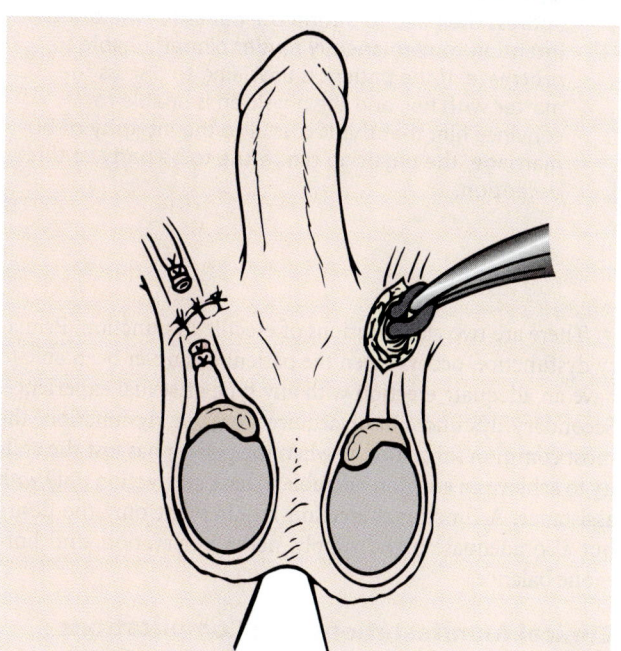

Fig. 52-6 Vasectomy procedure. The vas deferens is ligated or resected for the purpose of sterilization.

Sterilization

SITUATION

A 43-year-old male patient is requesting a vasectomy and informs the nurse that he does not wish to discuss this with his wife. The physician's policy is to have the spouse or partner sign a form acknowledging the patient's desire to be sterilized. This patient explains that while his wife wants to have more children, the one they already have is all he wants.

DISCUSSION

Physician practice rather than state law dictates the need for disclosure of the intent to sterilize a patient to that patient's spouse or significant other. Had the patient not informed the physician that he was married, there would be no issue. As it is, he can seek another physician to perform this procedure who has no such reservations, or he may choose to lie about his marital status. Women in most states are not required to prove that their husbands or significant others are aware of their intention to terminate a pregnancy, but the (intended) finality of a vasectomy is considered to be a different case. Professional ethics require that the nurse explain to the patient that he cannot have a vasectomy with this physician without obtaining the needed consultation with his wife. The patient would then be free to determine how to handle this problem.

ETHICAL AND LEGAL PRINCIPLES

- Patient autonomy would require that matters relating to reproduction be left to the privacy and discretion of the individual.
- Competent adults may legally choose to be sterilized for convenience or for medical reasons.
- Nonmaleficence and truth telling, however, would address the need to inform the patient's wife of his intention to permanently render himself unable to procreate. If the patient is unwilling to discuss the matter with her, and the physician is unable to convince him that this is crucial to the integrity of his marriage, the physician can refuse to be party to this deception.

There are two classifications of erectile dysfunction. Primary dysfunction occurs when the patient has never been able to have an adequate erection with any type of sexual experience. Secondary dysfunction, or acquired organic dysfunction, the most common form, occurs when the patient has lost the ability to achieve an erection or is able to have an erection only with assistance. A functional erection requires not only the desire but also adequate blood supply, nerve innervation, and hormone balance.

Clinical Manifestations and Complications

The causative factors for the disorder may be physiologic, psychologic, or both (Table 52-9). The major complication of this problem is that the man's inability to perform sexually can cause great distress in his interpersonal relationships and may interfere with his concept of himself as a man. Our society promotes images of a man being strong, capable, and sexually responsive. Table 52-10 lists normal age-related changes in sexual performance. Explanation of these age-related changes may be necessary to reassure an anxious older man regarding normal changes in his sexual abilities.

Diagnostic Studies

Rapid advances have been made in the diagnosis and treatment of erectile dysfunction. With the advent of modern technology, 80% to 90% of the causes are being attributed to physiologic reasons and can be determined by diagnostic studies. Diagnostic testing is now divided into primary and secondary levels based on findings during the initial assessment (Table 52-11). For primary testing, a complete medical history and physical examination is performed. In addition, self-administered, assessment- and treatment-related questionnaires have been developed and may prove useful as primary screening tools. For example, the International Index of Erectile Function (IIEF)[38] identifies a man's response to five key areas of male sexual function. These areas include erectile function, orgasmic function, sexual desire, intercourse satisfaction, and overall satisfaction. Intracavernosal vasoactive testing is done to help distinguish psychogenic from neurogenic or vascular causes of erectile dysfunction. In this test vasoactive agents such as papaverine, phentolamine (Regitine), or prostaglandin (PGE_1), are given to directly relax the smooth muscle of the corporal erectile tissue, causing an erection within 5 to 10 minutes. Failure of an erection to occur indicates a potential vascular etiology.

Secondary testing may include vascular flow studies (duplex Doppler, cavernosogram). Nocturnal penile tumescence may also be performed to distinguish a psychogenic from neurogenic or vascular cause. This test is based on the theory that normal erections occur during the rapid eye movement phase of sleep. The test involves recording of both sleep and penile changes.

Neurogenic factors can be evaluated using somatosensory evoked potential studies. In this test, electrical activity within the bulbocavernosa muscle is measured in response to stimulation of the penile skin. The presence of electrical activity following tactile stimulation suggests an intact sacral arc.

Collaborative Care

The treatment for erectile dysfunction is based on the cause.[37,39] Treatment of psychogenic erectile dysfunction should be carried out by a qualified therapist. The approach may be behavioral or psychologic, and in some patients it may also involve medical intervention to temporarily restore self-confidence. The goal of all erectile dysfunction therapy is to have the man and his partner develop a satisfactory sexual relationship, including good communication skills.

When the problem is physical, interventions are directed at correcting or eliminating the cause or restoring function by medical means. The results of these interventions are usually most satisfactory when both partners are involved in the deci-

Table **52-9** Risk Factors for Erectile Dysfunction

Anatomic
Congenital deformities of the penis (e.g., hypospadias)
Peyronie's disease

Cardiorespiratory
Angina pectoris
Atherosclerosis
Emphysema
Hypertension
Myocardial infarction
Post cardiac surgery

Drug Induced
5-alpha-reductase inhibitors (finasteride [Proscar])
Alcohol
Antiandrogens
Antilipidemic agents
Antihypertensives
Caffeine
Diuretics (chlorothiazide [Diuril]; spironolactone [Aldactone])
Drugs for Parkinson's disease (carbidopa-levodopa [Sinemet])
Estrogens
Major tranquilizers (diazepam [Valium]; alprazolam [Xanax])
Marijuana, cocaine, LSD
Narcotics
Nicotine neuroleptics (phenothiazine [Thorazine])
Tricyclic antidepressants (amitriptyline [Elavil])

Endocrine
Addison's disease
Diabetes mellitus
High levels of prolactin
Obesity
Pituitary tumor
Testosterone deficiency
Thyrotoxicosis

Genitourinary
Cystectomy
Hydrocele
Perineal or suprapubic prostatectomy
Phimosis
Post kidney transplant
Postpriapism
Prostatitis
Renal failure
Varicocele

Neurologic and nerve conduction
Central nervous system disorders
Cerbrovascular accident
Electroshock therapy
Multiple sclerosis
Parkinson's disease
Peripheral neuropathic conditions
Spina bifida
Sympathectomy
Trauma to the spinal cord
Tumors or transection of spinal cord

Psychogenic
Depression
Excessive stress in family, work, or interpersonal relationships
Fatigue
Fear of failure to perform

Vascular
Aortic aneurysm
Aortofemoral bypass
Atherosclerosis of pelvic blood vessels

GERONTOLOGIC DIFFERENCES IN ASSESSMENT
Table **52-10** Sexual Performance

1. Time lag between perceiving sexual opportunity and full erection
2. Diminished size and rigidity of the penis at full erection
3. Increased time interval to ejaculation
4. Changed nature of ejaculation with less spurting and lessened intensity of feeling
5. Shortened period between ejaculation and flaccidity
6. Increase in time to next reaction to sexual stimulation

*For almost all men by the age of 45 to 50 years.

sion-making process and have realistic expectations of the treatment. Many treatment options are available to the man experiencing vascular or neurogenic erectile dysfunction. Clinical practice guidelines on erectile dysfunction were developed by the American Urological Association.[40] Treat-ment recommendations include vasoactive drug therapy, vacuum constrictive devices, and penile prosthesis. Other invasive and experimental techniques are limited to research centers.

Nonsurgical Management

Drug therapy. Whenever possible, collaboration should occur between the primary physician providing the medical care and the urologist treating the erectile dysfunction. Elimi-nation of or substitution for a medication that causes erectile dysfunction is sometimes all that is necessary to alleviate the problem (see Table 52-9).

When there is an established diagnosis of testicular failure (hypogonadism), androgen replacement therapy may some-times be effective in improving erectile function. It should be given as an intramuscular injection of testosterone enanthate (Delatestryl) or testosterone cypionate (Virilon). Oral andro-gens that are currently available are not as effective. The effec-tiveness of testosterone supplementation for older men expe-riencing a normal, gradual decline is doubtful. Careful evaluation of the man's serum testosterone level and prostate

DIAGNOSTIC STUDIES

Table 52-11 Erectile Dysfunction

Primary
- Medical history and physical examination
- Detailed sexual history, including practices and techniques
- Psychosocial evaluation
- Testosterone levels
- Prostate-specific antigen
- Intracavernosal vasoactive testing

Secondary
- Hormone profile (e.g., prolactin, FSH, LH)
- Vascular flow studies (e.g., duplex Doppler, cavernosogram)
- Neurologic evaluation
- Sacral evoked potential test
- Nocturnal penile tumescence
- Tests to exclude unrecognized systemic disease: CBC, urinalysis, creatinine, lipid profile, FBS, thyroid function studies

FBS, fasting blood sugar; *FSH,* follicle stimulating hormone; *LH,* luteinizing hormone.

condition must precede introduction of this therapy. Administration of testosterone to a man with normal levels of hormone production may actually suppress the body's natural ability to produce testosterone. Testosterone is contraindicated in men with cancer of the prostate because of its ability to cause proliferation of the prostate cancer cells. For men with hyperprolactinemia, bromocriptine (Parlodel) therapy is often effective in normalizing the prolactin level and improving sexual functioning.

A major breakthrough in the treatment of erectile dysfunction has been in the area of penile vasoactive drug therapy. The medication enhances blood flow into the penile arteries. Until recently the only method available for administration was in the form of penile injections. These medications are now available in pill, gel, patch, pellet, and injection form. Current vasoactive medications include papaverine (topical gel or injection),[41,42] alprostadil (topical, transurethral pellet [e.g., MUSE], or injection),[43-47] phentolamine (Regitine) in combination with other vasoactive medications (injection), vasoactive intestinal peptide (injection), and sildenafil (Viagra, pill).[48]

The vasoactive medication dose is regulated on an individual basis to prevent side effects. Side effects may include penile pain, priapism, corporal fibrosis, fibrotic nodules, and hypotension. It is important to instruct patients carefully on the specific administration techniques and precautions for any of the vasoactive medications.

Home injection therapy instruction is given to those men who are suitable candidates for the therapy. The injection is nearly painless and generally begins to work in 20 to 30 minutes. Success rates have been high when there is adequate patient teaching and follow-up.[49-51] This treatment is not suitable for men with severe vascular problems, intolerance for

transient hypotension, severe psychiatric disease, poor manual dexterity, or poor vision or those receiving anticoagulant therapy. The man may discontinue treatment if he perceives a lack of spontaneity, has a needle phobia, or wants a more permanent treatment option.

The latest advances in treatment of erectile dysfunction are the oral vasoactive medications. The most widely prescribed medication is sildenafil (Viagra), a pill that increases smooth muscle relaxation in the penis by blocking specific enzymes.[52] Viagra is generally taken 30 to 60 minutes before engaging in sexual activity. The usual dose is 50 to 100 mg orally and has a success rate of approximately 70% to 80% for psychogenic causes, 50% to 60% in diabetes mellitus, and 40% to 50% in radical prostatectomy patients. It should be avoided in men using nitrates (antianginal agents) such as Isordil, nitroglycerin, Nitro-Bid, and Transderm Nitro and used cautiously in men with retinitis pigmentosa. Other oral medications under investigation include apomorphine (a parkinsonian drug), which affects brain chemistry, and Vasomax, an oral version of an injectable vasodilator.[52]

Aids or devices. Suction devices applied to the flaccid penis produce an erection by pulling blood up into the corporeal bodies. A penile ring or other device is placed around the base of the penis, causing vasoconstriction and preventing detumescence (subsidence of swelling). Special care must be taken in using these devices to prevent tissue damage. Suction devices are sometimes used in conjunction with intracorporeal injection therapy and in those patients with moderate to severe venous leaks of the penile veins.[53]

Alternative methods. Some patients do not require penetration for satisfactory sexual expression, and a vibrator or dildo (rubber penis) could be used by the partner. Patients experiencing temporary loss of erection or who are awaiting surgical interventions can use a variety of methods to achieve sexual satisfaction. Sexual counselors or therapists acting as consultants can provide support and suggest alternative forms of sexual expression.

Surgical Therapy

Penile implants. Penile implants have provided surgical management of erectile dysfunction for more than 25 years. The paired devices can be semirigid, malleable, or inflatable (Fig. 52-7).[54,55] They are implanted into the corporeal bodies to provide an erection firm enough for penetration. All implants provide a usable erection and should be chosen carefully based on the man's mental and physical capabilities, surgical risk factors, personal lifestyle, insurance, and financial resources. The main problems associated with penile prostheses are mechanical failure, infection, and erosions.

For essentially healthy men the surgical procedure may be performed on an outpatient basis, with patients being monitored by home care nurses. Complete recovery time varies from 4 to 6 weeks. Patients considered to be at high risk for complications include those with uncontrolled diabetes mellitus and those with severe circulatory problems.

Patients should be advised that none of the options will restore ejaculation or tactile sensations if they were absent before treatment. Sexual counseling is often recommended before and after treatment. The ability to please both partners enhances satisfaction levels.

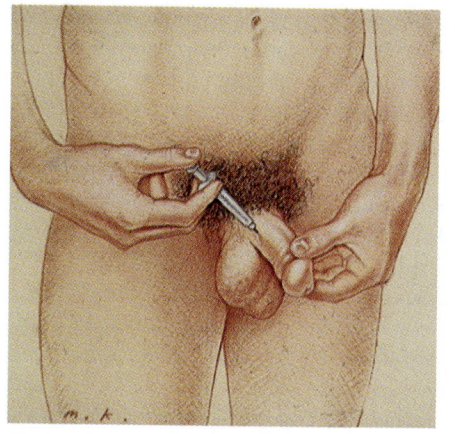
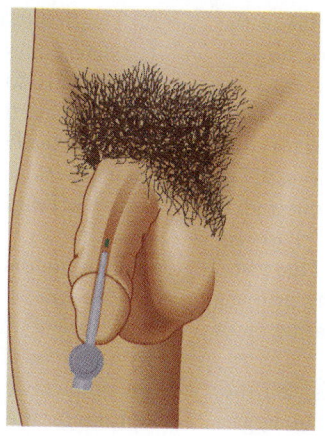
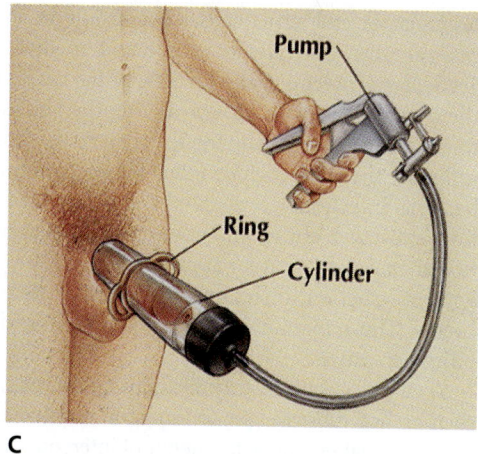
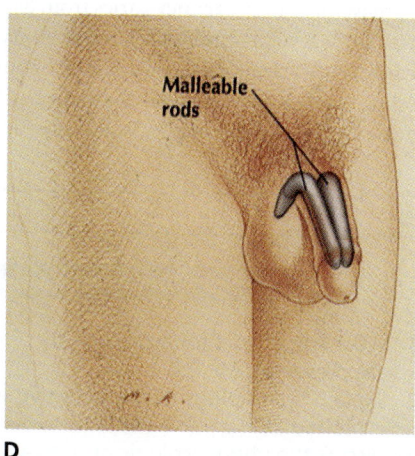
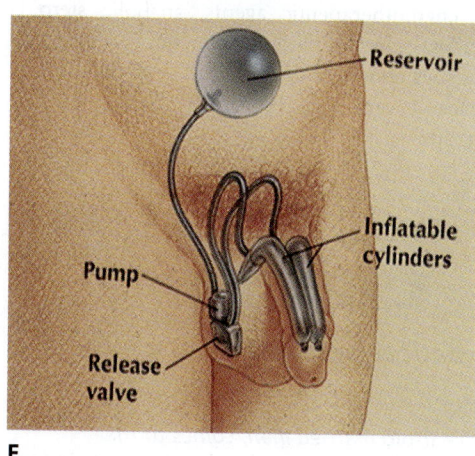

Fig. 52-7 A, Self-injection therapy involves injecting a medication directly into the penis. This increases blood flow and causes an erection. **B,** Intraurethral pellets are used to deliver drug therapy. **C,** With the vacuum device in place, blood can be drawn into the penis by means of a hand pump. This creates an erection. For intercourse, the ring is slipped to the base of the penis and the cylinder removed. **D,** A malleable implant is always erect but can be bent close to the body for concealment. **E,** Inflatable implants consist of cylinders in the penis, a small pump in the scrotum, and a reservoir in the lower abdomen. When activated, the pump fills the cylinders with fluid from the reservoir. A small release valve permits the fluid to drain back into the reservoir after intercourse.

NURSING MANAGEMENT: ERECTILE DYSFUNCTION

The man experiencing erectile dysfunction requires a great deal of emotional support for both himself and his partner. Men often do not feel comfortable discussing their problems with others because of society's expectations of a man's sexual abilities. The man may experience and demonstrate isolation from support systems, and he may also lose self-esteem, which can eventually lead to loss of role functions.[56]

The patient needs reassurance that confidentiality will be maintained. In conjunction with medical treatment, it often becomes necessary to provide counseling and therapy for the couple to establish realistic expectations and develop meaningful communication patterns. The majority of men wait an average of 2 years before seeking medical assistance. They are often highly motivated and expect immediate solutions to their problems. The health care team should provide a support system and accurate information as soon as possible.[56]

Nurses are in a unique position of conducting routine health assessments on men seeking any form of medical treatment. It provides an opportunity to ask not only general health questions but also those seldom-asked sexual function ones as well. Given the opportunity, most men do not hesitate to answer these questions when they know that someone cares and can provide them with answers.

INFERTILITY

In about one third of childless marriages in which children are desired, the primary cause of infertility is due to male factors.[56] Infertility can be caused by disorders of the hypothalamic-pituitary system, disorders of the testes, and abnormalities of the ejaculatory system.

The physical causes are generally divided into three categories: pre-testicular, testicular, and post-testicular. The pre-testicular or endocrine causes occur only in about 3% of the cases and can generally be treated with medication or surgery. Testicular problems make up 50% of the cases. Varicoceles are the major cause with 60% involving the left testis, 39% both testes, and only 1% involving the right testis. Other factors that influence the testes include infection (e.g., mumps virus, STDs, bacterial infections), congenital anomalies, medications, radiation, substance abuse, and environmental hazards.[57] Post-testicular causes account for approximately 5% to 7% of the cases, with obstruction, infection, or vasectomy being the primary causes. The remaining 40% are classified as idiopathic or of unknown causes.

A careful health history includes occupation; lifestyle issues such as hot tubs, weight training, or wearing tight undergarments; sexual practices; frequency of intercourse; and emotional factors such as stress levels and the desire for children. The use of drugs, such as chemotherapeutic agents, anabolic steroids (testosterone), sulfasalazine (Azulfidine), cimetidine (Tagamet), and recreational drugs, should be documented. A physical examination can disclose a varicocele, Peyronie's disease, or other physical abnormalities.

The first test in an infertility study is a semen analysis. The test determines the sperm concentration (count greater than 20 million/ml), forward progressive motility (at least 60% with a grade greater than 2), and morphology (at least 60% have normal oval head and long tail). Additional tests that may be helpful in determining the etiology include plasma testosterone and serum LH and FSH measurements. A test for sperm penetration abilities may also be done. The specific cause of infertility is often not determined.

The nurse should be concerned and tactful in dealing with the male patient undergoing infertility studies. For many men, fertility and masculinity are equated. The nurse must be sensitive to the problem of gender identity in the infertile man.[56] Treatment options for the man include medications,[58] conservative lifestyle changes (e.g., avoidance of scrotal heat, substance abuse, high stress), in vitro fertilization techniques, and corrective surgery. Achievement of pregnancy varies from 8% to 60% and ranges in cost from several hundred to several thousand dollars. Infertility can seriously strain a marriage, and the couple may require counseling and discussion of alternatives if conception is not achieved. (Female infertility is discussed in Chapter 51.)

CRITICAL THINKING EXERCISES

CASE STUDY

Benign Prostatic Hyperplasia

Patient Profile

Mr. R.K., a 71-year-old married man, comes to the emergency department because of an inability to void for the past 12 hours.

Subjective Data

- Complains of severe bladder pain and pressure
- Is very restless and agitated
- Relates history of three cans of beer at party the previous evening; has not voided since then

Objective Data

Physical Examination
- Has prostate enlargement on rectal examination
- Has hematuria and WBCs in urine
- Has palpable bladder above umbilicus

Laboratory Studies
- PSA: 8 ng/ml (normal: 0 to 4 ng/ml)

Collaborative Care

- Indwelling catheter inserted by a urology resident
- Mr. R.K. admitted to the hospital

Critical Thinking Questions

1. What risk factors for acute urinary retention and BPH are present in Mr. R.K.?
2. Explain the etiology of the objective symptoms Mr. R.K. exhibited.
3. Discuss the pharmacologic options available to Mr. R.K.
4. Discuss the invasive options available to Mr. R.K.
5. Mr. R.K. asks you about the effect of the various treatment options on his ability to have sex. How would you respond?
6. Write one or more appropriate nursing diagnoses based on the assessment data presented. Are there any collaborative problems?
7. On further assessment, you note that Mr. R.K. has a nursing diagnosis of decisional conflict. How would you help him resolve this conflict related to treatment options?

NURSING RESEARCH ISSUES

1. Is a man more likely to report problems related to prostatic enlargement directly to the health care provider or via a printed questionnaire?
2. What percentage of patients with prostatic enlargement have a concurrent urinary tract infection?
3. What is the best strategy to get men over 40 years of age to have an annual digital rectal examination?
4. What relaxation techniques are most effective in relieving bladder spasms after a transurethral or suprapubic prostatectomy?
5. How receptive are men with an erectile dysfunction to the idea of a prosthetic device to accomplish an erection?
6. What is the compliance rate for testicular self-examination at 3, 6, and 12 months following a training program for high school boys?
7. Does awareness of behaviors that can cause acute urinary retention in men with BPH alter the practice of these behaviors?

REVIEW QUESTIONS

The number of the question corresponds to the same-numbered objective at the beginning of the chapter.

1. A patient with BPH experiences hesitancy in initiating voiding and a feeling of incomplete bladder emptying. In assessing for complications related to these symptoms the nurse asks specifically about the presence of
   a. constipation.
   b. dysuria and urgency.
   c. gross blood in the urine.
   d. decreased force of the urinary stream.

2. Postoperatively a patient who has had a transurethral prostatectomy has continuous bladder irrigation with a three-way Foley with a 30 ml balloon and traction applied. The patient complains that he feels the urge to void even with the catheter in place. The nurse should
   a. hand irrigate the catheter to ensure that it is patent.
   b. deflate the catheter balloon to 10 ml to decrease bulk in the bladder.
   c. encourage the patient to try to have a bowel movement to relieve colon pressure.
   d. explain that this feeling is normal and that he should not try to urinate around the catheter.

3. In teaching health promotion related to early detection of prostate cancer the nurse advises that beginning at middle age men should have an annual
   a. urinalysis.
   b. rectal examination.
   c. prostatic ultrasound.
   d. prostatic acid phosphatase (PAP).

4. A patient scheduled for a suprapubic prostatectomy for prostate cancer expresses the fear that he will be impotent. In responding to the patient the nurse explains that
   a. sterility, but not impotence, is common with a suprapubic prostatectomy.
   b. the most common complication of this surgery is postoperative urinary retention.
   c. a penile implant may be an alternative to consider after he has recovered from his surgery.
   d. pain control will be a more important factor than sexual function in the long-term consideration of his condition.

5. The nurse advises the patient with chronic prostatitis that long-term management includes
   a. a permanent indwelling catheter.
   b. regular injection of sclerosing agents.
   c. sexual activities that result in ejaculation.
   d. aspiration or surgical drainage of abscesses.

6. Discharge teaching for the patient who has had a vasectomy includes explaining that
   a. the procedure blocks the production of sperm.
   b. an alternative form of contraception will be necessary for 6 to 8 weeks.
   c. the ejaculate will be about half the volume it was before the procedure.
   d. erectile dysfunction is temporary and will return with continued sexual activity.

7. A nursing measure that can decrease the patient's discomfort over care involving his reproductive organs includes
   a. relating his sexual concerns to his sexual partner.
   b. arranging to have only male nurses care for the patient.
   c. maintaining a nonjudgmental attitude toward his sexual practices.
   d. using only technical terminology when discussing reproductive function.

References

1. McConnell JD and others: *Benign prostatic hyperplasia: diagnosis and treatment. Clinical practice guideline no. 8,* AHCPR publ no 940582, Rockville, Md, 1994, Agency for Health Care Policy and Research, Public Health Service, US Department of Health and Human Services.

2. Prostate Health Council: *Enlarged prostate: BPH and male urinary problems,* Baltimore, 1998, American Foundation for Urologic Disease.

3. Reilly NJ: Benign prostatic hyperplasia. In Meredith CE, Karlowicz KA, editors: *Urologic nursing: a study guide,* New Jersey, 1995, Soc of Urol Nurs Assoc.

4. Barry MJ and others: A nationwide survey of practicing urologists: current management of benign prostatic hyperplasia and clinically localized prostate cancer, *Urology* 158:488, 1997.

5. Oesterling JE: Benign prostatic hyperplasia: medical and minimally invasive treatment options, *N Engl J Med* 332:99, 1995.

6. Albertsen PC: Prostate disease in older men: benign hyperplasia, *Hosp Pract* 32:61, 1997.

7. Campo B and others: Transurethral needle ablation (TUNA) of the prostate: a clinical and urodynamic evaluation, *Urology* 49:847, 1997.

*8. Bartkui TP, Goldfarb B, Trachtenberg J: Understanding microwave therapy as a treatment option for benign prostatic hyperplasia, *Urol Nurs* 17:53, 1997.

9. Ramsey EW, Miller PD, Parsons K: A novel transurethral microwave thermal ablation system to treat benign prostatic hyperplasia: results of a prospective multicenter clinical trial, *J Urol* 158:112, 1997.

10. Anderson RJ: Primary care management of benign prostatic hyperplasia, *Hosp Pract* 33:11, 1998.

11. Angelucci PA: Caring for patients with benign prostatic hyperplasia, *Nursing* 27:54, 1997.

12. Albertsen PC: Prostate disease in older men: cancer, *Hosp Pract* 32:159, 1997.

13. LaFollette SS, Reilly NJ: Cancer of the prostate. In Meredith CE, Karlowicz KA, editors: *Urologic nursing: a study guide,* New Jersey, 1995, Soc of Urol Nurs Assoc.

14. Powell IJ and others: Outcome of African American men screened for prostate cancer: the Detroit Education and Early Detection study, *J Urol* 158:146, 1997.

15. Choday GW and others: Results of conservative management of clinically localized prostate cancer, *N Engl J Med* 330:242, 1994.

16. Zincke H and others: Radical prostatectomy for clinically localized prostate cancer: long-term results of 1,143 patients from a single institution, *J Clin Oncol* 12:2254, 1994.

17. Catalona WJ, Basler JW: Return of erections and urinary continence following nerve sparing radical retropubic prostatectomy, *J Urol* 150:905, 1993.

18. Jonler M and others: Sequelae of radical prostatectomy, *Br J Urol* 74:352, 1994.

19. Lim AJ and others: Quality of life: radical prostatectomy versus radiation therapy for prostate cancer, *J Urol* 154:1420, 1995.

20. Litwin MS and others: Quality of life outcomes in men treated for localized prostate cancer, *JAMA* 273:129, 1995.

21. Helgason AR and others: Factors associated with waning sexual function among elderly men and prostate cancer patients, *J Urol* 158:155, 1997.

22. Bolla M and others: Improved survival in patients with locally advanced prostate cancer treated with radiotherapy and goserelin, *N Engl J Med* 337:295, 1997.

23. Brufsky A and others: Finasteride and flutamide as potency-sparing androgen-ablative therapy for advanced adenocarcinoma of the prostate, *Urology* 49:913, 1997.

24. Kirschenbaum A: Management of hormonal treatment effects, *Cancer* 75:1983, 1995.

*25. Jakobsson L, Hallberg IR, Loven L: Met and unmet nursing care needs in men with prostate cancer: an explorative study, *Eur J Cancer Care* 6:117, 1997.

*26. Davison BJ, Degner LF: Empowerment of men newly diagnosed with prostate cancer, *Cancer Nurs* 20:187, 1997.

27. Thin RN: Diagnosis of chronic prostatitis: overview and update, *Int J STD AIDS* 8:475, 1997.

28. Krieger JN and others: Chronic pelvic pains represent the most prominent urogenital symptoms of "chronic prostatitis," *Urology* 48:715, 1996.

29. Donovan DA, Nicholas PK: Prostatitis: diagnosis and treatment in primary care, *Nurse Pract* 22:144, 1997.

30. Pansadoro V and others: Prostate-specific antigen and prostatitis in men under fifty, *Eur Urol* 30:24, 1996.

31. Nickel JC, Sorensen R: Transurethral microwave thermotherapy for nonbacterial prostatitis: a randomized double-blind sham controlled study using new prostatitis specific assessment questionnaires, *J Urol* 155:1950, 1996.

32. McLachlan JA and others: Are estrogens carcinogenic during development of the testes? *AOMIS* 106:240, 1998.

33. Pont J and others: Chemotherapy should follow orchiectomy in high-risk patients, *J Clin Oncol* 14:441, 1996.

34. Leibovitch I and others: Delayed orchiectomy after chemotherapy for metastatic nonseminomatous germ cell tumors, *J Urol* 155:952, 1996.

35. Travis LB and others: Risk of second malignant neoplasms among long-term survivors of testicular cancer, *J Natl Cancer Inst* 89:1439, 1997.

36. Arai Y and others: Psychosocial aspects in long-term survivors of testicular cancer, *J Urol* 155:574, 1996.

37. Kim ED, Lipshultz LI: Advances in the treatment of organic erectile dysfunction, *Hosp Pract* 32:101, 1997.

38. Rosen RC and others: The international index of erectile function (IIEF): a multidimensional scale for assessment of erectile dysfunction, *Urology* 49:822, 1997.

39. Greiner KA, Weigel JW: Erectile dysfunction, *Am Fam Physician* 54:1675, 1996.

40. Montague DK and others: Clinical guidelines panel on erectile dysfunction: summary report on the treatment of organic erectile dysfunction. The American Urological Association, *J Urol* 156:2007, 1996.

41. Bechara A and others: Comparative study of papaverine plus phentolamine versus prostaglandin-E1 in erectile dysfunction, *J Urol* 157:2132, 1997.

42. Kim ED, el-Rashidy R, McVary KT: Papaverine topical gel for treatment of erectile dysfunction, *J Urol* 153:361, 1995.

*43. Kupecz D: Alprostadil for the treatment of erectile dysfunction, *Nurs Pract* 21:143, 1996.

44. Linet OI, Ogrine FG: Efficacy and safety of intracavernosal alprostadil in men with erectile dysfunction. The Alprostadil Study Group, *N Engl J Med* 334:873, 1996.

45. Kim ED, McVary KT: Topical prostaglandin-E1 for the treatment of erectile dysfunction, *J Urol* 153:182, 1995.

46. Padma-Nathan H and others: Treatment of men with erectile dysfunction with transurethral alprostadil, *N Engl J Med* 336:1, 1997.

47. Hellstrom WJ and others: A double-blind, placebo-controlled evaluation of the erectile response to transurethral alprostadil, *Urology* 48:851, 1996.

48. McMahon CG: A pilot study of the role of intracavernous injection of vasoactive intestinal peptide (VIP) and phentolamine mesylate in the treatment of erectile dysfunction, *Int J Impot Res* 8:233, 1996.

49. Truss MC and others: Intracavernous pharmacotherapy, *World J Urol* 15:71, 1997.

50. Sundaram CP and others: Long-term follow-up of patients receiving injection therapy for erectile dysfunction, *Urology* 49:932, 1997.

51. Riley AJ, Athanasiadis L: Impotence and its non-surgical management, *Br J Clin Pract* 51:99, 1997.

52. Boolel M and others: Sildenafil, a novel effective oral therapy for male erectile dysfunction, *Br J Urol* 78:257, 1996.

53. Soderdahl DW, Thrasher JB, Hansberry KL: Intracavernosal drug-induced erection therapy versus external vacuum devices in the treatment of erectile dysfunction, *Br J Urol* 79:952, 1997.

54. Shafik A: Hollow and fenestrated penile prosthesis: a new implant for treatment of impotence, *Arch Androl* 38:93, 1997.

55. Goldstein I and others: Safety and efficacy of mentor alpha-1 inflatable penile prosthesis implantation for impotence treatment, *J Urol* 157:833, 1997.

56. Meredith CE: Erectile dysfunction. In Karlowicz KA, editor: *Urologic nursing: principles and practice*, Philadelphia, 1995, Saunders.

57. Bigelow PL and others: Association of semen quality and occupational factors: comparison of case-control analysis and analysis of continuous variables, *Fertil Steril* 69:11, 1998.

58. Gregoriou O and others: Treatment of idiopathic oligozoospermia with an alpha-blocker: a placebo controlled, double-blind trial, *Int J Fertil Womens Med* 42:301, 1997.

Resources

National Prostate Cancer Coalition
1156 15th Street NW, Suite 905
Washington, DC 20005
202-463-9455
Fax: 202-463-9456
http://www.4npcc.org/

Prostate Cancer Home Page
c/o UMHS
1500 E. Medical Center Dr.
Ann Arbor, MI 48109
734-936-4000
http://www.cancer.med.umich.edu/prostcan/prostcan.html

For additional Internet resources, see the website for this book at www.mosby.com/MERLIN/medsurg_lewis

*Nursing research-based article.

PROBLEMS RELATED TO MOVEMENT AND COORDINATION

SECTION OUTLINE

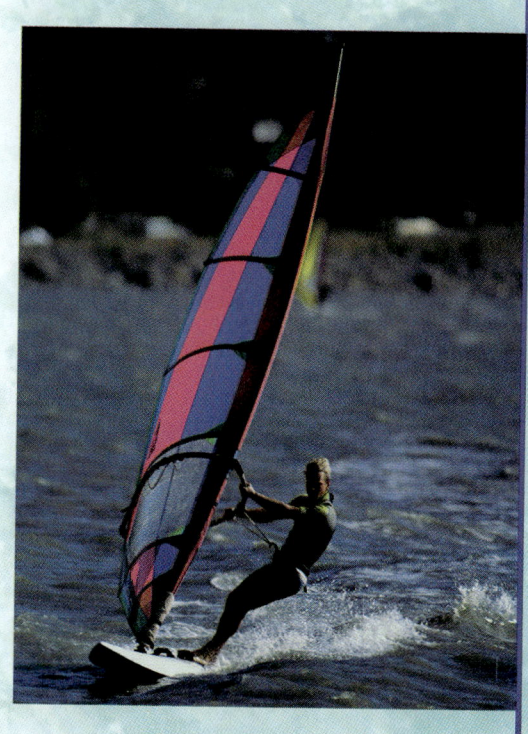

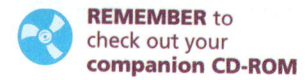
53

NURSING ASSESSMENT
Neurologic System

Judith M. Ozuna

www.mosby.com/MERLIN/medsurg_lewis

LEARNING OBJECTIVES

1. Describe the functions of neurons and neuroglia.
2. Explain the electrochemical aspects of nerve impulse transmission.
3. Explain the anatomic location and functions of the cerebrum, brainstem, cerebellum, spinal cord, peripheral nerves, and cerebrospinal fluid.
4. Identify the major arteries supplying the brain.
5. Describe the functions of the 12 cranial nerves.
6. Compare the functions of the two divisions of the autonomic nervous system.
7. Describe age-related changes in the neurologic system and differences in assessment findings.
8. Identify the significant subjective and objective data related to the nervous system that should be obtained from a patient.
9. Describe the techniques used in the physical assessment of the nervous system.
10. Differentiate normal from common abnormal findings of a physical assessment of the nervous system.
11. Describe the purpose, significance of results, and nursing responsibilities related to diagnostic studies of the nervous system.

STRUCTURES AND FUNCTIONS OF THE NERVOUS SYSTEM

The human nervous system is a highly specialized system responsible for the control and integration of the body's many activities. The nervous system can be divided into the central nervous system (CNS) and the peripheral nervous system (PNS). The CNS consists of the brain and spinal cord. The PNS consists of the cranial and spinal nerves and the peripheral components of the autonomic nervous system (ANS). Before considering higher-order structures and their functions, cellular elements and nerve impulse transmission are discussed.

Cells of the Nervous System

The nervous system is made up of two types of cells: neurons and neuroglia. Although neuroglial cells are more numerous, they are mainly supportive to the neuron, the primary functional unit of the nervous system. Neurons are generally non-mitotic; that is, they do not replicate and cannot replace themselves if they are irreversibly damaged. Neuroglia, however, are mitotic and can replicate themselves.

Neurons. The neurons of the nervous system come in many different shapes and sizes, but they all share common characteristics: (1) excitability, or the ability to generate a nerve impulse; (2) conductivity, or the ability to transmit the impulse to other portions of the cell; and (3) the ability to in-

fluence other neurons, muscle cells, and glandular cells by transmitting nerve impulses to them.

A typical neuron consists of a cell body, an axon, and several dendrites (Fig. 53-1). The cell body containing the nucleus and cytoplasm is the metabolic center of the neuron. Dendrites are short processes extending from the cell body. They receive nerve impulses from the axons of other neurons and conduct impulses toward the cell body. The nerve axon projects varying distances from the cell body, ranging from several micrometers to more than a meter. Its function is to carry nerve impulses to other neurons or to end organs. The end organs are smooth and striated muscles and glands. Axons may be myelinated or unmyelinated. Many axons present in the CNS and the PNS are covered by a segmentally interrupted myelin sheath composed of a white, lipid substance that acts as an insulator for the conduction of impulses. Generally, the smaller fibers are unmyelinated.

Neuroglia. Neuroglia, or glial cells, provide support, nourishment, and protection to neurons. They constitute almost half the brain and spinal cord mass and are 5 to 10 times more numerous than neurons. Different types of glial cells, including oligodendroglia, astrocytes, ependymal cells, and microglia, have specific functions. Oligodendroglia produce the myelin sheath of nerve fibers in the CNS (Schwann cells myelinate the nerve fibers in the periphery) and are primarily found in the white matter of the CNS. Astrocytes are found primarily in gray matter; however, their physiologic importance is not well understood. They are thought to provide structural support to neurons and their delicate processes, form the blood-brain barrier with the endothelium of the blood vessels, and play an indirect role in synaptic transmission (conduction of impulses between neurons). When the

Reviewed by Mary Baird, RN, MN, ARNP, Nurse Practitioner, Neuromuscular Associates, Olympia, Wash; Lecturer, School of Nursing, University of Washington, Seattle, Wash.

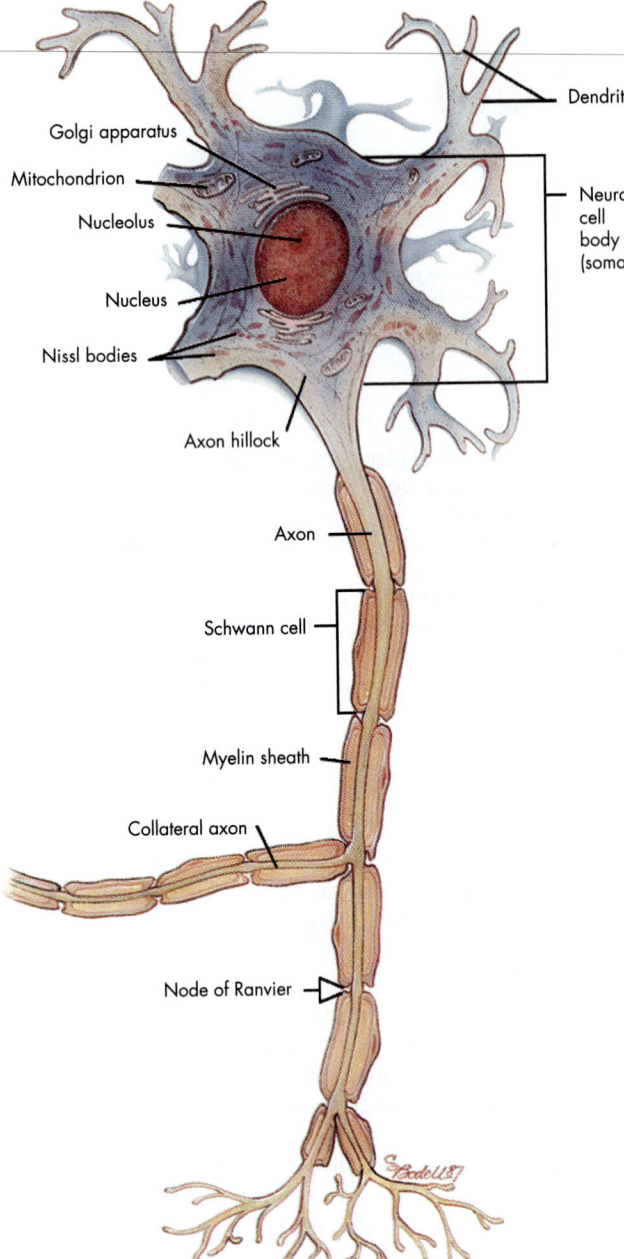

Fig. 53-1 Structural features of neurons: dendrites, cell body, and axons.

brain is injured, astrocytes act as phagocytes for neuronal debris. They help restore the neurochemical milieu and provide support for repair. Proliferation of astrocytes contributes to the formation of scar tissue (gliosis) in the CNS. Ependymal cells line the brain ventricles and aid in the secretion of cerebrospinal fluid. Microglia, a type of macrophage, are relatively rare in normal CNS tissue. They migrate to areas of CNS damage, act as phagocytes, and are important in host defense.

Most primary CNS tumors involve neuroglia. Primary malignancies involving neurons are rare because these cells are usually not mitotic.

Nerve Regeneration

Once a neuron dies, it is generally not replaced. If only the axon of the nerve cell is damaged, the cell attempts to repair itself. When damaged, all nerve cells attempt to grow back to their original destinations by sprouting many branches from the damaged ends of their axons. Unfortunately, axons in the CNS are less successful than peripheral axons in regenerating. This difference may be because of dense scar tissue that develops in the CNS and forms a barrier. Regenerating nerve fibers grow 4 mm per day.

In the PNS (outside the brain and the spinal cord), injured nerve fibers can successfully regenerate by growing within the protective myelin sheath of the supporting Schwann cells if the cell body is intact. The final result of nerve regeneration depends on the number of axon sprouts that join with the appropriate Schwann cell columns and reinnervate appropriate end organs.

Nerve Impulse

The purpose of a neuron is to initiate, receive, and process messages about events both within and outside the body. The initiation of a neuronal message (nerve impulse) involves the generation of an action potential. Once an action potential is initiated, a series of action potentials travels along the axon. When the impulse reaches the end of the nerve fiber, it is transmitted across the junction between nerve cells (synapse) by a chemical interaction involving neurotransmitters. This chemical interaction generates another set of action potentials in the next neuron. These events are repeated until the nerve impulse reaches its destination.

Action Potential. When nerve cells are in a resting (nonactive) state, the inside of the cell carries a negative electric charge relative to the outside of the cell. Sodium ions (Na^+) are in high concentration outside the cell, and potassium ions (K^+) are in high concentration inside the cell. The difference in electric charge across the cell membrane is termed the *resting membrane potential* (Fig. 53-2). An action potential occurs when a stimulus is of sufficient magnitude to alter the membrane potential.

During the action potential, the cell membrane becomes more permeable to Na^+, allowing the Na^+ to move readily into the cell. The resulting change in the voltage across the cell membrane is called *depolarization*. The inside of the cell temporarily becomes positive relative to the outside. After rapid depolarization, *repolarization* (the inside of the cell becoming negative relative to the outside) is facilitated by a slower increase in K^+ permeability, which in turn is caused by the depolarization associated with entry of Na^+ into the cell. The whole process of depolarization and repolarization of the nerve cell membrane takes only 1 to 2 milliseconds. With repeated action potentials the cells accumulate Na^+. An active metabolic process within the cell is required to move Na^+ out of and K^+ back into the cell. This metabolic process is accomplished by the Na^+-K^+ pump, which requires energy from the breakdown of adenosine triphosphate (ATP).

The action potential has an all-or-none quality; that is, once the cell depolarizes enough to cause an action potential, the size of the action potential is independent of the strength of the stimulus. When an action potential is initiated at one point

Resting membrane potential

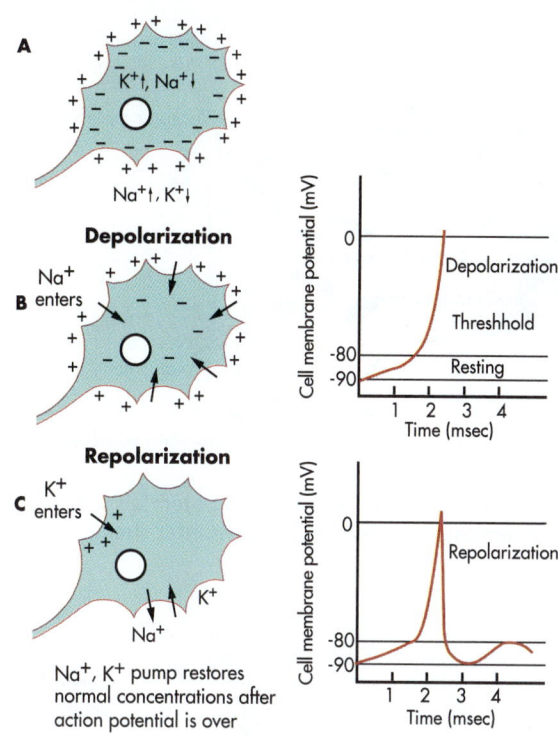

Fig. 53-2   **A,** Resting membrane potential. **B,** Depolarization. **C,** Repolarization.

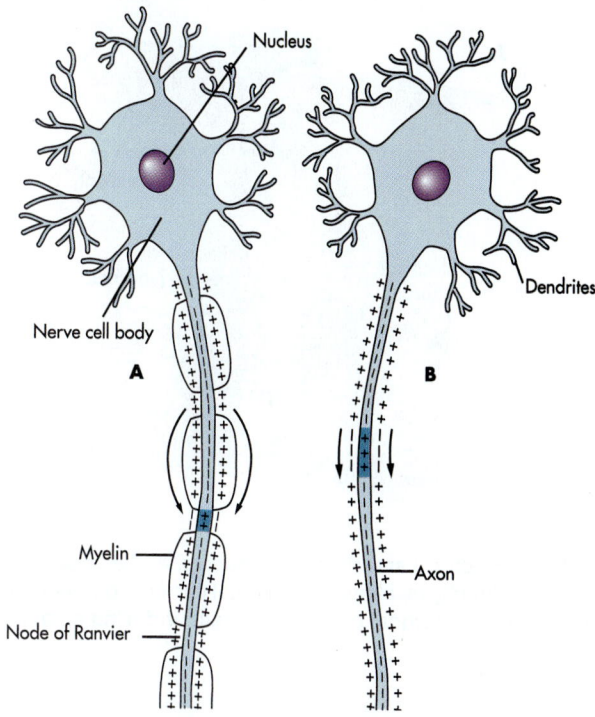

Fig. 53-3   **A,** Saltatory conduction in a myelinated nerve. **B,** Depolarization in an unmyelinated fiber.

of a neuron, it is transmitted along the axon without losing its intensity.

Because of its insulating capacity, myelination of nerve axons facilitates the conduction of an action potential. Many peripheral nerve axons have gaps, termed *nodes of Ranvier,* at regular intervals in the myelin sheath surrounding them. An action potential traveling down one of these axons hops from node to node without traversing the insulated membrane segment between nodes, making the action potential travel much faster than it would otherwise. This is called *saltatory (hopping) conduction.* In an unmyelinated fiber the wave of depolarization traverses the entire length of the axon, each portion of the membrane becoming depolarized in turn. Figure 53-3 compares nerve impulse transmission of myelinated and unmyelinated fibers.

Synapse. A synapse is the structural and functional junction between two neurons. It is the point at which the nerve impulse is transmitted from one neuron to another or from neuron to end or effector organ. The essential structures of synaptic transmission are a presynaptic terminal, a synaptic cleft, and a receptor site on the postsynaptic cell (Fig. 53-4). When a nerve impulse reaches the end of the axon (presynaptic terminal), it causes release of a chemical substance (neurotransmitter) from tiny vesicles within the axon terminal. This release depends on influx of calcium (Ca^+), initiated by depolarization of the nerve terminal. The neurotransmitter then crosses the microscopic space (synaptic cleft) between the two neurons and attaches to receptor sites of the receiving (postsynaptic) neuron. This causes a change in the permeability of the postsynaptic cell membrane to specific ions such as Na^+ and K^+ and a change in the electric potential of the membrane.

Neurotransmitters. Neurotransmitters are chemical agents involved in the transmission of an impulse across the synaptic cleft. Some neurotransmitters are excitatory: they cause an increase in Na^+ permeability at the postsynaptic cell membrane, increasing the likelihood that an action potential will be generated. This type of synaptic input results in an excitatory postsynaptic potential. Other neurotransmitters are inhibitory: they cause an increase in permeability of K^+ and chloride (Cl^-) ions, decreasing the likelihood that an action potential will be generated. This type of synaptic input results in an inhibitory postsynaptic potential.

Each of the hundreds to thousands of synaptic connections of a single neuron has an influence on that neuron. The net effect of the input is sometimes excitatory and sometimes inhibitory. In general, the net effect is dependent on the number of presynaptic neurons that are releasing neurotransmitters on the postsynaptic cell. A presynaptic cell that releases an excitatory neurotransmitter does not always cause the postsynaptic cell to depolarize enough to generate an action potential. However, when many presynaptic cells release excitatory neurotransmitters on a single neuron, the sum of their input is enough to generate an action potential. The presynaptic input can be summed by the number of presynaptic cells firing (spatial summation) or by the frequency of firing of a single presynaptic cell (temporal summation). Summation usually occurs by both events.

The effect of an excitatory or inhibitory neurotransmitter depends on which ion channels in the postsynaptic membrane are influenced by that neurotransmitter. In mammals, the neurotransmitters that are known to generally have an excitatory influence are acetylcholine, norepinephrine, serotonin, dopamine, glutamate, and histamine. The neurotransmitters that generally have an inhibitory influence are gamma-aminobutyric acid (GABA) and glycine.

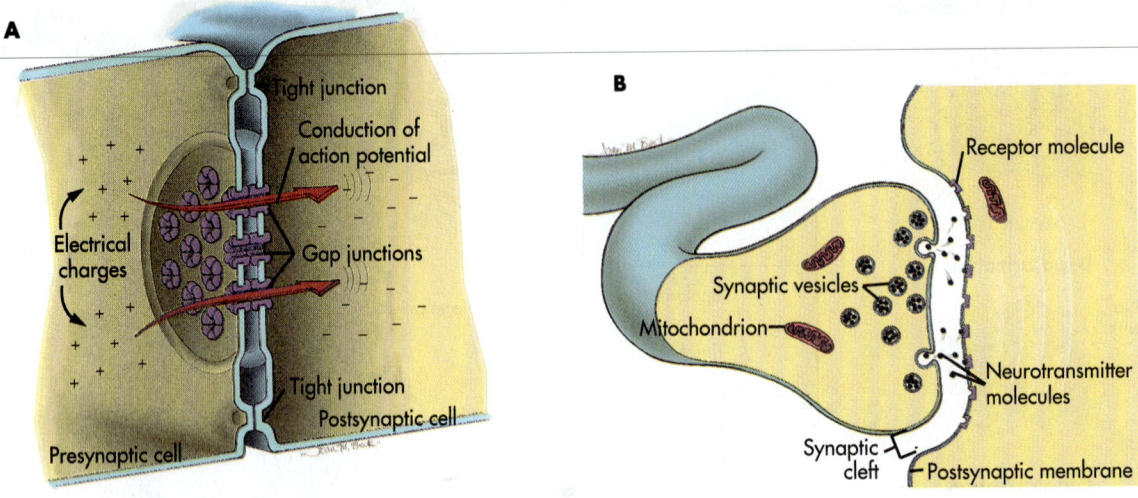

Fig. 53-4   Electrical and chemical synapses. **A,** Electrical synapses involve gap junctions that allow action potentials to move from cell to cell directly by allowing electrical current to flow between cells. **B,** Chemical synapses involve transmitter chemicals (neurotransmitters) that signal postsynaptic cells, inducing an action potential.

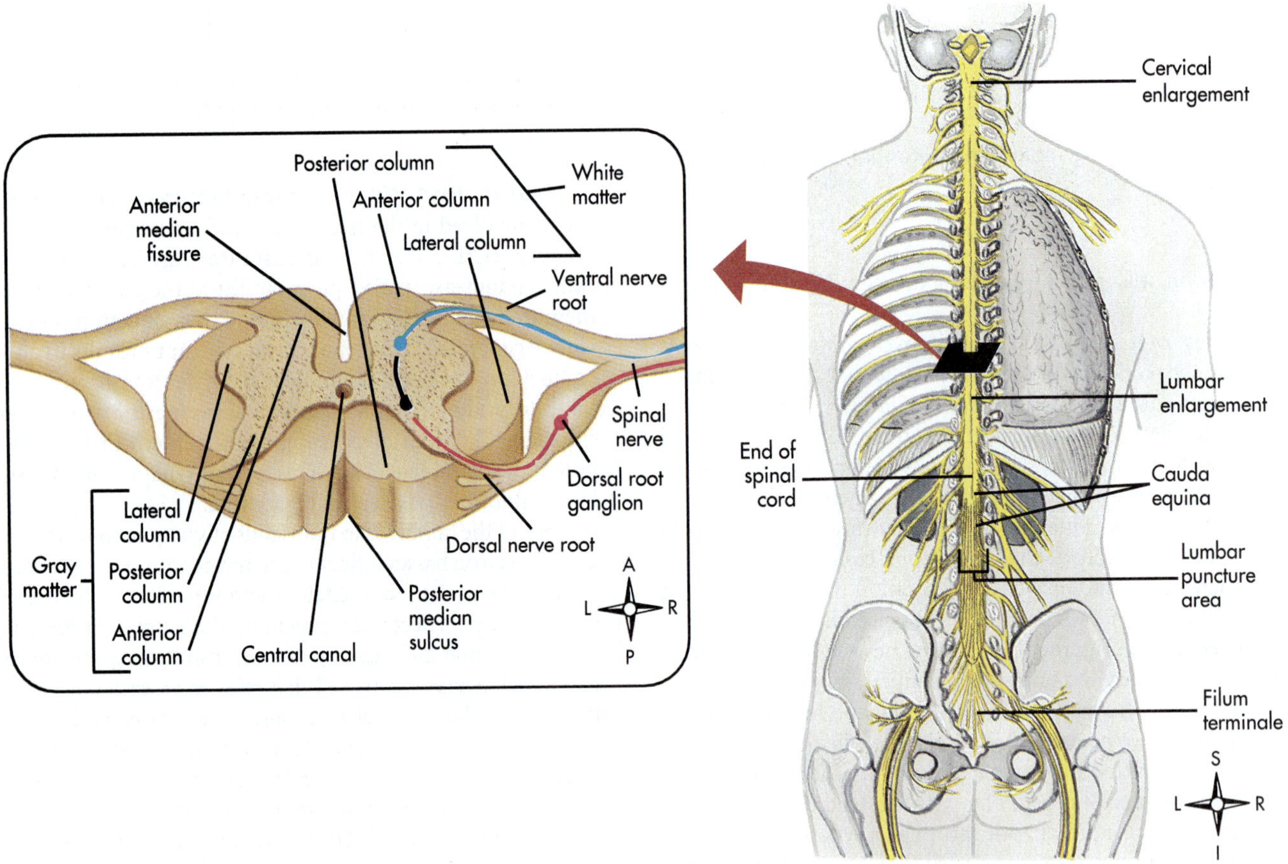

Fig. 53-5   Spinal cord. The inset illustrates a transverse section of the spinal cord shown in the broader view.

Neurotransmitters continue to combine with the receptor sites at the postsynaptic membrane until they are inactivated by enzymes, are taken up by the presynaptic endings, or diffuse away from the synaptic region. In addition, neurotransmitters can be affected by drugs and toxins, which can modify their function or block their attachment to receptor sites on the postsynaptic membrane. Enkephalins and endorphins are also considered neurotransmitters. These substances have opiate-like properties. They are found in multiple areas of the CNS and PNS and act to inhibit pain perception (see Chapter 9).

Central Nervous System

Major structural components of the CNS are the spinal cord and brain. The brain consists of the cerebral hemispheres, the cerebellum, and the brainstem.

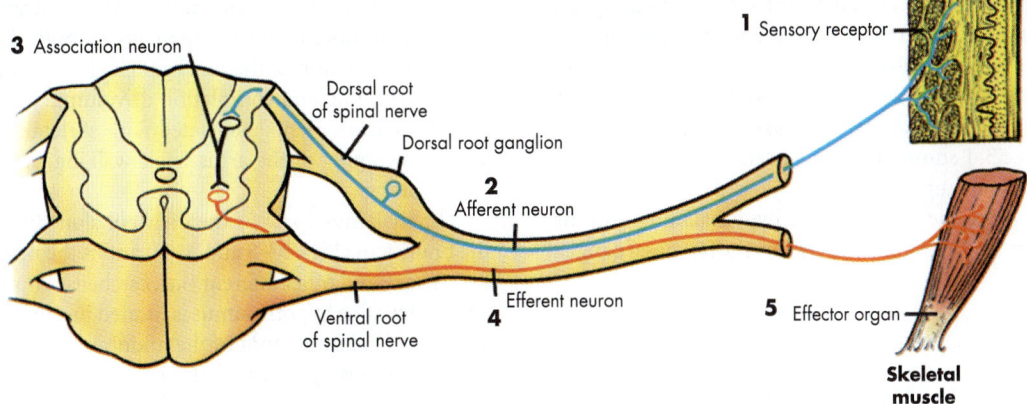

Fig. 53-6   Basic diagram of a reflex arc, including the (1) sensory receptor, (2) afferent neuron, (3) association neuron, (4) efferent neuron, and (5) effector organ.

Spinal Cord. The spinal cord is continuous with the brainstem and exits from the cranial cavity through the foramen magnum. A cross section of the spinal cord reveals gray matter that is centrally located in an H shape and is surrounded by white matter (Fig. 53-5). The gray matter contains the cell bodies of voluntary motor neurons and preganglionic autonomic motor neurons, as well as cell bodies of association neurons (interneurons). The white matter contains the axons of the ascending sensory and the descending (suprasegmental) motor fibers. The myelin surrounding these fibers gives them their white appearance. Specific ascending and descending pathways in the white matter can be identified. The spinal pathways or tracts are named for the point of origin and the point of destination (e.g., spinocerebellar tract [ascending], corticospinal tract [descending]). The major spinal pathways are presented in Fig. 53-5.

Ascending tracts. In general, the ascending tracts carry specific sensory information to higher levels of the CNS. This information comes from special sensory endings (receptors) in the skin, muscles and joints, viscera, and blood vessels, and enters the spinal cord by way of the dorsal roots of the spinal nerves. The fasciculus gracilis and the fasciculus cuneatus (commonly called the dorsal or posterior columns) carry information and transmit impulses concerned with touch, deep pressure, vibration, position sense, and kinesthesia (appreciation of movement, weight, and body parts). The spinocerebellar tracts carry subconscious information about muscle tension and body position to the cerebellum for coordination of movement. This information is not consciously perceived. The spinothalamic tracts carry pain and temperature sensations. Therefore the ascending tracts are organized by sensory modality, as well as by anatomy.

Although the functions of these pathways are generally accepted, other ascending tracts may also carry sensory modalities. The symptoms of various neurologic diseases suggest that additional pathways for touch, position sense, and vibration exist.

Descending tracts. Descending tracts carry impulses that are responsible for muscle movement. Among the most important descending tracts are the corticobulbar and corticospinal tracts, collectively termed the *pyramidal tract.* These tracts carry volitional (voluntary) impulses from the cortex to the cranial and peripheral nerves, respectively. Another group of descending motor tracts carries impulses from the extrapyra-midal system, which includes all motor systems (except the pyramidal system) concerned with voluntary movement. It includes descending pathways originating in the brainstem, the basal ganglia, and the cerebellum. The motor output exits the spinal cord by way of the ventral roots of the spinal nerves.

Lower and upper motor neurons. Lower motor neurons (LMNs) are the final common pathway through which descending motor tracts influence skeletal muscle, the effector organ for movement. The cell bodies of LMNs, which send axons to innervate the skeletal muscles of the arms, trunk, and legs, are located in the anterior horn of the corresponding segments of the spinal cord (e.g., cervical segments contain LMNs for the arms). LMNs for skeletal muscles of the eyes, face, mouth, and throat are located in the corresponding segments of the brainstem. These cell bodies and their axons make up the somatic motor components of the cranial nerves. LMN lesions generally cause weakness or paralysis, denervation atrophy, hyporeflexia or areflexia, and decreased muscle tone (flaccidity).

Upper motor neurons (UMNs) originate in the cerebral cortex and project downward. The corticobulbar tract ends in the brainstem, and the corticospinal tract descends into the spinal cord. These neurons influence skeletal muscle movement. UMN lesions generally cause weakness or paralysis, disuse atrophy, hyperreflexia, and increased muscle tone (spasticity).

Reflex arc. A *reflex* is defined as an involuntary response to a stimulus. The components of a monosynaptic reflex arc (the simplest kind of reflex arc) are a receptor organ, an afferent neuron, an effector neuron, and an effector organ (e.g., skeletal muscle). The afferent neuron synapses with the efferent neuron in the gray matter of the spinal cord. A reflex arc is shown in Fig. 53-6. More complex reflex arcs have other neurons (interneurons) in addition to the afferent neuron influencing the effector neuron. In the spinal cord, reflex arcs play an important role in maintaining muscle tone, which is essential for body posture.

Brain. The brain can be divided into three major components: the cerebrum, the brainstem, and the cerebellum.

Cerebrum. The cerebrum is composed of the right and left hemispheres. Both hemispheres can be further divided into four major lobes: frontal, temporal, parietal, and occipital (Fig. 53-7). These divisions are useful to delineate portions of the neocortex (gray matter), which makes up the outer layer of the cerebral hemispheres. Neurons in specific parts of the neocortex are essential for various highly complex and sophisticated aspects of mental functioning, such as language, memory, and appreciation of visual-spatial relationships.

The functions of the cerebrum are multiple and complex. Specific areas of the cerebral cortex are associated with specific functions. Table 53-1 summarizes the location and function of the parts of the cerebrum.

The basal ganglia, the thalamus, the hypothalamus, and the limbic system are also located in the cerebrum. The basal ganglia

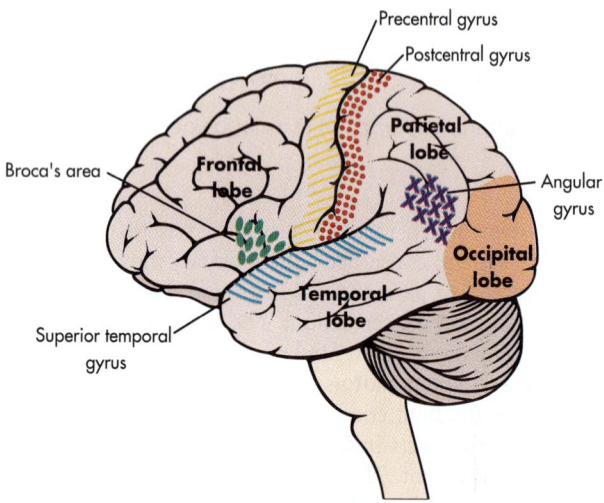

Fig. 53-7 Left hemisphere of cerebrum, lateral surface, showing major lobes and areas of the brain.

are a group of paired structures located centrally in the cerebrum and midbrain; most of them are on both sides of the thalamus. The function of the basal ganglia is to modulate the initiation, execution, and completion of voluntary movements and automatic movements associated with skeletal muscle activity, such as swinging of the arms while walking, swallowing saliva, and blinking.

The thalamus (part of the diencephalon) lies directly above the brainstem (Figs. 53-8 and 53-9) and is the major relay center for sensory and other afferent (i.e., cerebellar) inputs to the cerebral cortex. The hypothalamus is located just inferior to the thalamus and slightly in front of the midbrain. It regulates the autonomic nervous system and the endocrine system. The limbic system is, phylogenetically, an old part of the human cerebrum. It is located near the inner surfaces of the cerebral hemispheres (Fig. 53-10) and is concerned with emotion, aggression, feeding behavior, and sexual response.

Brainstem. The brainstem includes the midbrain, pons, and medulla (see Figs. 53-8 and 53-9). Ascending and descending fibers pass through the brainstem going to and from the cerebrum and cerebellum. The cell bodies, or nuclei, of cranial nerves III through XII are in the brainstem. Also located in the brainstem is the reticular formation, a diffusely arranged group of neurons and their axons that extends from the medulla to the thalamus and hypothalamus. The functions of the reticular formation include relaying sensory information, influencing excitatory and inhibitory control of spinal motor neurons, and controlling vasomotor and respiratory activity. The reticular activating system is part of a reticular formation and is the regulatory system for arousal, a component of consciousness.

Table **53-1** Location and Function of the Parts of the Cerebrum		
Part	**Location**	**Function**
Cortical areas		
Motor		
Primary	Precentral gyrus	Controls initiation of movement on opposite side of body
Supplemental	Anterior to precentral gyrus	Facilitates proximal muscle activity, including activity for stance and gait, and spontaneous movement and coordination
Sensory		
Somatic	Postcentral gyrus	Registers body sensations (e.g., temperature, touch, pressure, pain) from opposite side of body
Visual	Occipital lobe	Registers visual images
Auditory	Superior temporal gyrus	Registers auditory inputs
Association areas	Parietal lobe	Integrates somatic and special sensory inputs
	Posterior temporal lobe	Integrates visual and auditory inputs for language comprehension
	Anterior temporal lobe	Integrates past experiences
	Anterior frontal lobe	Controls higher-order processes (e.g., judgment, insight, reasoning, problem solving, planning)
Language		
Comprehension	Angular gyrus	Integrates auditory language (understanding of spoken words)
Expression	Broca's area	Regulates verbal expression
Basal ganglia	Near lateral ventricles of both cerebral hemispheres	Controls and facilitates learned and automatic movements
Thalamus	Below basal ganglia	Relays sensory and motor inputs to cortex and other parts of cerebrum
Hypothalamus	Below thalamus	Regulates endocrine and autonomic functions (e.g., feeding, sleeping, emotional and sexual responses)
Limbic system	Lateral to hypothalamus	Influences affective (emotional) behavior and basic drives such as feeding and sexual behavior

The vital centers concerned with respiratory, vasomotor, and cardiac function are located in the medulla. The brainstem also contains the centers for sneezing, coughing, hiccupping, vomiting, sucking, and swallowing.

Cerebellum. The cerebellum is located in the posterior part of the cranial fossa, along with the brainstem, under the occipital lobe of the cerebrum. The function of the cerebellum is to coordinate voluntary movement and to maintain trunk stability and equilibrium. It influences motor activity through its ax-onal connections to the motor cortex, brainstem nuclei, and their descending pathways. To perform these functions, the cerebellum receives information from the cerebral cortex, muscles, joints, and inner ear.

Ventricles and cerebrospinal fluid. Several supporting structures located within the CNS are important in regulating neuronal function and physical support of the brain. The ventricles are four fluid-filled cavities within the brain that connect with one another and with the spinal canal. The lower portion of the fourth ventricle becomes the spinal canal in the lower part of the brainstem. The spinal canal is located in the center and extends the full length of the spinal cord. Figure 53-11 shows the ventricles and the flow of cerebrospinal fluid in the CNS.

The ventricles and spinal canal are filled with an average of 135 ml of cerebrospinal fluid (CSF). CSF circulates within the subarachnoid space that surrounds the brain, brainstem, and spinal cord. This fluid provides cushioning for the brain and spinal cord, allows fluid shifts from the cranial cavity to the spinal cavity, and carries nutrients. The formation of CSF in the choroid plexus in the ventricles involves both passive diffusion and active transport of substances. CSF resembles an ultrafiltrate of blood. Although CSF is continually being formed, many physiologic factors influence its rate of absorption and formation.

The CSF circulates throughout the ventricles and seeps into the subarachnoid space surrounding the brain and spinal cord. It is absorbed primarily through the arachnoid villi (tiny projections into the subarachnoid space) and into the intradural venous sinuses and eventually into the venous system. The analysis of CSF composition provides useful diagnostic information relating to certain nervous system diseases. CSF pressure is sometimes measured in patients with actual or suspected intracranial diseases. Increases in intracranial pressure, indicated by increased CSF pressure, can lead to herniation of the brain and compression of vital brainstem structures. The signs marking this event are part of the herniation syndrome (see Chapter 54).

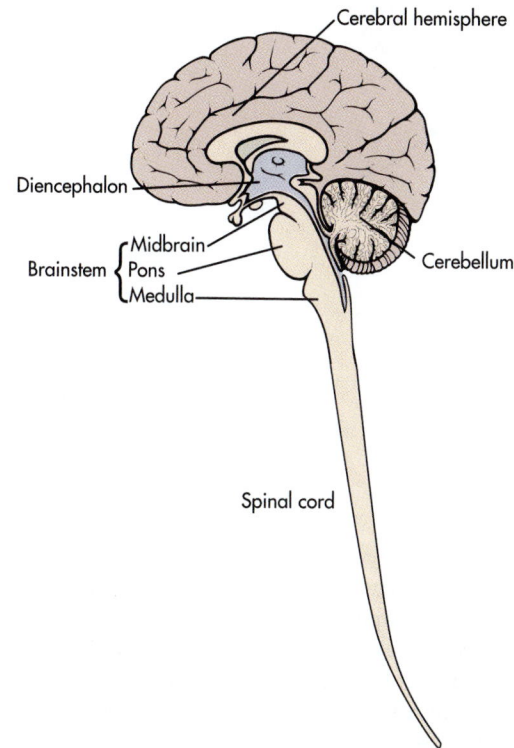

Fig. 53-8 Major divisions of the CNS.

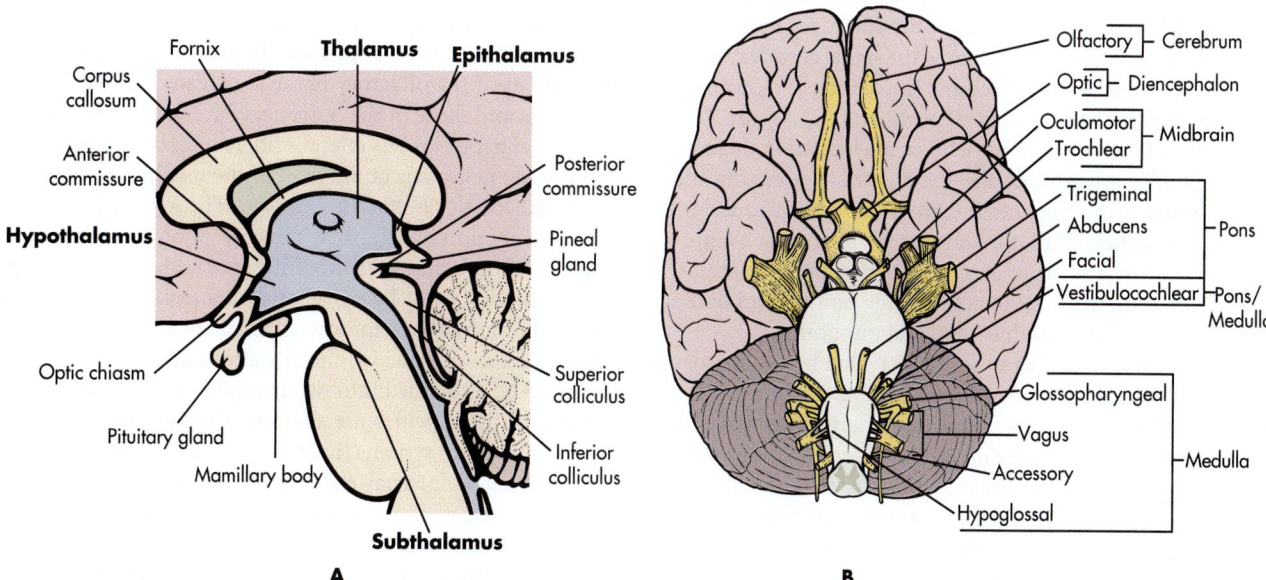

Fig. 53-9 **A,** The diencephalon (thalamus and hypothalamus) and **B,** cranial nerves.

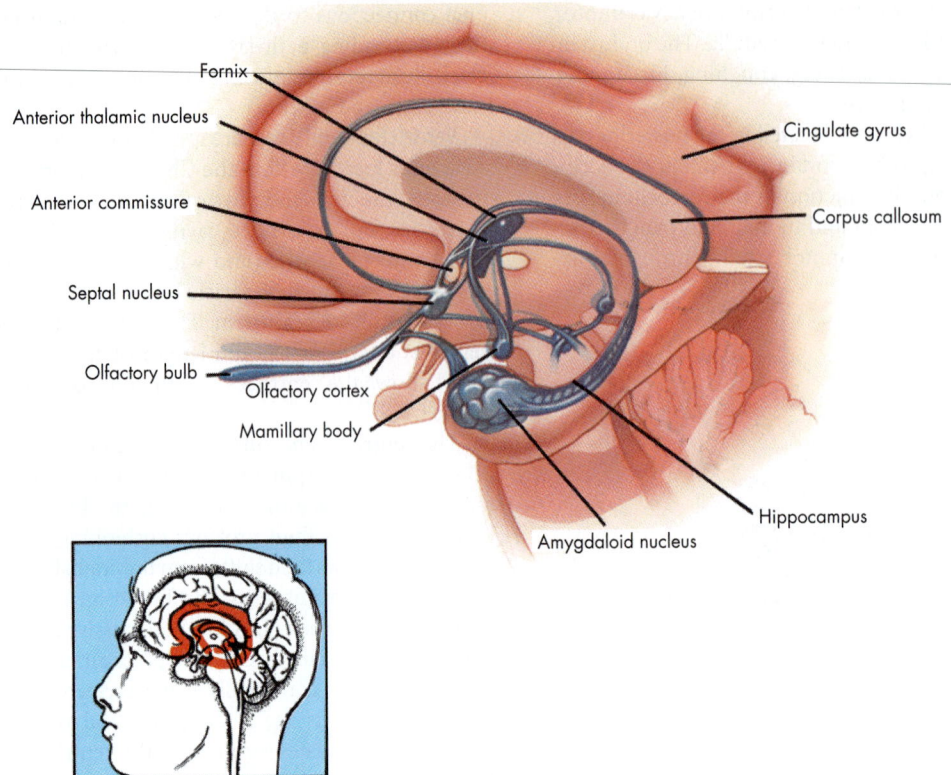

Fig. 53-10 Structures of the limbic system.

Peripheral Nervous System

The PNS includes all the neuronal structures that lie outside the CNS. It consists of the spinal and cranial nerves, their associated ganglia (groupings of cell bodies), and portions of the ANS.

Spinal Nerves. The spinal cord can be seen as a series of spinal segments, one on top of another. In addition to the cell bodies, each segment contains a pair of dorsal (afferent) sensory nerve fibers or roots and ventral (efferent) motor fibers or roots, which innervate a specific region of the neck, trunk, or limbs. This combined motor-sensory nerve is called a *spinal nerve* (Fig. 53-12). The cell bodies of the voluntary motor system are located in the anterior horn of the spinal cord gray matter. The cell bodies of the autonomic (involuntary) motor system are located in the anterolateral portion of spinal cord gray matter. The cell bodies of sensory fibers are located in the dorsal root ganglia just outside the spinal cord. On exiting the spinal column, each spinal nerve divides into ventral and dorsal rami, a collection of motor and sensory fibers that eventually goes to peripheral structures (e.g., skin, muscles, viscera). The sympathetic ganglia are attached to the ventral rami of the spinal nerves by gray and white rami communicans.

A dermatome is the area of skin innervated by the sensory fibers of a single dorsal root of a spinal nerve. A myotome is a muscle group innervated by the primary motor neurons of a single ventral root. These are simple components in the embryonic stage of human development. However, the dermatomes and myotomes of a given spinal segment overlap with those of adjacent segments in the adult because of the development of ascending and descending collateral branches of nerve fibers. The dermatomes give a general picture of somatic sensory innervation by spinal segments.

Cranial Nerves. The cranial nerves (CNs) are the 12 paired nerves composed of cell bodies with fibers that exit from the cranial cavity. Unlike the spinal nerves, which always have both afferent sensory and efferent motor fibers, some CNs have only afferent and some only efferent fibers; others have both. Table 53-2 summarizes the motor and sensory components of the CNs. Figure 53-9 shows the position of the CNs in relation to the brain and spinal cord. Just as the cell bodies of the spinal nerves are located in specific segments of the spinal cord, so are the cell bodies (nuclei) of the cranial nerves located in specific segments of the brain. Exceptions are the nuclei of the olfactory and optic nerves. The primary cell bodies of the olfactory nerve are located in the nasal epithelium, and those of the optic nerve are in the retina. CN XI is a spinal nerve, and its efferent fibers migrate upward before exiting the neuroaxis at the level of the medulla.

Autonomic Nervous System. The ANS governs involuntary functions of cardiac muscle, smooth (involuntary) muscle, and glands. Until recently it was thought that these functions could not be consciously controlled. However, research in biofeedback indicates that many of these "involuntary" functions can be voluntarily affected.[1]

The ANS is divided into two components, sympathetic and parasympathetic, which are anatomically and functionally different. These two systems function together to maintain a relatively balanced internal environment. The ANS is primarily considered an efferent system and consists of preganglionic nerves and postganglionic nerves.

The preganglionic cell bodies of the sympathetic nervous system (SNS) are located in spinal segments T1 through L2. The sympathetic ganglia, which contain the cell bodies of the

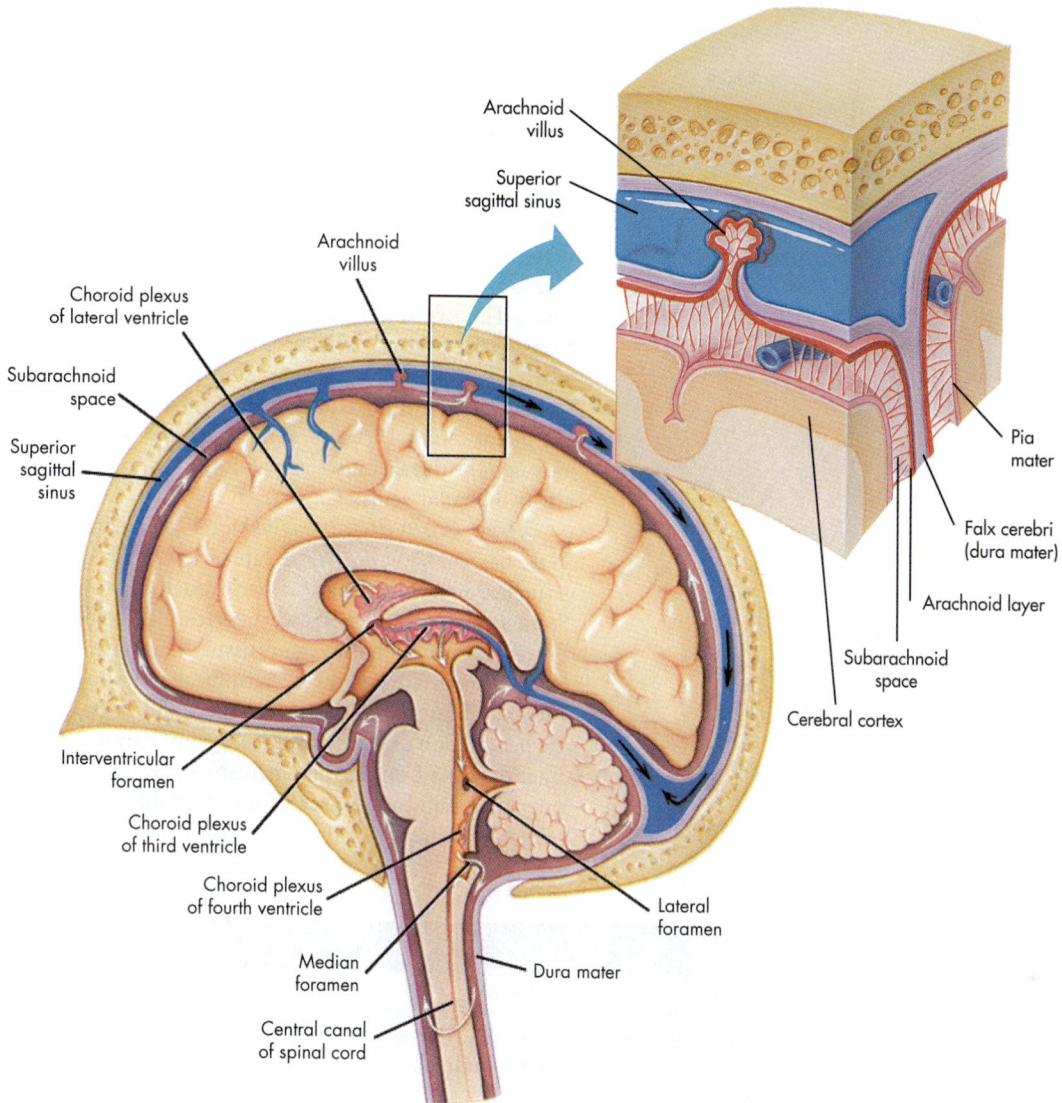

Fig. 53-11   Flow of cerebrospinal fluid. The fluid produced by filtration of blood by the choroid plexus of each ventricle flows inferiorly through the lateral ventricles, interventricular foramen, third ventricle, cerebral aqueduct, fourth ventricle, and subarachnoid space and to the blood.

postganglionic neurons, lie close to the spinal column, along the vertebral bodies in the rami communicans. These ganglia and the connecting nerves are called the *paravertebral chain.* The major neurotransmitter released by the postganglionic fibers of the SNS is norepinephrine, and the neurotransmitter released by the preganglionic fibers is acetylcholine.

In contrast, the preganglionic cell bodies of the parasympathetic nervous system (PSNS) are located in the brainstem and in the sacral spinal segments (S2 through S4). The parasympathetic ganglia are located in or near the structures that they innervate. Acetylcholine is the neurotransmitter released at both preganglionic and postganglionic nerve endings.

The ANS provides dual and often reciprocal innervation to many structures. For example, the SNS increases the rate and force of the heart contraction, and the PSNS decreases the rate and force. The SNS dilates bronchi and bronchioles of the lungs, and the PSNS constricts them. Some structures are in-

nervated by only one system (e.g., the hair follicles and the sweat glands, which are innervated only by the SNS). Table 53-3 compares the SNS and PSNS.

The result of SNS stimulation is activation of mechanisms required for the "fight or flight" response that occurs throughout the body. In contrast, the PSNS is geared to act in localized and discrete regions. It serves to conserve and restore the energy stores of the body.

Cerebral Circulation

The blood supply of the brain arises from the internal carotid arteries (anterior circulation) and the vertebral arteries (posterior circulation), which are shown in Fig. 53-13. Knowledge of the distribution of the major arteries of the brain and the area supplied is essential for understanding and evaluating the signs and symptoms of cerebrovascular disease and trauma.

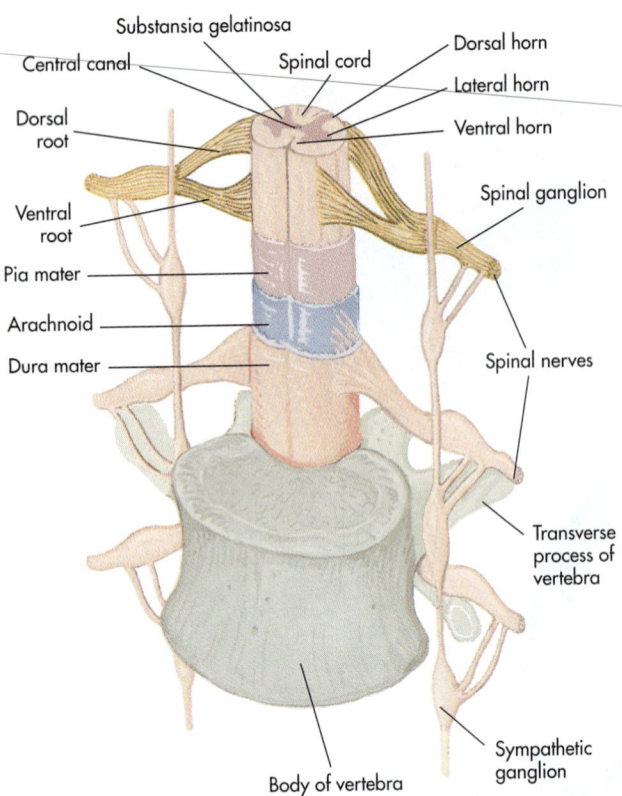

Substansia gelatinosa
Central canal
Spinal cord
Dorsal horn
Lateral horn
Ventral horn
Dorsal root
Ventral root
Pia mater
Arachnoid
Dura mater
Spinal ganglion
Spinal nerves
Transverse process of vertebra
Sympathetic ganglion
Body of vertebra

Fig. 53-12 Cross section of spinal cord showing attachments of spinal nerves and coverings of the spinal cord.

Each internal carotid artery supplies the ipsilateral hemisphere, whereas the basilar artery, formed by the junction of the two vertebral arteries, supplies structures within the posterior fossa (cerebellum and brainstem). The circle of Willis arises from the basilar artery and the two internal carotid arteries (Fig. 53-14). This vascular circle may act as a safety valve when differential pressures are present in these arteries. It also may function as an anastomotic pathway when occlusion of a major artery on one side of the brain occurs. In general, the two anterior cerebral arteries supply the medial portion of the frontal lobes. The two middle cerebral arteries supply the outer portions of the frontal, parietal, and superior temporal lobes. The two posterior cerebral arteries supply the medial portions of the occipital and inferior temporal lobes. Figure 53-13 shows the major cerebral arteries. Venous blood drains from the brain through the dural sinuses, which form channels that drain into the two jugular veins.

Blood-Brain Barrier. The blood-brain barrier is a physiologic barrier between blood capillaries and brain tissue. The structure of brain capillaries differs from that of other capillaries. Some substances that normally pass readily into most tissues are prevented from entering brain tissue. This barrier protects the brain from certain potentially harmful agents, while allowing nutrients and gases to enter. Because the blood-brain barrier affects the penetration of pharmaceutical agents, only certain drugs can enter the CNS from the bloodstream. Lipid-soluble compounds enter the brain easily, whereas water-soluble and ionized drugs enter the brain and spinal cord slowly. Damage to the blood-

Table **53-2**	**Cranial Nerves**	
Nerve	**Connection with Brain**	**Function**
I. Olfactory nerves and tract	Anterior ventral cerebrum	Sensory: from olfactory epithelium of superior nasal cavity
II. Optic nerve	Lateral geniculate body of the thalamus	Sensory: from retina of eyes
III. Oculomotor nerve	Midbrain	Motor: to four eye movement muscles and levator palpebrae Parasympathetic: smooth muscle in eyeball
IV. Trochlear nerve	Midbrain	Motor: to one eye movement muscle, the superior oblique
V. Trigeminal nerve		
Ophthalmic branch	Pons	Sensory: from forehead, eye, superior nasal cavity
Maxillary branch	Pons	Sensory: from inferior nasal cavity, face, upper teeth, mucosa of superior mouth
Mandibular branch	Pons	Sensory: from surfaces of jaw, lower teeth, mucosa of lower mouth, and anterior tongue Motor: to muscles of mastication
VI. Abducens nerve	Pons	Motor: to one eye movement muscle, the lateral rectus
VII. Facial nerve	Junction of pons and medulla	Motor: to facial muscles of expression and cheek muscle, the buccinator Sensory: taste from anterior two thirds of tongue
VIII. Vestibulocochlear nerve		
Vestibular branch	Junction of pons and medulla	Sensory: from equilibrium sensory organ, the vestibular apparatus
Cochlear branch	Junction of pons and medulla	Sensory: from auditory sensory organ, the cochlea
IX. Glossopharyngeal nerve	Medulla	Sensory: from pharynx and posterior tongue, including taste Motor: superior pharyngeal muscles
X. Vagus nerve	Medulla	Sensory: much of viscera of thorax and abdomen Motor: larynx and middle and inferior pharyngeal muscles Parasympathetic: heart, lungs, most of digestive system
XI. Accessory nerve	Medulla and superior spinal segments	Motor: to several neck muscles, sternocleidomastoid and trapezius
XII. Hypoglossal nerve	Medulla	Motor: to intrinsic and extrinsic muscles of tongue

Table 53-3 Effect of Sympathetic and Parasympathetic Nervous Systems

Visceral Effector	Effect of Sympathetic Nervous System*	Effect of Parasympathetic Nervous System†
Heart	Increase in rate and strength of heartbeat (β-receptors)	Decrease in rate and strength of heartbeat
Smooth muscle of blood vessels		
Skin blood vessels	Constriction (α-receptors)	No effect
Skeletal muscle blood vessels	Dilation (β-receptors)	No effect
Coronary blood vessels	Dilation (β-receptors), constriction (α-receptors)	Dilation
Abdominal blood vessels	Constriction (α-receptors)	No effect
Blood vessels of external genitals	Ejaculation (contraction of smooth muscle in male ducts [e.g., epididymis, ductus deferens])	Dilation of blood vessels causing erection in male
Smooth muscle of hollow organs and sphincters		
Bronchi	Dilation (β-receptors)	Constriction
Digestive tract, except sphincters	Decrease in peristalsis (β-receptors)	Increase in peristalsis
Sphincters of digestive tract	Contraction (α-receptors)	Relaxation
Urinary bladder	Relaxation (β-receptors)	Contraction
Urinary sphincters	Contraction (α-receptors)	Relaxation
Eye		
Iris	Contraction of radial muscle, dilation of pupil	Contraction of circular muscle, constriction of pupil
Ciliary	Relaxation, accommodation for far vision	Contraction, accommodation for near vision
Hairs (pilomotor muscles)	Contraction producing goose pimples or piloerection (α-receptors)	No effect
Glands		
Sweat	Increase in sweat (neurotransmitter, acetylcholine)	No effect
Digestive (e.g., salivary, gastric)	Decrease in secretion of saliva; not known for others	Increase in secretion of saliva and gastric HCl acid
Pancreas, including islets	Decrease in secretion	Increase in secretion of pancreatic juice and insulin
Liver	Increase in glycogenolysis (β-receptors), increase in blood glucose level	No effect
Adrenal medulla‡	Increase in epinephrine secretion	No effect

Modified from Thibodeau GA, Patton KT: *Anatomy and physiology*, ed 4, St Louis, 1999, Mosby.
*Neurotransmitter is norepinephrine unless otherwise stated.
†Neurotransmitter is acetylcholine unless otherwise stated.
‡Sympathetic preganglionic axons terminate in contact with secreting cells of the adrenal medulla. Thus the adrenal medulla functions as a "giant sympathetic postganglionic neuron."

brain barrier results in the penetration of drugs and other substances into brain tissue.

Protective Structures

Meninges. The meninges are three layers of protective membranes that surround the brain and spinal cord. The thick dura mater forms the outermost layer, with the arachnoid layer and pia mater being the next two layers. The falx cerebri is a fold of the dura that separates the two cerebral hemispheres and prevents expansion of brain tissue in situations such as the presence of a rapidly growing tumor or acute hemorrhage. The expanding brain must squeeze under this structure, causing displacement toward the side opposite the lesion. The tentorium cerebelli is a fold of dura that separates the cerebral hemispheres from the posterior fossa (which contains the brainstem and cerebellum). Expansion of mass lesions in the cerebrum forces the brain to herniate through the opening created by the brainstem. This is termed *tentorial herniation.*

The arachnoid layer is a delicate, impermeable membrane that lies between the thick dura mater and the pia mater and directly covers the brain and spinal cord. The subarachnoid space lies between the arachnoid layer and the pia mater. This space is filled with CSF. Structures passing to and from the brain and the skull or its foramina (holes through which blood vessels and nerves enter and exit the intracranial compartment) must pass through the subarachnoid space. Therefore all cerebral arteries and veins lie in this space, as do the cranial nerves. A larger subarachnoid space is present in the region of the third and fourth lumbar vertebrae, which is the area penetrated to obtain CSF during a lumbar puncture. (The spinal cord itself ends between the first and second lumbar vertebrae.)

Skull. The bony skull protects the brain from external trauma. It is composed of 8 cranial bones and 14 facial bones. The structure of the skull cavity explains the physiology of head injuries (see Chapter 54). Although the top and sides of the inside of the skull are relatively smooth, the bottom surface is uneven. It has many ridges, prominences, and foramina. The largest hole is the foramen magnum, through which the brainstem extends to the spinal cord. This foramen offers

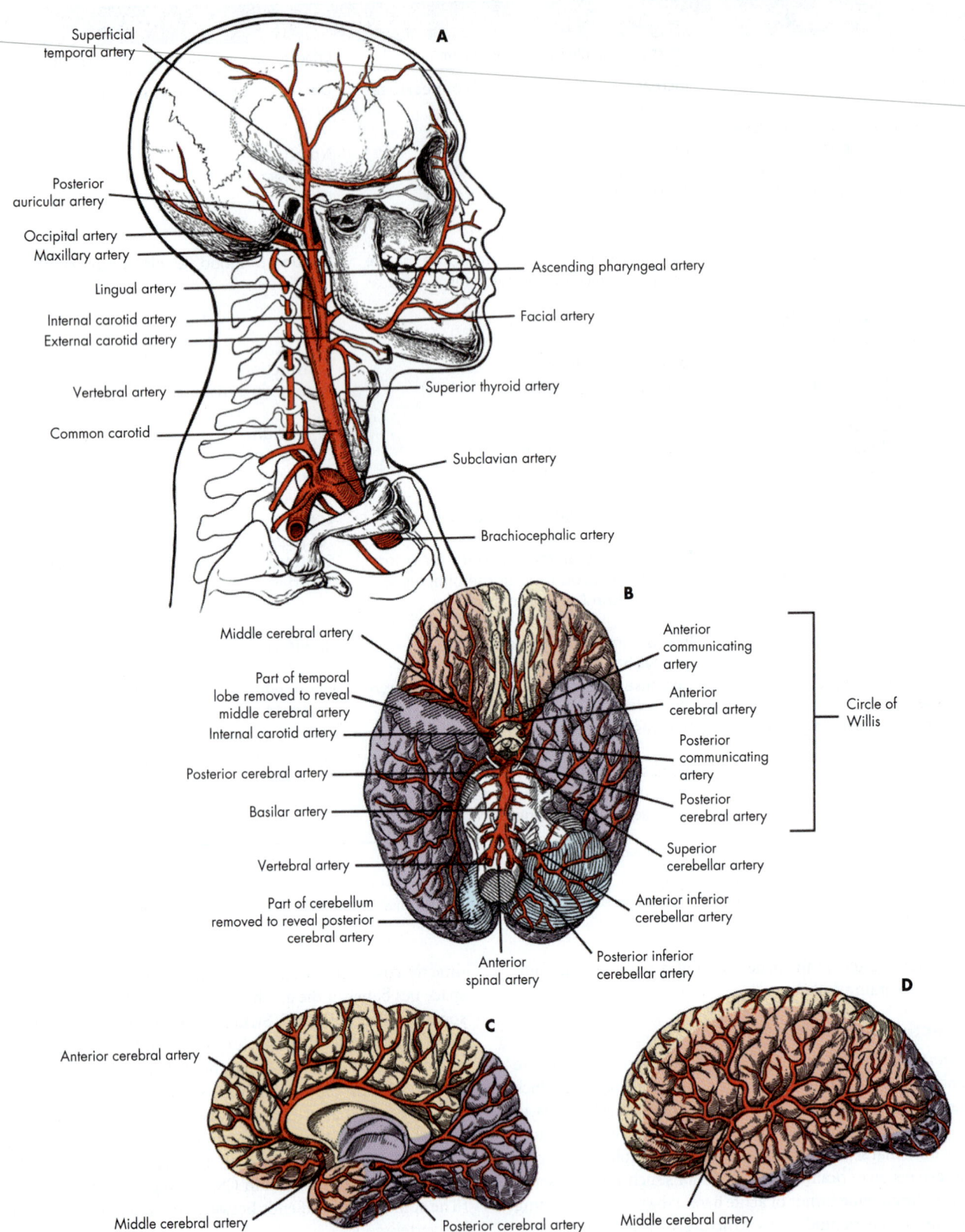

Fig. 53-13   Arteries of the head and neck. **A,** The brachiocephalic artery, the right common carotid artery, the right subclavian artery, and their branches. The major arteries to the head are the common carotid and vertebral arteries. **B,** Inferior view of the brain showing the vertebral, basilar, and internal carotid arteries and their branches. **C,** Medial view of the brain showing middle, anterior, and posterior cerebral arteries. **D,** Lateral view of the brain showing the distribution of the middle cerebral artery. **B to D,** Colors indicate brain regions supplied by various arteries—*yellow*, anterior cerebral; *orange*, middle cerebral; *purple*, posterior cerebral.

the only major space for the expansion of brain contents when increased intracranial pressure occurs.

Vertebral Column. The vertebral column protects the spinal cord, supports the head, and provides for flexibility. The vertebral column is made up of 33 individual vertebrae: 7 cervical, 12 thoracic, 5 lumbar, 5 sacral (fused into one), and 4 coccygeal (fused into one). Each vertebra has a central opening through which the spinal cord passes. The vertebrae are held together by a series of ligaments. Intervertebral disks oc-

cupy the spaces between vertebrae. Figure 53-15 shows the vertebral column in relation to the trunk.

GERONTOLOGIC CONSIDERATIONS

Effects of Aging on the Nervous System

Several parts of the nervous system are affected by aging. In the CNS loss of neurons occurs in certain areas of the brainstem, cerebellum, and cerebral cortex. This is a gradual process that begins in early adulthood. With loss of neurons there is widening or enlargement of the ventricles. Brain weight also decreases as a result of neuron loss. Cerebral blood flow and CSF production decline.[2]

In the PNS there are changes in the anterior horn cells and peripheral nerves, as well as the target organ, muscle. Degenerative changes in myelin cause a decrease in nerve conduction. Coordinated neuromuscular activity such as the maintenance of blood pressure in response to changing from a lying to a standing position is altered with aging. As a result older adults are more vulnerable to problems with orthostatic hypotension. Similarly, coordination of neuromuscular activity to maintain body temperature is also less efficient with aging. Older adults are less able to adapt to extremes in environmental temperature and are more vulnerable to both hypothermia and hyperthermia. Additional relevant changes associated with aging include decreases in memory, vision, hearing, taste, smell, vibration and position sense, muscle strength, and reaction time.

Changes in assessment findings result from age-related alterations in the various components of the nervous system. Age-related changes in the nervous system and differences in assessment findings are presented in Table 53-4.

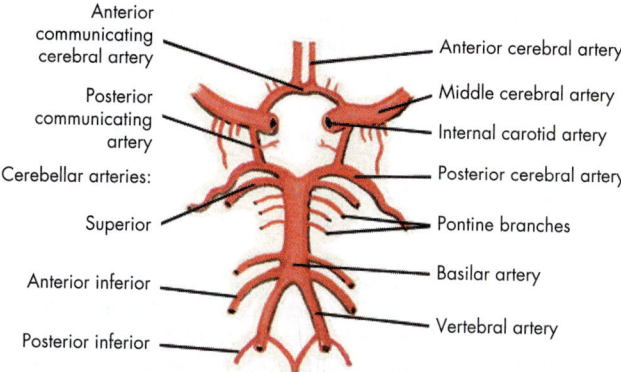

Fig. 53-14   Arteries at the base of the brain. The arteries that compose the circle of Willis are the two anterior cerebral arteries joined to each other by the anterior communicating cerebral artery and to the posterior cerebral arteries by the posterior communicating arteries.

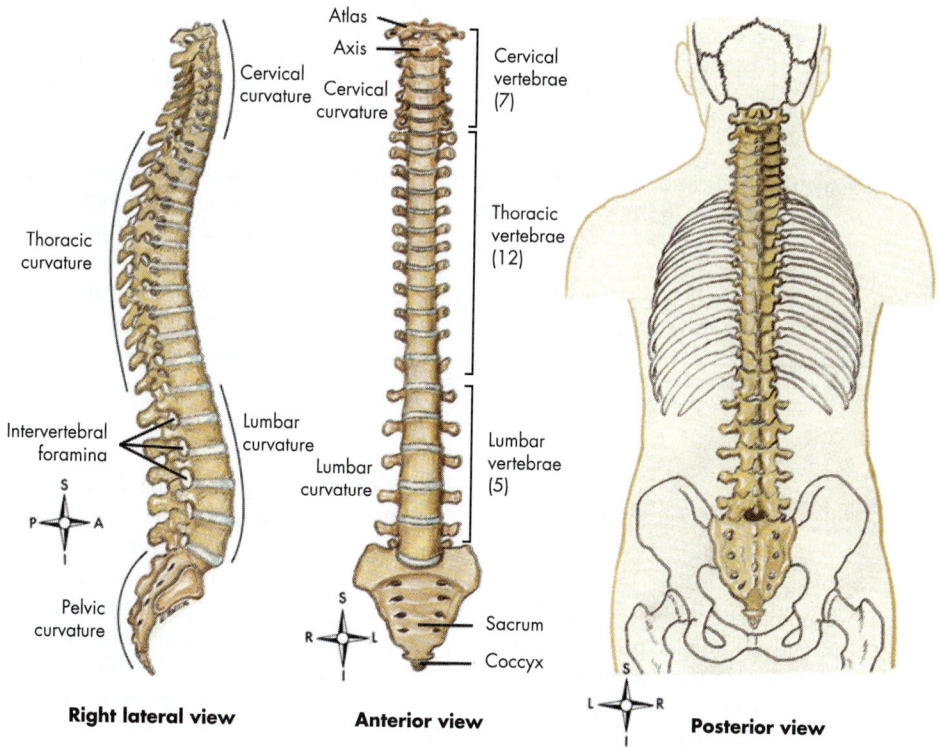

Fig. 53-15   The vertebral column (three views).

GERONTOLOGIC DIFFERENCES IN ASSESSMENT

Table 53-4   Nervous System

Component	Changes	Differences in Assessment Findings
Central Nervous System Brain	Reduction in cerebral blood flow and metabolism	Alterations in selected mental functioning
	Decrease in efficiency of temperature-regulating mechanism	Decrease in body temperature, impairment of ability to adapt to environmental temperature
	Decrease in neurotransmitter content, disruption in integration as result of loss of neurons	Repetitive movements, tremors
	Decrease in oxygen supply, changes in basal ganglia caused by vascular changes	Changes in gait and ambulation (e.g., extrapyramidal, Parkinson-like gait); diminished kinesthetic sense
Peripheral Nervous System Cranial and spinal nerves	Loss of myelin and decrease in conduction time in some nerves	Decrease in reaction time in specific nerves
	Cellular degeneration, death of neurons	Decrease in speed and intensity of neuronal reflexes
Functional Divisions Motor	Decrease in muscle bulk	Diminished strength and agility
	Decrease in electrical activity	Decrease in reactions and movement time
Sensory*	Decrease in sensory receptors caused by degenerative changes and involution of fine corpuscles of nerve endings	Diminished sense of touch; inability to localize stimuli; decrease in appreciation of touch, temperature, and peripheral vibrations
	Decrease in electrical activity	Slowing of or alteration in sensory reception
	Atrophy of taste buds	Signs of malnutrition, weight loss
	Degeneration and loss of fibers in olfactory bulb	Diminished sense of smell
	Degenerative changes in nerve cells in vestibular system of inner ear, cerebellum, and proprioceptive pathways in nervous system	Poor ability to maintain balance, widened gait
Reflexes	Possible decrease in deep tendon reflexes	Below-average reflex score
	Decrease in sensory conduction velocity as result of myelin sheath degeneration	Sluggish reflexes, slowing of reaction time
Reticular Formation Reticular activating system	Modification of hypothalamic function, reduction in stage IV sleep	Increase in frequency of spontaneous awakening together with tiredness, interrupted sleep, insomnia
Autonomic Nervous System SNS and PSNS	Morphologic features of ganglia, slowing of ANS responses	Orthostatic hypotension, systolic hypertension

*Specific changes related to the eye are in Table 19-1 and specific changes related to the ear are in Table 19-7.
ANS, autonomic nervous system; *PSNS,* parasympathetic nervous system; *SNS,* sympathetic nervous system.

ASSESSMENT OF THE NERVOUS SYSTEM

Subjective Data

Important Health Information

Past health history. Three points should be considered in taking the history of a patient with neurologic problems. The first is to avoid suggesting symptoms to the patient. Caution must be used not to suggest certain symptoms to the patient or ask leading questions such as "Is your headache throbbing?" or "Are you weak on the right side?" It is better to ask open-ended questions such as "What is your headache like?" or "Is there any-thing about your right side that bothers you?" A second point is that the mode of onset and the course of the illness are especially important aspects of the history. Often the nature of a neurologic disease process can be described by these facts alone, and the nurse should elicit all pertinent data in the history of the present illness, especially data related to the characteristics and progression of the symptoms. The third point is that because many neurologic diseases affect a patient's mental functioning, mental status must be accurately assessed before assuming that the history is factual. If the patient is not considered a reliable historian, the health history should be obtained from a person who has firsthand knowledge of the patient's problems and complaints. In many instances a health history cannot be obtained, and the clinician must proceed with only objective data.

The health history helps guide the approach for the neurologic examination; that is, it can direct the clinician toward the parts of the nervous system that need to be closely assessed. If the patient's primary complaint is dizziness, the examination may be focused on visual, vestibular, and cerebellar functions rather than on somatic motor and sensory functions.

Many complaints, including behavioral changes, alteration in level of consciousness, developmental problems, paroxysmal disorders, infectious processes, pain, motor or sensory aberrations, and trauma, should alert the clinician to the need for a detailed neurologic examination. In addition to being a primary complaint, neurologic problems often result from other problems, such as alcoholism or metastatic lesions.

When eliciting data about the health history, the nurse should ask the patient specific questions about diabetes mellitus, pernicious anemia, cancer, infections, thyroid disease, substance abuse, and hypertension because these conditions can affect the nervous system. Any hospitalizations, injuries, or surgeries related to the nervous system should be noted.

Medications. Particular attention should be given to eliciting a careful medication history, especially the use of sedatives, narcotics, tranquilizers, and mood-elevating drugs. If the patient experiences dizziness as a side effect of a medication, it should be noted. If the drug cannot be changed, the patient will need to be instructed in strategies to cope with dizziness and prevent falls.

Commonly, patients with chronic neurologic conditions will take medications to either treat the disease or manage symptoms. For example, many patients with neurologic problems will be taking antiseizure medications such as phenytoin (Dilantin), carbamazepine (Tegretol), and phenobarbital. The nurse should inquire about the occurrence of common side effects such as diplopia, drowsiness, ataxia, and mental slowing.

If the patient experiences headaches, the medications taken most commonly for the problem should be investigated. Many headache medications have potentially dangerous side effects such as gastric bleeding and coagulation abnormalities. The occurrence of these side effects should be noted.

Surgery or other treatments. The nurse should inquire about any surgery involving any part of the nervous system such as the head, spine, or sensory organs. If a patient had surgery, the date, cause, procedure, recovery, and current status should be investigated.

The perinatal history may reveal exposure to toxic agents such as viruses, alcohol, tobacco, drugs, and radiation, which are known to adversely influence the development of the nervous system. The history may reveal a difficult labor and delivery, which can cause brain damage as a result of hypoxia, forceps delivery, or Rh incompatibility. If the patient is elderly, this line of questioning may be unnecessary.

Growth and developmental history can be important in ascertaining whether nervous system dysfunction was present at an early age. The nurse should specifically inquire about major developmental tasks such as walking and talking. Success at school or identified problems in an educational setting are other important developmental data to gather. Often this information is not available when the older patient is interviewed. If the patient cannot provide a detailed developmental history, the nurse should proceed with the history gathering and avoid distressing the patient by further probing.

Functional Health Patterns. Key questions to ask a patient with a neurologic problem are presented in Table 53-5.

Health perception–health management pattern. The nurse should ask about the patient's health practices related to the nervous system, such as avoidance of substance abuse and smoking, maintenance of adequate nutrition, safe participation in physical and recreational activities, use of seat belts and helmets, and control of hypertension. The nurse should ask about previous hospitalizations for neurologic problems. A careful family history may determine whether the neurologic problem has a hereditary or congenital background. Specifically, the patient should be questioned about a family history of such disorders as epilepsy, amyotrophic lateral sclerosis, multiple sclerosis, Huntington's disease, muscular dystrophy, mental retardation, dementia, stroke, and cancer.

If the patient has an existing neurologic problem, the nurse should ask about how it affects daily living and the ability to carry out self-care. After a careful review of information, the nurse should ask someone who knows the patient well whether any mental or physical changes have been noticed in the patient. The patient with a neurologic problem may not be aware of it or may be unable to provide enough specific data to aid in the diagnosis.

Nutritional-metabolic pattern. Neurologic problems can result in problems of inadequate nutrition. Problems related to chewing, swallowing, facial nerve paralysis, and muscle coordination could make it difficult for the patient to ingest adequate nutrients. Also, certain vitamins such as thiamine (B_1), niacin, and pyridoxine (B_6) are essential for the maintenance and health of the CNS. Deficiencies in one or more of these vitamins could result in such nonspecific complaints as depression, apathy, neuritis, weakness, mental confusion, and irritability.

Elimination pattern. Bowel and bladder problems are often associated with neurologic problems, such as stroke, head injury, spinal cord injury, multiple sclerosis, and dementia. It is important to determine if the bowel or bladder problem was present before or after the neurologic event in order to plan appropriate interventions. Incontinence of urine and feces and urinary retention are the most common elimination problems associated with a neurologic problem. Careful documentation of the details of the problem, such as number of episodes, accompanying sensations or lack of sensations, and measures to control the problem, is important.

Activity-exercise pattern. Many neurologic disorders can cause problems in the patient's mobility, strength, and coordination. These problems can result in changes in the patient's usual activity and exercise patterns. Falls can also result from such problems. Many aspects of daily living such as getting out of a bed or chair, ambulating, preparing meals, and performing personal hygiene can be affected and should be assessed. The ability to perform fine motor tasks may be affected, which increases the possibility of personal injury.

Sleep-rest pattern. Sleep can be disrupted by many neurologically related factors. Discomfort from pain and inability to move and change to a position of comfort because of muscle weakness and paralysis could interfere with sound sleep. Hallucinations resulting from dementia or medications can also

HEALTH HISTORY

Table 53-5　Nervous System

Health Perception–Health Management Pattern
- What are your usual daily activities?
- Do you use any recreational drugs?*
- What safety practices do you perform in a car? On a motorcycle? On a bicycle?
- Do you have hypertension? If so, is it controlled?
- Have you ever been hospitalized for a neurologic problem?*
- How does it affect your daily living?

Nutritional-Metabolic Pattern
- Give a 24 hr dietary recall.
- Do you have any problems getting adequate nutrition because of chewing or swallowing difficulties, facial nerve paralysis, or poor muscle coordination?*
- Are you able to feed yourself?

Elimination Pattern
- Do you have incontinence of bowel or bladder? If yes, explain in detail the onset and pattern of the problem.
- What measures have you used to control the incontinence?
- Do you ever experience problems with hesitancy, urgency, retention?*
- Do you postpone defecation?*
- Does a neurologic problem make it difficult to reach a toilet when needed?
- Do you take any medication to manage neurologic problems? If so, what?

Activity-Exercise Pattern
- Describe any problems you experience with usual activities and exercise as a result of a neurologic problem.
- Do you have weakness or lack of coordination due to a neurologic problem?*
- Does a neurologic problem keep you from performing your personal hygiene needs independently?*

Sleep-Rest Pattern
- Describe any problems you have with sleep.
- If you have trouble falling asleep, what do you do about it? (Ask specifically about use of sleep-inducing medications.)

Cognitive-Perceptual Pattern
- Have you noticed any changes in your memory?*
- Do you experience vertigo, heat or cold sensitivity, numbness, or tingling?*
- Describe any pain you have experienced during the past 6 mo.
- Do you have any difficulty with verbal or written communication?*

Self-Perception–Self-Concept Pattern
- What effect has your neurologic problem had on how you feel about yourself? Your abilities? Your body?
- Describe your general emotional pattern.

Role-Relationship Pattern
- Have you experienced changes in roles such as spouse, parent, breadwinner because of neurologic disease?*
- How do you feel about these changes?

Sexuality-Reproductive Pattern
- Are you satisfied with sexual functioning? Describe any problems you experience related to your sexuality and sexual functioning.
- Are problems related to sexual functioning causing tension in an important relationship?*
- Do you feel the need for professional counseling related to your sexual functioning?*
- Do you use alternative methods of achieving sexual satisfaction?

Coping–Stress Tolerance Pattern
- Describe your usual coping pattern.
- Do you think your present coping pattern is adequate to meet the stressors of your neurologic problem?*
- Is your support system adequate to meet your needs? If not, what needs are unmet?

Value-Belief Pattern
- Describe any culturally specific beliefs and attitudes that may influence the treatment of this neurologic problem.

*If yes, describe.

interrupt sleep. The nurse should carefully document the sleep problem and the patient's methods of dealing with the problem.

Cognitive-perceptual pattern. Because the nervous system controls cognition and sensory integration, many neurologic disorders affect these functions. The nurse should assess memory, language, calculation ability, problem-solving ability, insight, and judgment. Often a structured mental status questionnaire will be used to evaluate these functions and provide baseline data.

Information about sensory changes related to hearing, sight, and touch should be sought. In addition, the patient should be questioned about problems with vertigo and sensitivity to heat and cold.

Ability to both use and understand language is a cognitive function that the nurse should also assess. Appropriateness of responses is a useful indicator of cognitive and perceptual ability.

Pain is a common event associated with many health problems. It is often the reason a patient seeks health care. A careful assessment of the patient's pain should be carried out (see Chapter 9).

Neurologic problems and their treatment can be complex and confusing. The patient's understanding and ability to carry out necessary treatments should be determined. Cognitive changes associated with the problem can also interfere with understanding and compliance.

Self-perception–self-concept pattern. Neurologic disease can drastically alter control over one's life and create dependency on others for daily needs. Also, the patient's physical appearance and emotional control can be affected. The nurse should ask about the patient's evaluation of self-worth, perception of abilities, body image, and general emotional pattern.

Role-relationship pattern. The patient should be asked if changes in roles, such as spouse, parent, or breadwinner, resulting from a neurologic problem have occurred. Physical impairments such as weakness and paralysis can alter or limit participation in usual roles and activities. Cognitive changes, however, can permanently change a person's ability to maintain previous roles. These changes can dramatically affect both the patient and significant others. Spousal relationships often change to dependent relationships.

Sexuality-reproductive pattern. The ability to participate in sexual activity should be assessed because many nervous system disorders can affect sexual response. Cerebral lesions may inhibit the desire phase or the reflex responses of the excitement phase. Brainstem and spinal cord lesions may partially or completely interrupt the connections between the brain and effector systems necessary for intercourse.

Neuropathies and spinal cord lesions that affect sensation, especially in the erotic zones, may decrease desire. Autonomic neuropathies and lesions of the sacral cord and cauda equina may prevent reflex activities of the sexual response. The nurse should determine if the patient and the spouse or significant other are satisfied with their sexual activity. The use or need for alternative methods of achieving sexual satisfaction should be explored. Despite neurologic-related changes in sexual functioning, many persons can achieve satisfying expression of intimacy and affection.

Coping–stress tolerance pattern. The physical sequelae of a neurologic problem can seriously strain a patient's coping patterns. Often the problem is chronic and may require that the patient learn new coping skills. The nurse should assess the patient's usual coping pattern to determine if coping skills are adequate to meet the stress of a problem.

When the problem is a decrease in cognitive functioning, both the patient and the caregiver can be seriously stressed. The nurse should assess for the potential for suicide, abuse, and burnout of the involved parties. The presence of an adequate support system in this type of situation should be assessed.

Value-belief pattern. Many neurologic problems have serious, long-term, life-changing effects. These effects can strain the patient's belief system and should be assessed. The nurse should also determine if any religious or cultural beliefs could interfere with the planned treatment regimen.

Objective Data

Physical Examination. The standard neurologic examination was developed by physicians and clinicians to help determine the presence, location, and nature of disease of the nervous system. The examination assesses six categories of functions: mental status, function of cranial nerves, motor function, cerebellar function, sensory function, and reflex function. The choice of particular parts of the examination depends on the purpose for which it is done. If a comprehensive baseline assessment of neurologic functioning is desired, all components of the examination are done. However, if a specific problem is to be evaluated, only certain components may be assessed. For example, if a patient's primary complaint is lack of feeling in the feet, the examination may be focused only on movement and sensation of the lower limbs. Similarly, if a patient comes into the emergency department after a head injury and is unconscious, a limited examination is conducted because the patient is not able to respond to verbal instructions.

A different approach to the neurologic examination has been proposed for nursing purposes. The primary purposes of the nursing neurologic examination are to determine the effects of neurologic dysfunction on daily living in relation to the patient's and the family's ability to cope with the neurologic deficits. Although the method of gathering data may be the same, the interpretation of the data is different from the medical model. The standard medical model of the neurologic examination can also be used for nursing purposes. Nurses and physicians share the responsibility for assessing life-threatening neurologic dysfunction.

Mental status. Assessment of mental status (cerebral functioning) gives an indication of how the patient is functioning as a whole and how the patient is adapting to the environment. It involves determination of complex and high-level cerebral functions that are governed by many areas of the cerebral cortex. Much of the area covered in this part of the examination is assessed during the history and therefore does not need to be evaluated further. For example, language and memory can be assessed when the patient is asked for details of the illness and significant past events. The patient's cultural and educational background should be taken into account when evaluating mental status.

The components of the mental status examination are as follows:

1. *General appearance and behavior.* This component includes motor activity, body posture, dress and hygiene, facial expression, and speech.
2. *State of consciousness.* The patient must be conscious before other functions can be determined. The nurse should note orientation to time, place, person, and situation, as well as memory, general knowledge, insight, judgment, problem solving, and calculation. Common questions are "Who were the last three presidents?" "What does 'a stitch in time saves nine' mean?" "Subtract 7 from 100, and keep subtracting 7." The nurse should consider whether the patient's plans and goals match the physical and mental capabilities.
3. *Mood and affect.* The nurse should note agitation, anger, depression, or euphoria and the appropriateness of these states. Questions should be directed to bring out the feelings of the patient.
4. *Thought content.* The nurse should note illusions, hallucinations, delusions, or paranoia.
5. *Intellectual capacity.* The nurse should note retardation, dementia, and intelligence.

Cranial nerves. Testing of each CN is an essential component of the neurologic examination (see Table 53-2).

Olfactory nerve. After determining that both nostrils are patent, the olfactory nerve (CN I) is tested by asking the patient to close one nostril, close both eyes, and sniff from a bottle containing coffee, spice, soap, or some other readily recognized odor. The same is done for the other nostril. Generally, olfaction is not tested unless the patient has some disturbance with smell. Chronic rhinitis, sinusitis, and heavy smoking can often decrease the sense of smell. Disturbance in ability to smell may be associated with a tumor involving the olfactory bulb, or it may be the result of a basilar skull fracture that has damaged the olfactory fibers as they pass through the delicate cribriform plate of the skull.

Optic nerve. Visual fields and visual acuity are assessed to test the function of the optic nerve (CN II). Visual fields are assessed by confrontation. The examiner, positioned directly opposite the patient, asks the patient to close one eye, look directly at the bridge of the examiner's nose, and indicate when an object (finger, pencil tip, head of pin) presented from the periphery of each of the four visual field quadrants is seen (Fig. 53-16). The same test is repeated for the other eye. The examiner is used as a control because both examiner and patient are sharing the same visual field. It is important to remember that the nasal side of the visual field is narrower because of the nasal

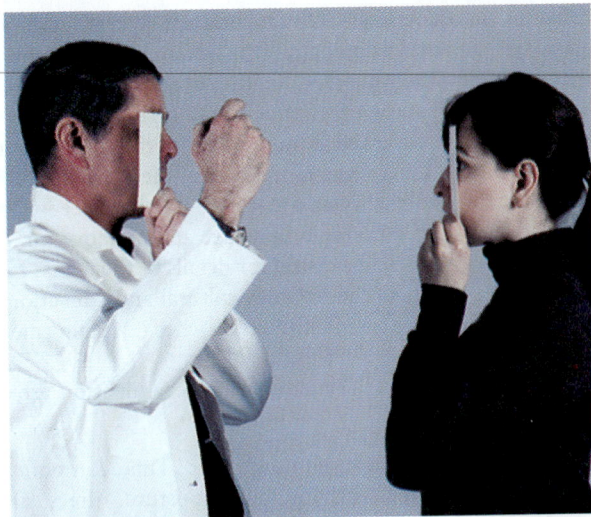

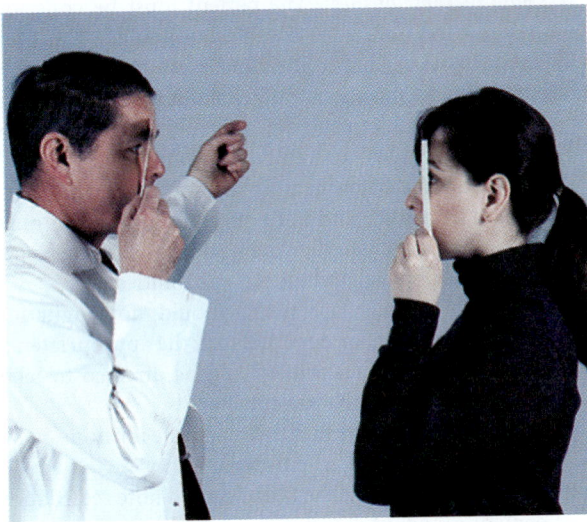

Fig. 53-16 Assessment of visual fields by gross confrontation.

bridge. Visual field defects may arise from lesions of the optic nerve, optic chiasm, or tracts that extend through the temporal, parietal, or occipital lobes. Visual field changes resulting from brain lesions are usually either a hemianopsia (one half of the visual field is affected), a quadrantanopsia (one fourth of the visual field is affected), or monocular.

Visual acuity is tested by asking the patient to read a Snellen chart from 20 feet away. The number on the lowest line that the patient can read with 50% accuracy is recorded. The patient who wears glasses should wear them during testing, unless they are used only for reading. The eyes should be tested individually and together. If a Snellen chart is not available, the patient should be asked to read newsprint for a gross assessment of acuity. The distance from the patient to the newsprint required for accurate reading should be recorded. Acuity may not be testable by these means if the patient does not read English or is aphasic.

Funduscopy reveals the physical condition of the optic disc (head of the optic nerve), as well as the retina and blood vessels. This procedure is routinely performed when the optic nerve is tested. Optic nerve atrophy and papilledema can be detected by this method.

Oculomotor, trochlear, and abducens nerves. Because the oculomotor (CN III), trochlear (CN IV), and abducens (CN VI) nerves all help move the eye, they are tested together. The patient is asked to follow the examiner's finger as it moves horizontally and vertically (making a cross) and diagonally (making an X). If there is weakness or paralysis of one of the eye muscles, the eyes do not move together, and the patient has a disconjugate gaze. The presence and direction of nystagmus (fine, rapid jerking movements of the eyes) is observed at this time, even though it is most often indicative of vestibulocerebellar problems.

Other functions of the oculomotor nerve are tested by checking for pupillary constriction and for convergence (eyes turning inward) and accommodation (pupils constricting with near vision). To test pupillary constriction, the examiner shines a light into the pupil of one eye and looks for ipsilateral constriction of the same pupil and contralateral (consensual) constriction of the opposite eye. The size and shape of the pupils are also noted. The optic nerve must be intact for this reflex to occur. Testing for pupillary constriction is an important component of the neurologic assessment of patients at risk for herniation syndrome (see Chapters 54 and 55). Because the oculomotor nerve exits at the top of the brainstem at the tentorial notch, it can be easily compressed by expanding mass lesions in the cerebral hemispheres. The result is a pupil that does not constrict to light; it may become dilated because the sympathetic input to the pupil acts unopposed. Convergence and accommodation are tested by having the patient focus on the examiner's finger as it moves toward the patient's nose. Another function of the oculomotor nerve is to keep the eyelid open. Damage to the nerve can cause ptosis (drooping eyelid), pupillary abnormalities, and eye muscle weakness.

Trigeminal nerve. The sensory component of the trigeminal nerve (CN V) is tested by having the patient identify light touch (cotton) and pinprick in each of the three divisions (ophthalmic, maxillary, and mandibular) of the nerve on both sides of the face. The patient's eyes should be closed during this part of the examination. The motor component is tested by asking the patient to clench the teeth and palpating the masseter muscles just above the mandibular angle. The corneal reflex test evaluates CN V and CN VII simultaneously. It involves applying a cotton wisp strand to the cornea. The sensory component of this reflex (corneal sensation) is innervated by the ophthalmic division of CN V. The motor component (eye blink) is innervated by the facial nerve (CN VII). This reflex is not normally tested in patients who are awake and alert because other tests evaluate these two nerves. However, for patients with a decreased level of consciousness, the corneal reflex test provides an opportunity to evaluate the integrity of the brainstem at the level of the pons because the fibers of CN V and CN VII have connections in this area.

Facial nerve. The facial nerve (CN VII) innervates the muscles of facial expression. Its function is tested by asking the patient to raise the eyebrows, close the eyes tightly, purse the lips, draw back the corners of the mouth in an exaggerated smile, and frown. The examiner should note any asymmetry in the facial movements because they can indicate damage to the facial nerve. Although taste discrimination of salt and sugar in the anterior two thirds of the tongue is a function of this nerve, it is not routinely tested unless a peripheral nerve lesion is suspected.

Acoustic nerve. The cochlear portion of the acoustic (vestibulocochlear) nerve (CN VIII) is tested by having the patient close the eyes and indicate when a ticking watch or the rustling of the examiner's fingertips is heard as the stimulus is brought closer to the ear. Each ear is tested individually, and the distance from the patient's ear to the sound source when first heard is recorded. This test identifies only gross deficits in hearing. For more precise assessment of hearing, an audiometer is used (see Chapter 19). The vestibular portion of this nerve is not routinely tested unless the patient complains of dizziness, vertigo, or unsteadiness or has auditory dysfunction. If this is the case, caloric testing, which is beyond the scope of routine testing, may be done.

Glossopharyngeal and vagus nerves. The glossopharyngeal and vagus nerves are tested together because both innervate the pharynx. The glossopharyngeal nerve (CN IX) is primarily sensory. In the gag reflex (bilateral contraction of the palatal muscles initiated by stroking or touching either side of the posterior pharynx or soft palate with a tongue blade), the sensory component is mediated by CN IX and the major motor component by the vagus nerve (CN X). It is important to assess the gag reflex in patients who have a decreased level of consciousness, a brainstem lesion, or a disease involving the throat musculature. If the reflex is weak or absent, the patient is in danger of aspirating food or secretions. The strength and efficiency of swallowing is important to test in these patients for the same reason. Another test for the awake, cooperative patient is to have the patient phonate by saying "ah" and to note the bilateral symmetry of elevation of the soft palate. Any asymmetry can indicate weakness or paralysis. Swallowing is also assessed by lightly holding the examiner's hands on either side of the patient's throat and asking the patient to swallow. Any asymmetry is noted.

Spinal accessory nerve. The spinal accessory nerve (CN XI) is tested by asking the patient to shrug the shoulders against resistance and to turn the head to either side against resistance. There should be smooth contraction of the sternomastoid and trapezius muscles. Symmetry, atrophy, or fasciculation of the muscle should also be noted.

Hypoglossal nerve. The hypoglossal nerve (CN XII) is tested by asking the patient to protrude the tongue. It should protrude in the midline. The patient should also be able to push the tongue to either side against the resistance of a tongue blade. Again, any asymmetry, atrophy, or fasciculation should be noted.

Motor system. The motor system examination includes assessment of bulk, tone, and power of the major muscle groups of the body, as well as assessment of balance and coordination. The examiner tests strength by asking the patient to push and pull against the resistance of the examiner's arm as it opposes flexion and extension of the patient's muscle. The patient should be asked to offer resistance at the shoulder, elbow, wrist, hips, knees, and ankles. The patient's grip strength can also be tested. Mild weakness of the upper extremities may be tested by having the patient extend both arms forward at shoulder height with palms up while the eyes are closed. Mild weakness of the arm is demonstrated by downward drifting of the arm or pronation of the palm (pronator drift). Any weakness or asymmetry of strength between the same muscle groups of the right and left side should be noted.

Tone is tested by passively moving the limbs through their range of motion; there should be a slight resistance to these movements. Abnormal tone is described as hypotonia (flaccidity) or hypertonia (spasticity). Involuntary movements (e.g., tics, tremor, myoclonus, athetosis, chorea, dystonia) should be noted.

Cerebellar function is tested by assessing balance and coordination. A good screening test for both balance and muscle strength is to observe the patient's stature (posture while standing) and gait. The examiner should note the pace and rhythm of the gait and observe the arm swing. (The arms should move symmetrically and in the opposite direction of the leg on the same side.) The patient's ability to ambulate is a key factor in determining the amount of nursing care that is needed and the risk of injury from falling. A patient with cerebellar disease may have an ataxic or staggering gait, in which the feet are placed wide apart and the steps are unsteady.

Coordination can be easily tested in several ways. The finger-to-nose test involves having the patient alternately touch the nose with the index finger, then touch the examiner's finger. The examiner repositions the finger while the patient is touching the nose so that the patient must adjust to a new distance each time the examiner's finger is touched. These movements should be performed smoothly and accurately. Other tests include asking the patient to pronate and supinate both hands rapidly and to do a shallow knee bend, first on one leg, and then on the other. Dysarthria or slurred speech should be noted because it is a sign of uncoordination of the speech muscles.

The heel-to-shin test involves having the patient place one heel on the opposite shin below the knee and moving the heel down the shin to the ankle. This is repeated for the other leg. These movements should flow smoothly without jerking or hesitation.

Sensory system. Several modalities are tested in the somatic sensory examination. Each modality is carried by a specific ascending pathway in the spinal cord before it reaches the sensory cortex.

There are some general guidelines for performing the sensory examination. The patient should always have the eyes closed to avoid visual clues. The examiner should avoid giving verbal cues such as "Is this sharp?" The sensory stimulus should be applied in such a way that the patient does not expect it; that is, the examiner should avoid rhythmic application of the stimulus. In the routine neurologic examination, sensory testing of the four extremities is sufficient. However, if a disturbance in sensory function of the skin is identified, the boundaries of that dysfunction should be carefully delineated.

Light touch. Light touch is usually tested first. The examiner gently strokes a cotton wisp over each of the four extremities and asks the patient to indicate when the stimulus is felt by saying "touch." (The sensory examination of the trigeminal nerve may be delayed until this time because the same material for testing sensation is used.)

Pain and temperature. Pain is tested by touching the skin with the sharp end of a pin. This stimulus is irregularly alternated with a simple touch stimulus with the dull end of the pin to determine whether the patient can distinguish the two stimuli. Extinction or inhibition is assessed by simultaneously stimulating opposite sides of the body symmetrically with either a pain or a touch stimulus. Normally, the simultaneous stimuli are perceived (sensed); perception of only one may indicate a parietal lobe lesion.

The sensation of temperature is tested by applying tubes of warm and cold water to the skin and asking the patient to identify the stimuli with the eyes closed. If pain sensation is intact, assessment of temperature sensation may be omitted because both sensations are carried by the same ascending pathways.

Vibration sense. Vibration sense is assessed by applying a vibrating C128 tuning fork to the fingernails and the bony

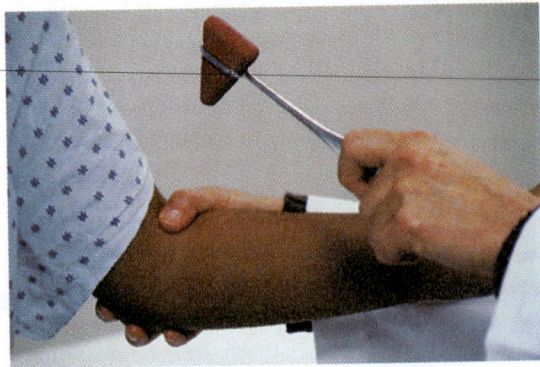

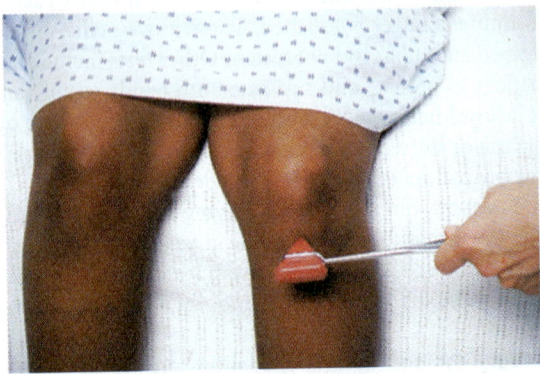

Fig. 53-17 The examiner strikes a swift blow over a stretched tendon to elicit a stretch reflex.

Table **53-6**	**Recording the Normal Neurologic Examination***

Mental Status
Alert and oriented, orderly thought processes, appropriate mood and affect

Cranial Nerves†
Smell intact to soap and coffee; visual fields full to confrontation; visual acuity 20/20 in both eyes; intact extraocular movements; no nystagmus; pupils equal, round, reactive to light and accommodation; intact facial sensation to touch and pinprick; facial movements full; intact gag and swallow reflexes; symmetric elevation of soft palate; full strength with head turning and shrugging of shoulders against resistance; midline protrusion of tongue

Motor System
Normal gait and station; normal tandem walk; negative Romberg test; normal and symmetric muscle bulk, tone, strength; smooth performance of finger-nose, heel-shin movements

Sensory System
Intact sensation to light touch, position sense, vibration, pinprick, heat and cold, two-point discrimination; intact stereognosis and graphesthesia

Reflexes‡
Biceps, triceps, brachioradialis, patellar, and Achilles tendon reflexes 2+ bilaterally; downgoing toes with plantar stimulation

*If some portion of the neurologic examination was not done, this should be indicated (e.g., "Smell not tested").
†May also be recorded as "CN I to XII intact."
‡May also be recorded as drawing of stick figure indicating reflex strength at appropriate sites.

prominences of the hands, legs, and feet with the patient's eyes closed. The examiner asks the patient if the vibration or "buzz" is felt. The examiner then asks the patient to indicate when the vibration ceases. The examiner stops the vibration with the hand as desired.

Position sense. Position sense is assessed by placing the thumb and forefinger on either side of the patient's forefinger or great toe and gently moving the finger up or down. The patient is asked to indicate the direction in which the digit is moved.

Another test of position sense of the lower extremities is the Romberg test. The patient is asked to stand with the feet together and then close his or her eyes. If the patient is able to maintain balance with the eyes open, but sways or falls with the eyes closed (i.e., a positive Romberg test), this may indicate disease in the posterior columns of the spinal cord. It is important that the nurse be aware of patient safety during this test.

Cortical sensory functions. Several tests evaluate cortical integration of sensory perceptions (which occurs in the parietal lobes). Two-point discrimination is assessed by placing the two points of a calibrated compass on the tips of the fingers and toes. The minimum recognizable separation is 4 to 5 mm in the fingertips and a greater degree of separation elsewhere. This test is important in diseases of the sensory cortex and in peripheral nerve disease.

Graphesthesia is tested by having the patient identify numbers traced on the palm of the hands. Stereognosis is tested by having the patient identify the size and shape of easily recognized objects (e.g., coins, keys, a safety pin) placed in the hands. Sensory extinction or inattention is evaluated by touching both sides of the body simultaneously. An abnormal response occurs when the patient perceives the stimulus only on one side. The other stimulus is "extinguished."

Reflexes. Tendons attached to skeletal muscles have receptors that are sensitive to stretch. A reflex contraction of the skeletal muscle occurs when the tendon is stretched. A simple muscle stretch reflex is initiated by briskly tapping the tendon of a stretched muscle, usually with a reflex hammer (Fig. 53-17). The response (muscle contraction of the corresponding muscle) is measured as follows: 0 = absent, 1 = weak response, 2 = normal response, 3 = exaggerated response, 4 = hyperreflexia with clonus. *Clonus*, an abnormal response, is a continued rhythmic contraction of the muscle after the stimulus has been applied.

In general, the biceps, triceps, brachioradialis, and patellar and Achilles tendon reflexes are tested. The examiner elicits the biceps reflex by placing the thumb over the biceps tendon in the antecubital space and striking the thumb with a hammer. The patient should have the arms partially flexed at the elbow with the palms up. The normal response is flexion of the arm at the elbow or contraction of the biceps muscle that can be felt by the examiner's thumb.

The triceps reflex is elicited by striking the triceps tendon above the elbow while the patient's arm is flexed. The normal response is extension of the arm or visible contraction of the triceps.

The brachioradialis reflex is elicited by striking the radius 3 to 5 cm above the wrist while the patient's arm is relaxed. The normal response is flexion and supination at the elbow or visible contraction of the brachioradialis muscle.

The patellar reflex is elicited by striking the patellar tendon just below the patella. The patient can be sitting or lying as long

COMMON ASSESSMENT ABNORMALITIES

Table 53-7 Nervous System

Finding	Description	Possible Etiology and Significance
Altered consciousness	Inability to speak, obey commands, open eyes appropriately with verbal or painful stimulus	Intracranial lesions, metabolic disorder, psychiatric disorders
Anisocoria	Inequality of pupil size	Lesion, injury, or intracranial pressure in area of midbrain
Agnosia	Inability to determine meaning or significance of sensory stimulus	Cerebral cortex lesion
Apraxia	Inability to perform learned movements, defect in motor planning	Cerebral cortex lesion
Aphasia	Loss of language faculty (language comprehension, language expression, or both)	Cerebral cortex lesion
Analgesia	Loss of pain sensation	Lesion in spinothalamic tract or thalamus, lack of or damage to sensory nerve endings
Anesthesia	Absence of sensation	Lesions in spinal cord, thalamus, sensory cortex, or peripheral sensory nerve
Hyperesthesia	Increase in sensation	
Hypoesthesia	Decrease in sensation	
Anosognosia	Inability to recognize bodily defect or disease	Lesions in right parietal cortex, common in right-brain stroke
Astereognosis	Inability to recognize form of object by touch	Lesions in parietal cortex
Ataxia	Lack of coordination of movement	Lesions of sensory or motor pathways, cerebellum; antiseizure drugs, sedative, hypnotic drug toxicity (including alcohol)
Muscle atrophy (disuse or denervation atrophy)	Wasting away or diminution in size of muscle	Suprasegmental (upper motor neuron) lesions, segmental (lower motor neuron) lesions
Bladder dysfunction		
Atonic (autonomous)	Absence of muscle tone and contractility, enlargement of capacity, no sensation of discomfort, overflow with large residual, inability to voluntarily empty or empty by reflex	Early stage of spinal cord injury
Hypotonic	More ability than atonic bladder but less than normal	Interruption of afferent pathways from bladder
Hypertonic	Increase in muscle tone, diminished capacity, reflex emptying, dribbling, incontinence	Lesions in pyramidal tracts (efferent pathways)
Diplopia	Double vision	Lesions affecting nerves of extraocular muscles, cerebellar toxicity
Dysarthria	Lack of coordination in articulating speech	Lesions in cerebellum or pathway of cranial nerves (including brainstem); antiseizure drug, sedative, or hypnotic drug toxicity (including alcohol)
Dyskinesia	Impairment of power of voluntary movement, resulting in fragmentary or incomplete movements	Disorders of basal ganglia, idiosyncratic reaction to psychotropic drugs
Dysphagia	Difficulty in swallowing	Lesions involving motor pathways of CN IX, X (including lower brainstem)
Extensor plantar response (Babinski's sign)	Upgoing toes with plantar stimulation	Suprasegmental or upper motor neuron lesion

Continued

as the leg being tested hangs freely. The normal response is extension of the leg with contraction of the quadriceps.

The Achilles tendon reflex is elicited by striking the Achilles tendon while the patient's leg is flexed at the knee and the foot is dorsiflexed at the ankle. The normal response is plantar flexion at the ankle.

Table 53-6 is an example of how to record a normal neurologic assessment. Common abnormal assessment findings of the neurologic system are presented in Table 53-7.

Nursing Approach. The premise of the nursing approach is that the primary purpose of nursing is to help patients cope effectively with deficits in self-care and in activities of daily living.

COMMON ASSESSMENT ABNORMALITIES

Table 53-7 Nervous System—cont'd

Finding	Description	Possible Etiology and Significance
Homonymous hemianopsia	Loss of vision in one side of visual field	Injury or lesions in area of optic tract or its radiations to occipital cortex
Hemiplegia	Paralysis on one side	Stroke and other lesions involving motor cortex
Nystagmus	Jerking or bobbing of eyes as they track moving object	Lesions in cerebellum, brainstem, vestibular system; antiseizure, sedative, hypnotic toxicity (including alcohol)
Ophthalmoplegia	Paralysis of eye muscles	Lesions in brainstem or CN III, IV, VI
Opisthotonus	Extreme arching of back with retraction of head	Meningitis, tonic phase of grand mal seizure
Papilledema	"Choked disc," swelling of optic nerve head	Increase in intracranial pressure
Paraplegia	Paralysis of lower extremities	Spinal cord transection or mass lesion (thoracolumbar region)
Quadriplegia	Paralysis of all extremities	Spinal cord transection or mass lesion (cervical region) or brainstem

Consequently, the neurologic examination should be viewed in terms of functional disabilities rather than dysfunction of component parts of the nervous system. The effects of the disabilities on the patient's potential for self-care, movement, and desired activities of daily living should be the focus. This includes understanding, communicating, remembering, seeing, speaking, feeling, moving, walking, and using integrated regulatory functions, such as elimination and temperature regulation. In addition, based on knowledge of the location of the problematic area and the functions it controls, the nurse should ask specific questions and perform certain examinations to determine what other effects the condition may have on daily functioning.

All functions of the nervous system can be categorized in six areas: consciousness, mentation, movement, sensation, integrated regulation, and coping with disability. Table 53-8 lists the functions involved in each of these categories and thus forms the basis of a nursing neurologic assessment.

DIAGNOSTIC STUDIES OF THE NERVOUS SYSTEM

Diagnostic studies provide important information to the nurse in monitoring the patient's condition and planning appropriate interventions. These studies are considered to be objective data. Diagnostic studies common to the nervous system are presented in Table 53-9.

Cerebrospinal Fluid Analysis

CSF analysis provides information about a variety of CNS diseases. Normal CSF fluid is clear, colorless, and free of red blood cells (RBCs) and contains little protein. Normal CSF values are listed in Table 53-10.

Lumbar Puncture. Lumbar puncture is the most common method of obtaining CSF for analysis. It is contraindicated in the presence of increased intracranial pressure or infection at the site of puncture.

Nurses often assist in this procedure because it is usually performed in the patient's room. Before the procedure, the nurse should have the patient empty the bladder. The patient

Table 53-8 Functional Categories in Nursing Neurologic Assessment

Consciousness
Arousal	Self-awareness

Mentation
Thinking	Language
Remembering	Problem solving
Perceiving	

Movement
Expressing (facial)	Transferring
Speaking	Eating (chewing, swallowing)
Walking	Blinking (combined movement and sensation)

Sensation
Seeing	Feeling (e.g., touch, temperature, pain, pressure, position, form, shape)
Smelling	
Hearing	

Integrated Regulatory Function
Eating (ingesting, digesting)	Circulation
Eliminating	Temperature control
Breathing	Sexual response
	Emotion

Coping with Disability
Self-care competence	Coping (e.g., adapting, supporting, growing)
Role competence	

should lie in the lateral recumbent position, with the back as near as possible to the edge of the bed. The nurse should assist the patient to draw up the knees to the abdomen and flex the head to the chest. This helps separate the vertebrae so that the needle can be inserted more easily.

Using strict sterile technique, the physician inserts a long needle below the third lumbar vertebra. This may cause some local discomfort. There is no danger of injuring the spinal cord, since the cord terminates between the first and second lumbar vertebrae. However, the patient may have some pain radiating

DIAGNOSTIC STUDIES

Table **53-9** | Nervous System

Study	Description and Purpose	Nursing Responsibility
Cerebrospinal Fluid Analysis		
▪ Lumbar puncture	CSF is aspirated by needle insertion in L3-4 or L4-5 interspace to assess many CNS diseases. (See Table 53-10.)	Assist patient to assume and maintain lateral recumbent position with knees flexed. Ensure maintenance of strict aseptic technique. Ensure labeling of CSF specimens in proper sequence. Keep patient flat for at least a few hours depending on physician preference. Encourage fluids. Monitor neurologic and VS. Administer analgesia as needed.
Radiologic		
▪ Skull and spine x-rays	Simple x-ray of skull and spinal column is done to detect fractures, bone erosion, calcifications, abnormal vascularity.	Explain that procedure is noninvasive. Explain positions to be assumed.
▪ Cerebral angiography	Serial x-ray visualization of intracranial and extracranial blood vessels is performed to detect vascular lesions and tumors of brain. Radiopaque contrast medium is used.	Withhold preceding meal. Explain that patient will have hot flush of head and neck when dye is injected. Administer premedication. Explain need to be absolutely still during procedure. Monitor neurologic and VS every 15-30 min first 2 hr, every hr next 6 hr, then every 2 hr for 24 hr. Maintain pressure dressing and ice to injection site. Maintain bed rest until patient is alert and VS are stable. Report any signs of change in neurologic status.
▪ Computed tomography (CT) scan	Computer-assisted x-ray of several levels or thin cross sections of body parts are done to detect problems such as hemorrhage, tumor, cyst, edema, infarction, brain atrophy, hydrocephalus.	Explain that procedure is noninvasive (if no dye used). Observe for allergic reaction and note puncture site (if dye used). Explain appearance of scanner. Instruct patient on need to remain absolutely still during procedure.
▪ Myelography	X-ray of spinal cord and vertebral column after injection of dye into subarachnoid space is used to detect spinal lesions (e.g., ruptured disk, tumor).	Administer preprocedure sedation as ordered. Instruct patient to empty bladder. Inform patient that test is performed with patient on tilting table that is moved during test. Encourage fluids. Monitor neurologic and VS.
▪ Magnetic resonance imaging (MRI)	Internal body parts are visualized by means of magnetic energy. No invasive procedures are required unless contrast material is used.	Screen patient for metal parts and pacemaker in body. Instruct patient on need to lie very still for up to 1 hr. Sedation may be necessary if patient is claustrophobic.
▪ Positron emission tomography (PET)	Measures metabolic activity of brain regions to assess cell death or damage. Uses radioactive compounds.	Explain procedure to patient. Explain that two IV lines will be inserted. Instruct patient not to take sedatives or tranquilizers. Empty bladder before procedure. May be asked to perform different activities during test.
Electrographic		
▪ Electroencephalography (EEG)	Electrical activity of brain is recorded by scalp electrodes to evaluate cerebral disease, CNS effects of systemic diseases, brain death.	Inform patient that procedure is painless and without danger of electric shock. Withhold stimulants. Inform that patient may be asked to perform various activities such as hyperventilation during test. Determine whether any medications (e.g., tranquilizers, antiseizure drugs) should be withheld. Resume medications after test. Assist patient to wash electrode paste out of hair.

Continued

DIAGNOSTIC STUDIES

Table **53-9**	Nervous System—cont'd	
Study	**Description and Purpose**	**Nursing Responsibility**
Electrographic—cont'd		
▪ Electromyography/ Nerve conduction	Electrical activity associated with nerve and skeletal muscle is recorded by insertion of needle electrodes to detect muscle and peripheral nerve disease.	Inform patient of slight discomfort associated with insertion of needles.
▪ Evoked potentials	Electrical activity associated with nerve conduction along sensory pathways is recorded by electrodes placed on skin and scalp. Stimulus generates the impulse. Procedure is used to diagnose disease, locate nerve damage, and monitor function intraoperatively.	Explain procedure to patient.
▪ Visual evoked potentials	Electrical activity in visual pathway is recorded with rapidly reversing checkerboard pattern on television screen. One eye is tested at a time.	Explain procedure to patient.
▪ Brainstem auditory evoked potentials	Electrical activity in auditory pathway is recorded with earphones that produce clicking sounds. One ear is tested at a time.	Explain procedure to patient.
▪ Somatosensory evoked potentials	Electrical activity in certain nerve pathways is recorded with mild electrical pulse (several per second).	Inform patient that stimulus may cause mild discomfort or muscle twitch.
Ultrasound		
▪ Carotid duplex studies	Sound waves determine blood flow velocity, which indicates presence of occlusive vascular disease.	Explain procedure to patient.
▪ Transcranial Doppler	Same technology as carotid duplex, but evaluates intracranial vessels.	Explain procedure to patient.

VS, vital signs.

Table **53-10**	Normal Cerebrospinal Fluid Values
Parameter	**Normal Value**
Specific gravity	1.007
pH	7.35
Appearance	Clear, colorless
RBCs	None
WBCs	0-8/μl (0-0.008/L)
Protein	
Lumbar	15-45 mg/dl (0.15-0.45 g/L)
Cisternal	15-25 mg/dl (0.15-0.25 g/L)
Ventricular	5-15 mg/dl (0.05-0.15 g/L)
Glucose	45-75 mg/dl (2.5-4.2 mmol/L)
Microorganisms	None
Opening pressure with lumbar puncture	60-150 mm H_2O

down the leg or muscle twitching if the spinal root is irritated by the needle. The nurse can assure the patient that this is temporary, and that the patient is not in danger of being paralyzed.

A manometer is attached to the needle, and CSF pressure is determined *after* the patient is asked to relax and extend the legs. If this is not done, the pressure appears abnormally high. CSF is withdrawn in a series of tubes and sent for analysis. Some examiners believe that the patient should be kept lying flat for at least a few hours after the procedure to avoid a spinal headache, which is presumably caused by loss of the cushioning effect of CSF as a result of leakage of CSF at the puncture site. The prone position may be effective in preventing CSF leakage. Other clinicians do not believe that the lying position is necessary because headache seems to develop in some patients despite precautions. Meningeal irritation (nuchal rigidity) or signs and symptoms of local trauma (e.g., hematoma, pain) may develop in some patients.

Radiologic Studies

Cerebral Angiography. Cerebral angiography is indicated when vascular lesions or tumors are suspected. A catheter is inserted into the femoral (sometimes brachial) artery. It is then passed up the artery to the aortic arch and into the base of a carotid or a vertebral artery for injection of radiopaque dye. A series of x-rays is taken in a timed sequence so that pictures of the arteries, smaller vessels, and veins can be obtained (Fig. 53-18). This study can help localize and determine the presence of abscesses, aneurysms, hematomas,

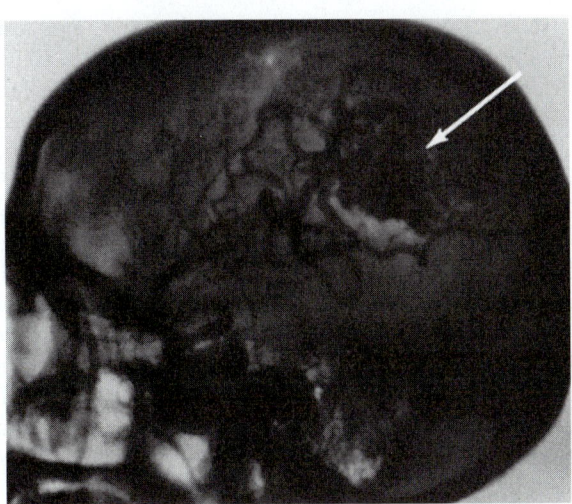

Fig. 53-18 Cerebral angiogram illustrating an arteriovenous malformation *(arrow)*.

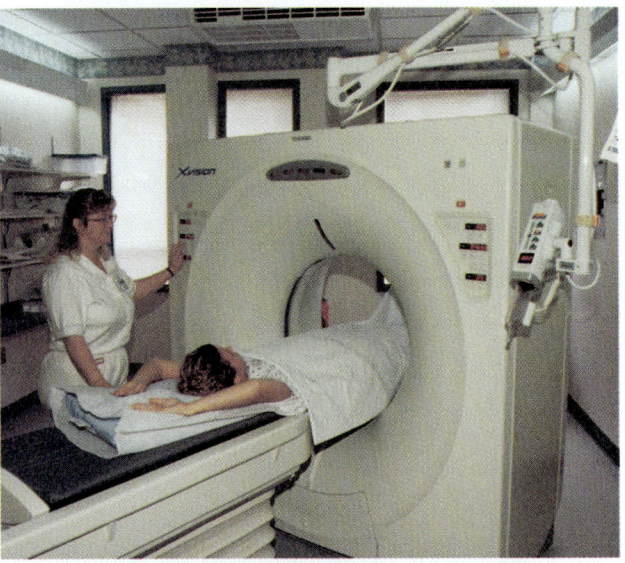

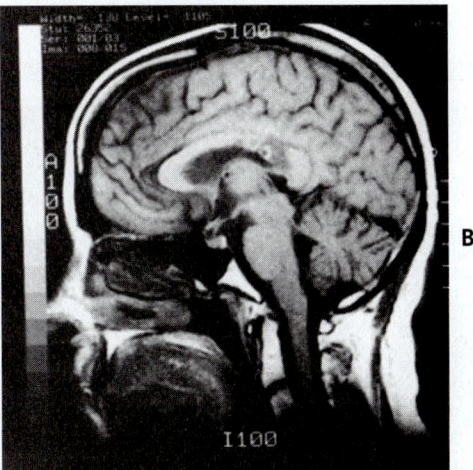

Fig. 53-19 **A,** Clinical setting for magnetic resonance imaging (MRI). **B,** Midline sagittal view of the brain using MRI.

arteriovenous malformations, arterial spasm, and certain tumors.

Because this is an invasive procedure, adverse reactions may occur. The patient may have an allergic (anaphylactic) reaction to the contrast medium. This reaction usually occurs immediately after injection of the contrast medium and may require emergency resuscitation measures in the procedure room. The most common precaution for nurses to take in caring for the patient after the return to the room is observation for bleeding at the catheter puncture site (usually the groin). A pressure dressing and ice are usually placed on the site to promote hemostasis and prevent swelling.

Computed Tomography. Computed tomography (CT) scan is a noninvasive procedure, although intravenous injection of contrast medium may be used to enhance visualization of the blood vessels and identify disruptions in the blood-brain barrier. CT scans can be done on an outpatient basis. A number of x-rays scanning different levels of the brain are compiled with computer assistance and presented in a series of black-and-white pictures. These pictures, which illustrate "slices" of the brain, can show hemorrhages, tumors, cysts, edema, infarction, brain atrophy, and hydrocephalus. CT scans do not illustrate structures in the posterior fossa and the base of the brain as clearly as does magnetic resonance imaging.

Magnetic Resonance Imaging. Magnetic resonance imaging (MRI) became available in the mid-1980s. Rather than using x-rays, this method involves two kinds of magnetism. The patient is placed within a giant magnetic field that aligns the protons of the hydrogen ions in the cells of the body (Fig. 53-19). Bursts of radio-frequency magnetism are introduced to flip the protons out of alignment. When the radio-frequency magnetism is turned off, the protons realign. The resulting magnetic field change is picked up by the machine and is processed by a computer. A vivid black-and-white picture of slices of the brain is then produced.

MRI is useful in evaluating brain and spinal cord edema, hemorrhage, infarction, blood vessels, neoplasms, and bone lesions. Intravenous injection of gadolinium is used to enhance the images obtained with MRI.[3] Because MRI yields greater contrast in the images of soft-tissue structures than does the CT scan, it is the diagnostic test of choice for many neurologic diseases.

Positron Emission Tomography. Positron emission tomography (PET) is used to determine regional metabolism in the brain. PET provides a noninvasive means of determining biochemical processes that occur in the brain. There is increased clinical use of PET scan to monitor select patients following cerebrovascular accident, Alzheimer's disease, epilepsy, and Parkinson' disease.

Myelography. Myelography is used to visualize the spinal column and the subarachnoid space when a spinal lesion is suspected. The most common lesion for which this test is used is a herniated or protruding intervertebral disk. Other lesions include spinal tumors, adhesions, syringomyelia, bony deformations, and arteriovenous malformations. The test involves x-rays of the spinal column after injection of the contrast medium into the subarachnoid space via a catheter. Water-soluble iodine dyes such as iopamidol (Isovue) are used most often because they are absorbed into the bloodstream and excreted by the kidneys.

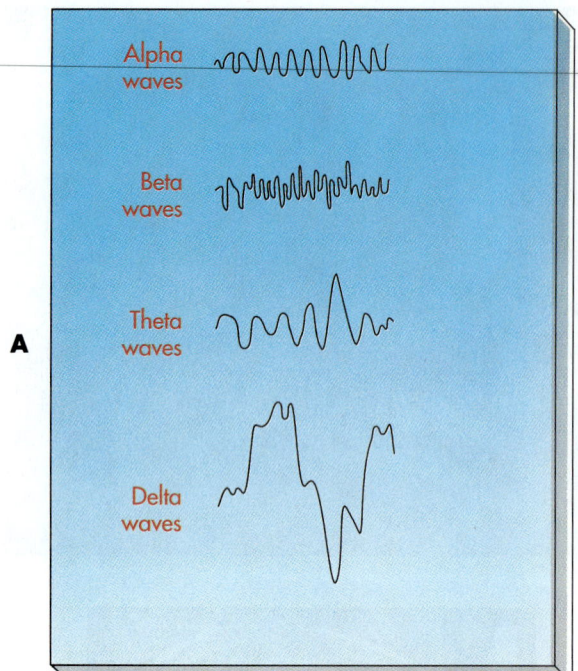

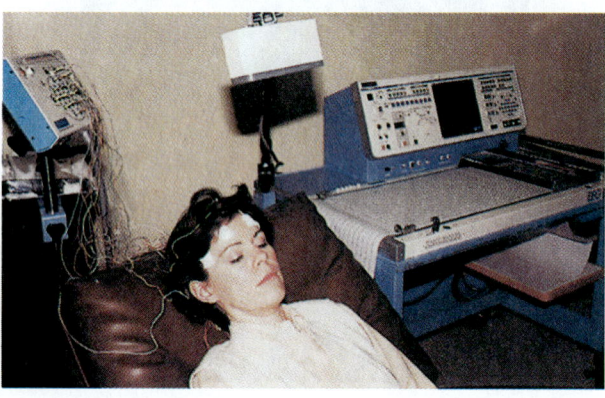

Fig. 53-20   The electroencephalogram (EEG). **A,** Examples of alpha, beta, theta, and delta waves seen on an EEG. **B,** Photograph showing a person undergoing an EEG test. Notice the scalp electrodes that detect voltage fluctuations within the cranium.

Preparation for this procedure is the same as for lumbar puncture. Before the dye is injected, patients must be asked whether they have any allergies, specifically whether they have had any anaphylactic or hypotensive episodes from other dyes. After myelography the patient should be flat for a few hours.

Headache is the most common complaint after myelography. It may be accompanied by nausea and occasionally by vomiting. The nurse should observe the patient for any changes in neurologic status and provide a quiet, comfortable environment after the procedure.

Electrographic Studies

Electroencephalography. The technique of electroencephalography (EEG) involves the recording of the electrical activity of the surface cortical neurons of the brain by 8 to 16 electrodes placed on specific areas of the scalp. This test is done to evaluate not only cerebral disease but also the CNS effects of many metabolic and systemic diseases and to determine brain death. Among the cerebral diseases assessed by EEG are epilepsy, mass lesions (e.g., tumor, abscess, hematoma), cerebrovascular lesions, and brain injury (Fig. 53-20). The procedure is noninvasive. Patients sometimes have the misconception that the recording electrodes will give them an electric shock. They should be assured that this is not true and that the procedure is similar to electrocardiography.

Electromyography and Nerve Conduction Studies. Electromyography (EMG) is the recording of electrical activity associated with innervation of skeletal muscle. The recording is displayed on a cathode-ray oscilloscope and may be played on a loudspeaker for simultaneous analysis. Needle electrodes are inserted into the muscle to record specific motor units because recording from the skin is not sufficient. Normal muscle at rest shows no electrical activity. Typical electrical activity occurs when the muscle contracts. This activity may be altered in diseases of muscle itself (e.g., myopathic conditions) or in disorders of muscle innervation (e.g., segmental or lower motor neuron lesions, peripheral neuropathic conditions). Fibrillations are spontaneous, independent contractions of individual muscle fibers that can be detected only by EMG. They appear on EMG 1 to 3 weeks after a muscle has lost its nerve supply.

Nerve conduction studies involve application of a brief electrical stimulus to a distal portion of a sensory or mixed nerve and recording the resulting wave of depolarization at some point proximal to the stimulation. For example, a stimulus can be applied to the forefinger and a recording electrode placed over the median nerve at the wrist. The time between the onset of the stimulus and the initial wave of depolarization at the recording electrode is measured. This is termed *nerve conduction velocity.* Damaged nerves have slower conduction velocities.

Evoked Potentials. Evoked potentials are recordings of electrical activity associated with nerve conduction along sensory pathways. The activity is generated by a specific sensory stimulus related to the type of study (e.g., checkerboard patterns for visual evoked potentials, clicking sounds for auditory evoked potentials, and mild electrical pulses for somatosensory evoked potentials). Electrodes placed on specific areas of the skin and scalp record the electrical activity, which is stored and averaged by a computerized instrument. A wave pattern appears on a screen and is printed on paper. Peaks in the wave pattern correspond to conduction of the stimulus through certain points along the sensory pathway (e.g., peripheral nerve, brainstem, cortical areas). Increases in the normal time from stimulus onset to a given peak (latency) indicate slowed nerve conduction or nerve damage. Indications for these tests include evaluation of the optic nerve in conditions such as multiple sclerosis (optic neuritis) and the vestibulocochlear nerve in acoustic neuroma.

Combined Doppler and Ultrasound (Duplex) Studies

Carotid Duplex. A carotid duplex study uses combined ultrasound and pulsed Doppler technology. A technician places a probe on the skin over the carotid artery and slowly moves the probe along the course of the common carotid to the bifurcation of the external and internal carotid arteries. The ultrasound signal emitted from the probe reflects off the moving blood cells within the vessel. The frequency of the reflected signal corresponds to the blood velocity. This response is amplified and is registered on a graphic record and also as sound. The graphic record registers blood velocity. Increased blood flow velocity can indicate stenosis of a vessel. Carotid duplex scanning is a noninvasive study that evaluates carotid occlusive disease.

Transcranial Doppler Sonography. Transcranial Doppler (TCD) sonography uses the same technology as carotid duplex studies, except that it records blood flow velocities of the intracranial blood vessels. The probe is placed on the skin at various "windows" in the skull (areas in the skull that have only a thin bony covering) in order to register velocities of the middle cerebral artery, anterior cerebral artery, posterior cerebral artery, terminal carotid artery, and occasionally the anterior and posterior communicating arteries. The temporal, orbital, and suboccipital sites are used. The ultrasound signal received is recorded graphically as a wave form. Peak blood flow velocities and systolic-diastolic ratios can be calculated from this information. TCD sonography is a noninvasive technique that is useful in assessing vasospasm associated with subarachnoid hemorrhage, altered intracranial blood flow dynamics associated with occlusive vascular disease, cerebral autoregulation, presence of emboli, and brain death.

REVIEW QUESTIONS

The number of the question corresponds to the same-numbered objective at the beginning of the chapter.

1. In a patient with a disease that affects the myelin sheath of nerves, such as multiple sclerosis, the glial cells that are affected are the
   a. microglia.
   b. astrocytes.
   c. oligodendroglia.
   d. ependymal cells.

2. A state of hypoxia alters the repeated action potentials necessary for transmission of nerve impulses because energy is required for
   a. repolarization of the cell membrane.
   b. creation of cell membrane permeability.
   c. movement of sodium into the nerve cell.
   d. maintenance of the resting membrane potential.

3. Drugs or diseases that impair the function of the extrapyramidal system may cause loss of
   a. sensations of pain and temperature.
   b. regulation of the autonomic nervous system.
   c. integration of somatic and special sensory inputs.
   d. automatic movements associated with skeletal muscle activity.

4. An obstruction of the anterior cerebral arteries will affect functions of
   a. visual imaging.
   b. balance and coordination.
   c. judgment, insight, and reasoning.
   d. visual and auditory integration for language comprehension.

5. Paralysis of lateral gaze indicates a lesion of cranial nerve
   a. II.
   b. III.
   c. IV.
   d. VI.

6. A result of stimulation of the parasympathetic nervous system is
   a. relaxation of the bladder.
   b. dilation of skin blood vessels.
   c. increased secretion of insulin.
   d. increased blood glucose levels.

7. Assessment of muscle strength of older adults cannot be compared with that of younger adults because
   a. stroke is more common in older adults.
   b. nutritional status is better in young adults.
   c. most young people exercise more than older people.
   d. aging leads to a decrease in muscle bulk and strength.

8. Data regarding mobility, strength, coordination, and activity tolerance are important for the nurse to obtain because
   a. many neurologic diseases affect one or more of these areas.
   b. patients are less able to identify other neurologic impairments.
   c. these are the first functions to be affected by neurologic disease.
   d. aspects of movement are the most important functions of the nervous system.

9. During neurologic testing the patient is able to perceive pain elicited by pinprick. Based on this finding the nurse may omit testing for
   a. position sense.
   b. patellar reflexes.
   c. temperature perception.
   d. heel-to-shin movements.

10. A patient's eyes jerk as they follow the nurse's moving finger. The nurse records this finding as
    a. nystagmus.
    b. normal tracking.
    c. ophthalmoplegia.
    d. ophthalmic dyskinesia.

11. Nursing responsibilities for lumbar puncture include
    a. ensuring the patient has a full bladder.
    b. placing the patient in the lateral recumbent position.
    c. straightening the patient's legs just before the puncture.
    d. having the patient cough when the needle has been inserted.

References

1. Bradley WG and others, editors: *Neurology in clinical practice*, ed 2, Boston, 1996, Butterworth-Heineman.
2. Haerer AF: *DeJong's the neurologic examination*, ed 5, Philadelphia, 1992, Lippincott.
3. Haines DE, editor: *Fundamental neuroscience*, New York, 1997, Churchill Livingstone.
4. Hickey JV: *The clinical practice of neurological and neurosurgical nursing*, ed 4, Philadelphia, 1997, Lippincott.
5. Mitchell PH and others: *Neurologic assessment for nursing practice*, Reston, Va, 1984, Reston.

For additional Internet resources, see the website for this book at **www.mosby.com/MERLIN/medsurg_lewis**

NURSING MANAGEMENT
54 Intracranial Problems

Mary E. Kerr

LEARNING OBJECTIVES

1. Define unconsciousness.
2. Explain the mechanisms of unconsciousness.
3. Describe the nursing management of the unconscious patient.
4. Define intracranial pressure, including normal values.
5. Identify the physiologic mechanisms of accommodation that maintain normal intracranial pressure.
6. Identify the common etiologies, clinical manifestations, and collaborative care of increased intracranial pressure.
7. Describe the nursing management of the patient with increased intracranial pressure.
8. Differentiate types of head injury by mechanism of injury, clinical manifestations, and treatments.
9. Describe the collaborative care and nursing management of head injury.
10. Compare the types, clinical manifestations, and collaborative care of intracranial tumors.
11. Identify the nursing diagnoses and nursing management of the patient with an intracranial tumor.
12. Describe the nursing management of the patient undergoing cranial surgery.
13. Compare the primary causes, collaborative care, and prognosis of common cerebral inflammatory problems.
14. Explain the general nursing management of the patient with a cerebral inflammatory problem.

UNCONSCIOUSNESS

Unconsciousness is an abnormal state in which the patient is unaware of self or environment.[1] Unconsciousness can range from a brief episode, such as fainting, to the prolonged unconsciousness of coma from which the person cannot be roused, even with vigorous external stimuli. Between these two extremes are degrees of unconsciousness varying in length and severity. Unconsciousness itself is not a diagnosis or a disease but rather a manifestation of a large number of pathophysiologic processes, including trauma, metabolic disturbances, mass lesions, and infections. Collaborative care is aimed at determining and correcting the cause of the unconsciousness, maintaining the bodily functions of the patient, supporting the vital functions, and protecting the patient from injury and the hazards of immobility.

Etiology

Consciousness involves two aspects: arousal and content. The arousal component of consciousness refers to a state of wakefulness dependent on the activity of the reticular activating system (RAS), a network of nerve fibers and cell bodies that is located in the reticular formation in the central part of the brainstem and has neural connections to many parts of the nervous system. An intact RAS can maintain a state of wakefulness, even in the absence of a functioning cortex. The content component of consciousness refers to the ability to reason, think, and feel and to react to stimuli with purpose and awareness. These activities are mediated by the cerebral hemispheres, commonly called the higher centers. Intellect and emotional functions are also controlled by these centers.

Interruption of impulses from the RAS or alteration of the functioning of the cerebral hemispheres can cause unconsciousness. Any condition that markedly alters the function of the hemispheres or that depresses or destroys the upper brainstem results in an impaired consciousness. Many specific etiologic events can result in unconsciousness. Causes can be grouped according to pathophysiologic mechanisms, such as supratentorial mass lesions, subtentorial mass lesions, destructive lesions, or metabolic and diffuse cerebral disorders (Table 54-1). Psychiatric disorders such as depression, catatonia, and schizophrenia can result in failure to respond to the environment.

Supratentorial mass lesions generally interfere with consciousness by compressing and shifting the cerebral contents and causing pressure on the upper brainstem containing the RAS. These lesions, occurring above the tentorium, may include those resulting from trauma (e.g., lacerations or contusions, subdural or epidural hematomas), subarachnoid hemorrhage, intracerebral hemorrhage or infarction, tumors, and abscesses. The most serious consequence of a supratentorial mass lesion is herniation of the cerebral hemisphere through the tentorial notch, causing compression of the brainstem. Another form of herniation can occur if the brain shifts laterally, forcing the cingulate gyrus under the falx and compressing the

Reviewed by Mary Lou Muwaswes, RN, MS, Clinical Nurse Specialist, San Francisco, Calif.

| Table **54-1** | Causes of Unconsciousness |

Supratentorial Mass Lesions
  Epidural hematoma
  Subdural hematoma
  Intracerebral hematoma
  Cerebral infarction
  Brain tumor
  Brain abscess

Subtentorial Lesions
  Brainstem infarction
  Brainstem tumor
  Brainstem hemorrhage
  Cerebellar hemorrhage
  Cerebellar abscess

Metabolic and Diffuse Cerebral Disorders
  Hypoxia or anoxia
  Postictal states and concussion
  Infection (meningitis, encephalitis)
  Subarachnoid hemorrhage
  Exogenous toxins
    Drug overdose
    Alcohol intoxication
    Lead poisoning
  Endogenous toxins and deficiencies
    Hypoglycemia
    Uremia
    Hepatic encephalopathy
    Thiamine deficiency

blood vessels and brain tissue of the opposite hemisphere. The end result of herniation is ischemia and irreversible infarction (see Fig. 54-5 later in this chapter).

Subtentorial masses or destructive lesions that occur below the tentorium interfere with consciousness by compressing or destroying the RAS above the midpons. Pontine or cerebellar hemorrhage, infarction, tumor, or abscess can affect the subtentorial area of the brain through direct brain compression, upward herniation through the tentorial notch, or downward herniation into the foramen magnum.

Metabolic and diffuse cerebral disorders of either intracranial or extracranial origin can cause alterations in the conscious state. These disorders can disturb cerebral metabolism and thus alter the regulation of cellular nutrition, electrolyte balance, oxygen and carbon dioxide regulation, and enzymatic functions. Specific metabolic problems that can cause unconsciousness include uremia, diabetes mellitus, hypoglycemia, alcohol intoxication, drug (e.g., barbiturate) overdose, and lead poisoning.

Regardless of the cause of the unconscious state, two pathophysiologic processes that affect cerebral metabolism generally occur: cerebral ischemia-anoxia and cerebral edema. The pathophysiologic problem common to all metabolic brain diseases is decreased oxygen uptake. Cerebral ischemia-anoxia, both focal and global, is managed by instituting measures to ensure adequate systemic circulation. Cerebral edema and the resulting increased intracranial pressure may be treated by hyperosmotic drugs and corticosteroids.

Psychiatric or psychogenic disorders can cause unconsciousness. Although the neurologic system is intact, the patient does not react to the environment. A psychiatric referral is appropriate when the possibility of organic disease has been ruled out.

Unconscious State

The patient's state of consciousness is defined by both the behavior and the pattern of brain activity recorded by an electroencephalogram (EEG). In the deepest state of unconsciousness, the patient does not respond to painful stimuli. Corneal and pupillary reflexes are absent. The patient cannot swallow or cough and is incontinent of urine and feces. The EEG pattern demonstrates decreased or absent neuronal activity. This patient is in a coma.

Behavior.   The nurse may find it helpful to conceptualize states of consciousness as a continuum. This continuum of electrical activity in the brain ranges from the hyperexcitable state of seizure to the hypoexcitable state of coma. The normal level of alertness is between these two states, with abnormalities ranging from slight disorientation to coma. A variety of terms have been used to describe points on the continuum, but they tend to be confusing. For example, the term *lethargy* has a variety of meanings. Rather than relying on these terms, the nurse must learn appropriate assessment techniques and describe the level of consciousness by noting the specific behaviors observed. When a deviation from the normal state of consciousness occurs, a more structured method of observation should be initiated. This type of systematic approach to nursing assessment is illustrated in Fig. 54-1 and consists of assessing the level of consciousness by the Glasgow Coma Scale (GCS) and by body functions.

Glasgow Coma Scale.   Because of the confusion and ambiguity that surround terms describing altered states of consciousness, the GCS was developed in 1974. The three areas assessed in this method correspond to the definition of *coma* as the inability of a patient to speak, obey commands, or open the eyes when a verbal or painful stimulus is applied.[2] Specific assessments evaluate the patient's response to varying degrees of stimuli. Three indicators of response are evaluated: (1) opening of the eyes, (2) the best verbal response, and (3) the best motor response (Table 54-2). Specific behaviors that are seen as responses to the testing stimulus in each of these three areas are given a numeric value and can be plotted on a graph. The clinician's responsibility is to elicit the best response on each of the scales: the higher the scores, the higher the level of brain functioning. The graph visually plots a place on the consciousness continuum to determine whether the patient is stable, improving, or deteriorating. The subscale scores are particularly important if a patient is untestable in one area. For example, severe periorbital edema may make eye opening impossible. The total GCS score is a sum of the numeric values assigned to each of the three areas evaluated. The highest GCS score is 15 for a fully alert person, and the lowest possible score is 3. A GCS score of 8 or less is generally indicative of coma.

The GCS offers several advantages in the assessment of the unconscious patient. It is specific and structured, allowing different clinicians to arrive at the same conclusion regarding the patient's status. It saves time for the assessor because the ratings are done with numbers rather than with lengthy descriptions. The GCS is also specific enough to discriminate between different or changing states.

The GCS is used to assess the arousal aspect of consciousness. Other components of the neurologic assessment include pupillary checks, extremity strength testing, and, if appropriate, corneal reflex testing.

Monitoring of Body Functions.   In addition to assessing the neurologic state of the unconscious patient, various body functions, such as respiration and elimination, also must

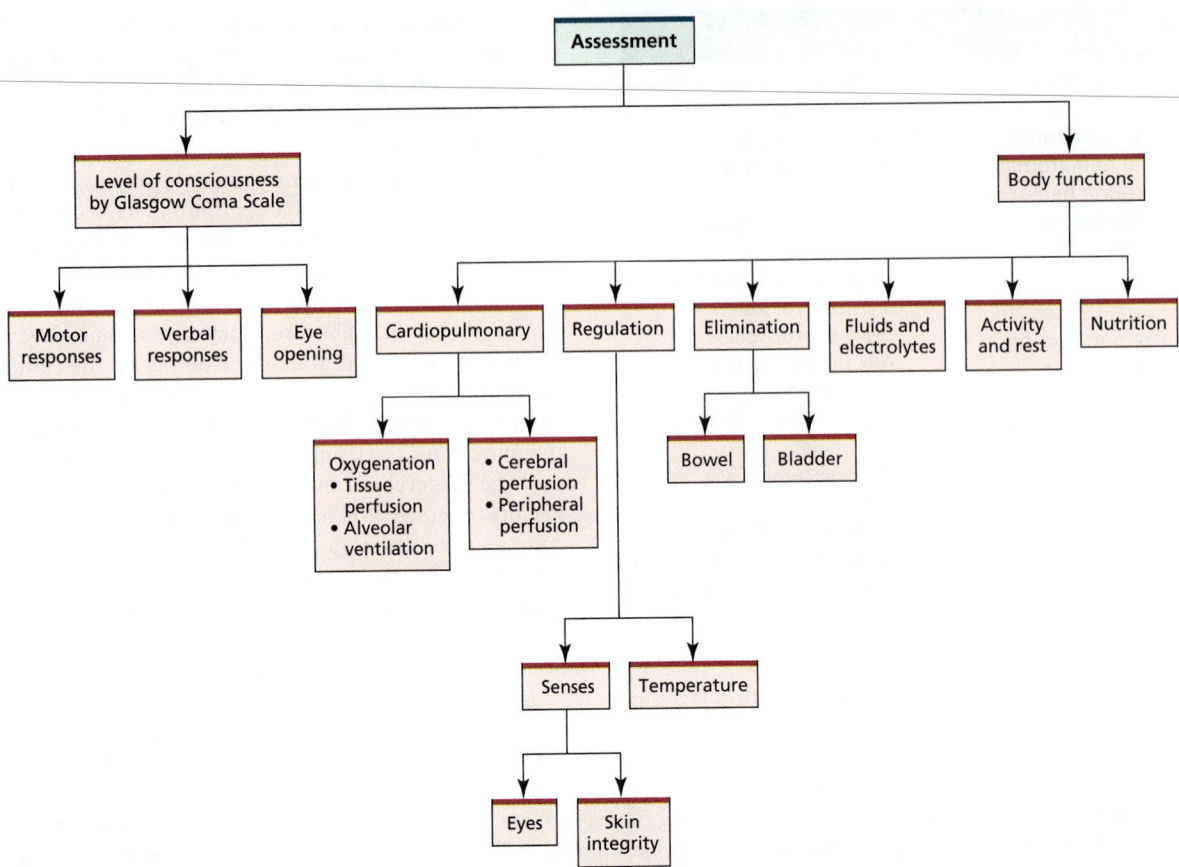

Fig. 54-1 A systematic approach to nursing assessment of the unconscious patient.

Table **54-2**	**Glasgow Coma Scale**		
Category of Response	**Appropriate Stimulus**	**Response**	**Score**
■ Eyes open	Approach to bedside	Spontaneous response	4
	Verbal command	Opening of eyes to name or command	3
	Pain	Lack of opening of eyes to previous stimuli but opening to pain	2
		Lack of opening of eyes to any stimulus	1
		Untestable	U
■ Best verbal response	Verbal questioning with maximum arousal	Appropriate orientation, conversant, correct identification of self, place, year, and month	5
		Confusion, conversant, but disorientation in one or more spheres	4
		Inappropriate or disorganized use of words (e.g., cursing), lack of sustained conversation	3
		Incomprehensible words, sounds (e.g., moaning)	2
		Lack of sound, even with painful stimuli	1
		Untestable	U
■ Best motor response	Verbal command (e.g., "raise your arm, hold up two fingers")	Obedience of command	6
		Localization of pain, lack of obedience but presence of attempts to remove offending stimulus	5
	Pain (pressure on proximal nail bed)	Flexion withdrawal,* flexion of arm in response to pain without abnormal flexion posture	4
		Abnormal flexion, flexing of arm at elbow and pronation, making a fist	3
		Abnormal extension, extension of arm at elbow usually with adduction and internal rotation of arm at shoulder	2
		Lack of response	1
		Untestable	U

*Added to the original scale by many centers.

be monitored (see Fig. 54-1). Adequate circulation and respiration are the most vital and should always be the first body functions evaluated.

INTRACRANIAL PRESSURE

Understanding the mechanisms associated with intracranial pressure (ICP) is important in caring for patients with many different neurologic problems. The skull is like a closed box with three essential volume components: brain tissue, blood, and cerebrospinal fluid (CSF) (Fig. 54-2). The total volume in the skull is 1900 ml. The intracellular and extracellular fluids of brain tissue make up approximately 78% of this volume. Blood in the arterial, venous, and capillary network makes up 12% of the volume, and the remaining 10% is the volume of the CSF. Under normal conditions, in which intracranial volume remains relatively constant, the balance between these components maintains the ICP. The modified Monro-Kellie doctrine explains the relatively constant volume of these three components within the rigid skull structure. If the volume added to the cranial vault equals the volume displaced from it, the total intracranial volume will not change.[3] This hypothesis is not applicable in situations in which the skull is not rigid (e.g., in neonates and in adults with unfused skull fractures).

Other factors that influence ICP under normal circumstances are changes in (1) arterial pressure, (2) venous pressure, (3) intraabdominal and intrathoracic pressure, (4) posture, (5) temperature (especially hypothermia), and (6) blood gases, particularly CO_2 levels. The degree to which these factors increase or decrease the ICP depends on the ability of the brain to accommodate to the changes.

Regulation and Maintenance of Intracranial Pressure

Normal Intracranial Pressure.
Normal ICP is the pressure exerted by the total volume from the three components within the skull: brain tissue, blood, and CSF. ICP can be measured in the ventricles, subarachnoid space, subdural space, epidural space, or brain parenchymal tissue using a water manometer or a pressure transducer. With the patient in the lateral recumbent position, the pressure is generally recorded at 60 to 150 mm H_2O with the use of the water manometer. When the patient is lying with a 30-degree elevation of the head and the pressure is measured intracranially, it is 0 to 15 mm Hg with the use of the pressure transducer. A sustained pressure above the upper limit is considered abnormal.

Normal Compensatory Adaptations.
In applying the modified Monro-Kellie doctrine, the body can compensate for changes in the volume of components of the skull to maintain a normal ICP. The body does this by making small changes in any of the three components. Initial compensatory mechanisms include increased CSF absorption, displacement of CSF into the spinal subarachnoid space, and collapse of the cerebral veins and dural sinuses. Other mechanisms that assist in compensation are (1) dispensability of the dura, (2) increased venous outflow, (3) decreased CSF production, (4) changes in intracranial blood volume through constriction and dilation, and (5) slight compression of brain tissue.[3]

Initially, an increase in volume produces no increase in ICP as a result of the compensatory mechanisms. However, these compensatory adaptations to changes in volume are limited,

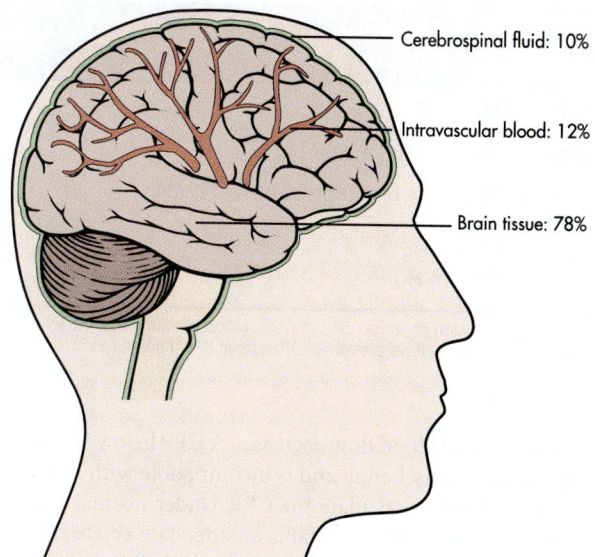

Cerebrospinal fluid: 10%

Intravascular blood: 12%

Brain tissue: 78%

Fig. 54-2   Components of the brain.

and as the volume increase continues, the ICP rises and decompensation occurs resulting in compression and ischemia.[3]

Cerebral Blood Flow

Cerebral blood flow (CBF) is the amount of blood in milliliters passing through 100 g of brain tissue in 1 minute. The global cerebral blood flow is approximately 50 ml per minute per 100 g of brain tissue. There is a difference in flow between the white and gray matter of the brain. The white matter has a slower blood flow, approximately 25 ml per minute per 100 g, and the gray matter has a faster blood flow, approximately 75 ml per minute per 100 g. The maintenance of blood flow to the brain is critical because the brain requires a constant supply of oxygen and glucose. The brain uses 20% of the body's oxygen and 25% of its glucose.

Autoregulation of Cerebral Blood Flow.
The brain has the ability to regulate its own blood flow in response to its metabolic needs in spite of wide fluctuations in systemic arterial pressure. *Autoregulation* is defined as the automatic alteration in the diameter of the cerebral blood vessels to maintain a constant blood flow to the brain during changes in systemic arterial pressure. The purpose of autoregulation is to ensure a consistent cerebral blood flow to provide for metabolic needs and to maintain cerebral perfusion pressure within normal limits. The lower limit of systemic arterial pressure at which autoregulation is effective in a normotensive person is a mean arterial pressure (MAP) of 50 mm Hg. Below this, cerebral blood flow decreases and symptoms of cerebral ischemia, such as syncope and blurred vision, occur. The upper limit of systemic arterial pressure at which autoregulation is effective is 150 mm Hg. When this pressure is exceeded, the vessels are maximally constricted. Thus further vasoconstrictor response is lost and the blood-brain barrier is disrupted; the result is an increase in ICP.

The cerebral perfusion pressure (CPP) is the pressure needed to ensure blood flow to the brain. CPP is equal to the MAP minus the ICP (CPP = MAP − ICP). This formula is clinically useful, although it does not consider the effect of systemic vascular resistance. As the CPP decreases, autoregulation

Table 54-3	Calculation of Cerebral Perfusion Pressure

$$CPP = MAP - ICP$$

$$MAP = DBP + \frac{1}{3}(SBP - DBP) \text{ or } \frac{SBP + 2(DBP)}{3}$$

Example: Systemic blood pressure = 122/84
   MAP = 97
   ICP = 12 mm Hg
   CPP = 85 mm Hg

CPP, cerebral perfusion pressure; *DBP*, diastolic blood pressure; *ICP*, intracranial pressure; *MAP*, mean arterial pressure; *SBP*, systolic blood pressure.

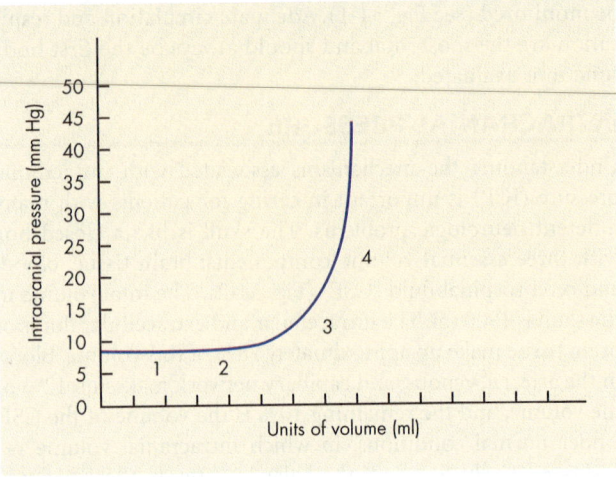

Fig. 54-3 Intracranial volume-pressure curve. (See text for descriptions of 1, 2, 3, and 4.)

fails and cerebral blood flow decreases. A CPP below 30 mm Hg results in cellular ischemia and is incompatible with life. Table 54-3 shows how to calculate the CPP. Under normal circumstances, autoregulation maintains an adequate cerebral blood flow and perfusion pressure by three physiologic mechanisms: changes in ICP, cerebral vasodilation, and metabolic factors.

Pressure Changes. The relationship of pressure to volume is depicted in the pressure-volume curve. The curve is affected by the brain's elastance and compliance. *Elastance* is the brain's ability to accommodate changes in volume. It represents the stiffness of the brain. With high elastance, large increases in pressure occur with small increases in volume.

$$\text{Elastance} = \text{Pressure/Volume}$$

Compliance is the inverse of elastance and is the expandability of the brain. It is represented as the volume increase for each unit increase in pressure. Low compliance is the same as high elastance. With low compliance, high changes in pressure result from small changes in volume.

$$\text{Compliance} = \text{Volume/Pressure}$$

The concept of the pressure-volume curve can be used to represent the stages of increased ICP (intracranial hypertension) (Fig. 54-3). At stage 1 on the curve, there is high compliance and low elastance. The brain is in total compensation, with accommodation and autoregulation intact. An increase in volume does not increase the ICP. At stage 2, the compliance is lower and elastance is increasing. An increase in volume places the patient at risk of increased ICP. At stage 3, there is high elastance and low compliance. Any small addition of volume causes a great increase in pressure. There is a loss of autoregulation, and there may be symptoms indicating increased ICP, such as systolic hypertension with an increasing pulse pressure, bradycardia, and slowing of respiratory rate (Cushing's triad). With the loss of autoregulation and the rise in the systolic blood pressure as a result of the Cushing response, decompensation occurs. The ICP passively mimics the blood pressure. Finally, when the patient is in stage 4, the ICP rises to terminal levels with little increase in volume. Herniation occurs as the brain tissue shifts from the compartment of greater pressure to a compartment of lesser pressure.

Factors Affecting Cerebral Blood Flow. Oxygen tension, carbon dioxide tension, and hydrogen ion concentration affect cerebral vessel tone. Cerebral arteries dilate when the cerebral oxygen tension falls below 50 mm Hg. This dilation decreases cerebral vascular resistance and increases cerebral blood flow in an effort to raise oxygen tension. If oxygen tension is not raised, anaerobic metabolism begins, resulting in an accumulation of lactic acid. In an acid environment, an increase in vasodilation and a further increase in blood flow occur. An increase in the partial pressure of arterial carbon dioxide ($PaCO_2$) is the most potent vasodilator. An increase in $PaCO_2$ relaxes the smooth muscles. This decreases cerebrovascular resistance and increases cerebral blood flow. A severely low arterial oxygen pressure (PaO_2) and a high hydrogen ion concentration (acidosis) are also potent cerebral vasodilators.[3]

Extreme cardiovascular changes such as asystole and pathophysiologic states such as diabetic coma can alter or abolish autoregulation globally. Trauma and tumors can alter autoregulation focally. When autoregulation is lost, cerebral blood flow is no longer maintained at a constant level but is directly influenced by changes in systemic blood pressure, hypoxia, or the effects of catecholamines. Increasing ICP can progress to loss of consciousness, changes in neurologic function, brain herniation, and death.

INCREASED INTRACRANIAL PRESSURE

Increased ICP is a life-threatening situation that results from an increase in any or all of the three components (brain tissue, blood, and CSF) of the skull. Cerebral edema is an important factor contributing to increased ICP.

Cerebral Edema

A variety of conditions are associated with cerebral edema (Table 54-4). Regardless of the cause, cerebral edema results in an increase in tissue volume that carries the potential for increased ICP. The extent and severity of the original insult are factors that determine the degree of cerebral edema.

Three types of cerebral edema have been distinguished: vasogenic edema, cytotoxic edema, and interstitial edema.[4] More than one type may result from a single insult in the same patient.[5]

Vasogenic Cerebral Edema. Vasogenic cerebral edema, the most common type of edema, occurs mainly in the white

Table **54-4**	Conditions Associated with Cerebral Edema

Mass lesions	**Vascular insult**
Neoplasm (primary and metastatic)	Infarct (thrombolic and embolic)
Abscess	Venous sinus thrombosis
Hemorrhage (intracerebral and extracerebral)	Anoxic and ischemic episodes
Head injuries	**Toxic or metabolic encephalopathic conditions**
Hemorrhage	
Contusion	Lead or arsenic intoxication
Posttraumatic brain swelling	Renal failure
Brain surgery	Liver failure
Infections	Reye's syndrome

matter and is attributed to changes in the endothelial lining of cerebral capillaries. These changes allow leakage of macromolecules from the capillaries into the surrounding extracellular space, resulting in an osmotic gradient that favors the flow of water from the intravascular to the extravascular space. A variety of insults, such as brain tumors, abscesses, and ingested toxins, may cause an increase in the permeability of the blood-brain barrier and produce an increase in the extracellular fluid volume. The speed and extent of the spread of the edema fluid are influenced by the systemic blood pressure, the site of the brain injury, and the extent of the blood-brain barrier defect. This edema may produce a continuum of symptoms ranging from focal neurologic deficits to disturbances in consciousness, including coma.

Cytotoxic Cerebral Edema. Cytotoxic cerebral edema results from local disruption of the functional or morphologic integrity of cell membranes and occurs most often in the gray matter. Cytotoxic cerebral edema develops from destructive lesions or trauma to brain tissue resulting in cerebral hypoxia or anoxia, sodium depletion, and syndrome of inappropriate antidiuretic hormone (SIADH). Cerebral edema results as fluid and protein shift from the extracellular space directly into the cells, with subsequent swelling and loss of cellular function.

Interstitial Cerebral Edema. Interstitial cerebral edema is the result of periventricular diffusion of ventricular CSF in a patient with uncontrolled hydrocephalus. It can also be caused by enlargement of the extracellular space as a result of systemic water excess (hyponatremia). Fluid moves into the cells to equilibrate with the hypo-osmotic interstitial fluid. Regardless of the cause of cerebral edema, manifestations of increased ICP result, unless compensation is adequate.

Mechanisms of Increased Intracranial Pressure

Sustained elevations of ICP, above the threshold of 20 mm Hg, are associated with a poor prognosis.[6] Increased ICP can be caused by several clinical problems, including a mass lesion, such as a hematoma, contusion, abscess, or rapidly growing tumor; cerebral edema associated with brain tumors, hydrocephalus, head injury, or brain inflammation; or metabolic insult. These cerebral insults may result in hypercapnia, cerebral

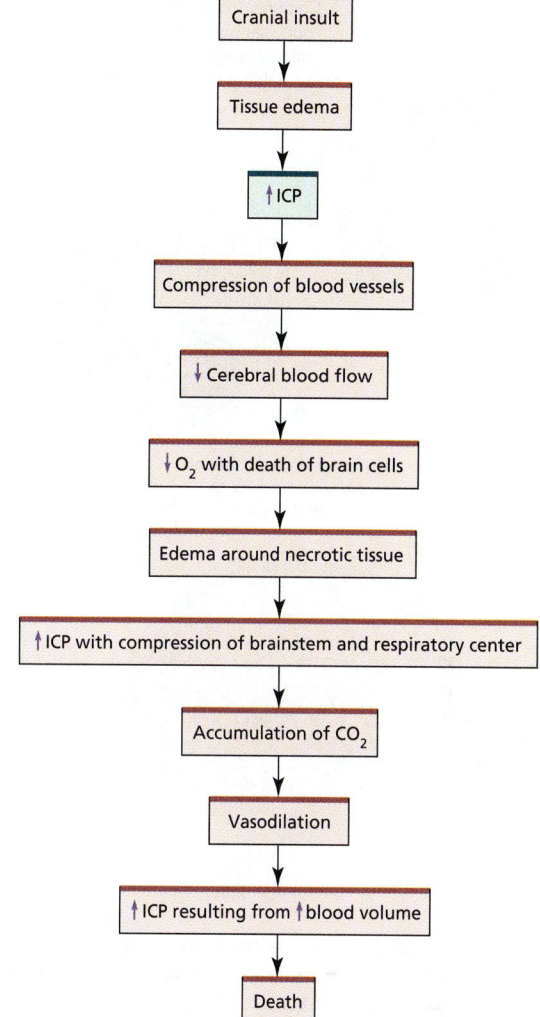

Fig. 54-4 Progression of increased intracranial pressure.

acidosis, impaired autoregulation, and systemic hypertension, which promote the formation and spread of cerebral edema. This edema distorts brain tissue, further increasing the ICP, which leads to even more tissue hypoxia and acidosis. Figure 54-4 illustrates the progression of increased ICP.

Unless there is a reduction in the ICP, the end result is brainstem compression. As the intracranial mass continues to increase, herniation of the brain from one compartment to another can occur.

Complications of Increased Intracranial Pressure

The major complications of uncontrolled increased ICP are inadequate cerebral perfusion and cerebral herniation (Fig. 54-5). The three major patterns of supratentorial brain shift are cingulate (lateral, beneath the falx) herniation, central or transtentorial (downward) herniation, and uncal (lateral and downward) herniation. These patterns are distinguished by the direction of the shift and by the cerebral structures involved. Regardless of the specific intracranial shift, displacement and herniation cause a potentially reversible pathophysiologic process to become irreversible. Ischemia and edema are further

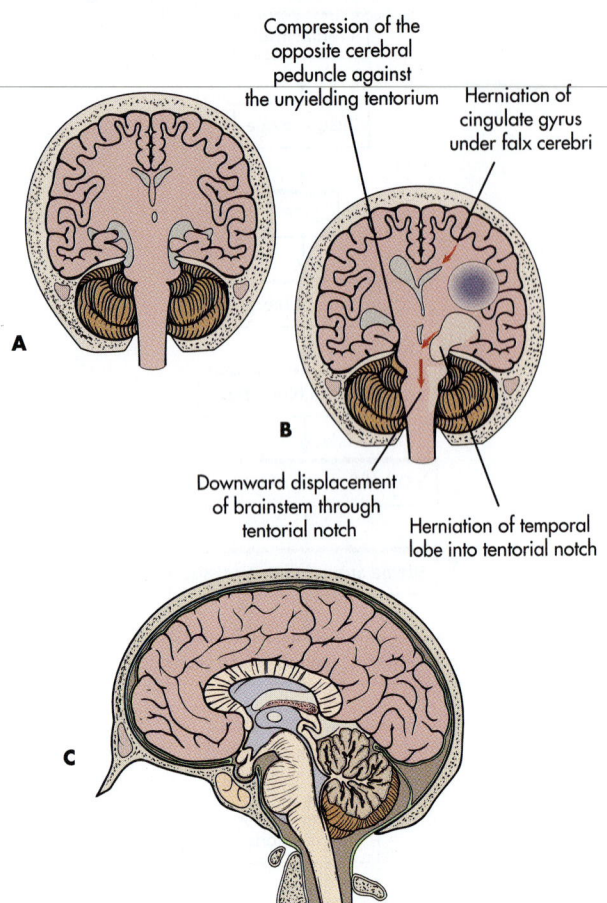

Compression of the opposite cerebral peduncle against the unyielding tentorium

Herniation of cingulate gyrus under falx cerebri

Downward displacement of brainstem through tentorial notch

Herniation of temporal lobe into tentorial notch

Fig. 54-5   Herniation. **A,** The normal relationship of intracranial structures. **B,** Shift of intracranial structures. **C,** Downward herniation of the cerebellar tonsils into the foramen magnum.

increased, compounding the preexisting problem. Compression of the brainstem and cranial nerves may be fatal. Figure 54-6 illustrates symptoms of supratentorial increased ICP from the early phase through herniation of the brain.

Subtentorial and infratentorial herniations force the cerebellum and brainstem downward through the foramen magnum. If compression of the brainstem is unrelieved, respiratory arrest may occur.

Clinical Manifestations

The clinical manifestations of increased ICP can take many forms, depending on the cause, location, and rate at which the pressure increase occurs. The earlier the condition is recognized and treated, the better the prognosis. The clinical manifestations of increased ICP associated with supratentorial lesions include the following:

1. *Change in level of consciousness.* The level of consciousness (LOC) is a sensitive and important indicator of the patient's neurologic status. The change in consciousness may be dramatic, as in coma, or subtle, such as a flattening of affect, change in orientation, or decrease in level of attention. Changes in LOC are a result of impaired cerebral blood flow, which affects the cells of the cerebral cortex and the RAS.

2. *Changes in vital signs.* Although the complex of increasing systolic pressure (widening pulse pressure), bradycardia with a full and bounding pulse, and irregular respiratory pattern (Cushing's triad) may be present, these symptoms often do not appear until ICP has been increased for some time or markedly increased suddenly (e.g., head trauma). Changes in vital signs are caused by increasing pressure on the thalamus, hypothalamus, pons, and medulla. A change in body temperature may also be noted.

3. *Ocular signs.* Compression of the oculomotor nerve (CN III) results in dilation of the pupil ipsilateral to the mass or lesion, sluggish or no response to light, inability to move the eye upward, and ptosis of the eyelid. These signs can be the result of a shifting of the brain from the midline, a process that compresses the trunk of CN III, paralyzing the pupil sphincter. A fixed, unilaterally dilated pupil is a neurologic emergency that indicates transtentorial herniation of the brain. Other cranial nerves may also be affected, such as the optic (CN II), trochlear (CN IV), and abducens (CN VI) nerves. Signs of dysfunction of these cranial nerves include blurred vision, diplopia, and changes in extraocular eye movements. Central herniation may initially manifest as sluggish but equal pupils. Uncal herniation may cause dilated unilateral pupil. Papilledema, a choked optic disc seen on retinal examination, is also seen and is a nonspecific sign that is associated with long-standing increased ICP.

4. *Decrease in motor function.* As the ICP continues to rise, the patient manifests changes in motor ability. A contralateral hemiparesis or hemiplegia may be seen, depending on the location of the source of the increased ICP. If painful stimuli to elicit a motor response are used, the patient may exhibit a localization to the stimuli or a withdrawal from it. Decorticate (flexor) and decerebrate (extensor) posturing may also be elicited by noxious stimuli (Fig. 54-7). A decorticate posture consists of internal rotation and adduction of the arms with flexion of the elbows, wrists, and fingers as a result of interruption of voluntary motor tracts. Extension of the legs may also be seen. A decerebrate posture may indicate more serious damage and results from disruption of motor fibers in the midbrain and brainstem. In this position, the arms are stiffly extended, adducted, and hyperpronated. There is also hyperextension of the legs with plantar flexion of the feet.

5. *Headache.* Although the brain itself is insensitive to pain, compression of other intracranial structures such as the walls of arteries and veins and the cranial nerves can produce headache. The headache is often continuous but worse in the morning. Straining or movement may accentuate the pain.

6. *Vomiting.* Vomiting, usually not preceded by nausea, is often a nonspecific sign of increased ICP. This is called *unexpected vomiting* and is related to pressure changes in the cranium. Projectile vomiting may also be seen and is related to increased ICP.

It is often difficult to identify increased ICP as the cause of coma. Loss of consciousness also confuses the interpretation of

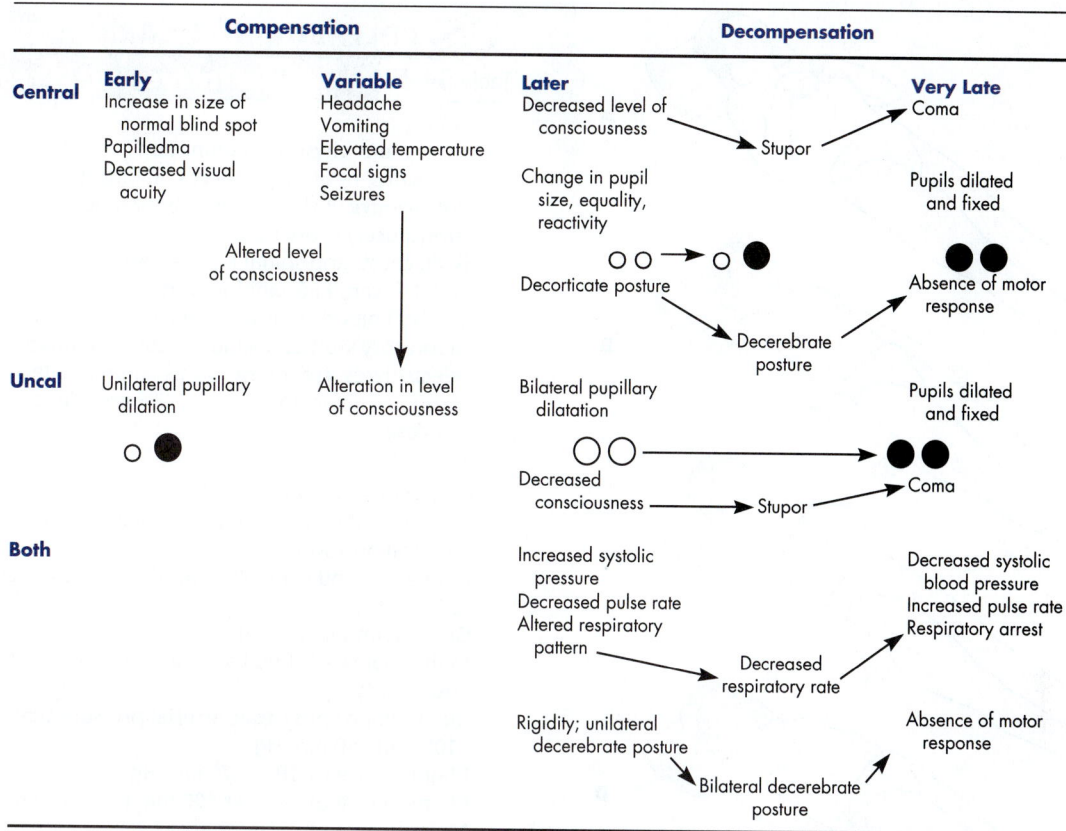

Fig. 54-6   Signs and symptoms of supratentorial increased intracranial pressure.

clinical signs, making it difficult to follow the progression of the increasing ICP.

Diagnostic Studies

Diagnostic studies are aimed at identifying the presence and the underlying cause of increased ICP (Table 54-5). Magnetic resonance imaging (MRI) and computed tomography (CT) have revolutionized the diagnosis of increased ICP. These tests are used to differentiate the many conditions that can cause increased ICP and to evaluate therapeutic options. Other tests that may be used include cerebral angiography, EEG, cerebral blood flow, transcranial Doppler studies, near-infrared spectroscopy for regional cerebral oxygenation, and evoked potential studies. Positron emission tomography (PET) may prove to be even more helpful in diagnosing the cause of increased ICP. In general, a lumbar puncture is not performed when increased ICP is suspected because of the possibility of cerebral herniation from the sudden release of the pressure in the skull from the area above the lumbar puncture.

Collaborative Care

The goals of collaborative care (see Table 54-5) are to identify and treat the underlying cause of increased ICP and to support brain function. A careful history is an important diagnostic aid that can direct the search for the underlying cause.

The emergency management of the patient with actual or potential increased ICP is important to prevent secondary injury to the brain (Table 54-6). Once the patient has been transported to a hospital, aggressive collaborative care is needed.

While the cause of increased ICP is being sought, the condition itself must be treated aggressively to interrupt the cycle. Ensuring adequate oxygenation to support brain function is the first step in the management of increased ICP. An endotracheal tube or tracheostomy may be necessary to maintain adequate ventilation. Arterial blood gas (ABG) analysis guides the oxygen therapy. The goal is to maintain the PaO_2 at 100 mm Hg or greater. It may be necessary to maintain the patient on a mechanical ventilator to ensure adequate oxygenation.

If the condition is caused by a mass lesion, such as a tumor or hematoma, surgical removal of the mass is the best management (see Intracranial Tumors later in this chapter). Nonsurgical intervention for the reduction of tissue volume related to cerebral tissue swelling and cerebral edema includes the use of diuretics and corticosteroids and fluid restriction.

Drug Therapy. Drug therapy plays an important part in the management of increased ICP. Osmotic and loop diuretics are used to reduce the volume of brain water. Corticosteroids are thought to control the vasogenic edema surrounding tumors and abscesses but appear to have limited value in the management of head-injured patients.[7]

Osmotic diuretics. Osmotically active agents have been used for more than 50 years to treat cerebral tissue swelling. The principle governing the use of hypertonic solutions is the removal of fluid from the cerebral tissues in response to a vascular osmotic gradient established between the brain and the intravascular compartment. To be effective, the agent must remain in the

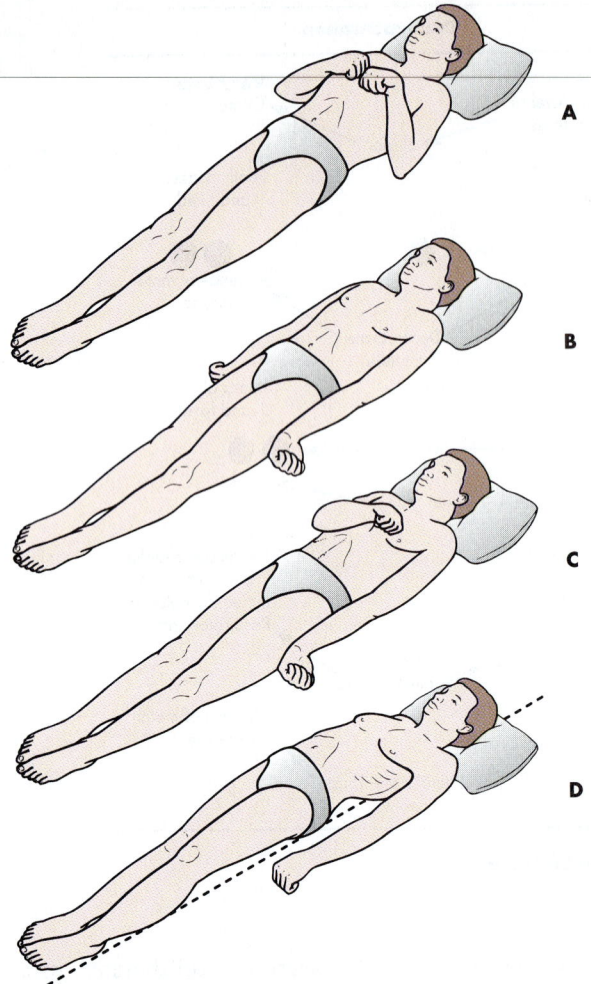

Fig. 54-7 Decorticate and decerebrate posturing. **A,** Decorticate response. Flexion of arms, wrists, and fingers with adduction in upper extremities. Extension, internal rotation, and plantar flexion in lower extremities. **B,** Decerebrate response. All four extremities in rigid extension, with hyperpronation of forearms and plantar extension of feet. **C,** Decorticate response on right side of body and decerebrate response on left side of body. **D,** Opisthotonic posturing.

COLLABORATIVE CARE

Table 54-5   Increased Intracranial Pressure

Diagnostic
 History and physical examination
 Vital signs, neurologic checks, ICP measurements (via intraventricular catheter, subdural bolt, or epidural transducer) every hour
 Skull, chest, and spinal x-ray studies
 MRI, CT scan, EEG, angiography
 Cerebral blood flow and velocity studies, PET
 Laboratory studies, including CBC, coagulation profile, electrolytes, creatinine, ABGs, ammonia level, general drug and toxicology screen, CSF protein, cells, and glucose
 ECG

Collaborative Therapy
 Elevation of head of bed to 30 degrees with head in a neutral position
 Intubation and controlled ventilation to $PaCO_2$ of 30 to 35 mm Hg
 Good pulmonary toilet
 Maintenance of fluid balance and assessment of osmolality
 Maintenance of systolic arterial pressure between 100 and 160 mm Hg
 Maintenance of CPP > 70 mm Hg
 Maintenance of PaO_2 at 100 mm Hg or greater
 Maintenance of normothermia
 Adequate sedation
 Drug therapy
  Osmotic diuretics (mannitol)
  Loop diuretics (furosemide [Lasix], ethacrynic acid [Edecrin])
  Corticosteroids (methylprednisone, dexamethasone [Decadron])
  GI ulcer prophylactics (H_2-receptor antagonist, e.g., cimetidine [Tagamet])
 ICP monitoring

ABGs, arterial blood gases; *CBC,* complete blood count; *CPP,* cerebral perfusion pressure; *CSF,* cerebrospinal fluid; *CT,* computerized tomography; *ECG,* electrocardiogram; *EEG,* electroencephalogram; *ICP,* intracranial pressure; *MRI,* magnetic resonance imaging; *PaCO₂,* partial pressure of arterial carbon dioxide; *PaO₂,* partial pressure of arterial oxygen; *PET,* positron emission tomography.

intravascular compartment. In cases of brain injury and damage to the blood-brain barrier, the osmotic withdrawal is from normal tissue, where the vessels and blood-brain barrier are intact, rather than from edematous tissue. The beneficial effects must therefore be attributed to a decrease in the bulk of the normal tissue. However, if a major disruption of the blood-brain barrier occurs, this form of therapy may be more harmful than beneficial, because the hypertonic solution can pass into the edematous tissue and lead to a rebound phenomenon.

Agents such as mannitol (Osmitrol), glycerol, and urea are available for use in osmotherapy. Mannitol (25%) is the most widely used agent and is given intravenously in doses ranging from 0.25 to 1 g/kg. For optimal effect, rapid administration with attention to preventing fluid overload is recommended. Mannitol acts to decrease the ICP in two ways: plasma expansion and osmotic effect. There is an immediate plasma-expanding effect whereby there is a reduction in the hematocrit and blood

viscosity that increases cerebral blood flow and cerebral oxygen delivery. The osmotic effect is delayed 15 to 30 minutes until gradients across cerebral vessels and tissues are reestablished. Thus the ICP is altered by a decrease in the total brain water content. Fluid and electrolyte status must be monitored when these drugs are used. Mannitol may be contraindicated if renal disease is present and if serum osmolality is elevated.[8]

Loop diuretics. Loop diuretics such as furosemide (Lasix), bumetanide (Bumex), and ethacrynic acid (Edecrin) may also be used in the management of increased ICP. These diuretics inhibit sodium and chloride reabsorption in the ascending limb of the loop of Henle and thus reduce blood volume and ultimately tissue volume. In addition these agents cause a reduction in the rate of CSF production, which also contributes to the reduction in ICP.[9]

Corticosteroid therapy. Corticosteroid therapy has been used extensively in the treatment of cerebral edema. The mode

+**EMERGENCY MANAGEMENT**

Table **54-6**	**Unconscious Patient**	
Etiology	**Assessment Findings**	**Interventions**

Trauma
  Head and neck trauma
Infection
  Meningitis
  Encephalitis
Poison
  Drug overdose
  Toxic exposure
  Carbon monoxide
Metabolic
  Diabetic coma
  Insulin shock
  Liver failure
  Uremia
  Cardiac arrest
  Cerebrovascular accident
	▪ Unresponsive to voice and pain
	▪ Dilated or pinpoint pupils, may be unreactive
	▪ Involuntary movements
	▪ Flaccidity or rigidity of muscles
	▪ Depressed or hyperactive reflexes
	▪ Decerebrate or decorticate posturing
	▪ Diaphoresis
	▪ Hyperthermia
	▪ Flushed, dry skin
	▪ Glasgow Coma Score <12
	▪ Abnormal vital signs
	▪ Arrhythmias
	▪ Odor of alcohol, acetone on breath
	▪ Track marks
	▪ Signs of trauma
	▪ Petechiae or rash
		Initial
		▪ Ensure patent airway.
		▪ Administer oxygen via nasal cannula or non-rebreather mask.
		▪ Establish IV access with one large-bore catheter and normal saline.
		▪ Administer IV naloxone if narcotic overdose suspected.
		▪ Administer thiamine to malnourished or known alcoholic patient to prevent Wernicke's encephalopathy.
		▪ Administer one vial 50% dextrose if blood glucose <60 mg/dl (3.3 mmol/L).
		▪ Prepare for IV insulin administration if glucose >400 mg/dl (22.2 mmol/L).
		▪ Elevate head of bed or position on side to prevent aspiration (unless trauma involved).
		Ongoing Monitoring
		▪ Monitor vital signs, level of consciousness, oxygen saturation, cardiac rhythm, Glasgow Coma Score, pupil size and reactivity, respiratory status.
		▪ Anticipate need for intubation if gag reflex is absent.
		▪ Anticipate gastric lavage if drug overdose is suspected.

of action of corticosteroids is not completely known. It is theorized that they act by their stabilizing effect on the cell membrane and by inhibiting the synthesis of arachidonic acid from cell membranes, thus preventing the formation of proinflammatory mediators.[9] Corticosteroids are also thought to improve neuronal function by improving cerebral blood flow and restoring autoregulation.

Dexamethasone (Decadron), a semisynthetic corticosteroid, is the most commonly used steroid. Corticosteroids are most beneficial in patients who have cerebral edema from vasogenic causes such as brain tumors with peritumoral edema. However, evidence for the efficacy of corticosteroid therapy in trauma or hemorrhage is limited. Clinical trials involving corticosteroid therapy in severe head injury were conducted in the 1980s. Overall these studies demonstrated that corticosteroid therapy did not improve outcomes. However, there were subpopulations that did improve, and these findings warrant further investigation.[10,11]

Complications associated with the use of corticosteroids include hyperglycemia, increased incidence of infections, and gastrointestinal (GI) bleeding. Patients receiving corticosteroids should concurrently be given antacids or histamine H_2 receptor blockers such as cimetidine (Tagamet) or famotidine (Pepcid) to prevent GI bleeding. Fluid intake should be monitored because of the potential for hyponatremia. Since hyperglycemia has also been associated with corticosteroid use, glucose levels of the blood and urine should be monitored regularly.

Other drug therapies. Drug therapy for reducing cerebral metabolism may be an effective strategy to control ICP. The reduction in the metabolic rate decreases the cerebral blood flow and therefore the ICP. High-dose barbiturates (e.g., pento-

barbital and thiopental) are used in patients with increased ICP refractory to treatment. Barbiturates produce a decrease in cerebral metabolism and a subsequent decrease in increased ICP. A secondary effect is a reduction in cerebral edema and production of a more uniform blood supply to the brain.[12] Capabilities to monitor the patient's ICP, blood flow, and metabolism should be available when this treatment is used. Other agents may also be used in the management of ICP. These include the antiseizure agent phenytoin (Dilantin) because seizures can further increase ICP.

Hyperventilation Therapy. In the past, aggressive hyperventilation ($PaCO_2$ <25 mm Hg) has been a mainstay treatment of elevated ICP. The lowering of the $PaCO_2$ leads to constriction of the cerebral blood vessels, reducing cerebral blood flow and thereby decreasing the ICP. More recent evidence suggests that aggressive hyperventilation increases the risk of focal cerebral ischemia and may adversely affect outcomes.[13] Prolonged aggressive hyperventilation therapy should be avoided in the absence of increased intracranial pressure, particularly during the first 24 hours following a head injury or when cerebral blood flow (CBF) is low. Brief periods of hyperventilation therapy may be useful for refractory intracranial hypertension.[13]

Nutritional Therapy. All patients must have their nutritional needs met, regardless of their state of consciousness or health. Early enteral feeding following brain injury improves outcomes.[14] The patient with increased ICP is in a hypermetabolic and hypercatabolic state and in need of glucose to provide the necessary fuel for the metabolism of the injured brain. If the patient cannot maintain an adequate oral intake, other means of meeting the nutritional requirements, such as enteral feedings or total parenteral nutrition, should be initiated. Nutritional replacements should begin within 3 days after injury in order to reach full nutritional replacement within 7 days after injury.[14] (Nutritional therapy is discussed in Chapter 38.) Because certain types of feedings are low in sodium, added salt may be necessary. In addition to added minerals, free water may also be needed to meet the fluid needs of the patient. Because malnutrition promotes continued cerebral edema, maintenance of optimal nutrition is imperative.

It is controversial as to whether patients should be maintained in a state of moderate dehydration. On one hand, moderate dehydration is thought to be effective in reducing cerebral edema; in this case fluids are restricted to 65% to 75% of normal requirements. However, the concern is that hypovolemia may result in a decrease in cardiac output and blood pressure, which may have an impact on cerebral perfusion and the amount of oxygen delivered to the brain. There is additional concern that dehydrated patients do not respond well to vasoactive drugs. Because of this the current therapy is directed at keeping patients normovolemic. The use of fluid restriction to reduce tissue volume should be evaluated on the basis of clinical factors such as urine output, insensible fluid loss, serum and urine osmolality, and the condition of the patient.

A lowering of serum osmolarity and an increase in cerebral edema occur if 5% dextrose in water is used for the administration of piggyback medications. If an intravenous (IV) drug routine is used, 0.45% or 0.9% sodium chloride is the preferred solution.

NURSING MANAGEMENT: INCREASED IN-TRACRANIAL PRESSURE

Regardless of the cause of unconsciousness, the unconscious patient is managed with the assumption that the ICP is increased or has the potential to increase. The primary goals of nursing management are to (1) prevent secondary cerebral damage, (2) maintain function, and (3) prevent complications secondary to immobility and decreased LOC.

■ Nursing Assessment

Subjective data about the unconscious patient can be obtained from family members or other persons who are familiar with the patient. Events preceding the unconscious state should be investigated. Figure 54-1 presents a systematic approach to the assessment of the unconscious patient. This information, together with data for the Glasgow Coma Scale (see Table 54-2), provides the base of knowledge on which a nursing care plan can be formulated.

Ongoing assessment and recording of the ICP is important for evaluating trends and responses to nursing care. Figure 54-8 illustrates a typical neurologic clinical flow sheet used to display a patient's neurologic status over time.

The general plan of the neurologic assessment is to evaluate the patient's mental status, cranial nerve functioning, motor functioning, sensory status, cerebellar functioning, and reflexes. This schema helps the nurse organize the assessment to gather the data needed (see Chapter 53 for a discussion of the neurologic assessment). If the patient is critically ill, an abbreviated neurologic assessment using the GCS, pupillary checks, and certain cranial nerve evaluations is made by the nurse on an ongoing basis.

The pupils are compared to one another for size, movement, and response (Fig. 54-9). If the oculomotor nerve is compressed by supratentorial pressure, the pupil on the affected side (ipsilateral) becomes larger until it fully dilates. If ICP continues to increase, both pupils dilate.

Pupillary reaction is tested with a flashlight. The normal reaction is brisk constriction when the light is shone directly into the eye. A consensual response (a slight constriction in the opposite pupil) should also be noted at the same time. A sluggish reaction can indicate early pressure on CN III. A fixed pupil shows no response to light stimulus, which usually indicates increased ICP.

Evaluation of other cranial nerves can be included in the neurologic check. Eye movements controlled by cranial nerves III, IV, and VI can be examined in the patient who is awake and can be used to assess the function of the brainstem. In the unconscious patient, extraocular eye movements are not specifically tested. Testing the corneal reflex gives information on the functioning of cranial nerves V and VII. If this reflex is absent, routine eye care should be initiated to prevent corneal abrasion (see Chapters 19 and 20).

Eye movements of the uncooperative or unconscious patient can be elicited by reflex with the use of head movements (oculocephalic) and caloric stimulation (oculovestibular) (see Chapters 19 and 20). To test the oculocephalic reflex (doll's head or doll's eyes phenomenon), the nurse rotates the patient's head briskly while holding the eyelids open. A positive response is movement of the eyes across the midline in the direction opposite that of the rotation. Next, the nurse quickly flexes and then extends the neck. Eye movement should be opposite to the direction of head movement—up when the neck is flexed and down when it is extended. Abnormal responses can aid in locating the intracranial lesion. This test should not be attempted if a cervical spine problem is suspected. (The oculovestibular reflex is discussed in Chapter 19.)

Motor strength is tested by asking the patient who is awake to squeeze the nurse's hands to compare strength in the hands. The palmar drift test is an excellent measure of strength in the upper extremities. The patient raises the arms in front of the body with the palmar surface facing upward. If there is any weakness in the upper extremity, the palmar surface turns downward and the arm drifts downward. Asking the patient to raise the foot from the bed or to bend the knees up in bed is a good assessment of lower extremity strength. All four extremities should be tested for strength and evaluated for any asymmetry in strength or movement.

The motor strength of the unconscious or uncooperative patient can be assessed by observation of spontaneous movement. If no spontaneous movement is possible, a pain stimulus should be applied to the patient, and the response should be noted. Resistance to movement during passive range-of-motion exercises is another measure of strength.

The vital signs, including blood pressure, pulse, respiratory rate, and temperature, should also be systematically

Neurologic Assessment Record

	Date ⟶																				
	Time ⟶																				
Eyes open	Spontaneously																		Eyes closed by swelling = C		
	To speech																				
	To pain																				
	None																				
Best verbal response	Oriented																		Endotracheal tube or tracheostomy = T		
	Confused																				
	Inappropriate																				
	Incomprehensible																				
	None																				
Best motor response	Obey commands																		Usually record the best arm response Agitated = A		
	Localize pain																				
	Flexion to pain																				
	Extension to pain																				
	None																				
Vital signs	Blood pressure																				
	Pulse																				
	Respiration																				
	Temperature																				
Pupils react = + No reaction = − Eye closed = C	**R** Size																				
	Reaction																				
	L Size																				
	Reaction																				
Limb movement	Right upper																				
	Right lower																				
	Left upper																				
	Left lower																				
	Intake																				
	Output																				

(left margin label: **Coma scale**)

Pupil scale (mm):
• 1   ● 6
• 2   ● 7
• 3   ● 8
• 4
• 5

Pupil scale (mm)

0. No evidence of muscle contraction.
1. Palpable muscle movement — no joint motion.
2. Complete motion without gravity.
3. Barely complete motion against gravity.
4. Complete motion against gravity with some resistance.
5. Complete motion against gravity with full resistance.
F — Abnormal flexion
E — Abnormal extension

Fig. 54-8 Neurologic clinical flow sheet.

recorded. The nurse must be aware of Cushing's triad, since this indicates severe increased ICP. Besides recording respiratory rate, the nurse should also note the respiratory pattern (Fig. 54-10).

■ Nursing Diagnoses

The nursing diagnoses are supported by the data obtained on assessment and include those associated with increased ICP and unconsciousness. Patients with one or both of these serious problems require the highest level of nursing care because they are usually totally dependent on the nurse. Nursing diagnoses related to the unconscious patient are presented in NCP 54-1.

■ Planning

The overall goals are that the patient with increased ICP and unconsciousness will (1) have decreased ICP to within normal limits, (2) maintain a patent airway, and (3) demonstrate normal fluid and electrolyte balance.

■ Nursing Implementation
Acute Intervention

Maintenance of respiratory function. Maintenance of a patent airway is critical in the patient with increased ICP and is a primary nursing responsibility. As the LOC decreases, the patient is at increased risk of airway obstruction from the tongue

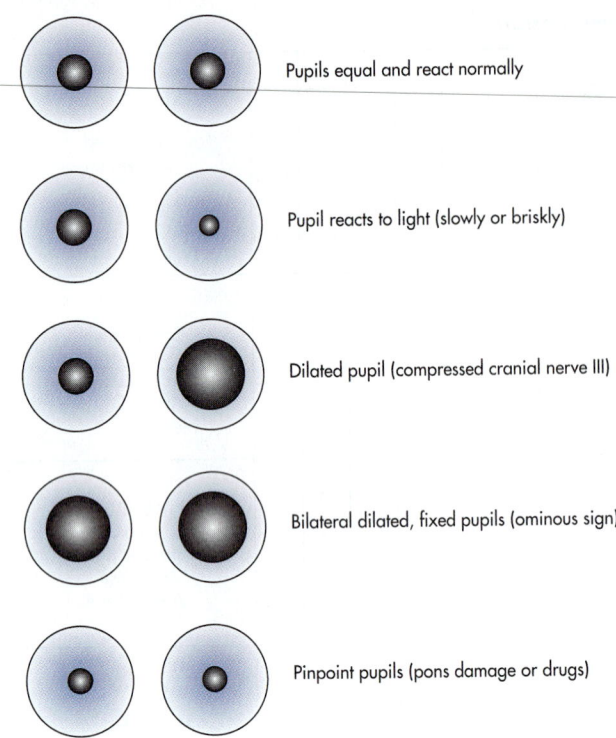

Fig. 54-9 Pupillary check for size and response.

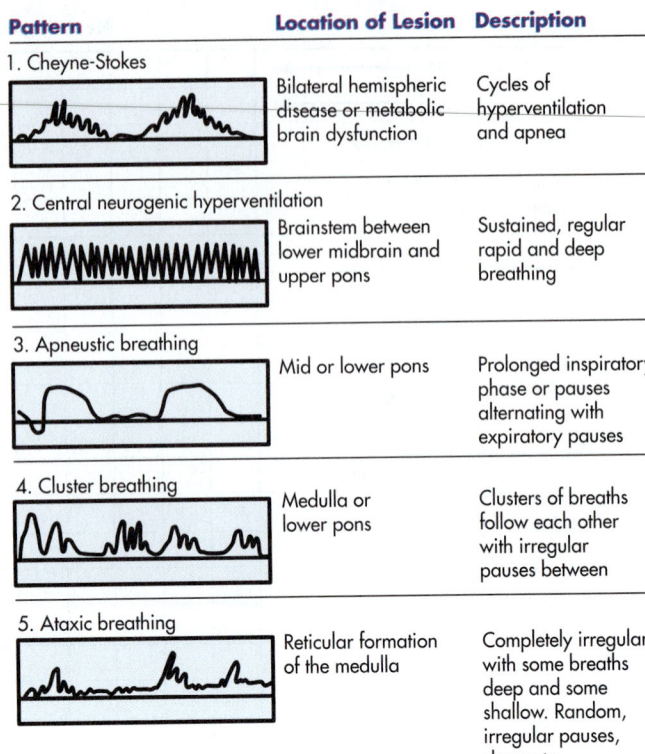

Fig. 54-10 Common abnormal respiratory patterns associated with coma.

dropping back and occluding the airway or from accumulation of secretions. Altered breathing patterns may become evident. Airway patency can be aided by keeping the patient lying on one side, with frequent position changes. Snoring sounds, which may indicate obstruction, should be noted. Accumulated secretions should be removed by suctioning, as needed. An oral airway facilitates breathing and provides an easier suctioning route in the comatose patient.

The nurse must use measures to prevent hypoxia and hypercapnia. Proper positioning of the head is important. Elevation of the head of the bed by 30 degrees enhances respiratory exchange and aids in decreasing cerebral edema. Suctioning and coughing can cause transient decreases in the PaO_2 and increases in the ICP. Suctioning should be kept to a minimum and should be less than 10 seconds in duration, with administration of 100% oxygen before and after to prevent decreases in the PaO_2.[15] To avoid cumulative increases in the ICP with suctioning, suctioning should be limited to two passes per suction procedure. Patients with elevated ICP are at risk for lower CPP during suctioning.[16]

Abdominal distention can interfere with respiratory function and should be prevented. Insertion of a nasogastric tube to aspirate the stomach contents can prevent distention, vomiting, and possible aspiration.

ABGs should be measured and evaluated regularly (see Chapter 24). The appropriate ventilatory support can be ordered on the basis of the PaO_2 and $PaCO_2$ values. The nurse should be aware if moderate hyperventilation ($PaCO_2$ of 30 to 35 mm Hg) is desired.

Unless the patient is on ventilatory support, the use of narcotic sedatives and opiates should be evaluated on an individual basis. Besides depressing respirations, these agents can also cloud the patient's LOC. A narcotic that does not increase the ICP, depress respiration, or cloud LOC should be selected to control pain. A nonnarcotic analgesic can be used in the patient with an increased ICP for an extended period of time. Agitation and restlessness should be evaluated, and appropriate drugs should be used, if indicated. Narcotics and opiates may be used in a patient on a mechanical ventilator who is also undergoing ICP monitoring. At times it may even be necessary to use paralytic agents such as pancuronium (Pavulon) or curare to ensure optimal ventilatory support (see Chapter 63). The patient should then be fully monitored.

Fluid and electrolyte balance. Fluid and electrolyte disturbances can have an adverse effect on ICP. IV fluids should be closely monitored with the use of a limited-volume device or a volume-control apparatus for accuracy. Intake and output, with insensible losses and daily weights taken into account, are important parameters in the assessment of fluid balance.

Electrolyte determinations should be made daily, and any abnormal values should be discussed with the physician. It is especially important to monitor serum glucose, sodium, potassium, and osmolality. Urinary output is monitored to detect problems related to diabetes insipidus (e.g., increased urinary output related to a decrease in antidiuretic hormone secretion) and SIADH, which results in decreased urinary output. Besides urinary output, the serum sodium and osmolality are also used to diagnose diabetes insipidus and SIADH. Diabetes insipidus may result in severe dehydration unless treated. The usual treatment is fluid replacement, vasopressin (Pitressin), or desmopressin acetate (DDAVP) (see Chapter 47). SIADH results in a dilutional hyponatremia that may produce cerebral edema, changes in LOC, seizures, and coma. (Treatment of SIADH is described in Chapter 47.)

54-1   NURSING CARE PLAN   UNCONSCIOUS PATIENT

Expected Patient Outcomes   Nursing Interventions and *Rationales*

NURSING DIAGNOSIS **Ineffective airway clearance** *related to* unconsciousness and inability to mobilize secretions *as manifested by* ineffective cough, inability to clear secretions, crackles on auscultation, thick secretions.

- Demonstration of increased air exchange as measured by ABGs within normal limits.
- Normal breath sounds in all lobes of the lungs.

- Maintain patient's side-lying position, keeping head of bed elevated *to prevent aspiration and tongue from blocking airway and to assist in decreasing cerebral edema.*
- Suction as needed *to remove accumulated secretions, reduce risk of aspiration, and ensure patent airway.*
- Perform chest physical therapy at least q4hr *to improve ventilation and prevent pulmonary complications.*
- Monitor patient for signs of decreased oxygenation, including changes in LOC, decreased PaO_2 or SaO_2, and increased respiratory rate and cyanosis *because low PaO_2 and a high hydrogen ion concentration (acidosis) are potent cerebral vasodilators that increase cerebral flow and may increase ICP.*

NURSING DIAGNOSIS **Altered tissue perfusion: cerebral** *related to* cerebral tissue swelling *as manifested by* mental state, intracranial pressure > 20 mm Hg, CPP < 60 mm Hg, decreased cerebral blood flow or oximetry.

- No further deterioration in LOC.
- ICP < 20 mm Hg, CPP > 60 mm Hg.
- Stable vital signs.

- Monitor patient's neurologic status at least every hour initially; assess level of consciousness and document *to evaluate patient's response to treatment and modify if necessary.*
- Monitor ICP and calculate CPP *to evaluate adequacy of cerebral blood perfusion, detect patient's response to treatment, and provide information necessary for clinical decisions.*
- Limit care activities that increase ICP (e.g., suctioning, hip flexion) *to prevent increases in ICP.*
- Provide comfort measures *because pain or agitation increases ICP.*
- Elevate head of bed 30 to 45 degrees *to facilitate reduction of cerebral edema.*
- Maintain the $PaCO_2$ at 30 to 35 mm Hg when ICP > 20 mm Hg *because CO_2 is a potent cerebral vasodilator and hyperventilation reduces $PaCO_2$.*
- Monitor level of cerebral oximetry and read cerebral blood flow reports *to ensure that global and regional cerebral oxygenation are maintained.*
- Monitor reactions to all medications (especially diuretics and sedatives) *to evaluate for signs (change in LOC) of reduced cerebral edema.*
- Calibrate and maintain intracranial monitoring device *to provide an accurate indicator of ICP.*

NURSING DIAGNOSIS **Altered nutrition: less than body requirements** *related to* hypermetabolism and inability to ingest food and fluids *as manifested by* inability to feed self, hyperthermia (>101° F [38.3° C]), metabolic needs in excess of intake, weight loss.

- Adequate caloric intake to maintain weight.
- Maintenance of weight within 5 lb (2.3 kg) of admission weight.

- Assess fluid status and document intake and output hourly initially *to evaluate adequacy of renal perfusion and indicators of fluid balance.*
- Assess skin turgor *as an indicator of fluid balance.*
- Monitor electrolytes *to identify electrolyte imbalances and initiate treatment.*
- Weigh patient daily *as an indicator of fluid balance and nutritional status.*
- Maintain oral fluid restrictions as ordered *because pharyngeal reflex may be absent and patient may be unable to swallow.*
- Evaluate swallowing abilities *to reduce risk of aspiration when oral intake is resumed.*
- Advance patient to high-protein, high-caloric feedings (enteral or oral) as indicated *to provide nutrients needed to prevent wasting and negative nitrogen balance.*
- Auscultate bowel sounds before feeding *to ensure presence of peristalsis.*
- Elevate head of bed during and after feedings *to reduce risk of regurgitation and aspiration.*
- Provide adequate free water if not contraindicated *to maintain a high fluid intake.*

Continued

54-1   **NURSING CARE PLAN**   **UNCONSCIOUS PATIENT**—continued

Expected Patient Outcomes   **Nursing Interventions and *Rationales***

NURSING DIAGNOSIS   **Risk for impaired skin integrity** *related to* nutritional deficit, self-care deficit, and immobility.

- Absence of skin breakdown.
- Intact skin.

- Assess skin frequently, especially over bony prominences and around genitalia and buttocks, *to identify potential or actual skin problems and initiate a plan of care.*
- Turn patient at least q2hr as indicated *because prolonged pressure decreases capillary circulation and leads to tissue hypoxia and necrosis.*
- Provide fluids *to prevent dehydration.*
- Use low-air-loss beds as indicated *to reduce pressure to bony prominences by distributing body weight evenly.*
- Cleanse all abrasions and lacerations; massage skin as indicated *to reduce risk of infection and stimulate circulation.*

NURSING DIAGNOSIS   **Risk of infection** *related to* immobility, invasive monitoring devices and lines, and compromised immune system.

- No wound infections.
- Normal temperature, white blood cell count, and chest x-ray.

- Assess for hyperthermia (temperature > 101° F [38.4° C]), exudate around catheter insertion sites (IV, indwelling, intracranial), lethargy, abnormal chest x-ray and breath sounds, foul-smelling urine *to determine if risk factors for infection are present.*
- Observe strict sterile technique when assisting with insertion and maintenance of ICP-monitoring devices and all invasive lines; maintain integrity of all closed systems *to prevent introduction of bacteria.*

Monitoring of intracranial pressure. In 1960 Lundberg refined a technique for the continuous monitoring of ICP by insertion of a catheter into the ventricles.[17] Over the last 35 years, the technology for monitoring ICP has improved greatly and is now regularly used in patients with suspected increased ICP who may benefit from treatment and in whom the underlying process is thought to be self-limiting. Patients with irreversible pathologic processes or advanced neurologic decline caused by primary or metastatic lesions may not be monitored. The measurement of ICP is valuable in detecting the early rise of ICP and the patient's response to treatment and in providing information necessary for clinical decisions.

There are four basic systems used to monitor ICP: a ventricular pressure monitoring system, a subarachnoid pressure monitoring system, an epidural pressure monitoring system, and an intraparenchymal pressure monitoring system. These methods are discussed in detail in Chapter 63.

Prevention of infection. Prevention of infection by use of strict aseptic technique during dressing changes or sampling of CSF is imperative. Maintenance of the intactness of the system is critical to ensure that the ICP readings are accurate, since treatment is initiated on basis of the level of the pressures.

Body position. The patient with increased ICP should be maintained in the head-up position. The nurse must take care to prevent extreme neck flexion, which can cause venous obstruction and contribute to increased ICP. The body position should be adjusted to decrease the ICP maximally and to improve the CPP. Traditional practice has been to elevate the head of the bed to at least 30 degrees, unless a concurrent cervical neck injury has been identified. Research now suggests there is

an inconsistent response of the ICP and the CPP to head elevation.[18,19] Elevation of the head of the bed reduces sagittal sinus pressure, promotes venous drainage from the head via the valveless jugular system, and decreases the vascular congestion that can produce cerebral edema. However, raising the head of the bed may decrease the CPP. There is no evidence, however, that head-of-bed elevation decreases cerebral tissue oxygenation. Careful evaluation of the effects of elevation of the head of the bed on both the ICP and the CPP is required. The bed should be positioned so that it lowers the ICP while maintaining the CPP and other indices of cerebral oxygenation.

Care should be taken to turn the patient with slow, gentle movements because rapid changes in position may increase the ICP. Continuous rotation bed therapy allows for frequent position changes and does not increase ICP.[20] Caution should be used to prevent discomfort in turning and positioning the patient because pain or agitation also increases pressure. Increased intrathoracic pressure also contributes to increased ICP by impeding the venous return; thus coughing, straining, and Valsalva's maneuver should be avoided. Extreme hip flexion should be avoided in order to decrease the risk of raising the intraabdominal pressure, which can restrict movement of the diaphragm and cause respiratory distress. The patient should be turned at least every 2 hours.

Decorticate or decerebrate posturing is a reflex response in some patients with increased ICP. Turning, skin care, and even passive range of motion can elicit the posturing reflexes. Attempts should be made to provide needed physical care activities to minimize complications of immobility, such as atelectasis and contractures. In cases of severe posturing reflexes, these

Table 54-7	Etiologic Factors for Increased Intracranial Pressure

- Hypercapnia ($PaCO_2$ >45 mm Hg)
- Hypoxemia (PaO_2 <60 mm Hg)
- Cerebral vasodilating agents (e.g., halothane, antihistamines)
- Valsalva's maneuver
- Body positions (e.g., prone position, flexion of neck, extreme hip flexion)
- Isometric muscle contractions
- Coughing or sneezing
- Rapid-eye-movement sleep
- Emotional upset
- Noxious stimuli
- Arousal from sleep
- Clustering of activities

activities may have to be done less frequently because posturing can cause increases in ICP.

Protection from injury and environmental management. The patient with increased ICP and a decreased LOC needs protection from self-injury. Confusion, agitation, and the possibility of seizures can put the patient at risk of injury. Restraints should be used judiciously in the agitated patient. If restraints are absolutely necessary to keep the patient from removing tubes or falling out of bed, they should be secure enough to be effective, and the skin area under the restraints should be observed regularly for irritation. Agitation may increase with the use of restraints, which indicates the need for other measures to protect the patient from injury. Light sedation with agents such as haloperidol (Haldol) or lorazepam (Ativan) may be needed. Having a family member stay with the patient may have a calming effect. For the patient with seizures or the patient at risk of seizure activity, seizure precautions should be instituted. They include padded side rails, an airway at the bedside, accurate and timely administration of antiseizure medications, and close observation.

The patient can benefit from a quiet, nonstimulating environment. The nurse should always use a calm, reassuring approach. Touching and talking to the patient, even one who is in a coma, is always an appropriate care approach. The nurse must create a balance between sensory deprivation and sensory overload for the patient with increased ICP.

Contributory factors to increased intracranial pressure. There is a relationship between nursing care activities and increases in ICP. Table 54-7 lists some of the factors that have been identified as contributors to increased ICP. Nurses should be alert to these factors and should attempt to minimize them. Nursing management of the patient with increased ICP is one of the most important aspects of the care provided these patients.

Psychologic considerations. Besides the carefully planned physical care provided patients with increased ICP, the nurse must also be aware of the psychologic well-being of the patients and their families. Anxiety over the diagnosis and the prognosis for the patient with neurologic problems can be distressing to the patient, the family, and the nursing staff. The nurse's competent and assured manner in performing the care needed

RESEARCH
IMPLICATIONS FOR NURSING PRACTICE

Impact of Critical Injury on the Family

Citation Leske JS, Jiricka MK: Impact of family demands and family strengths and capabilities on family well-being and adaptation after critical injury, *Am J Crit Care* 7:383, 1998.

Purpose To examine family demands, including prior stressors and severity of patient's injuries, and family strengths and capabilities, including hardiness, coping, problem solving, and on outcomes of family well-being and adaptation after critical illness.

Methods Family members of 21 intensive care unit (ICU) patients were interviewed using standardized questionnaires related to family demands, family strengths and capabilities, family resources, coping, problem-solving communication, and family adaptation outcomes. Patients were admitted to the ICU as a result of injuries from gunshot wounds or motor vehicle accident. The majority of the 21 patients were male (71%), and the majority of the 51 family members interviewed were female (73%).

Results and Conclusions There was no significant relationship between severity of the patient's injury and the family outcomes of well-being and adaptation. Increases in prior stressors, strains, and transitions were negatively related to family outcomes. In addition, family hardiness, resources, coping, and problem-solving communication were positively related to family adaptation scores.

Implications for Nursing Practice Nurses play an important role in helping families adjust to sudden, critical illness. In this role, the nurse must be aware of the negative impact of the patient's condition on the family so that planning for assistance of the family can be initiated. Vulnerable families should be identified early. Increased communication between the family members and health care providers may enhance understanding and decrease family tensions.

by the patient is reassuring to everyone involved. Short, simple explanations are appropriate and allow the patient and the family to acquire the amount of information they desire. There is a need for support, information, and education of both patients and families that begins with the traumatic event and continues for years after the event. The nurse should assess the family members' desire and need to assist in providing care for the patient and allow for their participation as appropriate.

■ Evaluation

The expected outcomes are that the unconscious patient will
- have ICP within normal limits
- maintain a patent airway
- exhibit no manifestations of infection
- demonstrate normal fluid and electrolyte and nutrition balance
- have no evidence of skin breakdown

Table **54-8**	Types of Skull Fractures	
Description		**Cause**
Linear		
Break in continuity of bone without alteration of relationship of parts		Low-velocity injuries
Depressed		
Inward indentation of skull		Powerful blow
Simple		
Linear or depressed skull fracture without fragmentation or communicating lacerations		Low to moderate impact
Comminuted		
Multiple linear fractures with fragmentation of bone into many pieces		Direct, high-momentum impact
Compound		
Depressed skull fracture and scalp laceration with communicating pathway to intracranial cavity		Severe head injury

Table **54-9**	Clinical Manifestations of Skull Fractures by Location
Location	**Syndrome or Sequelae**
Frontal fracture	Exposure of brain to contaminants through frontal air sinus; possible association with air in forehead tissue, CSF rhinorrhea, or pneumocranium
Orbital fracture	Periorbital ecchymosis (raccoon eyes)
Temporal fracture	Boggy temporal muscle because of extravasation of blood, benign oval-shaped bruise behind ear in mastoid region (Battle's sign), CSF otorrhea
Parietal fracture	Deafness, CSF or brain otorrhea, bulging of tympanic membrane caused by blood or CSF, facial paralysis, loss of taste, Battle's sign
Posterior fossa fracture	Occipital bruising resulting in cortical blindness, visual field defects; rare appearance of ataxia or other cerebellar signs
Basilar skull fracture	CSF or brain otorrhea, bulging of tympanic membrane caused by blood or CSF, Battle's sign, tinnitus or hearing difficulty, facial paralysis, conjugate deviation of gaze, vertigo

CSF, cerebrospinal fluid.

HEAD TRAUMA

Head injury includes any trauma to the scalp, skull, or brain. The term *head trauma* is used primarily to signify craniocerebral trauma, which includes an alteration in consciousness, no matter how brief.

Head trauma has a high potential for poor outcome.[21] Deaths from head injury trauma occur at three time points after injury: immediately after the injury, within 2 hours after injury, and approximately 3 weeks after injury.[22] The majority of deaths after a head injury occur immediately after the injury, either from the direct head trauma or from massive hemorrhage and shock. Deaths occurring within a few hours of the trauma are caused by progressive worsening of the head injury or from internal bleeding. An immediate note of changes in neurologic status and surgical intervention are critical in the prevention of deaths at this point. Deaths occurring 3 weeks or more after injury result from multisystem failure. Expert nursing care in the weeks following the injury are crucial in decreasing mortality. Factors that predict a poor outcome include the presence of an intracranial hematoma, increasing age of the patient, abnormal motor responses, impaired or absent eye movements or pupil light reflexes, early sustained hypotension, hypoxemia or hypercapnia, and ICP levels higher than 20 mm Hg.[22]

Statistics regarding the occurrence of head injuries are incomplete because many victims die at the scene of the accident or because the condition is considered minor and health care is not sought. An estimated 3 million persons suffer head injuries each year in the United States.[23] The mortality rate related to head injury is 19.3 per 100,000 persons in the United States and represents a 21% decline in fatalities related to head injury since 1976.[24] In the past, motor vehicle accidents and falls were the most common causes of head injury in both Canada and the United States. More recently, in the United States, deaths from motor vehicle accidents and falls have decreased while firearm-related head injury death rates have increased.[24] Other causes include assaults, sports-related injuries, and recreational accidents.

Types of Head Injuries

Scalp Lacerations. Scalp lacerations are the most minor of the head traumas. Because the scalp contains many blood vessels with poor constrictive abilities, most scalp lacerations are associated with profuse bleeding. The major complication associated with scalp laceration is infection.

Skull Fractures. Skull fractures frequently occur with head trauma. There are several ways to describe skull fractures: (1) linear or depressed; (2) simple, comminuted, or compound; and (3) closed or open (Table 54-8). Fractures may be closed or open, depending on the presence of a scalp laceration or extension of the fracture into the air sinuses or dura. The type and severity of a skull fracture depend on the velocity, the momentum, the direction of injuring agent, and the site of impact. Specific manifestations of a skull fracture are generally associated with the location of the injury (Table 54-9).

The location of the fracture alters the presentation of the clinical signs and symptoms. For example, a specialized type of linear fracture is seen when the fracture occurs at the base of the skull, a basilar skull fracture. This fracture generally crosses a sinus and tears the dura (e.g., the frontal or the temporal) and is associated with leakage of CSF. Rhinorrhea (CSF leakage from the nose) or otorrhea (CSF leakage from the ear) generally confirms that the fracture has traversed the dura (Fig. 54-11). Two methods of testing can be used to determine whether the fluid leaking from the nose or ear is CSF. The first method

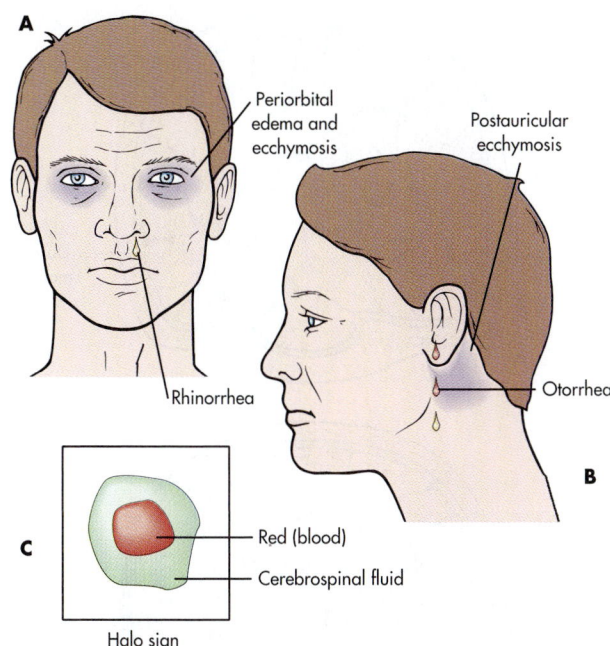

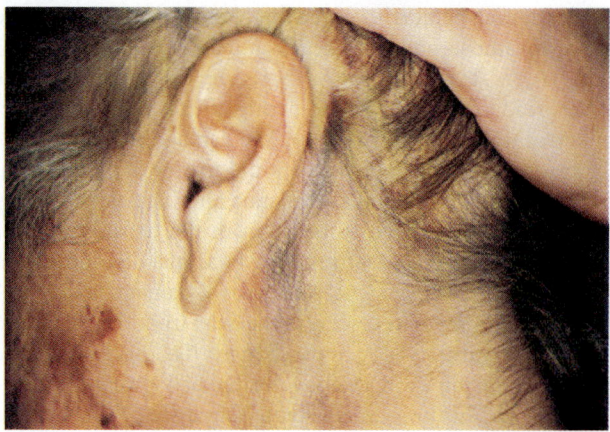

Fig. 54-12   Battle's sign.

Fig. 54-11   **A,** Raccoon eyes and rhinorrhea. **B,** Battle's sign (postauricular ecchymosis) with otorrhea. **C,** Halo or ring sign (see text).

is to test the leaking fluid with a Dextrostix or Tes-tape strip to determine whether glucose is present. CSF gives a positive reading for glucose. If blood is present in the fluid, however, testing for the presence of glucose is unreliable because blood contains glucose. In this event, the nurse should look for the "halo" or "ring" sign (Fig. 54-11, *C*). To perform this test, the nurse allows the leaking fluid to drip onto a white pad (4 × 4) or towel and observes the drainage. Within a few minutes the blood coalesces into the center, and a yellowish ring encircles the blood if CSF is present. The color, appearance, and amount of leaking fluid must be noted because both tests can give false-positive results.

The major potential complications of skull fractures are intracranial infections and hematoma, as well as meningeal and brain tissue damage. A frontal or orbital fracture may have CSF leakage along with periorbital ecchymosis (raccoon eyes). A basal skull fracture may result in ecchymosis of the mastoid process of the temporal bone (Battle's sign) (Fig. 54-11, *B*, and Fig. 54-12), conjunctival hemorrhage, or periorbital edema.

Minor Head Trauma. Brain injuries are categorized as being minor or major. Concussion (a sudden transient mechanical head injury with disruption of neural activity and a change in the LOC) is considered a minor head injury. The patient may not lose total consciousness with this injury.

Signs of concussion include a brief disruption in LOC, amnesia regarding the event (retrograde amnesia), and headache. The manifestations are generally of short duration. If the patient has not lost consciousness, or if the loss of consciousness lasts less than 5 minutes, the patient is usually discharged from the care facility with instructions to notify the physician if symptoms persist or if behavior changes are noted.

The postconcussion syndrome is seen anywhere from 2 weeks to 2 months after the concussion. Symptoms include persistent headache, lethargy, personality and behavior changes, shortened attention span, decreased short-term mem-

ory, and changes in intellectual ability. This syndrome can significantly affect the patient's abilities to perform the activities of daily living.

Although concussion is generally considered benign and usually resolves spontaneously, the symptoms may be the beginning of a more serious, progressive problem. At the time of discharge it is important to give the patient and the family instructions for observation and accurate reporting of symptoms or changes in neurologic status.

Major Head Trauma. Major head trauma includes contusions and lacerations. Both injuries represent severe trauma to the brain. Contusions and lacerations are generally associated with closed injuries.

A *contusion* is the bruising of the brain tissue within a focal area that maintains the integrity of the pia mater and arachnoid layers. A contusion develops areas of necrosis, infarction, hemorrhage, and edema. A contusion frequently occurs at the site of a fracture. With contusion, the phenomenon of coup-contrecoup injury is often noted. Damage from coup-contrecoup injury occurs because of mass movement of the brain inside the skull. Contusions or lacerations occur both at the site of the direct impact of the brain on the skull and at a secondary area of damage on the opposite side away from injury, leading to multiple contused areas. Bleeding around the contusion site is generally minimal, and the blood is reabsorbed slowly. Neurologic assessment demonstrates focal findings and a generalized disturbance in the LOC. Seizures are a common complication of brain contusion.

Lacerations involve actual tearing of the brain tissue and occur frequently in association with depressed and compound fractures and penetrating injuries. Tissue damage is severe, and surgical repair of the laceration is impossible because of the texture of the brain tissue. If bleeding is deep into the brain parenchyma, focal and generalized signs are noted.

When major head trauma occurs, many delayed responses are seen, including hemorrhage, hematoma formation, seizures, and cerebral edema. Intracerebral hemorrhage is generally associated with cerebral laceration. This hemorrhage manifests as a space-occupying lesion accompanied by unconsciousness, hemiplegia on the contralateral side, and a dilated pupil on the ipsilateral side. As the hematoma expands, symptoms of increased ICP become more severe. Prognosis is generally poor for the patient with a large intracerebral hemorrhage.

Subarachnoid hemorrhage and intraventricular hemorrhage can also occur secondary to head trauma.

Diffuse Axonal Injury.
Diffuse axonal injury (DAI) is widespread axonal damage occurring after a mild, moderate, or severe traumatic brain injury. The damage occurs primarily around axons in subcortical white matter of the cerebral hemispheres, basal ganglia, thalamus, and brainstem.[25] Initially, DAI was believed to occur from the tensile forces of trauma that sheared axons resulting in axonal disconnection. There is increasing evidence that axonal damage is not preceded by an immediate tearing of the axon from the traumatic impact but rather the trauma changes the function of the axon, resulting in axon swelling (axonal ballooning) and disconnection. This process takes approximately 12 to 24 hours to develop and may persist longer.

An MRI scan is more sensitive in detecting small DAI lesions than the CT scan because of the lack of gross pathologic changes in brain tissue. The clinical signs and symptoms, including a decreased LOC, increased ICP, decerebration or decortication, and global cerebral edema, are important indicators.

Complications

Epidural Hematoma.
An epidural hematoma results from bleeding between the dura and the inner surface of the skull. An epidural hematoma is a neurologic emergency and is usually associated with a linear fracture crossing a major artery in the dura, causing a tear. It can have a venous or an arterial origin. Venous epidural hematomas are associated with a tear of the dural venous sinus and develop slowly. With arterial hematomas, the middle meningeal artery lying under the temporal bone is frequently torn. Hemorrhage occurs into the epidural space, which lies between the dura and the inner surface of the skull (Fig. 54-13, *A*). Because this is an arterial hemorrhage, the hematoma develops rapidly and under high pressure. Symptoms typically include unconsciousness at the scene, with a brief lucid interval followed by a decrease in LOC. Other symptoms may be a headache, nausea and vomiting, or focal findings. Rapid surgical intervention to prevent cerebral herniation dramatically improves outcomes.[26] Patients over 65 years of age with increased ICP have a higher mortality rate than younger patients.[27]

Subdural Hematoma.
A subdural hematoma occurs from bleeding between the dura mater and the arachnoid layer of the meningeal covering of the brain. A subdural hematoma usually results from injury to the brain substance and its parenchymal vessels (Fig. 54-13, *B*). The veins that drain from the surface of the brain into the sagittal sinus are the source of most subdural hematomas. Because a subdural hematoma is usually venous in origin, the hematoma is much slower to develop into a mass large enough to produce symptoms. However, a subdural hematoma may be caused by an arterial hemorrhage, in which case it develops more rapidly. Subdural hematomas may be acute, subacute, or chronic (Table 54-10).

After the initial bleeding of the veins, a subdural hematoma may appear to enlarge over time as the breakdown products of the blood draw fluid into the subdural space to reach isotonicity. An acute subdural hematoma manifests signs within 48 hours of the injury. The signs and symptoms are similar to those associated with brain tissue compression in increased ICP

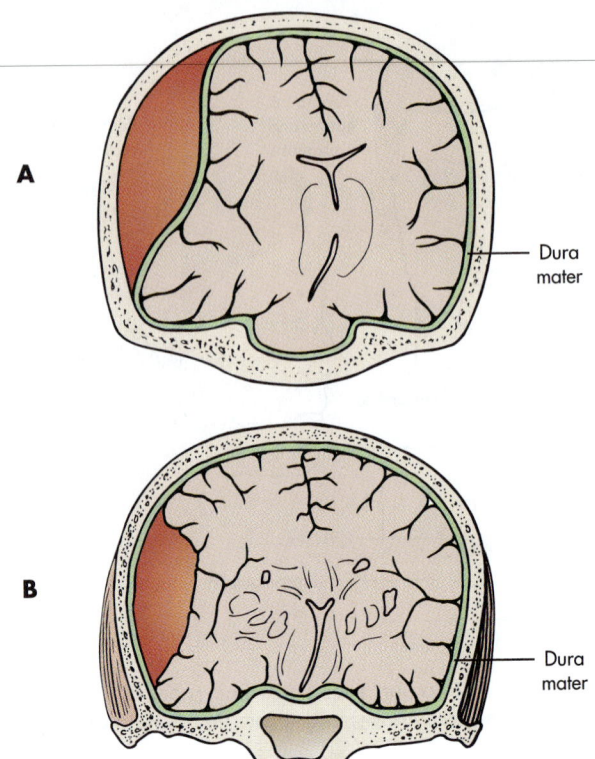

Fig. 54-13   A, Epidural hematoma in the temporal fossa, usually a result of laceration of the middle meningeal artery. **B,** Subdural hematoma, usually a result of laceration of the subdural veins.

and include decreasing LOC and headache. The patient appears drowsy and confused. The ipsilateral pupil dilates and becomes fixed. A subacute subdural hematoma usually occurs within 2 to 14 days of the injury. Failure to regain consciousness may point to this possibility.

A chronic subdural hematoma develops over weeks or months after a seemingly minor head injury. The peak incidence of chronic subdural hematoma is in the sixth and seventh decades of life when a potentially larger subdural space is available as a result of brain atrophy. With atrophy, the brain remains attached to the supportive structures, but tension is increased, and it is subject to tearing. The larger size of the subdural space also accounts for the presenting complaint to be the focal symptoms, rather than the signs of increased ICP. Chronic alcoholics are also prone to cerebral atrophy and subsequent development of subdural hematoma.

Delay in diagnosis in the older adult can be attributed to the fact that the symptoms mimic other health problems in persons of this age-group, such as vascular disease and senile dementia. Somnolence, confusion, lethargy, and memory loss are associated with health problems other than subdural hematoma. The patient has a history of head trauma in only 60% to 70% of cases.

Intracerebral Hematoma.
Intracerebral hematoma occurs from bleeding within the parenchyma and occurs in approximately 16% of head injuries. They usually occur within the frontal and temporal lobes possibly from the rupture of intracerebral vessels at the time of injury. A "burst" lobe is an intracerebral or intracerebellar hematoma that is an extension of a subarachnoid hemorrhage. This type of intra-

Table 54-10	Acute, Subacute, and Chronic Subdural Hematomas			
Occurrence after Injury	Progression of Symptoms	Treatment		Type of Trauma
Acute 24-48 hr	Immediate deterioration	Craniotomy, evacuation and decompression		Severe
Subacute 48 hr-2 wk	Initial unconsciousness, gradual improvement, deterioration over hours, dilation of pupils, ptosis	Evacuation and decompression		Severe
Chronic Weeks, months (>20 days)	Nonspecific, nonlocalizing progression; progressive alteration in LOC	Evacuation and decompression, membranectomy		Trivial, nonexistent, or forgotten (recollection of incident by only 60-70% of patients)

✚ EMERGENCY MANAGEMENT

Table 54-11	Head Injury	
Etiology	**Assessment Findings**	**Interventions**
Blunt Motor vehicle collision Pedestrian event Fall Assault Sports injury **Penetrating** Gunshot wound Arrow	**Surface Findings** • Scalp lacerations • Fracture or depressions in skull • Bruises or contusions on face, Battle's sign (bruising behind ears) • Raccoon eyes (dependent bruising around eyes) **Respiratory** • Central neurogenic hyperventilation • Cheyne-Stokes respirations • Decreased oxygen saturation • Pulmonary edema **Central Nervous System** • Unequal or dilated pupils • Asymmetric facial movements • Garbled speech, abusive speech • Confusion • Decreased level of consciousness • Combativeness • Involuntary movements • Seizures • Bowel and bladder incontinence • Flaccidity • Depressed or hyperactive reflexes • Decerebrate or decorticate posturing • Glasgow Coma Scale <12 • CSF leaking from ears or nose	**Initial** • Ensure patent airway. • Stabilize cervical spine. • Administer O_2 via nasal cannula or non-rebreather mask. • Establish IV access with two large-bore catheters to infuse normal saline or lactated Ringer's solution. • Control external bleeding with sterile pressure dressing. • Assess for rhinorrhea, otorrhea, scalp wounds. • Remove patient's clothing. **Ongoing Monitoring** • Maintain patient warmth using blankets, warm intravenous fluids, overhead warming lights, warm humidified oxygen. • Monitor vital signs, level of consciousness, O_2 saturation, cardiac rhythm, Glasgow Coma Score, pupil size and reactivity. • Anticipate need for intubation if gag reflex is absent. • Assume neck injury with head injury. • Administer fluids cautiously to prevent fluid overload and increasing ICP.

cerebral hematoma is thought to result from hemorrhage of supracortical vessels.

Diagnostic Studies and Collaborative Care

Skull x-rays are routinely ordered on any patient with a craniocerebral trauma. This is done to rule out a skull fracture. Skull x-rays are also useful in identifying orbital fractures and other facial fractures. CT scan and MRI are considered the best diagnostic tests to determine craniocerebral trauma. CT scan and MRI allow for rapid diagnosis and intervention. PET and evoked potential studies may also be used in the diagnosis and differentiation of head injuries. Transcranial Doppler studies allow for the measurement of cerebral blood flow velocity. In general, the diagnostic studies are similar to those used for a patient with increased ICP (see Table 54-5).

Emergency management of the patient with a head injury is presented in Table 54-11. In addition to measures to prevent secondary injury by treating cerebral edema and managing increased ICP, the principal treatment of head injuries is timely diagnosis and surgery if necessary. For the patient with concussion and contusion, observation and management of increased ICP are the primary management strategies.

The treatment of skull fractures is usually conservative. For depressed fractures and fractures with loose fragments, a craniotomy is necessary to elevate the depressed bone and remove the free fragments. If large amounts of bone are destroyed, the bone may be removed (craniectomy) and a cranioplasty will be needed at a later time (see Cranial Surgery later in this chapter).

In cases of acute subdural and epidural hematomas the blood must be removed. A craniotomy is generally performed to visualize the bleeding vessels so that the bleeding can be controlled. Burr-hole openings may be used in an extreme emergency for a more rapid decompression, followed by a craniotomy to stop all bleeding. A drain is generally placed postoperatively for several days to prevent any reaccumulation of blood.

NURSING MANAGEMENT: HEAD TRAUMA

■ Nursing Assessment

The patient with a head injury is always considered to have the potential for development of increased ICP. Increased ICP is associated with higher mortality rates and poorer functional outcomes.[28] The data collected generally include information gathered for the unconscious patient (see Fig. 54-1). The most important aspects of the objective data are noting the GCS score (see Table 54-2), monitoring the neurologic status (see Fig. 54-8), and determining whether a CSF leak has occurred.

■ Nursing Diagnoses

Nursing diagnoses for the patient who has sustained a head injury may include, but are not limited to, the following:

- Altered tissue perfusion: cerebral *related to* interruption of cerebral blood flow associated with cerebral hemorrhage, hematoma, and edema
- Hyperthermia *related to* increased metabolism, infection, and loss of cerebral integrative function secondary to possible hypothalamic injury
- Sensory/perceptual alterations *related to* cerebral injury and intensive care unit environment
- Pain *related to* headache, nausea, and vomiting
- Impaired physical mobility *related to* decreased LOC and treatment-imposed bed rest
- Risk for eye injury *related to* loss of protective reflexes
- Risk for infection *related to* environmental contamination secondary to open wound
- Anxiety *related to* abrupt change in health status, hospital environment, and lack of knowledge of seriousness of health problem
- Self-esteem disturbance *related to* altered appearance of head and face and dependence on others

■ Planning

The overall goals are that the patient with an acute head injury will (1) maintain adequate cerebral perfusion; (2) remain normothermic; (3) be free from pain, discomfort, and infection; and (4) attain maximal cognitive, motor, and sensory function.

■ Nursing Implementation

Health Promotion. One of the best ways to prevent head injuries is to prevent car and motorcycle accidents. The nurse can be active in campaigns that promote driving safety and can speak to driver education classes regarding the dangers of unsafe driving and of driving after drinking alcohol. The use of seat belts in cars and the use of helmets for riding on motorcycles are the most effective measures for increasing survival after accidents. Increasingly, individual states are passing legislation requiring the use of automobile safety devices for both children and adults. The wearing of protective helmets by lumberjacks, construction workers, miners, horseback riders, bicycle riders, and sky divers is also recommended. The nurse should be familiar with data on outcomes with and without safety devices in working with groups who oppose safety legislation as an infringement of personal freedom. Parents of young children should be educated in the proper use of car seats and restraints for their children. The nurse should also teach children about safety precautions for bicycle riding, skateboarding, and contact sports. Where appropriate parents and children should also be taught about the importance of handgun safety.

Acute Intervention. Action taken at the scene of the accident can have an important impact on the outcome of the head injury. Emergency management of head injury is discussed in Table 54-11. The general goal of nursing management of the head-injured patient is to maintain cerebral perfusion and prevention of secondary cerebral ischemia. Nursing care may initially consist of surveillance or monitoring for changes in neurologic status. This action is critically important because the patient's condition may deteriorate rapidly, necessitating emergency surgery. Appropriate preoperative and postoperative nursing interventions are initiated if surgery is anticipated.

The nurse should explain the need for frequent neurologic assessments to both the patient and the family. Behavioral manifestations associated with head injury can result in a frightened, disoriented patient who is combative and resists help. The nurse's approach should be calm and gentle. Restraints should be avoided if possible because they often produce agitation, which further increases ICP. A family member may be available to stay with the patient and thus prevent increasing anxiety and fear. Other teaching points are presented in Table 54-12.

The nurse should perform neurologic assessments at intervals, based on the patient's condition. The GCS is useful in assessing the level of arousal (see Table 54-2). Indications of a deteriorating neurologic state, such as a decreasing LOC or a lessening of motor strength, should be reported to the physician, and the patient's condition should be closely monitored.

The major focus of nursing care for the brain-injured patient relates to the unconscious state and increased ICP (see Nursing Management: Increased Intracranial Pressure earlier in this chapter). However, there may be specific problems that require nursing intervention.

Eye problems may include loss of the corneal reflex, periorbital ecchymosis and edema, and diplopia. Loss of the corneal reflex may necessitate administering lubricating eyedrops, taping the eyes shut, or suturing the eyelids to prevent abrasion. Periorbital ecchymosis and edema disappear spontaneously, but cold and, later, warm compresses provide comfort and hasten the process. Diplopia can be relieved by use of an eye patch.

Hyperthermia may occur from infection or injury to the hypothalamus. Increased metabolism secondary to hyperthermia increases metabolic waste, which in turn produces further cerebral vasodilation.

PATIENT & FAMILY HOME CARE

Table 54-12   Head Injury

Teaching guidelines for the patient and family during the initial 2-3 days following a head injury include the following:

1. Notify your health care provider immediately if experiencing signs and symptoms that may indicate complications:
   - Increased drowsiness (e.g., difficulty arousing, confusion)
   - Nausea and vomiting
   - Worsening headache or stiff neck
   - Seizures
   - Vision difficulties (e.g., blurring)
   - Behavior change (e.g., irritability, anger)
   - Motor problems (e.g., clumsiness, difficulty walking, slurred speech, weakness in arms or legs)
   - Sensory disturbances (e.g., numbness)
   - Decreased heart rate
2. Emphasize the importance of having someone stay with the patient.
3. Abstain from alcohol.
4. Check with your health care provider before taking medications that may increase drowsiness, including muscle relaxants, tranquilizers, and narcotic pain medications.
5. Avoid driving, using heavy machinery, contact sports, and warm baths.

If CSF rhinorrhea or otorrhea occurs, the nurse should inform the physician immediately. The patient should lie flat in bed unless this is contraindicated because of increased ICP. The head of the bed may be raised to decrease the CSF pressure so that a tear can seal. A loose collection pad may be placed under the nose or over the ear. No dressing should be placed into the nasal or ear cavities. The patient should be cautioned not to sneeze or blow the nose. Nasogastric tubes should not be used, and nasotracheal suctioning should not be performed on these patients.

Nursing measures specific to the care of the immobilized patient, such as those related to bladder and bowel function, skin care, and infection, are also indicated. Nausea and vomiting may be a problem and can be alleviated by antiemetic medication. Headache can usually be controlled with aspirin or small doses of codeine.

If the patient's condition deteriorates, intracranial surgery may be necessary (see Cranial Surgery later in this chapter). A burr-hole opening or craniotomy may be indicated, depending on the underlying injury that is causing the symptoms.

The patient is often unconscious before surgery, making it necessary for a family member to sign the consent form for surgery. This is a difficult and frightening time for the patient's family and requires sensitive nursing management. The suddenness of the situation makes it especially difficult for the family to cope.

The emergency nature of the surgery may prevent the usual careful preoperative preparation. The nurse should consult with the neurosurgeon to determine specific preoperative nursing measures.

Ambulatory and Home Care. Once the condition has stabilized, the patient is usually transferred for postacute rehabilitation management to prepare the patient for reentry into the community. As with any craniocerebral problem, there may be chronic problems related to motor and sensory deficits, communication, memory, and intellectual functioning. Many of the principles of nursing management of the patient with a stroke are appropriate (see Chapter 55). Conditions that may require nursing and collaborative management include poor nutritional status, bowel and bladder management, spasticity, dysphagia, neurogenic heterotopic ossification (overgrowth of bone), deep vein thrombosis, and communicating hydrocephalus. With time and patience, many of the chronic problems subside or disappear. The patient's outward appearance is not a good indicator of how well the patient will function in the home or work environment.

Seizure disorders are seen in approximately 5% of patients with a nonpenetrating head injury. The most vulnerable period of time for seizures to develop is during the first week after the head injury. In 25% of patients who develop a seizure disorder, the onset is at 4 or more years after the initial injury. Antiseizure agents are not used prophylactically but are generally instituted after a witnessed seizure or if an EEG demonstrates subclinical seizure activity. However, some clinicians recommend that antiseizure drugs be used during the first week and then be discontinued if no seizure activity is observed. Phenytoin (Dilantin) is the antiseizure drug of choice in posttraumatic seizure activity.

The mental and emotional sequelae of brain trauma are often the most incapacitating problems. It is estimated that more than 60% of patients with head injuries who have been comatose for more than 6 hours undergo some personality change. They may suffer loss of concentration and memory and defective memory processing. Personal drive may decrease; apathy and apparent laziness may increase. Euphoria and mood swings, along with a seeming lack of awareness of the seriousness of the injury, mark the affect of patients. The patient's behavior may indicate a loss of social restraint, judgment, tact, and emotional control.

Progressive recovery may continue for 6 months or more before a plateau is reached and a prognosis for recovery can be made. Specific nursing management in the posttraumatic phase depends on specific residual deficits.

In all cases the family must be given special consideration. They need to understand what is happening, and they must be taught appropriate interaction patterns. The nurse must give guidance and referrals for financial aid, child care, and other personal needs and must assist the family in involving the patient in family activities whenever possible. Assisting the patient and family in developing and maintaining hope and keeping communication open are strategies perceived as supportive by families.[29]

The family often has unrealistic expectations of the patient as the coma begins to recede. The family expects full return to pretrauma status. In reality, the patient experiences a reduced awareness and ability to interpret environmental stimuli. The nurse must prepare the family for the emergence of the patient from coma and must explain that the process of awakening often takes several weeks.

When the time for discharge planning arrives, the family and the patient may benefit from very specific posthospital instructions to avoid family-patient friction. Special "no" policies that may be appropriately suggested by the neurosurgeon, neuropsychologist, and nurse include *no* drinking of alcoholic beverages, *no* driving, *no* use of firearms, *no* work with hazardous implements and machinery, and *no* unsupervised smoking.[12] Family members, particularly spouses, go through role transition as the role changes from one of spouse to that of caregiver.[12]

■ Evaluation

The expected outcomes are that the head-injured patient will

- maintain normal cerebral perfusion pressure
- achieve maximal cognitive, motor, and sensory function
- experience no infection, hyperthermia, or pain

INTRACRANIAL TUMORS

Tumors within the cranial cavity cause approximately 2% of all deaths. It is estimated that in 1998 there were 17,400 primary brain cancers diagnosed in the United States.[30] The brain is also a frequent site for metastasis from other sites. Brain tumors rank fourth as cause of death from cancer in individuals 35 to 54 years of age.

Types

Tumors of the brain may be primary, arising from tissues within the brain, or secondary, resulting from a metastasis from a malignant neoplasm elsewhere in the body. Brain tumors are generally classified according to the tissue from which they arise. If malignant, the tumor is graded according to general cancer staging procedures. Brain tumors may be classified as those arising inside the brain substance (e.g., gliomas, vascular tumors) or those arising outside the brain substance (e.g., meningiomas, cranial nerve tumors). Glioblastoma multiforme is the most common tumor, followed by meningioma and astrocytoma. More than half of the intracranial tumors are malignant; they infiltrate the brain parenchyma and are not amenable to complete surgical removal. Other tumors may be histologically benign but are located such that complete removal is not possible. Brain tumors are more commonly seen in middle-aged persons, but they may occur at any age.

Unless treated, all intracranial tumors eventually cause death from increasing tumor volume leading to increased ICP. Brain tumors rarely metastasize outside the central nervous system (CNS) because they are contained by structural (meninges) and physiologic (blood-brain) barriers. Table 54-13 compares the major intracranial tumors. An astrocytoma is shown in Fig. 54-14.

Clinical Manifestations

The clinical manifestations of intracranial tumors are generally caused by the local destructive effects of the tumor, the resulting accumulation of metabolites, the displacement of structures, the obstruction of CSF flow, and the effects of edema and increased ICP on cerebral function. The rate of growth and the

Table **54-13**	**Major Intracranial Tumors**			
Tumor	**Tissue of Origin**	**% of Brain Tumors**	**Usual Locations**	**Malignant or Benign**
Gliomas				
Astrocytoma	Supportive tissue, glial cells and astrocytes	20	White matter of frontal and temporal lobes in adults, lateral cerebellar lobes in children	Moderately malignant, grades I and II
Glioblastoma multiforme	Primitive stem cell (glioblast)	20	Cerebral hemispheres	Highly malignant and invasive, grades III and IV
Oligodendroglioma	Glial cells and dendrites	2	Cerebral hemispheres, most in frontal lobe, some in basal ganglia and cerebellum	Benign (encapsulation and calcification)
Ependymoma	Ependymal epithelium	1	Lateral and fourth ventricles in children and young adults (usual)	Benign to highly malignant, most benign and encapsulated
Medulloblastoma	Supportive tissue	1	Posterior fossa, fourth ventricle, brainstem in children	Highly malignant and invasive, metastatic to spinal cord and remote areas of brain
Meningioma	Endothelial cells, fibrous tissue elements, transitional cells, angioblasts	20	Arachnoid villi, dura, half over convexity of hemisphere and half at base of hemisphere	Benign, encapsulation outside brain substance
Acoustic neuroma (neurofibroma)	Sheath of vestibular portion of CN VIII	5	Site between pons and cerebellum	Benign or low-grade malignancy, encapsulation
Pituitary adenoma	Pituitary glandular tissue	10	Pituitary gland	Usually benign
Vascular tumors Hemangioblastoma Arteriovenous malformation	Overgrowth of arteries and veins enlarging from feeder vessels	3	Parietal cortex near middle cerebral vessels	Benign
Metastatic tumors	Lungs, breast, kidney, thyroid, prostate	8	Cerebral cortex, diencephalon	Malignant

appearance of manifestations depend on the location, size, and mitotic rate of the cells of tissue of origin. Figure 54-15 illustrates the functional areas of the cerebral cortex and can be used as a guide to correlate local manifestations with the location of the tumor.

A wide range of possible clinical manifestations are associated with brain tumors with the classic feature being progressive manifestation of clinical symptoms. In some circumstances, a slight decrease in mental acuity may be the initial symptom. If left untreated, symptoms continue to progress to mental deterioration or a dramatic event such as a seizure. A brain tumor, as the tumor expands, may also produce manifestations of increased ICP from increased tumor volume, cerebral edema, or obstruction of the CSF pathways. Finally, manifestations may clearly indicate the location of the tumor by an alteration in the function controlled by the affected area (Table 54-14).

Complications

If the tumor mass obstructs the ventricles or occludes the outlet, ventricular enlargement (hydrocephalus) can occur. Surgical treatment is needed to relieve the pressure and involves placement of a ventriculoatrial or a ventriculoperitoneal shunt. A catheter with one-way valves is placed in the lateral ventricle and then tunneled through the skin to drain cerebrospinal fluid into the right atrium or the peritoneum. Rapid decompression of intracranial pressure can cause prostration and headache that may be prevented by gradually introducing the patient to the upright position. The patient should be instructed to avoid contact sports that may result in a blow to the valve or shearing

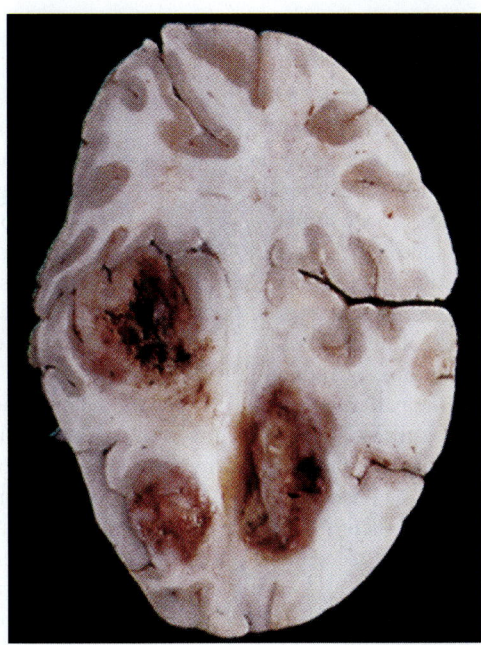

Fig. 54-14   Astrocytoma.

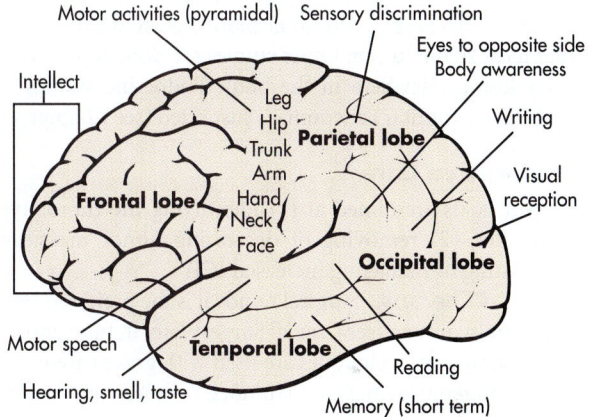

Fig. 54-15   Each area of the brain controls a particular activity.

Table **54-14**	Tumor Location and Associated Presenting Symptoms
Tumor Location	**Presenting Symptoms**
■ Cerebral hemisphere	
Frontal lobe (unilateral)	Unilateral hemiplegia; seizures; memory deficit; personality and judgment changes; visual disturbances
Frontal lobe (bilateral)	Symptoms associated with unilateral frontal lobe tumors; ataxic gait
Parietal lobe	Speech disturbance (if tumor is in the dominant hemisphere, inability to write, spatial disorders, unilateral neglect)
Occipital lobe	Blindness and seizures
Temporal lobe	Few symptoms; seizures, dysphagia
■ Subcortical	Hemiplegia; other symptoms may depend on area of infiltration
■ Meningeal tumors	Symptoms are associated with compression of the brain and depend on tumor location
■ Metastatic tumors	Headache, nausea or vomiting because of ICP; other symptoms depend on tumor location
■ Thalamus and sellar tumors	Headache, nausea, vision disturbances, papilledema, nystagmus occurs from an increase in ICP; diabetes insipidus may occur
■ Fourth ventricle and cerebellar tumors	Headache, nausea, and papilledema from increased ICP; ataxic gait and changes in coordination
■ Cerebellopontine tumors	Tinnitus and vertigo, deafness
■ Brainstem tumors	Headache upon awakening, drowsiness, vomiting, ataxic gait, facial muscle weakness, hearing loss, dysphagia, dysarthria, "crossed eyes" or other visual changes, hemiparesis
■ Spinal cord tumors	Depend on the nerves involved
	Cervical: pain, weakness or muscle wasting in arms, back, neck, or legs
	Thoracic area: pain accentuated with deep breathing and coughing, lack of bowel or bladder control may occur depending on tumor location

of the catheter. The physician should be notified if signs of increased ICP occur, such as decreasing level of consciousness, restlessness, headache, blurred vision, or vomiting without nausea. Signs of an infected shunt, such as high fever, persistent headache, and stiff neck, warrant investigation.

Diagnostic Studies

An extensive history and a comprehensive neurologic examination must be done in the workup of a patient with a suspected brain tumor. A careful history and physical examination may provide data with respect to location. Diagnostic studies are similar to those used for a patient with increased ICP (see Table 54-5). The sensitivity of MRI allows detection of very small tumors. Other diagnostic studies include CT scan, skull x-rays, cerebral angiography, EEG, brain scan, PET, lumbar puncture, and myelogram. CT and brain scanning are used to diagnose the location of the lesion. Newer diagnostic tools such as PET and MRI provide more reliable diagnostic information. The EEG is useful but of less importance. A lumbar puncture is seldom diagnostic and carries with it the risk of cerebral herniation. Angiography can be used to determine blood flow to the tumor and further localize the tumor. Other studies are done to rule out a primary lesion elsewhere in the body. Endocrine studies are helpful when a pituitary adenoma is suspected (see Chapter 47).

Collaborative Care

Treatment goals are aimed at (1) identifying the tumor type and location, (2) removing or decreasing tumor mass, and (3) preventing or managing increased ICP.

Surgical Therapy. Surgical removal is the preferred treatment for brain tumors (see Cranial Surgery later in this chapter). Stereotactic surgical techniques are used with greater frequency to biopsy and remove small brain tumors. However, the outcome of surgical therapy depends on the type, size, and location of the tumor. Meningiomas and oligodendrogliomas can usually be completely removed, whereas the more invasive gliomas and medulloblastomas can be only partially removed. Surgery reduces tumor mass, which decreases ICP and provides relief of symptoms with an extension of survival time. Tumors located in the deep central areas of the dominant hemisphere, the posterior corpus callosum, or the upper brainstem cause extensive neurologic damage and are considered inoperable.

Radiation and Chemotherapy. Radiation therapy lengthens survival in patients with malignant gliomas, especially when it is combined with partial surgical removal. Patients with less malignant tumors respond to radiation with a longer survival time and decreased recurrence of tumor. Cerebral edema and rapidly increasing ICP may be a complication of radiation therapy, but they can be managed with high doses of corticosteroids (dexamethasone [Decadron], prednisone, or methylprednisolone [Solu-Medrol]).

Normally the blood-brain barrier prohibits the entry of most drugs into the brain parenchyma. The most malignant tumors cause a breakdown of the blood-brain barrier in the area of the tumor, allowing chemotherapeutic agents to be used to treat the malignancy. A group of chemotherapeutic drugs called the nitrosoureas (e.g., carmustine [BCNU], lomustine [CCNU]) are particularly effective in treating brain tumors. Gliadel wafer (prolifeprosan 20 with carmustine), a biodegradable wafer implanted at the time of surgery, can deliver chemotherapy directly to the tumor site. Other drugs being used include methotrexate and procarbazine (Matulane). Two methods used to deliver chemotherapeutic drugs directly to the central nervous system are via an Ommaya reservoir and intrathecal administration. Brain tumors that cannot be totally removed may be treated with a combination of corticosteroids, surgery, radiation, and chemotherapy (see Chapter 14).

Many techniques to control and treat brain tumors are currently under investigation; these include radium implants into the tumor bed, local hyperthermia, and biologic therapy. Although progress in treatment has increased length and quality of survival of patients with gliomas, outcomes remain poor.

NURSING MANAGEMENT: INTRACRANIAL TUMOR

■ Nursing Assessment

The subjective and objective data of the patient with a brain tumor include the data the nurse collects for the unconscious patient. In addition to the assessment data listed in Fig. 54-8, the initial assessment should be structured to provide baseline data of the neurologic status and the information needed to design a realistic, individualized care plan. Areas to be assessed include the LOC and content of consciousness, motor abilities, sensory perception, integrated function (including bowel and bladder function), balance and proprioception, and the coping abilities of the patient and family. Watching a patient perform activities of daily living and listening to the patient's conversation are convenient ways to perform part of the neurologic assessment. Having the patient or the family explain the problem can be helpful in determining the patient's limitations and can also provide the nurse with information about the patient's insight into the problems. All initial data should be accurately recorded to provide a baseline for comparison to determine whether the patient's condition is improving or deteriorating.

Interview data are as important as the actual physical assessment. Questions concerning medical history, intellectual abilities and educational level, and history of nervous system infections and trauma should be asked. Determination of the presence of seizures, syncope, nausea and vomiting, pain, and headaches or other pain is important in planning care for the patient.

■ Nursing Diagnoses

Nursing diagnoses for the patient with a brain tumor may include, but are not limited to, the following:

- Altered tissue perfusion: cerebral *related to* cerebral edema
- Pain (headache) *related to* cerebral edema and increased ICP
- Self-care deficits *related to* altered neuromuscular function secondary to tumor growth and cerebral edema
- Anxiety *related to* diagnosis and treatment
- Potential complication: seizures *related to* abnormal electrical activity of the brain
- Potential complication: increased ICP *related to* presence of tumor and failure of normal compensatory mechanisms

■ Planning

The overall goals are that the patient with a brain tumor will (1) maintain normal ICP, (2) maximize neurologic functioning, (3) be free from pain and discomfort, and (4) be aware of the long-term implications with respect to prognosis and cognitive and physical functioning.

■ Nursing Implementation

A primary or metastatic tumor of the frontal lobe can cause behavioral and personality changes. Loss of emotional control, confusion, disorientation, memory loss, and depression may be signs of a frontal lobe lesion. These behavioral changes are often not perceived by the patient but can be disturbing and even frightening to the family. These changes can also cause a distancing to occur between the family and the patient. Assisting the family in understanding what is happening to the patient and supporting the family through this diagnostic phase are important roles for the nurse.

The confused patient with behavioral instability can be a challenge. Protecting the patient from self-harm is an important part of nursing care. At times when the patient manifests rage and aggression, the nurse must also be concerned about self-protection. Close supervision of activity, use of side rails, judicious use of restraints, padding of the rails and the area around the bed, and a calm, reassuring approach to care are all essential techniques in the care of these patients.

Perceptual problems associated with frontal lobe and parietal lobe tumors contribute to a patient's disorientation and confusion. Minimization of environmental stimuli, creation of a routine, and use of reality orientation can be incorporated into the care plan for the confused patient.

Seizures frequently occur with brain tumors. These are managed with antiseizure drugs. Seizure precautions should be instituted for the protection of the patient. Some behavioral changes seen in the patient with a brain tumor are a result of seizure disorders and can improve with control of the seizures by means of drugs (see Chapter 56).

Motor and sensory dysfunctions are problems that interfere with the activities of daily living. Alterations in mobility must be managed, and the patient should be encouraged to provide as much self-care as physically possible. Self-image often depends on the patient's ability to participate in care within the limitations of the physical deficits.

Language deficits can also occur in patients with brain tumors. Motor (expressive) or sensory (receptive) dysphasias may occur. The disturbance in communication can be frustrating for the patient and may interfere with the nurse's ability to meet the patient's needs. Attempts should be made to establish a communication system that can be used by both the patient and the staff.

Nutritional intake may be decreased because of the patient's inability to eat, loss of appetite, or loss of desire to eat. Assessing the nutritional status of the patient and ensuring adequate nutritional intake are important aspects of care. The patient may need encouragement to eat or, in some cases, may have to be fed orally, parenterally, by gastrostomy or nasogastric tube, or by total parenteral nutrition. The patient with a brain tumor who undergoes cranial surgery requires complex nursing care. This is discussed in the next section.

CRANIAL SURGERY

The cause or indication for cranial surgery may be related to a brain tumor, CNS infection (e.g., abscess), vascular abnormalities, craniocerebral trauma, epilepsy, and intractable pain (Table 54-15).

Table **54-15**	Indications for Cranial Surgery		
Indication	**Cause**	**Manifestations**	**Procedure**
Intracranial infection	Bacteria	Early findings: stiff neck, headache, fever, weakness, seizures; later findings: seizures, hemiplegia, speech disturbances, ocular disturbances, change in LOC	Excision or drainage of abscess
Hydrocephalus	Overproduction of CSF, obstruction to flow, defective reabsorption	Early findings: mental changes, disturbances in gait; later findings: memory impairment, urinary incontinence, increased tendon reflexes	Placement of ventriculoatrial or ventriculoperitoneal shunt
Intracranial tumors	Benign or malignant cell growth	Change in LOC, pupillary changes, sensory or motor deficit, papilledema, seizures, personality changes	Excision or partial resection of tumor
Intracranial bleeding	Rupture of cerebral vessels because of trauma or cardiovascular accident	Epidural: momentary unconsciousness; lucid period, then rapid deterioration; subdural: headache, seizures; pupillary changes	Surgical evacuation through burr holes or craniotomy
Skull fractures	Trauma to skull	Headache, CSF leakage, cranial nerve deficit	Debridement of fragments and necrotic tissue, elevation and realignment of bone fragments
Arteriovenous malformation	Congenital tangle of arteries and veins (frequently in middle cerebral artery)	Headache, intracranial hemorrhage, seizures, mental deterioration	Excision of malformation
Aneurysm repair	Dilation of weak area in arterial wall (usually near anterior portion of circle of Willis)	Before rupture: headache, lethargy, visual disturbance; after rupture: violent headache, decreased LOC, visual disturbances, motor deficit	Dissection and clipping of aneurysm

Table 54-16   Types of Cranial Surgery

Type	Description
■ Burr hole	Opening into the cranium with a drill; used to remove localized fluid and blood beneath the dura
■ Craniotomy	Opening into the cranium with removal of a bone flap and opening the dura to remove a lesion, repair a damaged area, drain blood, or relieve increased ICP
■ Craniectomy	Excision into the cranium to cut away a bone flap
■ Cranioplasty	Repair of a cranial defect resulting from trauma, malformation, or previous surgical procedure; artificial material used to replace damaged or lost bone
■ Stereotaxis	Precision localization of a specific area of the brain using a frame or a frameless system based on 3-dimensional coordinates; procedure is used for biopsy, radiosurgery, or dissection
■ Shunt procedures	Provide an alternate pathway to redirect cerebrospinal fluid from one area to another using a tube or implanted device; examples include ventriculoperitoneal shunt and Ommaya reservoir

Surgical Procedures

Various types of cranial surgical procedures are presented in Table 54-16.

Stereotactic Surgery. Stereotactic surgery is surgery targeted by three-dimensional coordinates identified through imagery (usually CT scan or MRI). These coordinates indicate where biopsy, radiosurgery, or dissection should occur. It is a procedure used frequently as part of the initial diagnostic workup. For example, stereotactic biopsy can be performed to obtain tissue samples for histologic examination. CT scan or MRI establish the sites for precise tumor sampling. With the patient under general or local anesthesia, the surgeon drills a burr hole or creates a bone flap for an entry site, and then introduces a probe and biopsy needle. Stereotactic procedures are being used with increasing frequency for removal of small brain tumors and abscesses, drainage of hematomas, ablative procedures for extrapyramidal diseases (e.g., Parkinson's), and repair of arteriovenous malformations. A major advantage of the stereotactic approach is a reduction in damage to surrounding tissue.

Stereotactic radiosurgery is a procedure that involves closed-skull destruction of an intracranial target using ionizing radiation focused with the assistance of an intracranial guiding device. The three radiosurgical techniques make use of a stereotactic Bragg peak proton beam, a linear accelerator, or a gamma knife. In the gamma knife procedure, a single, high dose of cobalt radiation is delivered to precisely targeted tumor tissue.

In combination with stereotactic procedures to identify and localize tumor sites, surgical lasers can be used to destroy tu-

mors. Stereotactic procedures are used to identify the tumor site. Three surgical lasers are currently used: the carbon dioxide, argon, and neodymium:yttrium-aluminum-garnet (Nd:YAG) lasers. All three work by creating thermal energy, which destroys the tissue on which it is focused. Laser therapy also provides the benefit of reducing damage to surrounding tissue.

Craniotomy. Depending on the location of the pathologic condition, a craniotomy may be frontal, parietal, occipital, temporal, or a combination of any of these. A set of burr holes is drilled, and a saw is used to connect the holes to remove the bone flap. Sometimes operating microscopes are used to magnify the site. After surgery the bone flap is wired or sutured. Sometimes drains are placed to remove fluid and blood. Patients are usually cared for in a critical care unit until stable.

NURSING MANAGEMENT: CRANIAL SURGERY
■ Nursing Assessment

The nursing assessment of the patient undergoing cranial surgery would be similar to that for the patient with increased ICP (see Nursing Management: Increased Intracranial Pressure earlier in this chapter) or that for the patient with an intracranial tumor (see Nursing Management: Intracranial Tumor earlier in this chapter).

■ Nursing Diagnoses

Nursing diagnoses for the patient with cranial surgery may include, but are not limited to, those presented in NCP 54-2.

■ Planning

The overall goals are that the patient with cranial surgery will (1) return to normal consciousness, (2) be free from pain and discomfort, (3) maximize neuromuscular functioning, and (4) be rehabilitated to maximum ability.

■ Nursing Implementation

Acute Intervention. The general preoperative and postoperative nursing care for the patient undergoing cranial surgery is similar, regardless of the cause. Nursing management is presented in NCP 54-2. The patient (if conscious and coherent) and the family will be gravely concerned about the potential physical and emotional problems that can result from surgery. The uncertainty regarding prognosis and outcome requires compassionate nursing care in the preoperative period.

Preoperative teaching is important in allaying the fears of the patient and the family and also in preparing them for the postoperative period. The patient and the family should be given general information concerning the type of operation that will be performed and what can be expected immediately after the operation. Explaining that the patient's hair will be shaved to allow for better exposure and prevention of contamination may prevent unnecessary concern over this task. The head is usually shaved in the operating room after induction of anesthesia. The family should also be informed that the patient will be taken to an intensive care unit or to a special care unit after the operation.

54-2 NURSING CARE PLAN PATIENT WITH CRANIAL SURGERY

Expected Patient Outcomes   **Nursing Interventions and *Rationales***

NURSING DIAGNOSIS   **Impaired gas exchange** *related to* decreased LOC and immobility *as manifested by* restlessness, irritability, abnormal ABGs.

- Patent airway.
- ABGs within normal limits.
- No respiratory distress.

- Assess all respiratory parameters q2hr for 72 hr, then every 4-8 hr *to provide a baseline for comparison to determine if breathing problem occurs.*
- Draw and evaluate ABGs regularly *to guide oxygen therapy and evaluate response to treatment.*
- Give oxygen by nasal catheter, prongs, or mechanical ventilator until ABGs are stable for at least 24-72 hr *to maintain stable cerebral oxygenation.*
- Encourage gentle coughing and turning and position patient on side with head slightly hyperextended if LOC is decreased *to improve ventilation, prevent atelectasis, and prevent aspiration of secretions or obstruction of airway.*
- Suction gently and for only <10-15 seconds duration when necessary *to minimize hypoxemia and avoid increasing ICP.*
- Hyperoxygenate before and after each coughing or suctioning session *to prevent hypoxia, which adversely affects cerebral perfusion.*
- Observe for gastric distention; insert nasogastric tube (if indicated) and maintain patency *to reduce pressure on the diaphragm and risk of aspiration.*
- Report any alterations in breathing patterns such as apnea or irregular and rapid ventilation *to ensure immediate medical intervention.*
- Be prepared for possible need for intubation *so mechanical ventilation can be started promptly if condition deteriorates.*

NURSING DIAGNOSIS   **Pain** *related to* craniotomy, position, and environmental stimuli *as manifested by* report of headache, holding head, pained expression.

- Decrease in complaints of pain.
- Expression of satisfaction with pain relief.

- Assess location, type, duration, degree, and severity of pain *to evaluate patient's need for and response to treatment.*
- Administer ordered analgesics *to decrease pain* and evaluate effects *to determine effectiveness of therapy.*
- Position as comfortably as possible *to relieve positional discomforts related to the location of incision.*
- Keep environment quiet, darken room, put cool cloth on patient's eyes *to promote comfort by reducing environmental stimuli.*

NURSING DIAGNOSIS   **Altered nutrition: less than body requirements** *related to* inability to feed self, difficulty swallowing, and decreased LOC *as manifested by* body weight 20% or more below ideal, poor muscle tone, low serum protein levels.

- Maintenance of weight.
- Normal serum protein and albumin levels.

- Evaluate ability to swallow *because feeding route is determined by swallowing ability.*
- Advance patient to high-protein, high-caloric, small, frequent feedings as tolerated *to prevent negative nitrogen balance and excessive weight loss and to prevent pressure on the diaphragm and feeling of bloating.*
- Feed patient if necessary *to ensure adequate nutritional intake if self-feeding is not possible.*
- If patient is unable to eat, use enteral tube feedings or total parenteral nutrition as ordered *to provide necessary fluids, electrolytes, calories, and protein until patient can eat.*

NURSING DIAGNOSIS   **Body image disturbance** *related to* physical appearance resulting from surgery *as manifested by* refusal to look at self or participate in self-care, crying, or anger about appearance; social withdrawal.

- Acceptance of temporary nature of appearance.
- Maintenance of normal activities.

- Encourage patient to express feelings about appearance *to enable patient to recognize and begin to deal with feelings.*
- Explain the rate of hair regrowth of $1/2$ - $3/4$ inch/month *so patient will have realistic expectation.*
- Provide information about wigs or hairpieces *so patient is aware of this alternative.*
- Encourage the use of scarves in women and hats in men *to boost their appearance and self-esteem and minimize embarrassment.*
- Reassure patient about self-worth *to bolster patient's self-esteem and coping ability.*

Continued

54-2   NURSING CARE PLAN   PATIENT WITH CRANIAL SURGERY—continued

| Expected Patient Outcomes | Nursing Interventions and *Rationales* |

NURSING DIAGNOSIS **Sensory-perceptual alterations** *related to* altered sensory reception, transmission, or integration secondary to neurologic surgery *as manifested by* possible disorientation; altered sight, hearing, taste, or smell; decreased LOC.

- Maintenance of highest possible level of interaction with environment.

- Assess patient's ability to speak, see, hear, taste, and smell *to enable appropriate planning of care.*
- Orient patient to surroundings; describe surroundings when sight is impaired *to increase patient's awareness and reduce anxiety and risk of injury.*
- Eliminate extraneous noise *to reduce anxiety and confusion caused by sensory overload.*
- Provide stimulation for all senses *to aid in retraining sensory pathways to integrate reception and interpretation of stimuli.*

NURSING DIAGNOSIS **Self-care deficits** *related to* decreased LOC, weakness, or postoperative status *as manifested by* inability or unwillingness to perform activities of daily living.

- All self-care needs met.

- Assess patient's self-care abilities *to determine level of care needed and plan appropriate interventions.*
- Provide for total self-care requirements of the patient, including hygiene and skin care and tube feeding or total parenteral nutrition, *to ensure that all activities of daily living needs are met.*
- Turn patient at least q2hr *to promote effective circulation and ventilation and to prevent skin breakdown.*
- Maintain indwelling catheter patency *to facilitate bladder emptying;* assess need for enema or suppository *to promote adequate bowel elimination.*
- Maintain range of motion of all joints *to prevent contractures.*
- Provide oral hygiene q2hr *to prevent stomatitis and promote comfort.*
- Keep patient's eyes closed or use artificial tears if unconscious or unable to blink *to prevent corneal damage.*

COLLABORATIVE PROBLEMS

| Nursing Goals | Nursing Interventions and *Rationales* |

POTENTIAL COMPLICATION **Increased ICP** *related to* cerebral edema.

- Monitor for signs of increased ICP.
- Report deviations from acceptable parameters.
- Carry out appropriate medical and nursing interventions.

- Assess for signs of increased ICP (e.g., altered LOC, headache, pupil inequality, decreased respirations and pulse rate, elevated systolic blood pressure with widened pulse pressure, swelling around surgical site, elevation of bone flap) *to enable immediate reporting and initiation of treatment.*
- Assess neurologic function immediately on patient's return from operating room *to establish baseline parameters.*
- Report significant changes *to enable prompt intervention and to prevent serious complications.*
- Calibrate and maintain ICP monitoring equipment in functioning condition *to ensure accurate readings.*
- Provide aseptic care of insertion site *to prevent infection and subsequent increase in ICP from exudate.*
- Administer diuretics and corticosteroids as ordered *to reduce cerebral edema.*
- Position patient with head of bed elevated to 30 degrees *to promote venous drainage from head, reducing cerebral edema.*
- Avoid neck and hip flexion *to prevent venous obstruction and decrease risk of increasing intraabdominal pressure, which restricts diaphragm movement, increasing $PaCO_2$, which increases cerebral blood flow and ultimately results in cerebral edema.*
- Prevent constipation and straining with defecation *to prevent increased ICP caused by Valsalva's maneuver.*
- Manage elevated temperature *because elevated temperature increases cerebral metabolism and causes increased ICP.*

Continued

54-2 NURSING CARE PLAN PATIENT WITH CRANIAL SURGERY—continued

Expected Patient Outcomes	Nursing Interventions and *Rationales*

POTENTIAL COMPLICATION CSF leak from nose or ears *related to* surgical incision.

- Monitor and report signs of CSF leak.
- Carry out appropriate medical and nursing interventions.

- Assess for clear or slightly yellow drainage from ears or nose *as indicators of CSF leaks, which increases risk for infection.*
- Test drainage for glucose or CSF ring, report to physician if positive *to confirm drainage is CSF.*
- Culture drainage of ears and nose *to rule out possibility of infectious drainage.*
- Do not plug nose or ears with cotton; use loose "snuffer" type of gauze dressing for comfort (change frequently) *to allow free drainage until injured area is repaired.*
- Watch for temperature elevation, irritability, headache, or nuchal rigidity and report immediately *because these are key indicators of meningitis.*
- Administer antibiotics if ordered *as treatment for infection.*

LOC, level of consciousness.

The primary goal of care after cranial surgery is prevention of increased ICP. The turning and positioning of the patient sometimes depends on the site of the operation. If the surgical approach is in the posterior fossa, the patient is generally kept flat or at a slight elevation (10 to 15 degrees). Lying on the back will be prevented as much as possible, and flexion of the neck will be avoided to protect the suture line. The maximum swelling in the operative area occurs within 24 to 48 hours after the surgery.

With an incision over the skull in the anterior or middle fossae, the patient will return from the operating room with the head elevated at an angle of 30 to 45 degrees. If a bone flap has been removed (craniectomy), care should be taken not to have the patient positioned on the operative side.

The dressing should be observed for color, odor, and amount of drainage. The physician should be notified immediately of any excessive bleeding or clear drainage. Checking drains for placement and assessing the area around the dressing are also important.

Frequent assessment of the neurologic status of the patient is essential during the first 48 hours. In addition to the neurologic functions, fluids, electrolyte levels, and osmolality are monitored closely to detect changes in sodium regulation, the onset of diabetes insipidus, or severe hypovolemia.

The dressing is usually in place for 3 to 5 days. Scalp care should include meticulous care of the incision to prevent wound infection. The area should be cleansed with povidone iodine (Betadine) or a similar antiseptic disinfectant. Cleansing should be followed by application of an antibiotic ointment according to procedure. Once the dressing is removed, use of an antiseptic soap for washing the scalp may also be beneficial. The psychologic impact of baldness can be alleviated by the use of a wig, turban, or cap after the incision has completely healed. For the patient who is receiving radiation, use of a sunblock and head covering should be advocated if any exposure to the sun is anticipated.

Ambulatory and Home Care. The rehabilitative potential for a patient after cranial surgery depends on the reason for the surgery, the postoperative course, and the patient's general state of health. Nursing interventions must be based on a realistic appraisal of these factors. An overall goal for the nurse is to foster independence for as long as possible and to the highest degree possible.

Specific rehabilitation potential cannot be determined until cerebral edema and increased ICP subside postoperatively. Care must be taken to maintain as much function as possible through measures such as careful positioning, meticulous skin and mouth care, regular range-of-motion exercises, bowel and bladder care, and adequate nutrition.

Referrals may be made to other specialists on the health care team. For example, the speech therapist may be helpful to the patient who has a speech problem. The needs and problems of each patient should be addressed individually because many variables affect the plan.

Mental and emotional residual deficits are often more difficult for the patient and the family to accept than are motor and sensory losses. The nurse can provide much help and support during the adjustment phase and in long-range planning.

The mental and physical deterioration of the patient, including seizures, personality disorganization, apathy, and wasting, is difficult for both family and health professionals to endure. Although progress is continuously being made to help the patient with a brain tumor by means of chemotherapy, conventional and interstitial radiation, and biologic therapies, the prognosis remains grim.

■ Evaluation

The expected outcomes are that the patient with an intracranial tumor will

- regain maximal cognitive, motor, and sensory function possible
- be free of infection
- have pain and discomfort alleviated

Table **54-17**	Cerebral Inflammatory Conditions		
	Bacterial Meningitis*	**Encephalitis**	**Brain Abscess**
Causative organisms	Bacteria (pneumococci, meningoccoci, streptococci)	Bacteria, fungi, parasites, herpes simplex virus (HSV) other viruses	Streptococci, staphylococci through bloodstream
CSF			
Pressure (normal, 60-150 mm H_2O)	Increased	Normal to slight increase with increased ICP	Increased
WBC count (normal, 0-8/μl)	>500/μl (mainly PMN)	<500/μl, PMN (early), lymphocytes (later)	25-300/μl (PMN)
Protein (normal, 15-45 mg/dl [0.15-0.45 g/L])	High	Slight increase	Normal
Glucose (normal, 45-75 mg/dl [2.5-4.2 mmol/L])	Low or absent	Normal	Low or absent
Appearance	Turbid, cloudy	Clear	Clear
Diagnostic studies	Gram's stain, smear, culture	Viral studies, MRI HSV DNA	CT scan, EEG, skull x-ray
Treatment	Antibiotics with sensitivity tests, supportive care, prevention of symptoms of ↑ ICP	Supportive care, prevention of symptoms of increased ICP, acyclovir (Zovirax) for HSV	Antibiotics, incision and drainage Supportive care

*Meningitis can also be caused by virus, yeast, and fungi.
PMN, polymorphonuclear cells; *WBC*, white blood cell.

INFLAMMATORY CONDITIONS OF THE BRAIN

Meningitis, encephalitis, and brain abscesses are the most common inflammatory conditions of the brain and spinal cord. Inflammation can be caused by bacteria, viruses, fungi, and chemicals (e.g., contrast media used in diagnostic tests or blood in the subarachnoid space) (Table 54-17). CNS infections may occur via the bloodstream, by extension from a primary site, by extension along cranial and spinal nerves, or in utero. Bacterial infections are the most common, and the organisms usually involved are *Streptococcus pneumoniae, Haemophilus influenzae, Neisseria meningitides, Staphylococcus aureus,* and *Meningococci.* The mortality rate is high, and 50% of the survivors experience long-term neurologic deficits. Bacterial meningitis carries the highest mortality rate and is considered a medical emergency.

MENINGITIS

Etiology and Pathophysiology

Meningitis is an acute inflammation of the pia mater and the arachnoid membrane surrounding the brain and the spinal cord. Therefore meningitis is always a cerebrospinal infection. The organisms usually gain entry to the CNS through the upper respiratory tract or the bloodstream, but they may enter by direct extension from penetrating wounds of the skull or through fractured sinuses in basal skull fractures.

Meningitis usually occurs in the fall, winter, or early spring and is often secondary to viral respiratory disease. Children under 6 years of age, older adults, and persons who are debilitated are more often affected than is the general population. *Streptococcus pneumoniae* causes about 30% of the infections.

The inflammatory response to the infection tends to increase CSF production, with a moderate increase in pressure. In bacterial meningitis the purulent secretion produced quickly spreads to other areas of the brain through the CSF. If this process extends into the brain parenchyma, or if a concurrent encephalitis is present, cerebral edema and increased ICP become more of a problem. All patients with meningitis must be observed closely for manifestations of increased ICP, which is thought to be a result of swelling around the dura, increased CSF volume, and endotoxins produced by the bacteria.

Clinical Manifestations

Fever, severe headache, nausea, vomiting, and nuchal rigidity (resistance to flexion of the neck) are key signs of meningitis. A positive Kernig's sign, a positive Brudzinski's sign (see Chapter 53), photophobia, a decreased LOC, and signs of increased ICP may also be present. Coma is associated with a poor prognosis and occurs in 5% to 10% of patients with bacterial meningitis. Seizures occur in 20% of all cases. With meningitis the headache becomes progressively worse and may be accompanied by vomiting and irritability. If the infecting organism is a meningococcus, a skin rash is common and petechiae may be seen.

Complications

The most common complication of meningitis is residual neurologic dysfunction. Cranial nerve dysfunction often occurs with cranial nerves III, IV, VI, VII, or VIII in bacterial meningitis. The dysfunction usually disappears within a few weeks. Hearing loss may be permanent after bacterial meningitis, but it is not a complication of viral meningitis.

Cranial nerve irritation can have serious sequelae. The optic nerve (CN II) is compressed by increased ICP. Papilledema is often present, and blindness may occur. When the oculomotor (CN III), trochlear (CN IV), and abducens (CN VI) nerves are irritated, ocular movements are affected. Ptosis, unequal pupils, and diplopia are common. Irritation of the trigeminal nerve (CN V) is evidenced by sensory losses and loss of the corneal reflex, and irritation of the facial nerve (CN VII) results in facial paresis. Irritation of the vestibulocochlear nerve (CN VIII) causes tinnitus, vertigo, and deafness.

Hemiparesis, dysphasia, and hemianopsia may also occur. These signs usually resolve over time. If resolution does not occur, a cerebral abscess, subdural empyema, subdural effusion, or persistent meningitis is suggested. Acute cerebral edema may occur with bacterial meningitis, causing seizures, CN III palsy, bradycardia, hypertensive coma, and death.

A noncommunicating hydrocephalus may occur if the exudate causes adhesions that prevent the normal flow of the CSF from the ventricles. CSF reabsorption by the arachnoid villi may also be obstructed by the exudate. Surgical implantation of a shunt is the only treatment.

A complication of meningococcal meningitis is the Waterhouse-Friderichsen syndrome. The syndrome is manifested by petechiae, disseminated intravascular coagulation, and adrenal hemorrhage. Disseminated intravascular coagulation is a serious complication of meningitis (see Chapter 29). It is the cause of death in about 1% of patients with meningitis.

Diagnostic Studies

A major diagnostic tool is examination of the CSF. Diagnosis is verified in 90% of the cases by a positive CSF culture. Variations in the CSF depend on the causative organism. Protein levels in the CSF are usually elevated and are higher in bacterial than in viral cases. Decreased CSF glucose concentration is common in bacterial meningitis and may be normal in viral meningitis. The CSF is purulent and turbid in bacterial meningitis; it may be the same or clear in viral meningitis. The predominant white blood cell type in the CSF during inflammatory disorders of the brain is polymorphonuclear cells (see Table 54-17). Specimens of blood, sputum, and nasopharyngeal secretions are taken for culture before the start of antibiotic therapy to identify the causative organism.

X-rays of the skull may demonstrate infected sinuses. CT scans are usually normal in uncomplicated meningitis. In other cases, CT scans may reveal evidence of increased ICP or hydrocephalus.

Collaborative Care

Rapid diagnosis based on history and physical examination is crucial because the patient is usually in a critical state when health care is sought. When meningitis is suspected, antibiotic therapy is instituted after the collection of specimens for cultures, even before the diagnosis is confirmed. Diagnostic measures include lumbar puncture and analysis of CSF. The fundus of the eye should be examined via ophthalmoscope for papilledema before lumbar puncture for identification of possible increased ICP.

Ampicillin, penicillin, and a third-generation cephalosporin, usually ceftriaxone (Rocephin) or cefotaxime (Claforan), are the drugs of choice for treating meningitis. These drugs are effective because of their ability to penetrate the blood-brain barrier. Collaborative care for cerebral inflammatory conditions is presented in Table 54-18.

COLLABORATIVE CARE

Table 54-18   Cerebral Inflammatory Problems

Diagnostic
History and physical examination
Analysis of CSF
CBC, coagulation profile, electrolyte levels, glucose, platelet count
Routine urinalysis
Blood cultures (twice)
Urine specific gravity (q4hr)
CT scan, MRI
EEG
Skull x-ray studies
Brain scan

Collaborative Therapy
Strict bed rest
IV fluids
Ampicillin, penicillin IV
Cefotaxime (Claforan), ceftriaxone (Rocephin)
Codeine for headache
Acetaminophen or aspirin for temperature above 100.4° F (38° C)
Hypothermia
Clear liquids as desired or tolerated
Phenytoin (Dilantin) IV
Furosemide (Lasix) or mannitol for diuresis

NURSING MANAGEMENT: MENINGITIS

■ Nursing Assessment

Initial assessment should include vital signs, neurologic evaluation, fluid intake and output, and evaluation of lung fields and skin. Fever, severe headache, nausea, vomiting, and nuchal rigidity are common presenting symptoms in the patient with meningitis.

■ Nursing Diagnoses

Nursing diagnoses for the patient with meningitis may include, but are not limited to, those presented in NCP 54-3.

■ Planning

The overall goals are that the patient with meningitis will have (1) return to maximal neurologic functioning, (2) resolution of infection, and (3) decreased pain and discomfort.

■ Nursing Implementation

Health Promotion. Prevention of respiratory infections through vaccination programs for pneumococcal pneumonia and influenza should be supported by nurses. In addition, early and vigorous treatment of respiratory and ear infections is important. Persons who have close contact with anyone who has meningitis should be given prophylactic antibiotics.

Acute Intervention. The patient with meningitis is usually acutely ill. The fever is high and head pain is severe. Irritation of the cerebral cortex may result in seizures. The

| 54-3 | NURSING CARE PLAN | **PATIENT WITH AN INFLAMMATORY CONDITION OF THE BRAIN** |

| **Expected Patient Outcomes** | **Nursing Interventions and *Rationales*** |

NURSING DIAGNOSIS **Sensory-perceptual alterations** *related to* decreased LOC *as manifested by* inaccurate interpretation of environment, signs of fear or anxiety, disorientation, restlessness, auditory or visual hallucinations.

- Minimal disorientation.
- Lack of evidence of agitation.

- Assess LOC *to determine extent of the problem.*
- Administer sedative medication as ordered *to reduce fear and anxiety.*
- Keep room quiet and lights dim; use calm, reassuring approach *to avoid stimulating or frightening the patient.*
- Do not use restraints *to avoid increasing patient's anxiety and initiating combative behavior.*
- Assist and support patient during uncomfortable or frightening diagnostic procedures; have family member at bedside when possible *to assist with orientation and reduce anxiety.*

NURSING DIAGNOSIS **Pain** *related to* headache, muscle and joint aches, and malaise *as manifested by* general discomfort of head, joints, and muscles; apathy; grimacing on movement.

- Satisfaction with pain relief.
- Increased participation in treatment plan.

- Administer mild analgesia as needed; assist patient to position of comfort in bed *to relieve pain.*
- Encourage gentle range-of-motion and leg exercises *to reduce joint stiffness and promote circulation.*
- Massage muscles as needed or requested *to promote comfort and show a caring attitude.*
- Control environment to encourage rest *because pain can be exhausting to the patient.*

NURSING DIAGNOSIS **Ineffective management of therapeutic regimen** *related to* possible sequelae of condition *as manifested by* motor or sensory problems, activity limitations.

- Satisfactory management of condition by self or others.

- Monitor for residual effects of condition such as vision, hearing, activity, and cognitive problems *to determine appropriate referrals.*
- Inform patient and others that residual problems often improve over time *to reduce anxiety.*
- Arrange for postdischarge care if required *so patient's needs are met.*

NURSING DIAGNOSIS **Hyperthermia** *related to* infection and abnormal temperature regulation by hypothalamus from increased ICP *as manifested by* increased temperature and chills.

- Normal body temperature.

- Carry out general measures of care for patient with a fever (see NCP 11-1).
- If prescribed, use hypothermia blanket to reduce temperature *because an elevated temperature increases brain metabolism and increases the risk of seizures or increased ICP.*
- Reduce temperature gradually *to prevent shivering, which can cause a rebound effect and raise rather than lower the temperature.*

COLLABORATIVE PROBLEMS

| **Nursing Goals** | **Nursing Interventions and *Rationales*** |

POTENTIAL COMPLICATION **Seizure activity** *related to* cerebral irritation.

- Monitor for seizure activity.
- Carry out appropriate medical and nursing interventions.
- Report and record any seizure activity.

- Monitor for seizure activity *so interventions can be initiated immediately.*
- Keep side rails up and padded *to protect patient if a seizure occurs.*
- Administer sedative and antiseizure medications as ordered *to control or prevent seizure activity.*
- Reduce fever *to decrease brain's oxygen demand.*
- Carry out interventions to treat underlying causes of inflammatory brain condition *to prevent seizure activity.*

POTENTIAL COMPLICATION **Increased ICP** *related to* presence of infectious exudate, increased production of CSF (see NCP 54-2).

changes in mental status and LOC depend on the degree of increased ICP. Assessment of vital signs, neurologic evaluation, fluid intake and output, and evaluation of lung fields and skin should be performed at regular intervals based on the patient's condition and recorded carefully.

Head pain and neck pain secondary to movement require attention. Codeine provides some pain relief without undue sedation for most patients. The patient should be assisted to a position of comfort, often curled up with the head slightly extended. The head of the bed should be slightly elevated, when permitted after lumbar puncture. A darkened room and a cool cloth over the eyes relieve the discomfort of photophobia.

For the delirious patient, additional low lighting may be necessary to decrease hallucinations. All patients suffer some degree of mental distortion and hypersensitivity and may be frightened and misinterpret the environment. Every attempt should be made to minimize environmental stimuli and the resulting exaggerated perception. Restraints should be avoided. Padded side rails with sheets tied to the four corners to keep the patient from getting out of bed may be used to prevent injury. Arm boards, secured with multiple layers of stretch gauze (e.g., Kerlix), protect the IV infusion site. The presence of a familiar person at the bedside has a calming effect. The nurse must be efficient with care but also should project an attitude of caring and of unhurried gentleness. The use of touch and a soothing voice to give simple explanations of activities is helpful. If seizures occur, appropriate observations should be made and protective measures should be taken. Antiseizure medications such as phenytoin (Dilantin) are administered as ordered. Problems associated with increased ICP are also managed (see Increased Intracranial Pressure earlier in this chapter).

Fever must be vigorously managed because it increases cerebral edema and the frequency of seizures. In addition, neurologic damage may result from an extremely high temperature over a prolonged time. Acetaminophen or aspirin may be used to reduce fever. However, if the fever is resistant to aspirin or acetaminophen, more vigorous means are necessary. If prescribed, an automatic cooling blanket may be used to reduce high fever. Care should be taken not to reduce the temperature too rapidly because shivering may result, causing a rebound effect and increasing the temperature. The extremities should be wrapped in sheepskin, soft towels, or a blanket covered with a sheet to protect them from "frostbite." Care of the skin should be frequent to prevent breaks in the skin. If a cooling blanket is not available or desirable, tepid sponge baths with water may be effective in lowering the temperature. The skin must be protected from excessive drying and injury.

Because high fever greatly increases the metabolic rate and thus insensible fluid loss, the patient should be assessed for dehydration and adequacy of fluid intake. Diaphoresis further increases fluid losses, which should be estimated and included in an intake and output record. Replacement fluids should be calculated as 800 ml/day for respiratory losses and 100 ml for each degree of temperature above 100.4° F (38° C). Supplemental feeding to maintain adequate nutritional intake via tube or oral feedings may be necessary. The designated antibiotic schedule must be followed to maintain therapeutic blood levels. Observations should be made for side effects of the drugs used.

In most cases, meningitis no longer requires isolation, with the exception of meningococcal meningitis. However, good aseptic technique is essential to protect the patient and the nurse.

Ambulatory and Home Care. After the acute period has passed, the patient requires several weeks of convalescence before normal activities can be resumed. In this period, good nutrition should be stressed, with an emphasis on a high-protein, high-caloric diet in small, frequent feedings.

Muscle rigidity may persist in the neck and the backs of the legs. Progressive range-of-motion exercises and warm baths are useful. Activity should be gradually increased as tolerated, but adequate bed rest and sleep should be encouraged. Quiet activities that are based on an assessment of individual interests should be encouraged to prevent boredom.

Residual effects are uncommon in meningococcal meningitis, but pneumococcal meningitis can result in sequelae such as dementia, seizures, deafness, hemiplegia, and hydrocephalus. Vision, hearing, cognitive skills, and motor and sensory abilities should be assessed after recovery, with appropriate referrals as indicated. Meningitis in infancy may have "silent" neurologic sequelae, which are manifested as learning and behavior problems when the child reaches school age.

Throughout the acute and convalescent periods the nurse should be aware of the anxiety and stress experienced by individuals close to the patient.

■ Evaluation

The expected outcomes are that the patient with meningitis will

- return to maximal neurologic function possible
- be free from pain and discomfort

ENCEPHALITIS

Encephalitis is an acute inflammation of the brain and is usually caused by a virus. Many different viruses have been implicated in encephalitis, some of them associated with certain seasons of the year and endemic to certain geographic areas. Epidemic encephalitis is transmitted by ticks and mosquitoes. Nonepidemic encephalitis may occur as a complication of measles, chickenpox, or mumps.

Encephalitis is a serious, and sometimes fatal, disease. Overall mortality rate ranges from 5% to 20%, with the highest mortality rate in encephalitis caused by herpes simplex virus (HSV) and the eastern and Venezuelan equine viruses. Unfortunately, HSV encephalitis is the most common form of viral encephalitis. Cytomegalovirus encephalitis is one of the common complications in patients with acquired immunodeficiency syndrome.[31]

Manifestations resemble those of meningitis, but they have a more gradual onset. They include headache, high fever, seizures, and a change in level of consciousness.

Early diagnosis and treatment of viral encephalitis are essential for favorable outcomes. Diagnostic findings related to viral encephalitis are shown in Table 54-17. Brain imaging techniques such as MRI and PET, along with polymerase chain reaction tests for the HSV DNA levels in CSF, allow for earlier detection of viral encephalitis.[31]

Collaborative and nursing management is symptomatic and supportive. Cerebral edema is a major problem, and diuretics (mannitol) and corticosteroids (dexamethasone [Decadron]) are used to control it. The disease is characterized by diffuse

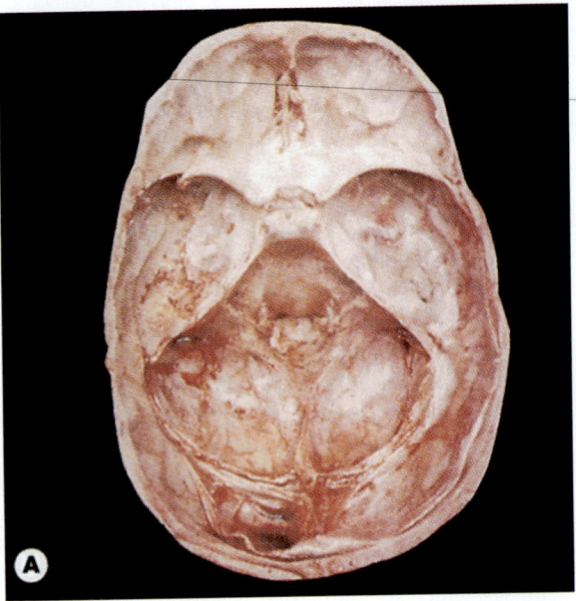
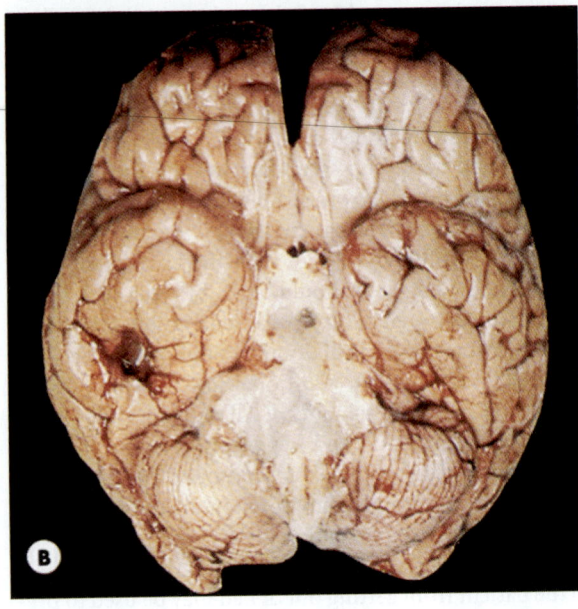

Fig. 54-16 **A,** Normal brain with most of dura intact. **B,** Brain with abscess.

CRITICAL THINKING EXERCISES

CASE STUDY

Head Injury

Patient Profile

Jason B., a 22-year-old unrestrained driver, was involved in a head-on collision. He was found at the scene of a motor vehicle accident trapped under the steering wheel of his car. He is admitted to the emergency department with a diagnosis of traumatic brain injury and open fracture of the right humerus and femur.

Subjective Data

- Paramedic reported that patient was unconscious at the scene, normotensive with Cheyne-Stokes respirations

Objective Data

At the Scene
- Slight decerebration with the left arm

In the Emergency Department
- Pupils equal, 2 mm, and fixed
- Vital signs within normal limits
- Glasgow Coma Scale = 5; ICP and CPP average 20 mm Hg and 60 mm Hg, respectively
- Fractured right femur and humerus
- Multiple lacerations and contusions

Diagnostic Studies
- Brain CT scan reveals fracture along lateral wall of right maxillary sinus, subarachnoid hemorrhage, generalized brain swelling, and slit ventricles

Critical Thinking Questions

1. What could be the cause of Mr. B.'s nonresponsive neurologic condition based on his initial clinical condition and CT scan?
2. Discuss conditions of the injury and the pathophysiologic changes that can occur from the injury in relation to Mr. B.'s neurologic status.
3. What do the signs and symptoms suggest for Mr. B.'s area of brain involvement?
4. What are the priority interventions based on the nursing assessment?
5. Write one or more appropriate nursing diagnoses based on the assessment data. Are there any collaborative problems?

NURSING RESEARCH ISSUES

1. What type of information and education do families need at each stage of recovery for the head-injured patient?
2. What are the temporal changes in brain compliance associated with mortality and poor functional outcomes?
3. Are there any age-related differences in brain compliance associated with poor outcomes?
4. What is the effect of nursing activities or interventions on intracranial pressure, cerebral perfusion pressure, cerebral blood flow, and cerebral tissue oxygenation?
5. What is the most valid noninvasive or continuous method for real-time monitoring of cerebral tissue perfusion and oxygenation?
6. What is the best method to sample cerebrospinal fluid from the ventricles without increased risk of infection?
7. Do neuromuscular blockers or other anesthetic agents (e.g., opioids, benzodiazepines) alter the patient's response to nursing care activities?
8. Do cognitive stimulation programs decrease the frequency of cognitive and behavior changes that occur after minor head injury?

damage to the nerve cells of the brain, perivascular cellular in-filtration, proliferation of glial cells, and increasing cerebral edema. The sequelae of encephalitis include mental deteriora-tion, amnesia, personality changes, and hemiparesis.

Acyclovir (Zovirax) and vidarabine (Vira-A) are used to treat encephalitis caused by HSV infection. Acyclovir has fewer side effects than vidarabine and is often the preferred treat-ment. Use of these antiviral agents has been shown to reduce mortality rates from 70% to 30%, although neurologic compli-cations may not be reduced.[32] Long-term symptoms include memory impairment, epilepsy, anosmia, personality changes, behavioral abnormalities, and dysphasia. For maximal benefit, antiviral agents should be started before the onset of coma.

BRAIN ABSCESS

Brain abscess is an accumulation of pus within the brain tissue that can result from a local or a systemic infection (Fig. 54-16). Direct extension from ear, tooth, mastoid, or sinus infection is the primary cause. Other causes for brain abscess formation in-clude septic venous thrombosis from a pulmonary infection, bacterial endocarditis, skull fracture, and a nonsterile neuro-logic procedure. Streptococci and staphylococci are the pri-mary infective organisms.

Manifestations are similar to those of meningitis and en-cephalitis and include headache and fever. Signs of increased ICP may include drowsiness, confusion, and seizures. Focal symptoms may be present and reflect the local area of the ab-scess. For example, visual field defects or psychomotor seizures are common with a temporal lobe abscess, whereas an occipital abscess may be accompanied by visual impairment and halluci-nations.

Antimicrobial therapy is the primary treatment for brain abscess. Other manifestations are treated symptomatically. If drug therapy is not effective, the abscess may need to be drained, or removed if it is encapsulated. In untreated cases, the mortality rate approaches 100%. Seizures occur in approxi-mately 30% of the cases. Nursing measures are similar to those for management of meningitis or increased ICP. If surgical drainage or removal is the treatment of choice, nursing care is similar to that described under cranial surgery.

Other infections of the brain include subdural empyema, osteomyelitis of the cranial bones, epidural abscess, and venous sinus thrombosis after periorbital cellulitis.

REVIEW QUESTIONS

The number of the question corresponds to the same-numbered ob-jective at the beginning of the chapter.

1. The nurse determines that a patient is unconscious when the patient
   a. has cerebral ischemia.
   b. responds only to painful stimuli.
   c. is unaware of self or environment.
   d. does not respond to verbal stimuli.

2. To evaluate levels of consciousness, the nurse uses the knowledge that consciousness involves
   a. adequate functioning of the autonomic nervous system.
   b. activation of a network of fibers located in the cere-bral cortex.
   c. an arousal component that functions if the cerebral cortex remains intact.
   d. the ability to reason, think, feel, and react to stimuli in a purposeful manner.

3. In caring for an unconscious patient the nurse
   a. pads the side rails for safety.
   b. frequently suctions the patient to stimulate coughing.
   c. places the patient on the side with the head of bed elevated.
   d. assesses motor and sensory status of the patient every 8 hours.

4. A patient with intracranial pressure monitoring has pres-sure of 12 mm Hg. The nurse understands that this pres-sure reflects
   a. a severe decrease in cerebral perfusion pressure.
   b. a decrease in the production of cerebrospinal fluid.
   c. the loss of autoregulatory control of intracranial pres-sure.
   d. a normal balance between brain tissue, blood, and cerebrospinal fluid.

5. Vasogenic cerebral edema increases intracranial pressure by
   a. shifting fluid in the gray matter.
   b. changes in the endothelial lining of cerebral capillaries.
   c. leaking molecules from the intracellular fluid to the capillaries.
   d. altering the osmotic gradient flow into the intravascu-lar component.

6. A patient with increased intracranial pressure is placed on mechanical ventilation to maintain PaO_2 at 100 mm Hg and $PaCO_2$ at 35 mm Hg. The rationale for this therapy is to
   a. increase cerebral blood flow.
   b. constrict cerebral blood vessels.
   c. remove fluid from cerebral tissues.
   d. decrease systemic blood pressure.

7. The nurse plans care for the patient with increased in-tracranial pressure with the knowledge that the best way to position the patient is to
   a. keep the head of the bed flat.
   b. maintain head alignment at 30 degrees.
   c. increase the head-of-bed angle to 30 degrees with pa-tient on left side.
   d. use a continuous-rotation bed to continuously change patient position.

8. The nurse is alerted to a possible acute subdural hematoma in the patient who
   a. has a linear skull fracture crossing a major artery.
   b. has focal symptoms of brain damage with no recollec-tion of a head injury.
   c. develops decreased level of consciousness and a headache within 48 hours of a head injury.
   d. has an immediate loss of consciousness with a brief lucid interval followed by decreasing level of con-sciousness.

9. During admission of a patient with a severe head injury to the emergency department, the nurse places the highest priority on assessment for
   a. patency of airway.
   b. presence of a neck injury.
   c. neurologic status with the Glasgow Coma Scale.
   d. cerebrospinal fluid leakage from the ears or nose.

10. A patient is suspected of having a cranial tumor. The signs and symptoms include memory deficits, visual distur-bances, weakness of right upper and lower extremities, and personality changes. The nurse recognizes that the tumor is most likely located in the
    a. frontal lobe.
    b. parietal lobe.
    c. occipital lobe.
    d. temporal lobe.

11. The nursing management of a patient with a brain tumor includes
    a. using diversion techniques to keep the patient stimulated and motivated.
    b. discussing with the patient methods to control inappropriate behavior.
    c. assisting and supporting the family in understanding any changes in behavior.
    d. limiting self-care activities until the patient has regained maximum physical functioning.

12. The primary goal of nursing care after a craniotomy is
    a. prevention of infection.
    b. ensuring patient comfort.
    c. avoiding need for secondary surgery.
    d. preventing increased intracranial pressure.

13. During assessment of the patient with meningitis, the most critical signs and symptoms for the nurse to note are
    a. headache, fever, nuchal rigidity.
    b. irritability, headache, anorexia.
    c. headache, fever, heart palpitations.
    d. nausea, vomiting, restlessness.

14. A nursing measure that is indicated to reduce the potential for seizures and increased intracranial pressure in the patient with meningitis is
    a. administering codeine for relief of head and neck pain.
    b. controlling fever with prescribed drugs and cooling techniques.
    c. keeping the room darkened and quiet to minimize environmental stimulation.
    d. maintaining the patient on strict bed rest with the head of the bed slightly elevated.

References

1. Plum F, Posner J: *The diagnosis of stupor and coma,* ed 3, Philadelphia, 1980, FA Davis.
2. Jennett B, Teasdale G: Aspects of coma after severe head injury, *Lancet* 23:878, 1977.
3. Cushing H: *Studies in intracranial physiology and surgery,* London, 1925, Oxford University Press.
4. Go KG: The normal and pathological physiology of brain water, *Adv Tech Stand Neurosurg* 23:47, 1997.
5. Betz AL, Crockard A: Brain edema and the blood-brain barrier. In Crockard A and others, editors: *Neurosurgery: the scientific basis of clinical practice,* Boston, 1992, Blackwell Scientific.
6. Ropper AH: Coma and acutely raised intracranial pressure. In Asbury AK and others, editors: *Diseases of the nervous system: clinical neurobiology,* Philadelphia, 1992, Saunders.
7. Gilman AG: *Goodman and Gilman pharmacological basis of therapeutics,* New York, 1993, McGraw-Hill.
8. Visweswaran P, Massin EK, Dubose TD: Mannitol-induced acute renal failure, *J Am Soc Nephrol* 8:1028, 1997.
9. Prough DS, DeWitt DS: Cerebral protection. In Chernow B, editor: *The pharmacologic approach to the critically ill patient,* ed 3, Baltimore, 1994, Williams & Wilkins.
10. Cooper PR and others: Dexamethasone and severe head injury. A prospective double-blind study, *J Neurosurg* 51:307, 1979.
11. Dearden NM and others: Effect of high-dose dexamethasone on outcome from severe head injury, *J Neurosurg* 64:81, 1986.
12. Hickey JV: *Neurological and neurosurgical nursing,* ed 4, Philadelphia, 1997, Lippincott.
13. Silvestri S, Aronson S: Severe head injury: prehospital and emergency department management, *Mt Sinai J Med* 64:329, 1997.
14. Roberts P: Nutrition in the head-injured patient, *New Horizons* 3:506, 1995.
15. Kerr ME and others: Effect of short-duration hyperventilation during endotracheal suctioning on intracranial pressure in severe head injured adults, *Nurs Res* 48:195, 1997.
16. Kerr ME and others: Head injured adults: recommendations for endotracheal suctioning, *J Neurosci Nurs* 25:86, 1993.
17. Lundberg N: Continuous recording and control of ventricular fluid pressure in neurosurgical practice, *Acta Psychiatr Neurol Scand* 36:1, 1960.
18. Unterberg AW and others: Multimodal monitoring in patients with head injury: evaluation of the effects of treatment on cerebral oxygenation, *J Trauma* 42(5 suppl):S32, 1997.
19. Simmons BJ: Management of intracranial hemodynamics in the adult: a research analysis of head positioning and recommendations for clinical practice and future research, *J Neuroscience Nurs* 29:44, 1997.
20. Tillett JM and others: Effect of continuous rotational therapy on intracranial pressure in the severely brain-injured patient, *Crit Care Med* 21:1005, 1993.
21. Quigley MR and others: Defining the limits of survivorship after very severe head injury, *J Trauma* 42:7, 1997.
22. Marmarou A and others: Impact of ICP instability and hypotension on outcome in patients with severe head trauma, *J Neurosurg* 75:S59, 1991.
23. National Safety Council: *Accident facts,* Chicago, 1997, National Safety Council.
24. Sosin DM, Sniezek JE, Waxweiler RJ: Trends in death associated with brain injury, *JAMA* 278:1778, 1995.
25. Povlishock JT: Traumatic brain injury: the pathobiology of injury and repair. In Gorio A, editor: *Neuroregeneration,* New York, 1993, Raven Press.
26. Walleck C: Patients with head injury and brain dysfunction. In Clochesy JM and others, editors: *Critical care nursing,* ed 2, Philadelphia, 1997, Saunders.
27. Celli P, Fruin A, Cervoni L: Severe head trauma. Review of factors influencing the prognosis, *Minerva Chir* 52:1467, 1997.
28. Rordorf G and others: Patients in poor neurological condition after subarachnoid hemorrhage: early management and long-term outcome, *Acta Neurochir* 139:1143, 1997.
29. Acorn S, Roberts E: Head injury: impact on the wives, *J Neurosci Nurs* 24:324, 1992.
30. Landis SH and others: Cancer statistics,1998, *CA Cancer J Clin* 48:6, 1998.
31. Wildemann B and others: Quantification of herpes simplex virus type 1 DNA in cells of cerebrospinal fluid of patients with herpes simplex virus encephalitis, *Neurology* 48:1341, 1997.
32. McGrath and others: Herpes simplex encephalitis treated with acyclovir: diagnosis and long term outcomes, *J Neurol Neurosurg Psychiatry* 63:321, 1997.

Resources

American Brain Tumor Association
2720 River Road
Des Plaines, IL 60018
847-827-9910
Fax: 847-827-9918
800-886-2282
http://www.abta.org

National Brain Tumor Association
Harvard Medical School
3725 North Talman Avenue
Chicago, IL 60618
http://neurosurgery.mgh.harvard.edu/

National Head Injury Foundation
333 Turnpike Road
Southborough, MA 01772
508-485-9950

For additional Internet resources, see the website for this book at **www.mosby.com/MERLIN/medsurg_lewis**

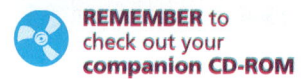
55 NURSING MANAGEMENT
Patient with a Stroke

Barbara Brillhart

www.mosby.com/MERLIN/medsurg_lewis

LEARNING OBJECTIVES

1. Describe the incidence of and risk factors for stroke.
2. Explain the mechanisms that affect cerebral blood flow.
3. Compare and contrast the pathophysiology of strokes caused by thrombosis, embolism, and intracranial hemorrhage.
4. Correlate the clinical manifestations of stroke with the underlying pathophysiology.
5. Describe diagnostic study abnormalities commonly found in patients with cerebrovascular accidents.
6. Describe the collaborative care, drug therapy, and dietary therapy of the stroke patient.
7. Describe the acute nursing management of the stroke patient.
8. Describe the rehabilitative nursing management of the stroke patient.
9. Explain the psychosocial impact of a stroke on the patient and family.

Cerebrovascular accident (*CVA*) (also referred to as stroke or "brain attack") is a broad term that includes a variety of disorders that influence blood flow to the brain and result in neurologic deficits. Proper functioning of the brain depends on an adequate blood supply to deliver oxygen and glucose for neuronal activity and to remove the end products of metabolism. CVAs result when there is inadequate supply of blood to the brain (cerebral ischemia) or cerebral hemorrhage within the brain. Regardless of the cause, the damaged brain no longer performs cognitive, sensory, motor, or emotional functions. The effects of the CVA may vary from minor to severe disability.

Stroke is the third most common cause of death and is the leading cause of serious, long-term disability in the United States and Canada. Strokes are considered a major public health problem in terms of mortality and morbidity; 500,000 to 600,000 persons experience CVAs annually. In the United States during 1995 there were approximately 158,000 deaths from CVA.[1] Approximately 31% of people who have an initial stroke die within 1 year. This percentage is higher among people age 65 and older. Permanent disability occurs in two thirds of the people having strokes. Although one third of individuals having a stroke die within 1 month of occurrence, 2 to 3 million people live with disability as a direct result of strokes. Rehabilitation is a realistic option for 90% of older adults who have had a stroke.

Strokes have significant economic effects on the patient, family, and community. The direct and indirect costs of strokes are estimated to be greater than $18 billion per year in the United States.[1] The majority of the cost for care of the patient who has experienced a CVA is provided by Medicare (72.8%) and Medicaid (8.7%). Self-pay (4.6%) and private insurance (1.9%) make up the rest of the financial support.[2] Disability, disruption of lives, and reduced quality of life for patients with a CVA cannot be calculated in terms of financial impact but in terms of human suffering and disruption of lives.

RISK FACTORS FOR STROKES

The risk factors associated with strokes can be divided into nonmodifiable and potentially modifiable. Risk for stroke increases for persons with more than one risk factor.

The nonmodifiable risk factors include gender, age, race, and heredity. The incidence of stroke is higher in men than women. The incidence of stroke increases with age until age 75. The occurrence rate in adults age 55 to 74 years is 15.1% as compared with 5.6% in those 75 years and older.[2] African-Americans experience a higher incidence of stroke that is associated with an increased incidence of hypertension. Persons with a family history of stroke or transient ischemic attacks (TIAs) are also considered at higher risk for stroke.[3]

Modifiable risk factors are those that can be potentially changed and thus reduce the risk of CVA. Lifestyle habits, including excessive alcohol consumption, cigarette smoking, obesity, diet high in fat content, and drug abuse, increase the risk for stroke. Many pathologic conditions also increase the risk for stroke and include cardiac disease, diabetes mellitus, hypertension, migraine headaches, hypercoagulability states (e.g., high serum fibrinogen levels, increased hematocrit), polycythemia, and sickle cell anemia. Approximately 9% of men and 18% of women who have had a myocardial infarction will have a stroke within 6 years. Control of hypertension is considered the most significant therapy in the prevention of strokes.[4] Women who smoke have a fivefold increased risk for

Reviewed by Karen March, RN, MN, CNRN, CCRN, Neuroscience Clinical Nurse Specialist, Harborview Medical Center, Seattle, Wash.

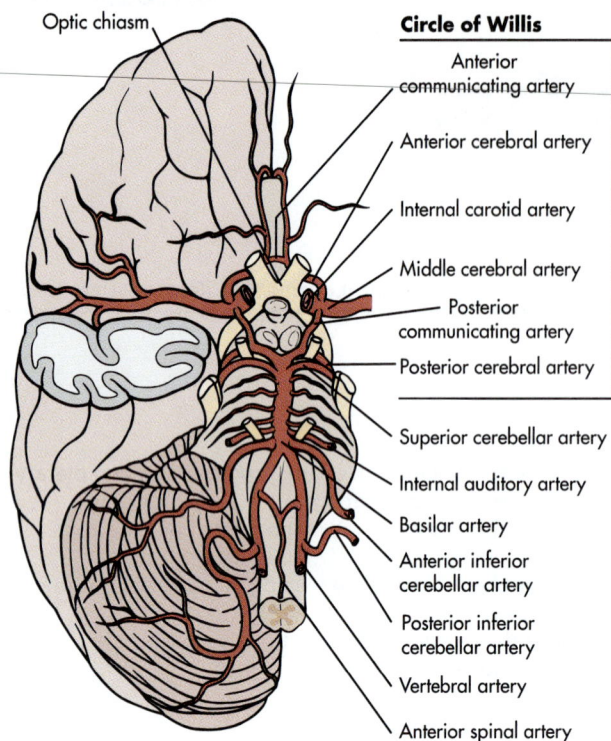

Fig. 55-1   Circle of Willis and vertebrobasilar circulation. Temporal lobes have been removed to show the course of the middle cerebral artery.

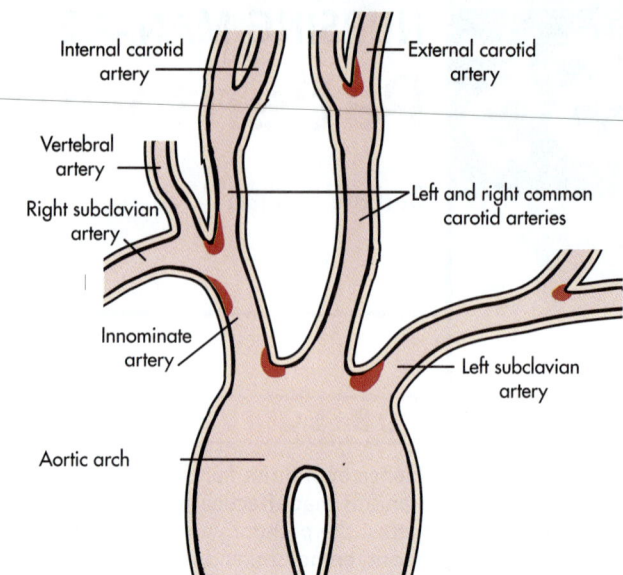

Fig. 55-2   Common sites for the development of atherosclerosis in extracranial and intracranial arteries. The main locations are just above the common carotid bifurcation (most common site) and the start of the branches from the aorta, innominate, and subclavian arteries.

stroke as compared with nonsmokers. If a woman smokes and uses estrogen-containing oral contraception, the risk for stroke increases.[5] Early treatment and management of these associated diseases and poor health habits will decrease the incidence of stroke.

ETIOLOGY AND PATHOPHYSIOLOGY
Regulation of Cerebral Blood Flow

Because neurons do not regenerate, the prevention of cerebral damage is necessary to prevent neurologic deficits. Blood flow must be maintained at 750 to 1000 ml/min (55 ml/100 g brain tissue) or 20% of the cardiac output to ensure optimal cerebral functioning. If blood flow to the brain is totally interrupted (e.g., cardiac arrest), neurologic metabolism is altered in 30 seconds, metabolism stops in 2 minutes, and cellular death occurs in 5 minutes.

The cerebrovascular system is highly adaptive. It maintains a constant blood flow to the brain in spite of significant changes in the systemic circulation. The factors that affect cerebral blood flow can be divided into extracranial and intracranial factors.

Extracranial Factors. The extracranial factors are primarily related to the circulatory system. They include systemic blood pressure, cardiac output, and viscosity of the blood. During activities of daily living (ADLs) there are great variations in local oxygen requirements. Alterations in cardiac output, vasomotor tone, and distribution of blood flow are effective in maintaining constant cerebral perfusion. The mean arterial blood pressure has to fall below 70 mm Hg or rise above 160 mm Hg before the cerebral blood flow is altered, and cardiac output has to be reduced by one third before cere-

bral blood flow is reduced. Changes in blood viscosity increase or decrease cerebral blood flow. Anemia increases cerebral blood flow and polycythemia reduces it.

Intracranial Factors

Metabolic factors. Metabolic alterations are important intracranial factors involved in the regulation of cerebral blood flow. Metabolic factors that result in vasodilation with restoration of blood flow toward normal include high carbon dioxide concentration and low oxygen tension. Carbon dioxide, however, is the most potent regulator of cerebral blood flow. An increase in hydrogen ion concentration also increases cerebral blood flow. Alone or in combination, these metabolic factors can maintain adequate cerebral blood flow in normal situations.

Blood vessels. The condition of the blood vessels supplying the brain also influences the cerebral blood flow (see Chapter 53). Many persons have congenital anomalies in the cerebrovascular system. These anomalies include tortuosity, coiling, kinking, and arteriovenous malformations. These congenital anomalies may interfere with cerebral blood flow and are common sites for the development of atherosclerotic diseases. Atherosclerosis from any cause increases resistance in the blood vessels and further reduces blood flow.

Collateral circulation (alternate flow to compensate for decreased blood flow) is another factor related to cerebral blood flow. Collateral circulation develops in response to a decrease in normal blood flow. The circle of Willis contains many collateral circulatory connections and is responsible for the greater part of collateral circulation (Fig. 55-1). These collateral vessels can maintain cerebral blood flow in the event of damage to the main blood supply. Individual differences in the state of the collateral circulation when a stroke occurs partly determine the degree of functional loss.

Intracranial pressure. Intracranial pressure is another factor that influences cerebral blood flow (see Chapter 54). Among

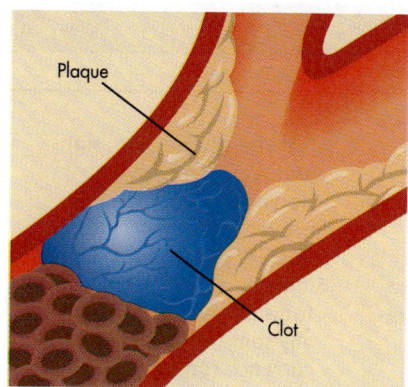

A. Thrombotic stroke. Cerebral thrombosis is a narrowing of the artery by fatty deposits called *plaque*. Plaque can cause a clot to form, which blocks the passage of blood through the artery.

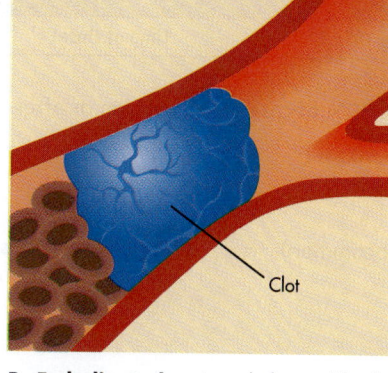

B. Embolic stroke. An embolus is a blood clot or other debris circulating in the blood. When it reaches an artery in the brain that is too narrow to pass through, it lodges there and blocks the flow of blood.

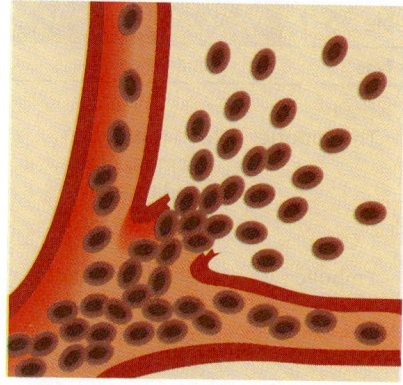

C. Hemorrhagic stroke. A burst blood vessel may allow blood to seep into and damage brain tissues until clotting shuts off the leak.

Fig. 55-3   Three types of stroke.

CULTURAL & ETHNIC CONSIDERATIONS

Cerebrovascular Disease

- A high mortality rate from CVAs exists among African-American men, possibly as a result of the high frequency of hypertension in this group.
- Ischemic strokes are twice as common among African-Americans as Caucasians.
- Hemorrhagic strokes are three times more common among African-Americans than Caucasians.

the causes of increased intracranial pressure are stroke, neoplasms, inflammation, trauma, and hydrocephalus. Increased intracranial pressure compresses the brain and reduces cerebral blood flow. Greatly reduced cerebral blood flow may result in cerebral infarction.

Both extracranial and intracranial factors may be involved in a stroke. The initial insult may be related to one or more of these factors. For example, when an intracranial hemorrhage occurs, the continuity of the vascular system is interrupted. The lost blood and cerebral edema secondary to the inflammatory process contribute to an increase in intracranial pressure. This interferes with cerebral perfusion, and carbon dioxide and hydrogen ion concentration increase, leading to a further dilation of cerebral vessels and increased intracranial pressure.

Atherosclerosis

Atherosclerosis, a common pathophysiologic process in stroke, is usually involved in the development of a thrombosis and is often implicated in strokes caused by emboli. (The role that atherosclerosis plays in the development of thrombosis and emboli is discussed in Chapter 32 and shown in Fig. 32-4.) Initially an abnormal infiltration of lipids occurs in the intima of the arteries. This fatty streak may develop into an atherosclerotic plaque. These plaques often develop where there is in-

creased turbulence in the blood, as at the bifurcation of an artery or a tortuous area (Fig. 55-2). Turbulence may later damage the atherosclerotic plaque, resulting in a loss of intimal continuity or ulceration. Platelet and fibrin aggregate on the roughened surface. Parts of the plaque may break off and travel to a narrower distal artery. Cerebral infarction occurs at the point where the blood supply is cut off.

TYPES OF STROKE

CVAs are classified as thrombotic, embolic, or hemorrhagic strokes based on their underlying pathophysiology (Fig. 55-3). Ischemic strokes result from a decreased blood flow to the brain secondary to partial or complete occlusion of an artery. They occur much more frequently than hemorrhagic strokes. The most common types of ischemic stroke are thrombotic and embolic (Table 55-1). Hemorrhagic strokes are generally the result of spontaneous bleeding into the brain tissue itself (intracerebral or intraparenchymal hemorrhage) or into the subarachnoid space or the ventricles (subarachnoid hemorrhage).

Thrombotic Stroke

Thrombosis is the formation of a blood clot or coagulation that results in the narrowing of the lumen of a blood vessel with eventual occlusion. It is the most common cause of cerebral infarction. Two thirds of the strokes caused by thrombosis are associated with hypertension or diabetes mellitus, both of which accelerate the atherosclerotic process. Additional risk factors associated with thrombotic strokes include oral contraceptives, coagulation disorders, polycythemia vera, arteritis, chronic hypoxia, and dehydration.

Thrombosis develops readily where atheromatous plaques have already narrowed blood vessels. The thrombus results in further narrowing of the vessel lumen and ultimately hypoperfusion, infarction, and ischemia. A cascade of biochemical events occurs, including release of excitatory amino acids (e.g., glutamate, glutamine).[6] Excitatory amino acids via their direct effects on neurons may further compromise the ability of neurons to survive the ischemia and infarction.

Table 55-1	Types of Stroke			
Type	**Gender/Age**	**Warning**	**Time of Onset**	**Course/Prognosis**
Ischemic				
Thrombotic	Men more than women, oldest median age	TIA (30-50% of cases)	During or after sleep	Stepwise progression, signs and symptoms develop slowly, usually some improvement, recurrence in 20-25% of survivors
Embolic	Men more than women	TIA (uncommon)	Lack of relationship to activity, sudden onset	Single event, signs and symptoms develop quickly, usually some improvement, recurrence common without aggressive treatment of underlying disease
Hemorrhagic				
Intracerebral	Slightly higher in women	Headache (25% of cases)	Activity (often)	Progression over 24 hr; poor prognosis, fatality more likely with presence of coma
Subarachnoid	Slightly higher in women, youngest median age	Headache (common)	Activity (often), sudden onset; Most commonly related to head trauma	Single sudden event usually, fatality more likely with presence of coma

TIA, transient ischemic attack.

Thrombotic strokes are preceded in 30% to 50% of cases by prodromal episodes (symptoms indicating onset of disease), which occur hours to months before the stroke. The prodromal symptoms are considered TIAs and usually last 5 to 30 minutes. Prodromal episodes leave no residual deficits. Prodromal episodes include paresis (decreased strength and motion of an extremity), aphasia (disturbance of language function), paralysis, mental confusion, or visual disturbances. These symptoms suggest involvement of the carotid arteries and middle cerebral arteries. Prodromal episodes that include dizziness, diplopia (double vision), numbness, impaired vision, headaches, or dysarthria (speech difficulty) may indicate involvement of vertebral and basilar arteries (vertebrobasilar system).

The thrombotic stroke is characterized by a pattern of (1) a single attack where symptoms occur over several hours, (2) intermittent progression toward a stroke occurring over hours to days, (3) partial stroke with permanent neurologic deficits, or (4) a series of TIAs followed by a stroke with permanent neurologic deficits. The extent of the stroke depends on rapidity of onset, the size of the lesion, and the presence of collateral circulation. The typical picture of the stroke is signs and symptoms that peak in severity within 72 hours as edema increases in the infarction areas of the brain. After resolution of edema, which usually occurs within 2 weeks, there is a decrease in signs and symptoms.

In summary, the patient with a thrombotic stroke typically has some prewarning manifestations (TIAs) that may be less serious if there is collateral blood circulation and may experience decreasing symptoms as the edema is resolved.

Embolic Stroke

Cerebral embolism is the occlusion of a cerebral artery by an embolus, resulting in necrosis and edema of the area supplied by the involved blood vessel. Embolism is the second most common cause of stroke. The majority of emboli originate in the endocardial (inside) layer of the heart, with plaques or tissue breaking off from the endocardium and entering the circulation. The emboli travel to smaller vessels and become a source of obstruction at areas of vascular narrowing or bifurcation. Emboli are associated with heart conditions such as atrial fibrillation, myocardial infarction, infective endocarditis, rheumatic heart disease, valvular prostheses, and atrial septal defects. Less common causes of emboli include air, fat from long bone (femur) fractures, amniotic fluid after childbirth, and tumors.

In general, the patient with an embolic stroke commonly has a rapid occurrence of severe clinical manifestations. Embolic strokes can affect any age-group. An embolic stroke secondary to rheumatic heart disease may involve young to middle-aged adults. An embolus arising from an atherosclerotic plaque is more common in older adults. A prodromal warning is less common with embolic than with thrombotic stroke. The onset of an embolic stroke is usually sudden and may or may not be related to activity. The patient usually maintains consciousness, although a headache may develop on the side where the embolus is lodged. Prognosis is related to the amount of brain tissue deprived of its blood supply. For example, embolic strokes most commonly affect the middle cerebral artery, which is a direct continuation of the internal carotid artery. The effects of the emboli are initially characterized by severe neurologic deficits, which can be temporary if the clot breaks up and allows blood to flow. Smaller emboli then continue to obstruct smaller vessels, which in turn involve smaller portions of the brain with fewer deficits noted. The embolic stroke often occurs so rapidly that the body does not have time to accommodate with the formation of collateral circulation. Recurrence of embolic stroke is common unless the underlying cause is aggressively treated.

Intracerebral Hemorrhage Stroke

Intracerebral hemorrhage is bleeding within the brain caused by a rupture of vessels that lasts from minutes to days. Intracerebral hemorrhage is commonly caused by hypertension. Other causes of intracerebral hemorrhage include brain tumors, trauma, thrombolytic drugs, and ruptured aneurysms. Hypertension and atherosclerosis cause degenerative changes in the walls of arteries, resulting in rupture and subsequent hemorrhage. Hemorrhage commonly occurs without prodromal symptoms and during periods of activity. The extent of the symptoms varies depending on the amount and duration of the bleeding. The blood within the closed area of the brain forms a fluid mass that imposes pressure on the brain tissue. The pressure in turn displaces brain tissue and decreases blood flow to the brain, which is associated with ischemia and infarction.

The most common sites of intracerebral hemorrhage are the putamen and internal capsule (50%), central white matter, thalamus, cerebellar hemispheres, and pons. Initially, the patient experiences a severe headache with nausea and vomiting. Clinical manifestations related to putaminal and internal capsule bleeding include weakness of one side, including the face, arm, and leg; slurred speech; and deviation of the eyes. Progression of manifestations related to a severe hemorrhage include hemiplegia, fixed and dilated pupils, abnormal body posturing, and coma. Thalamic hemorrhage results in hemiplegia with more sensory than motor losses. Bleeding into the subthalamic areas of the brain leads to disturbance with vision and eye movement. Cerebellar hemorrhages are characterized by severe headache, vomiting, loss of ability to walk, dysphagia, dysarthria, and eye movement disturbances. Hemorrhage in the pons is the most serious because basic life functions (e.g., respiration) are rapidly affected. In addition, hemorrhage in the pons can be characterized by hemiplegia leading to complete paralysis, coma, abnormal body posturing, fixed pupils, hyperthermia, and death.

The prognosis of intracerebral hemorrhage strokes is poor: 70% of patients die soon after the occurrence of the stroke. If the area of bleeding is minimal, prognosis is better because the small amount of hemorrhage can be resolved. In summary, the patient with intracerebral hemorrhage has no forewarning; has rapid, severe symptoms occurring with activity; and has a poor prognosis for recovery.

Subarachnoid Hemorrhage Stroke

The causes of subarachnoid hemorrhage include aneurysms (congenital or acquired weakness and ballooning of vessels), arteriovenous malformations, trauma, and hypertension. Aneurysms within the brain affect persons from 20 to 70 years of age. They are associated with atherosclerosis, trauma, hypertension, or congenital malformations and account for approximately 30,000 new cases of subarachnoid hemorrhage annually.[7] Occasionally, hemorrhages are related to medications such as anticoagulants, thrombolytics, and sympathomimetics. The patient may exhibit prodromal symptoms if the ballooning or dilation applies pressure to brain tissue. The aneurysm may also suddenly rupture, causing rapid neurologic changes. The majority (85%) of the aneurysms are in the circle of Willis. Aneurysms may be saccular or berry aneurysms ranging from a few millimeters to 20 to 30 millimeters in size or fusiform atherosclerotic aneurysms.

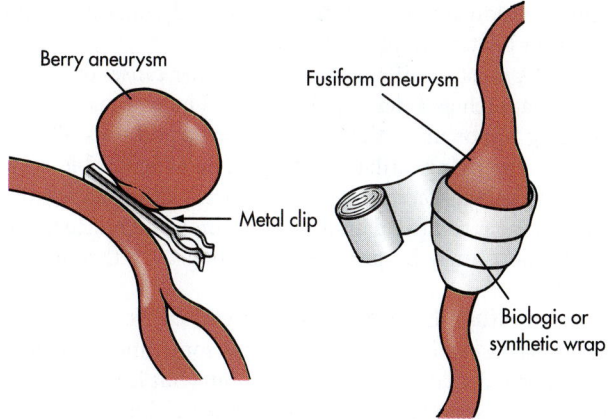

Fig. 55-4 Clipping and wrapping of aneurysms.

Headaches can be associated with a small amount of bleeding because of aneurysm leakage. Rupture of the aneurysm causes hemorrhage and pressure in the subarachnoid space, which may cause headache, lethargy, confusion, nausea, vomiting, fever, neck pain and backaches, paralysis, coma, and death.[7]

A massive hemorrhage is quantified as 30 to 50 ml of blood. Initially a clot forms at the site of a ruptured aneurysm. As the clot begins to dissolve and vasospasm subsides, the chance of renewed bleeding increases. Prognosis for patients with a subarachnoid hemorrhage is guarded because many patients (30%) experience another bleed within 2 weeks of the first occurrence. New surgical procedures, such as clipping and wrapping of aneurysms (Fig. 55-4), have decreased the death rate for these patients.

Temporal Development of Cerebrovascular Accident

The classification of temporal development of CVAs includes TIA, reversible ischemic neurologic deficit, stroke-in-evolution or progressing stroke, and completed stroke (stable stroke). Knowledge of this classification is useful in planning nursing care.

Transient Ischemic Attacks.
The TIA is characterized by brief episodes of neurologic manifestations, which clear completely in less than 24 hours.[7] The neurologic deficits present with TIAs disappear leaving no residual effects. Persons experiencing TIAs fall into three categories: one third never have another TIA, one third will have more than one TIA, and one third will experience a stroke.[8]

It is thought that TIAs are a result of microemboli from atherosclerotic plaques found in extracranial arteries that lead to temporary cerebral ischemia. Patients should consider TIAs as a warning sign of progressing cerebrovascular disease. The signs and symptoms of TIAs vary according to the part of the brain affected. The anatomic location of the neurologic deficit can be identified on the basis of clinical manifestations. If the carotid system is involved, the patient may report a temporary loss of vision in one eye, a transient hemiparesis, or a sudden inability to speak. Common manifestations of TIA related to vertebrobasilar insufficiency are tinnitus, vertigo, darkened or blurred vision, diplopia, ptosis, dysarthria, dysphagia, and unilateral or bilateral numbness or weakness.

A TIA must be differentiated from other causes of cerebral ischemia, such as a developing subdural hematoma or an increasing tumor mass. Cardiac monitoring and tests often reveal an underlying cardiac condition that is responsible for the clot formation. Medications that prevent platelet aggregation, such as aspirin, dipyridamole (Persantine), and anticoagulant medications, may be prescribed for long-term therapy after a TIA.

Reversible Ischemic Neurologic Deficit.   The term *reversible ischemic neurologic deficit* is sometimes used if the neurologic deficit remains after 24 hours but leaves no residual signs or symptoms after days to weeks. This is considered by some to be a completed stroke with minimal to no residual deficit.

Stroke-in-Evolution.   A stroke-in-evolution, or a progressing stroke, develops over a period of hours or days. This pattern of progression is most characteristic of an enlarging intraarterial thrombus. A stepwise or intermittent progression of deterioration of neurologic findings is common. The progression occurs because ischemic tissue becomes infarcted tissue. The manifestations of stroke-in-evolution do not resolve (as compared with TIAs) and leave residual neurologic effects.

Completed Stroke.   When the neurologic deficit remains unchanged over a 2- to 3-day period, the stroke is termed a *completed stroke* (stable stroke). An embolic stroke may demonstrate this characteristic from the onset. With the exception of stroke secondary to a ruptured aneurysm, a completed stroke signals readiness for more aggressive rehabilitative treatment. If a ruptured aneurysm is the suspected cause, activity may be restricted for as long as 3 to 4 weeks to reduce the possibility of rebleeding.

CLINICAL MANIFESTATIONS

A CVA ultimately affects many body functions, including neuromotor activity, elimination, intellectual function, spatial-perceptual alterations, personality and affect, sensation, and communication. The functions affected are directly related to the brain area perfused by the affected artery (Table 55-2). Manifestations related to right- and left-brain damage are shown in Fig. 55-5.

Neuromotor Function

Motor deficits are the most obvious effect of stroke. Problems associated with neuromotor function deficits include impairment of (1) mobility, (2) respiratory function, (3) swallowing and speech, (4) gag reflex, and (5) self-care abilities. The symptoms are caused by the destruction of motor neurons in the pyramidal pathway (nerve fibers from the brain and passing through the spinal cord to the motor cells). The characteristic motor deficits include loss of skilled voluntary movement (akinesia), impairment of integration of movements, alterations in muscle tone, and alterations in reflexes. The initial hyporeflexia (depressed reflexes) progresses to hyperreflexia (hyperactive reflexes) for most patients.

Motor deficits after a stroke follow characteristic patterns. Because of the pyramidal pathway crossing at the level of the medulla, a lesion on one side of the brain affects the motor function on the opposite side of the brain (contralateral). The

Table 55-2   Clinical Manifestations: Specific Cerebral Artery Involvement

Middle Cerebral Artery Involvement
Blockage of main stem
  Contralateral paralysis (hemiplegia)
  Contralateral anesthesia; loss of proprioception, fine touch, localization (hemiparesis)
  Dominant hemisphere: aphasia
  Nondominant hemisphere: neglect of opposite side, dysmetria
  Homonymous hemianopsia, conjugate gaze paralysis

Anterior Cerebral Artery Involvement
Occlusion of stem*
Occlusion distal to anterior to communicating artery
  Contralateral sensory and motor deficits of foot and leg
  Contralateral weakness of proximal upper extremity
  Urinary incontinence (possibly unrecognized by patient)
  Contralateral grasp and sucking reflexes may be present
  Apraxia
  Personality change: flat affect, loss of spontaneity, distractibility
  Possible cognitive impairment

Posterior Cerebral Artery Involvement†
Thalamogeniculate branch occlusion
  Contralateral sensory loss
  Temporary hemiparesis
  Homonymous hemianopsia
Paramedian branch occlusion: central midbrain and subthalamus
  Weber's syndrome: oculomotor nerve palsy and contralateral hemiplegia
Cortical occlusion: temporal and occipital lobes
  Incomplete homonymous hemianopsia
  Dominant hemisphere: dysphasia, anomia
  Nondominant hemisphere: disorientation
Upper basilar occlusion (bilateral)
  Visual disturbances (blindness, homonymous hemianopsia, visual hallucinations, apraxia of ocular movements)
  Anomia: objects and inability to count
  Possible memory loss

Vertebrobasilar Artery Involvement
Bilateral motor and sensory deficits of all extremities
Ipsilateral Horner's syndrome: miosis, ptosis, decreased sweating
Hoarseness
Dysphagia
Nystagmus, diplopia, blindness
Nausea, vomiting
Ataxia

*There is usually no problem if the stem is occluded near the anterior communicating artery because perfusion from the opposite side is maintained.
†The site of occlusion, the origin of the basilar arteries, and the arrangement of the circle of Willis are involved in the type of deficit seen. This can occur from a thrombus or embolus.

arms and legs of the affected side may be weakened or paralyzed to different degrees depending on which part of and to what extent the cerebral circulation was compromised. A stroke affecting the middle cerebral artery leads to a greater weakness in the upper extremity than the lower extremity. The

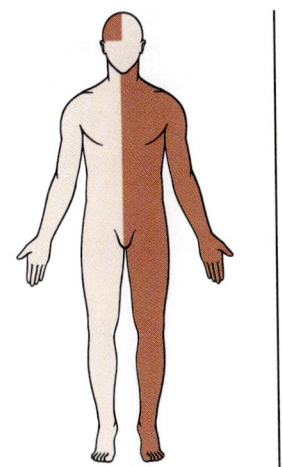
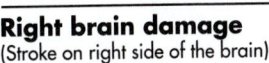
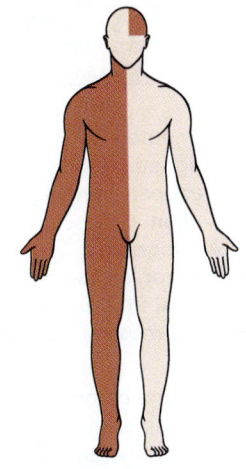

Right brain damage
(Stroke on right side of the brain)

- Paralyzed left side: hemiplegia
- Left-sided neglect
- Spatial-perceptual deficits
- Tends to deny or minimize problems
- Rapid performance, short attention span
- Impulsive, safety problems
- Impaired judgment
- Impaired time concepts

Left brain damage
(Stroke on left side of the brain)

- Paralyzed right side: hemiplegia
- Impaired speech/language aphasias
- Impaired right/left discrimination
- Slow performance, cautious
- Impaired speech/language
- Aware of deficits: depression, anxiety
- Impaired comprehension related to language, math

Fig. 55-5 Manifestations of right-sided and left-sided stroke.

affected shoulder tends to rotate internally, and the hip rotates externally. The affected foot is plantar flexed and inverted. An initial period of flaccidity may last from days to several weeks and is related to nerve damage. Spasticity of the muscles follows the flaccid stage and is related to interruption of upper motor neuron influence.

Communication

The left hemisphere is dominant for language skills in all right-handed persons and in the majority of left-handed persons. Language disorders involve the expression and comprehension of written and spoken words. The patient may experience aphasia (total loss of comprehension and use of language) when a stroke damages the dominant hemisphere of the brain. Dysphasia refers to dysfunction related to the comprehension or use of language and is due to partial disruption or loss. Patterns of dysphasia may differ as the stroke affects different portions of the brain. Dysphasias can be classified as nonfluent (minimal speech activity with slow speech that requires obvious effort) or fluent (speech is present, but contains little meaningful communication). Most dysphasias are mixed with impairment in both expression and understanding. A massive stroke may result in global aphasia, in which all communication and receptive function is lost.

Strokes affecting Wernicke's area of the brain exhibit symptoms of receptive aphasia when neither the sounds of speech nor its meaning can be understood. Damage to Wernicke's area impairs the patient's comprehension of both spoken and written language. Strokes affecting Broca's area of the brain cause expressive aphasia (difficulty in speaking and writing).

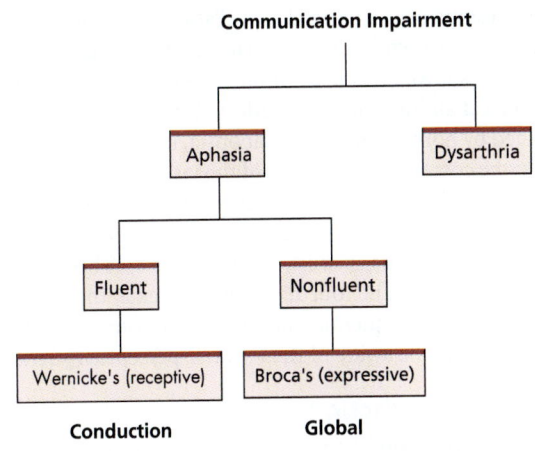

Fig. 55-6 Types of communication impairment common after stroke.

Many stroke patients also experience dysarthria, a disturbance in the muscular control of speech. Patients experience impairments with pronunciation, articulation, and phonation. Dysarthria does not affect the meaning of communication nor the comprehension of language by the patient, but it does affect the mechanics of speech. Some patients experience a combination of aphasia and dysarthria (Fig. 55-6).

Affect

Patients who have had a stroke may be unable to control their emotions. Their emotional response may be exaggerated or unpredictable. This situation is compounded by the depression associated with changes in body image and loss of function. In addition, they are frustrated related to mobility and communication problems. An example of unpredictable affect is as follows: A reserved professional engineer has returned home from the hospital following a stroke. During meals with his family, he becomes frustrated and begins to cry because of the difficulties involved in getting food into his mouth and chewing.

Intellectual Function

Both memory and judgment may be impaired as a result of stroke. These impairments are experienced with strokes affecting either side of the brain. A left-brain stroke is more likely to result in memory problems related to language. Patients with a left-brain stroke characteristically are very cautious in matters of judgment. The patient with a right-brain stroke tends to be impulsive and to move quickly. An example of behavior seen with right-brain stroke is the patient who tries to rise quickly from the wheelchair without locking the wheels or raising the foot rests. The patient with a left-brain stroke would move slowly and cautiously from the bed to the wheelchair. Patients with either type of stroke may experience difficulty in making generalizations, which interferes with their ability to learn.

Spatial-Perceptual Alterations

A stroke in the right side of the brain is more likely to cause deficits in spatial-perceptual orientation, although this can also occur with left-brain stroke. These spatial-perceptual deficits may be divided into four categories. The first is related to the patient's erroneous perception of self and illness. This deficit follows lesions of the parietal lobe. Patients may deny their illnesses or their own body parts. The second category concerns the patient's erroneous perception of self in space. The patient may neglect all input from the affected side. This may be compounded by homonymous hemianopsia, in which blindness occurs in the corresponding halves of the visual fields of both eyes. In addition, the patient has difficulty with spatial orientation, such as judgment of distances. The third spatial-perceptual deficit is agnosia, the inability to recognize an object by sight, touch, or hearing. The fourth deficit is apraxia, the inability to carry out learned sequential movements on command. Patients may or may not be aware of their spatial-perceptual alterations.

Elimination Function

Fortunately, most problems with urinary and bowel elimination occur initially and are transient. When a stroke affects one hemisphere of the brain, the prognosis for normal bladder function is excellent. The pathway between the bladder and the spinal cord remains intact, and partial sensation for bladder filling remains, as well as partial voluntary urination. Initially, the patient may experience frequency, urgency, and incontinence. Although motor control of the bowel is usually not a problem, patients are frequently constipated. Constipation is associated with immobility, weak abdominal muscles, dehydration, and diminished response to the defecation reflex. Both urinary and bowel elimination problems may also be related to the functional inabilities to express needs and inability to manage clothing.

DIAGNOSTIC STUDIES

After a stroke, various diagnostic studies are carried out in an effort to determine the cause and location of the stroke (Table 55-3). Tests are also done to guide decisions about therapeutic or surgical treatment. A computed tomography (CT) scan is the primary diagnostic test used after a stroke. It can indicate the size and location of the lesion. CT testing is also useful in differentiating between infarction and hemorrhage. Serial CT scans are often used to determine the effectiveness of treatment and to evaluate the course of healing.

Other diagnostic tests used in the diagnosis of stroke include magnetic resonance imaging (MRI), positron emission tomography (PET), and digital subtraction angiography (DSA). MRI uses a magnetic field instead of radiation to produce a picture of the brain that is similar to that of a CT scan. MRI is considered by some to be the best imaging method to differentiate hemorrhagic from nonhemorrhagic infarcts. The use of MRI in the diagnosis of stroke has increased significantly in recent years. Diffusion-weighted MRI, a more sensitive version of the MRI, shows greater sensitivity in delineating ischemic brain injury early after a stroke when CT and standard MRI may appear normal.[9]

PET shows the chemical activity of the brain and provides an excellent depiction of the extent of tissue damage after a stroke. Less active or diseased tissue appears darker than healthy, active cells. Major research efforts are aimed at perfecting this technique to aid in the diagnosis and treatment of brain disease.

DSA involves the intravenous (IV) or arterial injection of a contrast agent to produce good visualization of blood vessels in the neck and the large vessels of the circle of Willis. Intraarterial injection of contrast material has almost completely replaced IV DSA because the arterial approach requires a smaller bolus of contrast fluid and produces superior results. It is considered

---

DIAGNOSTIC STUDIES

Table 55-3   Cerebrovascular Accident

Diagnosis of CVA, Including Extent of Involvement
- Computed tomography scan
- Magnetic resonance imaging
- Electroencephalogram
- Radionuclide scan (brain scan)
- Angiography
- Positron emission tomography
- Digital subtraction angiography
- Cerebrospinal fluid analysis*

Evaluation of Etiology of CVA
- Cerebral blood flow
  Doppler ultrasonography
     Transcranial Doppler
     Carotid duplex
  Carotid angiography
- Cardiac assessment
  Electrocardiogram
  Cardiac enzymes
  Echocardiography
  Holter monitor (evaluation of arrhythmias)

*For cerebrospinal fluid testing, a lumbar puncture is avoided if elevation of intracranial pressure is suspected.

---

safer than cerebral angiography because less vascular manipulation is required. However, conventional intraarterial angiography is still needed for examination of intracranial arteries. Angiography is potentially dangerous because of the risks related to dislodging an embolus, causing vasospasm, or inducing further hemorrhage. Thus it is performed only when no other, safer test can provide the needed information.

Transcranial Doppler (TCD) ultrasonography measures the velocity of blood flow in the cerebral arteries. TCD has been shown to be effective in detecting microemboli and vasospasm. Certain neurodiagnostic tests such as skull x-rays, brain scan, lumbar puncture, and electroencephalogram (EEG) that were formerly used in the diagnosis of stroke are currently used much less. Although the skull x-ray is usually normal after a stroke, there may be a pineal shift with a massive infarction. A brain scan shows increased uptake of radioactive media in the infarcted area.

A lumbar puncture, although not performed routinely, may show a transient increase in leukocytes in the cerebrospinal fluid (CSF). The presence of blood in the CSF is indicative but not diagnostic of hemorrhage. A lumbar puncture is usually not done in the presence of increased intracranial pressure (ICP) because of the danger of herniation from a sudden decrease in pressure. An EEG may show low-voltage, slow-wave activity that is suggestive of ischemic infarction. If hemorrhage is the cause of the stroke, the EEG may show high-voltage slow waves. Arteriography can demonstrate areas of cervical and cerebrovascular occlusion, atherosclerotic plaques, and malformation of vessels. If the suspected cause of the stroke includes emboli from the heart, diagnostic cardiac tests should be done (see Table 55-3).

COLLABORATIVE CARE
Prevention

Primary prevention is a priority for reducing morbidity and mortality associated with CVAs (Table 55-4). The goals of

COLLABORATIVE CARE

Table 55-4 Cerebrovascular Accident

Diagnostic*
History and physical examination

Collaborative Therapy
Prevention
  Control of hypertension
  Control of diabetes mellitus
  No smoking
  Limit alcohol intake
  Platelet inhibitors (e.g., aspirin)
  Anticoagulation therapy for patients with atrial
    fibrillation
  Treatment of underlying cardiac problem
  Surgical interventions for patients with aneurysms at risk
    of bleeding
  Carotid endarterectomy
  Transluminal angioplasty
  Extracranial-intracranial bypass

Acute Care
  Maintenance of airway
  Fluid therapy
  Ischemic (thrombotic and embolic) CVA
    Tissue plasminogen activator (t-PA)
    Anticoagulation
  Ischemic and hemorrhagic CVA
    Treatment of cerebral edema
  Hemorrhagic CVA
    Surgical decompression if indicated
  Subarachnoid hemorrhage
    Surgical extirpation (dependent on size and location
      of hemorrhage)
  Embolic CVA
    Treatment of underlying cause

*Diagnostic studies are presented in Table 55-3.

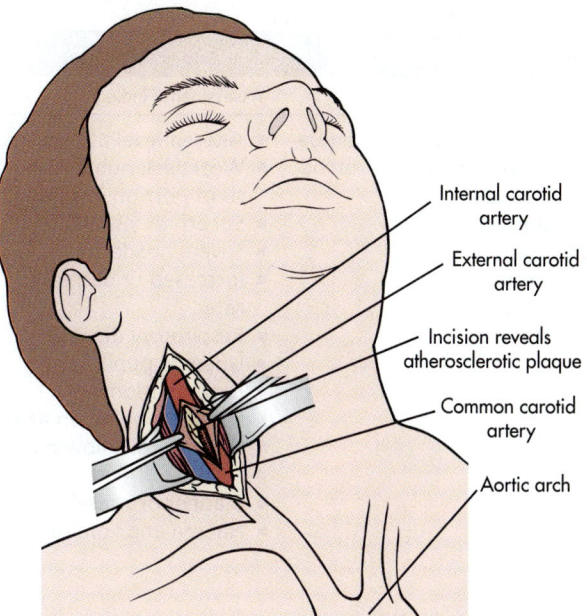

Fig. 55-7 Carotid endarterectomy. The atherosclerotic plaque in the internal carotid artery is removed to prevent impending cerebral infarction.

Labels: Internal carotid artery; External carotid artery; Incision reveals atherosclerotic plaque; Common carotid artery; Aortic arch

stroke prevention include health management for the well individual, management of modifiable risk factors, prevention of stroke for those with a history of TIA, and prevention of additional strokes for those who have had a CVA. Health management focuses on (1) healthy diet, (2) weight control, (3) regular exercise, (4) no smoking, (5) limiting alcohol consumption, and (6) routine health assessments. Patients with known risk factors such as diabetes mellitus, hypertension, obesity, high serum lipids, or cardiac dysfunction require close management of their illnesses. Postmenopausal women on estrogen therapy are less likely to experience a CVA as compared with women not on estrogen therapy.

Drug Therapy. Measures designed to prevent the development of a thrombus or embolus are also used in patients at risk. Low-dose aspirin is used prophylactically because of its antiplatelet effects. Studies have shown that daily aspirin use can reduce the risk of stroke in both men and women.[10] Dipyridamole (Persantine) 50 mg three times a day decreases platelet aggregation, which helps prevent thrombus and embolus formation. Daily use of platelet aggregation inhibitors such as ticlopidine (Ticlid) and clopidrogel (Plavix) has been shown to be as effective as aspirin in reducing the incidence of stroke.[11]

Surgical Therapy. Surgical interventions for the patient with TIAs from carotid disease include carotid endarterectomy (CEA), transluminal angioplasty, and extracranial-intracranial (EC-IC) bypass. In the CEA the atheromatous lesion is removed from the carotid artery to improve blood flow (Fig. 55-7). CEA surgery is associated with a reduction in stroke and vascular death.[12] This surgery is reserved for patients with occlusions of 70% to 99% of blood flow.

Transluminal angioplasty is the insertion of a balloon to open a stenosed artery to permit increased blood flow. This procedure has been used to treat patients with clinical manifestations related to stenosis in the vertebrobasilar or carotid arteries and their major branches. The risk of the angioplasty procedure is the possibility of dislodging emboli, which can travel to the brain or retina.

The EC-IC bypass is used for intracranial problems when the obstruction cannot be removed directly. The procedure usually involves anastomosing (surgically connecting) a branch of an extracranial artery to an intracranial artery just beyond an area of obstruction. Branches of the middle cerebral artery are most commonly used for the bypass surgery with the goal of increasing intracranial perfusion. Following the procedures these patients are at high risk for stroke and require close, long-term assessment and management (see Table 55-4).

Acute Care

The goals for collaborative care during the acute phase are preservation of life, prevention of further brain damage, and reduction in the level of disability. Treatment differs according to the type of stroke. Treatment also changes as the patient progresses from the acute phase to the rehabilitation phase of stroke.

The first goal is to maintain a patent airway because the airway may be compromised by decreased consciousness.[8] Interventions to maintain adequate oxygenation must be initiated immediately to prevent cerebral anoxia and permanent brain

Table 55-5 Stroke

Etiology	Assessment Findings	Interventions
Sudden vascular compromise causing disruption of blood flow to the brain Thrombosis Trauma Aneurysm Embolism Hemorrhage	■ Altered level of consciousness ■ Weakness, numbness, or paralysis of portion of body ■ Speech or visual disturbances ■ Severe headache ■ Increased or decreased heart rate ■ Respiratory distress ■ Unequal pupils ■ Hypertension ■ Facial drooping on affected side ■ Difficulty swallowing ■ Seizures ■ Bladder or bowel incontinence ■ Nausea and vomiting	**Initial** ■ Ensure patent airway. ■ Remove dentures. ■ Administer oxygen via nasal cannula or non-rebreather mask. ■ Establish IV access with normal saline to maintain BP. ■ Remove clothing. ■ Obtain CT scan immediately. ■ Position head midline. ■ Elevate head of bed 30 degrees if no symptoms of shock or injury. ■ Institute seizure precautions. ■ Anticipate thrombolytic therapy for ischemic stroke. **Ongoing Monitoring** ■ Monitor vital signs, level of consciousness, oxygen saturation, cardiac rhythm, Glasgow Coma Score, pupil size and reactivity. ■ Maintain patient warmth. ■ Reassure patient and family.

damage. Table 55-5 outlines the emergency management of the patient with a CVA. Common interventions for adequate oxygenation may include oxygen administration, artificial airway, intubation, and mechanical ventilation. The patient is monitored closely for signs of increasing neurologic deficit.

In response to both thrombotic and embolic strokes (ischemic strokes), a series of events termed the *ischemic cascade* occurs. During the initial period the ischemic area becomes discolored and soft. Around the core area of ischemia is a border zone termed *ischemic penumbra* that has marginal perfusion. The penumbra maintains function during an initial period of time following stroke, perhaps 3 to 6 hours, although the exact length is not known. If adequate blood flow is restored during the first 3 to 6 hours, the ischemic cascade is interrupted and less neurologic function will be lost. However, if the ischemic cascade is not interrupted, it continues producing neurologic deficits and disability. Therefore efforts are made to increase perfusion with the goal of reducing neurologic deficits.

Patients with ischemic strokes may be treated with hypervolemic hemodilution and volume expansion with crystalloids or colloids. The goal of treatment is to decrease blood viscosity, which promotes blood flow to the area of stroke.[7]

The fluid and electrolyte balance must be controlled carefully. The goal of fluid and electrolyte replacement generally is to keep the patient adequately hydrated to promote perfusion and decrease secondary injury. While the goal is to maintain perfusion to the brain, overhydration may further compromise perfusion by increasing cerebral edema. Adequate fluid intake during acute care via oral, IV, or tube feedings should be 1500 to 2000 ml/day.[13,14] Patients are monitored for urine output. If secretion of antidiuretic hormone (ADH) increases in response to the stroke, there is a decrease in urine output and an increase in fluid retention. IV solutions with glucose and water are avoided because these solutions are hypotonic and may further increase cerebral edema and intracranial pressure.[8] In addition, hyperglycemia may be associated with further brain damage. In general, individualized fluid and electrolyte replacement therapy decisions are based on the extent of intracranial edema, symptoms of increased intracranial pressure, central venous pressure levels, laboratory values for electrolytes, and intake and output.

Increased ICP is more likely to occur with hemorrhagic strokes, but it can occur with ischemic strokes. Increased ICP from cerebral edema usually peaks in 72 hours and may cause brain herniation. Management of increased ICP includes practices that enhance venous drainage, including elevation of head of the bed as ordered, maintenance of the head and neck in alignment, and avoidance of hip flexion. Efforts to limit cerebral tissue metabolism and thus vasodilation include avoidance of hyperthermia. Additional measures include treatment of pain, avoidance of hypervolemia, and management of constipation. Cerebrospinal fluid drainage may be used in some patients to reduce ICP. Diuretic medications, such as mannitol (Osmitrol) and furosemide (Lasix), may be used to decrease cerebral edema. Dexamethasone (Decradron, Hexadrol) may be used in patients with vasogenic cerebral edema.

A clinical pathway for care of the patient with CVA is provided on p. 1655.

Drug Therapy
Thrombolytic therapy. Recombinant tissue plasminogen activator (t-PA) is used to reestablish blood flow and prevent cell death for patients with ischemic strokes. A study by the National Institute of Neurological Disorders and Stroke (NINDS) found that patients who received IV t-PA within 3 hours of onset of stroke were 32% more likely to have minimal or no disability 3 months after the stroke.[1,15] Thrombolytic drugs such as t-PA act to produce localized fibrinolysis by binding to the fibrin in the thrombi. The lytic action of t-PA occurs as the plasminogen is converted to plasmin (fibrinolysin), whose enzymatic action digests fibrin and fibrinogen and thus lyses the clot. Because it is clot specific in its activation of the fibrinolytic

CLINICAL PATHWAY   Cerebrovascular Accident

Admit Date: _____   **DRG: 14**   **LOS: 4 days**   **Discharge Date:** _____

Pathway	ER—Day 1	Day 2	Day 3	Day 4
Critical Path Implemented				
Diagnostic Studies	■ CBC, sed rate ■ Chest x-ray ■ BMP ■ ECG ■ Lipid profile ■ CT of head ■ Progressive U/A without contrast ■ PT, PTT	■ PT if on Coumadin ■ Carotid duplex if indicated	■ PT if on Coumadin	■ PT if on Coumadin ■ Schedule further imaging as OP (CT, Angio, MRI)
Treatments	■ Telemetry (include ↑↓ parameters) ■ O₂____L/min via NC if indicated ■ Antiembolic stockings ■ Evaluate for high-risk pressure/ reduction therapy and place on bed	■ O₂____L/min NC→ ■ Telemetry	■ O₂____L/min NC→ ■ Consider D/C telemetry	■ D/C O₂ if appropriate for condition ■ D/C telemetry
IV/Meds	■ IV____@____cc/hr ■ Anticoagulation/antiplatelet Rx if indicated ■ Antihypertensives if indicated	→ → →	■ Adjust IV rate to accommodate PO/TF intake	■ Write transition orders for rehab/ECF
Consults	■ Physiatrist ■ Speech/language eval. ■ Neurology if ind. ■ Dysphagia eval. ■ Social Services ■ Nutrition services	■ PT: functional eval. ■ OT eval.: safety ■ ET: skin care		
Team Directives	( )Neuro assessment with LOC q4hr and prn; evaluate for risk for aspiration and sensorial changes. Use Glasgow Coma Scale. ( )Follow swallow program prescription to prevent aspiration. ( )Physical assessment q8hr and prn with close attention to respiratory system and skin integrity. ( )VS q4hr × 24hr, then q8hr × 24hr, then q shift and prn. ( )I & O, notify physician if UO < 600 cc/24 hr. Weigh on admission. ( )Skin care bid with daily reevaluation of skin risk assessment and implementation of appropriate interventions. ( )Assist with ADLs. Obtain BSC and overhead trapeze if indicated to assist with mobility and allow independence. ( )Monitor diagnostic study results and collaborate with the care team to further individualize the plan of care. ( )Provide emotional support and assist with reducing pt/family anxiety. (sign/date/time____/____/____, ____/____/____, ____/____/____, ____/____/____)			
Diet	■ NPO; transition to swallow program prescription as ordered→ →			
Activity and Safety	( )Active and passive ROM within pt's functional capability ( )Turn, cough, deep breathe q2hr; assist with IS if ordered ( )Assist with turning and positioning q2hr ( )Bed rest, elevate HOB 30° ____/____/____, ____/____/____, ____/____/____	( )Evaluate safety measures periodically and make necessary changes as neuro status changes ( )Reinforce PT activity protocol qid ( )Proper cushioning when OOB in chair ____/____/____, ____/____/____, ____/____/____		
Teaching Patient and Family	Instruct pt/family to call staff for assistance ( )Orient to environment, person, time (frequently if needed) ( )Initiate CVA (stroke) teaching plan ( )Explain tests and procedures to pt/family ( )Explain antiplatelet/anticoagulation Rx and precautions (sign/date/time)____/____/____, ____/____/____	( )Explain potential for surgical intervention (if it exists) ( )Explain need for long-term teaching in smoking cessation, cholesterol control, hypertension, weight reduction ____/____/____ ( )Teach stroke prevention strategies ____/____/____		
Transition Planning	( )Initial CM/SS evaluation to determine rehab needs ( )Review advance directives ____/____/____ ____/____/____	( )Rehab placement initiated ( )Risk evaluation referrals from admission database assessment initiated ____/____/____, ____/____/____	( )Outpatient and community support agencies identified and contacted; or pt/family have means to contact once in home setting ____/____/____	

Author: Molly Metzler, RN, BSN, for Nanticoke Health Services. Licensed by the Center for Case Management, South Natick, Mass, Nanticoke Health Services.   *Continued*

---

system, it is less likely to cause hemorrhage as compared with streptokinase or urokinase.

As stated previously, t-PA treatment is most effective if administered within 3 hours of the stroke occurrence as defined by the onset of clinical manifestations. Therefore the single most important factor is timing. Patients are screened carefully before treatment initiation. This includes blood tests for coagulation disorders, recent history of GI bleeding, and a CT or MRI scan to rule out hemorrhagic stroke.

The major side effect of t-PA is cerebral hemorrhage.[1,15] During the infusion of the drug the patient's vital signs are monitored to assess for improvement or deterioration related to intracerebral hemorrhage. Control of blood pressure is crit-

ical during treatment and for 24 hours following treatment. No anticoagulants or antiplatelet drugs are administered for 24 hours after t-PA treatment.

Currently other agents are being tested for their effectiveness during the acute phase. In a limited study, prourokinase (Proact I) has been shown to enhance vessel patency in patients when given within the first 6 hours of stroke symptoms.

Platelet inhibition/anticoagulant therapy. Patients with stroke caused by thrombi and emboli (ischemic strokes) may also be treated with platelet inhibitors and anticoagulants (after the first 24 hours if treated with t-PA) to prevent the formation of more clots. Common anticoagulants include heparin and warfarin (Coumadin, Panwarfin). Platelet inhibitors include

CLINICAL PATHWAY   Cerebrovascular Accident—continued

DRG: 14   LOS: 4 days

Meets Expected Outcomes (initial)	ER—Day 1	MET	NOT	Day 2	MET	NOT	Day 3	MET	NOT	Day 4	MET	NOT
Ineffective Airway Clearance: ■ RR changes ■ Inability to clear mucous secretions	■ Airway maintained_____/RC ■ Suctions easily if indicated_____/RC or N ■ Passive cooperation with TC and DB regimen_____/N ■ PT/family understand need for cough and deep breathing q2hr_____/RC or N			■ Performs C and DB exercises within limitations of function _____/RC or N ■ Pt. cooperating with pulmonary toilet regimen within functional capabilities _____/RC or N ■ Pt. using **IS** effectively _____/RC or N			■ Minimal adventitious breath sounds_____/RC or N ■ Pt. able to clear mucous secretions on own, or suctions easily_____/RC or N ■ Pt/family understand the need to continue **IS** after discharge or in subacute care facility_____/RC or N			■ No evidence of pulmonary infection_____/RC or N ■ Breath sounds clear_____/RC or N ■ **IS** sent with patient on discharge_____/RC or N		
Impaired Mobility: ■ Unable to perform purposeful movement ■ Hemiplegia ■ Limited ROM ■ Decreased muscle strength ■ Impaired coordination	■ Pt/family understand and cooperate with passive ROM_____/N ■ Skin integrity maintained clean, dry, and protected from pressure and rubbing_____/N ■ Pt.'s functional alignment maintained on air mattress or specialty bed_____/N			■ Functional mobility maintained_____/PT or N ■ No evidence of skin breakdown_____/N or ET ■ PT program initiated and pt/family understand the importance of early intervention to recovery_____/PT or N ■ Passive ROM keeping joints flexible_____/PT or N			■ Pt/family understand importance of maintaining long-term therapeutic exercise regimen_____/PT or N ■ Postdischarge rehab therapy arrangements in place_____/CM or N ■ No evidence of thromboembolic complications evident_____/N			■ Performing ADLs with assistance_____/N ■ Discharge environment safe for functional capabilities, or rehab placement procured_____/SS ■ Skin intact_____/N or ET		
Sensory-Perceptual Alteration: ■ Altered LOC ■ Inability to communicate needs ■ Impaired memory or intellectual capacity ■ Aphasia ■ Impaired awareness of bodily functions	■ Pt/family received and understand an explanation of care regimen and safety measures in place _____/N ■ Alternate form of communication devised and functional _____/N ■ Pt. responding to frequent reorientation to environment _____/N ■ Urinary cath patient (if indicated)_____/N			■ Pt/family starting to recognize physical limitations resulting from CVA_____/N ■ Pt able to communicate needs _____/N ■ Sensory-perceptual changes from CVA stabilizing_____/N ■ Bladder and bowel functions maintained with personal hygiene and pt's dignity in mind_____/N			■ LOC stabilized_____/N ■ Ability to communicate needs improving_____/N ■ Pt.'s response to reorientation to environment improving_____/N ■ Bladder and bowel function maintained with no S/S of infection_____/N			■ LOC stabilized for transfer to rehab facility or home care _____/N ■ Communication system explained to receiving rehab agency or home caregivers_____/N		
Emotional Lability: ■ Emotional outbursts ■ Inappropriate verbal and emotional responses ■ Changes in family processes from sudden-onset CVA	■ Explanation provided to family regarding inappropriate verbal and emotional responses from pt_____/N ■ Family beginning to identify the need to delegate responsibilities normally performed by pt to other family members_____/N			■ Family demonstrating effective coping skills with pt's inappropriateness_____/N ■ Family members begin to identify their internal support systems with help from staff _____/SS or CM or N ■ Community support agencies identified for pt's transitional care_____/SS or CM			■ Family activating their internal support network_____/SS or CM or N ■ Family members are able to share their feelings about illness in the family with each other_____/SS or CM or N ■ Community support systems discussed with pt/family_____/SS or CM			■ Family actively supporting each other_____/SS or CM or N ■ Family knows how to contact community support agencies after subacute care experience, or contact with appropriate agencies has been established before discharge _____/SS or CM		

Continued

Service

CM - Care management
ET - Ostomy/skin care
RC - Respiratory care
N - Nurse
PT - Physical therapy
NS - Nutrition services

RX - Pharmacist
SL - Speech/language
CCC - Primary RN clinical care coord.
SW - Social work
OT - Occupational therapy

HC - Home care
DR - Physician
Card - Cardiology
Rad - Radiology
Rehab - Cardiac, respiratory

CLINICAL PATHWAY Cerebrovascular Accident—continued

DRG: 14 LOS: 4 days

Meets Expected Outcomes (initial)	ER—Day 1	MET	NOT	Day 2	MET	NOT	Day 3	MET	NOT	Day 4	MET	NOT
Potential Nutritional Deficit: ■ Weight loss ■ Inadequate PO intake ■ Dysphagia ■ Poor muscle tone	■ Hydration/nutrition status maintained in homeostasis by IV/TF while pt unable to take or tolerate adequate PO fluids or nutrients____/NS or N			■ Weight stabilized____/NS or N ■ Pt cooperating with swallowing program prescribed to best of functional ability____/SLP or NS or N ■ Aspiration precautions explained to pt/family____/SLP or NS or N ■ Caloric and fluid needs being met____/NS or N			■ Pt. gaining strength____/NS or N ■ Weight stable____/NS or N ■ Pt/family understand aspiration precautions and know S/S of impending problems____/SLP or NS or N			■ Pt. tolerating and retaining appropriate fluid and caloric amounts to meet metabolic demands____/NS or N		
Knowledge Deficit: ■ Physiologic changes ■ Causes of CVA ■ Prevention measures ■ Rehabilitation ■ Safety measures ■ Precautions ■ Medications	■ Pt/family understand safety measures initiated____/N ■ Pt/family will understand the disease process of CVA____/N ■ Pt/family will understand some possible causes of CVA____/N			■ Pt/family will be able to understand and discuss the components of therapy for CVA____/N ■ Pt/family will understand how a CVA often leads to neurologic damage____/N			■ Pt/family will be able to identify usual impending S/S of stroke____/N ■ Pt/family will be able to identify prevention measures to reduce risk for further CVAs____/N ■ Pt/family understand medication regimen____/N			■ Pt/family know when and how to access their PCP and EMS____/N ■ Pt/family understand the importance of ongoing medical follow-up____/N		
Unmet Outcomes: (CCC Initials Required)	7-3 PM ( ) Resolved ( ) Planned /RN 3-7 PM ( ) Resolved ( ) Planned /RN 7-11 PM ( ) Resolved ( ) Planned /RN 11-7 AM ( ) Resolved ( ) Planned /RN			7-3 PM ( ) Resolved ( ) Planned /RN 3-7 PM ( ) Resolved ( ) Planned /RN 7-11 PM ( ) Resolved ( ) Planned /RN 11-7 AM ( ) Resolved ( ) Planned /RN			7-3 PM ( ) Resolved ( ) Planned /RN 3-7 PM ( ) Resolved ( ) Planned /RN 7-11 PM ( ) Resolved ( ) Planned /RN 11-7 AM ( ) Resolved ( ) Planned /RN			7-3 PM ( ) Resolved ( ) Planned /RN 3-7 PM ( ) Resolved ( ) Planned /RN 7-11 PM ( ) Resolved ( ) Planned /RN 11-7 AM ( ) Resolved ( ) Planned /RN		

aspirin, ticlopidine (Ticlid), clopidrogel (Plavix), and dipyridamole (Persantine).[3] IV heparin or low-molecular-weight heparin may be given in the situation of rapidly evolving strokes or strokes caused by emboli traveling from the heart. IV heparin is administered via continuous infusion, and the activated partial thromboplastin time is closely monitored.

Typically heparin is replaced by oral warfarin for long-term administration. Doses of warfarin are regulated by the results of the international normalized ratio (INR). The INR is a standardized measure of prothrombin time that adjusts for assay variations. The therapeutic dose is that which produces a value that is 2 to 3 times the normal level. Nurses must monitor the patient closely for hemorrhage or bleeding at other body sites while using anticoagulants and platelet inhibitors. A patient teaching guide for patients taking warfarin on a long-term basis is found in Table 36-15.

Anticoagulants and platelet inhibitors are contraindicated for patients with hemorrhagic strokes. The calcium channel blocker nimodipine (Nimotop) is given to patients with subarachnoid hemorrhage to decrease the effects of vasospasm and minimize tissue damage.[16] Calcium channel blockers inhibit the passage of calcium into brain cells during and after stroke. It is thought that excess intracellular calcium is harmful to brain tissue.

Acetylsalicylic acid (aspirin) is also used to prevent platelet aggregation at the site of the atherosclerotic plaque. The complications of aspirin include gastrointestinal bleeding with higher doses. Aspirin administration should be done cautiously if the patient has a history of peptic ulcer disease or is taking other anticoagulants.

Other drug therapies. Aspirin or acetaminophen (Tylenol) is given to treat hyperthermia. An elevation of as little as 1 degree of temperature can increase brain metabolism and further brain damage. The brain can tolerate hypoxia longer if the patient is hypothermic. Cooling blankets may be used cautiously to lower core temperatures. The nurse must closely monitor the patient's body temperature.

Approximately 15% of patients who experience a CVA will have seizures. Antiseizure medication, such as phenytoin (Dilantin), may be administered if seizure activity is present.[8] Prophylactic treatment with antiseizure medication is avoided unless seizure activity is present.

Investigation is ongoing to find potentially neuroprotective agents to prevent further ischemic damage in the infarcted area, including cells in the penumbra. Drugs that antagonize the action of excitatory neurotransmitters (e.g., glutamate) hold promise in the terms of protecting neurons from damage. Other agents include calcium channel blockers such as nimodipine and antagonists to nitric oxide.[15] Ultimately early treatment of stroke may involve drugs that increase blood flow and drugs that protect neurons from further ischemic damage.

Surgical Therapy. Surgical interventions for stroke include an immediate evacuation of blood occurring with strokes caused by aneurysm-induced hematomas or cerebellar hematomas larger than 3 cm. Subarachnoid hemorrhage is usually caused by a ruptured aneurysm. Approximately 20% of patients will have multiple aneurysms. Treatment of an aneurysm includes clipping the aneurysm (see Fig. 55-4) and removing the clot to prevent rebleeding into the brain.

Subarachnoid and intracerebral hemorrhage can involve bleeding into the ventricles of the brain. This situation produces hydrocephalus, which further damages brain tissue from increased intracranial pressure. The surgical procedure of ventriculostomy and drainage can give dramatic improvement in these situations.

Rehabilitation Care

After the stroke has stabilized for 12 to 24 hours, collaborative care shifts from the preservation of life to the lessening of disability and the attainment of optimal function. The patient may be evaluated by a physiatrist (a physician who specializes in physical medicine and rehabilitation). Depending on the patient's status, the patient's rehabilitation potential, and available resources, the patient may be transferred to a rehabilitation facility or unit. Other approaches for rehabilitation include outpatient therapy and home care–based rehabilitation.

As part of the long-term collaborative care after a stroke, various members of the health team may be involved in the effort to promote optimal function of the patient and the family. The exact composition of the team depends on the needs of the patient and family and the resources of the rehabilitation facility or institution (Fig. 55-8).

NURSING MANAGEMENT: STROKE

■ Nursing Assessment

Subjective and objective data that should be obtained from a person who has had a stroke are presented in Table 55-6. The nurse may be the initial health care professional to see a patient with a stroke. The primary assessment is focused on the cardiac and

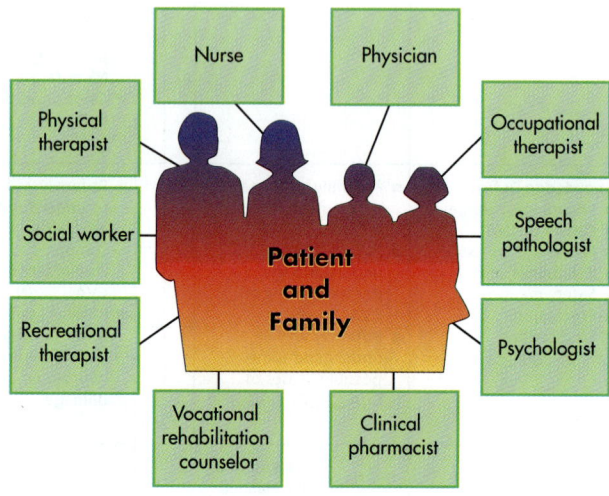

Fig. 55-8 Representative membership of the rehabilitation team.

NURSING ASSESSMENT

Table **55-6** | Stroke

Subjective Data

Important Health Information

Past health history: Hypertension; previous stroke, TIA(s), aneurysm, cardiac disease (including recent myocardial infarction), arrhythmias, congestive heart failure, valvular disease, infective endocarditis; hyperlipidemia, polycythemia, diabetes, gout

Medications: Use of oral contraceptives, use of and compliance with antihypertensive and anticoagulant agents

Functional Health Patterns

Health perception–health management: Positive family history; alcohol abuse, smoking

Nutritional-metabolic: Anorexia, nausea, vomiting; dysphagia, disturbances in taste and smell

Elimination: Change in bowel and bladder patterns

Activity-exercise: Loss of movement and sensation; syncope; weakness on one side; generalized weakness, easy fatigability

Cognitive-perceptual: Numbness, tingling of one side of the body; loss of memory; alteration in speech, language, problem-solving ability; pain; headache, possibly sudden and severe (hemorrhage); visual disturbances; denial of illness

Objective Data

General

Emotional lability, lethargy, apathy or combativeness, fever

Respiratory

Loss of cough reflex, labored or irregular respirations, tachypnea, rhonchi (aspiration), airway occlusion (tongue), apnea

Cardiovascular

Hypertension, tachycardia, carotid bruit

Gastrointestinal

Loss of gag reflex, bowel incontinence, decreased or absent bowel sounds, constipation

Urinary

Urinary frequency, urgency, incontinence

Neurologic

Contralateral motor and sensory deficits, including weakness, paresis, paralysis, anesthesia; unequal pupils, hand grasps; akinesia, aphasia (expressive, receptive, global), dysarthria (slurred speech), agnosias, apraxia, visual deficits, perceptual or spatial disturbances, altered level of consciousness (drowsiness to deep coma) and Babinski's sign, decreased followed by increased deep tendon reflexes, flaccidity followed by spasticity, amnesia, ataxia, personality change, nuchal rigidity, seizures

Possible Findings

Positive CT and MRI scans showing size, location, and type of lesion; positive Doppler ultrasonography and cerebral angiography

respiratory status of the patient and a brief neurologic assessment. If the patient is stable, the nursing history is obtained as follows: (1) description of the current illness with attention to initial symptoms, duration of symptoms, intermittent or continuous nature of symptoms, and changes of symptom characteristics; (2) history of similar symptoms previously experienced; (3) current medications; (4) history of associative illnesses such as hypertension; and (5) family history of stroke or cardiovascular diseases. This information would be gained through an interview of the patient, family members, significant others, or caregiver.

The secondary assessment should include a comprehensive neurologic examination of the patient. The neurologic screening examination includes the functional status of (1) level of consciousness, (2) cognition, (3) motor abilities, (4) cranial nerve function, (5) sensation, (6) proprioception, (7) cerebellar abilities, and (8) deep tendon reflexes. Serial documentation of the neurologic screening examination is essential to note progressing or diminishing status of the patient. The neurologic screen examination can be quickly evaluated and documented on a flow sheet and the Glascow Coma Scale for ease of patient assessment.

■ Nursing Diagnoses

Nursing diagnoses for the person with a stroke may include, but are not limited to, those presented in NCP 55-1.

55-1   NURSING CARE PLAN   PATIENT WITH A STROKE

Expected Patient Outcomes	Nursing Interventions and *Rationales*

NURSING DIAGNOSIS Altered tissue perfusion (cerebral) *related to* decreased cerebral blood flow secondary to thrombus, embolus, hemorrhage, edema, or spasm *as manifested by* intracranial pressure (ICP) >15 mm Hg for 15 to 30 seconds or longer, decreasing Glasgow Coma Scale (GCS) score, and altered respiratory pattern.

- ICP < 15 mm Hg.
- Stable and improving GCS.

- Assess ICP, level of consciousness (LOC), and breathing pattern at least hourly *to identify trends in patient's condition and to enable early notification of physician of significant changes.*
- Administer medications as prescribed *to decrease risk of further thrombus formation.*
- Implement measures, such as treating hypoxia, reducing pain, and maintaining patent urinary catheter, *to prevent increasing ICP.*

NURSING DIAGNOSIS Risk for ineffective airway clearance *related to* inability to raise secretions.

- Able to expectorate secretions.
- No respiratory distress.

- Assess for weak, ineffective cough; bronchial congestion; adventitious breath sounds; changes in color, amount, and consistency of sputum *to determine if risk factors are present.*
- Observe for increase in pulmonary secretions, changes in color of secretions, and temperature elevation *as indicators of pulmonary infection.*
- Auscultate lungs for breath sounds daily and as needed *to determine adequacy of respiratory excursion.*
- Suction as needed *to remove accumulated secretions.*
- Instruct patient and family in feeding program and emergency measures *to prevent aspiration and resultant respiratory distress.*

NURSING DIAGNOSIS Impaired physical mobility *related to* generalized weakness, muscle atrophy, or paralyzed extremities *as manifested by* decreased physical activity, limited range of motion, decreased muscle strength or control.

- Able to transfer and ambulate at maximal level of ability.
- Able to perform activities of daily living by self or with assistance.

- Assess and document range of motion, transfer abilities, and positioning ability *to determine extent of problem and plan appropriate interventions.*
- Administer passive or active range-of-motion exercises to affected extremities at least tid *to prevent unnecessary muscle atrophy and contractures.*
- Maintain alignment with support pillows and footboard according to procedures; teach and assist family and patient with positioning techniques *to prevent contractures.*
- Follow through with techniques for activities of daily living recommended by occupational or physical therapist *to help patient incorporate teaching from specialists into daily life and activities.*
- Encourage as much self-mobility as possible *to maintain physical activity at highest degree possible and to promote patient's sense of control.*

Continued

55-1   **NURSING CARE PLAN**   **PATIENT WITH A STROKE**—continued

| Expected Patient Outcomes | Nursing Interventions and *Rationales* |

NURSING DIAGNOSIS   **Impaired verbal communication** *related to* residual aphasia *as manifested by* refusal or inability to speak, word-finding problems, use of inappropriate words, inability to follow verbal directions.

- Able to communicate effectively.

- Assess exact communication deficits and strengths *to determine type of communication problem and plan appropriate interventions.*
- Intervene as appropriate.
- Use short, simple questions that elicit "yes" and "no" answers; speak slowly and allow adequate time for response *to avoid overwhelming patient with verbal stimuli.*
- Use gestures *to support verbal cues.*
- Teach specific techniques *to improve speech.*
- Speak slowly and use visual aids such as flash cards *to avoid frustration and anger from worsening problem.*

NURSING DIAGNOSIS   **Self-care deficits** *related to* motor weakness, paralysis, and loss of ability to effectively perform activities of daily living (ADLs) *as manifested by* observation or verbal report of inability to eat, bathe, use toilet, dress, or groom independently.

- Able to perform ADLs by self or with assistance from family or staff.

- Assess and document level of self-care *to determine extent of problem and plan appropriate interventions.*
- Encourage independence, provide supervision or assistance as needed *to avoid development of dependency.*
- Follow through with techniques for ADLs recommended by occupational or physical therapist *to help patient incorporate teaching from specialists and family.*

NURSING DIAGNOSIS   **Unilateral neglect** *related to* visual field cut and sensory loss on one side of body *as manifested by* consistent inattention to stimuli on affected side.

- Able to bring objects into field of vision.
- Scanning with eyes.
- Expression of satisfaction with vision.

- Assess and document amount of visual field impairment *to determine extent of problem and plan appropriate interventions.*
- Teach patient to turn head and scan environment.
- Early in care, approach patient on unaffected side; place objects in patient's field of vision; give physical and verbal cues to aid in path finding *to compensate for visual field deficits.*
- Later in care, approach patient on affected side *to encourage patient to turn head.*
- Provide visual stimulation *to promote use of full range of visual capabilities.*
- Use an eye patch *to prevent diplopia.*
- If corneal reflex is absent, protect affected eye to prevent injury.
- Teach family and patient to stimulate paralyzed limbs using touch and warm and cold stimuli *to promote reintegration with the whole body.*
- Encourage patient to use cue cards and mirrors *as reminder to survey her or his whole body for position, cleanliness, and appropriate dress.*

NURSING DIAGNOSIS   **Altered urinary elimination** *related to* impaired impulse to void or inability to reach toilet or manage tasks of voiding *as manifested by* incontinence and flow of urine at unpredictable times.

- Satisfactory urinary control by natural or artificial method.

- Assess and record patient's continent and incontinent voidings *to determine patterns and plan appropriate interventions.*
- Note color and character of urine daily and as needed *to ensure early detection of urinary tract infection and to prevent highly concentrated urine.*
- Provide fluid intake of 2000 ml/day unless contraindicated *to foster adequate elimination of dilute urine.*
- If indwelling catheter is used, give perineal cleansing and catheter care every shift and as needed *to avoid infection and ensure uninterrupted urinary flow.*
- Offer urinal or commode q2hr and as needed *to aid in establishing regular voiding pattern.*
- Assure patient of your willingness to assist with urinary problem *to avoid embarrassment and to demonstrate a caring attitude.*

Continued

55-1 NURSING CARE PLAN   PATIENT WITH A STROKE—continued

Expected Patient Outcomes   Nursing Interventions and *Rationales*

NURSING DIAGNOSIS Impaired swallowing *related to* weakness or paralysis of affected muscles *as manifested by* drooling, difficulty in swallowing, choking.

Expected Patient Outcomes	Nursing Interventions and Rationales
▪ No signs or symptoms of aspiration. ▪ Able to tolerate food and fluids without choking.	▪ Assess patient *to determine ability to swallow and presence of gag reflex.* ▪ Have patient sit upright for meals and for 30 minutes afterward *to use gravity to prevent aspiration.* ▪ Teach patient to take small bites and place food in unaffected side of mouth, keep chin down, and stroke throat *to stimulate swallowing.* ▪ After patient has eaten, check oral cavity for pocketed food and teach patient and family this technique *to prevent collection and putrefaction of food and resultant risk of infection.* ▪ Give thick shakes, foods with texture, and cold foods *to facilitate swallowing and minimize danger of choking.* ▪ If problem with sputum and saliva production, avoid milk products, *which increase production of mucus and saliva.* ▪ Give oral care after meals *to promote comfort and oral health.* ▪ Notify dietician of need to change food texture or fluids as needed.

NURSING DIAGNOSIS Self-esteem disturbance *related to* actual or perceived loss of function *as manifested by* expression of shame or guilt, increasing dependence on others, refusal to participate in self-care.

Expected Patient Outcomes	Nursing Interventions and Rationales
▪ Verbalization of feelings and concerns. ▪ Participation in appropriate socialization with family and staff. ▪ Setting of realistic goals.	▪ Encourage patient to verbalize feelings *to assess effect of stroke sequelae on self-esteem.* ▪ Spend time with patient using good listening techniques *to show a caring, concerned attitude, which fosters confidence in a relationship.* ▪ Establish achievable goals; explain all procedures and involve patient in planning goals; offer praise for every success and step of progress; involve patient as soon as possible in rehabilitation program *to promote sense of satisfaction and control and reduce frustration.* ▪ Refer for counseling or medical-psychiatric evaluation if indicated *so patient can have expert help with serious problems.*

NURSING DIAGNOSIS Risk for ineffective management of therapeutic regimen *related to* functional, cognitive, or communication limitations.

Expected Patient Outcomes	Nursing Interventions and Rationales
▪ Patient or family will make satisfactory arrangements to have patient's needs met on a daily basis.	▪ Assess degree of functional, cognitive, or communication limitations patient is experiencing *to determine teaching plan and arrange appropriate interventions.* ▪ Teach patient and family how to treat, prevent, and monitor for problems *so early intervention is ensured.* ▪ Evaluate plan *to determine if regimen is being followed or needs to be revised based on changing patient status or circumstances.*

▪ Planning

The patient, family, and nurse establish the goals of nursing care in a cooperative manner. These goals typically include that the patient will (1) maintain a stable or improved level of consciousness, (2) attain maximum physical functioning, (3) attain maximum self-care abilities and skills, (4) maintain stable body functions (e.g., bladder control), (5) maximize communication abilities, (6) maintain adequate nutrition, (7) avoid complications of stroke, and (8) maintain effective personal and family coping.

▪ Nursing Implementation

Health Promotion. To reduce the incidence of stroke, the nurse should focus teaching efforts toward stroke prevention for persons with known risk (e.g., patients with TIAs, hypertension, or diabetes mellitus). The significance of other potentially modifiable risk factors for the occurrence of stroke is unclear. However, control of risk factors implicated in coronary artery disease may indirectly help prevent stroke. (For the nurse's role in management of these risk factors, see Table 32-4.) In any health care setting and for the population as a whole, nurses can play a major role in the promotion of a healthy lifestyle. An overall program to prevent events such as stroke includes the recognition that people are responsible to some degree for their own health and for the health of future generations.

Another aspect of health promotion is teaching patients about when to seek health care for symptoms. Individuals

PATIENT & FAMILY TEACHING GUIDE

Table 55-7 Warning Signs of Stroke

Patients should be taught to seek help immediately if the following symptoms are present:

- Sudden weakness or numbness of the face, arm, or leg on one side of the body
- Sudden dimness or loss of vision, particularly in one eye
- Sudden difficulty speaking or trouble understanding speech
- Sudden severe headache with no known cause
- Unexplained dizziness, unsteadiness, or sudden falls, especially with any of the other symptoms

RESEARCH
IMPLICATIONS FOR NURSING PRACTICE

Early Recognition of Stroke

Citation Rosamond WD and others: Rapid response to stroke symptoms: the Delay in Accessing Stroke Healthcare (DASH) study, *Acad Emerg Med* 5:45, 1998.

Purpose To determine the factors that contribute to delays in seeking treatment for acute cerebral ischemic events.

Methods A prospective study was done using patients treated at the emergency department (ED) with clinical manifestations of stroke. Trained nurses using a structured interview talked with patients regarding delays in seeking health care. A total of 152 interviews were conducted.

Results and Conclusions The average delay in seeking health care from the onset of clinical manifestations to arrival at the ED for all patients with stroke-like symptoms was 3 hours with a range of 1.5 to 7.8 hours. The delay was less in those situations in which a witness first recognized that there was a serious change as compared with the patient self-identifying a problem. More rapid arrival in the ED was also associated with use of emergency medical services (EMS) by the patient. Most patients arrived within 3 hours when EMS was notified.

Implications for Nursing Practice Prompt treatment of ischemic strokes with thrombolytic drugs reduces the degree of neurologic impairment following a stroke. Therefore patients should be taught to seek health care immediately if they experience symptoms such as muscle weakness, visual disturbances, or swallowing problems. This study emphasizes the need for education of not only those at risk for a stroke but also their family members.

should be taught about early symptoms associated with stroke or TIA (Table 55-7).

Acute Intervention

Respiratory system. During the acute phase following a stroke the nursing priority is the management of the respiratory system. Stroke patients are particularly vulnerable to respiratory problems. Advancing age and immobility make them particularly susceptible to atelectasis and pneumonia. These patients are at high risk for aspiration pneumonia because of impaired consciousness or dysphagia. Problems commonly seen include poor chewing and swallowing, food pouching (food remaining in the buccal cavity of the mouth), and falling back of the tongue resulting in obstruction of the airway. Enteral tube feedings also place the patient at risk for aspiration pneumonia.

Nursing interventions to support adequate respiratory function are individualized to meet the needs of the patient. An oropharyngeal airway may be used in comatose patients to hold the tongue in place, prevent airway obstruction, and make suctioning accessible. In more prolonged situations, the oropharyngeal airway is replaced by a tracheostomy. Nasopharyngeal airways provide protection and access to the airway in patients with impaired consciousness. Nursing interventions include frequent assessment of airway patency and function, suctioning, patient mobility, positioning of the patient to prevent aspiration, and encouraging deep breathing. Patients who have an unclipped aneurysm may experience rebleeding and the possibility of further ICP increases with coughing exercises. Interventions related to maintenance of airway function are described in NCP 55-1.

Neurologic system. The patient's neurologic status must be monitored closely to detect changes suggesting stroke-in-evolution, extension of the stroke, increased intracranial pressure, or recovery from stroke symptoms. The Glasgow Coma Scale is used for neurologic assessment because it contains the essential factors of level of consciousness, mental status, pupillary responses, and movement and strength of extremities. (The Glasgow Coma Scale is shown in Table 54-2.) Vital signs are also closely monitored and documented. A decreasing level of consciousness is the earliest and most sensitive sign of increasing ischemia of the brain. Data from the nursing assessment are recorded on flow sheets to permit evaluation of neurologic status by the interdisciplinary team.

Cardiovascular system. Nursing goals for the cardiovascular system are aimed at maintaining homeostasis. Many patients with stroke have decreased cardiac reserves that are due to the secondary diagnoses of cardiac diseases. Cardiac efficiency is further compromised by fluid retention, overhydration, dehydration, and blood pressure variations. Fluids are retained because of increased production of ADH and aldosterone secondary to stress. Fluid retention plus overhydration can result in fluid overload. It can also increase cerebral edema and intracranial pressure. At the same time dehydration can add to the morbidity and mortality associated with stroke. Therefore the nurse should closely monitor intake and output. IV therapy is also carefully regulated.

Nursing interventions include (1) monitoring vital signs frequently; (2) monitoring cardiac rhythms; (3) calculating intake and output, noting imbalances; (4) regulating IV infusions; (5) adjusting the fluid intake to the individual needs of the patient; (6) monitoring lung sounds for crackles and rhonchi that indicate pulmonary congestion; and (7) monitoring heart sounds for murmurs or for S_3 or S_4 heart sounds. Hy-

ETHICAL DILEMMAS

Right to Die

SITUATION

A 93-year-old woman has had three strokes in the last 20 months. They have left her partially paralyzed and in need of full-time care. She has repeatedly told her home care nurse that she would not want to live if her condition worsened. She is now hospitalized for another stroke and her prognosis is the complete loss of physical functioning. She has tried to remove the feeding tube, which causes her discomfort. Responding to repeated questions of both the nurse and physician about whether she wants them to stop treatment and let her die, she has consistently answered yes.

DISCUSSION

Patients with severe life-threatening diseases or physical conditions may express concerns about not being kept alive. Providers should document these and encourage patients to execute advance directives while they are still able to do so. This patient had no advance directives but has witnesses to her repeated statements about not wanting to live like this. Competent adults have the right to refuse treatment, even if by doing so they hasten their own death. The health care providers should determine that she is competent and then ask several differently worded questions to clarify the patient's desire to die. Consistent responses would constitute the patient's desire to cease treatment, including artificial hydration and nutrition, in order to die.

ETHICAL AND LEGAL PRINCIPLES

- Competent adults have the legal right to choose to forego life-sustaining treatment, even if by doing so they hasten their death.
- The American Medical Association and other medical and nursing organizations support the ethical appropriateness of not imposing unwanted treatment on competent adults.
- By virtue of its delivery mechanism, artificial hydration and nutrition are considered to be medical treatments rather than simply the provision of food and water. The invasive nature of feeding tubes can be the grounds on which a patient refuses to continue this treatment.

pertension is sometimes seen following a stroke as the body attempts to increase cerebral blood flow.[8]

After a stroke, the patient is at risk for deep vein thrombosis in the weak or paralyzed lower extremity. This risk is related to immobility, loss of venous tone, and decreased muscle pumping activity in the leg. The most effective prevention is to keep the patient moving. Active range-of-motion exercises should be taught if the patient has voluntary movement in the affected extremity. For the patient with hemiplegia, passive range-of-motion exercises should be done several times a day. Additional measures often used to prevent deep vein thrombosis include positioning to minimize the effects of dependent edema and the use of elastic compression gradient stockings or support hose. Intermittent pneumatic compression stockings may be ordered for bedridden patients. The nursing assessment for deep vein thrombosis includes measuring the calf and thigh daily, observing swelling of the lower extremities, noting unusual warmth of the leg, and asking the patient about pain in the calf.

Musculoskeletal system. The nursing goal for the musculoskeletal system is to maintain optimal function. This is accomplished by the prevention of joint contractures and muscular atrophy. In the acute phase, range-of-motion exercises and positioning are important nursing interventions. Passive range-of-motion exercise is begun on the first day of hospitalization. If the stroke is due to subarachnoid hemorrhage, the movement is limited to the extremities. The patient is taught to actively exercise as soon as possible. Muscle atrophy secondary to lack of innervation and activity can develop within 1 month following stroke.

The paralyzed or weak side needs special attention when the patient is positioned. Each joint should be positioned higher than the joint proximal to it to prevent dependent edema. Specific deformities on the weak or paralyzed side that are characteristic of the patient with stroke include shoulder abduction; flexion contractures of the hand, wrist, and elbow; external rotation of the hip; and plantar flexion of the foot. Subluxation of the shoulder on the affected side is common and not preventable. However, careful positioning and moving of the affected arm may prevent the development of a painful shoulder condition. Immobilization of the affected upper extremity may precipitate a painful shoulder-hand syndrome.

Nursing interventions to optimize musculoskeletal function include (1) trochanter roll at the hip to prevent external rotation, (2) hand cones (not rolled wash clothes) to prevent hand contractures, (3) arm supports with slings and lap boards to prevent shoulder displacement, (4) avoidance of pulling the patient by the arm to avoid shoulder displacement, (5) footboards or high-topped tennis shoes to prevent footdrop, and (6) hand splints to reduce spasticity. Use of a footboard for the patient with spasticity is controversial. Rather than preventing plantar flexion (footdrop), the sensory stimulation of a footboard against the bottom of the foot increases plantar flexion. Likewise, there is disagreement whether hand splints facilitate or diminish spasticity. The decision regarding the use of footboard or hand splints is made on an individual patient basis.

Integumentary system. The skin of the patient with stroke is particularly susceptible to breakdown because of loss of sensation, diminished circulation, and immobility. The problem of skin integrity is compounded by the age of the patient, poor nutrition, dehydration, edema, and incontinence. The nursing plan for prevention of skin breakdown includes (1) pressure relief by position changes, special mattresses, or wheelchair cushions; (2) good skin hygiene; (3) emollients applied to dry skin; and (4) early mobility. The ideal position change schedule is side-back-side with a maximum duration of 2 hours for any position. Nurses should position the patient on the weak or paralyzed side for only 30 minutes. If an area of redness develops and does not return to normal color within 15 minutes of pressure relief, the epidermis and dermis are damaged. The damaged area should not be massaged because this may cause additional damage. Control of pressure is the single most important factor in both the prevention and treatment of skin breakdown. Vigilance and good nursing care are required to prevent pressure sores.

Gastrointestinal system. The stress of the illness contributes to a catabolic state that can interfere with recovery. Neurologic, cardiac, and respiratory problems are considered priorities in the acute phase of stroke. However, the nutritional needs of the patient require quick assessment and treatment. The patient may be initially on IV infusions to maintain fluid and electrolyte balance, as well as for administration of medications. Patients with severe impairment may require enteral or parenteral nutrition support. As the severity of stroke varies from mild to severe, individual assessment and planning for nutrition over time are necessary.

The first oral feeding should be approached with caution because the gag reflex may be impaired. Before initiation of feeding, the gag reflex may be assessed by gently stimulating the back of the throat with a tongue blade. If a gag reflex is present, the patient will gag spontaneously. If it is absent, the feeding should be deferred and exercises to stimulate swallowing should be started. The speech therapist or the occupational therapist is usually responsible for designing this program. However, the nurse may be called on to develop the program in some clinical settings.

To assess swallowing ability, the nurse should elevate the head of the bed to an upright position (unless contraindicated) and give the patient a small amount of crushed ice or ice water to swallow. If the gag reflex is present and the patient is able to swallow safely, the nurse may proceed with the feeding.

After careful assessment of swallowing, chewing, gag reflex, and pouching, oral feedings can be initiated. Mouth care before feeding helps stimulate sensory awareness and salivation and can facilitate swallowing. The patient should remain in a high Fowler's position, preferably in a chair with the head flexed forward for the feeding and for 30 minutes following feeding. Foods should be easy to swallow and provide enough texture, temperature (warm or cold), and flavor to stimulate a swallow reflex. Crushed ice can be used as a stimulant for swallowing. The patient is instructed to swallow and then swallow again. Pureed foods are not usually the best choice because they are often bland and too smooth and at room temperature by the time the patient is fed. Thin liquids are often difficult to swallow and may promote coughing. Milk products should be avoided because they tend to increase the viscosity of mucus and increase salivation. Food should be placed on the unaffected side of the mouth. The nurse should ensure that the atmosphere is unrushed and nonstressful. Each feeding must be followed by scrupulous oral hygiene because food tends to collect on the affected side of the mouth.

The most common bowel problem for the patient who has experienced a stroke is constipation. If the patient does not have a daily or every-other-day bowel movement, the patient should be checked for an impaction. In addition, if the patient has liquid stools, the patient should also be checked for stool impaction. Depending on the patient's fluid balance status and swallowing ability, fluid intake should be 1800 to 2000 ml/day and fiber intake up to 25 g/day. Physical activity also promotes bowel function. Laxative, suppositories, or stool softeners may be ordered if the patient does not respond to increased fluid and fiber.[17] Similarly, enemas are used only if suppositories and digital stimulation are ineffective because they cause vagal stimulation and increase ICP.

Table 55-8 **Communication with a Patient Who Has Aphasia**

1. Decrease environmental stimuli that may be distracting and disrupting to communication efforts.
2. Treat the patient as an adult.
3. Present one thought or idea at a time.
4. Keep questions simple or ask questions that can be answered with "yes" or "no."
5. Let the person speak. Do not interrupt. Allow time for the individual to complete thoughts.
6. Make use of gestures or demonstration as an acceptable alternative form of communication. Encourage this by saying "Show me. . ." or "Point to what you want."
7. Do not pretend to understand the person if you do not. Calmly say you do not understand and encourage the use of nonverbal communication, or ask the person to write out what he or she wants.
8. Speak with normal volume and tone.
9. Give the patient time to process information and generate a response before repeating a question or statement.
10. Allow body contact (e.g., the clasp of a hand or touching) as much as possible. Realize that touching may be the only way the patient can express feelings.
11. Organize the patient's day by preparing and following a schedule (the more familiar the routine, the easier it will be for the person with aphasia).
12. Do not push communication if the person is tired or upset. Aphasia worsens with fatigue and anxiety.

Urinary system. In the acute stage of stroke, the primary urinary problem is poor bladder control, resulting in incontinence. Efforts should be made to promote normal bladder function and avoid the use of indwelling catheters. If an indwelling catheter must be used initially, it should be removed as soon as the patient is medically and neurologically stable. Long-term use of the indwelling catheter is associated with urinary tract infections and delayed bladder retraining. An intermittent catheterization program may be used for patients with urinary retention because this procedure has less incidence of urinary infections. An alternative to intermittent catheterizations is the external catheter for male patients who are incontinent of urine. External catheters will not alleviate the problem of urine retention.

The bladder retraining program consists of (1) adequate fluid intake with the majority given between 8 AM and 7 PM; (2) scheduled toileting every 2 hours using bedpan, commode, or bathroom; and (3) noting signs of restlessness because this may indicate the need for urination.

Communication. During the acute stage of stroke, the nurses' role in meeting the psychologic needs of the patient is primarily supportive. An alert patient is usually anxious because of lack of understanding about what has happened and an inability to communicate or difficulty with communication. The patient is assessed both for the ability to speak and the ability to understand communication. The patient's response to simple questions can give the nurse a guideline for structuring explanations and instructions. If the patient cannot understand

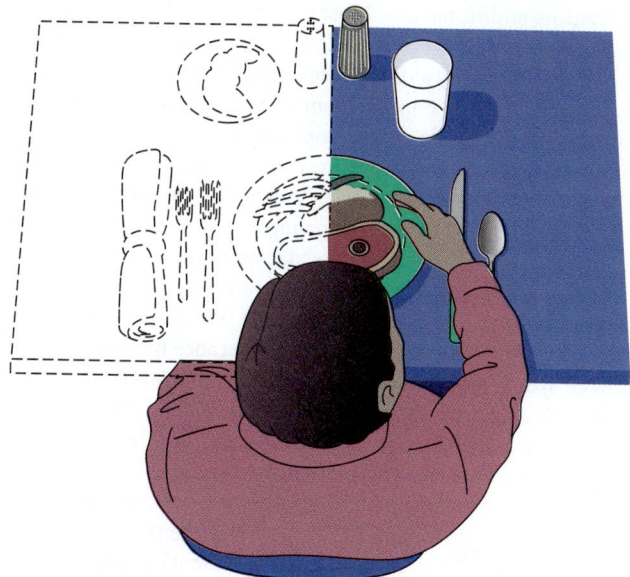

Fig. 55-9 Spatial and perceptual deficits in stroke. Perception of a patient with homonymous hemianopsia shows that food on the left side is not seen and thus is ignored.

words, gestures may be used to support verbal cues. It is helpful to speak slowly and calmly using simple words or sentences to enhance communication. The nurse must give the patient extra time to comprehend and respond to communication. The stroke patient with aphasia may easily be overwhelmed by verbal stimuli. (Guidelines for communicating with a patient who has aphasia are presented in Table 55-8.) Evaluation and treatment of language and communication deficits are often done by the speech pathologist after the patient has stabilized.

Sensory-perceptual alterations. Homonymous hemianopsia (blindness in the same half of each visual field) is a common problem after a stroke (Fig. 55-9). Persistent disregard of objects in part of the visual field should alert the nurse to this possibility. Initially, the nurse helps the patient to compensate by arranging the environment within the patient's perceptual field, such as arranging the food tray so that all foods are on the right side or the left side to accommodate for field of vision (see Fig. 55-9). Later, the patient learns to compensate for the visual defect by consciously attending or scanning the neglected side. The weak or paralyzed extremities are carefully noted for adequacy of dressing, for hygiene, and for trauma.

In the clinical situation it is often difficult to distinguish between a visual field cut and a neglect syndrome. Both problems may occur with strokes affecting either the right side or the left side of the brain. A person may be unfortunate enough to have both homonymous hemianopsia and a neglect syndrome, which increases the inattention to the weak or paralyzed side. A neglect syndrome results in decreased safety awareness and places the patient at high risk for injury. Immediately after the stroke, the nurse must anticipate potential safety hazards and provide protection from injury. Safety measures can include close observation of the patient by the nursing staff, elevating side rails, lowering the height of the bed, and video monitors. The use of restraints and soft vests is avoided because this may agitate the patient.

Other visual problems may include diplopia (double vision), loss of the corneal reflex, and ptosis (drooping eyelid), especially if the area of stroke is in the vertebrobasilar distribution. Diplopia is often treated with an eye patch. If the corneal reflex is absent, the patient is at risk for corneal abrasion and should be observed closely and protected against eye injuries. Corneal abrasion can be prevented with artificial tears or gel to keep the eyes moist. Ptosis is generally not treated because it usually does not inhibit vision.

Coping. A stroke is usually a sudden, extremely stressful event for the patient, close family members, and significant others. A stroke is often a family disease, affecting the family emotionally, socially, and financially, as well as changing roles and responsibilities within the family. An older couple may perceive the stroke as a very real threat to life and to accustomed lifestyle. Reactions to this threat vary considerably but may involve fear, apprehension, denial of the severity of stroke, depression, anger, and sorrow. During the acute phase of caring for the stroke patient and the family, nursing interventions designed to facilitate coping involve providing information and emotional support.

Explanations to the patient about what has happened and about diagnostic and therapeutic procedures should be clear and understandable. It will be particularly challenging to keep the aphasic patient adequately informed. Tone, demeanor, and touch may also be used to convey support.

The patient's family should be given a careful, detailed explanation of what has happened to the patient. However, if the family is extremely anxious and upset during the acute phase, explanations may have to be repeated at a later time. Because family members usually have not had time to prepare for the illness, they may need assistance in arranging care for family members or pets and for transportation and finances. A social services referral is often helpful.

Ambulatory and Home Care
Discharge planning. The patient is usually discharged from the acute care setting to home, an intermediate or long-term care facility, or a rehabilitation facility. Ideally, discharge planning with the patient and family starts early in the hospitalization and promotes a smooth transition from one care setting to another. The interdisciplinary team provides the guidance for the appropriate care required after discharge. If the patient requires a short- or long-term health care facility, the team can make appropriate referrals that allow time for family selection and arrangement of care. A critical factor in discharge planning is the patient's level of independence in performing ADLs. If the patient is returning home, the team can make referrals for needed equipment and services in preparation for discharge.

Nurses have an excellent opportunity to prepare the patient and family for discharge through education, demonstration and return demonstration, practice, and evaluation of self-care skills before discharge. Total care is considered in discharge planning: medications, nutrition, mobility, exercises, hygiene, and toileting. Follow-up care is carefully planned to permit continuing nursing, physical, occupational, and speech therapy, as well as medical care. Community resources should be identified to provide recreational activities, group support, spiritual assistance, respite care, adult day care, and home assistance based on the individual patient's needs.

Rehabilitation. *Rehabilitation* is the process of maximizing the patient's capabilities and resources to promote optimal functioning related to physical, mental, and social well-being. The goals of rehabilitation are to prevent deformity and maintain and improve function. Regardless of the care setting, ongoing rehabilitation is essential to maximize the patient's abilities.

The team approach to rehabilitation is used so the patient and family can benefit from the combined, expert care of the interdisciplinary team. The team must communicate and coordinate care to achieve the patient's and family's goals. The nurse is in a good position to facilitate this process and is often key to successful rehabilitation efforts. The patient's and family's participation in decision making during rehabilitation is essential to goal achievement after a stroke. The interdisciplinary team is composed of many members, including nurses, physicians, psychiatrist, physical therapist, occupational therapist, speech therapist, respiratory therapist, vocational therapist, recreational therapist, social worker, psychologist, pharmacist, and chaplains. Physical therapy focuses on mobility, progressive ambulation, transfer techniques, and equipment needed for mobility. Occupational therapy emphasizes retraining for skills of daily living such as eating, dressing, hygiene, and cooking. Occupational therapists are also skilled in cognitive and perceptual evaluation and training. Speech therapy focuses on speech, communication, cognition, and eating abilities.

Many of the nursing interventions outlined in the nursing care plan for the patient with stroke (see NCP 55-1) are initiated in the acute phase and continue throughout the rehabilitation phase of care. Some of the interventions are independent nursing actions, whereas others involve the entire rehabilitation team.

The rehabilitation nurse assesses the patient and family with attention to (1) rehabilitation potential of the patient, (2) physical status of all body systems, (3) presence of complications caused by the stroke or other chronic conditions, (4) cognitive status of the patient, (5) family resources and support, and (6) expectations of the patient and family related to the rehabilitation program.

The goals for rehabilitation of the patient with stroke are mutually set by the patient, family, nurse, and other members of the rehabilitation team. The rehabilitation goals typically include the following:

1. Learn techniques to self-monitor and maintain physical wellness
2. Demonstrate self-care skills
3. Exhibit problem-solving skills with self-care
4. Avoid complications associated with stroke
5. Establish and maintain a useful communication system
6. Maintain nutritional and hydration status
7. List community resources for equipment, supplies, and support
8. Establish flexible role behaviors to promote family cohesiveness

Musculoskeletal system. The nurse initially emphasizes the musculoskeletal functions of eating, toileting, and walking for the rehabilitation of the patient. The initial assessment consists of determining the stage of recovery of muscle function. If the muscles are still flaccid several weeks after the stroke, the prognosis for regaining function is poor and the focus of care is on preventing additional loss. Most patients begin to show signs of spasticity with exaggerated reflexes within 48 hours following the stroke. Spasticity at this phase of stroke denotes progress toward recovery. As improvement continues, small voluntary movements of the hip or shoulder may be accompanied by involuntary movements in the rest of the extremity (synergy). The final stage of recovery occurs when the patient has voluntary control of isolated muscle groups.

Interventions for musculoskeletal system advance in a manner of progressive activity. Balance training is the initial step and begins with the patient sitting up in bed or dangling on the edge of the bed. The nurse evaluates tolerance by noting dizziness or syncope caused by vasomotor instability. The next step is transferring from bed to chair or wheelchair. The chair is placed beside the bed so that the patient can lead with the stronger arm and leg. The patient sits on the side of the bed, stands, places the strong hand on the far wheelchair arm, and sits down. The nurse may either supervise the transfer or provide minimal assistance by guiding the patient's strong hand to the wheelchair arm, standing in front of the patient blocking the patient's knees with the nurse's knees to prevent knee buckling, and guiding the patient into a sitting position.

In some rehabilitation units the Bobath approach is used as a neurodevelopmental approach to mobility. The goal of the Bobath approach is to help the patient gain control over patterns of spasticity by inhibiting abnormal reflex patterns. Therapists and nurses use the Bobath approach to encourage normal muscle tone, normal movement, and promotion of bilateral function of the body. An example of the Bobath approach is to have the patient transfer into the wheelchair using the weak or paralyzed side and the stronger side to facilitate more bilateral functioning.

Supportive or assistive equipment, such as canes, walkers, and leg braces, may be needed on a short-term or long-term basis for mobility. The physical therapist usually selects and instructs the patient regarding the most appropriate supportive device(s) to meet individual needs. The nurse should incorporate physical therapy activities into the daily routine of the patient for additional practice and repetition of rehabilitation efforts.

Nutritional therapy. After the acute phase the registered dietician can assist in determining the appropriate daily caloric intake based on the patient's size, weight, and activity level. If the patient is unable to take in an adequate oral diet, enteral feedings via a nasogastric tube may be used. Most commercially prepared formulas provide about 1 calorie per milliliter. (Enteral feedings are described in Chapter 38.)

The nurse and speech therapist must assess the ability of the patient to swallow solids and fluids and adjust the diet appropriately. The registered dietician plans the diet type, texture, calorie count, and fluids to meet the patient's nutritional needs. The occupational therapist and nurse must evaluate the patient's ability to feed himself or herself and recommend assistive devices to allow for independent eating. Nurses are involved in the daily planning, implementation, and evaluation of the nutritional status of the patient.

The inability to feed oneself can be frustrating and may result in malnutrition and dehydration. Interventions to promote self-feeding include using the unaffected upper extremity to eat; employing assistive devices such as rocker knives, plate guards, and nonslip pads for dishes (Fig. 55-10); removing unnecessary items from the tray or table, which can reduce spills;

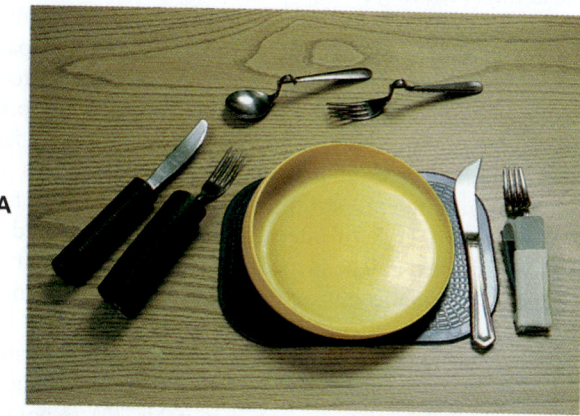

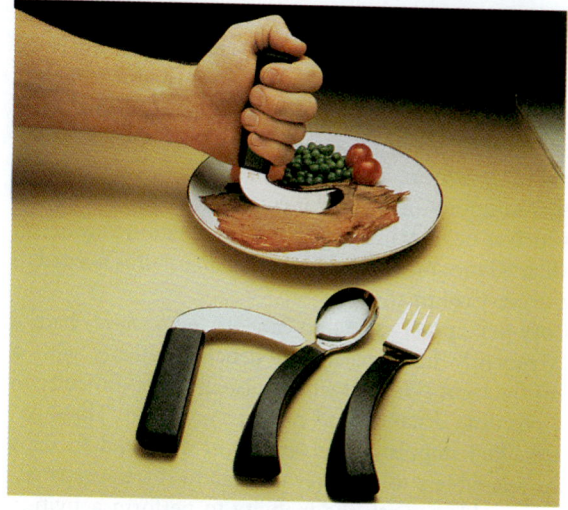

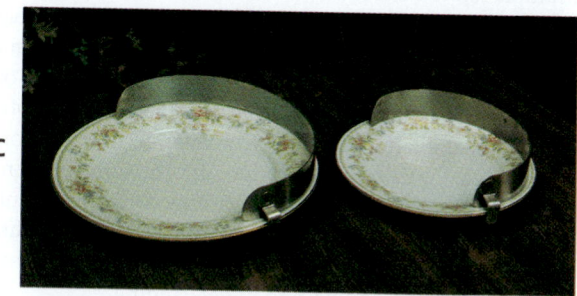

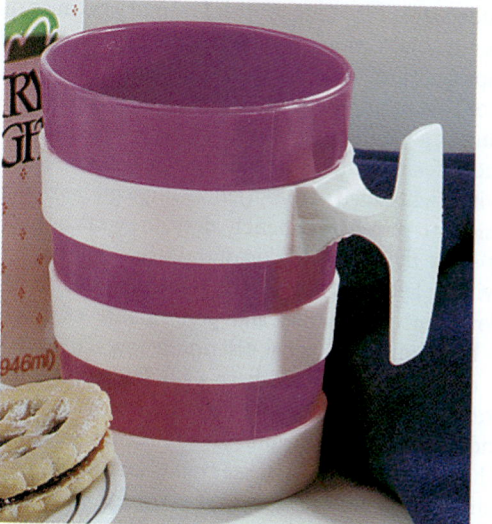

Fig. 55-10   Assistive devices for eating. **A,** The curved fork fits over the hand. The rounded plate helps keep food on the plate. Special grips and swivel handles are helpful for some persons. **B,** Knives with rounded blades are rocked back and forth to cut food. The person does not need a fork in one hand and a knife in the other. **C,** Plate guards help keep food on the plate. **D,** Cup with special handle.

and providing a nondistracting environment to decrease sensory overload and distraction. The effectiveness of the dietary program is evaluated in terms of maintenance of weight, adequate hydration, and patient satisfaction.

Elimination. A bowel management program is implemented for problems with bowel control, constipation, or incontinence. A high-fiber diet (see Table 40-9) and adequate fluid intake (2500 to 3000 ml) are usually recommended. Patients with stroke frequently have constipation, which responds to the following dietary management:

1. Fluid intake of 2500 to 3000 ml daily unless contraindicated
2. Prune juice (120 ml) or stewed prunes daily
3. Cooked fruit three times daily
4. Cooked vegetables three times daily
5. Whole-grain cereal or bread three to five times daily

The bowel management program for incontinence consists of placing the patient on the bedpan or bedside commode or taking the patient to the bathroom at a regular time daily to reestablish bowel regularity. A good time for the bowel program is 30 minutes after breakfast because eating stimulates the gas-

trocolic reflex and peristalsis. The time can be adjusted for individual bowel habits and preferred timing. Sitting on the commode or toilet promotes bowel elimination through both gravity and increased abdominal pressure. Stool softeners or suppositories may be ordered if the bowel program is ineffective in reestablishing bowel regularity. A glycerin suppository can be inserted 15 to 30 minutes before evacuation time to stimulate the anorectal reflex. The bisacodyl (Dulcolax) suppository is a chemical stimulant to the bowel and is used when other measures are ineffective. Ideally the suppository use is for short-term management.

Bladder function. The nurse often assists the patient with urinary difficulties or incontinence that may follow a stroke. Often the patient with stroke has functional incontinence, which is associated with communication difficulties, mobility problems, and dressing or undressing difficulties. Nursing interventions focused on urinary continence include (1) assessment for bladder distention by palpation; (2) offering the bedpan, urinal, commode, or toilet every 2 hours during waking hours and every 3 to 4 hours at night; (3) focusing the patient on the need to urinate with direct command; (4) assistance with clothing and mobility; (5) scheduling the majority of fluid intake between 7 AM and 7 PM; and (6) encouraging the usual position for urinating (standing for men and sitting for women). Short-term interventions for urinary incontinence may include indwelling catheters, intermittent catheterization, external catheters for men, or incontinent briefs. These are not long-term solutions for urinary incontinence because complications such as urinary infections or skin irritation may occur. A coordinated program by the entire nursing staff is needed to achieve urinary continence.

Sensory-perceptual system. Patients who have had a stroke frequently have perceptual deficits. Patients with a stroke on the right side of the brain usually have difficulty in judging position, distance, and rate of movement. These patients are often impulsive and impatient and tend to deny problems related to strokes. They may fail to correlate spatial-perceptual problems with the inability to perform activities, such as guiding a wheelchair through the doorway. The patient with a right-sided stroke is at higher risk for injury because of mobility difficulties. Directions for activities are best given verbally for comprehension. The task should be broken down to simple steps for ease of understanding. Environmental control such as less clutter, good lighting, and no obstacles aids in concentration and safer mobility. One-sided neglect is common for people with right-sided stroke (left hemiplegia), so the nurse may assist or remind the patient to dress the weak or paralyzed side or shave the forgotten side of the face.

Patients with a left-sided stroke (right hemiplegia) commonly are slower in organization and performance of tasks. They tend to have impaired spatial discrimination. These patients usually admit to deficits and have a fearful, anxious response to a stroke. Their behaviors are slow and cautious. Nonverbal cues and instructions are helpful for comprehension with patients who have had a left-sided stroke (right hemiplegia).

Affect. Patients who have had strokes often exhibit emotional responses that are not appropriate or typical for the situation. Patients may appear apathetic, depressed, fearful, anxious, weepy, frustrated, and angry. Some patients exhibit exaggerated mood swings, especially those with a stroke on the left side of the brain (right hemiplegia). The patient may be unable to control emotions and may suddenly burst into tears or laughter. This behavior is out of context and often is unrelated to the underlying emotional state of the patient. Nursing interventions for atypical emotional response are to (1) distract the patient who suddenly becomes emotional, (2) explain to the patient and family the reason for emotional outbursts, (3) maintain a calm environment, and (4) avoid shaming or scolding the patient during emotional outbursts.

Coping. The patient with a stroke may experience many losses, including sensory, intellectual, communicative, functional, role behavior, emotional, social, and vocational losses. The patient and family often go through the process of grief and mourning associated with the losses. Some patients experience long-term depression with symptoms such as anxiety, weight loss, loss of energy, poor appetite, and sleep disturbances.[18] In addition, the time and energy required to perform previously simple tasks can result in anger and frustration.

The patient and family need help with coping with the losses associated with stroke. The nurse may assist the coping by (1) supporting communication between the patient and family; (2) assisting with focusing on how stroke deficits will change lifestyle; (3) changing roles and responsibilities within the family; (4) being an active listener to allow the expression of fear, frustration, and anxiety; (5) including the family and patient in short- and long-term goal planning and patient care; and (6) supporting family conferences. Maladjusted dependence with inadequate coping occurs when the patient does not maintain optimal functioning for self-care, family responsibilities, decision making, or socialization. This situation can cause resentment from both the patient and family with a negative cycle of interpersonal dependency and control. Maladjusted independence occurs when the patient overestimates personal cognitive or physical capabilities and energy levels. These patients are at risk for injury.[19]

Family members must cope with three aspects of the patient's behavior: (1) recognition of behavioral changes resulting from neurologic deficits that are not changeable, (2) responses to multiple losses both by the patient and the family, and (3) behaviors that may have been reinforced during the early stages of stroke as continued dependency. The patient and family may express feelings of guilt over not living healthy lifestyles or not seeking professional help sooner. Family therapy is a helpful adjunct to rehabilitation. The patient and family need support and reassurance. Open communication, information regarding the total effects of stroke, education regarding stroke treatment, and therapy are helpful. Stroke support groups within rehabilitation facilities and in the community are helpful in terms of mutual sharing, education, coping, and understanding.

Sexual function. A patient who has had a stroke may be concerned about the loss of sexual function. Many patients are comfortable talking about their anxieties and fears regarding sexual function if the nurse is comfortable and open to the topic. The nurse may initiate the topic with the patient and spouse or significant other. Common concerns of sexual activity involving the patient with a stroke are impotence and the occurrence of another stroke during sex. Nursing interventions for sexual activity include education on (1) optional positioning of partners, (2) timing for peak energy times, and (3) patient and partner counseling.

Communication. Speech, comprehension, and language deficits are the most difficult problems for the patient and family. Speech therapists can assess and formulate a plan of care to support communication. The nurse can be a role model for communication with the patient who has aphasia. Nursing interventions that support communication include (1) frequent, meaningful communication; (2) allowing time for the patient to comprehend and answer; (3) using simple, short sentences; (4) using visual cues; (5) structuring conversation so that it permits simple answers by the patient; and (6) praising the patient honestly for improvements with speech.

Community integration. Traditionally, successful community integration following stroke may be difficult for the patient because of persistent problems with cognition, coping, physical deficits, and emotional lability that interfere with functioning. Older patients who have had a stroke often have more severe deficits and frequently experience multiple health problems. Advances in health care have resulted in an increased survival rate for patients with extensive stroke damage. Successful community integration can be redefined by the patient, family, and interdisciplinary health team as successful mobility, achievement of activities of daily living, and quality life with family and friends.

Community resources can be an asset to patients and their families. The National Stroke Association provides information, resources, referral services, and quarterly newsletters on stroke. The American Heart Association has information regarding stroke, hypertension, diet, exercise, and assistive devices. This association sponsors self-help groups in many areas. The Easter Seal Society provides wheelchairs and other assistive devices for stroke patients. Local groups can offer more daily assistance such as meals and transportation. These resources can be identified by nurse case managers, home health nurses, discharge planners, and clinical nurse specialists. (Resources are listed at the end of the chapter.)

GERONTOLOGIC CONSIDERATIONS

Stroke

Strokes are among the primary causes of death and disability among older adults. The highest incidence of stroke occurs among older adults. A stroke is a profound disruption for the life of an older person. The magnitude of disability and profound changes in total function can cause patients to wonder if they can ever return to their "old self." Changes in the totality of daily living require many disruptive changes because of current physical, emotional, perceptual, and cognitive deficits. Home management can be a challenge because often the patient has an elderly spouse caretaker who may also have health problems. There may be a limited number of family members (including adult children) who live in close proximity to the patient. This reduces the number of potential family caretakers. Middle-aged family members are becoming the "sandwich generation" caring for both old, ill parents and their own young families.

The nursing management of the older person who has had a stroke is a challenge. Skilled nursing care is obviously needed in the acute phase. However, the more demanding nursing challenge occurs in the rehabilitative phase in assisting the older patient to deal with residual deficits of stroke, as well as aging. These patients may become fearful and depressed because they think they may have another attack or die. The fear can become immobilizing and prevent effective rehabilitation.

There may be changes in the patient-spouse relationship. The dependency resulting from a stroke may be threatening to a previously stable marriage. The spouse may also have chronic medical problems that may affect the ability to take care of the stroke patient.

CRITICAL THINKING EXERCISES

CASE STUDY

Stroke

Patient Profile

John, a 76-year-old man, had a right-brain (left hemiplegic) stroke 2 months ago. Before the stroke, John, a retired engineer, had been an alert, involved person. He has been married for 40 years and has four adult children. He played golf and drove a car before the stroke. John has now returned home and is living with his wife. His past health history includes a 15 year history of hypertension, obesity, smokes one-half pack of cigarettes per day, moderate beer drinker, and had a myocardial infarction 5 years ago. He is eager to return to prior activity level.

Subjective Data

- Weakness in left arm and leg
- Speech difficulties, especially when tired
- Independent with ADLs
- Emotional instability and impulsive behaviors

Objective Data

Physical Examination

- Sensory impairment of the left side, especially the left hand
- Walks with a slight limp
- Slurred speech while using the phone or when fatigued
- Homonymous hemianopsia

Critical Thinking Questions

1. How does John's prior health history put him at risk for development of a stroke?
2. Are John's reported symptoms and behaviors typical of a person having a right-brain stroke?
3. How can John and his family address activity issues such as driving after the stroke?
4. What strategies might the home health nurse use to help John and his family cope with his emotional lability?
5. What lifestyle changes should John make to reduce the likelihood of another stroke?
6. How will homonymous hemianopsia affect John's hygiene, eating, driving, and golf game?
7. What factors should the nurse assess for in relation to further outpatient rehabilitation for John?
8. Based on the assessment data provided, write one or more nursing diagnoses. Are there any collaborative problems?

NURSING RESEARCH ISSUES

1. Determine the effectiveness of weight loss and stop smoking programs in reducing the incidence of strokes.
2. Examine the relationship between functional abilities and level of independence following a stroke.
3. Determine the effectiveness of nursing interventions to promote full-field visualization for patients with homonymous hemianopsia.
4. Examine the spouse-patient relationship and coping styles during the 6-month period following a stroke.
5. Examine the impact of stroke on socialization, quality of life, and loneliness.

One of the most difficult tasks in home management is helping the spouse or significant other who has to take care of the stroke patient. Living with these demands can be challenging for a younger person and can be even more so for the older spouse. The spouse may experience guilt if others try to help with care. The patient may not want anyone other than the spouse to provide care.

The nurse has the opportunity to aid the patient's and family's transition through acute hospitalization, rehabilitation, long-term care, and home care. The needs of the patient and family require continual nursing assessment, revision of interventions, and evaluation of changing health needs to optimize quality of life for the patient and family.

REVIEW QUESTIONS

The number of the question corresponds to the same-numbered objective at the beginning of the chapter.

1. Of the following patients the nurse recognizes that the one with the highest risk for a stroke is
   a. an obese 45-year-old Native-American.
   b. a 35-year-old Asian-American woman who smokes.
   c. a 32-year-old Caucasian woman on oral contraceptives.
   d. a 65-year-old African-American man with hypertension.

2. The factor related to cerebral blood flow that most often determines the extent of cerebral damage from a stroke is the
   a. amount of cardiac output.
   b. oxygen content of the blood.
   c. degree of collateral circulation.
   d. level of carbon dioxide in the blood.

3. Information provided by the patient that would help differentiate a thrombotic stroke from a hemorrhagic stroke includes
   a. a history of hypertension.
   b. a history of cardiac valvular disease.
   c. the type of early symptoms manifested.
   d. the patient's activity at the onset of symptoms.

4. A right-handed patient with hemiplegia and aphasia resulting from a stroke most likely has a lesion in the
   a. left frontal lobe.
   b. right brainstem.
   c. motor area of the right cerebrum.
   d. medial superior area of the paracentral lobule.

5. The nurse explains to the patient with a stroke who is scheduled for angiography that this test is used to determine the
   a. presence of increased ICP.
   b. site and size of the infarction.
   c. presence of blood in the CSF.
   d. patency of the cerebrovascular system.

6. A patient experiencing TIAs is scheduled for a carotid endarterectomy. The nurse explains that this procedure is done to
   a. promote cerebral blood flow to decrease cerebral edema.
   b. reduce the brain damage that occurs during a stroke-in-evolution.
   c. prevent a stroke by removing atherosclerotic plaques obstructing cerebral blood flow.
   d. provide a circulatory bypass around thrombotic plaques obstructing cranial circulation.

7. Nursing management of the patient with hemiplegia during the acute phase of a stroke includes
   a. using a footboard to prevent footdrop.
   b. positioning each joint higher than the proximal joint.
   c. performing passive range of motion on all limbs every 4 hours.
   d. maintaining the patient in a recumbent, side-lying position.

8. Bladder training in a male patient who has urinary incontinence after a stroke includes
   a. limiting fluid intake.
   b. keeping a urinal in place at all times.
   c. assisting the patient to stand to void.
   d. catheterizing the patient every 4 hours.

9. The most common response of the stroke patient to the change in body image is
   a. denial.
   b. depression.
   c. disassociation.
   d. intellectualization.

References

1. Kongable G: Code stroke: using t-PA to prevent ischemic brain injury, *AJN* 97:16BB, 1997.
2. *Statistical abstracts of the United States: the national data book,* ed 116, Washington, DC, 1996, US Department of Commerce, US Government Printing Office.
3. McCrory DC, Matchar DB: Stroke prevention: the emerging strategies, *Hosp Pract* 31:123, 1996.
4. Hennekens CH: Lessons from hypertension trials, *Am J Med* 104:50S, 1998.
5. Heinemann LA and others: Thromboembolic stroke in young women. A European case-control study on oral contraceptives, *Contraception* 57:29, 1998.
6. Sterz F and others: Possibilities of brain protection with tirilazad after cardiac arrest, *Semin Thromb Hemost* 22:105, 1996.
7. Hickey JV: *The clinical practice of neurological and neurosurgical nursing,* ed 4, Philadelphia, 1997, Lippincott.
8. Mower DA: Brain attack: treating acute ischemic CVA, *Nursing* 27:34, 1997.
9. Read SJ and others: Experience with diffusion-weighted imaging in an acute stroke unit, *Cerebrovasc Dis* 8:135, 1998.
10. Gonzalez ER: Antiplatelet therapy in atherosclerotic cardiovascular disease, *Clin Ther* 20:B18, 1998.
11. Diener HC: Antiplatelet drugs in secondary prevention of stroke, *Int J Clin Pract* 52:91, 1998.
12. Hallett JW and others: Comparison of North American Symptomatic Carotid Endarterectomy Trial and population-based outcomes for carotid endarterectomy, *J Vasc Surg* 27:845, 1998.
13. Kothari R: The biology of stroke and management of the stroke patient, *J Emerg Med Serv* 20:5, 1995.
14. Ball R: Treating stroke: new controversies in emergency care, *J Emerg Med Serv* 20:38, 1995.
15. Levine SR: Thrombolytic therapy for stroke: the new paradigm, *Hosp Pract* 32:57, 1997.
16. Moore K, Trifiletti E: Stroke: the first critical days, *RN* 57:22, 1994.
17. Hayn MA, Fisher TR: Stroke rehabilitation, *Nursing* 27:40, 1997.
18. Fowler S, Durkee CM, Webb DJ: Rehabilitating stroke patients in the acute care setting, *Medsurg Nurs* 5:327, 1996.
19. Brillhart B: Role-relationship pattern. In McCourt AE, editor: *The specialty practice of rehabilitation nursing: a core curriculum,* ed 3, Skokie, Ill, 1993, The Rehabilitation Nursing Foundation of the Association of Rehabilitation Nurses.

Resources

Academy of Aphasia (AA)
Boston Veterans Administration
Medical Center 116B
150 South Huntingdon Avenue
Boston, MA 02130
617-495-4342
http://cortex.neurology.umab.edu/academy/

American Association of Neuroscience Nurses (AANN)
218 North Jefferson Street, #204
Chicago, IL 60606
312-993-0043
http://www.aann.org/

American Brain Tumor Association
2720 River Road
Des Plaines, IL 60018
847-827-9910
800-886-2282
Fax: 847-827-9918
http://www.abta.org

Association of Rehabilitation Nurses (ARN)
4700 West Lake Avenue
Glenview, IL 60025-1485
847-375-4710
800-229-7530
Fax: 847-375-4777
http://www.rehabnurse.org/

Heart and Stroke Foundation of Canada
222 Queen Street, Suite 1402
Ottawa, Ontario K1P 5V9
CANADA
613-569-4361
Fax: 613-569-3278
http://www.hsf.ca/

Information Center for Individuals with Disabilities
Fort Point Place, First Floor
27-43 Wormwood Street
Boston, MA 02210-1606
617-727-5540

National Institute of Neurological and Communicative Disorders and Stroke
Division of Stroke and Trauma (grant applications)
Federal Building, Room 1016
7550 Wisconsin Avenue
Bethesda, MD 20892
301-496-4188

National Stroke Association
96 Inverness Drive East, Suite 1
Englewood, CO 80112-5112
303-649-9299
800-STROKES (787-6537)
Fax: 303-649-1328
http://www.stroke.org

Society for Neuroscience
11 Dupont Circle NW, Suite 500
Washington, DC 20036
202-462-6688
http://www.sfn.org/

Stroke Club International
805 12th Street
Galveston, TX 77550
409-762-1022

Stroke Foundation
898 Park Avenue
New York, NY 10021
800-367-1990

For additional Internet resources, see the website for this book at www.mosby.com/MERLIN/medsurg_lewis

56

NURSING MANAGEMENT
Chronic Neurologic Problems

Judith M. Ozuna

www.mosby.com/MERLIN/medsurg_lewis

LEARNING OBJECTIVES

1. Explain the potential impact of chronic neurologic disease on physical and psychologic well-being.
2. Compare and contrast tension-type, migraine, and cluster headaches in terms of etiology, clinical manifestations, and collaborative care and nursing management.
3. Describe the etiology, clinical manifestations, diagnostic studies, and collaborative management of epilepsy, multiple sclerosis, Parkinson's disease, and myasthenia gravis.
4. Explain the nursing role in the acute and chronic management of a patient with a chronic neurologic disease.
5. Describe the clinical manifestations and collaborative care of amyotrophic lateral sclerosis and Huntington's chorea.
6. Identify common physical complications in a patient who is immobilized by chronic neurologic disease.
7. Outline the major goals of treatment for the patient with a chronic, progressive neurologic disease.

Management of chronic neurologic diseases can be challenging for both the patient and the health care provider. Many neurologic disorders involve progressive deterioration in physical or mental capabilities, which can be devastating to the patient and the family. The patient may experience psychologic distress in the form of depression, fear, anxiety, anger, or withdrawal. This is compounded by changes in body image and self-esteem. In addition, the physical disabilities that result from degenerative diseases necessitate varying and sometimes extreme alterations in lifestyle, which add to the emotional trauma of the patient. Families are torn between their sense of obligation to care for the ill patient and the need to lead their own lives. They are simultaneously pushed and pulled by feelings of guilt, love, despair, hope, resentment, and empathy.

The challenge of chronic neurologic illness is equally great for health care providers. Many of these diseases have no cure. Therefore health care professionals can only attempt to alleviate physical symptoms, prevent complications, assist patients in maximizing self-care abilities in the face of neurologic deficits, and help them in the difficult task of adjusting to their illness. Nurses can and should greatly influence these aspects of management.

HEADACHE

Headache is probably the most common type of pain experienced by humans. Of all persons with headache, the majority have functional headaches, such as benign migraine or tension-type headaches; the remainder have organic headaches caused by significant intracranial or extracranial disease.

Not all tissues of the cranium are sensitive to pain. The pain-sensitive structures in the head include the venous sinuses, the dura (at the base of the brain near large blood vessels), cranial blood vessels, the three divisions of the trigeminal nerve (CN V), the facial nerve (CN VII), the glossopharyngeal nerve (CN IX), the vagus nerve (CN X), and the first three cervical nerves. Thus headache pain can arise from both intracranial and extracranial sources.

Headaches are classified based on the characteristics of the headache and the facial pain. The primary classifications include tension-type, migraine, and cluster headaches. Characteristics of these headaches are shown in Table 56-1. A patient may have more than one type of headache. The history and neurologic examination are diagnostic keys to determining the type of headache.

TENSION-TYPE HEADACHE

Tension-type headache is described as bilateral, dull, and non-pulsatile. Tension-type headache has been called muscle-contraction, tension, psychogenic, and rheumatic headache. It is the most common type of headache and is also considered the most difficult to treat. Tension-type headaches are often subcategorized as acute or episodic and chronic.

Etiology and Pathophysiology

It was originally thought that tension-type headache was the result of sustained and painful contraction of the muscles of the scalp and the neck. Recent evidence, however, does not support this mechanism in all patients with tension-type headaches. It

Reviewed by Patricia A. Blissett, RN, MSN, CCRN, CNRN, CCM, Staff Nurse, Neurosurgical Intensive Care Unit, Harborview Medical Center, Seattle, Wash.

Table 56-1	Comparison of Tension-type, Migraine, and Cluster Headaches		
Pattern	Tension-type	Migraine	Cluster
Site	Bilateral, bandlike pressure at base of skull, in face, or in both	Unilateral (in 60%), may switch sides, commonly anterior	Unilateral, radiating up or down from one eye
Quality	Constant, squeezing tightness	Throbbing, synchronous with pulse	Severe, bone-crushing
Frequency	Cycles for several years	Periodic; cycles of several months to years	May have months or years between attacks; attacks occur in clusters: one to three times a day over a period of 4-8 wk
Duration	Intermittent for months or years	Continuous for hours or days	30 to 90 min
Time and mode of onset	Not related to time	May be preceded by prodrome; onset after awakening; gets better with sleep	Nocturnal; commonly awakens patient from sleep
Associated symptoms	Palpable neck and shoulder muscles, stiff neck, tenderness	Nausea or vomiting, edema, irritability, sweating, photophobia, prodrome of sensory, motor, or psychic phenomena; family history (in 65%)	Vasomotor symptoms such as facial flushing or pallor, unilateral lacrimation, ptosis, and rhinitis

is likely that both increased pain sensitivity and muscle factors contribute to the etiology of tension-type headaches.

Clinical Manifestations

There is no prodrome (early manifestation of impending disease) in tension-type headache. The pain is usually bilateral, occurring most often in the back of the neck. It usually does not interfere with sleep. The pain is often described as a tight, squeezing, band-like pressure. It is sustained, chronic, dull, and persistent. The headaches may occur intermittently for weeks, months, or even years. Many patients can have a combination of migraine and tension-type headaches, with features of both headaches occurring simultaneously. Patients with migraine headaches may experience tension-type headaches between migraine attacks.

Diagnostic Studies

Careful history taking is probably the most important diagnostic tool for tension-type headache. Electromyography (EMG) may reveal sustained contraction of the neck, scalp, or facial muscles, but many patients may not show increased muscle tension with this test, even when the test is done during the actual headache. Conversely, patients with diagnosed migraine headaches may show increased muscle tension on EMG. If tension-type headache is present during physical examination, increased resistance to passive movement of the head and tenderness of the head and neck may be present.

MIGRAINE HEADACHE

Migraine headache is a benign, recurring headache characterized by unilateral or bilateral pain, a triggering event or factor, strong family history, and manifestations associated with neurologic and autonomic nervous system dysfunction. For some individuals migraine headaches begin in childhood or adolescence. A family history of migraine can be found in 65% of patients with migraine. Estimates of migraine prevalence in recent studies are about 6% in men and 15% to 18% in women.[1] Although migraine headaches have often been associated with patients who

are high achievers and who suppress expressions of aggression and hostility, no single personality type describes all patients who experience migraine headache.

Etiology and Pathophysiology

In the past it was thought that migraine headaches had a vascular origin and involved the intracranial and extracranial arteries of the head. The classic theory of migraine headaches is that the prodromal or aural phase is associated with vasoconstriction and decreased blood flow. The headache phase is associated with vasodilation and increased blood flow. Although the exact etiology of migraine headaches is not known, evidence now suggests that neurologic, vascular, and chemical factors are involved.[2] The neurogenic model of migraine implies that a stimulus can trigger the trigeminovascular system (trigeminal nerve and its connections to meningeal blood vessels) resulting in inflammation of the blood vessels and vasodilation, resulting in headache. The neurotransmitter serotonin appears to play an important role in migraine headache progression.

Migraine headaches, in many cases, have no known precipitating events. However, for other patients, the headache may be precipitated or triggered by stress, excitement, bright lights, menstruation, alcohol, or certain foods such as chocolate or cheese.

The aura of migraine is associated with "spreading depression," a wave of oligemia (diminished cerebral blood flow) beginning in the occipital lobe and spreading forward in the brain at a rate of 2 to 3 mm per minute. The progression of oligemia does not correlate with blood vessel supply, so it is unlikely to be generated by the blood vessels themselves.

Clinical Manifestations

There are two major types of migraine headaches: migraine without aura (formerly called common migraine) and migraine with aura (formerly called classic migraine). Migraine without aura is the most common type of migraine headache. The prodrome is not sharply defined, and it can involve psychic disturbances, gastrointestinal upset, and changes in fluid balance. The prodrome may precede the headache phase by several hours or several days. The headache itself may last several hours or days.

Migraine with aura occurs in only 10% of migraine headache episodes. The sharply defined aura may last for 10 to 30 minutes before the start of the headache and may include sensory dysfunction (e.g., visual field defects, tingling or burning sensations, or paresthesias), motor dysfunction (e.g., weakness, paralysis), dizziness, confusion, and even loss of consciousness. The classic preheadache symptom is perception of flashing lights in one quadrant of the visual field, often termed *scintillating scotomata*. This type of migraine headache usually peaks in 1 hour and may last several hours.

Clinical manifestations that occur in migraine with and without aura are generalized edema, irritability, pallor, nausea and vomiting, and sweating. During the headache phase, patients with migraine tend to "hibernate"; that is, they seek shelter from noise, light, odors, people, and problems. The headache is described as a steady, throbbing pain that is synchronous with the pulse. Although the headache is usually unilateral, it may switch to the opposite side in another episode. The diagnosis of migraine headache is usually made from the history. The neurologic and other diagnostic examinations are often normal.

CLUSTER HEADACHE

Cluster headache is one of the most severe forms of head pain. Cluster headache occurs less frequently than migraine (the cluster headache to migraine frequency is 1:10) and is more frequent in men than in women by a ratio of 5:1. The onset is usually between 30 and 60 years of age.

Etiology and Pathophysiology

Neither the cause nor the pathophysiology of cluster headache is fully known. The vasodilation that occurs in the affected part of the face is extracranial. The trigeminal nerve is implicated in the production of pain. Activation of this nerve causes release of substance P and other vasoactive substances that cause vasodilation, stimulation of afferent pain fibers, and neurogenic inflammation with extravasation of protein and platelets in the perivascular areas. The periodicity and the clocklike regularity of cluster headache indicate a dysfunction of the biologic clock mechanisms of the hypothalamus.[3] These headaches can also be triggered by alcohol ingestion.

Clinical Manifestations

The headache has an abrupt onset, usually without a prodrome. It peaks in 5 to 10 minutes and lasts 30 to 90 minutes. It is not uncommon for this type of headache to start at night, awakening the patient after a few hours of sleep. Headaches may recur several times a day over a period of several days, with each cluster lasting 2 to 3 months. It usually affects the upper face, the periorbital region, and the forehead on one side of the face and the head. The headache may not recur for months or years. The patient may also exhibit conjunctivitis, increased lacrimation (tearing), and nasal congestion on the side of the headache. Sweating may occur on the forehead of the affected side. A partial Horner's syndrome (miosis [constriction of the pupil] and ptosis [drooping of the eyelid on the affected side]) may be seen. The headache is described as deep, steady, and penetrating but not throbbing.

Unlike the patient with migraine, who seeks isolation and quiet, the patient with a cluster headache paces the floor, cries

out, does bizarre things, and resents being touched. The patient with a cluster headache does not experience the systemic manifestations that accompany a migraine headache, such as nausea or vomiting. As with migraine headaches, there are usually no complications.

Diagnostic Studies

The diagnosis of cluster headache is primarily based on the history. However, computed tomography (CT) scan, magnetic resonance imaging (MRI), or cerebral angiography may be performed to rule out an aneurysm, tumor, or infection.

OTHER TYPES OF HEADACHES

Although tension, migraine, and cluster headaches are by far the most common types of headaches, other types of headache can also occur. These headaches may be the first symptom of a more serious illness. Headache can accompany subarachnoid hemorrhage; brain tumors; other intracranial masses; arteritis; vascular abnormalities; trigeminal neuralgia (tic douloureux); diseases of the eyes, nose, and teeth; and systemic illness (e.g., bacteremia, carbon monoxide poisoning, mountain sickness, polycythemia vera). The symptoms vary greatly. Because of the variety of causes of headache, clinical evaluation must be thorough. It should include an evaluation of personality, life adjustment, environment, and family situation, as well as a comprehensive evaluation of physical status.

Collaborative Care: Headache

If no systemic underlying disease is found, therapy is directed toward the functional type of headache. Table 56-2 outlines the general workup for a patient with headache to rule out any intracranial or extracranial disease. Table 56-3 summarizes the current therapies for symptomatic relief of common headaches. These therapies include medications, meditation, yoga, biofeedback, and muscle relaxation training.

Biofeedback involves the use of physiologic monitoring equipment to give the patient information regarding muscle tension and peripheral blood flow (skin temperature of the fingers). The patient is trained to relax the muscles and raise the finger temperature and is given reinforcement (operant conditioning) in accomplishing these physiologic alterations.

DIAGNOSTIC STUDIES

Table 56-2 Patient with Headache

- Complete health history
- Clinical examination (often negative)
  - Inspect for local infections
  - Palpation for tenderness, hardened arteries, bony swellings
  - Auscultation for bruits over major arteries
- Routine laboratory studies to rule out underlying causes of headache
  - CBC
  - Electrolytes
  - Urinalysis
- CT scan of sinuses
- Special studies (e.g., CT scan, angiography, EMG, EEG, MRI)

CBC, complete blood count; *CT*, computed tomography; *EEG*, electroencephalography; *EMG*, electromyography; *MRI*, magnetic resonance imaging.

COLLABORATIVE CARE

Table 56-3   **Headache**

	Tension-type Headache	Migraine Headache	Cluster Headache
Diagnostic	History of neck and head tenderness, resistance to movement, EMG	History	History, thermography
Collaborative Therapy			
▪ Symptomatic	Nonnarcotic analgesics (aspirin, acetaminophen, ibuprofen) Analgesic combinations (butalbital [Fiorinal]) Muscle relaxants	Nonnarcotic analgesics (aspirin, acetaminophen, ibuprofen) Serotonin receptor agonist (sumatriptan [Imitrex], zolmitriptan [Zomig], naratriptan [Amerge], rizatriptan [Maxalt]) Alpha-adrenergic blockers (ergotamine tartrate [Ergomar]) Vasoconstrictors (isometheptene [Midrin]) Corticosteroids (dexamethasone)	Alpha-adrenergic blockers (ergotamine tartrate) Vasoconstrictors Oxygen
▪ Prophylactic	Tricyclic antidepressants (doxepin [Sinequan], amitriptyline [Elavil]) Beta-adrenergic blockers (propranolol [Inderal]) Biofeedback Muscle relaxation training Psychotherapy	Beta-adrenergic blockers (propranolol) Serotonin antagonists* (methysergide [Sansert]) Antidepressants (amitriptyline, imipramine) Calcium channel blockers (verapamil [Isoptin]) Divalproex (Depakote) Biofeedback Yoga Meditation Electric counterstimulation	Alpha-adrenergic blockers (ergotamine tartrate) Serotonin antagonists (methysergide) Corticosteroids (prednisone) Lithium Calcium channel blockers (verapamil) Divalproex (Depakote)

*Only for patients suffering from one or more severe headaches per week.
EMG, electromyography.

Acupuncture, acupressure, and hypnosis are successful innovative therapies that work well in some patients with headaches. Some patients can benefit from psychotherapy that is aimed at helping them recognize conflicts and deal with them more effectively. Treatments for tension-type headache include physical therapy (e.g., massage, hot packs, cervical collar), injection of local anesthetic into spastic muscles, and correction of faulty posture.

Drug Therapy

Tension-type headache. Drug treatment for tension-type headache usually involves a nonnarcotic analgesic (e.g., aspirin, acetaminophen) used alone or in combination with a sedative, a muscle relaxant, a tranquilizer, or codeine. However, many of these drugs have potentially dangerous side effects. The patient should be cautioned about the long-term use of aspirin and aspirin-containing drugs because they can cause gastric bleeding and coagulation abnormalities in susceptible patients. Long-term use of Fiorinal should be avoided because in addition to aspirin it contains a barbiturate (butalbital), which may be habit forming. Drugs containing acetaminophen (Tylenol, Phenaphen, Midrin) can cause kidney damage with chronic use and liver damage when combined with alcohol. Daily use of nonsteroidal antiinflammatory drugs (NSAIDs) can cause chronic daily headaches. Narcotics and benzodiazepines can cause addiction and habituation. Discontinuing an overused medication too abruptly can lead to withdrawal symptoms (analgesic rebound).

Migraine headache. Drug treatment of the acute migraine attack is aimed at terminating or decreasing the symptoms of the attack. Many people with mild or moderate migraine can obtain relief with aspirin or acetaminophen. Ergotamine (Ergomar) is often used when simple analgesics do not relieve headache. Ergotamine inhibits the reuptake of neuronally liberated norepinephrine into storage sites of the postganglionic nerve terminal of the sympathetic nervous system. This allows more norepinephrine to attach to alpha-adrenergic sites on smooth muscle in the artery wall, thereby causing prolonged vasoconstriction of cranial vessels. Ergotamine can be administered orally, sublingually, parenterally, rectally, or by inhalation. The usual dosage is 1 to 2 mg (oral or rectal) at the onset of the headache, followed by 2 mg within 1 hour. No more than 6 mg is given for any single attack. Dihydroergotamine mesylate is available as a nasal spray called Migranal. Other drugs that may relieve migraine headache include butalbital with aspirin or acetaminophen (Fiorinal, Fioricet), isometheptene with acetaminophen and dichloralphenazone (Midrin), and, in certain cases, narcotics.

Drugs that affect serotonin have been found to relieve migraine headaches. Sumatriptan (Imitrex), which is selective for vascular serotonin receptors, produces vasoconstriction and is used for the management of acute migraine headaches. In addition, sumatriptan inhibits the release of pain-producing inflammatory neuropeptides such as substance P, thus interfering with pain transmission. Sumatriptan can be given subcutaneously, orally, or nasally. It is a currently the drug of choice for acute management of migraine headaches. Newer agents that work via a serotonergic mechanism to constrict cerebral blood vessels include zolmitriptan (Zomig), naratriptan (Amerge), and rizatriptan (Maxalt). Similar to sumatriptan, these drugs can cause chest pain and are avoided in patients with heart disease.

A variety of drugs are used to prevent further tension-type and migraine attacks. Methysergide (Sansert) is an ergot alkaloid that competitively blocks serotonin receptors in the central and peripheral nervous systems. This drug has been found to be effective in the prevention of migraine headaches. However, because of side effects, including retroperitoneal, pulmonary, and cardiac fibrosis, the patient requires regular follow-up. It is recommended that a patient take a break ("drug holiday") every 4 to 6 months.

Other drugs taken daily to prevent recurrence of very severe or very frequent migraine headaches include β-adrenergic blockers (e.g., propranolol [Inderal], atenolol [Tenormin]), tricyclic antidepressants (e.g., amitriptyline [Elavil]), selective serotonin reuptake inhibitors (e.g., fluoxetine [Prozac]), calcium channel blockers (verapamil [Isoptin]), divalproex (Depakote), clonidine (Catapres), thiazides, and lithium.

Cluster headache. Because cluster headaches occur suddenly, often at night, and are not long lasting, drug therapy is not as useful as it is for the other types of headache. Prophylactic medications may include verapamil, lithium, ergotamine, divalproex (Depakote), or NSAIDs. Acute treatment of cluster headache is inhalation of 100% oxygen delivered at a rate of 7 to 9 L/min for 15 to 20 minutes, which may relieve headache by causing vasoconstriction. It can be repeated after a 5-minute rest. However, a drawback to this treatment is that the patient must have continuous access to the oxygen supply. Sumatriptan is also effective in treating acute cluster headache. Methysergide may be used prophylactically when the cluster headache recurs at a known time.

NURSING MANAGEMENT: HEADACHES

■ Nursing Assessment

Subjective and objective data that should be obtained from a patient with headache are presented in Table 56-4. Because the history provides the key to assessment of headache, it should include specific details of the headache itself, such as the location and type of pain, the onset, the frequency, the duration, the relation to events (emotional, psychologic, physical), and the time of day of the occurrence. Information about previous illnesses, surgery, trauma, allergies, family history, and response to medication should also be obtained. The nurse can suggest that the patient keep a diary of headache episodes with specific details. This type of record can be of great help in determining the type of headache and the precipitating events. If the patient has a history of migraine, tension-type, or cluster headaches, it is important to determine if the character, intensity, or location of the headache has changed. This may be an important clue as to the cause of the headache.

■ Nursing Diagnoses

Nursing diagnoses for the patient with headache may include, but are not limited to, those presented in NCP 56-1.

NURSING ASSESSMENT

Table 56-4 Headaches

Subjective Data

Important Health Information

Past health history: Hypertension, seizures, cancer, recent fall or trauma, cranial infection, craniotomy; cerebrovascular accident; asthma or allergies; mental illness; relationship of headache to overwork, stress, menstruation, exercise, food, sexual activity, travel, bright lights, or other noxious environmental stimuli

Medications: Use of hydralazine, bromides, nitroglycerin, ergotamine (withdrawal), nonsteroidal antiinflammatory drugs (in high daily doses), estrogen preparations, oral contraceptives, over-the-counter or prescription remedies

Surgery or other treatments: Craniotomy, sinus surgery, facial surgery

Functional Health Patterns

Health perception–health management: Positive family history; malaise

Nutritional-metabolic: Ingestion of alcohol, caffeine, cheese, chocolate, monosodium glutamate, aspartame, lunch meats (nitrites in cured meats), sausage, hot dogs, onions, avocados; anorexia, nausea, vomiting (migraine prodrome); unilateral lacrimation (cluster)

Activity-exercise: Vertigo, fatigue, weakness, paralysis, fainting

Sleep-rest: Insomnia

Cognitive-perceptual:

Migraine: aura; unilateral, severe, throbbing (possible switching of side) headache; visual disturbances; photophobia; phonophobia; dizziness; tingling or burning sensations

Cluster: unilateral and severe, nocturnal headache; nasal stuffiness

Tension-type: bilateral, band-like, dull and persistent, base of skull headache, neck tenderness

Self-perception–self-concept: Depression

Coping–stress tolerance: Stress, anxiety, irritability, withdrawal

Objective Data

General

Anxiety, apprehension

Integumentary

Cluster: forehead diaphoresis, pallor, unilateral facial flushing with cheek edema, conjunctivitis

Migraine: generalized edema (prodrome), pallor, diaphoresis

Neurologic

Horner's syndrome, restlessness (cluster), hemiparesis (migraine)

Musculoskeletal

Resistance of head and neck movement, nuchal rigidity (meningeal, tension-type), palpable neck and shoulder muscles (tension-type)

Possible Findings

Possible evidence of disease, deformity, or infection on brain imaging (CT, MRI), cerebral arteriogram, lumbar puncture, electroencephalogram, electromyography; nonspecific brain imaging or laboratory tests

56-1 NURSING CARE PLAN · PATIENT WITH HEADACHE

Expected Patient Outcomes **Nursing Interventions and *Rationales***

NURSING DIAGNOSIS · **Pain** *related to* headache *as manifested by* complaint of steady, throbbing, or severe crushing pain.

- Reduced pain.
- Satisfaction with pain relief.

- Assess pain intensity, characteristics, location, and duration *to determine appropriate interventions.*
- Encourage patient to keep a pain log including associated factors or precipitators *to provide patient some control in identifying and controlling factors that may precipitate headaches.*
- Encourage patient to learn and use alternative therapies such as meditation, yoga, biofeedback, and muscle-relaxation techniques *to supplement drug therapy and provide the patient with some sense of control over pain.*
- Support patient's use of counseling or psychotherapy *to enhance stress reduction.*
- Administer drugs as ordered *to reduce pain.**
- Monitor patient following administration of pain medication *to assess drug efficacy and identify adverse drug effects.*
- Provide a quiet, dimly lighted environment *to reduce stimuli that may trigger headaches.*
- Massage head/neck/shoulder area as tolerated *to relieve muscle tension and promote relaxation.*

NURSING DIAGNOSIS · **Anxiety** *related to* lack of knowledge about headache's etiology and ways to treat it *as manifested by* increased heart rate, insomnia, feeling of helplessness.

- Increased psychologic comfort and decreased anxiety.
- Effective coping mechanisms to manage anxiety.

- Assess level of anxiety *to determine appropriate interventions.*
- Encourage patient to verbalize concerns *because this reduces anxiety.*
- Teach relaxation techniques and coping strategies *to promote muscle relaxation and reduce anxiety.*
- Explain possible etiology of patient's specific headache type *to reduce patient's fear of unknown.*
- Reinforce physician's explanation of diagnostic tests *to relieve concerns about cause and seriousness of headache.*
- Discuss the physiologic dynamics of tension/anxiety *because knowledge about how these factors influence headache can help with management.*

NURSING DIAGNOSIS · **Hopelessness** *related to* chronic pain, alteration of lifestyle, and ineffective treatment modalities *as manifested by* expressions of extreme apathy and listlessness, lack of interest in doing usual activities.

- Expression of confidence in ability to function despite headaches.

- Assess patient's degree of hopelessness *to enable appropriate planning.*
- Explore patient's self-treatment of pain and alterations in lifestyle *to identify appropriateness and make appropriate adjustments.*
- Promote verbalization of fears and concerns *to convey empathy and correct patient's misconceptions.*
- Assist patient in identifying support systems that can be used *to bolster hopefulness.*
- Initiate referrals as indicated for counseling *to continue work on feeling of hopelessness.*

NURSING DIAGNOSIS · **Sleep pattern disturbance** *related to* pain *as manifested by* inability to maintain usual sleep pattern.

- Use effective strategies to get to and maintain sleep.
- Feeling rested.

- Assess patient's usual sleep pattern *to determine appropriate interventions.*
- Reduce external stimuli *to provide a calm environment conducive to sleep.*
- Use massage or relaxation techniques *to facilitate relaxation and sleep.*
- Schedule analgesia administration *so maximum effect for headache relief will coincide with bedtime.*
- Medicate for pain if patient awakens with headache pain *to foster return to sleep and pain-free awakening.*

*See Table 56-3.

Planning

The overall goals are that the patient with a headache will (1) have reduced or no pain, (2) experience increased comfort and decreased anxiety, (3) demonstrate understanding of triggering events and treatment strategies, and (4) use positive coping strategies to deal with chronic pain.

Nursing Implementation

Patients with chronic headache present a great challenge to health care providers. Headaches may result from an inability to cope with daily stresses. The most effective therapy may be to help patients examine their lifestyle, recognize stressful situations, and learn to cope with them more appropriately. Precipitating factors can be identified, and ways of avoiding them can be developed. Daily exercise, relaxation periods, and socializing can be encouraged, since each can help decrease the recurrence of headache. The nurse can suggest alternative ways of handling the pain of headache through techniques such as relaxation, meditation, yoga, and self-hypnosis.

In addition to using analgesics and analgesic combination drugs for the symptomatic relief of headache, the patient should be encouraged to use relaxation techniques because they are effective in tension-type and migraine headaches. The migraine sufferer often needs a quiet, dimly lit environment. Massage and moist hot packs to the neck and head can help a patient with tension-type headaches. The patient should learn about the medications prescribed for prophylactic and symptomatic treatment of headache and should be able to describe the purpose, action, dosage, and side effects of the medication. To prevent accidental overdose, the patient should make a written note of each dose of medication or headache remedy.

For the patient whose headaches are triggered by food, dietary counseling may be provided. The patient is encouraged to eliminate foods that may provoke headaches, such as vinegar, chocolate, onions, alcohol (particularly red wine), excessive caffeine, cheese, fermented or marinated foods, monosodium glutamate, and aspartame. Active challenge and provocative testing with specific foods may be necessary to determine the specific causative agents.[4] Patients should avoid smoking and exposure to triggers such as strong perfumes, volatile solvents, and gasoline fumes. Cluster headache attacks may occur at high altitudes with low oxygen levels during air travel. Ergotamine, taken before the plane takes off, may decrease the likelihood of these attacks. A teaching guide for the patient with a headache is listed in Table 56-5.

Evaluation

Expected outcomes for the patient with headache are addressed in NCP 56-1.

SEIZURE DISORDERS AND EPILEPSY

A *seizure* is a paroxysmal, uncontrolled electrical discharge of neurons in the brain that interrupts normal function. Seizures are frequently symptoms of an underlying illness. They may accompany a variety of disorders, or they may occur spontaneously without any apparent cause. Seizures resulting from

---

PATIENT TEACHING GUIDE
Table 56-5 | Headache

1. Avoid factors that can trigger a headache:
   Foods containing amines (cheese, chocolate), nitrites (meats such as hot dogs), vinegar, onions, fermented or marinated foods
   Monosodium glutamate
   Caffeine
   Nicotine
   Ice cream
   Alcohol (particularly red wine)
   Emotional stress
   Fatigue
   Medications such as ergot-containing and monoamine oxidase inhibitors
2. Able to describe the purpose, action, dosage, and side effects of medications taken
3. Able to self-administer sumatriptan subcutaneously if prescribed
4. Use stress-reduction techniques such as relaxation
5. Participate in regular exercise
6. Keep a diary or calendar of headaches and possible precipitating events
7. Contact health care provider if the following occur:
   - Symptoms become more severe, last longer than usual, or are resistant to medication
   - Nausea, vomiting, change in vision, or fever occur with the headache
   - Problems with medications

---

systemic and metabolic disturbances are not considered epilepsy if the seizures cease when the underlying problem is corrected. In the adult, metabolic disturbances that cause seizures include acidosis, electrolyte imbalances, hypoglycemia, hypoxia, alcohol and barbiturate withdrawal, dehydration, and water intoxication. Extracranial disorders that can cause seizures are heart, lung, liver, or kidney disease; systemic lupus erythematosus, diabetes mellitus; hypertension; and septicemia.

Epilepsy is a condition in which a person has spontaneously recurring seizures caused by a chronic underlying condition. Over 2 million people in the United States have epilepsy.[5] The incidence rates are high during the first year of life, decline through childhood and adolescence, plateau in middle age, and rise sharply again among the elderly.[5]

Etiology and Pathophysiology

The most common causes of epilepsy during the first 6 months of life are severe birth injury, congenital defects involving the central nervous system (CNS), infections, and inborn errors of metabolism. In patients between 2 and 20 years of age, the primary causative factors are birth injury, infection, trauma, and genetic factors. In individuals between 20 and 30 years of age, epilepsy usually occurs as the result of structural lesions, such as trauma, brain tumors, or vascular disease. After 50 years of age the primary causes of epilepsy are cerebrovascular lesions and metastatic brain tumors. Although many causes of epilepsy have been identified, three fourths of all epilepsy cases cannot be attributed to a specific cause and are considered idiopathic.

The role of heredity in the etiology of epilepsy has been difficult to determine because of the problem of separating hereditary from environmental or acquired influences. In addition, some families carry a predisposition to epilepsy in the form of an inherently low threshold to seizure-producing stimuli, such as trauma, disease, and high fever. For example, an inherently low seizure threshold may explain the reason some patients develop seizures after a head injury or similar insult, whereas others do not.

In recurring seizures (epilepsy) a group of abnormal neurons (seizure focus) seems to undergo spontaneous firing. This firing spreads by physiologic pathways to involve adjacent or distant areas of the brain. If this activity spreads to involve the whole brain, a generalized seizure occurs. The factor that causes this abnormal firing is not clear. Any stimulus that causes the cell membrane of the neuron to depolarize induces a tendency to spontaneous firing. Often the area of the brain from which the epileptic activity arises is found to have scar tissue (gliosis). The scarring is thought to interfere with the normal chemical and structural environment of the brain neurons, making them more likely to fire abnormally.

Repetitive electrical discharges from an epileptic focus in experimental animals can produce long-lasting and possibly permanent changes in neuron excitability, both locally and in distant areas of the brain. This effect is called *kindling,* and it presents an interesting and important implication for epilepsy in humans: seizures can beget more seizures. Clinical experience indicates that the longer a patient goes without good seizure control, the lower the likelihood that the seizures will be controllable. Therefore a vigorous attempt must be made to control recurring seizures.

Clinical Manifestations

The specific clinical manifestations of a seizure are determined by the site of the electrical disturbance. The preferred method of classifying epileptic seizures is the International Classification System proposed by Gastaut in 1970 and revised in 1981 (Table 56-6).[6,7] This system is based on the clinical and electroencephalographic manifestations of seizures. In this system, seizures are divided into two major classes: generalized and partial. Depending on the type, a seizure may progress through several phases, which include (1) the prodromal phase with signs or activity, which precede a seizure; (2) the aural phase with a sensory warning; (3) the ictal phase with full seizure; and (4) postictal phase, which is the period of recovery after the seizure.

Generalized Seizures. Generalized seizures are characterized by bilateral synchronous epileptic discharge in the brain from the onset of the seizure. Because the entire brain is affected at the onset of the seizures, there is no warning or aura. In most cases, the patient loses consciousness for a few seconds to several minutes.

Tonic-clonic seizures. The most common generalized seizure is the generalized tonic-clonic, or grand mal, seizure. This seizure is characterized by loss of consciousness and falling to the ground if the patient is upright, followed by stiffening of the body (tonic phase) for 10 to 20 seconds and subsequent jerking of the extremities (clonic phase) for another 30 to 40 seconds.

Table 56-6	International Classification of Epileptic Seizures

Generalized Seizures (bilaterally symmetric and without local onset)
Absence seizures, atypical absence seizures
Myoclonic seizures
Clonic seizures
Tonic seizures
Tonic-clonic seizures
Atonic seizures

Partial Seizures (local onset)
- Simple partial seizures (no impairment of consciousness)
  With motor symptoms
  With somatosensory or special sensory symptoms
  With autonomic symptoms
  With psychic symptoms
- Complex partial seizures (impairment of consciousness)
  Simple partial seizures with progression to impairment of consciousness
    With no other features
    With features of simple partial seizures
    With automatisms
  Impairment of consciousness at onset
    With no other features
    With features of simple partial seizures
    With automatisms

Unclassified Epileptic Seizures (inadequate or incomplete data)

Modified from Commission on Classification and Terminology of the International League against Epilepsy: Proposal for revised clinical and electroencephalographic classification of epileptic seizures, *Epilepsia* 22:489, 1981.

Cyanosis, excessive salivation, tongue or cheek biting, and incontinence may accompany the seizure.

In the postictal phase the patient usually has muscle soreness, is very tired, and may sleep for several hours. Some patients may not feel normal for several hours or days after a seizure. The patient has no memory of the seizure activity.

Typical absence seizures. The absence (petit mal) seizure usually occurs only in children and rarely continues beyond adolescence. This type of seizure may cease altogether as the child matures, or it may evolve into another type of seizure. The typical clinical manifestation is a brief staring spell that lasts only a few seconds, so it often occurs unnoticed. There may be an extremely brief loss of consciousness. When untreated, the seizures may occur up to 100 times a day.

The electroencephalogram (EEG) demonstrates a 3 Hz (cycles per second) spike-and-wave pattern that is unique to this type of seizure. Absence seizures can often be precipitated by hyperventilation and flashing lights.

Atypical absence seizures. Another type of generalized seizure is the staring spell accompanied by other signs and symptoms, including brief warnings, peculiar behavior during the seizure, or confusion after the seizure. The EEG demonstrates atypical spike-and-wave patterns, usually greater or less than 3 Hz.

Other types of generalized seizures. Other generalized seizures are myoclonic and akinetic seizures. A myoclonic seizure is characterized by a sudden, excessive jerk of the body or extremities. The jerk may be forceful enough to hurl the person to the ground. These seizures are very brief and may occur in clusters. The terms *akinetic* (arrest of movement), *atonic* (loss of tone), and *astatic* (loss of balance) have been used interchangeably to describe drop attacks or falling spells. This type of seizure involves either a tonic episode or a paroxysmal loss of muscle tone and begins suddenly with the person falling to the ground. Consciousness usually returns by the time the person hits the ground, and normal activity can be resumed immediately. Patients with this type of seizure are at a great risk of head injury and often have to wear protective helmets. A less severe akinetic seizure involves brief loss of muscle tone without falling.

Partial Seizures. Partial (focal) seizures are another major class of the International Classification System. Partial seizures begin in a specific region of the cortex, as indicated by the EEG and usually by the clinical manifestations. For example, if the discharging focus is located in the medial aspect of the postcentral gyrus, the patient may experience paresthesias and tingling or numbness in the leg on the side opposite the focus. If the discharging focus is located in the part of the brain that governs a particular function, sensory, motor, cognitive, or emotional manifestations may occur.

Partial seizures may be confined to one side of the brain and remain partial or focal in nature, or they may spread to involve the entire brain, culminating in a generalized tonic-clonic seizure. Any tonic-clonic seizure that is preceded by an aura or warning is a partial seizure that generalizes secondarily. Many tonic-clonic seizures that appear to be generalized from the outset may actually be secondary generalized seizures, but the preceding partial component may be so brief that it is undetected by the patient, the observer, or even on the EEG. Unlike the primary generalized tonic-clonic seizure, the secondary generalized seizure may result in a transient residual neurologic deficit postically. This is referred to as Todd's paralysis (focal paresis), which resolves after varying lengths of time.

Partial seizures are further divided into those with simple motor or sensory phenomena and those with complex symptoms (also called psychomotor seizures). Simple partial seizures with elementary symptoms do not involve loss of consciousness and rarely last longer than 1 minute. They may involve motor, sensory, or autonomic phenomena or a combination of these. The terms *focal motor, focal sensory,* and *jacksonian* have been used to describe seizures of the simple partial type.

Partial seizures with complex symptoms can involve a variety of behavioral, emotional, affective, and cognitive functions. The location of the discharging focus is usually in the temporal lobe, hence the term *temporal lobe seizure.* These seizures usually last longer than 1 minute and are frequently followed by a period of postictal confusion. Partial complex seizures are distinct from simple partial (focal motor, focal sensory) seizures in that they involve some alteration in consciousness. The sole manifestation of partial complex seizures may be clouding of consciousness or a confused state without any motor or sensory components. This type of attack is sometimes termed *temporal lobe absence.* There is rarely the complete loss of consciousness that is typical of the generalized absence attack, nor does the patient snap back to the preseizure state as does the patient who has had a generalized absence attack.

The most common complex partial seizure involves lip smacking and automatisms (repetitive movements that may not be appropriate). These are often called *psychomotor seizures.* The patient may continue an activity that was initiated before the seizure, such as counting out change or picking items from a grocery shelf, but after the seizure does not remember the activity performed during the seizure. Other automatisms are less organized, such as picking at clothing, fumbling with objects (real or imaginary), or simply walking away.

A variety of psychosensory symptoms may occur during a partial complex seizure, including distortions of visual or auditory sensations and vertigo. There may be alterations in memory, such as a feeling of having experienced an event before (déjà vu), or alterations in thought processes. Alterations in sexual functioning can vary from hyposexuality to hypersexuality. Many patients with temporal lobe seizures have decreased sexual drive or erectile dysfunction. However, some may experience sexual sensations during their seizures. This is because the abnormal electrical activity arises from the brain centers responsible for these sensations. Some experience increased sexual drive just after a seizure. In addition, some antiseizure medications can cause a decrease in sexual drive because of sedation. Others can cause erectile dysfunction.

Complications

Physical. *Status epilepticus* is a state in which seizures recur in rapid succession and the patient does not regain consciousness or normal function between seizures. It is the most serious complication of epilepsy and a neurologic emergency. Status epilepticus can involve any type of seizure. During repeated seizures the brain uses more energy than can be supplied. Neurons become exhausted and cease to function. Permanent brain damage may result. Tonic-clonic status epilepticus is the most dangerous because it can cause ventilatory insufficiency, hypoxemia, cardiac arrhythmias, hyperthermia, and systemic acidosis, all of which can be fatal.

Another complication of epilepsy is severe injury and even death from trauma suffered during a seizure. Patients who lose consciousness during a seizure are at greatest risk. Death can result from head injury incurred in a fall, from drowning in the bathtub, or from severe burns.

Psychosocial. Perhaps the most common complication of epilepsy is the effect it has on a patient's lifestyle. Although attitudes have improved in recent years, epilepsy still carries a social stigma. It used to be associated with supernatural powers, possession by the devil, and insanity. Today the stigma probably exists because the characteristics of seizures are in direct conflict with modern societal values of self-control, conformity, and independence. The patient with epilepsy may experience discrimination in employment and educational opportunities. Transportation may be difficult because of legal sanctions against driving in some states. The patient may develop ineffective methods of coping.

COLLABORATIVE CARE

Table 56-7 Seizures

Diagnostic
Complete history and physical examination
  Birth and development history
  Significant illnesses and injuries
  Family history
  Febrile seizures
  Comprehensive neurologic assessment
Seizure history
  Precipitating factors
  Antecedent events
  Seizure description (including onset, duration, frequency, postictal state)
Diagnostic studies
  CBC, urinalysis, electrolytes, creatinine, fasting blood glucose
  Lumbar puncture
  CT, MRI, PET scan
  Electroencephalography

Collaborative Therapy
Antiseizure medication (see Table 56-9)
Surgery (see Table 56-10)
Vagal nerve stimulation
Psychosocial counseling

PET, positron emission tomography.

Diagnostic Studies

The most useful diagnostic tools are accurate and comprehensive description of the seizures and the patient's health history (Table 56-7). The EEG is a useful diagnostic adjuvant to the history but only if it shows abnormalities. Abnormal findings help determine the type of seizure and help pinpoint the seizure focus. Unfortunately, only a small percentage of patients with epilepsy have abnormal findings on the EEG the first time the test is done. EEGs may need to be repeated often, or continuous EEG monitoring may be needed to detect abnormalities. Abnormal discharges may not occur during the 30 to 40 minutes of sampling during EEG, and the test may never indicate an abnormality. It is not a definitive test. Some patients who do not have epilepsy have abnormal patterns on their EEGs, whereas many patients with epilepsy have normal EEGs.

A complete blood count, serum chemistries, studies of liver and kidney function, and urinalysis should be done to rule out metabolic disorders. A CT or MRI scan should be done in any new-onset seizure to rule out a structural lesion. Cerebral angiography and positron emission tomography (PET) may be used in selected clinical situations.

Collaborative Care

Most seizures do not require professional emergency medical care because they are self-limiting and rarely cause bodily injury. However, if status epilepticus occurs, if significant bodily harm occurs, or if the event is a first-time seizure, medical care should be sought immediately. Table 56-8 summarizes emergency care of the patient with a generalized tonic-clonic seizure, the seizure most likely to warrant professional emergency medical care.

The diagnostic and collaborative care of seizure disorders are summarized in Table 56-7.

Drug Therapy. Epilepsy is treated primarily with antiseizure medication (Table 56-9). Therapy is aimed at preventing seizures, because cure is not possible. Medications generally act by stabilizing nerve cell membranes and preventing spread of the epileptic discharge. In about 70% of the patients epilepsy is controlled by medication. The primary goal of antiseizure drug therapy is to obtain maximum seizure control with a minimum of toxic side effects. The principle of drug therapy is to begin with a single drug and increase the dosage until seizures are controlled or toxic side effects occur. Serum levels of the drug should be monitored regularly. The therapeutic range for each drug indicates the serum level above which most patients experience toxic side effects and below which most continue to have seizures. Therapeutic ranges are only guides for therapy. If the patient's seizures are well controlled with a subtherapeutic level, the drug dose need not be increased. Likewise, if a drug level is above the therapeutic range and the patient has good seizure control without toxic side effects, the drug dose need not be decreased. If seizure control is not achieved with a single drug, a second drug is added.

The primary drugs for treatment of generalized tonic-clonic and partial seizures are phenytoin (Dilantin), carbamazepine (Tegretol), phenobarbital, primidone (Mysoline), and divalproex (Depakote). The primary drugs for treatment of absence, akinetic, and myoclonic seizures are ethosuximide (Zarontin), divalproex (Depakote), and clonazepam (Klonopin).

Four new antiepileptic drugs have recently been approved by the Food and Drug Administration (FDA). Gabapentin (Neurontin), lamotrigine (Lamictal), topiramate (Topamax), and tiagabine (Gabitril) are indicated for partial seizures and for secondary generalized seizures. These drugs are currently used as adjunctive therapy.

Felbamate (Felbatol) may be used to treat patients whose seizure disorders are refractory to other medications. However, its use is limited because it can cause aplastic anemia and liver toxicity.

Table 56-9 summarizes the known interactions of the major antiseizure drugs. Because many of these drugs (e.g., phenytoin, phenobarbital, ethosuximide, lomotrigine, topiramate) have a long half-life, they can be given in once- or twice-daily doses. This increases the patient's compliance with taking medication by simplifying the drug regimen and avoiding the need to take medication at work or school. Antiseizure drugs should not be discontinued abruptly because this can precipitate seizures.

During seizure activity, phenytoin will not immediately stop the seizure. Other agents such as benzodiazepines or phenobarbital may be given during an acute seizure.

Toxic side effects of antiseizure drugs involve the CNS and include diplopia, drowsiness, ataxia, and mental slowing. Neurologic assessment for dose-related toxicity involves testing the eyes for nystagmus, hand and gait coordination, cognitive functioning, and general alertness.

✚ EMERGENCY MANAGEMENT

Table **56-8**   Tonic-Clonic Seizures

Etiology	Assessment Findings	Interventions
Head Trauma Epidural hematoma Subdural hematoma Intracranial hematoma Cerebral contusion Traumatic birth injury **Drug-Related Process** Overdose Withdrawal of alcohol, opioids, antiseizure drugs Ingestion, inhalation **Infectious Processes** Meningitis Septicemia **Intracranial Event** Brain tumor Subarachnoid hemorrhage Stroke Hypertensive crisis Increased ICP secondary to clogged shunt **Metabolic Imbalance** Fluid and electrolyte imbalance Hypoglycemia **Medical Disorders** Heart, liver, lung, or kidney disease Systemic lupus erythematosus **Other** Cardiac arrest Idiopathic Psychiatric disorders High fever	■ Aura—peculiar sensations that precede seizure ■ Loss of consciousness ■ Bowel and bladder incontinence ■ Tachycardia ■ Diaphoresis ■ Warm skin ■ Pallor, flushing, or cyanosis ■ *Tonic phase*—continuous muscle contractions ■ *Hypertonic phase*—extreme muscular rigidity lasting 5 to 15 seconds ■ *Clonic phase*—rigidity and relaxation alternate in rapid succession ■ *Postictal phase*—lethargy, altered level of consciousness ■ Confusion and headache ■ Repeated tonic clonic seizures for several minutes	**Initial** ■ Ensure patent airway. ■ Assist ventilations if patient does not breathe spontaneously after seizure. Anticipate need for intubation if gag reflex absent. ■ Suction as needed. ■ Stay with patient until seizure has passed. ■ Protect patient from injury during seizure. *Do not restrain.* Pad side rails. ■ Establish IV access. ■ Anticipate administration of phenobarbital, phenytoin, or benzodiazepines (Valium, Versed, Ativan) to control seizures. ■ Remove or loosen tight clothing. **Ongoing Monitoring** ■ Monitor vital signs, level of consciousness, oxygen saturation, Glasgow Coma Scale, pupil size and reactivity. ■ Reassure and orient the patient after seizure. ■ Never force an airway between a patient's clenched teeth. ■ Give dextrose for hypoglycemia.

ICP, intracranial pressure.

DRUG THERAPY

Table **56-9**   Antiseizure Drugs

Generalized Tonic-Clonic and Partial Seizures
Phenytoin (Dilantin)
Carbamazepine (Tegretol)
Phenobarbital
Divalproex (Depakote)
Primidone (Mysoline)
Gabapentin (Neurontin)
Lamotrigine (Lamictal)
Topiramate (Topamax)
Tiagabine (Gabitril)

Absence, Akinetic, and Myoclonic Seizures
Ethosuximide (Zarontin)
Divalproex (Depakote)
Clonazepam (Klonopin)
Phenobarbital

Idiosyncratic side effects involve organs outside the CNS, including the skin (rashes), gingiva (hypertrophy), bone marrow (blood dyscrasias), liver, and kidneys. Nurses should be knowledgeable about these side effects so that patients can be informed and proper treatment can be instituted. A common idiosyncratic side effect of phenytoin is hypertrophy of the gingiva, especially in children and young adults. This can be limited by good dental hygiene, including regular toothbrushing and flossing. If gingival hypertrophy is extensive, the hypertrophied tissue may have to be surgically removed (gingivectomy), and phenytoin may have to be replaced by another antiseizure drug. Because phenytoin can also cause hirsutism in young people, other drugs are often used first.

Surgical Therapy. A significant number of patients whose epilepsy cannot be controlled with drug therapy are candidates for surgical intervention (Table 56-10). Surgery may be considered to control intractable seizures, prevent cerebral degeneration from repeated seizures, prevent toxic

Table 56-10 Surgical Procedures for Epilepsy

Type of Seizure	Surgical Procedure	Results
Complex partial seizure of temporal lobe origin	Resectioning of epileptogenic tissue	Absence of seizures 5 yr postoperatively in 55-70% of patients
Partial seizures of frontal lobe origin	Resectioning of epileptogenic tissue (if in resectable area)	Absence of seizures 5 yr postoperatively in 30-50% of patients
Generalized seizures (Lennox-Gastaut syndrome or drop attacks)	Sectioning of corpus callosum	Persistence of seizures, less violent, less frequent, less disabling events
Intractable unilateral multifocal epilepsy associated with infantile hemiplegia	Hemispherectomy or callosotomy	Reduction in seizure frequency and type, improvement in behavior

syndromes from long-term use of antiseizure drugs, and improve the quality of life.[8]

Not all types of epilepsy benefit from surgery. The benefits of surgery include cessation or reduction in frequency of the seizures. An extensive preoperative evaluation is important, including continuous EEG monitoring and other specific tests to ensure precise localization of the focal point. Before surgery is performed, three requirements must be met: (1) the diagnosis of epilepsy must be confirmed; (2) there must have been an adequate trial with drug therapy without satisfactory results; and (3) the electroclinical syndrome (type of seizure disorder) must be defined.[8]

Alternative Therapies. Biofeedback to control seizures is aimed at teaching the patient to maintain a certain brain-wave frequency that is refractory to seizure activity. This method is still in the experimental stage. Vagal nerve stimulation is a method of controlling or reducing seizures in poorly controlled patients by placement of electrodes around the left vagus nerve in the neck. An external generator is programmed to deliver intermittent electrical stimulation to the nerve. The exact mechanism of action is unknown, although the stimulation may interrupt synchronization of epileptic brain-wave activity. This method is currently used in only a small number of patients.

NURSING MANAGEMENT: SEIZURES

■ Nursing Assessment

Subjective and objective data that should be obtained from a patient with a seizure disorder are presented in Table 56-11. Data related to a specific seizure episode can be obtained from a witness.

■ Nursing Diagnoses

Nursing diagnoses for the patient with seizures may include, but are not limited to, those presented in NCP 56-2.

■ Planning

The overall goals are that the patient with seizures will (1) be free from injury during a seizure, (2) have optimal mental and physical functioning while taking antiseizure medication, and (3) have satisfactory psychosocial functioning.

■ Nursing Implementation

Health Promotion. Many cases of seizures can be prevented by promotion of general safety measures, such as the wearing of helmets in situations involving risk of head injury. Improved perinatal, labor, and delivery care have reduced fetal trauma and hypoxia and thereby have reduced brain damage leading to epilepsy. Children with fever should be treated quickly to avoid high temperatures, which may cause seizures.

The patient with epilepsy should practice good general health habits (e.g., maintaining a proper diet, getting adequate rest, and exercising). The patient should be helped to identify events or situations that precipitate the seizures and should be given suggestions for avoiding them or handling them better. Excessive alcohol intake, fatigue, and loss of sleep should be avoided, and the patient should be helped to handle stress constructively.

Acute Intervention. The nurse caring for a hospitalized patient with epilepsy or a patient who has had seizures as a result of metabolic factors has several responsibilities, including observation and treatment of the seizure, education, and psychosocial intervention.

When a seizure occurs, the nurse should carefully observe and record details of the event because the diagnosis and subsequent treatment often rest solely on the seizure description. All aspects of the seizure should be noted. What events preceded the seizure? When did the seizure occur? How long did each phase (aural [if any], ictal, postictal) last? What occurred during each phase?

Both subjective data (usually the only type of data in the aural phase) and objective data are important. Objective data should include the exact onset of the seizure (which body part was affected first and how), the course and nature of the seizure activity (loss of consciousness, tongue biting, automatisms, stiffening, jerking, total lack of muscle tone), the body parts involved and their sequence of involvement, and the presence of autonomic signs such as dilated pupils, excessive salivation, altered breathing, cyanosis, flushing, diaphoresis, or incontinence. Assessment of the postictal period should include a detailed description of the level of consciousness, vital signs, memory loss, muscle soreness, speech disorders (aphasia, dysarthria), weakness or paralysis, sleep period, and the duration of each sign or symptom.

During the seizure it is important to maintain a patent airway. This may involve supporting and protecting the head, turning the

NURSING ASSESSMENT

Table 56-11 Seizures

Subjective Data

Important Health Information

Past health history: Previous seizures, birth defects or injuries, anoxic episodes, CNS trauma, tumors, or infections; hypertension, cerebrovascular disease; metabolic disorders, alcoholism; exposure to metals and carbon monoxide; hepatic or renal failure; fever; pregnancy, systemic lupus erythematosus

Medications: Compliance with antiseizure medications; barbiturate or alcohol withdrawal; use and overdose of cocaine, amphetamines, lidocaine, theophylline, penicillin, lithium, phenothiazines, tricyclic antidepressants, benzodiazepines

Functional Health Patterns

Health perception–health management: Positive family history

Cognitive-perceptual: Headaches, aura, mood or behavioral changes before seizure; mentation changes; abdominal pain, muscle pain (postictal)

Self-perception–self-concept: Anxiety, depression; loss of self-esteem, social isolation

Sexuality-reproductive: Decreased sex drive, erectile dysfunction; increased sexual drive (postictal)

Objective Data

General

Precipitating factors, including severe metabolic acidosis or alkalosis, hyperkalemia, hypoglycemia, dehydration, or water intoxication

Integumentary

Bitten tongue, soft-tissue damage, cyanosis, diaphoresis (postictal)

Respiratory

Abnormal respiratory rate, rhythm, or depth; apnea (ictal); absent or abnormal breath sounds, possible airway occlusion

Cardiovascular

Hypertension, tachycardia or bradycardia (ictal)

Gastrointestinal

Bowel incontinence; excessive salivation

Urinary

Incontinence

Neurologic

Generalized

Tonic-clonic: loss of consciousness, muscle tightening then jerking, dilated pupils, hyperventilation, then apnea; postictal somnolence

Absence: altered consciousness (5-30 seconds), minor facial motor activity

Partial

Simple: aura, consciousness, focal sensory, motor, cognitive, or emotional phenomena (focal motor); unilateral "marching" motor seizure (jacksonian)

Complex: altered consciousness with inappropriate behaviors, automatisms, amnesia of event

Musculoskeletal

Weakness, paralysis, ataxia (postictal)

Possible Findings

Positive toxicology screen or alcohol level; altered serum electrolytes, acidosis or alkalosis, very low blood glucose level, elevated blood urea nitrogen or serum creatinine, liver function tests, ammonia; abnormal CT scan or MRI of head, lumbar puncture; epileptiform discharges on EEG

EEG, electroencephalogram.

patient to the side, loosening constrictive clothing, or easing the patient to the floor, if seated. The patient should not be restrained and no objects should be placed in the mouth. After the seizure the patient may require suctioning and oxygen may be needed.

A seizure can be a frightening experience for the patient and for others who may witness it. The nurse should assess the level of their understanding and provide information about how and why the event occurred. This is an excellent opportunity for the nurse to dispel many common misconceptions about seizures.

Ambulatory and Home Care. Prevention of recurring seizures is the major goal in the treatment of epilepsy. Because epilepsy cannot be cured, medication must be taken regularly and continuously, often for a lifetime. The nurse should ensure that the patient knows this, as well as the specifics of the medication regimen and what to do if a dose is missed. Usually the dose should be made up if the omission is remembered within 24 hours. The patient should be cautioned not to adjust medications without professional guidance because this can increase seizure frequency and even cause status epilepticus. The patient should be encouraged to report any medication side effects and to keep regular appointments with the health care provider.

Nurses play an important role in educating the patient and the patient's family. Guidelines for patient teaching are shown in Table 56-12. Nurses should teach family members and significant others the emergency management of tonic-clonic

seizures (see Table 56-8). They should be reminded that it is not necessary to call an ambulance or send a person to the hospital after a single seizure unless the seizure is prolonged, another seizure immediately follows, or extensive injury has occurred.

Patients with epilepsy also experience concerns or fears related to recurrent seizures, incontinence, or loss of self-control. The nurse provides support for the patient through education and by helping to identify coping mechanisms.

Perhaps the greatest challenge that epilepsy presents to the patient is adjusting to the personal limitations imposed by the illness. Discrimination in employment is the most serious problem facing the person with epilepsy. Patients can be informed that the Rehabilitation Act of 1973 was designed to protect handicapped persons (including those with epilepsy) from discrimination in employment. For issues relating to job discrimination, patients can be referred to the State Human Rights Commission or the State Department of Vocational Rehabilitation.

A variety of other resources can be offered to the patient with epilepsy who has a specific problem. If the nurse believes that associating with others who have epilepsy would be beneficial, the patient can be referred to the local chapter of the Epilepsy Foundation (EF), a voluntary agency that offers a variety of services to patients with epilepsy. The patient who is an eligible veteran can be referred to a Department of Veterans Affairs medical center that provides comprehensive care.

56-2 NURSING CARE PLAN   PATIENT WITH SEIZURES

Expected Patient Outcomes	Nursing Interventions and *Rationales*

NURSING DIAGNOSIS **Ineffective breathing pattern** *related to* neuromuscular impairment secondary to prolonged tonic phase of seizure or during postictal period *as manifested by* abnormal respiratory rate, rhythm, or depth.

- Appropriate rate, rhythm, and depth of respirations.

- Loosen constricting clothing *to avoid restricting breathing.*
- Assess breathing pattern, observing for labored respiration, tachypnea, bradypnea, dyspnea, apnea, and cyanosis *to determine if problem is present and extent of problem and to initiate appropriate interventions.*
- Provide manual ventilation or oxygen when necessary; be prepared to assist with endotracheal intubation *to maintain adequate oxygenation and prevent hypoxia.*
- Insert oral airway (if indicated) only after seizure activity has ceased *to prevent mouth and teeth injury from forcing airway between clamped teeth.*

NURSING DIAGNOSIS **Ineffective airway clearance** *related to* tracheobronchial obstruction *as manifested by* ineffective cough, inability to remove secretions, absence of or abnormal breath sounds.

- No airway obstruction.
- Clear breath sounds.

- Observe for signs of airway obstruction *to determine extent of problem and to plan appropriate interventions.*
- If vomiting occurs, turn patient's head gently to side and remove as much vomitus as possible after the seizure *to prevent aspiration of vomitus and subsequent interference with breathing.*
- Suction airway if necessary *to remove accumulated secretions.*
- Establish and maintain patent airway *to ensure adequate oxygenation.*

NURSING DIAGNOSIS **Risk for injury** *related to* seizure activity and subsequent impaired physical mobility secondary to postictal weakness or paralysis.

- No injury.
- Verbalization of knowledge of potential for injury during seizure.
- Arrangement of environment to minimize risk for injury.

- Assess for trauma to mouth, cheek, tongue, lips; abrasions, bruises; broken bones; burns *because these injuries may occur during seizure activity.*
- Assess for weakness, paralysis of one side of body, ataxia, fatigue, lethargy *as potential postictal risks for injury to plan appropriate interventions.*
- Do not permit smoking in bed *to prevent the patient from being burned by a bed fire if a seizure occurs.*
- If patient anticipates a seizure may occur, assist to a safe location or position; use seizure precautions as appropriate; remove potentially harmful objects from surrounding area; gently guide arm or leg movements *to prevent injury during a seizure.*
- Refrain from moving or restraining patient during a seizure *to prevent bone or soft-tissue injury.*
- Assist in determining whether operation of a motor vehicle or dangerous machinery is appropriate for patient *to assist patient in making the appropriate choice about driving.*

NURSING DIAGNOSIS **Ineffective individual coping** *related to* perceived loss of control and denial of diagnosis *as manifested by* verbalizations about not having epilepsy, lack of truth-telling regarding seizure frequency, noncompliant behavior.

- Acceptance of disorder as evidenced by using word *epilepsy* to describe illness.
- Acknowledgment that a seizure has occurred.

- Explore reasons for denial *to determine extent of problem and to plan appropriate interventions.*
- Implement and individualize teaching plan about causes and mechanisms of seizures, effectiveness of drugs in controlling seizures, inaccuracy of myths about epilepsy, avoidance of precipitating factors, state law regarding driving, pros and cons of medical ID tags, moderation in drinking and eating, exposure to stress, and avoidance of hazardous activities *to promote effective coping by providing facts.*

Continued

56-2 **NURSING CARE PLAN** **PATIENT WITH SEIZURES**—continued

Expected Patient Outcomes   **Nursing Interventions and *Rationales***

NURSING DIAGNOSIS **Self-esteem disturbance** *related to* diagnosis of epilepsy *as manifested by* anxiety, fear, social isolation, depression, role disturbance, altered family dynamics.

- Sharing of feelings about diagnosis.
- Identification of positive aspects about self.
- Appropriate interactions with others.

- Discuss patient's views about self in relation to seizures *to clarify effect of disease on self-concept.*
- Determine effect of seizures on daily activities and other activities important to patient *because major interference will likely affect self-concept.*
- Provide information about possible overprotection, community resources, and social stigmas that may be encountered *to improve self-concept by increasing sense of control.*
- Assist patient with explaining seizures and management to friends, school personnel, and employers *so these people can provide support and acceptance.*
- Advise patient about employment counseling and job retraining *because gainful employment usually improves self-concept.*

NURSING DIAGNOSIS **Ineffective management of therapeutic regimen** *related to* lack of knowledge about management of epilepsy *as manifested by* verbalization of lack of knowledge, inaccurate perception of health status, noncompliance with prescribed health behavior.

- Optimal seizure control.
- Therapeutic drug levels of antiseizure medication.
- Compliance with therapeutic regimen.

- Provide education to patient and family about seizure activity and therapeutic management including diagnosis, treatment, lifestyle adjustments, and community resources *so patient and family can make necessary lifestyle modifications to manage a chronic disease.*

PATIENT & FAMILY TEACHING GUIDE

Table 56-12 Seizures

The patient with a seizure disorder should be taught the following:

1. Medications must be taken as prescribed. Any and all side effects of medications should be reported to the health care provider. When necessary, blood drawings are done to ensure that therapeutic levels are maintained.
2. Use of nondrug techniques, such as relaxation therapy and biofeedback training to potentially reduce the number of seizures.
3. Availability of resources in the community.
4. Need to wear a Medic Alert bracelet, necklace, and identification card.
5. Avoidance of excessive alcohol intake, fatigue, and loss of sleep.
6. Regular meals and snack in between if feeling shaky, faint, or hungry.

Family members should be taught the following:

1. First aid treatment of tonic-clonic seizure. It is not necessary to call ambulance or send the patient to the hospital after a single seizure unless the seizure is prolonged, another seizure immediately follows, or extensive injury has occurred.
2. During an acute seizure, it is important to protect the patient from injury. This may involve supporting and protecting the head, turning the patient to the side, loosening constrictive clothing, and easing the patient to the floor, if seated.

The patient should be informed that medical alert bracelets, necklaces, and identification cards are available through the EF, local pharmacies, or companies specializing in identification devices (e.g., Medic Alert). However, the use of these medical identification tags is optional. Some patients have found them beneficial, but others have found them to be more a burden than a help because they prefer not to be identified as having epilepsy.

Social workers and welfare agencies can help with financial problems and living arrangements. State services for individuals with developmental disabilities include assistance with job training and placement for patients whose seizures are not well controlled. Sheltered housing and funding for special needs, such as medical and psychologic evaluation and transportation, are also offered. State agencies specializing in vocational rehabilitation services can offer vocational assessment, counseling, funding for training, and assistance with job placement. They can also offer financial assistance for transportation and medical costs that are necessary for vocational rehabilitation or job maintenance. If intensive psychologic counseling is needed, the nurse can refer the patient to a community mental health center.

The patient should be encouraged to learn more about epilepsy through self-education materials. The EF provides several information pamphlets and may facilitate support groups. Many agencies that offer services to epileptic patients, as well as local chapters of EF, have these available as teaching aids.

■ Evaluation

Expected outcomes for the patient with seizures are addressed in NCP 56-2.

MULTIPLE SCLEROSIS

Multiple sclerosis (MS) is a chronic, progressive, degenerative disorder of the CNS. It is not known exactly how many people have MS. Currently it is thought that there are approximately 250,000 to 350,000 people in the United States with MS diagnosed by a physician. Approximately 200 new cases are diagnosed each week. MS is five times more prevalent in temperate climates (between 45 and 65 degrees of latitude), such as those found in the northern United States, Canada, and Europe as compared with tropical regions. Age 15 seems to be critical in terms of risk for developing the disease. For example, if a person moves from a high-risk (temperate) to a low-risk (tropical) area before the age of 15, she or he will adopt the risk (in this case, low) of the new area and vice versa.[9] MS is considered a disease of young adults, with the onset usually being between 15 and 50 years of age. Women are affected more often than men.

MS primarily affects Caucasians of northern European descent, which means that the disease is associated with certain environmental and familial factors. African-Americans and Asians have a lower incidence of MS than do Caucasians.

Etiology and Pathophysiology

The cause of MS is unknown, although research findings suggest MS is related to infectious (viral), immunologic, and genetic factors and is perpetuated as a result of intrinsic factors (e.g., faulty immunoregulation). The susceptibility to MS appears to be inherited. First-, second-, and third-degree relatives of patients with MS are at a slightly increased risk. Multiple unlinked genes confer susceptibility to MS.

The role of precipitating factors such as exposure to pathogenetic agents in the etiology of MS is controversial. It is possible that their association with MS is random and that there is no cause-and-effect relationship. Possible precipitating factors include infection, physical injury, emotional stress, excessive fatigue, pregnancy, and a poorer state of health.

MS is characterized by chronic inflammation, demyelination, and gliosis (scarring) in the CNS. The primary neuropathologic condition is an immune-mediated inflammatory demyelinating process that some believe may be triggered by a virus in genetically susceptible individuals. Activated T cells responding to environmental triggers (e.g., infection) enter the CNS in increased numbers. These T cells, in conjunction with astrocytes, disrupt the blood-brain barrier, thereby promoting the entry of other immune mediators into the CNS. These factors, in combination, damage oligodendrocytes (cells that make myelin), resulting in demyelination. Macrophages are recruited and cause further cell damage.[10] The disease process consists of loss of myelin, disappearance of oligodendrocytes, and proliferation of astrocytes. These changes result in characteristic plaque formation, or sclerosis, with plaques scattered throughout multiple regions of the CNS.

Initially the myelin sheaths of the neurons in the brain and spinal cord are attacked (Fig. 56-1, *A* and *B*). Early in the disease the myelin sheath is damaged, but the nerve fiber is not affected and nerve impulses are still transmitted (Fig. 56-1, *C*). At this point the patient may complain of a noticeable impairment of function (e.g., weakness). However, the myelin can regenerate and the symptoms disappear, resulting in a remission.

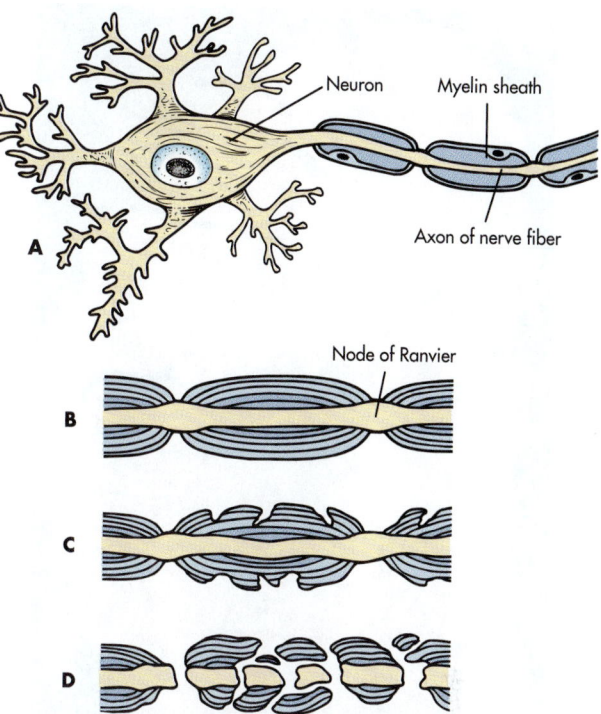

Fig. 56-1 Pathogenesis of multiple sclerosis. **A,** Normal nerve cell with myelin sheath. **B,** Normal axon. **C,** Myelin breakdown. **D,** Myelin totally disrupted; axon not functioning.

As the disease progresses, the myelin is totally disrupted, and the axon becomes involved (Fig. 56-1, *D*). Myelin is replaced by glial scar tissue, which forms hard, sclerotic plaques in multiple regions of the CNS (Fig. 56-2). Without myelin, nerve impulses slow down, and with destruction of nerve axons, impulses are totally blocked, resulting in permanent loss of function. In many chronic lesions, demyelination continues with progressive loss of nerve function.

Clinical Manifestations

Because the onset is often insidious and gradual, with vague symptoms that occur intermittently over months or years, the disease may not be diagnosed until long after the onset of the first symptom. The disease process has a spotty distribution in the CNS, so the signs and symptoms vary over time. The disease is characterized by chronic, progressive deterioration in some persons and by remissions and exacerbations in others. With repeated exacerbations, however, progressive scarring of the myelin sheath occurs, and the overall trend is progressive deterioration in neurologic function.

The clinical manifestations vary according to the areas of the CNS involved. Some patients have severe, long-lasting symptoms early in the course of the disease. Others may experience only occasional and mild symptoms for several years after onset. A classification scheme that identifies the various courses of MS has been developed.[10] *Relapsing-remitting MS* is characterized by clearly defined relapses with full recovery or with sequelae and residual deficit on recovery. *Primary-progressive MS* is characterized by disease progression from onset with occasional plateaus and temporary minor improvements. *Secondary-progressive MS* is characterized by a

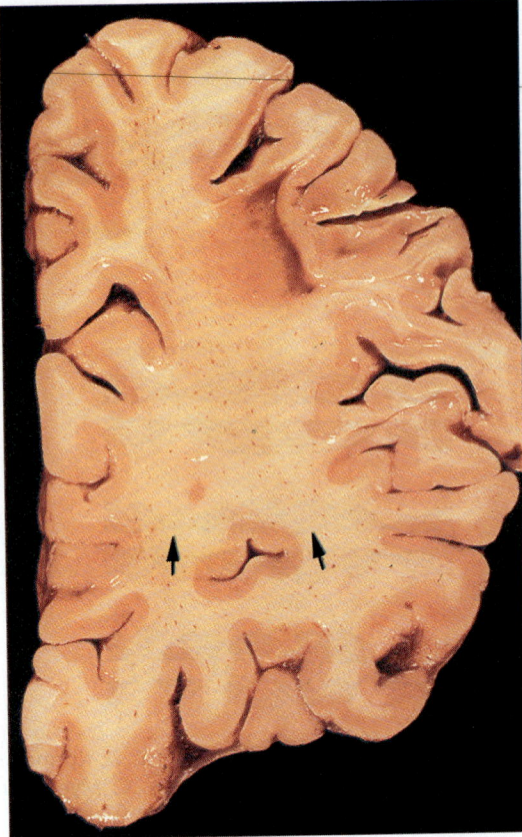

Fig. 56-2 Chronic multiple sclerosis. Demyelination plaque at gray-white junction and adjacent partially remyelinated shadow plaque *(arrow)*.

COLLABORATIVE CARE
Table **56-13** | Multiple Sclerosis

Diagnostic
History and physical examination
CSF analysis
Evoked response testing (also called evoked potential testing, e.g., SSEP—somatosensory evoked potential; AEP—auditory evoked potential; VEP—visual evoked potential)
CT scan
MRI

Collaborative Therapy
Drug Therapy*
Antiinflammatory
Immunosuppressants
Anticholinergics
Cholinergics
Muscle relaxants
Immunomodulators

Surgical Therapy
Thalamotomy (unmanageable tremor)
Neurectomy, rhizotomy, cordotomy (unmanageable spasticity)

*See Table 56-14.

relapsing-remitting initial course, followed by progression with or without occasional relapses, minor remissions, and plateaus. *Progressive-relapsing MS* is characterized by progressive disease from onset, with clear acute relapses, with or without full recovery; periods between relapses are characterized by continuing progression.

Common signs and symptoms of MS include motor, sensory, cerebellar, and emotional problems. Motor symptoms include weakness or paralysis of the limbs, trunk, or head, diplopia, scanning speech, and spasticity of the muscles that are chronically affected. Sensory symptoms include numbness and tingling and other paresthesias, patchy blindness (scotomas), blurred vision, vertigo, tinnitus, and decreased hearing. Cerebellar signs include nystagmus, ataxia, dysarthria, and dysphagia.

Bowel and bladder function can be affected if the sclerotic plaque is located in areas of the CNS that control elimination. Problems with defecation usually involve constipation rather than fecal incontinence. Urinary problems are variable. A common problem in MS patients is a spastic (uninhibited) bladder. This indicates a lesion above the second sacral nerve, which cuts off suprasegmental inhibiting influences on bladder contractility. As a result, the bladder has a small capacity for urine, and its contractions are unchecked. This is accompanied by urinary urgency and frequency and results in dribbling or incontinence. A flaccid (hypotonic) bladder indicates a lesion in the reflex arc governing bladder function. The bladder has a large capacity for urine because there is no sensation or desire to void,

no pressure, and no pain. Generally, there is urinary retention, but urgency and frequency may also occur with this type of lesion. Urinary problems cannot be adequately diagnosed and treated unless urodynamic studies are done.

Sexual dysfunction occurs in many persons with MS. Physiologic erectile dysfunction may result from spinal cord involvement in men. Women may experience decreased libido, difficulty with orgasmic response, painful intercourse, and decreased vaginal lubrication. Diminished sensation can prevent a normal sexual response in both sexes. The emotional effects of chronic illness and the loss of self-esteem also contribute to loss of sexual response.

MS has no apparent effect on the course of pregnancy, labor, delivery, or lactation. Some women with MS who become pregnant experience remission or an improvement in their symptoms during the gestation period. The hormonal changes associated with pregnancy appear to affect the immune system. However, during the postpartum period women are at greater risk for exacerbation of the disease.[11]

Although intellectual functioning generally remains intact, emotional stability may be affected. Persons may experience anger, depression, or euphoria. Signs and symptoms of MS are aggravated or triggered by physical and emotional trauma, fatigue, and infection.

The average life expectancy after the onset of symptoms is more than 25 years. Death usually occurs because of infective complications (e.g., pneumonia) of immobility or because of unrelated disease; occasionally, suicide is a cause.

Diagnostic Studies

Because there is no definitive diagnostic test for MS, diagnosis is based primarily on history and clinical manifestations (Table 56-13). Certain laboratory tests are currently used as adjuncts

DRUG THERAPY

Table 56-14 Multiple Sclerosis

Drug	Symptoms Relieved	Precautions	Side Effects	Educational Needs
Corticosteroids ACTH Prednisone Methylprednisolone	Exacerbations	Widespread effects on many enzymes and metabolic processes, few adverse effects with use for <1 mo at a time	Edema, mental changes (euphoria), weight gain, redistribution of body fat*	Restrict salt intake. Do not abruptly stop therapy. Know drug interactions.
Immunomodulators Beta-interferon (Betaseron) (Avonex)	Exacerbations	Monitor CBC, blood chemistries, and liver function tests every 3 mo	Flulike symptoms, local skin reactions, depression	Learn self-injection techniques, report side effects.
Glatiramer acetate (Copaxone)	Exacerbations	No laboratory monitoring required	Local skin reactions; chest pain; weakness	Learn self-injection techniques; report side effects.
Cholinergics Bethanecol (Urecholine) Neostigmine (Prostigmine)	Urinary retention (flaccid bladder)	History of hypotension, cardiac dysfunction, allergies, hyperthyroidism, stomach and intestinal problems; contraindication with adrenergic drugs (antiasthmatic drugs) because of possible induction of serious asthma attack (Urecholine only)	Hypotension, diarrhea, diaphoresis, salivation, muscle weakness	Consult physician before using other drugs.
Anticholinergics Propantheline (Pro-Banthine) Oxybutynin (Ditropan)	Urinary frequency† and urgency (spastic bladder)	History of glaucoma, prostatic hypertrophy, cardiac dysfunction, intestinal obstruction	Dry mouth, blurred vision, constipation, hypertension, flushing, urinary retention (too high of dose)	Consult physician before using other drugs, especially sleeping aids, antihistamines (possibly leading to potentiated effect).
Muscle Relaxants Diazepam (Valium)	Spasticity	History of narrow-angle glaucoma	Drowsiness, ataxia, fatigue	Avoid driving and similar activities because of CNS-depressant effects. Be aware of addictive potential; avoid long-term use. Avoid concomitant use of phenothiazines, narcotics, barbiturates, MAO inhibitors, other antidepressants.
Baclofen (Lioresal)	Spasticity	History of hypersensitivity and renal damage, contraindication in pregnancy, possible exacerbation of seizures in patients with epilepsy	Drowsiness, weakness	Do not abruptly stop therapy (possibly leading to hallucinations). Avoid driving and similar activities because of sedative effect. Avoid use with other CNS depressants; take with food or milk.

Continued

DRUG THERAPY

Table 56-14   Multiple Sclerosis—cont'd

Drug	Symptoms Relieved	Precautions	Side Effects	Educational Needs
Dantrolene (Dantrium)	Spasticity	History of respiratory or cardiac dysfunction, possible induction of abnormal liver function or hepatitis, contraindication with estrogen therapy because of predisposition of hepatotoxicity	Drowsiness, dizziness, malaise, fatigue, diarrhea	Avoid driving. Avoid use with tranquilizers and alcohol (possibly causing photosensitivity).
Tizanidine (Zanaflex)	Spasticity	History of hypersensitivity, possible liver injury, hypotension, bradycardia	Drowsiness, dry mouth, tiredness	Use with caution in women on oral contraceptives

*See Chapter 47 for effects of long-term corticosteroid therapy.
†Urodynamic studies must be done before institution of therapy because patients with MS have multiple lesions and type of bladder dysfunction cannot be diagnosed from symptoms alone.
ACTH, adrenocorticotropic hormone; *CBC,* complete blood count; *MAO,* monoamine oxidase.

to the clinical examination. In some patients, cerebrospinal fluid (CSF) analysis may show an increase in oligoclonal immunoglobulin G (IgG). The CSF also contains a high number of lymphocytes and monocytes. Evoked responses are often delayed in persons with MS because of decreased nerve conduction from the eye and the ear to the brain. MRI scan may be helpful, because sclerotic plaques as small as 3 to 4 mm in diameter can be detected. Characteristic white-matter lesions scattered through the brain or spinal cord are evident on such a scan.

Collaborative Care

Drug Therapy. Because there is no cure for MS, collaborative care is aimed at treating the disease process and providing symptomatic relief (see Table 56-13). The disease process is treated with drugs, and the symptoms are controlled with a variety of medications and other forms of therapy. Adrenocorticotropic hormone (ACTH), methylprednisolone, and prednisone are helpful in treating acute exacerbations of the disease, probably by reducing edema and acute inflammation at the site of demyelination. However, these medications do not affect the ultimate outcome or degree of residual neurologic impairment from the exacerbation. Immunosuppressive drugs, such as azathioprine (Imuran), cyclosporine (Sandimmune), and cyclophosphamide (Cytoxan), have been shown to produce some beneficial effects in patients with severe and relapsing MS. However, the potential benefits of these drugs in patients with MS must be counterbalanced against the potentially serious side effects. Table 56-14 summarizes the drugs that are commonly used for symptomatic treatment of MS.

Interferon β-1b (Betaseron) was the first drug aimed at controlling the disease rather than the symptoms. It was approved by the FDA in 1993 for ambulatory patients with exacerbating and remitting MS. Clinical trials with subcutaneous injections every other day have shown that the drug decreases the number of relapses and the number of new lesions seen on an MRI scan.[12] Since then two more drugs have become available for controlling the disease. Interferon β-1a (Avonex) is similar to interferon β-1b in efficacy. It is given intramuscularly once a week. Glatiramer acetate (Copaxone), formerly known as copolymer-1, is unrelated to interferon, but likewise reduces the number of relapses in MS. It is given subcutaneously every day.

Surgical Therapy. Spasticity is primarily treated with muscle relaxants (antispasmodic drugs). However, surgery (e.g., neurectomy, rhizotomy, cordotomy) or dorsal-column electrical stimulation may be required. Intention tremor that becomes unmanageable with medication is sometimes treated by stereotactic surgery on the thalamus. This involves selective destruction of the ventrolateral nucleus in the thalamus.

Other Therapies. Neurologic dysfunction sometimes improves with physical therapy, speech therapy, and hypothermia, which normalizes body temperature if it is above normal. Physical therapy is important in keeping the patient as functionally active as possible. The purpose of therapy is to relieve spasticity, increase coordination, and train the patient to substitute unaffected muscles for impaired ones. An especially beneficial type of physical therapy is water exercise (Fig. 56-3). Water gives buoyancy to the body and allows the patient to perform activities that would normally be impossible. In water, a patient experiences more control over the body.

Nutritional Therapy. Various nutritional measures that have been advocated in the management of MS include megavitamin therapy (cobalamin [vitamin B_{12}], vitamin C) and diets consisting of low-fat and gluten-free food and raw vegetables. These particular dietary measures have not come into widespread use because of lack of proof of their effectiveness.

A nutritious, well-balanced diet is essential. Although there is no standard prescribed diet, a high-protein diet with supplementary vitamins is often advocated. A diet high in roughage may help relieve the problem of constipation. Vitamins are merely supplemental and not curative.

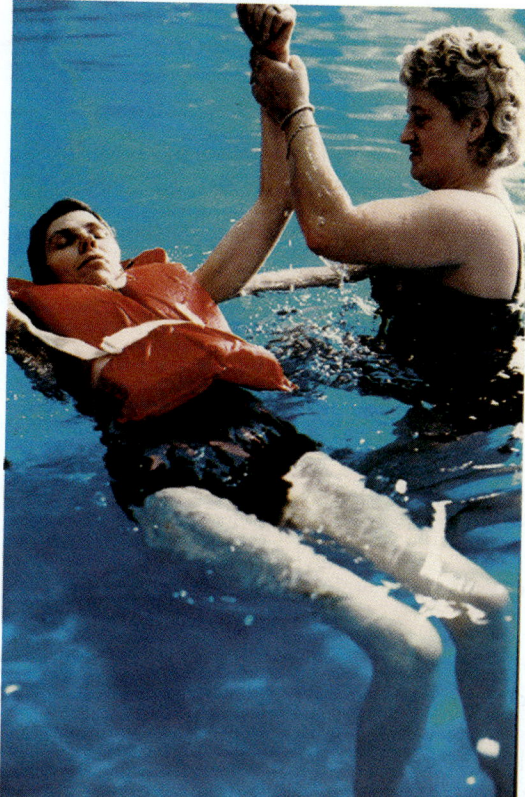

Fig. 56-3 Water therapy provides exercise and recreation for the patient with a chronic neurologic disease.

NURSING MANAGEMENT: MULTIPLE SCLEROSIS

■ Nursing Assessment

Subjective and objective data that should be obtained from a person with MS are presented in Table 56-15.

■ Nursing Diagnoses

Nursing diagnoses for the patient with MS may include, but are not limited to, those presented in NCP 56-3.

■ Planning

The overall goals are that the patient with MS will (1) maximize neuromuscular function, (2) maintain independence in activities of daily living for as long as possible, (3) optimize psychosocial well-being, (4) adjust to the illness, and (5) reduce factors that precipitate exacerbations.

■ Nursing Implementation

The patient with MS should be aware of triggers that may cause exacerbations or worsening of the disease. Exacerbations of MS are triggered by exogenous events, including infection (especially upper respiratory infections), trauma, immunization, delivery after pregnancy, stress, and change in climate. Of these the best documented are upper respiratory infections, delivery, and head trauma.[13] Each person responds differently to these triggers. The nurse should help the patient identify particular triggers and develop ways to avoid them or minimize their effects.

NURSING ASSESSMENT

Table 56-15   **Multiple Sclerosis**

Subjective Data

Important Health Information

Past health history: Recent or past viral infections or vaccinations, other recent infections, residence in cold or temperate climates, recent physical or emotional stress, pregnancy, exposure to extremes of heat and cold

Medications: Use of and compliance in taking corticosteroids, immunosuppressants, anticholinergics, antispasmodics

Functional Health Patterns

Health perception–health management: Positive family history; malaise

Nutritional-metabolic: Weight loss; difficulty in chewing, dysphagia

Elimination: Urinary frequency, urgency, dribbling or incontinence, retention; constipation

Activity-exercise: Generalized muscle weakness, muscle fatigue; tingling and numbness, ataxia (clumsiness)

Cognitive-perceptual: Eye, back, leg, joint pain; painful muscle spasms; vertigo; blurred or lost vision; diplopia; tinnitus

Sexuality-reproductive: Impotence, decreased libido

Coping–stress tolerance: Anger, depression, euphoria, social isolation

Objective Data

General

Apathy, inattentiveness

Integumentary

Pressure ulcers

Neurologic

Scanning speech, nystagmus, ataxia, tremor, spasticity, hyperreflexia, decreased hearing

Musculoskeletal

Muscular weakness, paresis, paralysis, spasms, foot dragging, dysarthria

Possible Findings

Reduction in T-suppressor cells, demyelinating lesions on MRI scans, increased IgG or oligoclonal banding in cerebrospinal fluid

---

The most common reasons for hospitalization of the patient with MS are for a diagnostic workup and treatment of an acute exacerbation. During the diagnostic phase the patient needs reassurance that even though there is a tentative diagnosis of MS, certain diagnostic studies must be done to rule out other neurologic disorders. The nurse should assist the patient in dealing with the anxiety caused by a diagnosis of a disabling illness. The patient with recently diagnosed MS may need assistance with the grieving process.

During an acute exacerbation the patient may be immobile and confined to bed for 2 to 3 weeks. The focus of nursing intervention at this phase is to prevent major complications of immobility, such as respiratory and urinary tract infections and pressure ulcers.

56-3 NURSING CARE PLAN PATIENT WITH MULTIPLE SCLEROSIS

Expected Patient Outcomes — **Nursing Interventions and *Rationales***

NURSING DIAGNOSIS **Impaired physical mobility** *related to* muscle weakness or paralysis and muscle spasticity *as manifested by* inability to ambulate, intermittent muscle spasms, pain associated with muscle spasms.

- Demonstration of use of adaptive devices.
- Maintenance of or increased strength of limbs.
- Decreased duration of muscle spasms.

- Use assistive devices as indicated *to decrease fatigue and to enhance independence, comfort, and safety.*
- Do active range-of-motion exercises at least twice per day *to prevent contractures and minimize muscle atrophy.*
- Encourage and assist with ambulation and transfer as indicated *to maintain mobility, promote independence, and provide for safety.*
- Change position of patient (if bedridden) at least q2hr *to prevent pressure ulcers and circulatory problems.*
- Administer medication as ordered *to reduce spasticity or to treat inflammatory response.*
- Perform stretching exercises every 6-8 hr *to relieve spasms and contracted muscles.*

NURSING DIAGNOSIS **Self-care deficits** *related to* muscle spasticity and neuromuscular deficits *as manifested by* inability to perform some or all activities of daily living.

- Maximum level of functioning.
- Activities of daily living needs met by self or others.

- Assess self-care problems *to plan appropriate interventions to meet care needs.*
- Promote use of appropriate assistive devices *so patient can maximally participate in self-care activities with minimum fatigue.*
- Counsel regarding need for homemaker services *to assist in meeting patient's needs, conserving energy, and promoting independence.*
- Perform or assist with activities of daily living only as indicated *to promote patient's independence.*
- Encourage independence when appropriate *to promote patient's sense of autonomy and control.*

NURSING DIAGNOSIS **Risk for impaired skin integrity** *related to* immobility, sensorimotor deficits, and inadequate nutrition.

- Intact skin.

- Assess skin for redness and irritation *to monitor changes in skin integrity and make appropriate plan for interventions.*
- Turn patient at least q2hr *to prevent pressure ulcers from developing.*
- Use circular massage of unreddened bony prominences with each turning *to improve circulation to these areas.*
- Provide high-protein diet *to promote healthy skin resistant to breakdown.*
- Cleanse back and buttocks if patient is incontinent *to prevent skin irritation and skin breakdown.*

NURSING DIAGNOSIS **Sensory-perceptual alterations** *related to* visual disturbances *as manifested by* blurred vision, decreased visual acuity, visual field defects, diplopia.

- Satisfactory visual function for activities of daily living.

- Orient patient to environment *to promote safety and to compensate for visual disturbances.*
- Patch alternate eyes *to alleviate diplopia.*
- Assess visual acuity monthly *to monitor increase or decrease in vision.*
- Maintain safe environment (e.g., side rails up, bed in low position) *to prevent injury.*
- Indicate visual impairment on chart, care plan, and over bed *to communicate visual problems to health team and foster continuity of care.*

NURSING DIAGNOSIS **Altered urinary elimination (retention)** *related to* sensorimotor deficits or inadequate fluid intake *as manifested by* posturination residual >50 ml, dribbling, bladder distention.

- Residual urine <50 ml.
- Maintenance of urinary continence.

- Administer cholinergic medications as ordered *to improve the muscle tone of bladder and facilitate emptying.*
- Follow intermittent catheterization protocol *to prevent distention or dribbling.*
- Use Credé maneuver or reflex stimulation (manual stimulation) *as an alternative method of emptying bladder.*
- Maintain fluid intake of 3000 ml/day *to dilute urine and reduce risk of urinary tract infection.*
- Teach patient signs and symptoms of urinary tract infection *to ensure early identification and treatment.*

Continued

56-3   NURSING CARE PLAN   PATIENT WITH MULTIPLE SCLEROSIS—continued

Expected Patient Outcomes	Nursing Interventions and *Rationales*

NURSING DIAGNOSIS   **Altered urinary elimination (incontinence)** *related to* sensorimotor deficits or possible urinary tract infection *as manifested by* incontinence, urgency, frequency.

- Urinary continence.

- Administer anticholinergic medications as ordered *to reduce urinary frequency and urgency.*
- Initiate bladder-training program *to help restore adequate bladder function.*
- Provide incontinence briefs *to ensure that patient is protected and will not be embarrassed by incontinence.*
- Maintain fluid intake of 3000 ml/day *to promote urinary output and aid in preventing infection.*

NURSING DIAGNOSIS   **Constipation** *related to* immobility, inadequate fluid intake, improper diet, and neuromuscular impairment *as manifested by* hard stool, decreased bowel sounds, infrequent or absent bowel movements.

- Regular bowel evacuation.

- Turn patient regularly; maintain activity to individual tolerance *because mobility enhances peristalsis.*
- Maintain fluid intake (3000 ml/day) *to promote normal stool consistency.*
- Use prune juice at same time of day *because dihydroxyphenyl isatin in prune juice has a laxative effect.*
- Encourage high-residue diet *to improve stool consistency and promote evacuation.*
- Administer stool softeners and suppositories as ordered *to promote regularity by improving stool consistency.*
- Initiate and maintain bowel program *to foster regular bowel elimination.*

NURSING DIAGNOSIS   **Sexual dysfunction** *related to* neuromuscular deficits *as manifested by* impotence, verbalization of problem, decreased libido.

- Verbalization of satisfaction with expression of sexuality.

- Initiate sexual counseling if indicated *because not all nurses have the education required for this type of counseling.*
- Suggest alternative methods of achieving sexual gratification *because sexual intercourse may not be possible due to neuromuscular deficits.*

NURSING DIAGNOSIS   **Self-esteem disturbance** *related to* prolonged debilitating condition *as manifested by* feelings of inadequacy, depression, fatigue, withdrawal.

- Maintenance of realistic self-concept in relation to disease.

- Focus on remaining abilities and maintaining independence *because a major part of self-concept is the ability to perform one's role functions.*
- Assist patient in grieving process *because progressive losses or changes in body function may interfere with resolution of grieving process.*
- Encourage patient to discuss effect of MS on self-concept *to clarify issues and identify coping behaviors.*
- Discuss importance of maintaining social interactions *to prevent social isolation, withdrawal, and negative self-concept.*

NURSING DIAGNOSIS   **Altered family processes** *related to* changing family roles, potential financial problems, and fluctuating physical condition *as manifested by* strained family relations, ineffective communication, verbalization of financial concerns.

- Open communication between family and patient.
- Able to seek outside assistance when indicated.
- Maintenance of adequate care.

- Facilitate open communication among family members *to help family understand behaviors that may be triggered by emotional or physical effects of MS.*
- Promote problem solving *to enable the family to handle the issues of long-term illness.*
- Refer for family and financial counseling (if indicated) *to provide additional help in coping with a chronic debilitating disease.*
- Educate family regarding fluctuating nature of disease *because lack of knowledge about MS affects ability to cope with the changes.*

Health Promotion for Women with Multiple Sclerosis

Citation Stuifbergen AK, Roberts GJ: Health promotion practices of women with multiple sclerosis, *Arch Phys Med Rehabil* 78:S3, 1997.

Purpose To examine health-promoting behaviors of women with multiple sclerosis (MS). The investigators hypothesized that health-promoting behaviors influence the relationship between severity of illness and quality of life.

Methods A community-based sample of women (*n* = 629) with MS completed a series of questionnaires focused on measures of illness-related disability, health-promoting behaviors (e.g., stress management, physical activity, nutrition), and quality of life. Results were compared with a community-based group of healthy women. In addition, women with MS were grouped by clinical course (e.g., benign sensory, relapsing-remitting, progressive, severe progressive) and compared on frequency of health-promoting behaviors.

Results and Conclusions As a group women with MS scored lower on physical activity but higher on stress management and interpersonal relationships than the control group. When grouped by severity of disease, women with benign sensory and relapsing-remitting MS were more likely to engage in physical activity and spiritual growth behaviors than women with progressive MS. The course of disease affects the health-promoting behaviors that women engage in, as do the severity of symptoms.

Implications for Nursing Practice The presence of a chronic disabling condition affects the degree to which women engage in health-promoting behaviors. Symptoms such as fatigue, weakness, and incoordination can affect the desire and ability to participate in physical activity. Women with MS should be encouraged to participate in physical activities that can be performed, such as yoga, tai-chi, and other stress-reducing activities.

Patient education should focus on building general resistance to illness, including avoiding fatigue, extremes of heat and cold, and exposure to infection. The last measure involves avoiding exposure to cold climates and to people who are sick, as well as vigorous and early treatment of infection when it does occur. It is important to teach the patient to (1) achieve a good balance of exercise and rest, (2) eat nutritious and well-balanced meals, and (3) avoid the hazards of immobility (contractures and pressure sores). Patients should know their treatment regimens, the side effects of medications and how to watch for them, and drug interactions with over-the-counter medications. The patient should consult a health care provider before taking nonprescription medications.

Bladder control is a major problem for many patients with MS. While anticholinergics may be beneficial for some patients to decrease spasticity, other patients may need to be taught self-catheterization (see Chapter 43). Bowel problems, particularly constipation, occur frequently in patients with MS. Increasing the dietary fiber may help some patients achieve regularity in bowel habits.

The patient with MS and the family must make many emotional adjustments because of the unpredictability of the disease, the need to change lifestyles, and the challenge of avoiding or decreasing precipitating factors. The National Multiple Sclerosis Society and its local chapters can offer a variety of services to meet the needs of patients with MS.

■ Evaluation

Expected outcomes for the patient with MS are addressed in NCP 56-3.

PARKINSON'S DISEASE

Parkinsonism is a syndrome that consists of a slowing down in the initiation and execution of movement (bradykinesia), increased muscle tone (rigidity), tremor, and impaired postural reflexes. Parkinson's disease, a form of parkinsonism, is named after James Parkinson, who, in 1817, wrote a classic essay on "shaking palsy," a disease whose cause is still unknown today. Many other disorders resemble this disease, but their causes are known. These include drug-induced parkinsonism, postencephalitic parkinsonism, and arteriosclerotic parkinsonism. The pathophysiology of these disorders, with the exception of drug-induced parkinsonism, is the same. Damage or loss of the dopamine-producing cells of the substantia nigra in the midbrain leads to depletion, in the basal ganglia, of dopamine that influences the initiation, modulation, and completion of movement and regulates unconscious autonomic movements (see Chapter 53). In cases of drug-induced parkinsonism the dopamine receptors in the brain are blocked.

Etiology and Pathophysiology

Parkinson's disease affects about 1.5% of the population in the United States over 65 years of age.[14] The disease shows no gender, socioeconomic, or cultural preference, and symptoms most commonly occur after 50 years of age. The average age of the patient with Parkinson's disease is 65 years. There is no apparent genetic cause and no known cure. The disease rarely occurs in African-Americans.

There are many causes of parkinsonism. Encephalitis lethargica, or type A encephalitis, has been clearly associated with the onset of parkinsonism. However, the incidence of postencephalitic parkinsonism has dwindled since the 1920s, when there was a large outbreak of this infectious illness. Parkinsonism-like symptoms have occurred after intoxication with a variety of chemicals, including carbon monoxide and manganese (among copper miners) and product of meperidine-analog synthesis. Drug-induced parkinsonism can follow reserpine (Hydropres), methyldopa (Aldomet), haloperidol (Haldol), and phenothiazine (Thorazine) therapy. Although patients with cerebrovascular disease may have parkinsonism-like

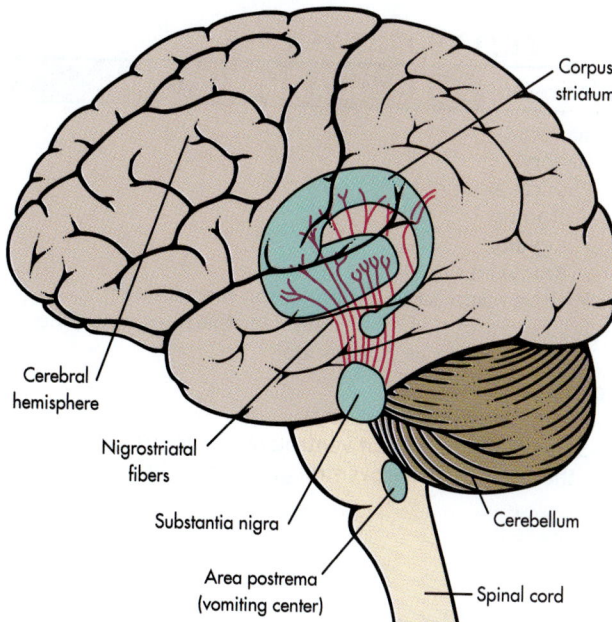

Fig. 56-4 Nigrostriatal disorders produce parkinsonism. Left-sided view of the human brain showing the substantia nigra and the corpus striatum (*shaded area*) lying deep within the cerebral hemisphere. Nerve fibers extend upward from the substantia nigra, divide into many branches, and carry dopamine to all regions of the corpus striatum.

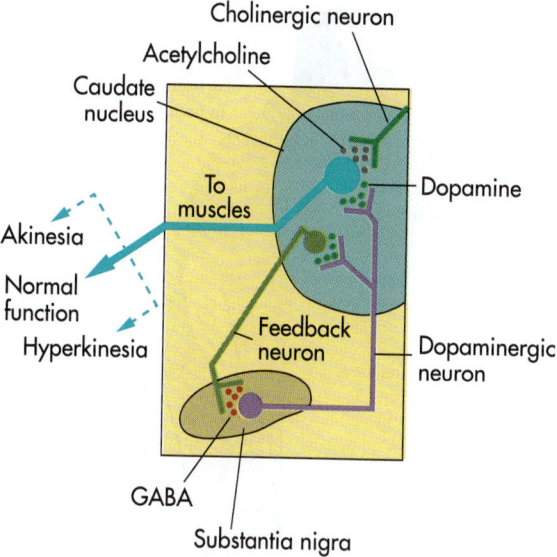

Fig. 56-5 Dopaminergic synaptic activity is mediated by dopamine. Cholinergic synaptic activity is mediated by acetylcholine. A balance between the two kinds of activity produces normal motor function. A relative excess of cholinergic activity produces akinesia and rigidity. A relative excess of dopaminergic activity produces involuntary movements. Neurons in the caudate nucleus contain gamma-aminobutyric acid (GABA) and possibly control dopaminergic neurons in the substantia nigra through a feedback pathway.

symptoms, there is little evidence that parkinsonism is caused by arteriosclerosis. Distinguishing arteriosclerosis from true Parkinson's disease is important for prognostic purposes. Patients with arteriosclerosis do not respond as well to treatment and are more likely to experience side effects of drug therapy. Most patients with parkinsonism have the degenerative or idiopathic form, for which the term *Parkinson's disease* is usually reserved.

The pathology of Parkinson's disease is associated with the degeneration of the dopamine-producing neurons in the substantia nigra of the midbrain (Figs. 56-4 and 56-5). It is hypothesized that there is normally a balance between acetylcholine (ACh) and dopamine (DA) in the basal ganglia. Any shift in the balance of activity (an increase in ACh or a decrease in DA) seems to lead to parkinsonism-like symptoms. Dopamine is a neurotransmitter that is essential for normal functioning of the extrapyramidal motor system, including control of posture, support, and voluntary motion. In Parkinson's disease the levels of DA-synthesizing enzymes and metabolites are reduced, and postmortem analysis of cross sections of the midbrain shows loss of the normal melanin pigment in the substantia nigra and loss of neurons. In addition, deficient amounts of gamma-aminobutyric acid (GABA), serotonin, and norepinephrine have been found in basal ganglia and in the substantia nigra.

Clinical Manifestations

The onset of Parkinson's disease is gradual and insidious, with a gradual progression and a prolonged course. In the beginning stages, only a mild tremor, a slight limp, or a decreased arm

swing may be evident. Later in the disease the patient may have a shuffling, propulsive gait with arms flexed and loss of postural reflexes. In some patients there may be a slight change in speech patterns. None of these alone is sufficient evidence for a diagnosis of the disease.

Because there is no specific diagnostic test for Parkinson's disease, the diagnosis is based solely on the history and the clinical features. A firm diagnosis can be made only when there are at least two of the three characteristic signs of the classic triad: tremor, rigidity, and bradykinesia (slow or retarded movement). Dementia occurs in up to 40% of patients with Parkinson's disease.[15,16] The ultimate confirmation of Parkinson's disease is a positive response to antiparkinsonian medication.

Tremor. Tremor, often the first sign, may be minimal initially, so the patient is the only one who notices it. This tremor can affect handwriting, causing it to trail off, particularly toward the ends of words. Parkinsonian tremor is more prominent at rest and is aggravated by emotional stress or increased concentration. The hand tremor is described as "pill rolling" because the thumb and forefinger appear to move in a rotary fashion as if rolling a pill, coin, or other small object. Tremor can involve the diaphragm, tongue, lips, and jaw but rarely causes shaking of the head. Unfortunately, in many people a benign essential tremor has mistakenly been diagnosed as Parkinson's disease. Essential tremor occurs during voluntary movement, has a more rapid frequency than parkinsonian tremor, and is often familial.

Rigidity. Rigidity, the second sign of the triad, is the increased resistance to passive motion when the limbs are moved through their range of motion. Parkinsonian rigidity

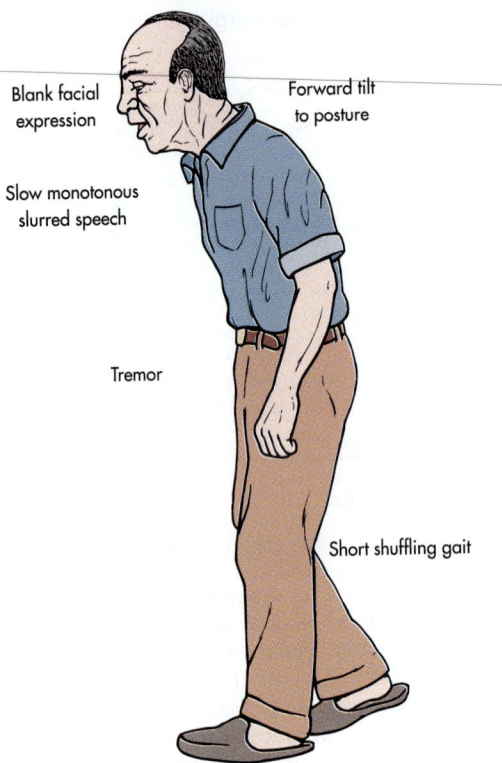

Blank facial expression

Forward tilt to posture

Slow monotonous slurred speech

Tremor

Short shuffling gait

Fig. 56-6 Characteristic appearance of a patient with Parkinson's disease.

COLLABORATIVE CARE

Table 56-16   Parkinson's Disease

Diagnostic
History
Physical examination
  Tremor
  Rigidity
  Bradykinesia
Positive response to antiparkinson medication*
Ruling out of side effects of phenothiazines, reserpine, benzodiazepines, haloperidol

Collaborative Therapy
Antiparkinson medication*
Surgical destruction of ventrolateral nucleus of the thalamus or posteroventral globus pallidus

*See Table 56-17.

is typified by a jerky quality, as if there were intermittent catches in the movement of a cogwheel, when the joint is moved. This is termed *cogwheel rigidity*. The rigidity is caused by sustained muscle contraction and consequently elicits a complaint of muscle soreness; feeling tired and achy; or pain in the head, upper body, spine, or legs. Another consequence of rigidity is slowness of movement, because it inhibits the alternating of contraction and relaxation in opposing muscle groups (e.g., the biceps and triceps).

Bradykinesia. Bradykinesia is particularly evident in the loss of automatic movements, which is secondary to the physical and chemical alteration of the basal ganglia and related structures in the extrapyramidal portion of the CNS. In the unaffected patient, automatic movements are involuntary and occur subconsciously. They include blinking of the eyelids, swinging of the arms while walking, swallowing of saliva, self-expression with facial and hand movements, and minor movement of postural adjustment. The patient with Parkinson's disease does not execute these movements, and there is a lack of spontaneous activity. This accounts for the stooped posture, masked facies ("deadpan" expression), drooling of saliva, and shuffling gait (festination) that are characteristic of a person with this disease. In addition, there is difficulty in initiating movement. Movements such as getting out of a chair cannot be executed unless they are consciously willed.

Complications

Many of the complications of Parkinson's disease are caused by the deterioration and loss of spontaneity of movement. Swallowing may become very difficult (dysphagia) in severe cases, leading to malnutrition or aspiration. General debilitation may lead to pneumonia, urinary tract infections, and skin breakdown. Mobility is greatly decreased. The gait slows, and turning is especially difficult. The gait usually consists of rapid, short, shuffling ministeps. The posture is that of the "old man" image, with the head and trunk bent forward and the legs constantly flexed (Fig. 56-6). The lack of mobility may lead to constipation, ankle edema, and, more seriously, contractures.

Orthostatic hypotension may occur in some patients, and along with loss of postural reflexes, may result in falls or other injury. Bothersome complications include seborrhea (increased oily secretion of the sebaceous glands of the skin), dandruff, excessive sweating, conjunctivitis, difficulty in reading, insomnia, incontinence, and depression.

Many of the apparent complications of Parkinson's disease are the result of side effects of medication, particularly levodopa. Dyskinesias (e.g., fidgeting movements of limbs) and weakness and akinesia (total immobility) may cause problems. These complications become apparent after prolonged levodopa therapy.

Collaborative Care

Because there is no cure for Parkinson's disease, collaborative management (Table 56-16) is aimed at relieving the symptoms.

Drug Therapy. Pharmacotherapy of Parkinson's disease is aimed at correcting an imbalance of neurotransmitters within the CNS. Antiparkinsonian drugs either enhance the release or supply of DA (dopaminergic) or antagonize or block the effects of the overactive cholinergic neurons in the striatum (anticholinergic). Levodopa with carbidopa (Sinemet) is often the first drug to be used. Levodopa is a precursor of dopamine and can cross the blood-brain barrier. It is converted to dopamine in the basal ganglia. Sinemet is the preferred medication because it also contains carbidopa, an agent that inhibits the enzyme dopa-decarboxylase in the peripheral tissues. This enzyme breaks down levodopa before it reaches the brain. The net result is that more levodopa reaches the brain, and therefore less drug is needed.

DRUG THERAPY

Table 56-17 Parkinson's Disease

Drug	Symptoms Relieved	Side Effects and Precautions
Dopaminergic		
Levodopa (L-dopa)	Bradykinesia, tremor, rigidity	Nausea, dyskinesia, hypotension, palpitations, arrhythmias; agitation, hallucinations, confusion (in older patient); avoidance of vitamin pills and diet high in vitamin B_6 (reversal of effect of levodopa); contraindicated in narrow-angle glaucoma
Levodopa/carbidopa (Sinemet)	Bradykinesia, tremor, rigidity	Less nausea but greater chance of dyskinesia, confusion, hallucinations; periodic check of BUN, AST, WBCs, Hct; contraindicated in melanoma, narrow-angle glaucoma, combination with MAO inhibitors, reserpine, methyldopa, guanethidine, antipsychotics
Bromocriptine mesylate (Parlodel)	Bradykinesia, tremor, rigidity	Orthostatic hypotension, nausea, vomiting, toxic psychosis, limb edema, phlebitis, dizziness, headache, insomnia
Pergolide (Permax)	Same as above	Same as above
Pramipexole (Mirapex)	Same as above	
Ropinirole (Requip)	Same as above	
Amantadine (Symmetrel)	Rigidity, akinesia	Nervousness, insomnia, confusion, hallucinations, dry mouth, nausea, edema, orthostatic hypotension
Anticholinergic		
Trihexyphenidyl (Artane)	Tremor	Dry mouth, blurred vision, constipation, delirium, anxiety, agitation, hallucinations; avoidance of drugs with similar actions, including over-the-counter drugs containing scopolamine or antihistamines (e.g., Sominex), antispasmodics (e.g., Donnatal, Bellergal), tricyclic antidepressants (Tofranil, Elavil, Norpramin, Vivactil)
Cycrimine (Pagitane)		
Procyclidine (Kemadrin)		
Benztropine (Cogentin)		
Biperiden (Akineton)		
Antihistamine		
Diphenhydramine (Benadryl)	Tremor, rigidity	Sedation, same precautions as for anticholinergic drugs
Orphenadrine (Disipal)		
Chlorphenoxamine (Phenoxene)		
Phenindamine (Thephorin)		
Monoamine Oxidase Inhibitor		
Selegiline (Eldepryl, Carbex)	Bradykinesia, rigidity, tremor	Similar to dopaminergic drugs

AST, aspartate aminotransferase; *BUN,* blood urea nitrogen; *Hct,* hematocrit; *MAO,* monoamine oxidase; *WBCs,* white blood cells.

During early-stage Parkinson's disease, if the symptoms are not severe, mild antiparkinsonian drugs (e.g., dopamine agonists such as bromocriptine [Parlodel] and pergolide [Permax]), can provide improvement in symptoms. Newer dopamine receptor agonists (ropinirole [Requip] and pramipexole [Mirapex]) have also been shown to be effective in improving symptoms of early Parkinson's disease.[17,18] These drugs directly stimulate dopamine receptors. When more moderate to severe symptoms are present, carbidopa/levodopa are added to the drug regimen. Other adjuvant agents include amantadine (Symmetrel), anticholinergic medications (trihexyphenidyl [Artane] or benztropine [Cogentin]), selegiline (Eldepryl, Carbex), and diphenhydramine (Benadryl).

Anticholinergic drugs are also used to manage Parkinson's disease. These drugs act by decreasing the activity of ACh and thus providing balance between cholinergic and dopaminergic

actions. Antihistamines (e.g., diphenhydramine [Benadryl]) with anticholinergic properties or propanolol (e.g., long-acting Inderal) are used to manage tremors. The antiviral agent amantadine (Symmetrel) is also an effective antiparkinsonian drug. Although its exact mechanism of action is not known, amantadine promotes the release of DA from neurons. Selegiline is a monoamine oxidase (MAO) inhibitor that is sometimes used in combination with Sinemet. By inhibiting MAO, the degradative enzyme for DA, the levels of DA are increased.

Table 56-17 summarizes the drugs commonly used in Parkinson's disease, the symptoms they relieve, and their common side effects. The use of only one drug is preferred, since there are fewer side effects and the medication is easier to adjust than when several drugs are used. Excessive amounts of dopaminergic drugs can lead to paradoxic intoxication (aggravation

NURSING ASSESSMENT

Table 56-18 Parkinson's Disease

Subjective Data	Objective Data
Important Health Information *Past health history:* CNS trauma, cerebrovascular disorders, exposure to metals and carbon monoxide, encephalitis *Medication:* Use of major tranquilizers, especially haloperidol (Haldol) and phenothiazines, reserpine, methyldopa **Functional Health Patterns** *Health perception–health management:* Fatigue *Nutritional-metabolic:* Excessive salivation, dysphagia; weight loss *Elimination:* Constipation, incontinence; excessive sweating *Activity-exercise:* Difficulty in initiating movements; frequent falls; loss of dexterity; micrographia (handwriting deterioration) *Sleep-rest:* Insomnia *Cognitive-perceptual:* Diffuse pain in head, shoulders, neck, back, legs, and hips; muscle soreness and cramping *Self-perception–self-concept:* Depression; mood swings, hallucinations	**General** Blank (masked) facies, slow and monotonous speech, infrequent blinking **Integumentary** Seborrhea, dandruff; ankle edema **Cardiovascular** Postural hypotension **Gastrointestinal** Drooling **Neurologic** Tremor at rest, first in hands (pill-rolling), later in legs, arms, face, and tongue; aggravation of tremor with anxiety, absence in sleep; poor coordination; subtle dementia, impaired postural reflexes **Musculoskeletal** "Cogwheel" rigidity, dysarthria, bradykinesia, contractures, stooped posture, shuffling gait **Possible Findings** Lack of specific tests, diagnosis on basis of history and physical findings and ruling out of other diseases

rather than relief of symptoms). Anticholinergic drugs can cause impaired erection and failure of ejaculation.

Surgical Therapy. Surgical procedures are aimed at relieving symptoms (e.g., tremor, rigidity) of Parkinson's disease. Surgical procedures such as thalamotomy, thalamic stimulation, and pallidotomy are often reserved for patients who are unresponsive to drug therapy or who have developed severe motor complications.[19,20] Stereotactic thalamotomy relieves tremor and to a lesser extent rigidity. However, bradykinesia and postural instability are not improved. It involves making a lesion in a specific region of the thalamus. Bilateral posteroventral pallidotomy relieves tremor, rigidity, and bradykinesia. The procedure involves making a lesion in a specific area between the medial and lateral segments of the globus pallidus.[19] Improvements in rigidity, tremor, dyskinesia, and dystonia have been shown. Chronic thalamic electrical stimulation has been used to reduce tremor and enhance motor function.[20]

Transplantation of fetal neural tissue into the caudate nucleus in an attempt to provide viable dopamine-producing cells to the brain has had variable results.[21] Fetal adrenal brain tissue transplantation has also been used with less promising results.[22]

Nutritional Therapy. Diet is of major importance to the patient with Parkinson's disease because malnutrition and constipation can be serious consequences of inadequate nutrition. Patients who have dysphagia and bradykinesia need appetizing foods that are easily chewed and swallowed. The diet should contain adequate roughage and fruit to avoid constipation. Food should be cut into bite-sized pieces before it is served, and it should be served on a warmed plate to preserve its appeal. Eating six small meals a day may be less exhausting than eating three large meals a day. Ample time should be planned for eating to avoid frustration and encourage independence.

NURSING MANAGEMENT: PARKINSON'S DISEASE

■ Nursing Assessment

Subjective and objective data that should be obtained from a person with Parkinson's disease are presented in Table 56-18.

■ Nursing Diagnoses

Nursing diagnoses for the patient with Parkinson's disease may include, but are not limited to, those presented in NCP 56-4.

■ Planning

The overall goals are that the patient with Parkinson's disease will (1) maximize neurologic function, (2) maintain independence in activities of daily living for as long as possible, and (3) optimize psychosocial well-being.

■ Nursing Implementation

Promotion of physical exercise and a well-balanced diet are major concerns for nursing care. Exercise can limit the consequences of decreased mobility, such as muscle atrophy, contractures, and constipation. The American Parkinson's Disease Association publishes a booklet, *Home Exercises for Patients with Parkinson's Disease*, that illustrates a variety of exercises; it can be used by family members and health professionals.

A physical therapist may be consulted to design a personal exercise program aimed at strengthening specific muscles. Overall muscle tone, as well as specific exercises to strengthen the muscles involved with speaking and swallowing, should be included. Although exercise will not halt the progress of the disease, it will bring the patient's motor function to an optimal level.

Because Parkinson's disease is a chronic degenerative disorder with no acute exacerbations, nurses should note that health teaching and nursing care are directed toward maintenance of

56-4 NURSING CARE PLAN PATIENT WITH PARKINSON'S DISEASE

| Expected Patient Outcomes | Nursing Interventions and *Rationales* |

NURSING DIAGNOSIS Impaired physical mobility *related to* rigidity, bradykinesia, and akinesia *as manifested by* difficulty in initiation of volitional movements.

- Safe ambulation.
- Maintenance of joint mobility.

- Assist with ambulation *to assess degree of impairment and to prevent injury.*
- Perform active range-of-motion (ROM) exercises to all extremities *to maintain joint ROM, prevent atrophy, and strengthen muscles.*
- Consult physical therapist or occupational therapist for aids *to facilitate activities of daily living (ADLs) and safe ambulation.*
- Evaluate tremor in relation to medication *to monitor patient's response and identify possible overdose.*
- Teach techniques to assist with mobility by instructing patient to step over imaginary line, rock from side to side to initiate leg movements *because these are helpful in dealing with "freezing" (akinesia) while walking.*

NURSING DIAGNOSIS Self-care deficits *related to* parkinsonian symptoms *as manifested by* inability to perform ADLs, need for assistive devices.

- Optimal independence in ADLs.
- Daily needs met by self or other.

- Encourage activities of daily living within limits of mobility *to prolong patient's independence.*
- Arrange patient's room *to facilitate optimal self-care.*
- Plan sufficient time for patient to perform self-care *because rigidity causes slowness of movement.*
- Provide assistance as needed *so patient's needs are met and frustration reduced.*
- Arrange occupational therapy consultation *to teach additional strategies for achieving ADLs and to minimize complications such as contractures.*
- Offer emotional support *to bolster patient's effort in coping with a chronic degenerative disease.*

NURSING DIAGNOSIS Impaired verbal communication *related to* dysarthria and tremor or bradykinesia *as manifested by* decreased amount of communication, slow and slurred speech, inability to move facial muscles, decreased tongue mobility, micrographia, inability to write.

- Development of communication method to meet needs.

- Allow sufficient time for communication *to reduce patient's frustration.*
- Encourage deep breaths before speaking.
- Consult speech therapist *to provide specialized guidance in care of the patient.*
- Provide alternative communication methods such as picture books or flash cards *since muscle involvement has impaired writing and speaking ability.*
- Massage patient's facial and neck muscles *to foster relaxation that can facilitate speech.*

NURSING DIAGNOSIS Constipation *related to* weakness of abdominal and perineal muscles, lack of exercise, and side effects of medication *as manifested by* hardened stool and decreased bowel sounds.

- Maintenance of regular bowel evacuation.

- Increase fluid intake to 3000 ml/day *to maintain soft stool.*
- Increase fiber in diet with every meal *to provide bulk to stool.*
- Increase mobility to tolerance *to stimulate peristalsis.*
- Give stool softeners, laxatives, suppositories as needed *to ensure regular bowel evacuation.*

NURSING DIAGNOSIS Altered nutrition: less than body requirements *related to* dysphagia *as manifested by* difficulty in swallowing and chewing, drooling, decreased gag reflex.

- Maintenance of satisfactory body weight.

- Carefully monitor swallowing ability during medication administration and mealtime *to evaluate patient's level of impairment and minimize risk of aspiration.*
- Provide soft-solid and thick-liquid diet *because these consistencies are more easily swallowed.*
- Massage patient's facial and neck muscles before meals *to reduce rigidity and enhance ability to chew and swallow.*
- Maintain patient in upright position for all meals *to reduce risk of aspiration.*
- Consult speech therapist and dietician *because they can provide specific plans to improve swallowing and intake.*

Continued

56-4 NURSING CARE PLAN **PATIENT WITH PARKINSON'S DISEASE**—continued

Expected Patient Outcomes	Nursing Interventions and *Rationales*

NURSING DIAGNOSIS Altered nutrition: less than body requirements—*continued*

- Maintain caloric counts and weekly weights *to evaluate patient's nutritional status and adjust plan if indicated.*
- Have suction available *to remove pooled secretions and prevent choking and aspiration.*

NURSING DIAGNOSIS Diversional activity deficit *related to* inability to perform usual recreational activities *as manifested by* boredom, lack of participation, restlessness, depression, hostility.

- Engagement in satisfying diversional activities. - Expression of acceptance of diminished capabilities.	- Assess patient's activity *to determine physical and emotional response to difficulties.* - Determine preferred diversional activities *so individual needs are considered.* - Adapt difficult activities when possible *so patient is able to continue performing activities.* - Initiate new activities within patient's capabilities, such as reading, *to replace activities patient can no longer perform.* - Encourage patient to discuss emotional response to decreasing capabilities *to provide opportunity to problem solve and demonstrate a caring attitude.*

NURSING DIAGNOSIS Sleep pattern disturbance *related to* medication side effects (e.g., hallucinations), anxiety, rigidity, and muscle discomfort *as manifested by* poor sleep history, inability to sleep uninterrupted, nightmares, vivid dreams or hallucinations, anxiety, rigidity, or muscle discomfort.

- Verbalization of feeling rested on awakening.	- Provide quiet environment *to promote uninterrupted sleep.* - Turn and position for comfort *because muscle soreness and inability to make minor postural changes as a result of bradykinesia may interfere with sleep.* - Provide passive ROM exercises to extremities *to alleviate rigidity that may interfere with sleep.* - Provide daytime stimulus to maintain wakefulness *to avoid excess napping, which prevents quality nighttime sleep.* - Offer support if hallucinations are present *to decrease anxiety, since levodopa may produce hallucinations.* - Give sleep medications as ordered *to facilitate sleep.*

good health, encouragement of independence, and avoidance of complications such as contractures.

Problems secondary to bradykinesia can be alleviated by relatively simple measures. The following are helpful hints for patients who tend to "freeze" while walking: consciously think about stepping over imaginary or real lines on the floor, drop rice kernels and step over them, rock from side to side, lift the toes when stepping, take one step backward and two steps forward. The patient should be assessed for the possibility of levodopa overdose because it is a common cause of akinesia "freezing." A brief period of dyskinesia, usually athetosis of the neck, should alert the nurse to this possibility.

Getting out of a chair can be facilitated by using an upright chair with arms and placing the back legs on small (2-inch) blocks. Other aspects of the environment can be altered. Rugs and excess furniture can be removed to avoid stumbling. An ottoman can be used to elevate the legs and avoid dependent ankle edema. Clothing can be simplified by the use of slip-on shoes and Velcro hook-and-loop fasteners or zippers on clothing, instead of buttons and hooks. An elevated toilet seat can facilitate getting on and off the toilet. The nurse should work closely with the patient's family in exploring creative adaptations that allow maximum independence and self-care.

■ Evaluation

Expected outcomes for the patient with Parkinson's disease are addressed in NCP 56-4.

MYASTHENIA GRAVIS

Myasthenia gravis (MG) is a disease of the neuromuscular junction characterized by the fluctuating weakness of certain skeletal muscle groups. The prevalence is estimated to be from 43 to 84 persons per million. The peak age at onset in women is 20 to 30 years. Women are affected slightly more often than men, although among patients with both thymoma and myasthenia gravis (15% of all persons with MG), the majority are men over the age of 50.

Etiology and Pathophysiology

MG is caused by an autoimmune process that results in production of antibodies directed against the ACh receptors and a reduction in the number of ACh receptor sites at the neuromuscular junction. This prevents ACh molecules from attaching and stimulating muscle contraction. Anti-ACh receptor antibodies are detectable in the serum of 70% to 85% of patients with MG. As a result of this process there is loss of muscle strength. Thymic tumors are found in about 15% of patients.

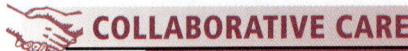

COLLABORATIVE CARE
Table 56-19 Myasthenia Gravis

Diagnostic
Complete history
Physical examination
   Fatigability with prolonged upward gaze (2-3 min)
   Muscle weakness
EMG
Tensilon test

Collaborative Therapy
Drugs
   Anticholinesterase agents
   Corticosteroids
   Immunosuppressive agents
Surgery (thymectomy)
Plasmapheresis

EMG, electromyography.

Although a viral infection is suspected as precipitating an attack, a single specific cause for all cases of MG has not been found.

Clinical Manifestations and Complications

The primary feature of MG is easy fatigability of skeletal muscle during activity. Strength is usually restored after a period of rest. The muscles most often involved are those used for moving the eyes and eyelids, chewing, swallowing, speaking, and breathing. The cell bodies of the neurons for these muscles are located in the brainstem. The muscles are generally the strongest in the morning and become exhausted with continued activity. Consequently, by the end of the day, muscle fatigue is prominent.

In more than 90% of the cases, the eyelid muscles or extraocular muscles are involved. Facial mobility and expression can be impaired. There may be difficulty in chewing and swallowing food. Speech is affected, and the voice often fades after a long conversation. The muscles of the trunk and limbs are less often affected. Of these, the proximal muscles of the neck, shoulder, and hip are more often affected than the distal muscles. No other signs of neural disorder accompany MG; there is no sensory loss, reflexes are normal, and muscle atrophy is rare.

The course of this disease is highly variable. Some patients may have short-term remissions, others may stabilize, and others may have severe, progressive involvement. Restricted ocular myasthenia, usually seen only in men, has a good prognosis. Exacerbations of MG can be precipitated by emotional stress, pregnancy, menses, secondary illness, trauma, temperature extremes, hypokalemia, ingestion of drugs with neuromuscular blocking properties, and surgery. In some cases the onset of MG occurs after one of these events.

The major complications of MG result from muscle weakness in areas that affect swallowing and breathing. Aspiration, respiratory insufficiency, and respiratory infection are the major complications. An acute exacerbation of this type is sometimes termed *myasthenic crisis.*

Diagnostic Studies

The simplest diagnostic test for myasthenia gravis is to have the patient look upward for 2 to 3 minutes. If the problem is MG, there will be an increased droop of the eyelids, so that the person can barely keep the eyes open. After a brief rest the eyes can open

again. Other tests may be used if the diagnosis is still in doubt. EMG may show a decrementing response to repeated stimulation of the hand muscles, indicative of muscle fatigue. Use of pharmacologic agents may also aid in the diagnosis. The Tensilon test in a patient with MG reveals improved muscle contractility after intravenous (IV) injection of the anticholinesterase agent edrophonium chloride (Tensilon). This test also aids in the diagnosis of cholinergic crisis (secondary to overdose of neostigmine). In this condition, Tensilon does not improve muscle weakness but may actually increase it. Atropine should be readily available to counteract Tensilon effects when it is used diagnostically.

Collaborative Care

Drug Therapy. The major forms of therapy for MG are anticholinesterase drugs, alternate-day corticosteroids, immunosuppressants, and plasmapheresis (Table 56-19). Anticholinesterase drugs are used in the management of MG. Acetylcholinesterase is the enzyme responsible for the breakdown of ACh in the synaptic cleft. Thus inhibition of this enzyme by an anticholinesterase inhibitor will prolong the action of ACh and facilitate transmission of impulses at the neuromuscular junction. Neostigmine (Prostigmin) and pyridostigmine (Mestinon) are the most successful drugs of this group. Tailoring the dose to avoid a myasthenic or cholinergic crisis often presents a clinical challenge. Because of the autoimmune nature of the disorder, corticosteroids (specifically prednisone) are used to suppress immunity. Cytotoxic drugs such as azathioprine (Imuran) and cyclophosphamide (Cytoxan) may also be used for immunosuppression.

Many drugs are contraindicated or must be used with caution in patients with MG. Classes of drug that should be cautiously evaluated before use include anesthetics, antiarrhythmics, antibiotics, quinine, antipsychotics, barbiturates and sedative-hypnotics, cathartics, diuretics, narcotics, muscle relaxants, thyroid preparations, and tranquilizers.

Surgical Therapy. Because the presence of the thymus gland in the patient with MG appears to enhance the production of ACh receptor antibodies, removal of the thymus gland results in improvement in a majority of patients. Thymectomy is indicated for almost all patients with thymoma, for patients with generalized MG between the ages of puberty and about 60 years, and for patients with purely ocular MG.[23]

Other Therapies. Plasmapheresis as a therapy for MG was first reported in 1976. This procedure involves separation of plasma from blood by a machine called a cell separator, which is connected to the patient by a vascular cannula. This process removes anti-ACh receptor antibodies. Plasmapheresis can yield a short-term improvement in symptoms and is indicated for patients in crisis or in preparation for surgery when corticosteroids must be avoided. (Plasmapheresis is discussed in Chapter 12.) Intravenous IgG has been used with some success. However, there have been no large, well-controlled, randomized prospective studies of this therapy in MG.[24]

NURSING MANAGEMENT: MYASTHENIA GRAVIS
■ Nursing Assessment

The nurse can assess the severity of MG by asking the patient about fatigability, what body parts are affected, and how severely they are affected. The patient's coping abilities and

Table **56-20**	Comparison of Myasthenic Crisis and Cholinergic Crisis	
	Myasthenic Crisis	**Cholinergic Crisis**
Causes	Exacerbation of myasthenia following precipitating factors or failure to take medication as prescribed or dose of medication too low	Overdose of anticholinesterase drugs resulting in increased ACh at the receptor sites, remission (spontaneous or after thymectomy).
Differential diagnosis	Improved strength after IV administration of anticholinesterase drugs; increased weakness of skeletal muscles manifesting as ptosis, bulbar signs (e.g., difficulty in swallowing, difficulty in articulating words), or dyspnea.	Weakness within 1 hr after ingestion of anticholinesterase; increased weakness of skeletal muscles manifesting as ptosis, bulbar signs, dyspnea; effects on smooth muscle include pupillary miosis, salivation, diarrhea, nausea or vomiting, abdominal cramps, increased bronchial secretions, sweating, or lacrimation

ACh, acetycholine.

understanding of the disorder should also be assessed. Some patients become so fatigued that they are no longer able to work or even ambulate.

Objective data should include respiratory rate and depth, oxygen saturation, arterial blood gas analyses, pulmonary function tests, and evidence of respiratory distress in patients with acute myasthenic crisis. Muscle strength of all face and limb muscles should be assessed, as should swallowing, speech (volume and clarity), and cough and gag reflexes.

■ Nursing Diagnoses

Nursing diagnoses for the patient with MG may include, but are not limited to, the following:

- Ineffective breathing pattern *related to* intercostal muscle weakness
- Ineffective airway clearance *related to* intercostal muscle weakness and impaired cough and gag reflex
- Impaired verbal communication *related to* weakness of the larynx, lips, mouth, pharynx, and jaw
- Altered nutrition: less than body requirements *related to* impaired swallowing, weakness, and inability to prepare food or feed self
- Sensory/perceptual alterations *related to* ptosis, decreased eye movements, and dysconjugate gaze
- Activity intolerance *related to* muscle weakness and fatigability
- Body image disturbance *related to* inability to maintain usual lifestyle and role responsibilities

■ Planning

The overall goals are that the patient with MG will (1) have a return of normal muscle endurance, (2) avoid complications, and (3) maintain a quality of life appropriate to disease course.

■ Nursing Implementation

The patient with MG who is admitted to the hospital usually has a respiratory tract infection or is in an acute myasthenic crisis. Nursing care is aimed at maintaining adequate ventilation, continuing drug therapy, and watching for side effects of therapy. The nurse must be able to distinguish cholinergic from myasthenic crisis (Table 56-20), because the causes and treatment of the two conditions differ greatly.

As with other chronic illnesses, care focuses on the neurologic deficits and their impact on daily living. A balanced diet with food that can be chewed and swallowed easily should be prescribed.

Semisolid foods may be easier to eat than solids or liquids. Scheduling doses of medication so that peak action is reached at mealtime may make eating less difficult. Diversional activities that require little physical effort and match the interests of the patient should be arranged. Education should focus on the importance of following the medical regimen, potential adverse reactions to specific drugs, planning activities of daily living to avoid fatigue, the availability of community resources, and the complications of the disease and therapy (crisis conditions) and what to do about them. Contact with the Myasthenia Gravis Foundation or an MG support group may be helpful and should be explored.

■ Evaluation

The overall expected outcomes are that the patient with MG will

- maintain optimal muscle function throughout the day
- be free from side effects of medication
- not experience complications from the disease
- maintain a quality of life appropriate to the disease course

ALZHEIMER'S DISEASE

Alzheimer's disease is a type of dementia that is characterized by progressive deterioration in memory and other aspects of cognition. Alzheimer's disease is increasingly recognized as one of the major health problems in the United States, particularly for persons over 65 years of age. It accounts for more than half of the cases of dementia (about 4 million cases). The major causes of progressive dementia are listed in Table 56-21.

Etiology and Pathophysiology

The etiology of Alzheimer's disease is still unclear, although age is the most important risk factor for developing it. Pathologic changes associated with Alzheimer's disease include neurofibrillary tangles and β-amyloid plaques in the cerebral cortex and hippocampus. The neuritic plaque is a cluster of degenerating axonal and dendritic nerve terminals that contain an abnormal protein (β-amyloid). Neurofibrillary tangles are seen in the cytoplasm of abnormal neurons (Fig. 56-7). These bundles of proteins are in the form of paired helical filaments. There is also an excessive loss of cholinergic neurons, particularly in regions essential for memory and cognition.

There has been much research on the possible genetic etiology of Alzheimer's disease. At least four chromosomes (1, 14, 19, and 21) are involved in some forms of familial Alzheimer's disease.[25] Inheritance of the apo E4 genotype (a gene responsi-

Table 56-21	Major Causes of Progressive Dementia	
Senile dementia, Alzheimer type		50%
Multiinfarct (arteriosclerotic)		10%
Combination of senile dementia and multiinfarct		15%
Communicating hydrocephalus		
Alcoholic or posttraumatic dementia		
Huntington's chorea		15%
Intracranial mass lesions		
Uncommon or in combination with other causes		10%
Chronic drug use, Creutzfeldt-Jakob disease, metabolic disease (thyroid, liver), nutritional deficits, degenerative disease (spinocerebellar, amyotrophic lateral sclerosis, parkinsonism, multiple sclerosis, Pick's disease, Wilson's disease, epilepsy), AIDS dementia, static postanoxic dementia		

Modified from Andreoli TE and others: *Cecil essentials of medicine,* ed 4, Philadelphia, 1997, Saunders.
AIDS, acquired immunodeficiency syndrome.

Table 56-22	Differentiation of Depression and Dementia of Alzheimer's Disease	
Characteristic	**Depression**	**Dementia**
Onset	Abrupt (weeks)	Insidious
Psychiatric history	Previous depression common	Usually no history
Mental status	Pervasive dysphoria	Flattening of affect
	Normal or impaired cognition	Impaired cognition
	Variable performance	Stable performance
	Variable memory disturbance	Serious effects on memory
Sleep disturbance	Initial and early-morning insomnia	Frequent awakenings
Somatic complaints	Often multiple	Often none
Self-image	Poor	Normal
Suicidal ideation	Present	Present early in disease, then absent
Treatment	High effectiveness of antidepressants	Very limited usefulness of antidepressants
Weight loss	Yes, with appetite disturbance	Not until late in disease

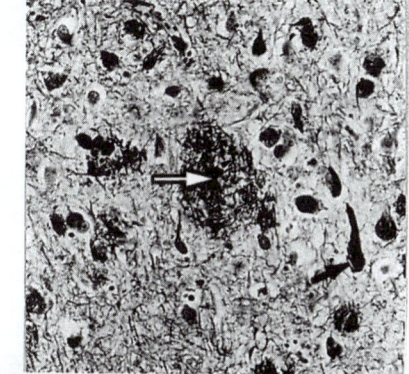

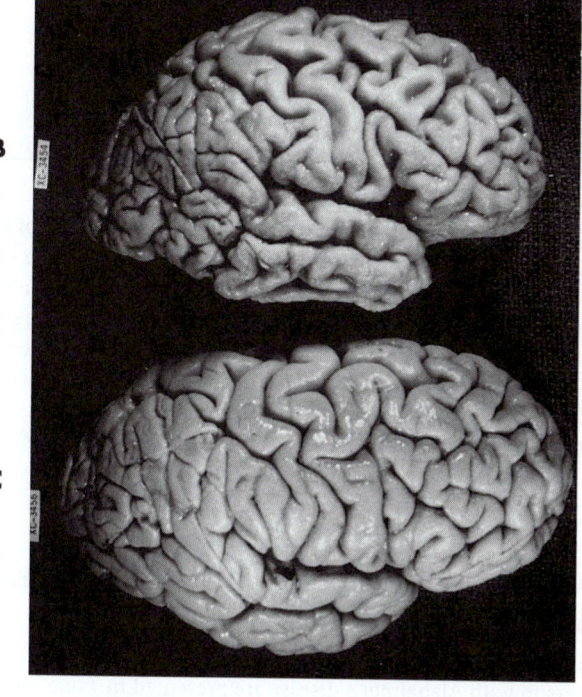

Fig. 56-7   Pathologic changes in Alzheimer's disease. **A,** Neuritic (mature) plaque with central amyloid core *(white arrow)* next to a neurofibrillary tangle *(black arrow).* **B,** Alzheimer's disease compared with **C,** age-matched and sex-matched control.

ble for making apolipoprotein) is a major genetic risk factor for developing Alzheimer's disease. There are also data to suggest that estrogen protects against the development of Alzheimer's. Estrogen may also slow the progression of Alzheimer's disease in those who already have it.[26] There is also recent interest in the role of NSAIDs in reducing the risk of Alzheimer's disease. Individuals who have a history of taking NSAIDs (e.g., ibuprofen) for other indications seem to have a lower risk of developing Alzheimer's disease.[26] However, long-term use of NSAIDs is associated with gastrointestinal and kidney problems.

Clinical Manifestations

An initial sign of Alzheimer's disease is a subtle deterioration in memory. Inevitably this progresses to more profound memory loss that interferes with the patient's ability to function. Recent events and new information cannot be recalled. Some patients develop psychotic symptoms. Personal hygiene deteriorates, as does the ability to maintain attention. Later in the disease, long-term memories cannot be recalled, and patients lose the ability to recognize family members. Eventually the ability to communicate and to perform activities of daily living is lost. The progression of the deterioration, which eventually leads to death, varies but can last as long as 20 years.

Alzheimer's disease must be distinguished from depression, a clinically similar condition, because depression is potentially reversible and often responds to appropriate treatment. A careful assessment can distinguish the two clinical conditions (Table 56-22).

Diagnostic Studies

The diagnosis of Alzheimer's disease is a diagnosis of exclusion.[27] When all other possible conditions that can cause mental impairment have been ruled out and the manifestations of dementia persist, the diagnosis of Alzheimer's disease can be made. A

DRUG THERAPY

Table 56-23   Alzheimer's Disease

Manifestation	Drugs	Side Effects
Depression	Tricyclic antidepressants (e.g., nortriptyline [Aventyl, Pamelor], amitriptyline [Elavil], imipramine [Tofranil], doxepin [Sinequan])	Orthostatic hypotension, sedation, dry mouth, constipation, urinary retention, blurry vision
	Nontricyclic antidepressant (e.g., trazodone [Desyrel])	Dry mouth, sedation, confusion
Psychoses and behavioral disturbances	Neuroleptics or antipsychotics (e.g., loxapine [Loxapac], haloperidol [Haldol])	Sedation, extrapyramidal effects, orthostatic hypotension, tardive dyskinesia
	Benzodiazepines (e.g., oxazepam [Serax], diazepam [Valium])	Sedation, confusion, disinhibition with paradoxic agitation, unsteady gait, dysarthria, incoordination
Anxiety	Benzodiazepines	Same as in psychoses and behavioral disturbances
Sleep disturbances	Benzodiazepines, neuroleptics	Same as in psychoses and behavioral disturbances
Decreased memory and cognition	Tacrine (Cognex)	Liver toxicity, nausea and vomiting
	Donepezil (Aricept)	Nausea, diarrhea, insomnia

NURSING ASSESSMENT

Table 56-24   Alzheimer's Disease

Subjective Data

Important Health Information

Past health history: Repeated head trauma, exposure to metals (especially aluminum), previous CNS infection

Medication: Use of any drug to mitigate symptoms (e.g., tranquilizers, hypnotics, antidepressants, antipsychotics)

Functional Health Patterns

Health perception–health management: Positive family history; emotional lability

Nutritional-metabolic: Anorexia, malnutrition, weight loss

Elimination: Incontinence

Activity-exercise: Poor personal hygiene; gait instability, weakness; inability to perform activities of daily living

Sleep-rest: Frequent nighttime awakening, daytime napping

Cognitive-perceptual: Forgetfulness, inability to cope with complex situations, difficulty with problem solving (early signs); depression, withdrawal, suicidal ideation (early)

Objective Data

General

Disheveled appearance, agitation

Neurologic

Early: Loss of recent memory; disorientation to date and time; flat affect; lack of spontaneity; impaired abstraction, cognition, and judgment; loss of remote memory; restlessness and agitation; inability to recognize family and friends; nocturnal wandering; repetitive behavior; loss of social graces; stubbornness, paranoia, belligerence

Advanced: Aphasia, agnosia, alexia (inability to understand written language), apraxia, seizures, limb rigidity, flexor posturing

Possible Findings

Diagnosis by exclusion, cerebral cortical atrophy on CT scan, poor scores on mental status tests, hippocampal atrophy on MRI scan

CT scan or an MRI scan may show brain atrophy and enlarged ventricles in the later stages of the disease, although this finding occurs in other diseases and can also be seen in normal persons. Neuropsychologic testing can help document the degree of cognitive dysfunction in the early stages.[27] The definitive diagnosis of Alzheimer's disease can be made only at autopsy, when the presence of neurofibrillary tangles is observed.

Collaborative Care

The collaborative care of Alzheimer's disease is aimed at improving or controlling decline in cognition and controlling the undesirable symptoms that the patient may exhibit. Table 56-23 details the manifestation of symptoms, the usual drug therapy, and the possible side effects of the prescribed drugs. It is important to be aware that these drugs do not significantly alter the course of the disease.

Recently drugs that inhibit the breakdown of acetylcholine in the brain and thereby enhance cognitive function have become available. In 1993 tacrine (Cognex), an acetylcholinesterase inhibitor, was approved for Alzheimer's disease. It slows the decline in cognitive function.[26,28] However, because of liver toxicity, frequent laboratory monitoring of liver function is required. Donepezil (Aricept) is also an acetylcholinesterase inhibitor. It does not require laboratory monitoring, can be given once a day, and has been shown to either mildly improve or stabilize cognitive decline in some people with Alzheimer's disease. Both drugs are used in the early and middle stages of Alzheimer's disease. These drugs do not cure Alzheimer's disease but rather slow the progression of symptoms.

NURSING MANAGEMENT: ALZHEIMER'S DISEASE

■ Nursing Assessment

Subjective and objective data that should be obtained from a person with Alzheimer's disease are presented in Table 56-24.

■ Nursing Diagnoses

Nursing diagnoses for Alzheimer's disease may include, but are not limited to, those presented in NCP 56-5.

56-5 NURSING CARE PLAN | PATIENT WITH ALZHEIMER'S DISEASE

Expected Patient Outcomes	Nursing Interventions and *Rationales*

NURSING DIAGNOSIS | **Altered thought processes** *related to* effects of dementia *as manifested by* loss of memory and cognitive deficits.

- Participation in care and social activities to maximum level of ability.

- Assess extent of cognitive deficits by direct contact with patient and information from family *to plan appropriate interventions.*
- Plan strategies to promote communication, increase self-esteem, and provide stimulation *to maximize patient's cognitive abilities.*
- Use reality orientation (early) and routine schedule *to promote memory and reduce confusion.*

NURSING DIAGNOSIS | **Self-care deficits** *related to* memory deficit and neuromuscular impairment *as manifested by* inability to independently and appropriately dress, bathe, groom, or toilet.

- Able to appropriately dress and groom self.
- Establishment of satisfactory toileting routine.
- Adequate nutritional intake.

- Assess self-care deficit and determine probable cause *to plan interventions specific to patient's unique problems.*
- Verbally remind (cue) patient of appropriate activity; demonstrate use of equipment (e.g., toothbrush, hairbrush, washcloth); lay out clothing daily *because memory loss impairs patient's ability to plan and complete specific sequential activities.*
- Continue to assess self-care capabilities and deficits, intervening when necessary, *because self-care abilities fluctuate and interventions must be revised regularly.*
- Toilet and change incontinence brief as scheduled *to prevent discomfort and skin excoriation and promote regularity.*
- Direct patient to feed self or feed patient if necessary *to ensure adequate food and fluid intake.*

NURSING DIAGNOSIS | **Sleep pattern disturbance** *related to* physical discomfort, environmental changes, excessive napping *as manifested by* erratic sleep patterns, nighttime wandering, daytime sleepiness.

- Reasonable periods of uninterrupted rest at appropriate times.

- Monitor patient's sleep pattern or get report from caregiver *to plan appropriate interventions.*
- Ensure that patient's physical needs are met related to bedtime (e.g., patient toileted, comfortable room temperature, quiet environment) *to prevent physical discomfort from interfering with quality sleep.*
- Adapt usual nightly habits such as bedtime, night-lights, warm milk *to provide as much continuity as feasible.*
- Reassure wakened patient and reorient in soft, soothing tone (e.g., "It's nighttime. It is time to go back to bed") *to avoid development of anxiety and fear.*
- Identify and initiate appropriate daytime diversional activities; plan and implement periods of physical activity during the day *because exercise reduces agitation, produces a calming effect, and promotes sleep at night.*

NURSING DIAGNOSIS | **Risk for injury** *related to* impaired judgment, possible gait instability, muscle weakness, and sensory-perceptual alteration.

- No injuries.

- Assess regularly for bruises, abrasions, broken bones, and burns *to determine presence of injury.*
- Monitor activity; maintain environment free from safety hazards *to decrease or prevent occurrence of injury.*
- Assess and record extent of physical limitation (if any) *so appropriate adjustments can be made in care routine and environment.*
- Provide assistance when necessary *so patient's needs are met.*
- Allow freedom in a safe environment *to give the patient a sense of autonomy.*

Continued

56-5 NURSING CARE PLAN PATIENT WITH ALZHEIMER'S DISEASE—continued

| Expected Patient Outcomes | Nursing Interventions and *Rationales* |

NURSING DIAGNOSIS Risk for violence: self or other-directed *related to* sensory overload, misinterpretation of environmental stimuli, lack of appropriate coping mechanisms, and unfamiliar environment.

- No self-directed or other-directed physical trauma.

- Monitor for indicators such as acting-out behavior, verbal threats, and agitation *to identify possibility of violent behavior and initiate appropriate nursing plan.*
- Decrease environmental stimuli; avoid giving patient tasks that prove frustrating *to avoid triggering violent behavior.*
- Ensure adequate sleep and rest periods *because tiredness and exhaustion can provoke violence.*
- Provide opportunities for patient to vent anxiety and frustration; use distraction *to prevent these emotions from escalating to a catastrophic reaction.*
- Observe and document in detail any catastrophic reaction and precipitating events *so interventions can be incorporated into care plan to prevent recurrence.*

NURSING DIAGNOSIS Ineffective individual coping *related to* depression in response to diagnosis of Alzheimer's disease *as manifested by* depression, withdrawal, fatigue, social isolation.

- Feeling valued as an individual.

- Assess for possibility and extent of depression *to develop appropriate interventions.*
- Provide opportunity for patient to verbalize feelings *to help clarify issues and show a caring attitude.*
- Facilitate communication between patient and family *to foster mutual understanding about relevant issues.*
- Provide appropriate diversional activities *to provide pleasurable activities to relieve depression.*
- Allow patient to make decisions regarding self-care and environment when possible *to increase sense of worth and control.*
- Refer for further evaluation and counseling if indicated.

NURSING DIAGNOSIS Risk for ineffective management of therapeutic regimen *related to* decreasing level of cognitive functioning and memory.

- Care needs met by self or others as condition deteriorates.

- Discuss with patient need to make plans for care as condition deteriorates *to ensure patient's wishes are respected and health needs are met.*
- Assist patient to make lifestyle adjustments such as labeling items and ceasing driving *to compensate for changing cognitive status and to live independently as long as possible.*

◼ Planning

The overall goals are that the patient with Alzheimer's disease will (1) maintain functional ability for as long as possible, (2) be maintained in a safe environment with a minimum of injuries, and (3) have personal care needs met.

◼ Nursing Implementation

Because traumatic brain injury is a risk factor for developing Alzheimer's disease, the nurse should promote safety in physical activities and driving. Depression should be recognized and treated early.

Although there is no current treatment for reversing Alzheimer's disease, there is a need for ongoing monitoring of both the patient with Alzheimer's disease and the patient's caregiver. An important nursing responsibility is to work collaboratively with the patient's physician to manage symptoms effectively as they change over time (see NCP 56-5). The nurse is often responsible for teaching the caregiver to perform the many tasks that are required to manage the care of the patient with Alzheimer's disease. The nurse must consider both the patient with Alzheimer's disease and the caregiver as patients with overlapping but unique problems. To aid in identifying the many problems of the caregiver, a nursing care plan for the caregiver of a person with Alzheimer's disease is presented (NCP 56-6).

Adult day care is one of the options available to the person with Alzheimer's disease. Although programs vary in size, structure, physical environment, and degree of experience of staff, the common goals of all day care programs are to provide respite for the family and a protective environment for the patient.

The middle stage of the disease is probably the most beneficial time for adult day care when the person with Alzheimer's disease can still benefit from stimulating activities that encourage independence and decision making in a protective

56-6 NURSING CARE PLAN CAREGIVER OF THE PATIENT WITH ALZHEIMER'S DISEASE

Expected Patient Outcomes   Nursing Interventions and *Rationales*

NURSING DIAGNOSIS **Caregiver role strain** *related to* grieving the family member's illness, change in role, and unrelieved caregiving *as manifested by* reported inadequate resources to provide care and worry about having to put the family member in a long-term care facility.

- Seeking of appropriate assistance by caregiver.
- Satisfactory care to the person with Alzheimer's disease.

- Assess health status of caregiver *to determine if health planning is needed.*
- Refer for medical evaluation when appropriate.
- Discuss effects of caregiving with the caregiver *to determine status of caregiver and to enable open discussion of needs.*
- Encourage visits from other family members or Alzheimer's support group member *to provide support and relief to caregiver as needed.*
- Acknowledge caregiver's fears of being unable to care for family member *to demonstrate empathy and awareness of this fear.*
- Provide financial or social service referrals *to assist caregiver with planning for long-term care.*
- Counsel and support caregiver if patient is placed in a long-term care facility *to allay guilt and reinforce services the patient now requires.*

NURSING DIAGNOSIS **Social isolation** *related to* diminishing social relationships, behavioral problems of patient with Alzheimer's disease, and underdeveloped social support system *as manifested by* feelings of abandonment and uselessness, behavior changes, inability to make decisions or concentrate.

- Satisfactory contact with significant others or members of a support group.

- Assess past social network and diversional activities *to determine size and scope of network and personal interests.*
- Assess social support system of family and willingness and ability to participate in care *to develop care alternatives.*
- Assist in planning respite care through this system or formal community resources *to enable caregiver to continue with important activities and social contacts.*
- Refer to social services *for realistic appraisal of financial resources for respite care and for linkage to community resources.*
- Provide information regarding available support groups (e.g., Alzheimer's Association) *because these groups can meet socialization, recreational, and educational needs of caregiver.*

NURSING DIAGNOSIS **Anxiety** *related to* uncertain outcome, perceived powerlessness, possible change in role functioning, erratic behavioral patterns of the person with Alzheimer's disease, risk for injury secondary to possible violent reactions of patient, and financial insecurity *as manifested by* tachycardia, hypertension, apprehension, helplessness, fear, irritability, forgetfulness, inability to concentrate.

- Decreased anxiety.
- Sense of control of situation.

- Assess past roles of patient with Alzheimer's disease and of caregiver *to determine extent of role changes required of caregiver.*
- Document changes in role expectations and refer to community resources or provide instruction as needed; assess knowledge of behavioral management techniques and instruct as appropriate; assist caregiver in problem-solving techniques; assist in looking at possible causes of catastrophic reactions, as well as indications of agitation that may indicate their onset, *to ensure that caregiver has skills to manage changing roles and patient status.*
- Refer to appropriate agencies as indicated for complete list of community resources and possible sources of financial aid *to relieve anxiety related to financial insecurity.*

Continued

56-6 NURSING CARE PLAN CAREGIVER OF THE PATIENT WITH ALZHEIMER'S DISEASE—continued

| Expected Patient Outcomes | Nursing Interventions and *Rationales* |

NURSING DIAGNOSIS Altered health maintenance *related to* unrelieved caregiving responsibilities, fatigue, and chronic stress *as manifested by* failure to care for self.

- Optimal health.
- Appropriate health practices for age and sex.

- Assess physical and emotional health status of caregiver *to determine if problem is present and to plan appropriate interventions.*
- Collaborate with caregiver in planning interventions in major identified problem areas *to prevent further deterioration of health.*
- Refer for additional evaluation if indicated.
- Assist with planning of continued care of patient *so that caregiver's personal health needs can be pursued.*
- Stress need for maintaining own health *to avoid increasing the complexity of the caregiving situation.*

NURSING DIAGNOSIS Ineffective family coping *related to* chronic and deteriorating nature of Alzheimer's disease, feelings of helplessness and hopelessness, increasing financial hardship, and disappearing support systems *as manifested by* verbalization of lack of help and hope in caring for family members, concern over finances, deteriorating emotional and physical health of caregiver.

- No evidence of inappropriate coping behaviors.

- Encourage family to discuss caregiving situation with one another *so consensus can be reached regarding plan of care.*
- Provide information on community resources such as day care, support groups, counseling, and respite care *to relieve stress and facilitate coping.*
- Encourage and support family in their caregiving efforts *to persons involved in a difficult situation.*
- Refer for assistance with financial concerns.
- Provide information on nature and course of Alzheimer's disease *so appropriate plans can be made for the patient based on accurate information.*

environment. The patient returns home tired, content, less frustrated, and ready to be with the family. The respite from the demands of care allows the family to be more responsive to the patient's needs.

Although adult day care may delay the transition, the demands on the caregiver eventually exceed the resources, and the person with Alzheimer's disease may be placed in a long-term care facility. Special units to care for persons with Alzheimer's disease are becoming increasingly common in long-term care settings. The nursing care needs of the patient with Alzheimer's disease change as the disease progresses, emphasizing the need for regular assessment, monitoring, and support. Regardless of the setting, the severity of the symptoms and the amount of care required intensify over time.

Patients with Alzheimer's disease are subject to acute and other chronic illnesses. Their inability to communicate health symptoms and problems places the responsibility for assessment and diagnosis on caregivers and health professionals. Hospitalization of the patient with Alzheimer's disease can be a traumatic event for both the patient and the caregiver and can precipitate a worsening of the disease.

Alzheimer's disease is a devastating disease that disrupts all aspects of personal and family life. Support groups for care-

givers and family members have been formed throughout the United States to provide an atmosphere of understanding and to give current information about the disease itself and related topics such as safety, legal, ethical, and financial issues. Nurses often receive personal and professional satisfaction in participating in such support groups.

■ Evaluation

Expected outcomes for the patient with Alzheimer's disease are addressed in NCP 56-5.

RESTLESS LEGS SYNDROME
Etiology and Pathophysiology

Restless legs syndrome (RLS) is characterized by sensory and motor abnormalities of, but not limited to, the legs. It has been estimated that between 3% and 8% of adults in the United States have RLS.[29] Although the exact cause of RLS is not known, there are epidemiologic data to support a genetic component, and it occurs in families. It has been associated with metabolic abnormalities associated with iron deficiency, uremia, or pregnancy. Up to 30% of patients receiving renal dialysis experience RLS. RLS resolves after kidney transplantation, supporting its relationship to uremia.

Clinical Manifestations

The severity of RLS ranges from infrequent minor discomfort to severe pain. Sensory symptoms often appear first and are manifested as an annoying and uncomfortable (but usually not painful) sensation in the legs. The sensation is often compared to the sensation of bugs creeping or crawling on the legs. The leg pain is localized within the calf muscles. Patients can also experience pain in the upper extremities and trunk. The discomfort occurs when the patient is sedentary and usually in the evening or at night. The pain at night can produce sleep disruptions and is often relieved by physical activity such as walking, stretching, rocking, or kicking. In the most severe cases, patients sleep only a few hours at night, resulting in daytime fatigue and disruption of the daily routine. The motor abnormalities associated with RLS consist of voluntary restlessness and stereotyped, periodic, involuntary movements. The involuntary movements usually occur during sleep. Symptoms are aggravated by fatigue. Over time, RLS advances to more frequent and more severe episodes.

Diagnostic Studies

RLS is a clinical diagnosis and is based in large part on the patient's history or the report of the bed partner related to nighttime activities. Polysomnography studies during sleep may be performed for the patient with RLS to distinguish the problem from other clinical conditions (e.g., sleep apnea) that can disturb sleep. The patient's history of diabetes mellitus and its management may provide information to determine whether paresthesias are due to peripheral neuropathy or RLS.

NURSING AND COLLABORATIVE MANAGEMENT: RESTLESS LEGS SYNDROME

The goal of collaborative management is to reduce patient discomfort and distress and to improve sleep quality. When RLS is secondary to uremia or iron deficiency, correction of these conditions will decrease symptoms. Nonpharmacologic approaches to RLS management include establishing regular sleep habits, providing adequate rest periods, encouraging exercise, and avoiding activities that cause symptoms. To promote sleep, caffeinated beverages should be avoided starting in the afternoon.

If nonpharmacologic measures fail to provide symptom relief, drug therapy may be started. The main drugs used in RLS are dopaminergic agents, opioids, and benzodiazepines. Dopaminergic agents such as carbidopa/levodopa (Sinemet) and dopamine agonists (pergolide [Permax], bromocriptine [Parlodel]) are the drugs of choice in treating RLS. These agents are effective in managing sensory and motor symptoms. Dopaminergic agents have a number of side effects, including hypotension and gastric irritation.

Opioids (e.g., oxycodone) in low doses have also been found to be effective in reducing the symptoms associated with RLS. The main side effect of opioids is constipation, so the patient may need to take a stool softener or laxative. Other agents that may be used include antiseizure medications such as gabapentin (Neurontin), divalproex (Depakote), lamotrigine (Lamictal), and carbamazepine (Tegretol).

OTHER NEUROLOGIC DISORDERS

AMYOTROPHIC LATERAL SCLEROSIS

Amyotrophic lateral sclerosis (ALS) is a rare progressive neurologic disorder characterized by loss of motor neurons. ALS usually leads to death within 2 to 6 years after diagnosis. This disease became known as Lou Gehrig's disease when the famous baseball player was stricken with it in the early 1940s. The onset is between 40 and 70 years of age, and two times as many men as women are affected.

For unknown reasons, motor neurons in the brainstem and spinal cord gradually degenerate in ALS (Fig. 56-8). The dead motor neuron cannot produce or transport vital signals to muscle. Consequently, electrical and chemical messages originating in the brain do not reach the muscles to activate them.

The primary symptoms are weakness of the upper extremities, dysarthria, and dysphagia. Muscle wasting and fasciculations result from the denervation of the muscles and lack of stimulation and use. Death usually results from respiratory infection secondary to compromised respiratory function. Unfortunately, there is no cure for ALS. Riluzole (Rilutek) was approved in 1997 to slow the progression of ALS.[30,31] This drug works to decrease the amount of glutamate (an excitatory neurotransmitter) in the brain. It was shown to delay the need for tracheostomy and to delay death by a few months in clinical trials.

The illness trajectory for ALS is devastating because the patient remains cognitively intact while wasting away. The challenge of nursing care is to support the patient's cognitive and emotional functions by facilitating communication, providing diversional activities such as reading and human companionship, and helping the person and family with advance care planning and anticipatory grieving related to loss of motor function and ultimately death.

HUNTINGTON'S DISEASE

Huntington's disease (HD) is a genetically transmitted, autosomal dominant disorder that affects both men and women of all races. The offspring of a person with this disease have a 50% risk of inheriting it. The diagnosis often occurs after the affected individual has had children. In the United States the incidence of HD is 1 in 15,000. Diagnosis in the past was based on family history and clinical symptoms. However, since the gene for HD has been discovered, one now can be tested for presence of the gene. People who are asymptomatic but who have a positive family history of HD face the dilemma of whether or not to get tested. If the test is positive, the person will develop HD, but when and to what extent the disease develops cannot be determined.

Like Parkinson's disease, the pathology of HD involves the basal ganglia and the extrapyramidal motor system. However, instead of a deficiency of DA, HD involves a deficiency of the

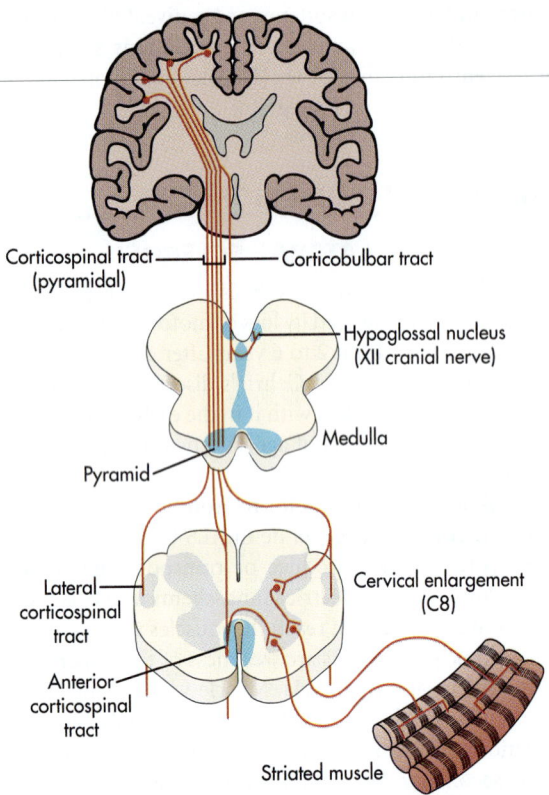

Fig. 56-8 Pathogenesis of amyotrophic lateral sclerosis. This disease is characterized by degeneration of the pyramidal tract and the motor cells in the anterior gray horns. In cases with corticobulbar involvement, the motor nuclei of cranial nerves V, VII, IX, X, XI, and XII also undergo degeneration.

neurotransmitters ACh and GABA. The net effect is an excess of DA, which leads to symptoms that are the opposite of those of parkinsonism. The clinical manifestations, the onset of which is between 35 and 45 years of age, are characterized by abnormal and excessive involuntary movements (chorea). These are writhing, twisting movements of the face, limbs, and body. The movements get worse as the disease progresses. Facial movements involving speech, chewing, and swallowing are affected and may cause aspiration and malnutrition. The gait deteriorates, and ambulation eventually becomes impossible. Perhaps the most devastating deterioration is in mental functions, which include intellectual decline, emotional lability, and psychotic behavior. Death usually occurs 10 to 20 years after the onset of symptoms.

Because there is no cure, collaborative care is palliative. Antipsychotic, antidepressant, and antichorea medications are prescribed and have some benefit. However, they do not alter the course of the disease. Surgical procedures involving transplantation of fetal striatal neural tissues are performed at some medical centers.[32] This disease presents a great challenge to health care professionals. The goal of nursing management is to provide the most comfortable environment possible for the patient and the family by maintaining physical safety, treating the physical symptoms, and providing emotional and psychologic support. Because of the choreic movements, caloric requirements are high. Patients may require as high as 4000 to 5000 calories per day to maintain body weight. As the disease progresses, meeting caloric needs becomes a greater challenge when the patient has difficulty swallowing and holding the head still. Depression and mental deterioration can also compromise nutritional intake.

CRITICAL THINKING EXERCISES

CASE STUDY

Multiple Sclerosis

Patient Profile

Ms. S., a 32-year-old Caucasian woman, born and raised in Minneapolis, was diagnosed with multiple sclerosis after an episode of numbness and tingling on the left side of her body. Two years ago she had an episode of optic neuritis in the right eye.

Subjective Data

- Difficulty seeing out of the right eye
- Numbness and tingling on the left side that worsens in hot weather
- Tires easily
- Used all sick days at work; concerned about losing her job and ability to care for 3-year-old son

Objective Data

Physical Examination
- Crying softly during interview
- Tense and anxious

Diagnostic Studies
- Prolonged visual evoked response in right eye
- MRI scan of head shows several plaques in white matter

Critical Thinking Questions

1. What is the pathogenesis of multiple sclerosis?
2. What precipitating factors for multiple sclerosis are present in Ms. S.'s life?
3. Why did it take so long for a definitive diagnosis to be made for Ms. S.?
4. What teaching plan should be developed for Ms. S.?
5. What treatment would be appropriate for Ms. S.?
6. Write one or more appropriate nursing diagnoses based on the assessment data presented. Are there any collaborative problems?

NURSING RESEARCH ISSUES

1. What kinds of physical activity can enhance functioning and well-being in patients with multiple sclerosis and Parkinson's disease?
2. How can caregivers of patients with Alzheimer's disease be helped to deal with their situation?
3. What are the most effective ways to assist patients with chronic neurologic problems to maintain a positive self-esteem?
4. What factors influence the quality of life for patients with epilepsy?
5. What can be done to promote self-efficacy in patients with chronic neurologic conditions?

REVIEW QUESTIONS

The number of the question corresponds to the same-numbered objective at the beginning of the chapter.

1. The emotional responses of the patient with a chronic neurologic disease are often
   a. symptoms of intellectual deterioration.
   b. absent in patients with cognitive impairment.
   c. a result of physical disability and changes in body image.
   d. reduced in patients who have family members to care for them.

2. The nurse plans care for the patient with a migraine headache based on the knowledge that during a migraine the patient is most likely to
   a. withdraw from stimuli.
   b. act out with bizarre behavior.
   c. seek out the company of others.
   d. experience painful facial spasms and tearing.

3. The triad of symptoms the nurse would expect to find during assessment of the patient with Parkinson's disease is
   a. spasticity, diplopia, tremor.
   b. tremor, rigidity, bradykinesia.
   c. ataxia, drowsiness, dysarthria.
   d. diplopia, tremor, bradykinesia.

4. Nursing intervention for the patient with MS is aimed at management of
   a. incontinence, tremor, seizures.
   b. chorea and mental deterioration.
   c. incontinence, depression, spasticity.
   d. intercostal muscle weakness and impaired swallowing.

5. During assessment of the patient with ALS the nurse would expect to find
   a. muscle wasting.
   b. emotional lability.
   c. mental deterioration.
   d. sensory loss in the extremities.

6. The nurse plans interventions for patients with chronic neurologic disease knowing that the most common cause of death in these patients as a result of their immobility is
   a. suicide.
   b. malnutrition.
   c. physical injury.
   d. respiratory infection.

7. A major goal of treatment for the patient with a chronic, progressive neurologic disease is
   a. reversal of pathophysiology.
   b. continuation of usual lifestyle.
   c. total remission of the disease.
   d. adjustment by patient and family to the disease.

References

1. Lipton RB, Stewart WF, Von Korff M: Burden of migraine: societal costs and therapeutic opportunities, *Neurology* 48(suppl 3):S4, 1997.
2. Goadsby PJ: Current concepts of the pathophysiology of migraine, *Neurol Clin* 15:27, 1997.
3. Kudrow L: Cluster headache and paroxysmal hemicrania. In Samuels M, Feske S, editors: *Office practice of neurology*, New York, 1996, Churchill Livingstone.
4. Blau JN: The effect of national lifestyles, *Cephalalgia* 18:23, 1998.
5. Hauser A: Epidemiology of seizure disorders and the epilepsies. In Santilli N, editor: *Managing seizure disorders*, Philadelphia, 1996, Lippincott-Raven.
6. Gastaut H: Clinical and electroencephalographical classification of epileptic seizures, *Epilepsia* 11:102, 1970.
7. Commission on Classification and Terminology of the International League Against Epilepsy: Proposal for the revised clinical and electroencephalographic classification of epileptic seizures, *Epilepsia* 22:249, 1981.
8. Behrens E and others: Surgical and neurological complications in a series of 708 epilepsy surgery procedures, *Neurosurgery* 41:1, 1997.
9. Health Information, National Institute of Neurological Disorders and Stroke, Bethesda, Md, NIH, 1998.
10. Lublin FD, Reingold SC: Defining the clinical course of multiple sclerosis, *Neurology* 46:907, 1996.
11. Confavreux C and others: Rates of pregnancy-related relapse in multiple sclerosis, *N Engl J Med* 339:285, 1998.
12. Khan OA, Hebel JR: Incidence of exacerbations in the first 90 days of treatment with recombinant human interferon beta-1b in patients with relapsing-remitting multiple sclerosis, *Ann Neurol* 44:138, 1998.
13. Edwards S and others: Clinical relapses and disease activity on magnetic resonance imaging associated with viral upper respiratory infections in multiple sclerosis, *J Neurol Neurosurg Psychiatry* 64:736, 1998.
14. Sudarsky LR: Parkinson's disease: recognition, diagnosis and management. In Samuels M, Feske S, editors: *Office practice of neurology*, New York, 1996, Churchill Livingstone.
15. Calne DB: Diagnosis and treatment of Parkinson's disease, *Hosp Pract* 30:83, 1995.
16. Scharre DW, Mahler ME: Parkinson's disease: making the diagnosis, selecting drug therapies, *Geriatrics* 49:14, 1994.
17. Schrag AE and others: The safety of ropinirole, a selective nonergoline dopamine agonist, in patients with Parkinson's disease, *Clin Neuropharmacol* 21:169, 1998.
18. Dooley M, Markham A: Pramipexole. A review of its use in the management of early and advanced Parkinson's disease, *Drugs Aging* 12:495, 1998.
19. Lozano AM, Lang AE: Pallidotomy for Parkinson's disease, *Neurosurg Clin North Am* 9:325, 1998.
20. Hariz GM and others: Assessment of ability/disability in patients treated with chronic thalamic stimulation for tremor, *Mov Disord* 13:78, 1998.
21. Lindvall O: Update on fetal transplantation: the Swedish experience, *Mov Disord* 13:83, 1998.
22. Fink JS: Transplantation in Parkinson's disease, *Artif Organs* 21:1199, 1997.
23. Urschel JD, Grewal RP: Thymectomy for myasthenia gravis, *Postgrad Med J* 74:139, 1998.
24. Lewis RA, Selwa JF, Lisak RP: Myasthenia gravis: immunological mechanisms and immunotherapy, *Ann Neurol* (suppl 1):S51, 1995.
25. Roses AD: Alzheimer's disease: the genetics of risk, *Hosp Pract* 33:51, 1997.
26. Smith AL, Whitehouse PJ: Progress in the management of Alzheimer's disease, *Hosp Pract* 34:151, 1998.
27. Adair JC: Is it Alzheimer's? *Hosp Pract* 34:35, 1998.
28. Kettl PA: Alzheimer's disease: an update, *Hosp Med* 33:12, 1997.
29. Hening WA: Restless legs syndrome: diagnosis and treatment, *Hosp Med* 33:54, 1997.
30. Miller RG: New approaches to therapy of amyotrophic lateral sclerosis, *West J Med* 168:262, 1998.
31. Riviere M and others: An analysis of extended survival in patients with amyotrophic lateral sclerosis treated with riluzole, *Arch Neurol* 55:526, 1998.
32. Kopyov OV and others: Safety of intrastriatal neurotransplantation for Huntingon's disease patients, *Exp Neurol* 149:97, 1998.

Resources

Alzheimer's Association
919 North Michigan Avenue, Suite 1000
Chicago, IL 60611-1676
312-335-8700
800-272-3900
Fax: 312-335-1110
http://www.alz.org

Alzheimer's Disease and Related Disorders Association
4709 Golf Road, Suite 1015
Skokie, IL 60076
708-933-1000

Alzheimer's Disease Education and Referral Center
ADEAR Center
PO Box 8250
Silver Spring, MD 20907-8250
800-438-4380
Fax: 301-495-3334
http://www.radiospace.com/adear.htm

Alzheimers.com
http://www.alzheimers.com/

American Association of Neuroscience Nurses (AANN)
218 North Jefferson Street, #204
Chicago, IL 60606
312-993-0043
http://www.aann.org/

Association of Rehabilitation Nurses
5700 Old Orchard Road, First Floor
Skokie, IL 60077
708-966-8673
Fax: 708-966-9418

Epilepsy Foundation
4351 Garden City Drive, 5th Floor
Landover, MD 20785-2267
301-459-3700
800-EFA-1000
Fax: 301-577-2684
http://www.efa.org

Huntington's Disease Society of America, Inc.
140 West 22nd Street, 6th Floor
New York, NY 10011-2420
212-242-1968
800-345-4372
Fax: 212-243-2443

Myasthenia Foundation
222 South Riverside Plaza
Suite 1540
Chicago, IL 60606-9524
312-258-0522
800-541-5454

National Foundation for Brain Research
1250 24th Street NW, Suite 300
Washington, DC 20037
202-293-5453
202-466-0585
http://www.brainnet.org/

National Headache Foundation
5252 Northwestern Avenue
Chicago, IL 60625
800-843-2256
Fax: 312-907-6278
http://www.headaches.org

National Institute of Neurological and Communicative Disorders and
  Stroke
Building 31, Room 8A52
9000 Rockville Pike
Bethesda, MD 20892
301-496-9746

National Multiple Sclerosis Society
800-Fight-MS (800-344-4867)
733 Third Avenue
New York, NY 10017
http://www.nmss.org/

National Parkinson Foundation, Inc.
1501 NW 9th Avenue/Bob Hope Road
Miami, FL 33136
305-547-6666
800-327-4545
Fax: 305-243-4403
http://www.parkinson.org

Parkinson's Disease Foundation
William Black Medical Research Building
Columbia Presbyterian Medical Center
650 West 168th Street
New York, NY 10032
212-923-4700

Restless Legs Foundation
4410 19th Street NW
Suite 201
Rochester, MN 55901-6624

For additional Internet resources, see the website for this book at
www.mosby.com/MERLIN/medsurg_lewis

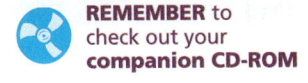

57

NURSING MANAGEMENT
Peripheral Nerve and Spinal Cord Problems

Diane H. Michalec

www.mosby.com/MERLIN/medsurg_lewis

LEARNING OBJECTIVES

1. Explain the etiology, clinical manifestations, collaborative care, and nursing management of trigeminal neuralgia and Bell's palsy.
2. Explain the etiology, clinical manifestations, collaborative care, and nursing management of Guillain-Barré syndrome, botulism, tetanus, and neurosyphilis.
3. Identify the population at risk for spinal cord injuries.
4. Describe the classification of spinal cord injuries and associated clinical manifestations.
5. Describe the clinical manifestations, collaborative care, and nursing management of spinal cord shock.

6. Correlate the clinical manifestations of spinal cord injury with the level of disruption and rehabilitation potential.
7. Describe the nursing management of the major physical and psychologic problems of the patient with a spinal cord injury.
8. Explain the types, clinical manifestations, collaborative care, and nursing management of spinal cord tumors.
9. Describe the effects of spinal cord injury on the older adult population.

CRANIAL NERVE DISORDERS

Cranial nerve disorders are commonly classified as peripheral neuropathies. The 12 pairs of cranial nerves are considered the peripheral nerves of the brain. The disorders usually involve the motor or sensory (or both) branches of a single nerve (*mononeuropathies*). Causes of cranial nerve problems include tumors, trauma, infections, inflammatory processes, and idiopathic (unknown) causes. Two cranial nerve disorders are trigeminal neuralgia (tic douloureux) and acute peripheral facial paralysis (Bell's palsy).

TRIGEMINAL NEURALGIA
Etiology and Pathophysiology

Trigeminal neuralgia (tic douloureux) is a relatively uncommon cranial nerve disorder with an estimated prevalence of 155 cases per million persons.[1] It is more commonly seen in women and usually begins in the fifth or sixth decade of life, but it may occur at any age. The trigeminal nerve is the fifth cranial nerve (CN V) and has both motor and sensory branches. The sensory branches are involved in trigeminal neuralgia, primarily the maxillary and mandibular branches (Fig. 57-1).[2]

Although no specific cause has been identified, major initiating pathologic events may include nerve compression by tor-

tuous arteries of the posterior fossa blood vessels, demyelinating plaques, herpes virus infection, infection of teeth and jaw, and a brainstem infarct.[3] The effectiveness of antiseizure drug therapy may be related to the ability of these drugs to stabilize the neuronal membrane and decrease paroxysmal afferent impulses of the nerve.[4]

Clinical Manifestations

The classic feature of trigeminal neuralgia is an abrupt onset of paroxysms of excruciating pain described as a burning, knifelike, or lightninglike shock in the lips, upper or lower gums, cheek, forehead, or side of the nose. Intense pain, twitching, grimacing, and frequent blinking and tearing of the eye occur during the acute attack (giving rise to the term *tic*). The attacks are usually brief, lasting only seconds to 2 or 3 minutes, and are generally unilateral. Recurrences are unpredictable; they may occur several times a day or weeks or months apart. After the refractory (pain-free) period, a phenomenon known as *clustering* can occur. Clustering is characterized by a cycle of pain and refractoriness that continues for hours.

The painful episodes are usually initiated by a triggering mechanism of light cutaneous stimulation at a specific point (*trigger zone*) along the distribution of the nerve branches. Precipitating stimuli include chewing, teeth brushing, a hot or cold blast of air on the face, washing the face, yawning, or even talking. Touch and tickle seem to predominate as causative triggers rather than pain or changes in temperature. As a result, the patient may eat improperly, neglect hygienic practices, wear a cloth over the face, and withdraw from interaction with other

Reviewed by Patricia A. Blissett, RN, MSN, CCRN, CNRN, CCM, Staff Nurse, Neurosurgical Intensive Care Unit, Harborview Medical Center, Seattle, Wash.

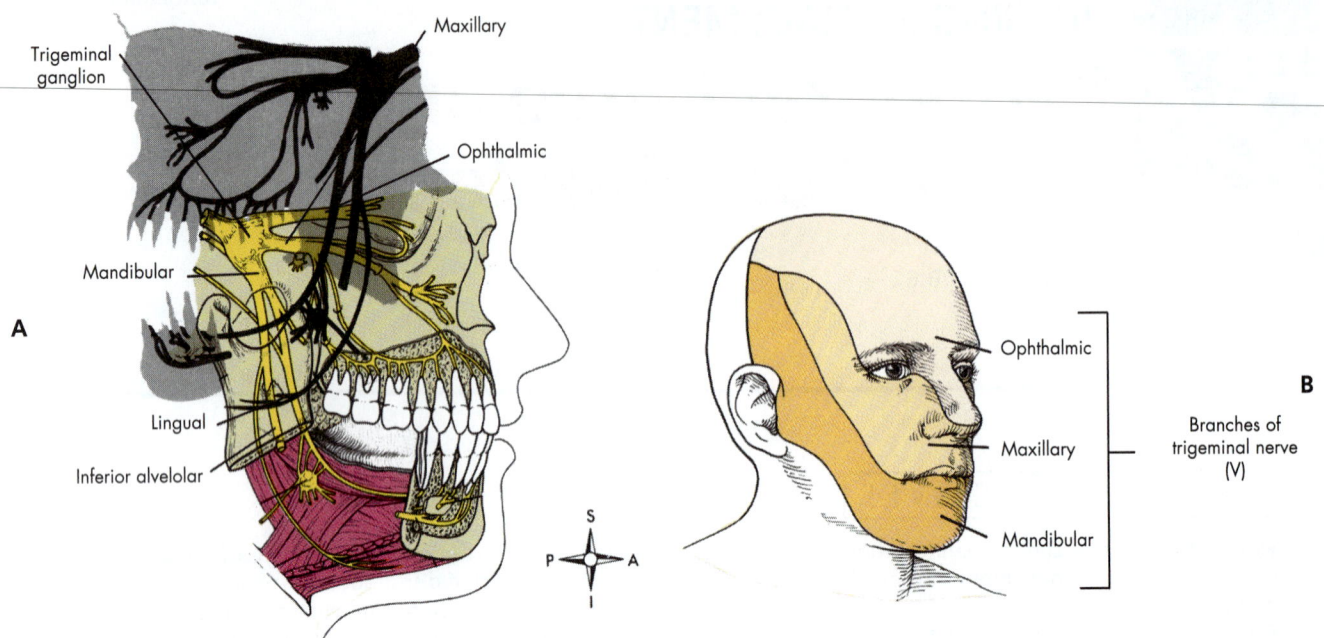

Fig. 57-1   A, Trigeminal (fifth cranial nerve and its three main divisions, the ophthalmic, maxillary, and mandibular nerves). **B,** Cutaneous innervation of the head.

COLLABORATIVE CARE

Table 57-1   Trigeminal Neuralgia

Diagnostic
  History and physical examination
  Brain or CT scan
  Audiologic evaluation
  EMG
  CSF analysis
  Arteriography
  Posterior myelography
  MRI

Collaborative Therapy
  Drug therapy (e.g., phenytoin [Dilantin] carbamazepine
    [Tegretol], valproic acid [Depakene])
  Local nerve blocking
  Biofeedback
  Surgical intervention (see Table 57-2)

CT, computed tomography; *CSF,* cerebrospinal fluid; *EMG,* electromyography; *MRI,* magnetic resonance imaging.

individuals. The patient may sleep excessively as a means of coping with the pain.

Although this condition is considered benign, the severity of the pain and the disruption of lifestyle can result in almost total physical and psychologic dysfunction or even suicide.

Diagnostic Studies

It is important to rule out other problems with similar manifestations, such as other forms of facial and cephalic neuralgias and pain arising from the sinuses, teeth, and jaws. In young patients with bilateral facial pain, a CT scan is performed to rule out any lesions or vascular abnormalities and a lumbar puncture and an MRI are done to rule out multiple sclerosis. A complete neuro-

logic assessment is done, although results are usually normal. Once the diagnosis is made, the goal of treatment is relief of pain either medically or surgically (Tables 57-1 and 57-2).

Collaborative Care

Drug Therapy. The majority of patients obtain adequate relief through antiseizure drugs such as carbamazepine (Tegretol), phenytoin (Dilantin), and valproate (Depakene). Carbamazepine is the most commonly prescribed. These drugs may prevent an acute attack or promote a remission of symptoms, although the mechanism by which they work is not known. Side effects of carbamazepine may include bone marrow suppression leading to blood abnormalities. Therefore, routine complete blood cell (CBC) counts are required. Because drug therapy may not provide permanent pain relief, some patients may seek continued help by numerous visits to otolaryngologists or from therapies such as acupuncture and megavitamins.

Conservative Therapy. Nerve blocking with local anesthetics is another treatment possibility. Local nerve blocking results in complete anesthesia of the area supplied by the injected branches. Relief of pain is temporary, lasting from 6 to 18 months. This treatment is usually tolerated well by older adults.

Biofeedback is another strategy that may be helpful for some patients. In addition to controlling the pain, the patient may experience a strong sense of personal control by mastering the technique and altering certain body functions.

Surgical Therapy. If a conservative approach is not effective, surgical therapy is available (see Table 57-2). *Percutaneous radiofrequency rhizotomy* (electrocoagulation) and *microvascular decompression* afford the greatest relief of pain. Percutaneous radiofrequency rhizotomy consists of placing a needle into the trigeminal rootlets that are adjacent to the pons and destroying the area by means of a radiofrequency

Table **57-2**	Surgical Interventions for Trigeminal Neuralgia	
Procedure	**Technique**	**Benefit**
Peripheral		
Glycerol injection into one or more branches of the trigeminal nerve	Chemical ablation	Total pain relief with sparing of touch and corneal reflex
Intracranial		
Retrogasserian rhizotomy	Temporal craniotomy (sectioning of sensory root in middle cranial fossa)	Permanent anesthesia (with adeptness, corneal reflex, touch)
Suboccipital craniotomy	Sectioning of sensory root of posterior fossa	Permanent anesthesia
Percutaneous radiofrequency rhizotomy	Destruction of sensory fibers by low-voltage current	Total pain relief, sparing of touch and corneal reflex (increased risk for sensory changes)
Microvascular decompression (Jannetta procedure)	Lifting of artery pressing on nerve root in posterior fossa with wedge of sponge, leading to removal of pressure at nerve-root entry zone or removing the involved vessel	Pain relief without loss of sensation
Gamma knife radiosurgery	Technique that uses high doses of radiation focused on the trigeminal nerve root using stereotactic localization	Pain relief 1 day to 4 months post-treatment; noninvasive; no loss of sensation

current. This can result in anesthesia of the face (although some degree of sensation may be retained) or trigeminal motor weakness. Irritation or inadvertent destruction of the ophthalmic branches of the nerve can result in loss of the corneal reflex. This procedure is easily performed with minimal risk to the patient and is based on the exchange of pain for numbness. It is tolerated well by older adults and avoids a major operative procedure in the high risk patient.[5]

Microvascular decompression of the trigeminal nerve is the most commonly used procedure for neuralgia. It is accomplished by displacing and repositioning blood vessels that appear to be compressing the nerve at the root-entry zone where it exits the pons. This procedure relieves pain without residual sensory loss, but it is potentially dangerous, as is any surgery near the brainstem. Microvascular decompression has a long-term success rate equal to or superior to percutaneous procedures without the higher rate of permanent neurologic sequelae. It is a safe operation with an almost negligible mortality and low morbidity in skilled hands.[6] Approximately 30% of patients experience a recurrence of symptoms within 6 years following surgery.[4]

Glycerol rhizotomy has become more popular in the last 10 years and is preferred over percutaneous radiofrequency rhizotomy. Glycerol rhizotomy consists of an injection of glycerol through the foramen ovale into the trigeminal cistern (Fig. 57-2). Glycerol rhizotomy is a more benign procedure with less sensory loss and fewer sensory aberrations than radiofrequency rhizotomy and with comparable or better pain relief.[7]

Gamma knife radiosurgery is a surgical treatment that is now available for the treatment of trigeminal neuralgia. Radiosurgery using the gamma unit provides precise radiation of the proximal trigeminal nerve identified on high resolution imaging. This image-guided approach has been useful for both patients with persistent pain after other surgeries and as a primary surgical option.[8]

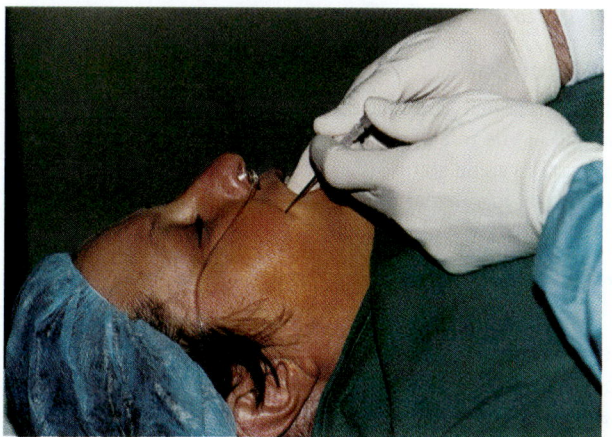

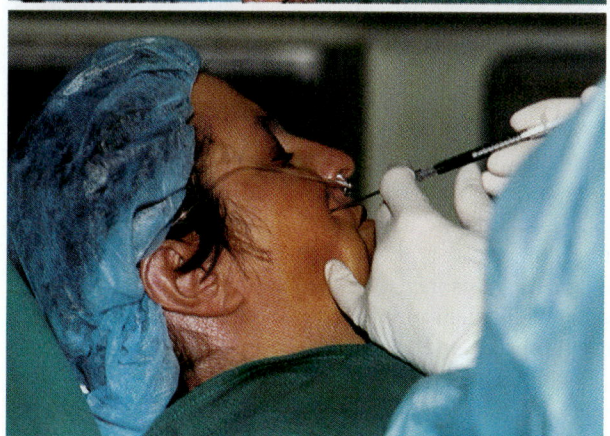

Fig. 57-2 A, Patient with trigeminal neuralgia having needle placed. **B,** Physician injecting glycerol.

NURSING MANAGEMENT: TRIGEMINAL NEURALGIA

■ Nursing Assessment

Assessment of the attacks, including the triggering factors, characteristics, frequency, and pain management techniques, helps the nurse plan for patient care. The nursing assessment should include the patient's nutritional status, hygiene (especially oral), and behavior (including withdrawal). Evaluation of the degree of pain and its effects on the patient's lifestyle, drug history, emotional state, and suicidal tendencies are other important factors.

■ Nursing Diagnoses

Nursing diagnoses for the patient with trigeminal neuralgia include, but are not limited to, the following:

- Pain *related to* inflammation or compression of the trigeminal nerve
- Altered nutrition: less than body requirements *related to* fear of triggering pain by eating or chewing
- Anxiety *related to* uncertainty of timing and initiating event of pain and uncertainty regarding effectiveness of pain-relieving treatments
- Altered oral mucous membrane *related to* unwillingness to practice oral hygiene measures secondary to potential for initiating pain
- Social isolation *related to* anxiety over pain attacks and desire to maintain nonstimulating environment

■ Planning

The overall goals are that the patient with trigeminal neuralgia will (1) be free of pain, (2) maintain adequate nutritional and oral hygiene status, (3) have minimal to no anxiety, and (4) return to normal or previous socialization and occupational activities.

■ Nursing Implementation

Health Promotion. Because the etiology of trigeminal neuralgia remains unknown, health promotion is directed at reducing recurrent episodes in those who have trigeminal neuralgia. Awareness and reduction of triggering events may be possible in some patients.

Acute Intervention. Pain relief is primarily obtained by the administration of the recommended drug therapy. The nurse should monitor the patient's response to therapy and note any side effects. Strong narcotics such as morphine should be used cautiously because of the potential for addiction over time. Alternative pain relief measures, such as biofeedback, should be explored for the patient who is not a surgical candidate and whose pain is not controlled by other therapeutic measures. Careful assessment of pain, including history, pain relief, and drug dependency, can assist in selecting appropriate interventions.

Environmental management is essential during an acute period to lessen triggering stimuli. The room should be kept at an even, moderate temperature and free of drafts. A private room is preferred during an acute period. The nurse must use care to avoid touching the patient's face or jarring the bed. Many patients prefer to carry out their own care, fearing that they will be inadvertently injured by someone else.

The nurse should instruct the patient about the importance of nutrition, hygiene, and oral care and convey understanding if previous neglect is apparent. The nurse should provide lukewarm water and soft cloths or cotton saturated with solutions not requiring rinsing for cleansing the face. A small, soft-bristled toothbrush or a warm mouthwash assist in promoting oral care. Hygiene activities are best carried out when analgesia is at its peak.

The patient will probably not engage in extensive conversation during the acute period. Alternative communication methods such as paper and pencil should be provided.

Food should be high in protein and calories and easy to chew. It should be served lukewarm and offered frequently. The diet should be individualized according to personal, cultural, and religious preferences. When oral intake is sharply reduced and the patient's nutritional status is compromised, a nasogastric tube is inserted on the unaffected side for nasogastric feedings.

The nurse is responsible for instruction related to diagnostic studies to rule out other problems, such as multiple sclerosis, dental or sinus problems, and neoplasms, and for preoperative teaching if surgery is planned. The nurse may also need to reinforce the surgeon's instructions related to postoperative expectations; appropriate teaching of postoperative activities depends on whether a craniotomy or a local procedure is planned. The patient needs to know that he or she will be awake during local procedures so that he or she can cooperate when corneal and ciliary reflexes and facial sensations are checked.

After the operation the patient's pain is compared with the preoperative level. The corneal reflex, extraocular muscles, hearing, sensation, and facial nerve function are evaluated frequently (see Chapter 53). If there is impairment of the corneal reflex, special attention must be paid to eye protection. This includes the use of artificial tears or eye shields. General postoperative nursing care after a craniotomy is appropriate if intracranial surgery is performed. (Nursing care related to craniotomy is discussed in Chapter 54.) Diet and ambulation should be increased according to the patient's progress or specific orders.

After a radiofrequency percutaneous electrocoagulation procedure, an ice pack is applied to the jaw on the operative side for 3 to 5 hours. To avoid injuring the mouth, the patient should not chew on the operative side until sensation has returned.

Ambulatory and Home Care. Regular follow-up care should be planned. The patient needs instruction regarding the dosage and side effects of medications. Although relief of pain may be complete, the patient should be encouraged to keep environmental stimuli to a moderate level and to use stress reduction methods. Herpes simplex infection (cold sores) can occur from manipulation of the gasserian ganglion. Treatment consists of antiviral agents such as acyclovir (see Chapter 22).

Long-term management after surgical intervention depends on the residual effects of the type of procedure. If anesthesia is present or the corneal reflex is altered, the patient should be taught to (1) chew on the unaffected side; (2) avoid hot foods or beverages, which can burn the mucous membranes; (3) check the oral cavity after meals to remove food particles; (4) practice meticulous oral hygiene and continue with semiannual dental visits; (5) protect the face against extremes of temperature; (6) use an electric razor; and (7) wear a protective eye shield.

The patient may have developed protective practices to prevent pain and may need counseling or psychiatric assistance in the readjustment, especially in reestablishing personal relationships. Some patients grieve the loss of the pain, especially if it had a special significance such as relieving guilt or anxiety.

Occasionally patients may have used their pain to manipulate family members and friends and may not adjust after successful relief of pain. Careful management in the rehabilitative period can prevent the patient from claiming continual pain for secondary gain (see Chapter 9).

■ Evaluation

The expected outcomes are that the patient with trigeminal neuralgia will

- report an improvement or relief from pain
- appear more comfortable and less anxious
- have normal facial sensation or expected paresthesias and anesthesias
- return to previous socialization and occupational activities

BELL'S PALSY
Etiology and Pathophysiology

Bell's palsy (peripheral facial paralysis, acute benign cranial polyneuritis) is a disorder characterized by a disruption of the motor branches of the facial nerve (CN VII) on one side of the face in the absence of any other disease such as a stroke. It can affect any age-group, but it is more commonly seen in the 20- to 60-year age range. Incidence rates in the United States are 23 cases per 100,000 persons annually.[9] Although the exact etiology is not known, there is evidence that reactivated herpes simplex virus (HSV) may be involved in the majority of cases.[10] The reactivation of the HSV causes inflammation, edema, ischemia, and eventual demyelination of the nerve, creating pain and alterations in motor and sensory function.

Bell's palsy is considered benign, with full recovery after 6 months in about 85% of patients, especially if treatment is instituted immediately. A small number of patients may have some residual effects. The remaining 15% of patients continue to be bothered by asymmetrical movement of facial muscles.[10]

Clinical Manifestations

The onset of Bell's palsy is often accompanied by an outbreak of herpes vesicles in or around the ear. Patients may complain of pain around and behind the ear. In addition, manifestations may include fever, tinnitus, and hearing deficit. The paralysis of the motor branches of the facial nerve typically results in a flaccidity of the affected side of the face, with drooping of the mouth accompanied by drooling (Fig. 57-3). An inability to close the eyelid, with an upward movement of the eyeball when closure is attempted, is also evident. A widened palpebral fissure (the opening between the eyelids), flattening of the nasolabial fold, and inability to smile, frown, or whistle are also common. Unilateral loss of taste is common. Decreased muscle movement may alter chewing ability, and although some patients may experience a loss of tearing, many patients complain of excessive tearing. The muscle weakness causes the lower lid to turn out, allowing overflow of normal tear production. Pain may be present behind the ear on the affected side, especially before the onset of paralysis. Interventions are primarily supportive until the patient has a return of function.

Complications

Complications can include psychologic withdrawal because of changes in appearance, malnutrition and dehydration, mucous

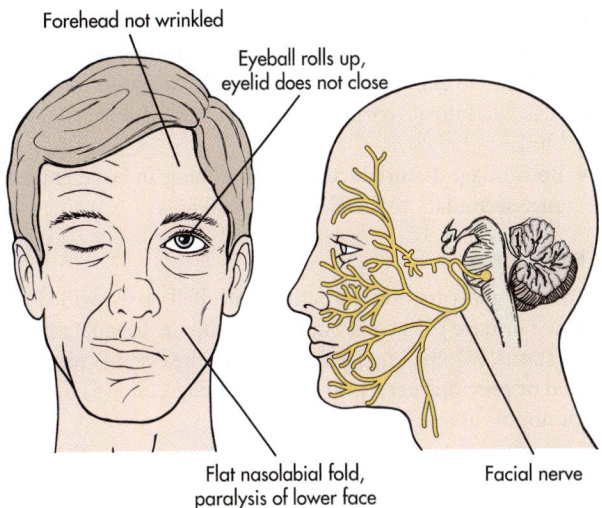

Forehead not wrinkled

Eyeball rolls up, eyelid does not close

Flat nasolabial fold, paralysis of lower face

Facial nerve

Fig. 57-3 Bell's palsy: facial characteristics.

membrane trauma, corneal abrasions, muscle stretching, and facial spasms and contractures.

Diagnostic Studies

The diagnosis of Bell's palsy is one of exclusion. There is no definitive test. The diagnosis and prognosis are indicated by observation of the typical pattern of onset and signs and the testing of percutaneous nerve excitability by electromyogram (EMG).

Collaborative Care

Methods of treatment for Bell's palsy include moist heat, gentle massage, and electrical stimulation of the nerve. Stimulation may maintain muscle tone and prevent atrophy. Care is primarily focused on relief of symptoms and prevention of complications.

Drug Therapy. Corticosteroids, especially prednisone, are started immediately, and the best results are obtained if corticosteroids are initiated before paralysis is complete. When the patient improves to the point that the corticosteroids are no longer necessary, they should be tapered off over a 2 week period. Usually, the corticosteroid treatment decreases the edema and pain, but mild analgesics can be used if necessary. Because the HSV is implicated in approximately 70% of cases of Bell's palsy, treatment with acyclovir (Zovirax), alone or in conjunction with prednisone, are used.[10] Newer drugs to treat HSV, including valacyclovir (Valtrex) and famciclovir (Famvir), have also been used in the management of Bell's palsy.

NURSING MANAGEMENT: BELL'S PALSY
■ Nursing Assessment

Early recognition of the possibility of Bell's palsy is important. Because HSV is a possible etiologic factor, any person who is prone to herpes simplex should be alerted to seek health care if pain occurs in or around the ear. Assessment of facial muscles for any signs of weakness should also be done (see Chapter 53). Careful recording of assessment data provides information related to the progress of the syndrome.

■ Nursing Diagnoses

The nursing diagnoses for the patient with Bell's palsy may include, but are not limited to, the following:

- Pain *related to* the inflammation of CN VII (facial)
- Altered nutrition: less than body requirements *related to* inability to chew secondary to muscle weakness
- Risk for injury (corneal abrasion) *related to* inability to blink
- Body image disturbance *related to* change in facial appearance secondary to facial muscle weakness

■ Planning

The overall goals are that the patient with Bell's palsy will (1) be pain free or have pain controlled, (2) maintain adequate nutritional status, (3) not experience injury to the eye, (4) return to normal or previous perception of body image, and (5) be optimistic about disease outcome.

■ Nursing Implementation

The patient with Bell's palsy does not usually require inpatient hospitalization. The following interventions are used throughout the course of the disease. Mild analgesics can relieve pain. Hot wet packs can reduce the discomfort of herpetic lesions, aid circulation, and relieve pain. The face should be protected from cold and drafts because trigeminal hyperesthesia may accompany the syndrome. Maintenance of good nutrition is important. The patient should be taught to chew on the unaffected side of the mouth to avoid trapping food and to enjoy the taste of food. Thorough oral hygiene must be carried out after each meal to prevent the development of parotitis, caries, and periodontal disease from accumulated residual food.

Dark glasses may be worn for protective and cosmetic reasons. Artificial tears (methylcellulose) should be instilled frequently during the day to prevent drying of the cornea. The eye should be inspected for the presence of eyelashes. Ointment and an impermeable eye shield can be used at night to retain moisture. In some patients, taping the lids closed at night may be necessary to provide protection. The patient is taught to report ocular pain, drainage, or discharge.

A facial sling may be helpful to support affected muscles, improve lip alignment, and facilitate eating. The facial sling is usually made and fitted by a physical or occupational therapist. Vigorous massage can break down tissues, but gentle upward massage has psychologic benefits even if physical effects other than the maintenance of circulation are questionable. When function begins to return, active facial exercises are performed several times a day.

The change in physical appearance as a result of Bell's palsy can be devastating. The patient must be reassured that a stroke did not occur and that chances for a full recovery are good. The patient's need for privacy should be respected, especially during meals, but the nurse's assistance in the patient's adjustment to the physical changes should not be delayed. Enlisting support from family and friends is important. It is important to share with the patient that most patients recover within about 6 weeks of the onset of symptoms.

■ Evaluation

The expected outcomes are that the patient with Bell's palsy

- will be free of pain
- will not experience any complications
- will return to previous perception of body image

POLYNEUROPATHIES

GUILLAIN-BARRÉ SYNDROME

Etiology and Pathophysiology

Guillain-Barré syndrome (Landry-Guillain-Barré-Strohl syndrome, postinfectious polyneuropathy, ascending polyneuropathic paralysis) is an acute, rapidly progressing, and potentially fatal form of polyneuritis. It affects the peripheral nervous system and results in loss of myelin (a segmental demyelination) and edema and inflammation of the affected nerves, causing a loss of neurotransmission to the periphery. With adequate supportive care, 85% of these patients recover completely from this disorder.[11]

The etiology of this disorder is unknown, but it is believed to be a cell-mediated immunologic reaction directed at the peripheral nerves. The syndrome is frequently preceded by immune system stimulation from a viral infection, trauma, surgery, viral immunizations, human immunodeficiency virus (HIV), or lymphoproliferative neoplasms. These stimuli are thought to cause an alteration in the immune system, resulting in sensitization of T lymphocytes to the patient's myelin, causing myelin damage. Demyelination occurs, and the transmission of nerve impulses is stopped or slowed down. The muscles innervated by the damaged peripheral nerves undergo denervation and atrophy. In the recovery phase, remyelination occurs slowly and returns in a proximal to distal pattern. The lymphocytes are basically normal and return to complete functioning after the illness.

The syndrome affects both genders equally and is more commonly seen in adults, although it is observed in all age-groups. Worldwide the incidence has varied from 0.4 to 1.7 cases per 100,000 persons per year. Guillain-Barré syndrome has an estimated annual cost of 2 to 3 billion dollars in the United States.[11]

Clinical Manifestations

Symptoms of Guillain-Barré syndrome usually develop 1 to 3 weeks after an upper respiratory or GI infection. Weakness of the lower extremities (evolving more or less symmetrically) occurs over hours to days to weeks, usually peaking about the fourteenth day. Distal muscles are more severely affected. *Paresthesia* (numbness and tingling) is frequent, and paralysis usually follows in the extremities. Hypotonia and areflexia are common, persistent symptoms. Objective sensory loss is variable, with deep sensitivity more affected than superficial sensations.

Autonomic nervous system dysfunction results from alterations in both the sympathetic and parasympathetic nervous systems. Autonomic disturbances are usually seen in patients with severe muscle involvement and respiratory muscle paralysis. The most dangerous autonomic dysfunctions include orthostatic hypotension, hypertension, and abnormal vagal responses (bradycardia, heart block, asystole). Other autonomic dysfunctions include bowel and bladder dysfunction, facial flushing, and diaphoresis. Patients may also have syndrome of inappropriate antidiuretic hormone (SIADH) secretion. SIADH is discussed further in Chapter 47. Progression of Guillain-Barré syndrome to include the lower brainstem involves the facial, abducens, oculomotor, hypoglossal, trigeminal, and vagus nerves (CN VII, VI, III, XII, V, and X, respectively). This involvement manifests itself through facial weakness, extraocular eye movement difficulties, dysphagia, and paresthesia of the face.

Pain is a common symptom in the patient with Guillain-Barré syndrome. The pain can be categorized as paresthesias, muscular aches and cramps, and hyperesthesias. Pain appears to be worse at night. Narcotics may be indicated for those experiencing severe pain. Pain may lead to a decrease in appetite and may interfere with sleep.

Complications

The most serious complication of this syndrome is respiratory failure, which occurs as the paralysis progresses to the nerves that innervate the thoracic area. Constant monitoring of the respiratory system by checking respiratory rate, depth, forced vital capacity, and negative inspiratory force provides information about the need for immediate intervention including intubation and mechanical ventilation. Respiratory or urinary tract infections (UTIs) may occur. Fever is generally the first sign of infection, and treatment is directed at the infecting organism. Immobility from the paralysis can cause problems such as paralytic ileus, muscle atrophy, deep vein thrombosis, pulmonary emboli, skin breakdown, orthostatic hypotension, and nutritional deficiencies.

Diagnostic Studies

Diagnosis is based primarily on the patient's history and clinical signs. Cerebrospinal fluid (CSF) is normal or has a low protein content initially, but after 7 to 10 days it shows an elevated protein level to 700 mg/dl (7 g/L) (normal protein is 15 to 45 mg/dl; 0.15 to 0.45 g/L) with a normal cell count. Electromyographic (EMG) and nerve conduction studies are markedly abnormal (reduced nerve conduction velocity) in the affected extremities.

Collaborative Care

Management is aimed at supportive care, particularly ventilatory support, during the acute phase. Plasmapheresis is used in the first 2 weeks of Guillain-Barré syndrome. In patients with severe disease treated within 2 weeks of onset, there is a distinct reduction in the length of stay, length of time on ventilator, and time required to resume walking. After 3 weeks of onset little value has been seen in plasmapheresis.[12] IV administration of high-dose immunoglobulin has also shown to be as effective as plasmapheresis and has the advantage of immediate availability and greater safety. Because of the ease of administering immunoglobulin, it is now being used more frequently than plasmapheresis. The costs of the two treatments are comparable.[11] Recovery is accelerated by early institution of plasmapheresis and IV therapy.[13] (Plasmapheresis is discussed in Chapter 12.) Corticosteroids and ACTH are used to suppress the immune response but appear to have little effect on the prognosis or duration of the disease.

Nutritional Therapy. Nutritional intake is compromised in the patient with Guillain-Barré syndrome. During the acute phase, the patient may experience difficulty swallowing because of cranial nerve involvement. Mild dysphagia can be managed by placing the patient in an upright position and flexing the head forward during feeding. For more severe dysphagia, tube feedings may be required. Patients who experience paralytic ileus or intestinal obstruction may require total parenteral nutrition. Later in the course of the disease, motor paralysis or weakness continue to affect the ability to self-feed. The patient's nutritional status, including body weight, serum albumin levels, and calorie counts, must be evaluated at regular intervals.

NURSING MANAGEMENT: GUILLAIN-BARRÉ SYNDROME

■ Nursing Assessment

Assessment of the patient is the most important aspect of nursing care during the acute phase. The nurse must monitor the ascending paralysis, assess respiratory function, monitor arterial blood gases (ABGs), and assess the gag, corneal, and swallowing reflexes during the routine assessment.

Monitoring blood pressure and cardiac rate and rhythm is also important during the acute phase because transient cardiac arrhythmias have been reported. Autonomic dysfunction is common and usually takes the form of bradycardia and arrhythmias. Orthostatic hypotension secondary to muscle atony may occur in severe cases. Vasopressor agents and volume expanders may be needed to treat the low blood pressure.

■ Nursing Diagnoses

Nursing diagnoses for the patient with Guillain-Barré syndrome may include, but are not limited to, the following:

- Inability to sustain spontaneous ventilation *related to* progression of disease process resulting in respiratory muscle paralysis
- Risk for aspiration *related to* dysphagia
- Pain *related to* paresthesias, muscle aches and cramps, and hyperesthesias
- Impaired verbal communication *related to* intubation or paralysis of the muscles of speech
- Fear *related to* uncertain outcome and seriousness of the disease
- Self-care deficits *related to* inability to use muscles to accomplish ADLs

■ Planning

The overall goals are that the patient with Guillain-Barré syndrome will (1) maintain adequate ventilation, (2) be free from aspiration, (3) be pain free or have pain controlled, (4) maintain an acceptable method of communication, (5) maintain adequate nutritional intake, and (6) return to usual physical functioning.

■ Nursing Implementation

The objective of therapy is to support body systems until the patient recovers. Respiratory failure and infection are serious threats. Monitoring the vital capacity and ABGs is essential. If the vital capacity drops to less than 800 ml (<15 ml/kg or two thirds of the patient's normal vital capacity) or the ABGs deteriorate, endotracheal intubation or tracheostomy may be done so that the patient can be mechanically ventilated (see Chapter 63). Meticulous suctioning technique is needed to prevent infection whether the patient has an endotracheal tube or tracheostomy. Thorough bronchial hygiene and chest physiotherapy help clear secretions and prevent respiratory deterioration. If fever develops, sputum cultures should be obtained to identify whether the respiratory tract is the source of the pathogen. Appropriate antibiotic therapy is then initiated.

A communication system must be established with the use of the patient's available abilities. This is extremely difficult if the disease progresses to involvement of the cranial nerves. At the peak of a severe episode the patient may be incapable of communicating. The nurse must explain all procedures before doing them and reassure the patient that muscle function will return.

Urinary retention is common for a few days. Intermittent catheterization is preferred to an indwelling catheter to avoid UTIs. However, for the acutely ill patient receiving a large volume of fluids (>2.5 L/day) indwelling catheterization may be safer to reduce overdistention of a temporarily flaccid bladder and to prevent vesicoureteral reflux. Physiotherapy is indicated early to help prevent problems related to immobility. Passive range-of-motion exercises and attention to body position help maintain function and prevent contractures. Patients who develop facial paralysis must receive meticulous eye care to avoid cornea irritation or damage (exposure keratitis).[13] Artificial tears should be instilled frequently during the day to prevent drying of the cornea. The eyes should be inspected for the presence of eyelashes. Ointment and an impermeable eye shield can be used at night to retain moisture.

Nutritional needs must be met in spite of possible problems associated with delayed gastric emptying, paralytic ileus, and potential for aspiration if the gag reflex is lost. In addition to checking for the gag reflex, nurses should note drooling and other difficulties with secretions, which may be more indicative of an inadequate gag reflex. Initially, tube feedings or parenteral nutrition may be used to ensure adequate caloric intake. Because of delayed gastric emptying, residual volumes of the feedings should be assessed at regular intervals or before feedings (see Chapter 38). Fluid and electrolyte therapy must be monitored carefully to prevent electrolyte imbalances. A bowel program should be initiated because constipation is a common problem related to diet changes, immobility, and decreased GI motility.

Throughout the course of the illness, the nurse needs to provide support and encouragement to the family and patient. Because residual problems and relapses are uncommon except in the chronic form of the disease, complete recovery can be anticipated although it is generally a slow process that takes months or years if axonal degeneration occurs.

BOTULISM
Etiology and Pathophysiology

Botulism is the most serious type of food poisoning. It is caused by GI absorption of the neurotoxin produced by *Clostridium botulinum*. This organism is found in the soil, and the spores are difficult to destroy. It can grow in any food contaminated with the spores. Improper home canning of foods is often the cause. It is thought that the neurotoxin destroys or inhibits the neurotransmission of acetylcholine at the myoneural junction, resulting in disturbed muscle innervation.

Clinical Manifestations

Symptoms are usually nausea, vomiting, and abdominal cramps, generally within 6 to 48 hours after consumption of the contaminated food. Neurologic manifestations develop rapidly over 2 to 4 days. They include difficulty in convergence of the eyes, photophobia, ptosis, paralysis of extraocular muscles, blurred vision, diplopia, dry mouth, sore throat, and difficulty in swallowing. Other manifestations include paralytic ileus, mild muscle weakness, seizures, and respiratory symptoms that can rapidly deteriorate to respiratory arrest and/or cardiac arrest. The course of the disease depends on the amount of toxin absorbed from the gut. If only a small amount is absorbed, symptoms are mild and recovery is complete. When large amounts are absorbed, death usually occurs in 4 to 8 days from circulatory failure, respiratory paralysis, or development of pulmonary complications.[14]

Because botulism is a reportable disease, local, state, and federal health agencies, particularly the Centers for Disease Control in Atlanta, must be notified.

Diagnostic Studies

Blood and CSF are obtained for studies to rule out other diseases. However, in botulism the blood and CSF results are normal.

Collaborative Care

Drug Therapy. The initial treatment of botulism is IV administration of botulinum antitoxin. Before administration of the antitoxin, an intradermal test dose for sensitivity to horse serum is given. If there are no reactions, the test dose is followed by daily doses of 50,000 units of botulism antitoxin IM until improvement begins.[11]

The GI tract is purged by laxatives, high colonic enemas, and gastric lavage to decrease the absorption of the toxin. Prophylactic penicillin may be ordered to halt the release of toxin in the GI tract.[15]

NURSING MANAGEMENT: BOTULISM
■ Nursing Implementation

Primary prevention is the goal of nursing management through educating consumers to be alert to situations that may result in botulism. Particular attention should be given to foods with a low acid content, which support germination and the production of botulin, a deadly poison. These foods include fish, vichyssoise, and peppers. All varieties of spores are destroyed by boiling for 10 minutes or maintaining a temperature of 176° F (80° C) for 30 minutes. Specific suggestions related to the preparation, storage, and use of food include the following:[11]

1. In home canning, the equipment manufacturer's directions should be followed. Only fresh fruits and vegetables (with all questionable spots removed) should be used. All containers and utensils must be cleansed, and the seal on the can or jar must be airtight. Canned foods should be stored properly in a cool, dry place.
2. A can with a swollen end should never be used; the swelling may be caused by gases from *Clostridium botulinum.*
3. If the food is forcefully expelled when a container is opened, it should be discarded immediately and the contents should not be tasted.
4. If the contents of a can look or smell bad after opening, the can should be discarded without tasting of the contents. Materials may be flushed down the toilet or disposed of in the garbage disposal if a large amount of water is used.

Nursing care during the acute illness is similar to that for Guillain-Barré syndrome. Supportive nursing interventions include rest, activities to maintain respiratory function, adequate nutrition, and prevention of loss of muscle mass. Because the recovery process is slow, the patient may develop problems related to a feeling of helplessness, boredom, and low morale.

TETANUS

Etiology and Pathophysiology

Tetanus (lockjaw) is an extremely severe polyradiculitis and polyneuritis affecting spinal and cranial nerves. It results from the effects of a potent neurotoxin released by the anaerobic bacillus *Clostridium tetani*. The toxin interferes with the function of the reflex arc by blocking of inhibitory transmitters at the presynaptic sites in the spinal cord and brainstem.[11] The spores of the bacillus are present in soil, garden mold, and manure. Thus *Clostridium tetani* enters the body through a traumatic or suppurative wound that provides an appropriate low-oxygen environment for the organisms to mature and produce toxin. Other possible sources include dental infection, injections of heroin, human and animal bites, frostbite, compound fractures, and gunshot wounds. The incubation period is usually 7 days but can range from 3 to 21 days, with symptoms frequently appearing after the original wound is healed. In general, the longer the incubation period, the milder the illness and the better the prognosis.

Worldwide the number of cases per year is estimated to be 1 million. Most victims are neonates born to unimmunized mothers in developing countries. In the United States about 100 to 200 cases occur each year and are due to infection of puncture wounds of the extremities by nails or splinters.[15] Of those reported cases the majority of patients are over the age of 59 years, suggesting inadequate immunization among older adults.[16] Mortality rates vary according to age, with infants and persons more than 50 years of age most seriously affected. Overall mortality rates range from 45% to 55%.

Clinical Manifestations

Manifestations of generalized tetanus include a feeling of stiffness in the jaw (*trismus*) or neck, slight fever, and other symptoms of general infection. Generalized tonic spasms occur because of the lack of reciprocal innervation. As the disease progresses, the neck muscles, back, abdomen, and extremities become progressively rigid. In severe forms, continuous tonic convulsions may occur with *opisthotonos* (extreme arching of the back and retraction of the head). Laryngeal and respiratory spasms cause apnea and anoxia. Additional effects are manifested by overstimulation of the sympathetic nervous system, including profuse diaphoresis, labile hypertension, episodic tachycardia, hyperthermia, and arrhythmias. The slightest noise, jarring motion, or bright light can set off the seizure. These seizures are agonizingly painful. Mortality is almost 100% in the severe form. Death is usually attributable to asphyxia or heart failure, the result of constantly recurring spasms. Residual injury, such as vertebral fracture, muscle contracture, and brain damage secondary to hypoxia, may be long-term consequences.

Collaborative Care

Serum electrolytes, CBC count, albumin, clotting factors, glucose, and ABGs are monitored. Cardiac function is monitored by electrocardiogram (ECG) and auscultation. As increasing numbers of nerve cells become involved, their inhibitory control over muscle activity decreases and symptoms develop.

Drug Therapy. The management of tetanus includes administration of tetanus toxoid booster (Td) and tetanus immune globulin (TIG) before the onset of symptoms to neutralize circulating toxins (see Table 64-8). Control of spasms is essential and is managed by deep sedation, usually with diazepam (Valium), barbiturates, or chlorpromazine (Thorazine). Chlorpromazine is also helpful in reducing hyperthermia. A 10-day course of penicillin is recommended to inhibit further growth of the organism.

Because of laryngospasm, a tracheostomy is usually performed early and the patient is maintained on mechanical ventilation. If sedation does not control seizures, skeletal muscle–paralyzing drugs such as d-tubocurarine (curare) are used. Pain is relieved by means of codeine or meperidine, often with the addition of promethazine (Phenergan). Any recognized wound should be debrided or an abscess drained. Antibiotics may be given to prevent secondary infections.

Nutrition is maintained through parenteral nutrition or nasogastric feeding. Even with the best of care, the mortality rate is 50%. Those who recover have a long convalescence that includes extensive physiotherapy.

NURSING MANAGEMENT: TETANUS

■ Nursing Implementation

Health teaching is aimed at ensuring tetanus prophylaxis, which is the most important factor influencing the incidence of this disease. Tetanus prevention and immunization protocols are summarized in Table 64-8. The patient should be taught that immediate, thorough cleansing of all wounds with soap and water is important in the prevention of tetanus. If an open wound occurs and the patient has not been immunized within 10 years, the primary care provider should be contacted so that a tetanus booster can be given.

If equine tetanus antitoxin is to be used, the patient should be tested for sensitivity. Administration of equine antitoxin is not recommended if sensitivity occurs; anaphylactic shock is potentially life threatening and desensitization is ineffective. The side effects of routine administration of the antitoxin are mild and include a sore arm, swelling at the site, and itching. Serious side effects rarely occur. Routine administration of a booster shot to an adequately immunized patient can cause arm swelling and lymphadenopathy.

Every patient should receive a written record of immunizations and be encouraged to complete the active immunization schedule. The patient's immunization history should be accurately recorded to protect the patient and care providers.

The acute nursing management of the patient with tetanus is aimed at supportive care based on the treatment of clinical manifestations. The patient should be placed in a quiet, darkened room insulated against noise. Judicious sedation should be given. Nursing care should be administered with the utmost caution to avoid triggering spasms. For example, the nurse should avoid unnecessary touching, use firm touching when necessary, avoid the use of linens to cover the patient, and maintain a slightly higher than normal ambient temperature. Nursing care related to tracheostomy and mechanical ventilation is given as appropriate. An indwelling urinary catheter may be used to prevent bladder distention and urinary reflux in the presence of spasms in the muscles of the pelvic floor. Attention must also given to skin care. The patient needs emotional support during the acute phase because the fear of death is real. The family also needs support and education.

NEUROSYPHILIS

Neurosyphilis (tertiary syphilis) is an infection of any part of the nervous system by the organism *Treponema pallidum.* It is the result of untreated or inadequately treated syphilis (see Chapter 50). The organism can invade the central nervous system (CNS) within a few months of the original infection. Except for causing some changes in the CSF, including increased white blood cells (WBCs) and protein and positive serologic reaction, the organism lies dormant for years. Untreated neurosyphilis, although not contagious, can be fatal. Penicillin therapy is effective for syphilitic meningitis, but the neurologic deficits remain.

Late neurosyphilis results from degenerative changes in the spinal cord (tabes dorsalis) and brainstem (general paresis). *Tabes dorsalis* (progressive locomotor ataxia) is characterized by vague, sharp pains in the legs; ataxia; "slapping" gait; loss of proprioception and deep tendon reflexes; and zones of hyperesthesia. *Charcot's joints,* which are characterized by enlargement, bone destruction, and hypermobility, also occur as a result of joint effusion and edema.

Dementia paralytica is an ongoing spirochetal meningoencephalitis that causes a general dissolution of mental and physical capabilities. It may mimic a number of major or minor psychoses. Management includes treatment with penicillin, symptomatic care, and protection from physical injury.

SPINAL CORD TRAUMA

Before World War II, the life expectancy for the person with a spinal cord injury ranged from months to 10 years from the onset of injury. The leading causes of death were renal failure and sepsis. Today, with improved treatment strategies (specifically, intermittent catheterization), even the very young patient with a spinal cord injury can anticipate a long life. The prognosis for life is generally only about 5 years less than for persons of the same age without spinal cord injury. The cause of premature death in the patient with quadriplegia is usually related to compromised respiratory function.

The disruption of individual growth and development, altered family dynamics, economic loss in terms of absence from work, and the high cost of rehabilitation or maintenance make spinal cord trauma a devastating problem. About 200,000 people in the United States today had traumatic spinal cord injuries and 6000 to 7000 people are newly injured each year.[17] The number of persons with spinal cord injuries living in the United States at any one time ranges from 183,000 to 203,000. The cost of spinal cord injury management is high. The average cost of care for a person with a high cervical injury is $417,067 in the first year and $74,707 in each subsequent year.[18]

Although many patients with spinal cord injuries can care for themselves with minimal assistance, a larger number are confined to nursing homes, care centers, and rehabilitation units. The loss to the workforce in terms of human potential is enormous.

Etiology and Pathophysiology

The population at risk for spinal cord injury is primarily young adult men between the ages of 15 and 30 years and those who are impulsive or risk takers in daily living. A history of numerous injuries before the cord injury is common. A high correlation exists between alcohol and drug abuse and spinal cord injury. Individuals at risk for spinal cord injury include motorcyclists, sky divers, football players, police officers, divers, and military personnel.

There has also been an increase in the number of older adult spinal cord injuries. Trauma has been called a young man's "disease," but when it happens in the older adult, trauma is often even more devastating. Besides having greater mortality, older adults with traumatic injuries as a group experience more complications than younger ones, and they are hospitalized longer. As the nation's population ages, the human and financial tolls of trauma in the elderly are certain to grow.[19] The most common causes of spinal cord injury include motor vehicle accidents, falls, gunshot wounds, and sports injuries.

Gunshot wounds is now listed as the third most common cause of spinal cord injuries in the United States. In large urban areas, gun shot wounds have recently surpassed falls as the second most common cause of spinal cord injuries.[20] The resulting spinal cord injury can be due to cord compression by bone displacement, interruption of blood supply to the cord, or traction resulting from pulling on the cord.

Initial Injury. The spinal cord is wrapped in tough layers of dura and is rarely torn or transected by direct trauma. Penetrating trauma, such as gunshot and stab wounds, can result in tearing and transection. The complete cord dissolution (previously thought to be transection) in severe trauma is related to autodestruction of the cord. Shortly after the injury, petechial hemorrhages are noted in the central gray matter of the cord. Hemorrhagic areas in the center of the spinal cord (gray matter) are grossly visible within 1 hour. Within 4 hours there may be infarction in the gray matter.[21]

Hemorrhage, edema, and metabolites act together to produce ischemia, which progresses to necrotic destruction of the cord. Figure 57-4 illustrates the cascade of events that follow spinal cord injury. The resulting hypoxia reduces the oxygen tension below the level that meets the metabolic needs of the cord. Lactate metabolites and an increase in vasoactive substances including norepinephrine, serotonin, and dopamine are noted. At high levels, these vasoactive substances cause vasospasms and hypoxia leading to subsequent necrosis. Unfortunately, the spinal cord has minimal ability to adapt to vasospasm.

By 24 hours, permanent damage has occurred because of the development of edema. Edema secondary to the inflammatory response is particularly harmful because of lack of space for tissue expansion. Therefore, resultant compression of the cord and extension of edema above and below the injury increase the ischemic damage. The end result is the same as mechanical severance of the cord.

The hemorrhagic necrosis causes the lesion to be complete after 48 hours, and any function of nerves that arise in and pass through this level is lost. Because additional edema extends the level of injury beyond the immediate level of destruction for 72 hours to 1 week, the exact extent of injury cannot be determined before that time.

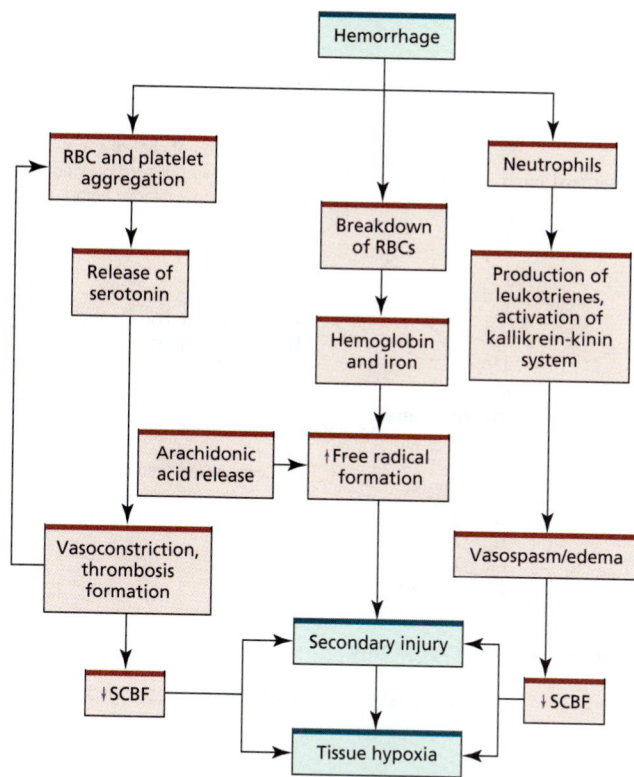

Fig. 57-4 Cascade of metabolic and cellular events that leads to spinal cord ischemia and hypoxia of secondary injury. *SCBF,* spinal cord blood flow. (Redrawn from Marciano FF and others: *BNI Quarterly* 11(2):6,1995. In McCance KL, Heuther SE: *Pathophysiology: the biologic basis for disease in adults and children,* St. Louis, 1998, Mosby.)

Spinal and Neurogenic Shock.

In addition to the discrete damage at the trauma site, the entire cord below the level of the lesion fails to function, resulting in spinal shock characterized by decreased reflexes and flaccid paralysis below the level of the injury. There is complete loss of motor and sensory function below the level of the lesion. Spinal shock usually occurs at the time of injury in response to severe damage to the cord and results in immediate depression of all cord functions. This affects musculoskeletal, bowel, and bladder function. Neurogenic shock characterized by hypotension, bradycardia, and warm, dry extremities also occurs. Loss of sympathetic innervation causes peripheral vasodilation, venous pooling, and a decreased cardiac output. These effects are generally associated with a cervical or high thoracic injury.

Spinal shock generally lasts for 7 to 10 days after onset but can last from weeks to months. Indications that spinal shock has ended include spasticity, reflex emptying of the bladder, and hyperreflexia. Active rehabilitation may begin in the presence of spinal shock.

Classification of Spinal Cord Injury

Spinal cord injuries are classified by the mechanism of injury, level of injury, or degree of injury.

Mechanisms of Injury.

The major mechanisms of injury are flexion, hyperextension, flexion-rotation, extension-rotation, and compression (Fig. 57-5). The flexion injury that includes dislocation is the most unstable of all injuries because the liga-

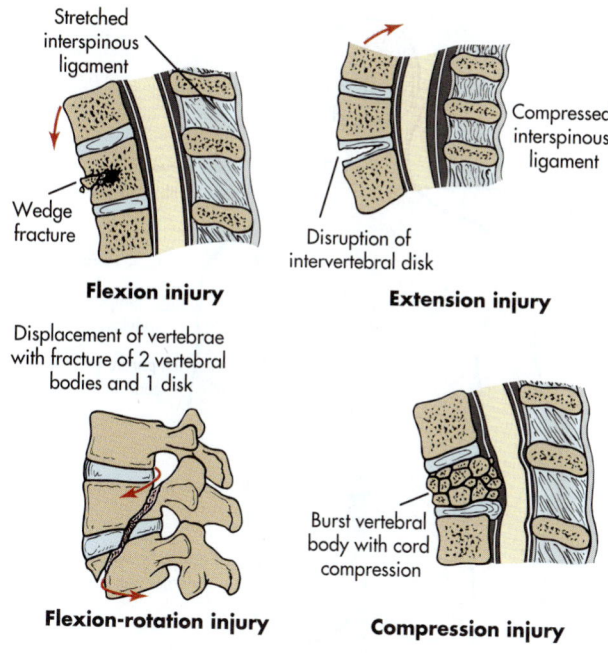

Fig. 57-5 Mechanisms of spinal injury.

mentous structures that stabilize the spine are torn. This injury is most often implicated in severe neurologic deficits.

Level of Injury.

The level of injury may be cervical, thoracic, or lumbar. Cervical and lumbar injuries are most common because these levels are associated with the greatest flexibility and movement.

Degree of Injury.

The degree of spinal cord involvement may be either complete or incomplete (partial). *Complete cord* involvement results in flaccid paralysis and total loss of sensory and motor function below the level of the lesion (injury). If the cervical cord is involved, paralysis of all four extremities (particularly the hands and forearms) occurs, resulting in quadriplegia. However, even with a cervical injury the arms are rarely completely paralyzed. If the thoracic or lumbar cord is damaged, the result is paraplegia. Figure 57-6 shows affected structures and functions at different levels of cord injury.

Incomplete cord lesion involvement (partial transection) results in a mixed loss of voluntary motor activity and sensation and leaves some tracts intact. The degree of sensory and motor loss varies depending on the level of the lesion and reflects the specific nerve tracts damaged and those spared. Four syndromes are associated with incomplete lesions: central cord syndrome, anterior cord syndrome, Brown-Séquard syndrome, and posterior cord syndrome.

Central cord syndrome. Damage in the cervical central cord is termed *central cord syndrome,* which is characterized by microscopic hemorrhage, edema of the central spinal cord, and compression on anterior horn cells (Fig. 57-7). Central cord syndrome is more common in older adults. Motor weakness is present in both the upper and lower extremities, but the weakness is much greater in the upper extremities than in the lower ones. It may change to a progressive lesion. Sensory dysfunction varies according to the site of injury or lesion. Bladder dysfunction is variable. This syndrome is frequently a result of hyperextension of an osteoarthritic spine. The extent of recovery

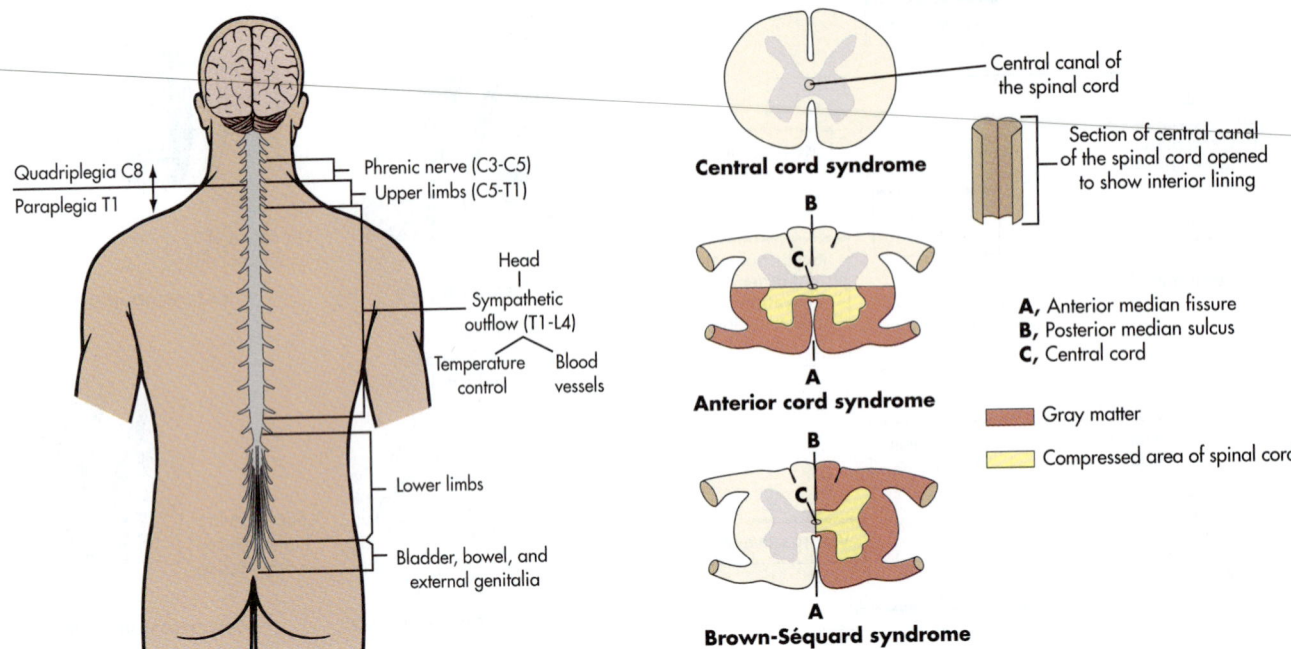

Fig. 57-6 Symptoms, degree of paralysis, and potential for rehabilitation depend on the level of the lesion.

Fig. 57-7 Syndromes associated with incomplete cord lesions.

depends on the resolution of edema and the intactness of the spinal cord tracts.

Anterior cord syndrome. *Anterior cord syndrome* is characterized by injury resulting in an acute compression of the anterior portion of the spinal cord, often a flexion injury (see Fig. 57-7). The spinal cord lesion is in the anterior two thirds of the cord. Compression is usually caused by a disk or bony fragment; it may also be caused by actual destruction of the anterior cord by an anterior spinal artery occlusion caused by ischemia or thrombus. Manifestations include immediate, complete motor paralysis from the site of the injury and below. *Hypoesthesia* (decreased sensation), decreased pain sensation, and loss of temperature occur below the level of injury. Because the posterior cord tracts are not injured, sensations of touch, position, vibration, and motion remain intact. Dorsal column function is preserved. If the syndrome is caused by the compression of the anterior cord from bony fragments, surgical decompression is indicated.

Brown-Séquard syndrome. *Brown-Séquard syndrome* is a result of transection or lesion of one half of the spinal cord (see Fig. 57-7). Brown-Séquard syndrome is usually caused by penetrating injuries, such as a gunshot wound or knife or possibly an acute ruptured disk. This syndrome is characterized by a loss of motor function (paralysis) and position and vibratory sense, as well as vasomotor paralysis on the same side (ipsilateral) and below the hemisection. The opposite (contralateral) side of the hemisection has loss of pain and temperature sensation below the level of the lesion or hemisection. Fibers that carry pain and temperature cross to the opposite side of the cord immediately after entering the cord and ascend, which accounts for the described symptoms.

Posterior cord syndrome. Less commonly seen is the *posterior cord syndrome*. This syndrome is associated with cervical

hyperextension trauma. It results from compression or damage to the posterior part of the spinal cord that contains the sensory neurons and position-sense capabilities. Generally the dorsal columns are damaged, resulting in loss of proprioception. However, pain, temperature sensation, and motor function below the level of the lesion remain intact.

Clinical Manifestations

The manifestations of spinal cord injury are generally the direct result of trauma that causes cord compression, ischemia, edema, and possible cord transection. Manifestations are related to the level and degree of injury. The patient with an incomplete lesion may demonstrate a mixture of symptoms. The higher the injury, the more serious the sequelae because of the proximity of the cervical cord to the medulla and brainstem. Movement and rehabilitation potential related to specific locations of the spinal cord injury are described in Table 57-3. In general, sensory function closely parallels motor function at all levels.

Immediate postinjury problems include maintaining a patent airway, adequate ventilation, and adequate circulating blood volume and preventing extension of cord damage.

Respiratory System. Cervical injury or fracture above the level of C4 presents special problems because of the total loss of respiratory muscle function. Mechanical ventilation is required to keep the patient alive. At one time the majority of these patients died at the scene of the injury, but with improved Emergency Medical Services more of these patients are surviving the initial events of their spinal cord injury. Injury or fracture below the level of C4 results in diaphragmatic breathing if the phrenic nerve is functioning. Even if the injury is below C4, spinal cord edema and hemorrhage can affect the function of the phrenic nerve and cause respiratory insufficiency. Hypoventilation almost always occurs with diaphragmatic respirations because of the decrease in vital capacity and tidal

Table **57-3**	Functional Level of Spinal Cord Disruption and Rehabilitation Potential	
Level of Injury	**Movement Remaining**	**Rehabilitation Potential**
Quadriplegia		
C1-C3		
Usually fatal injury, vagus nerve domination of heart, respiration, blood vessels, all organs below injury	Movement in neck and above, loss of innervation to diaphragm, absence of independent respiratory function	Ability to drive electric wheelchair equipped with portable respirator by using chin control or mouth stick, head-piece to stabilize head, lack of bowel and bladder control
C4		
Vagus nerve domination of heart, respirations, and all vessels and organs below injury	Sensation and movement above neck	Ability to drive electric wheelchair by using chin control or mouth stick, lack of bowel and bladder control
C5		
Vagus nerve domination of heart, respirations, and all vessels and organs below injury	Full neck, partial shoulder, back, biceps; gross elbow, inability to roll over or use hands; decreased respiratory reserve	Ability to drive electric wheelchair with mobile hand supports, ability to use powered hand splints (in some patients), lack of bowel and bladder control, feed self with setup and adaptive equipment
C6		
Vagus nerve domination of heart, respirations, and all vessels and organs below injury	Shoulder and upper back abduction and rotation at shoulder, full biceps to elbow flexion, wrist extension, weak grasp of thumb, decreased respiratory reserve	Ability to assist with transfer and perform some self-care, feed self with hand devices, push wheelchair on smooth, flat surface; lack of bowel and bladder control
C7-C8		
Vagus nerve domination of heart, respirations, and all vessels and organs below injury	All triceps to elbow extension, finger extensors and flexors, good grasp with some decreased strength, decreased respiratory reserve	Ability to transfer self to wheelchair, roll over and sit up in bed, push self on most surfaces, perform most self-care; independent use of wheelchair; ability to drive car with powered hand controls (in some patients); lack of bowel and bladder control
Paraplegia		
T1-T6		
Sympathetic innervation to heart, vagus nerve domination of all vessels and organs below injury	Full innervation of upper extremities, back, essential intrinsic muscles of hand; full strength and dexterity of grasp; decreased trunk stability, decreased respiratory reserve	Full independence in self-care and in wheelchair, ability to drive car with hand controls (in most patients), ability to use full body brace for exercise but not for functional ambulation, lack of bowel and bladder control
T6-T12		
Vagus nerve domination only of leg vessels, GI and genitourinary organs	Full, stable thoracic muscles and upper back; functional intercostals, resulting in increased respiratory reserve	Full independent use of wheelchair; ability to stand erect with full body brace, ambulate on crutches with swing (although gait difficult); inability to climb stairs; lack of bowel and bladder control
L1-L2		
Vagus nerve domination of leg vessels	Varying control of legs and pelvis, instability of lower back	Good sitting balance, full use of wheelchair
L3-L4		
Partial vagus nerve domination of leg vessels, GI and genitourinary organs	Quadriceps and hip flexors, absence of hamstring function, flail ankles	Completely independent ambulation with short leg braces and canes, inability to stand for long periods, bladder and bowel continence

GI, gastrointestinal.

volume, which occurs as a result of impairment of the intercostal muscles.

Cervical fractures or severe injuries cause a paralysis of abdominal musculature and frequently intercostal musculature; therefore the patient cannot cough effectively enough to remove secretions, leading to atelectasis and pneumonia. An artificial airway provides direct access for pathogens making bronchial hygiene and chest physiotherapy extremely important to reduce infection. Neurogenic pulmonary edema may occur secondary to a dramatic increase in sympathetic nervous system activity at the time of injury, which shunts blood to the lungs. In addition, pulmonary edema may occur in response to fluid overload.

Cardiovascular System. Any cord transection above the level of T5 greatly decreases the influence of the sympathetic nervous system. Bradycardia occurs as a result of the unopposed effect of the parasympathetic nervous system on the heart, and vasodilation results in hypotension. Cardiac monitoring is necessary. In marked bradycardia, appropriate medications to increase the heart rate and prevent hypoxemia are necessary. The peripheral vasodilation reduces the venous return of blood to the heart and subsequently decreases cardiac output, resulting in hypotension. IV fluids may resolve the problem, or vasopressor drugs may be required.

Urinary System. Urinary retention is a common development in acute spinal cord injuries and spinal shock. While the patient is in spinal shock the bladder is atonic and becomes overdistended. An indwelling catheter is inserted to drain the bladder. In the postacute phase the bladder can be hyperirritable, with a loss of inhibition from the brain resulting in reflex emptying. Consequently, the patient urinates small amounts frequently. However, the bladder may become distended because of inadequate emptying. Urinary retention increases the risk of infection. In addition, urinary calculi are more likely to develop in a distended bladder retaining urine. Catheterization is usually indicated. The indwelling catheter should be removed and intermittent catheterization should begin as early as possible.

Gastrointestinal System. If the cord transection has occurred above the level of T5, the primary GI problems are related to hypomotility. Decreased GI motor activity contributes to the development of paralytic ileus and gastric distention. A nasogastric tube for intermittent suctioning may relieve the gastric distention. The development of stress ulcers is common because of excessive release of hydrochloric acid in the stomach. Histamine H_2-receptor blockers, such as ranitidine (Zantac) and famotidine (Pepcid), are frequently used to prevent the occurrence of these ulcers during the initial phase. Other medications such as sucralfate (Carafate) and antacids may also be useful in prophylaxis. Intraabdominal bleeding may occur and is difficult to diagnose because no subjective signs such as pain, tenderness, and guarding are observed. Continued hypotension in spite of vigorous treatment and decreased hemoglobin and hematocrit may be indications of bleeding. Expanding girth of the abdomen may also be noted. Additional GI problems include gallstone formation, constipation, and fecal impaction.

Integumentary System. A major consequence of lack of movement is the potential for tissue breakdown in the area of denervation, which can occur quickly and can lead to major infection or sepsis. A certain degree of muscle atrophy occurs during the flaccid paralysis state, whereas contractures tend to occur during the spastic state.

Poikilothermism is the adjustment of the body temperature to the room temperature. This occurs in spinal cord injuries because the interruption of the sympathetic nervous system prevents peripheral temperature sensations from reaching the hypothalamus. Another factor is the reduction in heat generation because of minimal movement. With spinal cord disruption there is also decreased ability to sweat below the level of the lesion, which also affects the ability to regulate body temperature.

Metabolic Needs. Correcting an existing acid-base disturbance and maintaining acid-base balance promote the functions of other body systems. Nasogastric suctioning may lead to metabolic alkalosis, and decreased tissue perfusion may lead to acidosis. Electrolyte levels, including sodium and potassium, can be altered by gastric suctioning and must be monitored until suctioning is discontinued and a normal diet is resumed. A positive nitrogen balance and a high-protein diet help to prevent skin breakdown and infections and help to decrease the rate of muscle atrophy.

Peripheral Vascular Problems. Deep vein thrombosis (DVT) is a common problem accompanying spinal cord injury. It is more difficult to detect a DVT in a person with a spinal cord injury because the usual signs and symptoms such as pain, tenderness, and a positive Homans' sign will not be present.[18] Pulmonary embolism is one of the leading causes of death in patients with spinal cord injury. Techniques for assessment of DVT include Doppler examination, impedance plethysmography, and measuring leg and thigh girth.

Collaborative Care

The initial goals for the patient with a spinal cord injury are to sustain life and prevent further cord damage. Table 57-4 outlines the emergency management of the patient with a spinal cord injury. Systemic, neurogenic, and spinal cord shock must be treated. For injury at the cervical level, all body systems must be maintained until the full extent of the damage can be evaluated. Treatment of a spinal cord injury may be medical or surgical.

Collaborative care for the patient with a cervical injury is described in Table 57-5. The systemic support required by the patient is less intense for spinal cord injuries of the thoracic and lumbar vertebrae. Respiratory compromise is not as severe, and bradycardia is not a problem. Specific problems are treated symptomatically. After stabilization at the accident scene the person is transferred to a medical facility. A thorough assessment is done to specifically evaluate the degree of deficit and to establish the level and degree of injury. A history is obtained, with emphasis on how the accident occurred and the degree of disruption as perceived by the patient immediately after the accident. Assessment involves testing muscle groups rather than individual muscles. Muscle groups should be tested with and against gravity, alone and against resistance, and on both sides of the body. Spontaneous movement should be noted. The patient should be asked to move legs and then hands, spread fingers, extend wrists, and shrug shoulders. After assessment of motor status, a sensory examination including touch and pain as tested by pinprick should be carried out, starting at the toes and working upward. If time and conditions permit, position sense and vibration can also be assessed.

The types of accidents that cause spinal cord trauma can also result in head injury. The patient should therefore be assessed

✚ EMERGENCY MANAGEMENT

Table 57-4 Spinal Cord Injury

Etiology	Assessment Findings	Interventions
Blunt Compression, flexion, extension, or rotational injuries to spinal column Motor vehicle accidents Pedestrian accidents Falls Diving **Penetrating** Stretched, torn, crushed, or lacerated spinal cord Gunshot wounds Stab wounds	▪ Pain, tenderness, deformities, or muscle spasms adjacent to vertebral column ▪ Numbness, paresthesias ▪ Alterations in sensation: temperature, light touch, deep pressure, proprioception ▪ Weakness or heaviness in limbs ▪ Weakness, paralysis, or flaccidity of muscles ▪ Spinal shock ▪ Cuts, bruises, open wounds over head, face, neck, or back ▪ Neurogenic shock: hypotension, bradycardia, dry, flushed skin ▪ Bowel and bladder incontinence ▪ Urinary retention ▪ Difficulty breathing ▪ Priapism ▪ Diminished rectal sphincter tone	**Initial** ▪ Ensure patent airway. ▪ Stabilize cervical spine. ▪ Administer oxygen via nasal cannula or non-rebreather mask. ▪ Establish IV with two large-bore catheters and infuse normal saline or lactated Ringer's solution as appropriate. ▪ Assess for other injuries. ▪ Control external bleeding. ▪ Obtain cervical spine radiographs or CT scan. ▪ Prepare for stabilization with cranial tongs and traction. ▪ Administer high-dose methylprednisolone. **Ongoing Monitoring** ▪ Monitor vital signs, level of consciousness, oxygen saturation, cardiac rhythm, urine output. ▪ Keep warm. ▪ Monitor for urinary retention, hypertension. ▪ Anticipate need for intubation if gag reflex absent.

for signs of concussion and increased intracranial pressure (see Chapter 54). In addition, a careful assessment for musculoskeletal injuries and trauma to internal organs should be performed. Because there are no muscle, bone, or visceral sensations, the only clue to internal trauma with hemorrhage may be a rapidly falling hematocrit level. Urinary output is examined for hematuria, which is also indicative of internal injuries.

An x-ray is done to document the injury. The patient must be handled carefully before and during the x-ray procedure to prevent further injury. Respiratory, cardiac, urinary, and GI functions should be monitored closely. The patient may go directly to surgery following initial immobilization and stabilization or to the intensive care unit (ICU) for monitoring and management.

Surgical Therapy. The decision to perform surgery on a patient with a spinal cord injury often depends on the preference of a particular clinician. When cord compression is certain or the neurologic disorder progresses, benefit may be seen following immediate surgery.[17] Surgery stabilizes the spinal column. Other criteria used in the decision for early surgery include (1) evidence of cord compression, (2) progressive neurologic deficit, (3) compound fracture of the vertebrae, (4) bony fragments (may dislodge and penetrate the cord), and (5) penetrating wounds of the spinal cord or surrounding structures.

The more common surgical procedures include decompression laminectomy by anterior cervical and thoracic approaches with fusion, posterior laminectomy with the use of acrylic wire mesh and fusion, and insertion of stabilizing rods (e.g., Harrington rods for the correction and stabilization of thoracic deformities). (Specific surgical and nursing interventions for these techniques are discussed in Chapter 59.)

🤝 COLLABORATIVE CARE

Table 57-5 Cervical Cord Injury

Diagnostic
Complete neurologic examination
ABGs
Electrolytes, glucose, hemoglobin, and hematocrit levels
Urinalysis
Anteroposterior, lateral, and odontoid spinal x-ray studies
CT scan
Myelography
MRI
EMG to measure evoked potentials

Collaborative Therapy
Acute Care
Immobilization of vertebral column by skeletal traction
Maintenance of heart rate (e.g., atropine) and blood pressure (e.g., dopamine [Intropin])
Methylprednisone therapy to reduce edema
Insertion of nasogastric tube and attachment to suction
Intubation (if indicated by ABGs)
Oxygen by high humidity mask
Indwelling urinary catheter
Administration of IV fluids

Ambulatory/Home Care
Stress ulcer prophylaxis
Physical therapy (range-of-motion exercises)
Occupational therapy (splints, activities of daily living training)

ABGs, arterial blood gases.

NURSING ASSESSMENT

Table 57-6 Spinal Cord Injury

Subjective Data

Important Health Information

Past health history: Motor vehicle accident, sports injury, industrial accident, gunshot or stabbing injury, falls

Functional Health Patterns

Health perception–health management: Use of alcohol or recreational drugs; risk-taking behaviors

Activity-exercise: Loss of strength, movement, and sensation below level of injury; dyspnea, inability to breathe adequately

Cognitive-perceptual: Presence of tenderness, pain at or above level of injury; numbness, tingling, burning, twitching of extremities

Coping–stress tolerance: Fear, denial, anger, depression

Objective Data

General

Poikilothermia

Integumentary

Warm, dry, flushed extremities below level of injury (spinal shock)

Respiratory

Lesions at C1 to C3: apnea, inability to cough; lesions at C4: poor cough, diaphragmatic breathing, hypoventilation; lesions at C5 to T6: decreased respiratory reserve

Cardiovascular

Lesions above T5: bradycardia, hypotension, postural hypotension, absence of vasomotor tone

Gastrointestinal

Decreased or absent bowel sounds (paralytic ileus in lesions above T5), abdominal distention, constipation, fecal incontinence, fecal impaction

Urinary

Retention (for lesions between T1, L2); flaccid bladder (acute stages); spasticity with reflex bladder emptying (later stages)

Reproductive

Priapism, loss of sexual function

Neurologic

Complete: Flaccid paralysis and anesthesia below level of injury resulting in quadriplegia (for lesions above C8) or paraplegia (for lesions below C8), hyperactive deep tendon reflexes, bilaterally positive Babinski's test

Incomplete: Mixed loss of voluntary motor activity and sensations

Musculoskeletal

Muscle atony (in flaccid state), contractures (in spastic state)

Possible Findings

Location of level and type of bony involvement on spinal x-ray: lesion, edema, compression on CT scan and MRI; positive finding on myelogram

---

Drug Therapy. Vasopressor agents such as dopamine (Intropin) are employed in the acute phase as adjuvants to treatment. These agents are used to maintain the mean arterial pressure at a level greater than 80 to 90 mm Hg so that perfusion to the spinal cord is improved.

The National Acute Spinal Cord Injury Study II (NASCIS II) showed that methylprednisolone (MP), when administered early, resulted in an increased recovery of neurologic function. As a result of this study, MP is a standard of care and is administered IV bolus over 15 minutes. Dosing pauses for 45 minutes and then a maintenance dose of IV MP is started and infuses over the next 23 hours. Total dosing is completed over a 24 hour time period. MP, a blocker of lipid peroxidation by-products, has been found to improve blood flow and reduce edema in the spinal cord.[22] MP produces a number of effects that may account for the overall improvement noted in the spinal cord injured patient, including reduction of posttraumatic spinal cord ischemia, improvement of energy balance, restoration of extracellular calcium, improvement of nerve impulse conduction, and repression of the release of free fatty acids from spinal cord tissues.[23] MP is now a standard of comparison for future agents.

Currently a multicenter randomized trial NASCIS III is ongoing. The three purposes of this clinical trial are to determine (1) whether 48 hours of MP is as safe or safer than 24 hours, (2) whether tirilazad (Freedox) is a safe and effective substitution for MP, and (3) more precisely define the optimum time for drug administration. Tirilazad has been studied extensively in both spinal cord injury and brain injury. It inhibits both iron-dependent and independent lipid peroxidation. In vitro studies indicate that it has a stabilizing effect on cell membranes. Animal studies are ongoing and the drug looks promising as a treatment for acute spinal cord injuries.[23]

Pharmacologic properties and drug metabolism are altered in spinal cord injury; therefore, drug interactions may occur. For example, propoxyphene (Darvon) is believed to enhance vasodilation and possibly aggravate orthostatic hypotension, as well as act as an analgesic. The result may aggravate existing problems in the neurologically disabled patient. Drug-induced sedation can also mask a decreasing level of consciousness as a result of head injury or rising CO_2 levels with hypoventilation.

Pharmacologic agents are used to treat specific autonomic dysfunctions such as GI hyperactivity, bleeding, bradycardia, orthostatic hypotension, inadequate emptying of the bladder, and autonomic dysreflexia. The nurse must observe the response to these drugs and provide specific interventions when adverse reactions are seen.

NURSING MANAGEMENT: SPINAL CORD INJURY

■ Nursing Assessment

Subjective and objective data that should be obtained from a patient with a spinal cord injury are presented in Table 57-6.

■ Nursing Diagnoses

Nursing diagnoses for the patient with a spinal cord injury depend on the severity of the injury and the level of dysfunction. The nursing diagnoses for a patient with a spinal cord injury may include, but are not limited to, those presented in NCP 57-1. The care plan presented is for a patient with a complete cervical cord injury.

57-1 NURSING CARE PLAN   PATIENT WITH A SPINAL CORD INJURY*

| Expected Patient Outcomes | Nursing Interventions and *Rationales* |

NURSING DIAGNOSIS Impaired gas exchange *related to* muscle fatigue and retained secretions *as manifested by* decreased PaO$_2$ content, increased PaCO$_2$ concentration, fatigue, diminished breath sounds.

- ABGs within normal limits.
- Normal chest x-ray.
- Clear lungs on auscultation.
- Absence of respiratory distress.

- Maintain a patent airway *to prevent respiratory arrest.*
- Assess all respiratory parameters initially and at least q2hr *to determine extent of problem and plan appropriate interventions.*
- Monitor ABGs to determine oxygenation and ventilation status.
- Provide aggressive pulmonary toilet, including chest physiotherapy and quad-assist coughing q4hr *to facilitate the raising of secretions.*
- Assess strength of cough at least q4hr *to determine adequacy for raising secretions.*
- Suction as necessary *to remove accumulated secretions.*

NURSING DIAGNOSIS Inability to sustain spontaneous ventilation *related to* diaphragmatic fatigue or paralysis *as manifested by* dyspnea, increased use of accessory muscles, decreased PaO$_2$, increased PaCO$_2$.

- No signs of respiratory compromise.

- Provide chest physiotherapy *to mobilize secretions and prevent pneumonia.*
- Assist with application of mechanical ventilation *to support respiration.*
- Provide emotional support *as intubation and mechanical ventilation can be frightening.*

NURSING DIAGNOSIS Decreased cardiac output *related to* venous pooling of blood and immobility *as manifested by* hypotension, tachycardia, restlessness, oliguria, decreased pulmonary artery pressures.

- Adequate cardiac output.
- Stable blood pressure and pulse.
- Absence of arrhythmias.
- No complications such as venous thrombosis or pulmonary emboli.

- Monitor blood pressure and pulse at least q2hr initially; monitor cardiac rhythm *as indicators of cardiac status.*
- Administer dopamine (Intropin) or other vasopressor agents *to maintain mean blood pressure >80 mm Hg.*
- Apply pneumatic compression devices to calves and/or compression gradient stockings *to prevent venous pooling and thromboemboli.*
- Perform range-of-motion to all extremities at least q8hr *to cause muscle contractions, which aid in venous return.*
- Measure pulmonary artery wedge pressure and cardiac output as ordered *to evaluate circulatory status.*

NURSING DIAGNOSIS Impaired skin integrity *related to* immobility and poor tissue perfusion *as manifested by* reddened skin over bony prominences and at pin and tong sites.

- Intact skin.
- No pressure ulcers.

- Inspect all skin areas, especially over bony prominences, at least q2hr; observe area around pins or tongs for signs of breakdown or infection at least every shift *so interventions can be initiated promptly if a problem develops.*
- Turn patient at least q2hr; use kinetic treatment table or other specialty care devices as needed *to prevent development of pressure areas.*
- Ensure adequate nutritional intake *to maintain healthy skin resistant to breakdown.*
- Wash and dry patient's skin thoroughly *to prevent moisture from predisposing to skin breakdown.*
- Inform patient and family about risk of pressure ulcers *to empower them in participating in prevention measures.*

NURSING DIAGNOSIS Constipation *related to* the injury, inadequate fluid intake, diet low in roughage, and immobility *as manifested by* lack of bowel movement for more than 2 days, decreased bowel sounds, palpable impaction, hard stool or stool incontinence.

- Established bowel program.
- Bowel movement at least every other day.

- Auscultate bowel sounds at least q4hr; monitor abdominal distention *to determine if peristalsis is present.*
- Note any nausea and vomiting *as possible indicators of paralytic ileus.*
- Begin bowel program as soon as bowel sounds return and include suppository every other day and stool softeners *to establish a bowel routine as quickly as possible.*

Continued

57-1 **NURSING CARE PLAN** **PATIENT WITH A SPINAL CORD INJURY***—continued

| Expected Patient Outcomes | Nursing Interventions and *Rationales* |

NURSING DIAGNOSIS Constipation—*continued*

- Teach patient and family the bowel program *to ensure continuity of the program.*
- Ensure appropriate food and fluid intake *as bulk, fiber, and fluid are necessary to the success of a bowel program.*

NURSING DIAGNOSIS Urinary retention *related to* injury and limited fluid intake *as manifested by* lack of urine output, bladder distention, involuntary emptying of bladder (after spinal shock).

- No urinary retention or infection.
- Able to perform self-catheterization or Credé maneuver to empty bladder.

- Palpate bladder every shift *as loss of autonomic and reflex control of bladder and sphincter can cause distention.*
- Insert indwelling catheter during acute phase *to ensure continuous flow of urine preventing kidney reflux or possible bladder rupture.*
- Begin intermittent catheterization program when appropriate; teach patient and family intermittent catheterization using a clean technique *to avoid long-term use of indwelling catheter with high potential for infection.*
- Maintain accurate intake and output records *to evaluate balance.*
- Encourage fluids (2-4 L/day) *to maintain high volume of dilute urine*, which aids in preventing infection.
- Monitor BUN and creatinine levels, urine cultures, and WBC count *to monitor kidney function and presence of infection.*
- Teach Credé maneuver *to supplement intermittent catheterization or use alone for more complete emptying of the bladder.*

NURSING DIAGNOSIS Impaired physical mobility *related to* spinal cord injury, vertebral column instability, or forced immobilization by traction *as manifested by* inability to move purposefully, limited muscle strength, impaired coordination, impaired perception of position or presence of body parts.

- No complications of immobility.

- Assess motor and sensory function at least q4hr initially *to promptly detect deterioration of neurologic status.*
- Check traction to ensure that frames are secure and properly aligned and that weights are hanging freely *to ensure maintenance of vertebral column stability.*
- Promote good pulmonary function *as pulmonary complications are a common sequelae of immobility.*
- Use specialty bed or turn patient q1-2hr as ordered *to prevent prolonged pressure, which can lead to pressure ulcers.*
- Perform full range-of-motion to all extremities several times a day *to promote circulation and prevent contractures.*
- Use splints, foot boards, and trochanter rolls as appropriate *to prevent contractures and promote functional positioning.*
- Mobilize patient as soon as appropriate *to prevent hazards of immobility and provide encouragement to patient.*

NURSING DIAGNOSIS Risk for autonomic dysreflexia *related to* reflex stimulation of sympathetic nervous system.

- No occurrence of autonomic dysreflexia.
- Receive immediate and appropriate nursing or medical interventions if autonomic dysreflexia occurs.

- Assess for hypertension, bradycardia, severe headache, sweating, blurred vision, flushed feeling, nasal congestion *as signs of autonomic dysreflexia.*
- Reduce or eliminate noxious stimuli such as fecal impaction, urinary retention, tactile stimulation, and skin lesions by appropriate interventions *to prevent occurrence of autonomic dysreflexia.*
- If autonomic dysreflexia occurs, check for elevated blood pressure and administer antihypertensive medication as ordered; check for and correct possible sources of irritation such as a distended bladder or bowel; elevate head of bed immediately *to prevent a rupture of cerebral blood vessels or an increase in intracranial pressure.*

Continued

57-1 ▐ **NURSING CARE PLAN** **PATIENT WITH A SPINAL CORD INJURY***—continued

| Expected Patient Outcomes | Nursing Interventions and *Rationales* |

NURSING DIAGNOSIS Risk for autonomic dysreflexia—*continued*

- If nursing interventions do not reverse symptoms, notify physician so immediate medical interventions can be initiated *to prevent a life-threatening situation from developing.*
- Teach patient and family to recognize and treat autonomic dysreflexia *to reverse occurrence and prevent occurrence of status epilepticus, stroke, and possible death.*

NURSING DIAGNOSIS Altered nutrition: less than body requirements *related to* increased metabolic demand and inability to eat independently *as manifested by* weight loss >5.5 lb (2.5 kg) of admission weight and decreased serum albumin or protein.

- Weight loss <10 lb (4.5 kg).
- Normal values for serum protein and albumin.

- Assess nutritional status on admission *to provide baseline data.*
- Ensure enteral feedings given as ordered during acute phase *so nutrient intake is not interrupted.*
- When patient is eating, encourage high-protein, high-carbohydrate, high-calorie diet with high bulk *to counteract the severe catabolism that occurs with spinal cord injury and to promote bowel function.*
- Keep a caloric count and weigh patient at least weekly *to evaluate nutritional plan and continue or revise as necessary.*

NURSING DIAGNOSIS Sexual dysfunction *related to* inability to achieve erection or perceive pelvic sensations and lack of knowledge of alternate means of achieving sexual satisfaction *as manifested by* verbalization of problems in sexual dysfunction.

- Expression of satisfaction with sexual activities.
- Knowledgeable about variety of ways to achieve sexual expression.

- Establish an honest, caring relationship with patient and sexual partner *to encourage open discussion of sexual concerns.*
- Provide accurate information about effects of spinal cord injury on sexual functioning; encourage questions; suggest alternate methods and use of assistive devices to achieve sexual satisfaction *to provide important information to patient.*
- Discuss reflexogenic erection with men and vaginal lubrication techniques with women *as means of enhancing sexual satisfaction.*
- Refer for sexual counseling if indicated.

NURSING DIAGNOSIS Risk for injury *related to* sensory deficit and lack of self-protective abilities.

- No injuries.

- Assess environment for potentially injurious situations *to plan appropriate adjustments.*
- Use side rails; pad side rails; turn and transfer patient carefully with adequate assistance *as means of preventing patient injury.*
- Teach patient to anticipate possible injurious events *to develop a prevention mentality.*

NURSING DIAGNOSIS Altered family processes *related to* change in function of ill family member *as manifested by* poor communication patterns among family members, use of ineffective coping techniques (e.g., shouting, blaming, isolation), inability of family members to meet physical needs of family member.

- Family will maximize individual and collective strengths and meet patient's needs.

- Assess family dynamics related to roles and responsibilities *to determine problematic areas and strengths.*
- Encourage open communication among family members regarding long-term planning to meet patient's needs, including financial aspects *so ideas and concerns of all involved family members are considered.*
- Assist family members to understand patient's feelings *to strengthen patient's feeling of worth and support.*
- Assist family members to develop an action plan to meet patient's needs *to reduce sense of frustration and helplessness.*
- Coordinate an organized team approach *to help the patient and family cope with the complex changes.*

Continued

57-1 NURSING CARE PLAN **PATIENT WITH A SPINAL CORD INJURY***—continued

Expected Patient Outcomes	Nursing Interventions and *Rationales*

NURSING DIAGNOSIS **Risk for ineffective individual coping** *related to* loss of control over bodily functions and altered lifestyle secondary to paralysis.

- Verbalization of ability to cope with effects of spinal cord injury.

- Assess for prolonged use of inappropriate defense mechanisms, inability to accept permanence of prognosis, refusal to use available support services *to determine presence of risk factors for ineffective coping.*
- Offer support and acceptance of feelings; assist patient with problem solving *to bolster patient's confidence in ability to cope.*
- Encourage use of support systems *to discuss concerns.*
- Provide information *as knowledge of expectations can help patient cope with the future.*
- Teach patient healthy coping behaviors such as relaxation techniques to *prevent patient from practicing ineffective behaviors such as smoking, drinking, or angry outbursts.*

NURSING DIAGNOSIS **Body image disturbance** *related to* paralysis *as manifested by* expression of anger or other negative feelings, refusal to discuss changes in function, participate in social contacts, or look at body.

- Expression of feelings about self.
- Work through feelings to adaptation.

- Encourage discussion of feelings *to aid patient in venting and clarifying feelings.*
- Allow patient to grieve *as spinal cord injury results in a real loss, which requires adjustment through grieving.*
- Encourage social interaction *to foster sense of returning normalcy to life.*
- Assist family members in supporting patient *to enhance patient's sense of worth and value as a person.*
- Make referral for counseling as needed.

*This care plan is suitable for a patient with a high cervical injury caused by flexion-rotation. It can be modified for patients with less severe problems.

■ **Planning**

The overall goals are that the patient with a spinal cord injury will (1) maintain optimal level of neurologic functioning, (2) have minimal or no complications of immobility, and (3) return to home and the community at an optimal level of functioning.

■ **Nursing Implementation**

Health Promotion. Nursing interventions include identification of risk populations, counseling, and education. Support of local legislation related to seat belt use in cars, helmets for motorcyclists and bicyclists, child-safety seats, and tougher penalties for drunk-driving offenses is a professional responsibility. A coordinated community program for the training of emergency personnel is essential.

Acute Intervention. High cervical injury caused by flexion-rotation is the most complex spinal cord injury and is discussed in this section. Interventions for this type of injury can be modified for patients with less severe problems.

Immobilization. Proper immobilization of the neck involves the maintenance of a neutral or extension position. Sandbags, hard cervical collars, and backboards can be used to stabilize the neck to prevent lateral rotation of the cervical spine. The body should always be correctly aligned and turning should be performed so that the patient is moved as a unit (e.g., log-rolling)

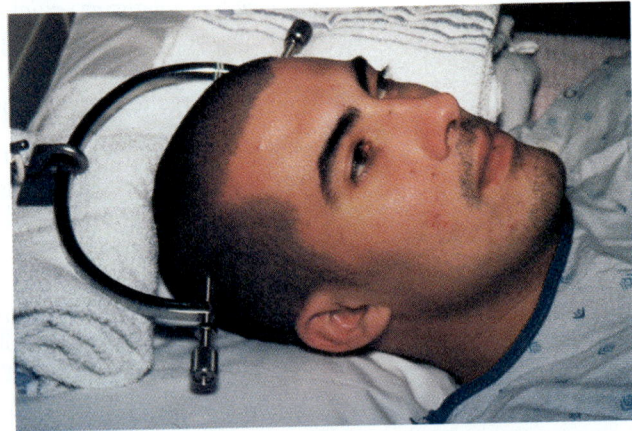

Fig. 57-8 Cervical traction is attached to tongs inserted in the skull.

to prevent movement of the spine. For cervical injuries, skeletal traction is usually provided by Crutchfield (Fig. 57-8), Vinke (Fig. 57-9), Gardner-Wells tongs, or other types of skull tongs. Traction is provided by a rope that is extended from the center of the tongs over a pulley and has weights attached at the end. Traction must be maintained at all times. One disadvantage of skull tongs is that the skull pins can be displaced. If this occurs,

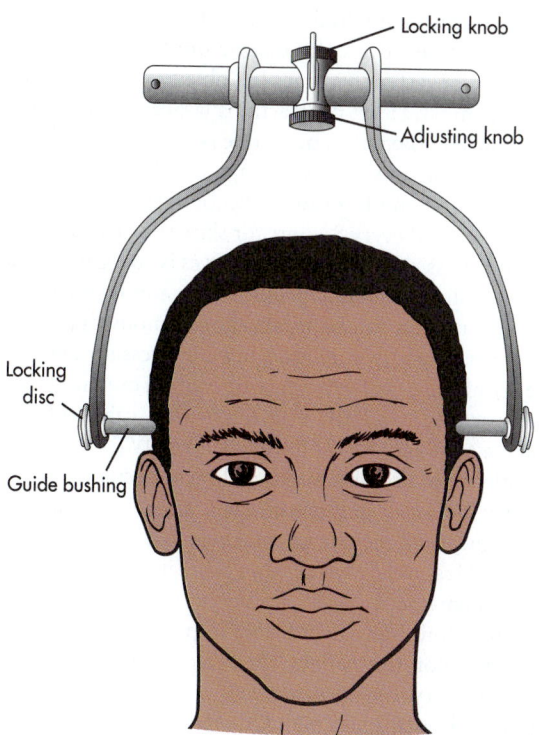

Fig. 57-9   Vinke tongs for cervical immobilization.

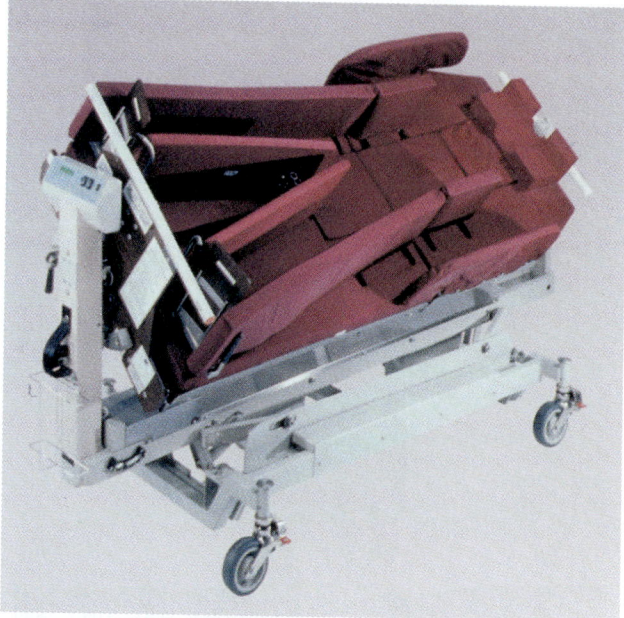

Fig. 57-10   Kinetic therapy treatment table.

the head should be held in a neutral or extended position and help should be summoned. Sandbags can be positioned to stabilize the head while the physician reinserts the tongs.

Infection at the sites of tong insertion is another potential problem. Preventive care includes cleansing the sites twice a day with normal saline solution and applying an antibiotic ointment, which acts as a mechanical barrier to the entrance of bacteria. The preventive care of insertion sites may vary depending on individual hospital standards of care.

Special frames and beds are often used in the management of the patient with a spinal cord injury. Equipment includes the Stryker frame and the Roto Rest® Delta bed (Fig. 57-10). The Stryker frame was developed in 1939 and was the first bed that afforded some benefits of mobilization. The Stryker frame bed uses a side-to-side lateral turn. The Roto Rest® Delta bed provides kinetic therapy using a continual side-to-side slow rotation 62 degrees laterally with the patient in constant motion. The bed allows a frequency of turns greater than 200 times per day. The bed is used to decrease the likelihood of pressure sores and cardiopulmonary complications. However, in some patients the turning can induce motion sickness and fear of falling out of bed when turned to the extremes. (Motion sickness is unlikely when automatic rather than manual turning is used.)

Depending on the type of injury and therapeutic interventions, the tongs and traction may be removed 2 to 4 weeks after injury. In a stable injury, halo traction may be applied. The removal of traction and application of a collar or halo traction device allows the patient to be more mobile and to begin active rehabilitation. The halo apparatus applies cervical traction by means of a jacket-like arrangement that allows greater mobility and wheelchair activity than other traction systems (Fig. 57-11).

Immobilization of the neck of the patient with a spinal cord injury prevents further injury, but the effects of immobility are profound. Meticulous skin care is critical because decreased sensation and circulation make the patient particularly susceptible to skin breakdown. Patients should be removed from backboards as soon as possible and cervical collars properly fitted or replaced with other forms of immobilization to prevent coccygeal and occipital area skin breakdown. It is important that areas under the halo vest or jacket be inspected to assess skin condition.

Respiratory dysfunction.   During the first 48 hours after injury, edema may increase the level of dysfunction and respiratory distress may occur. If the patient is exhausted from labored breathing or ABGs deteriorate (indicating inadequate oxygenation), endotracheal intubation or tracheostomy and mechanical ventilation should be initiated. Respiratory arrest is a possibility that requires careful monitoring of the respiratory system and prompt action should it occur. Pneumonia and atelectasis are potential problems because of reduced vital capacity and the loss of intercostal and abdominal muscle function, resulting in diaphragmatic breathing, pooled secretions, and an ineffective cough. The older adult has a more difficult time responding to hypoxia and hypercapnia and is extremely intolerant of hypoxia caused by lack of reserve. Therefore aggressive chest physiotherapy, adequate oxygenation, and proper pain management are essential to maximize respiratory function and gas exchange.[19] Other problems include nasal stuffiness and bronchospasms.

The nurse regularly assesses (1) breath sounds, (2) ABGs, (3) tidal volume, (4) vital capacity, (5) skin color, (6) breathing patterns (especially the use of accessory muscles), (7) subjective comments about the ability to breathe, and (8) the amount and color of sputum. A PaO_2 (partial pressure of oxygen in arterial blood) above 60 mm Hg and a $PaCO_2$ (partial pressure of

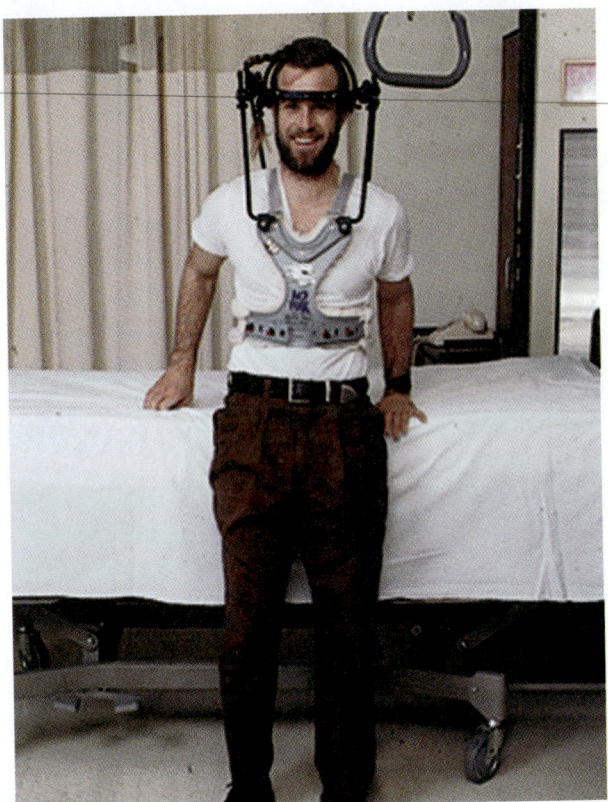

Fig. 57-11   Halo vest, Ace manufacturing design. Note the rigid shoulder straps and encompassing vest. Various vest sizes are available prefabricated. The halo ring, superstructure, and vest are magnetic resonance imaging (MRI)–compatible.

carbon dioxide in arterial blood) below 45 mm Hg are acceptable values in a patient with uncomplicated quadriplegia. The nurse should note the effect of the prone position because it can significantly reduce vital capacity and result in respiratory arrest. A patient who is unable to count to 10 out loud without taking a breath needs immediate attention.

In addition to monitoring activities, the nurse can intervene in maintaining ventilation. Oxygen is administered until ABGs stabilize. Chest physiotherapy and quad-assist coughing facilitate the raising of secretions. Quad-assist coughing stimulates the action of the ineffective abdominal muscles during the expiratory phase of a cough. The nurse places a fist or the heel of a hand between the umbilicus and xiphoid process and exerts firm pressure to the area (see Fig. 62-6). Tracheal suctioning should be performed if crackles or rhonchi are present. Incentive spirometry is an additional technique to improve the patient's respiratory status.

Cardiovascular instability. Because of unopposed vagal response, the heart rate is slowed, often to below 60 beats per minute. Any increase in vagal stimulation such as turning or suctioning can result in cardiac arrest. Loss of sympathetic tone in peripheral vessels results in chronic low blood pressure with potential postural hypotension. Lack of muscle tone to aid venous return can result in sluggish blood flow and predispose the patient to DVT.

Vital signs should be assessed frequently. If bradycardia is symptomatic, an anticholinergic medication such as atropine is administered. A temporary pacemaker may be inserted in some instances. Hypotension is managed with a vasopressor agent

such as dopamine and fluid replacement. In the older adult, the prevalence of cardiovascular disease must be considered. The cardiovascular system becomes less able to handle the stress of traumatic injury. Heart contractions weaken, and cardiac output is reduced. Maximum heart rate is also reduced.[19]

Compression gradient stockings can be used to prevent thromboemboli and to promote venous return. The stockings must be removed every 8 hours for skin care. The use of pneumatic compression devices for the calves is advocated, and they must be applied as soon as possible after admission and maintained throughout the hospitalization. Venous duplex studies may be performed before applying compression devices. The nurse should also perform range-of-motion exercises and heel-cord stretching regularly. The thighs and calves of the legs should be assessed every shift for signs of DVT.

Prophylactic use of heparin or low molecular weight heparin may be used to prevent DVT unless contraindicated. Contraindications include internal bleeding and recent surgery.

If blood loss has occurred from other injuries, the hemoglobin and hematocrit levels should be monitored and blood should be administered according to protocol. The nurse also should monitor the patient for indications of hypovolemic shock secondary to hemorrhage.

Fluid and nutritional maintenance. During the first 48 to 72 hours after the injury the GI tract may stop functioning (paralytic ileus) and a nasogastric tube must be inserted. Because the patient cannot have oral intake, fluid and electrolyte needs must be carefully monitored. Specific solutions and additives are ordered based on individual requirements. Once bowel sounds are present or flatus is passed, oral food and fluids can gradually be introduced. Because of severe catabolism, a high-protein, high-calorie diet is necessary for energy and tissue repair. In patients with high cervical cord injuries, swallowing must be evaluated before starting oral feedings. If the patient is unable to resume eating, total parenteral nutrition may be started to provide nutritional support.

Increased roughage should be included to promote bowel function. Some patients experience anorexia, which can be due to psychologic depression, boredom with institutional food, or discomfort at being fed (often by a hurried nurse). Some patients have a normally small appetite. Occasionally, refusal to eat is used as a means of maintaining control over the environment because of diminished or absent body control. If the patient is not eating adequately, the cause should be thoroughly assessed. On the basis of this assessment, a contract may be made with the patient using mutual goal setting regarding the diet. This gives the patient increased control of the situation and often results in improved nutritional intake. General measures such as providing a pleasant eating environment, allowing adequate time to eat (including any self-feeding the patient can achieve), encouraging the family to bring in special foods, and planning social rewards for eating may be useful. A calorie count should be kept and the patient's daily weight recorded as a means of evaluating progress. If feasible, the patient should participate in recording calorie intake. The nurse should avoid allowing the patient's nutritional intake to become a basis for a power struggle.

Bowel and bladder management. Urine is retained because of the loss of autonomic and reflex control of the bladder and sphincter. Because there is no sensation of fullness, overdistention of the bladder can result in reflux into the kidney with eventual renal failure. Bladder overdistention may even result

RESEARCH
IMPLICATIONS FOR NURSING PRACTICE

Bowel Function Following Spinal Cord Injury

Citation Kirk PM and others: Long-term follow-up of bowel management after spinal cord injury, *SCI Nursing* 14:56, 1997.

Purpose To describe bowel management programs, the prevalence of GI complaints, the impact of neurogenic bowel on life activities, and satisfaction with bowel management in patients with spinal cord injury.

Methods A telephone survey was used to ask 171 adults with spinal cord injury a series of questions related to bowel program, bowel function, and satisfaction. The mean duration of spinal cord injury for the participants was 8.9 years and their mean age was approximately 39 years.

Results and Conclusions In this sample, the most commonly reported bowel program was chemical rectal stimulation using laxatives. The average dietary fiber intake was 6.8 g per day. During the past year 90% of sample complained of GI problems such as constipation. Overall satisfaction with their bowel program was high.

Implications for Nursing Practice Constipation remains a problem for spinal cord injury patients long after the acute phase. In the patient with a spinal cord injury, constipation is related to a number of factors related to diet, mobility, and sensory and motor changes. Patients with spinal cord injury and their families need instructions related to diet (e.g., increase fiber), fluid intake, and other options (stool softeners, chemical laxatives) to enhance bowel function.

in rupture of the bladder. Consequently, an indwelling catheter is usually inserted as soon as possible after injury. Its patency must be ensured by frequent inspection and irrigation if warranted. In some institutions a physician's order is required for this procedure. Strict aseptic technique for catheter care is essential to avoid introducing infection. After the patient is stabilized, the best means of managing long-term urinary function is assessed. Usually the patient is started on an intermittent catheterization program. The patient is often maintained on a fluid restriction of 1800 to 2000 ml per day to facilitate a bladder training program. Urinary output is monitored closely.

UTIs are a common problem. A large fluid intake and the liberal use of juices such as cranberry, grape, and apple are used to prevent infections. When used in large quantities, these juices leave an acid ash in the urine, which discourages bacterial growth. Citrus juices are used sparingly. Ascorbic acid and a urinary antiseptic such as methenamine mandelate (Mandelamine) are sometimes given. The pH of the urine should be tested daily to evaluate acidity. If the appearance or odor of the urine is suspicious, a specimen is sent for culture. Age-related changes in renal function should be considered. The older adult is more likely to develop renal calculi and older men may have prostatic hyperplasia, which may interfere with urinary flow and complicate urinary management.[19]

Constipation is generally a problem during spinal shock because no voluntary or involuntary evacuation of the bowels occurs. Suppositories are used in combination with a laxative to assist in bowel evacuation. Enemas are used only if absolutely necessary because they can overdistend the rectum and create problems for initiating an effective bowel program.

Temperature control. Because there is no vasoconstriction, piloerection, or heat loss through perspiration below the level of injury, temperature control is largely external to the patient. Therefore the nurse needs to monitor the environment closely to maintain an appropriate temperature. Body temperature needs to be monitored regularly. The patient should not be overloaded with covers or unduly exposed (such as during bathing). If an infection develops, more extensive means of temperature control, such as a cooling blanket, may be necessary.

Stress ulcers. Stress ulcers are a problem for the patient with a spinal cord injury because of the physiologic response to severe trauma, psychologic stress, and high-dose corticosteroids. Peak incidence of stress ulcers is 6 to 14 days after injury. Stool and gastric contents are tested daily for blood, and the hematocrit is observed for a slow drop. When corticosteroids are given, they should be accompanied by antacids or food. Histamine H_2-receptor blockers, such as ranitidine (Zantac) and famotidine (Pepcid), may be given prophylactically to decrease the secretion of hydrochloric acid. Upper GI bleeding may also predispose to aspiration pneumonia.

Sensory deprivation. The nurse must compensate for the patient's absent sensations to prevent sensory deprivation. This is done by stimulating the patient above the level of injury. Conversation, music, strong aromas, and interesting flavors should be a part of the nursing care plan. Prism glasses are provided so that the patient can read and watch television. Every effort should be made to prevent the patient from withdrawing from the environment.

Patients with spinal cord injury often report altered sensorium and vivid dreams during the acute phase of their treatment. Whether this is due to drugs used to manage pain and anxiety is not known. Patients may also experience disrupted sleep patterns as a result of the hospital environment or post-traumatic stress disorder.

Reflexes. Once spinal cord shock is resolved, the return of reflexes may complicate rehabilitation. Lacking control from the higher brain centers, reflexes are inappropriate and often excessive. Erections can occur from a variety of stimuli, causing embarrassment and discomfort. Spasms ranging from mild twitches to convulsive movements below the level of the lesion may also occur. This reflex activity may be interpreted by the patient or family as a return of function, and the nurse must tactfully explain the reason for the activity. The patient may be informed of the positive use of these reflexes in sexual, bowel, and bladder retraining. Spasms may be relieved with the use of warm baths, whirlpool treatments, antispasmodics, and muscle relaxants. Peak spasticity occurs after 2 years, and if it is severe, destruction of the reflexes (cordotomy) may be necessary. This procedure compromises retraining and should only be done as a last resort.

Autonomic dysreflexia. *Autonomic dysreflexia* (hyperreflexia) is a massive uncompensated cardiovascular reaction mediated by the sympathetic nervous system. It occurs in response to visceral stimulation once spinal shock is resolved in patients with spinal cord lesions above T7. The condition is a

PATIENT & FAMILY HOME CARE GUIDE

Table 57-7 **Autonomic Dysreflexia**

Patient and family members must know the signs and symptoms of autonomic dysreflexia so that timely intervention can occur. These include the following:

- Sudden onset of acute headache
- Elevation in blood pressure and/or reduction in pulse rate
- Flushed face and upper chest (above the level of the lesion) and pale extremities (below the level of the lesion)
- Sweating above the level of the lesion
- Nasal congestion
- Feeling of apprehension

Immediate interventions include the following:

- Raise the person to a sitting position.
- Remove the stimulus (fecal impaction, kinked urinary catheter).
- Call the primary care provider if above actions do not relieve the signs and symptoms.

Efforts to decrease the likelihood of autonomic dysreflexia include the following:

- Maintain regular bowel function.
- If manual rectal stimulation is used, local anesthetics may reduce stimulation of autonomic dysreflexia.
- Monitor urine output.
- Wear a Medic-Alert bracelet indicating a history of autonomic dysreflexia.

Source: Autonomic hyperreflexia. In *Mosby's patient teaching guides,* St Louis, 1996, Mosby.

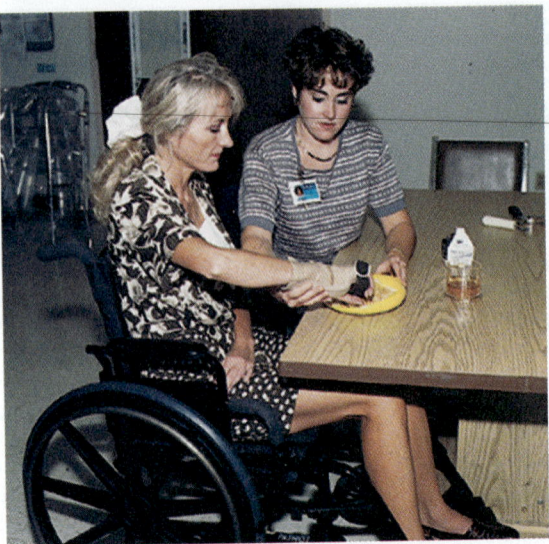

Fig. 57-12 A patient participating in occupational therapy using mobile arm supports and upper-extremity orthotics.

life-threatening situation that requires immediate resolution. If resolution does not occur, this condition can lead to status epilepticus, stroke, myocardial infarction, and even death.

The most common precipitating cause is a distended bladder or rectum, although any sensory stimulation may cause autonomic dysreflexia. Contraction of the bladder or rectum, stimulation of the skin, or stimulation of the pain receptors may also cause autonomic dysreflexia. Manifestations include hypertension (up to 300 mm Hg systolic), blurred vision, throbbing headache, marked diaphoresis above the level of the lesion, bradycardia (30 to 40 beats per minute), piloerection (erection of body hair) as a result of pilomotor spasm, nasal congestion, and nausea. It is important to measure blood pressure when a patient with a spinal cord injury complains of a headache.

The pathology of autonomic dysreflexia involves the stimulation of sensory receptors below the level of the cord lesion. The intact autonomic system below the level of the lesion responds to the stimulation with a reflex arteriolar vasoconstriction that increases blood pressure. Baroreceptors in the carotid sinus and the aorta sense the hypertension and stimulate the parasympathetic system. This results in a decrease in heart rate, but the visceral and peripheral vessels do not dilate because efferent impulses cannot pass through the cord lesion.

Nursing interventions in this serious emergency are elevation of the head of the bed 45 degrees, notification of the physician, and assessment to determine the cause. The most common cause is bladder irritation. Immediate catheterization to

relieve the distention may be necessary. Catheter irrigation performed slowly and gently may open a plugged catheter, or a new catheter may be inserted. A digital rectal examination should be performed only after application of an anesthetic ointment to decrease rectal stimulation and to prevent an increase of symptoms. The nurse should remove all skin stimuli such as constrictive clothing and tight shoes. If symptoms persist after the source has been relieved, an α-adrenergic blocker or an arteriolar vasodilator may be given. Careful monitoring must continue until the vital signs stabilize.

Patient and family must be taught the causes and symptoms of autonomic dysreflexia (Table 57-7). They must understand the life-threatening nature of this dysfunction and must know how to relieve the cause.

Ambulatory and Home Care. The physiologic and psychologic rehabilitation of the person with spinal cord injury is complex and involved. With physical and psychologic care and intensive and specialized rehabilitation, the patient with a spinal cord injury learns to function at the highest level of wellness. Special rehabilitation centers are available, but patients must demonstrate adequate motivation for self-care to be admitted.

Health care providers often consider spinal cord disability to be one of the most devastating of physical disabilities. However, patients with spinal cord injury are remarkably resourceful and possess an impressive resilience. Staff members often underestimate the patient's potential for independence. Misplaced sympathy and overidentification can compromise the nurse's attempt to give the involved and complex care required by the injured person for optimal rehabilitation. Recovery is prolonged, and nurses must learn to gauge progress in inches rather than miles. Skilled, persistent care draws on every known nursing intervention until the patient achieves a maximal level of independence.

Many of the problems identified in the acute period become chronic and continue throughout life. Rehabilitation focuses on refined retraining of physiologic processes. Braces, electronic wheelchairs, and mechanical devices are used to maximize the patient's remaining function (Fig. 57-12). Patient and

PATIENT & FAMILY HOME CARE GUIDE

Table **57-8** Halo Vest Care

The following are teaching guidelines for a patient with a halo vest:

- Inspect the pins on the halo traction ring. Report to health care provider if pins are loose or if there are signs of infection including redness, tenderness, swelling, or drainage at the insertion sites.
- Clean around pin sites carefully with hydrogen peroxide on a cotton swab. Repeat the procedure using water.
- Use alcohol swabs to cleanse pin sites of any drainage.
- Apply antibiotic ointment as prescribed.
- To provide skin care, have the patient lie down on a bed with his or her head resting on a pillow to reduce pressure on the brace. Loosen one side of the vest. Gently wash the skin under the vest with soap and water, rinse it, and then dry it thoroughly. At the same time, check the skin for pressure points, redness, swelling, bruising, or chafing. Close the open side and repeat the procedure on the opposite side.
- If the vest becomes wet or damp it can be carefully dried with a blow dryer.
- An assistive device (e.g., cane or walker) may be used to provide greater balance. Flat shoes should be worn.
- Turn the entire body, not just the head and neck, when trying to view sideways.
- In case of an emergency, keep a set of wrenches close to the halo vest at all times.
- Mark the vest strap such that consistent buckling and fit can be maintained.

Source: Halo vest care at home. In *Mosby's patient teaching guides,* St Louis, 1996, Mosby.

PATIENT & FAMILY HOME CARE GUIDE

Table **57-9** Skin Care for Patients with Spinal Cord Injuries

Skin breakdown is a potential problem following spinal cord injury. The following measures are used to decrease this possibility:

Change Position Frequently

- If in a wheelchair, lift self up and shift weight every 15 to 30 minutes.
- If in bed, a regular turning schedule (at least every 2 hours) that includes sides, back, and abdomen is encouraged to change position.
- Use special mattresses and wheelchair cushions.
- Use pillows to protect bony prominences when in bed.

Monitor Skin Condition

- Inspect skin frequently for areas of redness, swelling, and breakdown.
- Keep fingernails trimmed to avoid scratches and abrasions.
- If a wound develops, follow standard wound care management, which includes keeping wound open to air and applying treatments as prescribed.

Source: Skin care tips following spinal cord injury. In *Mosby's patient teaching guides,* St Louis, 1996, Mosby.

---

family teaching related to care of the halo vest are described in Table 57-8 and home care guidelines for skin care are presented in Table 57-9.

The patient with high cervical spinal cord injury has greatly increased mobility with phrenic nerve stimulators or electronic diaphragmatic pacemakers. Diaphragmatic pacemakers may allow the patient to become independent of mechanical ventilation. Today, ventilators are also reasonably portable, and ventilator-dependent quadriplegic patients can be mobile and somewhat independent. Although rehabilitation and the special equipment required are costly, many programs are funded by the state or federal governments.

If the patient can be successfully brought through the acute period, the patient's life can be fuller and richer than previously believed possible. Like other persons who have been close to death, some patients find that their lives are richer and more meaningful than before the injury. Unfortunately, other patients may not have such a positive future outlook. The nurse has a pivotal role in the coordinated efforts of the health team to influence a positive outcome.

Neurogenic bladder. Once spinal cord shock and the resulting bladder atony are resolved, the bladder is neurogenic. A neurogenic bladder is any type of bladder dysfunction related to abnormal or absent bladder innervation. It may lead to problems with residual urine, stone formation (urolithiasis), or

infection, and it is often associated with progressive renal deterioration and urinary incontinence. The network of fibers of the detrusor muscle forms the muscular wall of the bladder. The trigone is a small rectangular area near the bladder neck sometimes called the *internal sphincter.* The urogenital diaphragm or baseplate encircles the urethral opening completely and is sometimes called the *external sphincter.* Depending on the lesion, a neurogenic bladder may have no reflex detrusor contractions (*areflexic, flaccid*) or may have hyperactive reflex detrusor contractions (*hyperreflexic, spastic*). Common symptoms of a neurogenic bladder include urgency, frequency, incontinence, inability to void, and characteristics of obstruction.

Neurogenic bladder can be classified according to reflex detrusor activity, intravesical filling pressure, and continence function. Types of neurogenic bladder are outlined in Table 57-10. Diagnostic and collaborative care of neurogenic bladder are described in Table 57-11. The patient with a spinal cord injury and a neurogenic bladder requires a comprehensive program to manage bladder function. The program should include the following:

1. *Diagnostic evaluation:* After the patient's overall condition is stable with evidence of neurologic reflexes, a cystometrogram, an IV pyelogram, and a urine culture are taken.
2. *Drug therapy:* Drugs to increase the strength of bladder contractions (detrusor), acidify the urine, and relax the urethral sphincter are administered.
3. *Nutrition:* A low-calcium diet (1 g/day) is advocated to reduce the possibility of kidney and bladder stones.

Table 57-10	Types of Neurogenic Bladders		
Type	**Characteristics**	**Cause**	**Clinical Manifestations**
▪ Uninhibited	No inhibitions influence time and place of voiding	Corticospinal tract lesion; observed in CVA, multiple sclerosis, brain tumor, brain trauma	Incontinence, increased frequency, urgency
▪ Reflex	Bladder behaves as part of spinal reflex arc with no connection to brain	Lesion of motor and sensory fibers; occasionally seen in multiple sclerosis, pernicious anemia	Incontinence, urinary frequency, lack of sensation of bladder filling
▪ Autonomous	Bladder behaves autonomously, as if it were cut off from brain and spinal cord	Lesions of cauda equina, pelvic nerves, spina bifida	Incontinence, difficulty initiating micturition
▪ Motor paralysis	Bladder acts as if there were paralysis of all motor functions	Lower motor neuron lesion caused by trauma involving S2-S4	If sensory function intact, feels bladder distention and hesitancy; no control of micturition, resulting in overdistention of bladder and overflow incontinence
▪ Sensory paralysis	Bladder acts as if there were paralysis of all sensory modalities	Damage to sensory limb of bladder spinal reflex arc; seen in multiple sclerosis, diabetes mellitus, pernicious anemia	Poor bladder sensation, infrequent voiding, large residual volume

CVA, cerebrovascular accident.

COLLABORATIVE CARE

Table 57-11	Neurogenic Bladder

Diagnostic
  Neurologic examination
  Cystometrogram
  IV pyelogram
  Urine culture

Collaborative Therapy
Drug Therapy
  Increasing detrusor muscle strength (bethanechol [Urecholine])
  Acidification of urine (ascorbic acid [vitamin C])
  Urinary antiseptics (e.g., methenamine mandelate [Mandelamine])
  Relaxation of urethral sphincter

Nutrition
  Low-calcium diet (<1 g/day)
  Fluid intake at 1800-2000 ml/day

Urine Drainage
  Reflex training
  Intermittent catheterization
  Indwelling catheter
  Urinary diversion surgery

4. *Fluids:* A fluid intake of 1800 to 2000 ml per day must be maintained to prevent stone formation and to ensure adequate urine flow.
5. *Urine drainage:* The method used for urinary drainage depends on the condition of the patient; the preference of the physician, nursing staff, and patient; and the policy of the institution. Numerous drainage methods are possible, including reflex training, indwelling catheter, intermittent catheterization, and urinary diversion surgery.

Many factors are considered when selecting a bladder management strategy. These include upper extremity function, caregiver burden, and lifestyle choices.

With the return of the reflex arc, bladder function may be a reflex. However, because of the interruption in the pathways to the brain, the patient has no control over urination, which results in a bladder with a small capacity, hyperirritable detrusor muscle and sphincter, and loss of inhibition of the reflex by the brain. The patient or the nurse can use techniques such as the Credé and Valsalva maneuvers or a rectal stretch to facilitate complete emptying of the bladder. The Credé maneuver involves the exertion by the nurse or patient of downward pressure over the bladder with a pumping motion. This maneuver is only used in those patients with a lower motor neuron pattern bladder and may require a physician's order in some settings because it has the potential of stimulating autonomic dysreflexia in the patient with upper motor neuron disease. In the Valsalva maneuver, the patient inhales deeply, holds his or her breath, and bears down. The rectal stretch is the insertion of a gloved finger into the rectum, gently pulling to exert pressure on the sphincter to cause relaxation of the perineal floor. Combining the Valsalva maneuver with rectal stretch results in more complete emptying of the bladder. The patient should be regularly assessed for residual urine after reflex bladder emptying. It may take up to 3 to 5 days before residual urine is less than 100 ml. Many drugs affect urinary retention and thus should be assessed for their effects on residual volume. The ultimate goal for this technique is for the patient to not need a catheter.

The long-term use of an indwelling catheter should be carefully evaluated because of the associated high incidence of UTI, fistula formation, and diverticula. Adequate fluid intake and patency of the catheter should be ensured. The frequency of catheter changing ranges from 1 week to 1 month, depending on the type of catheter used and agency policy.

Intermittent catheterization is the recommended method of bladder management (see Chapter 43). Nursing assessment is important in selecting the time interval between catheterizations. Initially, catheterization is done every 4 hours. If less than 200 ml of urine is drained, the time interval may be extended. If 500 ml or more of urine is obtained, the time interval is shortened. An overdistended bladder can cause ischemia, which may predispose tissues to bacterial invasion and infection. Patients often experience diuresis at a regular time during a 24-hour period, which may necessitate an extra catheterization. The number of intermittent catheterizations per day is usually five or six.

Urinary diversion surgery may be necessary if the patient has repeated UTIs with renal involvement or repeated stones or if therapeutic intervention has been unsuccessful (see Table 43-19). Surgical treatment of neurogenic bladder includes bladder neck revision (sphincterotomy), bladder augmentation (augmentation cystoplasty), penile prosthesis, artificial sphincter, perineal ureterostomy, cystotomy, vesicotomy, and anterior urethral transplantation.

Bowel evacuation. Bowel evacuation needs careful management in the patient with a spinal cord injury because voluntary control of this function may be lost. The usual measures for preventing constipation include a high-fiber diet and adequate fluid intake (see Table 40-11). Patient and family teaching guidelines related to bowel management are presented in Table 57-12. However, these measures by themselves may not be adequate to stimulate evacuation. In addition, suppositories or digital stimulation by the nurse or patient may be necessary. In the patient with an upper motor neuron lesion, digital stimulation is necessary to promote defecation. Small-volume enemas and agents such as docusate sodium (Colace), bisacodyl (Dulcolax), and glycerin may also be used.

Valsalva maneuver and manual stimulation are useful in patients with lower motor neuron lesions. The Valsalva maneuver requires intact abdominal muscles, so it is used in those patients with injuries below T12. In general, a bowel movement every other day is considered adequate. However, preinjury patterns should be considered. Incontinence can result from too much stool softener or a fecal impaction.

Careful recording of bowel movements, including amount, time, and consistency, is important to the overall success of the program. Timing of defecation may also be an important factor. If bowel evacuation is planned for 30 to 60 minutes following the first meal of the day, this may enhance success by taking advantage of the gastrocolic reflex induced by eating.

Sexuality. Because the majority of patients with spinal cord injuries are men between 18 and 35 years of age, sexual rehabilitation is a major issue. It is important to remember that sexuality is an important issue regardless of the patient's age. To work with these patients, the nurse must have an awareness and an acceptance of personal sexuality, as well as knowledge of human sexual responses. When discussing sexual potential, the nurse should use scientific terminology rather than slang whenever possible. Knowledge of the level of the lesion is

PATIENT & FAMILY HOME CARE GUIDE

Table 57-12   Bowel Management After Spinal Cord Injury

The following are teaching guidelines for a patient with a spinal cord injury:

- Optimal nutritional intake includes:
  - 3 well-balanced meals each day
  - 2 servings from the milk group
  - 2 or more servings from the meat group, including beef, pork, poultry, eggs, fish
  - 4 or more servings from the vegetable and fruit groups
  - 4 or more servings from the bread and cereal group
- Fiber intake should be approximately 20 to 30 g per day. Gradually increase amount of fiber eaten over 1 to 2 weeks.
- Three quarts of fluid per day should be consumed unless contraindicated. Water or fruit juices should be used and caffeinated beverages such as coffee, tea, and cola should be avoided. Fluid softens hard stools; caffeine stimulates fluid loss through urination.
- Foods that produce gas (e.g., beans) or upper GI upset (spicy foods) should be avoided.
- Timing: A regular schedule for bowel evacuation should be established. A good time is 30 minutes after the first meal of the day.
- Position: If possible, an upright position with feet flat on the floor or a step stool enhances bowel evacuation. Staying on the toilet, commode, or bedpan for longer than 20 to 30 minutes causes skin breakdown. Based on stability, someone may need to stay with the patient.
- Activity: Exercise is important for bowel function. In addition to improving muscle tone, it also increases GI transit time and increases appetite. Muscles should be exercised. This includes stretching, range-of-motion, and position changing.
- Drug treatment: Laxatives, including suppositories, may be necessary to stimulate a bowel movement. However, these drugs can be habit-forming and thus should only be taken when necessary. Manual stimulation of the rectum may also be helpful in initiating defecation.

Source: Bowel management at home following spinal cord injury. In *Mosby's patient teaching guides,* St Louis, 1996, Mosby.

needed to understand the patient's potential for orgasm, erection, and fertility and the patient's capacity for sexual satisfaction (Table 57-13). All patients with spinal cord injuries generally lack perineal sensation during intercourse regardless of the type of lesion.

Reflex sexual function capability is possible if the patient has an upper motor neuron lesion. The presence of tone in the external rectal sphincter indicates an upper motor lesion. The absence of external rectal sphincter tone, bulbocavernosus reflex, or both indicates that the patient has lower motor neuron involvement and may be capable of psychogenic erection but not reflex erection. If ejaculation occurs, it may be retrograde into the bladder.

Table 57-13	Potential for Sexual Activity in Men with Spinal Cord Injuries	
Erection	**Ejaculation**	**Orgasm**
Upper Motor Neuron		
Complete		
Frequent (93%), reflexogenic only	Rare	Absent
Incomplete		
Most frequent (99%), reflexogenic (80%), reflexogenic and psychogenic (19%)	Less frequent (32%), after reflexogenic erection (74%), after psychogenic erection (26%)	Present (if ejaculation occurs)
Lower Motor Neuron		
Complete		
Infrequent (26%)	Infrequent (18%)	Present (if ejaculation occurs)
Incomplete		
Psychogenic and reflexogenic	Frequent (70%), after psychogenic and reflexogenic erections	Present (if ejaculation occurs)

The type of lesion determines the physical sexual response. Men with upper motor neuron lesions may have reflexogenic erections that are produced by reflex activity or external stimuli or that occur spontaneously. These spontaneous erections are often short lived and uncontrolled and cannot be maintained or summoned at the time of coitus. Orgasm and ejaculation are usually not possible for men with a complete upper motor neuron lesion.

Most patients with a complete lower motor neuron lesion are unable to have either psychogenic or reflexogenic erections. Patients with incomplete lower motor neuron lesions have the highest possibility of successful psychogenic erection with ejaculation, and up to 10% of these patients are fertile.

The woman of childbearing age with a spinal cord injury usually remains fertile, although orgasmic ability is lost. The injury does not affect the ability to become pregnant or to deliver normally through the birth canal.

Sexual rehabilitation for both men and women should begin informally after the acute phase of the injury has passed. Questions such as "Have you had an erection since your accident?" and "Have your menstrual periods continued since the accident?" are nonthreatening ways to introduce the topic of sexual functioning. The male patient may pose a question such as, "Can I ever be a man again?"

Open discussion with the patient is essential. This important aspect of rehabilitation should be handled by someone specially trained in sexual counseling. Unless this type of training has occurred, the nurse should not attempt to direct the plan for sexual rehabilitation.

The properly trained nurse works with the patient and partner to provide support during new relationships, with the emphasis on open communication. The nurse's educational role requires respect for every couple's personal standards of religious and cultural beliefs. Alternative methods of obtaining sexual satisfaction such as oral-genital sex (cunnilingus and fellatio) may be suggested. Explicit films (e.g., *Touching*) may also be used. This film demonstrates the sexual activities of a patient with paraplegia and a nondisabled partner. Graphics should be used cautiously because they may be too limiting or focus too much on the mechanics of sex rather than on the relationship.

Sexual activities may require more planning and be less spontaneous than before the injury. For example, an attendant may have to undress the patient and remove equipment. A relaxed atmosphere with music and perfume creates an attractive environment. Ample time for caressing, fondling, and kissing is essential. The partners should be encouraged to explore each other's erogenous areas, such as the lips, neck, and ears, which can arouse psychogenic erection or orgasm. Few demands should be made initially.

Care should be taken not to dislodge the indwelling catheter during sexual activity. If a Texas catheter is used, it should be removed before sexual activity and the patient should refrain from fluids. The bowel program should include evacuation the morning of sexual activity. The partner should be informed that an accident is always possible. The woman may need a water-soluble lubricant to supplement diminished vaginal secretions and facilitate vaginal penetration.

Menses may cease for as long as 6 months. If sexual activity is resumed, protection against an unplanned pregnancy is necessary. A normal pregnancy may be complicated by UTIs, anemia, and autonomic dysreflexia. Because uterine contractions are not felt, a precipitous delivery is always a danger. In men, fertility is reduced because of decreased number and motility of sperm and retrograde ejaculation of sperm into the bladder. For male patients desiring children, alternative methods include sperm harvesting and concentration, adoption, and artificial insemination.

Grief. Patients with spinal cord injuries are aware of the extent of injury and feel an overwhelming sense of loss. They are no longer in control and must depend on others for ADLs and for life-sustaining measures. Patients may believe that they are useless and burdens to their families. At a stage when independence is often of the greatest importance developmentally (the ages of 18 to 35 years), they are totally dependent on others.

The patient's response and recovery differ in some important aspects from those experiencing loss from amputation or terminal illness. First, regression can and does occur at different stages. Working through grief is a difficult, lifelong process with which the patient needs support and encouragement. With recent advances in rehabilitation, it is usual for the patient to be independent physically and discharged from the rehabilitation center before completion of the grief process. Another phenomenon involves that of triggering experiences, including new experiences such as marriage, that may recall earlier unresolved

Table 57-14	Mourning Process and Nursing Interventions in Spinal Cord Injury
Patient Behavior	**Nursing Intervention**
Shock and Denial Struggle for survival, complete dependence, excessive sleep, withdrawal, fantasies, unrealistic expectations	Use of meticulous nursing care. Be honest. Use simple diagrams to explain injury. Encourage patient to begin road to recovery.
Anger Refusal to discuss paralysis, decreased self-esteem, manipulation, hostile and abusive language	Coordinate care with patient and encourage self-care. Support family members; prevent alleviation of guilt by supporting dependency. Use humor liberally. Allow patient outbursts. Do not allow fixation on injury.
Depression Sadness, pessimism, anorexia, nightmares, insomnia, agitation, psychomotor retardation, "blues," suicidal preoccupation, refusal to participate in any self-care activities	Encourage family involvement and resources. Plan graded steps in rehabilitation to give success with minimal opportunity for frustration. Give cheerful and willing assistance with activities of daily living. Avoid sympathy. Use firm kindness.
Adjustment Planning for future, active participation in therapy, finding of personal meaning in experience and continuation of growth, return to premorbid personality	Remember that patients with spinal cord injuries have individual personalities. Balance support systems to encourage independence. Set goals with patient input. Emphasize potentials as achieved by others. Avoid use of clichés.

difficulties. Depending on the success of previous grief work, the new demand for grief work may be shortened or prolonged. The goal of recovery is related more to adjustment than to acceptance. Adjustment implies the ability to go on with living with certain limitations. Although the patient who is cooperative and accepting is easier to treat, the nurse should expect a wide fluctuation of emotions from a patient with a spinal cord injury. Depression may not be a component of the recovery process. Societal norms allow depression after severe loss and almost impose it on those confronted with death or radical lifestyle changes. However, every patient may not experience depression.

The nurse's role in grief work is to allow mourning as a component of the rehabilitation process. Table 57-14 summarizes the mourning process and appropriate nursing interventions. During the shock and denial stage the nurse reassures the patient and stresses the expertise of the entire health care team. During the anger stage, the nurse assists the patient in achievement of control over the environment, particularly by allowing the patient's input into the plan of care. The nurse should not respond to anger or manipulation or become involved in a power struggle with the patient. As self-care abilities increase, the patient's independence increases.

The patient's family also requires counseling to avoid promoting dependency in the patient through guilt or misplaced sympathy. The family is also experiencing an intense grieving process. A support group of family members and friends of patients with spinal cord injury can help increase family members' knowledge and participation in the grieving process, physical difficulties, rehabilitation plan, and the meaning of the disability in society.

During the stage of depression, the nurse must be patient, persistent, and maintain a sense of humor. Sympathy is not helpful. The patient should be treated in an adult manner and be involved in decision making about care, but the nurse must insist that the care be performed. A primary nurse relationship

is helpful, but the nurse needs some relief from the intense stress of continual interaction with the patient. Staff planning and sessions in which staff members can express their feelings are helpful in providing consistency of care. To achieve the stage of adjustment, the patient needs continual support throughout the rehabilitation in the forms of acceptance, affection, and caring. The nurse must be attentive when the patient needs to talk and sensitive to needs at the various stages of the grief process.

■ Evaluation

Expected outcomes for the patient with a spinal cord injury are presented in NCP 57-1 on p. 1729.

SPINAL CORD TUMORS

Etiology and Pathophysiology

Tumors that affect the spinal cord account for 0.5% to 1% of all neoplasms. These tumors are classified as primary (arising from some component of cord, dura, nerves, or vessels) or secondary (from primary growths in the breast, thyroid, lung, kidney, and other sites). The thoracic and lumbar spine, including the sacrum, are the most commonly affected areas. Spinal cord tumors are further classified as extramedullary (outside the spinal cord), including extra- and intradural, or intramedullary (within the spinal cord) (Fig. 57-13, Table 57-15). Extramedullary tumors compose 90% of all spinal cord tumors. Neurofibromas, meningiomas, gliomas, and hemangiomas are the most frequently occurring neoplasms.

Because many of these tumors are slow growing, their symptoms stem from the mechanical effects of slow compression and irritation of nerve roots, displacement of the cord, or gradual obstruction of the vascular supply. The slowness of growth does not cause autodestruction as in traumatic lesions. Therefore complete functional restoration is possible when the tumor is removed, except with the intradural-intramedullary tumors.

Most metastatic tumors are extradural lesions.[24] Tumors that commonly metastasize to the spinal epidural space are those that spread to bone, such as carcinomas of the breast, lung, prostate, and kidney.

Clinical Manifestations

The most common early symptom of a spinal cord tumor outside the cord is pain in the back with radicular pain simulating intercostal neuralgia, angina, or herpes zoster. The location of the pain depends on the level of compression. The pain worsens with activity, coughing, straining, and lying down. Sensory disruption is later manifested by coldness, numbness, and tingling in an extremity or in several extremities, slowly progressing upward until it reaches the level of the lesion. Impaired sensation of pain, temperature, and light touch precedes a deficit in vibration and position sense that may progress to complete anesthesia. Motor weakness accompanies the sensory distur-

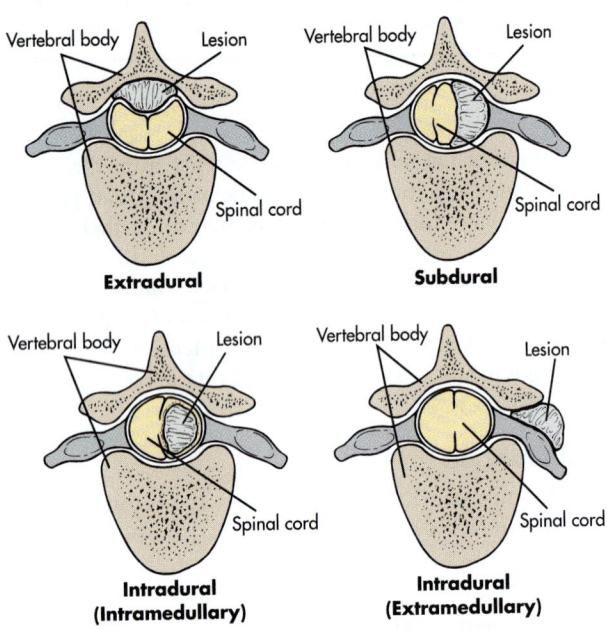

Fig. 57-13   Types of spinal cord tumors.

bances and consists of slowly increasing clumsiness, weakness, and spasticity. The sensory and motor disturbances are ipsilateral to the lesion. Bladder disturbances are marked by urgency with difficulty in starting the flow and progressing to retention with overflow incontinence.

Manifestations of intradural spinal tumor develop as progressive damage to the long spinal tracts, producing paralysis, sensory loss, and bladder dysfunction. Pain can be severe as a result of compression of spinal roots or vertebrae.

NURSING AND COLLABORATIVE MANAGEMENT: SPINAL CORD TUMORS

Extradural tumors are seen early on routine spinal x-rays, whereas intradural and intramedullary tumors require MRI or CT scans for detection. CSF analysis may reveal tumor cells. The cord is decompressed after removal of the tumor by a laminectomy. More than 85% of primary neoplasms are benign and can be completely resected; 90% of patients recover without residual problems.

Compression of the spinal cord is an emergency. Relief of the ischemia related to the compression is the goal of therapy. Corticosteroids are generally prescribed immediately to relieve tumor-related edema. Dexamethasone (Decadron) is usually used, often in large doses.

Treatment for nearly all spinal cord tumors is surgical removal. The exception is the metastatic tumor that is sensitive to radiation and that has caused only minimal neurologic deficits in the patient.[24] In general, tumors of the extradural or intradural-extramedullary group can be completely removed surgically. Intramedullary tumors offer a less favorable prognosis; however, exploration and removal is usually attempted.

Radiation therapy after the operation is fairly effective. Maximum permissible tissue dose is given over 6 to 8 weeks. Chemotherapy has also been used in conjunction with radiation therapy.

Relief of pain and return of function are the ultimate goals of treatment. Nurses must be aware of the neurologic status of the patient before and after treatment. Ensuring that the patient receives pain medication as needed is an important nursing responsibility. Depending on the amount of neurologic dysfunction exhibited, the patient may need to be cared for as though recovering from a spinal cord injury.

Table **57-15**	**Classification of Spinal Cord Tumors**		
Type	**Incidence**	**Treatment**	**Prognosis**
Extradural From bones of spine, in extradural space, or in paraspinal tissue	20-50% of all intraspinal tumors, mostly malignant metastatic lesions	Relief of cord pressure by surgical laminectomy, radiation, chemotherapy, or combination approach	Poor
Intradural Extramedullary Within dura mater outside cord	Most frequent of intradural tumors (40%), mostly benign meningiomas and neurofibromas	Complete surgical removal of tumor (if possible), partial removal followed by radiation	Usually very good if lack of damage to cord from compression
Intradural Intramedullary	Least frequent of intradural tumors (5-10%)	Partial surgical removal, radiation therapy (resulting in only temporary improvement)	Very poor

CRITICAL THINKING EXERCISES

CASE STUDY

Spinal Cord Injury

Patient Profile

Samuel D., a 25-year-old-male, is admitted to the emergency department with the diagnosis of a cervical spinal cord injury. Samuel was swimming at a neighbor's backyard pool. He dove into the shallow end, striking his head on the bottom of the pool. His friends noticed that he did not resurface and they brought him to the side of the pool. They maintained neck immobilization until the rescue crews arrived.

Subjective Data

- Is awake and alert
- Has complaints of neck pain
- Is anxious and asking why he cannot move his legs
- Is asking to see his family

Objective Data

Physical Examination
- Weak biceps movement
- No triceps movement
- Gross elbow movement present
- Decreased sensation from the shoulders down
- No bladder or bowel control
- BP 90/56; pulse 56; respirations 32 and labored

Diagnostic Studies
- X-rays revealed C5 fracture dislocation

Collaborative Care

- Placed in tongs and traction in the emergency department
- Started on methylprednisolone in the emergency department
- Admitted to intensive care unit

Critical Thinking Questions

1. What nursing activities would be a priority on Samuel D.'s arrival in the intensive care unit?
2. What physiologic problems are causing Samuel D. to have hypotension and bradycardia?
3. What would the first line of treatment be for Samuel D.'s hypotension and bradycardia?
4. What signs and symptoms would indicate respiratory distress and what physiologic problem would cause respiratory distress in Samuel D.'s injury state?
5. What can the nurse do to decrease Samuel D.'s anxiety?
6. Based on the assessment data provided, write one or more nursing diagnoses. Are there any collaborative problems?

NURSING RESEARCH ISSUES

1. What is the best method of education in the prevention of spinal cord injuries?
2. What is the best method to prevent skin breakdown?
3. What type of support or education is best for the families of patients with spinal cord injuries to help them cope with their situation?
4. What nursing interventions enhance self-care in the patient with a spinal cord injury?
5. What is the best method of preventing UTIs in the spinal cord injured patient?
6. Examine the relationship between the functional ability of spinal cord injury and quality of life.

REVIEW QUESTIONS

The number of the question corresponds to the same-numbered objective at the beginning of the chapter.

1. During assessment of the patient with trigeminal neuralgia the nurse should
   a. inspect all aspects of the mouth and teeth.
   b. lightly palpate the affected side of the face for edema.
   c. ask the patient to describe factors that initiate an episode.
   d. test for temperature and sensation perception on the face.
2. During routine assessment of a patient with Guillain-Barré syndrome the nurse finds the patient to be short of breath. The patient's respiratory distress is caused by
   a. immobility resulting from ascending paralysis.
   b. elevated protein levels in the CSF.
   c. degeneration of motor neurons in the brainstem and spinal cord.
   d. paralysis ascending to the nerves that stimulate the thoracic area.
3. The person most likely to sustain a spinal cord injury is a
   a. 35-year-old male tennis player.
   b. 75-year-old male with heart disease.
   c. 19-year-old male who rides a motorcycle.
   d. 60-year-old female with multiple sclerosis.
4. A patient is admitted to the ICU with a C7 spinal cord injury and diagnosed with Brown-Séquard syndrome. On physical examination the nurse would most likely find
   a. upper extremity weakness only.
   b. complete motor and sensory loss below C7.
   c. ipsilateral motor loss and contralateral sensory loss below C7.
   d. loss of position sense and vibration in both lower extremities.
5. A patient is admitted to the hospital with a spinal cord injury following an automobile accident. The nurse recognizes that the pathophysiology of indirect spinal cord trauma involves
   a. initial infarction of the white matter of the cord.
   b. mechanical transection of the cord by the trauma.
   c. necrotic destruction of the cord from hemorrhage and edema.
   d. release of epinephrine leading to massive vasodilation of spinal cord vessels.

6. A rehabilitation goal for the patient with an injury at the C5 level includes
   a. feeding self with hand devices.
   b. driving an electric wheelchair.
   c. assisting with transfer activities.
   d. controlling bowel and bladder functions.
7. A patient with a C7 spinal cord injury undergoing rehabilitation tells the nurse he must have the flu because he has a bad headache and nausea. The initial action of the nurse is to
   a. call the physician.
   b. check the patient's temperature.
   c. take the patient's blood pressure.
   d. palpate the patient's bladder for distention.
8. The most common early symptom of a spinal cord tumor is
   a. urinary incontinence.
   b. back pain that worsens with activity.
   c. paralysis below the level of involvement.
   d. impaired sensation of pain, temperature, and light touch.

References

1. DeMarco JK, Hesselink JR: Trigeminal neuropathy, *Neurosurg Clin N Am* 8:1, 1997.
2. Brown JA: The trigeminal complex, *Neurosurg Clin N Am* 8:1, 1997.
3. Lange DJ, Trojaburg W, Roland LP: Peripheral and cranial nerve lesion. In Rowland LP, editor: *Merritt's textbook of neurology,* ed 9, Baltimore, 1995, Williams & Wilkins.
4. MacFarlane BV and others: Chronic neuropathic pain and its control by drugs, *Pharmacol Ther* 75:1, 1997.
5. McConoghy DJ: Trigeminal neuralgia: a personal review and nursing implications, *J Neurosci Nurs* 26:85, 1994.
6. Lovely TJ, Jannetta PJ: Microvascular decompression for trigeminal neuralgia, *Neurosurg Clin N Am* 8:1, 1997.
7. Jho HD, Lunsford LD: Percutaneous retrogasserian glycerol rhizotomy, current techniques and results, *Neurosurg Clin N Am* 8:1, 1997.
8. Kondziolka D and others: Gamma knife radiosurgery for trigeminal neuralgia, *Neurosurg Clin N Am* 8:1, 1997.
9. Hashisaki GT: Medical management of Bell's palsy, *Compr Ther* 23:715, 1997.
10. Billue JS: Bell's palsy: an update on idiopathic facial paralysis, *Nurse Pract* 22:88, 1997.
11. Adams RD, Victor M, Ropper AH, editors: *Principles of neurology,* ed 6, New York, 1997, McGraw-Hill.
12. Koski CL: Guillian-Barré syndrome and chronic inflammatory demyelinating polyneuropathy: pathogenesis and treatment, *Semin Neurol* 14:123, 1994.
13. Lange DJ, Latov N, Trojabor W: Acquired neuropathies. In Rowland LP, editor: *Merritt's textbook of neurology,* ed 9, Baltimore, 1995, Williams & Wilkins.
14. Hui YH and others, editors: *Foodborne disease handbook,* New York, 1994, Marcel Dekker.
15. Miller JR: Bacterial toxins. In Rowland LP, editor: *Merritt's textbook of neurology,* ed 9, Baltimore, 1995, Williams & Wilkins.
16. Dworkin R, Leggett J: Gram positive bacillary infections and clostridial infections. In Stein JH, editor: *Internal medicine,* ed 5, St Louis, 1998, Mosby.
17. Marotta JT: Spinal injury. In Rowland LP, editor: *Merritt's textbook of neurology,* ed 9, Baltimore, 1995, Williams & Wilkins.
18. Wirtz KM, LaFavor KM, Ang R: Managing chronic spinal cord injury: issues in critical care, *Crit Care Nurse* 16:4, 1996.
19. Stamatos CA and others: Meeting the challenge of the older trauma patient, *AJN* 96:5, 1996.
20. Heary RF and others: Steroids and gun shot wounds to the spine, *Neurosurgery* 41:3, 1997.
21. Hickey JV: *The clinical practice of neurological and neurosurgical nursing,* ed 4, Philadelphia, 1997, Lippincott.
22. Segator M, Way C: Neuroprotection after spinal cord injury: state of the science, *Sci Nursing* 14:8, 1997.
23. Rhoney DH and others: New pharmacological approaches to acute spinal cord injuries, *Pharmacotherapy* 16:3, 1996.
24. McCormick PC, Fetell MR: Spinal tumors. In Rowland LP, editor: *Merritt's textbook of neurology,* ed 9, Baltimore, 1995, Williams & Wilkins.

Resources

American Association for Rehabilitation Therapy (AART)
PO Box 6412
Gulfport, MS 39506

American Association of Spinal Cord Injury Nurses (AASCIN)
75-20 Astoria Boulevard
Jackson Heights, NY 11370-1177
718-803-3782
Fax: 718-803-0414
http://www.aascin.org/default.html

American Congress of Rehabilitation Medicine
4700 W Lake Avenue
Glenview, IL 60025
847-375-4725
Fax: 847-375-4777
http://www.acrm.org/

American Paralysis/Spinal Cord Hotline
2201 Argonne Drive
Baltimore, MD 21218
800-526-3456
800-638-1733 (in Maryland)

Amyotrophic Lateral Sclerosis Association
21021 Ventura Blvd, Suite 321
Woodland Hills, CA 91364
818-990-2151
http://www.alsa.org

Guillain-Barré Syndrome Foundation International
PO Box 262
Wynnewood, PA 19096
610-667-0131
Fax: 610-667-7036
http://www.webmast.com/gbs/

Myasthenia Gravis Foundation
53 West Jackson Blvd, Suite 909
Chicago, IL 60604
800-541-5454
312-258-0522
Fax: 312-258-0461
http://www.med.unc.edu/mgfa/

National Rehabilitation Information Center
8455 Colesville Road, Suite 935
Silver Spring, MD 20910
301-588-9284
http://www.naric.com/naric/index.html

National Spinal Cord Injury Association
8300 Colesville Road, Suite 551
Silver Spring, MD 20910
301-588-6959
800-962-9629
http://www.spinalcord.org/

Paralyzed Veterans of America
801 18th Street NW
Washington, DC 20006
202-872-1300
800-424-8200 x619 or x620
202-416-7619 or 7620
http://www.pva.or

For additional Internet resources, see the website for this book at **www.mosby.com/MERLIN/medsurg_lewis**

58 NURSING ASSESSMENT
Musculoskeletal System

Susan C. Ruda

www.mosby.com/MERLIN/medsurg_lewis

LEARNING OBJECTIVES

1. Describe the gross anatomic and microscopic composition of bone.
2. Explain the classification system of joints and movements at synovial joints.
3. Describe the types and structure of muscle tissue.
4. Describe the functions of cartilage, muscles, ligaments, tendons, fascia, and bursae.
5. Describe age-related changes in the musculoskeletal system and differences in assessment findings.
6. Identify the significant subjective and objective data related to the musculoskeletal system that should be obtained from a patient.
7. Describe the appropriate techniques used in the physical assessment of the musculoskeletal system.
8. Differentiate normal from abnormal findings of a physical assessment of the musculoskeletal system.
9. Describe the purpose, significance of results, and nursing responsibilities related to diagnostic studies of the musculoskeletal system.

The ability to perform complex and precise movements permits human beings to interact and adapt to the environment. Proper functioning of the musculoskeletal system makes such movements possible. The musculoskeletal system consists of bones, muscles, joints, cartilage, ligaments, tendons, fascia, and bursae.

The musculoskeletal system is particularly vulnerable to external forces. These forces can cause alteration in the structure of bone or soft connective tissue, resulting in functional disruption. The consequences may be deformity, alteration of body image, alteration in mobility, pain, or permanent disability. These problems may produce long-term health problems that interfere with activities of daily living and quality of life.

STRUCTURES AND FUNCTIONS OF THE MUSCULOSKELETAL SYSTEM

Bone

Function. The main functions of the musculoskeletal system are support, protection of vital organs, movement, blood cell production, and mineral storage.[1] Bone forms the body's supporting framework. Without this support, the body would collapse. Bone also allows the body to bear weight. The musculoskeletal system is important in protecting underlying vital organs and tissues. For example, the skull protects the brain, the vertebrae protect the spinal cord, and the rib cage protects the lungs and heart. Bones serve as a point of attachment for muscles; muscles are anchored to bones by tendons. Bone acts as a lever for muscles, and joints serve as fulcrums.

Movement occurs as a result of muscle contractions applied to these levers. Bone also serves as a site for storage of inorganic minerals such as calcium and phosphorus. Cancellous bone contains hematopoietic tissue for the production of blood cells and platelets.

Gross Structure. Bone is a dynamic tissue that changes form and substance continually. It is composed of organic material (collagen) and inorganic material (calcium, phosphate). The internal and external growth and remodeling of bone are continuous processes.

Bone is classified according to structure as compact (dense) or cancellous (spongy). In compact bone, cylinder-shaped structural units (haversian systems) fit closely together, giving a dense consistency to the bone structure.[2] In cancellous bone, there are many open spaces between thin processes and networks of bone tissue. The networks are filled with either red or yellow marrow.

The anatomic structure of bone can best be visualized by the typical long bone (e.g., femur) (Fig. 58-1). Each long bone consists of an epiphysis, articular cartilage, a diaphysis, periosteum, and a medullary (marrow) cavity.

The epiphysis is located at each end of a long bone and is composed of cancellous bone. It is the location for muscle attachment and provides stability for the joint. Articular cartilage covers the ends of the bone and provides a smooth surface for joint movement.

The diaphysis is the main shaft of bone. It provides the bone with structural support and is composed of compact bone. The metaphysis is the flared area between the epiphysis and the diaphysis. During bone development it contains the growth zones. In the adult the metaphysis is joined to the epiphysis. The epiphyseal plate, or growth zone, is the cartilaginous area that

Reviewed by Dennis Ross, RN, PhD, Professor of Nursing, Castleton State College, Castleton, Vt; Nursing Faculty, Regents College, Albany, NY.

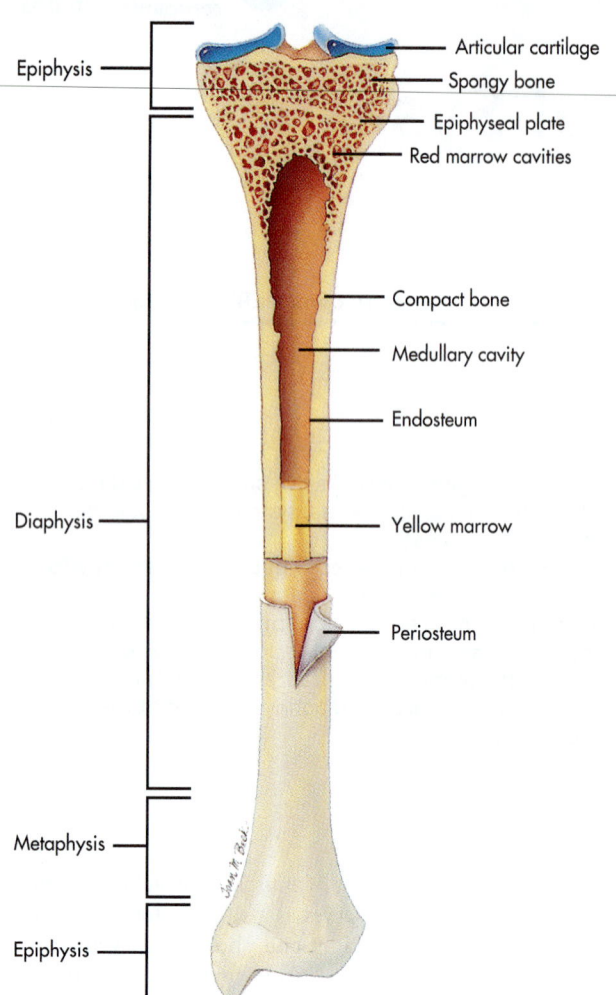

Epiphysis

Articular cartilage
Spongy bone
Epiphyseal plate
Red marrow cavities

Compact bone

Medullary cavity

Endosteum

Diaphysis

Yellow marrow

Periosteum

Metaphysis

Epiphysis

Fig. 58-1   Longitudinal section of a long bone.

actively produces bone and results in longitudinal growth in children. Injury to the epiphyseal plate in a growing child can cause significant problems, such as altered growth of the extremity. In the adult, this plate will harden to mature bone, and longitudinal growth will cease.

The periosteum is fibrous connective tissue that covers the bone. Musculotendinous fibers attach to the outer layer of the periosteum. The inner layer of the periosteum contains osteoblasts (bone-forming cells), which are essential for transverse bone growth and fracture repair.

The medullary (marrow) cavity is in the center of the diaphysis. In the adult, the medullary cavity of long bones contains yellow bone marrow, which is mainly adipose tissue. In the growing child, red bone marrow in the medullary cavity is actively involved in hematopoiesis. In the adult, hematopoiesis normally occurs only in the red bone marrow of the skull, ribs, sternum, pelvis, vertebrae, and proximal ends (epiphyses) of the humerus and femur.

Microscopic Structure. The three types of bone cells are osteoblasts, osteocytes, and osteoclasts. *Osteoblasts* synthesize organic bone matrix (collagen) and are the basic bone-forming cells. *Osteocytes* are the mature bone cells. *Osteoclasts* function in the breakdown of bone tissue and participate in bone remodeling. *Bone remodeling* is the removal of old bone by

osteoclasts (resorption) and the deposition of new bone by osteoblasts (ossification). The inner layer of bone is primarily made up of osteoblasts with a few osteoclasts.

Bone is a special kind of connective tissue in which organic matter (collagen) has become mineralized. The structural unit of compact bone is the haversian system (Fig. 58-2). It consists of lamellae, which are concentric layers of calcified collagen matrix that enclose a long canal (haversian system). The main function of the haversian system is to transport blood to bone tissue. Blood vessels from the periosteum travel through Volkmann's canals to the blood vessels of the haversian system.

Osteocytes (mature bone cells) lie in small spaces termed *lacunae* between lamellae. Canaliculi (tiny canals) extend from the lacunae to connect the osteocytes to one another and to the haversian system.

Types.   The skeleton consists of 206 named bones. These bones are classified according to shape as long, short, flat, or irregular.

Long bones are characterized by a central shaft (diaphysis) and two epiphyseal ends (see Fig. 58-1). Examples include the femur, humerus, and radius. Short bones are characterized by cancellous bone covered by a thin layer of compact bone. Examples include the carpals and tarsals.

Flat bones are characterized by two layers of compact bone separated by a layer of cancellous bone. Examples include the ribs, skull, scapula, and sternum. The spaces in the cancellous bone contain bone marrow. Irregular bones have a variety of shapes and sizes. Examples include the vertebrae, sacrum, and mandible.

Joints

A *joint* (articulation) is a place where two bones come together. Joints hold bones firmly together while permitting movement between them. Joints are commonly classified according to their degree of movement (Fig. 58-3).

The diarthrodial (synovial) type, the most common joint, consists of a cavity between the articular surfaces of the bones that make up the joint (Fig. 58-4). The ends of the bone are covered with articular (hyaline) cartilage. A capsule of connective tissue (the fibrous or joint capsule) joins the two bones together, forming a cavity. The capsule is lined by a synovial membrane, which secretes a thick synovial fluid to lubricate the joint and reduce friction. Types of diarthrodial joints are shown in Fig. 58-5. Structures surrounding the joint (periarticular tissues) provide support for joint function (e.g., ligaments and tendons).

Cartilage

Cartilage is a rigid connective tissue that functions to support soft tissue and provides the articular surface for joint movement. It protects underlying tissues. The cartilage that makes up the epiphyseal plate is also essential for the growth of long bones before physical maturity is reached.

Cartilage is avascular and therefore is nourished by the diffusion of material from capillaries in adjacent connective tissue. Cartilage cells are slow to reproduce because of the lack of a direct blood supply, which explains why damaged cartilage heals slowly.

The three types of cartilage tissue are hyaline, elastic, and fibrous. Hyaline cartilage, the most common, contains a moderate amount of collagen fibers. It is found in the trachea,

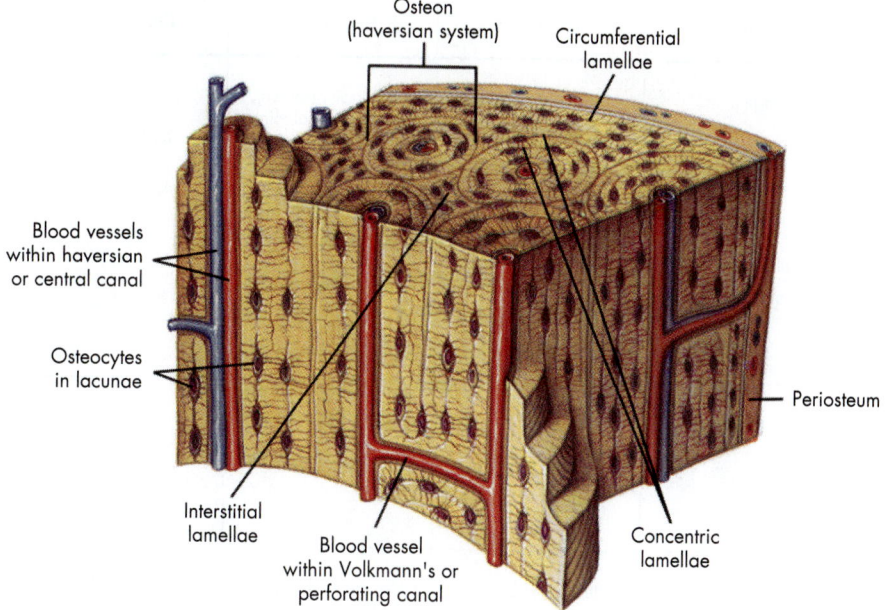

Fig. 58-2   Structure of compact bone showing haversian system.

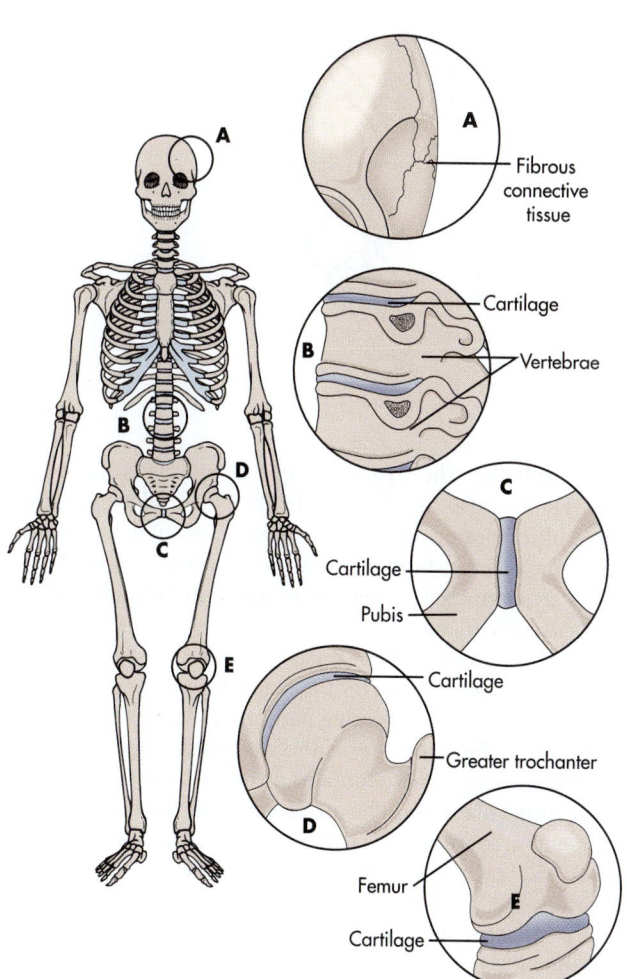

Fig. 58-3   Classification of joints. **A, B, C,** Synarthrotic (immovable) and amphiarthrotic (slightly movable) joints. **D, E,** Diarthrodial (freely movable) joints.

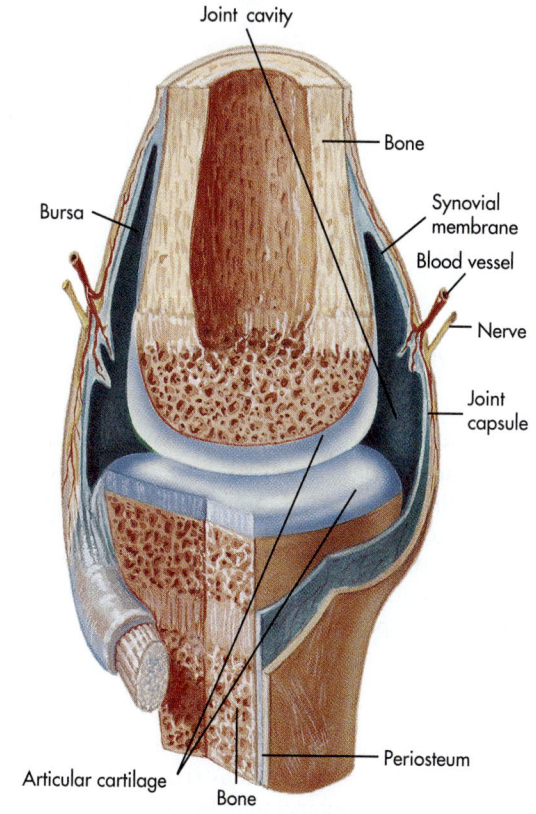

Fig. 58-4   Structure of a synovial joint.

Joint	Movement	Examples	Illustration
Hinge joint	Flexion, extension	Elbow joint (shown), interphalangeal joints, knee joint	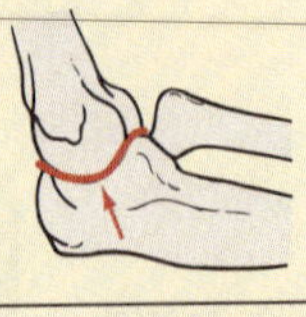
Ball and socket (spheroidal)	Flexion, extension; adduction, abduction; circumduction	Shoulder (shown), hip	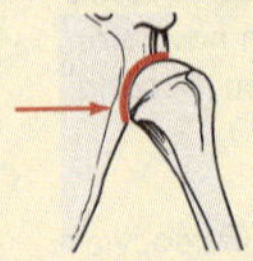
Pivot (rotary)	Rotation	Atlas-axis, proximal radioulnar joint (shown)	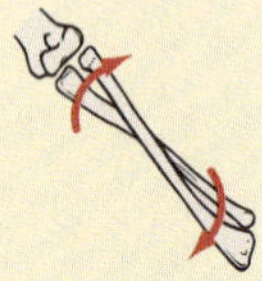
Condyloid	Flexion, extension; abduction, adduction; circumduction	Wrist joint (between radial and carpals) (shown)	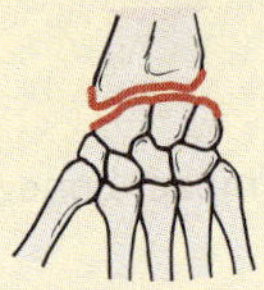
Saddle	Flexion, extension; abduction, adduction; circumduction, thumb-finger opposition	Carpometacarpal joint of thumb	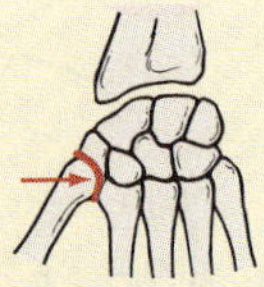
Gliding	One surface moves over another surface	Between tarsal bones, sacroiliac joint, between articular processes of vertebrae, between carpal bones (shown)	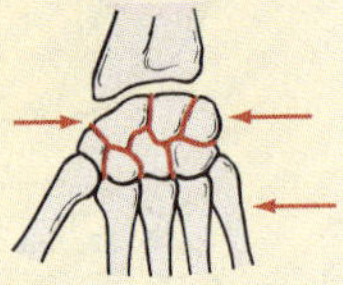

Fig. 58-5   Types of diarthrodial joints.

bronchi, nose, and articular surfaces of bones. Elastic cartilage, which contains collagen and elastic fibers, is more flexible than hyaline cartilage. It is found in the ear, epiglottis, and larynx. Fibrocartilage, which consists mostly of collagen fibers, is a tough tissue that often functions as a shock absorber. It is found between the vertebral disks and in the knee. Fibrocartilage also forms a protective cushion between the bones of the pelvic girdle.

Muscle

Types. The three types of muscle tissue are cardiac (striated, involuntary), smooth (nonstriated, involuntary), and skeletal (striated, voluntary) muscle. Cardiac muscle is found in the heart. Its contractions provide the major force for propelling blood through the circulatory system. Cardiac muscle contracts spontaneously. Smooth muscle is found in the walls of hollow structures such as airways, the gastrointestinal (GI) tract, urinary bladder, uterus, and some blood vessels. Smooth muscle contraction is modulated by neuronal and hormonal influences. Skeletal muscle requires neuronal stimulation for contraction. Skeletal muscle composes the largest mass of tissue in the body and is the focus of the following discussion.

Structure. The structural unit of muscle is the muscle cell, which is also called a muscle fiber. Skeletal muscle fibers are multinucleated cylinders that range in length and diameter from several millimeters to several centimeters. Muscle fibers are composed of myofibrils, which in turn are made up of contractile filaments.

Under a microscope, skeletal muscle shows alternating banding, which accounts for the striated appearance.[3] This appearance is due to a repeating pattern of filaments seen in the myofibrils. The sarcomere is the contractile unit of the myofibrils. Each sarcomere contains myosin (thick) filaments and actin (thin) filaments. The arrangement of the thin and thick filaments accounts for the banding. As thick and thin filaments slide past each other, the sarcomeres shorten and muscle shortens.

Contractions. Skeletal muscle contractions are responsible for the functions of posture, movement, and facial expressions. Isometric contractions increase the tension within a muscle but do not produce movement. Repeated isometric contractions make muscles grow larger and stronger. Isotonic contractions produce movement. Most contractions are a combination of tension generation (isometric) and shorten-

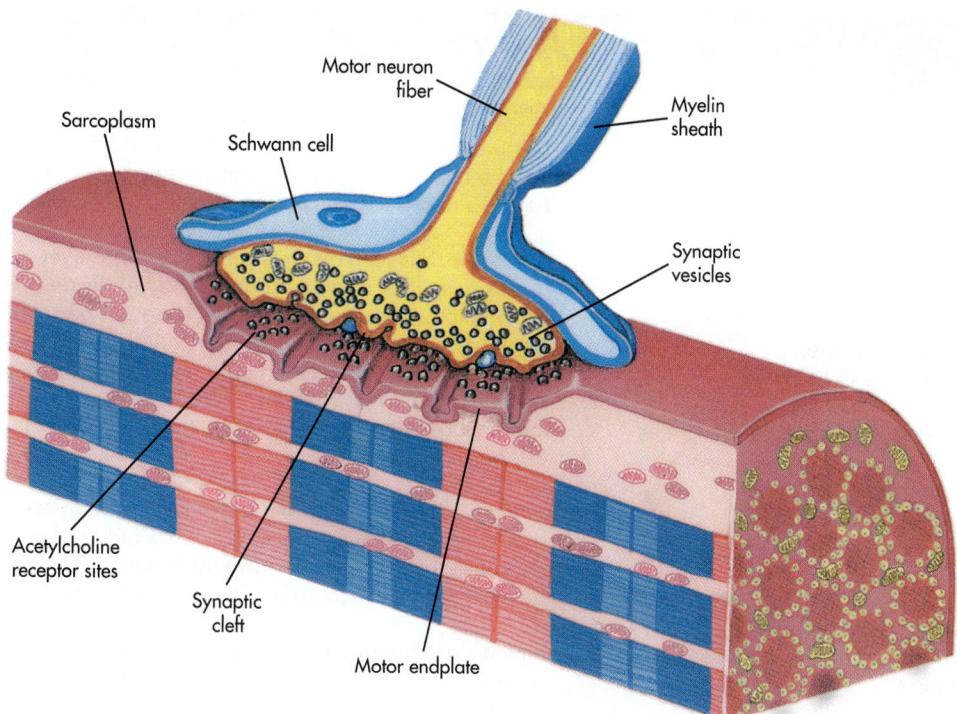

Fig. 58-6   Neuromuscular junction.

ing (isotonic). Without muscle contraction there is atrophy (decrease in size), and with increased muscle activity there is hypertrophy (increase in size).

Skeletal muscle produces other types of contractions that have little to do with functional posture and movement. They are a twitch contraction (a quick contraction in response to a single stimulus) and a tetanic contraction (a more sustained twitch).

Neuromuscular Junction. Skeletal muscles require a nerve supply in order to contract. The nerve fiber and the skeletal muscle fibers it supplies are called a *motor end plate*.[4] The junction between the axon of the nerve cell and the muscle cell it supplies is called the *myoneural* or *neuromuscular junction* (Fig. 58-6).

When acetylcholine is released from the motor end plate of the neuron, it diffuses across the neuromuscular junction and binds with receptors on the muscle fiber. In response to this stimulation, the sarcoplasmic reticulum releases calcium ions into the cytoplasm. The presence of these ions triggers the contraction in the myofibrils.

Energy Source.   The energy source used in muscle fiber contractions comes from adenosine triphosphate (ATP). ATP is synthesized by cellular oxidative metabolism in numerous mitochondria located close to the myofibrils. A second energy source is creatine phosphate, which supplies phosphate to rephosphorylate ATP. Creatine phosphate is synthesized and stored in muscle tissue.

Ligaments and Tendons

Ligaments and tendons are both composed of dense, fibrous connective tissue. This type of connective tissue contains large numbers of collagen fibers that are closely packed. Tendons attach muscles to bones. They are an extension of the muscle sheath that attaches to the periosteum. Ligaments connect bones to bones at joints (e.g., the knee joint). They permit movement while providing stability.

Fibrous connective tissue has a relatively poor blood supply. Although the tissue can repair itself after injury, it is usually a slow process. For example, a sprain, which is the stretching or tearing of the ligaments, may require a long time to heal.[5]

Fascia

Fascia is the term used for layers of connective tissue. It is classified as either superficial or deep. Superficial fascia is the loose connective tissue located immediately under the skin. Deep fascia (dense, fibrous connective tissue) is found surrounding muscle, between muscles, and surrounding the bundles that bind muscles, nerves, and blood vessels together.

Fascia separates one muscle from another to permit independent muscle action. It allows gliding of one muscle over another. In addition, fascia provides strength to muscle tissues.

Bursae

Bursae are small sacs of connective tissue lined with synovial membrane and synovial fluid. They are commonly located at bone prominences such as the joint. Bursae function as cushions to relieve pressure between the moving parts and prevent friction (see Fig. 58-4). For example, they are found between the patella and the skin (prepatellar bursa), between the olecranon process and the skin (olecranon bursa), between the head of the humerus and the acromion process (subacromial bursa), and between the lower portion of the gluteus maximus muscle and the bony ischial tuberosity (submuscular bursa). Bursitis (inflammation of the bursa) may be caused by mechanical injury to the bursa or excessive use of a joint.

GERONTOLOGIC DIFFERENCES IN ASSESSMENT

Table 58-1 Prevention of Common Musculoskeletal Problems in the Older Adult

Activity	Rationale
■ Use of ramps in buildings and at street corners instead of steps	Stair-walking motion may create enough stress on fragile bones to cause a hip fracture. Use of ramps may prevent falls.
■ Elimination of scatter rugs in the home	These are notorious for causing falls and fractures.
■ Response to pain and discomfort of osteoarthritis	
Resting in reclining position	Osteoarthritis is seen on x-ray of most persons over age 50 and causes pain. Rest is the most useful way to decrease discomfort.
Use of plain or enteric-coated aspirin or nonsteroidal antiinflammatory	Aspirin and other antiinflammatory drugs (as prescribed by physician) diminish inflammation of joints and reduce pain.
Use of a walker or cane to help with walking	Assistance decreases stress on inflamed joints and thus decreases discomfort. Use may prevent falls.
■ Eating amount and kind of foods to prevent excess weight gain	Obesity adds stress to bones, which may predispose patient to osteoarthritis.
■ Regular and frequent exercise	
Activities of daily living	Activities of daily living provide range-of-motion exercise, which should be done four times a day; 100% range of motion is not as critical as the ability to perform usual and preferred activities.
Hobbies (e.g., jigsaw puzzles, needlework, model building)	These exercise distal joints and prevent stiffness.
Walking short distances daily with shoes that give good support	Some weight-bearing exercise is essential and should be done two or three times daily. Good shoes provide for safety and promote comfort.
■ Gradual initiation of all activities	Starting gradually promotes optimal coordination. When a patient rises slowly to a standing position, dizziness and hence falls and fractures can be prevented.

GERONTOLOGIC CONSIDERATIONS

Effects of Aging on the Musculoskeletal System

Many of the functional problems of the aging adult are due to changes of the musculoskeletal system. Many of these changes begin in early adulthood, but obvious signs of musculoskeletal impairment may not appear until later in adulthood. These alterations may affect posture, function, and gait and lead to an increase in falls. They affect the older adult's lifestyle and activities of daily living, ranging from discomfort and decreased ability to perform activities of daily living to severe, chronic pain and immobility.[6]

Numerous age-related changes affect the bones, muscles, joints, and connective tissue. The bone remodeling process is altered, resulting in increased bone resorption and decreased osteoblastic activity. These alterations in bone density are a major factor in osteoporosis (see Chapter 59). Muscle functioning declines because of a decrease in muscle mass and strength.[7] Almost 30% of the muscle mass is lost by the eighth decade of life. An age-related loss in the motor neurons that control skeletal muscle movement also occurs. Joints, tendons, and ligaments harden over time, resulting in less flexible and rigid movement.[8] Joints become stiff.

In addition to the usual musculoskeletal assessment with a particular emphasis on exercise practices, the nurse should determine the impact of age-related changes of the musculoskeletal system on the functional status of the older patient. Functional limitations that are accepted by older adults as a normal part of aging can often be halted or reversed with appropriate preventive strategies (Table 58-1). Age-related changes in the musculoskeletal system and differences in assessment findings are presented in Table 58-2.

ASSESSMENT OF THE MUSCULOSKELETAL SYSTEM

Correct diagnosis depends on an accurate patient history and a thorough examination. A musculoskeletal assessment can be made on a specific body part, as part of a general physical examination, or as an examination in itself. Judgment must be used on the basis of the patient's problem in selecting all or part of the components of the musculoskeletal history and physical examination. Accidents often result in trauma to the musculoskeletal system and require a thorough assessment. If the injury is serious or life threatening, only pertinent information related to the accident is obtained, and a complete assessment is deferred.

Complaints that should alert the nurse to obtain subjective and objective data related to the musculoskeletal system include joint or muscle pain, joint swelling, decreasing strength or function, change in size of an extremity or muscle, deformity, spasms, crepitation, changes in sensation, stiffness, and changes in gait. Health history questions presented in Table 58-3 should be asked when a musculoskeletal problem is noted.

Subjective Data

Important Health Information

Past health history. Certain illnesses are known to affect the musculoskeletal system either directly or indirectly. The patient should be questioned specifically about a history of tuberculosis, poliomyelitis, diabetes mellitus, gout, inflammatory and degenerative arthritis, hemophilia, parathyroid problems, rickets, osteomalacia, scurvy, osteomyelitis or soft tissue infection, fungal infection of the bones or joints, and neuromuscular disabilities. If the patient has a history of any of these problems, a detailed account of the illness should be obtained. In addition, the patient should be questioned about

Table 58-2 **Musculoskeletal System**

Changes	Differences in Assessment Findings
Muscle	
Decreased number and diameter of muscle cells, replacement of muscle cells by fibrous connective tissue	Decreased muscle strength and bulk, abdominal protrusion, muscle flabbiness
Loss of elasticity in ligaments and cartilage	Decreased fine motor activity, decreased agility
Reduced ability to store glycogen; decreased ability to release glycogen as quick energy in times of stress	Slowed reaction times, slowing of most muscle neuronal reflexes, slowing of impulse conduction along motor units, easy fatigability
Joints	
Erosion of articular cartilage, possible direct contact between bone ends	Manifestations of osteoarthritis, joint stiffness, possible crepitation on movement of joints, pain with range-of-motion movements
Overgrowth of bone around joint margins (osteophytes)	Heberden's nodes in fingers (especially in women), limited mobility in affected joints
Loss of water from disks between vertebrae, narrowing of joint vertebral spaces	Loss of height, back pain, joint subluxation
Bone	
Decrease in bone mass	Dowager's hump (kyphosis) caused by compression of vertebral bodies
	Decreased height

possible sources of secondary bacterial infections, such as ears, tonsils, teeth, sinuses, or genitourinary tract, which can result in osteomyelitis.

Medications. The patient should be questioned carefully regarding prescription and over-the-counter drugs used to treat a musculoskeletal problem. Information on the reason for taking the medication, its name, the dose and frequency, length of time it was taken, its effect, and any side effects should be obtained. Specific inquiry should be made related to skeletal muscle relaxants, antirheumatoid agents, nonsteroidal antiinflammatory drugs, narcotics, and systemic corticosteroids. The patient should be questioned about GI distress or a bleeding ulcer if antiinflammatory agents have been taken.

In addition to drugs taken for treatment of a musculoskeletal problem, the patient should be questioned about drugs that can have detrimental effects on this system. These drugs include antiseizure drugs (osteomalacia), phenothiazines (gait disturbances), corticosteroids (abnormal fat distribution, avascular necrosis, and decreased bone and muscle mass), and potassium-depleting diuretics (muscle cramps and weakness). Amphetamines and caffeine intake can cause a generalized increase in motor activity. Older women should be questioned about their menopausal status, the use of hormone replacement therapy, and calcium and vitamin D supplementation.

Surgery or other treatments. Information should be obtained about hospitalizations that were necessitated by a musculoskeletal problem. The reason for the hospitalization, the date and duration, and the treatment should be carefully documented. Specifics of any surgical procedure and postoperative course should also be obtained. If there was a period of prolonged immobilization, the possible development of osteoporosis and muscle atrophy should be considered. The patient should also be questioned about emergency treatment related to musculoskeletal disorders and injuries.

Functional Health Patterns. The use of functional health patterns aids the nurse in organizing the data and formulating diagnoses based on data collected about the muscu-

loskeletal system. Table 58-3 summarizes the health history questions to ask in relation to functional health patterns.

Health perception–health management pattern. The nurse should ask about the patient's health practices related to the musculoskeletal system, such as maintenance of a normal body weight, avoidance of excessive stress on muscles and joints, and the use of proper body mechanics when lifting objects.[9]

The patient should be specifically questioned about immunizations related to tetanus and polio. The most current date and reaction to a tuberculin skin test should also be obtained.

Food or contact allergies are of little consequence in relation to musculoskeletal problems. However, the general malaise often associated with allergic reactions may manifest in musculoskeletal stiffness and lethargy. Allergic reactions to drugs used to treat musculoskeletal problems can interfere with therapy, and an alternative treatment may have to be employed if the allergic reaction is severe.

The list of minor and major injuries of the musculoskeletal system can be extensive in the patient who is a good historian. It includes documentation of fractures, sprains, strains, and dislocations. The information should be recorded chronologically and should include the following:

1. Mechanism of the injury (twist, crush, stretch)
2. Circumstances related to the injury
3. Diagnostic evaluations
4. Methods of treatment
5. Duration of treatment
6. Current status related to the injury
7. Need for assistive devices
8. Interference with activities of daily living

A three-generation family history should be obtained related to rheumatoid arthritis, degenerative joint disease, gout, osteoporosis, and scoliosis because these problems have a familial predisposition.

Safety practices can play a role in the patient's predisposition for certain injuries and illnesses. Specific questions should be

HEALTH HISTORY

Table 58-3 Musculoskeletal System

Health Perception–Health Management Pattern
- Describe your usual daily activities.
- Do you experience any difficulties performing these activities?* Describe what you do when you experience difficulty in dressing, feeding yourself, performing basic hygiene, or maintaining your home.
- Do you use any mechanical assistive devices?* Do you have to lift heavy objects? If so, describe how you do this.
- Describe any specialized equipment you use or wear when you work or exercise that helps protect you from injury.
- What type of safety precautions do you take?
- Do you take any medications to manage your musculoskeletal problem? If so, what is/are the name(s) of the medication? When did you have your last tetanus and polio immunization? When were you last tested for tuberculosis?

Nutrition-Metabolic Pattern
- Give a 24 hr diet recall. Do you take supplemental vitamins or minerals? (Ask specifically about calcium and vitamin D supplements.)
- What is your weight? Have you had a recent change in your weight?*

Elimination Pattern
- Does your musculoskeletal problem make it difficult for you to reach the toilet in time?* Do you experience constipation related to immobility?
- Do you need any assistive devices or equipment to achieve satisfactory toileting?*

Activity-Exercise Pattern
- Do you have any limitations in your activities of daily living because of a musculoskeletal problem?*
- Describe your usual exercise pattern. Do you experience symptoms related to your musculoskeletal system before, during, or after exercising?*

- Are you able to move all your joints comfortably through full range of motion? Describe any limitations in mobility.
- Do you require assistance in moving or in doing activities of daily living?*
- Do you use any prosthetic or orthotic devices?*

Sleep-Rest Pattern
- Do you experience any difficulty sleeping because of a musculoskeletal problem?* Do you require frequent position changes at night? Why?
- Do you wake up at night because of musculoskeletal pain?*

Cognitive-Perceptual Pattern
- Describe any musculoskeletal pain you experience. How do you manage your pain?

Self-Perception–Self-Concept Pattern
- Describe how changes in your musculoskeletal system (posture, walking, muscle strength) or the ability to do certain things have affected how you feel about yourself. How have these changes affected your lifestyle?

Role-Relationship Pattern
- Do you live alone?
- Describe how your family or others assist you with your musculoskeletal problems.
- Describe the effect of your musculoskeletal problem on your work and on your social relationships.

Sexuality-Reproductive Pattern
- Describe the effect of your musculoskeletal problem on your sexual activity. How do you feel about this?

Coping–Stress Tolerance Pattern
- Describe how you deal with the problems such as pain or immobility that have resulted from your musculoskeletal problem.

Value-Belief Pattern
- Describe any cultural or religious beliefs that may influence the treatment of your musculoskeletal problem.

*If yes, describe.

---

asked about safety practices of the patient as they relate to the job environment, recreation, and exercise. For example, if the patient is a jogger, the type of shoes worn and the jogging surface used should be investigated. The high incidence of trauma to the musculoskeletal system requires a careful investigation in the area of safety practices. Identification of problems in this area will direct the plan for patient education.

Nutritional-metabolic pattern. The patient's recounting of a typical day's diet can provide clues to areas of nutritional concern in relation to the musculoskeletal system. Obesity predisposes people to ligamentous instability, particularly in the lower back region. It also adds stress to weight-bearing joints such as the knees and hips. The maintenance of normal weight is an important patient goal.

Abnormal nutritional states can predispose individuals to specific musculoskeletal problems such as osteoporosis, osteomalacia, and rickets. Adequate amounts of vitamins C and D, calcium, and protein are essential for a healthy, intact musculoskeletal system. The nurse should also evaluate the patient's ability to tolerate lactose in milk products.

Elimination pattern. The patient's ability to ambulate adequately to reach a toileting facility should be assessed. A mus-

culoskeletal problem could be an etiologic factor in functional incontinence of bladder and bowel. Also, immobility secondary to a musculoskeletal problem can result in constipation. The patient should be asked if an assistive device such as an elevated toilet seat or grab bar is necessary to accomplish toileting.

Activity-exercise pattern. A detailed account of the type, duration, and frequency of activities related to exercise and recreation should be obtained and assessed regarding adequacy and predisposition to musculoskeletal problems. This information can be obtained when the patient recounts a typical day. Daily, weekend, and seasonal patterns should be compared because occasional or sporadic exercise can be more problematic than regular exercise. Many musculoskeletal problems can affect the patient's activity-exercise pattern. The nurse should question the patient about limitations of movement, pain, weakness, clumsiness, crepitus, or any change in the bones or joints that interfere with daily activities.

Extremes of activity related to occupation can affect the musculoskeletal system. A sedentary occupation does not allow for maintaining muscle flexibility and strength. Jobs that require extreme effort and use of the body for heavy lifting and pushing can result in damage to the joints and supporting structures of the body. The nurse should inquire about job-related injuries to the musculoskeletal system, the amount of time lost from work, and the treatments used.

Sleep-rest pattern. Musculoskeletal disorders might require frequent position changes at night. Discomfort may also interfere with a normal sleep pattern. The patient should be questioned about sleep patterns and how they have been altered. If the patient recounts that a musculoskeletal problem is interfering with sleep, further inquiry should be made related to the type of bedding, pillows used, sleeping partner, and sleeping positions.

Cognitive-perceptual pattern. Any pain experienced by the patient as a result of a musculoskeletal problem should be fully explored and documented. Pain assessment conducted over time can assist in determining the effectiveness of the treatment plan. The patient should be asked what measures are used at home to control pain. Other complaints that could cause a problem either directly or indirectly through pain include joint swelling, decreasing strength, and changes in sensation.

Self-perception–self-concept pattern. Many musculoskeletal problems are chronic and deforming. Such changes can have a serious impact on the patient's body image and sense of personal worth. An account of how the patient feels about these changes should be addressed by the nurse.

Role-relationship pattern. Musculoskeletal problems that affect mobility or result in a chronic pain syndrome can seriously affect the patient's roles and responsibilities, such as spouse, parent, and worker. Also, such problems can affect the ability to seek and maintain meaningful social and personal relationships. These problems should be assessed and documented during the history.

If the patient lives alone, the possibility of maintaining this living arrangement in the future should be assessed in light of the problem and rehabilitation potential. The degree of assistance from family, friends, and organized caregivers should also be determined.

Sexuality-reproductive pattern. Musculoskeletal problems and the resulting pain or potential for pain can greatly affect the patient's ability to obtain sexual satisfaction. This area must be sensitively assessed so the patient feels comfortable in relating sexual problems related to pain, movement, and positioning.

Coping–stress tolerance pattern. Mobility limitations and pain, both acute and chronic, can be serious stressors that affect the patient's coping ability. The nurse must recognize the potential for ineffective coping (both patient and family or significant other) and gather adequate data to determine if a musculoskeletal problem is causing a coping problem.

Objective Data

Physical Examination. The primary methods used in the physical examination of the musculoskeletal system include inspection and palpation. The data gathered from a careful health history will provide the nurse with clues about areas on which to concentrate the examination.

Inspection. Inspection begins during the nurse's initial contact with the patient. The nurse should observe the patient for any apparent asymmetry and for sitting and standing posture, gait, general body build, and configuration of the muscles. The nurse should be particularly aware of limitations in the patient's ability to perform normal activities such as dressing, toileting, and eating.

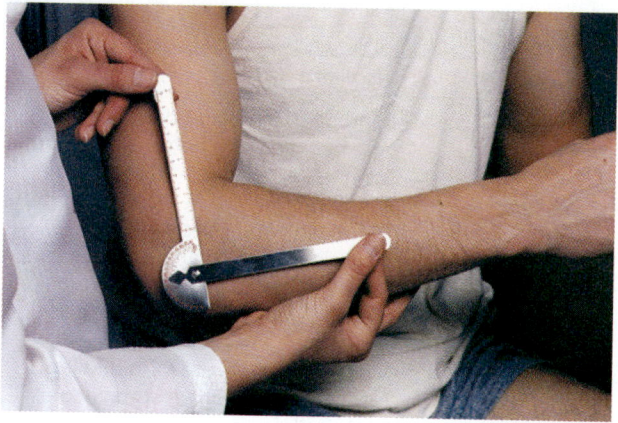

Fig. 58-7 Measurement of joint motion with a goniometer.

The condition of the skin is observed for general color, scars, or overt signs of previous injury or operations. A systematic inspection is performed starting at the head and neck and proceeding to the upper extremities, the lower extremities, and the back. Although the order is not of great importance, the regular use of a systematic approach is important to avoid missing important aspects of the examination. The nurse should specifically inspect for joint motion and asymmetry of movement, swelling, deformity, masses, and evidence of limb-length or muscle-size discrepancies. The patient's opposite body part is used for comparison when an abnormality is suspected.

Palpation. Any area that has aroused concern because of a subjective complaint or has been noted on inspection should be carefully palpated. The examiner's hands should be warm to prevent muscle spasm, which can interfere with identification of essential landmarks or soft-tissue structures. Palpation of the soft tissues, including muscles and joints, enables the examiner to evaluate skin temperature, local tenderness, swelling, and crepitation. It is important to establish the relationship of adjacent structures and to evaluate the general contour, abnormal prominences, and local landmarks. The usual sequence is to begin at the neck and proceed cephalopedally (head to toe) to examine the neck, shoulders, elbows, wrists, hands, back, hips, knees, ankles, and feet. Both superficial and deep palpation are usually performed consecutively.

Movement. When examining joint movement, the nurse must carefully evaluate passive and active range of joint motion. Normally the active and passive joint motions are similar. There are three range-of-motion categories: passive, active, and functional. Passive range of motion occurs when someone else moves the patient's joints through their range of motion. Caution is required when testing passive joint motion because of the possibility of injury to the underlying soft-tissue structures. Manipulation must cease immediately if pain or resistance is encountered. Active range of motion means the patient actively moves his or her own joints through their normal range of motion. Functional range of motion is assessed by asking the patient if the activities of daily living, such as eating and bathing independently, are performed with assistance or not at all. The patient may require an assistive device such as a cane, wheelchair, or walker, which should be noted.

Joint motion is most accurately measured by a goniometer, which measures the amount of bending or angles of the joints (Fig. 58-7). Specific degrees of range of motion of all joints are

Table 58-4 Movement at Synovial Joints

Movement	Description
Flexion	Bending of joint that decreases angle between two bones; shortening of muscle length
Extension	Bending of joint that increases angle between two bones
Hyperextension	Extension in which angle exceeds 180 degrees
Abduction	Movement of part away from midline
Adduction	Movement of part toward midline
Pronation	Turning of palm downward or sole outward
Supination	Turning of palm upward or sole inward
Circumduction	Combination of flexion, extension, abduction, and adduction resulting in circular motion of body part
Rotation	Movement about longitudinal axis
Inversion	Turning of sole inward toward midline
Eversion	Turning of sole outward away from midline

usually not measured unless a musculoskeletal problem has been identified. A less accurate but nevertheless valuable method is to compare the range of motion of one extremity with the range of motion on the opposite side. The most common movements that occur at the synovial joints are listed in Table 58-4.

Measurement. Limb length and circumferential measurement of muscle mass are often obtained when subjective problems or length discrepancies are noted. For example, leg length measurements are obtained when gait disorders are observed. Limb length is measured between two bony prominences and compared with the similar measurement of the opposite extremity. Muscle mass is measured circumferentially at the largest area of the mass. When recording measurements, the nurse should record the exact location at which the measurements were obtained (e.g., the quadriceps muscle is measured 15 cm above the patella). This informs the next examiner of the exact area to be measured and ensures consistency in future examinations.

Muscle-strength testing. The strength of individual muscles or groups of muscles is graded in performance of movements during contraction against applied resistance (Table 58-5). The examiner should instruct the patient to apply resistance to the force exerted by the examiner. For example, the examiner tries to pull the bent arm down while the patient tries to raise it. Muscle strength should also be compared with the strength of the opposite extremity. Subtle variations in muscle

Table 58-5 Muscle Strength Scale

0—No detection of muscular contraction
1—A barely detectable flicker or trace of contraction
2—Active movement of body part with elimination of gravity
3—Active movement against gravity
4—Active movement against gravity and some resistance
5—Active movement against full resistance without evident fatigue (normal muscle strength)

Table 58-6 Normal Physical Assessment of the Musculoskeletal System

Full range of motion of all joints
No joint swelling, deformity, or crepitation
Normal spinal curvatures
No tenderness on palpation of spine
No muscle atrophy or asymmetry
Muscle strength of 5

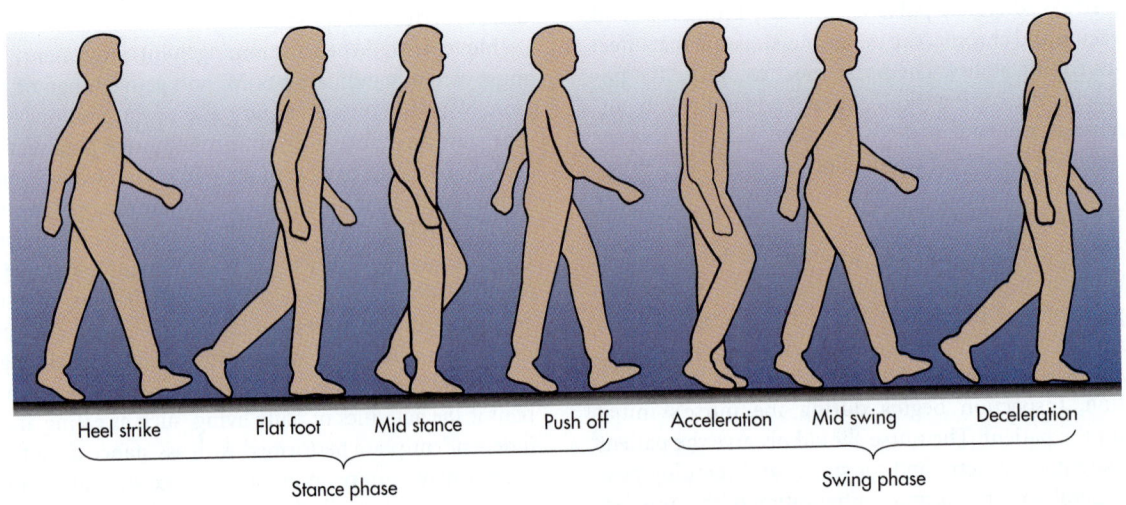

Heel strike   Flat foot   Mid stance   Push off   Acceleration   Mid swing   Deceleration

Stance phase   Swing phase

Fig. 58-8 Phases of gait. (Modified from DeLisa J, Gans B: *Rehabilitation medicine principles,* ed 2, Philadelphia, 1993, JB Lippincott.)

strength may be noted when comparing the patient's dominant side with the nondominant side.[9]

Gait. The nurse assesses gait by having the patient walk across the room and back. The normal gait is divided into two separate phases: the stance phase and the swing phase (Fig. 58-8). The two occur simultaneously: while one limb is in stance phase, the other is in swing phase. Musculoskeletal and neurologic problems can result in gait abnormalities.

Other. Assessment of reflexes is discussed in Chapter 53. Table 58-6 is an example of how to record a normal physical assessment of the musculoskeletal system. Common abnormal assessment findings of the musculoskeletal system are presented in Table 58-7.

DIAGNOSTIC STUDIES OF THE MUSCULOSKELETAL SYSTEM

Diagnostic studies provide important information to the nurse in monitoring the patient's condition and planning appropriate interventions. These studies are considered to be objective data. Table 58-8 contains diagnostic studies common to the musculoskeletal system.

Radiologic Studies

The most common diagnostic study used to assess musculoskeletal problems is an x-ray examination. Radiologic studies are important to establish the presence of a musculoskeletal problem and to follow its progress and the effectiveness of treatment.

A standard x-ray study is a film produced by the action of x-rays emitted from a cathode tube diphotosensitive surface. X-rays can be thought of as shadows of structures, particularly bony structures. Bones are more dense than other tissues and do not allow the x-ray to penetrate. The standard x-ray develops dense areas as white.

The anteroposterior and lateral views are the most commonly used standard x-ray perspectives. Because disk and cartilage structures are not visible on standard x-rays, special x-rays (diskograms, arthrograms) involving the use of contrast media can be used to visualize them.

Magnetic Resonance Imaging

Magnetic resonance imaging (MRI) is a diagnostic study that is useful in diagnosing numerous musculoskeletal disorders.

COMMON ASSESSMENT ABNORMALITIES

Table 58-7 Musculoskeletal System

Finding	Description	Possible Etiology and Significance
Ankylosis	Scarring within a joint leading to stiffness or fixation	Chronic joint inflammation
Atrophy	Wasting of muscle, characterized by decrease in circumference and flabby appearance and resulting in decrease in function and muscle tone	Prolonged disuse, contracture, immobilization, muscle denervation
Contracture	Resistance to movement of muscle or joint as result of fibrosis of supporting soft tissues	Shortening of muscle or ligament structure, tightness of soft tissue, immobilization, incorrect positioning
Crepitation	Crackling sound or grating sensation as result of friction between bones	Fracture, chronic inflammation, dislocation
Effusion	Fluid in joint possibly with swelling and pain	Trauma, especially to knee
Felon	Abscess occurring in pulp space (tissue mass) of distal phalanx of finger as a result of infection	Minor hand injury, puncture wound, laceration
Ganglion	Small, fluid-filled synovial cyst usually on dorsal surface of wrist and foot	Degeneration of connective tissue close to tendons and joints leading to formation of small cysts
Hypertrophy	Increase in size of muscle as result of enlargement of existing cells	Exercise, increased androgens, increased stimulation or use
Kyphosis (round back)	Anteroposterior or forward bending of spine with convexity of curve in posterior direction; common at thoracic and sacral levels	Poor posture, tuberculosis, chronic arthritis, growth disturbance of vertebral epiphysis, osteoporosis
Lordosis	Deformity of spine resulting in anteroposterior curvature with concavity in posterior direction; common in lumbar spine	Secondary to other deformities of spine, muscular dystrophy, obesity, flexion contracture of hip, congenital dislocation of hip
Pes planus	Flatfoot	Congenital condition, muscle paralysis, mild cerebral palsy, early muscular dystrophy
Scoliosis	Deformity resulting in lateral curvature of spine	Idiopathic or congenital condition, fracture or dislocation, osteomalacia, functional condition
Subluxation	Partial dislocation of joint	Instability of joint capsule and supporting ligaments (e.g., from trauma, arthritis)
Valgus	Angulation of bone away from midline	Alteration in gait, pain, abnormal erosion of articular cartilage
Varus	Angulation of bone toward midline	Alteration in gait, pain, abnormal erosion of articular cartilage

DIAGNOSTIC STUDIES

Table 58-8 Musculoskeletal System

Study	Description and Purpose	Nursing Responsibility
Radiologic Studies		
▪ Standard x-ray	An x-ray is taken to determine density of bone. Study evaluates structural or functional changes of bones and joints. In anteroposterior view, x-ray beam passes from front to back, allowing one-dimensional view; lateral position provides two-dimensional view.	Avoid excessive exposure of patient and self. Before procedure, remove any radiopaque objects that can interfere with results. Explain procedure to patient.
▪ Arthrogram	Study involves injection of contrast medium or air into joint cavity, which permits visualization of joint structures. Joint movement is followed with series of x-rays.	Assess patient for possible allergy to contrast medium, including iodine or seafood. Explain procedure. Prepare area to be injected aseptically.
▪ Diskogram	An x-ray of cervical or lumbar intervertebral disk is done after injection of contrast dye into nucleus pulposus. Study permits visualization of intervertebral disk abnormalities.	Same as for arthrogram. May be performed in surgery.
▪ Sinogram	An x-ray is taken after injection of contrast dye into sinus tract (deep draining wound). Study visualizes course of sinus and tissues involved.	Same as for arthrogram.
▪ Tomogram	Multiple x-ray views of body region are focused at successively deeper layers of tissue lying in predetermined planes. Study focuses on certain tissues, eliminating or blurring surrounding structures. Technique is useful in locating bone destruction, small body cavities, foreign bodies, and lesions overshadowed by opaque structures.	Inform patient that procedure is painless.
▪ Computed tomography (CT) scan	An x-ray beam is used with a computer to provide a three-dimensional picture. It is used to identify soft-tissue abnormalities, bony abnormalities, and various musculoskeletal trauma.	Inform patient that procedure is painless. Inform patient of importance of remaining still during procedure.
▪ Magnetic resonance imaging (MRI)	Radio waves and magnetic field are used to view soft tissue. Study is especially useful in the diagnosis of avascular necrosis, disk disease, tumors, osteomyelitis, ligament tears, and cartilage tears. Patient is placed inside scanning chamber. Gadolinium may be injected into a vein to enhance visualization of the structures. Open MRI does not require the patient to be placed inside a chamber.	Inform patient that it is painless. Be aware that it is contraindicated in patient with aneurysm clips, metallic implants, pacemakers, electronic devices, hearing aids, shrapnel, and extreme obesity. Ensure that patient has no metal on clothing (e.g., snaps, zippers, jewelry, credit cards). Convert IV to heparin lock. Inform patient of importance of remaining still throughout examination. Inform patients who are claustrophobic that they may experience symptoms during examination. Administer antianxiety agent (if indicated and ordered). Open MRI may be indicated for obese patient or patient with large chest and abdominal girth or severe claustrophobia. Open MRI may not be available at all facilities.
Bone Mass Measurements		
▪ Radiogrammetry, radiodensitometry	Study evaluates bone mass of metacarpals. A very low dose of radiation is used.	Explain procedure to patient. Inform patient that procedure is painless.
▪ Single-photon absorptiometry (SPA)	Low-dose radiation scanner measures mostly peripheral cortical bone at distal radius or midradius. Study is not useful for follow-up because of slow changes in cortical bone.	Same as above.

Continued

DIAGNOSTIC STUDIES

Table **58-8** | **Musculoskeletal System—cont'd**

Study	Description and Purpose	Nursing Responsibility
Bone Mass Measurements—cont'd		
▪ Dual-photon absorptiometry (DPA)	Technique measures mixed trabecular and cortical bones at sites such as hip and lumbar spine. It can be used to calculate total body calcium concentration.	Same as above.
▪ Dual-energy x-ray absorptiometry (DEXA)	Technique measures bone mass of spine, femur, forearm, and total body. Considered to be fast and precise with low dose of radiation.	Same as above.
Radioisotope Studies		
▪ Bone scan	Technique involves injection of radioisotope (usually sodium pertechnate) that is taken up by bone. Camera scans entire body (front and back), and recording is made on paper. Degree of uptake is related to blood flow to bone. Increased uptake is seen in osteomyelitis, osteoporosis, primary and metastatic malignant lesions of bone, and with certain fractures. Decreased uptake is seen in areas of avascular necrosis.	Give calculated dose of radioisotope 2 hr before procedure. Ensure that bladder is emptied before scan. Inform patient that procedure requires 1 hr while patient lies supine and that no pain or harm will result from isotopes. Be aware that no follow-up scans are required.
Endoscopy		
▪ Arthroscopy	Study involves insertion of arthroscope into joint (usually knee) for visualization of structure and contents. It can be used for exploratory surgery (removal of loose bodies and biopsy) and for diagnosis of abnormalities of meniscus, articular cartilage, ligaments, or joint capsule. Other structures that can be visualized through the arthroscope include the shoulder, elbow, wrist, and ankle.	Inform patient that procedure is performed in operating room with strict asepsis and that either local or general anesthesia is used. After procedure, cover wound with sterile dressing. Wrap leg from midthigh to midcalf with compression dressing for 24 hr for knee arthroscopy. Instruct patient to limit activity for a few days.
Mineral Metabolism		
▪ Alkaline phosphatase	This enzyme, produced by osteoblasts of bone, is needed for mineralization of organic bone matrix. Elevated levels are found in healing fractures, bone cancers, osteoporosis, osteomalacia, and Paget's disease. *Normal:* 20-90 U/L (0.3-1.5 μkat/L).	Obtain blood samples by venipuncture. Observe venipuncture site for bleeding or hematoma formation. Inform patient that procedure does not require fasting.
▪ Calcium	Bone is primary organ for calcium storage. Calcium provides bone with rigid consistency. Decreased serum level is found in osteomalacia, renal disease, and hypoparathyroidism; increased level is found in hyperparathyroidism, some bone tumors. *Normal:* 9-11 mg/dl (2.3-2.7 mmol/L).	Same as above.
▪ Phosphorus	Amount present is indirectly related to calcium metabolism. Decreased level is found in osteomalacia; increased level is found in chronic renal disease, healing fractures, osteolytic metastatic tumor. *Normal:* 2.8-4.5 mg/dl (0.9-1.5 mmol/L).	Same as above.
Serologic Studies		
▪ Rheumatoid factor (RF)	Study assesses presence of autoantibody (rheumatoid factor) in serum. Factor is not specific for rheumatoid arthritis and is seen in other connective tissue diseases, as well as in a small percentage of normal population. *Normal:* negative or titer <1:20.	Same as above.

Continued

DIAGNOSTIC STUDIES

Table 58-8   Musculoskeletal System—cont'd

Study	Description and Purpose	Nursing Responsibility
Serologic Studies—cont'd		
■ Erythrocyte sedimentation rate (ESR)	Study is nonspecific index of inflammation. Study measures rapidity with which red blood cells settle out of unclotted blood in 1 hr. Results are influenced by physiologic factors, as well as diseases. Elevated levels are seen with any inflammatory process (especially rheumatoid arthritis, rheumatic fever, osteomyelitis, and respiratory infections). *Normal:* <20 mm/hr. Some gender variation.	Observe venipuncture site for bleeding or hematoma formation. Inform patient that procedure does not require fasting.
■ Lupus erythematosus (LE) cells	Lupus erythematosus cells are seen in about 80% of cases of systemic lupus erythematosus. Normally no lupus erythematosus cells are present.	Obtain blood from patient and have blood smear made on slide. Observe venipuncture site for bleeding or hematoma formation.
■ Antinuclear antibody (ANA)	Study assesses presence of antibodies capable of destroying nucleus of body's tissue cells. Finding is positive in 95% of patients with systemic lupus erythematosus and may also be positive in individuals with scleroderma or rheumatoid arthritis and in a small percentage of normal population.	Observe venipuncture site for bleeding or hematoma formation. Inform patient that procedure does not require fasting.
■ Anti-DNA antibody	Study detects serum antibodies that react with DNA. It is the most specific test for systemic lupus erythematosus.	Same as above.
■ Complement	Complement, a normal body protein, is essential to both immune and inflammatory reactions. Complement components used up in these reactions are depleted. Subsequent test applied to serum yields little or no serum complement components. Complement depletions may be found in patients with rheumatoid arthritis or systemic lupus erythematosus.	Same as above.
■ Uric acid	End product of purine metabolism is normally excreted in urine. Although not specific, levels are usually elevated in gout. *Normal:* male 4.5-6.5 mg/dl (268-387 μmol/L); female 2.5-5.5 mg/dl (149-327 μmol/L).	Same as above.
■ C-reactive protein (CRP)	Study is used to diagnose inflammatory diseases, infections, and active widespread malignancy. CRP is synthesized by the liver and is present in large amounts in serum 18-24 hr after onset of tissue damage. *Normal:* negative.	Same as above.
■ Human leukocyte antigen (HLA)-B27	Antigen present in disorders such as ankylosing spondylitis and variants of rheumatoid arthritis.	Same as above.
Muscle Enzymes		
■ Creatine kinase (CK)	Highest concentration is found in skeletal muscle. Increased values are found in progressive muscular dystrophy, polymyositis, and traumatic injuries. *Normal:* men 5-55 U/L (0.1-0.9 μkat/L); women 5-35 U/L (0.01-0.6 μkat/L).	Same as above.
■ Aldolase	Study is useful in monitoring muscular dystrophy and dermatomyositis. *Normal:* 1.0-7.5 U/L (16.7-125 nkat/L).	Same as above.

Continued

DIAGNOSTIC STUDIES

Table 58-8 | Musculoskeletal System—cont'd

Study	Description and Purpose	Nursing Responsibility
Muscle Enzymes—cont'd		
■ Aspartate aminotransferase (AST) or serum glutamic-oxaloacetic transaminase (SGOT)	Enzyme is found in skeletal muscle but is primarily an enzyme of cardiac and hepatic cells. *Normal:* 15-45 U/L (0.12-0.67 μkat/L).	Observe venipuncture site for bleeding or hematoma formation. Inform patient that procedure does not require fasting.
Invasive Procedures		
■ Arthrocentesis	Incision or puncture of joint capsule is done to obtain samples of synovial fluid from within joint cavity or to remove excess fluid. Local anesthesia and aseptic preparation are used before needle is inserted into joint and fluid aspirated. Study is useful in diagnosis of joint inflammation.	Inform patient that procedure is usually done at bedside or in examination room. Send samples of synovial fluid to laboratory for examination (if indicated). After procedure apply compression dressing and have patient rest joint for 8-24 hr. Observe for leakage of blood or fluid on dressing.
■ Electromyogram (EMG)	Study evaluates electrical potential associated with skeletal muscle contraction. Long, small-gauge needles are inserted into certain muscles. Needle probes are attached to leads that feed information to electromyogram machine. Recordings of electrical activity of muscle are traced on audiotransmitter, as well as on oscilloscope and recording paper. Study is useful in providing information related to lower motor neuron dysfunction and primary muscle diseases.	Inform patient that procedure is usually done in electromyogram laboratory while patient lies supine on special table. Keep patient awake to cooperate with voluntary movement. Inform patient that procedure involves some discomfort from needle insertion. Avoid administration of stimulants and sedatives 24 hr before procedure.
Miscellaneous		
■ Thermography	Technique uses infrared detector, which measures degree of heat radiating from skin surface. Study is useful in investigation of cause of inflamed joints and in following up patient's response to antiinflammatory drug therapy.	Inform patient that procedure is painless and noninvasive.
■ Plethysmography	Study records variations in volume and pressure of blood passing through tissues. Test is nonspecific and quantitative.	Inform patient that procedure is painless and noninvasive.
■ Somatosensory evoked potential (SSEP)	Study evaluates evoked potential of muscle contractions. Electrodes are placed on skin and provide recordings of electrical activity of muscle. Study useful in identifying subtle dysfunction of lower motor neuron and primary muscle disease. SSEP measures nerve conduction along pathways not accessible by electromyogram. Transcutaneous or percutaneous electrodes are applied to the skin and help identify neuropathy and myopathy.	Inform patient that procedure is similar to electromyogram but does not involve needles. Electrodes are applied to the skin.

Radio waves and magnetic fields are used to construct soft-tissue and bone images. It is advantageous in determining soft-tissue disorders, including cartilage and ligament tears and herniated disks, but it also can be helpful in diagnosing bone disorders such as avascular necrosis, tumors, and multiple myeloma.

Arthroscopy

Endoscopy of the joints involves the use of an arthroscope for direct visualization of the interior of a joint cavity.[5] It is performed in the operating room under sterile conditions. After local or general anesthesia has been administered, a large-bore needle is inserted into the joint and the joint is distended with saline solution (Fig. 58-9). The arthroscope is inserted and the joint cavity is examined. Photographs or videotapes can be made through the scope, and a biopsy of the synovium or cartilage can be obtained. The procedure is particularly useful in the diagnosis of disorders of the knee and shoulder. It can also be used in procedures involving other joints, such as the wrist, elbow, and ankle. Tears in cartilage and other repairs can be made through the arthroscope (arthroscopic surgery), thus eliminating the need for a more extensive incision and surgical procedure.

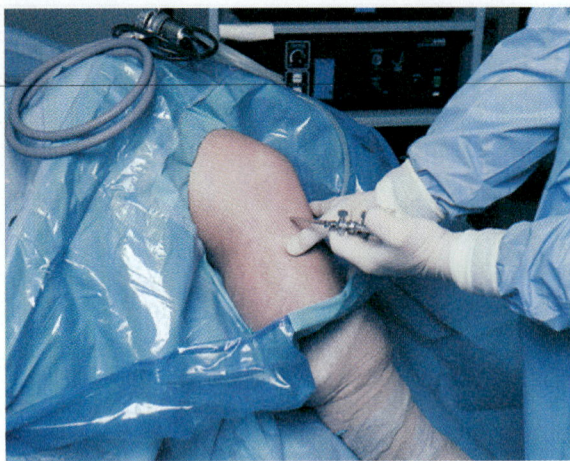

Fig. 58-9 Arthroscopy of a knee.

Arthrocentesis and Synovial Fluid Analysis

An arthrocentesis is usually performed to obtain synovial fluid for examination. It may also be used to instill medications and remove fluid from joints to relieve pain. After the skin has been cleaned, a local anesthetic is instilled. An 18-gauge or larger needle is inserted into the joint, and fluid is aspirated. The appropriate container must be readily available for laboratory analysis of the aspirated fluid. The fluid is examined grossly for volume, color, clarity, viscosity, and mucin clot formation. Normal synovial fluid is clear, light yellow, and scanty (1 to 3 ml). Fluid from a septic joint may be purulent and thick, or gray and thin. In gout the fluid may be whitish yellow. Blood may be aspirated if there is hemarthrosis because of injury. The mucin clot test indicates the character of the protein portion of the synovial fluid. Normally a white, ropelike mucin clot is formed. In an inflammatory process the clot breaks apart easily and fragments.

The fluid is examined microscopically for cell count and identification of the cells. The normal white blood cell (WBC) count is less than 200 cells/μl with fewer than 25% neutrophils and no bacteria. The WBC count and protein are increased in an inflammatory process. The presence of uric acid crystals may indicate gout.

Muscle Enzymes

Muscle enzymes are released from injured or dead muscle cells. Determinations of muscle enzyme values are used to distinguish between muscle weakness that is due to nerve innervation problems and dystrophic disease of the muscle itself. The level of enzymes reflects the progress of the disorder and the effectiveness of treatment. Aspartate aminotransferase (AST) (also known as serum glutamic-oxaloacetic transaminase[SGOT]) levels are the least sensitive indicators of muscle disease, and creatine kinase (CK) levels are the most sensitive. Enzyme levels are also helpful in determining hepatic and cardiac disease.

Serologic Studies

Approximately 85% of people with rheumatoid arthritis and related diseases have an autoantibody known as rheumatoid factor in their serum. This autoantibody is usually of the IgM class, although it may be IgG. The test used to determine the presence of this factor is the latex fixation test. Latex particles are coated with aggregated immunoglobulin G. If serum containing rheumatoid factor is mixed with these latex particles, it reacts with the latex particles and causes agglutination. An estimation of the titer is obtained by performing serial dilutions of the serum.

REVIEW QUESTIONS

The number of the question corresponds to the same-numbered objective at the beginning of the chapter.

1. The bone cells that function in the breakdown of bone tissue (resorption) are called
   a. osteoids.
   b. osteocytes.
   c. osteoclasts.
   d. osteoblasts.
2. While performing passive range of motion for a patient, the nurse puts a hinge joint through the movements of
   a. rotation.
   b. flexion and extension.
   c. flexion, extension, abduction, and adduction.
   d. flexion, extension, abduction, adduction, and circumduction.
3. The nurse teaches a patient with a leg immobilized in traction to prevent muscle atropy in the affected leg by performing
   a. twitch contractions.
   b. tetanic contractions.
   c. isotonic contractions.
   d. isometric contractions.
4. A patient with bursitis of the shoulder asks the nurse what the bursa does. The nurse's response is based on the knowledge that bursae
   a. connect bone to bone.
   b. separate muscle from muscle.
   c. lubricate joints with synovial fluid.
   d. relieve friction between moving parts.
5. The decreased agility found during assessment of the older adult is caused by the age-related change of
   a. decrease in bone mass.
   b. erosion of articular cartilage.
   c. loss of elasticity in ligaments and cartilage.
   d. decrease in number and diameter of muscle cells.
6. While obtaining subjective assessment data related to the musculoskeletal system it is particularly important for the nurse to ask about family history in the patient with
   a. osteomyelitis.
   b. osteomalacia.
   c. low back pain.
   d. rheumatoid arthritis.
7. When grading muscle strength the nurse records a score of 2 indicating
   a. active movement against gravity.
   b. a barely detectable flicker of contraction.
   c. active movement with elimination of gravity.
   d. active movement against full resistance without evident fatigue.
8. A normal assessment finding of the musculoskeletal system is
   a. muscle strength of 4.
   b. a lateral curvature of the spine.
   c. angulation of bone toward midline.
   d. simultaneous occurrence of stance and swing phase of gait.

9. A patient is scheduled for an electromyogram. The nurse explains that this diagnostic test involves
   a. placement of long, thin needles into the muscles.
   b. placement of electrodes on the skin to record electrical activity of muscles.
   c. measurement of the heat of muscle contractions radiating from the skin surface.
   d. administration of a calculated dose of radioisotope 2 hours before the procedure.

■

References

1. Thompson JM and others, editors: *Mosby's clinical nursing*, ed 4, St Louis, 1997, Mosby.
2. Thibodeau GA, Patton KT: *Anatomy and physiology*, ed 4, St Louis, 1999, Mosby.
3. Guyton AC, Hall JE, editors: *Textbook of medical physiology*, ed 9, Philadelphia, 1996, Saunders.
4. *Mastering geriatric care*, Springhouse, Penn, 1997, Springhouse.
5. Beare PG, Myers JL, editors: *Adult health nursing*, ed 3, St Louis, 1998, Mosby.
6. Browstein B, Bronner S, editors: *Functional movement in orthopaedic and sports physical therapy*, New York, 1997, Churchill Livingstone.
7. Lueckenotte A, editor: *Gerontologic nursing*, St Louis, 1996, Mosby.
8. Ebersole P, Hess P, editors: *Toward healthy aging*, ed 5, St Louis, 1998, Mosby.
9. Potter PA, Perry AG, editors: *Fundamentals of nursing*, ed 4, St Louis, 1997, Mosby.
10. McCance KL, Huether SE, editors: *Pathophysiology: the biologic basis for disease in adults and children*, ed 3, St Louis, 1998, Mosby.

Resources

Resources for this chapter are listed after Chapter 59 on p. 1818.

59

NURSING MANAGEMENT
Musculoskeletal Problems

Susan C. Ruda

www.mosby.com/MERLIN/medsurg_lewis

LEARNING OBJECTIVES

1. Explain the etiology, pathophysiology, clinical manifestations, and collaborative care of soft-tissue injuries, including strains, sprains, dislocations, subluxations, bursitis, carpal tunnel syndrome, repetitive strain injury, and muscle spasms.
2. Describe the sequential events involved in fracture healing.
3. Explain common complications associated with fracture injury and fracture healing.
4. Differentiate among open reduction, closed reduction, traction, and cast immobilization regarding purpose, complications, and nursing management.
5. Describe the neurovascular assessment of an injured extremity.
6. Describe the collaborative care and nursing management of patients with specific fractures.
7. Describe the pathophysiology, collaborative care, and nursing management of osteomyelitis.
8. Describe the indications for and collaborative care and nursing management of amputation.
9. Describe the types, pathophysiology, clinical manifestations, and collaborative care of bone cancer.
10. Differentiate between the causes and characteristics of acute and chronic low back pain.
11. Describe the conservative and surgical treatments of low back pain.
12. Describe the postoperative nursing management of a patient who has undergone spinal surgery.
13. Explain the etiology and collaborative care of common foot disorders.
14. Describe the etiology, pathophysiology, clinical manifestations, and management of metabolic bone disorders.

The most common cause of musculoskeletal problems is injury from accidents resulting in fracture, dislocations, and associated soft-tissue injuries. Although most of these injuries are not fatal, the cost in terms of pain, disability, medical expense, and lost wages is enormous. For all ages, accidents are exceeded only by heart disease, cancer, and strokes as a cause of death. Accidents are the leading cause of death in children and young adults.

The nurse has an important role in educating the public about the basic principles of safety and accident prevention. The morbidity associated with accidents can be significantly reduced if people are aware of environmental hazards, use existing safety equipment, and apply safety and traffic rules. In the industrial setting, the nurse should educate employees and employers about the use of proper safety equipment and avoidance of hazardous working situations.

In the home environment, falls account for many musculoskeletal injuries. Preventive education should be directed toward the importance of wearing shoes with functional soles and heels, avoidance of wet or slippery surfaces, careful placement of throw rugs, and removal of obstacles from the pathway of high risk individuals such as persons with gait instability or visual or cognitive impairment.

Reviewed by Dennis Ross, RN, PhD, Professor of Nursing, Castleton State College, Castleton, Vt; Nursing Faculty, Regents College, Albany, NY.

SOFT-TISSUE INJURIES

Soft-tissue injuries include sprains, strains, dislocations, and subluxation. These common injuries are usually caused by trauma. The increase in the number of people who have committed themselves to maintaining a regular fitness program or participate in sports has contributed to the increased incidence of soft-tissue injuries.[1] Common sports-related injuries are summarized in Table 59-1. Most sport injuries result from direct trauma or contusion or indirect stretch injury.[1]

SPRAINS AND STRAINS

Sprains and strains are the two most common types of injury affecting the musculoskeletal system. These injuries are usually associated with abnormal stretching or twisting forces that may occur during vigorous activities.

A *sprain* is an injury to ligamentous structures surrounding a joint, usually caused by a wrenching or twisting motion. A sprain is classified according to the amount of ligament fibers torn. A first-degree sprain involves tears of only a few fibers resulting in mild tenderness and slight swelling. A second-degree sprain is partial disruption of the involved tissue with more swelling and tenderness. A third-degree sprain is a complete tearing of the ligament. A gap in the muscle may be apparent or felt through the skin if the muscle is torn. Because these areas are rich in nerve endings, the injury can be extremely painful. The most common areas of sprains occur in the ankle

Table 59-1	Common Sports-Related Injuries	
Injury	**Definition**	**Treatment**
Impingement syndrome	Entrapment of soft-tissue structures under coracoacromial arch of the shoulder	NSAIDs; rest until symptoms decrease and then gradual range-of-motion and strengthening exercises
Rotator cuff tear	Tear within muscle or ligaments of shoulder	If minor tear, rest, NSAIDs, and gradual mobilization with range-of-motion and strengthening exercises If major tear, surgical repair
Shin splints	Inflammation along tibial shaft from tearing away of tendons caused by improper shoes, overuse, or running on hard pavement	Rest, ice, NSAIDs, proper shoes; gradual increase in activity; if pain persists, x-ray should be done to rule out stress fracture of tibia
Tendinitis	Inflammation of tendon in upper or lower extremity as a result of overuse or incorrect use	Rest, ice, NSAIDs; gradual return to sport activity; protective brace (orthosis) may be necessary if symptoms recur
Ligament injury	Tearing or stretching of ligament; usually occurs as a result of direct blow; characterized by sudden pain, swelling, and instability	Rest, ice, NSAIDs; protection of affected extremity by use of brace; if symptoms persist, surgical repair may be necessary
Meniscal injury	Injury to fibrocartilage of the knee characterized by popping, clicking, or tearing sensation, swelling	Rest, ice, NSAIDs; gradual return to regular activities; if symptoms persist, surgical arthroscopy to diagnose and repair meniscal injury may be necessary

NSAIDs, nonsteroidal antiinflammatory drugs.

and wrist. A *strain* is a stretching of a muscle and its fascial sheath.

The clinical manifestations of sprains and strains are similar and include pain, edema, decrease in function, and bruising. Pain aggravated by continued use is common. Edema develops in the injured area because of minute hemorrhages within the disrupted tissues and the ensuing inflammatory response. Usually the patient will recount a history of traumatic injury, possibly of a twisting nature, or recent exercise activity.

Minor sprains and strains are usually self-limiting, with full function returning within 3 to 6 weeks. A severe sprain can result in an avulsion fracture, in which the ligament pulls loose a fragment of bone. Alternatively, the joint structure may become unstable and result in subluxation or dislocation. At the time of injury, hemarthrosis (bleeding into a joint space or cavity) or disruption of the synovial lining may occur. An acute strain may involve partial or complete rupture of a muscle.

X-rays of the affected part are usually taken to rule out a fracture or widening of the joint structure. Surgical repair may be necessary if the injury is significant enough to produce severe disruption of ligamentous or muscle structures, fracture, or dislocation.

NURSING MANAGEMENT: SPRAINS AND STRAINS

■ Nursing Implementation

Health Promotion. The use of elastic support bandages or adhesive tape wrapping before beginning a vigorous activity is thought to reduce the occurrence of sprains. However, some physicians do not support preventive wrapping or taping because it may predispose the athlete to injury. Stretching and

warm-up exercises before vigorous activity significantly reduce sprains and strains.

Preconditioning exercise protects an inherently weak joint, because slow stretching is tolerated better by biologic tissues than is quick stretching. Warm-up exercises "prelengthen" potentially strained tissues by avoiding the quick stretch often encountered in sports. Warm-up exercises also increase the temperature of muscle, which increases the speed of cell metabolism and the speed of nerve impulse transmission. The increased metabolism contributes to better oxygenation of muscle fiber during work. Stretching is also thought to improve kinesthetic awareness, thus lessening the chance of uncoordinated movement.

Acute Intervention. If an injury occurs, the immediate care focuses on (1) rest and limitation of movement, (2) application of ice to the injured area, (3) compression of the involved extremity, (4) elevation of the extremity, and (5) analgesia as necessary (Table 59-2). Movement should be limited and the extremity rested as soon as pain is felt. Unless the injury is severe, prolonged rest is usually not necessary. Cold in several forms can be used to produce hypothermia to the involved part. Physiologic changes that occur in soft tissue as a result of the use of cold include vasoconstriction, reduction in transmission of nerve impulses, and reduction in conduction velocity. These changes result in analgesia and anesthesia, reduction of muscle spasm without changes in muscular strength or endurance, reduction of local edema and inflammation, and reduction of local metabolic requirements. Few unwanted side effects accompany the use of cold to treat a soft-tissue injury. Cold is most useful when applied immediately after the injury has occurred. Ice applications should not exceed 20 to 30 minutes per application, allowing a "warm-down" time of 10 to 15 minutes between applications.

Compression also helps limit swelling, which, if left uncontrolled, could lengthen healing time. An elastic compression

✚ EMERGENCY MANAGEMENT

Table 59-2   Acute Soft-Tissue Injury

Etiology	Assessment Findings	Interventions
Falls Direct blows Crush injury Motor vehicle collisions Sports injuries	■ Edema ■ Ecchymosis ■ Pain, tenderness ■ Decreased sensation with severe edema ■ Decreased pulse, coolness, and capillary refill ■ Decreased movement ■ Pallor ■ Shortening or rotation of extremity ■ Inability to bear weight when lower extremity involved ■ Decreased function with upper-extremity involvement ■ Muscle spasms	**Initial** ■ Ensure airway, breathing, and circulation. ■ Assess neurovascular status of involved limb. ■ Elevate involved limb. ■ Apply compression bandage unless dislocation present. ■ Apply ice packs to affected area. ■ Immobilize affected extremity in the position found. ■ Anticipate x-rays of injured extremity. ■ Give analgesia as necessary. ■ Administer tetanus prophylaxis if skin integrity broken. **Ongoing Monitoring** ■ Monitor for changes in neurovascular status. ■ Eliminate weight bearing when lower extremity involved. ■ Anticipate compartment pressure monitoring if neurovascular status changes.

bandage can be wrapped around the injured part. The bandage is too tight if numbness is felt in the area or there is cramping or additional pain or swelling beyond the edge of the bandage. The bandage can be left in place for 30 minutes and then removed for 15 minutes.

The injured part should be elevated above the heart level to help drain excess fluid from the area and impede further edema. The injured part should be elevated even during sleep. Mild analgesia such as aspirin, ibuprofen, or acetaminophen may be necessary to manage patient discomfort.

After the acute phase (usually lasting 24 to 48 hours), warm, moist heat can be applied to the affected part to reduce swelling and provide comfort. Heat applications should not exceed 20 to 30 minutes, allowing a "cool down" time between applications. Nonsteroidal antiinflammatory drugs (NSAIDs) may be recommended to decrease edema and pain. The patient is encouraged to use the limb provided that the joint is protected by means of casting, taping, or splinting. Movement of the joint maintains nutrition to the cartilage, and muscle contraction speeds circulation and resolution of the hematoma.

Ambulatory and Home Care. With the exception of treatment in the emergency department following the injury, sprains and strains are treated in the outpatient setting. The patient should be instructed in the use of ice and elevation for 24 to 72 hours after injury to reduce edema. The use of mild analgesics to promote comfort should be encouraged. Use of an elastic wrap may provide additional support during activity. To prevent reinjury, the patient should learn proper measures of prevention.

The physical therapist may help provide added comfort by means of specialized techniques, such as ultrasound. The therapist may also teach the patient exercises to perform to strengthen shortened muscles.

DISLOCATION AND SUBLUXATION

A *dislocation* is a severe injury of the ligamentous structures that surround a joint. It results in the complete displacement or separation of the articular surfaces of the joint. A *subluxation* is a partial or incomplete displacement of the joint surface. The clinical manifestations of a subluxation are similar to those of a dislocation but are less severe. Treatment of subluxation is similar to that of a dislocation, but subluxation requires less healing time.

Dislocations characteristically result from overwhelming forces transmitted to the joint that cause a disruption of the soft tissues surrounding the joint. The joints most frequently dislocated in the upper extremity include the thumb, elbow, and shoulder. In the lower extremity, the hip is vulnerable to dislocation occurring as a result of severe trauma, often associated with motor vehicle accidents (Fig. 59-1). The patella may dislocate because of instability of the ligaments surrounding the knee.

The most obvious clinical manifestation of a dislocation is asymmetry of the musculoskeletal contour. For example, if a hip is dislocated, the limb is shorter on the affected side. Additional manifestations include local pain, tenderness, loss of function of the injured part, and swelling of the soft tissues in the region of the joint. The major complications of a dislocated joint are open joint injuries, intraarticular fractures, fracture dislocation, avascular necrosis, and damage to adjacent neurovascular tissue.

X-ray studies are performed to determine the extent of shifting of the involved structures. The joint may also be aspirated to determine the presence of blood (hemarthrosis) or fat cells. Fat cells from the synovial fluid indicate probable intraarticular fracture.

NURSING AND COLLABORATIVE MANAGEMENT: DISLOCATION

A dislocation requires prompt attention. The longer the joint remains unreduced, the greater is the possibility of avascular necrosis (bone cell death as a result of inadequate blood supply). The hip joint is particularly susceptible to avascular necrosis. The first goal of management is to realign the dislocated

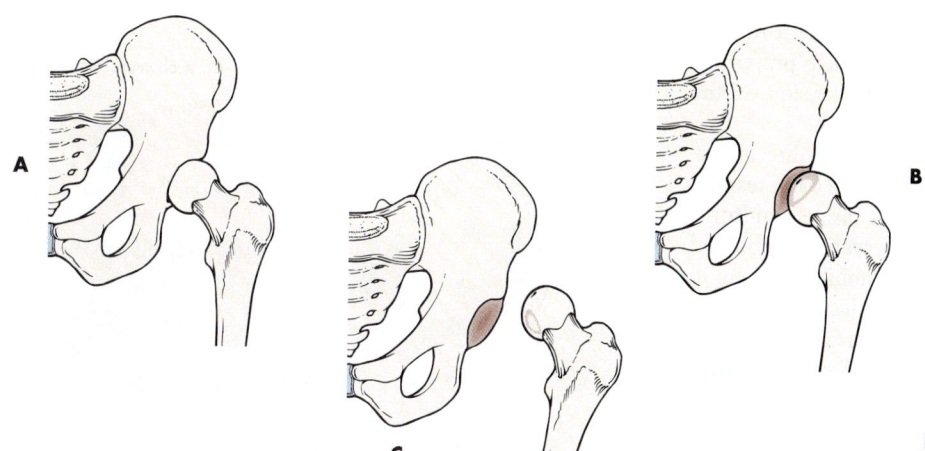

Fig. 59-1 Soft-tissue injury of the hip. **A,** Normal. **B,** Subluxation (partial dislocation). **C,** Dislocation.

portion of the joint in its original anatomic position. This can be accomplished by a closed reduction, which may be performed under local or general anesthesia. Anesthesia is often necessary to produce muscle relaxation so that the bones can be manipulated. In some situations, surgical open reduction may be necessary. After reduction, the extremity is usually immobilized by taping or using a sling to allow the torn ligaments and capsular tissue time to heal. Observation is indicated for the patient with a posterior sternoclavicular dislocation because delayed intrathoracic complications, such as pneumothorax or subclavian vessel injury, may occur.[2]

Nursing management of subluxation or dislocation is directed toward relief of pain and support and protection of the injured joint. After the joint has been reduced and immobilized, motion is usually restricted. A carefully regulated rehabilitation program can prevent the formation of contractures. The patient should not stretch the joint beyond its limits because the torn capsule and ligament heal in a shortened position with fibrous scar tissue that is not as strong as the original tissue. An exercise program slowly and methodically restores the joint to its original range of motion without causing another dislocation. The patient should gradually return to normal activities.

A patient who has dislocated a joint may be at greater risk to experience repeated dislocations because the joint has been weakened by shortened ligaments and scar tissue. Activity restrictions of the affected joint may be imposed to decrease the risk of repeatedly dislocating the joint.

CARPAL TUNNEL SYNDROME

Carpal tunnel syndrome is a condition caused by compression of the median nerve beneath the transverse carpal ligament within the narrow confines of the carpal tunnel located at the wrist (Fig. 59-2). This condition frequently is due to pressure from trauma or edema caused by inflammation of a tendon (tenosynovitis), neoplasm, rheumatoid synovial disease, or soft-tissue masses such as ganglia. Carpal tunnel syndrome occurs most frequently in middle-aged or postmenopausal women. This syndrome is associated with occupations that require continuous wrist movement (e.g., butchers, musicians, hair stylists, secretaries, carpenters, computer operators).

The clinical manifestations of carpal tunnel syndrome are weakness (especially of the thumb), pain and numbness, or im-

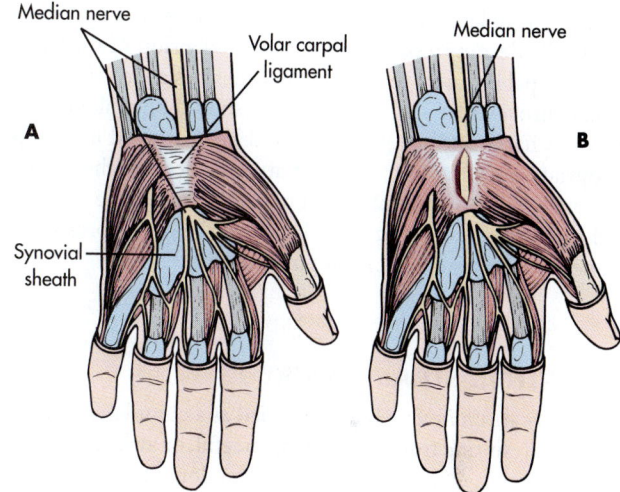

Fig. 59-2 **A,** Wrist structures involved in carpal tunnel syndrome. **B,** Decompression of median nerve.

paired sensation in the distribution of the median nerve, and clumsiness in performing fine hand movements. Numbness and tingling may be present that awaken the patient at night. Holding the wrist in acute flexion for 60 seconds will produce tingling and numbness over the distribution of the median nerve, the palmar surface of the thumb, the index finger, the middle finger, and part of the ring finger. This is known as a positive Phalen's sign. Tapping gently over the area of the inflamed median nerve may reproduce the paresthesia. This is known as a positive Tinel's sign. In late stages there is atrophy of the thenar muscles around the base of the thumb. This syndrome can result in recurrent pain and eventual dysfunction of the hand.

NURSING AND COLLABORATIVE MANAGEMENT: CARPAL TUNNEL SYNDROME

Prevention of carpal tunnel syndrome involves educating employees and employers to identify risk factors. Adaptive devices such as wrist splints may be worn to hold the wrist in slight dorsiflexion to relieve pressure on the median nerve. Special keyboard pads that help prevent repetitive pressure on the median nerve are available for computer operators to help prevent or reduce carpal tunnel syndrome by decreasing tension on the carpal tunnel.

Collaborative care of carpal tunnel syndrome is directed toward relieving the underlying cause of the nerve compression. The early symptoms associated with carpal tunnel syndrome can usually be relieved by stopping the aggravating action and by placing the hand and wrist at rest by immobilizing them in a hand splint. If the cause is inflammation, injection of hydrocortisone directly into the carpal tunnel may provide relief. The patient's sensation may be impaired. Therefore the patient should be instructed to avoid hazards such as extreme heat because of the risk of thermal injury. Nursing care of the patient with carpal tunnel syndrome usually occurs in the office or outpatient setting. The patient may be required to consider occupational changes because of discomfort and sensory and functional changes.

If the problem continues, the median nerve may have to be surgically decompressed by longitudinal division of the transverse carpal ligament under regional anesthesia (see Fig. 59-2). The neurovascular status of the hand should be evaluated before discharge and the patient should be instructed in the appropriate assessments to perform at home because the surgery is usually done on an outpatient basis. Endoscopic carpal tunnel release is a new procedure in which the decompression is done through a small incision puncture site.

REPETITIVE STRAIN INJURY

Repetitive strain injury (RSI) is defined as a cumulative trauma disorder resulting from prolonged, forceful, or awkward movements. Repeated movements strain tendons, ligaments, and muscles, causing tiny tears that become inflamed. If the tissues are not given time to heal properly, scarring can occur. Blood vessels of the arms and hands may become constricted, depriving tissues of vital nutrients and causing an accumulation of factors such as lactic acid. Without intervention, tendons and muscles can deteriorate and nerves become hypersensitive. At this point even the slightest movement can cause pain.

In addition to the repetitive movements, other factors related to RSI include poor posture and positioning, ill-fitting furniture, a badly designed keyboard, and a heavy workload. The result is damage to the muscles, tendons, and nerves of the neck, shoulder, forearm, and hand. Symptoms of RSI include pain, weakness, numbness, or impairment of motor function. Persons most often affected by RSI include musicians, dancers, electricians, butchers, and, most commonly, keyboard operators.[3]

RSI is becoming a serious public health problem. Reported incidence has risen from 1% to 4% in less than 10 years. It is theorized that the increase is due to increased productivity, an increased number of women in the workforce, and a heightened awareness of RSI in the media and health care system.[4] It is expected that the number of cases of RSI will continue to increase as computers become more commonplace.

RSI can be prevented through education, ergonomics (consideration of the interaction of humans and their work environment), and appropriate job design. Once diagnosed, the treatment of RSI consists of avoidance of the precipitating ac-

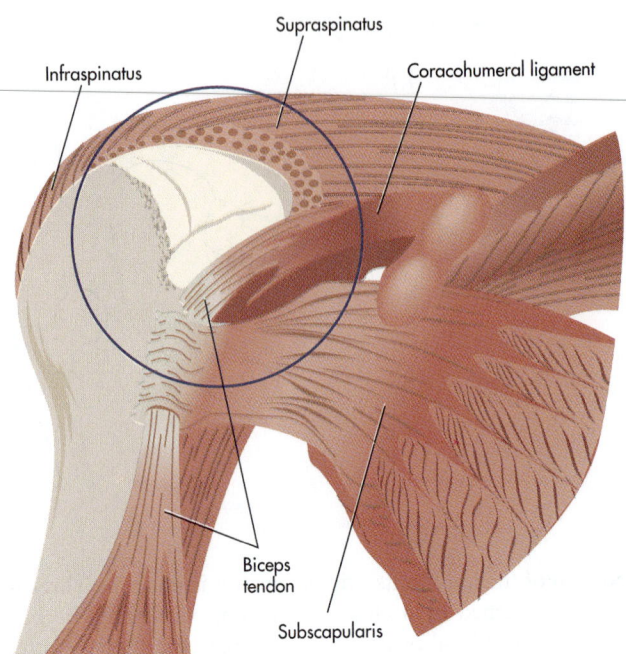

Fig. 59-3   Massive rotator cuff tear.

tivity, physical therapy, and careful use of analgesia. In most cases, the muscle and tendon damage associated with RSI cannot be surgically repaired.

ROTATOR CUFF INJURIES

The rotator cuff is a complex of four muscles in the shoulder: supraspinatus, infraspinatus, teres minor, and subscapularis. These muscles act to stabilize the humeral head in the glenoid fossa and rotate the humerus.[5]

A tear in the rotator cuff may occur as a gradual, degenerative process resulting from aging, poor posture, repetitive stress (especially overhead arm motions), or using an arm to break a fall[6] (Fig. 59-3). Young adults are more prone to experience a tear as a result of trauma such as a fall, lifting a heavy object, or throwing a ball.

Patients with a rotator cuff injury will complain of shoulder pain and cannot initiate or maintain abduction of the arm or shoulder. An X-ray alone is usually not much benefit in diagnosing a rotator cuff injury. A tear can be confirmed by arthrogram or magnetic resonance imaging (MRI).[7]

The patient may be treated conservatively with rest, ice and heat, NSAIDs, periodic corticosteroid injections into the joint, and physical therapy. If the patient does not respond to conservative treatment or if a complete tear is present, a surgical repair may be necessary. Surgical repair may be done through the arthroscope. If an extensive tear is present, open repair may be necessary. An immobilization device such as a sling or more commonly a shoulder immobilizer may be used for several weeks after surgery.[8] Exercises and physical therapy begin within a few days of surgery.

MENISCUS INJURY

The meniscus is the fibrous cartilage in the knee and other joints. Meniscus injuries are closely associated with ligament

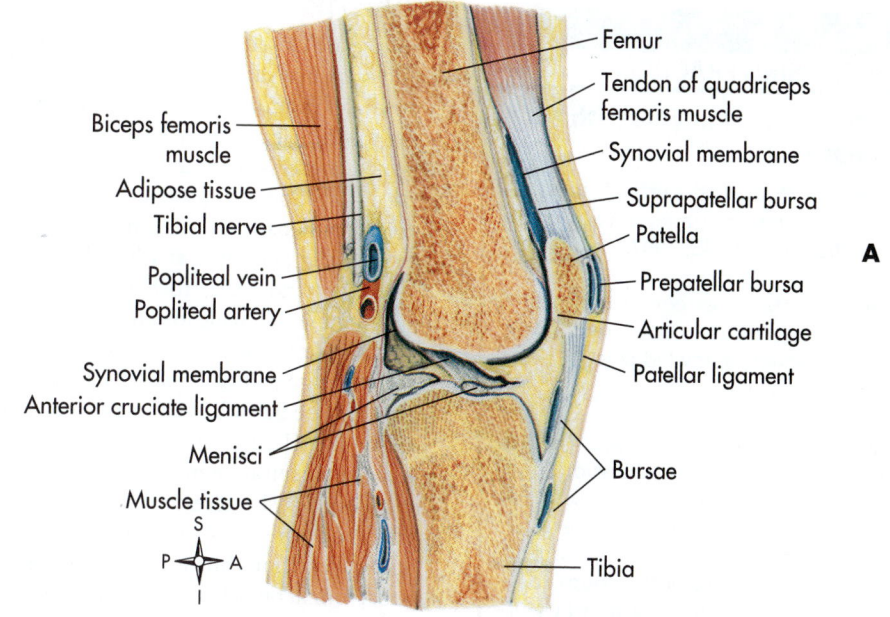

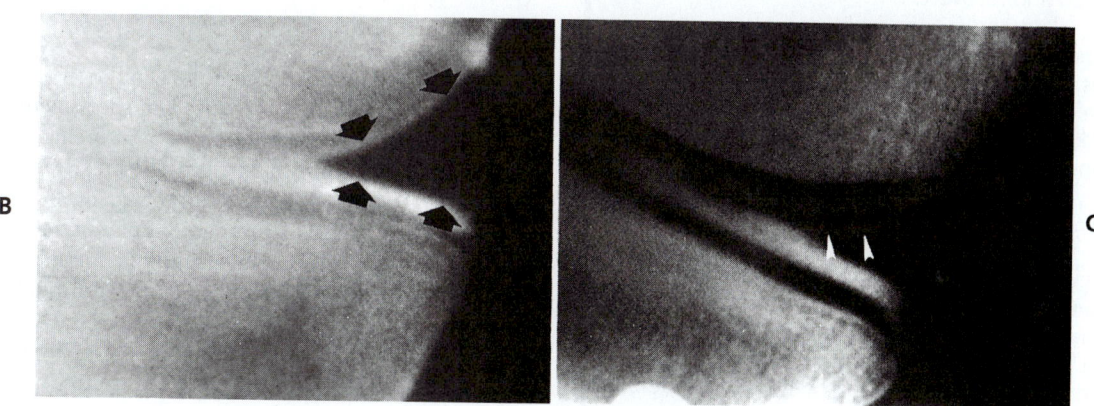

Fig. 59-4 **A,** Sagittal section through knee joint. Knee arthrogram. **B,** Normal medial meniscus. Spot film shows normal triangular shape of meniscus *(arrows)*. **C,** Linear tear of medial meniscus *(arrowheads)*.

sprains commonly occurring in athletes engaged in sports such as basketball, rugby, football, soccer, and hockey. These activities produce a rotational stress when the knee is in a flexed position and the foot is fixed. A blow to the knee can cause the meniscus to be trapped between the femoral condyles and the plateau of the tibia, resulting in a torn meniscus (Fig. 59-4). A causal relationship exists between occupations that require working in a squatting or kneeling position and meniscus injuries.

Meniscus injuries alone do not usually cause chronic edema because cartilage is avascular and aneural. However, a torn meniscus may be suspected when local tenderness or pain is reported. Pain is elicited by abduction or adduction of the leg at the knee. The usual clinical picture is a feeling by the patient that the knee is unstable and a report that the knee may click and lock periodically. Quadriceps atrophy is evident if the injury has been present for some time. Degenerative joint disease can occur if a damaged, roughened meniscus is not surgically removed.

An arthrogram or arthroscopy or both can diagnose knee problems. MRI is beneficial in confirming the diagnosis before arthroscopy is used. MRI has eliminated the use of an arthrogram as a diagnostic tool in many cases.

NURSING AND COLLABORATIVE MANAGEMENT: MENISCUS INJURY

Because meniscal injuries are commonly caused by sports-related activity, athletes should be educated about warm-up activities. Proper stretching may make the patient less prone to meniscal injury when a fall or twisting occurs. Examination of the acutely injured knee should occur within 24 hours of injury. Initial care of this type of injury involves application of ice, immobilization, and partial weight bearing with crutches. Most meniscal injuries are treated in an outpatient setting. The patient should be allowed to ambulate as tolerated. Crutches may

RESEARCH

IMPLICATIONS FOR NURSING PRACTICE

Effectiveness of Education in Patients with Total Knee Arthroplasty

Citation Lin P, Lin L, Lin J: Comparing the effectiveness of different education programs for patients with total knee arthroplasty, *Orthop Nurs* 16:43, 1997.

Purpose To compare the differences between patients having two different types of educational programs on subsequent outcomes of anxiety, knowledge level, exercise performance, and recovery.

Methods A quasi-experimental design was used. The experimental group (n = 30) received preadmission (outpatient) and preoperative (hospital) teaching with the control group (n = 30) receiving only preoperative teaching. Mean subject age was 69 years. In the preoperative and postoperative phases both groups completed questionnaires related to anxiety and knowledge about arthroplasty. Data were also collected postoperatively on regularity and accuracy of exercises performed and recovery.

Results and Conclusions There were no significant differences between the two groups in preoperative anxiety. The experimental group had a significantly higher level of knowledge and performed exercises more regularly and correctly than subjects in the control group. Recovery as evidenced by flexion of the operative knee joint was significantly higher in the experimental group.

Implications for Nursing Practice Preoperative teaching alone may not be effective in reducing anxiety and increasing patient knowledge about impending surgery. The nurse should begin teaching the patient before hospital admission with repeated preoperative instruction before surgery. The extra time allowed for learning may be especially helpful for older patients who are in an unfamiliar hospital environment. Providing teaching before hospital admission when anxiety is lower may facilitate improved patient outcomes.

be necessary. Use of an immobilizer during the first few days protects the knee.

After acute pain has decreased, gradual increases in flexion and strengthening help return the patient to full functioning. Physical therapy may be needed to help the patient strengthen muscles before returning to sport activities. Surgical repair or excision of part of the meniscus (meniscectomy) may be necessary. Frequently this can be done by arthroscopy.

Use of the laser for arthroscopy is being investigated. It is used to vaporize the exposed tissue in an area where precise cutting and ablation of tissue is needed during an arthroscopy. The value of the laser for arthroscopic surgery is undergoing clinical research.[9]

BURSITIS

Bursae are closed sacs that are lined with synovial membrane and contain a small amount of synovial fluid. They are located at sites of friction, such as between tendons, bones, and overlying joints. A bursa may become inflamed (bursitis) from repeated or excessive trauma or friction, gout, rheumatoid arthritis, or infection. The primary clinical manifestations of bursitis are warmth, pain and swelling, and limited range of motion in the affected part. Sites at which bursitis commonly occurs include the hand, knee, trochanter, shoulder, and elbow.

Attempts are made to determine and correct the cause of the bursitis. Rest is often the only treatment needed. Icing the area will decrease pain and may reduce inflammation. The affected part may be immobilized in a compression dressing or plaster splint. NSAIDs may be recommended to reduce inflammation and pain. Aspiration of the bursal fluid and injection of hydrocortisone may be necessary. If the bursa wall has become thickened and continues to interfere with normal joint function, surgical excision (bursectomy) may be necessary. For example, subacromial bursal thickening causes pain and loss of range of motion on abduction of the shoulder. Septic bursae usually require surgical drainage.

MUSCLE SPASMS

Local muscle spasms are a common condition often associated with excessive everyday activities and sports activities. Injury to a muscle results in inflammation and edema, which stimulates free nerve endings, resulting in muscle excitation and spasm. The spasms produce additional pain, creating a repetitive cycle. The clinical manifestations of muscle spasm include pain, palpable muscle mass in spasm, tenderness, diminished range of motion of the affected site, and limitation of daily activities.

A careful history should be taken and a physical examination should be performed to rule out central nervous system (CNS) problems. Muscle spasms can be managed with drug therapy, physical therapy, or both. A physical therapy program might include the use of heat or ice, supervised exercise, massage, hydrotherapy, local heat-producing applications (oil of wintergreen), ultrasound (deep heat), manipulation, and bracing. Drugs used for treatment of local muscle spasm include mild analgesics, NSAIDs, and skeletal muscle relaxants.

FRACTURES

Classification

A *fracture* is a disruption or break in the continuity of the structure of bone. Traumatic injuries account for the majority of fractures, although some fractures are secondary to a disease process (pathologic fractures). Fractures are described and classified according to (1) type (Fig. 59-5), (2) communication or noncommunication with the external environment (Fig. 59-6), and (3) location of fracture (Fig. 59-7). Fractures are also described as stable or unstable. A stable fracture occurs when some of the periosteum is intact across the fracture and either external or internal fixation has rendered the fragments stationary. Stable fractures are usually transverse, spiral, or greenstick. An unstable fracture is grossly displaced

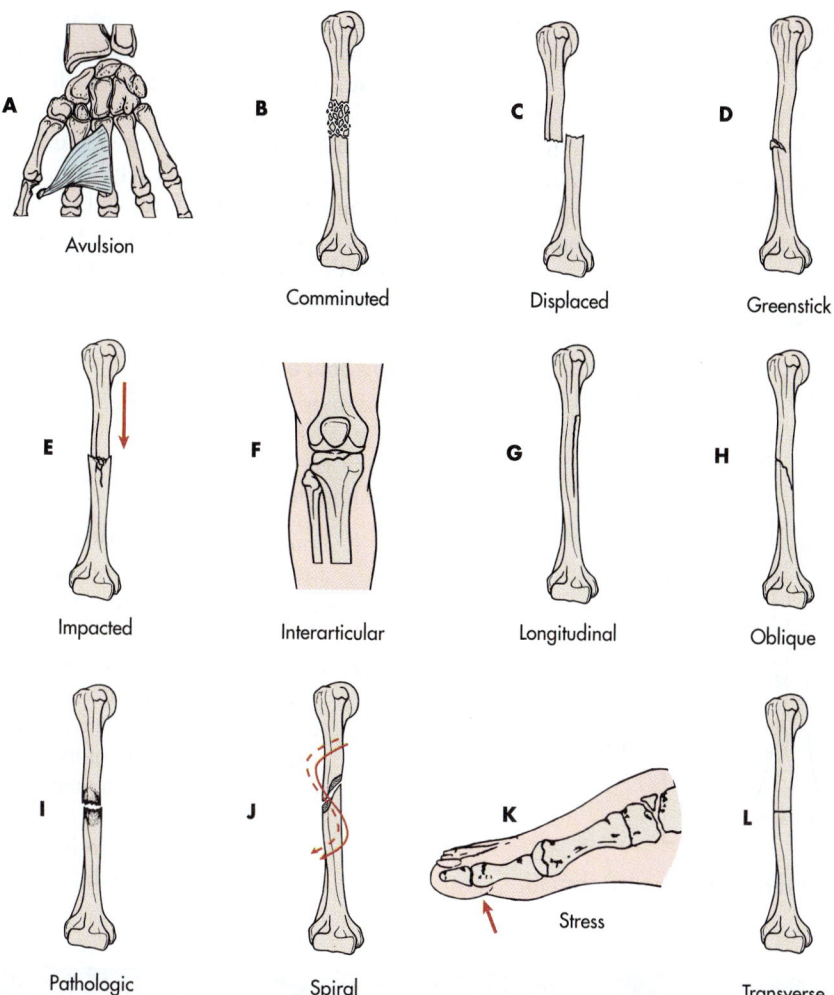

Fig. 59-5 Types of fractures. **A,** An avulsion is a fracture of bone resulting from the strong pulling effect of tendons or ligaments at the bone attachment. **B,** A comminuted fracture is a fracture with more than two fragments. The smaller fragments appear to be floating. **C,** A displaced (overriding) fracture involves a displaced fracture fragment that is overriding the other bone fragment. The periosteum is disrupted on both sides. **D,** A greenstick fracture is an incomplete fracture with one side splintered and the other side bent. **E,** An impacted fracture is a comminuted fracture in which more than two fragments are driven into each other. **F,** An interarticular fracture is a fracture extending to the articular surface of the bone. **G,** A longitudinal fracture is an incomplete fracture in which the fracture line runs along the longitudinal axis of the bone. The periosteum is not torn away from the bone. **H,** An oblique fracture is a fracture in which the line of the fracture extends in an oblique direction. **I,** A pathologic fracture is a spontaneous fracture at the site of a bone disease. **J,** A spiral fracture is a fracture in which the line of the fracture extends in a spiral direction along the shaft of the bone. **K,** A stress fracture is a fracture that occurs in normal or abnormal bone that is subject to repeated stress, such as from jogging or running. **L,** A transverse fracture is a fracture in which the line of the fracture extends across the bone shaft at a right angle to the longitudinal axis.

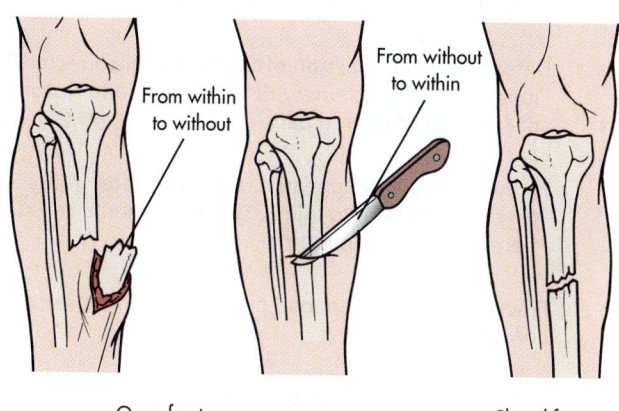

Fig. 59-6 Fracture classification according to communication.

during injury and is a site of poor fixation. Unstable fractures are usually comminuted or oblique.

Clinical Manifestations

The patient's history indicates injury associated with numerous signs and symptoms, including immediate localized pain, decreased function, and inability to use the affected part (Table 59-3). The patient guards and protects the part against move-

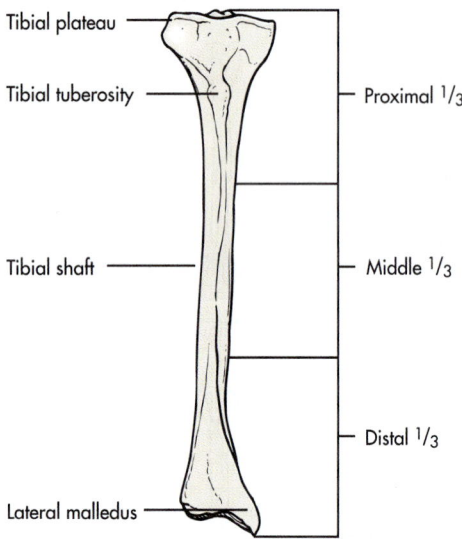

Fig. 59-7   Fracture classification according to location.

ment. The fracture may not be accompanied by obvious bone deformity. If a fracture is suspected, the affected part should be immobilized in the position in which it is found. Unnecessary movement increases soft-tissue damage and may convert a closed fracture to an open fracture or involve adjacent neurovascular structures. Careful management is particularly important for fractures through the epiphyseal plate in children. If fixation is not solid, the long bone may cease its longitudinal growth at all or part of the epiphyseal plate, causing a limb-length discrepancy.

Fracture Healing

It is important to understand the principles of fracture healing (Fig. 59-8) to provide appropriate therapeutic interventions. Bone goes through a remarkable reparative process of self-healing (termed *union*) that occurs in the following stages:

1. *Fracture hematoma.* When a fracture occurs, bleeding and edema create a hematoma, which surrounds the ends of the fragments. The hematoma is extravasated blood that changes from a liquid to a semisolid clot.
2. *Granulation tissue.* During this stage active phagocytosis absorbs the products of local necrosis. The hematoma converts to granulation tissue. Granulation tissue (consisting of young blood vessels, fibroblasts, and osteoblasts) produces the basis for a new bone substance called *osteoid.*
3. *Callus formation.* As minerals (calcium, phosphorus, and magnesium) are deposited in the osteoid, it forms

Table 59-3 Clinical Manifestations of Fracture	
Manifestation	**Significance**
Edema and Swelling Disruption of soft tissues or bleeding into surrounding tissues	Unchecked edema in closed space can occlude circulation and damage nerves (i.e., there is a risk of acute compartment syndrome).
Pain and Tenderness Muscle spasm as result of involuntary reflex action of muscle, direct tissue trauma, increased pressure on sensory nerve, movement of fracture parts	Pain and tenderness encourage splinting of fracture with reduction in motion of injured area.
Muscle Spasm Protective response to injury and fracture	Muscle spasms may displace nondisplaced fracture or prevent it from reducing spontaneously.
Deformity Abnormal position of bone as result of original forces of injury and action of muscles pulling fragment into abnormal position; seen as a loss of normal bony contours	Deformity is cardinal sign of fracture; if uncorrected, it may result in problems with bony union and restoration of function of injured part.
Ecchymosis Discoloration of skin as result of extravasation of blood in subcutaneous tissues	Ecchymosis usually appears several days after injury and may appear distal to injury. The nurse should reassure patient that process is normal.
Loss of Function Disruption of bone, preventing functional use	Fracture must be managed properly to ensure restoration of function.
Crepitation Grating or crunching together of bony fragments, producing palpable or audible crunching sensation	Examination of crepitation may increase chance for nonunion if bone ends are allowed to move excessively.

an unorganized network of bone that is woven about the fracture parts. Callus is primarily composed of cartilage, osteoblasts, calcium, and phosphorus. It usually begins to appear by the end of the first week after injury. Evidence of callus formation can be verified by x-ray.

4. *Ossification.* Ossification of the callus begins within 2 to 3 weeks after the fracture and continues until the fracture has healed. This stage is marked by ossification of the callus that is sufficient to prevent movement at the fracture site when the bones are gently stressed. However, the fracture is still evident on x-ray. During this stage of clinical union the patient can be converted from skeletal traction to a cast or the cast can be removed to allow limited mobility.

5. *Consolidation.* As callus continues to develop, the distance between bone fragments diminishes and eventually closes. This stage is called *consolidation,* and ossification continues. It can be equated with radiographic union.

6. *Remodeling.* Excess tissue is absorbed in the final stage of bone healing, and union is completed. Gradual return of the injured bone to its preinjury structural strength and shape occurs. Remodeling of bone is enhanced as it responds to physical stress. Initially, stress is provided through exercise. Weight bearing is gradually introduced. New bone is deposited in sites subjected to stress and resorbed at areas where there is little stress. Radiographic union occurs when there is x-ray evidence of complete bony union.

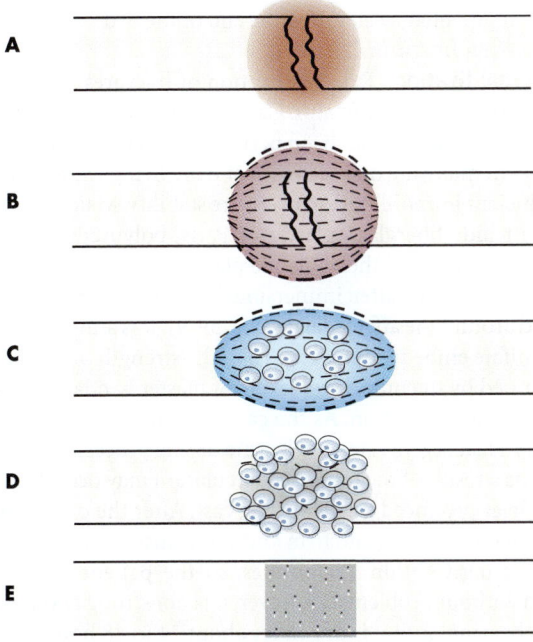

Fig. 59-8 Bone healing (schematic representation). **A,** Bleeding at broken ends of the bone with subsequent hematoma formation. **B,** Organization of hematoma into fibrous network. **C,** Invasion of osteoblasts, lengthening of collagen strands, and deposition of calcium. **D,** Callus formation: new bone is built up as osteoclasts destroy dead bone. **E,** Remodeling is accomplished as excess callus is reabsorbed and trabecular bone is laid down.

Many factors, such as age, initial displacement of the fracture, site of the fracture, and blood supply to the area, influence the time required for fracture healing to be complete. Fracture healing may not occur in the expected time (delayed union) or may not occur at all (nonunion). The ossification process is arrested by causes such as inadequate immobilization and reduction, excess movement, infection, and poor nutrition. Healing time for fractures increases with age. For example, an uncomplicated midshaft fracture of the femur heals in 3 weeks in a newborn and requires 20 weeks in an adult. Table 59-4 summarizes complications of fracture healing.

Electrical stimulation is used successfully to stimulate bone healing in some situations of nonunion or delayed union. The electric current acts by modifying cell behavior causing bone remodeling.[10] The underlying mechanism for electrically induced bone remodeling remains unknown. It is thought to be related to negative electrical fields attracting positive ions such as calcium. The electrodes are semiinvasive, noninvasive, or surgically implanted. Patient motivation and adherence to prescribed stimulator use must be high because the treatment can take up to 10 hours a day for many months.[11]

Collaborative Care

The overall goals of fracture treatment are (1) anatomic realignment of bone fragments known as reduction, (2) immobilization to maintain realignment, and (3) restoration of function of the injured part. Table 59-5 summarizes the collaborative care of fractures.

Fracture Reduction

Manipulation or closed reduction. Manipulation is a nonsurgical, manual realignment of bone fragments to their previous anatomic position. Traction and countertraction are manually applied to the bone fragments to restore position, length, and alignment. Closed reduction is usually performed under local or general anesthesia. After reduction or manipulation, the injured part is immobilized by traction, casting, external fixation, splints, or orthoses (braces) to maintain alignment until healing occurs.

Open reduction. Open reduction is the correction of bone alignment through a surgical incision. It frequently includes internal fixation of the fracture with the use of wire, screws, pins, plates, intramedullary rods, or nails. The type and location of the fracture, age of patient, and concurrent disease, as well as the result of attempted closed reduction by means of traction, may influence the decision to use open reduction. The chief disadvantages of this form of treatment are the possibility of infection and the complications associated with anesthesia.

If open reduction with internal fixation (ORIF) is used for intraarticular fractures (involving joint surfaces), early initiation of range of motion of the joint is indicated. Machines that provide continuous passive motion (CPM) to various joints are now available. Use of such machines can result in prevention of intraarticular adhesions, faster reconstruction of the subchondral (beneath cartilage) bone plate, more rapid healing of the articular cartilage, and possibly decreased incidence of later posttraumatic arthritis. If open reduction is used, early ambulation may be initiated in some instances for patients with lower-extremity fractures. Early ambulation decreases the risk of complications related to prolonged immobility while also facilitating healing with gradually increasing increments of stress.

Table 59-4   Complications of Fracture Healing

Problem	Description
Delayed union	Fracture healing progresses more slowly than expected; healing eventually occurs.
Nonunion	Fracture fails to heal properly despite treatment, resulting in fibrous union or pseudoarthrosis.
Malunion	Fracture heals in expected time but in unsatisfactory position, possibly resulting in deformity or dysfunction.
Angulation	Fracture heals in abnormal position in relation to midline of structure (type of malunion).
Pseudoarthrosis	This type of nonunion occurs at fracture site in which false joint is formed on shaft of long bones. It is a fracture site that failed to fuse (neoarthrosis). Each bone end is covered with fibrous scar tissue.
Posttraumatic osteoporosis	This condition represents loss of mineral (bone substance) as result of immobilization or disuse.
Refracture	New fracture occurs through original fracture site.
Myositis ossificans	This condition is a response to muscle hemorrhage caused by trauma. The hematoma ossifies. Response may occur in arm, elbow, and thigh.

COLLABORATIVE CARE

Table 59-5   Fractures

Diagnostic
 History and physical examination
 X-ray examination
 CT scan or MRI

Collaborative Therapy
Fracture Reduction
 Manipulation
 Open reduction
 Closed reduction
 Traction devices
  Skin traction
  Skeletal traction

Fracture Immobilization
 Casting
 External fixation
 Internal fixation
 Maintenance traction

Open Fractures
 Surgical debridement and irrigation
 Tetanus immunization
 Prophylactic antibiotic therapy
 Immobilization

CT, computed tomography; *MRI,* magnetic resonance imaging.

Traction. Traction devices apply a pulling force on the fractured extremity and result in realignment. The two most common types of maintenance traction are skin traction and skeletal traction. Skin traction is generally used for short-term treatment (48 to 72 hours) until skeletal traction or surgery is possible. Tape, boots, or splints are applied directly to the skin to maintain alignment, assist in reduction, and help diminish muscle spasms in the injured part. The traction weights are usually limited to 5 to 10 lb (2.3 to 4.5 kg). Skeletal traction, generally in place for longer periods of time, is used to align injured bones and joints or to treat joint contractures and congenital hip dysplasia. It provides a long-term pull that keeps the injured bones and joints aligned. To establish skeletal traction, the physician inserts a pin or wire into the bone, either partially or completely, to align and immobilize the injured body part. Weight for skeletal traction ranges from 5 to 45 lb (2.3 to 20.4 kg).

When traction is used to treat fractures, the forces are usually exerted on the distal fragment to obtain alignment with the proximal fragment. Several types of traction are used for this purpose (Table 59-6). Fracture alignment depends on the correct positioning and alignment of the patient while the traction forces remain constant. For extremity traction to be effective, forces must be pulling in the opposite direction (countertraction) to prevent the patient from sliding to the end or side of the bed. Countertraction is commonly supplied by the patient's body weight or may be augmented by elevating the end of the bed.

Fracture Immobilization

External fixation. External fixation of fractures is achieved by a cast or an external fixator. Casting is a common treatment after closed reduction has been performed. It allows the patient to perform many normal activities of daily living while providing sufficient immobilization to ensure stability. Major cast materials include fiberglass, plaster of Paris, polyurethane, thermoplastic resins, and thermolabile plastic.

Plaster of Paris, after immersion in water, is wrapped and molded around the affected part (Fig. 59-9). It is anhydrous calcium sulfate embedded in gauze roll. The strength of the cast is determined by the number of layers of plaster bandage and the technique of application. As the cast dries, it recrystallizes and hardens. Heat is generated during the drying process. Increased edema as a result of the increased circulation may occur as a result of heat produced by the drying cast. After the cast is completely dry, it is strong and firm and can withstand stresses. The plaster is hard within 15 minutes, so the patient can move around without problems. However, it is not strong enough for weight bearing until it is dry (after about 24 to 48 hours).

Thermolabile plastic (Orthoplast) and thermoplastic resins (Hexcelite) are molded to fit the torso or extremity after being heated in warm water. Polyurethane, which is formed from polyester and cotton fabric impregnated with a chemical, is water activated by immersing in cool water to start the chemical process. Casts made of this fiberglass tape are frequently used because they are lightweight and relatively waterproof and support earlier mobilization. They are appropriate in cases in

Table 59-6 Common Types of Traction

Type	Indications	Nursing Implications
Skin		
Buck's	Used for many conditions affecting hip, femur, knee, or back. It is generally used for temporary immobilization and stabilization of fractured hips or fractures of the femoral shaft. It can be unilateral or bilateral. May also be used to correct knee and hip joint contractures.	All assessments should be at least q4hr. Assess for altered neurovascular status caused by original injury or the application of the bandages used in Buck's traction. Especially note decreased peripheral vascular flow and peroneal nerve deficit by assessing for ability to dorsiflex toes and foot, and for changes in sensation in the first webspace between the great and second toes. Pressure from the elastic wrap may result in pressure necrosis, especially over bony prominences and areas prone to pressure (anterior tibial border, fibular head, both malleoli, Achilles tendon, calcaneus, and dorsum of the foot). In addition, assess for an allergic reaction to the adhesive material, rotation of the extremity, and constant traction and countertraction forces.
Russell's	Used for fractures of femur or hip.	Same as above. An additional area prone to pressure necrosis is the area over the hamstring tendons in the popliteal space.
Bryant's	Used for fractures of the femur, fractures in small children, and stabilization of hip joints in children under 2 yr or 30 lb (14 kg) in weight.	Be aware that with traction in place, buttocks should just clear the mattress. Check for undue pressure over the outer head and neck of fibula, dorsum of foot, Achilles tendon, scapulae, and shoulders. Check that bandages or boot has not slipped. Be aware that these are usually removed for skin care and assessment q4hr.

Continued

Table 59-6 Common Types of Traction—cont'd

Type	Indications	Nursing Implications
Skin—cont'd		
Pelvic belt (or girdle)	Used for sciatica, muscle spasms (low back), and minor fractures of the lower spine.	Check for security of the pelvic belt. Check frequently for skin irritation over iliac crests and in the intergluteal fold. Use measures to prevent skin breakdown. Check and adjust pelvic belt straps so that they are unrestricted and equal in length. Secure the straps with adhesive tape. Use a footboard to prevent footdrop. Maintain the correct angle of pull of the traction. Be aware that the physician orders the type of countertraction.
Pelvic sling traction	Used for pelvic fractures to provide compression for a separated pelvic girdle.	The sling should keep the pelvis just above the surface of the bed. Assess for pressure necrosis and skin irritation q4hr; especially assess for pressure over the iliac crests, intergluteal fold, and greater trochanters. Monitor for soiling of the sling and change as needed; use a fracture bedpan for toileting. Limit use of trapeze since it will reduce compressive force from the sling. Use alternating air pressure mattress or other pressure dispersing devices; provide frequent back care.
Circumferential Head halter	Used for soft-tissue disorders and degenerative disk disease of the cervical spine. It is not commonly used for unstable fractures of the cervical spine.	Assess for alignment with trunk, areas of local pressure over the ears and mandibular joints and under the chin and occipital area, and pain or dysfunction in the temporomandibular joint. Patients may be permitted to remove traction for meals; if not, provide a liquid or mechanical soft diet to reduce temporomandibular joint pain. Since this traction is commonly used in the home, ensure patients can demonstrate safe and effective setup, application, and use of the traction before discharge.

Skeletal

Overhead arm (90°–90°)

Commonly used for immobilization of fractures and dislocations of the upper arm and shoulder.

Be aware that the shoulder and elbow joint are maintained at 90° angles. Assess for pressure necrosis beneath the sling, especially over bony prominences. Assess distal neurovascular status; because of exposure, skin temperature may be cool and thus not indicative of decreased perfusion. Perform assessments q4hr. Inspect the pin site and perform pin site care according to hospital policy.

Lateral arm

Commonly used in immobilization of fractures and dislocations of the upper arm and shoulder.

Inspect the pin site and perform pin site care according to hospital policy. Assess neurovascular status.

Balanced suspension traction

Used for injury or fracture of the femoral shaft of the femur, acetabulum, hip, tibia, or any combination of these.

Be aware that this traction uses half-ring Thomas splint (1) and Pearson attachment (2) and that suspension of the extremity and direct skeletal traction are applied. This allows raising of the buttocks off the bed for bedpan use and skin care without altering the line of traction. Use nursing assessments so that countertraction is maintained (e.g., position patient high in bed so that feet do not press on foot of bed, do not elevate the head of the bed >25° if it causes continual movement toward foot of the bed). Encourage self-help in patient's performance of activities of daily living, movement in bed with help of trapeze, and flexion and extension of affected foot to prevent footdrop. Assess for pressure necrosis in areas contacted by the traction, especially the greater trochanter, ischial tuberosity, hamstring tendons, fibular head, and both malleoli. Assess distal neurovascular status q4hr. Inspect the pin site and perform pin site care according to hospital policy.

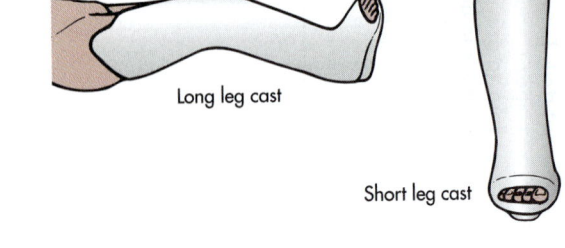

Fig. 59-9 Common casts used in treatment of disorders of the musculoskeletal system.

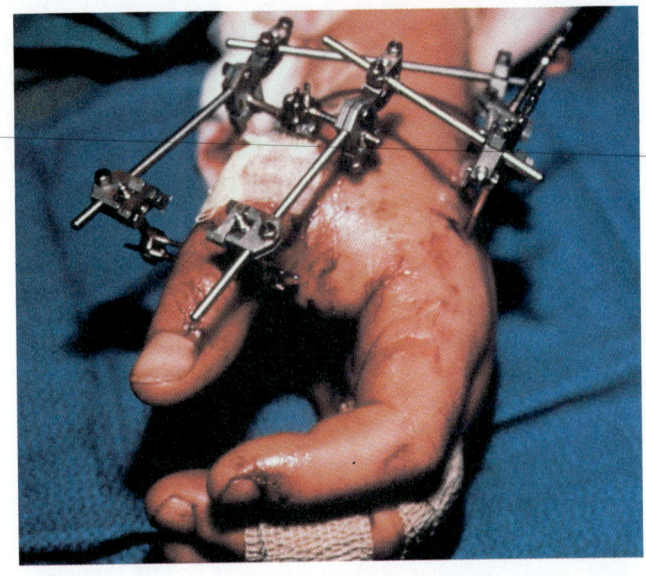

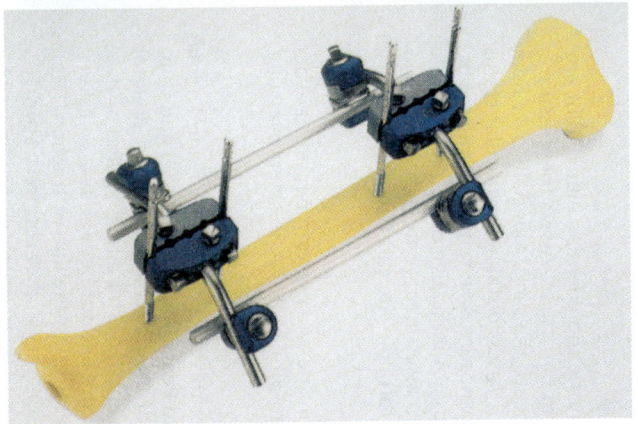

Fig. 59-10 External fixators. **A,** Mini Hoffman system in use on hand. **B,** Hoffman II on the tibia (standard system).

which severe edema is not present or when multiple cast changes are not anticipated.

An external fixator is a metallic device composed of metal pins that are inserted into the bone and attached to external rods to stabilize the fracture while it heals. It can be used to apply traction or to compress fracture fragments and to immobilize reduced fragments when the use of a cast or other traction is not appropriate. The external device holds fracture fragments in place much like surgically implanted internal devices do. The external fixator is attached directly to the bones by percutaneous pins (Fig. 59-10). Assessment for pin loosening and infection is critical. Infection signaled by exudate, redness, tenderness, and pain may require removal of the device. An external fixator used to treat fractures with associated soft-tissue trauma facilitates wound care.

External fixator devices can also be used as part of a limb-lengthening process for patients who have a significant leg-length discrepancy. The pins connected to these fixators are turned regularly as part of a prescribed regimen.

Types of casts (see Fig. 59-9). Immobilization of an acute fracture or soft-tissue injury of the upper extremity is frequently accomplished by use of (1) the sugar-tong splint, (2) the posterior splint, (3) the short arm cast, and (4) the long arm cast. The sugar-tong splint is typically used for acute wrist injuries or injuries that may result in significant swelling. Plaster splints are applied to the well-padded forearm, beginning at the phalangeal joints of the hand and extending up the dorsal aspect of the forearm around the distal humerus and then extending down the volar aspect of the forearm to the distal palmar crease. The splinting material is wrapped with either elastic bandage or bias stockinette. The major advantage of the sugar-tong cast and posterior splint are avoidance of the circumferential effects of a nonelastic cylinder cast, because these devices allow for swelling.

The short arm cast is frequently used for the treatment of stable wrist or metacarpal fractures. An aluminum finger splint can be fabricated into the short arm cast for concurrent treatment of phalangeal injuries. The short arm cast is a circular cast extending from the distal palmar area to the proximal forearm. This cast provides wrist immobilization and permits unrestricted elbow motion.

The long arm cast is commonly used for stable forearm or elbow fractures and unstable wrist fractures. It is similar to the short arm cast but extends to the proximal humerus, restricting motion in the wrist and elbow. Nursing measures should be directed toward supporting the extremity and reducing the effects of edema by maintaining extremity elevation with a sling. However, when a hanging arm cast is used for a proximal humerus fracture, elevation or a supportive sling are contraindicated because hanging provides traction and promotes fracture healing.

When a sling is used, the nurse must ensure that the axillary area is well padded to prevent skin maceration associated with direct skin-to-skin contact. Placement of the sling should not put undue pressure on the posterior neck. Movement of the fingers (unless contraindicated) should be encouraged to enhance the pumping action of veins to decrease edema. The nurse should also encourage the patient to actively move non-immobilized joints of the upper extremity to prevent stiffness and contractures.

The body jacket cast is frequently used for immobilization and support for stable spine injuries of the thoracic or lumbar spine. This cast is applied around the chest and abdomen and extends from above the nipple line to the pubis. After application of the cast, the nurse must assess the patient for the development of *cast syndrome*. This condition occurs if the body cast is applied too tightly and the cast compresses the superior mesenteric artery against the duodenum. The patient generally complains of abdominal pain, abdominal pressure, nausea, and vomiting. The abdomen should be assessed for bowel sounds (a window may be left over the umbilicus). Treatment includes gastric decompression with a nasogastric tube and suction. The cast may need to be removed or split. Nursing assessment also includes observation of respiratory status, bowel and bladder function, and areas of pressure over the bony prominences, especially the iliac crest. During the time required for the cast to dry, the nurse should reposition the patient every 2 to 3 hours to promote even cast drying and to relieve pressure and discomfort.

The hip spica cast is used in treating femoral fractures, especially in children. The purpose of the hip spica cast is to immobilize the affected extremity and the trunk securely. It includes two casts joined together: (1) the body jacket cast and (2) the long leg cast. The location of the femoral fracture will determine whether the thigh of the unaffected extremity will have to be immobilized to restrict rotation of the pelvis and possible hip motion on the side of the femur fracture. The hip spica cast extends from above the nipple line to the base of the foot (single spica) and may include the opposite extremity up to an area above the knee (spica and a half) or both extremities (double spica).

The nurse should assess the patient with a hip spica cast for the same problems that are associated with the body jacket cast. During the initial drying stage the patient should not be placed in the prone position, because the cast may break. The patient should be slightly turned from side to side and supported with pillows. When the patient is repositioned, the support bar joining the thighs must never be used to assist in moving, since the bar can break and cause cast disruption. After the cast has dried, the nurse (with assistance) can turn the patient to the prone position and provide pillow support under the chest and immobilized extremity. Skin care around the cast edges and the areas not encompassed by plaster is important to prevent any pressure sores. The nurse should instruct the patient in the positioning activities required to get on and off the bedpan. A fracture bedpan may be used to provide comfort and ease the movement of getting on and off the bedpan. After the hip spica cast has dried sufficiently, the patient may be instructed in ambulation techniques by the physical therapist.

Injuries to the lower extremity are frequently immobilized by either a long leg, short leg, or cylinder cast or a Jones dressing. The usual indications for applying a long leg cast are an unstable ankle fracture, soft-tissue injuries, a fractured tibia, and knee injuries. The cast usually extends from the base of the toes to the groin and gluteal crease. The short leg cast can be used for a variety of conditions but is usually used for stable ankle and foot injuries. A cylinder cast is used for knee injuries or fractures. The cast extends from the groin to the malleoli of the ankle. A Jones dressing is composed of significant padding materials (absorption dressing and sheet wadding), anterior or posterior and lateral splints, and an elastic wrap or bias-cut stockinette. The Jones dressing, like the sugar-tong splint, is used for knee fractures or surgery when there is a risk of significant edema. After the application of a lower-extremity cast or dressing, the extremity should be elevated with pillows above the heart level for the first 24 hours. After the initial phase, the casted extremity should not be placed in a dependent position because of the possibility of excessive edema.

Initially, no weight can be put on the injured extremity. Later, a walking heel or cast shoe may be added to the cast if the patient will be allowed to bear weight and walk on the affected leg. Following cast application, the nurse should observe for signs of pressure, especially in the regions of the heel, anterior tibial border, fibular head, and malleoli.

Internal fixation. Internal fixation devices are surgically inserted at the time of realignment. Examples of internal fixation devices include pins, plates, and screws. They are biologically inert metal devices such as stainless steel, vitallium, or titanium that are used to realign and maintain bony fragments. Proper alignment is evaluated by x-ray studies at regular intervals.

Maintenance traction. Maintenance traction is initiation or continuation of traction and countertraction. A continuous pulling force can be applied directly to bone with wires and pins (skeletal traction) or can be applied indirectly by weights that are attached to the skin with slings, belts, adhesive straps, or boots (skin traction). Skin traction is usually applied directly to the extremity by adhesive material that is wrapped circumferentially with a bandage or slings, belts, or a special splint that is attached to a rope with a weight. Skin traction for extremities is applied for a short time and usually consists of not more than 7 to 10 lb (3.2 to 4.5 kg) of traction weight because of skin intolerance to pressure. Pelvic or cervical skin traction may require heavier weights applied intermittently. Skeletal traction is usually indicated when the traction forces are expected to exceed 10 lb (4.5 kg) or when traction will be used for a long time. Use of too much weight to maintain traction can result in delayed union or nonunion. The major disadvantages of skeletal traction are infection in the area of bone where the skeletal pin has been inserted and the consequences of prolonged immobility necessitated by skeletal traction.

Open fracture. An open fracture involves communication to or from the fracture through the skin, formerly termed *compound fracture*. Tetanus prevention should be ensured with tetanus toxoid or tetanus antitoxin for a patient who has not been immunized. A broad-spectrum antibiotic (such as the cephalosporins) is usually used prophylactically. A decision on whether to close the wound or leave it open is based on the degree of contamination and the time elapsed before initiation of treatment. Infection is the greatest risk of an open fracture.

The overall long-term goal of treatment is the union of the fracture and return of the patient to the preinjury level of functioning as soon as possible. Discharge planning should include referral to the appropriate human service agency for assistance in the transition to the home environment.

Drug Therapy. Patients with fractures often experience varying degrees of pain associated with muscle spasms. These spasms are caused by involuntary reflexes that result from edema following muscle injury. Muscle relaxants, such as carisoprodol (Soma), cyclobenzaprine (Flexeril), or methocarbamol (Robaxin), may be prescribed for relief of pain associated with muscle spasms.

Common side effects associated with muscle relaxants are drowsiness, lassitude, headache, weakness, fatigue, blurred vision, ataxia, and gastrointestinal upset. Hypersensitivity reactions may include skin rash or pruritus. Ingestion of large doses of muscle relaxants may cause hypotension, tachycardia, or respiratory depression. The possible habituating effects associated with long-term use and the potential for abuse must be carefully considered.

Some physicians do not advocate the use of muscle relaxants for relief of muscle spasms. Their rationale is that the reflex spasm will continue as long as the precipitating pain persists. If the pain is controlled by use of appropriate analgesia, the muscle spasms will cease.

Nutritional Therapy. Proper nutrition is an essential component of the reparative process in injured tissue. An adequate energy source is needed to promote muscle strength and tone, build endurance, and enhance ambulation and gait-training skills. The patient's dietary requirements must include ample protein (e.g., 1 g per kilogram of body weight), vitamins (especially D, B, and C), and calcium to ensure optimal soft-tissue and bone healing. Low serum protein levels and vitamin C deficiencies interfere with tissue healing. Immobility and callus formation increase calcium needs. Three well-balanced meals a day will usually provide the necessary nutrients. The well-balanced meal should be supplemented by a fluid intake of 2000 to 3000 ml/day to promote optimal bladder and bowel function. Adequate fluid and a high-fiber diet with fruits and vegetables will prevent constipation. If immobilized in a body jacket or hip spica bandage, the patient should be instructed not to overeat to avoid abdominal pressure and cramping.

NURSING MANAGEMENT: FRACTURES

■ Nursing Assessment

A brief history of the accident, mechanism of injury, and the position in which the victim was found can be obtained from the patient or witnesses. As soon as possible, the patient should be transported to an emergency department where a thorough assessment and treatment can be initiated (Table 59-7). Subjective and objective data that should be obtained from an individual with a fracture are presented in Table 59-8.

Special emphasis must be focused on the region distal to the site of injury. The involved extremity should be compared with the uninvolved extremity. Clinical findings must be documented before fracture treatment is initiated to avoid doubts about whether a problem discovered later was missed during the original examination or was caused by the treatment. Misdiagnosis may result from failure to consider clinical procedures as the cause of a patient's complaints.

Neurovascular Assessment. Many musculoskeletal injuries have the potential of causing neurovascular injuries. Such events as the original trauma, application of a cast or constrictive dressing, or poor positioning can cause nerve or vascular damage, usually distal to the injury. One method to use for a neurovascular assessment is to consider the five *P*s: *pain, pulses, pallor, paresthesia,* and *paralysis.*

The nurse should carefully assess the location, quality, and intensity of the pain of the affected extremity. Pain unrelieved by medication could be an early sign of compartment syndrome. The pulses on both the affected and injured extremity should be compared to identify differences in rate or quality. A diminished or absent pulse distal to the injury can indicate vascular insufficiency.

Paresthesia (abnormal sensation, such as numbness or tingling) can be evaluated by comparing the patient's sensations above and below the injury. Comparison of the sensations felt between the injured and uninjured extremity should also be made. Changes in sensation such as decreased sensation, hypersensation, numbness, tingling, or loss of sensation may be reported by the patient.

Next, color (pallor) and temperature changes in the area of nerve distribution of the affected extremity should be assessed. Pallor or a cold extremity below the injury could indicate arterial insufficiency. A warm, bluish extremity could indicate poor venous return. Capillary refill should also be checked. A compressed nailbed should return to its original color within 3 seconds. Comparisons should be made between the injured and uninjured extremities.

The final assessment of a neurovascular assessment is to check for paralysis or decreased motor strength. Range of motion and strength can be compared between the two extremities. Reduced motion or strength in the injured extremity can alert to problems with the motor portion of the involved nerves.

Patients should be instructed to report any changes in strength, sensation, color, temperature, or pain in the fractured extremity.

■ Nursing Diagnoses

Nursing diagnoses for the patient with a fracture may include, but are not limited to, those presented in NCP 59-1.

■ Planning

The overall goals are that the patient with a fracture will (1) have no associated complications, (2) obtain satisfactory pain relief, and (3) achieve maximal rehabilitation potential.

■ Nursing Implementation

Health Promotion. The public should be educated to take appropriate safety precautions to prevent injuries while at home, at work, when driving, or when participating in sports. Nurses should be vocal advocates for personal actions known to reduce injuries such as regular use of seat belts,

✚**EMERGENCY MANAGEMENT**

Table **59-7** Fractured Extremity

Etiology	Assessment Findings	Interventions
Blunt Motor vehicle collision Pedestrian event Falls Direct blows Forced flexion or hyperextension Twisting forces **Penetrating** Gunshot **Other** Pathologic conditions Violent muscle contractions (seizures)	▪ Deformity (loss of normal bony contours) or unnatural position of affected limb ▪ Edema and ecchymosis ▪ Muscle spasm ▪ Tenderness and pain ▪ Loss of function ▪ Numbness, tingling, loss of distal pulses ▪ Grating (crepitus) ▪ Open wound over injured site, exposure of bone	**Initial** ▪ Treat life-threatening injuries first. ▪ Ensure airway, breathing, and circulation. ▪ Control external bleeding with direct pressure or sterile pressure dressing. ▪ Splint joints above and below fracture site. ▪ Check neurovascular status distal to injury before and after splinting. ▪ Elevate injured limb if possible. ▪ Do *not* attempt to straighten fractured or dislocated joints. ▪ Do *not* manipulate protruding bone ends. ▪ Apply ice packs to affected area. ▪ Obtain x-rays of affected limb. ▪ Administer tetanus prophylaxis if skin integrity is violated. ▪ Mark location of pulses to facilitate repeat assessment. ▪ Splint fracture site, including joints above and below fracture site. **Ongoing Monitoring** ▪ Monitor vital signs, level of consciousness, oxygen saturation, peripheral pulses, and pain. ▪ Monitor for compartment syndrome characterized by excessive pain, pain with passive stretch, pallor, paresthesia, paralysis, pulselessness. ▪ Monitor for fat embolism (dyspnea, chest pain).

NURSING ASSESSMENT

Table **59-8** Fracture

Subjective Data	Objective Data
Important Health Information *Past health history:* Traumatic injury; long-term repetitive forces (stress fracture); bone or systemic diseases, prolonged immobility (pathologic fracture) *Medications:* Use of corticosteroids (pathologic fractures); analgesics *Surgery or other treatments:* First aid treatment of fracture **Functional Health Patterns** *Health perception–health management:* Estrogen replacement therapy, calcium supplementation *Activity-exercise:* Loss of motion or weakness of affected part; muscle spasms *Cognitive-perceptual:* Sudden and severe pain in affected area; numbness, tingling, loss of sensation distal to injury; chronic pain that increases with activity (stress fracture)	**General** Apprehension, guarding of injured site **Integumentary** Skin lacerations, pallor and cool skin or bluish and warm skin distal to injury; ecchymosis, hematoma, edema at site of fracture **Cardiovascular** Reduced or absent pulse distal to injury, decreased skin temperature, delayed capillary refill **Neurologic** Paresthesias, decreased or absent sensation, hypersensation **Musculoskeletal** Restricted or lost function of affected part, local bony deformities, abnormal angulation, shortening, rotation, crepitation; muscle weakness **Possible Findings** Localization and extent of fractures on x-ray, bone scans, tomograms, CT scan, or MRI

59-1 NURSING CARE PLAN PATIENT WITH A FRACTURE

Expected Patient Outcomes	Nursing Interventions and *Rationales*

NURSING DIAGNOSIS Risk for peripheral neurovascular dysfunction *related to* nerve compression.

- Has normal neurovascular examination.

- Assess for signs and symptoms of peripheral neurovascular dysfunction such as pain in affected extremity that is unrelieved by medication, paresthesias, pain on passive movement, weakness, cool temperature, pallor, diminished pulses *to ensure early recognition and intervention.*
- Elevate extremity above heart level *to reduce edema by promoting return circulation to heart.* (Note: If compartment syndrome is suspected, elevate extremity no higher than heart level.)
- Apply ice compresses as ordered *to reduce edema and provide comfort.* (Note: If compartment syndrome is suspected, remove ice because it may exacerbate decreased tissue perfusion.)
- Notify physician immediately if patient complains of increasing pain that is unrelieved by medication *because this may indicate neurovascular impairment, which can result in significant injury if unrelieved.*
- Teach patient the signs of peripheral neurovascular dysfunction *to enable patient participation in care.*

NURSING DIAGNOSIS Pain *related to* edema, movement of bone fragments, and muscle spasms *as manifested by* complaints of pain, guarding, moaning, crying, restlessness.

- Tolerable or no pain.
- Satisfaction with plan for pain relief.

- Gently and correctly position fractured extremity *to minimize pain and prevent bone displacement.*
- Assess site for constriction or pressure caused by immobilization apparatus *to prevent skin or neurovascular injury.*
- Use a pain scale *to assess pain and evaluate effectiveness of interventions.*
- Give patient analgesics or muscle relaxants as indicated *to relieve pain and promote muscle relaxation.*
- Elevate, apply ice (if prescribed), and support affected extremity *to reduce edema and promote comfort.*
- Be alert for pain that is not diminished after analgesic is administered *since this may indicate an impending compartment syndrome.*

NURSING DIAGNOSIS Risk for infection *related to* disruption of skin integrity and presence of environmental pathogens secondary to open fracture or external fixation pins.

- No evidence of wound infection.

- Assess fracture or pin insertion points for blistering, tenting discoloration, and drainage *as indicators of infection.*
- Use aseptic technique when providing pin or wound care or when performing dressing change *to prevent cross-contamination and possible introduction of infection.*
- Obtain culture of wound if infection is suspected *to identify infective organism.*
- Administer antibiotics as ordered *to provide prophylaxis or treatment of diagnosed infection.*
- Monitor temperature q2hr *because fever may reflect developing sepsis.*

NURSING DIAGNOSIS Risk for impaired skin integrity *related to* immobility and presence of cast.

- No evidence of skin breakdown.

- Examine potential pressure areas q4hr *to assess condition of skin.*
- Petal cast edges *to prevent skin abrasion or cast crumbs from falling beneath the cast.*
- Turn patient q2hr *to reduce pressure over bony prominences.* Use special pressure mattresses for prolonged bed rest.
- Assess exposed skin areas of traction sites for signs of infection or irritation *because improper positioning of traction devices can cause localized pressure necrosis.*
- Seek medical attention if cast becomes loose *to prevent rotation, flexion, and skin abrasion.*
- Instruct patient not to insert items (e.g., hangers or forks) into cast to scratch self *because these may cause tissue injury.*
- Instruct patient to report areas of warmth, pain, burning, or moisture beneath the cast; foul odor from cast ends; or areas of new or increasing drainage on cast surfaces.

Continued

59-1 NURSING CARE PLAN PATIENT WITH A FRACTURE—continued

Expected Patient Outcomes	Nursing Interventions and *Rationales*

NURSING DIAGNOSIS Ineffective management of therapeutic regimen *related to* lack of knowledge regarding muscle atrophy, exercise program, and cast care *as manifested by* questioning of long-term effect of casting and cast care, activity restrictions.

- Minimal loss of muscle bulk of affected extremity.
- Verbalization of confidence in ability to follow prescribed discharge plan.

- Instruct patient on home care measures related to exercise, cast care, and prevention of complications *so patient can carry out prescribed discharge plan.*
- Explain factors that contribute to atrophy; emphasize relationship of inactivity to muscle atrophy *so patient will exercise involved extremity to maximum allowed and will not be alarmed at appearance of extremity when cast is removed.*
- Provide written instructions of prescribed exercise.

NURSING DIAGNOSIS Impaired walking *related to* ineffective use of crutches *as manifested by* inability to move about independently.

- Crutches correctly used to move about as needed.

- Teach gait-training principles to patient (non–weight-bearing gait status unless otherwise ordered by physician); sit with feet over edge of bed, stand with no weight on affected extremity, measure and adjust crutches *to promote mobility according to patient's abilities.*
- Start gait training on parallel bars *because this increases patient's confidence.*
- Ensure gait is compatible with weight-bearing status *to prevent malalignment.*
- Cooperate with physical therapist regarding exercise and gait training *to reinforce plan and to provide unified approach to patient.*

COLLABORATIVE PROBLEMS

Nursing Goals	Nursing Interventions and *Rationales*

POTENTIAL COMPLICATION Fat embolism *related to* fracture of a long bone.

- Monitor for embolic phenomena.
- Report abnormal findings.
- Carry out appropriate medical and nursing interventions.

- Monitor for changes in mental status caused by hypoxemia; symptoms of acute respiratory distress syndrome such as mild agitation, confusion, chest pain, tachypnea, cyanosis, dyspnea, apprehension, tachycardia, and decreased PaO_2; and petechiae on upper trunk and axillae *to enable prompt identification and reporting to physician.*
- As indicated, assess oxygen saturation with oximetry and report O_2 saturation $\leq 92\%$.
- Initiate oxygen therapy if indicated.
- Maintain immobilization of long bone fractures *to reduce the occurrence of fat embolism.*
- Be alert to patient's verbalization of a feeling of impending doom *because this is frequently a premonitory sign.*
- Provide emergency respiratory support as needed *to prevent respiratory arrest.*

---

driving within posted speed limits, stretching before exercise, use of protective devices (helmets, knee, wrist, and elbow pads), and not combining drinking and driving.

Elderly patients should be encouraged to participate in moderate exercise to aid in the maintenance of muscle strength and balance. To reduce falls, their living environment should be examined to rule out the use of scatter rugs, to ensure adequate footwear and lighting, and to clear paths to bathrooms for nighttime use. The nurse should also stress the importance of adequate calcium and vitamin D intake.

Acute Intervention. Patients with fractures may be treated in an emergency department or a physician's office and released to home care, or they may require hospitalization for varying amounts of time. Specific nursing measures de-

pend on the type of treatment used and the setting in which patients are placed.

Preoperative management. If surgical intervention is required to treat the fracture, patients will need preoperative preparation. In addition to the usual preoperative nursing measures (see Chapter 16), the nurse should inform patients of the type of immobilization device that will be used and the expected activity limitations. Patients must be assured that their needs will be met by the nursing staff until they can again meet their needs. Assurance that pain medication will be available, if needed, is often beneficial.

Proper skin preparation is an important part of preoperative preparation. The protocol for skin preparation varies among agencies and may be the responsibility of the nurse.

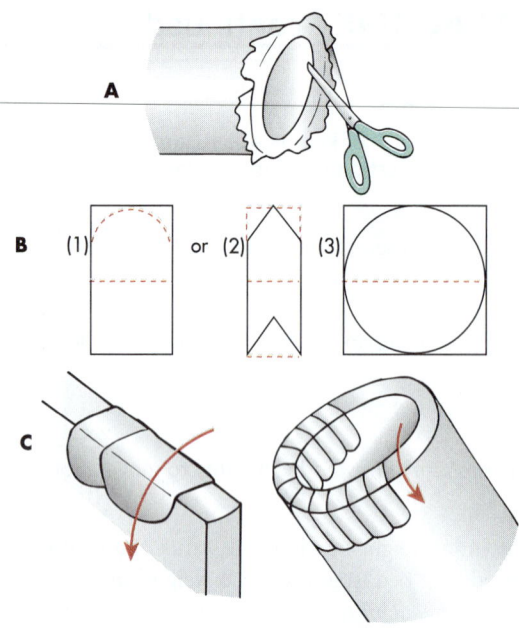

Fig. 59-11   Finishing edges of cast with waterproof adhesive strips. **A,** The cast must be thoroughly dry. The nurse trims the excess sheet wadding and stretches the stockinette over the cast edge (when possible). **B,** Several strips (petals) of waterproof adhesive tape (2-inch-wide strips for wide areas and 1-inch-wide strips for small areas, each 1 inch long) are made in advance. **C,** The uncut end of the tape is placed beneath the cast edge. Each succeeding petal overlaps the previous one by one-half inch, ensuring a smooth cast edge. A family member can help, and this can be done at home as needed.

The aim of skin preparation is to clean the skin and remove debris and hair to reduce the possibility of infection. Careful attention to this preoperative treatment can influence the postoperative course.

Postoperative management. In general, postoperative nursing care and management is directed toward monitoring vital signs and applying the general principles of postoperative nursing care (see Chapter 18). Frequent neurovascular assessments of the affected extremity are necessary to detect subtle changes. Any limitations of movement or activity related to turning, positioning, and extremity support should be monitored closely. Pain and discomfort can be minimized through proper alignment and positioning. Dressings or casts should be carefully observed for any overt signs of bleeding or drainage. A significant increase in size of the drainage area should be reported. If a wound drainage system is in place, the patency of the system and the volume of drainage should be regularly assessed. Whenever the contents of a drainage system are measured or emptied, the nurse should use sterile technique to avoid contamination. Additional nursing responsibilities depend on the type of immobilization used. A blood salvage and reinfusion system that allows for recovery and reinfusion of the patient's own blood may be used. The blood is retrieved from a joint space or cavity and the patient receives this blood in the form of an autotransfusion.[12]

Cast care. Immediately after a plaster cast is applied, there is a short period of exothermic reaction, during which heat is

released from the plaster. The patient should be alerted to this occurrence, since it can increase edema. Evaporation of water and dissipation of heat from the cast can be hastened by exposing the cast to room air. A fresh cast should never be covered with a blanket because air cannot circulate and heat builds up in the cast. The patient should be turned every 2 hours to reduce continuous pressure and promote even drying of the cast. The drying process is usually complete within 24 to 72 hours. During the drying period the cast should not be subjected to any wetness, soiling, or abnormal stresses that can cause weakening or a break in the cast. It should be carefully handled by the palms of the hands rather than with the fingertips to avoid indentations that will dry and become potential pressure areas. Once the cast is thoroughly dry, the edges may need to be finished if it is rough to avoid skin irritation from rough spots or cast "crumbs" falling into the cast and causing irritation or pressure necrosis (Fig. 59-11).

Regardless of the type of material of which it is made, a cast can interfere with circulation and nerve function from being applied too tightly or because of excessive edema after application. Thus frequent neurovascular assessments of the immobilized extremity are critical. The patient must be taught about signs of cast complications so that they can be reported promptly. Elevation of the extremity above the level of the heart to promote venous return and applications of ice to control or prevent edema are measures frequently used during the initial phase of immobilization. The nurse should instruct the patient to exercise joints above and below the cast. Pulling out cast padding and scratching or placing foreign objects inside the cast is forbidden because it predisposes the patient to skin breakdown and infection.

Other measures.   If the patient is immobilized as a result of the fracture, the nurse must plan care to prevent the occurrence of constipation and renal calculi. Constipation can be prevented by activity and maintenance of a high fluid intake (more than 2500 ml/day) and a diet high in bulk and roughage (fresh fruit and vegetables). If these measures are not effective in maintaining the patient's normal bowel pattern, stool softeners, laxatives, or suppositories may be necessary. Maintaining a regular time for elimination despite bed rest aids in promoting regularity.

Renal calculi can develop as a result of bone demineralization caused by immobilization. The resulting hypercalcemia causes a rise in urine pH and stone formation resulting from the precipitation of calcium. Unless contraindicated, a fluid intake of 2500 ml/day is recommended. Cranberry juice or ascorbic acid (500 mg/day) may be recommended to acidify the urine and prevent calcium precipitation. (Renal calculi are discussed in Chapter 43.)

Rapid deconditioning of the circulatory system can occur as a result of bed rest, resulting in orthostatic hypotension. Unless contraindicated, these effects can be diminished by permitting the patient to sit on the side of the bed, allowing the patient's lower limbs to dangle over the bedside, and performing standing transfers. When the patient is allowed to increase activity, careful evaluation should be made to assess for orthostatic hypotension.

Traction.   The nurse is responsible for patient comfort and safety while traction is used and for ensuring proper functioning of the traction equipment. The equipment should be regularly examined for frayed ropes, loose knots, ropes out of the groove of the pulley, pulley clamps not fastened firmly to the bed frame, and weights not hanging freely.

When slings are used with traction, the nurse should inspect the skin area that is exposed in and near the sling regularly. Pressure over a bony prominence or a wrinkled area can impair blood flow, causing injury to the peripheral neurovascular structures. Skeletal traction pin sites must be observed for signs of infection. Pin site care varies according to the preference of the physician but usually includes regular removal of exudate with hydrogen peroxide, rinsing pin sites with sterile saline, drying of the area with sterile gauze, and application of antibiotic ointment.

External rotation of the hip can occur when skin traction is used on the lower extremity. The nurse can correct this position by placing a pillow, sandbag, or rolled-up drawsheet along the greater trochanteric region of the femur. When traction is used, the nurse should ensure that the patient's body is always correctly aligned. Generally, the patient should be in the center of the bed in a supine position. Incorrect alignment can result in increased pain, nonunion, or malunion.

To offset some of the problems associated with prolonged immobility, the nurse should discuss specific patient activity with the physician. If exercise is permitted, the nurse should encourage participation by the patient in a simple exercise regimen within activity restrictions. Activities that the patient should participate in include frequent position changes, range-of-motion exercises of unaffected joints, deep breathing exercises, isometric exercises, and use of the trapeze bar (if permitted) to raise oneself off the bed for linen changes and use of the bedpan. These activities should be performed several times each day.

Active exercises that move uninvolved joints through the range of motion are the preferred activity, if allowed. Frequent exercise of the trunk and extremities is an excellent stimulus to deep breathing. Active, resistive exercise (isotonic) of uninvolved extremities helps reduce deconditioning from prolonged immobility.

Ambulatory and Home Care

Cast care. Because many fractures are casted in an outpatient setting, the patient often requires only a short hospitalization or none at all. Therefore patient education is an important nursing responsibility to prevent complications. In addition to specific instructions for cast care and recognition of complications, the nurse should encourage the patient to contact the clinic or care provider should questions arise. Table 59-9 summarizes patient instructions for cast care. The nurse should validate the patient's understanding of these instructions before discharge from the clinic or hospital.

Psychosocial problems. Short-term rehabilitative goals are directed toward the transition from dependence to independence in performing simple activities of daily living and preservation or increasing strength and endurance. Long-term rehabilitative goals are aimed at preventing problems associated with musculoskeletal injury (Table 59-10). An important part of nursing care during the rehabilitative phase is assisting the patient to adjust to any problems caused by the injury (e.g., separation from family, financial impact of medical care, loss of income from inability to work). The nurse must exhibit gentleness, support, and encouragement and should actively listen to the patient's fears.

PATIENT TEACHING GUIDE

Table 59-9 Cast Care

Do Not
- Get cast wet*
- Remove any padding
- Insert any foreign object inside cast
- Bear weight on new cast for 48 hr (not all casts are made for weight bearing; check with health care provider when unsure)
- Cover cast with plastic for prolonged periods

Do
- Apply ice directly over fracture site for first 24 hr (avoid getting cast wet by keeping ice in plastic bag and protecting cast with cloth)
- Check with physician before getting cast wet†
- Dry cast thoroughly after exposure to water
  - Blot dry with towel
  - Use hair dryer on low setting until cast is thoroughly dry
- Elevate extremity above level of heart for first 48 hr
- Move joints above and below cast regularly
- Report signs of possible problems to health care provider
  - Increasing pain
  - Swelling associated with pain and discoloration of toes or fingers
  - Pain during movement
  - Burning or tingling under cast
  - Sores or foul odor under the cast
- Keep appointment to have fracture and cast checked

*Plaster of Paris cast.
†Synthetic cast.

Ambulation. The physical therapist often assumes primary responsibility for directing the patient during the strengthening phase of care. The nurse must know the overall goals of physical therapy in relation to the patient's abilities, needs, and tolerance. Mobility training and instruction in the use of assistive aids constitute one of the major areas of responsibility of the physical therapist. The patient with lower extremity dysfunction is usually started in mobility training when able to sit in bed and dangle the feet over the side. This activity should be done two or three times for 10 to 15 minutes, with the nurse assisting as necessary. As endurance increases, the patient is instructed in the techniques of transferring from bed to chair. Progressive ambulation is usually started with parallel bars and progresses to ambulatory assistive devices. When the patient begins to ambulate, the nurse must know the weight bearing allowed for the affected extremity and the correct technique if the patient is using an assistive device. There are different degrees of weight-bearing ambulation: (1) non–weight-bearing ambulation, (2) partial–weight-bearing ambulation, and (3) full–weight-bearing ambulation.

Assistive devices. Devices for ambulation range from a cane, which can relieve up to 40% of the weight normally borne by a lower limb, to a walker or crutches, which allow complete non–weight-bearing ambulation. The decision about which

Table 59-10   Problems Associated with Injury of the Musculoskeletal System

Problem	Description	Nursing Considerations
Muscle atrophy	Decreased muscle mass normally occurs as a result of disuse following prolonged immobilization.	An isometric muscle-strengthening exercise regimen within the confines of the immobilization device assists in reducing the amount of atrophy. Muscle atrophy interferes with and prolongs the rehabilitation process.
Contracture	Abnormal condition of joint characterized by flexion and fixation. Caused by atrophy and shortening of muscle fibers or by loss of normal elasticity of skin over a joint. Related to improper support and positioning of a joint.	This condition can be prevented by frequent position change, correct body alignment, and active-passive range-of-motion exercises several times a day. Contracture of a joint immobilized for a long time with a cast is common. Intervention requires gradual and progressive stretching of the muscles or ligaments in the region of the joint.
Footdrop	Plantar-flexed position of the foot (footdrop) occurs when the Achilles tendon in the ankle shortens because it has been allowed to assume an unsupported position. This may signify damage to the peroneal nerve.	Nursing management of the patient with long-term injuries must include preventive measures by supporting the foot in a neutral position. Once footdrop has developed, ambulation and gait training may be significantly hindered.
Pain	Frequently associated with fractures, edema, and muscle spasm; pain varies in intensity from mild to severe and is usually described as aching, dull, burning, throbbing, sharp, or deep.	Important causal factors of pain include incorrect positioning and alignment of the extremity, incorrect support of the extremity, sudden movement of the extremity, and immobilization device that is applied too tightly or in an incorrect position, constrictive dressings, motion occurring at the fracture site, and psychosocial factors. Pain is a valuable assessment parameter, and the underlying causes should be determined so that corrective nursing action can be taken before analgesics are administered.
Muscle spasms	Caused by involuntary muscle contraction after fracture and may last as long as several weeks. Pain associated with muscle spasms is often intense. The duration varies from several seconds to several minutes.	Nursing measures to reduce the intensity of the muscle spasms are similar to the corrective actions for pain control. The area involved in muscle spasms should not be massaged. Thermotherapy, especially heat, may reduce muscle spasm.

device is appropriate for a patient involves weighing the need for maximum stability and safety versus maneuverability, which is required in small spaces such as bathrooms and buses. The decision is made more easily by discussing with patients the requirements of their lifestyles and determining the device with which each patient feels most secure and independent.

The technique for using assistive devices varies. The involved limb is usually advanced at the same time or immediately after the advance of the device. The uninvolved limb is advanced last. In almost all cases, canes are held in the hand opposite the involved extremity.

The common gait patterns with assistive devices are the two-point gait, the four-point gait, the swing-to gait, and the swing-through gait:

- *Two-point gait.* Crutch on one side advances simultaneously with the opposite foot; gait is also used with cane ambulation.
- *Four-point gait.* A slower version of the two-point gait, each "point" is advanced separately.
- *Swing-to gait.* Both crutches are advanced together, followed by the lifting of both lower limbs to the same place; this gait is also used with walkers.

- *Swing-through gait.* This gait is similar to the swing-to gait, but the patient swings body past the crutches.

A belt should be placed around the patient's waist to provide stability during the learning stages. The nurse should discourage the patient from reaching for furniture or relying on another person for support. When there is inadequate upper limb strength or poorly fitted crutches, the patient bears weight at the axilla rather than at the hands, endangering the neurovascular bundle that passes across the axilla. If verbal coaching does not correct the problem, the patient should be kept from further ambulation until strength is adequate.

Patients who must ambulate without weight bearing require sufficient upper limb strength to lift their own weight at each step. Since the muscles of the shoulder girdle are not accustomed to this work, they require vigorous and diligent training in preparation for this task. Push-ups, pull-ups using the overhead trapeze bar, and lifting weights develop the triceps and biceps. Straight-leg raises and quadriceps-setting exercises strengthen the quadriceps.

Counseling and referrals. During the rehabilitative process the patient's family assumes an important role in the provision and follow-through of long-term care plans. The family must be instructed in the techniques of strength and endurance exercises, assistance with mobility training, and promoting activities that enhance the quality of daily living. Sexual counseling should be included in discharge planning. Unless nurses have specific preparation for sexual health counseling, they should remember that wrong answers may be more harmful than no answers. For referral purposes, nurses must know whether sexual activity is compatible with the degree of injury and whether any immobilization or support devices are necessary.

■ Evaluation

The expected outcomes for a patient with a fracture are presented in NCP 59-1.

COMPLICATIONS OF FRACTURES

The majority of fractures heal without complications. If death occurs after a fracture, it is usually the result of damage to underlying organs and soft tissue or from complications of the fracture or immobility. Complications of fractures may be either direct or indirect. Direct complications include problems with bone union, avascular necrosis, and bone infection. Indirect complications of fractures are associated with blood vessel and nerve damage resulting in conditions such as compartment syndrome, venous thrombosis, fat embolism, and traumatic or hypovolemic shock. Although most musculoskeletal injuries are not life threatening, open fractures or fractures accompanied by severe blood loss and fractures that damage vital organs (such as the lung or bladder) are medical emergencies requiring immediate attention.

Infection

Open fractures and soft-tissue injuries have a high incidence of infection. An open fracture usually results from the impact of severe external forces. The soft-tissue injury often has more serious consequences than the fracture. Devitalized and contaminated tissue is an ideal medium for many common pathogens, including gas-forming (anaerobic) bacilli. Treatment of infections is costly in terms of extended nursing and medical care and treatment and loss of patient income. Infection may be present for a long time. (Osteomyelitis is discussed later in this chapter.)

Collaborative Care

Open fractures require surgical intervention. The wound is cleaned by extensive irrigation, usually with sterile normal saline, and any gross contaminants are mechanically removed. Contused, contaminated, and devitalized tissue such as muscle, subcutaneous fat, skin, and fragments of bone are surgically excised (debridement). The extent of the soft-tissue damage determines whether the wound will be closed at the time of surgery, whether closed suction drainage will be used, and whether skin grafting will be necessary. Depending on the location and extent of the fracture, reduction may be maintained by a cast or by traction. During surgery the open wound may be irrigated with antibiotic solution. During the postoperative phase the patient may have antibiotics administered intravenously or orally usually for 7 to 10 days. Antibiotics, in con-

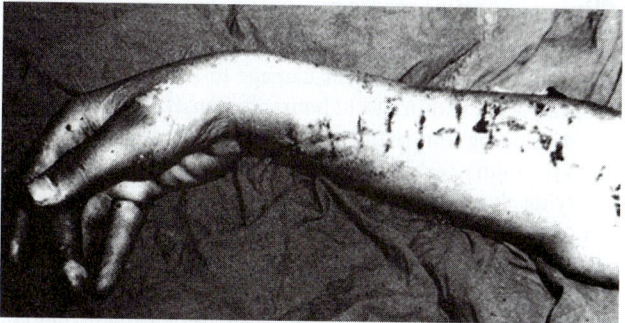

Fig. 59-12 Volkmann's ischemic contracture of the forearm following acute compartment syndrome secondary to a supracondylar fracture of the humerus. Note the incision line of an unsuccessful fasciotomy.

junction with aggressive surgical management, have greatly reduced the occurrence of infection.

Compartment Syndrome

Compartment syndrome is the compression of structures within closed compartments of the upper and lower extremities formed by fascial sheaths or bone. A closed compartment may also be created by an externally applied circumferential dressing, splint, or cast.[13] Normally there is some increase in edema as a result of soft-tissue injury in the general region of the injury. If edema continues, there may be an increase of pressure within the closed spaces of the tissue compartments. This can create sufficient pressure to obstruct circulation and cause venous occlusion, which increases edema. Eventually arterial flow is compromised, resulting in inadequate circulation to the extremity or ischemia. As ischemia continues, muscle and nerve cells are destroyed over time, and fibrotic tissue replaces the healthy tissue. Contracture and loss of function can occur. Delay in diagnosis and treatment can result in irreversible muscle and nerve ischemia.[14] This produces a functionally useless or severely impaired extremity.

Compartment syndrome is associated with fractures or extensive soft-tissue damage or crush injury in an extremity. The forearm and lower leg are the most common sites of compartment syndrome. Fractures of the distal humerus and proximal tibia are the most common fractures associated with compartment syndrome. In the upper extremity this condition is referred to as *Volkmann's ischemic contracture* (Fig. 59-12) and in the lower extremity as *anterior tibial compartment syndrome,* although the underlying pathophysiology is similar.

Although compartment syndrome is frequently associated with fractures, it should be noted that it can occur in situations when the soft tissue has been disrupted such as persons who have experienced severe burns, crush injuries, wringer injuries, venomous bites, or revascularization procedures. Prolonged pressure on a muscle compartment may occur when someone is trapped under a heavy object or a person's limb is trapped beneath the body due to an obtunded state such as drug or alcohol overdose. It has even been known to occur as the result of massive infiltration of intravenous fluids. An acute form of exertional compartment syndrome may occur after intensive exercise.[15]

Clinical Manifestations

Early recognition and treatment of compartment syndrome is essential to avoid permanent damage to muscles and nerves. This can occur within 4 to 12 hours after onset. The earliest sign of a developing compartment syndrome is progressive pain distal to the injury that is not relieved by the usual analgesics. The overlying skin may appear normal because surface vessels are not occluded. In addition to the inability to actively extend the digits, pain results from passive extension of the digits. Other symptoms that develop as the condition progresses include numbness and tingling, tenseness of the compartment, pain on passive stretch of muscle traveling through the compartment, loss of sensation, loss of function, pallor, coolness of the extremity, and diminished or absent peripheral pulses. Absence of a peripheral pulse is an ominous late sign that indicates severe disturbance of circulation. Regular neurovascular assessments should be performed on all patients with fractures, but especially those with injury of the distal humerus or proximal tibia or soft-tissue disruption in these areas.

Because of the possibility of muscle damage, urine output should be assessed. Myoglobin, released from damaged muscle cells, can be trapped in renal tubules because of its high molecular weight. Large amounts of myoglobinemia may result in acute renal failure. Common signs of myoglobinuria are (1) dark urine associated with a positive benzidine test in the absence of hematuria and (2) the manifestations associated with acute renal failure (see Chapter 44).

Collaborative Care

Prompt, accurate diagnosis of compartment syndrome is critical. Prevention or early recognition is the key. Because elevation may raise venous pressure, the extremity should not be elevated above the heart level. Similarly, ice may result in vasoconstriction and exacerbate compartment syndrome. Ice should not be used in patients with suspected compartment syndrome. It may also be necessary to remove or loosen the bandage or cast or to reduce traction weight to prevent edema formation.

Treatment is often a fasciotomy of the involved compartment. The fasciotomy is left open for several days to ensure edema formation has subsided. Infection is a potential problem following a fasciotomy.[16] Severe compartment syndrome may require amputation to decrease myoglobinemia or to replace a functionally useless extremity with a more effective prosthesis.

Venous Thrombosis

The veins of the lower extremities and pelvis are highly susceptible to thrombus formation after fracture, especially hip fracture. Precipitating factors are venous stasis caused by incorrectly applied casts or traction, local pressure on a vein, or immobility. Venous stasis is aggravated by inactivity of the muscles that normally assist in the pumping action of venous return of blood in the extremities. In addition to wearing compression gradient stockings (antiembolism hose) and using sequential compression devices, the patient should be instructed to move the fingers or toes of the affected extremity against resistance and to perform range-of-motion exercises on the unaffected lower extremities. Because of the high risk of venous thrombosis in the immobile patient, prophylactic anticoagulant medication such as aspirin, warfarin, or heparin may be or-

dered. Low-molecular-weight heparin (e.g., enoxaparin [Lovenox]) has recently been shown to be more effective in preventing venous thrombosis than warfarin.[17] Because it has a predictable dose response, there is no need to provide follow-up monitoring of prothrombin time. Assessment and management of venous thrombosis is discussed in Chapter 36.

Fat Embolism Syndrome

Fat embolism syndrome (FES) occurs in 0.5% to 2% of patients with fractures of long bones and up to 10% of patients with multiple fractures associated with pelvic injuries. FES is a contributory factor in many deaths associated with fractures. The fractures that most frequently cause FES are those of the femur, ribs, tibia, and pelvis. FES has also been known to occur following total joint replacement, spinal fusion, liposuction, crush injuries, and bone marrow transplantation. Two theories related to the origin of fat emboli exist. One theory suggests that fat is released from the marrow of injured bone. It is driven out by an increase in intramedullary pressure and enters the circulation through draining veins traveling to pulmonary capillaries, where it lodges. Some fat droplets traverse the capillary bed to enter systemic circulation and embolize to other organs such as the brain. The other theory postulates that catecholamines released at the time of trauma mobilize free fatty acids from the adipose tissue, causing loss of chylomicron emulsion stability. The chylomicrons form large fat globules that lodge in the lungs. This is possibly due to some biochemical change initiated by injury. The tissues of the lungs, brain, heart, kidneys, and skin are most frequently affected.

Clinical Manifestations

Early recognition of FES is crucial in preventing a potentially lethal course. Initial manifestations usually occur 24 to 48 hours after injury.[18] Severe forms have occurred within hours of injury. The fat globules transported to the lungs cause a hemorrhagic interstitial pneumonitis that produces signs and symptoms of acute respiratory distress syndrome (ARDS), such as chest pain, tachypnea, cyanosis, dyspnea, apprehension, tachycardia, and decreased partial pressure of arterial oxygen (PaO_2). All of these symptoms are caused by poor oxygen exchange. Because they are frequently the presenting symptoms, changes in the mental status as a result of hypoxemia are important to recognize. Memory loss, restlessness, confusion, elevated temperature, and headache prompt further investigation so that CNS involvement is not mistaken for alcohol withdrawal or acute head injury. The continued change in level of consciousness and petechiae located around the neck, anterior chest wall, axilla, buccal membrane, and conjunctiva of the eye help distinguish fat emboli from other problems. Petechiae result from intravascular thromboses caused by decreased oxygenation.

The clinical course of a fat embolus may be rapid and acute. Frequently the patient expresses a feeling of impending disaster. In a short time, skin color changes from pallor to cyanosis, and the patient may become comatose. No specific laboratory examinations are available to aid in the diagnosis. However, certain diagnostic abnormalities may be present. These include fat cells in the blood, urine, or sputum; a decrease of the PaO_2 to less than 60 mmHg; ST segment changes on electrocardiogram (ECG); a decrease in the platelet count and hematocrit

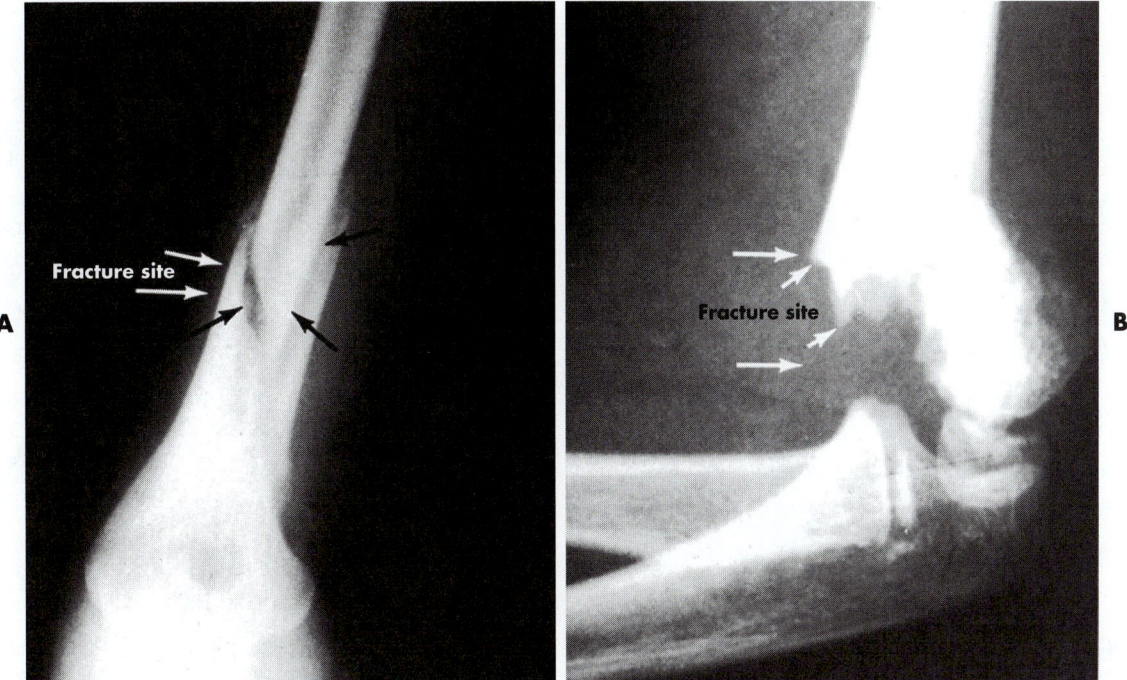

Fig. 59-13 **A,** Supracondylar fracture of the humerus. This type of injury results in the formation of a large hematoma. **B,** Fracture of distal shaft of humerus.

levels; and a prolonged prothrombin time. A chest x-ray may reveal areas of pulmonary infiltrate or multiple areas of consolidation. This is sometimes referred to as the *snowstorm effect.*

Collaborative Care

Treatment for fat embolism is directed at prevention. Careful immobilization of a long bone fracture is probably the most important factor in the prevention of fat embolism. Management of FES is essentially symptom related and supportive.[19] It includes maintaining adequate fluid intake, correction of acidosis, and replacement of any blood loss. Coughing and deep breathing should be encouraged. The patient should be repositioned as little as possible before fracture immobilization or stabilization because of the danger of dislodging more fat droplets into the general circulation. Use of corticosteroids to prevent or treat fat embolism is controversial.[20,21] Oxygen is administered to treat hypoxia. Intubation or intermittent positive pressure breathing may be considered if a satisfactory PaO$_2$ cannot be obtained with supplemental oxygen alone. Some patients may develop pulmonary edema, acute respiratory distress syndrome (ARDS), or both, leading to an increased mortality rate. Most patients survive FES with few sequelae.[18]

TYPES OF FRACTURES

Colles' Fracture

A *Colles' fracture* is a fracture of the distal radius and is one of the most common fractures in adults. The styloid process of the ulna may be involved as well. The injury usually occurs when the patient attempts to break a fall on an outstretched hand. This type of fracture most frequently occurs in women over age 50 whose bones are osteoporotic. The clinical manifestations of Colles' fracture are pain in the immediate area of injury, pro-

nounced swelling, and dorsal displacement of the distal fragment (dinner-fork deformity). This may appear as a bump on the wrist. The major complication associated with a Colles' fracture is vascular insufficiency as a result of edema.

A Colles' fracture is usually managed by closed manipulation of the fracture and immobilization by either a sugar-tong splint or a long arm cast. The elbow must be immobilized to prevent wrist supination and pronation. Nursing management should include measures to prevent or reduce edema and frequent neurovascular assessment. Support and protection of the extremity should be provided, along with encouragement of active movement of the thumb and fingers. This type of movement helps reduce edema and increases venous return. The patient should be instructed to perform active movements of the shoulder to prevent stiffness or contracture.

Fracture of the Humerus

Fractures involving the shaft of the humerus are a common injury among young and middle-aged adults. The prominent clinical manifestations are an obvious displacement of the humerus shaft, shortened extremity, abnormal mobility, and pain (Fig. 59-13). The major complications associated with fracture of the humerus are radial nerve injury and vascular injury to the brachial artery as a result of laceration, transection, or spasm.

The treatment for a fracture of the humerus depends on the location and displacement of the fracture. Treatment may include a hanging arm cast, a shoulder immobilizer, or the sling and swathe, which is a type of immobilization that prevents glenohumeral movement. The swathe encircles the trunk and humerus as an additional binder. It is often used for surgical repairs and shoulder dislocation.

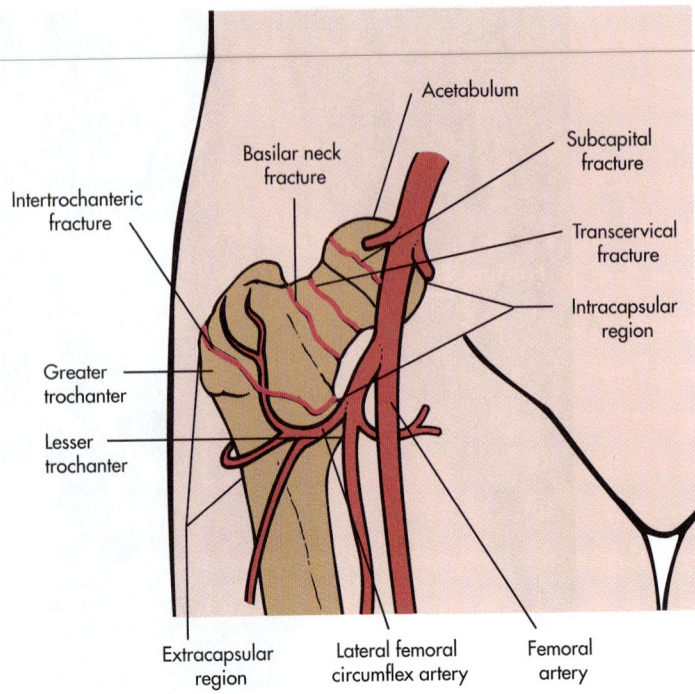

Fig. 59-14 Femur with location of various types of fracture.

When these devices are used, the head of the bed should be elevated to assist gravity in reducing the fracture. The arm should be allowed to hang freely when the patient is sitting and standing. Nursing care should include measures to protect the axilla and prevent skin maceration by placing lightly powdered absorbable dressing pads in the axilla and changing them twice daily or as needed. Skin or skeletal traction may be used for purposes of reduction and immobilization.

During the rehabilitative phase an exercise program geared toward improving strength and motion of the injured extremity is extremely important. This should include assisted motion of the hand and fingers. The shoulder can also be exercised if the fracture is stable, which prevents stiffness.

Fracture of the Pelvis

Pelvic fractures are usually caused by vehicular or skiing accidents. Older adult patients may sustain this injury from a fall. Although only a small percentage of all fractures are pelvic fractures, this type of injury accounts for 5% to 20% of the mortality rate from fractures. Preoccupation with associated injuries at the time of an accident may result in neglect of pelvic injuries. Pelvic fractures may cause serious intraabdominal injury such as colon laceration, paralytic ileus, hemorrhage, and laceration of the urethra, bladder, or colon.

Physical examination demonstrates local swelling, tenderness, deformity, unusual pelvic movement, and ecchymosis. The neurovascular status of the lower extremities and manifestations of associated injuries should be assessed. Pelvic fractures are diagnosed and classified by x-ray study. They may range from simple undisplaced fractures to more serious fracture dislocations with the potential for serious complications.

Treatment of a pelvic fracture depends on the severity of the injury. Bed rest for stable pelvic fractures is maintained from a few days to 6 weeks. More complex fractures may be treated with pelvic sling traction, skeletal traction, hip spica casts, ex-

ternal fixation, open reduction, or a combination of these methods. Internal fixation of a pelvic fracture may be necessary if the fracture is displaced. Extreme care in handling or moving the patient is important to prevent serious injury from a displaced fracture fragment. Because a pelvic fracture can damage other organs, assessment of bowel and urinary tract function and distal neurovascular status are important in early nursing activities for this patient.

The patient should be turned only when specifically ordered by the physician. Back care is provided while the patient is raised from the bed either by independent use of the trapeze or with adequate assistance. Weight bearing on the affected side should be avoided until healing is complete. If the pelvic fracture is undisplaced, the patient is usually allowed to ambulate using a walker or crutches to distribute the weight bearing between the upper and lower extremities.

Fracture of the Hip

Hip fractures are a common trauma in older adults. More than 250,000 hip fractures occur annually.[22] A hip fracture may be expected to occur more frequently in women than in men older than 65 years because of osteoporosis. It is estimated that 14% to 36% of patients who experience a hip fracture will die within 1 year of injury because of medical complications caused by the fracture or resulting immobility. More than 25% of the survivors lose their ability to walk independently, and 60% do not regain their preinjury level of ambulation.[23]

Fractures that occur within the capsule are called *intracapsular* fractures. Intracapsular fractures are further identified by a name taken from their specific location: (1) subcapital, (2) transcervical, and (3) basilar neck. These fractures are often associated with osteoporosis and minor trauma. *Extracapsular* fractures occur below the capsule and are termed *intertrochanteric* if they occur in a region between the greater and lesser trochanter. They are termed *subtrochanteric* if they occur in the region below the trochanter (Fig. 59-14). Extracapsular fractures are usually caused by severe direct trauma or a fall.

Clinical Manifestations

The clinical manifestations of hip fractures are external rotation, muscle spasm, shortening of the affected extremity, and severe pain and tenderness in the region of the fracture site. Displaced femoral neck fractures cause serious disruption of the blood supply to the femoral head, which can result in avascular necrosis.

Collaborative Care

Surgical repair is the preferred method of managing intracapsular and extracapsular hip fractures. Surgical treatment permits the patient to be out of bed sooner and decreases the major complications associated with immobility. In contrast, treatment with traction requires 12 to 16 weeks of immobilization for healing to occur, even if the blood supply to the region is intact. Initially the affected extremity may be temporarily immobilized by either Buck's or Russell's traction until the patient's physical condition is stabilized and surgery can be performed. Traction also helps relieve painful muscle spasms.

Intracapsular fractures are usually repaired with the use of an endoprosthesis to replace the femoral head (Fig. 59-15, *A*). Extracapsular fractures are usually pinned (Fig. 59-15, *B*). The principles of patient care for these procedures are similar.

The intracapsular fracture is slow to heal because of interruptions in blood supply. When avascular necrosis appears imminent, the surgeon may elect to resect the femoral head and neck and insert a femoral head prosthesis. A variety of devices in the form of compression screws and plates, nails, and pins are available to the surgeon for the purpose of repairing a hip fracture by pinning.

NURSING MANAGEMENT: HIP FRACTURE

■ Preoperative Management

Because older adults are most prone to hip fractures, chronic health problems must often be considered when planning treatment. Diabetes mellitus, hypertension, cardiac decompensation, pulmonary disease, and arthritis are chronic problems that may complicate clinical status. Surgery may be delayed for a brief time until the patient's general health is stabilized.

Before surgery, severe muscle spasms can increase pain. These spasms are managed by appropriate analgesics or muscle relaxants, comfortable positioning unless contraindicated, and properly adjusted traction if it is being used.

Careful preoperative patient teaching can affect future mobility. The patient should know the method and frequency for exercising the unaffected leg and both arms. The patient should also be shown how to use the trapeze bar and the opposite side rail to assist in changing positions. Practice in getting out of bed and transferring to a chair should be discussed and demonstrated before surgery. The family should be informed about the patient's weight-bearing status after surgery. Plans for discharge should be discussed, and arrangements should be initiated well before the actual discharge date.

■ Postoperative Management

The initial postoperative management of a patient following surgical repair of hip fracture is similar to that for any older sur-

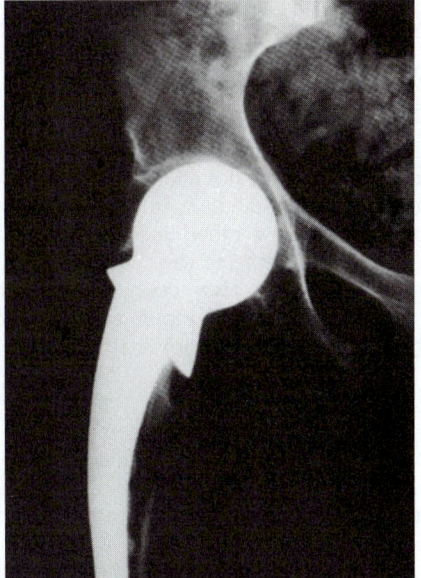

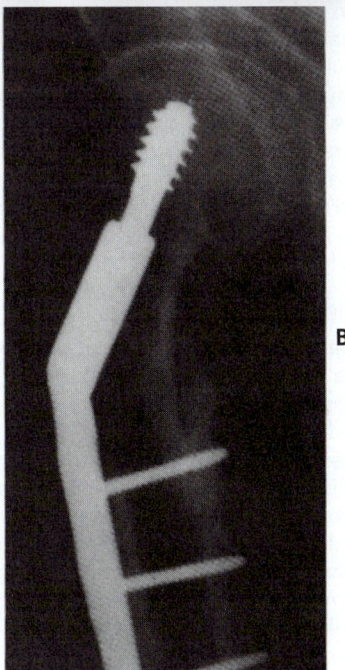

Fig. 59-15 Types of internal fixation for a hip fracture. **A,** Femoral head endoprosthesis. **B,** Type of hip compression screw with side plate.

gical patient. The nurse must monitor vital signs and intake and output, supervise respiratory activities such as deep breathing and coughing, administer pain medication cautiously, and observe the dressing and incision for signs of bleeding and infection. Specific nursing interventions for the patient with a fracture of the hip are described in NCP 59-2.

In the early postoperative period there is a potential for neurovascular impairment. The nurse should assess the patient's toes for (1) ability to move and weakness, (2) warmth and color, (3) sensation and absence of paresthesia, (4) distal pulses and capillary refill, and (5) edema, which may develop after the patient is out of bed. Edema is alleviated by elevation of the leg whenever the patient is in a chair. The pain resulting from poor

ETHICAL DILEMMAS

Premature Discharge of Patient

SITUATION

An 83-year-old patient with a total hip replacement is to be discharged from the hospital because of diagnosis-related group (DRG) standards for the number of days in the hospital. The nurse knows that the patient lives alone, has no relatives to care for him, and is unable to manage at this stage in his recovery with the limited home care available to him. Should the nurse request that the patient not be discharged at this time?

DISCUSSION

Third-party payer procedures for determining reimbursement for medical care are a means to determine reimbursement, *not* medical diagnoses. They are based on standards of medical care and pooled patient information rather than an individual patient's history and the physician's orders. In his current condition, this patient does not seem to have access to appropriate home care. If discharge planning is unable to find suitable care or to arrange transfer to an intermediate nursing facility, it would be unethical to discharge him. Both the physician and a hospital administrator should be involved in the plans for this patient to guarantee that appropriate care will be extended beyond the hospital. If it is not, the hospital might be liable for any medical consequences of the patient's inadequate care.

ETHICAL AND LEGAL PRINCIPLES

- Medicare began basing payment for short-term hospitalization on a DRG system in 1983, but not all facilities receiving Medicare reimbursement are covered under this system.
- Facilities may extend the length of stay beyond the DRG-alloted time, but the reimbursement for the patient will be reduced for the additional days.
- Medical decisions may not be ethically or legally made based on profit or reimbursement concerns. Concerns about reimbursement procedures and social policy should not be expressed in individual patient care contexts.

alignment of the affected extremity can be reduced by keeping pillows (or an abductor splint) between the knees when the patient is turning to either side. Sandbags and pillows are also used to prevent external rotation. If an endoprosthesis was placed, these patients are at risk for hip dislocation.

The physical therapist usually supervises active-assistance exercises for the affected extremity and ambulation when the surgeon permits it. Ambulation usually begins on the first or second postoperative day. The nurse should monitor the patient's ambulation status for proper crutch walking or use of the walker. The patient must be able to use crutches or a walker before discharge.

Complications associated with femoral neck fracture include nonunion, avascular necrosis, dislocation, and degenera-

tive arthritis. As a result of an intertrochanteric fracture, the affected leg may be shortened.

If the hip fracture has been treated by insertion of a femoral head prosthesis, measures to prevent dislocation must always be used (Table 59-11). The patient and family must be fully aware of positions and activities that predispose the patient to dislocation (greater than 90 degrees of flexion, adduction, or internal rotation). Many daily activities may reproduce these positions (e.g., putting on shoes and socks, crossing the legs or feet while seated, assuming the side-lying position incorrectly, standing up or sitting down while the body is flexed relative to the chair, sitting on low seats—especially low toilet seats). Until the soft tissue surrounding the hip has healed sufficiently to stabilize the prosthesis these activities must be avoided, usually for at least 6 weeks. Sudden severe pain, a lump in the buttock, limb shortening, and external rotation indicate prosthesis dislocation. This requires a closed reduction or open reduction to realign the femoral head in the acetabulum.

In addition to teaching the patient and family how to prevent prosthesis dislocation, the nurse should (1) place a large pillow between the patient's legs when turning, (2) keep leg abductor splints on the patient except when bathing, (3) avoid extreme hip flexion, and (4) avoid turning the patient on the affected side until approved by the surgeon.

If the hip fracture is treated by pinning, dislocation precautions are not necessary. The patient is usually encouraged to be out of bed on the first postoperative day. Weight bearing on the involved extremity varies. Weight bearing of especially fragile fractures may be restricted until x-ray examination indicates adequate healing, usually within 6 to 12 weeks.

The nurse must assist both the patient and the family in adjusting to the restrictions and dependence imposed by the hip fracture. Depression can easily occur, but creative nursing care and awareness of the problem can do much to prevent it. The patient and family may need to be informed about community referral services that can assist in the postdischarge rehabilitation phase. Hospitalization averages 4 days. Patients frequently require care at a skilled nursing facility or rehabilitation facility for a few weeks before returning home. Regular follow-up care after discharge including home health nursing should be arranged. Recovery can take up to a year.[22]

■ Evaluation

The expected outcomes for the patient with fracture of the hip are presented in NCP 59-2.

■ GERONTOLOGIC CONSIDERATIONS

Hip Fracture

Factors that contribute to the occurrence of a hip fracture in older adults include a propensity to fall, inability to correct a postural imbalance, orientation of the fall, adequacy of local tissue shock absorbers (e.g., fat and muscle bulk), and underlying skeletal strength. Several factors have been identified in older persons that increase their risk of falling. These include gait and balance problems, decreased vision and hearing, decreased reflexes, orthostatic hypotension, and medication use.[23] Leading hazards of falls are loose rugs and slippery or

59-2 NURSING CARE PLAN PATIENT WITH FRACTURE OF THE HIP

Expected Patient Outcomes	Nursing Interventions and *Rationales*

NURSING DIAGNOSIS Pain *related to* edema, movement of bone fragments, muscle spasms, and ineffective pain relief or comfort measures *as manifested by* guarding, moaning, crying, restlessness, rating pain as >2 on a scale of 1 through 5.

- Decrease in or absence of pain.
- Satisfaction with pain relief (rates pain as 2 or less on scale of 1 through 5).

- Align and position extremity and patient correctly *to reduce pressure on nerves and tissue.*
- Gently position or turn *to prevent muscle spasm and malalignment of bone fragments.*
- Maintain constant traction forces *to reduce muscle spasm and maintain alignment of bone.*
- Administer analgesics, nonsteroidal antiinflammatory agents, and muscle relaxants as indicated *to reduce pain, edema, and muscle spasms.*
- Use a pain scale to assess pain and evaluate pain-control interventions.

NURSING DIAGNOSIS Risk for peripheral neurovascular dysfunction *related to* edema, concurrent injury of adjacent neurovascular structures from fracture fragment, or hematoma formation (see NCP 59-1).

NURSING DIAGNOSIS Impaired physical mobility *related to* decreased muscle strength, or pain *as manifested by* inability to purposefully move, limited joint range of motion, inability to bear weight, presence of immobilization device.

- Sufficient muscle strength to participate in gait-training program.
- Optimal level of function with ambulatory assistive device.

- Cooperate with physical therapist in muscle-strengthening program *to maximize patient's progress in rehabilitation.*
- Teach and assist patient in exercise program; include resistive strengthening exercises of uninvolved lower and both upper limbs, elbow extension, shoulder depressors, and knee and hip extension *to develop strength in all extremities preparatory to initiation of ambulation.*
- Provide written instructions for exercises for patient to refer to as needed.
- Assist patient in standing at side of bed with abductor pillow (if indicated) using non–weight bearing (if indicated) on affected leg *to increase mobility.*
- Encourage quadriceps exercises, arm-strengthening exercises, and abdominal and gluteal contraction exercises *to develop muscle strength, which will help with rehabilitation.*
- Be aware that ordered weight-bearing status of involved extremity must be maintained unless changed by physician *because soft tissue surrounding hip requires about 3 to 5 months of healing to sufficiently stabilize the endoprosthesis.*
- Get patient out of bed and into chair, usually within 24 to 48 hours after surgery, *to reduce the complications associated with immobility.*
- Instruct and assist patient with transfer from bed to chair *to prevent accidental falling and improper movements, which could cause endoprosthesis dislocation or hip malalignment.*

NURSING DIAGNOSIS Risk for wound infection *related to* exposure to environmental pathogens and surgical procedure.

- No evidence of wound infection.

- Assess wound site for erythema, local warmth, tenderness, edema, and drainage; monitor temperature q4hr *to identify fever as an indication of infection and initiate appropriate interventions.*
- Teach patient the signs and symptoms of infection and the need to promptly report them.
- Obtain wound culture, if indicated, *to identify infecting organism.*
- Administer antibiotics as ordered *for prophylaxis or to treat infection.*
- Use sterile technique when changing dressings or providing wound care *to minimize the risk of cross-contamination.*

Continued

59-2 NURSING CARE PLAN PATIENT WITH FRACTURE OF THE HIP—continued

Expected Patient Outcomes	Nursing Interventions and *Rationales*

NURSING DIAGNOSIS **Ineffective management of therapeutic regimen** *related to* injury, surgery, and lack of knowledge of postdischarge care *as manifested by* verbalization of concern by patient or caregiver regarding ability to care for patient after discharge, lack of knowledge regarding postdischarge care.

■ Verbalization by patient and family of confidence in ability to manage postdischarge care.	■ Assess home environment *to identify needed modifications such as elevated toilet seat, height of shelves, steps, scatter rugs, low chairs.* ■ Teach patient and family about proper ambulation, diet, medications, wound care, and physician follow-up *to reduce risk of injury, promote proper wound healing, and foster effective rehabilitation.* ■ Inform about symptoms to report to physician such as fever, signs of wound infection, severe pain, cognitive changes *because these are indicators of complications that require prompt treatment.* ■ Teach patient and family positions and activities to avoid such as putting on shoes and socks, crossing legs while seated, sitting on low seats *because these may cause dislocation of prosthesis.* ■ Refer for home care as needed *because this resource can provide additional therapy and other assistance.* ■ Provide written information that reviews preceding information and provide phone numbers to call with any questions.

COLLABORATIVE PROBLEMS

Nursing Goals	Nursing Interventions and *Rationales*

POTENTIAL COMPLICATION **Thromboembolic complications** *related to* immobility.

■ Monitor for thromboembolic complications. ■ Report abnormal findings. ■ Carry out appropriate medical and nursing interventions.	■ Monitor for coolness, paleness, edema, and distended veins of the distal lower extremity *to detect decreased venous return.* ■ Monitor for local warmth, edema, erythema, increased circumference, pain over the area, and systemic low-grade fever (<101° F [38° C]) *to detect thrombophlebitis.* ■ Instruct patient in the need for fluid intake to exceed 2500 ml/day *to reduce hemoconcentration.* ■ Apply antiembolism hose *to reduce venous pooling and promote venous return.* ■ Provide ordered anticoagulant therapy prophylaxis (i.e., heparin, warfarin, aspirin, or low-molecular-weight heparin) as prescribed *to reduce thrombus formation.* ■ Monitor for tachypnea, tachycardia, changes in mental status, voiced feelings of "impending doom," decreased O_2 saturation by oximetry, chest pain, dyspnea, and orthopnea *to detect thromboembolism.*

uneven surfaces. Approximately 75% of all falls occur indoors. Many falls are associated with getting in or out of a chair or bed. Falls to the side, the most common type in the frail elderly, are more likely to result in a hip fracture than a forward fall.

Two important factors influencing the amount of force imposed on the hip are the presence of energy-absorbing soft tissue over the greater trochanter and the state of leg muscle contraction at the time of the fall. Since many elderly have poor muscle tone these are important factors in the severity of a fall. Finally, elderly women often have osteoporosis and accompanying low bone density, which increases the risk of hip fracture.

Targeted interventions to reduce hip fractures in the elderly include a variety of strategies. Calcium and vitamin D supplementation, estrogen replacement, and drug therapy have been shown to decrease bone loss or increase bone density and decrease the likelihood of fracture.[24] (See section on osteoporosis

later in this chapter.) Nurses must be vigilant in planning interventions for the elderly that are known to reduce the incidence of hip fracture.

FEMORAL SHAFT FRACTURE

Femoral shaft fracture is a common injury occurring particularly in young adults. Severe direct force is required to produce this injury, since the femur can bend slightly before actual fracture occurs. The force exerted to cause the fracture frequently causes damage to the adjacent soft-tissue structures. These injuries may be more serious than the bone injury. Displacement of the fracture fragments frequently results in open fracture and increased soft-tissue damage. This can result in considerable blood loss (1 to 1.5 L).

The clinical manifestations of a fracture of the femoral shaft are usually obvious. They include marked deformity and angu-

PATIENT & FAMILY TEACHING GUIDE

Table 59-11   Femoral-Head Prosthesis

Do Not

- Force hip into greater than 90 degrees of flexion*
- Force hip into adduction
- Force hip into internal rotation
- Cross legs
- Put on own shoes or stockings until 8 wk after surgery without adaptive device (e.g., long-handled shoehorn or stocking-helper)
- Sit on chairs without arms to aid rising to a standing position*

Do

- Use toilet elevator on toilet seat*
- Place chair inside shower or tub and remain seated while washing
- Use pillow between legs for first 8 wk after surgery when lying on "good" side or when supine*
- Keep hip in neutral, straight position when sitting, walking, or lying*
- Notify surgeon if severe pain, deformity, or loss of function occurs*
- Inform dentist of presence of prosthesis before dental work so that prophylactic antibiotics can be given

*These precautions may also apply after a hip pinning.

lation, shortening of the extremity, inability to move either the hip or knee, and pain. The common complications associated with fracture of the femoral shaft include fat embolism, nerve and vascular injury, and problems associated with union, open fracture, and soft-tissue damage.

Initial management is directed toward stabilization of the patient and immobilization of the fracture. Treatment may consist of skeletal traction via a tibial pin and balanced suspension traction. Traction continues for 8 to 12 weeks. The nurse must encourage the patient to perform exercises and range-of-motion activities for the uninvolved extremities and joints to discourage deconditioning. The physician determines when active exercise can be instituted on the affected extremity. When there is sufficient clinical evidence of bone union, a hip spica or long leg cast may be applied.

Internal fixation is another way to manage a femoral fracture. It is carried out with an intramedullary rod, compression plate, and screws or side plate with an intercondylar nail. Internal fixation is frequently the preferred treatment because it reduces hospital stay and the complications associated with prolonged bed rest. Other indications for internal fixation are failure to obtain satisfactory reduction by nonsurgical methods and multiple associated injuries. In some instances the surgically repaired femur may be supported by suspension traction for 3 to 4 days to prevent excessive movement of the extremity and to control rotation; non–weight-bearing gait training is then begun. Fractures associated with extensive soft-tissue injury may be treated with external fixation.

Promotion and maintenance of strength in the affected extremity usually include gluteal and quadricep isometric

exercises. It is important to ensure performance of range-of-motion and strengthening exercises for all uninvolved extremities in preparation for ambulation. The patient may be immobilized in a hip spica cast and gradually progress to an articulating cast brace or may be allowed to begin non–weight-bearing activities with an ambulatory assistive device. Full weight bearing is usually restricted until there is x-ray evidence of bony union of the fracture fragments.

FRACTURE OF THE TIBIA

Although the tibia is vulnerable to injury because it lacks anterior muscle covering, strong force is required to produce a fractured tibia. As a result, soft-tissue damage, devascularization, and open fracture are frequent. Other complications associated with tibial fractures are compartment syndrome, fat embolism, problems associated with bony union, and possible infection associated with open fracture.

The recommended management for closed tibial fracture is closed reduction followed by immobilization in a long leg cast. Open reduction may be achieved with intramedullary rods or compression plate. With either method of reduction, emphasis is placed on maintaining the strength of the quadriceps.

The neurovascular status of the affected extremity must be assessed at least every 2 hours during the first 48 hours. Patients are instructed to perform active range-of-motion exercises with all uninvolved extremities, as well as exercises for the upper extremities, to build the strength required for crutch walking. When the physician has determined that the patient is ready for gait training, the patient is instructed in the principles of crutch walking. The patient may be on non–weight-bearing status for 6 to 12 weeks depending on healing. When fracture healing has progressed sufficiently, a walking heel is applied to the cast and full weight bearing is allowed.

STABLE VERTEBRAL FRACTURES

A stable fracture of the vertebral column is usually caused by motor vehicle accidents, falls, diving, or athletic injuries. A stable fracture is one in which the fracture or the fragment is not likely to move or cause spinal cord damage. This type of injury is frequently confined to the anterior element (vertebral body) of the spinal column in the lumbar region. It involves the cervical and thoracic regions less frequently. The vertebral bodies are usually protected from displacement by the intact spinal ligaments.

Most patients with spinal fractures have stable fractures and experience only brief periods of disability. However, if the ligamentous structures are significantly disrupted, dislocation of the vertebral structures may occur, resulting in instability and injury to the spinal cord (unstable fracture). These injuries may require surgery. The most serious complication of vertebral fractures is fracture displacement, which can cause damage to the spinal cord (see Chapter 57). Although stable vertebral fractures are not associated with abnormal spinal cord pathology, all spinal injuries should initially be considered unstable and potentially serious until diagnostic tests and the physician determine that the fracture is stable.

The most common injury to the vertebral body is the compression type of fracture caused by excessive vertical load, such as a severe fall on the buttocks or injury resulting from sudden flexion that forces the spine beyond its normal range of motion.

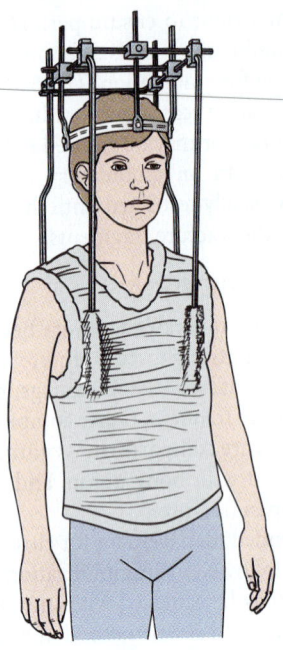

Fig. 59-16   Halo apparatus attached to a body jacket cast. It may also be attached to a brace. A halo vest can be used in treatment of a cervical spine injury or following cervical spine surgery.

Table **59-12**	**Clinical Manifestations of Facial Fractures**
Fracture	**Clinical Manifestation**
Frontal bone	Rapid edema that may mask underlying fractures
Periorbital	Possible frontal sinus involvement, entrapment of ocular muscles
Nasal	Displacement of nasal bones, epistaxis
Zygomatic arch	Depression of zygomatic arch
Maxilla	Segmental motion of maxilla
Mandible	Dental fractures, bleeding, limited motion of mandible

The patient usually complains of pain and tenderness in the affected region of the spine. Compression fractures are associated with a gibbous deformity (flexion angulation of several vertebrae). This deformity may be noted during the physical examination. In patients with osteoporosis, several vertebral levels may be involved as evidenced by a dowager's hump (abnormal backward curvature of cervical spine). Bowel and bladder dysfunction may be an indication of an interruption of the autonomic nervous system or injury to the spinal cord.

The overall goal in management of stable fractures of a vertebral body is to keep the spine in good alignment until union has been accomplished. Many nursing interventions are aimed at assessing for the possibility of spinal cord trauma. Vital signs and bowel and bladder function should be evaluated regularly, as should the motor and sensory status of the peripheral nerves distal to the injured region. Any deterioration in the patient's neurovascular status should be promptly reported.

Treatment includes support, heat, and traction. The patient is usually placed in a standard hospital bed with firm support from the mattress or a bedboard. The aim is to support the spinal column, relax muscles, and release any compression on nerve roots. Heat and traction may be used to relieve muscle spasms resulting from the fracture. Traction may also be used to reduce and immobilize fracture fragments. A trapeze is not usually allowed because its use disrupts spinal alignment. Both an upright position and turning of the torso are prohibited. When turning, the patient should be taught to keep the spine straight by turning shoulders and pelvis together. Nursing assistance is necessary for the patient to learn how to turn in this "logrolling" fashion. Several days after the initial injury, the physician may apply a specially constructed orthotic device (e.g., Milwaukee, Jewett, or Taylor braces), a jacket cast, or a removable corset if there is no evidence of neurologic deficit.

If the fracture is in the cervical spine, a cervical collar may be worn by the patient. Some cervical fractures are immobilized by use of a halo vest (Fig. 59-16). This consists of a plastic jacket or cast fitted about the chest and attached to a halo that is held in place by skeletal pins inserted into the cranium. These devices immobilize the spine in the fracture area but allow patient mobility. The patient is discharged after (1) regaining ambulation skills, (2) learning care of the cast or orthotic device, and (3) learning how to cope with interferences in safety and security imposed by injury and treatment.

MAXILLOFACIAL FRACTURES

Any bone of the face can be fractured as a result of trauma. Fractures can occur as a result of collision with another person or object, fighting, or blunt trauma. The primary concern after facial injury is to establish and maintain a patent airway and to provide adequate ventilation by removal of foreign material and blood. Suctioning may be necessary. An artificial airway (tracheostomy) may be needed if a patent airway cannot be maintained. Hemorrhage is controlled by pressure packing. Cervical spine injuries are common. All patients with maxillofacial injuries should be treated as though they have a cervical injury until proven otherwise by examination and testing. Table 59-12 describes the clinical manifestations of more common facial fractures.

Concurrent soft-tissue injury often makes assessment of a facial injury difficult. Oral and maxillofacial examinations should be performed after the patient has been stabilized and any life-threatening situations have been treated. Careful assessment is made for entrapment of ocular muscles and cranial nerve involvement.

An x-ray documents the extent of the injury. Computed tomography (CT) imaging helps differentiate between bone and soft tissue and gives a more specific view of the fracture.[25]

Injury to the eye must be suspected when a facial injury occurs, particularly if the injury is near the orbit. If a global rupture is suspected the examination is stopped and a protective shield is placed over the eye until examined by the ophthalmologist. Signs of global rupture include brown tissue (iris or ciliary body) on the surface of the globe or penetrating through a laceration with an eccentric or teardrop-shaped pupil.[26] Specific treatment of a facial fracture depends on the site and extent of the fracture and the associated soft tissue injury. Immobilization or surgical stabilization may be necessary. (Mandibular fractures are discussed in Chapter 39.)

The patient who sustains a facial fracture requires sensitive nursing care, since alteration in appearance after the trauma may be drastic. Edema and discoloration subside with time, but concurrent soft-tissue injuries may result in permanent scarring. Attention to maintenance of a patent airway and adequate nutrition are ongoing concerns of the nurse throughout the recovery period. Suction should always be available to maintain a patent airway for these patients.

OSTEOMYELITIS

Etiology and Pathophysiology

Osteomyelitis is an infection of bone by direct or indirect invasion by an organism. In children, long bones are most commonly affected whereas the vertebrae are more commonly affected in adults. Direct entry results from contamination as a result of an open fracture or surgery. Indirect inoculation results from a blood-borne infection from a distant site such as teeth, infected tonsils, diabetic ulcers, or furuncles. The most common infecting organism is *Staphylococcus aureus*. Aerobic gram-negative bacteria alone or mixed with gram-positive organisms are often found.[27] The course and virulence of osteomyelitis are influenced by the blood supply to the affected bone. The widespread use of antibiotics in conjunction with surgical treatment has significantly reduced the mortality rate associated with osteomyelitis. However, the incidence and morbidity remain relatively unchanged because new, drug-resistant strains of organisms, such as methicillin-resistant *Staphylococcus aureus* (MRSA), have developed.

The indirect-entry (also called hematogenous) type of osteomyelitis most frequently affects growing bone in boys and is associated with local trauma. The most common sites of indirect-entry osteomyelitis are the long bones of the leg, although any bone can be involved.

The direct-entry type of osteomyelitis can occur at any age when there is an open wound. After gaining entrance to the bone by way of the arterial blood supply, the bacteria lodge in an area of bone in which circulation slows, usually the metaphysis. The locus of bacteria grows, resulting in an increase in pressure because of the nonexpanding container of tubular bone. This increasing pressure eventually leads to ischemia and vascular compromise. Once ischemia occurs, the bone dies. The area of devitalized bone eventually separates from the surrounding living bone, forming *sequestra*. These sequestra form havens for bacteria, and chronic osteomyelitis develops.

Once formed, a sequestrum continues to be an infected island of bone, surrounded by pus and difficult to reach by blood-borne antibiotics or leukocytes. It may enlarge and serve as a source of bacteria for spread to other sites, including the lungs and brain. Two situations are possible. The sequestrum may extrude through a defect in tubular bone; however, this is hindered by the formation of new bone laid down by the elevated periosteum called *involucrum* (Fig. 59-17). Once outside the bone, the sequestrum may revascularize and undergo removal by normal defense processes. The other possibility is surgical removal. Unless resolved naturally or surgically, the necrotic sequestrum may develop a sinus tract, resulting in chronic purulent wound drainage.

Clinical Manifestations

Acute osteomyelitis refers to the initial infection or an infection of less than 1 month in duration. The clinical manifestations of acute osteomyelitis are both systemic and local. Systemic man-

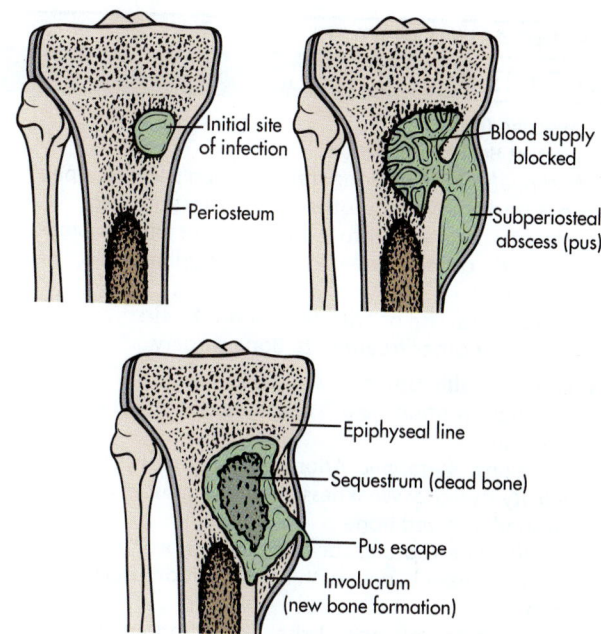

Fig. 59-17 Development of osteomyelitis infection with involucrum and sequestrum.

ifestations include fever, night sweats, chills, restlessness, nausea, and malaise. Local manifestations include severe bone pain that is unrelieved by rest and worse with activity; swelling, tenderness, and warmth at infection site; and restricted movement of affected part. Later signs include drainage from sinus tracts to the skin and fracture site.

Chronic osteomyelitis refers to a bone infection that persists for longer than 4 weeks or an infection that has failed to respond to the initial course of antibiotic therapy. Chronic osteomyelitis can represent either a continuous, persistent problem or a process of exacerbations and quiescence. It results from inadequately treated acute osteomyelitis. Pus accumulates, causing ischemia of the bone. Over time, granulation tissue turns to scar tissue. This avascular scar tissue provides an ideal site for bacterial growth and is impenetrable to antibiotics.

Diagnostic Studies

Wound culture determines the causative organism. A bone or tissue biopsy is the definitive way to determine the causative agent. The patient's blood or sequestrum cultures are frequently positive. An elevated blood leukocyte count and sedimentation rate may also be found. Radiologic signs suggestive of osteomyelitis usually do not appear until 10 days to weeks after the appearance of clinical symptoms, by which time the disease will have progressed. Radionuclide bone scans can establish the diagnosis within 24 to 72 hours.[28] MRI and CT scans may be used to help identify the boundaries of the infection. Gallium scans and indium scans may also prove useful in some instances.

Collaborative Care

Vigorous antibiotic therapy is the treatment of choice for acute osteomyelitis, as long as ischemia has not yet occurred. Wound cultures or bone biopsy should be taken before antibiotic therapy is initiated so that the specific antibiotic therapy can be determined by sensitivity studies. If antibiotic therapy is not

Table 59-13 Osteomyelitis

Subjective Data

Important Health Information

Past health history: Bone trauma, open fracture, open or puncture wounds, other acute infections (e.g., streptococcal sore throat, bacterial pneumonia, sinusitis, skin or tooth infection, chronic urinary tract infection)

Medications: Use of analgesics or antibiotics

Surgery or other treatments: Bone surgery

Functional Health Patterns

Health perception–health management: IV drug abuse; malaise

Nutritional-metabolic: Anorexia, weight loss; chills

Activity-exercise: Weakness, paralysis, muscle spasms around affected bone

Cognitive-perceptual: Local tenderness over affected area, increase in pain with movement of affected bone

Coping–stress tolerance: Irritability, withdrawal, dependency, anger

Objective Data

General

Restlessness; high, spiking temperature; night sweats

Integumentary

Diaphoresis; erythema, warmth, edema at infected bone

Musculoskeletal

Restricted movement; wound drainage; spontaneous fractures

Possible Findings

Leukocytosis, positive blood and wound cultures, elevated erythrocyte sedimentation rate; rarefaction with presence of sequestrum and involucrum on x-rays, radionuclide bone scans, CT, and MRI

---

acin (Floxin) are effective agents for the treatment of some forms of osteomyelitis. IV antibiotics are delivered via a central venous catheter or peripherally inserted central catheter (PICC). IV antibiotic therapy may be started in the hospital and continued in the home for 4 to 6 weeks or as long as 3 to 6 months.[29]

Surgical removal of the infection may be necessary. Myocutaneous flaps or skin and bone grafting may be necessary if destruction is extensive. Antibiotic-impregnated bead chains may be surgically implanted at the time of debridement to aid in combating the infection. Infection may occur in the presence of a foreign body such as an implant or an orthopedic device such as a plate or a total joint prosthesis. It may be necessary to remove the device to effectively treat the infection.[30] Infection and bone destruction may be so extensive that amputation of the extremity may be necessary to preserve life or improve the quality of life.

NURSING MANAGEMENT: OSTEOMYELITIS

The nursing management of the patient with osteomyelitis is challenging and demanding. A prolonged hospital or long-term care facility stay may be required to ensure that adequate remission has been achieved. Extended home care with frequent home visits by nurses is currently a more common mode of therapy.

■ Nursing Assessment

Subjective and objective data that should be obtained from an individual with osteomyelitis are presented in Table 59-13.

■ Nursing Diagnoses

Nursing diagnoses for the patient with osteomyelitis may include, but are not limited to, those presented in NCP 59-3.

■ Planning

The overall goals are that the patient with osteomyelitis will (1) have satisfactory pain and fever control, (2) not experience any complications associated with osteomyelitis, (3) cooperate with the treatment plan, and (4) maintain a positive outlook on the outcome of the disease.

■ Nursing Implementation

Health Promotion. Patients with artificial implants such as a total joint replacement or metallic bone implants should be educated about methods to reduce the risk of osteomyelitis. Some physicians recommend prophylactic doses of antibiotics for procedures such as teeth cleaning, colonoscopy, or vaginal examinations.

Acute Intervention. The involved extremity should be handled carefully to avoid excessive manipulation, which increases pain and may cause pathologic fracture. Sterile dressings are used to contain the exudate from draining wounds. Besides protecting the wound area, dressings are also used as adjuncts in the mechanical debridement of devitalized tissue from the wound site when they are removed. Types of dressings used include dry, sterile dressings, dressings saturated in saline or antibiotic solution, and wet-to-dry dressings. Soiled dressings should be handled carefully to prevent cross-contamination of the wound or spread of the infection to other patients. When the dressing is changed, sterile technique is essential; it should always include sterile dressing sets, gloves, and surgical cap, gown, and mask to reduce wound contamination from external sources.

---

started early in the course of the illness, surgical debridement and decompression are necessary to relieve pressure within the bone and prevent ischemia. Some type of immobilization for the affected part is usually indicated. Pathologic fractures may occur because of weakened, devitalized bone. Soft-tissue and bone healing occur slowly in the presence of infection, and subsequent deformity of the extremity may develop.

Treatment for chronic osteomyelitis includes surgical removal of poorly vascularized tissue and dead bone and extended use of antibiotics.[28] After surgical debridement of devitalized and infected tissue, the wound may be closed, and a suction irrigation system for removal of any devitalized tissues remaining in the wound area is inserted. Intermittent or constant irrigation of the affected bone with antibiotics may be initiated. Hyperbaric oxygen therapy may be used as an adjunctive therapy for chronic osteomyelitis where available, especially when associated with pressure necrosis or diabetic ulcers.

Treatment for chronic osteomyelitis previously involved an extended hospital stay for intravenous (IV) antibiotic treatment or stabilization of the patient and discharge with IV antibiotics. Most oral antibiotics have limited success rate because of poor penetration into organic bone. Ciprofloxacin (Cipro) and oflox-

59-3 NURSING CARE PLAN PATIENT WITH OSTEOMYELITIS

Expected Patient Outcomes	Nursing Interventions and *Rationales*

NURSING DIAGNOSIS Pain *related to* inflammatory process secondary to infection *as manifested by* guarding, moaning, crying, restlessness, altered muscle tone, decreased activity, rating pain as >2 on a scale of 1 through 5.

- Decrease in or absence of pain.
- Satisfaction with pain relief.

- Assess location and severity of pain and previous pain-relieving measures *to plan appropriate interventions.*
- Use a pain scale *to assess pain and evaluate effectiveness of interventions.*
- Give analgesics as indicated *to relieve pain.*
- Instruct patient to request analgesia *before pain becomes severe.*
- Avoid activities that increase circulation, such as exercise or application of heat, *to prevent increasing edema and subsequent pain.*
- Use gentle handling and support when moving extremity *to reduce pain and prevent pathologic fractures.*
- Utilize the prescribed immobilization device and maintain patient's body in correct alignment and positioning *to prevent unusual position or muscle stretching from increasing pain.*
- Restrict ambulation or teach patient to use assistive device (e.g., crutches) *to prevent pathologic fracture, pain, and increased stress on bone.*
- Elevate extremity *to reduce swelling and provide comfort.*
- Instruct patient in nonpharmacologic methods of pain control such as auditory, visual, or tactile distraction; rhythmic breathing; guided imagery; thermotherapy *to augment or reduce the need for analgesics.*

NURSING DIAGNOSIS Hyperthermia *related to* infection *as manifested by* fever, restlessness, diaphoresis, chills.

- Normal temperature.
- Minimal discomfort.
- Absence of chilling or dehydration.

- Take temperature q4hr *to determine presence of elevated temperature and to monitor patient's response to treatment.*
- Provide cool environment, light clothing and bedding, antipyretic drugs as ordered, and sponge bath or tub bath *to increase patient's comfort and reduce temperature.*
- Offer fluids every hour *to prevent dehydration from insensible fluid loss.*
- When chilled, cover with light blankets.

NURSING DIAGNOSIS Impaired physical mobility *related to* pain, immobilization devices, and weight-bearing limitations *as manifested by* inability or unwillingness to move purposefully within environment.

- Consistent increase in mobility and range of motion with minimal pain or discomfort.

- Assist patient as needed *to reduce patient's frustration with impaired mobility and prevent injury.*
- Explain the rationale for immobilization *to foster the patient's cooperation.*
- Increase mobility as ordered and tolerated *to maintain muscle function and strength.*
- Provide assistive devices (e.g., pick-up stick, long-handled shoe horn, stocking helpers) *to increase independence in ADLs and activity.*

NURSING DIAGNOSIS Ineffective management of therapeutic regimen *related to* lack of knowledge regarding long-term management of osteomyelitis *as manifested by* verbalization of concern regarding home care by patient or family members, need to learn new knowledge or skills for home management.

- Verbalization of confidence in self or caregiver's ability to carry out home management routine.

- Provide information and instruction regarding wound care, aseptic technique, and dressing disposal *to reduce risk of cross-contamination and encourage wound healing.*
- Review medication regimen including schedule, name, dosage, purpose, and side effects *because long-term antibiotic therapy is required.*
- Stress importance of proper diet, rest, physician follow-up, and physical rehabilitation *to facilitate wound healing and reduce risk of chronic osteomyelitis.*
- Provide written instructions about the preceding information along with a phone number to call with any questions.

Good body alignment and frequent position changes prevent complications associated with immobility and promote comfort. Flexion contracture, especially of the hip or knee, is a common sequela of osteomyelitis of the lower extremity because the patient frequently positions the affected extremity in a flexed position to promote comfort. This can cause the development of contracture, which may progress to a deformity. Footdrop can develop quickly in the lower extremity if the foot is not correctly supported. A splint is frequently applied to the involved extremity in an attempt to maintain immobilization, support, and comfort. The patient should be instructed to avoid any activities such as exercise or heat application that increase circulation and serve as stimuli to the spread of infection.

The patient should also be taught potential complications of antibiotic therapy and the need to report symptoms as early as possible. This includes hearing deficit and fluid retention associated with the aminoglycosides (e.g., tobramycin [Nebcin], neomycin) and jaundice, photosensitivity, and hepatotoxicity with cephalosporins (e.g., cefazolin [Ancef]).

Patients are frightened and discouraged because of the serious nature of the disease, systemic illness, pain, and the length and cost of treatment. Continued psychologic support is an integral part of nursing management.

Ambulatory and Home Care. With the introduction of various intermittent venous access devices, IV antibiotics can be administered to the patient in a nursing home or home setting. If at home, the patient and family must be instructed on the proper care and management of the venous access device. They must also be taught how to administer the antibiotic and the need for follow-up laboratory testing. Periodic home nursing visits provide the family with a resource on correct technique, which relieves anxiety. If there is an open wound, dressing changes may be necessary. The patient may require supplies and instruction in the technique.

If the osteomyelitis becomes chronic, patients need physical and psychologic support for a prolonged period. They may become suspicious and hostile toward the care providers when treatment plans do not effect a cure. Well-informed patients are better able to participate in decisions and cooperate in treatment plans.

■ Evaluation

The expected outcomes for the patient with osteomyelitis are presented in NCP 59-3.

AMPUTATION

During the past 20 years, major advances have been made in surgical amputation techniques, prosthetic design, and rehabilitation programs. These advances are enabling amputees to return to productive and satisfying social roles. There are an estimated 400,000 amputees in the United States, with an annual increase of 20,000. The middle and older age-groups have the highest incidence of amputation because of the effects of peripheral vascular disease, especially atherosclerosis and vascular changes related to diabetes mellitus. Traumatic injury is the usual cause for amputation in the younger adult. Amputation is required more often in persons engaged in hazardous occupations. The incidence in men is greater, since men are more often involved in such occupations. Amputation may also be indi-

COLLABORATIVE CARE

Table 59-14 **Amputation**

Diagnostic
  Physical examination
    Physical appearance of soft tissues
    Skin temperature
    Sensory function
    Presence of peripheral pulses
  Arteriography
  Thermography
  Plethysmography
  Transcutaneous ultrasonic Doppler recordings

Collaborative Therapy
Medical
  Appropriate management of underlying disease
    process
  Stabilization of trauma victim
Surgical
  Appropriate type of amputation, leaving as long a
    residual limb as possible
  Residual limb management
    Immediate prosthetic fitting
    Delayed prosthetic fitting
Rehabilitation
  Coordination of prosthesis-fitting and gait-training
    activities
  Coordination of muscle-strengthening and physical
    therapy regimens

cated for certain types of bone cancer affecting an extremity (e.g., osteogenic sarcoma).

Clinical Indications

The clinical features that indicate the need for an amputation depend on the underlying diseases or trauma. Common indications for amputation include circulatory impairment resulting from a peripheral vascular disorder, traumatic and thermal injuries, malignant tumors, uncontrolled or widespread infection of the extremity, and congenital disorders. These conditions may manifest as loss of sensation, inadequate circulation, pallor, sweating, and local or systemic infection. Although pain is often present, it is not usually the primary reason for an amputation. The underlying problem dictates whether the amputation is performed as elective or emergency surgery.

Diagnostic Studies

The types of diagnostic studies done depend on the underlying problem that makes the amputation necessary (Table 59-14). An elevated white blood cell (WBC) count may be indicative of infection. Vascular studies such as arteriography provide information about the circulatory status of the extremity.

Collaborative Care

The potential for revascularization surgery rather than amputation can be assessed on the basis of vascular studies. If amputation is to be considered "elective," the patient's general health is carefully assessed. Chronic illnesses and infection are monitored closely. The patient and family should be helped to un-

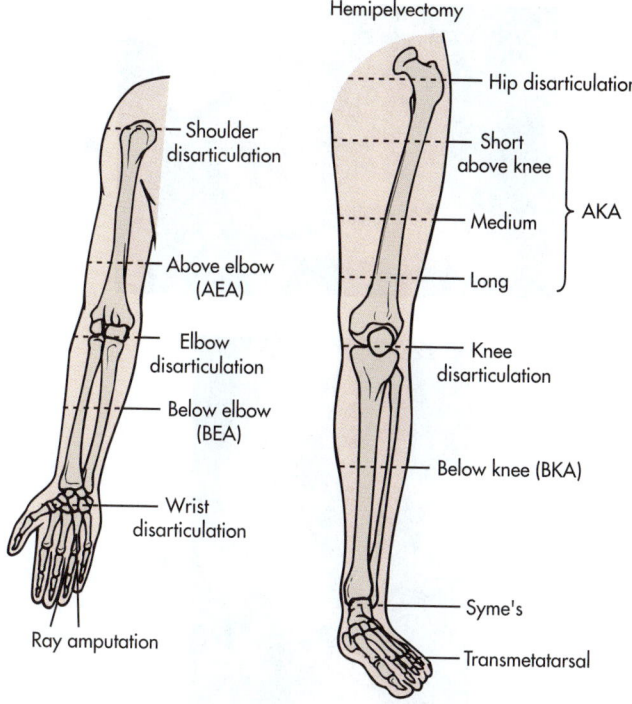

Fig. 59-18 Location and description of amputation sites of the upper and lower extremities. *AKA*, above the knee amputation.

derstand the need for the amputation and be assured that rehabilitation can result in an active, useful life. If the amputation is done on an emergency basis as a result of trauma, the management is physically and emotionally more complicated.

The goal of amputation surgery is to preserve extremity length and function while removing all infected, pathologic, or ischemic tissue. This improves the possibility of good prosthetic, cosmetic, and functional satisfaction. (Levels of amputation of upper and lower extremities are illustrated in Fig. 59-18.) The type of amputation depends on the reason for the surgery. A closed amputation is performed to create a weight-bearing residual limb (or stump); an anterior skin flap with dissected soft-tissue padding covers the bony part of the residual limb. The skin flap is sutured posteriorly so it will not be positioned in a weight-bearing area. Special care is necessary to prevent the accumulation of drainage, which can produce pressure and harbor infection. *Disarticulation* is an amputation performed through a joint. A Syme's amputation is a form of disarticulation at the ankle. An *open amputation* leaves a surface on the residual limb that is not covered with skin. This type of surgery is generally indicated for control of actual or potential infection. The wound is usually closed later by a second surgical procedure or closed by skin traction surrounding the residual limb. This type of amputation is often referred to as a *guillotine amputation.*

NURSING MANAGEMENT: AMPUTATION
■ Nursing Assessment

Preexisting illnesses must be adequately assessed since most amputations are performed because of vascular problems. Assessment of the vascular and neurologic status is an important part of this assessment process (see Chapters 30 and 53).

■ Nursing Diagnoses

Nursing diagnoses for the patient with an amputation may include, but are not limited to, the following:

- Body image disturbance *related to* amputation and impaired mobility
- Impaired skin integrity *related to* immobility and improperly fitted prosthesis
- Pain *related to* phantom limb sensation
- Impaired physical mobility *related to* amputation of lower limb

■ Planning

The overall goals are that the patient with an amputation will (1) have relief from the underlying health problem, (2) have satisfactory pain control, (3) reach maximum rehabilitation potential with the use of a prosthesis (if indicated), (4) cope with the body image changes, and (5) make satisfying lifestyle adjustments.

■ Nursing Implementation

Health Promotion. Most lower-limb amputations result from peripheral vascular disease, and most upper-limb amputations result from severe trauma. This knowledge directs patient education related to prevention of amputation. Control of causative illnesses such as peripheral vascular disease, diabetes mellitus, chronic osteomyelitis, and pressure ulcers can eliminate or delay the need for amputation. Patients with these problems should be taught to carefully examine their lower extremities daily for signs of potential problems. If the patient cannot assume this responsibility, a family member should be instructed in the procedure. Patients and their families should be instructed to report problems such as change in skin color or temperature, decrease or absence of sensation, tingling, pain, or the presence of a lesion to the health care provider.

Instruction in proper safety precautions in recreation and in the performance of hazardous work is a nursing responsibility of major importance, especially for occupational health nurses. Preventing limb mutilation and subsequent amputation is one of the serious consequences of trauma avoided through such instruction.

Acute Intervention. The nurse must recognize the tremendous psychologic and social implications of a lower-limb amputation for the patient. The disruption in body image caused by an amputation often causes a patient to go through psychologic stages similar to the grieving process of death. Allowing the patient to go through a grieving process or period of depression and recognizing it as a normal consequence of the amputation may do much to aid the patient's acceptance of the amputation. The patient's family must also be helped to work through the process to arrive at a realistic and positive attitude about the future. The reasons for an amputation and the rehabilitation potential depend on age, diagnosis, occupation, personality, resources, and support systems.

Preoperative management. Before surgery, the nurse should reinforce information the patient and family have received about the reasons for the amputation, the proposed prosthesis, and the mobility training program. In addition to the usual preoperative instructions, the patient undergoing an amputation has special education needs. To meet these needs, the nurse must know the level of amputation, the type of postsurgical dressing to be applied, and the type of prosthesis planned. The patient should receive instruction in the performance of upper-extremity exercises such as push-ups in bed or the wheelchair to promote arm strength. This is essential for later crutch walking and gait training. If possible, the nurse should instruct the patient in the technique of crutch walking and the type of gait that will be used after surgery and during gait training with the prosthesis. General postoperative nursing care should be discussed, including positioning, support, and residual limb care. If a compression bandage is to be used after surgery the patient should be instructed about its purpose and how it will be applied. If an immediate prosthesis is planned, the general ambulation program should be discussed.

The patient should be warned that she or he may feel as though the amputated limb is still present after surgery. This phenomenon, termed *phantom sensation* (a sensation of aching, tingling, or itching of the amputated limb), usually disappears but may cause patients grave concern unless they are forewarned. If pain was present in the affected limb preoperatively, the patient may experience phantom limb pain postoperatively. The patient may have feelings of coldness and heaviness or cramping, shooting, burning, or crushing pain. Often, the patient may be extremely anxious about this pain because the patient knows the limb is gone but still feels pain in it. Usually, phantom limb pain goes away in time, although it can become chronic. The pain is a real sensation to the patient and interventions should be provided for relief. As recovery and ambulation progress, phantom limb sensation usually subsides.

Postoperative management. General postoperative care for the patient who has had an amputation depends largely on the patient's general state of health, the reason for the amputation, and the patient's age. Nursing care must be individualized on the basis of these factors. For example, an older adult patient needs particularly careful monitoring of respiratory status; a victim of a motor vehicle accident may need careful neurologic monitoring.

Prevention and detection of complications are important nursing responsibilities during the postoperative period. Careful monitoring of the patient's vital signs and dressing can alert the nurse to hemorrhage in the operative area. Careful attention to sterile technique during dressing changes reduces the potential for wound infection and subsequent interruption of rehabilitation.

If an immediate postoperative prosthesis has been applied, the nurse must monitor vital signs carefully, since the surgical site is heavily covered and may not be visible. A surgical tourniquet must always be available for emergency use. If hemorrhage occurs, the surgeon should be notified immediately and efforts to control the hemorrhage should begin at once.

The surgeon must decide the type of prosthetic fitting that will be used after surgery. An immediate prosthetic fitting, often called the immediate postsurgical fitting or the immediate postoperative fitting, is done in the operating room after the amputation (Fig. 59-19). A rigid, cast-like bandage is applied around the closed residual limb with a prosthetic pylon and an ankle-foot assembly. While the patient is still anesthetized, the prosthetic pylon and ankle-foot assembly are aligned and adjusted to provide a smooth gait and to avoid excessive pressure on the residual limb area. A strap is placed on the proximal anterior surface of the rigid plaster bandage and attached to a waistband to prevent slippage. The main advantages of this de-

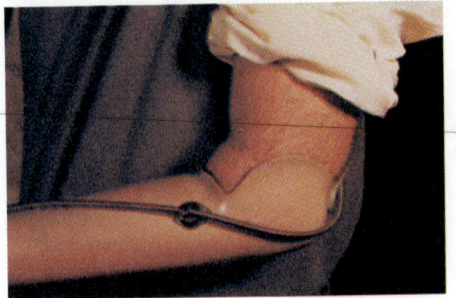

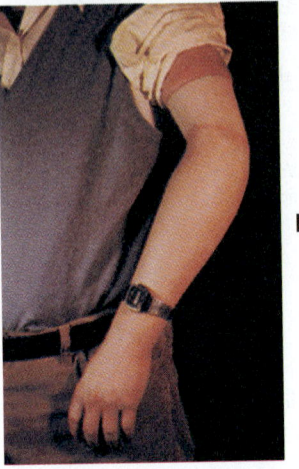

Fig. 59-19 Two types of prosthesis. **A,** Traditional fiberglass. **B,** New materials and techniques have made possible fabrication of prosthetic sockets that are light, soft, flexible, and secure.

vice are reduction of edema and the psychologic benefit of early ambulation. A disadvantage is the inability to directly visualize the surgical site.

The delayed prosthetic fitting may be the best choice for certain patients. Patients who have had amputations above the knee or below the elbow, older adults, debilitated individuals, and those with infection usually have delayed prosthetic fittings. The appropriate time for use of a prosthesis depends on satisfactory healing of the residual limb, as well as on the general condition of the patient. A temporary prosthesis may be used for partial weight bearing once the sutures are removed. Barring any problems, patients can bear full weight on permanent prostheses by approximately 3 months after amputation.

Not all patients are candidates for a prosthesis. It is important that the surgeon discuss ambulation possibilities frankly with the patient and family. The seriously ill or debilitated patient may not have the energy required to use a prosthesis. Mobility with a wheelchair may be the most realistic goal for this type of patient.

Collaborative care also includes the direction and coordination of the rehabilitation program for the amputee. Success depends on the physical and emotional health of the patient. Chronic illness and debilitation complicate aggressive rehabilitation efforts.

Flexion contractures may delay the rehabilitation process. The most common and debilitating contracture is hip flexion. Hip adduction contracture is rare. Patients should avoid sitting in a chair with hips flexed or having pillows under the surgical extremity to prevent flexion contractures. Unless specifically

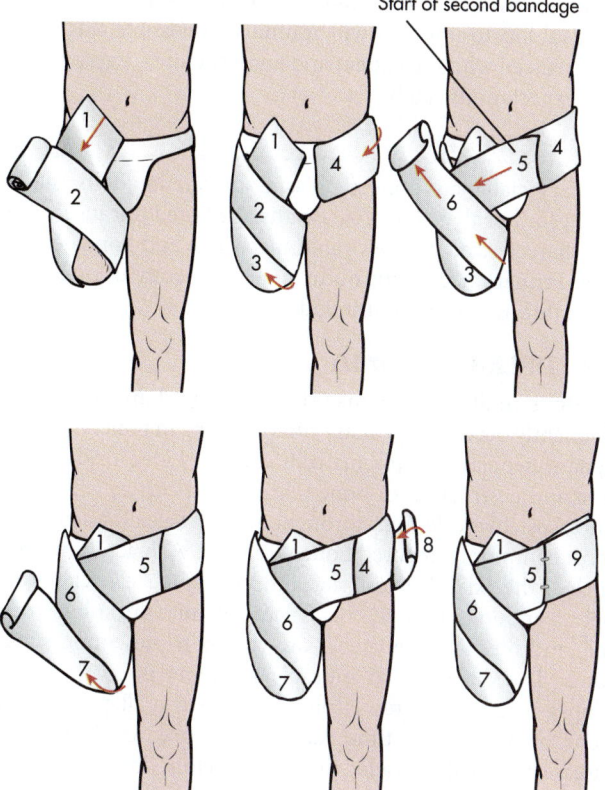

Start of second bandage

Fig. 59-20 Bandaging for the above-the-knee amputation residual limb. Figure-eight style covers progressive areas of the residual limb. Two elastic wraps are required.

contraindicated, patients should lie on their abdomen for 30 minutes three to four times each day and position the hip in extension while prone.

Proper residual limb bandaging fosters shaping and molding for eventual prosthesis fitting (Fig. 59-20). The physician usually orders a compression bandage to be applied immediately after surgery to support the soft tissues, reduce edema, hasten healing, minimize pain, and promote residual limb shrinkage and maturation. This bandage may be an elastic roll applied to the residual limb or a residual limb shrinker, which is an elastic stocking that fits tightly over the residual limb and lower trunk area.[31]

The compression bandage is initially worn at all times except during physical therapy and bathing. The bandage is taken off and reapplied several times daily, and care is taken so that it is applied snugly but not so tight as to interfere with circulation. Shrinker bandages should be washed and changed daily. It is recommended that the patient have two residual limb shrinker bandages so one can be worn while the other is being washed. After healing has occurred, the residual limb is bandaged only when the patient is not wearing the prosthesis. The patient should be instructed to avoid dangling the residual limb over the bedside to minimize edema formation.

As the patient's overall condition improves, the nurse begins instruction in the principles and techniques of transferring from bed to chair and back. Active exercises and conditioning are essential in developing ambulation skills. The exercise regimen is normally started under the supervision of the physician and the physical therapist. The nurse must have a clear understanding of

the exercise regimen to reinforce it and ensure that the exercises are performed correctly. Active range-of-motion exercises of all joints should be started as soon after surgery as the patient's pain level and medical status permit. In preparation for mobility, the patient should increase triceps and shoulder strength and lower limb support and learn balance of the altered body. The loss of the weight of a limb requires adaptation of the patient's proprioceptive mechanisms to prevent falls and frustration.

Crutch walking is started as soon as patients are physically able. If they have had immediate postsurgical fitting, orders related to weight bearing must be carefully followed to avoid disruption of the skin flap and delay of the training process. Initial periods of ambulation should not exceed 5 minutes to prevent dependent edema.

Before discharge, the patient and family need careful instruction related to residual limb care, ambulation, prevention of contractures, recognition of complications, exercise, and follow-up care. Table 59-15 outlines patient teaching following an amputation.

Ambulatory and Home Care. When the healing has occurred satisfactorily and the residual limb is well molded, the patient is ready for fitting a prosthesis. Walking with a below-the-knee prosthesis requires 40% additional energy, and an above-the-knee prosthesis requires 60% more energy. Matching a patient with a suitable prosthesis involves many factors, including age, general health, intelligence, motivation, occupation, and finances. After the physician makes the recommendation, the patient is referred to a prosthetist, who initially makes a mold of the residual limb and measures landmarks for the fabrication of the prosthesis. The molded residual limb socket allows the residual limb to fit snugly into the prosthesis. The residual limb is covered with a residual limb stocking to ensure good fit and prevent skin breakdown. The residual limb may continue to shrink, causing a loose fit, in which case a new socket has to be fabricated. The patient may need to have the prosthesis adjusted to prevent rubbing and friction between the residual limb and the socket. Excessive movement of a loose prosthesis can cause severe skin irritation and breakdown.

The prosthesis is fitted by the prosthetist, who may also train the amputee to use it. It is important for the nurse to be familiar with the training program to encourage and assist the patient. Learning to use a prosthesis is frustrating, and the patient may easily become discouraged. The nurse must continually offer support until the patient is able to manage alone.

Artificial limbs become an integral part of the patient's body image. Proper care ensures their long life and useful functioning. The patient should be instructed to clean the prosthesis socket daily with a mild soap and rinse thoroughly to remove irritants. The leather and metal parts of the prosthesis should not get wet. The patient should be encouraged to have regular maintenance of the prosthesis. Consideration of the condition of the shoe is also necessary. A badly worn shoe alters the gait and may cause damage to the prosthesis.

Referral to a community health nurse can foster optimal physical and emotional adjustment. The family should be instructed on ambulation and transfer techniques and proper residual limb care.

■ Evaluation

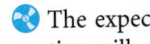 The expected outcomes are that the patient with an amputation will

- accept changed body image and integrate changes into lifestyle
- have no evidence of skin breakdown
- have reduction or absence of pain
- become mobile within limitations imposed by amputation

Special Considerations in Upper-Limb Amputation

The emotional implications of an upper-limb amputation are often more devastating than those for lower-limb amputation. The enforced dependency brought about by one-handedness is both frustrating and humiliating to many patients. Because most upper-extremity amputations result from trauma, the patient has also not had the opportunity to adjust psychologically to an amputation or to participate in the decision-making process.

Both immediate and delayed prosthetic fittings are possible for the below-the-elbow amputee. Prosthetic fitting is delayed for the above-the-elbow amputee. The usual functional prosthesis is the arm and hook. A cosmetic hand is available but has limited functional value. As with the lower-limb prosthesis, patient motivation and endurance are major factors toward a satisfactory outcome.

■ GERONTOLOGIC CONSIDERATIONS

Amputation

If a lower limb amputation has been performed on an older adult, the patient's previous ability to ambulate may affect the extent of recovery. Use of a prosthesis requires a significant amount of energy for ambulation. Older adults whose general health is weakened by disorders such as cardiac or pulmonary problems may not be candidates for prosthesis use. This patient's ability to ambulate will be limited. If possible, this should be discussed with the patient and family before surgery so realistic expectations can be set.

BONE CANCER

Primary malignant bone neoplasms are rare in adults and account for less than 1% of all deaths attributed to cancer. They are characterized by their rapid metastasis and bone destruction. Primary neoplasms occur most frequently during childhood through young adulthood.

MULTIPLE MYELOMA

In adults, multiple myeloma (plasma cell myeloma) is the most frequently occurring primary tumor arising in bone. It is a malignant neoplasm of plasma cells causing widespread infiltration and destruction of bone marrow and cortex, which produces osteolytic lesions throughout the skeletal system. The most commonly involved bones are those with active marrow, such as the axial skeleton, sternum, ribs, spine, clavicles, skull, pelvis, and long bones.[32] Back pain, anemia, thrombocytopenia, and bleeding tendencies are common presenting symptoms. The diagnosis of multiple myeloma is confirmed by biopsy or bone marrow aspiration. The overall prognosis is poor, because by the time diagnosis has been confirmed, the disease has usually invaded the axial skeleton. Chemotherapeutic treatment of multiple myeloma has limited usefulness; it is primarily directed toward suppressing plasma cell growth. Radiation therapy may be helpful in reducing pain. Corticosteroids are commonly used in conjunction with melphalan (Alkeran), vincristine (Oncovin), or doxorubicin (Adriamycin). (Multiple myeloma is also discussed in Chapter 29.)

OSTEOGENIC SARCOMA

Osteogenic sarcoma (osteosarcoma) is a primary neoplasm of bone that is extremely malignant and is characterized by rapid growth and metastasis. It usually occurs in the metaphyseal region of the long bones of the extremities, particularly in the regions of the distal femur, proximal tibia, and proximal humerus, as well as the pelvis. Osteogenic sarcoma is the most common malignant bone tumor affecting children and young adults; its highest incidence is in the 10- to 25-year-old age-group. It occurs most commonly in males. Secondary osteosarcoma is known to occur in adults over age 60 and is most commonly associated with Paget's disease.

The clinical manifestations of osteogenic sarcoma are usually associated with a past history of minor injury and gradual onset of pain and swelling, especially around the knee. The injury does not cause the neoplasm but rather serves to bring the preexisting condition to medical attention. The neoplasm grows rapidly and produces a noticeable increase in the size of the general region, which can restrict joint motion if the lesion is close to a joint structure. The diagnosis is confirmed from biopsied tissue specimens, elevation of serum alkaline phosphatase and calcium levels, x-ray, CT scan, and MRI findings.

Major advances continue to be made in the treatment of osteosarcoma. Preoperative (neoadjuvant) chemotherapy is used to decrease tumor size. As a result limb-salvage procedures, including a wide surgical resection of the tumor, are being used more frequently. Amputation may be necessary depending on the size and location of the tumor. Current use of adjunct chemotherapy following amputation has increased the projected 5-year survival rate to 60%.[33]

OSTEOCLASTOMA

True osteoclastoma (giant cell tumor) is a destructive tumor that arises in the cancellous ends of long bones in young adults. Most (98%) of these variant giant cell tumors are benign. Giant cell tumors most commonly occur between the ages of 20 and 35. The common sites are the distal ends of the femur, proximal tibia, and distal radius. The giant cell tumor is a locally destructive lesion, the growth of which extends from a few months to several years. The clinical manifestations are usually swelling, local pain, and some disturbances in joint function. X-ray evidence of giant cell tumor is variable but usually reveals local areas of bone destruction and eventual expansion of the bone ends. Treatment initially includes biopsy to establish the diagnosis, followed by surgical curettage of the lesion with bone grafting. After treatment there is a greater than 50% chance of recurrence. Recurrent giant cell tumors may subsequently make amputation necessary. Advances in chemotherapy have improved the rate of survival.

EWING'S SARCOMA

Ewing's sarcoma is the fourth most common primary malignant neoplasm of bone, occurring most frequently in male patients under the age of 30. This neoplasm is characterized by rapid growth within the medullary cavity of long bone, especially the femur, humerus, pelvis, tibia, and ribs. Metastasis occurs early, and the most frequent site is the lungs. The use of radiation, surgical excision, and chemotherapy has increased the 5-year survival rate to 70%. Common manifestations are progressive local pain, swelling, palpable soft-tissue mass, noticeable increase in size of the affected part, fever, and leukocytosis. Initially, x-rays show periosteal bone destruction. Treatment usually involves radiation therapy and wide surgical resection of the tumor or amputation. Chemotherapeutic agents commonly used are cyclophosphamide (Cytoxan), vincristine (Oncovin), ifosfamide (Ifex), and doxorubicin (Adriamycin). New chemotherapeutic techniques hold promise of improvement in survival rates. Surgical resection of the tumor has helped decrease the rate of recurrence.[34]

METASTATIC BONE LESIONS

The most common type of malignant bone tumor occurs as a result of metastasis from a primary tumor. Common sites for the primary tumor include the breast, intestinal tract, lungs, prostate, kidney, ovary, and thyroid. The metastatic bone lesion is commonly found in the vertebrae, pelvis, femur, humerus, or ribs. Pathologic fractures at the site of metastasis are common because of weakening of the involved bone.

Once a primary lesion has been identified, bone scans are often done to detect the presence of metastatic lesions before they are visible on x-ray. It is important to note that metastatic bone lesions may occur at any time (even years later) following diagnosis and possible treatment of the primary tumor. Metastasis to the bone should be suspected in any patient who has local pain to the bone and a past history of cancer. Treatment may be palliative and consists of pain management and radiation. Surgical stabilization of the fracture may be indicated if there is a fracture or pending fracture. Prognosis depends on the extent of metastasis and location.

NURSING MANAGEMENT: BONE CANCER

■ Nursing Assessment

The patient with bone cancer should be assessed for the location and severity of pain. Weakness caused by anemia and increased debility may also be noted. Swelling at the involved site and decreased joint function, depending on the tumor site, should also be monitored.

■ Nursing Diagnoses

Nursing diagnoses for the patient with bone cancer may include, but are not limited to, the following:

- Pain *related to* the disease process, inadequate pain medication, or comfort measures
- Impaired physical mobility *related to* disease process, pain, weakness, and debility
- Body image disturbance *related to* possible amputation, deformity, swelling, and effects of chemotherapy
- Anticipatory grieving *related to* poor prognosis of the disease
- Risk for injury (pathologic fracture) *related to* disease process and inadequate handling or positioning of affected body part

■ Planning

The overall goals are that the patient with bone cancer will (1) have satisfactory pain relief; (2) maintain preferred activities as long as possible; (3) demonstrate acceptance of body image changes resulting from chemotherapy, radiation, and surgery; (4) be free from injury; and (5) verbalize a realistic idea of disease progression and prognosis.

■ Nursing Implementation

Health Promotion. The nurse should teach the public to recognize the warning signs of bone cancer, including swelling, bone pain of unexplained origin, limitation of joint function, and changes in skin temperature. As with all forms of cancer, health promotion should stress the importance of periodic health examinations.

Acute Intervention. Nursing care of the patient with a malignant bone neoplasm does not differ significantly from the care given to the patient with a malignant disease of any other body system. However, special attention is required to reduce the complications associated with prolonged bed rest and to prevent pathologic fractures. The patient is often reluctant to participate in therapeutic activities because of weakness and fear of pain. Regular rest periods should be provided between activities. Careful handling of the affected extremity is important to prevent pathologic fractures. As with all forms of cancer, health promotion should stress the importance of periodic health examinations.

Ambulatory and Home Care. The nurse must be able to assist the patient in accepting the guarded prognosis associated with neoplasms of the bone. Inability to accomplish age-specific developmental tasks can increase the frustrations with this condition. General principles related to cancer nursing are applicable (see Chapter 14). Special attention is necessary for the problems of pain and dysfunction, chemotherapy, and specific surgery such as spinal cord decompression or amputation.

■ Evaluation

The expected outcomes are that the patient with bone cancer will

- have minimal to no pain
- have no falls
- have no pathologic fractures
- accept changes in body image
- have maximal functional ability

LOW BACK PAIN

Etiology and Pathophysiology

Low back pain is common and has probably affected about 80% of adults in the United States at least once during their lifetime. In industry, low back pain is responsible for more lost working hours than any other medical condition and represents one of the nation's most costly health problems. Each year about 18 million visits are made to physicians for treatment of this condition.[35]

Several risk factors are associated with low back pain, including lack of muscle tone and excess weight, poor posture, smoking, and stress. Jobs that require repetitive heavy lifting, vibration (such as a jackhammer operator), and prolonged periods of sitting are also associated with low back pain.

Pain in the lumbar region is a common problem because this area (1) bears most of the weight of the body, (2) is the most flexible region of the spinal column, (3) contains nerve roots that are vulnerable to injury or disease, and (4) has an inherently poor biomechanical structure.

Low back pain is most often due to a musculoskeletal problem. However, other causes such as metabolic, circulatory, gynecologic, urologic, or psychologic problems, which may refer pain to the lower back, must not be overlooked. The causes of low back pain of musculoskeletal origin include (1) acute lumbosacral strain, (2) instability of lumbosacral bony mechanism, (3) osteoarthritis of the lumbosacral vertebrae, (4) intervertebral disk degeneration, and (5) herniation of the intervertebral disk. Of these, the most common cause is mechanical strain of paravertebral muscles. Herniation of the nucleus pulposus is another common cause of low back pain.

Acute Low Back Pain

Acute low back pain is usually associated with some type of activity that causes undue stress on the tissues of the lower back. Often symptoms do not appear at the time of injury but develop later because of gradual increase in paravertebral muscle spasms. Few definitive diagnostic abnormalities are present with paravertebral muscle strain. The straight-leg raise test may produce pain in the lumbar area without radiation along the sciatic nerve.

Collaborative Care

If the muscle spasms are not severe, the patient may be treated on an outpatient basis with a combination of the following: (1) analgesics, (2) NSAIDs, (3) muscle relaxants (e.g., cyclobenzaprine [Flexeril]), and (4) use of a corset. A corset prevents rotation, flexion, and extension of the lower back.

If the spasms and pain are severe, a brief period of rest at home may be necessary. Since paravertebral muscle spasms are worse when the patient is upright, bed rest is the prime treatment for severe acute low back pain. Bathroom privileges are usually allowed. Bed rest is maintained until the patient can

---

NURSING ASSESSMENT

Table 59-16 | **Low Back Pain**

Subjective Data

Important Health Information

Past health history: Acute or chronic lumbosacral strain, osteoarthritis, degenerative disk disease, obesity

Medications: Use of analgesics, muscle relaxants, nonsteroidal antiinflammatory drugs, corticosteroids, over-the-counter remedies

Surgery or other treatments: Previous back surgery, epidural corticosteroid injections

Functional Health Patterns

Health perception–health management: Smoking, lack of exercise

Nutritional-metabolic: Obesity

Activity-exercise: Poor posture, muscle spasms; activity intolerance

Elimination: Constipation

Sleep-rest: Interrupted sleep

Cognitive-perceptual: Pain in back, buttocks, or leg associated with walking, turning, straining, coughing, leg raising; numbness or tingling of legs, feet, toes

Role-relationship: Occupation requiring heavy lifting, vibrations, or extended driving

Objective Data

General

Guarded movement

Neurologic

Depressed or absent Achilles tendon reflex; positive straight-leg raise test

Musculoskeletal

Tense, tight paravertebral muscles on palpation, decreased range of motion of spine

Possible Findings

Localization of site of lesion on myelogram, CT scan, or MRI; determination of nerve irritation on electromyography

---

move and turn from side to side with minimal discomfort. At this time, gradually increasing activity is initiated. When the patient is comfortable on oral pain medication, a progressive physical therapy program is begun to regain mobility and strength in lower back structures.

If conservative treatment is ineffective and the cause of the pain is nerve root irritation, an epidural corticosteroid injection may be performed. A needle is inserted into the epidural space and a corticosteroid and local anesthetic are injected. Epidural corticosteroids have been shown to decrease pain, speed return of function, and improve objective neurologic signs. These injections are most effective in patients with acute rather than chronic pain and patients with radicular pain who are not candidates for surgery. Epidural injections typically consist of a series of one to three injections over a span of several days to several weeks.

NURSING MANAGEMENT: ACUTE LOW BACK PAIN

■ Nursing Assessment

Subjective and objective data that should be obtained from the patient with low back pain are summarized in Table 59-16.

59-4 NURSING CARE PLAN PATIENT WITH LOW BACK PAIN

Expected Patient Outcomes	Nursing Interventions and *Rationales*

Acute Management

NURSING DIAGNOSIS **Pain** *related to* herniated nucleus pulposus, muscle spasms, and ineffective comfort measures *as manifested by* verbalization of back pain on movement, guarded movements, palpable muscle spasm, decreased physical activity, rating pain as >2 on a scale of 1 through 5.

- Reduction or absence of pain and muscle spasms.
- Expression of satisfaction with pain relief (rates pain as 2 or less on scale of 1 through 5).

- Assess location, severity, and circumstances of pain *to plan appropriate interventions.*
- Use a pain scale and evaluate pain relief interventions *to assess pain and treatment measures.*
- Enforce decreased activity *to reduce paravertebral muscle spasms and resulting pain.*
- Keep head of bed elevated 20 degrees and knee of bed flexed *to promote comfort by reducing stress on lower back muscles.*
- Maintain pelvic traction, correctly aligned, as ordered *to reduce muscle spasm.*
- Apply moist heat or ice to lower back *to reduce pain and muscle spasm.*
- Administer analgesics, nonsteroidal antiinflammatory drugs, or muscle relaxants as ordered; document effect *to promote comfort and evaluate effectiveness.*

NURSING DIAGNOSIS **Impaired physical mobility** *related to* pain *as manifested by* limited active joint range of motion (ROM), movement restrictions, muscle spasms.

- Unrestricted gait.
- Ambulation within normal limits.
- Resumption of previous level of mobility.
- Performance of prescribed exercises.

- Have patient perform ROM and muscle-strengthening exercises daily *to strengthen the supporting muscles and maintain all joints in normal ROM.*
- Start ambulation program and progress with assistance *to promote gradual and progressive return to previous mobility level.*
- Avoid having patient bend, sit, or lift *to prevent back strain and increased pain.*
- Report leg or back pain and change in sensation *because these are indicators of severe lumbosacral intravertebral pressure and sciatic nerve involvement.*
- Provide written instructions that describe each exercise and activity and a phone number to call with any questions.

Chronic Management

NURSING DIAGNOSIS **Chronic pain** *related to* progression of problem *as manifested by* verbal report or evidence of pain longer than 6 months in duration.

- Development of effective methods of managing pain.
- Expression of satisfaction with pain control measures.

- Assess variety and effectiveness of pain management techniques *to determine extent of problem and develop appropriate interventions.*
- Use a pain scale *to assess pain and to evaluate pain control interventions.*
- Instruct patient and family about home care and alternative methods of pain control, including use of heat, transcutaneous electrical nerve stimulation, and massage, *to provide information about supplementary methods of pain management.*
- Avoid strenuous activities, *which increase pain.*
- Assist in identifying activities that exacerbate pain *to make adjustments in lifestyle so that pain is reduced.*

NURSING DIAGNOSIS **Ineffective individual coping** *related to* effects of chronic pain on lifestyle *as manifested by* verbalization of inability to cope, irritability, tension, inability to meet role expectations, altered participation in social events, ineffective or inappropriate use of defense mechanisms.

- Return to previous levels of work and lifestyle or successfully adapt to lifestyle changes.

- Explain factors that may contribute to development of maladaptive coping behavior *to communicate information and a caring attitude.*
- Explain how to develop therapeutic coping skills and activities that enhance self-esteem and social interaction *to foster effective coping behaviors and adjustment to chronic pain condition.*
- Discuss chronic nature of pain and need for lifestyle adjustments to patient *to avoid repeated and demoralizing attempts to eliminate pain.*

Continued

59-4 NURSING CARE PLAN PATIENT WITH LOW BACK PAIN—continued

| Expected Patient Outcomes | Nursing Interventions and *Rationales* |

NURSING DIAGNOSIS Ineffective management of therapeutic regimen *related to* lack of knowledge regarding posture, exercises, body mechanics, and weight reduction *as manifested by* lack of necessary knowledge to participate in treatment plan, inadequate understanding or inaccurate follow-through of previous instructions.

- Use of proper body mechanics at all times.
- Maintenance of weight within normal limits.
- Maintenance of activity and ambulation appropriate to age and state of health.

- Assess body mechanics *to identify incorrect techniques and intervene appropriately.*
- Instruct patient on proper body mechanics and use of firm mattress or bedboard *to reduce risk of reinjury, provide back support, and maintain proper body alignment.*
- Assess for decreasing muscle strength *to identify complications and modify care plan.*
- Refer to physical therapist for low back exercises *to develop abdominal and paravertebral muscle strength to provide increased support.*
- Encourage activity and ambulation within limitations *to maintain physical mobility and minimize sick-role behaviors.*
- Teach about weight reduction or refer to dietician if indicated *because increased abdominal weight puts strain on low back.*

NURSING DIAGNOSIS Body image disturbance *related to* impaired mobility and chronic pain *as manifested by* negative statements about body, change in social involvement or relationships, statements of hopelessness.

- Positive self-image.

- Provide psychologic support, active listening, and encouragement *to prevent development of negative body image.*
- Assist patient in becoming as independent as possible *to prevent assumption of sick role.*
- Refer to local support groups or psychologic evaluation *to provide therapeutic adjustment.*

■ Nursing Diagnoses

Nursing diagnoses for the patient with low back pain may include, but are not limited to, those presented in NCP 59-4.

■ Planning

The overall goals are that the patient with low back pain will (1) have satisfactory pain relief, (2) avoid constipation secondary to medication and immobility, (3) learn back-sparing practices, and (4) return to previous level of activity within prescribed restrictions.

■ Nursing Implementation

Health Promotion. The nurse is a significant role model and teacher for patients with low back problems. As a role model, the nurse should use proper body mechanics at all times. This should be a primary consideration when teaching patients and care providers transfer and turning techniques. The nurse should assess the patient's use of body mechanics and offer advice when activities that could produce back strain are used (Table 59-17).

Some health care providers refer patients with back pain to a program called "Back School." It is a formal program usually taught by health professionals such as physicians, nurses, and physical therapists. It is designed to teach the patient how to minimize back pain and avoid repeat episodes of low back pain. Tips for prevention of back injury are listed in Table 59-17. Exercises to strengthen the back are presented in Table 59-18.

Patients are also advised to maintain appropriate body weight. Excess body weight places extra stress on the lower

PATIENT TEACHING GUIDE

Table 59-17 Low Back Problems

Do Not
- Lean forward without bending knees
- Lift anything above level of elbows
- Stand in one position for prolonged time
- Sleep on abdomen or on back or side with legs out straight
- Exercise without consulting health care provider if having severe pain
- Exceed prescribed amount and type of exercises without consulting health care provider

Do
- Prevent lower back from straining forward by placing a foot on a step or stool during prolonged standing
- Sleep in a side-lying position with knees and hips bent
- Sleep on back with a lift under knees and legs or on back with 10-inch-high pillow under knees to flex hips and knees
- Sit in a chair with knees higher than hips and support arms on chair or knees
- Exercise 15 min in the morning and 15 min in the evening regularly; begin exercises with a 2- or 3-min warm-up period by moving arms and legs, by alternately relaxing and tightening muscles; exercise slowly with smooth movements as directed by a physical therapist
- Avoid chilling during and after exercising
- Maintain appropriate body weight
- Use a lumbar roll or pillow for sitting

PATIENT TEACHING GUIDE

Table 59-18   Back Exercises

Knee-to-chest lift (to stretch hip, buttocks, lower back muscles)
- Lie on back on the floor with knees bent and feet flat on floor.
- Draw both knees up to chest.
- Place both hands around knees and pull them firmly against chest. Hold for 30 seconds.
- Lower legs and return to starting position.
- Repeat 5-10 times.

Simple leg lift
- Lie flat on back on floor with left knee bent and left foot flat on floor.
- Raise right leg as high as comfortably possible.
- Hold for 5 counts.
- Slowly return leg to floor.
- Bend right knee and put right foot flat on floor.
- Raise left leg and hold for 5 counts.
- Repeat 5-10 times for each leg.

Double leg lift
- Lie flat on back.
- Slowly lift legs until feet are 12 inches from the floor.
- Keep legs straight and hold this position for 10 counts.
- Lower legs to floor.
- Repeat 5 times.

Pelvic tilt
- Lie flat on back on floor with knees bent and feet flat on the floor.
- Firmly tighten your buttock muscles.
- Hold for 5 counts.
- Relax buttocks.
- Repeat 5-10 times.
- Be sure to keep lower back flat against floor.

Half sit-ups (to strengthen abdominal muscles)
- Lie flat on floor on back with knees bent, feet flat on floor, and hands on chest.
- Slowly raise head and neck to top of chest.
- Reach both hands forward and place them on knees.
- Hold for 5 counts.
- Return to starting position.
- Repeat 5-10 times.

Elbow props (to extend lower back)
- Lie face down with your arms beside your body and your head turned to one side.
- Stay in this position for 2-5 minutes, making sure that you relax completely.
- Remain face down and prop yourself on your elbows.
- Hold this position for 2-3 minutes.
- Return to starting position and relax for 1 minute.
- Repeat 5-10 times.

Hip tilts
- Lie flat on back with knees bent.
- Slowly bend legs and hips to one side as far as possible.
- Bend to other side.
- Repeat 5 times.

Toe touches
- Stand straight and relaxed.
- Lower head and body and try to touch floor with fingertips.
- Keep knees straight.
- Do not jerk or lunge toward floor.
- Bend only as far as you can.
- Repeat 5 times.

From Canobbio MM: *Mosby's handbook of patient teaching,* St Louis, 1996, Mosby.

back and weakens the abdominal muscles that support the lower back.

The position assumed while sleeping is also important in preventing low back pain. Sleeping in a prone position should be avoided because it produces excessive lumbar lordosis, placing excessive stress on the lower back. A firm mattress is recommended. The patient should sleep in either a supine or side-lying position with the knees and hips flexed to prevent unnecessary pressure on support muscles, ligamentous structures, and lumbosacral joints. Patients should be educated about the necessity to avoid or cease smoking. Nicotine has been shown to decrease circulation to the disks, and a causal relationship exists between smoking and some types of low back pain.[36,37]

Acute Intervention. The primary nursing responsibilities in acute low back pain are to assist the patient to maintain activity limitations, promote comfort, and educate the patient about the health problem and appropriate exercises. Other nursing interventions are summarized in NCP 59-4. Use of analgesics, nonsteroidal antiinflammatory agents, thermo-

therapy (ice and heat), and muscle relaxants to promote comfort is incorporated into the plan of care.

Muscle stretching and strengthening exercises may be part of the management plan. Although the actual exercises are often taught by the physical therapist, it is the nurse's responsibility to ensure that the patient understands the type and frequency of exercise prescribed, as well as the rationale for the program.

Ambulatory and Home Care. The goal of management is to make an episode of acute low back pain an isolated incident. If the lumbosacral mechanism is unstable, repeated episodes can be anticipated. The lumbosacral spine may be unable to meet the demands placed on it without strain because of factors such as obesity, poor posture, poor muscular support, advancing age, or local trauma. Intervention is aimed at strengthening the supporting muscles by exercise and the use of a corset to limit extremes of movement. In addition, weight reduction decreases the mechanical demands on the lower back.

Persistent use of poor body mechanics may result in repeated episodes of low back pain. If the strain is work related, occupational counseling may be necessary. The frustration, pain, and disability imposed on the patient with low back pain require emotional support and understanding care by the nurse.

■ Evaluation

The expected outcomes for the patient with low back pain are presented in NCP 59-4.

Chronic Low Back Pain

Etiology and Pathophysiology

The causes of chronic low back pain include degenerative disk disease, lack of physical exercise, prior injury, obesity, structural and postural abnormalities, and systemic disease. Structural degeneration of the intervertebral disk results in degenerative disk disease manifested by low back pain. This degeneration can also occur in the cervical spine area. The degeneration results in intervertebral narrowing and a lessening of the efficiency of the intervertebral disks in acting as shock absorbers. This inefficiency causes small tears in the annulus fibrosis, which predisposes the patient to herniated nucleus pulposus. As the stresses on the degenerated disk continue and eventually exceed the strength of the disk, herniation of the intervertebral disk may result. Nuclear material from the intervertebral disk herniates and may compress or place tension on a cervical lumbar or sacral spinal nerve root (Fig. 59-21).

Clinical Manifestations

The most common feature of a lumbar herniated intervertebral disk is back pain with associated buttock and leg pain along the distribution of the sciatic nerve (radiculopathy). (Specific manifestations based on the level of lumbar disk herniation are summarized in Table 59-19.) The straight-leg raise test may be positive. Back or leg pain may be reproduced by raising the leg and flexing the foot at 90 degrees. Low back pain from other causes may not be accompanied by leg pain.

Reflexes may be depressed or absent, depending on the spinal nerve root involved. Paresthesia or muscle weakness in the legs, feet, or toes may be reported by the patient. If the disk ruptures in the cervical area, the clinical manifestations are stiff neck, shoulder pain radiating to the hand, and paresthesias and sensory disturbances of the hand.

Diagnostic Studies

X-rays are done to note any structural defects. A myelogram, MRI, or CT scan is helpful in localizing the site of herniation. A diskogram may be necessary if other methods of diagnosis are unsuccessful. An electromyogram (EMG) of the extremities can be performed to determine the severity of nerve irritation caused by herniation or to rule out other pathology such as peripheral neuropathy.

Collaborative Care

Degenerative disk disease is managed conservatively with rest, limitation of extremes of spinal movement (corset), local heat or ice, ultrasound, transcutaneous electrical nerve stimulation (TENS), and NSAIDs. If herniation of the disk occurs, more

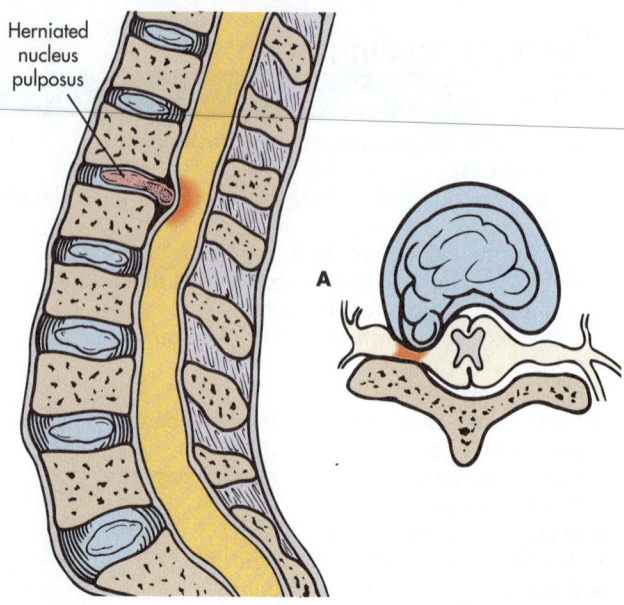

Fig. 59-21 Compression of spinal cord caused by herniation of nucleus pulposus into spinal cord. **A,** Pressure on nerves as they leave the spinal canal.

aggressive treatment may be indicated (Table 59-20). Conservative treatment sometimes results in a healing over of the herniated area with a decrease in the pain of nerve root irritation. Muscle relaxants may be used to decrease muscle spasms. Once the symptoms subside, back strengthening exercises are begun. The patient should be educated in principles of good body mechanics. Extremes of flexion and torsion are strongly discouraged. Most patients with herniated disks recover with a conservative treatment plan. However, if conservative treatment is unsuccessful, radiculopathy becomes progressively worse, or there is documented loss of bowel or bladder control (cauda equina), surgery may be indicated.

Surgical Therapy. A *percutaneous laser diskectomy* is a surgical procedure using a tube that is passed through the retroperitoneal soft tissues to the lateral border of the disk with the aid of fluoroscopy. Laserization is performed to the herniated portion of the disk.[38] Small stab wounds are used, and minimal blood loss occurs during the procedure. The long-term effects of this procedure are being investigated.

A *diskectomy* is another type of surgical procedure that may be performed to decompress the nerve root.[39] It involves the partial removal of the lamina to allow access to the intervertebral disk. *Microsurgical diskectomy* is a version of the standard diskectomy in which the surgeon uses a microscope to allow better visualization of the disk and disk space during surgery to aid in the removal of the herniated portion.

The traditional and most common procedure performed is a *laminectomy*. It involves the surgical excision of part of the posterior arch of the vertebra (referred to as the lamina) to gain access to part or all of the protruding disk to remove it.

A *spinal fusion* may be performed if an unstable bony mechanism is present. The spine is stabilized by creating an ankylo-

Table 59-19	Neurologic Assessment of Herniated Intervertebral Disk*			
Intervertebral Level	Subjective Pain	Affected Reflex	Motor Function	Sensation
L3-L4	Back to buttocks to posterior thigh to inner calf	Patellar	Quadriceps, anterior tibialis	Inner aspect of lower leg, anterior part of thigh
L4-L5	Back to buttocks to dorsum of foot and big toe	None	Anterior tibialis, extensor halucis longus, gluteus medius	Dorsum of foot and big toe
L5-S1	Back to buttocks to sole of foot and heel	Achilles	Gastrocnemius, hamstring, gluteus maximus	Heel and lateral foot

*A disk herniation can involve pressure on more than one nerve root.

COLLABORATIVE CARE
Table 59-20   Herniated Intervertebral Disk

Diagnostic
History
Physical examination with emphasis on neurologic deficits and straight-leg raising
CT scan
MRI
Myelogram
Diskogram
EMG
Somatosensory evoked potential

Collaborative Therapy
Conservative
Restricted activity
Medication
  Analgesics
  Nonsteroidal antiinflammatory drugs
  Muscle relaxants (e.g., cyclobenzaprine [Flexeril])
Diathermy
Thermotherapy
Physical therapy

Surgical
Laminectomy with or without spinal fusion
Diskectomy
Percutaneous lateral diskectomy
Spinal fusion with or without instrumentation

EMG, electromyogram.

Table 59-21   Postoperative Assessment Following Lumbar Surgery

Sensation*
Assess sensation of extremities for paresthesia in all appropriate neurotomes.

Movement*
Assess ability to move all extremities.

Muscle Strength*
Assess for any weakness of the extremities.

Wound
Assess dressing for drainage and note amount, color, characteristics.

Pain
Document location of the pain.
Ask patient to rate the pain on a scale of 1 to 5, with 1 being no pain and 5 being worst pain.
Evaluate pain after analgesia has been administered.

*Postoperative findings should be compared with preoperative assessments. It is not unusual for the patient to continue to experience these symptoms after surgery. Symptoms gradually decrease over several months.

sis (fusion) of contiguous vertebrae with a bone graft from the patient's fibula or iliac crest or donated bone. If vertebral instability exists, metal fixation with rods, plates, or screws may be implanted at the time of spinal surgery to provide more stability and decrease vertebral motion.

NURSING MANAGEMENT: SPINAL SURGERY

Patients who have undergone spinal surgery require vigilant postoperative care. Nursing implementation is aimed at maintaining proper alignment of the spine at all times until healing has occurred. Flat bed rest may be maintained for 1 to 2 days depending on the extent of surgery. Logrolling patients when turning is essential to maintain proper body alignment. Pillows can be used under the thighs of each leg when supine and be-

tween the legs when in side-lying positions to provide comfort and ensure alignment.

Severe muscle spasms in the surgical area can be managed with medication and with correct turning and positioning. The patient often fears turning or any movement that increases pain by straining the surgical area. The nurse must offer reassurance to the patient that the proper technique is being used to maintain body alignment. Sufficient staff should be available to move the patient without undue pain or strain on staff members or the patient.

Because the spinal canal may be entered during surgery, there is potential for spinal fluid leakage. Severe headache or leakage of cerebrospinal fluid (CSF) on the dressing should be reported immediately. CSF appears as clear or slightly yellow drainage on the dressing. It has a high glucose concentration and will be positive for glucose when a dipstick test is done. The amount and characteristics of drainage should be noted.

Frequent monitoring of peripheral neurologic signs of the extremities is a routine postoperative nursing responsibility after spinal surgery. Movement of arms and legs and assessment of sensation should be unchanged when compared with the preoperative status. Table 59-21 summarizes a lumbar laminectomy assessment appropriate for the patient who has undergone back surgery. These assessments are repeated every 2 to 4 hours during the first 48 hours after surgery, and findings are compared with the preoperative assessment. Paresthesias, such as numbness and tingling, may not be relieved immediately after surgery. Any new muscle weakness or paresthesias should be documented and reported to the surgeon immediately.

Paralytic ileus and interference with bowel function may occur for several days and may manifest as nausea, abdominal distention, and constipation. The nurse should assess whether the patient is passing flatus, has bowel sounds in all quadrants, and has a flat, soft abdomen.

Adequate bladder emptying may be altered because of activity restrictions, narcotics, or anesthesia. If allowed by the surgeon, men should be encouraged to dangle or stand to urinate. Patients should use the commode or ambulate to the bathroom when allowed to promote adequate emptying of the bladder. The nurse should ensure that privacy is maintained. It is necessary to clarify whether the patient can be allowed up to the bathroom without the corset or brace. Intermittent catheterization or an indwelling catheter may be necessary for patients who have difficulty urinating.

Loss of sphincter tone or bladder tone may be indicative of nerve damage. Incontinence or difficulty evacuating the bowel or bladder must be monitored closely and reported to the surgeon.

Activity prescriptions vary with surgeons, but the patient who has had spinal surgery usually ambulates early in the postoperative period. It is a nursing responsibility to know the specific orders related to activity for any patient.

In addition to the nursing care appropriate for a patient who has had a laminectomy, there are other nursing responsibilities if the patient has also had a spinal fusion. Because a bone graft is usually involved, the postoperative healing time is prolonged compared with that of a laminectomy. Immobilization over an extended time may be necessary. A rigid orthosis (thoracic-lumbar-sacral orthosis or chairback brace) is often used during the period of immobilization. Some surgeons require that the patient be taught to put it on and take it off by logrolling in bed, whereas others allow their patients to apply the brace in a sitting or standing position. The nurse should verify the preferred method before initiating this activity. The extended immobilization required by a spinal fusion carries with it all the potential problems related to this inactive state.

In addition to the primary surgical site, the donor site for the bone graft must be regularly assessed. The posterior iliac crest is the most commonly used donor site, although a rib or fibula may also be used. The donor site usually causes greater postoperative pain than the fused area. The donor site is bandaged with a pressure dressing to prevent excessive bleeding. If the donor site is the fibula, neurovascular assessments of the extremity are a postoperative nursing responsibility. Any restrictions on activity such as exercise should be clarified with the physician.

As the bone graft heals, the patient must adjust to the permanent immobility at the graft or fusion site. Instruction in proper body mechanics is essential and should be evaluated during the hospital stay.

The patient should be instructed to avoid sitting or standing for prolonged periods. Activities that should be encouraged include walking, lying down, and shifting weight from one foot to the other when standing. The patient should learn to mentally think through an activity before starting any potentially injurious task such as bending, lifting, or stooping. Any twisting movement of the spine is contraindicated. The thighs and knees, rather than the back, should be used to absorb the shock of activity and movement. A firm mattress or bedboard is essential.

NECK PAIN

Causes of neck pain are similar to those of the low back. Patients have symptoms of neck pain and possible pain radiating into the arm and hand. They also may have weakness or paresthesia of the arm and hand. Diagnosing the cause of neck pain is done by x-ray, MRI, CT scan, and myelogram. An EMG of the upper extremities is done to diagnose cervical radiculopathy.

Types of surgery done on the neck are similar to those done on the lower back with the exception that either posterior or anterior approaches may be used. These include a diskectomy, laminectomy, and spinal fusion. If surgery is done on the cervical spine, the nurse must be alert for symptoms of spinal cord edema such as respiratory distress and a worsening neurologic status of the upper extremities. After surgery, the patient's neck is immobilized in either a soft or hard cervical collar.

COMMON FOOT PROBLEMS

The foot is the platform that provides support for the weight of the body and absorbs considerable shock in ambulation. It is a complicated structure composed of bony structures, muscles, tendons, and ligaments. It can be affected by (1) congenital conditions, (2) structural weakness, (3) traumatic injuries, and (4) systemic conditions such as diabetes mellitus and rheumatoid arthritis. Abnormalities of the foot affect over 80 million persons in the United States. Much of the pain, deformity, and disability associated with foot disorders can be directly attributed to or accentuated by improperly fitting shoes, which cause crowding and angulation of the toes and inhibition of the normal movement of foot muscles. The purposes of footwear are to (1) provide support, foot stability, protection, shock absorption, and a foundation for orthoses; (2) increase friction with the walking surface; and (3) treat foot abnormalities. (Table 59-22 summarizes common foot problems and their treatment.)

NURSING MANAGEMENT: COMMON FOOT PROBLEMS

Health Promotion. Well-constructed and properly fitted shoes are essential for healthy, pain-free feet. Fashion styles, especially for women, often influence selection of footwear instead of considerations of comfort and support. Patient education should stress the importance of having a shoe that conforms to the foot rather than to current fashion trends. The shoe must be long enough and wide enough to prevent crowding of the toes and forcing of the great toe into a position of hallux valgus. At the metatarsal head the width of the shoe should be sufficient to allow free movement of the foot muscles and permit bending of the toes. The shank of the shoe should be rigid enough to give optimal support. The height of the heel should be realistic in relation to the purpose for which the shoe is worn. Ideally, the heel of the shoe should not rise more than 1 inch higher than the forefoot support.

Table 59-22 Common Foot Problems

Disorder	Definition	Treatment
Common Disorders		
Forefoot		
Hallux valgus (bunion)	Painful deformity of great toe consisting of lateral angulation of great toe toward second toe, bony enlargement of medial side of first metatarsal head, and formation of bursa or callus over bony enlargement	Conservative treatment includes wearing shoes with wide forefoot or "bunion pocket" and use of bunion pads to relieve pressure on bursal sac. Surgical treatment is removal of bursal sac and bony enlargement and correction of lateral angulation of great toe; may include temporary or permanent internal fixation.
Hallux rigidus	Painful stiffness of first metatarsophalangeal joint caused by osteoarthritis or local trauma	Conservative treatment includes intraarticular corticosteroids and passive manual stretching of first metatarsophalangeal joint. A shoe with a stiff sole decreases pain in the joint during walking. Surgical treatment is joint fusion or arthroplasty with silicone rubber implant.
Hammertoe	Deformity of second through fifth toes, including dorsiflexion of metatarsophalangeal joint, plantar flexion of proximal interphalangeal joint, and callus on dorsum of proximal interphalangeal joint and end of involved toe; complaints related to hammertoe include burning on bottom of foot and pain and difficulty in walking when wearing shoes	Conservative treatment consists of passive manual stretching of proximal interphalangeal joint and use of metatarsal arch support. Surgical correction consists of resection of base of middle phalanx and head of proximal phalanx and bringing raw bone ends together. Kirschner wire maintains straight position.
Morton's neuroma (Morton's toe or plantar neuroma)	Neuroma in web space between third and fourth metatarsal heads, causing sharp, sudden attacks of pain and burning sensations	Surgical excision is the usual treatment.
Midfoot		
Pes planus (flatfoot)	Loss of metatarsal arch causing pain in foot or leg	Symptoms are relieved by use of resilient longitudinal arch supports. Surgical treatment consists of triple arthrodesis or fusion of subtalar joint.
Pes cavus	Elevation of longitudinal arch of foot resulting from contracture of plantar fascia or bony deformity of arch	Treatment is manipulation and casting (in patients younger than 6 yr of age); surgical correction is necessary if it interferes with ambulation (in patients older than 6 yr of age).
Hindfoot		
Painful heels	Complaint of heel pain with weight bearing, common cause of plantar bursitis or calcaneal spur in adult	Corticosteroids are injected locally into inflamed bursa and sponge rubber heel cushion is used; surgical excision of bursa or spur is performed.
Local Problems		
Corn	Localized thickening of skin caused by continual pressure over bony prominences, especially metatarsal head, frequently causing localized pain	Corn is softened with warm water or preparations containing salicylic acid and trimmed with razor blade or scalpel. Pressure on bony prominences caused by shoes is relieved.
Soft corn	Painful lesion caused by bony prominence of one toe pressing against adjacent toe; usual location in web space between toes; softness caused by secretions keeping web space relatively moist.	Pain is relieved by placing cotton between toes to separate them. Surgical treatment is excision of projecting bone spur (if present).
Callus	Similar formation to corn but covering of wider area and usual location on weight-bearing part of foot	Same as for corn.
Plantar wart	Painful papillomatous growth caused by virus that may occur on any part of skin on sole of foot	Excision with electrocoagulation or surgical removal is done; ultrasound may also be used.

Acute Intervention. Many foot problems require surgery. When surgery is performed, the foot is usually immobilized by a bulky dressing, short leg cast, slipper (plaster) cast, or a platform "shoe" that fits over the dressing and has a rigid sole (known as a bunion boot). The foot should be elevated with the heel off the bed to help reduce discomfort and prevent edema. The neurovascular status should be assessed frequently during the immediate postoperative period. Depending on the type of surgery, pins or wires may extend through the toes, or a protective splint that extends over the end of the foot may be in place. Care must be taken not to jar these devices and cause pain. The devices may interfere with or preclude assessment for movement. The nurse should be aware that sensation may be difficult to evaluate, since postoperative pain can interfere with the patient's ability to differentiate pain caused by the surgical procedure from pain resulting from nerve pressure or circulatory impairment.

The type and extent of surgery determine the degree of ambulation allowed. Crutches or canes may be necessary. The patient may experience pain or a throbbing sensation when starting ambulation. The nurse should reinforce instructions given by the physical therapist and ensure that the patient does not develop a faulty gait pattern such as walking on the heels in an attempt to avoid excessive pain or pressure. The nurse must reinforce the importance of walking with an erect posture and with proper weight distribution. Dysfunction of gait or continued pain should be reported to the physician. The nurse should instruct the patient on the importance of frequent rest periods with the foot elevated.

Ambulatory and Home Care. Foot care should include daily hygienic care and the wearing of clean stockings. Stockings should be long enough to avoid wrinkling and the development of pressure areas. Trimming toenails straight across helps prevent ingrown toenails and reduces the possibility of infection. Persons with impaired circulation or diabetes mellitus require detailed instruction to prevent serious complications associated with blisters, pressure areas, and infections (see Table 46-25 for guidelines for foot care).

■ **GERONTOLOGIC CONSIDERATIONS** ■

Foot Problems

The older adult is prone to developing foot problems because of poor circulation, atherosclerosis, and decreased sensation in the lower extremities. This is especially a problem for older patients with diabetes mellitus. A patient may develop an open wound but not feel it because of altered sensation. This may be the result of peripheral vascular disease or diabetic neuropathy. Older adults should be instructed to inspect their feet daily and report any open wounds or breaks in the skin to their physician. If left untreated, wounds may become infected, lead to osteomyelitis, and require surgical debridement. If infection becomes widespread, amputation may be necessary.

METABOLIC BONE DISEASES

Normal bone metabolism is dependent on adequate intake, absorption, and use of calcium, phosphorus, protein, and vitamins. When there is dysfunction in any of these critical factors, generalized reduction of bone mass may result.

OSTEOMALACIA

Osteomalacia is an uncommon disorder of adult bone associated with vitamin D deficiency, resulting in decalcification and softening of bone. This disease is the same as rickets in children except that the epiphyseal growth plates are closed in the adult. Vitamin D is required for the absorption of calcium from the intestines. Insufficient vitamin D intake can interfere with the normal mineralization of bone, causing failure or insufficient calcification of bone, which results in softening of bone, bone pain, and deformities. Etiologic factors in the development of osteomalacia include lack of exposure to ultraviolet rays, gastrointestinal malabsorption, extensive burns, chronic diarrhea, pregnancy, kidney disease, and medications such as phenytoin (Dilantin).

The most common clinical feature of osteomalacia is persistent skeletal pain, especially while bearing weight. Other clinical manifestations include low back pain, progressive muscular weakness, weight loss, and progressive deformities of the spine (kyphosis) or extremities. Fractures are common and demonstrate delayed healing when they occur.

Laboratory findings commonly associated with osteomalacia are decreased serum calcium or phosphorus levels and elevated serum alkaline phosphatase. X-ray examination may demonstrate the effects of generalized bone demineralization, especially loss of calcium in the bones of the pelvis and the presence of associated bone deformity. Looser's transformation zones (ribbons of decalcification in bone found on x-ray) are diagnostic of osteomalacia. Significant osteomalacia may exist without demonstrable x-ray changes.

Collaborative care of osteomalacia is directed toward correction of the underlying cause. Vitamin D (cholecalciferol) is usually supplemented, and the patient often shows a dramatic response. Calcium or phosphorus intake may also be supplemented.

OSTEOPOROSIS

Osteoporosis, or porous bone, is a condition characterized by low bone mass and structural deterioration of bone tissue, leading to increased bone fragility. This metabolic bone disease is the major cause of fractures (especially hip, spine, and wrist) in postmenopausal women and older adults in general.[40] Osteoporosis is increasing in incidence because more people are surviving to an older age. At least 25 to 35 million persons in the United States have some degree of osteoporosis, and with the projected increase in life expectancy, this number is expected to grow. In the United States, the total cost of osteoporosis in terms of medical care, nursing home fees, and loss of income is estimated to exceed 10 billion dollars.[40,41]

Osteoporosis is eight times more common in women than in men for several reasons: (1) women tend to have lower calcium intake than men throughout their lives (men between 15 and 50 years of age consume twice as much calcium as women); (2) women have less bone mass because of their generally smaller frame; (3) resorption begins at an earlier age in women and is accelerated at menopause; (4) pregnancy and breastfeeding deplete a woman's skeletal reserve unless calcium intake is adequate; and (5) longevity increases the likelihood of osteoporosis, and women live longer than men. Although osteoporosis is more common in women than men, it is important to realize that men can also develop osteoporosis.

Table **59-23**   **Risk Factors for Osteoporosis**

- Female gender
- Thin, small framed
- Family history of osteoporosis
- Diet low in calcium
- Caucasian or Asian-American
- Excessive use of alcohol
- Cigarette smoking
- An inactive lifestyle
- Long-term use of corticosteroids, thyroid replacements, or antiseizure medications
- Postmenopausal, including early or surgically induced menopause
- History of anorexia nervosa or bulimia, chronic liver disease, or malabsorption

From National Osteoporosis Foundation: *Position paper: current perspectives on diagnosis, prevention, and treatment of osteoporosis,* Washington, DC, 1995, The Foundation.

Etiology and Pathophysiology

Risk factors for osteoporosis are female gender, increasing age, family history of osteoporosis, Caucasian or Asian race, small stature, anorexia, oophorectomy, sedentary lifestyle, and insufficient dietary calcium.[42] Increased risk is associated with cigarette smoking and alcoholism, and decreased risk is associated with adequate physical activity and fluoride and vitamin D ingestion (risk factors for osteoporosis are listed in Table 59-23). Family history is the predominant risk factor in men.

Peak bone mass (maximum bone tissue) is achieved during adolescence. It is determined by a combination of four major factors: hereditary, nutrition, exercise, and hormone function. Heredity may be responsible for up to 70% of peak bone mass. Bone loss from midlife (age 35 to 40 years) onward is inevitable, but the rate of loss varies. At menopause, women experience rapid bone loss with reduced rates after 8 to 10 years.[43]

Bone is continually being deposited by osteoblasts and resorbed by osteoclasts, a process called remodeling. Normally the rates of bone deposition and resorption are equal to each other so that the total bone mass remains constant. In osteoporosis, bone resorption exceeds bone deposition. Although resorption affects the entire skeletal system, osteoporosis occurs most commonly in the bones of the spine, hips, and wrists. Over time, wedging and fractures of the vertebrae produce gradual loss of height and a humped back known as dowager's hump or kyphosis. The usual first signs are back pain or spontaneous fractures. The loss of bone substance causes the bone to become mechanically weakened and prone to either spontaneous fractures or fractures from minimal trauma.

Specific diseases associated with osteoporosis include intestinal malabsorption, kidney disease, rheumatoid arthritis, advanced alcoholism, cirrhosis of the liver, and diabetes mellitus. Many medications can contribute to bone loss, including corticosteroids, antiseizure drugs (phenytoin [Dilantin]), aluminum-containing antacids, heparin, isoniazid (INH), and tetracycline.[44] At the time a medicine is prescribed, the patient should be informed of this possible side effect. Long-term corticosteroid use is a major contributor to osteoporosis. When a corticosteroid is taken, there is a disproportionate loss of trabecular or cancellous bone.

Genetic factors influence bone mass. A genetic marker, the vitamin D receptor (VDR) gene, has been linked to bone density. The VDR gene is responsible for constructing the receptors that assist cells to use vitamin D, a vitamin important to bone and calcium metabolism. Persons with a specific VDR genotype may have significantly lower bone density. This relationship remains under investigation.[45] Identification of a person's genotype could allow targeted interventions at an early age for persons genetically at risk for the development of osteoporosis.

Clinical Manifestations

Osteoporosis is often called the "silent disease" because bone loss occurs without symptoms. People may not know they have osteoporosis until their bones become so weak that a sudden strain, bump, or fall causes a hip, vertebral, or wrist fracture. Collapsed vertebrae may initially be manifested as back pain, loss of height, or spinal deformities such as kyphosis or severely stooped posture.

Diagnostic Studies

Osteoporosis often goes unnoticed because it cannot be detected by conventional x-ray until more than 25% to 40% of calcium in the bone is lost. Serum calcium, phosphorus, and alkaline phosphatase levels usually are normal, although alkaline phosphatase may be elevated after a fracture. Bone minimal density (BMD) measurements are used to measure the bone density. BMD assesses the mass of bone per unit volume, or how tightly the bone is packed. (BMD measurements are presented in Table 58-8.) One of the most common studies is dual-energy x-ray absorptiometry (DEXA), which measures bone density in the spine, hips, and forearm (the most common sites of fractures resulting from osteoporosis). DEXA studies are also useful to evaluate changes in bone density over time and to assess the effectiveness of treatment.

NURSING AND COLLABORATIVE MANAGEMENT: OSTEOPOROSIS

Collaborative care of osteoporosis focuses on proper nutrition, calcium supplementation, exercise, and medication (Table 59-24). Prevention and treatment of osteoporosis focuses on adequate calcium intake (1000 mg/day in premenopausal women and postmenopausal women taking estrogen, and 1500 mg/day in postmenopausal women who are not receiving supplemental estrogen). If dietary intake of calcium is inadequate, supplemental calcium should be taken.[46] Foods that are high in

COLLABORATIVE CARE
Table 59-24 Osteoporosis

Diagnostic
History and physical examination
Serum calcium, phosphorus, and alkaline phosphatase
Bone mineral densitometry

Collaborative Therapy
Calcium supplements (see Table 59-26)
Vitamin D supplements
Diet high in calcium (see Table 59-25)
Exercise program
Estrogen replacement therapy
Calcitonin
Biphosphonates
  Etidronate (Didronel)
  Alendronate (Fosamax)
Raloxifene (Evista)

NUTRITIONAL THERAPY
Table 59-25 Sources of Calcium

Food	Calcium (mg)
1 cup milk	
Buttermilk	285
Chocolate	284
Whole	291
Low-fat	300
Skim	302
Half and half	254
Evaporated, canned	657
Egg nog	330
1 oz cheese	
American	174
Blue	150
Brie	52
Camembert	110
Cheddar	130
Cottage	130
Mozzarella	207
Parmesan	390
Swiss	272
8 oz yogurt	415
1 cup ice cream	176
Soft serve	272
3 oz seafood	
Salmon	167
Sardines with bones	372
Shrimp	98
Oysters	113
1 med stalk cooked broccoli	158
1 cup cooked spinach	200
1 cup cooked mustard greens	193
1 cup turnip greens	252
1 cup cooked collard greens with stems	289
1 cup bok choy	250
1 cup kale	206
Bonus Sources	
1 cup almonds	304
1 cup hazelnuts	240
1 tbs blackstrap molasses	137
Poor Sources	
Egg	28
1 cup cabbage	44
1 oz cream cheese	23
3 oz beef, pork, poultry	10
Apple, banana	10
½ grapefruit	20
1 med potato	14
1 med carrot	14
¼ head lettuce	27

calcium content include whole and skim milk, yogurt, turnip greens, cottage cheese, ice cream, sardines, and spinach (Table 59-25). The amount of elemental calcium varies in different calcium preparations (Table 59-26). Calcium supplementation inhibits age-related bone loss; however, no new bone is formed.

Vitamin D is important in calcium absorption and function and may have a role in bone formation. Most people get enough vitamin D from the diet or naturally through synthesis in the skin from exposure to sunlight. However, supplemental vitamin D (400 to 800 IU) may be recommended for older adults, those who are homebound, and those who get minimal sun exposure. Many calcium supplements also have vitamin D.

Moderate amounts of exercise are important to build up and maintain bone mass. Exercise also increases muscle strength, coordination, and balance. The best exercises are weight-bearing exercises that force an individual to work against gravity. These exercises include walking, hiking, weight training, stair climbing, tennis, and dancing. Walking is preferred to high-impact aerobics or running, both of which may put too much stress on the bones of patients with osteoporosis.

Cigarette smoking and excess alcohol intake are risk factors for osteoporosis. Regular consumption of 2 to 3 ounces of alcohol a day may increase the degree of osteoporosis, even in young men and women. Patients should be instructed to quit smoking and cut down on alcohol intake to decrease the likelihood of losing bone mass.

Although loss of bone cannot be significantly reversed, further loss can be prevented if the patient follows a regimen of calcium and vitamin D supplementation, exercise, estrogen replacement, and alendronate (Fosamax) or raloxifene (Evista), if indicated. Efforts should be made to keep patients with osteoporosis ambulatory to prevent further loss of bone substance as a result of immobility. Treatment also involves protecting areas of potential pathologic fractures; for example, a corset can be used to prevent vertebral collapse.

Drug Therapy. Estrogen replacement therapy after menopause is used to prevent osteoporosis. Although the exact mechanism for the protective function of estrogen is not known, it is believed that estrogen inhibits osteoclast activity, leading to decreased bone resorption and preventing both cortical and trabecular bone loss. Estrogen replacement therapy is most effective when combined with calcium. The greatest benefit of estrogen is probably in the first 10 years after menopause. Transdermal estrogen treatment has been shown to be effective in the treatment of postmenopausal women with established osteoporosis. (See Chapter 51 for further discussion of estrogen replacement therapy.)

Calcitonin is secreted by the thyroid gland and inhibits osteoclastic bone resorption by directly interacting with active

Table 59-26	Elemental Calcium Content of Various Oral Calcium Preparations
Calcium Preparation	**Elemental Calcium Content**
Calcium carbonate (Tums 500)	500 mg/tablet
Calcium carbonate + 5 μg vitamin D₂ (Os-Cal 250)	250 mg/tablet
Calcium gluconate	40 mg/500 mg
Calcium carbonate	400 mg/g
Calcium lactate	80 mg/600 mg
Calcium citrate	40 mg/300 mg

osteoclasts. Calcitonin (Calcimar) is available as intramuscular, subcutaneous, and intranasal forms. The nasal form is easy to administer, and patients should be taught to alternate nostrils daily. Nasal dryness and irritation are the most frequent side effects. Administration of the intramuscular or subcutaneous form of the medication at night has been shown to decrease the side effects of nausea and facial flushing. Nausea does not occur with the nasal spray. When calcitonin is used, calcium supplementation is necessary to prevent secondary hyperparathyroidism.[42]

Biphosphonates inhibit osteoclast-mediated bone resorption, thereby increasing bone mineral density and total bone mass.[44] This group of drugs includes etidronate (Didronel), alendronate (Fosamax), pamidronate (Aredia), risendronate (Actonel), clodronate (Bonefos), and tiludronate (Skelid). The most commonly used biphosphonate drug in treating osteoporosis is alendronate. Patients should be instructed on the proper administration of alendronate to aid in its absorption. It should be taken after rising in the morning with a full glass of water. The patient should not eat or drink anything for 30 minutes after taking it. The patient should also be instructed not to lie down after taking the medication. These precautions have been proven to decrease gastrointestinal side effects (especially esophageal irritation) and increase absorption.

Another type of drug used in treating osteoporosis is selective estrogen receptor modulators, such as raloxifene (Evista). This drug mimics the effect of estrogen on bone by reducing bone resorption without stimulating the tissues of the breast or uterus. Raloxifene in postmenopausal women significantly increases bone mineral density.[47] The most commonly reported side effects are leg cramps and hot flashes. Unlike estrogen, it does not relieve menopausal symptoms or have a cardiovascular protective function.

Medical management of patients receiving corticosteroids includes prescribing the lowest possible dose of the drug, as well as calcium and vitamin D supplementation and estrogen replacement in postmenopausal women. If osteopenia is evident on bone densitometry, treatment with bisphosphonate agents, such as alendronate (Fosamax), should be considered.

PAGET'S DISEASE

Paget's disease (osteitis deformans) is a skeletal bone disorder in which there is excessive bone resorption followed by replacement of normal marrow by vascular, fibrous connective tissue and new bone that is larger, disorganized, and weaker. It occurs most often after the fourth decade of life and most commonly in men. It is characterized by deformities of bone caused by un-

explained abnormal focal remodeling and resorption of bone, fibrotic changes, and remodeling with structurally uneven bone. The regions of the skeleton commonly affected are the pelvis, long bones, spine, ribs, sternum, and cranium. The cause of Paget's disease is unknown, although a viral etiology has been proposed.[48]

In milder forms of Paget's disease, patients may remain free of symptoms, and the disease may be discovered incidentally on x-ray or serum chemistry. The initial clinical manifestations are usually insidious development of skeletal pain (which may progress to severe intractable pain), complaints of fatigue, and progressive development of a waddling gait. Patients may complain that they are becoming shorter or that their heads are becoming larger. Serum alkaline phosphatase levels are markedly elevated in advanced forms of the disease. X-rays may demonstrate that the normal contour of the affected bone is curved and the bone cortex is thickened, especially the weight-bearing bones and cranium. Pathologic fracture is the most common complication of Paget's disease and may be the first indication of the disease. Other complications include malignant osteosarcoma, fibrosarcoma, and benign giant cell tumors.

Collaborative care of Paget's disease is usually limited to symptomatic and supportive care and correction of secondary deformities by either surgical implementation or braces. Bone resorption, relief of acute symptoms, and lowering the serum alkaline phosphatase levels may be significantly influenced by the administration of calcitonin, which inhibits osteoclastic activity. Response to calcitonin therapy is not permanent and often stops when therapy is discontinued.[48] Biphosphonates, such as alendronate (Fosamax), tiludronate (Skelid), risedronate (Actonel) and pamidronate (Aredia), are nonhormonal agents that are effective in reducing the bone resorption in Paget's disease.[48] Radiation therapy and local surgical procedures such as periosteal stripping may be used for the control of the patient's pain.

A firm mattress should be used to provide back support and to relieve pain. The patient may be required to wear a corset or light brace to relieve back pain and provide support when in the upright position. The patient should be proficient in the correct application of such devices and know how to regularly examine areas of the skin for friction damage. Activities such as lifting and twisting should be discouraged. Good body mechanics are essential. Analgesics and muscle relaxants may be administered to relieve pain. A properly balanced nutritional program is important in the management of metabolic disorders of bone, especially pertaining to vitamin D, calcium, and protein, which are necessary to ensure the availability of the components for bone formation. Prevention measures such as patient education, use of an assistive device, and environmental changes should be actively pursued to prevent falls and subsequent fractures.

GERONTOLOGIC CONSIDERATIONS

Metabolic Bone Diseases

Osteoporosis and Paget's disease are common in older adults. Patients should be instructed in proper nutritional management to prevent further bone loss such as that occurring from osteoporosis.

Because metabolic bone disorders increase the possibility of pathologic fractures, the nurse must use extreme caution when the patient is turned or moved. It is important to keep the

CRITICAL THINKING EXERCISES

CASE STUDY

Osteoporosis

Patient Profile

Mrs. Green is a 52-year-old cafeteria worker who had a total hysterectomy and salpingo-oophorectomy for removal of a benign ovarian cyst 3 years ago.

Subjective Data

- Experiences chronic, mild lumbar pain and tenderness that radiates to her right hip and the lateral thigh
- Had a stress fracture in wrist 6 months ago
- Regular walking offers some relief
- Reports no noticeable loss of height
- Has maternal history of osteoporosis
- On corticosteroids past 6 years for Addison's disease
- Drinks socially—two alcoholic beverages per day
- Dislikes dairy products

Objective Data

- Is Asian-American, 5 ft 6 in tall, 116 lb

Diagnostic Studies

- Bone mass/density tests show decreased bone mineral density at spine and hip
- Laboratory tests reveal normal serum calcium, phosphorus, and alkaline phosphatase levels

Collaborative and Nursing Management

- Conjugated equinine estrogen—0.625 mg PO daily
- Alendronate (Fosamax)—10 mg PO daily
- Calcium supplements—1200 mg PO daily
- Increase calcium intake from food
- Reduce alcohol intake
- Maintain regular exercise program

Critical Thinking Questions

1. What risk factors made Mrs. Green prone to develop osteoporosis?
2. Why does regular exercise help Mrs. Green's symptoms?
3. What is the purpose of prescribing estrogen replacement for Mrs. Green?
4. What educational teaching should the nurse provide to Mrs. Green regarding alendronate?
5. How might the nurse assist Mrs. Green in increasing her intake of calcium?
6. Based on the assessment data presented, write one or more nursing diagnoses. Are there any collaborative problems?

NURSING RESEARCH ISSUES

1. What is the most effective technique of providing pin care for a patient in skeletal traction?
2. What body image and self-concept issues does a patient who has undergone an amputation experience?
3. Are casual and weekend athletes using proper protective gear to prevent injury? How compliant are these individuals?
4. Have postoperative orthopedic complications (e.g., deep vein thrombosis, dislocations) increased with shorter length of hospital stay?
5. Do nurses' pain medication–dispensing behaviors change in relation to the orthopedic patient's mental status: alert (able to communicate needs) versus demented (unable to communicate needs)?
6. What home health nursing interventions are most effective for increasing mobility in the patient recovering from a hip fracture?
7. Do nurses recognize the signs and symptoms of fat embolism and acute compartment syndrome?
8. What factors are important for the nurse to address in helping an adolescent female increase her calcium intake?

patient as active as possible to retard demineralization of bone resulting from disuse or extended immobilization. A supervised exercise program is an essential part of the treatment program. If the patient's condition permits, ambulation without causing fatigue must be encouraged.

REVIEW QUESTIONS

The number of the question corresponds to the same-numbered objective at the beginning of the chapter.

1. The nurse suspects an ankle sprain when a patient at the urgent care center
   a. is hit by another soccer player on the field.
   b. has ankle pain after running a 10-mile race.
   c. drops a 10 lb weight on his lower leg at the health club.
   d. has a twisting injury while running bases during a baseball game.
2. The nurse explains to a patient with a distal tibial fracture returning for a 3-week checkup that healing is indicated by
   a. callus formation.
   b. complete union of bone.
   c. presence of granulation tissue.
   d. formation of a hematoma at the fracture site.
3. A patient with a stable, closed fracture of the humerus caused by trauma to the arm has a temporary splint with bulky padding applied with an elastic bandage. The nurse suspects compartment syndrome and notifies the physician when the patient experiences
   a. pain at the fracture site.
   b. increasing edema of the limb.
   c. muscle spasms of the lower arm.
   d. pain when the nurse passively extends the fingers.
4. A patient with a comminuted fracture of the femur is to have an open reduction with internal fixation (ORIF) of the fracture. The nurse explains that ORIF is indicated when
   a. a cast would be too large to provide normal mobility.
   b. the patient is able to tolerate long-term immobilization.
   c. adequate alignment cannot be obtained by other methods.
   d. the patient cannot tolerate the discomfort of a closed reduction.

5. An indication of a neurovascular problem noted during assessment of the patient with a fracture is
   a. exaggeration of extremity movement.
   b. petechiae on the head and upper thorax.
   c. purulent drainage at the site of an open fracture.
   d. decreased sensation distal to the fracture site.

6. A patient with symphysis pubis and pelvic rami fractures should be monitored for
   a. sudden thirst.
   b. changes in urinary output.
   c. a palpable lump in the buttock.
   d. sudden decrease in blood pressure.

7. A patient with osteomyelitis is treated with surgical debridement followed by continuous irrigation of the affected bone with antibiotics. In responding to the patient who asks why oral or IV antibiotics cannot be used alone, the nurse explains that
   a. the irrigation is necessary to wash out dead tissue and pus from the infected area.
   b. the ischemia and bone death associated with osteomyelitis is frequently impenetrable to most antibiotics carried by the blood.
   c. there are not effective oral or IV antibiotics to treat *S. aureus,* the most common cause of osteomyelitis.
   d. an irrigation can penetrate involucrum created by the infection and prevent bacterial seeding to other tissue.

8. During the postoperative period, the patient with an above-the-knee amputation should be instructed that the residual limb should not be routinely elevated because
   a. the flexed position can promote hip flexion contracture.
   b. this position reduces the development of phantom pain.
   c. this position promotes clot formation at the incision site and thigh.
   d. unnecessary movement of the extremity can cause wound dehiscence.

9. A patient with an osteogenic sarcoma of the left femur has a nursing diagnosis of risk for injury: pathologic fracture related to bone tissue changes. The nursing management of this patient is primarily directed toward
   a. preventing pain.
   b. relieving edema.
   c. increasing physical mobility.
   d. supporting and positioning the leg.

10. In identifying people at risk for back injuries the nurse recognizes that the person at greatest risk for low back pain is a
   a. long-distance truck driver.
   b. 100 lb aerobics instructor.
   c. 62-year-old widow who walks daily.
   d. 25-year-old newborn nursery nurse.

11. The primary nursing responsibility in caring for a patient with acute low back pain associated with severe pain and muscle spasms is
   a. positioning the patient on the abdomen with the legs extended.
   b. teaching exercises such as straight-leg raises to decrease pain.
   c. providing pain medication to promote exercise and ambulation.
   d. assisting the patient to maintain activity restrictions with a gradual increase in activity.

12. In caring for the patient after a spinal fusion, the nurse recognizes that interventions for this surgery differ from a simple laminectomy in that
   a. body alignment is maintained by the fusion procedure.
   b. earlier ambulation is permitted because the spine is more stabilized.

   c. the donor site for the bone graft may be more painful than the spinal incision.
   d. teaching regarding body mechanics and prevention of future back injuries is not as critical.

13. Before discharge from the same-day surgery unit, the nurse instructs the patient who has had a surgical correction of bilateral hallux valgus to
   a. rest frequently with the feet elevated.
   b. soak the feet in warm water several times a day.
   c. walk primarily on the heels to relieve pressure on the toes.
   d. expect the feet to be numb for several days postoperatively.

14. The nurse advises the patient with early osteoporosis to
   a. lose weight.
   b. stop smoking.
   c. eat a high-protein diet.
   d. start swimming for exercise.

References

1. Best TM: Soft tissue injuries and muscle tears, *Clin Sports Med* 16:419, 1997.
2. Jobe FW and others, editors: *Operative techniques in upper extremity sports injuries,* St Louis, 1996, Mosby.
3. English CJ and others: Relations between upper limb soft tissue disorders and repetitive movements at work, *Am J Ind Med* 27:75, 1995.
4. Brogmus GE, Sorock GS, Webster BS: Recent trends in work-related cumulative trauma disorders of the upper extremities in the United States: an evaluation of possible reasons, *J Environ Med* 38:401, 1996.
*5. Heveron B, Kaempffe FA: Tears of the rotator cuff, *Orthop Nurs* 14:38, 1995.
6. Mayo Clinic: Rotator cuff injuries, *Mayo Clin Health Lett* 16:1, 1998.
7. Guckel C, Nidecker A: Diagnosis of tears in rotator cuff injuries, *Eur J Radiol* 25:168, 1997.
8. McFarland EG and others: Shoulder immobilization devices, *Orthop Nurs* 16:66, 1997.
9. Verdonk R: Alternative treatments for meniscal injuries, *J Bone Joint Surg Br* 79:866, 1997.
10. Scott G, King JB: A prospective double-blind trial of electrical capacitive coupling in the treatment of non-union of long bones, *J Bone Joint Surg* 76A:820, 1994.
11. Brighton CT and others: Tibial nonunion treated with direct current, capacitive coupling of bone graft, *Clin Orthop Relat Res* 321:223, 1995.
12. Salmond SW, Mooney NE, Verdisco LA, editors: *NAON core curriculum for orthopaedic nursing,* ed 3, Pitman, NJ, 1996, Anthony Jannetti.
13. Wilson SC and others: A simple method to measure compartment pressures using an intravenous catheter, *Orthopedics* 20:403, 1997.
14. Resnick D, Goergen T, Pathria M: Traumatic, iatrogenic, and neurogenic diseases. In Resnick D, editor: *Bone and joint imaging,* ed 2, Philadelphia, 1996, Saunders.
15. Gwynne DP, Theis J: Acute compartment syndrome due to closed muscle rupture, *Aust N Z J Surg* 67:227, 1997.
16. Thelan L and others, editors: *Critical care nursing diagnosis and management,* ed 3, St Louis, 1998, Mosby.
17. Colwell CW and others: Efficacy and safety of enoxaparin versus unfractionated heparin for prevention of deep venous thrombosis after elective knee arthroplasty, *Clin Orthop Relat Res* 321:19, 1995.
18. Johnson MJ, Lucas GL: Fat embolism syndrome, *Orthopedics* 19:41, 1996.
19. Hager CA, Brncick N: Fat embolism syndrome: a complication of orthopaedic trauma, *Orthop Nurs* 17:41, 1998.
20. Richards RR: Fat embolism syndrome, *Can J Surg* 40:334, 1997.
21. Bulger EM and others: Fat embolism syndrome: A 10-year review, *Arch Surg* 132:435, 1997.
22. Mayo Clinic: Hip fractures, *Mayo Clin Health Lett* 16:2, 1998.
23. Ebersole P, Hess P, editors: *Toward healthy aging: human needs and nursing response,* ed 5, St Louis, 1998, Mosby.
24. Reichel W, editor: *Care of the elderly: clinical aspects of aging,* ed 4, Baltimore, 1995, Williams & Wilkins.

25. Magee D: *Orthopedic physical assessment,* ed 3, Philadelphia, 1997, Saunders.
26. Feliciano DV, Moore EE, Mattox KL, editors: *Trauma,* ed 3, Stamford, Conn, 1996, Appleton & Lange.
27. Reese RE, Betts RF, editors: *A practical approach to infectious diseases,* ed 4, Boston, 1996, Little, Brown.
28. Hellman D: Arthritis and musculoskeletal disorders. In Tierney L, McPhee S, Papadakis M, editors: *Medical diagnosis and treatment,* ed 36, Stanford, Conn, 1997, Appleton & Lange.
29. Keen J, Swearingen P: *Critical care nursing consultant,* St Louis, 1997, Mosby.
30. Mourad L: Alterations of musculoskeletal function. In McCance KL, Huether SE, editors: *Pathophysiology: the biologic basis for disease in adults and children,* ed 3, St Louis, 1998, Mosby.
31. Yetzer EA: Helping the patient through the experience of an amputation, *Orthop Nurs* 15:45, 1996.
32. Wiernik PH and others, editors: *Neoplastic diseases of the blood,* ed 3, New York, 1996, Churchill Livingstone.
33. Vander Griend RA: Osteosarcoma and its variants, *Orthop Clin North Am* 27:575, 1996.
34. Vlasak R, Sim FH: Ewing's sarcoma, *Orthop Clin North Am* 27:591, 1996.
35. Kuritzky L: Steps in the management of low back pain, *Hosp Pract* 31:109, 1996.
36. Chase J: Outpatient management of low back pain, *Orthop Nurs* 11:11, 1992.
37. Leboeuf-Yde C, Yashin A, Lauritzen T: Does smoking cause low back pain? Results from a population-based study, *J Manipulative Physiol Ther* 19:99, 1996.
38. Nerubay J, Caspi I, Levinkopf M: Percutaneous carbon dioxide laser nucleolysis with 2- to 5-year followup, *Clin Orthop Relat Res* 337:45, 1997.
39. Bigos S, Nordin M, Leger D: Treatment of the acutely injured worker. In Nordin M, Andersson G, Pope M, editors: *Musculoskeletal disorders in the work place, principles and practice,* St Louis, 1997, Mosby.
*40. Hunt AH: The relationship between height change and bone mineral density, *Orthop Nurs* 15:57, 1996.
41. Kessenich CR, Rosen CJ: Vitamin D and bone status in elderly women, *Orthop Nurs* 15:67, 1996.
42. Kessenich C: Preventing and managing osteoporosis, *AJN* 97:16B, 1997.
43. Tucci JR and others: Effect of three years of oral alendronate treatment in postmenopausal women with osteoporosis, *Am J Med* 101:488, 1996.
44. Jackson R: Forestalling fracture in osteoporosis, *Hosp Pract* 32:77, 1997.
45. Vandevyver C and others: Influence of the vitamin D receptor gene alleles on bone mineral density in postmenopausal and osteoporotic women, *J Bone Mineral Res* 12:241, 1997.
46. Barzel U: Osteoporosis: taking a fresh look, *Hosp Pract* 31:59, 1996.
47. Balfour JA and others: Raloxifene, *Drugs Aging* 12:335, 1998.
48. Weinstein R: Advances in the treatment of Paget's bone disease, *Hosp Pract* 32:63, 1997.

*Nursing research-based article.

Resources

American Academy of Orthopedic Surgeons
6300 North River Road
Rosemont, IL 60018-4262
847-823-7186
800-346-AAOS
Fax: 847-823-8125
http://www.aaos.org

American College of Sports Medicine
PO Box 1440
401 W Michigan Street
Indianapolis, IN 46202
317-637-9200
Fax: 317-634-7817
http://www.acsm.org

Amputees In Motion
PO Box 2703
Escondido, CA 92033
619-454-9300
http://www.usinter.net/wasa/sandiego1.html

Calcium Information Center
Clinical Nutrition and Research Unit
Division of Nephrology, Hypertension, and Clinical Pharmacology
Oregon Health Sciences University
3314 SW U.S. Veterans Hospital Road
Portland, OR 97201
800-321-2681

Muscular Dystrophy Association
3561 East Sunrise Avenue
Tucson, AZ 85718
602-529-2000
http://www.mdausa.org/

National Amputation Foundation
38-40 Church St
Malverne, NY 11565
516-887-3600
http://www.va.gov/vso/naf.htm

National Arthritis/Musculoskeletal and Skin Diseases Information Clearinghouse
9000 Rockville Pike
Bethesda, MD 20892-2350
800-283-7800
http://www.nih.gov/niams/

National Association of Orthopaedic Nurses, Inc. (NAON)
East Holly Avenue
Box 56
Pitman, NJ 08071-0056
609-256-2310
Fax: 609-589-7463
naon@mail.ajj.com
http://naon.inurse.com

National Easter Seal Society
70 East Lake Street
Chicago, IL 60601
312-726-6200
http://www.easter-seals.org

National Fibromyalgia Research Association
PO Box 500
Salem, OR 97302
http://www.teleport.com/~nfra/

National Osteoporosis Foundation
1150—17th Street NW, Suite 500
Washington, DC 20036-4603
202-223-2226
800-223-9994
http://www.nof.org/

Older Women's League
666 Eleventh Street SW, Suite 700
Washington, DC 20001
202-783-6686
800-TAKE-OWL
http://www.womenconnect.com/

For additional Internet resources, see the website for this book at **www.mosby.com/MERLIN/medsurg_lewis**

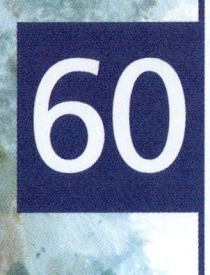
NURSING MANAGEMENT

60

Arthritis and Connective Tissue Diseases

Melissa Bush

www.mosby.com/MERLIN/medsurg_lewis

LEARNING OBJECTIVES

1. Describe the pathophysiology, clinical manifestations, and collaborative care of osteoarthritis, rheumatoid arthritis, gout, systemic lupus erythematosus, and systemic sclerosis.
2. Describe the clinical manifestations and management of juvenile rheumatoid arthritis, human leukocyte antigen–associated rheumatic diseases, septic arthritis, polymyositis, dermatomyositis, and fibromyalgia.
3. Compare and contrast the sequence of events leading to joint destruction in osteoarthritis and rheumatoid arthritis.
4. Compare and contrast osteoarthritis with rheumatoid arthritis related to clinical manifestations, treatment, and prognosis.
5. Identify the nursing management of arthritis and related rheumatic disorders.
6. Describe the types of reconstructive surgery associated with arthritis and related rheumatic disorders.
7. Identify the preoperative and postoperative teaching and collaborative care of the patient having reconstructive surgery associated with arthritis and related rheumatic disorders.
8. Describe the drug therapy and related nursing considerations associated with arthritis and related rheumatic disorders.
9. Identify psychologic and sociocultural issues of the patient with rheumatic disease and the appropriate nursing strategies that meet these needs.
10. Identify the importance of the interdisciplinary team approach to comprehensive management of rheumatic disorders.

OSTEOARTHRITIS

Osteoarthritis (OA), also known as *degenerative joint disease* (DJD), is a slowly progressive disorder of articulating joints, particularly weight-bearing joints, and is characterized by degeneration of articular cartilage. The damage from OA is confined to the joints and surrounding tissues. Clinical manifestations include joint pain, stiffness, and limited range of motion (ROM). Radiographically, the disease is characterized by joint-space narrowing, subchondral sclerosis, and osteophyte (bony outgrowth) formation. There is a wide spectrum of disease severity, ranging from annoying and uncomfortable symptoms to significantly disabling disease.

The most significant risk factor for OA is age. It is estimated that nearly one third of all adults have x-ray evidence of degenerative joint disease, with the incidence increasing to 60% to 80% by age 60. Because only one half of these adults experience significant symptoms, joint pain and functional disability should not be considered a normal finding in aging persons.

Reviewed by Debra A. Bancroft, RN, MSN, FNP-C, Nurse Practitioner, Rheumatic Disease Center, Milwaukee, Wisc; and Sharon G. Childs, RN, MS, CRNP, CS, CEN, ONC, Orthopedic Clinical Specialist, Johns Hopkins Hospital, Assistant Professor, Johns Hopkins University, Baltimore, Md.

OA is generally distributed throughout the peripheral and central joints.[2]

Etiology and Pathophysiology

OA may occur as a primary idiopathic or secondary disorder.[1] The cause of primary OA is unknown. Although both primary and secondary OA are influenced by multiple factors (e.g., metabolic, mechanical, genetic, chemical), secondary OA has an identifiable precipitating event, such as previous trauma, fractures, infection, or congenital deformities, that is believed to predispose the person to later degenerative changes.

Degenerative changes over time cause the normally smooth, white, translucent joint cartilage to become yellow and opaque, with rough surfaces and areas of malacia (softening). As the layers of cartilage become thinner, bony surfaces are drawn closer together. As the cartilage breaks down, fissures may appear and fragments of cartilage become loose. Inflammation of the synovial membrane secondary to cartilage breakdown may follow. As the articular surface becomes totally denuded of cartilage, subchondral bone increases in density and becomes sclerotic (eburnated). New bone outgrowths (osteophytes) are formed at joint margins and at the attachment sites of ligaments and tendons.

There are several possible causes for cartilage deterioration, which is an active process. The enzyme hyaluronidase, which is normally found in the synovial fluid, may be responsible for digestion of proteoglycans via cracks in the surface layer of articular cartilage. Another possible cause is that inadequate nutrition of the cartilage may result in cartilage degeneration. Because cartilage is avascular, nutrients are provided by the synovial fluid. DNA synthesis, which is normally absent in adult articular cartilage, is active in OA tissue and appears to be directly proportional to disease severity.[3]

Specific predisposing factors such as excessive use of or stress on a joint have been identified as accelerating osteoarthritic changes (e.g., in the knees of football players and the feet and ankles of ballet dancers). Genetic factors influence the development of Heberden's nodes, which involve a single autosomal gene, dominant in women and recessive in men. (Heberden's nodes are discussed later.)

Other factors that influence the development of OA include congenital structural defects (e.g., Legg-Calvé-Perthes disease [osteochrondritis of head of femur in children]), metabolic disturbances (e.g., diabetes mellitus, acromegaly), repeated intraarticular hemorrhage (e.g., hemophilia), neuropathic arthropathies (Charcot's joints), and inflammatory and septic arthritis.

Clinical Manifestations

Systemic. Systemic manifestations, such as fatigue or fever, are not present in OA. Other organ involvement is absent as well, which is an important differentiation between OA and inflammatory joint disorders such as rheumatoid arthritis.[4]

Joints. Articular manifestations are related to the particular joint involved. The patient has pain on motion and weight bearing that is generally relieved by rest. In advanced disease, sleep may be disrupted by joint pain. As cartilage (which does not contain nerve endings) is worn away, direct irritation and pressure occur on the nerves of subchondral bone. Pain is most often caused by swelling and stretching of soft tissue structures surrounding the joint and not by the arthritic joint itself. Increasing pain is accompanied by progressive loss of function. Overall body coordination and posture may be affected as a result of the pain and loss of mobility.

Unlike pain, which is typically provoked by activity, joint stiffness occurs after periods of rest or static position. The symptoms related to OA are often aggravated by rising humidity and falling barometric pressure. Crepitation (grating sensation caused by the rubbing together of abnormal joint surfaces) on motion and malalignment of the extremity may be noted on physical examination. Advanced disease is characterized by

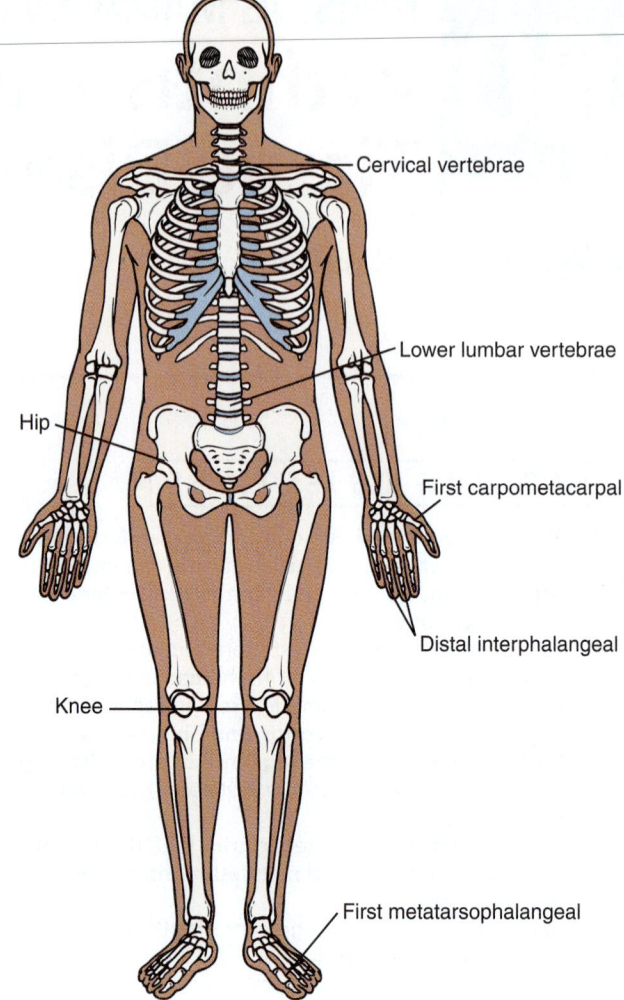

Fig. 60-1 Joints most frequently involved in osteoarthritis.

gross deformity and subluxation (partial dislocation) caused by deterioration of cartilage, collapse of subchondral bone, and extensive bony overgrowth.

Joints are usually affected asymmetrically. The joints most frequently involved are the distal and proximal interphalangeal joints of the fingers, first carpometacarpal joint, hips, knees, first metatarsophalangeal joint, and lower lumbar and cervical vertebrae (Fig. 60-1). Degenerative changes are rarely seen in metacarpophalangeal joints, elbows, or shoulders.

Nodules. Heberden's nodes are another common manifestation of OA, particularly in women with primary OA. These nodes are reactive bony overgrowths located at the distal interphalangeal joints (Fig. 60-2). Heberden's nodes are palpable protuberances that are often associated with flexion and lateral deviation of the distal phalanx, occur more frequently in women, and tend to appear in families. Bouchard's nodes, seen less commonly in OA, involve the proximal interphalangeal joints.

Heberden's nodes and Bouchard's nodes may cause redness, swelling, tenderness, and aching. They often begin in one finger and spread to others. Although there is usually no significant loss of function caused by the bony enlargements, the patient is often distressed by the resulting disfigurement of the hands. Little can be done to prevent the occurrence of these nodes.

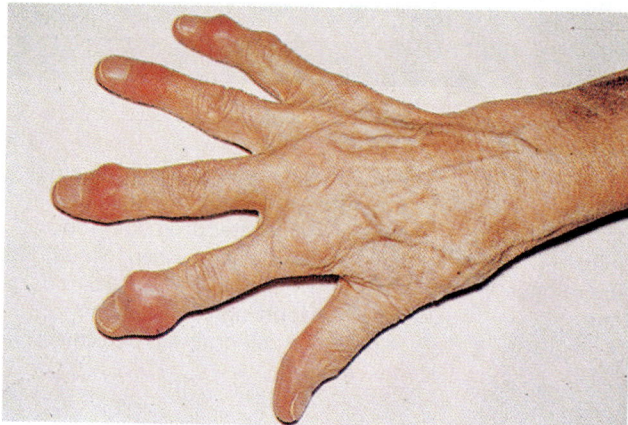

Fig. 60-2   Heberden's nodes.

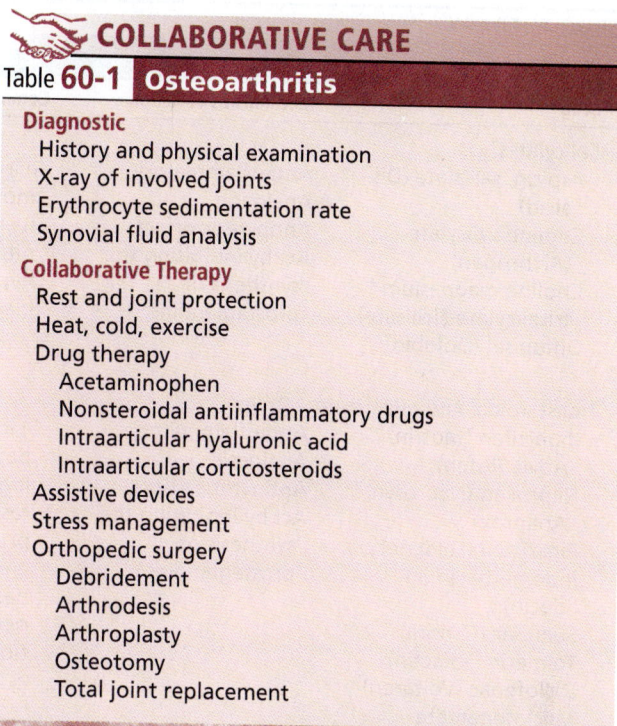

🤝 **COLLABORATIVE CARE**

Table **60-1**   **Osteoarthritis**

Diagnostic
  History and physical examination
  X-ray of involved joints
  Erythrocyte sedimentation rate
  Synovial fluid analysis
Collaborative Therapy
  Rest and joint protection
  Heat, cold, exercise
  Drug therapy
    Acetaminophen
    Nonsteroidal antiinflammatory drugs
    Intraarticular hyaluronic acid
    Intraarticular corticosteroids
  Assistive devices
  Stress management
  Orthopedic surgery
    Debridement
    Arthrodesis
    Arthroplasty
    Osteotomy
    Total joint replacement

Hips.   OA of the hips may be extremely disabling. Congenital or structural abnormalities are frequent causes. This problem occurs more frequently in men than in women and may be unilateral or bilateral. Hip pain may be perceived as pain in the groin, buttock, or medial side of the thigh or knee, so the patient may find it difficult to localize the problem correctly. Pain on motion or on weight bearing may become progressively severe, and pain on rest may ensue. Sitting down is difficult, as is rising from a chair when the hips are lower than the knees. The patient learns to sit in a high seat with firm support and arm rests. Eventually, loss of ROM is significant, with pronounced limitation of extension and internal rotation.

Knees.   Softening of the posterior surface of the patella (chondromalacia patellae) is seen most commonly in young people. Degeneration of the weight-bearing surfaces of the femoral and tibial condyles is usually seen in older women and is associated with limitation of motion, crepitus, and flexion deformity. Obesity has been implicated in OA of the knee in women, which is possibly the result of mechanical stress.

Vertebral Column.   OA in the spine may produce localized symptoms of stiffness and pain. Degenerative disease of the intervertebral disks results as the nucleus pulposus deteriorates, becoming brittle and inelastic. Herniation of the degenerating nucleus most often occurs posteriorly or laterally, compressing a nerve root and causing muscle spasm or radicular pain. Another type of OA of the vertebral column involves development of degenerative disease of the intervertebral (apophyseal) joints, which generally follows disk disease by a number of years. Marginal osteophytes (spurs) also appear at vertebral attachments of the anulus, periosteum, and longitudinal ligaments. These osteophytes may fuse and limit ROM, or they may press against intervertebral foramina, producing symptoms of nerve root compression. Although rare, osteophyte formation in the posterior aspect of the cervical spine may produce vascular compression on the vertebrobasilar arteriole system producing insufficiency, resulting in intermittent dizziness, visual disturbances, headaches, and ataxia.

Diagnostic Studies

In late OA disease, x-rays show joint space narrowing, bony sclerosis, spur formation, and subluxation in some cases. X-ray changes do not always correlate with the degree of pain experienced by the patient. The patient may be completely free of symptoms, despite significant radiologic joint space narrowing. Conversely, some patients have severe pain with only moderate x-ray changes. No specific laboratory abnormalities are useful in the diagnosis of OA. The erythrocyte sedimentation rate (ESR) is normal except in instances of erosive OA, when moderate ESR elevation may be noted. Synovial fluid aspirated from an involved joint may be increased in volume but is clear yellow and viscous. Analysis of the fluid reveals little or no sign of inflammation.

Collaborative Care

There is no specific treatment for OA. Therapy is aimed at pain control, prevention of progression and disability, and restoration of joint function (Table 60-1). Once the diagnosis is confirmed, the patient should be assured that OA is likely to remain confined to a few joints and does not generally cause crippling. However, if joint destruction is extensive and pain is severe, surgery may be an option. Possible surgical procedures are listed in Table 60-1.

Drug Therapy.   New guidelines for the management of OA were developed in 1995.[5,6] First-line therapy starts with acetaminophen 1 g up to four times daily. Topical agents such as capsaicin cream may be used alone or in conjunction with acetaminophen. This cream, made from chili peppers, causes depletion of substance P from nerve endings, thus blocking pain signals to the brain. Various strengths are available and must be used regularly for maximal effect. A generally short-lived burning sensation may accompany initial use. If response to these methods is suboptimal, low-dose ibuprofen (Motrin, Advil) 400 mg up to four times daily or nonacetylated salicylates are subsequently used.

Second-line therapy used in OA consists of nonsteroidal antiinflammatory drugs (NSAIDs) at full doses (Table 60-2). NSAIDs block the production of prostaglandins from arachidonic acid by inhibiting the production of cyclooxygenase (COX) (see Fig. 11-7). Concerns have been raised regarding

DRUG THERAPY

Table 60-2 Rheumatic Disorders

Drug	Mechanisms of Action	Common Side Effects	Nursing Considerations
Salicylates Aspirin, salsalate (Disalcid) Choline salicylate (Arthropan) Choline magnesium trisalicylate (Trilisate) Diflunisal (Dolobid)	Antiinflammatory Analgesic Antipyretic effect Act by inhibiting the synthesis of prostaglandins*	GI irritation (ulcer and hemorrhage), hypersensitivity, salicylism (nausea, tinnitus, dizziness, hyperpnea), prolonged bleeding time	When drug is taken for antiinflammatory effect, discontinue if pain decreases. Administer drug with food, milk, antacids as prescribed, or full glass of water or use enteric-coated aspirin. Report signs of bleeding (e.g, tarry stool, bruising, petechiae, melena).
Nonsteroidal Antiinflammatory Drugs Ibuprofen (Motrin, Advil, Rufen) Naproxen (Naprosyn, Anaprox) Piroxicam (Feldene) Indomethacin (Indocin) Sulindac (Clinoril) Tolmetin (Tolectin) Diclofenac (Voltaren) Meclofenamate (Meclomen) Celecoxib (Celebrex)[†] Rofecoxib (Vioxx)[†]	Antiinflammatory Analgesic Antipyretic effect Act by inhibiting the synthesis of prostaglandins*	GI irritation, including dyspepsia, nausea and vomiting, GI bleeding, dizziness, rash, headache, tinnitus, prolonged bleeding time, elevated serum transaminases, drug-induced nephrotoxicity, exacerbation of asthma	Administer drug with food, milk, or antacids as prescribed. Report signs of bleeding, edema, skin rashes, persistent headaches, or visual disturbances. Monitor elevations in BP.
Nonnarcotic Analgesics Acetaminophen (Tylenol)	Analgesic Antipyretic effect	Rash, urticaria, hepatotoxicity, leukopenia	Advise patient that concomitant use of alcohol may cause liver damage. Teach patient not to exceed recommended dosage.
Capsaicin cream (Zostrix, Capzacin P)	Topical analgesic, depletes substance P from nerve endings thereby interrupting pain signals to the brain	Localized burning sensation, erythema	Must be used regularly over time for maximal effect. Aloe vera cream may moderate burning sensation. Fatty substance such as butter or milk will deactivate action of cream. Available in several strengths.
Tramadol (Ultram)	Analgesic, centrally acting, binds to opioid receptors	Dizziness, nausea, constipation, headache, GI bleeding, somnolence, vomiting, pruritus, dyspepsia	Not recommended with concomitant MAO inhibitors. Advise patient to make position changes slowly, because orthostatic hypotension may occur. May potentiate seizure risk with MAO inhibitors, tricyclics, or neuroleptics. Administer with antiemetic to prevent nausea and vomiting.
Narcotic Analgesics Propoxyphene with acetaminophen or aspirin (Darvocet, Darvon) Codeine with acetaminophen or aspirin (Tylenol #3 or #4, Empirin #3 or #4) Hydrocodone with acetaminophen or aspirin (Lorcet, Lortab, Vicodin) Oxycodone with acetaminophen or aspirin (Oxycontin, Percodan, Percocet, Tylox)	Analgesic	Constipation, arrhythmias, dizziness, sedation, nausea, headache, vomiting, rash; respiratory depression or hepatotoxicity with overdosage	Advise patient regarding potential for constipation. Report signs of bleeding with products containing aspirin. Monitor CBC and liver function tests. Administer with antiemetic if nausea occurs. Teach patient and family to report any CNS or respiratory changes.

Continued

DRUG THERAPY

Table **60-2** **Rheumatic Disorders—cont'd**

Drug	Mechanisms of Action	Common Side Effects	Nursing Considerations
Corticosteroids			
Intraarticular Injections			
Methylprednisolone acetate (Depo-Medrol) Triamcinolone (Aristospan)	Antiinflammatory Analgesic Act by inhibiting the synthesis of prostaglandins*	Local osteoporosis, tendon rupture, and neuropathic arthropathy from repeated injection. Possibility of local infection.	Use strict aseptic technique as joint fluid is removed and corticosteroids are injected. Inform patient that joint may feel worse immediately after injection. Inform patient that improvement lasts weeks to months after injection and that weight bearing should be minimized for 2-6 wk after injection.
Systemic			
Hydrocortisone sodium succinate (Solu-Cortef) Methylprednisolone succinate sodium (Solu-Medrol) Dexamethasone (Decadron) Prednisone Triamcinolone (Aristocort)	Antiinflammatory Analgesic	Cushing's syndrome, including fluid retention, GI irritation, osteoporosis, insomnia, hypertension, psychosis, diabetes mellitus, acne, menstrual irregularities, hirsutism, risk of infection, bruising	Use only when symptoms persist with less potent antiinflammatory drugs or in life-threatening situations. Administer for limited time only, tapering dose slowly. Be aware that exacerbation of symptoms occurs with abrupt withdrawal. Monitor blood pressure, weight, CBC, and potassium. Limit sodium intake. Report signs of infection. Instruct patient to report corticosteroid use to surgeon or dentist to avoid postoperative adrenal insufficiency.
Immunosuppressive Agents			
Azathioprine (Imuran)	Acts as an immunosuppressant by inhibiting purine metabolism and decreasing DNA, RNA, and protein	GI irritation and ulceration, alopecia, oral lesions, dermatitis, blood dyscrasia, bone marrow depression, general increase in susceptibility to infection	Be aware of teratogenic potential that cautions against use for children or women of childbearing age. Monitor CBC, platelets, and urinalysis values. Be aware that drug should be used with great caution in patients with hepatic or renal impairment and should not be used in patients with a history of malignant tumors.
Cyclophosphamide (Cytoxan)	Acts as an immunosuppressant by crosslinking DNA and RNA strands and inhibiting the synthesis of protein	GI irritation and ulceration, alopecia, oral lesions, dermatitis, blood dyscrasia, bone marrow depression, oncogenicity, hemorrhagic cystitis, sterility	Be aware that therapy is limited to patients not responsive to conventional therapy. Monitor CBC, platelets, and urinalysis values. Be aware of teratogenic potential that cautions against use for children or women of childbearing age. Inform patient that contraception should be used during therapy. Use usually limited to treatment of rheumatoid vasculitis.
Cyclosporine (Sandimmune, Neoral)	Acts as an immunosuppressant by inhibiting T lymphocytes	Hypertension, tremor, hepatotoxicity, nephrotoxicity, hyperkalemia, increased susceptibility to infection, nausea, and vomiting	Be aware drug should be used with caution in patients with hepatic or renal impairment. Monitor CBC and liver function tests. Administer with meals for GI upset.

Continued

DRUG THERAPY

Table 60-2   Rheumatic Disorders—cont'd

Drug	Mechanisms of Action	Common Side Effects	Nursing Considerations
Immunosuppressive Agents—cont'd			
Methotrexate (Rheumatrex)	Acts as an immunosuppressant by inhibiting the metabolism of folic acid, thus inhibiting the synthesis of RNA and DNA	GI irritation, photosensitivity, oral lesions, hepatic toxicity, blood dyscrasia, infertility	Monitor CBC, liver function tests, and serum creatinine. Instruct patient to avoid alcoholic beverages and report signs of jaundice. Be aware of teratogenic potential that cautions against use for children or women of childbearing age. Inform patient that contraception should be used during and 3 mo after treatment.
Sulfasalazine (Azulfidine)	Acts as an antiinflammatory/immunosuppressant by causing release of adenosine at sites of inflammation thereby increasing secretion of IL-10 and decreasing T cell function	Rash, yellow-orange skin color, neutropenia, thrombocytopenia, fever, GI irritation, dizziness, photosensitivity, headache, myelosuppression	Monitor CBC and liver function tests. Avoid sun exposure. Also used in patient with inflammatory bowel conditions.
Remission-Inducing Agents			
Chrysotherapy Parenteral Gold sodium thiomalate (Myochrysine) Aurothioglucose (Solganal) Oral Auranofin (Ridaura)	Unknown, inflammatory-suppressive effect, possibly due to inhibition of macrophage function, complement activation, and prostaglandin synthesis	Parenteral: Dermatitis, pruritus, stomatitis, blood dyscrasia, nephrotoxicity, diarrhea Oral: Less toxic than parenteral; GI irritation, mucocutaneous, hematopoietic system, and kidney complications	Parenteral: Test blood and urine regularly. Check urine for blood and protein before each dose and delay injection until negative. Mix drug well and give deep intramuscular injection in buttocks. Inform patient that symptomatic improvement is not expected for 3-6 mo and that therapy may be continued indefinitely. Oral: Institute new oral therapy with bulking agents. Do not taper oral dosage; be aware that laboratory testing is less frequent with oral drug. Instruct women to not become pregnant while receiving chrysotherapy. Less toxic and less effective than parenteral gold.
Antimalarials Chloroquine (Aralen) Hydroxychloroquine (Plaquenil)	Unknown, but it has the ability to bind and alter DNA-modifying effect	Nausea, abdominal discomfort, rash, asymptomatic retinopathy, corneal opacity, headache, dizziness, blood dyscrasia	Inform patient that ophthalmologic examination including slit-lamp studies is required every 6-12 mo. Instruct patient to take drug with meals, milk, or antacid as prescribed, to report all skin eruptions and visual disturbances, and to avoid excessive sun exposure. Monitor CBC and liver enzyme values periodically. Instruct patient to discuss condition with physician before pregnancy and breastfeeding.

Continued

possible negative effects of long-term NSAID treatment on cartilage metabolism, particularly in older patients. Gastrointestinal (GI) side effects also commonly occur with the use of NSAIDs. This has led to use of misoprostol (Cytotec) to prevent NSAID-induced GI effects. Arthrotec, a combination of misoprostol and the NSAID diclofenac (Voltaren), is available.

Newer NSAIDs offer the advantage of a once- or twice-daily regimen, which improves compliance (see Table 60-2 for a list of drugs used in the management of OA). When given in equivalent antiinflammatory dosages, all NSAIDs are comparable in efficacy but vary widely in cost. Individual responses and side effects of NSAIDs are variable. Aspirin, no longer

DRUG THERAPY

Table 60-2 Rheumatic Disorders—cont'd

Drug	Mechanisms of Action	Common Side Effects	Nursing Considerations
Remission-Inducing Agents—cont'd			
Penicillamine (Cuprimine, Depen)	Unknown, disease-modifying effect	Blood dyscrasias, glomerulonephropathy, myasthenia gravis, rashes, GI irritation, diarrhea, pruritus	Give drug on empty stomach before meals (not with). Monitor CBC, urinalysis, and liver function values. Report fever, sore throat, chills, bruising, or bleeding. Be aware that drug is contraindicated with gold therapy. Instruct women to not become pregnant while taking drug.
Tetracyclines (minocycline, doxycycline)	Unclear, possibly anti-inflammatory, immunomodulatory, and chondroprotective effects in addition to antibacterial properties.	GI irritation, rash, photosensitivity, blood dyscrasias, hepatotoxicity	Monitor renal and liver function tests in long-term use. May increase digoxin levels. Antacids, iron, zinc, calcium, and magnesium reduce absorption.

*See Fig. 11-7.
†Cyclooxygenase—two inhibitors that are less likely to cause GI problems than traditional NSAIDs.
CBC, complete blood count; *IL*, interleukin; *MAO*, monoamine oxidase.

common in treatment, should not be used in combination with NSAIDs because both inhibit platelet function and prolong bleeding time.

A new generation of NSAIDs, COX-2 inhibitors, has recently been approved by the FDA. These drugs include celecoxib (Celebrex) and rofecoxib (Vioxx). They work by inhibiting cyclooxygenase-2 (COX-2) without affecting cyclooxygenase-1 (COX-1), an enzyme that primarily protects the stomach lining. Traditional NSAIDs are nonspecific inhibitors of both COX-1 and COX-2. The major advantage of COX-2 inhibitors as compared to traditional NSAIDs is that they are less likely to cause GI problems, such as ulcers and bleeding.

Intraarticular injections of corticosteroids are used to treat a symptomatic flare of OA. Systemic use of corticosteroids should be avoided because they may accelerate the disease process. The use of oral glucosamine sulfate and chondroitin sulfate as dietary supplements has become popular among individuals with OA.[7] However, concerns remain that well-controlled studies of significant length have not been done. These agents are not currently recommended by the Arthritis Foundation.

A newly approved treatment for OA of the knee uses intraarticular injections of synthetic and naturally occurring hyaluronic acid derivatives (Orthovisc, Synvisc, Artz, and Hyalgan). Although the exact mechanisms of action are unknown, these compounds appear to have some antiinflammatory benefits and a short-term lubricant effect.[7] In addition, an analgesic effect may be possible through the direct buffering effect of hyaluronic acid on synovial nerve endings, and a stimulating effect on synovial lining cells may produce normal hyaluronic acid.

Nutritional Therapy. There is no specific diet for OA except one that maintains optimal health. If a patient is overweight, a weight-reduction program becomes an important part of the total treatment plan. Body weight is magnified five times through the hips and three times through the knees. The additional strain of extra pounds can greatly increase pain and loss of function in OA. Furthermore, heavy thighs lead to malalignment at the knee, increasing wear on the medial aspect. (Chapter 38 discusses ways to assist the patient in attaining and maintaining a healthy body weight.)

NURSING MANAGEMENT: OSTEOARTHRITIS

■ Nursing Assessment

Nursing assessment of the patient with OA should include careful documentation of the nature, location, severity, and frequency of joint pain and stiffness. The extent to which these symptoms affect the patient's ability to perform activities of daily living should also be assessed. Successful and unsuccessful pain-relieving practices should be noted. Physical examination of the affected joint or joints includes assessment of tenderness, swelling, limitation of movement, and crepitation. It is useful to compare the involved joint with the same joint on the opposite side of the body if that joint is not affected.

■ Nursing Diagnoses

Nursing diagnoses for the patient with OA may include, but are not limited to, the following:

- Pain *related to* physical activity and lack of knowledge of pain self-management techniques
- Sleep pattern disturbance *related to* pain
- Impaired physical mobility *related to* weakness, stiffness, or pain on ambulation
- Self-care deficits *related to* joint deformity and pain with activity
- Altered nutrition: more than body requirements *related to* intake in excess of energy output
- Self-esteem disturbance *related to* changing social and work roles

Table **60-3** **Joint Protection and Energy Conservation**

- Maintain good posture and proper body mechanics.
- Maintain normal weight.
- Use assistive devices, if indicated.
- Avoid positions of deviation and stress.
- Find less stressful ways to perform tasks.
- Avoid tasks that cause pain.
- Develop organizing and pacing techniques.
- Avoid forceful repetitive movements.

■ Planning

The overall goals are that the patient with OA will (1) balance rest and activity; (2) use joint-protection measures (Table 60-3) to improve activity tolerance; (3) modify the home and work environment to include work-saving and joint-protecting assistive devices; (4) use pharmacologic and nonpharmacologic pain management techniques to achieve satisfactory pain control (see Chapter 9); and (5) perform ROM, muscle-strengthening, and aerobic exercise regularly.

■ Nursing Implementation

Health Promotion. Prevention of primary OA is not possible. However, preventive education may include elimination of excessive strain on joints by reduction of occupational and recreational hazards and nutritional counseling for weight reduction. Community education may include proper body mechanics of lifting and good posture. Athletic instruction and physical fitness programs should include safety measures that protect and reduce trauma to the joint structures. Congenital conditions, such as Legg-Calvé-Perthes disease, that are known to predispose to the development of OA should be treated promptly.

Acute Intervention. The person with OA is most troubled by pain, stiffness, limitation of function, and the frustration of coping with these physical difficulties on a daily basis. The older adult may believe that OA is an inevitable part of the aging process and that nothing can be done to ease the discomfort and related disability.

Usually a patient with OA is treated on an outpatient basis by a team of arthritis professionals including a personal physician or rheumatologist, a nurse, an occupational therapist, and a physical therapist. Health assessment questionnaires are helpful tools to pinpoint areas of difficulty for the patient with arthritis and target those areas for which specific interventions can then be developed.[8] These questionnaires may also be updated periodically to monitor the effectiveness of therapy. Hospitalization is usually necessary only if joint surgery or osteotomy is planned.

Medications are administered for the relief of pain and inflammation, if present. Nonpharmacologic pain management includes massage, application of heat (thermal packs) and cold (ice packs), relaxation, and guided imagery. Once an acute flare has subsided, a physical therapist can provide valuable assistance in planning an exercise program.

The hospital or home health nurse or family should assist the patient with activities of daily living as necessary and help the patient plan rest periods during the day. The patient needs sufficient time to move stiff, painful joints, especially when arising in the morning or after any period of sustained inactivity. Proper body alignment should be maintained at all times.

Patient education related to OA is an important nursing responsibility that should be carried out regardless of the care setting. Teaching should include information about the nature and treatment of the disease, pain management, correct posture and body mechanics, correct use of assistive devices such as a cane or walker, principles of joint protection and energy conservation (see Table 60-3), and a therapeutic exercise program. Home management goals must be individualized to meet the patient's needs, and family and social support should be included in goal setting and education.

Ambulatory and Home Care. After the diagnosis of OA and the initial educational efforts have been completed, the nurse should assist the patient in developing long-term strategies in managing the disease. The patient should be assured that OA is a localized disease and that severe deforming arthritis is not the usual course.

Safety measures in the home and work environment are important. These measures include removing scatter rugs, providing rails at stairs and bathtub, using night-lights, and wearing well-fitting supportive shoes. Assistive devices such as canes, walkers, elevated toilet seats, and grab bars reduce joint load and promote safety.

Splints may be prescribed to rest and stabilize painful or inflamed joints. Soft collars or cervical traction may be used at home for cervical OA. Stiff, painful hands can be relieved by warm-water soaking, contrast baths, or paraffin.[9] If swelling is more diffuse, stretch gloves can be worn at night to provide relief. Sexual counseling helps the patient and significant other to enjoy physical closeness by learning to adapt positions, alter timing, and increase awareness of partner's needs. Analgesics may be helpful when taken before activities.

Management of the chronic pain and loss of function of affected joints continue to be a primary concern. Nonpharmacologic techniques such as meditation, relaxation, and transcutaneous electric nerve stimulation (TENS) are particularly suited to chronic pain management (see Chapter 9). The nurse should be open to helping the patient and family to develop creative new approaches to pain relief. The practice of tai chi, for example, can increase mobility through gentle stretching and provides a calming effect with its focus on breathing and emotional centering. Nursing interventions should assist the patient and family to overcome feelings of helplessness and encourage active participation in managing chronic symptoms. The correct combination of joint protection, exercise (range of motion, isotonic, and isometric), heat or cold therapy, and medication can restore self-esteem and improve physical functioning. An aerobic exercise program, such as walking or aerobic aquatics, is also important.[10]

■ Evaluation

The expected outcomes are that the patient with osteoarthritis will

- experience adequate amounts of rest and activity
- use joint protection and energy conservation measures
- achieve satisfactory pain control
- maintain joint flexibility and muscle strength through ROM, aquatic, or aerobic exercises

RHEUMATOID ARTHRITIS

Rheumatoid arthritis (RA) is a chronic, systemic disease characterized by recurrent inflammation of the diarthrodial joints and related structures. It is frequently accompanied by a variety of extraarticular manifestations, such as rheumatoid nodules, arteritis, neuropathy, scleritis, pericarditis, lymphadenopathy, and splenomegaly.[11] RA is characterized by periods of remission and exacerbation of disease activity. The course of illness varies, ranging from episodes of illness separated by periods of remission to a more continuous, progressive disease.[12] Mortality rates are higher with severe disease.[13]

Of the approximately 6 million Americans who have RA, 75% are women. Although RA can occur at any age, it most often occurs in women of childbearing age.[14] There are no geographic or ethnic predispositions. RA is considered a significant national health problem in terms of its potential for chronic disability.

Etiology and Pathophysiology

The cause of RA is unknown. Whether a single causative factor is responsible or multiple factors are involved is unclear. Several etiologies are possible:

1. *Infection.* Research continues to probe the possibility of specific infectious pathogens, such as Epstein-Barr virus, parvovirus, and mycobacteria, which may trigger the process.

2. *Autoimmunity.* Although no virus particles have been identified, it is likely that an antigenic stimulus such as a virus leads to the formation of an abnormal immunoglobulin G (IgG). RA is characterized by the presence of autoantibodies against this abnormal IgG. The autoantibodies to this altered IgG are termed *rheumatoid factors*, and they combine with IgG to form immune complexes that deposit in the joints, blood vessels, and pleura. Complement is activated and an inflammatory response results (see Chapter 11). Neutrophils are attracted to the site of inflammation and release proteolytic enzymes that can damage articular cartilage and basement membranes of blood vessels and pleura.

   Joint changes are characterized by chronic inflammation with the presence of inflammatory cells and mediators. The infiltrating macrophages are activated and release a variety of cytokines, including interleukin-1 and interleukin-6, tumor necrosis factor (TNF), and colony-stimulating factor[15] (see Table 12-4). The activity of these cytokines accounts for many of the features of rheumatoid synovitis, including the synovial tissue inflammation, synovial proliferation, cartilage and bone damage, and systemic manifestations of RA.

3. *Genetic factors.* Certain familial factors may influence the expression of the disease. An increased prevalence of a human leukocyte antigen (HLA) known as the HLA-DR4 occurs in 65% of persons with RA. Persons in this group seem to experience a particularly crippling form of the disease. It is possible that the presence of this HLA and perhaps other genetic factors increase genetic susceptibility to an unidentified environmental antigen, such as a virus, which may then initiate the disease process (see Chapter 12).

4. *Other factors.* Metabolic and biochemical abnormalities, nutritional and environmental factors, and occupational and psychosocial influences may play a part in the cause or expression of the disease, but their contribution is entirely speculative.

The pathogenesis of RA is more clearly understood than its etiology. If unarrested, the disease progresses through four stages:

1. *First stage.* The unknown etiologic factor initiates joint inflammation, or synovitis, with swelling of the synovial lining membrane and production of excess synovial fluid.

2. *Second stage.* Pannus (inflammatory granulation tissue) is formed at the juncture of the synovium and cartilage. This extends over the surface of the articular cartilage and eventually invades the joint capsule and subchondral bone.

3. *Third stage.* Tough fibrous connective tissue replaces pannus, occluding the joint space. Fibrous ankylosis results in decreased joint motion, malalignment, and deformity.

4. *Fourth stage.* As fibrous tissue calcifies, bony ankylosis may result in total joint immobilization.

Clinical Manifestations

Joints. RA typically develops insidiously. Nonspecific manifestations such as fatigue, anorexia, weight loss, and generalized stiffness may precede the onset of arthritic complaints. The stiffness becomes more localized after weeks to months. Some patients report a history of a precipitating stressful event such as infection, work stress, physical exertion, childbirth, surgery, or emotional upset. However, there is no scientific evidence to correlate these events with the onset of RA.

Specific articular involvement is manifested clinically by pain, stiffness, limitation of motion, and signs of inflammation (heat, swelling, and tenderness). Joint symptoms are generally bilaterally symmetric and frequently affect small joints of the hands (proximal interphalangeal and metacarpophalangeal) and feet (metatarsophalangeal), as well as larger peripheral joints, including wrists, elbows, shoulders, knees, hips, ankles, and jaw. The cervical spine may be affected, but the axial spine is generally spared. Early shoulder involvement is common in the older adult. Table 60-4 compares the manifestations of RA and OA.

The patient characteristically has joint stiffness on arising in the morning and after periods of inactivity. This morning stiffness may last for 30 minutes to several hours or more, depending on disease activity. Metacarpal and proximal interphalangeal joints are typically swollen. The fingers may become spindle shaped from synovial hypertrophy and thickening of the joint capsule (Fig. 60-3). Joints become tender, painful, and warm to the touch. The pain is more pronounced on motion, varies in intensity, and may not be proportional to the degree of inflammation. Tenosynovitis frequently affects the extensor and flexor tendons around the wrists, producing manifestations of carpal tunnel syndrome and making it difficult to grasp objects.

As disease activity progresses, inflammation and fibrosis of the joint capsule and supporting structures may lead to deformity and disability. Atrophy of muscles and destruction of tendons around the joint cause one articular surface to slip past the

Table 60-4 | **Comparison of Rheumatoid Arthritis and Osteoarthritis**

Parameter	Rheumatoid Arthritis	Osteoarthritis
Age	Young and middle-aged	Usually >40 yr of age
Gender	Female more often than male	Same incidence
Weight	Weight loss	Usually overweight
Illness	Systemic manifestations	Local joint manifestations
Affected joints	PIPs, MCPs, MTPs, wrists, elbows, shoulders, knees, hips, cervical spine	DIPs, first CMCs, thumbs, first MTPs, knees, spine, hips; asymmetric, one or more joints
	Usually bilateral	
Effusions	Common	Uncommon
Nodules	Present	Heberden's nodes
Synovial fluid	Inflammatory	Noninflammatory
X-rays	Osteoporosis, narrowing, erosions	Osteophytes, subchondral cysts, sclerosis
Anemia	Common	Uncommon
Rheumatoid factor	Positive	Negative
Sedimentation rate	Elevated	Normal except in erosive osteoarthritis

CMC, carpometacarpal; *DIP,* distal interphalangeal; *MCP,* metacarpophalangeal; *MTP,* metatarsophalangeal; *PIP,* proximal interphalangeal.

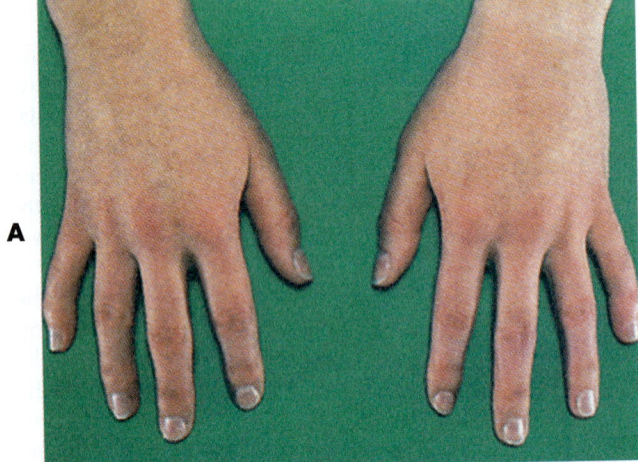

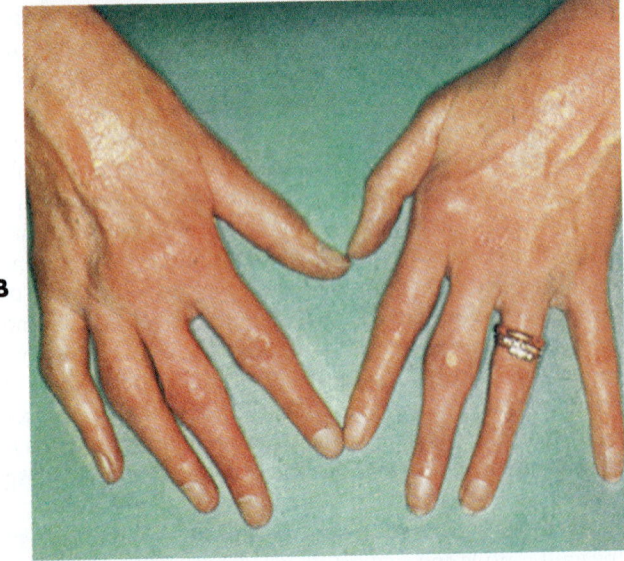

Fig. 60-3 Rheumatoid arthritis of the hand. **A,** Early stage. **B,** Moderate involvement.

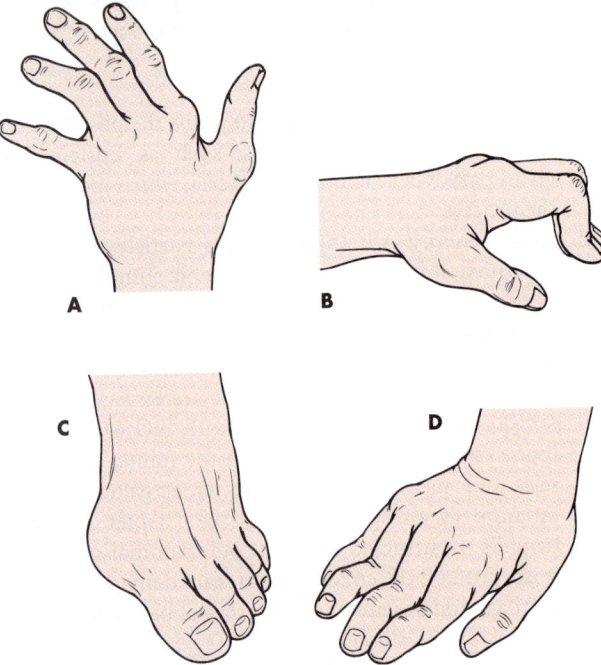

Fig. 60-4 Typical deformities of rheumatoid arthritis. **A,** Ulnar drift. **B,** Boutonnière deformity. **C,** Hallux valgus. **D,** Swanneck deformity.

other (subluxation). Typical deformities of the hand include ulnar drift, swan-neck, and boutonnière deformities (Fig. 60-4). Metatarsal-head subluxation and hallux valgus (bunion) may cause pain and walking disability.

Extraarticular Manifestations. Rheumatoid nodules are present in 25% to 50% of all people with RA and are probably the most common extraarticular finding. Small-vessel vasculitis is considered to be the initiating event in the formation of these nodules. The nodules appear subcutaneously as firm, nontender masses and are usually found on olecranon bursae or along the extensor surface of the forearm. Nodules at the base of the spine and back of the head are common in older adults. Nodules develop insidiously and can persist or regress spontaneously. They are usually not removed because of the high probability of recurrence unless they are signifi-

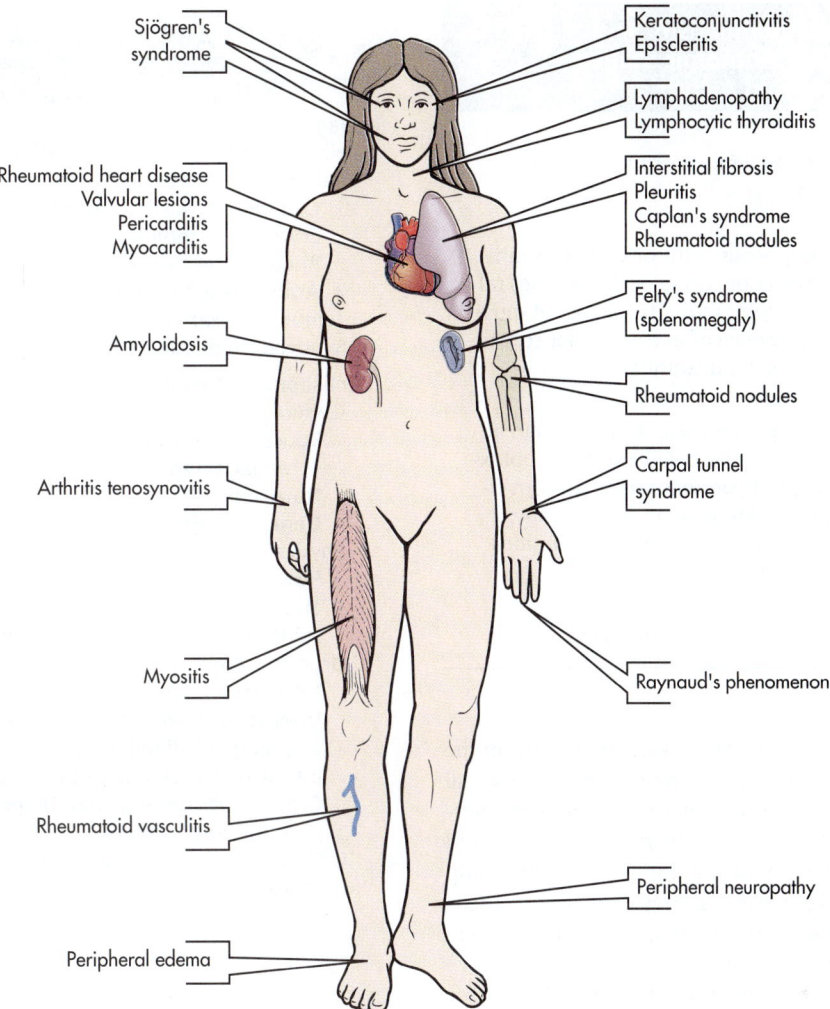

Fig. 60-5 Extraarticular manifestations of rheumatoid arthritis.

cantly disabling. Nodules may also appear on the eye or lungs; these indicate active disease and a poor prognosis.

Vasculitis (inflammation of blood vessels) may be responsible for a variety of systemic complications, including peripheral neuropathy, myopathy, cardiopulmonary involvement, and ischemic ulcerations of the skin. Figure 60-5 shows extraarticular manifestations of RA.

Complications
Potential complications of RA include infection, osteoporosis, and amyloidosis. Spinal cord compression may occur from instability of articulations in the cervical spine.

Diagnostic Studies
Although no single laboratory test is conclusive, several findings are helpful in diagnosing RA in conjunction with the history and physical examination.[16] Moderate anemia is common. The erythrocyte sedimentation rate (ESR) is elevated in 85% of patients and is useful in monitoring the response to therapy. Serum rheumatoid factor is present in titers greater than 1:160 in nearly 80% of individuals with RA. Antinuclear antibody and lupus cell tests may be positive in a smaller percentage of patients.

Synovial fluid analysis may show increased volume and turbidity but decreased viscosity of the fluid. The white blood cell (WBC) count of synovial fluid is elevated (often as high as 30,000/μl [30×10^9/L]) and consists predominantly of neutrophils. Inflammatory changes in the synovium can be confirmed by tissue biopsy.

X-ray findings (which are not specifically diagnostic) may reveal only bone demineralization and soft-tissue swelling during the early stage of the disease. Later, narrowing of the joint space, destruction of articular cartilage, erosion, subluxation, and deformity are present. Malalignment and ankylosis occur in advanced disease. Table 60-5 describes the anatomic stages of RA.

Collaborative Care
Care of the patient with RA begins with a comprehensive program of drug therapy and education. Physical comfort is promoted by NSAIDs and rest. The patient and family are educated about the disease process and home management strategies. Compliance with drug therapy includes correct administration, reporting of side effects, and frequent medical and laboratory follow-up visits. Physical therapy maintains joint motion and muscle strength. Occupational therapy develops upper-extremity function and encourages joint protection through the use of splinting, pacing techniques, and assistive devices.

Table **60-5**	American Rheumatism Association Anatomic Stages of Rheumatoid Arthritis

Stage I—Early
No destructive changes on x-ray, possible x-ray evidence of osteoporosis

Stage II—Moderate
X-ray evidence of osteoporosis, with or without slight bone or cartilage destruction, no joint deformities (although possibly limited joint mobility), adjacent muscle atrophy, possible presence of extraarticular soft tissue lesions (e.g., nodules, tenovaginitis)

Stage III—Severe
X-ray evidence of cartilage and bone destruction in addition to osteoporosis; joint deformity, such as subluxation, ulnar deviation, or hyperextension, without fibrous or bony ankylosis; extensive muscle atrophy; possible presence of extraarticular soft tissue lesions (e.g., nodules, tenosynovitis)

Stage IV—Terminal
Fibrous or bony ankylosis, criteria of stage III

An individualized treatment plan considers the nature of the disease activity, joint function, age, gender, family and social roles, and response to previous treatment. Collaborative therapy generally includes education, therapeutic exercise, rest, and drug therapy (Table 60-6). A caring, long-term relationship with an arthritis health care team promotes the patient's self-esteem and hope and discourages the use of unproven remedies, which waste money and time.

Drug Therapy. The concepts regarding drug therapy for RA have changed considerably in recent years. In the past, patients were maintained on high doses of aspirin or NSAIDs for several years until there was x-ray evidence of characteristic bone erosions. Now a more aggressive drug therapy approach that is initiated earlier is more common because the erosive, destructive process begins within the first 2 years of disease.

Many rheumatologists are now using a disease-modifying agent (such as methotrexate) early in the course of the disease. A disease-modifying agent is a drug that has the potential to lessen the permanent effects of RA such as joint deformity. The damaging effects of the disease may be prevented or postponed by this plan. The exact time to introduce a disease-modifying drug varies among clinicians. Some start treatment when the patient has been symptomatic for only a few weeks. Others prefer to wait several months until the diagnosis is confirmed by x-ray and laboratory findings or the patient has sustained symptomatic arthritis. At this time there is no way to differentiate patients with mild disease from the larger group whose disease may be relentlessly progressive.[17] The least toxic agent, alone or in combination, that is likely to be effective is usually the drug chosen for initial therapy. Table 60-2 lists drugs commonly used in the treatment of RA.

For patients with mild disease, hydroxychloroquine (Plaquenil) is often prescribed initially. It is one of the safest of the disease-modifying drugs. The most common side effects of this drug are nausea, abdominal discomfort, and rash. The possibility of rare, irreversible retinal degeneration caused by deposition of this drug in the pigment layer of the retina requires

COLLABORATIVE CARE

Table **60-6**	**Rheumatoid Arthritis**

Diagnostic
History and physical examination
Laboratory studies
    Complete blood cell count
    Erythrocyte sedimentation rate
    Rheumatoid factor
    Antinuclear antibody profile
Joint x-ray examination
Synovial fluid analysis

Collaborative Therapy
General
    Education, including disease process and management
    Nutrition
    General health measures
Physical
    Rest, including local joint, systemic, and emotional
    Therapeutic exercise
    Joint protection and energy conservation
Drug therapy
    Nonsteroidal antiinflammatory drugs
    Disease-modifying drugs such as hydroxychloroquine, gold, penicillamine
    Intraarticular or systemic corticosteroids
    Cytotoxic drugs (e.g., azathioprine, methotrexate, cyclophosphamide)
Orthopedic surgery, especially reconstructive joint replacement

---

ophthalmologic examination before therapy and at 6-month intervals. A low dose of prednisone may be given with or instead of hydroxychloroquine.

Corticosteroid therapy can be used to aid in symptom control. Intraarticular injections are administered for a flare-up of the disease in one or two joints. Pain in the joint may increase for 1 to 2 days after injection because of the irritation by the medication. Alternatively, intramuscular injections of methylprednisolone (Solu-Medrol), for example, may be useful if several joints are affected. Pain and swelling are usually relieved for 1 to 6 weeks.

Bridge therapy (5 to 10 mg orally of the prescribed corticosteroid daily for 4 to 6 weeks) is used until one of the longer-acting drugs, such as hydroxychloroquine, gold, or D-penicillamine (Cuprimine), has been used long enough to suppress disease activity. Burst corticosteroid therapy, used for a severe articular flare, consists of high-dose (e.g., 40 to 60 mg) corticosteroids, which are then quickly tapered in 7 to 14 days. Pulse therapy (Solu-Medrol, at dosages of no more than 1 g per day intravenously for 3 days) is used to achieve fast control of inflammation and results in fewer side effects over the long term as a result of taking a smaller daily dose. Regardless of the regimen, high-dose or long-term corticosteroid therapy carries a high risk of drug dependency and serious side effects (see Chapter 47).

For patients with moderate to severe disease with symmetric joint involvement and a positive rheumatoid factor assay, a more aggressive drug regimen may be initiated. Usually methotrexate is the first drug of choice. The rapid antiinflammatory effect of methotrexate reduces clinical symptoms in days to weeks. Side effects include bone marrow suppression and hepatotoxicity. Methotrexate therapy requires frequent laboratory monitoring, including CBC and chemistry panel. A sustained, nonprogressive cough may be related to methotrexate therapy and should be evaluated with pulmonary function testing.[18] Avoidance of alcohol is often advised because it can increase the toxicity of methotrexate and confound liver enzyme elevations.

Gold therapy may be considered for patients who do not respond to methotrexate. Gold has an antiinflammatory action and may decrease phagocytosis and lysosomal activity.[19] It is usually given in a weekly injection for 5 months, then biweekly or monthly to sustain the clinical effects. Although the serious side effects of proteinuria and cytopenia are uncommon, gold therapy often causes minor side effects, such as skin rashes, mouth sores, and GI problems, particularly diarrhea.

Azathioprine (Imuran) or D-penicillamine (Cuprimine) may be used if the patient does not respond to either methotrexate or gold therapy. Azathioprine and penicillamine may cause mild pancytopenia.

There is increased interest in combination therapy to treat RA, although it is still somewhat controversial. Combinations include methotrexate plus sulfasalazine (Azulfidine) and hydroxychloroquine plus sulfasalazine, among others.[20] Multiple agents may provide a synergistic effect and more adequately control symptoms.

Although new drug regimens are being used with increasing frequency, aspirin and NSAIDs are still commonly used. Aspirin is often used in high dosages of 4 to 6 g per day (10 to 18 tablets) in divided doses to obtain a blood level of 15 to 30 mg/dl. Enteric-coated aspirin is absorbed in the small intestine and is often used to prevent gastric irritation. Enteric-coated tablets have a special covering to prevent them from disintegrating in the stomach and may require higher doses than regular tablets. The ability to obtain serum salicylate levels, unavailable with other NSAIDs, is helpful in individualizing treatment programs and evaluating compliance.

NSAIDs have antiinflammatory, analgesic, and antipyretic properties. Although many NSAIDs are potent inhibitors of inflammation, they do not appear to alter the natural history of RA. Although some relief from NSAIDs may be noted within days of the start of treatment, it takes approximately 2 to 3 weeks for full effectiveness to be demonstrated. NSAIDs may be used when patients are intolerant to high doses of aspirin. NSAIDs that are taken only once or twice a day may improve patient compliance.

There are significant but subtle differences in the mechanisms of action, effectiveness in various diseases, and other properties of the different NSAIDs. The unpredictable differences in effectiveness in various patients make it worthwhile to try different NSAIDs if the first drug does not work satisfactorily in a given patient. NSAIDs are often used in conjunction with disease-modifying drugs for their antiinflammatory effect.

The newer generation of NSAIDs, Cox-2 inhibitors, are effective in RA as well as OA. These include celecoxib (Celebrex) and rofecoxib (Vioxx) (see p. 1825).

Relatively new drugs used in the treatment of RA include leflunomide (Arava) and etanercept (Enbrel). Leflunomide inhibits the proliferation of activated lymphocytes, which are linked to the inflammation and pathophysiology of RA. Leflunomide slows joint deterioration and is well tolerated by patients. Leflunomide is contraindicated in pregnant women or women of childbearing age who are not using reliable birth control methods.

Etanercept is a biologically engineered copy (using recombinant DNA technology) of the tumor necrosis factor (TNF) cell receptor. This soluble TNF receptor binds to TNF in circulation before TNF can bind to its cell surface receptor. TNF, a naturally occurring cytokine, once bound to its cell receptor promotes inflammation. This drug is given two times per week as a subsutaneous injection. Etanercept may be especially effective in patients who have not responded to other therapies.

Nutritional Therapy. There is no special diet for RA. However, balanced nutrition is important. The fatigue, pain, depression, limited endurance, and limitation of mobility that may accompany RA may interfere with the patient's appetite and ability to shop for and prepare food, resulting in weight loss. The occupational therapist may help the patient to modify the home environment and to use assistive devices to make food preparation easier. Although patients are vulnerable to fad claims for improvement through health foods and vitamins, there is little credible research evidence for their use.

Corticosteroid therapy or immobility secondary to pain may result in unwanted weight gain. A sensible weight loss program consisting of balanced nutrition and exercise reduces stress on arthritic joints. Limited sodium intake may help minimize fluid gain caused by sodium retention. Corticosteroids also increase the appetite, resulting in a higher caloric intake. Even the most compliant patient becomes distressed as Cushing's syndrome signs and symptoms, such as moon face and redistribution of fatty tissue to the trunk, change the body's appearance. The patient must be encouraged to continue a balanced diet and not to alter corticosteroid dose or stop therapy abruptly. Weight slowly adjusts to normal several months after cessation of therapy.

GERONTOLOGIC CONSIDERATIONS

Arthritis

The prevalence of rheumatic disease in older adults is high, and the disease is accompanied by problems unique to this age-group. The most problematic areas related to rheumatic disease in older adults include the following:

1. The high incidence of OA expected in older adults often keeps the clinician from considering the presence of other rheumatic diseases.
2. Age alone causes changes in serologic profiles, making interpretation of laboratory values such as rheumatoid factors and sedimentation rates more difficult.
3. Multidrug regimens common to the older adult can result in iatrogenic arthritis.
4. Nonorganic musculoskeletal pain syndromes and weakness may be related to depressive reactions and physical inactivity.
5. Rheumatic diseases, such as systemic lupus erythematosus, that commonly manifest in younger adults can occur in older adults, but often in milder form.
6. Residual effects of rheumatic disease are present for long periods and must be managed.

Aging brings many physical and metabolic changes that may increase the older patient's sensitivity to both the therapeutic and toxic effects of some drugs. The use of NSAIDs with a

NURSING ASSESSMENT

Table 60-7 Rheumatoid Arthritis

Subjective Data

Important Health Information

Past health history: Epstein-Barr or other viral infections; presence of precipitating factors such as emotional upset, infections, overwork, childbirth, surgery; pattern of remissions and exacerbations

Medications: Use of aspirin, NSAIDs, corticosteroids, gold salts, penicillamine

Surgery or other treatments: Any joint surgery

Health Patterns

Health perception–health management: Positive family history for rheumatoid arthritis, malaise, ability to comply with therapeutic regimen

Nutritional-metabolic: Anorexia, weight loss; dry mucous membranes of mouth and pharynx

Activity-exercise: Morning stiffness and joint swelling, muscle weakness, difficulty walking, fatigue

Cognitive-perceptual: Paresthesias of hands and feet; numbness, tingling, loss of sensation; symmetric joint pain and aching that increases with motion or stress on joint

Objective Data

General

Lymphadenopathy, fever

Integumentary

Keratoconjunctivitis; subcutaneous rheumatoid nodules on forearm, elbows; skin ulcers; shiny, taut skin over involved joints; peripheral edema

Cardiovascular

Symmetric pallor and cyanosis of fingers (Raynaud's phenomenon); distant heart sounds, murmurs, arrhythmias (rheumatoid heart disease)

Respiratory

Chronic bronchitis, tuberculosis, histoplasmosis, fibrosing alveolitis

Gastrointestinal

Splenomegaly (Felty's syndrome)

Musculoskeletal

Symmetric joint involvement with swelling, erythema, heat, tenderness, and deformities; enlargement of proximal phalangeal and metacarpophalangeal joints; limitation of joint movement; muscle contractures, muscle atrophy

Possible Findings

Positive rheumatoid factor, elevated ESR, anemia; increased WBC in synovial fluid; evidence of osteoporosis, joint space narrowing, and bony erosion and deformity on x-ray

ESR, erythrocyte sedimentation rate.

shorter half-life requiring more frequent dosing may produce fewer side effects in the older patient with altered drug metabolism. The common occurrence of polypharmacy makes the use of multidrug therapy in RA particularly problematic in the older adult because of the increased likelihood of untoward drug interactions. Particular care should be taken when the older adult takes NSAIDs because of their increased propensity for side effects, particularly GI and renal toxicity. If such therapy is necessary, a cytoprotective agent such as misoprostol (Cytotec) should be considered.[21] The frequency of taking medication and the complexity of the drug regimen should be simplified as much as possible to increase compliance in the older adult, particularly for the patient without regular assistance.

A major concern of treatment in the older patient relates to the use of corticosteroid therapy. Corticosteroid-induced osteopenia adds to the problem of age-related and inactivity-related osteoporosis and can increase the occurrence of pathologic fractures, especially compression fractures of vertebrae. Corticosteroid-induced myopathy can be minimized or prevented by an age-appropriate exercise program. Although important for all age-groups, an adequate support system for the older adult is a critical factor in compliance with the management program, which should include nutritional planning, exercise, general health maintenance, and appropriate pharmacotherapy.

NURSING MANAGEMENT: RHEUMATOID ARTHRITIS

■ Nursing Assessment

Subjective and objective data that should be obtained from the patient with RA are presented in Table 60-7.

■ Nursing Diagnoses

Nursing diagnoses for the patient with RA may include, but are not limited to, those presented in NCP 60-1.

■ Planning

The overall goals are that the patient with RA will (1) have satisfactory pain relief, (2) have minimal loss of functional ability of the affected joints, (3) participate in planning and carrying out the therapeutic regimen, (4) maintain a positive self-image, and (5) perform self-care to the maximum amount possible.

■ Nursing Implementation

Health Promotion. Prevention of RA is not possible at this time. However, community education programs should include information concerning the symptoms of RA to promote early diagnosis and treatment. Many publications for the public are available through the Arthritis Foundation (see Resources at end of this chapter).

Acute Intervention. The primary objectives in the management of RA are reduction of inflammation, relief of pain, preservation of joint function, and prevention or correction of joint deformity. These may be approached by a comprehensive program of daily antiinflammatory medication, rest, joint protection, therapeutic heat, exercise, and thorough patient and family teaching. The nurse is an integral member of the health team, working closely with the physician, physical and occupational therapists, and social worker to restore function and to help the patient make lifestyle adjustments to chronic illness (Fig. 60-6).

The newly diagnosed patient with RA may be hospitalized for control of acute inflammation, evaluation of systemic in-

60-1 NURSING CARE PLAN PATIENT WITH RHEUMATOID ARTHRITIS

| Expected Patient Outcomes | Nursing Interventions and *Rationales* |

NURSING DIAGNOSIS **Chronic pain** *related to* joint inflammation, overuse of joint, and ineffective pain or comfort measures *as manifested by* complaints of pain and limited joint function; hot, swollen, painful joints of more than 6 months duration.

- Decreased pain, swelling, and erythema of joints.

- Assess location, severity, and precipitators of pain *to plan appropriate interventions.*
- Encourage decreased activity, increased rest, and supportive resting splints for affected joints *to decrease stress on joints and resulting pain during acute flare-ups of disease.*
- Teach self-administration of antiinflammatory medications as prescribed, including names, actions, side effects, dose, and administration of prescribed drugs.
- Use relaxation techniques *to reduce physical and emotional stress;* protective techniques *that limit stress to joints;* and nonpharmacologic pain strategies (e.g., heat or cold application, meditation, massage) *to reduce pain.*

NURSING DIAGNOSIS **Impaired physical mobility** *related to* joint pain, stiffness, and deformity *as manifested by* limitation of joint motion, strength, and endurance; inability to perform routine activities of daily living.

- Increased ROM and function.
- Decreased stiffness.
- Ability to perform activities of daily living.
- Minimal deformity.

- Apply moist heat to affected joints (e.g., paraffin bath, hot packs, warm shower) *to relieve stiffness and increase mobility.*
- Encourage ROM exercises *to prevent unnecessary mobility restriction;* reduce frequency if pain and swelling are present *to prevent joint destruction when active disease is present.*
- Schedule morning care and procedures later in the day *after morning stiffness subsides.*
- Teach patient to use assistive devices *to promote independence.*
- Encourage flexibility, strengthening, and conditioning exercises in water or on land *to increase joint motion, flexibility, muscle strength, and endurance.*
- Instruct patient on correct application of resting splints, selection of properly fitting footwear, maintenance of proper posture and body alignment, and selection and use of assistive devices *to prevent or limit joint deformity.*

NURSING DIAGNOSIS **Fatigue** *related to* exacerbation of disease activity, anemia, drug side effects, sleep disturbance, or depression *as manifested by* verbilization of overwhelming lack of energy and decreased activity tolerance.

- Improved stamina and endurance.
- Better quality of sleep.
- Good eating habits.

- Assess causative factors and degree of fatigue *to plan appropriate activities.*
- Balance activity with rest periods.
- Encourage regular general physical exercise such as walking, bicycling, or swimming to patient's level of tolerance *to prevent deconditioning and foster a positive attitude.*
- Teach energy conservation techniques *to enable continued activity.*
- Review nutrition and sleep patterns *to determine if adjustments could prevent fatigue.*

NURSING DIAGNOSIS **Body image disturbance** *related to* chronic disease activity, long-term treatment, deformities, stiffness, and inability to perform usual activities *as manifested by* social withdrawal, flat affect, altered self-concept, reduced sexual interest.

- Acceptance of body changes.
- Maintenance of interest in life.

- Allow patient to express feelings about disease *to determine extent of problems and plan appropriate interventions.*
- Offer psychologic support to patient and family *to prevent unnecessary or excessive emotional response to disease.*
- Provide sexual counseling *because sexual problems and concerns can have a serious impact on body image.*
- Reassure patient of self-worth *so a positive body image is fostered in spite of distressing physical manifestations.*

Continued

60-1 NURSING CARE PLAN   PATIENT WITH RHEUMATOID ARTHRITIS—continued

| Expected Patient Outcomes | Nursing Interventions and *Rationales* |

NURSING DIAGNOSIS Ineffective management of therapeutic regimen *related to* complexity of chronic health problem, pain, and fatigue *as manifested by* questioning management plan, self-doubt about ability to manage disease, ability to perform activities for only short periods.

- Expression of increased confidence in ability to manage disease.
- Ability to describe treatment plan.
- Expression of satisfaction with pain and fatigue management.

- Assess patient's knowledge of disease *to plan appropriate interventions.*
- Include patient's family members in discussion of disease management *to increase their sense of control and to increase patient's sense of support.*
- Evaluate patient's understanding through verbalization and demonstration *to ensure correct understanding of disease management.*
- Focus on patient's problems of pain and fatigue *because these are major deterrents to successful disease management and must be addressed.*
- Assist patient to recognize need for ongoing therapy and to resist false advertising and unproven remedies *so only proven methods of treatment will be used.*

NURSING DIAGNOSIS Altered family processes *related to* patient's inability to function secondary to chronic illness and complexity of treatment regimen *as manifested by* changes in family, social, and occupational roles; dysfunctional family dynamics.

- Successful adjustment to disease activity by patient and family.
- Vocational rehabilitation or modification.

- Help patient and family identify appropriate coping strategies *to foster adjustment to changes in function and role responsibilities.*
- Refer patient to community vocational centers *for work adjustment or retraining.*
- Encourage professional family counseling *because unresolved serious family problems can interfere with successful disease management.*

NURSING DIAGNOSIS Self-care deficits *related to* disease progression, weakness, and contracture *as manifested by* inability to perform activities of daily living (ADLs).

- Completion of ADLs independently or with assistance.
- Expression of satisfaction with how self-care needs are met.

- Assess patient's ability to perform ADLs *to plan appropriate interventions.*
- Assist patient with ADLs as necessary *to ensure all needs are met.*
- Provide assistive devices or refer to occupational therapist where appropriate *to compensate for contractures and weakness so patient can perform as many self-care activities as possible.*
- Encourage patient to pace activities *to foster maximum independence with minimal fatigue.*

---

volvement, and comprehensive education by the health team. Hospitalization may also be necessary for patients with extraarticular complications or advanced disease requiring reconstructive surgery for disabling deformities.

Nursing intervention begins with a careful assessment of physical needs (joint pain, swelling, ROM, and general health status), psychosocial needs (family support, sexual satisfaction, emotional stress, financial constraints, vocation and career limitations), and environmental needs (transportation, home or work modifications). After the identification of problems and potential problems, a carefully planned program for rehabilitation and education can be coordinated by the nurse for the health care team.

Suppression of inflammation is most effectively achieved through the administration of antiinflammatory or disease-modifying agents. Careful attention to timing sustains a therapeutic level and reduces early-morning stiffness. Education centers around the action and side effects of each drug prescribed and the importance of laboratory monitoring when necessary. Many patients with RA are taking several different drugs. The nurse must make the drug regimen as clear and sim-

ple as possible. High-dose intravenous (IV) corticosteroids (pulse therapy) require careful observation for changes in blood pressure, peripheral edema, and signs of congestive heart failure.

Nonpharmacologic relief of pain may include the use of therapeutic heat and cold, rest, relaxation techniques, joint protection (see Tables 60-3 and 60-8), biofeedback (see Chapter 8), transcutaneous electrical nerve stimulation (see Chapter 9), and hypnosis. Assessment for individual differences and preference allows the nurse to help the patient and family set goals that promote optimal comfort.

Lightweight splints are sometimes used to rest an inflamed joint and prevent deformity from muscle spasms and contractures. These splints should be removed, skin care given, ROM exercises performed, and splints reapplied as prescribed. The occupational therapist may help identify self-help devices that can assist in activities of daily living.

Morning care and procedures should be planned around the patient's morning stiffness. Sitting or standing in a warm shower, sitting in a tub with warm towels around the shoulders, or simply soaking the hands in a basin of warm water may help

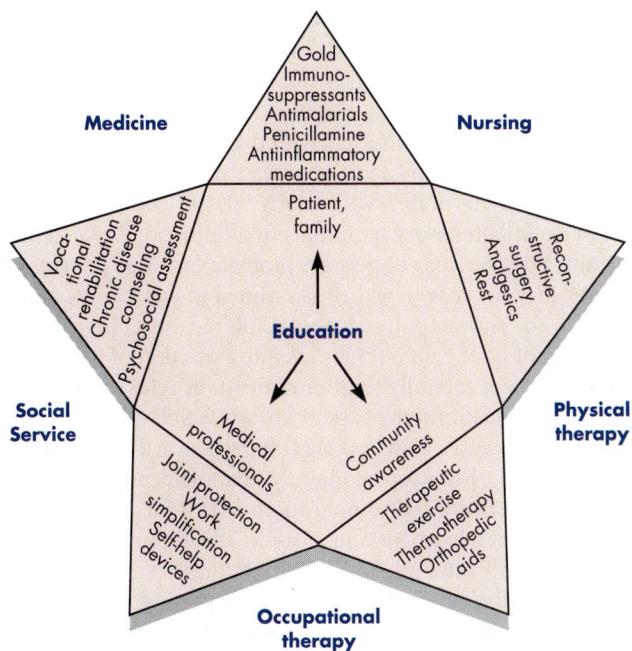

Fig. 60-6   Team approach to the management of rheumatoid arthritis.

PATIENT TEACHING GUIDE

Table **60-8**   **Protection of Small Joints**

1. Avoid positions of deformity.
   - Press water from a sponge instead of wringing.
2. Use strongest joint available for any task.
   - When rising from chair, push with palms rather than fingers.
   - Carry laundry basket in both arms rather than with fingers.
3. Distribute weight over many joints instead of stressing a few.
   - Slide objects instead of lifting them.
   - Hold packages close to body for support.
4. Change positions frequently.
   - Do not hold book or grip steering wheel for long periods without resting.
   - Avoid grasping pencil or cutting vegetables with knife for extended periods.
5. Avoid repetitious movements.
   - Do not knit for long periods.
   - Rest between rooms when vacuuming.
6. Modify chores to avoid stress on joints.
   - Avoid heavy tasks.
   - Sit on stool instead of standing.

relieve joint stiffness and allow the patient to more comfortably perform activities of daily living. Careful skin care should be offered, particularly if the patient is confined to bed.

The professional nurse acts as liaison between the patient, family, and other members of the health team, coordinating services and evaluating the patient's understanding of the total home management program (see NCP 60-1).

Ambulatory and Home Care

Rest. Regularly scheduled rest periods alternated with activity throughout the day help relieve fatigue and pain and minimize excessive weight bearing.[22] The amount of rest necessary varies according to the severity of the disease and each patient's limitations. Total bed rest is rarely necessary and should be avoided to prevent stiffness and immobility. Even a patient with mild disease may require daytime rest in addition to 8 to 10 hours of sleep at night. The nurse should help the patient identify ways to modify daily activities because overexertion can lead to fatigue and a flare-up in disease activity. For instance, the patient may tolerate meal preparation more easily if the patient sits on a high stool in front of the sink. Patients should rest before becoming exhausted. The nurse should assist the patient to pace activities and set priorities on the basis of realistic goals.

Good body alignment while resting is important. A firm mattress or bedboard should be used. Positions of extension should be encouraged, and positions of flexion should be avoided. Lying prone for half an hour twice daily is recommended. Pillows should never be placed under the knees. A small, flat pillow may be used under the head and shoulders. Splints and casts may be helpful in maintaining proper alignment and promoting rest, especially when joint inflammation is present.

Joint protection. Protecting joints from stress is an important part of the therapeutic regimen for RA. Nursing intervention includes helping the patient identify ways to modify tasks.

Each patient must learn less stressful ways that put less stress on joints to accomplish routine activities. The emphasis is on changing the way the task is done and on work simplification techniques.

Energy conservation requires careful planning. Work should be done in short periods with scheduled rest breaks to avoid fatigue (pacing). Chores should be spread through the week rather than concentrated (e.g., all cleaning should not be done on the weekend). Activities should be organized to avoid running up and down stairs. Carts should be used to carry things. Materials used often should be stored in a convenient, easily reached area. Time-saving and joint-protective devices (e.g., electric can opener) should be used if possible. Chores should be delegated to other family members.

The nurse should instruct the patient with arthritis to protect the small joints from stress. Assessment of the patient's performance of tasks at work, in the hospital, and in the home identifies activities that must be revised. Joint-saving activities should be reinforced. Table 60-8 lists sample activities that protect small joints.

Patient independence may be increased by occupational therapy training with assistive devices that help simplify tasks, such as built-up utensils, buttonhooks, modified drawer handles, lightweight plastic dishes, and raised toilet seats. Wearing shoes with Velcro fasteners and clothing with buttons or a zipper down the front instead of the back makes dressing easier. A cane or a walker offers support and relief of pain when walking. A platform-wheeled walker minimizes strain on the small joints of the hands and wrists. The Arthritis Foundation offers many programs to assist people with rheumatologic disorders and is an excellent resource for additional suggestions related to self-care.[23]

Daily heat and exercise. Heat and cold therapy help relieve stiffness, pain, and muscle spasm. Application of ice may be beneficial in an acute episode ("flare"), and moist heat appears to offer better relief of chronic stiffness. Superficial heat sources such as heating pads, moist hot packs, paraffin baths, whirlpool baths, and warm baths or showers relieve stiffness before therapeutic exercises. The modality should be selected according to disease severity, ease of application, and cost. Cold therapy effectively relieves joint and muscle pain. Easy home applications include plastic bags of frozen vegetables (peas or corn), which can easily mold around the shoulder, wrists, or knees, or "icing" the skin proximally or distally to a painful joint with ice cubes or small paper cups of frozen water. Heat and cold can be used as often as desired as long as the heat application does not exceed 20 minutes at one time and the cold application does not exceed 10 to 15 minutes at one time.[24] The nurse should alert the patient to the possibility of a burn, especially if a heat-producing liniment is used with another external heat device.

Individualized exercise is an integral part of the treatment plan. This program is usually developed by a physical therapist and includes exercises to improve flexibility, strength, and endurance. The nurse should reinforce compliance with the program and ensure that the exercises are being done correctly. Inadequate joint movement can result in progressive joint immobility and muscle weakness; overaggressive exercise can result in increased pain, inflammation, and joint damage.

Gentle ROM exercises are usually done daily to keep the joints functional. The nurse should emphasize that usual daily activities do not provide adequate exercise to maintain joint motion. Careful adherence to the prescribed exercise program should be a prime goal of the teaching program. The patient should have the opportunity to practice the exercises with supervision. Warm-water (78° to 86° F [25° to 30° C]) aquatic exercises allow easier ROM because of the buoyancy of the water.[25] Aerobic conditioning programs have been shown to improve the physical fitness levels of patients with arthritis. During an acute inflammatory episode, exercise should be limited to one or two repetitions of ROM.

Psychologic support. Self-management and adherence to an individualized home program are contingent on a thorough understanding of RA, the nature and course of the disease, and the objectives of treatment. In addition, the patient's perception of the disease and value system must be considered. Chronic pain or loss of function may make the patient vulnerable to fad claims of false advertising and unproven remedies.

A treatment program tailored to individual problems and lifestyle increases adherence. The nurse can help the patient recognize common fears and concerns faced by all people living with a chronic illness. Evaluation of the family support system is important. The patient is constantly threatened by problems of limited function and fatigue, loss of self-esteem, altered body image, and fear of disability and deformity. Alterations in sexuality should be discussed. Financial planning may be necessary. Community resources such as a home care nurse, homemaker services, and vocational rehabilitation may be considered. Self-help groups are beneficial for some patients. Self-management classes are available in many communities.

JUVENILE RHEUMATOID ARTHRITIS

Juvenile rheumatoid arthritis (JRA), a major rheumatic disease of youth, is defined as RA beginning before 16 years of age. It may be classified on the basis of the type of onset: systemic, pauciarticular, or polyarticular.[26] The last form most closely resembles adult RA; the others may represent other types of arthritis with onset during childhood. Children as young as 6 months of age may be affected, with the peak ages at onset between 1 and 5 years and again between 9 and 12 years. Prognosis is generally favorable, with nearly 70% of children having few or no inflammatory symptoms by adulthood. Residual deformity, however, may be a severe problem for some patients.

JRA may occur with arthritis confined to one joint (pauciarticular) or several (polyarticular). Children most often do not complain of joint pain but may assume a position of flexion to minimize pain, carefully limit movement, or refuse to walk at all. A more constitutional variant known as Still's disease (systemic onset) causes high-spiking fever, vague arthralgias, generalized rash, hepatosplenomegaly, lymphadenopathy, and pleuritis or pericarditis. Complications of JRA include retarded growth and development and chronic, asymptomatic (and at times vision-threatening) eye inflammation.

The criterion for the diagnosis of JRA is persistent arthritis of one or more joints for at least 6 consecutive weeks, provided certain other similar disorders are ruled out. High-spiking fever, generalized lymphadenopathy, and splenomegaly are more common in children than in adults with RA. Leukocytosis is common, whereas rheumatoid factor is present in only 15% of those affected. NSAIDs suppress inflammation in the majority of cases. Chrysotherapy (treatment with gold salts) can be used for arthritis unresponsive to NSAIDs. Corticosteroids are avoided when possible because of their effect on growth.

Nursing intervention requires an individualized written home program with emphasis on compliance. The family is best counseled about the course and prognosis of their child's arthritis according to the onset classification. Daily participation in a planned physical training program encourages full ROM and muscle strengthening and does not strain affected joints. Swimming, bicycling, and dance therapy are better than running, jumping, and kicking. Growth and development should be documented. Slit-lamp ophthalmologic examinations must be done routinely for those children at highest risk for developing ocular complications.

The school nurse should be involved in the child's care. Early-morning classes and stair climbing may be difficult for the child with arthritis. Parents are encouraged to treat the child as normally as possible, avoiding infantilizing or overprotecting. An experienced multidisciplinary health care team can help the child and family meet the challenges of social and personality development. A family-oriented rather than a child-oriented approach is critical for the optimal management of JRA.

DISEASES ASSOCIATED WITH HLA-B27

An unusually high frequency of HLA-B27 is found in patients with ankylosing spondylitis, psoriatic arthritis, and Reiter's syndrome, known as the seronegative spondyloarthritides.[27] (Human leukocyte antigens [HLA] and their relationship to autoimmune diseases are discussed in Chapter 12.) The common characteristics of the spondyloarthropathies are (1) predilection for involvement of sacroiliac joints and spine; (2) oligoarticular asymmetric arthritis; (3) enthesopathy (e.g., plantar fasciitis, Achilles tendinitis); (4) absence of rheumatoid factor and autoantibodies; (5) extraarticular disease in characteristic sites (e.g., eye, heart, skin, mucous membranes); (6) male predominance; and (7) a strong association with the HLA antigen B27.[28] Detection of this marker is an important aid to early diagnosis of these diseases.

ANKYLOSING SPONDYLITIS

Ankylosing spondylitis (AS) is a chronic inflammatory disease that primarily affects the sacroiliac joints, apophyseal and costovertebral joints of the spine, and adjacent soft tissues. Approximately 90% of Caucasian patients with AS are positive for HLA-B27. The disease typically appears in adolescence or young adulthood.

AS is prevalent in both sexes, with progressive disease more common in men. Because women tend to have more peripheral joint involvement, the diagnosis is often delayed or missed.[29] There appears to be a definite familial tendency, and the disease is unusual in African-Americans.

Etiology and Pathophysiology

The cause of AS is unknown. Genetic predisposition appears to play an important role in the disease pathogenesis, but the precise mechanisms are unknown. Environmental factors and infectious agents are also suspected. Inflammation in joints and adjacent tissue causes the formation of granulation tissue and eroding vertebral margins, resulting in spondylitis. Calcification tends to follow the inflammation process, leading to bony ankylosis.

Clinical Manifestations and Complications

The patient typically has lower back pain, stiffness, and limitation of motion that is worse during the night and in the morning but improves with mild activity. General constitutional features such as fever, fatigue, anorexia, and weight loss are rarely present. Other symptoms depend on the stage of the disease and include arthritis of the shoulders, hips, and knees and occasional ocular inflammation (iritis).

Involvement of costovertebral joints leads to a decrease in chest expansion. Advancing kyphosis leads to a bent-over posture, and compensating hip-flexion contractures may occur. There is pronounced impairment of neck motion in all directions. Extraskeletal involvement may include iritis, aortic valvular regurgitation, and apical pulmonary fibrosis.

Diagnostic Studies

Changes on x-rays may not become apparent for months to years after the onset of symptoms. When abnormalities are present, they include sacroiliac joints that show pseudowidening of the joint space and later obliteration with ankylosis. New bone formation (syndesmophytes) may be spotty or generalized (classic "bamboo spine"). ESR, alkaline phosphatase, and creatine kinase (CK) levels are usually elevated. Tissue typing is positive for HLA-B27 in the majority of patients.

Collaborative Care

Prevention of AS is not possible. However, families with diagnosed HLA-B27–positive rheumatic diseases should be alert to signs of low back pain and arthritis symptoms so early treatment can be initiated.

Care of the patient is aimed at maintaining maximal skeletal mobility. Proper posture is important in all activities. Although drugs do not halt the progression of the disease, NSAIDs, such as diclofenac (Voltaren) and indomethacin (Indocin), can reduce inflammation, which makes proper posture easier. Disease-modifying agents such as sulfasalazine (Azulfidine) or methotrexate are sometimes used to control symptoms and delay disease progression. Surgery to correct extreme flexion deformities may be performed in certain cases. A total hip replacement is done for patients with crippling hip ankylosis.

NURSING MANAGEMENT: ANKYLOSING SPONDYLITIS

Nursing responsibilities for the patient with AS include education about the nature of the disease and principles of therapy. A home management program consists of local heat and exercise and proper use of medications. Baseline ROM including chest expansion (using breathing exercises) should be assessed by the nurse. Smoking cessation should be a goal because the risk for lung complications is increased in those with reduced chest expansion. Pain should be managed by appropriate medication, heat, massage, and gentle exercise. Application of moist heat should be followed by ROM exercises and daily chest expansion and deep-breathing exercises. A continuing physical therapy program incorporating gentle, graded stretching and strengthening exercises preserves ROM and improves thoracolumbar flexion and extension. Excessive physical exertion during periods of active inflammation should be discouraged. Proper positioning at rest is essential. The mattress should be firm, and pillows must be avoided. The patient should sleep on the back and avoid positions that encourage flexion deformity. Postural training emphasizes avoiding forward flexion (e.g., leaning over a desk); heavy lifting; and prolonged walking, standing, or sitting. Sports that facilitate natural stretching, such as swimming and racquet games, should be encouraged. Family counseling and vocational rehabilitation are important.

PSORIATIC ARTHRITIS

Psoriatic arthritis can be defined as an association of clinically apparent psoriasis with inflammatory polyarthritis. Psoriatic skin changes may precede or follow articular symptoms. Approximately 10% to 15% of persons with psoriasis have such an arthritis, which is generally mild, with intermittent flare-ups affecting only a few peripheral joints. However, a severe erosive form is also seen. Certain x-ray findings such as asymmetric distribution and resorption of tufts of the distal phalanges of hands, feet, and metatarsal bones help distinguish psoriatic arthritis from RA. Patients with psoriasis are likely to get spondylitis, which is associated with an 80% frequency of HLA-B27 positivity. Hyperuricemia often accompanies the disease. Forms of treatment include splinting, joint protection, and physical therapy. Although gold therapy has recently been used with success for the treatment of psoriatic arthritis, methotrexate continues to be one of the most effective agents for both cutaneous and articular manifestations.

REITER'S SYNDROME

Reiter's syndrome is a self-limiting disease associated with arthritis, urethritis, conjunctivitis, and mucocutaneous lesions.

Although the exact etiology is unknown, Reiter's syndrome appears to be a reactive arthritis after certain enteric (e.g., *Shigella*) or venereal (e.g., *Chlamydia trachomatis*) infections. The disease usually affects males, and 85% of patients with Reiter's syndrome are positive for HLA-B27, which provides evidence for a genetic predisposition. Few other laboratory abnormalities occur, although the ESR may be elevated.

The arthritis of Reiter's syndrome tends to be asymmetric, frequently involving the weight-bearing joints of the lower extremities and sometimes the lower part of the back. Arthralgias usually begin 1 to 3 weeks after the appearance of the initial infection. The full attack may be accompanied by fever and other constitutional complaints, including anorexia with considerable weight loss, and may prove highly debilitating. Soft-tissue manifestations commonly include Achilles tendinitis.

Prognosis is favorable, with most patients recovering after 2 to 16 weeks. Joints heal completely, and many patients have complete remission with full joint function. About one half of the patients, however, have recurring acute attacks; others follow a chronic course, having continued synovitis and progression of x-ray changes closely resembling those of AS. Progressive disease may result in major disability. Treatment is symptomatic, and joint inflammation is treated with NSAIDs.

SEPTIC ARTHRITIS

Septic arthritis (infectious or bacterial arthritis) is caused by invasion of the joint cavity with microorganisms. Various bacteria are commonly responsible, including *Staphylococcus aureus, Streptococcus hemolyticus, Diplococcus pneumoniae,* and *Neisseria gonorrhoeae.* Factors increasing the risk of such infections include previous joint trauma or arthritic disease, diseases of decreased host resistance such as leukemia and diabetes mellitus, treatment with corticosteroids or immunosuppressive drugs, and serious chronic illness. Infants, young children, and older adults appear to be more frequently affected, with the exception of gonococcal arthritis, which affects sexually active young adults. A site of active infection is often responsible for bacteremia (microorganisms reaching the bloodstream), leading to hematogenous seeding of joints.

Inflammation of the joint cavity causes severe pain, erythema, and swelling of one or several joints. Large joints, such as the knee and the hip, are most frequently involved. Fever or shaking chills often accompany articular symptoms because bacterial entry into a joint is usually by the hematogenous route from a primary site of infection. Precise diagnosis is made by aspiration of the joint and culture of the synovial fluid. Blood cultures for aerobic and anaerobic organisms should be obtained.

Septic arthritis is a medical emergency that requires prompt diagnosis and treatment to prevent joint destruction. Parenteral antibiotic administration is maintained until there are no clinical signs of active synovitis or inflammation in the joint fluid. Infections may respond to treatment within 2 weeks or take as long as 4 to 8 weeks, depending on the causative organism. Open surgical drainage may be required.

Nursing intervention includes assessment and monitoring of joint inflammation, pain, and fever. Immobilization of affected joints to control pain is often achieved by resting splints or traction. Gentle ROM exercises should be done. Strict aseptic technique should be used during assistance with joint aspiration procedures. The necessity of antibiotics should be explained, and the importance of their continued use should be stressed. Support should be offered to the patient requiring repeated arthrocentesis or operative drainage. The extent of joint damage is generally related to the invading microorganism and the time between infection onset and initiation of effective treatment.

LYME DISEASE

Lyme disease is a spirochetal infection caused by *Borrelia burgdorferi* and transmitted by the bite of an infected tick. It was first identified in 1975 in Lyme, Connecticut, after an unusual clustering of arthritis in children.[30] It is the most common vector-borne disease in the United States.[31] The tick is no bigger than a poppy seed and typically feeds on mice, dogs, cats, cows, horses, raccoons, deer, and humans. Wild animals do not exhibit the illness, but clinical Lyme disease does occur in domestic animals. The peak season for human infection is during the summer months.

The most characteristic clinical symptom is a skin lesion, erythema migrans (EM), which occurs at the site of the tick bite in 80% of patients. This lesion begins as a red macule or papule that slowly expands to form a large round lesion with a bright red border and central clearing. The EM lesion is often accompanied by other acute symptoms, such as fever, chills, headache, stiff neck, and migratory joint and muscle pain. If not treated, Lyme disease can progress in several weeks or months to (1) severe arthritis; (2) atrioventricular conduction defects, bradycardia, or myocarditis; and (3) neurologic abnormalities, including meningitis, facial palsy, and radiculoneuropathy.

Diagnosis is based on clinical manifestations, history of exposure in an endemic area, and a positive serologic test for *B. burgdorferi.* Other illnesses are frequently misdiagnosed as Lyme disease, particularly chronic fatigue syndrome and fibromyalgia. Serologic testing for antibodies to *B. burgdorferi* is available. Most U.S. cases occur in three endemic areas: along the northeastern coast from Maryland to Massachusetts; in the midwestern states of Wisconsin and Minnesota; and along the northwestern coast of northern California and Oregon.

Active lesions can be treated with antibiotic therapy. Oral doxycycline or amoxicillin is often effective in early-stage infection and in prevention of later stages of the disease. More diffuse infection may require 20 to 30 days of therapy. Intravenous ceftriaxone (Rocephin) is used for cardiac or neurologic abnormalities. Lyme disease arthritis usually responds to oral antibiotic therapy. However, in genetically susceptible persons, chronic arthritis of the knees may not respond to either oral or IV antibiotics. It usually resolves eventually, although it may take several years. LYMErix is a new vaccine for Lyme disease that was recently approved by the FDA.[32] The vaccine is given in three doses over a two-month period. This vaccine is recommended for individuals at high risk. Patient education for the prevention of Lyme disease in endemic areas is outlined in Table 60-9.

HUMAN IMMUNODEFICIENCY VIRUS INFECTION AND ARTHRITIS

A variety of inflammatory arthritis conditions have been reported in the presence of human immunodeficiency virus (HIV) infection.[33,34] The pathogenesis of these disorders is unknown. With suppression of the CD4[+] lymphocytes, oppor-

PATIENT & FAMILY TEACHING GUIDE

Table 60-9   Prevention of Lyme Disease (Endemic Areas)

- Avoid walking through tall grasses and low brush.
- Mow grass and remove brush along paths, buildings, and campsites.
- Move woodpiles and bird feeders away from house.
- Wear long pants or nylon tights of tightly woven, light-colored fabric so that ticks can be easily seen.
- Tuck pants into boots or long socks, tuck long-sleeved shirts into pants, and wear closed shoes when hiking.
- Check often for ticks crawling from legs to open skin.
- Thoroughly inspect and wash clothes.
- Spray insect repellent containing DEET on skin or permethrin on clothes, especially on lower extremities.
- Have pets wear tick collars, inspect them often, and do not allow them on furniture or beds.
- Remove attached ticks with tweezers (not fingers). Grasp tick's mouth parts as close to skin as possible and gently pull straight out. Do not twist or jerk.
- Dispose of tick in alcohol or flush down toilet. Do not crush with fingers.
- Wash bitten area with soap and water and apply antiseptic. Wash hands.
- See a doctor immediately if flulike symptoms or "bull's-eye" rash appears within a few weeks after removal of tick.

DEET, NN, diethyl-M-toluamide.

Table 60-10   Associated Conditions Leading to Hyperuricemia

Acidosis or ketosis
Alcoholism
Atherosclerosis
Cytotoxic drugs
Diabetes mellitus
Drug-induced renal impairment
Hyperlipidemia
Hypertension
Intrinsic renal disease
Malignant disease
Myeloproliferative disorders
Obesity
Sickle cell anemia

tunistic organisms cause infectious arthritis, osteomyelitis, and polymyositis. RA and SLE generally improve as immunodeficiency develops. However, rheumatic diseases associated with HLA-B27 appear to become more severe in HIV-infected patients. For example, progressive, erosive upper-extremity joint disease occurs in Reiter's syndrome, and psoriatic arthritis exhibits a generalized, pustular rash. A Sjögren's-type syndrome, diffuse infiltrative lymphocytosis syndrome, has been identified as a response to HIV infection in children and adults with specific HLA typing. Vasculitis may be responsible for unexplained multisystem disease, arthritis, or fever of unknown origin in HIV-infected patients. Antirheumatic therapy may be effective for short periods but may impair cellular immunity and promote exacerbations of underlying infections.

GOUT

Gout is characterized by recurrent attacks of acute arthritis in association with increased levels of serum uric acid. It may be classified as primary or secondary. In primary gout a hereditary error of purine metabolism leads to the overproduction or retention of uric acid. Secondary gout may be related to another acquired disorder (Table 60-10) or may be the result of medications known to inhibit uric acid excretion. Secondary gout may also be caused by medications that increase the rate of cell death, such as the chemotherapeutic agents used in treating leukemia.

Primary gout occurs predominantly (90%) in middle-aged men, with almost no incidence in premenopausal women. Frequency of hyperuricemia is increased in the families of patients with primary gout. Although some races have been identified as having a low incidence of gout, people of the same race living in another country may exhibit higher mean serum uric acid levels, indicating that both genetic and environmental factors contribute to the etiology.

Etiology and Pathophysiology

Uric acid is the major end product of the catabolism of purines and is primarily excreted by the kidneys. Thus hyperuricemia may be the result of increased purine synthesis, decreased renal excretion, or both. About half the patients with primary gout can be shown to produce excessive amounts of uric acid. Folklore has long associated excesses of food and drink with acute attacks of gouty arthritis. Although high dietary intake of purine alone has relatively little effect on uric acid levels, it is clear that hyperuricemia may result from prolonged fasting or excessive alcohol drinking because of increased production of keto acids, which then inhibit normal renal excretion of uric acid.

Clinical Manifestations and Complications

In the acute phase, gouty arthritis may occur in one or more joints but usually less than four. Affected joints may appear dusky or cyanotic and are extremely tender. Inflammation of the great toe (podagra) is most commonly the initial involvement and occurs in 75% of all patients. Other joints affected are the midtarsal, ankle, knee, and wrist joints and the olecranon bursa. Acute gouty arthritis is usually precipitated by events such as trauma, surgery, alcohol ingestion, or systemic infection. Onset of symptoms is usually rapid, with swelling and pain peaking within several hours, often accompanied by low-grade fever. Individual attacks usually subside, treated or untreated, in 2 to 10 days. The affected joint returns entirely to normal, and patients are often free of symptoms between attacks.

Chronic gout is characterized by multiple joint involvement and deposits of sodium urate crystals called *tophi.* These are typically seen in the synovium, subchondral bone, olecranon bursa, and vertebrae; along tendons; and in the skin and cartilage (Fig. 60-7). Tophi are rarely present at the time of the initial attack and are generally noted only many years after the onset of disease.

The severity of gouty arthritis is variable. The clinical course may consist of infrequent mild attacks or multiple severe

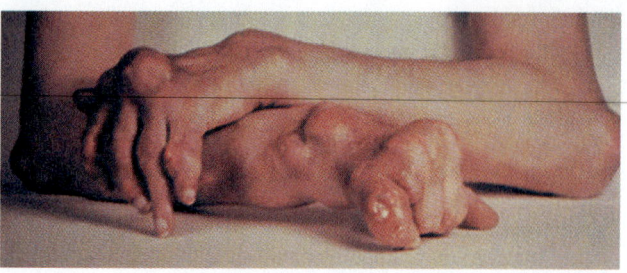

Fig. 60-7 Tophaceous gout. (Reprinted from the Clinical Slide Collection on the Rheumatic Diseases, copyright 1991, 1995, 1997. Used by permission of the American College of Rheumatology. In Seidel HM and others: *Mosby's guide to physical examination,* ed 4, St. Louis, 1999, Mosby.)

episodes associated with a slowly progressive disability. In general, the higher the serum uric acid level, the earlier the appearance of tophi and the greater the tendency toward more frequent and severe episodes of acute gout. An elevated serum uric acid alone does not indicate gout, even when joint symptoms are present, because high serum uric acid levels are found in a variety of diseases. Gout can be diagnosed unequivocally only when urate crystals are found in joint fluid.

Chronic inflammation may result in joint deformity. Destruction of the cartilage may predispose the joint to secondary OA. Tophaceous deposits may be large and unsightly and may perforate overlying skin, producing draining sinuses that often become secondarily infected. Excessive uric acid excretion may lead to kidney or urinary tract stone formation. Pyelonephritis associated with intrarenal sodium urate deposits and obstruction may contribute to renal disease.

Diagnostic Studies

The diagnosis can be established by finding monosodium urate monohydrate crystals in the synovial fluid of an inflamed joint or tophus. In another goutlike syndrome, termed *pseudogout,* nonurate (calcium pyrophosphate dihydrate) crystals are identified in synovial fluid analysis. Serum uric acid levels are almost always elevated to 8 mg/dl (476 (mol/L) or higher. Specimens for 24-hour urine uric acid levels are obtained to control for daily fluctuations in urate concentrations and are important in determining whether the patient undersecretes or overproduces uric acid. Hyperuricemia is not specifically diagnostic of gout because increased levels may be related to a variety of drugs or may exist as a totally asymptomatic abnormality in the general population.

Collaborative Care

Care of the patient with gout (Table 60-11) has several goals. The first is to terminate an acute attack. This is accomplished by the use of an antiinflammatory agent such as colchicine. Future attacks are prevented by a maintenance dose of colchicine, weight reduction if necessary, avoidance of alcohol and high-purine foods, and the use of drugs to reduce the serum urate concentration. Treatment is also aimed at preventing the formation of uric acid kidney stones and other associated conditions such as hypertriglyceridemia and hypertension.

Drug Therapy. Acute gouty arthritis is treated with one of three types of antiinflammatory agents: colchicine, NSAIDs, or corticosteroids. Corticosteroids should be re-

COLLABORATIVE CARE
Table 60-11 | Gout

Diagnostic
History and physical examination
Family history of gout
Presence of monosodium urate monohydrate crystals in synovial fluid
Elevated serum uric acid levels
Elevated 24 hr urine for uric acid levels

Collaborative Therapy
Joint immobilization
Local application of heat or cold
Joint aspiration and intraarticular corticosteroids
Drug therapy
    Nonsteroidal antiinflammatory drugs
    Colchicine
    Probenecid (Benemid)
    Allopurinol (Zyloprim)
Dietary avoidance of food/fluids with high purine content (e.g., anchovies, liver, wine/beer)

served for cases in which colchicine and NSAIDs are contraindicated or ineffective.

Although medication does not prevent recurrent attacks of gout, it can control its symptoms in 75% of gout attacks, particularly with prompt treatment. Oral administration of colchicine generally produces dramatic pain relief within 24 to 48 hours. Colchicine has diagnostic merit in that a good response to treatment gives further evidence for the diagnosis of gout. Prophylactic doses of colchicine reduce the frequency of attacks but do not alter the serum uric acid level.

For many years the standard therapy for hyperuricemia has been a uricosuric drug (e.g., probenecid [Benemid]), which acts by increasing urinary uric acid excretion through inhibiting tubular reabsorption of urates. Aspirin inactivates the effect of uricosurics, resulting in urate retention, and should be avoided while patients are taking probenecid and other uricosuric drugs. Acetaminophen can be used safely if analgesia is required.

Adequate urine volume must be maintained to prevent precipitation of uric acid in the renal tubules. Allopurinol (Zyloprim), which blocks the production of uric acid, may control the serum level and is particularly useful in patients with uric acid stones or renal impairment, in whom uricosuric drugs may be ineffective or dangerous. Regardless of which drug or combination of drugs is prescribed, it is essential that the concentration of serum uric acid be checked regularly to monitor the effectiveness of treatment.

Nutritional Therapy. Dietary restrictions may include limiting the use of alcohol and of foods high in purine (see Table 43-11). However, medication can generally control the situation without necessitating these limitations. Obese patients should be instructed in a carefully planned weight-reduction program.

NURSING MANAGEMENT: GOUT

Acute gouty arthritis may be prevented by maintenance of the serum uric acid at normal levels. Nursing intervention is directed at supportive care of the inflamed joints. Bed rest may be appropriate, with affected joints properly immobilized. The limitation of motion and degree of pain should be assessed. Treatment effectiveness should be documented. Special care is taken to avoid causing pain to an inflamed joint by careless handling. Involvement of a lower extremity may require use of a cradle or footboard to protect the painful area from the weight of bedclothes.

The patient and the family should understand that hyperuricemia and gouty arthritis are chronic problems that can be controlled with careful adherence to a treatment program.[35] Thorough explanations should be given concerning the importance of drug therapy and the need for periodic determination of blood uric acid levels. The patient should be able to demonstrate knowledge of precipitating factors that may cause an attack, including overindulgence in the intake of calories, purines, and alcohol; starvation (fasting); medication use (e.g., aspirin, diuretics); and major medical events (e.g., surgery, myocardial infarction).

SYSTEMIC LUPUS ERYTHEMATOSUS

Systemic lupus erythematosus (SLE) is a chronic multisystem inflammatory disease of connective tissue that often involves the skin, joints, serous membranes (pleura, pericardium), kidneys, hematologic system, and central nervous system (CNS).[36] SLE is characterized by its variability within and among persons, with a chronic unpredictable course of exacerbations of disease activity alternating with periods of remission. The clinical presentation of SLE ranges from a mild to a serious illness, with a tendency to acute exacerbations precipitated by several factors. Individuals with SLE can now live a normal life span.

The true incidence of SLE is unknown, but the rate appears to be increasing. It is unknown whether this increase is a reflection of heightened diagnostic awareness or a true increase in frequency.[37] The general prevalence of SLE is approximately 1 in 2100. Women have a higher incidence of SLE than men. The disease occurs three times more often in African-American than in Caucasian women.[38] Because of the difficulty in diagnosing SLE, the incidence and prevalence of the disease may be much higher than statistics indicate.

Etiology and Pathophysiology

The etiology of SLE is unknown. However, factors implicated in the etiology of SLE include genetic predisposition, sex hormones, race, environmental factors (e.g., ultraviolet radiation, drugs, chemicals), viruses and infections, stress, and immunologic abnormalities. SLE is a disorder of immunoregulation. Autoimmune reactions are directed against constituents of the cell nucleus, particularly DNA. In SLE, autoantibodies are produced against nuclear antigens (DNA, histones, ribonucleoproteins, and nucleolar factors), cytoplasmic antigens (ribosomal and cardiolipin), and blood cell surface antigens (WBCs, red blood cells [RBCs], and platelets). When autoantibodies bind to their specific antigens, complement activation occurs. Accumulation of immune complexes within the blood vessel walls and subsequent complement activation leads to a condition called lupus vasculitis. The ensuing ischemia within the blood vessel walls gradually leads to the thickening of the internal lin-

ing, fibrinoid degeneration, and thrombus formation. The specific manifestations of SLE depend on which cell types or organs are involved.

The overaggressive antibody response is related to B cell hyperactivity accompanied by multiple abnormalities in immunoregulation. Examples of these include decreased T-suppressor cells and diminished interleukin-2 production.[39]

Although studies have shown the importance of heredity in the development and expression of SLE, the susceptibility genes are largely unknown.[40] The major histocompatibility complexes HLA-DR2, HLA-DR3, and HLA-DR4 show significant associations with SLE.

Hormones are known to play a role in the etiology of SLE. A disproportionate number of females have SLE. In addition, there is a tendency for the disease to worsen in the immediate postpartum period. Healthy women are more immunologically reactive than healthy men because estrogens enhance immune reactivity, whereas androgens suppress it. It is thought that estrogens produce their effect through their impact on suppressor T cells, which normally regulate B cell reactivity. In the absence of the T cell regulatory function, the antibody production by the B cells continues.[41] In addition, it has been determined that the type of lymphocytes varies between women and men. Women have slightly higher proportions of T-helper cells (which increase immune reactivity) and lower proportions of T-suppressor cells (which decrease immune reactivity) than men.[42] These factors may contribute to a woman's increased potential for acquiring autoimmune diseases. Onset or exacerbation of disease symptoms sometimes occurs after the onset of menarche, with the use of oral contraceptives, and during and after pregnancy.

SLE may also be precipitated or aggravated by certain drugs such as procainamide (Pronestyl), hydralazine (Apresoline), and a number of antiseizure agents. Sulfonamides (e.g., Bactrim) should not be used in patients with SLE because they can cause a flare-up of the condition. Oral contraceptives may also aggravate the disease and should be used cautiously. Some foods, such as alfalfa sprouts, celery, parsley, and shiitake or reishi mushrooms, should be avoided for the same reason.

Clinical Manifestations and Complications

SLE is extremely variable in its severity, ranging from a relatively mild disorder to a rapidly progressive one affecting many organ systems (Fig. 60-8). There is no characteristic pattern of progressive organ involvement, nor is it predictable which systems may become affected. Theoretically, any organ can be affected by the accumulation of the circulating immune complexes. However, cutaneous and muscle tissue, the lining of the lungs, the heart, nervous tissue, and the kidneys are most commonly affected. SLE is characterized by alternating periods of remission and exacerbation. General constitutional complaints include fever, weight loss, arthralgia, and excessive fatigue and may precede an exacerbation of disease activity.

Dermatologic Manifestations. The most common cutaneous feature of SLE is an erythematous rash that can occur on the face, neck, and extremities. The classic butterfly rash, which is distributed across the bridge of the nose and cheeks, occurs in about 40% of patients (Fig. 60-9). The rash may appear as discoid (coin-like) lesions or as a diffuse maculopapular rash; it may occur anywhere on the body but is

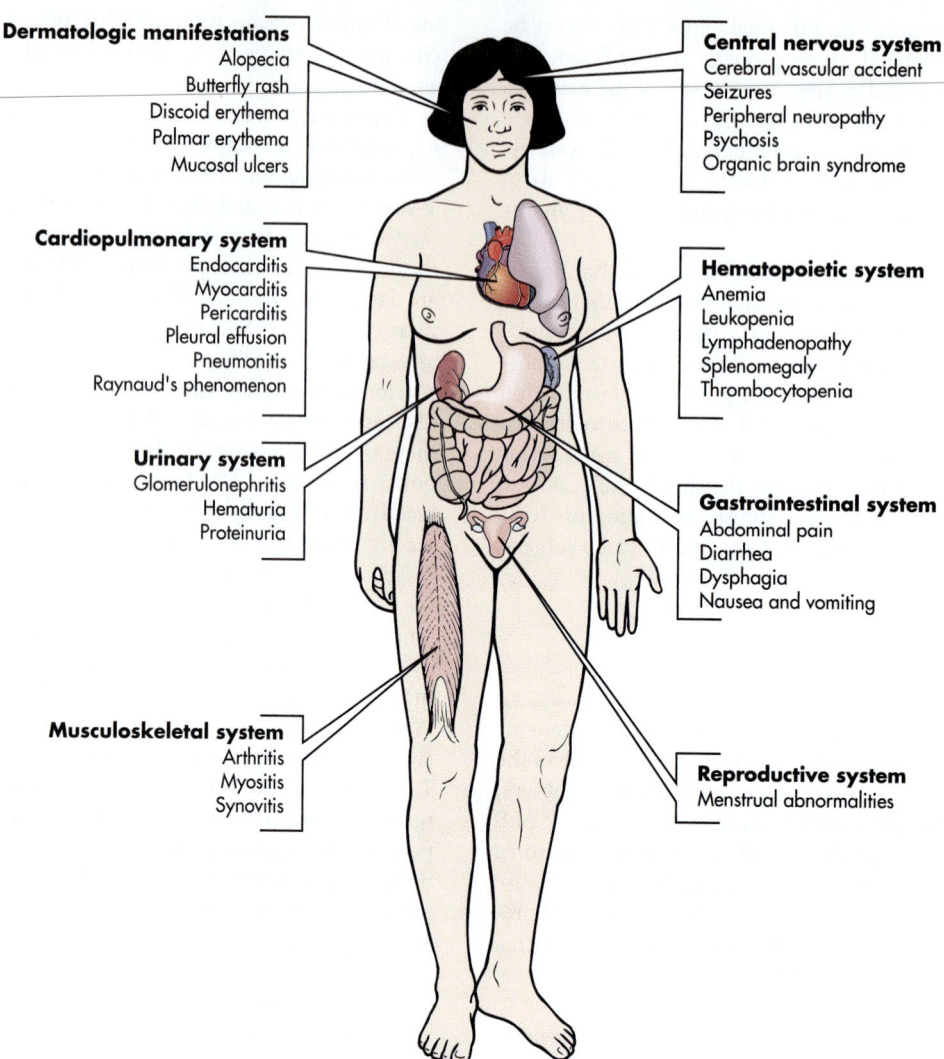

Dermatologic manifestations
Alopecia
Butterfly rash
Discoid erythema
Palmar erythema
Mucosal ulcers

Cardiopulmonary system
Endocarditis
Myocarditis
Pericarditis
Pleural effusion
Pneumonitis
Raynaud's phenomenon

Urinary system
Glomerulonephritis
Hematuria
Proteinuria

Musculoskeletal system
Arthritis
Myositis
Synovitis

Central nervous system
Cerebral vascular accident
Seizures
Peripheral neuropathy
Psychosis
Organic brain syndrome

Hematopoietic system
Anemia
Leukopenia
Lymphadenopathy
Splenomegaly
Thrombocytopenia

Gastrointestinal system
Abdominal pain
Diarrhea
Dysphagia
Nausea and vomiting

Reproductive system
Menstrual abnormalities

Fig. 60-8 Multisystem involvement in systemic lupus erythematosus.

most frequently seen on the face and chest. A small number of patients have persistent lesions, photosensitivity, and mild systemic disease. This syndrome is referred to as *subacute cutaneous lupus.*[43]

Exposure to sunlight and to other sources of ultraviolet radiation can cause a severe skin reaction and may precipitate a flare-up of disease activity in persons who are photosensitive.[44] Ulcers of the oral or nasopharyngeal membranes occur in up to one third of patients with SLE. Transient diffuse or patchy hair loss (alopecia) is common, with or without underlying scalp lesions. The hair may grow back during remission. The scalp becomes dry, scaly, and atrophied.

Musculoskeletal Problems. Polyarthralgia with morning stiffness is often the patient's first complaint and may precede the onset of multisystem disease by many years. Arthritis occurs in 95% of all patients with SLE at some time in the disease course. Joint symptoms are typically migratory, producing pain without objective signs of inflammation. Lupus-related arthritis is generally nonerosive, but it may cause deformities such as swan-neck appearance of the hands, ulnar deviation, and subluxation with hyperlaxity of the joints.

Only about 15% to 35% of SLE patients test positive for rheumatoid factor.[45]

Cardiopulmonary Problems. Pericarditis is present in nearly one fourth of patients with SLE and is usually associated with myocardial disease. Patients treated with corticosteroids have a higher incidence of atherosclerosis. Pleurisy with or without effusion is seen in nearly 50% of patients at some time during the illness, and pulmonary function studies are abnormal in 90%. Raynaud's phenomenon occurs in 20% of patients. Cardiovascular involvement is an ominous sign of advanced disease and contributes significantly to the morbidity and mortality seen in SLE.

Renal Problems. Clinical evidence of renal involvement is present in nearly one half of patients with SLE and includes microscopic hematuria, excessive cellular casts in the urine sediment, proteinuria, and elevation of serum creatinine level. Kidney involvement varies in degree but may eventually end in renal failure. Regardless of whether renal manifestations are evident, nearly all patients with SLE show renal histologic abnormalities in renal biopsy studies or autopsy results. Lupus nephritis is the leading cause of death in SLE.[46]

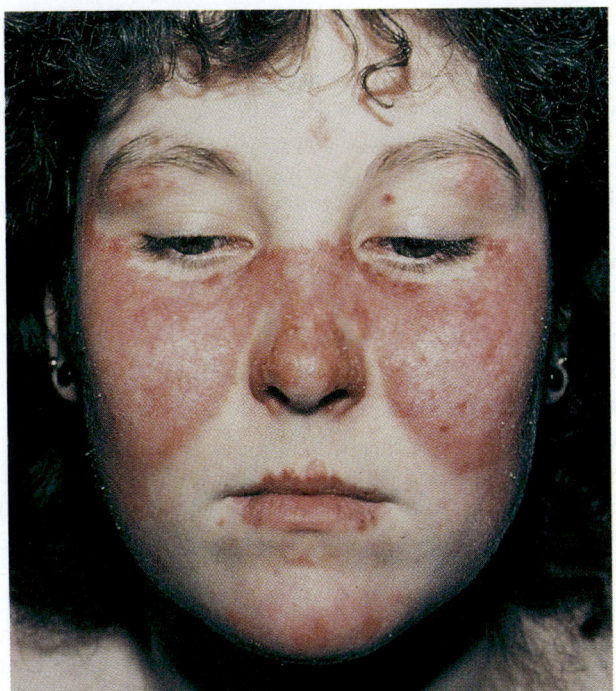

Fig. 60-9   Butterfly rash of systemic lupus erythematosus.

Table **60-12**	Criteria for Diagnosis of Systemic Lupus Erythematosus*

Malar rash
Discoid rash
Photosensitivity
Oral ulcers
Arthritis: nonerosive, involvement of two or more joints
Serositis: pleuritis or pericarditis
Renal disorder: proteinuria or cellular casts in urine
Neurologic disorder: seizures or psychosis
Hematologic disorder: hemolytic anemia, leukopenia, lymphopenia, or thrombocytopenia
Immunologic disorder: positive lupus cell preparation; anti-DNA antibody or antibody to Sm nuclear antigen; false-positive serologic tests for syphilis
Antinuclear antibodies

*A person is classified as having SLE if four or more of the criteria are present, serially or simultaneously, during any interval of observation. Revised criteria by a subcommittee of the American College of Rheumatology are used for the purpose of *classification* in population surveys, *not* for the diagnosis of individual patients.
Sm, Smith.

Clinical factors, including blood pressure, urinalysis, serum creatinine levels, serum complement levels, and autoantibodies to DNA, should be monitored carefully and frequently over prolonged periods because renal involvement in the early stages is usually asymptomatic.

Central Nervous System Problems. CNS involvement ranks close behind kidney disease and infection as a leading cause of death in SLE. Seizures are the most common neurologic manifestation and occur in as many as 15% of patients with SLE by the time of diagnosis. They are generally controlled by corticosteroids or antiseizure therapy.

Organic brain syndrome, another recognized CNS manifestation of SLE, may result from the deposition of immune complexes within brain tissue. It is characterized by disordered thought processes, disorientation, memory deficits, and psychiatric symptoms such as severe depression and psychosis. Recovery from organic brain disease is expected, although some residual impairment may result. Occasionally a cerebrovascular accident (stroke) or aseptic meningitis may be attributable to SLE. It is difficult to differentiate neuropsychiatric SLE from non-SLE neurologic problems.

Hematologic Problems. The formation of antibodies against blood cells, such as erythrocytes, leukocytes, thrombocytes, and coagulation factors, is one of the most common features of SLE. Anemia (98%), mild leukopenia (80%), and thrombocytopenia (36%) are often present.[47] Some patients show a tendency to bleed whereas others show a tendency toward blood clots. In addition, SLE patients have positive antinuclear antibodies.

Infection. Patients with SLE appear to have increased susceptibility to infections, possibly related to defects in their ability to phagocytize invading bacteria, deficiencies in production of antibodies, and the immunosuppressive effect of many antiinflammatory drugs. Infection, a major cause of death, has an incidence of 30%. Pneumonia is most common. Fever should be considered serious because it may indicate an underlying infectious process rather than lupus activity alone. However, it is not unusual for patients with SLE to have low-grade fevers of 99° to 100° F (37.2° to 37.8° C).

Diagnostic Studies

The diagnosis of SLE is based on the history, physical examination, and laboratory findings (Table 60-12). A variety of abnormalities may be present in the blood, including elevated ESR, increased gamma-globulin levels, anemia, decreased WBC and platelet counts, electrocardiogram (ECG) or chest x-ray evidence of pericarditis or pleural effusion, and a false-positive serologic test for syphilis. Abnormalities in urine sediment (cellular casts, proteinuria), reduced serum complement levels (C3 and CH 50), and tissue specimens demonstrating changes compatible with SLE are other confirmatory findings.

The lupus erythematosus cell prep is the presence of neutrophils with phagocytized inclusions of IgG antibody to DNA. It is a nonspecific test for SLE and is positive in other rheumatologic diseases.

Antinuclear antibodies (ANA), autoantibodies against nuclear antigens, have been detected in 99% of persons with SLE. Although extremely sensitive, ANA is not specific for SLE because it is present in 5% of normal persons and 38% of all persons more than 60 years of age. Anti-DNA is found most commonly in SLE and is rarely seen in other rheumatic diseases. Anti-Sm antibody, an antibody to the Smith nuclear antigen, is a definitive serologic marker for SLE and is not demonstrated in other rheumatic diseases.[48] About 15% to 35% of SLE patients test positive for rheumatoid factor.[45]

Collaborative Care

The rate of spontaneous remission in SLE is high. Corticosteroids remain the mainstay for treatment of severe illness. Their use should be reserved for acute generalized exacerbation

COLLABORATIVE CARE
Table 60-13 Systemic Lupus Erythematosus

Diagnostic
History and physical examination
Lupus cell preparation
Antibodies
   Anti-DNA antibody
   Anti-Sm antibody
   Antinuclear antibody (ANA)
Complete blood cell count
Urinalysis
X-ray of affected joints
Chest x-ray
Complement levels (CH50, C3)
ECG

Collaborative Therapy
NSAIDs
Antimalarials (e.g., hydroxychloroquine [Plaquenil])
Corticosteroids for exacerbations and severe disease
Immunosuppressive drugs
   Cyclophosphamide (Cytoxan)
   Azathioprine (Imuran)

Sm antibody, Smith antibody.

or serious organ involvement, although a reduced maintenance dosage is sometimes used. Immunosuppressive drugs may be used for symptoms that are resistant to or to reduce the need for long-term corticosteroid therapy (Table 60-13). Efficacy of treatment is most appropriately monitored by serial serum complement levels and anti-DNA titers. Simpler and less costly tests such as ESR or C-reactive protein levels may also help in monitoring treatment effectiveness.

An improving prognosis of SLE may be the result of earlier diagnosis, prompt recognition of serious organ involvement, and better therapeutic regimens. Survival is influenced by several factors, including age, race, gender, socioeconomic status, accompanying morbid conditions, and severity of disease. For example, childhood-onset SLE accounts for nearly 20% of all cases and has a higher incidence of lupus nephritis (up to 80%) than in other age-groups.

Drug Therapy. Medications are prescribed to suppress inflammation and the immune system. The type of medication used depends almost entirely on disease activity. Aspirin or other NSAIDs may reduce mild symptoms such as fever and arthritic complaints. GI upset and tinnitus should be reported. Antimalarial drugs, such as hydroxychloroquine (Plaquenil), may be used to improve skin and musculoskeletal problems, but eye examinations must be scheduled periodically during this therapy because visual loss is a rare but a serious side effect.[49] Topical corticosteroid preparations and intralesional corticosteroid injections are effective treatments for skin lesions.

Corticosteroids are potent antiinflammatory medications used for acute generalized exacerbations of SLE and for the treatment of serious involvement of vital organs, including hematologic abnormalities. As clinical and laboratory values improve, the dosages are gradually tapered.

Patient teaching must include indications for use and proper administration of corticosteroids and possible side effects (see Chapter 47). The patient should understand that abrupt cessation may precipitate recurrence of disease activity. Immunosuppressive drug therapy such as azathioprine (Imuran) and cyclophosphamide (Cytoxan) is often used in life-threatening situations for symptoms unresponsive to more conservative treatment. Close monitoring is necessary to minimize drug toxicity.

NURSING MANAGEMENT: SYSTEMIC LUPUS ERYTHEMATOSUS
■ Nursing Assessment

As in the majority of rheumatic diseases, the chronic and unpredictable nature of SLE presents many challenges to the patient and family. The physical, psychologic, and sociocultural problems associated with the long-term management of SLE require the varied approaches and skills of the multidisciplinary health care team.

Subjective and objective data that should be obtained from a patient with SLE are presented in Table 60-14. The extent to which pain and fatigue influence activities of daily living must be evaluated. A developmental approach focuses on age-appropriate educational and counseling issues, such as personal relationships, family planning, occupational responsibilities, and recreational activities.

■ Nursing Diagnoses

Nursing diagnoses for the patient with SLE may include, but are not limited to, those presented in NCP 60-2.

■ Planning

The overall goals are that the patient with systemic lupus erythematosus will (1) have satisfactory pain relief, (2) comply with therapeutic regimen to achieve maximum symptom management, (3) avoid activities that induce disease exacerbation, and (4) maintain a positive self-image.

■ Nursing Implementation

Health Promotion. Prevention of SLE is not possible at this time. Education of health professionals and the community may promote a clearer understanding of the disease and earlier diagnosis and treatment.

Acute Intervention. During an exacerbation, patients may become abruptly and dramatically ill. Nursing intervention includes accurately recording the severity of symptoms and documenting the response to therapy. Fever pattern, joint inflammation, limitation of motion, location and degree of discomfort, and fatigability should be specifically assessed. The patient's weight and fluid intake and output should be monitored because of the fluid-retention effect of corticosteroids and the possibility of renal failure. Collection of 24-hour urine samples for protein and creatinine clearance may be ordered. The nurse should observe for signs of bleeding that result from drug therapy, such as pallor, skin bruising, petechiae, or tarry stools.

NURSING ASSESSMENT

Table 60-14 Systemic Lupus Erythematosus

Subjective Data

Important Health Information

Past health history: Exposure to ultraviolet radiation, drugs, chemicals, viral infections; physical or psychologic stress; states of increased estrogen activity, including early onset of menarche, pregnancy, and postpartum period; pattern of remissions and exacerbations

Medications: Use of oral contraceptives, procainamide (Pronestyl), hydralazine (Apresoline), isoniazid (INH), antiseizure drugs, antibiotics (possibly precipitating symptoms of SLE); corticosteroids, NSAIDs

Functional Health Patterns

Health perception–health management: Family history of SLE or immunologic disorders; frequent infections; malaise

Nutritional-metabolic: Weight loss, oral and nasal ulcers; nausea and vomiting; xerostomia (salivary gland dryness), dysphagia; photosensitivity with rash; frequent infections

Elimination: Decreased urine output; diarrhea or constipation

Activity-exercise: Morning stiffness; joint swelling and deformity; shortness of breath, dyspnea; excessive fatigue

Sleep-rest: Insomnia

Cognitive-perceptual: Visual disturbances; vertigo; headache; polyarthralgia; chest pain (pericardial, pleuritic); abdominal pain; joint pain; pain, throbbing, coldness of fingers with numbness and tingling

Sexuality-reproductive: Amenorrhea, irregular menstrual periods

Coping–stress tolerance: Depression, withdrawal

Objective Data

General

Fever, lymphadenopathy, periorbital edema

Integumentary

Alopecia; dry, scaly scalp; keratoconjunctivitis, malar "butterfly" rash, palmar or discoid erythema, urticaria, periungal erythema, purpura, or petechiae; leg ulcers

Respiratory

Pleural friction rub, decreased breath sounds

Cardiovascular

Vasculitis; pericardial friction rub; hypertension, edema, arrhythmias, murmurs; bilateral, symmetric pallor and cyanosis of fingers (Raynaud's phenomenon)

Gastrointestinal

Oral and pharyngeal ulcers; splenomegaly

Neurologic

Facial weakness, peripheral neuropathies, papilledema, dysarthria, confusion, hallucination, disorientation, psychosis, seizures, aphasia, hemiparesis

Musculoskeletal

Myopathy, myositis, arthritis

Possible Findings

Positive lupus cell preparation, elevated ANA titers, presence of anti-DNA, Sm-nuclear, and antinuclear antibodies; decreased T-suppressor lymphocyte count, elevated gamma globulin; anemia, leukopenia, thrombocytopenia; increased erythrocyte sedimentation rate; increased serum creatinine; proteinuria, microscopic hematuria, cellular casts in urine; pericarditis or pleural effusion evident on chest x-ray

ANA, antinuclear antibody

Careful assessment of neurologic status includes observation for visual disturbances, headaches, personality changes, seizures, and forgetfulness. Psychosis may indicate CNS disease or may be the effect of corticosteroid therapy. Irritation of the nerves of the extremities (peripheral neuropathy) may produce numbness, tingling, and weakness of the hands and feet. Less frequently a stroke may result.

The nurse must explain the nature of the disease and modes of therapy and prepare the patient for numerous diagnostic procedures. Emotional support for the patient and family is essential.

Ambulatory and Home Care. Nursing interventions must emphasize health teaching and home management. The patient must understand that even perfect adherence to the treatment plan is not a guarantee against exacerbation because the course of the disease is unpredictable. However, a variety of factors may encourage exacerbation, such as fatigue, sun exposure, emotional stress, infection, drugs, and surgery. Nursing interventions should be directed toward assisting the patient and family to eliminate or minimize exposure to precipitating factors (Table 60-15). Patient understanding and cooperation are important to this goal.

Lupus and pregnancy. For the best outcome for the female patient with SLE, pregnancy should be planned with the cooperation of the primary physician and obstetrician at a point when the disease activity is minimal.[50] Only women with serious renal, cardiac, or CNS involvement should be counseled against pregnancy. Exacerbation is common during the postpartum period. Therapeutic abortion offers the same risk of postdelivery exacerbation as carrying the fetus to term.

Fetal risks include increased rates of miscarriage, prematurity, and stillbirth. Neonatal lupus, an uncommon occurrence, is characterized by rash, transient lupus antibodies, or congenital complete heart block. The presence of antiphospholipid antibodies in the mother may be predictive of placental insufficiency and thrombosis and have been correlated with repeated miscarriage and intrauterine fetal death. Regular clinical and laboratory monitoring is essential for the pregnant woman with SLE.

Psychosocial issues. The patient with SLE confronts many psychosocial issues. Disease onset may be vague, and SLE is often undiagnosed for long periods of time. The nurse should counsel the patient and family that SLE has a good prognosis for the majority of persons. Men are often embarrassed that they have a "woman's disease." Families are anxious about hereditary aspects and want to know whether their children will also have SLE. Many couples require pregnancy and sexual counseling. Individuals making decisions about marriage and

60-2 NURSING CARE PLAN PATIENT WITH SYSTEMIC LUPUS ERYTHEMATOSUS

Expected Patient Outcomes   **Nursing Interventions and *Rationales***

NURSING DIAGNOSIS **Fatigue** *related to* disease process *as manifested by* lack of energy, inability to maintain usual routine.

- Completion of priority activities.
- Pacing of activities.
- Verbalization of having more energy.

- Analyze energy level patterns *to plan daily activities.*
- Assist patient to prioritize activities *to establish preferred daily routine.*
- Teach energy conservation techniques such as sitting at kitchen sink, enlisting aid of others *to accomplish as much as possible with a minimum of energy expenditure.**
- Include family in planning *to increase patient's sense of support and family's understanding of patient's disease and related problems.*
- Teach patient techniques such as meditation, yoga *to provide patient with stress-reducing strategies.*
- Encourage patient to rest regularly and as needed *to temporarily reverse effect of fatigue.*

NURSING DIAGNOSIS **Pain** *related to* disease process and inadequate comfort measures *as manifested by* complaints of joint pain, lack of relief from pain-relieving measures; reduction of activity to avoid exacerbating pain.

- Expression of satisfaction with pain relief measures.
- Performance of activities of daily living without pain.

- Assess pain location and severity *to plan appropriate interventions.*
- Administer analgesia as ordered and monitor effect; teach joint protection measures; apply heat or cold as individually determined *to relieve pain.*
- Use nonpharmacologic pain interventions such as relaxation and visual imagery *to replace or supplement analgesics.*

NURSING DIAGNOSIS **Body image disturbance** *related to* changes in physical appearance *as manifested by* verbalization of dissatisfaction with physical appearance, lack of participation in hygiene and grooming practices.

- Increased self-interest and participation in self-care.
- Expression of positive comments about self.

- Discuss realistic expectations of physical changes *to help patient make plans to maximize physical assets and minimize problematic areas.*
- Encourage interest in hygiene and grooming and teach ways to use cosmetics creatively *because these activities improve body image and sense of control.*
- Encourage discussion about feelings and positive attributes *to reduce patient's sense of isolation and poor body image and redirect self-focus to positive attributes.*

NURSING DIAGNOSIS **Impaired skin integrity** *related to* photosensitivity, skin rash, and alopecia *as manifested by* rash anywhere on body, butterfly rash on face, hair loss, areas of ulceration on fingertips.

- Limitation of direct exposure to sun and use of sunscreens.
- No open skin lesions.
- Strategies to cope with alopecia.

- Assess and monitor location and progression of rash *to plan appropriate interventions.*
- Administer medications and apply ointments as ordered *to control skin manifestations.*
- Keep skin clean and dry *to avoid secondary infections.*
- Avoid unprescribed ointments *because these often exacerbate existing conditions.*
- Discuss need to limit direct sun exposure and use of sunscreens and sun-protective clothing when outdoors *because sun exacerbates skin and systemic manifestations.*

NURSING DIAGNOSIS **Activity intolerance** *related to* arthralgia, weakness, and fatigue *as manifested by* inability or unwillingness to ambulate or engage in physical activity, dyspnea, abnormal response to activity (e.g., increased pulse, respiratory rate).

- Expression of satisfaction with activity pattern.
- Pacing of activities to match level of tolerance.

- Monitor vital signs when ambulating *because an increasing pulse and respiratory rate may indicate a need to allow patient to rest.*
- Pace activities and allow periods of rest between activities *to promote recuperation and to foster maximum participation in activities.*
- Encourage patient to assist in setting activity schedule *to allow patient a sense of control and to foster cooperation with the plan.*
- Provide bed rest during exacerbation *to conserve energy for vital activities.*
- Provide ROM exercises q4hr to unaffected joints *to prevent development of stiffness and contractures.*
- Encourage use of assistive devices *to minimize energy expenditure.*

Continued

60-2 NURSING CARE PLAN PATIENT WITH SYSTEMIC LUPUS ERYTHEMATOSUS
—continued

Expected Patient Outcomes	Nursing Interventions and *Rationales*

NURSING DIAGNOSIS **Altered nutrition: less than body requirements** *related to* anorexia, fatigue, oral ulcerations, and side effects of medication *as manifested by* weight loss, poor appetite, inability or unwillingness to eat adequate food to meet nutritional requirements.

- Maintenance of weight.
- Intake of sufficient quantity and quality of food to meet daily needs.

- Assess food preferences and include them in meal planning when possible *to promote adequate intake and patient's sense of control.*
- Offer small, frequent meals *to foster adequate intake by reducing fatigue and bloating associated with larger meals.*
- Provide oral hygiene before and after meals *to increase patient comfort and prevent causing or exacerbating oral ulcerations.*
- Monitor pertinent laboratory values such as hemoglobin, electrolytes, and protein levels *because lowered levels can indicate inadequate intake.*
- Encourage family to bring in favorite foods *to increase patient's intake and as a gesture of love and caring.*

NURSING DIAGNOSIS **Ineffective management of therapeutic regimen** *related to* lack of knowledge of long-term management of disease *as manifested by* questions about SLE or incorrect answers to questions by patient or family, use of unproven remedies.

- Expression of confidence in ability to manage SLE over time and in home environment.

- Teach patient about disease process, including chronic management, *to increase probability of successful long-term management.*
- Include family in teaching activities *to provide caregivers support during exacerbation and increase their sense of involvement.*
- Discuss need to wear Medic Alert bracelet *to alert uninformed health care providers in time of emergency.*
- Teach patient to report signs and symptoms of complications such as fever, edema, decreased urine output, chest pain, and dyspnea *to ensure early intervention.*
- Inform patient of availability of assistance from Lupus Foundation and Arthritis Foundation *to provide additional sources of information and support.*

*See Tables 60-3 and 60-8.

✎ PATIENT & FAMILY TEACHING GUIDE
Table 60-15 Systemic Lupus Erythematosus

1. Education on the disease process
2. Names of medications and actions, side effects, dosage, and administration
3. Energy-conservation and pacing techniques
4. Daily heat and exercise program (for arthralgia)
5. Avoidance of physical and emotional stress, overexposure to ultraviolet light, and unnecessary exposure to infection
6. Regular medical and laboratory follow-up
7. Marital counseling, if necessary
8. Referral resources to community and health care agencies

SLE, yet pain and fatigue are cited most frequently as interfering with quality of life. Friends and relatives are confused by the patient's complaints of transient joint pain and overwhelming fatigue. Pacing techniques and relaxation therapy can help keep the patient actively involved. Daily planning should include recreational and occupational activities. Children and young adults find sun restrictions and physical limitations particularly difficult to follow. SLE may also have a negative effect on the patient's self-esteem and body image.[51] Nursing interventions should assist the patient in developing and accomplishing reasonable goals toward improving mobility, energy levels, and self-esteem.[52]

■ **Evaluation**

The expected outcomes for the patient with SLE are presented in NCP 60-2.

SYSTEMIC SCLEROSIS

Systemic sclerosis (SS), or *scleroderma*, is a disorder of connective tissue characterized by fibrotic, degenerative, and occasion-

careers worry about how SLE will interfere with their plans. The nurse may have to educate teachers, employers, and co-workers.

The obvious physical effects of skin rashes, discoid lesions, and alopecia may cause social isolation for the patient with

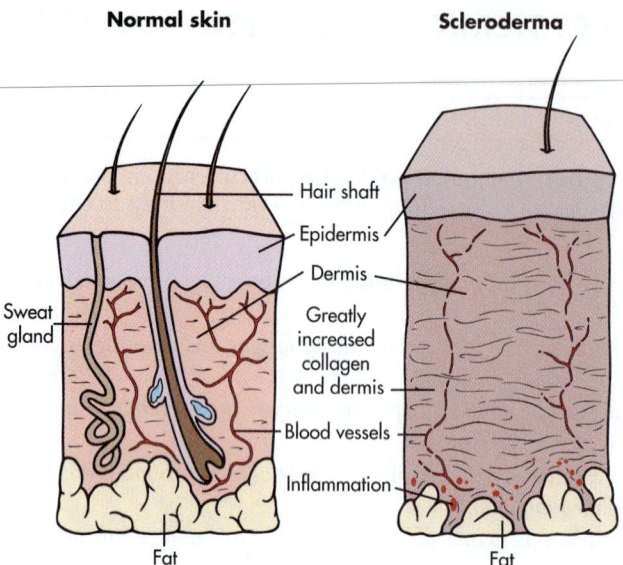

Fig. 60-10   Scleroderma skin changes.

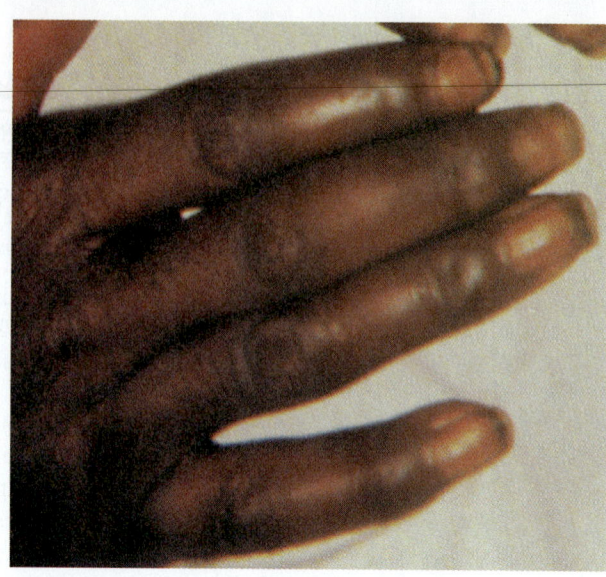

Fig. 60-11   Hand of a patient with systemic sclerosis showing sclerodactyly.

ally inflammatory changes in the skin, blood vessels, synovium, skeletal muscle, and internal organs. Skin thickening and tightening are the cardinal features. The disease may range from a diffuse cutaneous thickening with rapidly progressive and fatal visceral involvement to a more benign variant called CREST syndrome (*c*alcinosis, *R*aynaud's phenomenon, *e*sophageal hypomotility, *s*clerodactyly [skin change of the fingers], and *t*elangiectasia [macule-like angioma on the skin]).[53] (Raynaud's phenomenon is explained in Chapter 36.)

SS affects women three times more frequently than men, with the female-to-male ratio increasing to 15:1 during the childbearing years. SS has been reported in all races but is more common in African-Americans than Caucasians. Although symptoms may begin at any time, the usual age at onset is between 30 and 50 years. SS affects approximately 250,000 people in the United States.

The disease course of SS is variable. Persons with CREST syndrome have limited disability and the longest survival rates, although they are at higher risk for pulmonary hypertension. Myocardial and renal involvement adversely affect the outcome in diffuse disease.

Etiology and Pathophysiology

The exact cause of SS remains unclear. Possible links include environmental toxin exposure to vinyl chloride, epoxy resins, and trichloroethylene. Occupational silica dust exposure has been associated with an increased incidence of systemic sclerosis.[54] Vibrational tool exposure may be another factor involved in the development of this disorder. Collagen, the protein that gives normal skin its strength and elasticity, is overproduced (Fig. 60-10). Widespread systemic disease may be the result of primary vessel injury or immune dysregulation. Disruption of the cell is followed by platelet aggregation, myointimal cell proliferation, and fibrosis. Proliferation of collagen disrupts the normal functioning of internal organs, such as the lungs, kidney, heart, and GI tract.

Clinical Manifestations

Raynaud's Phenomenon.   Raynaud's phenomenon (paroxysmal vasospasm of the digits) occurs in nearly 98% of patients with SS and is the most common initial complaint in CREST syndrome. Patients have diminished blood flow to the fingers and toes on exposure to cold (blanching or white phase), followed by cyanosis as hemoglobin releases oxygen to the tissues (blue phase), and then erythema on rewarming (red phase). The color changes are often accompanied by numbness and tingling. Raynaud's phenomenon may precede the onset of systemic disease by months, years, or even decades.

Skin and Joint Changes.   Symmetric painless swelling or thickening of the skin of the fingers and hands may progress to diffuse scleroderma of the trunk. In CREST syndrome skin thickening is generally limited to the fingers and face. The skin loses elasticity and becomes taut and shiny, producing the typical expressionless facies with tightly pursed lips. The hands may be affected by sclerodactyly in which the fingers are in a semiflexed position, with tightened skin to the wrist (Fig. 60-11). Polyarthralgias and morning stiffness may be early symptoms. Tendon friction rubs may be present.

Internal Organ Involvement.   Esophageal hypomotility causes frequent reflux of gastric acid, causing heartburn and substernal dysphagia for solid foods. If swallowing becomes difficult, the patient often decreases food intake and loses weight. GI complaints also include abdominal distention, diarrhea, malodorous floating stools (malabsorption syndrome) as a result of small-bowel disease, and constipation secondary to colonic involvement.

Lung involvement includes pleural thickening, pulmonary fibrosis, and pulmonary function abnormalities. Pulmonary hypertension is seen almost exclusively in CREST syndrome.

Primary heart disease consists of pericarditis, pericardial effusion, and cardiac arrhythmias. Myocardial fibrosis resulting in congestive failure occurs most frequently in those persons with diffuse SS.

COLLABORATIVE CARE

Table 60-16 Systemic Sclerosis

Diagnostic
History and physical examination
Antinuclear antibody titers
Nail-bed capillary microscopy
X-rays of chest, hands
Upper or lower GI series (or both)
Skin or visceral biopsy
Urinalysis (proteinuria, hematuria, casts)

Collaborative Therapy
Vasodilator drugs
  Calcium channel blockers
  Reserpine (Serpasil)
Antiinflammatory drugs
  Aspirin
  NSAIDs
  Penicillamine (Cuprimine)
  Corticosteroids
Antihypertensive drugs
Physical therapy

Renal disease is a major cause of death in SS. Malignant arterial hypertension associated with rapidly progressive and irreversible renal insufficiency is often present. Recent improvements in dialysis, bilateral nephrectomy in patients with uncontrollable hypertension, and kidney transplantation have offered some hope to patients with renal failure.

Diagnostic Studies

Blood studies may reveal a mildly elevated ESR and occasionally hypergammaglobinemia. The presence of ANA is observed in almost all persons with SS. Autoantibody Scl-70 has been reported in diffuse SS; anticentromere antibody is associated with the CREST syndrome. Nail-bed capillary microscopy characteristically shows capillary loop dilation with limited disease and dilation with avascular areas in patients with diffuse disease.[55] If renal involvement is present, urinalysis may show proteinuria, microscopic hematuria, and casts. X-ray evidence of subcutaneous calcification, digital tuft resorption, distal esophageal hypomotility, or bilateral pulmonary fibrosis is diagnostic of SS. Pulmonary function studies reveal decreased vital capacity. Skin biopsy shows dermal collagen thickening, condensation, or homogenization.

Collaborative Care

The collaborative care of SS (Table 60-16) offers no specific treatment with long-term effects. Care is directed toward attempts to prevent or treat secondary complications of involved organs. Various drugs such as antiinflammatory agents, D-penicillamine (Cuprimine), minocycline, and colchicine have been used with varying degrees of success.

Physical therapy helps maintain joint mobility and preserve muscle strength. Occupational therapy assists the patient in maintaining functional abilities. Gastroesophageal reflux may be treated by antacids and periodic dilation of the esophagus. (Gastroesophageal reflux is discussed in Chapter 39.)

Drug Therapy. No specific drugs or combination of drugs has been proven effective as treatment for SS. Cortico-steroids are generally reserved for patients with myositis or overlap syndromes (e.g., mixed connective tissue disease). D-penicillamine increases the solubility of dermal collagen and may cause thinning of the skin, but it has many side effects. Minocycline may improve symptoms, particularly collagen thickening. Colchicine is being used to inhibit the accumulation of collagen, but evidence is still insufficient to prove its therapeutic worth. The use of immunosuppressive agents is under investigation.

Raynaud's phenomenon can be treated with supportive measures, including oral (e.g., niacin) or topical vasodilating drugs (e.g., nitroglycerin ointment) applied to fingers and toes. However, calcium channel blockers (nifedipine [Adalat, Procardia] and diltiazem [Cardizem]) are the treatment of choice for Raynaud's phenomenon.[56] Reserpine (Serpasil), an adrenergic blocking agent, increases blood flow to the fingers. Iloprost, a prostaglandin that promotes vasodilation, is also used to treat Raynaud's phenonomen in SS.[57]

Infected ulcers of the fingertips may be treated by soaking with hyaluronidase and using bacterial antibiotic ointment. Joint symptoms may be relieved by aspirin and other NSAIDs. Antacids and H_2 receptor antagonists (e.g., cimetidine [Tagamet]) may be useful for heartburn. Combinations of antihypertensive medications, including hydralazine (Apresoline), minoxidil (Loniten), captopril (Capoten), propranolol (Inderal), and methyldopa (Aldomet), have been used in the treatment of hypertension.

NURSING MANAGEMENT: SYSTEMIC SCLEROSIS

Because prevention is not possible, nursing intervention often begins during a hospitalization for diagnostic purposes. Vital signs, weight, intake and output, respiratory function, and joint ROM should be assessed daily as indicated by specific symptoms to plan appropriate care. Emotional stress and a cold environment may aggravate Raynaud's phenomenon. Patients with SS should not have finger-stick blood testing done because of compromised circulation and poor healing of the fingers. Diagnostic studies should be thoroughly explained. The nurse can help the patient resolve feelings of helplessness by providing information about the illness and encouraging active participation in planning care.

Health teaching is a major nursing concern as the patient and family begin to live with this disease. Obvious changes in the face and hands lead to poor self-image and loss of mobility and function. The patient must actively carry out therapeutic exercises at home. The nurse should reinforce heat therapy, the use of assistive devices, and organization of activities to preserve strength and reduce disability.

Hands and feet should be protected from cold exposure and possible burns or cuts that might heal slowly. Smoking should be avoided because of its vasoconstricting effect. Signs of infection should be reported. Lotions may help alleviate skin dryness and cracking, but they must be rubbed in for an unusually long time because of the thickness of the skin.

Dysphagia may be reduced by eating small, frequent meals, chewing carefully and slowly, and drinking fluids. Heartburn may be minimized by using antacids 45 to 60 minutes after each meal and by sitting upright for 30 to 45 minutes after eating. Using additional pillows or raising the head of the bed on blocks may help reduce nocturnal gastroesophageal reflux.

Job modifications are often necessary because stair climbing, typing, writing, and cold exposure may pose particular problems. The patient may become socially withdrawn as skin tightening alters the appearance of the face and hands. Some people must wear gloves to protect fingertip ulcers and to provide extra warmth. Sensitive areas on fingertips resulting from ulcers or calcinosis may require padded utensils or special assistive devices to reduce discomfort. Dining out may become a socially embarrassing event because the patient's small mouth, difficulty swallowing, and reflux make eating less enjoyable. Daily oral hygiene must be emphasized, or neglect may lead to increased tooth and gingival problems. The patient needs a dentist who is familiar with SS and can deal with a small oral aperture. Psychologic support reduces stress and may positively influence peripheral motor response. Biofeedback training and relaxation techniques can reduce tension, improve sleeping habits, and raise the temperature of the fingers and toes.

Sexual dysfunction resulting from body changes, pain, muscular weakness, limited mobility, decreased self-esteem, and decreased vaginal secretions may require sensitive counseling by the nurse. Specific suggestions based on individual patient assessment should be offered.[58]

POLYMYOSITIS AND DERMATOMYOSITIS

Polymyositis and *dermatomyositis* are diffuse inflammatory myopathies of striated muscle, producing symmetric weakness usually most severe in the proximal muscles (e.g., trunk, shoulders, and hips). These disorders occur twice as frequently in women as in men. Onset of the disease occurs most frequently in the fifth and sixth decades of life. The incidence is slightly greater than that of muscular dystrophy in adults. Some cases of myositis are associated with an underlying malignant disease. In this situation the myositis is a paraneoplastic syndrome.

Etiology and Pathophysiology

The exact cause of polymyositis and dermatomyositis is unknown. Theories include the presence of an infectious agent, a hypersensitivity response, and cell-mediated immune system abnormalities.

Clinical Manifestations and Complications

Muscular. The patient usually experiences an insidious onset of proximal muscle weakness over a period of several months, primarily of the shoulders, neck, and pelvic girdle. The patient may have difficulty rising from a chair or bathtub, climbing stairs, combing the hair, or reaching into a high cupboard. Neck muscles may become so weak that the patient is unable to raise the head from the pillow. Muscle discomfort or tenderness is uncommon. Muscle examination reveals an inability to move against resistance or even gravity. Weak pharyngeal muscles may produce dysphagia and dysphonia (nasal or hoarse voice).

Dermal. The typical skin rash appears as a dusky erythema of the face, neck, shoulders, anterior part of the chest, upper part of the back, and arms and occurs in nearly 40% of patients with muscular disease. A heliotrope (lavender hue) rash over the eyelids and periorbital edema are nearly pathognomonic for dermatomyositis.[59] The rash is prominent on the extensor surfaces of the forearms, elbows, knuckles, periungual areas, knees, and ankles. A scaly, red, often raised rash on the knuckles is the Gottron's rash of dermatomyositis, which may easily be confused with that of psoriasis or seborrheic dermatitis. Hyperemia and telangiectasias are often present at the nail beds.

Other Manifestations. Nearly half of the patients with polymyositis have mild or transient arthritis and Raynaud's phenomenon. "Cotton-wool" patches can occur in the retina. Calcinosis, contractures, and muscle atrophy may occur with advanced disease. Aspiration pneumonia may result from weak pharyngeal muscles. Childhood dermatomyositis appears to have a more progressive, crippling course. Dermatomyositis diagnosed in men older than 40 years of age is more frequently associated with concurrent malignant disease. In severe cases, deglutition impairment and cardiorespiratory complications, such as pulmonary fibrosis and conduction defects, contribute to mortality.

Diagnostic Studies

Elevations in serum muscle enzymes (creatine kinase, aldolase, and aspartate aminotransferase) are valuable in determining the diagnosis and response to treatment. Circulating autoantibodies designated anti-Jo (antibodies to histidyl tRNA synthetase) are now recognized to be highly disease specific in patients with inflammatory myopathies.[60] Elevation of ESR is expected with active disease. The electromyogram shows polyphasic, short-duration potentials, fibrillation, and positive-spike waves. Muscle biopsy reveals necrosis, degeneration, regeneration, and interstitial chronic inflammatory cell infiltration (primarily lymphocytes).

Collaborative Care

Polymyositis and dermatomyositis can be treated with some success by the use of corticosteroids and, occasionally, immunosuppressive drugs. Improvement is generally achieved with prompt institution of corticosteroid therapy, and dosage is usually reduced as clinical improvement is noted. Relapses are common. Topical corticosteroids may be applied to the skin rash. Patients who respond poorly to corticosteroids may improve with immunosuppressives (e.g., intermittent IV or daily oral cyclophosphamide [Cytoxan]). Corticosteroid therapy may cause potassium to be released from damaged muscle cells and to be lost in the urine. Supplemental dietary potassium (e.g., from orange juice, bananas) is encouraged. Corticosteroid-induced myopathy may complicate long-term therapy. Immunosuppressive agents such as methotrexate, azathioprine (Imuran), and cyclophosphamide are used for their corticosteroid-sparing effect, allowing functional improvement with reduction in corticosteroid dosage.

Physical therapy can be helpful and should be tailored to the activity of the disease. Massage and passive movement are appropriate during active disease, with more aggressive exercises reserved for periods when disease activity is minimal, as evidenced by low serum enzyme levels.

A careful search for possible malignant lesions should be undertaken for the patient more than 40 years of age. If malignant disease is found, it should be treated appropriately. Complete remission of dermatomyositis may occur if the malignant lesion is removed.

NURSING MANAGEMENT: POLYMYOSITIS AND DERMATOMYOSITIS

Although prevention is not possible, greater recognition of polymyositis and its insidious onset resembling muscular dystrophy may favorably influence prognosis by more rapid diagnosis and institution of therapy.

Nursing interventions should include assessment of muscular weakness and limitation of motion. The nurse should maintain the patient on bed rest and assist the patient with activities of daily living when extreme weakness is present. Special attention is provided at mealtime to prevent aspiration. The nature of the disease and modes of therapy should be thoroughly reviewed, and the diagnostic tests should be explained. Understanding that the benefits of therapy are often delayed is important; for example, weakness may increase during the first few weeks of corticosteroid therapy.

The patient should have a thorough understanding of the chronic nature of this disorder, the usefulness and the side effects of all prescribed medications, and the importance of regular medical care and serial laboratory testing. The nurse should provide guidelines for conserving energy by means of organizing activities and pacing techniques. Daily ROM exercises are encouraged to prevent contractures. When active inflammation is not evident, muscle-strengthening (repetitive) exercises may be started. Home care will be necessary during the acute phase of polymyositis because profound muscle weakness renders the patient unable to carry out activities of daily living. Homemaker services, visiting nurses, and family caregivers are needed to assist the patient in routine hygiene, meal preparation and eating, and ambulation.

OVERLAPPING FORMS OF CONNECTIVE TISSUE DISEASE

Patients having a combination of clinical features of several rheumatic diseases are described as having *overlapping* or *mixed connective tissue disease*. Although this combination was believed to be a distinct clinical disorder, follow-up revealed evolution primarily to SLE or SS. This early undifferentiated or transitional form of connective tissue disease has a typical serologic pattern, including high titer of speckled pattern of ANA (a type of ANA), high levels of antibody to ribonuclease-sensitive extractable nuclear antibody, and autoantibodies to ribonucleoprotein.

SJÖGREN'S SYNDROME

Sjögren's syndrome is characterized by autoantibodies to two protein-RNA complexes termed *SS-A/Ro* and *SS-B/La*. The clinical manifestations are caused by inflammation and dysfunction of the exocrine glands, particularly the salivary and lacrimal glands.[61]

More than 90% of the patients are women, and half have RA or another connective tissue disease. Dry mouth can complicate the differential diagnosis in older women. Decreased tearing leads to a "gritty" sensation in the eyes, burning, and photosensitivity. Dry mouth produces buccal membrane fissures, dysphagia, and frequent dental caries. Dry nasal and respiratory passages are common and can result in a cough. Often the parotid glands are enlarged. Other exocrine glands may also be affected; for example, vaginal dryness may lead to dyspareunia.

Histologic study reveals lymphocyte infiltration of salivary and lacrimal glands, but the disease may become more generalized and involve lymph nodes, bone marrow, and visceral organs (pseudolymphoma). Extraglandular proliferation may become frankly malignant (e.g., lymphoma). Rheumatoid and antinuclear factors are present in the majority of patients. Anemia, leukopenia, hypergammaglobulinemia, and elevated ESR are usually found.

Ophthalmologic examination (Schirmer's test), salivary flow rates, and lower lip biopsy of minor salivary glands confirm the diagnosis. The treatment is symptomatic, including (1) instillation of artificial tears as often as necessary to maintain adequate hydration and lubrication, (2) surgical punctal occlusion, and (3) increased fluids with meals. Dental hygiene is important. Pilocarpine (Salagen) can be used to treat symptoms of dry mouth. Increased humidity at home may reduce respiratory infections. Vaginal lubrication with a water-soluble product such as K-Y jelly may increase comfort during intercourse. Corticosteroids and immunosuppressive drugs are indicated for treatment of pseudolymphoma.

FIBROMYALGIA

Fibromyalgia (FM) is a musculoskeletal chronic pain syndrome of unknown etiology.[62] It is characterized by fatigue, stiffness, myalgias, arthralgias, headaches, irritable bowel syndrome, and sleep disturbance. Temporomandibular joint dysfunction, premenstrual symptoms, and mitral valve prolapse may also accompany the disorder. Cognitive disturbances such as memory problems ("brain fog") or difficulty concentrating are common. Depression, anxiety, and feelings of hopelessness often result because of the chronic nature of FM. There is a 50% association of FM and irritable bowel syndrome.[63] FM is seen most commonly in women, with the highest incidence occurring in women age 50 years and older.[63]

Although the etiology and pathogenesis of FM are not known, clinicians have speculated that the syndrome is a result of referred pain from deep structures (pain amplification), a pain-spasm cycle, repetitive stress to the muscle, or reactivation of a latent virus.[64] It is known that FM has a powerful stress-related component that needs attention for long-lasting resolution.

The diagnosis of FM is made by the presence of typical symptoms and the location of *tender points*. Eighteen points, tender in normal people, have been identified that are hypersensitive in persons with FM. The diagnostic criterion for FM is a history of widespread pain and the presence of at least 11 consistent tender points on digital palpation.[65] FM may be localized to a specific region of the body (often termed *myofascial pain*) or generalized with migratory tender points. Myofascial pain most often involves the posterior neck, low back, shoulders, and chest.

The treatment of FM is symptomatic and requires a high level of patient motivation. The nurse can play a key role in educating the patient to be an active participant in the therapeutic regimen. Pain, aching, and tenderness can be helped by rest, and NSAIDs are effective for some patients. Stress, fatigue, and sleep disturbances can be helped by low-dose tricyclic antidepressants (e.g., amitriptyline [Elavil], imipramine [Tofranil], or

RESEARCH

IMPLICATIONS FOR NURSING PRACTICE

Health of Women with Fibromyalgia

Citation Schaefer KM: Health patterns of women with fibromyalgia, *J Adv Nurs* 26:565, 1997.

Purpose To improve understanding of fibromyalgia from the perspective of women who are living with this disease.

Methods The sample included eight women diagnosed with fibromyalgia ranging in age from 27 to 46 years old. Women completed a health diary for 3 months related to how they were living with their fibromyalgia on a daily basis. Demographic information was also collected.

Results and Conclusions Aches and pains were the most common symptom patterns. For most women pain was the worst when the weather was damp or cool. All women used complementary approaches to supplement care with relaxation and heat the most effective. Narrative data from diaries revealed six qualitative themes: (1) pain as mental and physical, (2) fear of pain interferes with ability to do things, (3) suffering results from doing things out of the ordinary, (4) knowing oneself helps control illness, (5) stress affects how one feels, and (6) doing pleasant things helps ease discomfort.

Implications for Nursing Practice Patient diaries can help identify disease symptom patterns and assist the nurse in developing helpful interventions. Diaries can also empower patients by giving back some control over their disease. Patients can anticipate times when they will feel worse and learn what interventions help most. Complementary approaches to pain management should be offered and reinforced by the health care team. The nurse should support the uniqueness of each woman's experience in living with this disease.

trazodone [Desyrel]), muscle relaxants, stress management and stress-reduction techniques, deep relaxation, and a healthful diet. Zolpidem (Ambien) is useful in more recalcitrant cases of sleep disturbance, and clonazepam (Klonopin) may help restless legs syndrome, but both can be habit forming. Selective serotonin reuptake inhibitor antidepressants (e.g., paroxetine [Paxil] and sertraline [Zoloft]) may alleviate pain and fatigue. Participation in a safe, moderate exercise program (e.g., swimming, walking) is one of the most beneficial approaches for reducing FM symptoms. In addition, gentle stretching exercises, yoga, massage therapy, or tai chi may be helpful.

Many parameters of FM except morning stiffness improve on cyclobenzaprine (Flexeril), a muscle relaxant that is a tricyclic derivative. Opioids are rarely used because of the addiction potential. Tramadol (Ultram) acts at the same receptor sites as narcotic analgesics but is thought to have less addiction potential. Subcutaneous injections of lidocaine, cortisone, or both, or even sterile saline, directly into tender points may temporarily relieve pain, but risks are associated with this invasive procedure.

Because of the chronic nature of FM and the need to maintain an ongoing rehabilitation program, the patient with FM needs consistent support from the nurse and other members of the health care team. The most successful treatment approaches combine physical fitness, stress-reduction programs, and psychologic counseling (individual or group).

COMMON JOINT SURGICAL PROCEDURES

Surgery plays an important role in the treatment and rehabilitation of patients with various forms of arthritis, conditions related to trauma, and other painful conditions resulting in functional disability. Joint replacement surgery is the most common orthopedic operation performed on older adults. Significant advances in the field of reconstructive surgery have resulted in improvements in prosthetic design, materials, and surgical techniques that provide significant relief of pain and deformity and improve function and joint motion for patients with arthritis.

Indications

Surgery is aimed at relieving pain, improving joint motion, correcting deformity and malalignment, reducing vertical loads and shear stresses, and removing intraarticular causes of erosion. Pain is one of the primary reasons for joint surgery. In addition to the effects of chronic pain on the physical and emotional well-being of the patient, any movement of the painful joint is often avoided. If this lack of movement is not corrected, contraction with permanent limitation of motion often occurs. Limitation of motion at any joint can be demonstrated on physical examination and by joint-space narrowing on radiologic examination.

There may also be a slow loss of cartilage in affected joints, which may be related to loss of motion. Synovitis can cause tendon damage, resulting in rupture or subluxation of the joint and subsequent loss of function. Continuing disease activity may cause loss of cartilage and bony surface and result in mechanical barriers to movement requiring surgical intervention.

Types of Joint Surgeries

Synovectomy. Synovectomy (removal of synovial membrane) is used as a prophylactic measure and as a palliative treatment of RA. Removal of synovial membrane, thought to be the location of the basic pathologic changes in joint destruction, helps prevent further progression of joint damage. A synovectomy is best performed early in the disease process to prevent serious destruction of joint surfaces. Removal of the thickened synovium prevents extension of the inflammatory process into the adjacent cartilage, ligaments, and tendons.

It is impossible to surgically remove all the synovium in a joint. The underlying disease process is still present and will again affect the regenerating synovium. However, the disease appears to be milder after synovectomy, and definite improvement in pain, weight bearing, and ROM can be expected. Common sites for this surgery include the elbow, wrist, and fingers. Synovectomy in the knee is done less frequently because knee joint replacement techniques are usually used.

Osteotomy. An osteotomy is performed by removing or adding a wedge or slice of bone to change its alignment and shift weight bearing, thereby correcting deformity and relieving pain. Cervical osteotomy may be used to correct defor-

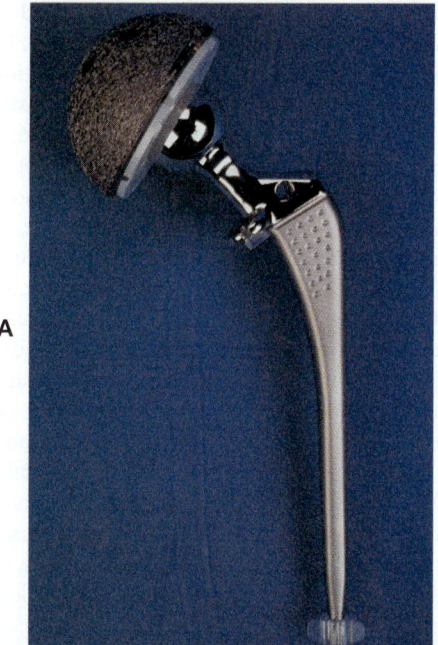

A

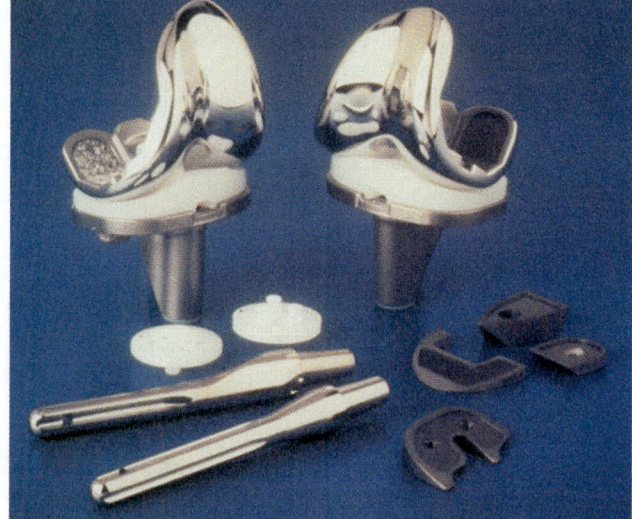

B

Fig. 60-12 Total joint replacements. **A,** Hip. **B,** Knee.

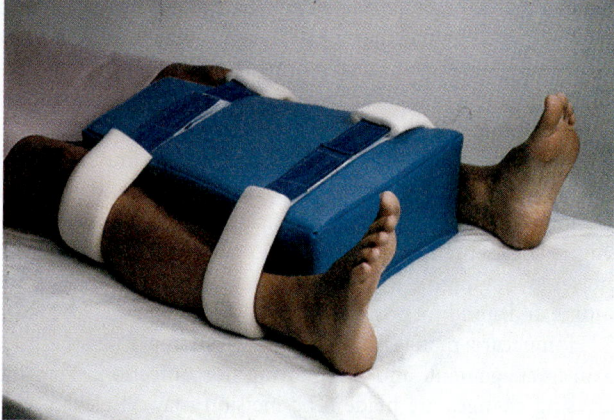

Fig. 60-13 Maintaining postoperative abduction following total hip replacement.

Weight bearing is permitted following knee arthroscopy. Because this is done as an outpatient procedure, patient education includes monitoring for signs of infection, managing pain, and restricting excessive activity for 24 to 48 hours.

Arthroplasty. *Arthroplasty* is the reconstruction or replacement of a joint. This surgical procedure is performed to relieve pain, improve or maintain ROM, and correct deformity—conditions that can result from OA, RA, avascular necrosis, congenital deformities or dislocations, and other systemic problems. There are several types of arthroplasty, including replacement of part of a joint, surgical reshaping of the bones of the joints, and total joint replacement. Innovative procedures and prosthetic devices offer exciting possibilities for reconstructive joint surgery (Fig. 60-12). Replacement arthroplasty is available for the elbow, shoulder, phalangeal joint of the finger, hip, knee, ankle, and foot.[66]

Hip. Total hip replacement is undoubtedly the most important advancement in reconstructive surgery of the twentieth century and has provided significant relief of pain and improvement of function for patients with arthritis. Hip reconstruction is frequently used in the treatment of patients with RA and OA, as well as for fractures of the hip.

Implants are often "cemented" in place with polymethylmethacrylate, which bonds to the bone. With time, a significant number of femoral components loosen and require revision. Because of this risk, total hip replacement is recommended for less active, older adults. More recently, "cementless" arthroplasties have been used. They provide long-term implant stability by facilitating biologic ingrowth of new bone tissue into the porous surface coating of the prosthesis. A patient with a high activity potential and a life expectancy of 25 years or more is an excellent candidate for an uncemented prosthesis.

In both types of arthroplasties, extremes of internal rotation, adduction, and 90-degree flexion of the hip must be avoided for 4 to 6 weeks postoperatively. A foam abduction pillow is sometimes placed between the legs to prevent dislocation of the new joint (Fig. 60-13). Elevated toilet seats and platforms under chairs at home are necessary. Tub baths and driving a car are not allowed for 4 to 6 weeks. An occupational therapist may teach the patient to use assistive devices such as reach bars ("reachers") to avoid bending over to pick something off the floor, long-handled shoehorns, or sock pullers. The knees must

mity in some patients with ankylosing spondylitis. A halo and body jacket are worn until fusion occurs (3 or 4 months). Subtrochanteric or femoral osteotomy may provide some relief of pain and improve motion in selected patients with hip osteoarthritis. Osteotomy has proven ineffective in patients with inflammatory joint disease. Osteotomy of the knee provides relief of pain in selected patients, but advanced joint destruction is usually corrected by joint replacement surgery. The postoperative care is similar to the treatment of an internal fixation of a fracture at a comparable site (see Chapter 59). The osteotomy is usually fixed by internal wires, screws and plates, bone grafts, or an external fixator.

Debridement. *Debridement* is the removal of degenerative debris such as loose bodies, osteophytes, joint debris, and degenerated menisci from a joint. This procedure is usually performed on the knee or the shoulder using a fiberoptic arthroscope. A compression dressing is applied postoperatively.

be kept apart; the patient must never cross the legs or twist to reach behind. Physical therapy is initiated 1 day postoperatively with ambulation and weight bearing with a walker for cemented prosthesis and partial weight bearing on the operative side for uncemented prosthesis.

Exercises are designed to restore strength and muscle tone in the hip muscles essential to improved function and range of motion. These include quadriceps setting, gluteal muscle setting, leg raises in supine and prone positions, and abduction exercises (swinging the leg out but never crossing midline) from supine and standing positions.

Home care management includes nursing assessment of pain management and monitoring for infection. Periodic dressing changes are made. The incision may be closed with metal staples, which are removed at the surgeon's office. Prothrombin times will be drawn weekly and anticoagulation adjusted accordingly if warfarin is used. Enoxaparin (Lovenox), a low-molecular-weight heparin, is administered subcutaneously and can be given at home by the patient or family member. An advantage of enoxaparin is that it does not require daily blood monitoring of the patient's coagulation status. The patient should be instructed to use prophylactic antibiotics before dental appointments or procedures that might put the patient at risk for bacteremia.

A physical therapist will assess range of motion, ambulation, and compliance with the exercise regimen.[67] The patient will gradually increase the number of repetitions of exercises, add weights to ankles, swim, and may eventually use a stationary bicycle to tone quadriceps and improve cardiovascular fitness. High-impact exercises and sports, such as jogging and tennis, may loosen the implant and should be avoided. The elderly adult may require rehabilitation at an extended care facility until able to function independently.

A clinical pathway for care of the patient with primary total hip replacement is provided on p. 1855.

Knee. Unremitting pain and instability as a result of severe destructive deterioration of the knee joint is the main indication for knee arthroplasty. The presence of osteoporosis may necessitate bone grafting to augment defects and to correct bone deficiencies. Either part or all of the knee joint may be replaced with a metal and plastic prosthetic device. A compression dressing is used to immobilize the knee in extension immediately after the operation. This is removed before discharge and may be replaced with a knee immobilizer or posterior plastic shell, which maintains extension during ambulation and at rest for about 4 weeks.

Great emphasis is placed on postoperative exercising, and dislocation is not a problem. Isometric quadricep setting begins the first day after surgery. The patient progresses to straight-leg raises and gentle ROM to increase muscle strength and obtain 90-degree knee flexion. Active flexion exercises through the use of a passive-motion machine postoperatively promotes earlier joint mobility and shortens hospitalization. Full weight bearing is begun before discharge. An active home exercise program involves progressive ROM, muscle strengthening, and stationary bicycle exercising.

Finger joints. A silicone rubber arthroplastic device is used to help restore function in the fingers of the patient with RA. The goal of hand surgery is primarily to restore function related to grasp, pinch, stability, and strength rather than to correct cosmetic deformity. The metacarpophalangeal and proximal interphalangeal joints are most commonly involved. Ulnar deviation is often present, which results in severe functional limitations of the hand. Before surgery the patient is instructed in hand exercises, including flexion, extension, abduction, and adduction of the fingers. Postoperatively, the hand is kept elevated with a bulky dressing in place. The operative area and the hand should be checked for sensation, temperature, pulse, and signs of infection. Once the dressing is removed, a guided splinting program is initiated. The success of the surgery depends largely on the postoperative treatment plan, which is often carried out under the direction of an occupational therapist. The patient is discharged with splints to use while sleeping and hand exercises to perform for 10 to 12 weeks at least three to four times a day. The patient is also instructed to avoid lifting heavy objects.

Elbows and shoulders. Although available, total replacement of elbow and shoulder joints is not as common as other forms of arthroplasty. Shoulder replacements are used in patients with severe pain because of RA, OA, necrosis, or an old trauma. The shoulder replacement is usually considered if the patient has adequate surrounding muscle strength and bone stock. If joint replacement is necessary for both elbow and shoulder, the elbow is usually done first because a severely painful elbow interferes with the shoulder rehabilitation program.

Significant pain relief has been achieved following arthroplasty, with 90% of patients having no pain at rest or minimal pain with activity. Functional improvements have resulted in better hygiene and increased ability to perform activities of daily living in most patients. Rehabilitation is longer and more difficult than with other joint surgeries.

Arthrodesis. Arthrodesis is the surgical fusion of a joint. This procedure is indicated only if articular surfaces are too severely damaged or infected to allow joint replacement or for reconstructive surgery failures. Arthrodesis relieves pain and provides a stable but immobile joint. The fusion is usually accomplished by removal of the articular hyaline cartilage and the addition of bone grafts across the joint surface. The affected joint must be immobilized until bone healing has occurred. Common areas of fusion are the wrist, ankle, cervical spine, lumbar spine, and the metatarsophalangeal joint of the great toe.

Complications of Joint Surgery

Infection is a serious complication of joint surgery, particularly joint replacement surgery. The most common causative organisms are gram-positive aerobic streptococci and staphylococci. Infection almost always leads to pain and loosening of the prosthesis, generally requiring extensive surgery. Efforts to reduce the incidence of infection include the use of specially designed hypersterile operating rooms with laminar air flow and prophylactic antibiotic administration.

Deep vein thrombosis is another potentially serious complication after selected joint surgeries, particularly those involving the lower extremities. Prophylaxis such as aspirin, warfarin, or pneumatic compression of the legs is usually instituted. Patients may be followed postoperatively with venous Doppler ultrasound to detect proximal deep vein thrombosis, the source of most pulmonary emboli. The peak incidence of pulmonary embolus is bimodal, occurring on the fourth and fourteenth postoperative day.

MR
Patient Name
Diagnosis
Procedure
Procedure Data

_____

Function	Activity	PreOp __/__	Or Day __/__	PostOp #1 __/__	Post Day #2 __/__	PostOp #3 __/__
Hemostasis Thromboembolic Prophylaxis	Lab Work	PT/CBC, U/A Type and cross one unit PRBC (send 10 cc clot)	PT at 4 P.M. Heme Panel *(See Left Side Panel)	PT at 6 A.M. Heme Panel*	PT at 6 A.M. Heme Panel*	PT at 6 A.M. Heme Panel*
Heme Panel Hgb/Hct and Total	Assessment	Assess for transfusion	Assess for transfusion Criteria < 11 anticipate blood loss with autogolous unit expiration	Assess for transfusion See Criteria	Assess for transfusion See Criteria	Assess for transfusion See Criteria
WBC w/o DIFF Hgb/Hct RBC Indices Total WBC W/DIFF Quant. Platelets		Assess for sequential compression device if cannot anticoagulate	< 10 active bleeding anticipated mod/massive bleeding marginal cardiac reserve/O$_2$ capacity < 9 above criteria suspected bone marrow suppression < 8 MD discretion			
	Medications	No NSAIDs 10-14 days preop	If on Coumadin maintain INR at 1.5-2.0 or low-molecular-weight heparin 30 mg SC bid No NSAIDs	If on Coumadin adjust to protime or low-molecular-weight heparin 30 mg SC bid NO NSAIDs	In on Coumadin adjust to protime or low-molecular-weight heparin 30 mg SC bid NO NSAIDs	If on Coumadin adjust to protime or low-molecular-weight heparin 30 mg SC bid NO NSAIDs
	Treatments	Measure for thigh-high TEDS and tape to chart for OR	APPLY TEDS	APPLY TEDS	APPLY TEDS	APPLY TEDS
	Education	Anticoagulant instructions		Anticoagulant Instructions		
	Clinical Outcomes			No DVT or PE, stable Hgb and Hct No hemorrhagic complications	No DVT or PE, stable Hgb and Hct No hemorrhagic complications	No DVT or PE, stable Hgb and Hct No hemorrhagic complications
Pain Management	Assessment		Pain assessment q4hr while awake	Pain assessment q4hr while awake	Pain assessment q4hr while awake	Pain assessment q4hr while awake
	Medication		If motor deficit, contact anesthesia to evaluate. If inadequate pain relief, contact anesthesia to adjust dose PCA (if no epidural)	If motor deficit, contact anesthesia to evaluate D/C epidural / PCA after afternoon PT session Start oral meds q4hr around the clock	Oral meds q4hr after PM PT Change oral meds to prn	Oral meds q4hr Change oral meds to prn
	Clinical Outcomes		Adequate pain relief (pain scale score ____)	Adequate pain relief (self-report scale)	Adequate pain relief (self-report scale)	Adequate pain relief (self-report scale)
Wound Management	Assessment			Wound drainage	Wound drainage	Wound drainage
	Treatment			Service to D/C drain and collection devices when clotted or <100 cc in 8 hr for 2 shifts Surgical service to change OR dressing	Change dressing daily and prn if excessive drainage	Change dressing daily and prn if excessive drainage
	Medications	Ancef (Use Vancomycin if allergic PCN)	Start Ancef IV in OR 1 hour before incision then Ancef 1 g q8hr × 3 doses (Vancomycin if allergic to PCN)	Keflex PO if Foley is continued Septra DS if PCN allergic	Keflex PO if Foley is continued Septra DS if PCN allergic	
	Clinical Outcomes	No hematoma/dehiscence/infection	No hematoma/dehiscence/infection	No hematoma/dehiscence/ infection	No hematoma/dehiscence/infection	No hematoma/dehiscence/infection Wound dry and intact Afrebile (Temp <100.0)

Continued

From Rush-Presbyterian St. Luke's Medical Center.

Function	Activity	PreOp __/__	Or Day __/__	PostOp #1 __/__	Post Day #2 __/__	PostOp #3 __/__
General	Test	CXR, ECG if > 40 yr old SMA 18, hepatitis B profile if no autologous blood donation				
	Consults	Internal medicine consult CRC for discharge assessment				
	Medications		Compazine in PAR	Colace qAM Compazine PRN for nausea	Colace qAM Compazine PRN for nausea	Colace qAM Compazine PRN for nausea
	Assessments		Skin assessment, I & O q8hr, VS q4hr Circulation and neuro checks q2hr × 8 hr then q4hr × 4 hr	Skin assessment, I & O q8hr, VS q4hr Circulation and neuro checks q4hr	Skin assessment, I & O q8hr, VS q8hr Circulation and neuro checks q8hr	Skin assessment, I & O q8hr, VS q8hr Circulation and neuro checks q8hr
	Treatments		Introduce Inspiratory spirometer Encourage pt to use spirometer q1hr	Inspiratory spirometer q1hr	Inspiratory spirometer q4hr	Inspiratory spirometer q4hr
	Diet	NPO	Administer IV fluids as ordered Clear liquid diet as tolerated	Change IV to heplock Advance diet	D/C heplock after antibiotics completed General diet	General diet
	Elimination		Order raised toilet seat if 5'4" or taller Foley with epidural	Prune juice prn D/C Foley 4-6 hr after epidural D/C	Prune juice prn Fleet enema prn	Prune juice prn Fleet enema prn
	Education	Preop standards of care	Reinforce hip precautions			
	Clinical Outcomes		Braden Score > 17 No IV restarts needed	Braden Score >17	Braden Score >17	Braden Score > 17 Tolerate general diet Chest clear to auscultation Voids freely
	Discharge Planning		Nursing to notify CRC for discharge assessment	CRC to review case		CRC to make home arrangements for: Blood draws for PT Physical therapy and other services PRN Transfer to outside rehabilitation facility or ECF on selected patients
Rehabilitation	Consults		PT (physical therapy) OT (occupational therapy)	Physical med and rehab consults on selected pts		OT to see patient before discharge
	Assessments			Pain assessment pre-physical therapy	Pain assessment pre-physical therapy	Pain assessment pre-physical therapy
	Treatments		Regular pillow for abduction Hip flexion not to exceed 90 degrees No adduction of operated leg No internal rotation of operated leg	Regular pillow for abduction Hip flexion not to exceed 90 degrees No adduction of operated leg No internal rotation of operated leg	Regular pillow for abduction Hip flexion not to exceed 90 degrees No adduction of operated leg No internal rotation of operated leg	Regular pillow for abduction Hip flexion not to exceed 90 degrees No adduction of operated leg No internal rotation of operated leg
	Activity		Trapeze on bed Dangle at bedside late PM	Bathroom, chair, and ambulation when approved by PT For cemented or hybrid THR: - WBAT - crutches or walker For cementless THR: - touchdown weight bearing For all THR: - active/passive abduction per surgical protocol On nursing unit - Assist with ADLs PRN - Up to chair for dinner	Bathroom, chair, and ambulation when approved by PT Move trapeze to end of bed after PM PT session On unit Up to chair for dinner Ambulate in hallway with assistive device in accordance with PT note	Bathroom, chair, and ambulation when approved by PT On unit Up to chair for dinner Ambulate in hallway with assistive device
	Education	Hip precautions Home preparation for discharge	Reinforce postop teaching with patient and family	Transfer techniques		Home exercise program Hip precautions
	Clinical Outcomes	No hip dislocation	No hip dislocation Patient tolerates activities	Pain control adequate to participate in PT No hip dislocation Patient tolerates activities	Pain control adequate to participate in PT No hip dislocation Patient tolerates activities	Pain control adequate to participate in PT No hip dislocation Independent gait with appropriate device Independent transfers

Collaborative Care

Preoperative Management. As surgical techniques and care improve, more patients with chronic diseases such as RA are being considered as surgical candidates. The primary goal of preoperative assessment is to identify risk factors associated with postoperative complications so that nursing strategies can be implemented that promote optimal positive outcomes. A careful history will include previous medical diagnosis and complications such as diabetes and thrombophlebitis, pain tolerance and management preferences, current functional status and expectations following surgery, and level of social support and home care needs after discharge. The patient should be free from evidence of infection and acute joint inflammation. If lower-extremity surgery is planned, upper extremity muscle strength and joint function are assessed to determine the type of assistive devices needed postoperatively for ambulation and activities of daily living. Preoperative education informs the patient and family of the expected hospital course and postoperative management at home and readies them for a lifestyle that is compatible with the intrinsic capabilities of the prosthetic components so that prosthesis longevity can be maximized.

Postoperative Management. Postoperatively, a neurovascular assessment of the affected extremity is done to assess nerve function and circulatory status. Anticoagulation therapy, analgesia, and parenteral antibiotics are administered. In general, the affected joint is exercised and ambulation is encouraged as early as possible to prevent complications of immobility. Specific protocols vary according to patient, type of prosthesis, and surgeon preference.

The hospital stay after arthroplasty is about 3 to 5 days depending on the patient's course and need for physical therapy. Physical therapy and ambulation enhance mobility, build muscle strength, and reduce the risk of thrombus formation. If the patient is on Coumadin, therapy starts on the day of surgery and continues for 3 weeks with a prothrombin time (PT) done twice weekly. For those on enoxaparin, therapy starts 24 to 36 hours after surgery and continues for 3 weeks postoperatively. Daily monitoring of the patient's coagulation status is not necessary with enoxaparin therapy. The decision to use Coumadin or enoxaparin depends on many factors, including the patient's age and overall state of health.

60-3 NURSING CARE PLAN — PATIENT WITH JOINT REPLACEMENT SURGERY

Expected Patient Outcomes	Nursing Interventions and *Rationales*

Acute Intervention

NURSING DIAGNOSIS **Impaired physical mobility** *related to* pain, stiffness, and surgical procedure *as manifested by* difficulty in ambulating, inability to participate in physical rehabilitation, guarded movement.

▪ Functional ROM of joint.	▪ Assess effect of surgery on patient's mobility *to plan appropriate interventions.* ▪ Maintain proper positioning *to prevent dislocation or other complications.* ▪ Begin exercise program as directed *to minimize mobility impairment and stiffness.* ▪ Collaborate with physical and occupational therapist *to increase patient compliance and promote continuity of exercise.* ▪ Give pain medication before exercise *to decrease discomfort from exercise and increase patient participation.*

NURSING DIAGNOSIS **Self-care deficits** *related to* restrictions imposed by joint surgery, pain, weakness *as manifested by* inability to perform part or all of activities of daily living (ADLs).

▪ ADLs met satisfactorily by patient or caregivers.	▪ Assess patient's ability to perform ADLs *to plan appropriate assistance.* ▪ Assist as necessary *to ensure all basic needs are met.* ▪ Assure patient of your willingness to assist with ADLs postoperatively *to relieve anxiety related to feelings of helplessness.* ▪ Assure patient that self-care abilities will be resumed with time *to decrease anxiety over dependency.*

NURSING DIAGNOSIS **Ineffective management of therapeutic regimen** *related to* lack of knowledge of follow-up care *as manifested by* expression of concern with ability to care for self after discharge, frequent questioning about follow-up care, lack of plan for follow-up care.

▪ Confidence in ability to manage self-care after discharge and to make necessary lifestyle changes.	▪ Instruct patient on usual follow-up protocol, including activity limitations, medications, follow-up visit, signs of infection, and dislocation, *to prepare patient for self-care and decision making.* ▪ Assist patient to identify activities that require modification *so appropriate modification can be made.* ▪ Refer for vocational counseling *so expert guidance is available if necessary.* ▪ Initiate a nurse referral *to monitor the long-term exercise program at home.*

Continued

60-3 NURSING CARE PLAN PATIENT WITH JOINT REPLACEMENT SURGERY —continued

Expected Patient Outcomes	Nursing Interventions and *Rationales*

NURSING DIAGNOSIS Risk for peripheral neurovascular dysfunction *related to* edema and dislocated prosthesis.

▪ Palpable peripheral pulses. ▪ Warm extremities.	▪ Assess nerve and circulatory status q1hr first 24 hr, then every 2-4 hr *to determine if problem is present so treatment can be initiated promptly.* ▪ Notify surgeon immediately if abnormalities are noted *so interventions are started without delay.* ▪ Initiate measures such as cold packs and elevation of affected part *to minimize edema.* ▪ Carry out measures to prevent dislocation *because this can be a cause of neurovascular dysfunction.* ▪ Teach patient to report signs of neurovascular dysfunction such as paresthesia, coldness, pallor, excessive pain, swelling of affected extremity or body area *so treatment is not delayed.*

COLLABORATIVE PROBLEMS

Nursing Goals	Nursing Interventions and *Rationales*

POTENTIAL COMPLICATION

	Dislocation of prosthesis *related to* improper movement or activity.
▪ Monitor and report signs of joint dislocation. ▪ Carry out appropriate medical and nursing interventions.	▪ Monitor for pain in affected joint, loss of function, shortening or malalignment of extremity *to determine if dislocation has occurred.* ▪ Instruct patient on safe positions and activities; use assistive devices (e.g., raised toilet seat) as indicated *to avoid extremes of movement, which can cause dislocation.* ▪ Reinforce instructions of physical therapists *to foster confidence in plan and prevent misunderstanding.* ▪ Teach signs of dislocation to report (e.g., pain, loss of function, deformity) *so treatment is initiated promptly.*

POTENTIAL COMPLICATION

	Thrombophlebitis *related to* surgery and immobilization.
▪ Monitor and report signs of thrombosis. ▪ Carry out appropriate medical and nursing interventions.	▪ Monitor for redness, swelling, and tenderness or pain of the extremity *to recognize and report signs of thrombophlebitis.* ▪ Apply elastic compression stockings and instruct patient to perform isotonic exercises such as quadriceps setting, ankle rolling, and pushing on footboard *to promote circulation and prevent clot formation.* ▪ Provide adequate parenteral and oral fluids *to prevent dehydration and thrombus formation.* ▪ Instruct the patient in the importance of home exercise *to prevent venous stasis.* ▪ Instruct the patient and caregivers in the proper administration and follow-up of oral anticoagulation medications *to prevent side effects of under- or over-anticoagulation.*

NURSING MANAGEMENT: JOINT SURGERY

The nursing management of the patient undergoing joint surgery begins with preoperative teaching and realistic goal setting. It is important that the patient understands and accepts the limitations of the proposed surgery and realizes that it will not remove the underlying disease process. Postoperative procedures such as turning, deep breathing, use of bedpan and bedside commode, and use of abductor pillows should be explained and opportunities for practice provided. The patient should be reassured that pain relief will be available. Patient-controlled analgesia such as intravenous ketorolac (Toradol) and morphine sulfate can be helpful postoperatively, as can intramuscular ketorolac. A preoperative visit from a physical therapist allows practice of postoperative exercises and measurement for crutches or other assistive devices. The spirit of respect and cooperation displayed between the physical therapist and the nurse can do much to reassure an anxious patient.

Discharge planning begins immediately. The duration of the hospital stay and the expected postoperative events should be discussed so that the patient and family can plan ahead. The home environment should be assessed for safety (e.g., presence of scatter rugs and electrical cords) and accessibility. (Are the bathroom and bedroom on the first floor? Are door frames wide enough to accommodate a walker?) Social support must be assessed. Is a friend or family member available to assist the patient in the home? Will the patient require homemaker or meal services? The elderly patient may need the rehabilitation services of an extended care facility for a few weeks postoperatively to progressively develop independent living skills. Specific nursing interventions related to joint surgery are summarized in NCP 60-3.

Patient teaching includes instructions on reporting complications, including infection (e.g., fever, increased pain, drainage) and dislocation of the prosthesis (pain, loss of function, shortening or malalignment of an extremity). The home

CRITICAL THINKING EXERCISES

CASE STUDY

Systemic Lupus Erythematosus

Patient Profile

Nicole is a 30-year-old married woman who is seen at the rheumatology clinic following a recent 2-week vacation to Australia.

Subjective Data

- Works in a flower shop
- Complains of migratory joint pain, overwhelming fatigue, and a facial rash
- Is 6 months pregnant
- Has Raynaud's phenomenon when she works in the refrigerator room stocking flowers
- Had episode of pleurisy at age 21
- Fears something is horribly wrong with her
- Is afraid to take medication because of pregnancy

Objective Data

Physical Examination

- Malar rash
- Swelling of third and fourth metacarpophalangeal joints of both hands
- Dry, scaly scalp
- Pain on motion of both wrists, shoulders, and knees with no obvious swelling

Diagnostic Studies

- WBC count 4000/μl (4×10^9/L)
- Platelets 100,000/μl (150×10^9/L)
- Complement (C3) 60 mg/dl (0.6 g/L)
- Positive ANA and antiphospholipid antibodies

Collaborative Care

- Diagnosed with systemic lupus erythematosus
- Started on prednisone 10 mg daily

Critical Thinking Questions

1. How might the nurse explain the pathophysiology of systemic lupus erythematosus to Nicole?
2. How might the vacation have influenced the symptoms that she is currently experiencing?
3. What are some home and work modifications that the nurse can suggest to Nicole that will reduce her symptoms?
4. Discuss the types of prenatal and postpartal considerations essential in caring for Nicole.
5. What other sources of information regarding systemic lupus erythematosus might the nurse suggest to Nicole and her family?
6. Based on the assessment data presented, write one or more nursing diagnoses. Are there any collaborative problems?

NURSING RESEARCH ISSUES

1. What is the relationship between social support systems and quality of life for people with SLE?
2. What are the needs of the family when the patient is diagnosed with SLE?
3. Is gender a factor in the experience of arthritic pain?
4. What are effective measures that the nurse can institute to improve patient compliance with arthritis home management programs?
5. Are the coping strategies of younger patients diagnosed with systemic sclerosis different from those of older patients?

care nurse acts as the liaison between the patient and the surgeon, monitoring for postoperative complications, assessing comfort and ROM, and facilitating improvements in functional performance.

REVIEW QUESTIONS

The number of the question corresponds to the same-numbered objective at the beginning of the chapter.

1. In teaching a patient with SLE about the disorder the nurse uses the knowledge that the pathophysiology of SLE includes
   a. production of autoantibodies directed against constituents of cellular DNA.
   b. an autoimmune reaction resulting in degeneration, necrosis, and fibrosis of muscle fibers.
   c. deposition in tissues of immune complexes formed from IgG autoantibodies reacting with IgG.
   d. chronic inflammation and cytokine activity, which results in synovial proliferation and cartilage and bone damage.

2. An important nursing intervention in caring for the patient with ankylosing spondylitis is to teach the patient
   a. thoracic stretching and ROM exercises to prevent deformity.
   b. to sleep on the side with the legs flexed and supported with pillows.
   c. to prevent enteric and venereal infections that precipitate recurring attacks.
   d. that continuous therapeutic blood levels of nonsteroidal antiinflammatory drugs can limit the progression of the disease.

3. In assessing the joints of a patient with rheumatoid arthritis the nurse understands that the joints are damaged by
   a. the development of Heberden's nodes in the joint capsule.
   b. the deterioration of cartilage by the enzyme hyaluronidase.
   c. invasion of pannus into the joint capsule and subchondral bone.
   d. bony ankylosis following inflammation of the joints in HLA-B27–positive individuals.

4. Assessment data noted by the nurse in the patient with osteoarthritis commonly include
   a. elevated ESR.
   b. significant morning stiffness.
   c. progressive joint pain with activity.
   d. symmetric swelling of metacarpophalangeal joints.

5. When teaching the patient with arthritis the nurse should instruct the patient to
   a. avoid foods high in fat and calories.
   b. use cold applications to increase mobility in stiff joints.
   c. balance regularly scheduled rest periods with periods of activity.
   d. prevent any movement of affected joints during an acute inflammatory attack.

6. A patient with rheumatoid arthritis is scheduled for an arthroplasty. The nurse explains that the purpose of this procedure is to
   a. fuse a joint and reduce pain.
   b. prevent further joint damage.
   c. assess the extent of joint damage.
   d. replace the joint and improve function.

7. The nurse teaches a patient recovering from a total hip replacement that it is important to avoid
   a. sleeping on the abdomen.
   b. sitting with the legs crossed.
   c. abduction exercises of the affected leg.
   d. bearing weight on the affected leg for 6 weeks.

8. The nurse planning education for the patient with rheumatoid arthritis who is on multiple drug therapy includes information related to the need to
   a. use aspirin only on a prn basis for pain relief.
   b. use birth control during and 3 months following gold therapy.
   c. have frequent laboratory monitoring while taking methotrexate.
   d. stop taking any corticosteroids as soon as symptoms are relieved.

9. A patient with SLE has a nursing diagnosis of body image disturbance related to change in physical appearance. An appropriate nursing intervention for the patient is to
   a. discourage the patient from talking about her appearance.
   b. teach the patient creative uses of cosmetics in hygiene and grooming.
   c. enlist the support of family members to reassure the patient that she is valued.
   d. refer the patient for sexual counseling since sexual problems affect body image.

10. The most effective way to manage the health care needs of the patient with arthritis is to
    a. provide round-the-clock nursing care.
    b. let the family take over the patient's workload.
    c. explore the patient's spiritual response to pain.
    d. endorse the skills of a multidisciplinary health care team.

References

1. Hellmann D: Arthritis and musculoskeletal disorders. In Tierney L and others, editors: *Current medical diagnosis and treatment*, ed 36, Stamford, Conn, 1997, Appleton & Lange.
2. McCance K, Huether S: *Pathophysiology: biologic basis for disease in adults and children*, ed 3, St Louis, 1998, Mosby.
3. Kraus VB: Pathogenesis and treatment of osteoarthritis, *Med Clin North Am* 81:1, 1997.
4. Greidinger EL, Hellman DB: Arthritis: what to emphasize on the rheumatologic exam, *Consultant* 35:1609, 1995.
5. Griffin MR and others: Practical management of osteoarthritis: integration of pharmacologic and non-pharmacologic measures, *Arch Fam Med* 4:1049, 1995.
6. Hochberg MC, Altman RD, Brandt KD: Guidelines for the medical management of osteoarthritis, *Arthritis Rheum* 38:11, 1995.
7. Lozada CJ, Altman RD: Chondroprotection in osteoarthritis, *Bull Rheum Dis* 46:7, 1997.
8. McDowell I, Newell C: *Measuring health: a guide to rating scales and questionnaires*, ed 2, New York, 1996, Oxford University Press.
9. Torburn L: Principles of rehabilitation, *Prim Care* 23:2, 1996.
10. Stein MC, Griffin MR, Brandt KD: Osteoarthritis. In Wegener S and others, editors: *Clinical care in the rheumatic diseases*, Atlanta, 1996, American College of Rheumatology.
11. O'Dell JR, Pischel KD, Weinblatt M: Rheumatoid arthritis: what's new in treatment, *Patient Care* 31:5, 1997.
12. Ross C: A comparison of osteoarthritis and rheumatoid arthritis: diagnosis and treatment, *Nurse Pract* 22:9, 1997.
13. Callahan LF, Pincus T: Mortality in rheumatic diseases, *Arthritis Care Res* 8:229, 1995.
14. Mayo Clinic: Rheumatoid arthritis, *Mayo Clin Health Lett* 15:6, 1997.
15. Ali H and others: Mechanisms of inflammation and leukocyte activation, *Med Clin North Am* 81:1, 1997.
16. Dearborn JT, Jergesen HE: The evaluation and initial management of arthritis, *Prim Care* 23:2, 1996.
17. Lipsky PE, Jain R: Treatment of rheumatoid arthritis, *Med Clin North Am* 81:1, 1997.
18. Schnabel A and others: Sustained cough in methotrexate therapy for rheumatoid arthritis, *Clin Rheumatol* 15:277, 1996.
19. Skidmore-Roth L: *Nursing drug reference*, St Louis, 1998, Mosby.
20. O'Dell JR and others: Treatment of rheumatoid arthritis with methotrexate alone, sulfasalazine, and hydroxychloroquine or a combination of all three medications, *N Engl J Med* 334:20, 1996.
21. Silverstein FE and others: Misoprostol reduces serious gastrointestinal complications in patients with rheumatoid arthritis receiving nonsteroidal antiinflammatory drugs, *Ann Intern Med* 123:241, 1995.
22. Pigg JS: Rheumatoid arthritis: how allied health professionals can help, *J Musculoskel Med* 12:2, 1995.
23. Boutaugh MC, Brady TJ: Quality of life programs of the Arthritis Foundation, *Orthop Nurs* 15:5, 1996.
24. Veeser PI, editor: Patient education: treating arthritis, *Nurse Pract* 22:4, 1997.
25. Hall J and others: A randomized and controlled trial of hydrotherapy in rheumatoid arthritis, *Arthritis Care Res* 9:3, 1996.
26. Erlandson M: Rheumatic diseases in childhood. In Wegener S and others, editors: *Clinical care in the rheumatic diseases*, Atlanta, 1996, American College of Rheumatology.
27. Halverson PB: The spondyloarthropathies, *Orthop Nurs* 16:4, 1997.
28. Khan MA: Ankylosing spondylitis: clinical features. In Klippel JH, Dieppe PA, editors: *Rheumatology*, St Louis, 1995, Mosby.
29. Wollenhaupt J, Hoffmann A: HLA-B27 associated diseases. In Zierhut M, Thiel HJ, editors: *Immunology of the joint and the eye*, Boston, 1996, Butterworth Heinemann.
30. Verdon ME, Sigal LH: Recognition and management of Lyme disease, *Am Fam Physician* 56:2, 1997.
31. Schlesinger P: Lyme disease: an update, *Hospital Medicine* 34:26, 1998.
32. Jancin B: Give Lyme disease vaccine over a 2-month period, *Skin and Allergy News* 30:10, 1998.
33. Itescu S: Rheumatic aspects of acquired immunodeficiency syndrome, *Curr Opin Rheumatol* 8:4, 1996.
34. Gomez-Reino JJ, Carreira PE: Inflammation and HIV infection: a friendly connection, *Lancet* 348(suppl II):24, 1996.
35. Calin A: Managing hyperuricemia and gout: challenges and pitfalls, *J Musculoskel Med* 12:2, 1995.
36. Pisetsky DS, Gilkeson G, St Clair EW: Systemic lupus erythematosus: diagnosis and treatment, *Med Clin North Am* 81:1, 1997.
37. Ward MM, Pyun E, Studensk S: Long-term survival in systemic lupus erythematosus, *Arthritis Rheum* 38:2, 1995.
38. Howser RL: Nursing care of a patient with lupus cerebritis, *DCCN* 15:5, 1996.
39. Llorente L and others: Dysregulation of interleukin-10 production in relatives of patients with systemic lupus erythematous, *Arthritis Rheum* 40:8, 1997.
40. Tsao B and others: The genetic basis of systemic lupus erythematosus, *Proc Assoc Am Physicians* 110:113, 1998.

41. Clark J and others: B-lymphocyte hyperactivity in families of patients with systemic lupus erythematosus, *J Autoimmun* 9:59, 1996.

42. Petri M: Systemic lupus erythematosus. In Rich RR, editor: *Clinical immunology: principles and practice*, St Louis, 1996, Mosby.

43. Wallace DJ, Metzger AL: Systemic lupus erythematosus: clinical aspects and treatment. In Koopman WJ, editor: *Arthritis and allied conditions*, ed 13, Baltimore, 1997, Williams & Wilkins.

44. Tebbe B, Orfanos CE: Epidemiology and social impact of skin disease in lupus erythematosus, *Lupus* 6:96, 1997.

45. Peter JB, Reyes HR: *Use and interpretation of tests in rheumatology*, Santa Monica, 1996, Specialty Laboratories.

46. Lefkowith JB, Gilkeson GS: Nephritogenic autoantibodies in lupus, *Arthritis Rheum* 39:6, 1996.

47. Panush RS, Schur PH: Is it lupus? *Bull Rheum Dis* 46:6, 1997.

48. Sanchez-Guerrero J and others: Utility of anti-SM, anti-RNP, anti-Ro/SS-A and anti-La/SS-B (extractable nuclear antigens) detected by enzyme-linked immunosorbent assay for the diagnosis of systemic lupus erythematosus, *Arthritis Rheum* 39:6, 1996.

49. Levy GD and others: Incidence of hydroxychloroquine retinopathy in 1207 patients in a large multicenter outpatient practice, *Arthritis Rheum* 40:8, 1997.

50. Wallace DJ, Metzger AL: Systemic lupus erythematosus. In Koopman WJ, editor: *Arthritis and allied conditions*, ed 13, Baltimore, 1997, Williams & Wilkins.

51. Failla S and others: Adjustment of women with systemic lupus erythematosus, *Appl Nurs Res* 9:2, 1996.

52. Kostyak LR: Systemic lupus erythematosus. In Goreczny AJ, editor: *Handbook of health and rehabilitation psychology*, New York, 1995, Plenum Press.

53. Mitchell H, Bolster MB, LeRoy EC: Scleroderma and related conditions, *Med Clin North Am* 81:1, 1997.

54. Seibold JR: Connective tissue diseases characterized by fibrosis. In Kelley WN and others, editors: *Textbook of rheumatology*, ed 5, Philadelphia, 1997, Saunders.

55. Casale R, Buonocore M, Matucci-Cerinic M: Systemic sclerosis (scleroderma): an integrated challenge in rehabilitation, *Arch Phys Med Rehab* 78:7, 1997.

56. Pope J: Treatment of systemic sclerosis, *Rheum Dis Clin North Am* 22:893, 1996.

57. Kremer JM: Nutrition and rheumatic diseases. In Kelley WN and others, editors: *Textbook of rheumatology*, ed 5, Philadelphia, 1997, Saunders.

58. Dale KG: Intimacy and rheumatic diseases, *Rehabil Nurs* 21:1, 1996.

59. Wortmann RL: Inflammatory diseases of muscle and other myopathies. In Kelley WN and others, editors: *Textbook of rheumatology*, ed 5, Philadelphia, 1997, Saunders.

60. Vazquez-Abad D, Rothfield NF: Sensitivity and specificity of anti-Jo-1 antibodies in autoimmune diseases with myositis, *Arthritis Rheum* 39:2, 1996.

61. Manthorpe R, Asmussen K, Oxholm P: Primary Sjögren's syndrome: diagnostic criteria, clinical features, and disease activity, *J Rheumatol Suppl* 24:50, 1997.

62. Boisset-Pioro MH, Esdaile JM, Fitzcharles MA: Sexual and physical abuse in women with fibromyalgia syndrome, *Arthritis Rheum* 38:2, 1995.

63. Gordon S, Morrison C: Fibromyalgia and its primary care implications, *Medsurg Nurs* 7:207, 1998.

64. Wolfe F and others: The prevalence and characteristics of fibromyalgia in the general population, *Arthritis Rheum* 38:19, 1995.

65. Yunus MB: Fibromyalgia syndrome: blueprint for a reliable diagnosis, *Consultant* 36:1260, 1996.

66. Brewster N, Lewis P: Joint replacement for arthritis, *Aust Fam Physician* 27:21, 1998.

67. Enloe LF and others: Total hip and knee replacement treatment programs: a report using consensus, *J Orthop Sports Phys Ther* 23:3, 1996.

Resources

Arthritis Foundation
1330 West Peachtree Street
Atlanta, GA 30309
404-872-7100
800-283-7800
http://www.arthritis.org/

Association of Rheumatology Health Professionals
American College of Rheumatology
1800 Century Place, Suite 250
Atlanta, GA 30345
404-633-3777
Fax: 404-633-1870
http://www.rheumatology.org/arhp/

Lupus Foundation of America, Inc.
1300 Piccard Drive, Suite 200
Rockville, MD 20850-4303
301-670-9292
800-558-0121
http://internet-plaza.net/lupus/

National Arthritis and Musculoskeletal and Skin Diseases
Information Clearinghouse
National Institutes of Health
1 AMS Circle
Bethesda, MD 20892-3675
301-495-4484
Fax: 301-587-4352
http://www.nih.gov/niams/healthinfo/info.htm

Scleroderma Foundation, Inc.
89 Newbury Street, Suite 201
Danvers, MA 01923
978-750-4499
800-722-HOPE
Fax: 978-750-9902
http://www.scleroderma.org/

Scleroderma International Foundation
1725 York Avenue, #29F
New York, NY 10128
212-427-7040

Scleroderma Research Foundation
Pueblo Medical Commons
2320 Bath Street, Suite 307
Santa Barbara, CA 93105
800-441-CURE
http://www.srfcure.org/

Spondylitis Association of America
511 N. La Cienega, Suite 216
Los Angeles, CA 90048
800-777-8189
http://www.spondylitis.org/jas.htm

United Scleroderma Foundation
PO Box 399
Watsonville, CA 95077
800-722-4673
408-728-2202

For additional Internet resources, see the website for this book at **www.mosby.com/MERLIN/medsurg_lewis**

NURSING CARE IN SPECIALIZED SETTINGS

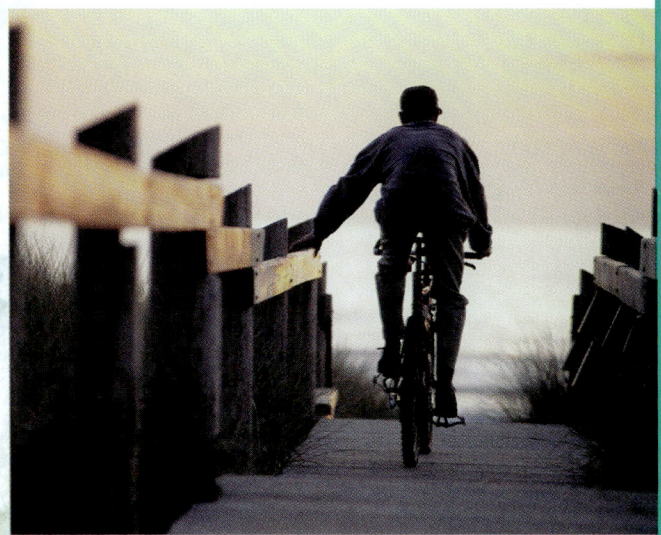

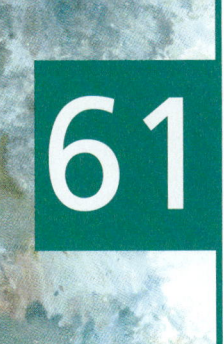

61

NURSING MANAGEMENT
Shock and Multiple Organ Dysfunction Syndrome

Julie M. Dax & Cynthia L. Hermey

www.mosby.com/MERLIN/medsurg_lewis

LEARNING OBJECTIVES

1. Define shock.
2. Differentiate among the three major classifications of shock in relationship to cause and precipitating factors.
3. Describe the pathophysiology and clinical manifestations of shock, systemic inflammatory response syndrome, and multiple organ dysfunction syndrome.
4. Describe the effects of shock, systemic inflammatory response syndrome, and multiple organ dysfunction syndrome on the major body systems.
5. Compare the collaborative care, drug therapy, and nursing management of patients with the different types of shock.
6. Discuss the nursing management of the patient with multiple organ dysfunction syndrome.

Shock, systemic inflammatory response syndrome (SIRS), and multiple organ dysfunction syndrome (MODS) are serious and interrelated complications. Shock is a complex pathophysiologic process that often leads to the development of SIRS and MODS (Fig. 61-1). This chapter provides a comprehensive overview of shock and then a discussion of SIRS and MODS.

SHOCK

Shock is a clinical syndrome characterized by an inadequate supply of oxygen and nutrients to cells from impaired tissue perfusion. Shock has many signs and symptoms and may be precipitated by a variety of etiologic factors. Although the cause and initial presentation of various types of shock differ, the physiologic responses to cellular hypoxia are the same, leading to the same sequence of events if shock is not recognized and treated early.[1] The challenge is to recognize early manifestations of impending shock and intervene quickly and appropriately to prevent further progression to MODS or death.

It is important to note that shock cannot be defined solely in terms of hypotension, because shock may be manifested in the absence of hypotension. Conversely, hypotension may occur in the absence of shock.

The morbidity and mortality rates associated with shock are extremely difficult to determine. It is estimated that the financial impact of patients in shock is between 10 and 20 billion dollars annually. For all types of shock, older adults have a greater mortality rate than younger adults. Sepsis has increased by 137% in the last decade and is the thirteenth leading cause of death, the tenth leading cause of death in the elderly, and the most common cause of death in critical care units. The mortality rate related to sepsis remains between 40% and 60%. It is predicted that the incidence and mortality rate of sepsis will continue to increase over the coming years as more immunocompromised patients enter the health care system.[2,3]

Although the intensive care unit (ICU) may be the only environment where a critically ill patient can be sustained, it is an environment in which there is a high risk for infection and an increasing prevalence of multidrug-resistant microorganisms. It is a major nursing responsibility to institute the highest standards of asepsis in caring for patients who are vulnerable to infection, especially immunocompromised patients.

CLASSIFICATION OF SHOCK

Although there have been many attempts to classify shock, none has been totally satisfactory. Table 61-1 presents one classification system that lists common types of shock and precipitating factors. This classification is based on the three primary mechanisms responsible for adequate circulation: (1) vascular tone (distributive shock), (2) the ability of the heart to pump (cardiogenic shock), and (3) intravascular volume (hypovolemic shock). In all shock states, the etiology should be considered because each shock state has its own specific causes. Patients may have more than one form of shock simultaneously. For example, hypovolemic shock and septic shock may coexist. Table 61-2 compares the hemodynamic effects of the three types of shock. (Hemodynamic monitoring is discussed in Chapter 63.)

Reviewed by Rebecca Fruge, RN, MN, Clinical Nurse Specialist and Coordinator, English Trimester Nursing Program, InterAmerican University–Metropolitan Campus, San Juan, Puerto Rico; and Susan B. Stillwell, RN, MSN, Clinical Associate Professor, College of Nursing, Arizona State University, Tempe, Ariz.

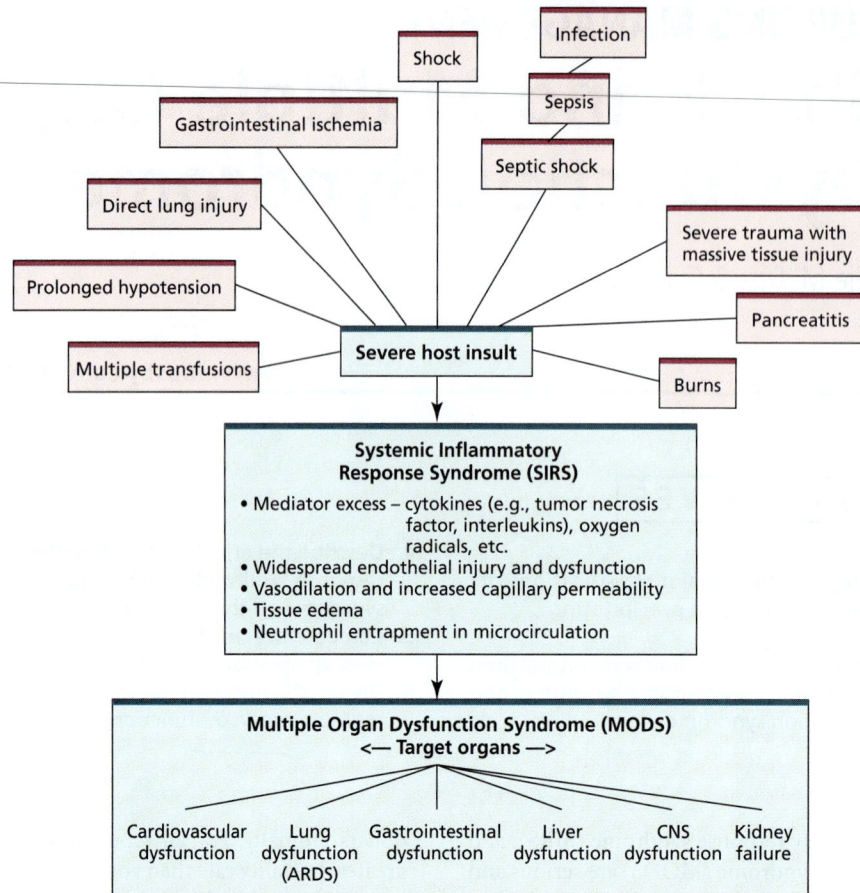

Fig. 61-1   Relationship of shock, systemic inflammatory response syndrome, and multiple organ dysfunction syndrome. *ARDS,* acute respiratory distress syndrome; *CNS,* central nervous system.

Table **61-1**	**Classification and Precipitating Factors of Shock**

Distributive Shock
Neurogenic Shock
- Injury and disease to the spinal cord at or above T_6
- Spinal anesthesia, deep general anesthesia, or epidural block
- Vasomotor center depression (severe pain, drugs, hypoglycemia)

Septic Shock
- Infection (urinary tract, respiratory tract, septic abortion, postpartum, invasive procedures [especially urologic procedures], and indwelling lines and catheters)
- At-risk patients: older adults, patients with chronic diseases (diabetes, cancer, HIV/AIDS), patients receiving immunosuppressive therapy, malnourished or debilitated patients

Anaphylactic Shock
- Contrast media
- Drugs (especially antimicrobials)
- Insect bites/stings
- Anesthetic agents
- Foods/food additives
- Vaccines
- Environmental agents (pet dander, molds, pollens)

Hypovolemic Shock
Absolute Hypovolemia
- Loss of whole blood (hemorrhage from trauma or surgery, GI bleeding)
- Loss of plasma (burn injuries)
- Loss of other body fluids (vomiting, diarrhea, excessive use of diuretics or laxatives, diaphoresis, diabetes insipidus, diabetic ketoacidosis)

Relative Hypovolemia
- Pooling of blood (ascites, peritonitis, bowel obstruction)
- Internal bleeding (fracture of long bones, ruptured spleen, hemothorax, severe pancreatitis, femoral arterial punctures, or catheters in patients on anticoagulant therapy)
- Massive vasodilation (as can occur in conditions that cause distributive shock)

Cardiogenic Shock
- Primary ventricular dysfunction (acute myocardial infarction, cardiac surgery)
- Arrhythmias
- Structural problems (septal rupture, papillary muscle rupture, ventricular aneurysm, cardiomyopathy)
- Obstructive causes (pericardial tamponade, pericardial diseases, tension pneumothorax, acute valvular damage, pulmonary embolism)

AIDS, acquired immunodeficiency syndrome; *HIV,* human immunodeficiency virus.

Table 61-2	Hemodynamic Effects of Shock, Systemic Inflammatory Response Syndrome, and Multiple Organ Dysfunction Syndrome									
Type	HR	Pulse Pressure	BP	SVR	PVR	CVP	PAP	PAWP	CO	SvO₂
Hypovolemic shock	↑	↓	↓	↑	↑	↓	↓	↓	↓	↓
Cardiogenic shock	↑	↓	↓	↑	↑	≈↑	↑	↑	↓	↓
Anaphylactic shock	↑	↓	↓	↓	≈↑	↓	↓	↓	↓	↓
Neurogenic shock	↓	↓	↓	↓	≈	↓	↓	↓	↓	↓
Septic shock	↑	↓	↓	↓	≈↑	↓	↑≈↓	↓	↑	↑≈↓
SIRS	↑	≈	≈	↓	≈↑	↓	↑≈↓	↓	↑	↑≈↓
MODS	↑	≈	≈	↓	↑	↓	↑≈↓	↓≈↑	↓	↑

KEY: ↓ decrease; ↑ increase; ≈ no change.
NOTE: Hemodynamic effects in some illnesses are quite variable. The hemodynamic findings in MODS depend on the system failing.
BP, blood pressure; *CO*, cardiac output; *CVP*, central venous pressure; *HR*, heart rate; *MODS*, multiple organ dysfunction syndrome; *PAP*, pulmonary artery pressure; *PAWP*, pulmonary artery wedge pressure; *PVR*, pulmonary vascular resistance; *SIRS*, systemic inflammatory response syndrome; *SvO₂*, mixed venous oxygen saturation; *SVR*, systemic vascular resistance.

Distributive Shock

Distributive shock includes three types of shock: neurogenic, septic, and anaphylactic. In distributive shock, relative hypovolemia occurs when vasodilation increases the size of the vascular space and results in altered distribution of the blood volume rather than actual loss of volume. This type of shock is often complicated by loss of intravascular fluid from increased capillary permeability, resulting in decreased blood flow to tissues. In distributive shock, there is no change in the blood volume but rather a decrease in the vascular tone.

Neurogenic Shock. Neurogenic shock is caused by massive vasodilation without compensation as a result of impairment of autonomic nervous system function and loss of sympathetic vasoconstrictor tone in the vascular smooth muscle. This massive vasodilation causes pooling of the blood in the venous vasculature, decreased venous return to the heart, decreased cardiac output (CO), and eventually inadequate tissue perfusion (Fig. 61-2). Typically, the patient with neurogenic shock has hypotension and bradycardia. Hypotension is the result of the vasodilation, and the decreased heart rate (HR) is caused by the increased vagal tone from the now unopposed parasympathetic nervous system.

Several precipitating factors can lead to neurogenic shock (see Table 61-1). Disease or injury to the spinal cord above or at the T6 level is the most common cause because transmission of sympathetic nerve impulses to peripheral blood vessels is interrupted. After spinal cord injury, neurogenic shock (sometimes called spinal shock) can last from hours to weeks. (Spinal shock is discussed in Chapter 57.)

Spinal anesthesia can also block the transmission of impulses from the sympathetic nervous system. Depression of the vasomotor center of the medulla as a result of drugs can also decrease vasoconstrictor tone of peripheral blood vessels.

Septic Shock. The definitions and clinical indicators related to the septic-SIRS continuum are presented in Table 61-3. Bacteria, fungi, parasites, viruses, and other causes may cause infection leading to sepsis. Sepsis is SIRS caused by an infection; SIRS is a systemic inflammatory response to a variety of causes, including burn injury, trauma, and pancreatitis (see Fig. 61-1). Severe sepsis is sepsis that is accompanied by organ dysfunction. Septic shock is sepsis with hypotension despite adequate fluid resuscitation.[4]

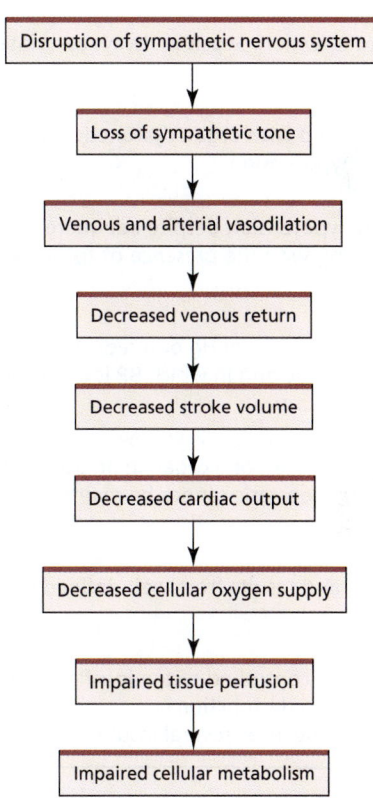

Fig. 61-2   The pathophysiology of neurogenic shock.

Sepsis is most commonly caused by gram-negative bacteria but is increasingly occurring secondary to staphylococcal, streptococcal, fungal, and protozoan infections. Toxic shock syndrome is an example of gram-positive shock resulting from *Staphylococcus aureus*. (Toxic shock syndrome is discussed in Chapter 51.) Causes of septic shock are listed in Table 61-1.

Gram-negative bacteria are responsible for more than one half of the cases of septic shock.[5] When gram-negative bacteremia occurs, endotoxin, a component of the gram-negative bacteria cell wall, triggers a cascade of host inflammatory responses that produce the major detrimental effects seen in

Table **61-3**	Definitions of Terms Related to Sepsis and Organ Failure

Infection
Disease caused by invasion of body by pathogenic organisms.

Bacteremia
Presence of viable bacteria in the blood. Demonstrated by positive blood culture.

Systemic Inflammatory Response Syndrome (SIRS)
Systemic inflammatory response to a variety of insults. Manifested by two or more of the following:
Temperature >100.4° F (38° C) or <97° F (36° C)
Heart rate >90 beats/min
Respiratory rate >20 breaths/min or $PaCO_2$ <32 mm Hg
White blood cell count >12,000 cells/μl or <4000 cells/μl or >10% immature (band) neutrophils

Sepsis
SIRS due to infection. Sepsis is always associated with SIRS.

Severe Sepsis
Sepsis associated with organ dysfunction, hypoperfusion, or hypotension.

Septic Shock
Sepsis with hypotension despite adequate fluid resuscitation along with the presence of tissue perfusion abnormalities.

Hypotension
A systolic BP of <90 mm Hg or a reduction of >40 mm Hg from baseline and in which BP is not adequate for normal perfusion.

Multiple Organ Dysfunction Syndrome
Failure of more than one organ in an acutely ill patient such that homeostasis cannot be maintained without intervention.

Primary MODS
Occurs early and results from well-defined illness or injury.

Secondary MODS
Results from uncontrolled systemic inflammation with resultant organ dysfunction.
Develops latently after several insults.

Myocardial depressant factor works together with TNF, PAF, and other mediators to suppress myocardial contractility. Myocardial depression is almost always present despite an initial rise in CO.

The clinical presentation of septic shock is often subtle, especially in the older, debilitated, or malnourished patient. The blood pressure (BP) is usually low, but the skin is warm and dry because of the vasodilation. In the early stage of septic shock, the patient may have urine output of up to 100 ml/hr.

The survivors of septic shock typically have resolved their high CO and low SVR in the first 24 hours. Cardiovascular parameters that are associated with a high mortality rate include persistent elevation in both HR and CO with low SVR and refractory hypotension for more than 24 hours.

Septic shock is more common among older persons, who often have debilitating chronic diseases and weakened immune systems. The increased longevity of patients with complex, chronic diseases has increased the number of patients who are at risk for developing severe infection and subsequent complications. The rise in the incidence of sepsis is largely due to advances in health care and technology and the rise in the number of immunocompromised patients.

Anaphylactic Shock. Anaphylactic shock is an acute and life-threatening allergic reaction. It is an immediate hypersensitivity reaction that causes massive vasodilation and increased capillary permeability, causing microvascular leakage throughout the body. Anaphylactic shock can lead to respiratory failure, as a result of laryngeal edema or severe bronchospasm, and circulatory failure, as a result of massive vasodilation.[8] (Anaphylactic shock is discussed in Chapter 12.) Generally, the severity of an anaphylactic reaction is directly related to how rapid the onset of symptoms occurs.

A patient can develop a severe allergic reaction, possibly leading to anaphylactic shock, after ingesting or being injected with an antigen to which the person has previously been sensitized. Parenteral administration of an antigen is the route most likely to cause anaphylaxis. However, oral, topical, and inhalation routes of administration of an antigen have been known to cause anaphylactic reactions. Examples of substances that can cause anaphylactic shock are listed in Table 61-1.

Hypovolemic Shock

Hypovolemic shock occurs when there is a loss of intravascular fluid volume. In hypovolemic shock the volume is inadequate to fill the vascular space. Loss of intravascular volume can be divided into absolute causes and relative causes (see Table 61-1). The external loss of fluid from the body is defined as *absolute hypovolemia*. Internal fluid shifting from the intravascular to the extravascular space (interstitial, intracellular, or cavitary space) is defined as *relative hypovolemia*.

In hypovolemic shock the vascular compartment has not changed, but the volume of blood or plasma has decreased. Loss of fluid results in decreased venous return to the heart, decreased stroke volume, decreased CO, circulatory insufficiency, and eventually inadequate tissue perfusion (Fig. 61-4). In hypovolemic shock there is no decrease in the pumping ability of the heart or dilation of the vascular space. The fluid that is lost may be either whole blood, plasma, or water and electrolytes.

In relative hypovolemia, fluid has not left the body, but has shifted out of the intravascular space and is unavailable for cir-

sepsis. (A comparable cell-wall substance from gram-positive bacteria or fungi can similarly trigger this cascade.[2]) When endotoxin binds to monocytes and macrophages, it stimulates the release of mediators, including tumor necrosis factor (TNF) and interleukin-1 (IL-1). These mediators stimulate the release or activation of other mediators, including platelet-activating factor (PAF), prostaglandins, leukotrienes, thromboxane A_2, kinins, and complement[6] (Table 61-4). These factors are responsible for widespread vasodilation and increased capillary permeability, resulting in decreased systemic vascular resistance (SVR) and normal or high CO because of the decreased peripheral resistance (Fig. 61-3). Endotoxins cause the release of histamine, which results in increased capillary permeability and further decreases circulating blood volume.[7]

Table **61-4**	**Mediators of Sepsis, Systemic Inflammatory Response Syndrome, and Multiple Organ Dysfunction Syndrome**
Mediator	**Action**
Endotoxin (component of gram-negative bacterial cell wall)	Stimulation of monocytes, macrophages, and neutrophils to produce cytokines
Interleukin-1	Vasodilation, increased capillary permeability
Tumor necrosis factor	Endothelial injury, vasodilation, increased capillary permeability
Hageman factor	Activation of intrinsic clotting system
Prekallikrein	Production of bradykinin
Bradykinin	Vasodilation, increased capillary permeability, leukocyte chemotaxis
Complement components C3a, C5a	Neutrophil aggregation, release of toxic oxygen radicals, histamine release, vasodilation, increased capillary permeability
Prostaglandins	Vasodilation, decreased platelet aggregation
Platelet activating factor	Platelet aggregation with resultant microvascular stasis; decreased renal perfusion, decreased coronary blood flow, decreased cardiac output
Histamine	Vasodilation, increased capillary permeability
Catecholamines	Inotropic stimulation; altered regional blood flow; increased blood glucose
Cortisol	Gluconeogenesis, hyperglycemia
Myocardial depressant factor	Decreased cardiac contractility and output

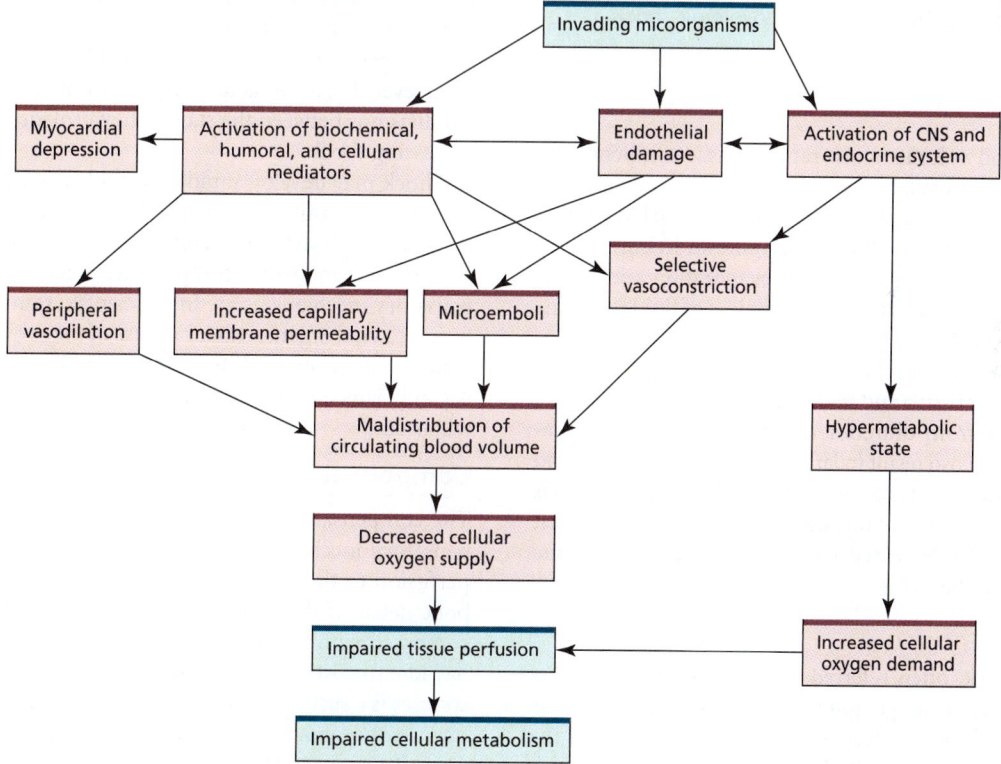

Fig. 61-3   The pathophysiology of septic shock.

culation. Increased capillary permeability can cause pooling of fluid in the interstitial or intracavitary spaces (third spacing). This loss of fluid from the intravascular space causes increased viscosity of the blood and sludging of blood components (microsludging). This, in turn, can block capillaries and venous return, as well as contribute to an increased SVR and decreased tissue perfusion. In addition, the loss of intravascular volume will decrease venous return to the heart and cardiac output.

The most common cause of absolute hypovolemia is hemorrhage (an excessive loss of whole blood). The amount of blood loss that results in shock depends on the efficiency of a person's compensatory mechanisms and the rapidity of blood loss. A healthy adult can compensate for a sudden loss of up to 15% (750 ml in a 70 kg man, 500 ml in a 60 kg woman) of the total blood volume, primarily using sympathetic nervous system–mediated vasoconstriction. However, if greater than

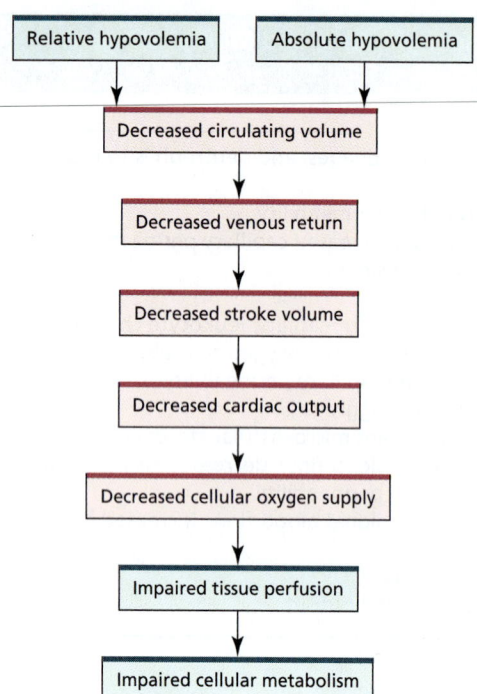

Fig. 61-4   The pathophysiology of hypovolemic shock.

15% of the blood volume is lost rapidly, these compensatory mechanisms begin to fail.

Other common causes of hypovolemic shock include burns, loss of gastrointestinal (GI) fluids, and diuresis. In burn injury there is a direct loss of fluid through evaporation and an increased capillary permeability that causes loss of fluid to the interstitial spaces. GI fluid losses usually occur secondary to severe vomiting, diarrhea, or excessive drainage from a nasogastric tube or fistula and results in a loss of water and electrolytes. Diuresis from diuretics, diabetes insipidus, and diabetes mellitus may also result in large losses of fluid volume and electrolytes. Susceptibility to shock as a result of these factors is generally related to age. Infants and the elderly are at highest risk because of the decreased efficiency of their physiologic compensatory mechanisms.

Cardiogenic Shock

Cardiogenic shock, often referred to as pump failure, occurs when the heart can no longer pump blood efficiently to all parts of the body and the CO is decreased. There is no decreased intravascular volume or vasodilation. Conversely, the vascular space vasoconstricts and further decreases the CO.

Cardiogenic shock is usually the result of left ventricular dysfunction. However, the right ventricle can also be involved. Damage to the ventricles, especially the left, results in failure of the pumping chambers and blood backs up. In right ventricular dysfunction, blood is backed up into the systemic circulation. Left ventricular dysfunction (1) results in decreased cardiac output to the systemic circulation and (2) causes blood to back up into the pulmonary circulation, resulting in pulmonary congestion (Fig. 61-5). A vicious cycle develops as the SVR increases in response to the decreased CO. The failing heart now has to pump harder against a higher systemic resistance.

The most common cause of cardiogenic shock is an acute myocardial infarction (MI). Cardiogenic shock occurs when at least 40% of the left ventricular myocardium has been damaged by infarction.[5] This damage to the myocardium can occur after one massive MI, or it may be cumulative as a result of several smaller MIs occurring over a period of time. With the infarcted muscle, there is a decrease in myocardial compliance and therefore a decrease in contractility. Thus decreased functioning of the left ventricle occurs, as evidenced by decreased CO and BP. There is then less arterial pressure to perfuse the coronary arteries. This continued decrease in coronary perfusion causes increased ischemia of the myocardium, leading to a larger infarction, less contractility, arrhythmias, and metabolic acidosis. These conditions further reduce the effective functioning of the left ventricle.

Other causes of cardiogenic shock are listed in Table 61-1. Regardless of the cause, the extent of pump failure depends on the degree of heart muscle impairment and the adequacy of compensatory mechanisms.

STAGES OF SHOCK

Shock is a dynamic event in which several different processes may be occurring at the same time. In addition, the patient may progress toward death or toward recovery over widely varying time periods. Regardless of the cause, shock can be divided into three stages: (1) compensated stage, (2) progressive stage, and (3) irreversible or refractory stage. Although there are no clear-cut divisions between the stages, they provide a framework for discussing shock.

Shock may develop rapidly or gradually, depending on the severity of the initial insult and the adequacy of compensatory mechanisms. If these mechanisms can maintain adequate arterial pressure and CO, a compensated stage is reached. If compensatory mechanisms are insufficient to restore effective perfusion to vital organs, either because of the severity of the initial insult or its prolonged duration, clinical evidence of reduced organ perfusion and progression through the stages of shock will occur.[9]

Compensated Stage

The compensated stage is the reversible stage in which compensatory mechanisms are effective in maintaining adequate perfusion to the vital organs. In this stage, most of the metabolic needs of the body continue to be met. The stage can be compared with the fight-or-flight response in which the body has identified that it is in danger. The end result of these responses is a sustained stress response. The pathophysiologic sequence of events occurring during this stage is detailed in Fig. 61-6. If promptly treated, the patient will recover with no or minimal organ damage.

Pathophysiology

Regardless of the cause of shock, the body attempts to compensate for a decrease in tissue perfusion in a variety of ways. First, a reduction in mean arterial pressure will inhibit baroreceptor activity, resulting in stimulation of the vasomotor center in the medulla, causing activation of the sympathetic nervous system and release of epinephrine from the medulla and norepinephrine from nerve endings. Stimulation of alpha-adrenergic receptors causes selective peripheral vasoconstriction. Blood flow to the heart and brain is maintained, and blood flow to the

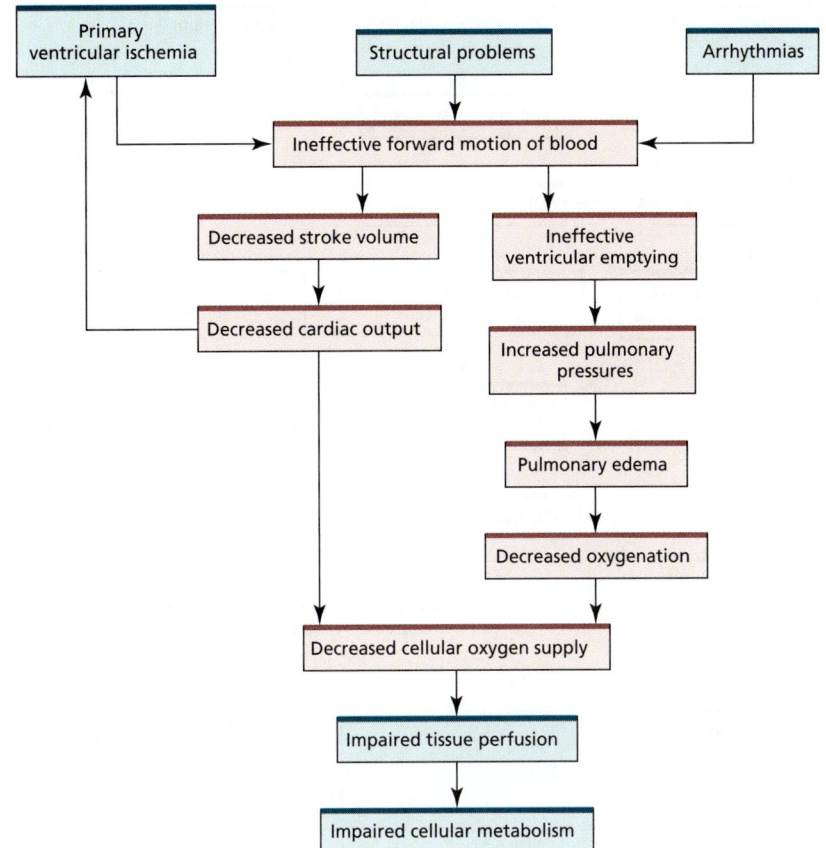

Fig. 61-5   The pathophysiology of cardiogenic shock.

kidneys, GI tract, lungs, muscles, and skin is decreased. Beta-adrenergic receptor stimulation causes a mild increase in HR and force of myocardial contraction, resulting in increased CO. This sympathetic stimulation also causes dilation of the coronary arteries, increasing the O_2 delivery to the myocardium, which now has an increased oxygen demand from the increase in heart rate and contractility.

The decrease in blood flow to the kidneys stimulates the release of renin into the blood where it activates angiotensinogen to produce angiotensin I, which is then converted to angiotensin II (see Fig. 42-6). Angiotensin is a strong vasoconstrictor, causing arterial and venous constriction. The net result is increased venous return to the heart and an increase in BP. Angiotensin also stimulates the adrenal cortex to release aldosterone, which results in sodium reabsorption by the kidneys. The increased sodium raises the serum osmolarity and stimulates the release of antidiuretic hormone (ADH). (ADH is also released when there is decreased blood flow to the posterior pituitary.) The action of ADH results in increased water reabsorption by the kidneys, increased blood volume, and increased venous return to the heart.

A decrease in arterial pressure also causes a similar decrease in capillary hydrostatic pressure. When the hydrostatic pressure no longer exceeds the colloidal osmotic pressure, fluid moves from the interstitial space to the intravascular space. This fluid shift may add sufficient volume to the vascular space to maintain normal arterial pressure without the aid of other compensatory mechanisms.

Venous return is increased by the combination of vasoconstriction and hormonal changes. Increased venous return, as

well as increased HR and myocardial contractility, results in increased CO, maintenance of BP, and adequate tissue perfusion.

Clinical Manifestations

The clinical manifestations of the compensated stage of shock may be subtle and can be easily overlooked (Table 61-5). One of the most reliable signs of the compensatory stage is the patient's level of consciousness. Subtle changes in sensorium, usually in the form of restlessness, irritability, or apprehension, are frequently observed and are probably caused by hypoxia of brain cells. Sedation at this time may be contraindicated because it may mask important neurologic signs.

During this stage, the resting supine BP may be slightly decreased or normal for the patient. For this reason, the BP may not be a useful indicator at this stage. However, a narrowing of the pulse pressure (difference between systolic and diastolic blood pressure) is a classic sign of compensatory shock. Orthostatic hypotension (a decrease in systolic BP of at least 15 mm Hg when a patient is raised from a flat position to an upright, sitting position [90 degrees]) is significant and indicates absolute or relative volume depletion.

The heart rate in the compensatory stage is moderately increased. The pulse is likely to be bounding (in septic shock) or thready because of peripheral vasoconstriction. Respirations increase in rate and depth in an attempt to compensate for decreased cardiac output, resulting in respiratory alkalosis. Urine output may begin to decrease because of reduced renal perfusion and the action of ADH. Because of extravascular volume depletion and decreased secretion of saliva secondary to peripheral vasoconstriction, the patient may complain of thirst.

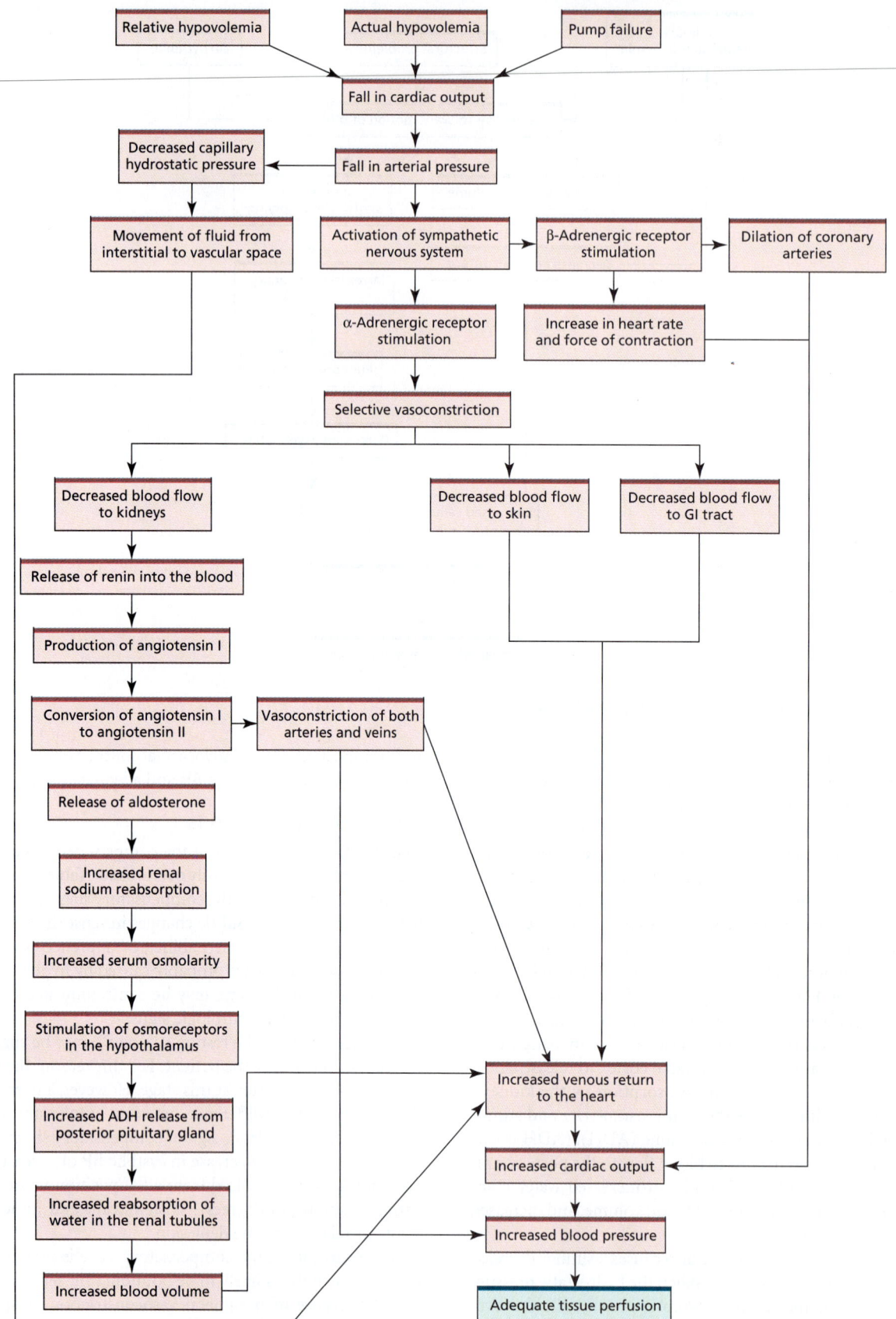

Fig. 61-6 Compensated stage: reversible stage during which compensatory mechanisms are effective and homeostasis is maintained.

Table **61-5**	**Clinical Manifestations Correlated with Stage of Shock**		
Clinical Manifestations	**Compensated Stage**	**Progressive Stage**	**Irreversible or Refractory Stage**
Neurologic Status			
Level of consciousness	Restlessness, irritability, and apprehension	Listlessness or agitation; apathy, confusion, alteration or decrease in response to painful stimuli	Unconsciousness, absent reflexes likely
Orientation	Oriented, verbal	Orientation possible, slowed speech	Confusion and disorientation with slurred, incoherent speech
Cardiovascular Status			
Heart rate	Increased (20 beats/min above patient's normal)	Tachycardia (rate of >100 beats/min), often irregular	Slow and irregular
Peripheral pulses	Bounding (septic shock) or thready	Weak, thready, may be absent	Absent
Blood Pressure			
Systolic	Normal or slight decrease	Hypotension <90 mm Hg with decrease in pulse pressure	Falling to unobtainable
Diastolic	Normal or slight increase	Falling	Approaching zero
Respiratory Status			
Rate	Greater than patient's normal rate	Rapid (>20/min)	Slow
Depth	Deeper than normal	Shallow	Shallow with irregular rhythm such as Cheyne-Stokes or Biot's respirations
Renal Status			
Urine output	Slight decrease but within normal limits	Oliguria (<0.5 ml/kg/hr) with increase in specific gravity	≤18 ml/hr, progressing to anuria with proteinuria
General Status			
Appearance of skin	Pale and cool (warm and flushed in septic shock)	Cold and clammy, cyanosis possible	Cold, clammy, cyanotic, and mottled
Body temperature	Decrease, normal, or increase	Usually subnormal (subnormal or elevated in sepsis)	Significant decrease
Degree of thirst	Normal or slight increase	Marked increase	Severe increase if patient conscious
Bowel sounds	Normal or hypoactive	Hypoactive or absent	Absent

The skin will be cool and pale (except in sepsis where the skin may be warm and dry). Bowel sounds will often be hypoactive because of decreased peristalsis, and abdominal distention can occur.

Associated with the sympathetic nervous system response is the secretion of large amounts of catecholamines from the adrenal medulla. Catecholamines enhance the cellular metabolism of the brain and heart. Catecholamines also stimulate the liver to undergo glycogenolysis, releasing its glycogen stores in the form of glucose. In addition, the pancreatic release of insulin is suppressed. Therefore the brain, which does not require insulin for glucose utilization, has large quantities of glucose available for metabolism.

Progressive Stage

During the progressive stage of shock, compensatory mechanisms are becoming ineffective and may even be detrimental to the patient. The pathophysiologic sequence of events occurring during this stage is outlined in Fig. 61-7. Aggressive management is necessary at this stage to reverse the shock state. Im-

paired cell function, altered capillary dynamics, and altered systemic circulation are the hallmarks of this stage.

Pathophysiology

When shock is not detected and the precipitating cause is not corrected during the earlier stages, a massive sympathetic nervous system response occurs. Profound vasoconstriction of most vascular beds occurs with some peripheral vessels possibly becoming totally occluded. Renal ischemia leads to further activation of the renin-angiotensin mechanism, causing even more pronounced vasoconstriction. Despite the attempt of the body to increase CO by increasing the heart rate and myocardial contractility, there is a net decrease in CO. This decreased CO and profound peripheral vasoconstriction lead to tissue hypoxia, which causes the cells to undergo anaerobic metabolism. A by-product of anaerobic cellular metabolism is lactic acid production. Metabolic acidosis results from the accumulation of lactic acid and impaired renal excretion of acids. As the shock state progresses, the rise in the lactic acid level will often correlate with the severity of the shock state. Severe acidosis (pH less

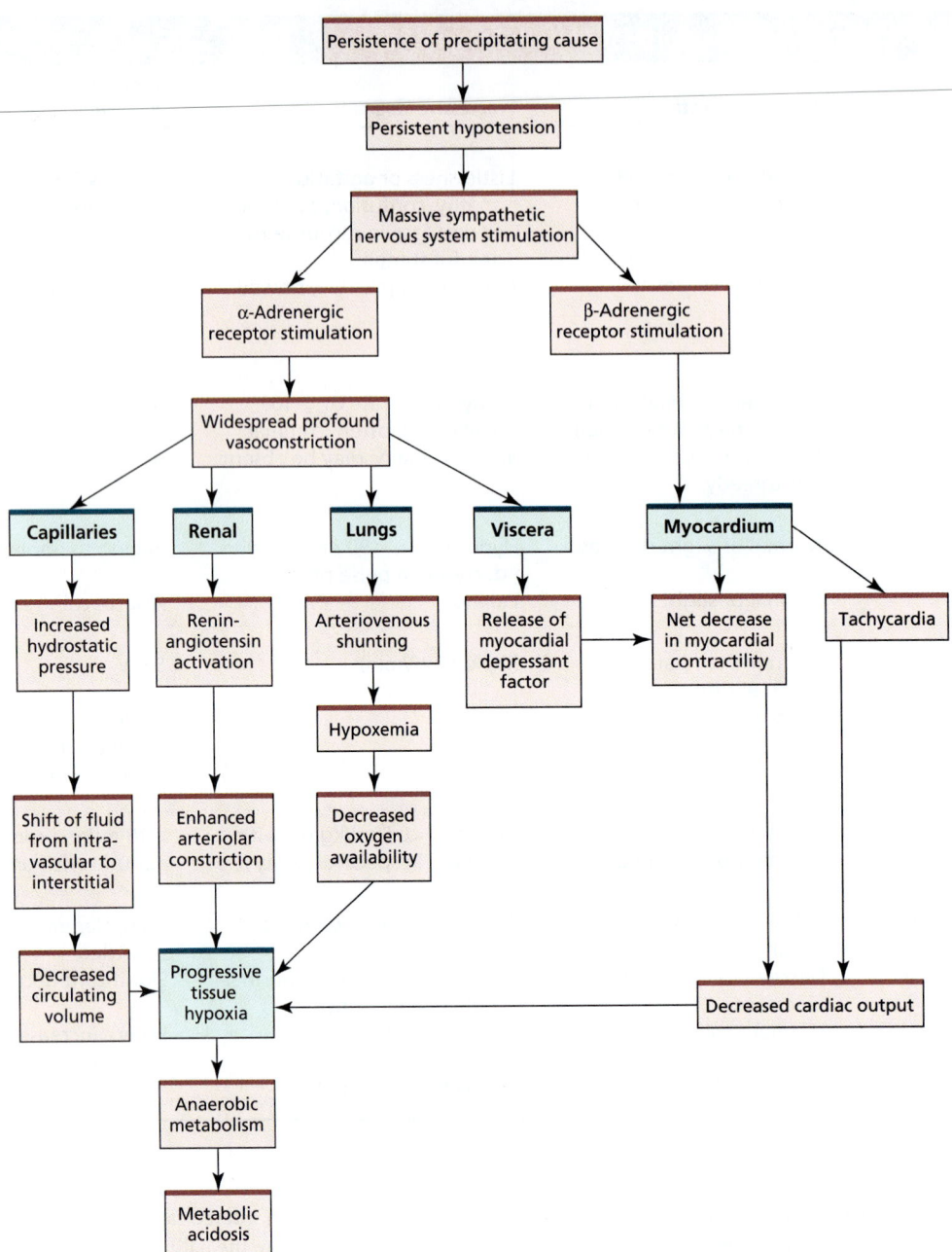

Fig. 61-7 Progressive stage: compensatory mechanisms are becoming ineffective and fail to maintain perfusion to vital organs.

than 7.20) has a direct depressant effect on cardiac function by impairing calcium metabolism within myocardial cells.

Clinical Manifestations

The clinical manifestations of the progressive stage of shock are presented in Table 61-5. The patient demonstrates listlessness, apathy, and confusion. A decreased response to painful stimuli may be observed.

When the BP begins to fall, the patient is no longer in compensated shock. Regardless of the previous normal BP, a systolic pressure below 80 mm Hg or a reduction of greater than 25% in the hypertensive patient is considered to be significant, as well as the increasingly narrow pulse pressure. The narrowed pulse pressure is indicative of decreased stroke volume caused by a decrease in systolic pressure. Because of the severe periph-

eral vasoconstriction, BPs taken with cuff pressures are likely to be inaccurate. Therefore intraarterial monitoring may be used to provide more reliable pressure readings.

Tachycardia is more evident during this stage of shock, and the pulse is weak and thready. However, older adults and patients who are receiving beta-adrenergic blockers may show little change in their heart rate. Other cardiovascular effects of shock during the progressive stage are shown in Table 61-5.

Respirations increase in rate in an attempt to compensate for tissue hypoxia and metabolic acidosis. Urine output decreases and may fall below 0.5 ml/kg per hour, indicating inadequate renal perfusion, which can lead to acute renal failure. The lips and oral mucosa are dry, and the patient may continue to complain of thirst. The skin is cold, pale, and clammy, with slow capillary refill. There may be cyanosis

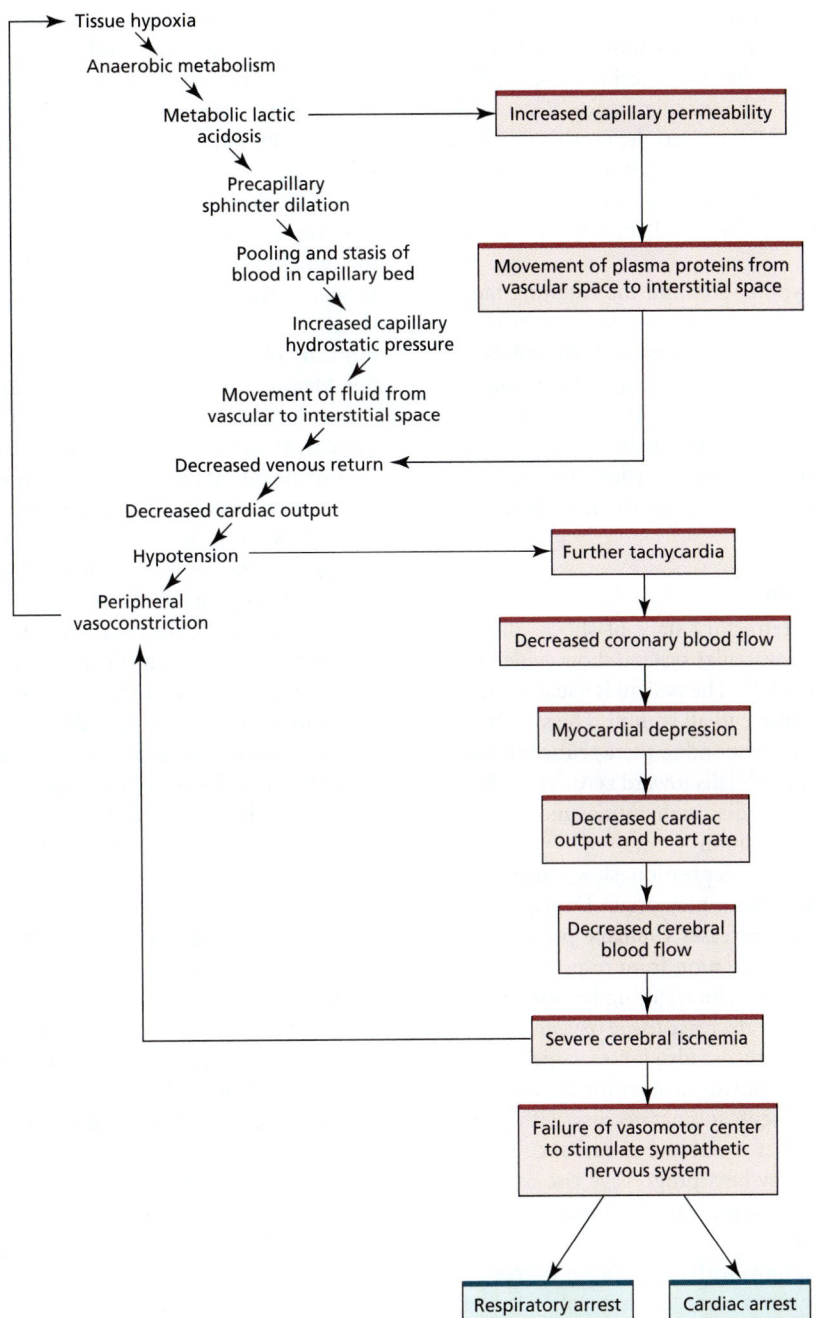

Fig. 61-8 Irreversible or refractory stage: compensatory mechanisms are not functioning or are totally ineffective, leading to multiple organ dysfunction syndrome.

caused by tissue hypoxia. Body temperature is usually low, except in septic shock.

Irreversible or Refractory Stage

The irreversible or refractory stage of shock is the stage during which compensatory mechanisms are either nonfunctioning or totally ineffective. Cellular necrosis and MODS may occur. Attempts to restore the BP have failed, and death becomes imminent. Occasionally patients may be resuscitated from this stage, only to die 7 to 14 days later as a result of the massive cellular death related to MODS.

Pathophysiology

As shock progresses, the sympathetic nervous system activity can no longer compensate to maintain homeostasis. Thus one of the major compensatory mechanisms has failed. There is pooling and sludging of the blood because of the lack of vasomotor tone. Thrombosis of the small blood vessels occurs. Increased vascular permeability and oliguria also occur.

Tissue hypoxia resulting from peripheral vasoconstriction and decreased CO makes it necessary for cells to continue to metabolize anaerobically (Fig. 61-8). The accumulation of lactic acid and other acid metabolites in the body's tissues contributes to cell death. The acid environment also contributes to increased capillary permeability and dilation of the precapillary sphincters. Increased capillary permeability allows fluid and plasma proteins to leave the vascular space. Because the venules remain constricted and the arterioles are dilated, blood pools in the capillary bed. This also causes fluid to move out of the vascular space. The loss of fluid from the vascular space leads to hypotension, and a vicious cycle of decompensation ensues.

As shock progresses, hypotension and the resulting tachycardia decrease coronary blood flow leading to myocardial depression, which further decreases CO. Cerebral blood flow can no longer be maintained, and severe cerebral ischemia occurs. The body cannot maintain vasoconstriction for long with the vicious cycle repeating itself. Consequently, failure of the medullary vasomotor center then occurs, which results in loss of sympathetic tone. The result is respiratory or cardiac arrest and death.

Clinical Manifestations

During the irreversible or refractory stage of shock, all body systems, especially the cardiovascular system, show evidence of decompensation (see Table 61-5). The patient is usually unconscious and may be unresponsive to all stimuli. The systolic BP continues to fall and does not respond to therapeutic interventions to raise it. The diastolic BP falls toward zero. The HR becomes progressively slower. Cardiac arrhythmias may develop because of an ischemic myocardium.

Because of respiratory center depression, slow, shallow respirations with an irregular rhythm may occur. Damage to the pulmonary endothelial cells increases capillary permeability. Pulmonary edema and hypoventilation from respiratory muscle fatigue impair gas exchange. The resulting hypoxemia and respiratory acidosis will further decrease tissue oxygen delivery.

Ischemia of the intestinal mucosa also increases permeability, allowing bacteria and their toxins to enter the bloodstream. Renal ischemia may result in acute tubular necrosis with altered fluid and electrolyte and other metabolic disturbances. Urine output is minimal. There may be a progressive rise in serum creatinine and blood urea nitrogen (BUN) levels, indicating some degree of renal failure.

The skin is cold and clammy, with a significant decrease in temperature. Cyanosis may be present and is usually observed in the lips, mucous membranes, and nail beds. However, it may be more obvious in the palms, soles, and palpebral conjunctiva (inside the eyelid) of dark-skinned patients.

DIAGNOSTIC STUDIES

The history and physical examination provide initial clues leading to a diagnosis of shock and identifying the person at high risk for shock. A history of a recent event that may be associated with shock (e.g., trauma, infection, crushing chest pain, pancreatitis) is significant. Changes in sensorium and a decreased level of consciousness reported by others also are important considerations. During the physical examination, it is important to observe for the clinical manifestations of shock. Of particular importance is the immediate overall impression of central nervous system (CNS) function, which is a measure of cerebral perfusion. Also, the status of the cuta-

neous vascular bed is noted because it may be indicative of impaired peripheral tissue perfusion. In the surgical patient it is important to observe dressings and tubes for the appearance of bleeding. The output of nasogastric tubes and urinary catheters may also provide important clues as to the source of fluid loss.

In addition to the history interview and physical examination, various diagnostic studies (Tables 61-6 and 61-7) are used to confirm the diagnosis and assist in identifying the cause of shock, as well as to monitor the progression and severity of shock.[10] An arterial line and a pulmonary artery catheter, or both, are placed for accurate, ongoing hemodynamic monitoring. Measurements of hemodynamic pressures, flows, and arterial and mixed venous oxygen can be used to guide fluid replacement and drug therapy. A chest x-ray may reveal thoracic trauma or pulmonary changes consistent with shock or acute respiratory distress syndrome (ARDS). Continuous monitoring of heart rate and rhythm is useful for early detection of changes in the patient's cardiopulmonary status. A 12-lead electrocardiogram (ECG) and cardiac monitor may indicate alterations in cardiac electrical activity. Accurate measurement of the BP of the patient in shock is critical, since the level of systemic pressure greatly influences the adequacy of tissue blood flow and myocardial oxygen demands. Auscultatory and noninvasive blood pressure measurements with a sphygmomanometer in the patient in shock may be grossly inaccurate, especially when vasoconstriction is present. Arterial blood gases (ABGs) are important to detect any acid-base abnormalities. Pulse oximetry and ABGs are used to assess the oxygenation status of the patient. An indwelling urinary catheter is placed in the bladder to measure urine output, which is an indicator of renal perfusion.

Hypoperfusion predisposes to impaired oxidative metabolism. Tissue hypoxia predisposes to anaerobic metabolism with a buildup of lactic acid. Therefore lactate is a marker of anaerobic metabolism. A lactate level of greater than 3 mEq/L (3 mmol/L) indicates significant hypoperfusion. Sequential measurements demonstrating continually decreasing levels of lactate are usually a good prognostic sign, whereas high stable or increasing levels are usually an ominous sign.

Base deficit (the amount of base needed to correct the pH back to normal) has been found to be a good indicator of the severity of bleeding and shock in trauma patients. Base deficits may be tracked to assess the effectiveness of therapy.

GENERAL COLLABORATIVE CARE: SHOCK

The critical factor in management of shock is early recognition and treatment (see Table 61-7). Prompt intervention can alter the shock process and prevent the development of the refractory stage and death.[10] Successful management of shock depends on the ability to do the following:

1. Identify the patient at high risk for shock
2. Diagnose shock swiftly and accurately
3. Eliminate or treat the primary cause
4. Initiate therapy to correct pathologic changes, modify the systemic response, and enhance tissue perfusion
5. Protect target organs from dysfunction
6. Provide supportive care

DIAGNOSTIC STUDIES

Table **61-6** Abnormalities in Shock and Multiple Organ Dysfunction Syndrome

Diagnostic Study	Abnormal Finding	Significance of Abnormality
Blood		
Red blood cell count, hematocrit, hemoglobin	Normal	■ Remains within normal limits in shock because of relative hypovolemia and pump failure and in hemorrhagic shock before fluid restoration
	Decreased	■ Decreases in hemorrhagic shock after fluid resuscitation when fluids other than blood are used
	Increased	■ Increases in nonhemorrhagic shock as a result of actual hypovolemia because fluid lost does not contain erythrocytes
DIC screen		
Fibrin split products	Increased	■ Acute DIC can develop within hours to days after an initial assault on the body (i.e., shock)
Fibrinogen level	Decreased	
Platelet count	Decreased	
PTT and PT	Prolonged	
Thrombin time	Increased	
D-dimer	Increased	
BUN	Increased	■ Indicates impaired kidney function caused by hypoperfusion as a result of severe vasoconstriction or occurs secondary to catabolism of cells (e.g., trauma)
Serum creatinine	Increased	■ Indicates impaired kidney function caused by hypoperfusion as a result of severe vasoconstriction; is more sensitive indicator of renal function than BUN
Blood glucose	Increased	■ Occurs in early shock because of breakdown of liver glycogen to glucose in response to sympathetic nervous system stimulation
	Decreased	■ Occurs because of depleted glycogen stores with hepatocellular dysfunction possible as shock progresses
Serum electrolytes		
Sodium	Increased	■ Occurs early in shock because of increased secretion of aldosterone, causing renal retention of sodium
	Decreased	■ May occur iatrogenically when excess hypotonic fluid is administered after fluid loss
Potassium	Increased	■ Occurs when cellular death liberates intracellular potassium; also occurs in acute renal failure and in the presence of acidosis
	Decreased	■ Occurs early in shock because of increased secretion of aldosterone, causing renal excretion of potassium
Calcium	Decreased	■ Sometimes occurs after rapid infusion of large amounts of citrated blood; also occurs secondary to respiratory alkalosis of early shock
	Increased	■ Occurs secondary to lactic acidosis, permitting increased ionization of calcium
Arterial blood gases	Respiratory alkalosis	■ Occurs early in shock secondary to hyperventilation
	Metabolic acidosis	■ Occurs later in shock when organic acids, such as lactic acid, accumulate in blood from anaerobic metabolism
Base deficit	>−6	■ Indicates acid production secondary to hypoperfusion
Blood cultures	Growth of organisms	■ May grow organisms in patients who are in septic shock
Lactate	Increased	■ Usually increases once significant hypoperfusion has occurred with impaired oxygen utilization at the cellular level
Liver enzymes (AST, ALT, LDH)	Increased	■ Elevations confirm liver cell destruction in progressive stage of shock
Urine		
Specific gravity	Increased	■ Occurs secondary to the action of ADH
	Fixed at 1.010	■ Occurs in renal failure

ADH, antidiuretic hormone; *ALT,* alanine aminotransferase; *AST,* aspartate aminotransferase; *BUN,* blood urea nitrogen; *DIC,* disseminated intravascular coagulation; *LDH,* lactate dehydrogenase; *PT,* prothrombin time; *PTT,* partial thromboplastin time.

COLLABORATIVE CARE

Table **61-7**   Shock

Diagnostic

- History and physical examination
- Diagnostic studies (see Table 61-6)
- Placement of CVP, pulmonary artery catheter, arterial line (as indicated)
- Chest x-ray
- Twelve-lead ECG and cardiac monitor
- Identification of precipitating cause (if possible)

Collaborative Therapy

General Measures

- Establishment of a patent airway and administration of oxygen; careful monitoring of oxygenation
- Intubation and mechanical ventilation
- Placement of peripheral IV lines with large-gauge catheters
- Stabilization of BP with fluid replacement (blood, blood products, colloids, crystalloids, or autotransfusion) or drug therapy (see Table 61-10)
- Treatment of cardiac arrhythmias
- Placement of indwelling urinary catheter
- Nutritional support (enteral or parenteral nutrition)
- Emotional support of patient and family

Specific Measures

Hypovolemic Shock

- Control of bleeding (surgery, if indicated)
- Reduction of fluid loss from vomiting, diarrhea, and diuresis
- Volume replacement and blood/blood products (if necessary)
- Discontinue thrombolytics and anticoagulants (as indicated)

Cardiogenic Shock

- Correction of arrhythmias
- Cardiac catheterization with coronary angioplasty or stenting
- Administration of inotropic agents (e.g., dopamine [Intropin]) to increase cardiac contractility

- Careful fluid administration if patient is volume depleted (monitor PAWP)
- Reduction of workload of heart by decreasing afterload with vasodilator drugs (e.g., nitroglycerin)
- IABP to increase coronary perfusion and decrease afterload (if indicated)
- Use of ventricular assist device
- Emergency cardiac surgery or cardiac transplantation

Distributive Shock

Neurogenic Shock

- Treatment according to cause (e.g., pain relief, management of hypoxemia)
- Correction of underlying cause (if possible)
- Careful administration of fluid
- Administration of dopamine for hypotension and bradycardia (as indicated)
- Administration of phenylephrine (Neo-Synephrine) or norepinephrine (Levophed) to increase SVR

Anaphylactic Shock

- Maintenance of patent airway
- Administration of epinephrine for vasoconstriction, bronchodilation, and block histamine
- Administration of fluid
- Administration of inhaled albuterol (Proventil) for bronchodilation (aminophylline if ineffective)
- Administration of aerosolized epinephrine for laryngeal edema
- Administration of diphenhydramine (Benadryl) to counteract effects of histamine
- Administration of vasopressors (e.g., norepinephrine [Levophed]) as indicated

Septic Shock

- Administration of fluid
- Collection of cultures to identify organism
- Use of vasopressors (e.g., norepinephrine [Levophed]) to support BP as indicated
- Administration of appropriate antibiotics
- Control of temperature

CVP, central venous pressure; *ECG*, electrocardiogram; *IABP*, intraaortic balloon pump; *PAWP*, pulmonary artery wedge pressure; *SVR*, systemic vascular resistance.

Emergency care of the patient in shock is important and greatly increases the patient's chance of survival. The emergency care of the patient in shock is presented in Table 61-8.

The patient should be treated in an ICU and have continuous ECG and hemodynamic monitoring. A general goal is to maintain the mean arterial BP greater than 60 mm Hg.

Oxygen and Ventilatory Assistance

Management of shock begins by ensuring that the patient has an adequate airway. This may be accomplished solely by hyperextension of the neck (unless contraindicated by possibility of spinal cord injury). Placement of an endotracheal (ET) tube may be necessary. The patient requires mechanical ventilation to provide adequate ventilation and to decrease the work of breathing. In addition, it is essential that the patient in shock receive sufficient supplemental oxygen to maintain oxygen saturation above 90% or arterial oxygen pressure (PaO$_2$) at 60 mm Hg or higher and to avoid hypoxemia.

Oxygen delivery is dependent on CO, hemoglobin, oxygenation saturation of hemoglobin, mean arterial pressure, and circulating blood volume. Methods to optimize oxygen delivery include increasing the cardiac output (with drug therapy, fluid replacement), increasing the hemoglobin (with blood products), and increasing the oxygen saturation (supplemental oxygen, mechanical ventilation as necessary). Mean arterial pressure and circulating blood volume are optimized by fluid replacement and drugs. Oxygen utilization is decreased by sedation and analgesics and using antipyretics in hyperthermic patients. Nursing care must be provided as gently as possible and spaced out to provide recovery between interventions.

Patient Position

In terms of the patient's cardiovascular status, the recommended position for the treatment of shock (after neck and spine injuries have been ruled out) is supine with the legs elevated to an angle of 45 degrees. The trunk should be horizon-

✚**EMERGENCY MANAGEMENT**

Table 61-8 Shock

Etiology*	Assessment Findings	Interventions

Surgical
  Postoperative bleeding
  Ruptured ectopic
    pregnancy or
    ovarian cyst
  Ruptured organ/vessel
  Gastrointestinal
    bleeding
  Esophageal varices
  Vaginal bleeding
  Aortic dissection
 	
Medical
  Myocardial infarction
  Dehydration
  Addisonian crisis
  Diabetes insipidus
  Sepsis
  Diabetes mellitus
  Pulmonary embolus
 	
Trauma
  Ruptured or lacerated
    vessel or organ
  Fractures
  Multisystem or
    multiorgan injury
	■ Decreased level of consciousness
	■ Restlessness
	■ Anxiety
	■ Weakness
	■ Rapid, weak, thready pulse
	■ Arrhythmia
	■ Hypotension
	■ Narrowed pulse pressure
	■ Cool, clammy skin (warm skin in sepsis)
	■ Tachypnea, dyspnea, or shallow,
	  irregular respirations
	■ Decreased oxygen saturation
	■ Extreme thirst
	■ Nausea and vomiting
	■ Chills
	■ Feeling of impending doom
	■ Pallor
	■ Cyanosis
	■ Obvious hemorrhage or injury
	■ Temperature elevation (in sepsis)
		Initial
		■ Establish and maintain patent airway.
		■ Administer high-flow oxygen (100%) by
		  non-rebreather mask.
		■ Anticipate need for intubation.
		■ Stabilize cervical spine as appropriate.
		■ Establish IV access with two large-bore
		  catheters and begin fluid resuscitation with
		  crystalloids (lactated Ringer's, normal
		  saline).
		■ Control external bleeding with direct
		  pressure or pressure dressing.
		■ Assess for life-threatening injuries (e.g.,
		  hemothorax, cardiac tamponade, liver
		  laceration, pelvic fractures.)
		■ Consider vasopressor therapy only after
		  hypovolemia has been corrected.
		■ Insert an indwelling urinary catheter and
		  nasogastric tube.
		■ Treat arrhythmias.
		
		Ongoing Monitoring
		■ Monitor vital signs, level of consciousness,
		  cardiac rhythm, oxygen saturation, and
		  urine output.

*Other etiologies of shock are listed in Table 61-1.

tal, the head at the level of the chest, and the knees straight. The Trendelenburg's (head-down) position should be avoided in shock because it may (1) initiate aortic and carotid sinus reflexes, causing impaired cerebral blood flow and decreased jugular venous outflow; (2) cause the abdominal organs to press against the diaphragm, thus limiting respiratory excursion and contributing to respiratory distress; (3) decrease filling of the coronary arteries, causing myocardial ischemia; and (4) cause an increase in intracranial pressure in the presence of a head injury. Pneumatic antishock garments should also be avoided because they can increase pressure on the abdomen and decrease diaphragm excursion.

Fluid Replacement

Because shock (with the exception of cardiogenic shock) almost always involves a decreased effective circulating blood volume, the cornerstone of shock therapy is volume expansion by intravenous (IV) administration of appropriate fluids, either crystalloids, colloids, blood products, or a combination[11] (Table 61-9). At least two large-gauge IV catheters should be inserted immediately into large, easily accessible arm veins before severe vasoconstriction occurs and IV access becomes difficult. Crystalloids are electrolyte solutions that are either hypotonic, hypertonic, or isotonic relative to plasma. However, in the critically ill patient approximately two thirds of the volume will diffuse out of the vascular space because of increased capillary permeability and reduced oncotic pressure. Therefore large amounts of crystalloids are needed for adequate volume replacement.[12] Because of the expansion of the interstitial space

following large amounts of crystalloid administration, the development of systemic edema is common.

Colloids usually remain in the intravascular space because of the size of the molecules. The osmotic pressure of these solutions draws fluid into the intravascular space, expanding the intravascular volume. Colloids are extremely effective volume expanders. Colloids are used in the treatment of shock when plasma protein loss is excessive, as in burn shock and peritonitis.

It is important to replace blood with blood or blood products to maintain the hemoglobin for promoting the delivery of oxygen to the tissues to occur. If needed, packed cells or whole blood is administered as soon as available once blood loss has been stopped. The patient's hemoglobin should be used as a guide for blood administration, because 1 U will raise the hemoglobin level about 1 g/dl. (Blood transfusions are discussed in Chapter 29.)

The choice of fluid for volume expansion remains controversial. Neither crystalloids nor colloids are the perfect fluid replacement. However, it is generally accepted that isotonic crystalloids, such as normal saline, are used in the initial resuscitation of shock.[13] Lactated Ringer's solution should be used cautiously in all shock situations because the lactate levels will increase further, and the failing liver cannot convert lactate to bicarbonate. Furthermore, several medications and all blood products are incompatible with lactated Ringer's solution. Crystalloids may be the only fluid used in volume replacement when neither blood nor serum proteins have been lost, as in shock resulting from GI fluid loss. Fluid replacement in cardiogenic shock should be done cautiously, and

RESEARCH
IMPLICATIONS FOR NURSING PRACTICE

Use of Trendelenburg's Position

Citation Ostrow CL: Use of the Trendelenburg position by critical care nurses: Trendelenburg survey, *Am J Crit Care* 6:172, 1997.

Purpose To assess the degree of use of the Trendelenburg's position by critical care nurses, the clinical uses of this position, and the sources of knowledge and beliefs of nurses about the efficacy of the position.

Methods A survey was mailed to 1000 nurses whose names were randomly selected from the membership list of the American Association of Critical Care Nurses. The survey consisted of 17 questions about the frequency of use of the Trendelenburg's position and the reasons for use.

Results and Conclusions The return rate was 49.4%. Ninety-nine percent of the respondents had used the Trendelenburg's position, and 80% had used the modified Trendelenburg's position, mostly for treatment of hypotension. Most used this intervention as an independent nursing action, and most learned about these positions from their nursing education, nurse colleagues, supervisors, and physicians. Eighty percent of the respondents believed that use of the Trendelenburg's position improves hypotension almost always or sometimes.

Implications for Nursing Practice According to this study, the use of the Trendelenburg's position in critical care nursing is widespread. However, there is no scientific evidence indicating that changing a patient's body position to the Trendelenburg's position (head lower than feet) or the modified Trendelenburg's position (only the legs elevated) significantly improves blood pressure or low cardiac output. The results of this study provide evidence that tradition-based therapy still underlies some interventions used in the care of critically ill patients and that some nurses may be relying on an outdated knowledge base that is not supported by the current literature.

---

colloids should not be used because of the osmotic pull of fluid into the vascular space, further decreasing the ability of the heart to pump. The amount and type of fluid given are based on the patient's response to treatment. This can be assessed by observing the BP, pulse, urine output, skin perfusion, lung sounds, hemodynamic parameters, and sensorium.

Ideally fluid replacement should be monitored with a pulmonary artery catheter to determine the pulmonary artery wedge pressure (PAWP) and the CO. The physical assessment of the patient is an important indicator of the patient's fluid status. Complications of excessive volume replacement, such as pulmonary edema and postresuscitation hypertension, can be treated with diuretics. If the patient does not have a pulmonary artery catheter, a urine output of 1 ml/kg per hour will usually indicate adequate fluid replacement. If, after fluid replacement, the cardiac output is still low, an inotropic agent with vasopressor activity such as dopamine (Intropin) or a vasopressor such

as norepinephrine (Levophed) should be administered. Dobutamine (Dobutrex) is an inotropic agent with no vasopressor activity and could be added after adequate vasoconstriction has occurred.

The patient who has sustained a major hemorrhage requires rapid, massive fluid volume and blood replacement, which can exceed the patient's normal blood volume. Complications of massive volume infusion include hypothermia (from cold blood) and coagulopathy (from hemodilution of clotting factors). All blood products and IV solutions should be warmed to prevent hypothermia. Commercial devices are available that warm solutions, as well as provide pumps for rapid infusion. Clotting factor values (see Table 61-6) should be closely monitored.

Acid-Base Imbalance

Frequent monitoring of ABGs allows the physician to prescribe therapy to correct acid-base imbalances. This may be accomplished through the use of fluid administration and mechanical ventilation. Lactic acidosis resolves rapidly once circulating blood volume has been restored. Sodium bicarbonate is used only when the pH is below 7.20. At this point inotropic and vasopressor drugs are ineffective because of the profound acidosis.

Cardiac Arrhythmias

Arrhythmias may cause rapid, profound shock. As a general rule, prompt treatment of the arrhythmia will abolish the shock. Treatment of cardiac arrhythmias is discussed in Chapter 34.

COLLABORATIVE CARE: SPECIFIC TYPES OF SHOCK

In addition to general management of shock, there are specific interventions for different types of shock (see Table 61-7).

Hypovolemic Shock

The major treatment priority for hypovolemic shock is rapid fluid volume replacement. Each patient must be carefully monitored during fluid administration. The patient has probably received adequate volume replacement when the CO, hemoglobin, ABGs, and BP return to the acceptable range and urine output is at least 0.5 ml/kg per hour. Blood and blood products are needed for hemorrhagic shock. Autotransfusion (collection and administration of patient's own blood) may be used in patients with hemorrhage from trauma, especially chest trauma. Because control of bleeding is essential, surgical intervention may be required.

Cardiogenic Shock

The first goal in the management of cardiogenic shock is early restoration of coronary artery blood flow to the myocardium. Cardiac catheterization with coronary angioplasty or stenting is performed as soon as possible. Catheterization may also reveal the extent of myocardial compromise and may unmask surgically treatable mechanical lesions (e.g., septal rupture, papillary muscle rupture). Thrombolytic therapy may be used if cardiac catheterization is unavailable or delayed.

The intraaortic balloon pump (IABP) is a circulatory assist device that is inserted into the femoral, axillary, or subclavian

Table 61-9 Fluid Therapy in Shock and Multiple Organ Dysfunction Syndrome

Fluid Type	Mechanism of Action	Type of Shock	Nursing Implications
Crystalloids			
Isotonic ■ 0.9% NaCl ■ Lactated Ringer's (LR)	Fluid primarily remains in the intravascular space, increasing intravascular volume	Used for initial volume replacement in most types of shock	Monitor patient closely for circulatory overload. LR should not be used in patients with liver failure.
Hypertonic ■ Hypertonic saline (3%)	Draws intracellular and interstitial fluid into the intravascular space, increasing intravascular volume	Hypertonic saline may be indicated for shock from hemorrhage or burns	Carefully monitor serum sodium levels and serum osmolarity.
Colloids (Plasma Volume Expanders)			
■ Human serum albumin (5%, 25%)	Can increase intravascular volume up to five times within 30-60 minutes	All types of shock except cardiogenic	Monitor for circulatory overload. Mild side effects of chills, fever, and urticaria may develop. More expensive than other colloids.
■ Plasma protein fraction	Has albumin as primary component; similar action to that of albumin	All types of shock	May cause greater hypersensitivity reactions than albumin.
■ Hetastarch (Hespan)	Made from starch and acts as volume expander and is at least as effective as albumin; can exert osmotic effect for up to 36 hours	All types of shock	May be 50% less costly than albumin. Use cautiously in patients with congestive heart failure, renal failure, or bleeding disorders (because of anticoagulant effect).
■ Dextran Dextran 40 Dextran 70	Hyperosmotic glucose polymer; similar degrees of volume expansion with dextran 40 and dextran 70; longer duration of action with dextran 70	Limited use because of side effects including reducing platelet adhesion, diluting clotting factors	Increases risk of bleeding. Important to monitor patient for allergic reactions and acute renal failure.
Blood			
■ Whole blood/packed cells	Replaces blood loss, increases oxygen-carrying capability, improves oxygenation of tissues	All types of shock if hemoglobin is <12 g/dl (120 g/L)	Same precautions as any blood administration (see Chapter 29).

artery and placed in the aorta, just distal to the aortic arch (see Chapter 63). The goal of this intervention is to decrease the systemic vascular resistance and thus left ventricular workload, while increasing diastolic pressure resulting in increased coronary and cerebral blood flow. Another type of circulatory assist device is a ventricular assist device (VAD). Ventricular assist devices may be used on a temporary basis for the cardiogenic shock patient or as a bridge while awaiting cardiac transplantation if the treatable lesion cannot be repaired immediately. (IABPs and VADs are discussed in Chapter 63.) Cardiac transplantation is an option for a small and select group of patients with cardiogenic shock.

Cardiogenic shock requires hemodynamic monitoring. If the patient is volume depleted, fluid is replaced cautiously. The goal of drug therapy is to increase cardiac contractility while decreasing afterload and thus the workload of the heart. Inotropic and vasodilator agents (Table 61-10) are commonly used. In addition, diuretics used to decrease preload are indicated if the patient is volume overloaded, and arrhythmias should be aggressively treated.

Septic Shock

In septic shock, the source of infection must be identified and treated with antimicrobial therapy, surgical drainage, or both. The specific organisms causing septic shock are frequently not identified when patients have this illness. Therefore broad-spectrum, antimicrobial therapy must be instituted until the specific organisms are identified through culture and sensitivity testing. Usually two broad-spectrum antibiotics, including an aminoglycoside, are used.[2]

Rapid infusion of large amounts of fluid, including both crystalloids and colloids, are used in treating septic shock. Hemodynamic monitoring of pulmonary artery pressure (PAP), PAWP, and CO is often necessary because of the increased risk

DRUG THERAPY

Table 61-10   Shock and Multiple Organ Dysfunction Syndrome

Drug	Mechanism of Action	Type of Shock	Nursing Implications
Sympathomimetics*			
Dobutamine (Dobutrex)	Primarily stimulates β_1-adrenergic receptors with minimal β_2 and α-adrenergic effects. Increases myocardial contractility. Causes mild vasodilation, decreasing SVR.	Cardiogenic shock in absence of profound hypotension (<80 mm Hg systolic).	Do not give with sodium bicarbonate. Observe for hypotension, arrhythmias, and tachycardia at higher doses.
Dopamine (Intropin)	Is precursor of epinephrine and norepinephrine. Has dose-dependent actions. Stimulates α- and β-adrenergic receptors, causing peripheral vaso-constriction and positive inotropic effect. Increases renal perfusion at low doses only.	All types of shock, especially with decreased SVR; often used with nitroglycerin for cardiogenic shock.	Administer drug through central venous catheter or large peripheral vein (infiltration may cause tissue damage). Monitor for hypotension, tachycardia, and arrhythmias. Be aware that intravascular volume should be adequate.
Epinephrine (Adrenalin)	Stimulates α- and β-adrenergic receptors. Counteracts effects of histamine. Causes bronchodilation and peripheral vasoconstriction, elevating BP. Positive inotropic effect.	All types of shock; drug of choice for ana-phylactic shock.	Observe for cardiac arrhythmias, dyspnea, and pulmonary edema.
Norepinephrine (Levophed)	Stimulates α- and β-adrenergic receptors, causing marked vaso-constriction, as well as inotropic and chronotropic effects.	All types, especially shock from decreased SVR. Reserved for patients with hypotension unre-sponsive to fluids and dopamine.	Best administered through a central venous line. Closely monitor rapid fluctuations in BP and urine output (severe decrease in renal perfusion may occur). Be aware that drug may also cause reflex bradycardia.
Phenylephrine (Neo-Synephrine)	Predominately stimulates α-adrenergic receptors, causing vasoconstriction.	Shock resulting from relative hypovolemia, neurogenic shock.	Observe for reflex bradycardia and ventricular ectopy.
Phosphodiesterase Inhibitor			
Milrinone (Primacor)	Produces inotropic action, increasing CO. Directly relaxes vascular smooth muscles, decreasing preload and afterload.	Cardiogenic shock unresponsive to initial drug therapy.	An initial bolus is administered before beginning the continu-ous IV infusion. Monitor for arrhythmias and hypotension.
Vasodilators			
Nitroglycerin (Tridil, Nitrol)	Primarily acts as venous vasodilator. Dilates veins and arteries at higher doses.	Cardiogenic shock, with inotropic agent.	Monitor BP carefully. Observe for reflex tachycardia. Be aware that headache is common. Use non-PVC tubing and glass bot-tle to prevent drug absorption.
Nitroprusside (Nipride)	Acts as a potent vasodilator on veins and arteries. May increase or decrease CO depending on the extent of preload and afterload reduction.	Primarily cardiogenic shock with increased SVR and preload and afterload; decreased CO, with inotropic drug, such as dopamine.	Closely monitor for hypotension and reflex tachycardia. Admin-ister only with D_5W and protect solution from light. Be aware that thiocyanate toxicity and cyanide poisoning may occur when used for >72 hr.
Morphine sulfate	Is narcotic analgesic and acts as potent venodilator (decreases preload) with some arterial dilation (decreased afterload)	Primarily cardiogenic shock (to decrease preload).	Monitor carefully for hypoten-sion and respiratory depression. Have naloxone (Narcan) at bedside.

Continued

DRUG THERAPY

Table 61-10   Shock and Multiple Organ Dysfunction Syndrome—cont'd

Drug	Mechanism of Action	Type of Shock	Nursing Implications
Corticosteroids Dexamethasone (Decadron) Hydrocortisone (Solu-Cortef) Methyl-prednisolone (Solu-Medrol)	Inhibit inflammatory process, stabilizes lysosomal membranes, reduces capillary permeability, reduces release of chemical mediators in the septic process, and promotes sodium retention.	Serious cases of anaphylactic shock; adrenal insufficiency.	Monitor patient for GI bleeding and hypotension. Be aware that these drugs may make control of diabetes difficult and may cause slow wound healing and predisposition to infection.

*All sympathomimetic drugs are incompatible with sodium bicarbonate.

for multiple system involvement with shock. Therefore these patients have an increased risk of developing fluid overload and cardiac failure. Assessment is important because subtle changes can rapidly occur, and the patient's condition can rapidly deteriorate. If tissue perfusion is inadequate, inotropic and vasopressor drugs (primarily dopamine or norepinephrine) are indicated to improve the blood flow and oxygen delivery.

Antibiotics may not be effective once septic shock has developed, because the harmful effects of the endotoxins and mediators continue even after the bacteria are dead. The current antibiotic therapy for septic shock reverses the effects in only some of the patients. Currently, research is being done using human monoclonal antibodies against various mediators of septic shock. These include antibodies to TNF, endotoxin, and IL-1.[2] To date results have been disappointing. Research is also being conducted regarding the use of continuous renal replacement therapy in removing the endotoxins and mediators from the bloodstream mechanically. (Renal replacement therapies are discussed in Chapter 44.)

Anaphylactic Shock

Full-blown anaphylactic shock is dramatic, and immediate drug intervention is required. Epinephrine is the drug of choice to treat anaphylactic shock. It causes peripheral vasoconstriction and bronchodilation and blocks the effect of histamine. Attention to the airway is important, because the patient can quickly develop respiratory failure from laryngeal edema or bronchoconstriction. Nebulized bronchodilators (e.g., albuterol [Proventil]) are highly effective. Aerosolized epinephrine can be used to treat laryngeal edema. Aminophylline may also be used when bronchoconstriction is severe. Endotracheal intubation or tracheostomy may be necessary to maintain a patent airway. Hypotension results from the leakage of fluid out of the intravascular space as a result of increased vascular permeability and peripheral vasodilation. Aggressive fluid replacement (usually with colloids) is necessary. Diphenhydramine (Benadryl) is used to counteract the effects of massive histamine release. However, it is not effective for the life-threatening vasodilation or bronchoconstriction. Corticosteroids may be administered if hypotension persists.

Neurogenic Shock

Neurogenic shock has multiple causes, and therefore the treatment varies. Fluid replacement for blood pressure maintenance and tissue perfusion is extremely important. Careful monitor-

ing of the patient during fluid administration is important to prevent the patient from developing pulmonary edema as a result of volume overload. Sympathomimetic and vasopressor drug therapy may be indicated to increase BP through vasoconstriction and to increase heart rate.

Drug Therapy: Shock

The primary purpose of drugs used in the treatment of shock is correction of the poor tissue perfusion. These drugs are administered intravenously. Drugs used in the treatment of shock are presented in Table 61-10.

Sympathomimetic Drugs. Many of the drugs used in the treatment of shock have an effect on the sympathetic nervous system. Drugs that mimic the action of the sympathetic nervous system are termed *sympathomimetic*. The effects of these drugs are mediated through action of the α-adrenergic or β-adrenergic receptors. The various drugs differ in their relative α-adrenergic and β-adrenergic effects. (Table 31-1 discusses sympathetic nervous system receptors.)

Many of the sympathomimetic drugs cause peripheral vasoconstriction and are referred to as vasopressor drugs (e.g., epinephrine, norepinephrine). At high doses these vasopressor drugs have the potential to cause severe peripheral vasoconstriction and to further jeopardize tissue perfusion, either directly or indirectly. The increased SVR increases the workload of the heart and can be detrimental to a patient in cardiogenic shock, causing further myocardial damage. Use of vasopressor drugs is generally reserved for patients who have been unresponsive to other therapy. Adequate volume replacement must be administered before the use of any vasopressor drug, because peripheral vasoconstrictor effects in patients with low blood volume cause further reduction in tissue perfusion.

The goals of vasopressor therapy are to achieve and maintain a mean arterial blood pressure of 70 to 80 mm Hg, which ensures improved perfusion to key organs. The sympathomimetic drug of choice for cardiogenic shock is norepinephrine if the systolic BP is less than 70 mm Hg; dobutamine is added when the systolic BP is greater than 90 mm Hg.[14] Norepinephrine and dopamine are the drugs of choice for hypovolemic shock and distributive shock.

Vasodilator Drugs. Some patients in shock show evidence of excessive vasoconstriction and poor tissue perfusion in spite of volume replacement and normal or even high systemic pressures. This is especially true of patients in cardiogenic shock. Although generalized sympathetic vasoconstriction is a useful compensatory mechanism for maintaining systemic pressure, excessive constriction can reduce tissue blood flow and increase the workload of the heart. The rationale for using vasodilator therapy for a patient in shock is to break the deleterious cycle in which widespread vasoconstriction causes a decrease in CO and BP, resulting in further sympathetic-induced vasoconstriction.

The goal of vasodilator therapy, as in vasopressor therapy, is to maintain a mean arterial blood pressure of 70 to 80 mm Hg. It is also important to closely monitor PAP and mean arterial pressure so that fluid administration can be increased or the dose of the vasodilating drug decreased if a serious fall in BP occurs. The vasodilator agent most often used for the patient in cardiogenic shock is nitroglycerin. In noncardiogenic shock vasodilation may be enhanced with nitroprusside (Nipride).

Corticosteroids. IV corticosteroids may be helpful in anaphylactic shock if significant symptoms continue after 1 to 2 hours of aggressive therapy. Although corticosteroids do not have an effect in neurogenic shock, methylprednisolone is used in spinal cord injury to prevent secondary spinal cord damage caused by the release of chemical mediators (see Chapter 57). Corticosteroids are not used in the treatment of other types of shock except in patients with suspected adrenal insufficiency. The use of these immunosuppressant agents may actually increase the incidence of secondary infections in patients with septic shock.[2]

Antibiotics. Antibiotics are always used in the treatment of septic shock. Susceptibility to infection is increased in all patients with prolonged shock of nonseptic etiology. Broad-spectrum prophylactic antibiotic therapy may be indicated because of the high prevalence of nosocomial organisms in critical care units. Methods to prevent nosocomial infections include hand washing, aseptic technique when managing invasive lines and tubes, instituting enteral feeding as soon as possible, elevating the head of the bed to prevent gastric reflux of enteral feedings to the lung, and frequent mouth care. Before antibiotic therapy is begun, specimens of the blood, urine, wound exudate, and sputum should be obtained for culture and sensitivity studies. The organisms that most frequently cause septic shock are gram-negative bacteria. Antibiotic therapy should never be delayed. Unless appropriate antibiotics are started within 24 hours of the beginning of shock, the mortality rate is greatly increased.

Nutritional Therapy: Shock

Protein-calorie malnutrition is one of the primary manifestations of hypermetabolism in shock. Nutrition is vital to decreasing morbidity. Some type of nutrition should be implemented within the first 24 hours. Generally, parenteral feeding is used only if enteral feedings have failed, are contraindicated, or fail to meet the patient's caloric requirements. (Total parenteral nutrition and enteral tube feedings are discussed in Chapter 38.) The patient is started on a continuous drip of very small amounts of enteral feeding. Early enteral feedings are thought to enhance perfusion of the GI tract and prevent translocation of gut bacteria.[15]

A patient in shock should be weighed daily on the same scale at the same time of day. If the patient experiences a significant weight loss, dehydration should be ruled out before additional calories are provided parenterally. Large weight gains are common because of third spacing of fluids. Therefore daily weights

may function more as an indicator of fluid status than caloric needs and balance. Serum protein, nitrogen balance, BUN, serum glucose, and serum electrolytes are all used to assess nutritional status.

NURSING MANAGEMENT: SHOCK
■ Nursing Assessment

Subjective and objective data that should be obtained from a person with shock are presented in Table 61-11. Initial assessment of the patient in shock, or impending shock, need not be extensive. The assessment should focus on the evaluation of the indicators of tissue perfusion, including level of consciousness, skin, vital signs, and urine output. Although a continual decline in the patient's level of consciousness indicates a further reduction in cerebral blood flow and a worsening of the shock state, some patients in shock may remain fully conscious. As shock progresses, severe arterial vasoconstriction continues to decrease perfusion to the skin and kidneys. Therefore the skin becomes colder and mottled and the urine output declines to eventual anuria. The BP may not be a reliable indicator of the severity of shock. Changes from the baseline vital signs are important to evaluate and document.

■ Planning

The overall goals are that the patient in shock will have (1) adequate tissue perfusion, (2) normal BP for the patient, (3) return of organ function, and (4) no complications related to shock.

■ Nursing Diagnoses

Nursing diagnoses for the patient with shock may include, but are not limited to, those presented in NCP 61-1.

■ Nursing Implementation

Health Promotion. It is important for nurses to become involved in the prevention of shock. To prevent shock, the nurse must first identify persons who are at risk. In general, the very old; the very young; persons with chronic, debilitating disease; and the immunocompromised are at an increased risk. More specifically, any person who sustains surgical or accidental trauma is at high risk of shock resulting from hemorrhage, spinal cord injury, burn injury, and the conditions listed in Table 61-1.

Any patient who is at risk for decreased oxygen delivery or tissue hypoxia is at risk for the development of shock. Implementation of the nursing process is essential to help prevent shock after a susceptible individual has been identified. A thorough baseline nursing assessment and frequent ongoing assessments to monitor and detect changes in the patient's condition are the initial nursing actions. Identification of pertinent nursing diagnoses, implementation of appropriate nursing interventions, and evaluation of these actions should follow. Health education is important to prevent the onset of diseases that may result in shock. For example, regular exercise and cessation of smoking may help decrease the risk of MI.

A person with an acute MI, especially an anterior wall MI, is at risk for cardiogenic shock. All patients with symptoms of angina or MI should be encouraged to seek medical attention immediately. The primary goal for the patient with an acute MI is to limit the size of the infarction. This is done by attempting

NURSING ASSESSMENT

Table 61-11   Shock and Multiple Organ Dysfunction Syndrome

Subjective Data

Important Health Information

Past health history: MI, pulmonary embolism, infection, spinal cord injury, hemorrhage, trauma, burns, diabetes mellitus, dehydration, congestive heart failure, valvular dysfunction, pancreatitis, intestinal obstruction, use of tampons, severe reaction to insect bites or stings or blood products

Medications: Severe reaction to any drugs, vaccines, contrast dye, general anesthesia; drug overdose (including insulin); immunosuppressive agents

Surgery or other treatments: Any major surgical procedure, especially involving extensive blood or fluid loss

Functional Health Patterns

Nutritional-metabolic: Thirst, nausea, vomiting, abdominal cramps; chills

Activity-exercise: Weakness, dizziness, fainting, palpitations, dyspnea, productive or nonproductive cough

Elimination: Decreased urinary output, diaphoresis

Cognitive-perceptual: Pruritus; chest pain

Coping–stress tolerance: Apprehension, anxiety, irritability

Objective Data

General

Normal, decreased, or increased (septic shock) body temperature; external evidence of bleeding

Integumentary

Pale, cool, moist skin or warm, flushed skin (septic and anaphylactic shock); dry lips and mucosa; urticaria, rash, and angioedema (anaphylaxis); cyanosis (late)

Respiratory

Rapid, deep respirations, may progress to slow, shallow, irregular respirations; wheezes, crackles, absence of breath sounds, choking, coughing (anaphylaxis)

Cardiovascular

Tachycardia with weak, thready pulse, may progress to slow, irregular pulse with pulse deficit; orthostatic hypotension, narrowing pulse pressure, progressive hypotension; slow capillary refill; flat neck veins (except in cardiogenic shock); abnormal heart sounds; arrhythmias

Gastrointestinal

Diminished or absent bowel sounds

Urinary

Progressive decrease in urinary output

Neurologic

Irritability, restlessness progressing to lethargy, agitation, stupor, coma; slurred speech progressing to disoriented, incoherent speech; decreased response to painful stimuli and absence of reflexes; pupils normal size progressing to dilation and minimal or absent response to light

Possible Findings

Altered serum electrolytes, decreased hemoglobin and hematocrit, leukocytosis, hypoxemia, and hypocapnia or hypercapnia; respiratory alkalosis and metabolic acidosis; increased creatinine and BUN; increased cardiac enzymes (cardiogenic); elevated liver enzymes; elevated lactate levels; positive wound, blood, and body fluid cultures; abnormal chest and abdominal x-rays and ECG

---

to increase coronary artery perfusion and decrease the workload of the heart through rest, drug therapy, thrombolytic therapy, and coronary artery angioplasty.

A person with a severe allergy to such substances as drugs, shellfish, and insect bites may develop anaphylactic shock. The risk of anaphylactic shock can be decreased if the patient is carefully questioned about allergies before administering a new drug (even if the patient has received this drug in the past) or before undergoing a diagnostic procedure involving the use of an IV dye. Patients with severe allergies should wear a Medic Alert tag and report their allergies to their health care providers. These patients should also be instructed about the availability of special kits that contain equipment and medication for the treatment of acute hypersensitivity reactions.

Careful monitoring of fluid balance can help prevent hypovolemic shock. Intake and output, daily body weights, and drainage from wounds and tubes must be carefully calculated and documented. Immediate control of hemorrhage is essential.

An immunocompromised person may develop an opportunistic infection that may rapidly develop into shock. A patient who is at risk of sepsis must be carefully monitored for signs of infection. Limitation of portals of entry into the body, including IV lines and indwelling catheters, is important. Aseptic technique must be used with all invasive procedures.[16] Frequent hand washing is essential. Care must be taken to clean all equipment and other items that are used on more than one patient.

Acute Intervention. The nursing role in the acute stages of shock involves (1) monitoring the patient's ongoing physical and emotional status to detect subtle changes in the patient's condition, (2) planning and implementing nursing interventions and therapy, (3) evaluating the patient's response to therapy, and (4) providing emotional support to the patient and significant others. Nursing responsibilities also include judging when it is necessary to alert other health team members to changes in the patient's status that may require reevaluation of treatment. Therefore reassessment, as often as the patient's condition warrants it, is important (see NCP 61-1).

As care is begun, it is essential for the nurse to obtain the following brief history from the patient or another knowledgeable person:

1. Description of the events leading to the shock condition
2. Time of onset and duration of symptoms
3. Health history, especially medications and allergies
4. Care received before hospital admission
5. Date of last tetanus immunization, if shock is a result of trauma
6. Patient's religious faith
7. Presence of Medic Alert tag

Neurologic status. Neurologic checks, including orientation and level of consciousness, should be performed at least every hour. The patient's neurologic status is the best indicator

61-1   NURSING CARE PLAN   PATIENT IN SHOCK

Expected Patient Outcomes	Nursing Interventions and *Rationales*

NURSING DIAGNOSIS   Decreased cardiac output *related to* shock state *as manifested by* increased diastolic, decreased systolic BP; postural hypotension; tachycardia; weak, thready pulse; flat neck veins; low CVP and PAWP; thirst and dry mucous membranes; urinary output <0.5 ml/kg/hr; altered mentation; arrhythmias; tachypnea; hypoxemia; pallor or cyanosis; cool, clammy skin.

- Normal BP (for patient).
- HR 60-110 beats/min and regular.
- Strong peripheral pulses.
- Normal CVP (1-8 mm Hg) and PAWP (6-12 mm Hg).
- Warm, dry, pink skin.
- Urinary output >0.5 ml/kg/hr.
- Normal mentation.
- Respiratory rate >12 and <20 breaths/min.
- SaO_2 ≥90%.

- Monitor vital signs, CVP, pulmonary artery pressures every 15 min to 1 hr *to monitor patient's status and detect fluid deficits or excesses.*
- Administer crystalloids, colloids, or blood *to restore blood and fluid volume to maintain perfusion of vital organs.* Assess response.
- Titrate drug therapy (as indicated) to support BP *to maintain perfusion.*
- Record accurate intake and output of vital organs *to monitor fluid balance status.*
- Monitor laboratory and x-ray findings *to evaluate patient's response to treatment.*
- Keep patient at normal body temperature *to prevent an increase in metabolic need for O_2 and increased CO_2 production.*
- Administer oxygen *to keep SaO_2 ≥90%.*

NURSING DIAGNOSIS   Fear and anxiety *related to* severity of condition *as manifested by* verbalization of anxiety about condition and fear of death, or withdrawal with no communication; restlessness; sleeplessness; increase in heart and respiratory rate.

- Verbalization of anxieties and fears.
- Verbalization of reduced anxiety.

- Acknowledge expressed fear and anxiety *to validate patient's feelings.*
- Demonstrate concern and respect for patient.
- Try to draw out patient if withdrawn *to encourage verbalization and discussion of fears.*
- Seek out significant other's perception of situation *to enlist help.*
- Maintain calm and reassuring demeanor and environment *to reduce patient's anxieties and oxygen need.*
- Explain interventions, patient status, and equipment simply and honestly *to reduce patient's fear of the unknown and assist patient in making informed decisions.*
- Teach simple relaxation techniques *to aid in stress reduction.*

COLLABORATIVE PROBLEMS

Nursing Goals	Nursing Interventions and *Rationales*

POTENTIAL COMPLICATION   Organ ischemia/dysfunction *related to* decreased tissue perfusion.

NEUROLOGIC ISCHEMIA/DYSFUNCTION

- Monitor for signs of neurologic ischemia.
- Report deviations from acceptable parameters.
- Carry out medical and nursing interventions.

- Perform neurologic assessment every hour including assessment of changes in mentation or level of consciousness *to provide information regarding status of cerebral blood flow.*
- Record and report any changes *to guide selection of appropriate interventions.*
- Closely observe and protect confused patient from injury *to prevent falls and accidents.*
- Take measures to minimize noise *to control sensory input and allow for rest.*

RENAL ISCHEMIA/DYSFUNCTION

- Monitor for signs of renal ischemia.
- Report deviations from acceptable parameters.
- Carry out medical and nursing interventions.

- Monitor for urine output <0.5 ml/kg/hr, increase in urine specific gravity, elevation in serum BUN and creatinine, abnormal serum electrolytes, low urine sodium, protein and blood in urine, metabolic acidosis *to assess renal function.*
- Insert indwelling catheter *to accurately measure urinary output.*
- Take daily weights *to monitor fluid status and evaluate renal function.*
- Administer fluids and drug therapy as ordered and assess results *to maintain adequate renal perfusion.*
- Monitor signs and symptoms of fluid overload *to identify a possible complication of overtreatment.*

Continued

| 61-1 | **NURSING CARE PLAN** | **PATIENT IN SHOCK**—continued |

Nursing Goals	Nursing Interventions and *Rationales*

GASTROINTESTINAL ISCHEMIA/DYSFUNCTION

▪ Monitor for signs of GI ischemia. ▪ Report deviations from acceptable parameters. ▪ Carry out medical and nursing interventions.	▪ Monitor for presence of abdominal pain, distention, nausea, vomiting, anorexia, diarrhea, thirst, absent or diminished bowel sounds *to assess GI status.* ▪ Monitor bowel sounds q4hr. ▪ Measure intake and output *to determine fluid balance.* ▪ Initiate parenteral or enteral nutrition as soon as possible.

PERIPHERAL VASCULAR ISCHEMIA/DYSFUNCTION

▪ Monitor for signs of peripheral vascular ischemia. ▪ Report deviations from acceptable parameters. ▪ Carry out appropriate medical and nursing interventions.	▪ Monitor for presence of cool, pale, or cyanotic extremities; diminished or absent peripheral pulses; pain, tingling, or numbness in extremities; necrotic or gangrenous extremities; poor capillary refill *as indicators of peripheral vascular ischemia.* ▪ Report any changes in peripheral perfusion *so treatment can be initiated promptly.* ▪ Prevent pressure ulcers *because they can develop quickly when immobility is combined with tissue ischemia.* ▪ Keep patient warm and dry *to promote comfort and prevent vasoconstriction.*

RESPIRATORY ISCHEMIA/DYSFUNCTION

▪ Monitor for signs of respiratory distress. ▪ Report deviations from acceptable parameters. ▪ Carry out appropriate medical and nursing interventions.	▪ Monitor for the following: altered respiratory rate and depth, dyspnea, use of accessory muscles, cyanosis, adventitious breath sounds, cough, abnormal chest x-ray *to assess for respiratory distress.* ▪ Initiate oxygen and maintain SaO_2 ≥90% *to ensure adequate oxygenation.* ▪ Monitor ABGs *to evaluate gas exchange in the lungs and acid-base balance.* ▪ Auscultate and record breath sounds q1-2hr to determine presence of crackles, wheezes, and decreased or unequal breath sounds *as indicators of impaired respirations.* ▪ Assist patient to deep breathe *to open up alveoli and improve gas exchange.* ▪ Suction as needed *to remove secretions patient cannot remove independently.* ▪ Maintain patent airway and prepare for possible mechanical ventilation.

CVP, central venous pressure; *PAWP*, pulmonary artery wedge pressure.

of cerebral blood flow. The nurse should be alert to clinical manifestations that may indicate neurologic involvement, such as changes in behavior, restlessness, overalertness, blurred vision, agitation, confusion, and paresthesias.

Attempts should be made to orient the patient to time, place, person, and situation. If the patient is in an ICU, orientation to the environment is particularly important. Measures such as minimizing noise and light levels should be taken to control sensory input. A day-night cycle of activity and rest should be maintained as much as possible. Sensory overload and disruption of the patient's diurnal cycle may contribute to an altered neurologic status, especially if the patient is elderly.

Cardiovascular status. Much of the therapy for shock is based on information about the patient's cardiovascular status. Until the patient is stable, the heart rate, BP, central venous pressure (CVP), and pulmonary artery pressures (if available) should be determined every 15 minutes. (Hemodynamic monitoring is discussed in Chapter 63.) Once the patient is stable, the PAWP should be obtained only as often as needed to avoid

complications associated with balloon inflation. The PAWP most accurately reflects left ventricular function, especially in the presence of lung problems (e.g., pulmonary embolism, chronic lung disease) when the pulmonary artery pressure is often elevated. Trends in pulmonary artery pressures and other hemodynamic parameters are more important than the individual numbers themselves. In addition, care should be taken to avoid dependence on these numbers. It should be remembered that direct physical assessment of the patient is extremely valuable.

The patient's ECG should be continuously monitored to detect arrhythmias that may result from the shock itself or the medications used in treatment. Heart sounds should be assessed for quality and the presence of an S_3 or S_4 sound or murmurs. The presence of an S_3 sound in an adult usually indicates heart failure. The frequency of this monitoring is decreased as the patient's condition improves.

In addition to carrying out these measures, which are necessary to monitor the patient's cardiovascular status, the nurse must administer the prescribed therapy that is designed to correct the patient's impaired cardiovascular status. The response to fluid and medication administration must be assessed every 15 minutes. Appropriate adjustments should be made as needed. After the patient is stable, medications are slowly weaned.

Respiratory status. The respiratory status of the patient in shock must be frequently assessed to ensure adequate oxygenation and early detection of respiratory complications, as well as to provide data regarding the patient's acid-base status. The rate, depth, and rhythm of respirations are initially monitored every 15 to 30 minutes. Increased rate and depth provide information regarding the patient's attempts to correct metabolic acidosis. Breath sounds should be assessed every hour for the development of crackles, which can indicate the presence of fluid buildup in the lungs.

Pulse oximetry, a noninvasive method, is used to continuously monitor oxygen saturation. Pulse oximetry consists of a microprocessor and a probe that attaches to the patient's ear, finger, toe, or nose. Pulse oximetry using a finger or toe may not be accurate in an advanced shock state because of poor peripheral circulation. In this situation, the ear or nose should be used to increase accuracy. ABGs provide definitive information on oxygenation status and acid-base balance. Initial interpretation of ABGs is often the nurse's responsibility. A PaO_2 below 60 mm Hg (in the absence of chronic lung disease) indicates the presence of hypoxemia and the need for the administration of higher oxygen concentrations or for a different method of oxygen administration. A low $PaCO_2$ in the presence of a low pH and a low bicarbonate level indicates that the patient's hyperventilation is attempting to compensate for the metabolic acidosis. A rising $PaCO_2$ in the presence of a persistently low pH indicates the need for intubation and mechanical ventilation.

Most patients in shock will be intubated and on mechanical ventilation. Maintaining a patent airway and monitoring for ventilator-related complications are important. (Mechanical ventilation is discussed in Chapter 63.)

Renal status. Hourly measurements of urinary output are essential in assessment of the adequacy of renal perfusion. An indwelling catheter is inserted to facilitate measurements. Urine output of less than 0.5 ml/kg per hour may indicate inadequate perfusion of the kidneys. BUN and serum creatinine determinations are used as guides to assess renal function. Serum creatinine is a better indicator of renal function because BUN levels can be influenced by the catabolic state of the patient.

Body temperature and skin changes. In the presence of an elevated or subnormal temperature, tympanic or pulmonary arterial temperatures should be obtained hourly. If normal, the temperature should be monitored only every 4 hours. The patient should be kept comfortably warm with the use of light covers and the control of environmental temperature. If the patient's temperature rises above 101.5° F (38.6° C), this condition may be treated with medication such as acetaminophen suppositories, tepid sponge baths, removal of some covers, or a hypothermia blanket (in some situations). Nonsteroidal antiinflammatory drugs (e.g., ibuprofen) decrease body temperature. It is important to treat a fever (greater than 101.5° F [38.6° C]) because an elevated temperature and shivering cause an increased metabolic need for oxygen and increased carbon dioxide production.

Skin color should be assessed for pallor, flushing, and cyanosis. Diaphoresis or piloerection should be noted. In addition, the rapidity of capillary refill should be assessed as an indicator of peripheral perfusion.

Gastrointestinal status. Bowel sounds should be auscultated at least every 4 hours, and abdominal distention should be assessed. Serial measurements of abdominal girth may be indicated. If a nasogastric tube is used, the drainage should be measured as part of the fluid output and tested for occult blood. If the patient has a bowel movement, the stool should be checked for occult blood.

Personal hygiene. Hygiene is especially important to the patient in shock because impaired tissue perfusion predisposes to infection and skin breakdown. However, bathing and other nursing measures must be carried out judiciously because a patient in shock has major problems with oxygen delivery to tissues. Nursing measures must be performed with the least fatiguing method possible and spaced to allow adequate recovery. Using an alternating-pressure or other special foam mattress, turning the patient every 1 to 2 hours, and positioning the patient in good body alignment help prevent pressure ulcer formation. The patient in shock frequently is hemodynamically unstable, and repositioning may result in a worsening of vital signs. The nurse must use clinical judgment in determining priorities of care. Passive ROM should be performed three to four times per day to maintain joint mobility if the patient can tolerate it.

Oral care for the patient in shock is essential because mouth breathing is common and mucous membranes may be dry in the volume-depleted patient. In addition, the intubated patient usually has difficulty swallowing, resulting in pooled secretions in the mouth. A water-soluble lubricant applied to the lips prevents drying and cracking. Moist swabbing of the tongue and oral mucosa with saline solution or diluted mouthwash is also beneficial. Lemon glycerin swabs should not be used because they can cause drying of the mucosa.

Emotional support. The effects of the patient's anxiety and fear in the face of this critical, life-threatening situation are frequently overlooked or underestimated. Anxiety and fear may aggravate respiratory distress and increase catecholamine secretion. It is important for the nurse to remember that compassionate understanding is as essential as scientific and technical expertise in the total care of a patient in shock.

In planning and implementing the nursing care of the patient in shock, the nurse should assess the patient's anxiety. Medication to decrease anxiety is a common mode of therapy. However, in some shock situations, sedation may be contraindicated. Continuous infusions of a benzodiazepine (e.g., lorazepam [Ativan]), a narcotic (e.g., morphine), and occasionally a neuromuscular blocking agent (e.g., vecuronium [Norcuron]) are extremely helpful in decreasing pain, anxiety, and oxygen utilization.

The nurse should talk to the patient, even if the patient is intubated or appears comatose. If the intubated patient is capable of writing, a magic slate or a pencil and paper should be provided. The patient should also receive simple explanations of procedures before they are carried out, as well as information regarding the current plan of care and its rationale. If the patient asks questions about progress and prognosis, simple and honest answers should be given.

Privacy should be provided as much as possible, but the patient should be assured that assistance is readily available should it be required. The call bell should be in reach. In addition, joking and "kidding around" among health care personnel should be kept to a minimum or occur where the patient and family cannot hear it. This type of behavior can often lead the patient to believe that staff members are having too much fun to be available to provide adequate care. Furthermore, conversations about the patient should not take place where the patient can overhear them. Such conversations can constitute a violation of the patient's confidentiality or may be misinterpreted in a way that causes the patient unnecessary distress. Hearing is often the last sense to go, and even if the patient cannot respond, he or she may still be able to hear.

Many patients desire the comfort of a priest, rabbi, or minister. The nurse should offer to call a member of the clergy rather than wait for the patient or family to express a wish for spiritual counseling.

Family and significant others have a therapeutic effect on the patient. To perform this role, they need support and comfort. Family and significant others (1) link the patient to the outside world, (2) facilitate decision making and advise the patient, (3) assist with activities of daily living, and (4) provide safe, caring, familiar relationships for the patient.[17]

The family primarily needs to be kept informed of the patient's condition with reassurance that capable, compassionate personnel are taking care of their loved one. If possible, the same nurse should continue to care for the patient to decrease anxiety, avoid confusing contradictions, and increase trust. Should the prognosis become increasingly grave, the patient's family should be given support when making difficult decisions regarding continuation of life support. The nursing staff must support the family's decisions and facilitate realism. Family members and friends should be shown where they can wait and where a telephone can be found.

Family time with the patient should be facilitated rather than hindered, provided this time is perceived as a comfort by the patient. The nurse should explain in simple terms the purpose of tubes and machines surrounding the patient, and the family should be informed of what they may and may not touch. They should be encouraged to touch their loved one and to perform simple comfort measures. Privacy should be ensured as much as possible. The patient is much more likely to receive comfort from a loved one than from the nurse.

Ambulatory and Home Care. Rehabilitation of the patient in shock necessitates prevention or early treatment of complications and correction of the precipitating cause. The nurse should continue to assess the patient for indications of complications throughout the recovery period. These complications include such problems as chronic renal failure following acute tubular necrosis or the development of fibrotic lung disease as a result of ARDS (see Chapters 44 and 62).

■ **Evaluation**

Expected outcomes for the patient with shock are addressed in NCP 61-1.

SYSTEMIC INFLAMMATORY RESPONSE SYNDROME AND MULTIPLE ORGAN DYSFUNCTION SYNDROME

Systemic inflammatory response syndrome (SIRS) is an abnormal host response to a variety of insults and is characterized by generalized inflammation in organs remote from the initial insult. Normally the inflammatory process is contained within a confined environment. (Inflammation is discussed in Chapter 11.) If the inflammation is not contained, SIRS (a widespread systemic inflammatory response) occurs that is deleterious to organ function.[18] Clinical conditions that predispose to SIRS are presented in Fig. 61-1. When SIRS is the result of infection, the term *sepsis* is used.

Multiple organ dysfunction syndrome (MODS) results from SIRS and is a progressive failure of more than one organ. Transition from the hypermetabolic state of SIRS to clinically defined MODS does not occur in a clear-cut manner because these two entities represent a continuum. In addition, it is difficult to measure organ dysfunction in its early stage. Furthermore, not all patients with SIRS develop MODS.

In MODS, organ dysfunction can be a direct result of the insult (primary MODS) or can manifest latently secondary to a widespread systemic inflammation and involve organs not directly affected in the initial insult (secondary MODS). Examples of primary MODS include the immediate consequences of trauma (e.g., pulmonary contusion, aspiration or inhalation injury). A common cause of secondary MODS is sepsis. Patients can experience both primary and secondary MODS.[5]

Etiology and Pathophysiology

Initiating Events. Bacteria are common causes and can release toxins that initiate the systemic inflammatory response. Exotoxins are released from certain bacteria (e.g., *S. aureus* and *Clostridium perfringens*). Endotoxins originate from the cell walls of gram-negative bacteria (e.g., *Escherichia coli, Pseudomonas*). These substances often have direct toxic effects and can activate cellular and humoral immune responses, and ultimately cause sepsis, SIRS, or MODS. Other clinical conditions that predispose to SIRS and MODS are presented in Fig. 61-1.

Whatever the stimulus, the cause of SIRS and MODS seems to be an uncontrollable systemic inflammatory response mediated by a variety of factors (see Table 61-4). Activation of one mediator leads to activation of another.[19]

When the inflammatory process is not controlled, consequences may occur that can lead to SIRS and MODS. These include activation of inflammatory cells and release of mediators, direct damage to the vascular endothelium, and hypermetabolism. During SIRS endothelial cells are common targets for white blood cell–derived mediators, which cause endothelial destruction and increased vascular permeability. Inflammatory mediators causing endothelial damage include endotoxin, TNF, IL-1, PAF, and many others (see Table 61-4). Organ perfusion may be compromised by hypotension, microemboli, or redistributed or shunted blood flow. Cellular metabolism may be impaired even if adequate oxygen is delivered.

Organ and Metabolic Dysfunction. The lungs are highly vulnerable to mediator-induced injury and are generally the first organ system affected in SIRS and MODS. Acute lung injury manifests as ARDS and generally occurs 1 to 3 days after the initial injury. (ARDS is discussed in Chapter 62.) ARDS is accompanied by a hypermetabolic response.

Cardiovascular changes include myocardial depression and vasodilation. Vasodilation results in decreased systemic vascular resistance (decreased afterload) and decreased blood pressure. The baroreceptor reflex causes release of inotropic (increasing force of contraction) and chronotropic (increasing heart rate) factors that enhance cardiac output. For a while, blood pressure may be maintained but at a higher heart rate and cardiac output. Increases in capillary permeability result in shifting of albumin and fluid from the vascular space, which further diminishes preload. The patient is warm and tachycardic with a high cardiac output and a low systemic vascular resistance. Mixed venous oxygen saturation may be abnormally high because the patient is perfusing areas not consuming much oxygen (e.g., skin, nonworking muscle) while other areas may have blood shunted away from them. Eventually, either perfusion of vital organs becomes insufficient or the cells are unable to use oxygen and their function is compromised. As MODS progresses, cardiac failure develops.

Neurologic dysfunction commonly manifests as mental changes with SIRS and MODS. Acute alteration in mental status can be an early sign of SIRS. The patient may become confused and agitated, combative, disoriented, lethargic, or comatose. These changes may be due to hypoxemia or impaired perfusion. Mediators may damage neuronal tissue directly or indirectly via capillary leakage and related tissue damage. This in turn may produce cerebral edema resulting in increased intracranial pressure.

Peripheral neurologic dysfunction also occurs in patients with MODS, possibly from edema and hypoxia of the peripheral nerves. Clinical findings may be obvious (e.g., severe weakness) or subtle (e.g., difficulty weaning from mechanical ventilation).

Renal failure may result from prerenal causes (impaired perfusion) or from direct damage to renal tubular cells (acute tubular necrosis [ATN]). The frequent use of nephrotoxic drugs (see Table 42-2) for critically ill patients also increases the risk of ATN.

Failure of the coagulation system manifests as disseminated intravascular coagulation (DIC). DIC results in simultaneous microvascular clotting and bleeding because of the depletion of clotting factors and platelets and excessive fibrinolysis. (DIC is discussed in Chapter 29.)

Initially leukocytosis generally occurs. This is especially true if MODS is caused by an infectious agent. Hematopoiesis is impaired, causing anemia, leukopenia, and thrombocytopenia.

Impaired GI circulation may diminish motility, causing paralytic ileus. The GI system is extremely vulnerable to ischemia. Hypoperfusion damages the normal GI mucosa. Following injury the potential for translocation of GI luminal bacteria into the systemic circulation is thought to be increased.[15] This mechanism may be a source of additional activators (e.g., bacteria and endotoxin). Mucosal ischemia results in an increased incidence of gastric and duodenal ulcer formation, and places the patient at risk for GI bleeding.

Liver dysfunction may result in clinical evidence of bleeding, jaundice, hypoglycemia, and lactic acidosis. The patient develops hypoproteinemia because of a shift in the liver activity toward production of acute phase proteins. The serum level of liver enzymes is increased because of ischemic hepatitis, and the prothrombin time is prolonged.

Metabolic changes are pronounced. SIRS and MODS trigger a hypermetabolic response. Glycogen stores are rapidly converted to glucose. Catecholamines and glucocorticoids result in hyperglycemia and insulin resistance. Once glycogen is gone, amino acids are converted to glucose, depleting protein stores. Fatty acids are mobilized for fuel. The net result is a catabolic state, and lean body mass is lost. If hepatic insufficiency is severe, hypoglycemia occurs. Serum protein and albumin levels are generally low because of the catabolic state, leakage of these substances across capillary membranes, and altered liver production.

Electrolyte imbalances, which are common, are related to hormonal and metabolic changes and fluid shifts. These changes exacerbate mental status changes, neuromuscular dysfunction, and cardiac arrhythmias. Antidiuretic hormone results in water retention and hyponatremia. Aldosterone increases urinary potassium loss, and the patient becomes hypokalemic. Catecholamines cause potassium to move into the cell, increasing hypokalemia. Hypokalemia is associated with arrhythmias and muscle weakness. Metabolic acidosis results from impaired tissue perfusion, hypoxia, and a shift to anaerobic metabolism with a related increase in hydrogen ion production. Progressive renal dysfunction also causes an increase in metabolic acidosis. Hypocalcemia, hypomagnesemia, and hypophosphatemia are common.

Clinical Manifestations of SIRS and MODS

The clinical manifestations and laboratory findings of SIRS include the following:

1. Temperature greater than 100.4° F (38° C) or less than 97° F (36° C)
2. Heart rate greater than 90 beats per minute
3. Respiratory rate greater than 20 breaths per minute or $PaCO_2$ less than 32 mm Hg
4. White blood cell count greater than 12,000 cells/μl or less than 4000 cells/μl or greater than 10% immature (band) neutrophils

SIRS is present when two or more of these four clinical manifestations are present (see Table 61-3). The patient may also demonstrate hypotension, confusion, hyperglycemia, and thrombocytopenia. Manifestations range from mild signs and symptoms to circulatory collapse.

Early signs and symptoms of SIRS vary widely. Most patients initially have mild restlessness or confusion, hyperthermia, tachycardia, some increase in fluid requirements, tachypnea with mild respiratory alkalosis, oliguria with reduced responsiveness to diuretics, abdominal distention, and hyperglycemia or increased glucose requirements.

In fully developed sepsis or SIRS the patient appears acutely sick and unstable. Confusion worsens to lethargy or stupor. Cardiac output is greatly increased, the heart rate is rapid, and the skin is warm. Although large volumes of fluid are required to maintain preload, cardiac output tends to be low because of third spacing. Maintaining blood pressure requires volume expansion and vasoactive and cardiotonic drugs. Mixed venous oxygen saturation may be increased because of failure to effi-

Table **61-12**	Clinical Evidence of Organ Dysfunction

Cardiovascular Failure
Heart rate <55 beats/min
Mean arterial pressure <50 mm Hg or systolic blood pressure <60 mm Hg
Ventricular tachycardia or fibrillation
Cardiac index <2.0 L/min/m^2
Serum pH <7.25 with a PaCO$_2$ <50 mm Hg

Respiratory Failure
Severe dyspnea
Respiratory rate <6 or >50 breaths/min
Chest x-ray with decreased lung volumes and bilateral diffuse patchy infiltrates
PaCO$_2$ ≥50 mm Hg
Crackles, wheezes
PaO$_2$/FIO$_2$ <200
Ventilatory dependence >72 hr

Renal Failure
Urine output <0.5 ml/kg/hr
BUN ≥100 mg/dl (35.7 mmol/L)
Serum creatinine ≥3.5 mg/dl (309 μmol/L)

Central Nervous System Failure
Glasgow Coma Scale ≤6 (in absence of sedation)
Hypothermia or hyperthermia
Cardiovascular failure
Respiratory depression

Hematologic Failure
White blood cell count ≤1000/μl (1 × 10^9/L)
Platelets ≤20,000/μl (20 × 10^9/L)
Hematocrit ≤ 20% (.20)
Bleeding studies prolonged

Hepatic Failure
Presence of both of the following:
Serum bilirubin ≥6 mg/dl (102.6 μmol/L)
Prothrombin time >4 sec over control in the absence of systemic anticoagulation

Pancreatic Failure
Elevated serum lipase and amylase
Elevated serum glucose (often resistant to insulin administration)

Gastrointestinal Failure
Mucosal erosion on endoscopy
Perforation
Upper or lower GI bleeding
Diarrhea
Paralytic ileus

BUN, blood urea nitrogen; *FIO$_2$*, fraction of inspired O$_2$; *PaCO$_2$*, partial arterial pressure of CO$_2$; *PaO$_2$*, partial arterial pressure of O$_2$.

Table **61-13**	Progression of Multiple Organ Dysfunction Syndrome*

Days after Precipitating Event or Insult
1-4 Days
Low grade fever
Tachycardia
Dyspnea
Altered mental status
Hyperdynamic/hypermetabolic state
Lungs first to fail—acute respiratory distress syndrome

6-10 Days
Hyperdynamic/hypermetabolic state increases
Bacteremia
Signs of liver and renal failure

10-14 Days
Liver and renal failure more severe
Gastrointestinal system fails
Cardiovascular collapse

15-21 Days
Multiple organ dysfunction syndrome

21-28 Days
Death occurs

*This is a possible sequence of events.

In advanced SIRS and MODS, the patient is unstable and appears close to death. The patient may lose consciousness. Vasopressors and inotropic agents are needed to maintain blood pressure. The patient will be grossly edematous (anasarca). Mixed venous oxygen saturation may rise because of problems with tissue oxygen delivery or may fall if the patient has severe arterial hypoxemia. The patient may be hypercapneic despite aggressive ventilation and have a combined metabolic and respiratory acidosis. The patient may become anuric and require renal replacement therapy. Liver enzyme and bilirubin levels increase. Lactic acidosis worsens. Coagulopathy becomes impossible to correct.

Multiple organs can fail. Criteria for organ system failure are presented in Table 61-12. A prototype progression of MODS is presented in Table 61-13.

NURSING AND COLLABORATIVE MANAGEMENT: SIRS AND MODS

The prognosis of SIRS and MODS is poor, with estimated mortality rates at 90% to 95% when three or more organs fail.[3] Therefore the most important goal is to prevent the development of SIRS and MODS.[19] An important component of the nursing role is vigilant assessment to detect early signs of deterioration or organ dysfunction.

Collaborative care for patients with SIRS or MODS focuses on (1) prevention and treatment of infection, (2) maintenance of tissue oxygenation, (3) nutritional and metabolic support, and (4) appropriate support of individual failing organs.

■ Prevention and Treatment of Infection

Aggressive avoidance, early detection, and prompt treatment of infection are important to eliminate the source of inflammation. If there is an infection, it is important to quickly di-

ciently distribute blood to working organs. The patient is tachypneic, hypocapnic, and possibly hypoxemic, especially if ARDS develops. There is oliguria progressing to renal failure. The GI tract, especially the stomach and colon, is adynamic, and enteral feedings are poorly tolerated. Stress ulceration may occur. As the liver is compromised, bilirubin levels increase and the patient may appear jaundiced. The prothrombin time is prolonged. The patient may develop thrombocytopenia progressing to DIC. Stress-related hormones are high, resulting in increased catabolism and hyperglycemia.

ETHICAL DILEMMAS

Entitlement to Treatment

SITUATION

A 35-year-old European tourist had a hang gliding accident while touring the United States. He was taken to the regional trauma center for treatment of internal injuries, loss of blood, and severe pelvic fractures. He has become septic with a rare organism, is now in renal failure, and has acute respiratory distress syndrome. Despite a 5% to 6% chance of survival, his wife and parents want all possible measures to be taken.

DISCUSSION

The patient, who is not a U.S. resident or citizen, intentionally participated in a (potentially) dangerous activity when he had no insurance coverage. According to federal law, a patient may not be refused admission to an emergency department for acute care. His family believes that his condition entitles him to treatment. His overall prognosis is grim, but his individual condition can be treated with modern technology and expensive drug therapy. There is still a question about the futility of continuing his treatment. The hospital may be left with an enormous uncompensated bill for this patient whether or not he survives. Many hospitals suffer the same dilemma with U.S. residents and citizens who are unable to pay for their treatment.

ETHICAL AND LEGAL PRINCIPLES

- Under the Emergency Medical Treatment and Labor Act (also known as COBRA), hospitals receiving federal money under Medicaid and Medicare must provide emergency screening and treatment in order to stabilize a patient before transferring to another facility.
- The Hill-Burton Act requires states to provide sufficient hospitals and necessary services for those unable to pay.
- Medically futile treatment need not be offered by the hospital. If the family or patient demands obviously futile treatment, the medical team should seek clarification of the goals of such treatment (i.e., recovery, survival, continuing biologic existence, nonabandonment of the patient.) There is no legal right to require medical treatment in cases where the treatment goals cannot be met.

agnose it. Sometimes infections may be difficult to identify. Known infections should be treated with specific agents. If the organism is not known, therapy should begin with broad-spectrum antibiotics and then changed to indicated antibiotics when the organism is identified. Early, aggressive surgery is recommended to remove necrotic tissue (e.g., early debridement of burn tissue) that may provide a culture medium for microorganisms. Aggressive pulmonary management, including early ambulation, can decrease infection. Strict asepsis can decrease infections related to intraarterial lines, endotracheal tubes, urinary catheters, IV lines, and other invasive procedures.

Patients may become infected even when infection control procedures are stringent. Critically ill patients may infect themselves. For example, bacterial contamination of the respiratory tract and development of pneumonia can result from colonization of GI tract bacteria. In some cases infections are thought to be due to systemic invasion by GI bacteria, which are able to penetrate the mucosal barrier following ischemia of the GI tract. Selective decontamination of the GI tract and pharynx has been used to reduce infection but does not alter morbidity or mortality rates from MODS. Another approach to this problem is to institute early enteral feedings, which may enhance perfusion of the GI tract. The induction and maintenance of enteral feedings improves the GI mucosal barrier and decreases the incidence of bacterial and endotoxin translocation.[15,20]

Maintenance of Tissue Oxygenation

Hypoperfusion and resultant hypoxemia frequently occur in patients with SIRS or MODS. These patients have greater O_2 needs and decreased O_2 supply to the tissues. Interventions that decrease O_2 demand and increase O_2 delivery are essential. Decreasing O_2 demand may be accomplished by sedation, mechanical ventilation, analgesia, and rest. Oxygen delivery may be increased by maintenance of a normal hematocrit and PaO_2, positive end-expiratory pressure, increasing preload or myocardial contractility to enhance cardiac output, or reducing afterload to increase cardiac output. Throughout treatment, the ICU nurse must assess the intensity of symptoms, stability of the patient, and potential for recovery. The nurse should discuss the treatment progress with the patient and family.

Nutritional and Metabolic Needs

Hypermetabolism in SIRS or MODS can result in profound weight loss, cachexia, and organ failure. Protein-calorie malnutrition is one of the primary manifestations of hypermetabolism and MODS. Total energy expenditure is increased 1.5 to 2.0 times the normal metabolic rate. Plasma transferrin and prealbumin levels are monitored to indicate hepatic protein synthesis.

The goal of nutritional support is to preserve organ function. Providing adequate nutrition decreases morbidity and mortality rates in patients with SIRS and MODS. The enteral route is preferable to parenteral nutrition and may limit bacterial translocation. If the enteral route cannot be used, parenteral nutrition is used. (Enteral and parenteral nutrition are discussed in Chapter 38.)

Support of Failing Organs

Support of any failing organ is a primary goal of therapy. The patient with ARDS requires oxygen therapy and mechanical ventilation (see Chapter 62). DIC should be treated appropriately (see Chapter 29). Renal failure may require renal replacement therapy (see Chapter 44). Continuous renal replacement therapy is better tolerated than dialysis, especially in a patient with hemodynamic instability.

Research in SIRS and MODS

Monoclonal antibodies and antagonists have been developed against a number of different mediators, including TNF, endotoxin, IL-1, PAF, and bradykinin. Preliminary results have not been encouraging. Thus continued research with this approach will be necessary before effective clinical therapy becomes available to control sepsis or an excessive inflammatory response.[19,21]

CRITICAL THINKING EXERCISES

CASE STUDY

Shock

Patient Profile

Mr. S., a 25-year-old man, was an unrestrained driver involved in a motor vehicle crash. He was found face down 15 feet from his car. There were no passengers. The windshield was broken and the car was found up against a tree. Mr. S. was found conscious and moaning. He was taken to the emergency department (ED).

Subjective Data

- States that he cannot breathe
- Complains of abdominal pain

Objective Data

Physical Examination

- Cardiovascular: BP 84/70; apical pulse 120 but no radial or brachial pulses palpable; carotid pulse present but weak
- Lungs: respiratory rate 35/min; labored breathing with severe respiratory distress; asymmetric chest wall movement; absence of breath sounds on left side
- Abdomen: slightly distended and painful to palpation

Diagnostic Studies

- Chest x-ray: hemopneumothorax and rib fractures on left side
- Hematocrit: 28%

Collaborative Care

- In the ED, placement of chest tube, which drained bright red blood

Surgical Procedure

- Splenectomy
- Repair of torn thoracic artery

Critical Thinking Questions

1. What type of shock was present in Mr. S.? What clinical manifestations did he display?
2. What were the causes of Mr. S.'s shock? What are other causes of this type of shock?
3. What are the initial nursing responsibilities for Mr. S.?
4. What continual nursing assessment parameters are essential for this patient?
5. Based on the assessment data presented, write one or more nursing diagnoses. Are there any collaborative problems?

NURSING RESEARCH ISSUES

1. What is the patient's ability to understand what is being said and happening as the shock state worsens?
2. Compare the cognitive status of patients in different stages of shock.
3. What nursing measures can be implemented to conserve oxygen and decrease oxygen utilization in patients with shock or MODS?
4. What patient positions improve oxygenation and circulatory status?
5. Compare the accuracy of blood pressure monitoring devices to detect the blood pressure changes in shock: invasive arterial monitoring compared with noninvasive devices.

REVIEW QUESTIONS

The number of the question corresponds to the same-numbered objective at the beginning of the chapter.

1. *Shock* is best defined as
   a. cardiovascular collapse.
   b. loss of sympathetic tone.
   c. inadequate tissue perfusion.
   d. blood pressure less than 90 mm Hg systolic.

2. A 78-year-old man has confusion and temperature of 104° F (40° C). He is a diabetic with purulent drainage from his right great toe. His hemodynamic findings are BP 90/40; HR 110; respiratory rate 42 and shallow; CO 6L/min; and PAWP 4 mm Hg. This patient's presentation of symptoms is most likely indicative of
   a. septic shock.
   b. hypovolemic shock.
   c. cardiogenic shock.
   d. anaphylactic shock.

3. A patient in shock is very pale and has a falling blood pressure with tachycardia; a weak, thready pulse; and shallow respirations at a rate of 24 per minute. The nurse recognizes that the patient is in
   a. the compensated phase of shock.
   b. the progressive phase of shock.
   c. the refractory phase of shock.
   d. multiple organ dysfunction syndrome.

4. The effect that shock has on the body includes
   a. sympathetic nervous system activation that results in stimulation of adrenergic receptors.
   b. massive vasoconstriction in the heart and brain that causes stimulation of the renin-angiotensin system.
   c. a heart rate that is usually slow and irregular in the compensatory stage because of parasympathetic nervous stimulation.
   d. decreased tissue perfusion that causes the cells to undergo aerobic metabolism, leading to the development of lactic acidosis.

5. Appropriate treatment modalities for the management of cardiogenic shock include
   a. dopamine to increase myocardial contractility.
   b. corticosteroids to stabilize the cell wall in the infarcted area.
   c. vasopressors to increase systemic vascular resistance.
   d. plasma volume expanders such as albumin to decrease an elevated preload.

6. The most accurate assessment parameters for the nurse to use to determine adequate tissue perfusion in the patient with MODS are
   a. blood pressure, pulse, and respirations.
   b. breath sounds, blood pressure, and body temperature.
   c. pulse pressure, level of consciousness, and pupillary response.
   d. level of consciousness, urine output, and skin color and temperature.

■

References

1. Hill KA, Suter RE: Shock: recognition and care, *JEMS* 21:38, 1996.
2. Sundaresan R, Sheagren JN: Current understanding and treatment of sepsis, *Infect Med* 12:261, 1995.
3. Wadhwa J, Sood R: Multiple organ dysfunction syndrome, *Natl Med J India* 10:277, 1997.
4. Members of the American College of Chest Physicians/Society of Critical Care Medicine Consensus Conference Committee: Definitions for sepsis and organ failure and guidelines for the use of innovative therapies in sepsis, *Crit Care Med* 20:864, 1992.
5. Thelan LA and others: *Critical care nursing: diagnosis and management,* ed 3, St Louis, 1998, Mosby.
6. Koch T: Origin and mediators involved in sepsis and the systemic inflammatory response syndrome, *Kidney Int (Suppl)* 64:S66, 1998.
7. Bone RC, Grodzin CJ, Balk RA: Sepsis: a new hypothesis for pathogenesis of the disease process, *Chest* 112:235, 1997.
8. James JM: Anaphylaxis: multiple etiologies—focused therapy, *J Ark Med Soc* 93:281, 1996.
9. Fink M: Shock: an overview. In Rippe J and others: *Intensive care medicine,* ed 3, Boston, 1996, Little, Brown.
10. Pearl RG: Treatment of shock—1998, *Anesth Analg* (suppl):75, 1998.
11. Kreimeier U, Peter K: Strategies of volume therapy in sepsis and systemic inflammatory response syndrome, *Kidney Int (Suppl)* 64:S75, 1998.
12. Conte MA: Fluid resuscitation in the trauma patient, *CRNA* 8:31, 1997.
13. Sandrock J: Treating traumatic hypovolemia: which fluid to choose? *Nursing* 98:32cc1, 1998.
14. Marino PL: The ICU book, ed 2, Baltimore, 1998, Williams & Wilkins.
15. Lemaire LC and others: Bacterial translocation in multiple organ failure: cause or epiphenomenon still unproven, *Br J Surg* 84:1340, 1997.
16. Tasota FJ and others: Protecting ICU patients from nosocomial infections: practical measures for favorable outcomes, *Crit Care Nurse* 18:54, 1998.
17. Leske JS: Needs of relatives of critically ill patients: a follow-up, *Heart Lung* 15:189, 1990.
18. Nystrom PO: The systemic inflammatory response syndrome: definitions and aetiology, *J Antimicrob Chemother* 41(suppl A):1, 1998.
19. Baue AE: Multiple organ failure, multiple organ dysfunction syndrome, and systemic inflammatory response syndrome, *Arch Surg* 132:703, 1997.
20. Campbell IT: Can body composition in multiple organ failure be favorably influenced by feeding? *Nutrition* 13(suppl):79S, 1997.
21. Horn KD: Evolving strategies in the treatment of sepsis and systemic inflammatory response syndrome (SIRS), *Q J Med* 91:265, 1998.

Resources

Resources for this chapter are listed after Chapter 63 on p. 1957.

62

NURSING MANAGEMENT
Respiratory Failure

Patricia J. Davies & Leslie A. Hoffman

LEARNING OBJECTIVES

1. Explain the physiologic mechanisms that result in hypoxemic or hypercapnic respiratory failure, including acute respiratory distress syndrome (ARDS).
2. Differentiate between early and late clinical manifestations of respiratory failure.
3. Describe the nursing and collaborative management of the patient with hypoxemic or hypercapnic respiratory failure.
4. Describe nursing and collaborative management for the patient with ARDS.
5. Identify complications that may result from acute respiratory failure and measures to prevent or reverse these complications.

ACUTE RESPIRATORY FAILURE

The major function of the respiratory system is gas exchange, which involves the transfer of oxygen (O_2) and carbon dioxide (CO_2) between the atmosphere and the blood (Fig. 62-1). Respiratory failure results when one or both of these gas-exchanging functions are inadequate. For example, insufficient O_2 is transferred to the blood or inadequate CO_2 is removed from the lungs. Inadequate O_2 transfer results in hypoxemia, which is manifested by a decrease in arterial O_2 tension (PaO_2) and a decrease in arterial O_2 saturation (SaO_2). Insufficient CO_2 removal results in hypercapnia, which is manifested by an increase in arterial CO_2 tension ($PaCO_2$).[1] Changes in PaO_2, $PaCO_2$, and SaO_2 can be assessed using arterial blood gases. Pulse oximetry can be used to measure SaO_2 (see Chapter 24). Respiratory failure is not a disease; it is a condition that occurs as a result of one or more diseases involving the lungs or other body systems (Tables 62-1 and 62-2).

Respiratory failure can be classified as hypoxemic or hypercapnic (Fig. 62-2). Hypoxemic respiratory failure is also referred to as oxygenation failure because the primary problem is inadequate O_2 transfer.[1] Although no universal definition exists, hypoxemic respiratory failure is commonly defined as a PaO_2 of 60 mm Hg or less when the patient is receiving an inspired O_2 concentration of 60% or greater. This definition incorporates two important concepts: (1) the PaO_2 is at a level that indicates danger of inadequate O_2 saturation of hemoglobin; and (2) this PaO_2 level exists despite administration of supplemental O_2 at a percentage (60%) that is about three times that in room air (21%).

Hypercapnic respiratory failure is also referred to as ventilatory failure because the primary problem is insufficient CO_2 removal. Hypercapnic respiratory failure is commonly defined as a $PaCO_2$ above normal (greater than 45 mm Hg) in combination with acidemia (pH less than 7.35). This definition incorporates three important concepts: (1) the $PaCO_2$ is higher than normal; (2) there is evidence of the body's inability to compensate for this increase (acidemia); and (3) the pH is at a level where a further decrease may lead to severe acid-base imbalance. (See Chapter 15 for a discussion of acid-base balance.) Many patients experience both hypoxemic and hypercapnic respiratory failure.

Etiology and Pathophysiology

Hypoxemic Respiratory Failure. Common diseases and conditions that cause hypoxemic respiratory failure are listed in Table 62-1. Four physiologic mechanisms may cause hypoxemia and subsequent hypoxemic respiratory failure: (1) mismatch between ventilation ($\dot{V}$) and perfusion ($\dot{Q}$), commonly referred to as $\dot{V}/\dot{Q}$ mismatch; (2) shunt; (3) diffusion limitation; and (4) hypoventilation. The most common causes are $\dot{V}/\dot{Q}$ mismatch and shunt.[1,2]

$\dot{V}/\dot{Q}$ mismatch. In the normal lung, the volume of blood perfusing the lungs each minute (4 to 5 L) is approximately equal to the amount of fresh gas that reaches the alveoli each minute (4 to 5 L). In a perfectly matched system, each portion of the lung would receive about 1 ml of air for each 1 ml of blood flow. This match of ventilation and perfusion would result in a $\dot{V}/\dot{Q}$ ratio of 1:1 (e.g., 1 ml of air per 1 ml of blood), which is expressed as $\dot{V}/\dot{Q} = 1$. Ventilation is ideally matched with perfusion.[3]

Reviewed by Susan B. Stillwell, RN, MSN, Clinical Associate Professor, College of Nursing, Arizona State University, Tempe, Ariz; and Janet T. Crimlisk, RN, MS, NP, CS, Pulmonary Clinical Nurse Specialist, Adult Nurse Practitioner, Boston Medical Center, Boston, Mass.

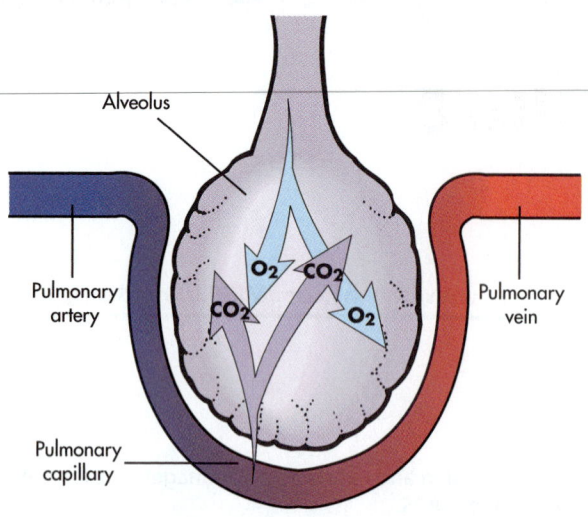

Fig. 62-1   Normal gas exchange unit in the lung.

Glossary Of Abbreviations

ARTERIAL BLOOD MONITORING

ABGs	Arterial blood gases
pH	Negative log of the free hydrogen ion [H^+]
PaO_2	Partial pressure of oxygen in arterial blood
$PaCO_2$	Partial pressure of carbon dioxide in arterial blood
SaO_2	Oxygen saturation in arterial blood measured by ABGs
SpO_2	Oxygen saturation in arterial blood measured by pulse oximetry

OXYGEN AND LUNG FUNCTION MONITORING

FIO_2	Fraction of inspired oxygen concentration
FRC	Functional residual capacity (volume of air in lung at end of expiration)
PEEP	Positive end-expiratory pressure (pressure in lungs at end of expiration)
PEFR	Peak expiratory flow rate (maximum airflow during a forced expiration)
$\dot{V}/\dot{Q}$	Ventilation/perfusion ratio (relationship of ventilation to perfusion in the lungs)
V_E	Minute ventilation (product of tidal volume times respiratory rate)
V_T	Tidal volume (volume of air inspired with each breath)

Although this example presumes that ventilation and perfusion are ideally matched in all areas of the lung, this situation does not normally exist. Although there is overall matching of ventilation to perfusion within the normal lung, there is some regional mismatch. At the lung apex, $\dot{V}/\dot{Q}$ ratios are greater than 1 (more ventilation than perfusion). At the lung base, $\dot{V}/\dot{Q}$ ratios are less than 1 (less ventilation than perfusion). The net effect is a close overall match, since changes at the lung apex balance changes at the base (Fig. 62-3, p. 1898).

Table 62-1	Types of Respiratory Failure and Common Causes

Hypoxemic Respiratory Failure*	Hypercapnic Respiratory Failure*
Respiratory System	**Respiratory System**
Acute respiratory distress syndrome	Asthma
Respiratory distress syndrome of the newborn	COPD
	Cystic fibrosis
Pneumonia	**Central Nervous System**
Cardiac System	Brainstem infarction
Cardiogenic pulmonary edema	Sedative and narcotic overdose
Pulmonary Vascular System	Severe head injury
	Chest Wall
Massive pulmonary embolism (e.g., thrombus emboli or fat emboli)	Flail chest
	Kyphoscoliosis
	Massive obesity
	Neuromuscular System
	Amyotrophic lateral sclerosis
	Phrenic nerve injury
	Cervical cord injury
	Guillain-Barré syndrome
	Poliomyelitis
	Muscular dystrophy
	Multiple sclerosis

*This list is not all inclusive.
COPD, chronic obstructive pulmonary disease.

Many diseases and conditions alter overall $\dot{V}/\dot{Q}$ matching and thus cause $\dot{V}/\dot{Q}$ mismatch (Fig. 62-4, p. 1899). The most common are those in which increased secretions are present in the airways (e.g., chronic obstructive pulmonary disease [COPD]) or alveoli (e.g., pneumonia) or when bronchospasm is present (e.g., asthma). $\dot{V}/\dot{Q}$ mismatch may also result when alveoli collapse (atelectasis). In these conditions, secretions or bronchospasm limit airflow (ventilation) to alveoli but have no effect on blood flow (perfusion) to the gas exchange units. The consequence is $\dot{V}/\dot{Q}$ mismatch. A pulmonary embolus causes the opposite change. The embolus limits blood flow but has no effect on airflow to the alveoli, again causing $\dot{V}/\dot{Q}$ mismatch. O_2 therapy is usually effective in reversing hypoxemia caused by $\dot{V}/\dot{Q}$ mismatch because not all gas exchange units are affected. O_2 therapy increases the PaO_2 in blood leaving normal gas exchange units, thus causing a higher than normal PaO_2. The well-oxygenated blood mixes with poorly oxygenated blood, raising the overall PaO_2 of blood leaving the lungs.

Shunt. Shunt occurs when blood exits the heart without being exposed to O_2. A shunt can be viewed as an extreme $\dot{V}/\dot{Q}$ mismatch (see Fig. 62-4). There are two types of shunt: anatomic and intrapulmonary. An anatomic shunt occurs when blood passes through an anatomic channel in the heart (e.g., a ventricular septal defect or a patent ductus arteriosus) and therefore does not pass through the lungs. An intrapulmonary shunt occurs when blood flows through the pulmonary capillaries without participating in gas exchange. Intrapulmonary shunt is seen in conditions in which the alveoli fill with fluid (e.g., acute respiratory distress syndrome [ARDS]

Table 62-2   Predisposing Factors for Acute Respiratory Failure

Predisposing Factors	Mechanisms of Respiratory Failure
Airways and Alveoli	
Acute respiratory distress syndrome	Direct lung injury from aspiration of gastric contents, diffuse infection, near-drowning, toxic gas inhalation, or airway contusion. Indirect lung injury from sepsis syndrome, severe nonthoracic trauma, or cardio-pulmonary bypass. Fluid enters the interstitial space and, ultimately, the alveoli markedly impairing gas exchange. The result is an initial ↓ in PaO_2 and later ↑ in $PaCO_2$.
Asthma	Bronchospasm escalates in severity rather than responding to therapy. Bronchospasm, edema of the bronchial mucosa, and plugging of small airways with secretions greatly reduce airflow. Work of breathing increases, causing respiratory muscle fatigue. ↓ PaO_2 and ↑ $PaCO_2$.
Chronic obstructive pulmonary disease	Alveoli are destroyed by protease-antiprotease imbalance or respiratory infection or an exacerbation of COPD escalates in severity rather than responding to therapy. Secretions obstruct airflow. Work of breathing increases and causes respiratory muscle fatigue. ↓ PaO_2 and ↑ $PaCO_2$.
Cystic fibrosis	Abnormal Na^+ and Cl^- transport produces secretions that are viscous, poorly cleared, and therefore a foci for infection. Over time the airways become clogged with viscous, purulent, often greenish-colored sputum. Secretions obstruct airflow. Repeated infections destroy alveoli. Work of breathing increases, causing respiratory muscle fatigue. ↓ PaO_2 and ↑ $PaCO_2$.
Central Nervous System	
Narcotic or other drug overdose	Respirations slowed by drug effect. Insufficient CO_2 is excreted, resulting in an increase in $PaCO_2$.
Brainstem infarction, head injury	Medulla cannot alter respiratory rate in response to change in $PaCO_2$
Chest Wall	
Flail chest	Fractures prevent normal rib cage expansion resulting in inadequate gas exchange.
Kyphoscoliosis	Change in spinal configuration compresses the lungs and prevents normal expansion of the chest wall.
Massive obesity	Weight of the chest and abdominal contents prevents normal rib cage movement.
Neuromuscular Conditions	
Cervical cord injury, phrenic nerve injury	Neural control is lost preventing use of the diaphragm, the major muscle of respiration. As a consequence, the patient inspires a smaller tidal volume, which predisposes to ↑ $PaCO_2$.
Amyotrophic lateral sclerosis (ALS), Guillain-Barré, muscular dystrophy, multiple sclerosis, poliomyelitis	Respiratory muscle weakness or paralysis occurs preventing normal CO_2 excretion. Dysfunction may be slowly progressive (muscular dystrophy, multiple sclerosis), progressive with no potential of recovery (ALS), rapid with good expectation of recovery (Guillain-Barré), or stable for extended periods of time (poliomyelitis).

and pulmonary edema).[1] O_2 therapy may be ineffective in increasing the PaO_2 if hypoxemia is due to shunt because (1) blood passes from the right to the left side of the heart without passing through the lungs (anatomic shunt); or (2) the alveoli are filled with fluid, which prevents gas exchange (intrapulmonary shunt). Patients with shunt are usually more hypoxemic than patients with $\dot{V}/\dot{Q}$ mismatch, and they may require mechanical ventilation to improve gas exchange.

Diffusion limitation. Diffusion limitation occurs when gas exchange across the alveolar-capillary membrane is compromised by a process that thickens or destroys the membrane (Fig. 62-5). Pulmonary capillary blood flow may be reduced as a result of obstruction or destruction of vessels such as severe emphysema or recurrent pulmonary emboli. Some diseases cause the alveolar-capillary membrane to become thicker (fibrotic), which slows gas transport. These diseases include pul-

monary fibrosis, interstitial lung disease, and ARDS. Diffusion limitation is more likely to cause hypoxemia during exercise than at rest. During exercise, blood moves more rapidly through the lungs. Because transit time is increased, red blood cells are in the lungs for a shorter time, decreasing the time for diffusion of O_2 across the alveolar-capillary membrane. The classical sign of diffusion limitation is hypoxemia that is present during exercise but not at rest.

Alveolar hypoventilation. Alveolar hypoventilation is a generalized decrease in ventilation that results in an increase in the $PaCO_2$ and a consequent decrease in PaO_2. Hypoventilation may be the result of lung disease, central nervous system (CNS) disease, chest wall dysfunction, or neuromuscular disease. Although alveolar hypoventilation is primarily a mechanism of hypercapnic respiratory failure, it is mentioned here because it can cause hypoxemia.

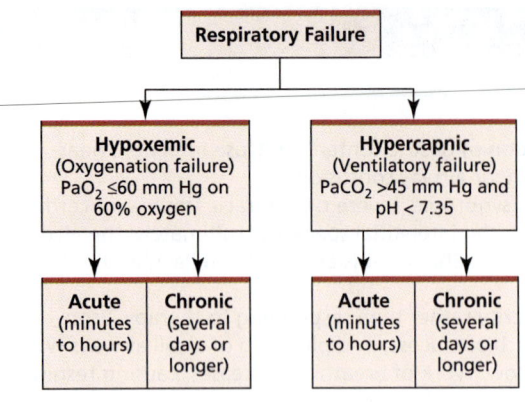

Fig. 62-2 Classification of respiratory failure.

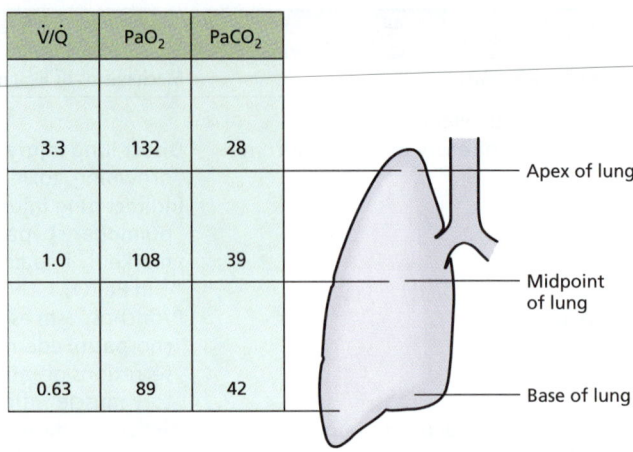

V̇/Q̇	PaO₂	PaCO₂
3.3	132	28
1.0	108	39
0.63	89	42

Fig. 62-3 Regional $\dot{V}/\dot{Q}$ differences in the normal lung. At the lung apex, the $\dot{V}/\dot{Q}$ ratio is 3.3, at the midpoint 1.0, and at the base 0.63. This difference causes the PaO_2 to be higher at the apex of the lung and lower at the base. Values for $PaCO_2$ are the opposite (i.e., lower at the apex and higher at the base). Blood that exits the lung is a mixture of these values.

Interrelationship of mechanisms. Frequently, hypoxemic respiratory failure is caused by a combination of two or more of the following: $\dot{V}/\dot{Q}$ mismatch, shunting, diffusion limitation, and hypoventilation. The patient with acute respiratory failure secondary to pneumonia may have a combination of $\dot{V}/\dot{Q}$ mismatch and shunt because the inflammation, edema, and hypersecretion of exudate within the bronchioles and terminal respiratory units obstruct the airways ($\dot{V}/\dot{Q}$ mismatch) and fill the alveoli with exudate (shunt). The patient with cardiogenic pulmonary edema or ARDS may have a combination of shunt and $\dot{V}/\dot{Q}$ mismatch because some alveoli are completely filled with fluid from edema (shunt) and others are partially filled with fluid ($\dot{V}/\dot{Q}$ mismatch).

Hypercapnic Respiratory Failure. Hypercapnic respiratory failure results from an imbalance between ventilatory supply and ventilatory demand. Ventilatory supply is the maximum ventilation (gas flow in and out of the lungs) that the patient can sustain without developing respiratory muscle fatigue. Ventilatory demand is the amount of ventilation needed to keep the $PaCO_2$ within normal limits. Normally, ventilatory supply far exceeds ventilatory demand. As a consequence, individuals with normal lung function can engage in strenuous exercise, which greatly increases CO_2 production without an elevation in $PaCO_2$. Patients with lung disease do not have this advantage. However, considerable dysfunction is typically present before ventilatory demand exceeds ventilatory supply.

When ventilatory demand exceeds ventilatory supply, the $PaCO_2$ can no longer be sustained within normal limits and hypercapnia occurs. Hypercapnia reflects substantial lung dysfunction.[1] Hypercapnic respiratory failure is sometimes called pump failure because the primary problem is the inability of the respiratory system to expel (pump out) sufficient CO_2 to maintain a normal $PaCO_2$. Hypercapnic respiratory failure may also be described as acute on chronic respiratory failure since the episode of respiratory failure represents an acute decompensation in a patient whose underlying lung function has deteriorated to the point that some degree of decompensation is always present (chronic respiratory insufficiency).

Many different diseases can cause a limitation in ventilatory supply (see Tables 62-1 and 62-2). These diseases can be grouped into four categories: (1) abnormalities of the airways and alveoli, (2) abnormalities of the CNS, (3) abnormalities of the chest wall, and (4) neuromuscular conditions.[1]

Airways and alveoli. Patients with asthma, emphysema, chronic bronchitis, and cystic fibrosis are at high risk for hypercapnic respiratory failure because the underlying pathophysiology of these conditions results in airflow obstruction and air trapping.

Central nervous system. A variety of problems may suppress the drive to breathe. A common example is an overdose of a narcotic or other respiratory depressant drug. A brainstem infarction or severe head injury may also interfere with normal function of the respiratory center in the medulla. Patients with these conditions are at risk for respiratory failure because the medulla does not alter the respiratory rate in response to a change in $PaCO_2$.

Chest wall. A variety of conditions may prevent normal movement of the chest wall and hence limit lung expansion. In patients with flail chest, fractures prevent the rib cage from expanding normally. In patients with kyphoscoliosis, the change in spinal configuration compresses the lungs and prevents normal expansion of the chest wall. In patients with massive obesity, the weight of the chest and abdominal contents may limit lung expansion. Patients with these conditions are at risk for respiratory failure because these dysfunctions limit lung expansion or diaphragmatic movement and consequently gas exchange.

Neuromuscular conditions. Various types of neuromuscular diseases may result in respiratory muscle weakness or paralysis (see Table 62-1). Patients with these conditions are at risk for respiratory failure because the respiratory muscles are weakened or paralyzed as a consequence of the underlying neuromuscular condition. Therefore they are unable to maintain normal $PaCO_2$ levels.

Ventilatory failure with normal lung function. In three of these categories (CNS, chest wall, neuromuscular conditions), respiratory failure may occur despite the presence of normal lungs. Respiratory failure occurs because the medulla, respiratory muscles, or chest wall is not functioning normally. The patient may have no damage to lung tissue but may be unable to inspire a tidal volume sufficient to expel CO_2 from the lungs.

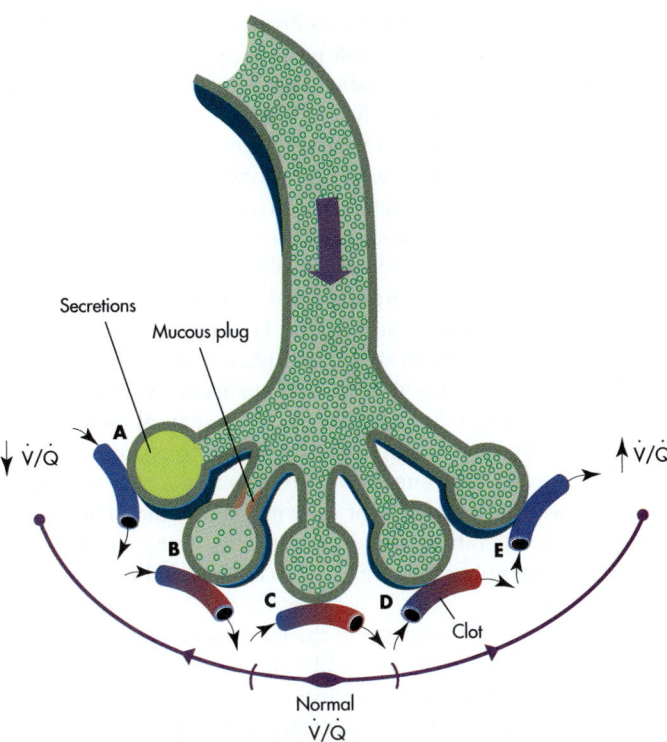

Fig. 62-4 Range of ventilation to perfusion ($\dot{V}/\dot{Q}$) relation-ships. *A* =absolute shunt, no ventilation because of fluid filling the alveoli; *B* = $\dot{V}/\dot{Q}$ mismatch, ventilation partially compro-mised by mucus in the airway; *C* = normal lung unit; *D* = $\dot{V}/\dot{Q}$ mismatch, perfusion partially compromised by emboli ob-structing blood flow; *E* = dead space, no perfusion because of obstruction of the pulmonary capillary.

Tissue Oxygen Needs. It is important to remember that even though the definition of respiratory failure is deter-mined by the PaO_2 and $PaCO_2$, the major threat of respiratory failure is inability to meet tissue O_2 needs. This inability may occur as a result of inadequate tissue O_2 delivery or because the tissues are unable to use the O_2 delivered to them. Tissue O_2 de-livery is determined by the amount of O_2 carried in the hemo-globin, as well as cardiac output. Therefore respiratory failure places the patient at greater risk if there is coexisting cardiac problems or anemia. Failure of O_2 utilization most commonly occurs as a result of septic shock. In this situation, adequate O_2 may be delivered to the tissues, but an abnormally high amount of O_2 returns in the venous blood indicating that it is not being extracted at the tissue level. (Shock is discussed in Chapter 61.)

Clinical Manifestations

Respiratory failure may develop suddenly (minutes or hours) or gradually (several days or longer). A sudden decrease in PaO_2 or a rapid rise in $PaCO_2$ implies a serious condition, which can rapidly become a life-threatening emergency. An ex-ample is the patient with asthma who develops severe bron-chospasm and a marked decrease in airflow, resulting in a res-piratory arrest. A more gradual change in PaO_2 and $PaCO_2$ is better tolerated because compensation can occur. An example is the patient with COPD who develops a progressive increase in $PaCO_2$ over several days following the onset of a respiratory infection. Because the change occurred over several days, there is time for renal compensation (e.g., retention of bicarbonate),

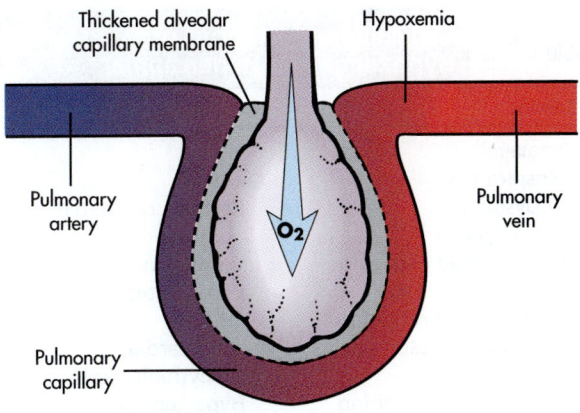

Fig. 62-5 Diffusion limitation. Exchange of CO_2 and O_2 cannot occur because of the thickened alveolar-capillary membrane.

which will minimize the change in pH. The patient has com-pensated respiratory acidosis.[4] (See Chapter 15 for a discussion of renal compensation for acid-base disorders.)

Manifestations of respiratory failure are related to the extent of change in PaO_2 or $PaCO_2$, the rapidity of change (acute ver-sus chronic), and the ability to compensate to overcome this change. When the patient's compensatory mechanisms fail, res-piratory failure occurs. Because clinical manifestations are vari-able, it is important to monitor arterial blood gas (ABG) values or use pulse oximetry to evaluate the extent of change. How-ever, these cannot substitute for clinical assessment.

The nurse may detect manifestations of respiratory failure that are specific (arise from the respiratory system) or nonspe-cific (arise from other body systems) (Table 62-3). An under-standing of the significance of these manifestations is critical to the ability to detect the onset of respiratory failure and effec-tiveness of treatment.

Restlessness, confusion, and combative behavior suggest in-adequate delivery of O_2 to the brain. Such changes are seen early because the brain is highly sensitive to a decrease in O_2 de-livery. Tachycardia and mild hypertension are also early signs. Such changes indicate an attempt by the heart to compensate for decreased O_2 delivery. A severe morning headache suggests that hypercapnia may have occurred during the night. At night the respiratory rate is slower and less $PaCO_2$ may be removed by the lungs. Rapid, shallow breaths suggest that the tidal vol-ume may be inadequate to remove CO_2 from the lungs. Cyanosis is an unreliable indicator of hypoxemia and is a late sign of respiratory failure because it does not occur until hy-poxemia is severe (PaO_2 45 mm Hg or less).

Hypoxemia versus Hypoxia. Hypoxemia occurs when the amount of O_2 in arterial blood is less than the normal value (see Chapter 24 for normal values). Hypoxia occurs when the PaO_2 has fallen sufficiently to cause signs and symp-toms of inadequate oxygenation (see Table 62-3). Hypoxemia can lead to hypoxia if not corrected. If hypoxia or hypoxemia is severe, the cells must shift from aerobic to anaerobic me-tabolism. Anaerobic metabolism uses more fuel and produces less energy and is less efficient than aerobic metabolism. The waste product of anaerobic metabolism, lactic acid, is more difficult to remove from the body than CO_2 because lactic acid has to be buffered with sodium bicarbonate. When the body does not have adequate amounts of sodium bicarbonate

Table 62-3	Clinical Manifestations of Hypoxemia and Hypercapnia*	
Specific	**Nonspecific**	

Hypoxemia

Respiratory	**Cerebral**
Dyspnea	Restless, combative
Tachypnea	behavior
Prolonged expiration	Confusion
(I:E = 1:3, 1:4)	Coma (late)
Intercostal retraction	**Cardiac**
Accessory respiratory	Tachycardia
use	Arrhythmias (late)
Paradoxic breathing	Hypertension
(late)	Hypotension (late)
Cyanosis (late)	**Other**
↓ SpO_2 (<80%)	Fatigue
	Unable to speak with-
	out pausing to breathe

Hypercapnia

Respiratory	**Cerebral**
Dyspnea	Morning headache
↓ Respiratory rate or	Disorientation
rapid rate with	Progressive somnolence
shallow respirations	Coma (late)
↓ Tidal volume	**Cardiac**
↓ Minute ventilation	Arrhythmias
	Neuromuscular
	Muscle weakness
	Tremor, seizures (late)
	Other
	Pursed-lip breathing
	Use of tripod position

*List is not all inclusive.

to buffer the lactic acid produced by anaerobic metabolism, metabolic acidosis and cell death occur.

Hypoxia and metabolic acidosis have adverse effects on the vital organs, especially the heart and CNS. The heart tries to compensate for the decreased O_2 level in the blood by increasing the heart rate and cardiac output. As the PaO_2 decreases and acidosis increases, the heart muscle may be unable to function and arrhythmias may occur, resulting in a further decrease in PaO_2. Permanent brain damage may occur because of O_2 deprivation. Renal function may also be impaired, and sodium retention, edema formation, acute tubular necrosis, and uremia may occur. Gastrointestinal system alterations include tissue ischemia, increased permeability of the intestinal wall, and possible translocation of bacteria into the circulation.

Specific Clinical Manifestations The patient may have a rapid, shallow breathing pattern or a respiratory rate that is slower than normal. Both changes predispose to insufficient CO_2 removal. The patient may increase the respiratory rate in an effort to blow off accumulated CO_2. This breathing pattern requires a substantial amount of work and predisposes to respiratory muscle fatigue. A change from a rapid rate to a slower rate in a patient in acute respiratory distress suggests tiring and the possibility of respiratory arrest.

The position that the patient assumes is an indication of the effort associated with breathing. The patient may be able to lie down (mild distress), be able to lie down but prefer to sit (mod-

erate distress), or be unable to breathe unless sitting upright (severe distress). A common position is to sit with the arms propped on the overbed table. This position, called the tripod position, helps decrease the work of breathing because propping the arms increases the anterior-posterior diameter of the chest and changes pressure in the thorax. Pursed-lip breathing may be used. This strategy causes an increase in SaO_2 because it slows respirations, allows more time for expiration, and prevents the small bronchioles from collapsing, thus facilitating air exchange. (Pursed-lip breathing is discussed in Chapter 27.)

The person who is working hard to breathe may be able to speak only a few words at a time between breaths. The ability of the patient to speak without pausing to breathe is an indication of the severity of dyspnea. The patient may speak in sentences (mild or no distress), phrases (moderate distress), or words (severe distress). The number of words is also a clue (e.g., how many words can the patient say without pausing to breathe?). The patient may have "three-word" or "two-word" dyspnea, signifying that only two or three words can be said before pausing to breathe.

There may be a change in the inspiratory (I) to expiratory (E) (I:E) ratio. Normally, the I:E ratio is 1:2, which means that expiration is twice as long as inspiration. In patients in respiratory distress, the ratio may increase to 1:3 or 1:4. This change signifies airflow obstruction and that more time is required to empty the lungs.

The nurse may observe retraction (inward movement) of the intercostal spaces or the supraclavicular area and use of the accessory muscles during inspiration or expiration. Use of the accessory muscles signifies moderate distress. Paradoxic breathing indicates severe distress. Normally, the thorax and abdomen move outward on inspiration and inward on exhalation. During paradoxic breathing, the abdomen and chest move in the opposite manner—outward during exhalation and inward during inspiration. Paradoxic breathing results from maximal use of the accessory muscles of respiration. The patient may be diaphoretic from the work associated with breathing.

The nurse's assessment may result in early detection of manifestations associated with respiratory insufficiency, allowing therapy to be instituted before the patient experiences respiratory failure. Patients with end-stage (severe) chronic lung disease may have low PaO_2 values or elevated $PaCO_2$ levels as their "normal" baseline. It is especially important to monitor specific and nonspecific signs of respiratory failure in patients with COPD because a small change can cause significant decompensation (see Table 62-3). Any deterioration in mental status, such as combative behavior, confusion, or decreased level of consciousness, should be reported immediately since this change may indicate the onset of rapid deterioration in clinical status and the need for mechanical ventilation.

Diagnostic Studies

The most common diagnostic study used to determine respiratory failure is ABGs.[5] ABG analysis is used to determine the levels of $PaCO_2$, PaO_2, and blood pH. An indwelling catheter may be inserted into an artery for monitoring pressures. This arterial line can be used to obtain frequent arterial blood gases. Pulse oximetry is frequently used for monitoring of oxygenation status, but in respiratory failure, ABGs are necessary to obtain both oxygenation (PaO_2) and ventilation ($PaCO_2$) status.

NURSING ASSESSMENT

Table 62-4 Acute Respiratory Failure

Subjective Data

Important Health Information

Past health history: Chronic lung disease; previous hospitalizations related to lung disease; thoracic or spinal cord trauma; extreme obesity, altered consciousness

Medications: Use of oxygen, inhalers, home nebulization, over-the-counter medications; immunosuppressant therapy, CNS depressants

Surgery or other treatments: Previous intubation and mechanical ventilation; recent thoracic or abdominal surgery

Functional Health Patterns

Health perception–health management: Smoking (pack-years)

Nutritional-metabolic: Anorexia, bloatedness, heartburn; weight gain or loss; decreased appetite; diaphoresis

Activity-exercise: Fatigue, dizziness; dyspnea at rest or with activity, wheezing, cough (productive or nonproductive); sputum (volume, color, viscosity); palpitations, swollen feet

Sleep-rest: Changes in sleep pattern

Cognitive-perceptual: Headache, chest pain or tightness

Coping–stress tolerance: Anxiety, depression

Objective Data

General

Restlessness, agitation

Integumentary

Pale, cool, clammy skin or warm flushed skin; peripheral and central cyanosis; peripheral dependent edema

Respiratory

Shallow, increased respirations progressing to decreased rate; use of accessory muscles with evidence of retractions, altered I/E ratio; increased diaphragmatic excursion or asymmetric chest expansion; asynchronous respirations; tactile fremitus, crepitus, or deviated trachea on palpation; resonant, hyperresonant, or dull percussion note; absent, diminished, or adventitious breath sounds; bronchial or bronchovesicular sounds heard in other than normal location, inspiratory stridor, pleural friction rub

Cardiovascular

Tachycardia progressing to bradycardia, arrhythmias, extra heart sounds (S_3, S_4); bounding pulse; hypertension progressing to hypotension; pulsus paradoxus; jugular vein distention; pedal edema

Gastrointestinal

Abdominal distention with tympany; ascites, epigastric tenderness, hepatojugular reflex

Neurologic

Somnolence, confusion, slurred speech, tremors, seizures, coma; asterixis, decreased deep tendon reflexes; papilledema

Possible Findings

↑↓ pH, ↑↓ $PaCO_2$, ↓ PaO_2, ↓ SaO_2, ↓ PEFR, ↓ tidal volume, ↓ forced vital capacity, ↓ minute ventilation, ↓ negative inspiratory force; altered values of serum electrolytes, hemoglobin, and hematocrit; abnormal findings on chest x-ray; abnormal pulmonary artery and pulmonary artery wedge pressures

---

Other diagnostic studies that may be done include a chest x-ray, complete blood cell count, serum electrolytes, urinalysis, and electrocardiogram (ECG). Cultures of the sputum and blood are obtained as necessary to determine sources of possible infection. If pulmonary embolus is suspected, a ventilation/perfusion ($\dot{V}/\dot{Q}$) lung scan or pulmonary angiography may be done. Although not commonly done in acute situations, pulmonary function tests may be performed.

In severe respiratory failure, measurement of cardiac output and mixed venous blood gases by a pulmonary artery catheter (see Chapter 63) is important in determining the amount of blood flow to tissues and the response to treatment. Pulmonary artery, pulmonary artery wedge, and left atrial pressures are monitored to determine whether the accumulation of fluid in the lungs is the result of cardiac or pulmonary problems. These parameters also are monitored to determine the response of the lung and heart to hypoxemia and the patient's response to therapy. (Hemodynamic monitoring is discussed in detail in Chapter 63.)

NURSING AND COLLABORATIVE MANAGEMENT: ACUTE RESPIRATORY FAILURE

Because many different problems cause respiratory failure, specific care of these patients varies. This section will discuss general assessment and collaborative care measures that apply to patients with acute respiratory failure. In acute care settings there is often an overlap of function between nursing and other members of the health care team.

■ Nursing Assessment

Subjective and objective data that should be obtained from the patient with acute respiratory failure are presented in Table 62-4.

■ Nursing Diagnoses

Nursing diagnoses for the patient with acute respiratory failure include, but are not limited to, those presented in NCP 62-1.

■ Planning

The overall goals are that the patient in acute respiratory failure will have (1) ABG values within the patient's baseline, (2) baseline breath sounds, (3) no dyspnea or dyspnea at patient's baseline, and (4) effective cough and ability to clear secretions.

■ Respiratory Therapy

The major goals of respiratory care for acute respiratory failure include maintaining adequate oxygenation and ventilation. This goal is accomplished through cooperative efforts of the medical, nursing, and respiratory care team. The therapy used includes O_2 therapy, mobilization of secretions, and positive pressure ventilation (Table 62-5).

62-1 **NURSING CARE PLAN** **PATIENT WITH ACUTE RESPIRATORY FAILURE***

Expected Patient Outcomes   Nursing Interventions and *Rationales*

NURSING DIAGNOSIS **Ineffective airway clearance** *related to* excessive secretions, decreased level of consciousness, presence of an artificial airway, neuromuscular dysfunction, and pain *as manifested by* difficulty in expectorating sputum, presence of rhonchi or crackles, ineffective or absent cough.

- No abnormal breath sounds (e.g., rhonchi, crackles).
- Normal baseline breath sounds.
- Presence of effective cough.
- Easy expectoration of sputum.

- Assess patient's ability to cough *to determine need for assistance in secretion removal.*
- Implement assistive coughing strategies *to promote secretion removal.*
- Position patient with head of bed elevated at least 45 degrees or in the tripod position *to promote maximal chest expansion and cough effects.*
- Humidify O_2 if over 3 L/min *to prevent drying of the mucosa.*
- Perform tracheobronchial suctioning if cough is ineffective or if artificial airway is present *to remove secretions and improve oxygenation.*
- Perform chest physiotherapy *to enhance removal of secretions.*
- Splint any abdominal or chest incision with pillow *to reduce pain and allow for improved inspiratory efforts.*
- Turn every 2 hours *to prevent stasis of secretions and promote optimal ventilation.*
- Ensure adequate fluid intake of 2-3 L/day *to liquefy secretions.*
- Administer prescribed routine and as needed bronchodilator and mucolytic medications *to promote better airflow and secretion removal.*

NURSING DIAGNOSIS **Ineffective breathing pattern** *related to* neuromuscular impairment of respirations, pain, anxiety, decreased level of consciousness, respiratory muscle fatigue, and bronchospasm *as manifested by* respiratory rate <12 or >24 breaths/min, alterated I/E ratio, irregular breathing pattern, use of accessory muscles, asynchronous thoracoabdominal movement, wheezing, apnea.

- Respiratory rate, depth, and rhythm within normal limits for patient.
- Synchronous thoracoabdominal movement.
- Use of accessory muscles appropriate for level of activity.

- Monitor for increased or decreased respiratory rate, periods of apnea, decreased inspiratory depth, and alternating rocking movement between chest and abdomen *to assess for presence of inability to sustain ventilation.*
- Position patient with head of bed elevated at least 45 degrees or in a tripod position *to promote diaphragmatic excursion.*
- Place oral or nasal airway and Ambu bag at the bedside *because airway support may be needed in the event of severely impaired ventilation or apnea.*
- Provide comfort measures (e.g., analgesics, positioning) *to reduce anxiety and promote patient cooperation.*
- Anticipate the need for possible application of NIPPV or intubation with mechanical ventilation *to maintain adequate oxygenation and ventilation.*

NURSING DIAGNOSIS **Risk for fluid volume excess** *related to* increases in peripheral or pulmonary fluid.

- Normal breath sounds.
- Decreased or absent peripheral edema.
- Normal pulmonary artery or pulmonary artery wedge pressures.

- Assess for manifestations of fluid volume excess such as abnormal breath sounds (crackles), weight gain, jugular venous distention, peripheral or sacral edema *to identify if problem is present.*
- Monitor fluid status by I & O measurements, daily weights, and pulmonary artery or pulmonary artery wedge pressures *to monitor for changes in systemic fluid volume.*
- Restrict fluid intake and administer diuretics as ordered *to prevent or reduce fluid overload.*

NURSING DIAGNOSIS **Anxiety** *related to* dyspnea, intubation, severity of illness, loss of personal control and uncertain outcome *as manifested by* increased heart rate, respiratory rate, and blood pressure; agitation, restlessness; verbalization of anxiety.

- Decreased anxiety.
- Relaxed demeanor.
- Increased sense of personal control.
- Verbalization of hopeful attitude toward outcome.

- Perform interventions in a calm, assured manner *to decrease patient's anxiety.*
- Reassure patient of competence of caregivers *to encourage patient relaxation.*
- Answer questions simply and honestly *to provide patient with needed information for decision making.*
- Teach and demonstrate to patient relaxation techniques of slow pursed-lip breathing, progressive relaxation, and guided imagery *to promote restoration of control over breathing.*
- Administer and evaluate effectiveness of any prescribed antianxiety medication.

Continued

62-1 NURSING CARE PLAN PATIENT WITH ACUTE RESPIRATORY FAILURE*
—continued

Expected Patient Outcomes   Nursing Interventions and *Rationales*

NURSING DIAGNOSIS **Impaired gas exchange** *related to* alveolar hypoventilation, intrapulmonary shunting, $\dot{V}/\dot{Q}$ mismatch, and diffusion impairment *as manifested by* hypoxemia or hypercapnia.

- PaO_2 and $PaCO_2$ within normal ranges for patient.
- Normal breath sounds.

- Monitor for clinical manifestations of hypoxemia and hypercapnia *to detect systemic manifestations of decreased oxygen and increased carbon dioxide.*
- Administer oxygen as ordered *to increase PaO_2 and SaO_2 levels.*
- Monitor ABGs for PaO_2 below 60 mm Hg, SaO_2 below 90%, and $PaCO_2$ above 50 mm Hg *to assess pulmonary gas exchange.*
- Place the patient on continuous pulse oximetry *to assess for increases or decreases in blood oxygen levels.*
- Monitor the apical heart rate for irregular rhythm, tachycardia, bradycardia, and cardiac arrhythmias on the cardiac monitor *because hypoxemia may precipitate cardiac arrhythmias.*
- Teach and encourage pursed-lip breathing *to improve gas exchange.*
- Anticipate the need for ventilatory support *to improve oxygenation and ventilation status.*
- Withhold sedative drugs unless discussed with physician *because they can depress respirations.*
- Administer narcotic antagonists (e.g., naloxone [Narcan]) as ordered *to reverse respiratory depression resulting from narcotic administration.*

NURSING DIAGNOSIS **Altered nutrition: less than body requirements** *related to* poor appetite, shortness of breath, presence of artificial airway, decreased energy level, and increased caloric requirements *as manifested by* weight loss, weakness, muscle wasting, dehydration, poor muscle tone, poor skin integrity.

- Maintenance of weight or weight gain.
- Serum albumin and protein within normal ranges.

- Provide high-protein, high-calorie, enteral or parenteral nutrition as ordered *to meet increased nutritional requirements.*
- If able to take nutrition orally, provide six small meals per day *to decrease oxygen energy expenditure during digestion.*
- Provide between-meal nutritional supplements *to maintain adequate caloric intake.*
- Maintain the ordered oxygen delivery device during meals *to prevent shortness of breath and blood oxygen desaturation while eating.*
- Monitor for signs of CO_2 increase with parenteral nutrition *because carbohydrates may increase CO_2 levels in patients with hypercapnia.*

*The nursing care for the patient on mechanical ventilation is presented in NCP 63-2 and discussed in Chapter 63.
NIPPV, noninvasive positive pressure ventilation.

Oxygen Therapy. The primary goal of O_2 therapy is to correct hypoxemia. If hypoxemia is secondary to $\dot{V}/\dot{Q}$ mismatch, supplemental O_2 administered at 1 to 3 L/min by nasal cannula or 24% to 32% by simple face mask should improve the PaO_2 and SaO_2. Hypoxemia secondary to an intrapulmonary shunt is usually not responsive to high O_2 concentrations and the patient will usually require positive pressure ventilation (PPV). PPV offers a means of providing O_2 therapy, decreasing the work of breathing, and reducing respiratory muscle fatigue. In addition, the positive pressure may assist in opening collapsed airways and decreasing shunt. (Mechanical ventilation is discussed in Chapter 63.)

The type of O_2 delivery system chosen for the patient in acute respiratory failure should (1) be tolerated by the patient, since anxiety caused by feelings of claustrophobia related to the face mask or dyspnea may prompt the patient to remove the O_2 device; and (2) maintain a PaO_2 at 55 to 60 mm Hg or more and SaO_2 at 90% or more at the lowest O_2 concentration possible. High O_2 concentrations eliminate the nitrogen normally present in the alveoli, causing instability and atelectasis. O_2 toxicity, a condition that results in fibrotic changes in the alveoli, may also occur. In intubated patients, exposure to 60% or greater O_2 for longer than 48 hours poses a significant risk for O_2 toxicity. In nonintubated patients, the risk is less clear. (O_2 delivery devices are discussed in Chapter 27.)

Additional risks of O_2 therapy are specific to the patient with chronic hypercapnia such as the patient with COPD. Chronic hypercapnia may blunt the response of chemoreceptors in the medulla, a condition termed *CO_2 narcosis.* In this situation, respirations are stimulated by hypoxia. If the PaO_2 is

COLLABORATIVE CARE

Table 62-5   Acute Respiratory Failure

Diagnostic
History and physical examination
Arterial blood gases
Pulse oximetry
Chest x-ray
CBC
Serum electrolytes and urinalysis
ECG
Blood and sputum cultures (if indicated)
PAP, PAWP, LAP

Collaborative Therapy
Respiratory Therapy
O_2 therapy
Mobilization of secretions
   Effective coughing
   Hydration/humidification
   Chest physical therapy
   Airway suctioning
Positive pressure ventilation
   Noninvasive positive pressure ventilation
   Intubation with mechanical ventilation

Drug Therapy
Relief of bronchospasm (e.g., metaproterenol
   [Alupent])
Reduction of airway inflammation (corticosteroids)
Reduction of pulmonary congestion (e.g., furosemide
   [Lasix])
Treatment of pulmonary infections
Reduction of severe anxiety and restlessness (e.g., lor-
   azepam [Ativan])

Medical Supportive Therapy
Management of the underlying cause of respiratory
   failure
Maintenance of adequate cardiac output
Maintenance of adequate hemoglobin concentration

Nutritional Therapy
Parenteral nutrition support
Enteral nutrition support

CBC, complete blood count; *LAP,* left atrial pressure; *PAP,* pulmonary artery pressure; *PAWP,* pulmonary artery wedge pressure.

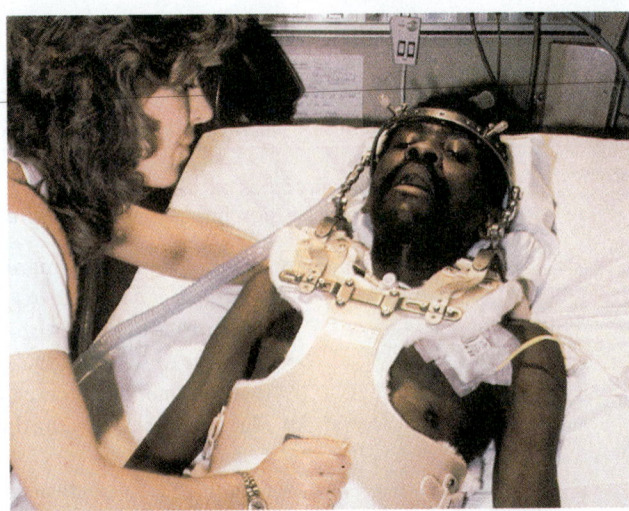

Fig. 62-6   Augmented cough. Augmented coughing is performed by placing the hand on the abdominal musculature below the xiphoid process. As the patient ends a deep inspiration and begins the expiration, the hand should be moved forcefully downward, increasing abdominal pressure, resulting in a forceful cough.

Effective coughing and positioning. If secretions are obstructing the airway, the patient should be encouraged to cough. The patient with a neuromuscular weakness, from the disease or exhaustion, may not be able to generate sufficient airway pressures to produce an effective cough. Augmented coughing (quad coughing) may be of benefit to these patients. Augmented coughing is performed by placing the palm of the hand or hands on the abdomen below the xiphoid process (Fig. 62-6). As the patient ends a deep inspiration and begins the expiration, the hands should be moved forcefully downward, increasing abdominal pressure and facilitating the cough. This measure helps increase expiratory flow and thereby facilitate secretion clearance.

Some patients may benefit from therapeutic cough techniques. Huff coughing is a series of coughs performed while saying the word "huff." This technique prevents the glottis from closing during the cough. Patients with COPD generate higher flow rates with a huff cough than is possible with a normal cough. The huff cough is effective in clearing only the central airways, but it may assist in moving secretions upward. The staged cough also assists secretion mobilization. To perform the staged cough, the patient sits in a chair, breathes three or four times in and out through the mouth, and coughs while bending forward and pressing a pillow inward against the diaphragm.

Positioning the patient either by elevating the head of the bed to at least 45 degrees or by using a reclining chair or chair bed may help maximize thoracic expansion, thereby decreasing dyspnea and improving secretion mobilization. A sitting position improves pulmonary function and assists in venous pooling. Lateral or side-lying positioning may be used in patients with disease involving only one lung. This position, termed *down with the good lung,* allows for improved $\dot{V}/\dot{Q}$ matching in the affected lung. The patient should be side lying if there is any possibility that the tongue will obstruct the airway or that aspi-

suddenly increased, the patient will no longer be hypoxemic, will have no stimulus to breathe, and may experience a respiratory arrest. Patients with chronic hypercapnia should receive O_2 through a low-flow device such as a nasal cannula at 1 to 2 L/min or a Venturi mask at 24% to 28%. They should be closely monitored for changes in mental status and respiratory rate, and ABG results, until their PaO_2 level has reached their normal value.

Mobilization of Secretions. Retained pulmonary secretions may cause or exacerbate acute respiratory failure by blocking movement of O_2 into the alveoli and pulmonary capillary blood. Secretions can be mobilized through effective coughing, adequate hydration and humidification, chest physical therapy, and suctioning.

ration may occur. An oral or nasal airway should be kept at the bedside for use if necessary.

Hydration and humidification. Thick and viscous secretions are difficult to raise and should be thinned. Adequate fluid intake (2 to 3 L per day) is necessary to keep secretions thin and easy to expel. If the patient is unable to take sufficient fluids orally, intravenous (IV) hydration will be used. An appropriate humidification device is an adjunct in secretion management. Aerosols of sterile normal saline, administered by a nebulizer, may be used to liquefy secretions. Aerosol therapy may induce bronchospasm and severe coughing causing a decreased PaO_2. Mucolytic agents such as nebulized acetylcysteine (Mucomyst) mixed with a bronchodilator may be used to thin secretions but as a side effect may also cause airway erythema and bronchospasm. Therefore it is used only in special situations.

Chest physical therapy. Chest physical therapy is indicated in patients who produce more than 30 ml of sputum per day. If tolerated, postural drainage, percussion, and vibration to the affected lung segments may assist in moving secretions to the larger airways where they may be removed by coughing or suctioning. Because positioning may affect oxygenation, patients may not tolerate head-down or lateral positioning because of extreme dyspnea or hypoxemia caused by $\dot{V}/\dot{Q}$ mismatch. (Chest physical therapy is discussed in Chapter 27.)

Airway suctioning. If the patient is unable to expectorate secretions, nasopharyngeal, oropharyngeal, or nasotracheal suctioning (blind suctioning without a tracheal tube in place) is indicated. Suctioning through an artificial airway, such as endotracheal or tracheostomy tubes, may also be performed (see Chapters 25 and 63). A mini-tracheostomy (or mini-trach) may be used to suction patients who have difficulty mobilizing secretions and when blind suctioning is difficult or ineffective. The mini-trach is a 4 mm indwelling plastic cuffless cannula inserted through the cricothyroid membrane. It is used to instill sterile normal saline solution to elicit a cough and to perform suctioning with a no. 10 French catheter. Contraindications for a mini-trach include an absent gag reflex, history of aspiration, and the need for long-term mechanical ventilation.[6]

Positive Pressure Ventilation. If intensive measures fail to improve ventilation and oxygenation and the patient continues to exhibit manifestations of acute respiratory failure, ventilatory assistance may be initiated. PPV may be provided invasively through endotracheal or nasotracheal intubation or noninvasively through a nasal or face mask. Patients who require PPV are typically cared for in a critical care unit. (See Chapter 63 for a discussion of artificial airways and mechanical ventilation.)

Noninvasive positive pressure ventilation (NIPPV) may be used as a treatment for patients with acute or chronic respiratory failure.[7,8] During NIPPV a mask is placed over the patient's nose or nose and mouth and the patient breathes spontaneously while PPV is delivered (Fig. 62-7). With NIPPV it is possible to decrease the work of breathing without the need for endotracheal intubation. Bilevel positive airway pressure (BiPAP® Ventilatory Support System) is a form of NIPPV in which different positive pressure levels are set for inspiration and expiration (see Fig. 62-7). Continuous positive airway pressure (CPAP) is another form of NIPPV in which a constant positive pressure is delivered to the airway during inspiration and expiration.

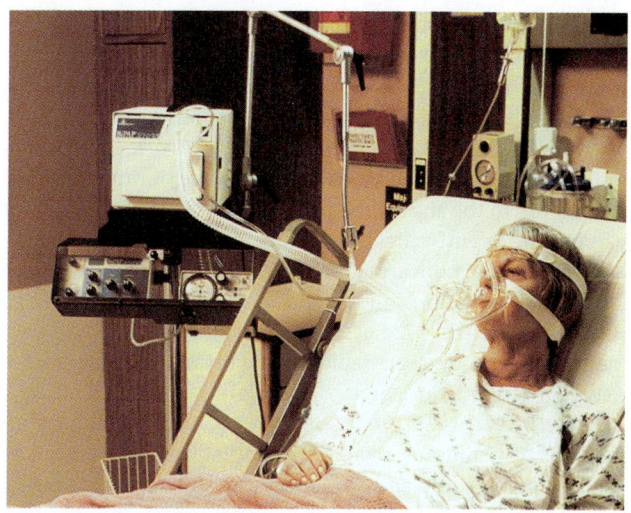

Fig. 62-7 Noninvasive bilevel positive pressure ventilation. A mask is placed over the nose or nose and mouth. Positive pressure from a mechanical ventilator assists the patient's breathing efforts, decreasing the work of breathing.

NIPPV is most useful in managing chronic respiratory failure in patients with chest wall and neuromuscular disease (see Table 62-1). NIPPV has been used in patients with hypoxemic respiratory failure (ARDS, cardiogenic pulmonary edema), but with less success. NIPPV may also be used for patients who refuse endotracheal intubation but still desire some palliative ventilatory support (e.g., patients with end-stage COPD).[9] NIPPV is not appropriate for the patient who has absent respirations, excessive secretions, a decreased level of consciousness, high O_2 requirements, facial trauma, or hemodynamic instability.

■ Drug Therapy

Goals of drug therapy for patients in acute respiratory failure include relief of bronchospasm, reduction of airway inflammation and pulmonary congestion, treatment of pulmonary infection, and reduction of severe anxiety and restlessness.

Relief of Bronchospasm. Alveolar ventilation will be increased with relief of bronchospasm. Short-acting bronchodilators, such as metaproterenol (Alupent) and albuterol (Ventolin), are frequently administered to reverse bronchospasm using either a handheld nebulizer or a metered-dose inhaler with a spacer.[10] In acute bronchospasm these drugs may be given at 30- to 60-minute intervals until it can be determined that a response is occurring. If severe bronchospasm continues, IV aminophylline may be administered. The bronchodilator effects of these medications can sometimes cause a worsening of arterial hypoxemia by redistributing the inspired gas to areas of decreased perfusion. Administering the bronchodilator with an O_2-enriched gas mixture usually alleviates this effect. (See Chapter 27 for nursing management related to bronchodilators.)

Reduction of Airway Inflammation. Corticosteroids may be used in conjunction with bronchodilating agents when bronchospasm and inflammation are present. Inhaled corticosteroids are not used for acute respiratory failure, because they require 4 to 5 days before optimum therapeutic effects are seen. However, IV corticosteroids (e.g., methylprednisolone) have an immediate onset of action.

Reduction of Pulmonary Congestion.
Pulmonary interstitial fluid can occur as a consequence of direct or indirect injury to the alveolar capillary membrane (e.g., ARDS) or from right or left ventricular failure, and therefore can be either cardiac or noncardiac in origin. The result is decreased alveolar ventilation and hypoxemia. IV diuretics (e.g., furosemide [Lasix]) are used to decrease the pulmonary congestion caused by heart failure. Digitalis may also be used if left ventricular failure or atrial fibrillation is present.

Treatment of Pulmonary Infections.
Pulmonary infections (pneumonia, acute bronchitis) result in excessive mucus production and inflamed, fluid-filled, or collapsed alveoli. Alveoli that are fluid filled or collapsed cannot participate in gas exchange. Pulmonary infections can either cause or exacerbate acute respiratory failure. IV antibiotics are frequently administered to inhibit bacterial growth. Chest x-rays are performed to determine the location and extent of a suspected infectious process. Sputum cultures are used to determine the type of organisms causing the infection and their sensitivity to antimicrobial medications.

Reduction of Severe Anxiety and Restlessness.
Anxiety, restlessness, and agitation result from cerebral hypoxia. In addition, fear caused by the inability to breathe and a sense of loss of control may exacerbate anxiety. Agitation and anxiety increase O_2 consumption, which may worsen the degree of hypoxemia. Several nursing strategies can assist the patient in reducing the level of anxiety (see NCP 62-1).

Low-dose sedation (e.g., lorazepam [Ativan]) may be used to decrease anxiety because continued agitation will increase the patient's work of breathing and therefore O_2 consumption. Patients receiving any sedative medication must be monitored for respiratory depression. In the critical care setting sedation and neuromuscular paralysis are commonly used for severely restless and agitated patients in acute respiratory failure who breathe asynchronously with mechanical ventilation. These medications inhibit patient breathing efforts and patient awareness of surroundings, thereby allowing the ventilator to provide optimum ventilation.

■ Medical Supportive Therapy
Therapeutic goals and interventions to maximize O_2 delivery and treat the underlying cause of the respiratory failure are essential to improving the patient's oxygenation and ventilation status. The primary goal is to treat the underlying cause of the respiratory failure.[11] Other goals include maintaining an adequate cardiac output and hemoglobin concentration.

Treating the Underlying Cause.
Interventions are directed toward reversing the disease process that resulted in the development of acute respiratory failure. Patients with hypoventilation can be diagnosed and treated rapidly. Patients with $\dot{V}/\dot{Q}$ mismatch, shunting, or diffusion limitation are managed differently depending on the underlying cause. In all patient situations, monitoring treatment effects and ABG results is a continuous process.

Maintaining Adequate Cardiac Output.
Cardiac output reflects the blood flow reaching the tissues. Blood pressure is an important indicator of the adequacy of cardiac output. Usually a systolic blood pressure of at least 90 mm Hg is adequate to maintain perfusion to the vital organs. (See Chapter 30 for a discussion of cardiac output.) If the systolic blood pressure is at least 90 mm Hg, changes in mental status may be attributed to the level of O_2 and CO_2 rather than decreased cerebral perfusion. Decreased cardiac output is treated by administration of IV fluids, medications, or both. (See Chapter 61 for a discussion of drugs used in decreased cardiac output and shock.)

Maintaining Adequate Hemoglobin Concentration.
Hemoglobin is the primary carrier when delivering O_2 to the tissues. If the patient is anemic, tissue O_2 delivery will be compromised. A hemoglobin concentration of 9 to 10 g/dl (90 to 100 g/L) or greater typically ensures adequate O_2 saturation of the hemoglobin. The patient should be monitored for sites of blood loss and transfused with packed red blood cells if an adequate hemoglobin concentration cannot be maintained.

■ Nutritional Therapy
Maintenance of protein and energy stores is especially important in patients who experience acute respiratory failure because nutritional depletion causes a loss of muscle mass, including the respiratory muscles, and may prolong recovery. During the acute manifestations of respiratory failure, the risk of aspiration typically prevents oral nutritional intake. Enteral or parenteral nutrition may therefore be administered. When the acute manifestations subside, the patient may resume oral intake as tolerated.

■ Evaluation
The expected outcomes for the patient with acute respiratory failure are presented in NCP 62-1.

GERONTOLOGIC CONSIDERATIONS

Respiratory Failure
Older adults are at higher risk of developing respiratory failure because of the reduction in ventilatory capacity that accompanies aging, especially if other risk factors are present. In older adults, the PaO_2 falls further and the $PaCO_2$ rises to a higher level before the respiratory system is stimulated to alter the rate and depth of breathing. This delayed response predisposes to the development of respiratory failure.

ACUTE RESPIRATORY DISTRESS SYNDROME

ARDS is a sudden and progressive form of acute respiratory failure in which the alveolar capillary membrane becomes damaged and more permeable to intravascular fluid (Fig. 62-8). The alveoli fill with fluid, resulting in severe dyspnea, hypoxemia refractory to supplemental O_2, reduced lung compliance, and diffuse pulmonary infiltrates.

The incidence of ARDS in the United States is estimated at more than 150,000 cases annually. Despite supportive therapy, the mortality rate from ARDS is approximately 50%. Patients who have both gram-negative septic shock and ARDS have a mortality rate of 70% to 90%.[12]

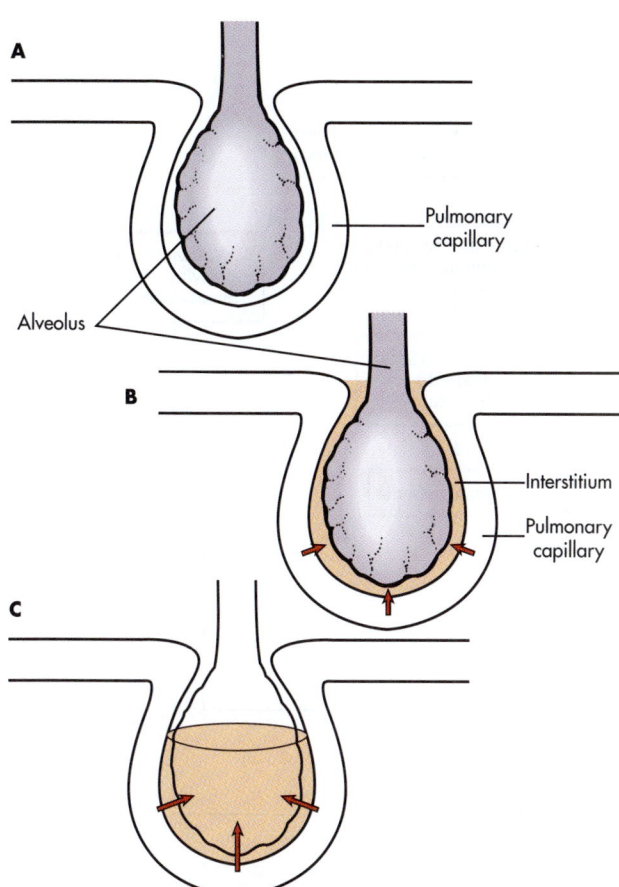

Fig. 62-8 Stages of edema formation in acute respiratory distress syndrome. **A,** Normal alveolus and pulmonary capillary. **B,** Interstitial edema occurs with increased flow of fluid into the interstitial space. **C,** Alveolar edema occurs when the fluid crosses the blood-gas barrier.

Etiology and Pathophysiology

Table 62-6 lists conditions that predispose patients to the development of ARDS. The two risk factors most commonly associated with ARDS are gram-negative septic shock and aspiration of gastric contents. Patients with multiple risk factors are 3 to 4 times more likely to develop ARDS.[13]

Direct lung injury may cause ARDS (Fig. 62-9), or ARDS may develop as a consequence of the systemic inflammatory response syndrome (SIRS) (see Fig. 61-1). SIRS may have an infectious or a noninfectious etiology and is characterized by widespread inflammation or clinical responses to inflammation following a variety of physiologic insults, including severe trauma, gut ischemia, injury to the lung, and sepsis.[14] ARDS may also develop as a consequence of multiple organ dysfunction syndrome (MODS). MODS results from organ system dysfunction that progressively increases in severity and ultimately results in multisystem organ failure. (SIRS and MODS are discussed in Chapter 61.)

An exact cause for the damage to the alveolar-capillary membrane is not known. However, the pathophysiologic changes of ARDS are thought to be due to stimulation of the inflammatory and immune systems, which causes an attraction of neutrophils to the pulmonary interstitium.[15] The neutrophils cause a release

Table **62-6**	Conditions Predisposing to Acute Respiratory Distress Syndrome

Direct Lung Injury
- Aspiration of gastric contents or other substances
- Near-drowning
- Inhalation of toxic substances
- Viral/bacterial pneumonia
- Chest trauma
- Embolism: fat, air, amniotic fluid
- Oxygen toxicity
- Radiation pneumonitis

Indirect Lung Injury
- Sepsis (especially gram-negative infection)
- Severe pancreatitis
- Multiple blood transfusions
- Multiple trauma/fractures
- Severe head injury
- Disseminated intravascular coagulation
- Shock states
- Nonpulmonary systemic diseases
- Cardiopulmonary bypass
- Anaphylaxis
- Narcotic drug abuse

of biochemical, humoral, and cellular mediators (Table 62-7) that produce changes in the lung, including increased pulmonary capillary membrane permeability, destruction of elastin and collagen, formation of pulmonary microemboli, and pulmonary artery vasoconstriction (see Fig. 62-9). (These mediators are discussed in Chapters 11 and 12.)

The pathophysiologic changes in ARDS are divided into three phases: (1) injury or exudative phase, (2) reparative or proliferative phase, and (3) fibrotic phase.

Injury or Exudative Phase. The injury or exudative phase occurs approximately 1 to 7 days (usually 24 to 48 hours) after the initial direct lung injury or host insult. Neutrophils adhere to the pulmonary microcirculation, causing damage to the vascular endothelium and increased capillary permeability. In the earliest phase of injury, there is engorgement of the peribronchial and perivascular interstitial space, which produces interstitial edema. Next, fluid from the interstitial space crosses the alveolar epithelium and enters the alveolar space. Intrapulmonary shunt develops because the alveoli fill with fluid and blood passing through them cannot be oxygenated (see Figs. 62-4 and 62-8).

Alveolar type I and type II cells (which produce surfactant) are damaged by the changes caused by ARDS. This damage, in addition to further fluid and protein accumulation, results in surfactant dysfunction. The function of surfactant is to maintain alveolar stability by decreasing alveolar surface tension and preventing alveolar collapse. Decreased synthesis and inactivation of surfactant causes the alveoli to become unstable and collapse (atelectasis). Widespread atelectasis further decreases lung compliance, compromises gas exchange, and contributes to hypoxemia.

Also during this stage, hyaline begins to line the alveolar membrane. These hyaline membranes are thought to result from the exudation of high-molecular-weight substances (particularly fibrinogen) in the edema fluid. Hyaline membranes

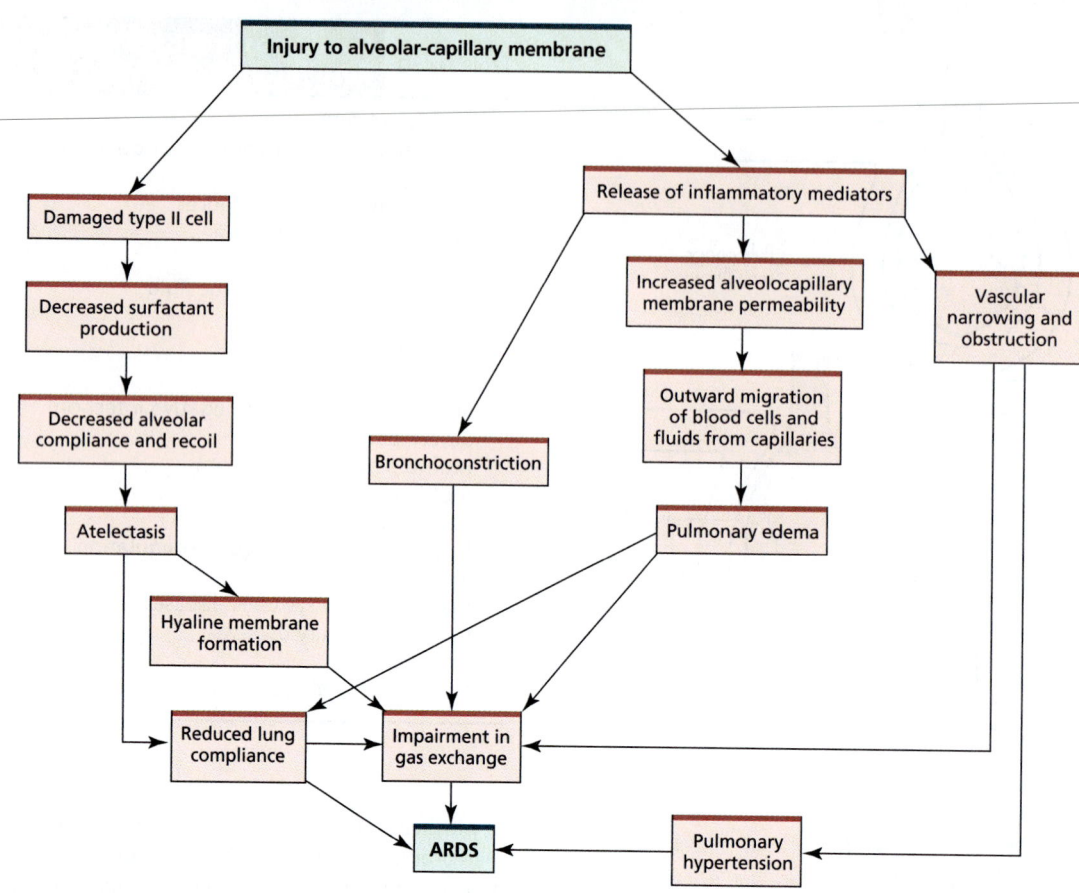

Fig. 62-9 Pathophysiology of ARDS.

Table **62-7**	Mediators of Acute Lung Injury

Complement component C5a
Neutrophil products, including proteases and O_2 radicals
Monocyte and macrophage products, including tumor necrosis factor, interleukin-1, and colony-stimulating factor
Arachidonic acid metabolites, including prostaglandins and leukotrienes
Coagulation products, including kallikreins, kinins, fibrin degradation products, and plasminogen-activating factor
Histamine
Serotonin
Endotoxin
Elastase
Collagenase

contribute to the development of fibrosis and atelectasis, leading to a decrease in gas exchange capability and lung compliance.

The primary pathophysiologic changes that characterize the injury or exudative phase of ARDS are interstitial and alveolar edema (noncardiogenic pulmonary edema) and atelectasis.[16] Severe $\dot{V}/\dot{Q}$ mismatch and shunting of pulmonary capillary blood result in hypoxemia unresponsive to increasing concentrations of O_2 (refractory hypoxemia). Diffusion limitation, caused by hyaline membrane formation, further contributes to the severity of the hypoxemia. As the lungs become less com-pliant because of decreased surfactant, pulmonary edema, and atelectasis, the patient must generate higher airway pressures to inflate "stiff" lungs. Reduced lung compliance greatly increases the patient's work of breathing.

Hypoxemia and the stimulation of juxtacapillary receptors in the stiff lung parenchyma (J reflex) initially cause an increase in respiratory rate and decrease in tidal volume. This breathing pattern increases CO_2 removal, producing respiratory alkalosis. Cardiac output increases in response to hypoxemia, a compensatory effect to increase pulmonary blood flow. However, as atelectasis, pulmonary edema, and pulmonary shunt increase, compensation fails, and hypoventilation, decreased cardiac output, and decreased tissue O_2 perfusion eventually occur.

Reparative or Proliferative Phase. The reparative or proliferative phase begins 1 to 2 weeks after the initial lung injury. During this phase, there is an influx of granulocytes, monocytes, and lymphocytes and fibroblast proliferation as part of the inflammatory response. The injured lung has an immense regenerative capacity after acute lung injury. The proliferative phase is complete when the diseased lung becomes characterized by dense, fibrous tissue. Increased pulmonary vascular resistance and pulmonary hypertension may occur in this stage because the presence of fibroblasts and inflammatory cells obliterate the pulmonary vasculature. Lung compliance continues to decrease as a result of interstitial fibrosis. Hypoxemia worsens because of the thickened alveolar membrane, causing diffusion limitation and shunting. If the

Table **62-8**	Diagnostic Findings in Acute Respiratory Distress Syndrome

Hypoxemia
  PaO_2 <50 mm Hg on FIO_2 >40% with PEEP >5 cm H_2O
Chest X-ray
  New bilateral interstitial and alveolar infiltrates
Pulmonary Artery Wedge Pressure
  ≤18 mm Hg and no evidence of heart failure
Predisposing Condition
  Identification of a predisposing condition for ARDS within 48 hours of clinical manifestations

Table **62-9**	Complications Associated with Acute Respiratory Distress Syndrome

Infection
  Nosocomial pneumonia
  Catheter-related infection
  Sepsis (bacteremia)
Respiratory complications
  Pulmonary emboli
  Pulmonary barotrauma (e.g., pneumothorax, pneumomediastinum, subcutaneous emphysema)
  O_2 toxicity
  Pulmonary fibrosis
Gastrointestinal complications
  Stress ulceration and hemorrhage
  Paralytic ileus
  Pneumoperitoneum

Renal complications
  Acute renal failure
Cardiac complications
  Arrhythmias
  Decreased cardiac output
Hematologic complications
  Anemia
  Thrombocytopenia
  Disseminated intravascular coagulation
ET intubation complications
  Laryngeal ulceration
  Tracheal ulceration
  Tracheal malacia
  Tracheal stenosis

reparative phase persists, widespread fibrosis results. If the proliferative phase is arrested, the lesions resolve.

Fibrotic Phase. The fibrotic phase occurs approximately 2 to 3 weeks after the initial lung injury. This phase is also called the chronic or late phase of ARDS. By this time the lung is completely remodeled by sparsely collagenous and fibrous tissues. There is diffuse scarring and fibrosis, resulting in decreased lung compliance. In addition, the surface area for gas exchange is significantly reduced because the interstitium is fibrotic, and therefore hypoxemia continues. Pulmonary hypertension results from pulmonary vascular obliteration and fibrosis.

Clinical Progression

Progression of ARDS varies among patients. Some persons survive the acute phase of lung injury; pulmonary edema resolves and complete recovery occurs in a few days. The chance for survival is poor in patients who enter the fibrotic (chronic or late) stage, which requires long-term mechanical ventilation. It is not known why injured lungs repair and recover in some patients, and in others ARDS progresses. Several factors seem to be important in determining the course of ARDS, including the nature of the initial injury, extent and severity of coexisting diseases, and the pulmonary complications.

Clinical Manifestations

The initial presentation of ARDS is often insidious. At the time of the initial injury, and for several hours to 1 to 2 days afterward, the patient may not experience respiratory symptoms, or the patient may exhibit only dyspnea, tachypnea, cough, and restlessness. Chest auscultation may be normal or reveal fine, scattered crackles. ABGs usually indicate mild hypoxemia and respiratory alkalosis caused by hyperventilation. Respiratory alkalosis results from hypoxemia and the stimulation of juxtacapillary receptors. The chest x-ray may be normal or exhibit evidence of minimal scattered interstitial infiltrates. Edema may not show on the x-ray until there is a 30% increase in fluid content in the lung.

As ARDS progresses, symptoms worsen because of increased fluid accumulation and decreased lung compliance. Respiratory discomfort becomes evident as the work of breathing increases. Tachypnea and intercostal and suprasternal retractions may be present. Pulmonary function tests in ARDS reveal decreased compliance and decreased lung volumes, particularly a decreased functional residual capacity (FRC). Tachy-

cardia, diaphoresis, changes in sensorium with decreased mentation, cyanosis, and pallor may be present. Chest auscultation usually reveals scattered to diffuse crackles and rhonchi. The chest x-ray demonstrates diffuse and extensive bilateral interstitial and alveolar infiltrates. A pulmonary artery catheter may be inserted. Pulmonary artery wedge pressure does not increase in ARDS since the cause is noncardiogenic (not related to cardiac function). Pulmonary edema that is caused by cardiac dysfunction will cause an increase in pulmonary artery wedge pressure.

Refractory hypoxemia, despite increased FIO_2 by mask, cannula, or endotracheal tube, is a hallmark of ARDS. ABGs may initially demonstrate a normal or decreased $PaCO_2$ despite severe dyspnea and hypoxemia. Hypercapnia signifies that hypoventilation is occurring, and the patient is no longer able to maintain the level of ventilation needed to provide optimum gas exchange.

As ARDS progresses it is associated with profound respiratory distress requiring endotracheal intubation and PPV. The chest x-ray is often termed *whiteout* or *white lung,* because consolidation and coalescing infiltrates are widespread throughout the lungs, leaving few recognizable air spaces. Pleural effusions may also be present. Severe hypoxemia, hypercapnia, and metabolic acidosis, with symptoms of target organ or tissue hypoxia, may ensue if prompt therapy is not instituted.

No precise criteria define ARDS. ARDS is considered to be present if the patient has hypoxemia, a chest x-ray with new bilateral interstitial or alveolar infiltrates, a pulmonary artery wedge pressure of 18 mm Hg or less or no evidence of heart failure, and a predisposing condition consistent for ARDS within 48 hours of clinical manifestations (Table 62-8).

Complications

Complications may develop as a result of ARDS itself or its treatment. (Table 62-9 lists the common complications of

COLLABORATIVE CARE

Table 62-10 Acute Respiratory Distress Syndrome

Diagnostic*
Collaborative Therapy

Respiratory Therapy
O₂ administration
Prone positioning
Medical ventilation with PEEP

Supportive Therapy
Identification and treatment of underlying cause
Hemodynamic monitoring
Inotropic/vasopressor medications
    Dopamine (Intropin)
    Dobutamine (Dobutrex)
Diuretics
Intravenous fluid administration

*See Table 62-8.

ARDS.) The major cause of death in ARDS is MODS, often accompanied by sepsis. The organs most commonly involved are the kidneys, liver, and heart. The systems most often involved are the CNS, hematologic, and gastrointestinal systems.

Nosocomial Pneumonia. A frequent complication of acute respiratory failure is nosocomial pneumonia, occurring in 20% of mechanically ventilated patients, and in as many as 68% of patients with ARDS. Risk factors include impaired host defenses, contaminated medical equipment, invasive monitoring devices, aspiration of gastrointestinal contents, and colonization of the respiratory tract. Strategies to prevent nosocomial pneumonia include infection control measures (e.g., strict hand washing and sterile technique during endotracheal suctioning) and elevating the head of the bed more than 30 degrees to prevent aspiration. (See Chapter 26 for discussion of pneumonia.)

Barotrauma. Barotrauma or volutrauma may result from rupture of overdistended alveoli during mechanical ventilation. The high peak airway pressures that may be required in patients with ARDS predispose to this complication. Barotrauma results in the presence of alveolar air in locations where it is not usually found. This can lead to pulmonary interstitial emphysema, pneumothorax, subcutaneous emphysema, pneumoperitoneum, pneumomediastinum, and tension pneumothorax. (See Chapter 26 for discussion of pneumothorax.) To avoid barotrauma, the patient with ARDS is sometimes ventilated with smaller tidal volumes, resulting in higher $PaCO_2$. This method of mechanical ventilation is termed *permissive hypercapnia* because the $PaCO_2$ is allowed (permitted) to rise above normal limits.

Stress Ulcers. Critically ill patients with acute respiratory failure are at high risk for stress ulcers. Bleeding from stress ulcers occurs in 30% of patients with ARDS who require PPV, a higher incidence than other causes of acute respiratory failure. Management strategies include correction of predisposing conditions such as hypotension, shock, and acidosis. Prophylactic management includes antacids, histamine-receptor blockers (e.g., cimetidine [Tagemet] or ranitidine [Zantac]), sucralfate, and enteral nutrition.

Renal Failure. Renal failure can occur from decreased renal tissue oxygenation as a result of hypotension, hypoxemia, or hypercapnia. Renal failure may also be caused by administration of nephrotoxic drugs (e.g., aminoglycosides), which are used to treat infections associated with ARDS.

NURSING AND COLLABORATIVE MANAGEMENT: ACUTE RESPIRATORY DISTRESS SYNDROME

The collaborative care for acute respiratory failure (see Table 62-4) is applicable to ARDS. The following section discusses additional collaborative care measures for the patient with ARDS (Table 62-10). Patients with ARDS are commonly cared for in critical care units. The nursing care plan for acute respiratory failure (see NCP 62-1) is applicable to patients with acute respiratory failure.

■ Nursing Assessment

Because ARDS causes acute respiratory failure, the subjective and objective data that should be obtained from a person with ARDS are the same as that for acute respiratory failure (see Table 62-4.) Abnormal findings on physical examination are indications that ARDS has progressed beyond the initial stages.

■ Nursing Diagnoses

Nursing diagnoses for the patient with ARDS may include, but are not limited to, those described for acute respiratory failure (see NCP 62-1).

■ Planning

The overall goals are that the patient with ARDS will have (1) PaO_2 within limits of normal for age or baseline values, (2) SaO_2 greater than 90%, (3) patent airway, and (4) clear lungs on auscultation.

■ Respiratory Therapy

Oxygen Administration. The primary goal of O_2 therapy is to correct hypoxemia. O_2 administered via a simple face mask or nasal cannula is usually inadequate to treat refractory hypoxemia. Masks with high-flow systems that deliver higher O_2 concentrations are initially used to maximize O_2 delivery. SpO_2 is continuously monitored to assess the effectiveness of O_2 therapy. The general standard for O_2 administration is to give the patient the lowest concentration that results in a PaO_2 of 60 mm Hg or greater. When the FIO_2 exceeds 60% for more than 48 hours, the risk for O_2 toxicity increases. Patients with ARDS commonly need intubation with mechanical ventilation because the PaO_2 cannot otherwise be maintained at acceptable levels.

Mechanical Ventilation. Endotracheal intubation and mechanical ventilation provide additional respiratory support. However, even with these interventions it may be necessary to maintain the FIO_2 at 60% or greater to maintain the PaO_2 at 60 mm Hg or greater. During mechanical ventilation, it is common to apply positive end-expiratory pressure (PEEP) at 5 cm H_2O to compensate for loss of glottic function caused by the presence of the endotracheal tube.[17] In patients with ARDS, additional PEEP is often used. PEEP is a ventilatory maneuver that applies positive pressure to the airway and lungs at the end of exhalation. Without PEEP, pressure in the chest becomes equal to atmospheric pressure (zero) at the end of exhalation. When PEEP is applied, the lung is kept partially expanded, which prevents the alveoli from totally collapsing. PEEP is typically applied in 3 to 5 cm H_2O increments until oxygenation is adequate with FIO_2 of 60% or less. The mechanism of action of PEEP is related to its ability to increase FRC and recruit (open up) collapsed alveoli. PEEP may improve $\dot{V}/\dot{Q}$ in respiratory units that collapse at low airway pressures, allowing the FIO_2 to be lowered.[18]

If hypoxemic failure persists in spite of high levels of PEEP, alternative modes and therapies may be used. These include pressure support ventilation, pressure release ventilation, pressure control ventilation, inverse ratio ventilation, high frequency ventilation, and permissive hypercapnia (low tidal volumes that allow $PaCO_2$ to increase slowly, maintaining normal pH and low airway pressures). (See Chapter 63 for a discussion of mechanical ventilation.) Extracorporeal membrane oxygenation (ECMO) and extracorporeal CO_2 removal ($ECCO_2R$) pass blood across a gas-exchanging membrane outside the body and then return oxygenated blood back to the body. $ECCO_2R$ with low-frequency PPV allows the lung to heal while the lung is not functional.

Prone Positioning.
Some patients with ARDS demonstrate a marked improvement in PaO_2 when turned from the supine to prone position (e.g., PaO_2 70 mm Hg supine, PaO_2 90 mm Hg prone) with no change in inspired O_2 concentration. The response may be sufficient to allow a reduction in inspired O_2 concentration or PEEP.

In the early phases of ARDS, edema fluid moves freely throughout the lung. Because of gravity, this fluid pools in dependent regions of the lung. As a consequence, some alveoli are fluid filled (dependent areas), whereas others are air filled (nondependent areas). In addition, when the patient is supine the heart and mediastinal contents place more pressure on the lungs than in the prone position, which changes pleural pressure and predisposes to atelectasis. If the patient is turned from supine to prone, air-filled, nonatelectatic alveoli in the dorsal (upper) portion of the lung become dependent. Perfusion may be better matched to ventilation, causing less $\dot{V}/\dot{Q}$ mismatch. Not all patients respond to prone positioning with an increase in PaO_2, and there is no reliable way of predicting who will respond. Prone positioning is typically reserved for patients with refractory hypoxemia who do not respond to other strategies to increase PaO_2.[19,20] When this positioning is used, there must be a plan in place for immediate positioning for cardiopulmonary resuscitation in the event of a cardiac arrest.

■ Medical Supportive Therapy

Maintenance of Cardiac Output and Tissue Perfusion.
Patients on PPV and PEEP frequently experience decreased cardiac output. One cause is decreased venous return, which results from the PEEP-induced increase in intrathoracic pressure. Cardiac output may also be decreased by impaired contractility and decreased preload. Continuous hemodynamic monitoring is essential to detect these changes and titrate therapy. An arterial catheter is inserted to permit continuous monitoring of blood pressure and to withdraw blood for ABGs. A pulmonary artery catheter is normally inserted to allow monitoring of pulmonary artery pressure and

pulmonary artery wedge pressures (which indicate the fluid status of the left side of the heart) and cardiac output. If the cardiac output falls, it may be necessary to administer crystalloid fluids or colloid solutions or to lower PEEP. Use of inotropic drugs such as dobutamine (Dobutrex) or dopamine (Intropin) may also be necessary. (See Chapter 63 for discussion of hemodynamic monitoring.)

The hemoglobin level is usually kept at levels of more than 9 to 10 g/dl (90 to 100 g/L) with an oxygen saturation of 90% or greater (when PaO_2 is more than 60 mm Hg). Packed red blood cells may be administered to increase O_2-carrying capacity of the blood.

Maintenance of Fluid Balance.
Maintenance of fluid balance is precarious in the patient with ARDS. Leaky capillaries increase fluid in the lungs and cause pulmonary edema. At the same time, the patient may be volume depleted and therefore prone to hypotension and decreased cardiac output from mechanical ventilation and PEEP. Controversy exists as to the benefits of fluid replacement with crystalloids versus colloids. Critics of colloid replacement believe that proteins of colloid fluid may leak into the pulmonary interstitium, exacerbating the movement of proteinaceous fluid into the alveoli. Advocates of colloid replacement believe that colloids help keep fluid from leaking into the alveoli. The pulmonary artery wedge pressure is kept as low as possible without impairing cardiac output. The patient is usually placed on mild fluid restriction, and diuretics are used as necessary. Pulmonary artery wedge pressures, intake and output, and daily weights are monitored to assess the patient's fluid status.

■ Evaluation

The expected outcomes for the patient with ARDS are similar to those for a patient with acute respiratory failure and are presented in NCP 62-1.

Trends and Research in ARDS Management

Pharmacologic agents to treat ARDS have been researched extensively. Monoclonal antibodies are being studied for their effects in binding endotoxin and interleukins, thus limiting or preventing mediator-induced damage to the alveolar capillary endothelium. Prostaglandin E_1 (PGE_1), a vasodilator, is being studied for its use in decreasing systemic and pulmonary vascular resistance.[21] Inhaled nitric oxide (NO) is another vasodilator currently being studied for its effects on decreasing pulmonary artery pressure and improving oxygenation.[22,23] Surfactant (a lipid-protein complex produced by alveolar type II cells), which decreases surface tension and maintains lung compliance, is also being used in ARDS.[24] Surfactant replacement therapy has been effective in respiratory distress syndrome in infants. The use of partial liquid ventilation in the ARDS patient on mechanical ventilation is under investigation. A liquid fluorocarbon is instilled into the lung. This liquid keeps the alveoli open and has a high carrying capacity for O_2. Both actions help improve O_2 movement across the alveolus into the pulmonary blood.[25]

The use of corticosteroids in the acute phase of ARDS has not proven beneficial. However, the use of corticosteroids in the chronic phases of ARDS may be indicated if the patient is not responding to conventional treatment.[26]

CRITICAL THINKING EXERCISES

CASE STUDY

Acute Respiratory Distress Syndrome

Patient Profile

Mr. J. is a 35-year-old man who was admitted 32 hours ago to a general surgical unit after surgery for multiple gunshot wounds in the abdomen. The surgical procedure involved extensive abdominal surgery to repair a perforated colon, remove bullets, and repair a torn mesenteric artery. During transport to the hospital and during surgery his systolic blood pressure dropped to 70 mm Hg. Ten units of packed red blood cells and 6 L of normal saline were administered intravenously to restore blood loss and volume. He is receiving 60% oxygen through an aerosol face mask. He is being monitored with a cardiac monitor and pulse oximeter. He has a central intravenous catheter in place and is receiving 0.9% normal saline intravenously at 125 ml per hour. A urinary catheter is in place.

Subjective Data

- Complains of shortness of breath, inability to lie flat, and diffuse abdominal pain

Objective Data

Physical Assessment
- General: alert, well-nourished man who appears restless and anxious; head of bed elevated 45 degrees; skin cool with moderate diaphoresis

- Respiratory: no accessory muscle use, retraction, paradoxic breathing; respiratory rate 28 breaths/min; SpO_2 88%; fine crackles at lung bases
- Cardiovascular: blood pressure 100/60 mm Hg; cardiac monitor shows sinus tachycardia at 120 beats/min, which correlates with his apical pulse rate; temperature 101° F (38° C) orally
- Gastrointestinal: surgical dressing dry and intact; sharp pain on palpation over incisional area
- Urologic: urinary catheter draining concentrated urine

Diagnostic Findings
- Chest x-ray shows scattered interstitial infiltrates compatible with an ARDS pattern as interpreted by the radiologist

Critical Thinking Questions

1. How does the pathophysiology of ARDS predispose to the development of refractory hypoxemia?
2. What clinical manifestations does Mr. J. exhibit that support a diagnosis of ARDS?
3. What are the possible causes of ARDS in Mr. J.?
4. What are the possible complications Mr. J. is at risk for developing secondary to ARDS?
5. What respiratory care interventions might be implemented to improve Mr. J's hypoxemia?
6. Based on the assessment data presented, write one or more appropriate nursing diagnoses. Are there any collaborative problems?

REVIEW QUESTIONS

The number of the question corresponds to the same-numbered objective at the beginning of the chapter.

1. Hypercapnic respiratory failure can be caused by
   a. ARDS.
   b. asthma.
   c. pneumonia.
   d. pulmonary emboli.
2. An early sign of acute respiratory failure is
   a. restlessness.
   b. coma.
   c. cyanosis.
   d. paradoxic breathing.
3. The oxygen delivery system chosen for the patient in acute respiratory failure should
   a. always be a low-flow device, such as a nasal cannula.
   b. correct the PaO_2 to a normal level as quickly as possible.
   c. administer positive pressure ventilation to prevent CO_2 narcosis.
   d. maintain the PaO_2 at 55 to 60 mm Hg or greater at the lowest O_2 concentration possible.
4. The most common early clinical manifestations of ARDS that the nurse may observe are
   a. dyspnea and tachypnea.
   b. hypotension and tachycardia.
   c. cyanosis and apprehension.
   d. respiratory distress and frothy sputum.

5. Maintenance of fluid balance in the patient with ARDS involves
   a. hydration using colloids.
   b. administration of surfactant.
   c. mild fluid restriction and diuretics as necessary.
   d. keeping the hemoglobin at levels of 15 to 16 g/dl (150 to 160 g/L).

References

1. Grippi MA: Respiratory failure: an overview. In Fishman AP and others, editors: *Fishman's pulmonary diseases and disorders*, ed 3, New York, 1998, McGraw-Hill.
2. Pierson DJ: Normal and abnormal oxygenation: physiology and clinical syndromes, *Respir Care* 38:587, 1993.
3. Misasi R, Keyes JL: Matching and mismatching ventilation and perfusion in the lung, *Crit Care Nurse* 16:23, 1996.
4. Panettieri RA, Murray RK: *Chronic obstructive pulmonary disease*. In Fishman AP, editor: *Pulmonary diseases and disorders: companion handbook*, ed 3, New York, 1998, McGraw-Hill.
5. Syabbalo N: Measurement and interpretation of arterial blood gases, *Br J Clin Pract* 51:173, 1997.
6. Callaghan SP and others: Minitracheostomy: an alternative to "blind" endotracheal suctioning, *DCCN* 13:38, 1994.
7. Clark HE, Wilcox PG: Noninvasive positive pressure ventilation in acute respiratory failure or chronic obstructive pulmonary disease, *Lung* 175:143, 1997.
8. Abou-Shala N, Meduri U: Noninvasive mechanical ventilation in patients with acute respiratory failure, *Crit Care Med* 24:705, 1996.

9. Freichels T: Palliative ventilatory support: use of noninvasive positive pressure ventilation in terminal respiratory insufficiency, *Am J Crit Care* 3:6, 1994.

10. Karpel JP and others: Emergency treatment of acute asthma with albuterol metered-dose inhaler plus holding chamber, *Chest* 112:348, 1997.

11. Zuege DJ, Whitelaw WA: Management of acute respiratory failure in chronic obstructive pulmonary disease, *Curr Opin Pulmonary Med* 3:190, 1997.

12. *American Lung Association fact sheet*, New York, *ARDS*, 1997, American Lung Association.

13. Volman K: Adult respiratory distress syndrome mediators on the run, *Crit Care Nurs Clin North Am* 6:2, 1994.

14. Luce JM: Acute lung injury and the acute respiratory distress syndrome, *Crit Care Med* 26:369, 1998.

15. Shanley TP, Warner RL, Ward PA: The role of cytokines and adhesion molecules in the development of inflammatory injury, *Molecular Medicine Today* 1:40, 1995.

16. Thelan LA and others: *Critical care nursing: diagnosis and management*, ed 3, St Louis, 1998, Mosby.

17. Cawley MJ and others: Mechanical ventilation and pharmacologic strategies for acute respiratory distress syndrome, *Pharmacotherapy* 18:140, 1998.

18. Moore FA, Haenel JB: Ventilatory strategies for acute respiratory failure, *Am J Surg* 173:53, 1997.

19. Volman K: Prone positioning for the ARDS patient, *DCCN* 16:4, 1997.

20. Shapiro R, Broccard A: Patient positioning in respiratory disease, *Clinical Pulmonary Medicine* 4:45, 1997.

21. Lackmann B, Heulitt M: New therapies in respiratory failure, *Controversies in Critical Care* 3:2, 1997.

22. Kalweit S: Inhaled nitric oxide in the ICU, *Crit Care Nurse* 17:26, 1997.

23. Kalweit S: Inhaled nitric oxide in the ICU, *Crit Care Nurse* 17:26, 1998.

24. Baudouin SV: Surfactant medication for acute respiratory distress syndrome, *Thorax* 52(suppl 3):S9, 1997.

25. Dirkes S: Liquid ventilation: new frontiers in the treatment of ARDS, *Crit Care Nurse* 16:53, 1996.

26. Honig EG, Ingram RH: Acute respiratory distress syndrome. In Fauci and others, editors: *Harrison's principles of internal medicine*, ed 14, New York, 1998, McGraw-Hill.

Resources

Resources for this chapter are listed after Chapter 63 on p. 1957.

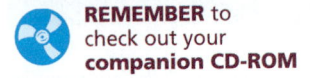
63 NURSING MANAGEMENT
Critical Care

Eleanor F. Bond & Julie Dax

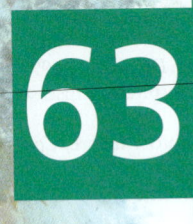

www.mosby.com/MERLIN/medsurg_lewis

LEARNING OBJECTIVES

1. Describe the critical care unit.
2. Describe the critical care nurse.
3. Identify common problems and needs of patients in critical care units and related nursing management.
4. Identify common problems and needs of families of patients in critical care units and related nursing management.
5. Describe the principles of hemodynamic monitoring and related nursing management.
6. Describe the types, indications, potential complications, and nursing management of ventricular assist devices.
7. Describe the purpose, indications, and function of intra-aortic balloon pumps and related nursing management.
8. Describe the types and potential complications of endotracheal intubation.
9. Discuss the nursing management of the patient who requires endotracheal intubation.
10. Describe the indications for and modes of mechanical ventilation and related nursing management.
11. Describe the principles of intracranial pressure monitoring.
12. Identify strategies for management of patients with increased intracranial pressure.

CRITICAL CARE NURSING

Critical Care Units

Critical care units or intensive care units are designed to meet the special needs of acutely and critically ill patients. The concept of clustering the most acutely ill is not new. Florence Nightingale recommended grouping acutely ill patients together.[1] During poliomyelitis and tuberculosis pandemics in the middle of the twentieth century, special units were established, equipped with technical equipment to manage the airway and ventilate the patient, and staffed by specialized care providers. During World War II and the Vietnam War, trauma units were developed for battle casualties.

In the 1960s technologic developments allowed for more accessible monitoring of the electrocardiogram (ECG), arterial and central venous pressures, and arterial blood gases. Coronary care units were developed for patients with acute myocardial infarction. In these units patients were continually monitored for cardiac arrhythmias. Nurses followed protocols to aggressively manage arrhythmias. By the 1970s the intensive care unit (ICU) was a standard component of most general hospitals. Since that time, technical advances have continued at a rapid pace, bringing improved monitoring capabilities and new strategies to manage life-threatening problems.

The term *critical care nursing* is often used interchangeably with the term *ICU nursing*. The critical care nurse is responsi-

ble for diagnosing life-threatening conditions and instituting appropriate treatment. Technology and equipment available in the ICU are extensive and continually evolving. In ICUs the capability exists to continuously monitor ECG, blood pressure, cardiac output, ventilation, intracranial pressure, oxygenation, and temperature. More advanced monitoring devices allow for the measurement of stroke volume, ejection fraction, end-tidal carbon dioxide, and oxygen consumption. Patients may be receiving continual support from mechanical ventilators, ventricular assist devices, or dialysis machines. A typical critical care patient unit is illustrated in Fig. 63-1. Some common abbreviations used in ICUs are given in Table 63-1.

Critical Care Nurse

The critical care nurse cares for patients and the families of patients with acute and unstable physiologic problems in an environment equipped for technically advanced methods of assessing and managing patient problems. The American Association of Critical Care Nurses (AACN) defines *critical care nursing* as that specialty dealing with human responses to life-threatening problems. Critical care nursing requires knowledge of physiology, pathophysiology, pharmacology, and the ability to use advanced technology to accurately measure physiologic parameters. The nurse provides ongoing assessment and early recognition and management of complications while fostering healing and recovery. Appropriate actions by an astute nurse can prevent complications. The nurse must also be able to provide psychologic support to the patient and the family. To be effective the critical care nurse must be able to communicate clearly and work as a team member.

Reviewed by Susan B. Stillwell, RN, MSN, Clinical Associate Professor, College of Nursing, Arizona State University, Tempe, Ariz.

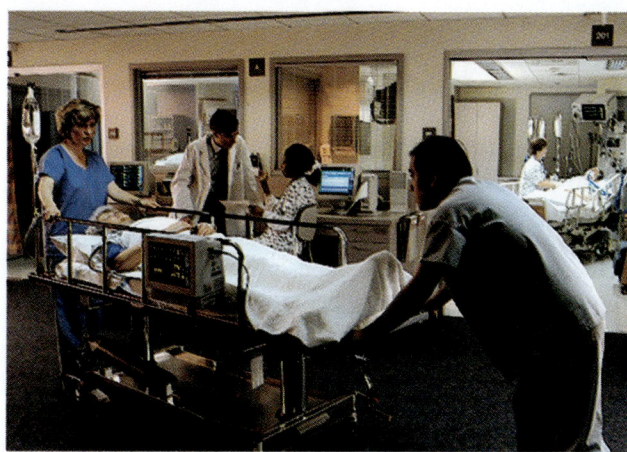

Fig. 63-1 Typical intensive care unit.

Table 63-1	Abbreviations Commonly Used in the Intensive Care Unit
Abbreviation	**Term**
ABP	Arterial blood pressure
CI	Cardiac index
CO	Cardiac output
CVP	Central venous pressure
FIO$_2$	Fraction of inspired oxygen
IABP	Intraaortic balloon pump
MAP	Mean arterial pressure
MRB	Manual resuscitation bag
PA	Pulmonary artery
PAS, PAD	PA systolic (pressure), PA diastolic (pressure)
PAWP	Pulmonary artery wedge pressure
PVR	Pulmonary vascular resistance
SpO$_2$	Percent oxygen saturation of hemoglobin measured by pulse oximetry
SvO$_2$	Percent oxygen saturation of hemoglobin in mixed venous blood (i.e., in the PA)
SV	Stroke volume
SVR	Systemic vascular resistance
VAD	Ventricular assist device

Nursing practice in the ICU often follows a primary care model with the patient cared for by a limited group of nurses who become thoroughly familiar with the patient's condition and the needs of the patient and the family. The ICU nurse spends most working hours near the patient's bedside. Specialization in ICU nursing usually requires formal training and mentored clinical practice, which is usually followed by an internship.

Certification in critical care nursing (CCRN) is offered by the AACN Certification Corporation. The designation requires registered nurse certification, clinical experience, and successful completion of a written test. Additional experience and testing or education are required for recertification. CCRN certification designates competency and not advanced practice. It does not require a master's degree and is not a basis for prescriptive authority.

Advanced practice critical care nurses generally have a graduate (master's or doctorate) degree. These nurses are employed as patient and staff educators, consultants, administrators, researchers, or practitioners. The critical care clinical nurse specialist role traditionally includes aspects of each of these role components. An important emerging role is the acute care nurse practitioner. These master's-prepared nurses provide advanced, comprehensive care to selected critically ill patients and their families. The acute care nurse practitioner is prepared to conduct comprehensive health assessments, order and interpret diagnostic tests, diagnose and treat health problems and disease-related symptoms, prescribe and evaluate drugs and treatments, and coordinate care during transitions in settings. They may practice independently (e.g., providing comprehensive care to the chronically critically ill) or collaboratively (e.g., providing symptom management in conjunction with physician specialists).

Critical Care Patient

A patient is generally admitted to the ICU for one of three reasons. First, the patient may be physiologically unstable, requiring advanced and sophisticated clinical judgments by the nurse or physician. Second, the patient may be at risk for serious complications and require frequent and often invasive physical assessment. Third, the patient may require intensive and complicated nursing support such as the use of life support technology and invasive monitoring equipment such as ventricular assist devices, mechanical ventilation, renal dialysis, and hemodynamic monitoring.

ICU patients can be clustered by disease condition (e.g., neurology) or age-group (e.g., pediatrics). ICU patients are sometimes clustered by acuity (e.g., acute and unstable versus technology dependent but stable). The patient with myocardial ischemia or infarction or respiratory distress is commonly treated in the ICU, as is the patient with acute neurologic impairment, after cardiac surgery, or after major organ transplantation. Trauma ICUs treat the critically injured. The patient with a medical emergency (e.g., sepsis, diabetic ketoacidosis, drug overdoses, poisonings, thyroid, adrenal, or hematologic crises) is often treated in a medical ICU. The patient with a serious underlying condition may be monitored in the ICU while receiving care for unrelated conditions. The patient who is not expected to recover is not treated in an ICU. The ICU should not be used to treat the patient in a persistent coma, nor should ICU care be used to prolong the natural process of death.

Despite the emphasis on caring for the patient who can survive, death is common in ICU patients. A review of British adult ICU admissions (excluding patients with burns or cardiac surgery) showed that 32.5% of patients died in the hospital.[2] Similar rates were reported in Canada.[3] Nonsurvivors were older and had longer ICU stays. However, even patients at relatively low risk such as those with asthma and drug overdoses had high death rates (greater than 10%). Often death occurred following transfer from ICU to the general hospital units, suggesting a need for caution and coordination of care in transferring patients from ICUs.

Progressive care units have recently been established as a graded option, intermediate between the ICU and the general hospital ward.[4] Generally patients in the progressive care unit are at risk for serious complications, but their risk is lower than that of ICU patients. Patients may require cardiac telemetry monitoring or slow weaning from mechanical ventilation. Progressive care units offer an opportunity to reduce health care costs and provide a calmer and quieter care environment.

Common Problems of Critical Care Patients. The patient admitted into the ICU is at risk for complications and special problems. Invasive devices carry a risk of infection, particularly in the immunocompromised patient. Sepsis and multiple organ dysfunction syndrome may follow (see Chapter 61). Other special problems for ICU patients include anxiety, dependency, impaired communication, sensory-perceptual problems, and sleep difficulties.

Anxiety. Patients commonly find the ICU frightening. Frequently patients are at risk of dying and fear death. Many patients and families feel uncomfortable in the ICU environment with its equipment, high noise and light levels, and intense pace of activity. Pain and sleeplessness enhance anxiety, as do immobilization, loss of control, and impaired communication.[5] Some patients become acutely stressed by the ICU experience and others experience chronic posttraumatic stress disorder (PTSD), characterized by intrusive memories, irritability, and difficulty concentrating. In one study 25% of patients treated in the ICU for acute respiratory distress syndrome experienced PTSD.[6] Patients experienced PTSD even when they could not remember details of the ICU experience.

The nurse can assist the patient and family with their feelings of anxiety by encouraging them to express concerns, ask questions, and state their needs. The nurse should explain equipment and procedures. The nurse may be able to structure the patient's surrounding environment in a way that may decrease anxiety. For example, family members can be encouraged to bring in photographs and personal items. Flexible visiting schedules may diminish the patient's anxiety.[5] Judicious use of sedation may blunt some of the acute and chronic stress-related conditions.

Dependency. Patients in the ICU commonly are unable to perform self-care activities such as eating, bathing, and oral hygiene. The patient may lack control over bodily functions such as elimination and breathing. The patient is frequently dependent on the nursing staff for access to food, liquids, the bedpan, and other needed items. In addition, the ICU patient is frequently connected to equipment and placed on bed rest. The degree of dependency experienced by an ICU patient can be distressing. Although the highest priority is the safety of the patient, the nurse should provide as much autonomy as the patient's condition allows. Family members can be taught to assist the patient with activities of daily living.

Impaired communication. Inability to communicate can be a distressing problem for the patient who may be unable to speak because of the use of paralyzing drugs or an endotracheal tube. As part of any procedure the nurse should explain what will happen or is happening to the patient. When the patient cannot speak, the nurse should explore alternative methods of communication, including the use of devices such as picture boards, notepads, magic slates, or computer keyboards. When speaking with the patient, the nurse should look directly at the patient and use hand gestures when appropriate.

Nonverbal communication is important. The ICU is characterized by high levels of procedure-related touch and decreased affection-related or comfort-related touch. Patients have different levels of tolerance for being touched, possibly related to cultural background and personal history. It may be appropriate to provide comforting touch with ongoing evaluation of the patient's response. Often the ICU nurse encourages the family to touch and talk with the patient.

Sensory-perceptual problems. Transient sensory-perceptual changes are common in ICU patients. Approximately 50% of patients treated in the ICU experience decreased orientation and impaired cognition.[7] The combination of changes in mentation (e.g., hallucinations, delusions) and behavior (e.g., shouting, hitting) has been inappropriately labeled *ICU psychosis.* The patient is not psychotic, but is suffering from delirium and may demonstrate confusion, irritability, and inappropriate behavior.[8] Factors predisposing the patient to sensory-perceptual changes include sleep deprivation, anxiety, sensory overload, stress, and many drugs. Physical conditions such as hypoxemia and electrolyte disturbances can produce similar symptoms, including confusion and irritability. Potassium, calcium, and magnesium imbalances are common in the critically ill patient, and each can result in altered cognition.

The task of the ICU nurse is to identify predisposing factors, whether they be physiologic, psychologic, or environmental, and attempt to improve the patient's mental clarity and cooperation with therapy. Helpful strategies include correction of contributing oxygenation, perfusion, and electrolyte problems. The use of clocks and calendars may help the patient remain oriented. Although symptoms may be managed pharmacologically with a sedative, hypnotic, or psychotropic (e.g., haloperidol [Haldol]) medication, these drugs may decrease the patient's ability to interact with family members. This may deprive patients and families of what may be the short and precious time remaining to discuss intimate and important issues.

Sensory overload can also result in patient distress and anxiety. Noise levels are particularly high in the ICU.[9] The "meaning" of a noise may determine its stressfulness with meaningful noise being less stressful. The nurse can limit noise and assist the patient in understanding noises that cannot be prevented. Conversation is a particularly stressful noise, especially when the discussion concerns the patient and is conducted in the presence of, but without participation from, the patient. The nurse can eliminate this source of stress by identifying better places for discussing the patient and by including the patient in the discussion. The nurse can also limit noise levels directly by muting phones, setting alarms appropriate to the patient's condition, and eliminating unnecessary alarms. For example, the nurse should silence the blood pressure alarms while manipulating invasive lines, and then reactivate the alarms when the procedures are complete. Similarly, ventilator alarms should be transiently silenced during endotracheal suctioning. Overhead paging should be limited in patient care areas. Music should be played only if it comforts the patient.

Sleep problems. Nearly all ICU patients experience serious sleep disturbances.[10] Patients may have difficulty falling asleep or have disrupted sleep because of frequent monitoring or treatment procedures.[11,12] Drugs such as sedatives and hypnotics may result in disturbed sleep patterns, including reductions in slow wave and rapid eye movement (REM) sleep.[13] Sleep disturbance is a significant stressor in the ICU, contributing to impaired cognition and possibly affecting recovery. The ICU nurse can structure the environment to promote patient sleep. Strategies include clustering activities, scheduling rest, making physiologic measurements without changing the patient's position, limiting noise, and promoting comfort and relaxation.

Issues Related to Family Members

When someone becomes critically ill, loved ones and family should not be forgotten. Family members play a valuable role in recovery and should be considered as members of the health care team. They can contribute to the patient's well-being by doing the following:[14]

1. Providing a link to the patient's personal life (e.g., news of family, friends, and job) to which the nurse has no access
2. Advising the patient in health care decisions because they know the patient better than the nursing staff
3. Helping with activities of daily living (e.g., bathing, oral suctioning)
4. Having a positive, loving, and caring presence

To be effective in caring for their loved one, family members need guidance and support from the nurse. The experience of having a friend or family member in the ICU is physically and emotionally difficult. Families of the critically ill are usually anxious about the patient's condition and prognosis. They have concerns regarding the patient's pain and other discomforts. They may question the quality of care that the patient is receiving. In addition, it is common for families to experience anxiety regarding the financial issues related to planning and providing care in the next phases of the illness. The family will typically be experiencing disruption of their daily routines to support the patient. They may be far from their own home, routines, and supportive friends and family members. During these difficult times, they are often asked to make critical decisions.

Lack of information is a source of anxiety for the family.[15] The nurse should assess the family's understanding of the patient's status, goals, treatments, and prognosis and provide information as appropriate. The first time the family member visits it is important for the nurse to prepare the family member for the experience by briefly describing the patient's appearance, condition, treatments, tubes, and equipment. Families should be told what to expect regarding the environment (sounds, noise, odors). It is helpful if the nurse can accompany the family members as they enter the room. They should be encouraged to participate in the patient's care. The nurse should observe the responses of both the patient and family. Sometimes the family may cease to be therapeutic and may tire the patient who is reluctant to tell them to leave. Another problem may be a family member whose own needs are neglected because of a sense of obligation to stay with the patient. The nurse should ensure that the patient's needs are being met and intervene with the family as needed. Family members who are exhausted, sleep deprived, anxious, and fearful are in no position to provide support to the patient. Rather than a rigid open or closed visiting policy, each patient should have a plan tailored to the patient's and family's needs.

The family needs information about the way in which the patient's care is managed and decisions are made. The family should have the opportunity to be involved in decision making. The family should also be invited to meet the health care team members, including physicians, dietician, respiratory therapist, social worker, and physical therapist. The nurse should evaluate the appropriateness of including family members in multidisciplinary care conferences. It helps family members to accept and cope with problems if they observe that providers are caring and competent, decisions are deliberate, and they themselves have the opportunity to help shape the course of care.

While working with families, the ICU nurse should assess the response of the family to the stress. Their feelings should be acknowledged and accepted. They should be supported in their decisions. Institutional support personnel, such as chaplains, social workers, and psychologists, may be helpful in assisting the family and patient to adjust. The extent to which the family is involved and supported will in turn affect the patient's clinical course in the ICU.

HEMODYNAMIC MONITORING

Hemodynamic monitoring refers to measurement of pressure, flow, and oxygenation of blood within the cardiovascular system. Both invasive (internally placed devices) and noninvasive (external devices) measurements are made in the ICU. Values commonly measured include systemic and pulmonary arterial pressures, central venous pressure (CVP), pulmonary artery wedge pressure (PAWP), cardiac output, and oxygen saturation of the hemoglobin of arterial blood (SaO_2) and mixed venous blood (SvO_2). From these measurements the clinician calculates several values, including the resistance of the systemic and pulmonary arterial vasculature and oxygen content, delivery, and consumption. When these data are integrated with clinical assessment data, the nurse can derive a better picture of the patient's hemodynamic status and the effect of therapy. It is important that all measures be made with attention to technical aspects. False or inaccurate data are potentially misleading and thus dangerous.

Hemodynamic Terminology

Cardiac Output. *Cardiac output* (CO) is the volume of blood pumped by the heart in 1 minute. Although minor beat-to-beat changes may occur, generally the left and right ventricles pump the same volume. The volume pumped with each heartbeat is the *stroke volume*. Stroke volume times heart rate equals CO. Blood pressure, the force exerted by blood on the vessel wall, is determined by CO and the forces opposing blood flow. The opposition to blood flow offered by the vessels is called *systemic vascular resistance* or *pulmonary vascular resistance*. Stroke volume (and thus CO and blood pressure) is determined by preload, afterload, and contractility (see Chapters 30 and 31). Understanding these concepts and relationships is essential for the ICU nurse. In addition, the nurse must understand the effects of manipulation of each of these variables. Normal values for hemodynamic variables are given in Table 63-2.

Preload. *Preload* is the volume within a cardiac chamber at the end of diastole. Unfortunately, chamber volumes are difficult to obtain. Instead, various pressures are used to estimate volume. Left ventricular preload is called *left ventricular end-diastolic pressure*. PAWP, a measure of pulmonary capillary pressure, reflects left ventricular end-diastolic pressure under normal conditions (i.e., when there is no mitral valve pathology, intracardiac defect, or arrhythmia). CVP, measured in the right atrium or in the vena cava close to the heart, is the right ventricular preload or right ventricular end-diastolic pressure when there is no tricuspid valve pathology.

Table **63-2**	Hemodynamic Parameters at Rest
Indicators	**Normal Range**

Preload	
Right atrial pressure (RAP) or central venous pressure (CVP)	2-8 mm Hg
Pulmonary artery wedge pressure (PAWP) or left atrial pressure (LAP)	6-12 mm Hg
Pulmonary artery diastolic pressure	4-12 mm Hg
Afterload	
Pulmonary vascular resistance (PVR) = (mean pulmonary artery pressure [PAP] − mean pulmonary artery wedge pressure [PAWP]) × 80/cardiac output	<250 dyne sec/cm^5
Pulmonary vascular resistance index (PVRI) × 80 = pulmonary vascular resistance (PVR) × body surface area	160-380 dyne sec m^2/cm^5
Systemic vascular resistance (SVR) = (mean arterial pressure − central venous pressure) × 80/cardiac output	800-1200 dyne sec/cm^5
Systemic vascular resistance index (SVRI)=(systemic vascular resistance) × body surface area	1970-2390 dyne sec m^2/cm^5
Mean arterial pressure (MAP) = diastolic blood pressure + ⅓ pulse pressure*	70-105 mm Hg
Mean pulmonary artery pressure (PAP) = pulmonary artery diastolic pressure + ⅓ pulmonary artery pulse pressure*	10-20 mm Hg
Other	
Stroke volume = (cardiac output × 1000)/heart rate	60-150 ml/beat
Stroke volume index = (cardiac index × 1000)/heart rate	30-65 ml/beat/m^2
Heart rate	60-100 beats/min
Cardiac output = stroke volume × heart rate	4-8 L/min
Cardiac index = cardiac output/body surface area	2.2-4.0 L/min/m^2
Arterial hemoglobin oxygen saturation	92-99%
Mixed venous hemoglobin oxygen saturation	60-80%

*This formula is an approximation because it does not take into consideration the heart rate. The monitor looks at the area under the pressure curve, as well as the heart rate, to calculate MAP and PAP.

The effects of preload are based on muscle fiber length. The greater the stretch of the heart muscle at the end of diastole, the greater the force of the next contraction. As preload increases, force generated in the following contraction increases, thus stroke volume and CO increase. The greater the preload, the greater the myocardial (heart muscle) stretch, and the greater the oxygen requirement of the myocardium. Hence, increases in CO via increased preload require increased delivery of oxygen to the myocardium. It should be remembered that the change in stroke volume with preload comes about because of stretching of the heart muscle. However, the clinical measurement made is not a direct measurement of the muscle length; the measurement made is pressure at the time of the peak stretch (end-diastole). The pressure indirectly indicates the amount of stretch and the volume. The pressure is also important because it indicates pressure in the blood vessels of the lung or in the blood returning to the heart. Preload can be increased by fluid administration and decreased by diuresis.

Afterload. Afterload refers to the forces opposing ventricular ejection. These forces include systemic arterial pressure, the resistance offered by the aortic valve, and the mass and density of the blood to be moved. Clinically, although the measures fail to include all the components of afterload, systemic vascular resistance and arterial pressure are indices of left ventricular afterload. Similarly, pulmonary vascular resistance and pulmonary arterial pressure are indices of right ventricular afterload. Increased afterload results in a decreased CO. CO can be increased by decreasing afterload (i.e., decreasing forces opposing contraction). When afterload is reduced, myocardial oxygen needs are decreased. Thus CO is increased and myocardial oxygen requirements are decreased. Therapies directed at reducing afterload are used in the management of heart failure (see Chapter 33).

Contractility. Contractility describes the strength of contraction. Contractility is said to increase when preload is not changed, yet the heart contracts more forcefully. Contractility is increased by epinephrine, norepinephrine, isoproterenol (Isuprel), dopamine, dobutamine (Dobutrex), digitalis-like drugs, calcium, and milrinone (Primacor). These agents are termed *positive inotropes.* Contractility is diminished by *negative inotropes,* such as acidosis and certain drugs (e.g., barbiturates, alcohol, procainamide [Pronestyl], calcium channel blockers, beta-adrenergic blockers). Increased contractility results in increased stroke volume and increased myocardial oxygen requirements. There are no direct clinical measures of cardiac contractility. To indirectly determine contractility, the ICU nurse measures the patient's preload (PAWP) and CO and graphs the results. If preload, heart rate, and afterload remain constant, yet CO changes, contractility is altered. Contractility is diminished in the failing heart.

Vascular Resistance. Systemic vascular resistance (SVR) is the resistance of the systemic vascular bed. Pulmonary vascular resistance (PVR) is the resistance of the pulmonary vascular bed. SVR and PVR are calculated as indicated in Table 63-2.

Principles of Invasive Pressure Monitoring

Invasive lines are commonly used in the ICU to measure systemic and pulmonary blood pressures. Components of a typical invasive arterial pressure monitoring system are illustrated

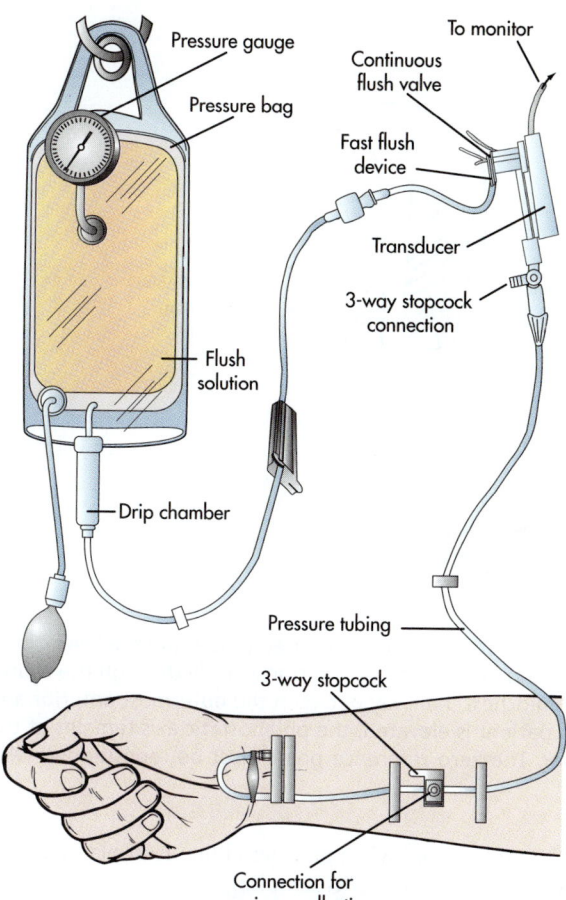

Fig. 63-2 Components of a pressure monitoring system. The cannula, shown entering the radial artery, is connected via pressure (nondistensible) tubing to the transducer. The transducer converts the pressure wave into an electronic signal. The transducer is wired to the electronic monitoring system, which amplifies, conditions, displays, and records the signal. Stopcocks are inserted into the line for specimen withdrawal and for referencing and zero-balancing procedures. A flush system consisting of a pressurized bag of intravenous fluid, tubing, and a flush device is inserted into the line. The flush system provides continuous slow (approximately 3 ml hourly) flushing and provides a mechanism for fast flushing of lines. All items except the electronic monitoring system are commonly disposable equipment.

in Fig. 63-2. Catheter, pressure tubing, flush system, and usually the transducer are disposable.

To accurately measure pressure, equipment must be referenced and zero balanced and dynamic response characteristics optimized. Referencing means positioning the monitoring equipment so that the zero reference point is at the vertical level of the left atrium of the heart. The port of the stopcock nearest the transducer is usually the zero reference for the transducer. To place this level with the left atrium, the nurse uses an external landmark, the phlebostatic axis. To identify the phlebostatic axis, two imaginary planes are drawn with the patient supine (Fig. 63-3). One plane is midchest, halfway between the outermost anterior and posterior surfaces. The second plane is transverse through the fourth intercostal space at the sternum. The phlebostatic axis is the intersection of the two planes. Once the

phlebostatic axis is identified, it is marked on the patient's chest with a permanent marker. The port of the stopcock nearest the transducer is positioned level with the phlebostatic axis.

Zeroing confirms that when pressure within the system is zero, the equipment reads zero. Most transducers in common current use are disposable and have little zero drift; thus once-per-shift zeroing is recommended.

Optimizing dynamic response characteristics involves checking that the equipment reproduces without distortion a signal that changes rapidly. Optimizing dynamic response characteristics is performed once per shift. It involves checking that the equipment reproduces a distortion-free signal.

In addition to performing these procedures each shift, they are repeated each time a major component in the monitoring system is changed, the recording system is moved, or unusual readings are obtained.

Steps in measuring pressure with an invasive line are given in Table 63-3. Pressure measurements can be obtained from both digital and printed analog outputs, but accurate readings are best obtained from a printed pressure tracing at the end-expiration point. Initial readings are made with the patient flat. Unless the patient's blood pressure is extremely sensitive to orthostatic changes, values at modest degrees of backrest elevation (up to 30 degrees) are generally equivalent to measurements with the patient flat.[16] After confirming that values are similar whether the backrest is flat or slightly elevated, subsequent measurements can be made with the backrest slightly elevated. Thus it is not necessary to reposition the patient for each pressure reading. However, it is necessary to move the zero reference stopcock to keep it positioned at the phlebostatic axis. Consistent landmarks for the left atrium have not been identified for the side-lying position. Thus pressures are not obtained in side-lying positions.

Types of Invasive Pressure Monitoring

Arterial Blood Pressure. Continuous arterial pressure monitoring is indicated for patients experiencing hypotension or increased intracranial pressure, receiving vasoactive drugs (e.g., sodium nitroprusside, dopamine [Intropin]), or requiring frequent arterial blood sampling (e.g., for arterial blood gases [ABGs]). A 20-gauge, 1.5 in (3.8 cm) plastic catheter is typically used to cannulate a peripheral artery such as the radial, brachial, dorsalis pedis, or femoral. The catheter can be inserted percutaneously or via cutdown. It is important that the insertion site be immobilized by an arm board so that the catheter line is not dislodged and lines are not kinked.

Measurements. The nurse can use the arterial line to obtain systolic, diastolic, and mean blood pressure (Fig. 63-4). The arterial waveform provides useful information. In heart failure, the systolic upstroke may be slower. In volume depletion, systolic pressure varies greatly with mechanical ventilation, diminishing during inspiration. In severe congestive heart failure, systolic amplitude does not vary with ventilation. With arrhythmias it is useful to observe simultaneous ECG and pressure tracings. Arrhythmias that significantly diminish arterial pressure are more urgent than those that cause only a slight decrease in systolic amplitude.

Complications. Arterial lines carry the risk of hemorrhage, infection, thrombus formation, and distal circulatory occlusion. Hemorrhage is most likely to occur when the

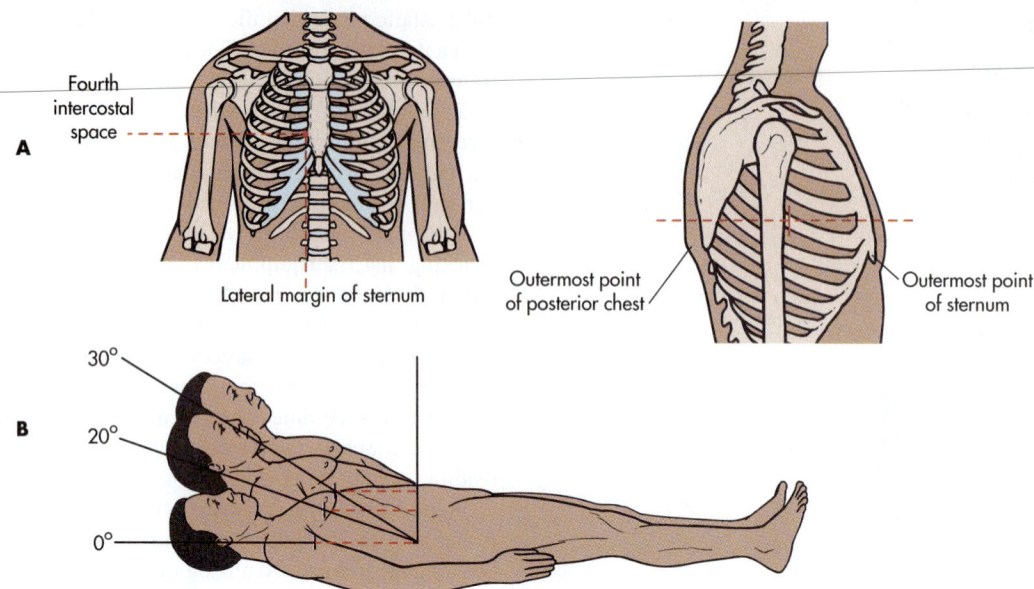

Fig. 63-3   Identification of the phlebostatic axis. **A,** The phlebostatic axis is an external landmark used to identify the level of the atrium in the supine patient. The phlebostatic axis is defined as the intersection of a plane drawn transversely through the fourth intercostal space at the sternum and a frontal plane drawn through the midchest, halfway between the outermost anterior and outermost posterior points of the chest. **B,** As the backrest of the supine patient is elevated, the phlebostatic axis remains at the same anatomic location, becoming progressively elevated from the floor. The zero reference point must be repositioned with changes in backrest elevation to keep it at the phlebostatic level.

Table **63-3**	Measurement of Blood Pressure with Invasive Lines

1. Explain the procedure to the patient.
2. Inactivate the high-pressure and low-pressure alarms for the duration of the procedure.
3. Identify and mark the phlebostatic axis on the patient's chest (mid–anterior-posterior chest at the fourth intercostal space [see Fig. 63-3]).
4. Position the patient supine and flat, or if appropriate, elevated up to 30°.
5. Confirm that the zero reference (port of the stopcock nearest the transducer) is placed at the level of the phlebostatic axis. It may be helpful to use a carpenter's level.
6. Observe the monitor tracing and assess the quality of the tracing. Check dynamic response.
7. Obtain an analog printout, if available, and measure the pressures of interest at end expiration. If no printout is available, freeze the tracing on the oscilloscope screen and use the cursor to measure the pressures at end expiration.
8. Reset the high-pressure and low-pressure alarms.
9. Record the pressure measurements promptly, including (if available) the printout marked to identify the points read.

catheter becomes dislodged or the line becomes disconnected. To avoid this serious complication, the nurse uses Luer-Lok connections and always activates (and records activation of) the low-pressure alarm. Thus if the pressure in the line falls (as it would when the line is disconnected), an alarm sounds immediately, allowing prompt repair of the problem. Pressure is always monitored when an arterial line is in place, even if the line was placed for ABG sampling.

Infection is a risk with any invasive line. The nurse should inspect the insertion site for inflammation and exudate and monitor the patient for signs of systemic infection. When infection occurs, the catheter, tubing, flushing apparatus, and transducers must be changed.

Circulatory impairment can result from formation of a thrombus around the catheter, release of an embolus, spasm, or occlusion of the circulation by the catheter. Before inserting a line into the radial artery, Allen's test should be performed to confirm that ulnar circulation is sufficient to sustain the hand. In this test, pressure is applied to the radial and ulnar arteries simultaneously. The patient is instructed to open and close the hand repeatedly. The hand should blanch. The nurse then releases the pressure on the ulnar artery while compressing the radial artery. If pinkness fails to return within 6 seconds, the ulnar artery is insufficient, indicating that the radial artery should not be used for line insertion.

Once the catheter is inserted, the nurse should evaluate the circulation distal to the arterial insertion site hourly. The limb with compromised arterial flow will appear cool and pale, with capillary refill greater than 3 seconds. There may be symptoms of neurologic impairment, such as tingling or paresthesia. Circulatory impairment can result in loss of a limb and is an emergency. In addition, the nurse should maintain the continuous flush irrigation system.

Pulmonary Artery Flow-Directed Catheter. Pulmonary artery (PA) pressure monitoring is used to guide acute-phase management in patients with complicated cardiac and intravascular volume problems (Table 63-4). PA diastolic (PAD) pressure and PAWP are sensitive indicators of fluid volume status and cardiac function. PAD pressure and

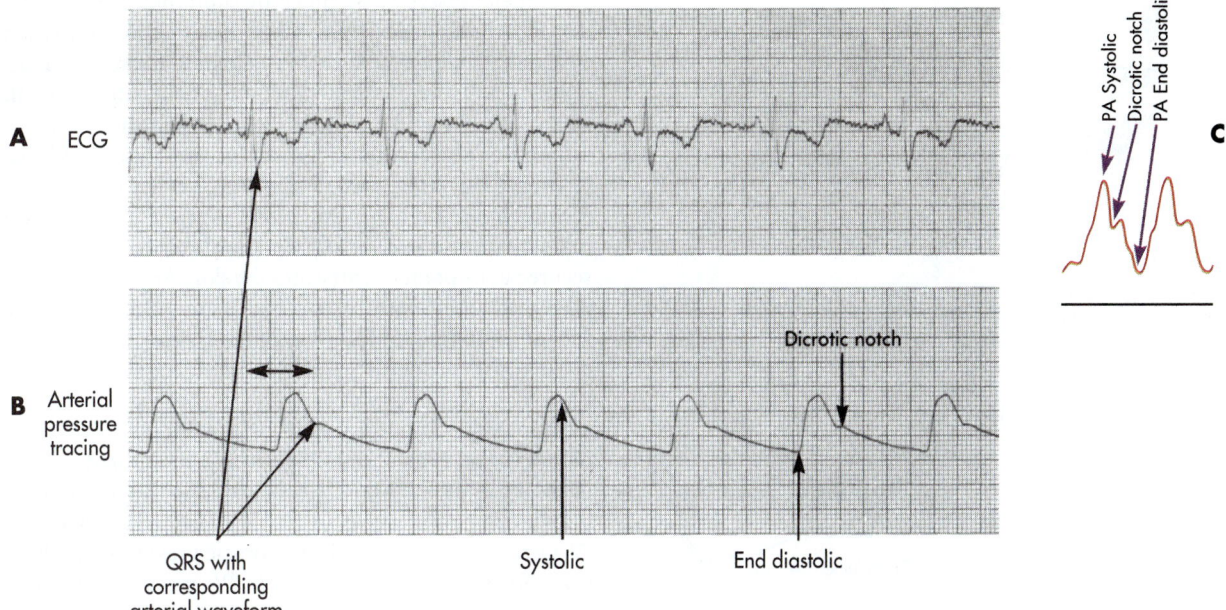

Fig. 63-4 **A,** Simultaneously recorded electrocardiogram tracing and **B,** systemic arterial pressure tracing. **C,** Pulmonary artery waveform. Systolic pressure is the peak pressure. The dicrotic notch indicates aortic valve closure. Diastolic pressure is the lowest value before contraction. Mean pressure is the average pressure over time calculated by the monitoring equipment. *PA,* pulmonary artery.

Table **63-4**	Clinical Indications for Pulmonary Artery Catheterization

- Acute respiratory distress syndrome
- Acute respiratory failure in patients with chronic obstructive pulmonary disease
- Cardiac tamponade
- Cardiogenic or noncardiogenic pulmonary edema
- Complex fluid imbalance (burns, sepsis)
- Evaluation of circulatory syndromes (mitral valve regurgitation and intraventricular shunts)
- Intraaortic balloon support
- Myocardial infarction with left ventricular failure or cardiogenic shock
- Perioperative fluid imbalance in high risk patients
- Septic and hypovolemic shock
- Vasoactive pharmacologic support

PAWP are increased in fluid volume overload and heart failure. They are decreased with volume deficit. Fluid therapy based on PA pressure allows restoration of fluid balance while avoiding overcorrection of the problem. Monitoring PA pressures can allow precise therapeutic manipulation of preload, which allows CO to be maintained without placing the patient at risk for pulmonary edema.

A PA flow-directed catheter (e.g., Swan-Ganz) is used to measure PA pressures, including PAWP. The standard PA catheter is no. 7 French, 43 in (110 cm) long, with four lumens (Fig. 63-5). When properly positioned, the distal lumen (catheter tip) is within the pulmonary artery (Fig. 63-6). This lumen is used to monitor PA pressures and withdraw mixed venous blood specimens (e.g., to evaluate oxygen saturation). The distal lumen is surrounded by a balloon connected to an exter-

nal valve via a second lumen. Balloon inflation has two purposes: (1) to allow moving blood to float the catheter forward and (2) to allow PAWP measurement. The third and fourth lumens are proximal, with exit ports in the right atrium. These are used for measurement of CVP, infusion of fluid and drugs, injection of fluid for CO determination, and withdrawal of blood specimens. The larger of the two proximal lumens is used for blood specimen collection. Often, when the patient is receiving total parenteral nutrition (TPN), the smaller proximal lumen is reserved for TPN infusion and is not interrupted for blood testing or injections. A thermistor located near the distal tip is wired to an external connector. The thermistor allows monitoring of core temperature and is used in the thermodilution method of measuring CO.

In addition to these relatively standard and common features of the PA flow-directed catheter, catheters with other features are available. One modification is the inclusion of an atrial electrode, useful in recording the atrial ECG or pacing the heart. Another common modification is inclusion of a fiberoptic sensor in the distal tip that detects mixed venous oxygen saturation. Another type of catheter provides continuous measurement of right ventricular volume and ejection fraction, while another catheter provides continuous CO monitoring. The pulmonary artery catheter sheath usually has a side port that serves as another intravenous line. Most catheters also have a plastic "sleeve" connected to the sheath, which permits manipulation of the catheter without breaking sterility.

Pulmonary artery catheter insertion. Before pulmonary artery catheter insertion, the nurse notes the patient's electrolyte, acid-base, oxygenation, and coagulation status. Imbalances such as hypokalemia, hypomagnesemia, hypoxemia, or acidosis can make the heart more irritable and increase the risk of ventricular arrhythmia during catheter insertion. Coagulopathy increases the risk of hemorrhage. The nurse prepares

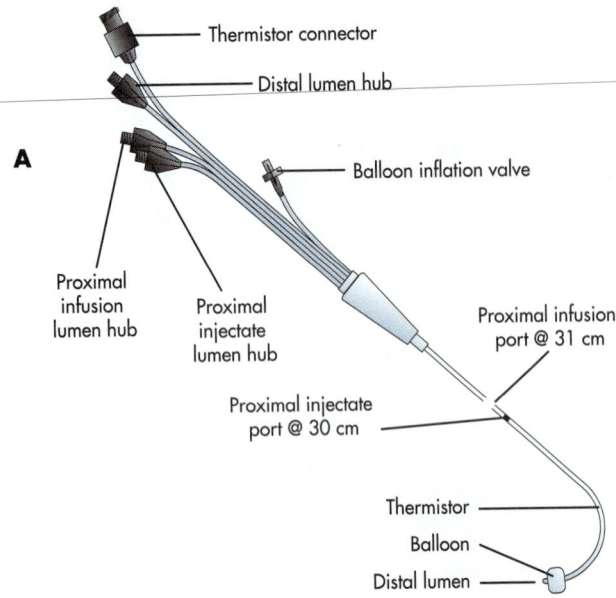

A

Thermistor connector

Distal lumen hub

Balloon inflation valve

Proximal infusion lumen hub

Proximal injectate lumen hub

Proximal infusion port @ 31 cm

Proximal injectate port @ 30 cm

Thermistor

Balloon

Distal lumen

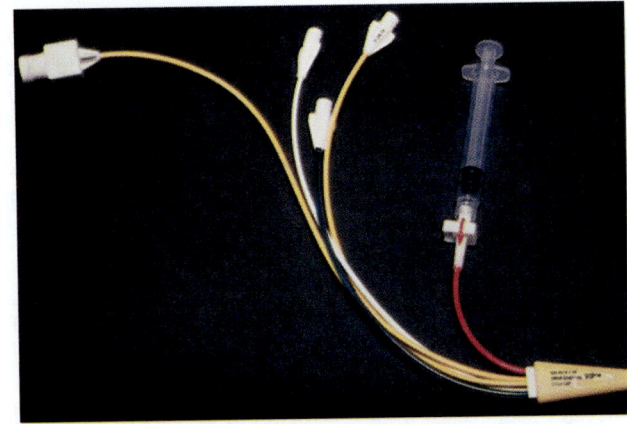

B

Fig. 63-5   Venous infusion port pulmonary artery (PA) catheter. **A,** The illustrated catheter has four lumens. When properly positioned, the distal lumen exit port is in the PA and the proximal lumen ports are in the right atrium. The distal and one of the proximal ports are used to measure PA and central venous pressures, respectively. A balloon surrounds the catheter near the distal end. The balloon inflation valve is used to inflate the balloon with air to allow reading of the pulmonary artery wedge pressure. A thermistor located near the distal tip senses PA temperature and is used to measure thermodilution cardiac output when solution cooler than body temperature is injected into a proximal port. **B,** Actual catheter.

for the procedure by preparing the monitor, cables, and flush and infusion solutions. The system is zero referenced to the phlebostatic axis. The patient is prepared for the procedure by explaining what will happen, and informed consent is obtained. The patient is positioned supine with the head of the bed tilted downward if tolerated.

The PA catheter is inserted through a sheath percutaneously into a deep peripheral vein using surgical asepsis. Venous cutdown is rarely required. Internal jugular, subclavian, antecubital, or femoral veins are acceptable insertion sites. The line is then advanced through the venous system to the heart.

Catheter insertion is guided by continuously observing the distal port (catheter tip) waveform on the monitor. When the tip reaches the right atrium, the balloon is inflated with the recommended volume of air. The catheter is floated through the tricuspid valve into the right ventricle and then through the pulmonic valve and into the PA. Once a typical PAWP tracing (see Fig. 63-6) is observed, the balloon is deflated. Following insertion, a chest x-ray is obtained to confirm the position. To maintain the catheter in its proper position, the catheter is then secured at its point of entry into the skin. An occlusive dressing is applied and changed according to unit protocol. It is necessary to monitor the ECG continuously during insertion because of the risk for arrhythmias, particularly when the catheter reaches the right ventricle.

Pulmonary artery pressure measurements. Systolic, diastolic, and mean pressures are routinely monitored. PA systolic is the peak pressure and PA diastolic is the lowest pressure point. Mean PA pressure is the time-weighted average. Because PA ports are in the chest, intrathoracic pressures alter PA pressure. To produce consistent data, PA measurements are obtained at the end of expiration.

The measurement of PAWP is obtained by slowly inflating the balloon with 1.5 ml of air while observing the distal lumen pressure tracing. Before inflation the pressure tracing visualized on the monitor looks like an arterial tracing, with a systolic peak, dicrotic notch, and then the diastolic low point. As the line becomes "wedged," the tracing changes shape and amplitude. The typical wedged waveform is characterized by two small waves, the A and V waves. The A wave indicates atrial contraction. The A wave is followed by the X descent, indicating atrial relaxation. Then the V wave is seen during the interval between the T and P waves of the ECG. The V wave indicates venous inflow into the atrium when the mitral valve is closed and the ventricle is contracting. The V wave is followed by the Y descent, indicating the emptying of the atrium when the mitral valve opens and ventricular filling.

When the tracing changes from arterial to atrial, the catheter is said to be wedged and PAWP is measured at the end of expiration. When measuring the wedge pressure, the balloon should be inflated for less than four respiratory cycles. There is danger of rupture of the pulmonary artery if the balloon is inflated too long or if the catheter migrates distally into a smaller vessel. This is suspected when less than 1.25 ml is needed to wedge the tracing, or an "overwedge" tracing is obtained. Readings should be acquired from an analog strip pressure recording, and the strip should be placed into the patient's record. If a printout of the tracing is not available, the readings should be taken from the monitor using the cursor.

Central venous or right atrial pressure measurement. CVP is a measurement of right ventricular preload. It can be measured with a PA catheter using one of the proximal lumens. Occasionally a CVP line may be placed. CVP is measured as a mean pressure at the end of expiration. CVP waveforms (Fig. 63-7) are similar to PAWP waveforms. Although the PA diastolic pressure and PAWP are more sensitive indicators of fluid volume status, CVP also reflects fluid volume problems. An elevated CVP indicates right ventricular failure or volume overload. A low CVP indicates hypovolemia.

Thermodilution cardiac output measurement. CO is frequently monitored in patients with hemodynamic instability.

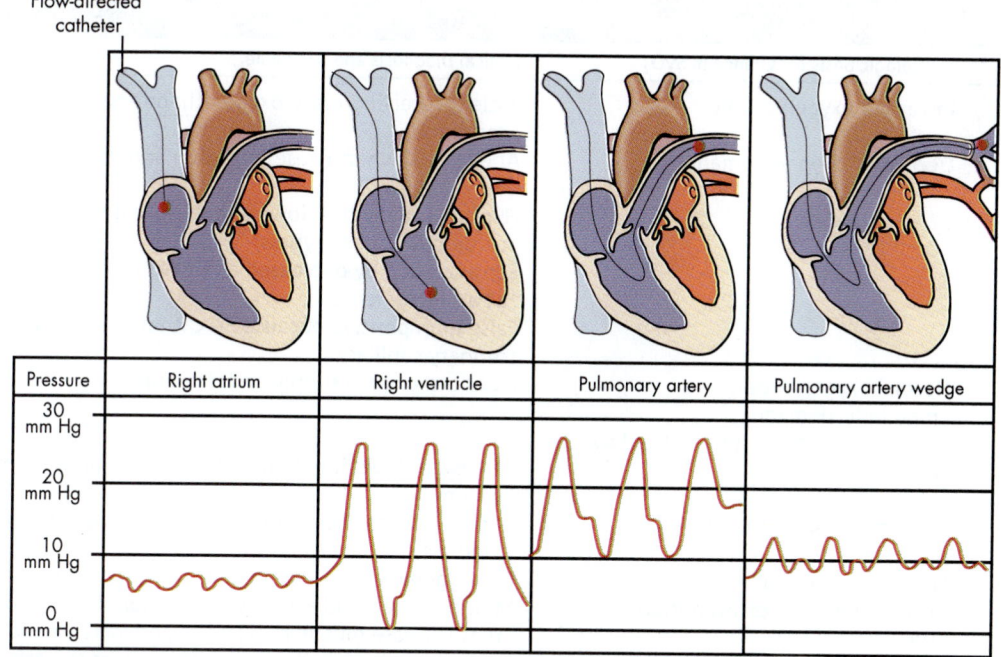

Fig. 63-6 Position of the pulmonary artery flow-directed catheter during progressive stages of insertion with corresponding pressure waveforms.

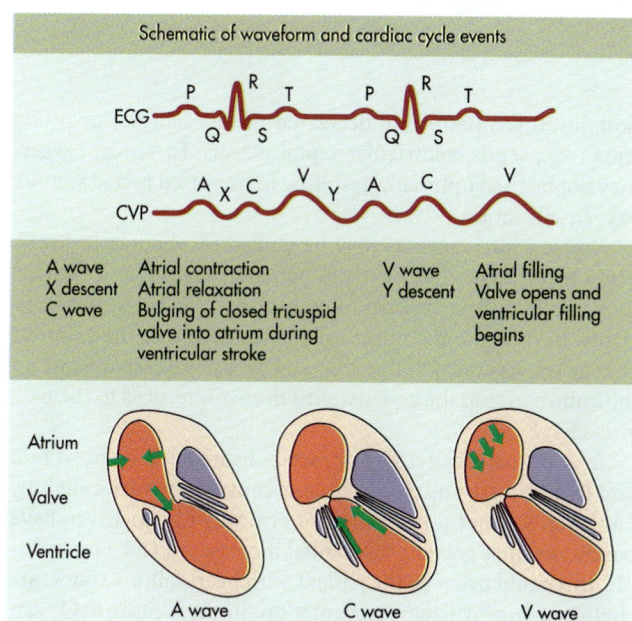

Fig. 63-7 Cardiac events that produce the CVP waveform with A, C, and V waves. A wave represents atrial contraction. X descent represents atrial relaxation. C wave represents the bulging of the closed tricuspid valve into the right atrium during ventricular systole. V wave represents atrial filling. Y descent represents opening of the tricuspid valve and filling of the ventricle.

Normal resting CO is 4 to 8 L per minute and varies with body size. Cardiac index (CI) is CO divided by body surface area. Cardiac index can be compared among individuals of varying body sizes. The normal cardiac index is 2.2 to 4.0 L/min/m². The CO is decreased in conditions such as hypovolemia, car-

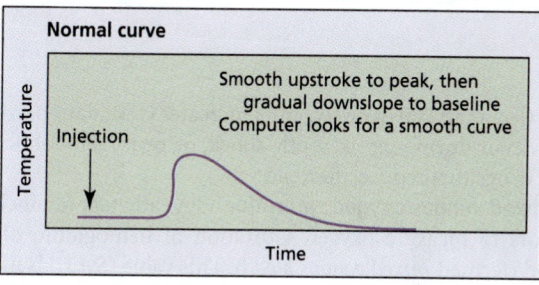

Fig. 63-8 Normal cardiac output curve. Cardiac output is calculated from the temperature change in the pulmonary artery when a fixed volume of a cool solution is injected into the proximal port in the right atrium. The nurse should visualize the curve and make sure that it is smooth. The larger the curve, the smaller the cardiac output.

diogenic shock, and heart failure. Under normal conditions, CO increases with exercise. Increases in CO at rest indicate a hyperdynamic state seen with fever or sepsis.

The PA catheter is commonly used to measure CO by thermodilution. With this technique, a known amount of solution (saline or 5% dextrose in water) of known temperature (room temperature or chilled) is injected rapidly into the right atrial lumen of the PA catheter. The drop in blood temperature is detected by a thermistor embedded in the catheter tip in the pulmonary artery. The CO computer is programmed to calculate the CO from the temperature waveform. The larger the curve, the smaller the CO (Fig. 63-8).

SVR can be calculated each time CO is measured. The formula for calculating SVR is shown in Table 63-2. Normal SVR is 800 to 1200 dyne sec/cm⁵. Increased SVR indicates vasoconstriction from shock, increased release or administration of epinephrine or norepinephrine, or left ventricular failure. A low

Table 63-5   Clinical Interpretation of SvO₂ Measurements

SvO₂ Measurement	Physiologic Basis for Change in SvO₂	Clinical Diagnosis and Rationale
High SvO₂ (80-95%)	Increased oxygen supply	Patient receiving more oxygen than required by clinical condition
	Decreased oxygen demand	Anesthesia, which causes sedation and decreased muscle movement.
		Hypothermia, which lowers metabolic demand (e.g., with cardiopulmonary bypass)
		Sepsis caused by decreased ability of tissues to use oxygen at a cellular level
		False high positive because PA catheter is wedged in a pulmonary capillary
Normal SvO₂ (60-80%)	Normal oxygen supply and metabolic demand	Balanced oxygen supply and demand
Low SvO₂ (less than 60%)	Decreased oxygen supply caused by: Low hemoglobin	Anemia or bleeding with compromised cardiopulmonary system
	Low arterial saturation (SaO₂)	Hypoxemia resulting from decreased oxygen supply or lung disease
	Low cardiac output	Cardiogenic shock caused by left ventricular pump failure
	Increased oxygen consumption (VO₂)	Metabolic demand exceeds oxygen supply in conditions that increase muscle movement and increase metabolic rate, including physiologic states such as shivering, seizures, and hyperthermia and nursing interventions such as obtaining bedscale weight and turning

From Thelan LA and others, editors: *Critical care nursing: diagnosis and management,* ed 3, St Louis, 1998, Mosby.

SVR (less than 800 dyne sec/cm⁵) indicates vasodilation, which may occur during sepsis, septic shock, or neurogenic shock or with drugs that reduce afterload.

Mixed venous oxygen saturation. PA catheters can include sensors to measure oxygen saturation of hemoglobin of PA blood (termed *mixed venous blood*). This value (SvO₂) is useful in determining the adequacy of tissue oxygenation. SvO₂ reflects the dynamic balance between oxygenation of the arterial blood, tissue perfusion, and tissue oxygen consumption. SvO₂, when considered in conjunction with the arterial oxygen saturation, is useful in analyzing hemodynamic status and response to treatments or activities (Table 63-5). Normal SvO₂ at rest is 60% to 80%.

Sustained decreases and increases in SvO₂ must be analyzed carefully. Decreased SvO₂ may indicate decreased arterial oxygenation, low CO, low hemoglobin, or increased oxygen consumption. If the SvO₂ falls, the nurse determines which of these four factors has changed. The nurse can observe for a change in arterial oxygenation by monitoring pulse oximetry or ABG analysis. Tissue perfusion can be grossly assessed by noting CO and organ function indicators (mentation, urine output, skin color). If arterial oxygenation, hemoglobin, and tissue perfusion are unchanged, a fall in SvO₂ indicates increased oxygen consumption, which could result from an increased metabolic rate, pain, movement, or fever. If oxygen consumption increases without a comparable increase in CO, more oxygen is extracted from the blood and SvO₂ falls. Similarly, when CO falls but arterial oxygenation and oxygen consumption are unchanged, the SvO₂ falls.

Increased SvO₂ is also clinically significant and may indicate a clinical improvement (e.g., increased arterial oxygen satura-

tion, improved perfusion, decreased metabolic rate) or problems (e.g., sepsis, ventricular septal defect). In sepsis, oxygen may not be used optimally, resulting in increased mixed venous oxygen saturation.

Nursing interventions may be guided by changes in SvO₂. The nurse might note that the patient's heart rate increased moderately during repositioning but that the SvO₂ remained stable. In this case the nurse might conclude that the position change was tolerated. If the SvO₂ had dropped, this would be an indication to stop the activity until the SvO₂ returns to the previous level.

In many cases as activity or metabolism increases, heart rate and CO increase and SvO₂ remains constant or varies slightly. However, it is not uncommon for critically ill patients to have conditions that prevent substantial increases in CO. For example, this could occur in the patient with heart failure, shock, arrhythmias, or cardiac transplantation. In these cases, SvO₂ can provide a useful indicator of the balance between oxygen consumption and perfusion.

Complications with pulmonary artery catheters. Like arterial catheters, PA catheters are associated with an increased risk of thrombus and embolus formation, and the PA catheter is continuously flushed with a slow infusion of saline solution to prevent thrombus formation. If a thrombus begins to form, the waveform appears blunted.

Infection and sepsis are serious problems associated with PA catheters. Careful surgical asepsis for insertion and maintenance of the catheter and tubing line is mandatory to prevent infection. The skin is cleaned according to unit procedure, usually with an iodine preparation. The insertion site is covered with a sterile occlusive dressing. The nurse should monitor the patient for local and systemic signs of infection (e.g., redness and exudate at the insertion site, fever, increased white blood cell count). The PA catheter must be removed if there are local or systemic signs of infection. To reduce the risk of infection, PA catheters should not be left in place any longer than necessary.

Air embolus is another risk associated with PA catheters. Air embolus can be caused by balloon rupture or by injection of air into the lumen of a ruptured balloon. The nurse decreases the risk of embolus by injecting only the prescribed volume of air into the balloon. Catheters are checked for balloon leak before insertion; defective catheters are not used. If the nurse observes that the catheter cannot be wedged or that injected air does not flow back into the syringe, the catheter should be so labeled and the physician notified. The nurse should use Luer-Lok connections on all pressure line connections. For lines that are used to monitor pressure, the nurse sets the low alarm limit to activate if the pressure in the line drops substantially. Any time the line must be opened to change the apparatus, the nurse closes the line to the patient via clamping or stopcocks.

The patient with a PA catheter is at risk for pulmonary infarction or PA rupture from the following causes: (1) the balloon may rupture, releasing fragments that could embolize; (2) balloon inflation may obstruct blood flow; (3) the catheter may advance into a wedge position, obstructing blood flow; and (4) a thrombus could form and embolize. To reduce the risk of pulmonary infarction and rupture, the balloon must never be inflated with more than 1.5 ml. The balloon must not be left inflated for more than four breaths (except during insertion). PA pressure waveforms are monitored continuously for evidence of catheter occlusion, dislocation, or spontaneous wedging. The pressure tracing will be blunted if the catheter starts to be occluded. The pressure tracing will appear wedged if the PA catheter advances and becomes spontaneously wedged. In each of these cases, the catheter must be immediately repositioned.

Ventricular arrhythmias can occur during PA catheter insertion or removal or if the tip migrates back from the PA to the right ventricle. The catheter should be repositioned, usually by the physician.

Noninvasive Arterial Oxygenation Monitoring.

Pulse oximetry is a noninvasive and continuous method of determining arterial oxygenation. Oxygenated and reduced (desaturated) hemoglobin absorb light differently. The pulse oximeter estimates the arterial oxygen saturation by detecting the differences in the light absorption by the two forms of hemoglobin. A light-emitting diode (LED) in the probe tip emits light at two specific wavelengths. The light is transmitted through the capillary bed of a finger or earlobe to a photodetector. Arterial hemoglobin is normally 95% to 100% saturated with oxygen.

A common use for pulse oximetry is to determine the effectiveness of oxygen therapy. By continuously monitoring with the pulse oximeter, there is less need for ABG sampling. Decreased arterial saturation indicates inadequate oxygenation of the blood in the pulmonary capillaries. This may be corrected by increasing the fraction of inspired oxygen (FIO_2). Similarly, the nurse uses the pulse oximeter to monitor how the patient tolerates a decreased FIO_2. Continuous monitoring of oxygenation is also useful to monitor the patient's response to changes in position and treatments. For example, the nurse might note that arterial saturation falls when the patient is positioned in a left lateral recumbent position. The nurse could then plan position changes that pose less risk for the patient.

Pulse oximetry may be inaccurate in the setting of (1) vasoconstriction from hypoperfusion or hypothermia, (2) patient movement, or (3) bright ambient light. Placing the probe on the earlobe or bridge of the nose may solve the problem of hypoperfusion. Obtaining readings only during rest will solve the second problem. Covering the probe with a towel will solve the third problem.

NURSING MANAGEMENT: HEMODYNAMIC MONITORING

Assessment of hemodynamic status requires integration of data from many sources and comparison of the data over time. Observations include the patient's general appearance, skin color, vital signs, and organ function. The nurse should begin with the patient's general appearance. Does the patient appear weak, tired, exhausted? There may be too little cardiac reserve to sustain minimum activity. Changing skin color or temperature may indicate decreased CO. If the patient is bleeding and developing shock, blood pressure might initially be relatively stable, yet the patient may become increasingly pale and cool from peripheral vasoconstriction. The nurse can confirm suspicion of impending shock by noting the SVR, which would increase in these circumstances. Conversely, the patient may remain warm and pink yet develop tachycardia and blood pressure instability. These features are characteristic of septic shock. The suspicion can be confirmed with measurements of CO, which would initially increase with septic shock, and of SVR, which would decrease.

The heart rate is often a useful indicator of the hemodynamic state. As tissue perfusion becomes compromised, heart rate increases. Although heart rates of 100 beats per minute are common among stressed, compromised, critically ill patients, further increases in heart rate may indicate compromised perfusion. In patients in whom heart rate cannot increase, such as those with atrioventricular block, the SvO_2 can be a useful indicator of impending compromise.

In addition to high technology measurements available to the ICU nurse, simple observations may provide useful insights into the patient's hemodynamic status. Mental clarity may reflect cerebral perfusion. Urine output may reflect renal perfusion. The patient with diminished gastrointestinal perfusion may develop hypoactive or absent bowel sounds and may have nausea and vomiting when gastrointestinal motility is impaired by a lack of perfusion. By carefully monitoring the patient, the astute nurse is able to recognize early clues and manage problems before they escalate.

CIRCULATORY ASSIST DEVICES

Mechanical circulatory assist devices, such as the intraaortic balloon pump (IABP) and left ventricular assist device (VAD), are used to decrease cardiac work and improve organ perfusion in patients with heart failure when conventional drug therapy is no longer adequate. The type of device used depends on the extent and nature of the myocardial problem and the

Table **63-6**	Indications and Contraindications for the Intraaortic Balloon Pump

Indications

Unstable angina (when medications have failed)
Severe cardiac disease as a bridge to cardiac transplant
Acute myocardial infarction with any of the following:*
    Ventricular aneurysm accompanied by ventricular arrhythmias
    Acute ventricular septal defect
    Acute mitral valve regurgitation
    Cardiogenic shock
    Continuing chest pain
Preoperative, intraoperative, and postoperative open heart surgery (e.g., aneurysectomy, revascularization, or valve replacement); often used to wean from cardiopulmonary bypass

Contraindications

Irreversible brain damage
Terminal or untreatable diseases of any major organ system
Ruptured or dissecting aortic or thoracic aneurysm
Generalized peripheral vascular disease (may prevent placement of balloon)
Incompetent aortic valve (considered an *absolute* contraindication)

*Allows time for emergency angiography and corrective cardiac surgery to be performed.

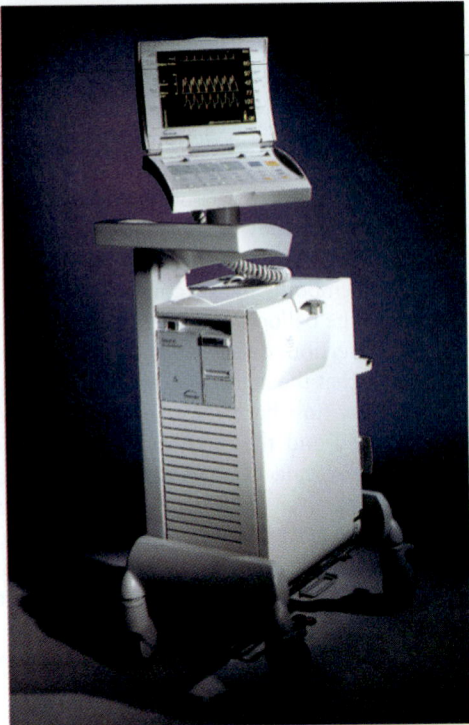

Fig. 63-9 Intraaortic balloon pump machine.

capabilities of the institution and staff. Circulatory assist devices provide interim support in three types of situations: (1) the left ventricle requires support while recovering from acute injury; (2) the heart requires surgical repair (e.g., a ruptured septum) but the patient must be stabilized and preparations made for the procedure; and (3) the patient in end-stage heart failure awaits cardiac transplantation. All circulatory assist devices decrease left ventricular workload, increase myocardial perfusion, and augment circulation. The most commonly used device is the IABP, and thus most ICU nurses encounter patients receiving IABP support. Several types of VADs are available, and additional devices are under development.

Intraaortic Balloon Pump

The IABP provides temporary circulatory assistance to the compromised heart by reducing afterload (via reduction in systolic pressure) and augmenting the aortic diastolic pressure. Table 63-6 lists clinical conditions for which the IABP is used. The IABP consists of a sausage-shaped balloon, a pump that inflates and deflates the balloon, control devices for synchronizing the balloon inflation to the cardiac cycle, and fail-safe devices (Figs. 63-9 and 63-10). The balloon is inserted percutaneously or surgically into the femoral artery, advanced toward the heart, and positioned in the descending thoracic aorta just below the left subclavian artery. Following placement, the position is confirmed with an x-ray. A pneumatic device cyclically fills the balloon with helium during diastole and deflates it just before systole. The ECG is used to trigger deflation on the R wave and inflation on the T wave. The arterial pressure tracing is used to refine timing. IABP support is referred to as *counterpulsation* because the timing of balloon inflation is opposite to ventricular contraction.

Effects of Counterpulsation. The balloon is rapidly inflated at the start of diastole, immediately after aortic valve closure, partially occluding the aorta (see Fig. 63-10). Displaced blood is forced forward into the extremities and back into the coronary arteries and main branches of the aortic arch. Diastolic arterial pressure rises (diastolic augmentation), increasing coronary artery perfusion pressure and perfusion of vital organs. The rise in coronary artery perfusion pressure causes an increase in blood flow to the myocardium. The balloon is rapidly deflated just before systole. The suddenly created vacuum causes aortic pressure to drop. With aortic resistance to left ventricular ejection reduced (reduced afterload), the left ventricle empties more easily and completely. As with other types of afterload reduction, the stroke volume increases, yet the myocardial oxygen consumption decreases. Hemodynamic effects of the IABP are summarized in Table 63-7.

Complications with Intraaortic Balloon Pumps. Complications are common with the IABP.[17-19] Vascular injuries such as dislodging of plaque, arterial dissection, and compromised distal extremity circulation are common, occurring in 3% to 65% of cases. Thrombus and embolus formation add to the risk of distal circulatory compromise. Peripheral nerve damage can occur, particularly when a cutdown is performed for insertion. To reduce these risks, hourly neurovascular assessment is necessary. Because the balloon pumping can cause physical destruction of platelets, mild thrombocytopenia is common and coagulation status indicators are monitored. Displacement of the balloon can occlude the left subclavian, renal, or mesenteric arteries. Patients on IABP therapy are prone to infection, as is any patient with invasive lines. Insertion site infection or sepsis caused by an unknown source necessitates catheter removal.

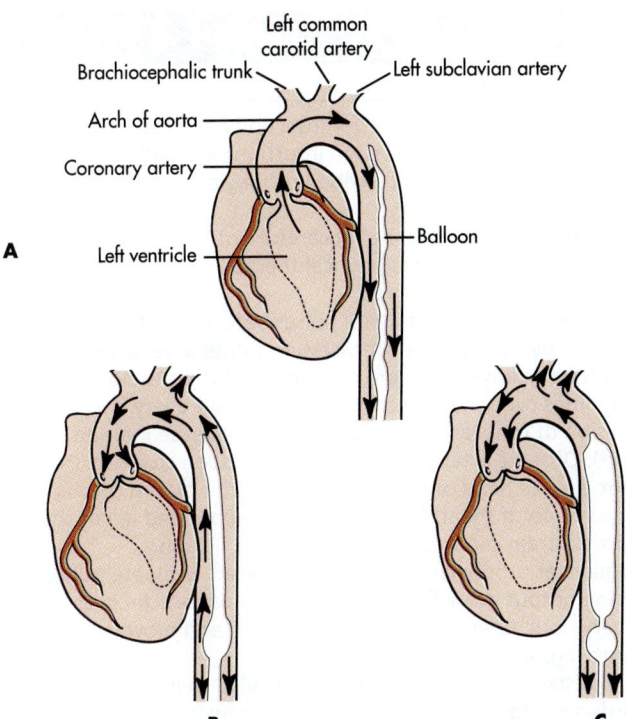

Fig. 63-10 Intraaortic balloon pump. **A,** During systole the balloon is deflated, which facilitates ejection of the blood into the periphery where systemic arterial resistance vessels are perfused. **B,** In early diastole, the balloon begins to inflate. **C,** In late diastole, the balloon is totally inflated, which augments aortic pressure and increases the coronary perfusion pressure with the end result of increased coronary and cerebral blood flow.

Mechanical complications are rare but may occur. Improper timing of balloon inflation may cause increased afterload, decreased CO, myocardial ischemia, and increased myocardial oxygen use and must be immediately corrected by the nurse. If the balloon develops a leak, the catheter must be changed immediately to avoid a gas embolus. Signs of a leak include less effective augmentation and blood backing up into the catheter. A malfunction of the balloon or console triggers fail-safe alarms and automatic shutdown of the unit.

The patient with an IABP is relatively immobile, limited to side-lying or supine positions with the head of the bed elevated no more than 30 to 40 degrees. The leg in which the catheter is inserted must not be flexed at the hip. The patient may be receiving ventilatory support and will likely have multiple invasive lines that increase the challenge of comfortable positioning. The patient may experience sleeplessness and anxiety. Adequate sedation, pain relief, skin care, and comfort measures are required.

As the patient improves, he or she is "weaned" from the IABP; that is, circulatory support provided by the IABP is gradually reduced. Weaning involves reducing the pumping to every second or third beat or decreasing augmentation pressure until the IABP catheter is removed. Even if the patient is stable without IABP, pumping is continued every third or fourth beat until the line is removed. This reduces the risk of thrombus formation around the catheter. Detailed, frequent hemodynamic assessment continues to be required during the weaning phase.

Table 63-7	Hemodynamic Effects of Intraaortic Balloon Pumps

Effects of Inflation During Diastole
Increased diastolic pressure (may exceed systolic pressure)
Increased pressure in the aortic root during diastole
Increased coronary perfusion pressure
Improved oxygen delivery to the myocardium
  Decreased angina pain
  Decreased electrocardiographic evidence of ischemia
  Decreased ventricular ectopy

Effects of Deflation During Systole
Decreased afterload
Decreased peak systolic pressure
Decreased myocardial oxygen consumption
Increased stroke volume, possibly associated with:
  Improved sensorium
  Warmed skin
  Increased urine output
  Decreased heart rate
Increased forward flow of blood, decreasing preload
  Decreased PA pressures, including PAWP
  Decreased crackles

NURSING MANAGEMENT: INTRAAORTIC BALLOON PUMP

The patient with an IABP requires highly skilled nursing care. Detailed cardiovascular assessment, including measurement of vital signs, hemodynamic pressures, CO, cardiac auscultation, and cardiac rhythm evaluation, is performed frequently. Assessments of myocardial ischemia (indicated by T-wave inversion, ST segment changes, chest pain) skin color and temperature, mentation, urine output, and bowel sounds are also performed at regular intervals. It is expected that with continuing IABP treatment these parameters should improve. Nursing management of IABP complications is presented in Table 63-8.

Ventricular Assist Devices

The VAD provides longer-term support for the failing heart (usually days to months) and allows more mobility than the IABP. There are several types of VAD. VADs work by being inserted into the path of the flowing blood to augment or replace the ventricle. For example, a typical arrangement would shunt the blood from the left atrium or ventricle into the VAD and then into the aorta. Other arrangements allow biventricular support. The types of VAD are listed in Table 63-9. A typical VAD is illustrated in Fig. 63-11.

Failure to wean from cardiopulmonary bypass after surgery has been the primary indicator for VAD support. Increasingly the VAD is used to support patients with ventricular failure caused by myocardial infarction and patients awaiting cardiac transplantation. A VAD is a temporary device with the capability to partially or totally support circulation until the heart recovers or a donor heart can be obtained. Cannula sites depend on the type of device used. For support of the right side of the heart, the right atrium and PA are cannulated. The left

Table **63-8**	Nursing Management: Potential Complications of the Intraaortic Balloon Pump
Potential Complication	**Nursing Management**
Site infection from invasive lines	Use strict aseptic technique for insertion and dressing changes for all lines. Cover all insertion sites with occlusive dressings. Administer prescribed prophylactic antibiotic for entire course of therapy.
Pneumonia associated with immobilization	Reposition patient q2hr, being careful not to displace balloon. If patient requires physical therapy of the chest, avoid introducing an ECG artifact.
Arterial trauma caused by insertion or displacement of balloon	Evaluate and mark peripheral pulses before insertion of balloon to use as baseline for assessing pulses after insertion. After insertion of balloon, evaluate perfusion to both extremities every hour. Measure urine output every hour (occlusion of renal arteries causes severe decrease in urine output). Observe arterial waveforms for sudden changes. Do not elevate head of bed higher than 30° if placed through a sheath; 40° if sheathless. Do not flex cannulated leg at the hip. Restrain cannulated leg to prevent flexion.
Thromboembolism caused by trauma, balloon obstruction of blood flow distal to catheter	Administer prophylactic heparin if ordered. Evaluate pulses, urine output every hour. Evaluate level of consciousness every hour. Check circulation, sensation, and movement in both legs every hour.
Hematologic complications caused by platelet aggregation along the balloon (decrease in platelets possible)	Administer Rheomacrodex (low-molecular-weight dextran) if ordered. Monitor coagulation status, hematocrit, and platelet count.
Hemorrhage from insertion site	Check site for bleeding every hour. Observe vital signs for hypovolemia with each vital sign check

Table **63-9**	Ventricular Assist Devices			
Type	**Example**	**Use**	**Description**
Centrifugal	Biomedicus	Univentricular or biventricular support	Blood is diverted to a cone-shaped pump head where blades rotate and propel blood back through return cannula via continuous (nonpulsatile) flow
Rotary	Hemopump	LV support	A propeller housed in the LV cannula draws blood from the LV and propels it into the aorta
Pneumatic	Thoratec	Univentricular or biventricular support	External pulsatile pump that uses a pressurized air sac to eject blood through outflow cannula
	Abiomed BVS 5000	Univentricular or biventricular support	A two-chamber external pump with bladders that fill by gravity; blood pumps are positioned at a level relative to the patient
	TCI Heartmate	LVAD	A pneumatically driven, totally implantable pump with external drive console
Electric	Novacor	LVAD	An electrically driven pulsatile pump that is implanted in an upper abdominal quadrant
	TCI Heartmate Vented Electric	LVAD	Totally implantable pump, powered by two 12-volt batteries or a direct power source
Cardiopulmonary support	Bard CPS	Emergency resuscitation (e.g., supported angioplasty)	Femoral-femoral bypass; venous blood delivered to centrifugal pump that passes through normothermic heat exchanger to membrane oxygenator and back to patient

Modified from Thelan LA and others, editors: *Critical care nursing: diagnosis and management,* ed 3, St Louis, 1998, Mosby.
LA, left atrium; *LV,* left ventricle; *LVAD,* left ventricular assist device; *PA,* pulmonary artery; *RA,* right atrium; *RVAD,* right ventricular assist device.

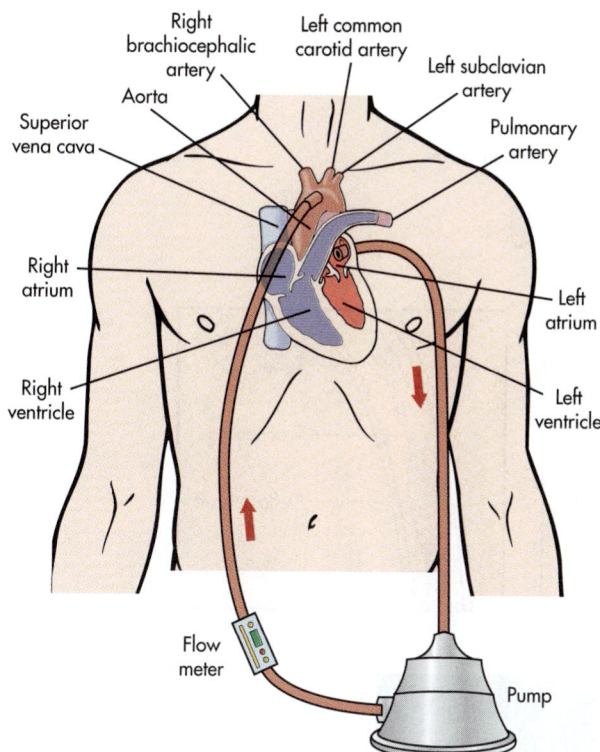

Fig. 63-11 Schematic diagram of a left ventricular assist device.

ventricular apex can be cannulated for left ventricular devices. Cannulation may occur at the bedside with femoral percutaneous technique or femoral cutdown. Direct cannulation of the atria and great vessels occurs in the operating room through a sternotomy.

Patient selection is critical. Three groups are recognized as potential candidates: (1) postcardiotomy patients, (2) those awaiting cardiac transplantation, and (3) patients with acute myocardial infarction in cardiogenic shock. Exclusion criteria include (1) significant aortic valve insufficiency, (2) major cerebrovascular accident, (3) body surface area less than 1.5 m^2, (4) sepsis, (5) life-limiting comorbid conditions (such as chronic renal failure, metastatic cancer, severe hepatic disease), and (6) comorbid conditions that would pose technical difficulties (coagulopathy, blood dyscrasia, certain infectious diseases, severe pulmonary disease).[20] Device selection depends on the institution and physician approval to use investigational or Food and Drug Administration (FDA)–approved devices.

Nursing care of the patient with a VAD is similar to that of the patient with an IABP. The patient is observed for bleeding, cardiac tamponade, ventricular failure, infection, arrhythmias, renal failure, hemolysis, and thromboembolism. The patient requires nutritional support. Unlike the patient with an IABP, who must remain in bed with limited position change, the patient with VAD is usually mobile and requires an activity plan.

Ideally, patients with VAD recover either through ventricular improvement or transplantation. However, many patients do die. Both the patient and family require psychologic support. Nursing care should include the family as much as possible. Other members of the health care team, such as social workers or clergy, should be notified to help the family and friends.

When the ventricle improves or transplantation occurs, the patient is taken to the operating room where the VAD is removed. Cannula sites are packed and wounds are closed. Usual wound care is followed after the patient is returned to the ICU.

The results of mechanical circulatory assist device use have been encouraging. With the development of new mechanical pumps that will act as biologic donor hearts and as cardiac replacements, nursing care will be a challenge.

ARTIFICIAL AIRWAYS

The patient in the ICU often requires mechanical assistance to maintain airway patency. An artificial airway is created by inserting a tube into the trachea, bypassing upper airway and laryngeal structures. A tube is placed into the trachea via the mouth or nose past the larynx (endotracheal [ET] intubation) or through the neck structures (tracheostomy). ET intubation is more common in ICU patients. It can be performed quickly without taking the patient to surgery. Tracheostomy is accomplished surgically and is used when the need for an artificial airway is more long term. Endotracheal tubes are illustrated in Fig. 63-12. Tracheostomies are discussed in Chapter 25 and illustrated in Fig. 25-6.

Indications for an artificial airway are to (1) prevent or relieve upper airway obstruction, (2) decrease aspiration when the patient lacks airway protection reflexes, (3) facilitate secretion removal when the patient cannot effectively clear the airway, and (4) provide a closed system for positive pressure mechanical ventilation. The patient who requires an artificial airway is often in acute respiratory distress and may have an altered level of consciousness.

Endotracheal Tubes

Endotracheal intubation can be performed by inserting the tube into the trachea through the mouth (oral intubation) or through the nose (nasal intubation). In oral intubation the endotracheal tube is passed through the mouth and vocal cords and into the trachea with the aid of a laryngoscope or bronchoscope. In nasal intubation, insertion is performed by manipulating the tube through the nose, nasopharynx, and vocal cords.

Oral ET intubation is the procedure of choice for most emergencies because the airway can be secured rapidly. Compared with the nasal route, a larger-diameter tube can be used for oral intubation. With a larger-bore tube, work of breathing is reduced because there is less airway resistance. It is easier to remove secretions and perform fiberoptic bronchoscopy if needed.

There are disadvantages of oral ET intubation. It is difficult to place an oral tube if head and neck mobility are limited. Salivation is increased and swallowing is difficult. A bite block or oral airway is used to stop the patient from biting and kinking the tube. The tube and bite block are taped to the face. Mouth care is a challenge. Finally, the larger tubes used in oral intubation are associated with laryngeal trauma and subglottic stenosis, particularly in smaller individuals (women).

Nasal ET intubation is sometimes preferred because it is more stable than the oral tube and more difficult to dislodge. It can be placed "blindly," that is, without visualizing the larynx, and thus is indicated when head and neck manipulation is risky. The nasal tube may be uncomfortable for some patients

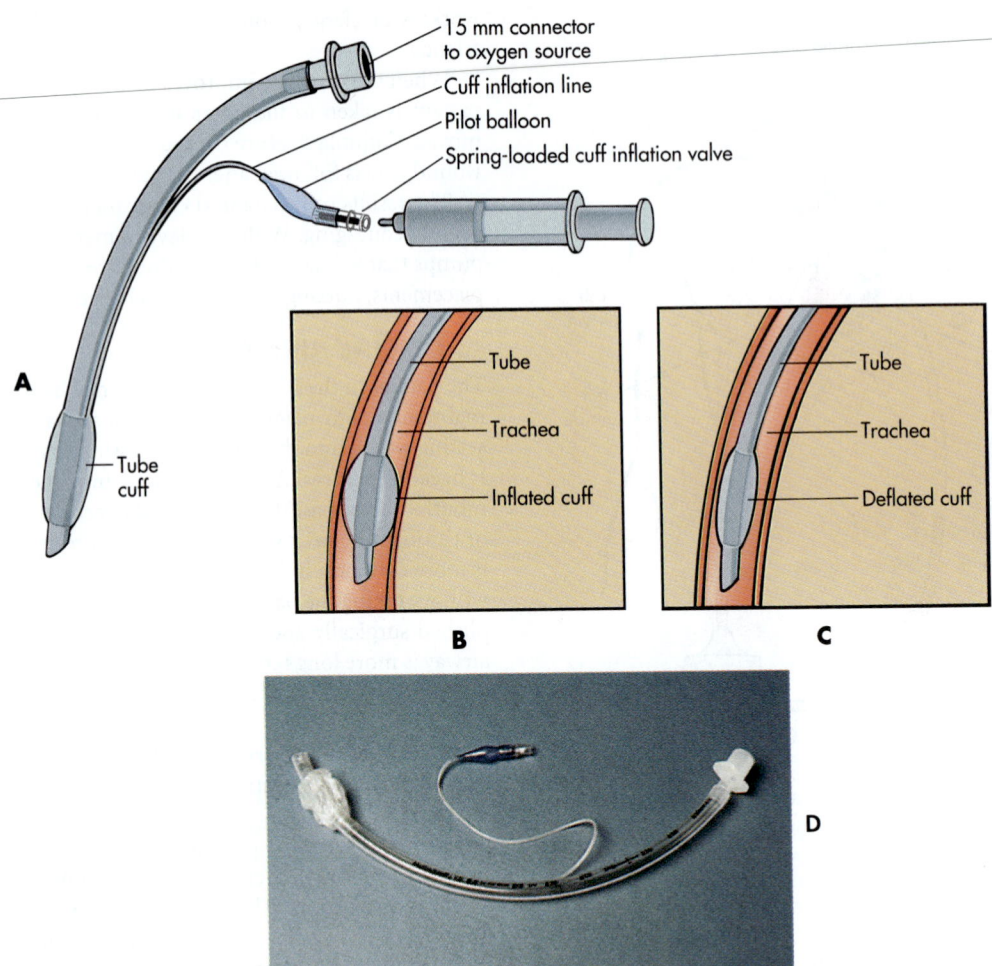

15 mm connector
to oxygen source
Cuff inflation line
Pilot balloon
Spring-loaded cuff inflation valve

A

Tube
cuff

Tube
Trachea
Inflated cuff

B

Tube
Trachea
Deflated cuff

C

D

Fig. 63-12   Endotracheal tube. **A,** Parts of an endotracheal tube. **B,** Tube in place with the cuff inflated. **C,** Tube in place with the cuff deflated. **D,** Photo of tube before placement.

because it presses on the septum, whereas others may prefer it because there is no need for a bite block and mouth care is more easily accomplished. However, nasal ET tubes are more subject to kinking than oral tubes; the work of breathing is greater because the longer, narrower tube offers more airflow resistance; and suctioning and secretion removal are more difficult. Nasal tubes have been linked with increased sinus infection incidence, which may be a source of sepsis.[21]

Tracheostomy Tubes

Tracheostomy tubes are used if the artificial airway will be needed for a long time (more than 4 to 6 weeks). Upper airway damage is minimized and patient comfort maximized when a tracheostomy is performed early in the course of treatment. The patient may be able to eat and to speak with some types of tracheostomy tubes. Secretion removal is easier and the work of breathing less than with ET intubation. There is debate regarding when to perform a tracheotomy in the patient with an ET tube. The situation varies with the patient, physician, and institution. Some institutions use ET intubation in patients for up to 6 weeks without harmful sequelae. Tracheostomy tubes and related nursing management are discussed in Chapter 25. Types of tracheostomy tubes are listed in Table 25-5 and illustrated in Fig. 25-6.

Endotracheal Intubation Procedures

Before intubation, the nurse should ensure that the patient is properly oxygenated. The nurse should explain why ET intubation is necessary, the procedure involved, and sensations (gagging, a feeling of suffocation) that may be experienced during the procedure. The nurse should also explain that because of the inflated cuff, it will not be possible to talk when the tube is in place, but speech will be possible after the tube is removed.

The nurse should assemble and check the equipment to be used during the procedure, remove the patient's dentures or partial plates, and administer medication as ordered. Premedication varies, depending on the patient's health status. In the operating room, premedication may include intravenous barbiturates (to induce sleep) and a neuromuscular blocking agent. In ICUs, premedication often includes a topical anesthetic spray such as 4% lidocaine. A sedative-hypnotic and amnestic (e.g., midazolam [Versed]) is used if the patient is agitated, disoriented, or combative. A rapid-onset narcotic such as fentanyl (Sublimaze) may be used to blunt the pain of laryngoscopy and intubation. A paralytic drug such as succinylcholine [Anectine] may be used to prevent movement. Atropine may be used to limit secretions. In emergency situations, intubation is commonly performed without premedication because the patient may be unconscious.

If oral intubation is selected, the patient is positioned so that the mouth, pharynx, and trachea are in relatively direct alignment. The patient is placed supine with the head extended and the neck flexed ("sniffing position"). The head must not hang over the edge of the bed. The lower jaw is held forward. The person performing the procedure (usually a physician or nurse practitioner) uses a laryngoscope to visualize the vocal cords and pass the ET tube through the mouth over the vocal cords into the trachea. Nasal intubation can be accomplished blindly without the patient moving the head and neck. For nasal intubation it may be helpful to have the patient extrude the tongue. The patient is preoxygenated with 100% oxygen via a manual resuscitation bag (MRB). Each insertion attempt is limited to 30 seconds. Pulse oximetry is helpful during intubation to assess hypoxemia.

Following tube insertion, the cuff is inflated, placement confirmed, and the tube secured. The nurse must immediately auscultate the chest to confirm bilateral breath sounds and observe to confirm bilateral chest expansion. The tube is secured with tape and bite block as needed. A chest x-ray is immediately obtained to confirm tube placement at 3 to 5 cm above the carina in the adult, about halfway between the vocal cords and carina. This position allows the patient to move the neck without dislodging the tube or causing it to enter the right mainstem bronchus.

Once proper positioning is confirmed with x-ray, the tube is marked where it exits the nose or mouth ("exit mark") and securely fixed in position. The tubing is cut to remove excess. To fix the oral tube in position, a bite block is used. Adhesive tape is placed on each cheek. A second, longer piece of tape is placed over the first piece; the free ends are split and wrapped around the tube and bite block. The bottom tape remains in place, and only the top piece is changed if necessary. The nasal tube is similarly taped to the side of the cheeks. In the event of facial injuries, it is possible to use ties made of umbilical tape rather than adhesive tape to secure the nasal tube. Several commercial devices are available to assist in securing ET tubes.

Following intubation, the patient might require suctioning. Oral suctioning is almost always needed because the patient cannot swallow normally. Tracheal suctioning may be needed because few patients can cough with sufficient vigor. Following intubation, the nurse should auscultate over the central airways. Coarse rhonchi suggest that secretions are present, which should be removed by suctioning or coughing (see Table 63-11).

The ET tube is connected either to humidified air, oxygen, or a mechanical ventilator. ABGs should be sampled 10 to 20 minutes after intubation to determine oxygenation and ventilation status. ABG values are reviewed and used to guide oxygenation and ventilation changes. Pulse oximetry provides useful continuous monitoring of arterial oxygenation.

NURSING MANAGEMENT: ARTIFICIAL AIRWAY

Nursing responsibilities for the patient with an artificial airway include (1) maintaining correct tube placement, (2) maintaining proper cuff inflation, (3) maintaining and monitoring ventilation status (includes oxygenation and acid-base status), (4) maintaining tube patency, (5) assessing for complicatons, (6) providing mouth care and rotating the tube placement, and (7) fostering comfort and communication. Nursing care for the patient with an artificial airway is presented in NCP 63-1.

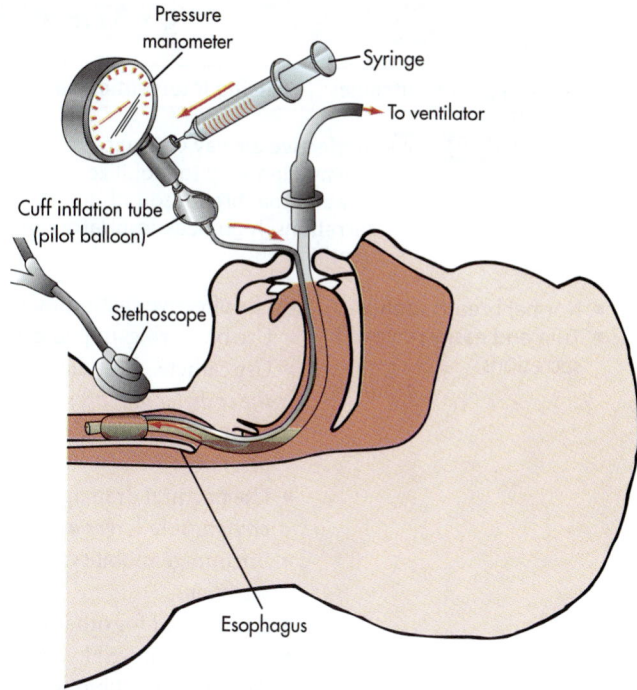

Fig. 63-13 Technique to inflate cuff and check cuff pressure. The cuff is inflated until no leak is heard at peak inspiratory pressure (end of ventilator inspiration). A stethoscope is then placed over the trachea or, for spontaneously breathing patients, after a deep breath or inhalation with a manual resuscitation bag. A manometer is used to verify that the pressure is within the recommended range (<20 mm Hg).

■ Maintaining Correct Tube Placement

The nurse must monitor and maintain tube placement. If the ET tube is not inserted to a sufficient depth, the tube can be dislodged from the trachea and terminate in the pharynx or enter the esophagus. If the tube is inserted too deeply, it can enter the right mainstem bronchus with the result that only the right lung receives ventilation. The nurse monitors tube position by confirming that the exit mark on the tube remains at the point of exit from the body. The nurse observes for symmetric rise and fall of both sides of the chest and auscultates to confirm bilateral breath sounds. If the ET tube is not positioned properly, this is an emergency. The nurse stays with the patient, maintains the airway, supports ventilation, and secures the appropriate assistance to immediately reposition the tube. It may be necessary to ventilate the patient with a manual resuscitation bag (MRB). If a malpositioned tube is not repositioned, no oxygen will be delivered to the lungs or the entire tidal volume will be delivered to one lung, placing the patient at risk for pneumothorax.

■ Maintaining Proper Cuff Inflation

The cuff is an inflatable, pliable sleeve encircling the outer wall of the ET tube. The inflated cuff stabilizes and seals the ET tube within the trachea. It prevents escape of ventilating gases. However, the cuff can cause pressure damage to the trachea wall. To avoid damage, the cuff is inflated a minimal amount and pressure in the cuff is measured and monitored. Normal capillary perfusion is estimated at 30 mm Hg. To ensure adequate tracheal perfusion, cuff pressure is kept well below this level, not to exceed 20 mm Hg (Fig. 63-13).

63-1   NURSING CARE PLAN   PATIENT WITH AN ARTIFICIAL AIRWAY*

Expected Patient Outcomes   Nursing Interventions and *Rationales*

NURSING DIAGNOSIS **Ineffective airway clearance** *related to* presence of artificial airway, accumulation of secretions in airways, inability to mobilize secretions and drying of mucous membranes *as manifested by* presence of abnormal breath sounds (crackles), frequent or absent cough, presence of thick or copious secretions, high peak inspiratory pressures on ventilator or frequent high-pressure alarm sounds on ventilator.

- Normal breath sounds.
- Thin and easily removed secretions.

- Use effective suctioning technique (see Table 63-11) *to prevent tissue damage.*
- Use blunt ring-tipped catheters *to diminish trauma to trachea and bronchi.*
- Use catheter with diameter $<^1/_2$ tube diameter *to allow space for air to move in or out around the catheter and prevent lung collapse.*
- Limit negative suction pressure (-80 to -120 mm Hg) *to prevent excess buildup of negative pressure.*
- Use postural drainage, vibration, and percussion maneuvers when indicated *to help move secretions into larger airways.*
- Encourage mobility; change patient's position at least q2hr as tolerated *to prevent pooling of secretions.*
- Assess need for other measures *to facilitate liquefication and mobilization of secretions.*
- Keep patient well hydrated; provide warm (98.6° F [37° C]) humidified gases for ventilation.
- Administer antibiotics as prescribed *to treat infection.*
- Administer aerosolized bronchodilators (if indicated) *to treat bronchospasm and reduce bronchial narrowing.*
- Auscultate breath sounds q2-4hr *to monitor effectiveness of interventions.*

NURSING DIAGNOSIS **Risk for infection** *related to* exposure to pathogens and loss of normal protective barrier to infection.

- No evidence of infection.
- Negative sputum cultures.

- Observe for change in color, quantity, odor, and viscosity of sputum; difficulty in suctioning secretions; increase in cough; fever; chills; diaphoresis; abnormal breath sounds (e.g., crackles, wheezing); tachycardia; deterioration of ABGs; flushing of skin; elevated WBC count; evidence of infiltrate or atelectasis on chest x-ray; positive sputum cultures *to determine if infection is present or developing.*
- Obtain sputum culture and order sensitivity test if secretions become purulent or tenacious, change color, or become odorous *to diagnose infectious agent.*
- Keep head of bed elevated (especially if receiving enteral nutrition) *to prevent aspiration.*
- Keep ventilator tubing cleared of condensed water *to eliminate source of infection.*
- Use sterile technique with suctioning (see Table 63-11) *to reduce the risk of infection.*
- Suction oropharynx *to remove pooled secretions.*

NURSING DIAGNOSIS **Risk for injury** *related to* suctioning, potential for aspiration of gastric secretions, right mainstem intubation, esophageal intubation, accidental extubation, mechanical obstruction or kinking of ET tube, and irritation from artificial airway.

- Maintenance of tube alignment.
- No accidental extubation.
- No aspiration.
- No gastric contents in trachea.
- No tracheal trauma.

- Assess for progressive hypoxemia, tachycardia, tachypnea, increase in BP, cyanosis, absent or unilateral breath sounds, dyspnea *to identify signs of ineffective ventilation.*
- Monitor for inability to ventilate patient with ventilation bag, inability to introduce suction catheter into ET tube, misplacement of ET tube on chest x-ray, high peak airway pressures and frequent high airway pressure alarms, aspiration of gastric contents, frequent suctioning *as indicators of ineffective respirations.*
- Use bite block or oral airway *to keep patient from biting tube and obstructing tube opening.*
- Move patient with care if connected to ventilator *to avoid traction on ET tube from ventilator tubing.*

Continued

63-1 | NURSING CARE PLAN | PATIENT WITH AN ARTIFICIAL AIRWAY*—continued

Expected Patient Outcomes	Nursing Interventions and *Rationales*

NURSING DIAGNOSIS **Risk for injury** —*continued*

- Mark tube with india ink or indelible marker at teeth, gums, or nose insertion point *as indicator of proper positioning.*
- Auscultate breath sounds immediately after intubation, q4hr, and as needed *to ensure correct placement and effective ventilation.*
- Ensure that chest x-ray is done immediately after intubation and whenever serious question of tube position arises *to validate correct placement.*
- Restrain patient with wrist restraints *to prevent inadvertent extubation.*

NURSING DIAGNOSIS **Risk for aspiration** *related to* presence of artificial airway.

- No occurrence of aspiration.

- Elevate head of bed and keep cuff inflated during tube feedings or while patient is eating *to prevent aspiration.*
- Use small-bore feeding tubes for enteral nutrition *to minimize pressure on esophagus.*
- Add food coloring to feedings *to make identification of aspiration easier.*
- If patient is eating, encourage anteflexion of head *to open esophagus wider.*
- Position patient in side-lying position (never flat on back) *if danger of aspiration is high.*

NURSING DIAGNOSIS **Altered oral mucous membrane** *related to* tissue trauma caused by presence of artificial airway, dry mouth, increased oral secretions, or frequent mechanical stimulation with suction catheter *as manifested by* presence of red, shiny, edematous mucosa of mouth; stomatitis; coated or encrusted oral ulcers.

- Pink, moist, intact mucous membranes.
- Absence of lesions, crusts, hard debris.

- With bite block or oral airway removed, gently brush mouth and teeth with toothbrush, toothette, or swab with normal saline every 2 hours while awake *to provide comfort and to maintain integrity of oral mucosa.*
- Apply lubricant to lips *to protect lips from drying.*
- Maintain ventilator thermostat at 98.6° F (37° C) *to ensure that adequate humidity and warmth are being applied by mechanical ventilator or O_2 source.*
- Check cascade water level on ventilator *to ensure that respiratory gases are continually humidified.*

NURSING DIAGNOSIS **Risk for ineffective breathing pattern** *related to* possible upper airway damage secondary to cuffed ET tube.

- Maintenance of normal integrity of upper airway structures.
- Able to phonate and swallow adequately within 1 week after extubation.

- Monitor for tachypnea, tachycardia, decreased breath sounds, inspiratory stridor, use of accessory muscles, inability to phonate, hoarseness, sore throat, cough, swallowing difficulties after extubation *to identify signs of ineffective breathing pattern.*
- Use smallest-diameter ET tube that will support effective ventilation *to minimize tracheal trauma.*
- Use only low-pressure cuffs for intubation *to minimize tracheal and laryngeal damage.*
- Use minimal leak or minimal occluding volume (MOV) technique and cuff pressures of <20 mm Hg (or 27 cm H_2O) *to prevent tracheal dilation, which may lead to esophageal compression, causing aspiration and difficulty in swallowing.*
- Stabilize tube, tubing, and patient's head when turning *to prevent tracheal tissue trauma.*
- Deflate cuff when mechanical ventilator not required for ventilation *to relieve pressure on the trachea.*
- Immediately after extubation, monitor patient closely *for signs of respiratory distress secondary to laryngeal edema and other signs of upper airway damage.*

Continued

63-1 NURSING CARE PLAN PATIENT WITH AN ARTIFICIAL AIRWAY*—continued

| Expected Patient Outcomes | Nursing Interventions and *Rationales* |

NURSING DIAGNOSIS Impaired verbal communication *related to* inability to speak secondary to intubation *as manifested by* inability to speak.

- Effective method of communicating basic needs.

- Provide patient with paper and pencil, magic slate, alphabet board, symptom board, or computer *to have an alternative means of communication.*
- Learn to read patient's body language, facial expression, and signals *to ease patient's efforts to communicate.*
- Attempt to anticipate patient's needs *to decrease frustration.*
- Provide easily accessible call light or bell *to enable patient to call for assistance.*
- Explain temporary nature of problem and that patient will have no vocalization with ET tube in place and will be hoarse after intubation *to inform patient and relieve anxiety.*
- Acknowledge that inability to speak can be frustrating *to empathize with patient.*
- Instruct family in effective strategies for communication with patient.

NURSING DIAGNOSIS Altered nutrition: less than body requirements *related to* possible inability to take nourishment orally, increased caloric demands secondary to clinical condition, and need for mechanical ventilation *as manifested by* loss of more than 10% of body weight (see NCP 62-1 for nursing interventions related to this diagnosis).

*Nursing care plan for the patient with a tracheostomy is presented in NCP 25-5.

Most cuffs are inflated by injecting air into the fine-bore tubing leading to the cuff. If an air leak is heard, the nurse adds air to the cuff following the minimal occluding volume technique, outlined in the next paragraph. The nurse measures and records cuff pressure after intubation and once every 8 hours to confirm that the cuff is properly inflated.

The steps in cuff inflation are as follows: (1) inflate the cuff to minimal occluding volume (MOV) by adding air until no leak is heard at peak inspiratory pressure (end of ventilator inspiration) when a stethoscope is placed over the trachea; (2) for the spontaneously breathing patient, inflate until no sound is heard after a deep breath or after inhalation with an MRB; (3) use a manometer to verify that cuff pressure is less than 20 mm Hg; and (4) record cuff pressure value in the chart. See Table 63-10 for nursing management of endotracheal tubes and monitoring of cuff pressure.

■ Maintaining and Monitoring Ventilation and Oxygenation

The patient with an ET tube is vigilantly monitored for adequate oxygenation status by monitoring ABGs, clinical condition, and oximetry of arterial or mixed venous blood. Periodic ABGs are analyzed to give objective information regarding oxygenation. In addition, the nurse monitors for clinical signs of hypoxemia, such as dusky skin coloring, confusion, irritability, and cardiac arrhythmias. Continuous pulse oximeter (SpO_2) detects hypoxemia and is especially helpful in the patient with low hemoglobin who is unlikely to become dusky or with a dark complexion, and at night when room lighting is low. SpO_2 greater than 95% is generally desired. Lower values are expected in patients with obstructive pulmonary disease. PA catheters with a device to monitor oxygen saturation of the mixed venous blood hemoglobin in the pulmonary artery (SvO_2) can give an indirect indication about the patient's oxygenation status. A drop in SvO_2 may indicate a drop in arterial oxygenation,

CO, or oxygen demand. Mixed venous values are observed for a substantial drop in value.

Indicators of ventilation include arterial PCO_2, end-tidal PCO_2 (capnography), and clinical assessment data. Arterial PCO_2 is the best indicator of alveolar hypoventilation (elevated PCO_2, respiratory acidosis) or hyperventilation (low PCO_2, respiratory alkalosis). The PCO_2 at the end of expiration in the normal patient is equivalent to the arterial PCO_2 and can indicate ventilation status. However, in patients with unusually large dead space, unusually prolonged expiration, or serious mismatch between ventilation and perfusion, capnography is inaccurate. The patient who is hyperventilating will be breathing rapidly and deeply and may experience circumoral and peripheral numbness and tingling. The patient who is hypoventilating will be breathing shallowly or slowly and may appear dusky.

■ Maintaining Tube Patency by Suctioning

Suctioning an ET or tracheostomy tube is performed to remove secretions from the central airways. The procedure is performed as needed and not routinely. Dyspnea, increased ventilator peak-inspiratory pressures, activation of the ventilator pressure alarm, and noisy or gurgling respirations suggest the presence of secretions. Auscultation of coarse rhonchi over the central airways confirms the presence of secretions. Peripheral crackles are not an indication for suctioning. Suctioning has been suggested as a means of inducing a cough, but this is not recommended.[22]

When the presence of secretions is confirmed, the nurse encourages the patient to move the secretions by coughing. The patient may be able to expel the secretions or advance them into the ET tube for removal. If the secretions cannot be moved or expelled by the patient, suctioning is indicated. Coughing will be induced if the suction catheter touches the carina. Two recommended procedures for suctioning the patient with an artificial airway are described in Table 63-11.

Table **63-10**	Characteristics and Nursing Management of Endotracheal Tubes
Characteristics	**Nursing Management**
When properly inflated, low-pressure, high-volume cuff distributes cuff pressure over large area, minimizing pressure on tracheal wall.	▪ Inflate the cuff to MOV by slowly injecting air into the cuff until no leak is heard at peak inspiratory pressure (end of ventilator inspiration), when a stethoscope is placed over the trachea (Fig. 63-13). If the patient is breathing spontaneously, inflate cuff until no sound is heard after deep breath or during inhalation with MRB. Verify pressure is within accepted range with a manometer. Record value in chart. ▪ Monitor and record cuff pressure q8hr using above technique. Cuff pressure should be ≤20 mm Hg or ≤25 cm H_2O to allow adequate tracheal capillary perfusion. If needed, remove or add air to the pilot tubing using a syringe and stopcock. Afterward, verify cuff pressure is within accepted range with manometer. ▪ Report inability to keep the cuff inflated or need to use progressively larger volumes of air to keep cuff inflated. Potential causes include tracheal dilation at the cuff site or a crack or slow leak in the housing of the one-way inflation valve. If the leak is caused by tracheal dilation, the physician may intubate the patient with a larger tube. Cracks in the inflation valve may be temporarily managed by clamping the small-bore tubing with a hemostat. The tube should be changed within 24 hr. ▪ Assess for signs of respiratory distress when a fenestrated cannula is first used. If this occurs, the cap should be removed, the inner cannula replaced, and the cuff reinflated. ▪ Monitor cuff pressure q8hr as noted above.

Table **63-11**	Suctioning Procedures for a Patient on a Mechanical Ventilator

General Measures

1. Wash hands.
2. Apply eye protection (shield or goggles) and clean (nonsterile) glove to nonsterile hand.
3. Explain procedure, purpose, and sensations to patient.
4. Prepare all equipment:
    Check negative suction pressure (usual range between –80 and –120 mm Hg).
    Pour sterile normal saline solution into sterile container.
    Turn on O_2 flow to bag ventilator to 15 L.
    Place manual resuscitation bag (MRB) on bed.
    Open suction catheter and glove packages. Suction catheter should be no wider than half the diameter of artificial airway.

One-Person Method

1. Pause ventilator alarms.
2. Disconnect patient from ventilator.
3. Preoxygenate with 100% O_2* and hyperventilate patient with MRB or ventilator breaths 3-6 times (done before and after suctioning).
4. Connect patient to ventilator.
5. Put on sterile glove and pick up catheter with sterile hand.
6. Connect catheter to suction tubing, using sterile hand for catheter and nonsterile hand for suction tubing.
7. Disconnect patient from ventilator.
8. Using nonsterile hand, stabilize artificial airway and hold catheter suction regulator.
9. Insert catheter gently, swiftly, and without suction with sterile hand.
10. When resistance is met, pull back catheter 1-2 cm without suction.
11. Begin depressing suction vacuum regulator in an on-off (intermittent) fashion with nonsterile hand while rotating catheter in sterile hand between thumb and forefinger.
12. Swiftly remove catheter. Each suctioning pass should not exceed 15 sec.
13. Rinse catheter in sterile saline between suctioning passes as necessary.
14. With nonsterile hand, reconnect patient to ventilator.
15. Depress manual breath or sigh button (if activated) on ventilator to hyperventilate or ventilate patient.[†]
16. Let patient equilibrate for 30 sec to 1 min or as needed.
17. Rinse catheter with sterile normal saline solution.
18. Repeat procedure as needed.
19. Place patient back on ventilator.
20. Suction oropharynx.
21. Discard catheter.
22. Hyperventilate and oxygenate via MRB or ventilator for three to six breaths.
23. Assess patient's tolerance to suctioning (continuous observation of the patient during entire suctioning procedure is necessary).
24. Confirm that ventilator alarms are reactivated.

Two-Person Method

1. First person hyperventilates and preoxygenates before, between, and after suctions; stabilizes airway.
2. Second person suctions as in one-person method.

*Use O_2 concentration of 60% or less for patients with chronic hypercapnia who are breathing spontaneously.
[†]As nurse becomes more adept at suctioning, bag ventilation may be done with nonsterile hand between suctioning passes. Ideally, it is better for two persons to be present during suctioning so one person can bag ventilate the patient while the other person does the suctioning. (One nurse with one hand on the bag ventilator can generate up to 800 ml and with two hands up to 1000 ml.)

Complications associated with suctioning include hypoxemia, arrhythmias, mucosal damage, pneumothorax, contamination and infection, retained secretions, discomfort, and anxiety. Hypoxemia occurs when oxygen-enriched gas is sucked from the lungs along with secretions. Other causes of hypoxemia include irritation-induced bronchospasm and microatelectasis resulting from aspiration of intrapulmonary air. Arterial oxygen tension may be reduced by 10 to 39 mm Hg with ET suctioning.[23]

Hypoxemia is prevented by preoxygenation, postoxygenation, hyperinflation, and limiting each suction pass to 10 to 15 seconds. If pulse oximetry is used, SpO_2 can be assessed throughout the suctioning procedure. Saturations greater than 95% are desired. If SvO_2 monitoring is available, it provides an indirect indication about the patient's oxygenation status. During suctioning, the patient is observed for tachycardia, arrhythmias, hypertension, diaphoresis, and pallor or graying of mucous membranes. If these occur, the patient should be ventilated with an MRB or placed back on the ventilator until equilibration occurs before another suction pass is attempted. In spontaneously breathing patients with chronic hypercapnia (e.g., patients with chronic obstructive pulmonary disease [COPD]) an MRB with 35% to 60% oxygen is used. The patient is assessed to confirm spontaneous ventilation after the suctioning procedure. There is some evidence that patients are more stable hemodynamically when ventilator-delivered preoxygenation is used.[23]

Causes of cardiac arrhythmias during suctioning include hypoxemia resulting in myocardial hypoxia, vagal stimulation caused by tracheal irritation, and sympathetic nervous system stimulation caused by anxiety, discomfort, or pain. Arrhythmias include tachycardia; bradycardia; premature atrial, junctional, or ventricular beats; and asystole. Suctioning should be halted if serious arrhythmias develop. The patient should be slowly ventilated via MRB with 100% oxygen until the arrhythmia subsides. Excessive suctioning should be avoided in patients with hypoxemia or bradycardia.

Tracheal mucosal damage may occur because of excessive suction pressures, overly vigorous catheter insertion, and the characteristics of the suction catheter itself. The presence of blood streaks or tissue shreds in aspirated mucus indicates that mucosal damage has occurred. Mucosal damage increases the risk of infection. Trauma to the mucosa can be prevented by the following precautions:

1. Use blunt or ring-tipped catheters with side holes.
2. Lubricate the catheter tip with sterile saline solution.
3. Stabilize the ET tube throughout the procedure.
4. Insert the catheter gently and quickly without suction.
5. Limit negative suction to −80 to −120 mm Hg.
6. Withdraw catheter 1 to 2 cm before applying suction (to prevent adhering to mucosa).
7. Apply intermittent suction as the catheter is removed.
8. Gently rotate the catheter during removal.

Although rare, pneumothorax can occur when a large catheter is inserted into a small-diameter artificial airway. If there is inadequate space for air to move in or out around the catheter, the lung may collapse or microatelectasis may occur when vacuum is applied. To prevent this, the suction catheter should not occupy more than half the internal diameter of the tube being suctioned. Suction should be maintained at −80 to −120 mm Hg. Intermittent suction should be used when removing the catheter.

Secretions may be thick and difficult to suction because of inadequate hydration, inadequate humidification, infection, or inaccessibility of the left mainstem bronchus or lower airways. Chest physical therapy and having the patient turn and cough before suctioning may help move secretions into larger airways. If the patient is inadequately hydrated, oral or intravenous fluids should be administered. If the airway is inadequately humidified, the inspired gases should be prewarmed to body temperature and hydrated with sterile water. If infection causes thick mucus, the patient should be placed on appropriate antibiotics.

The patient may experience anxiety during suctioning because of the inability to breathe, choking, or not knowing what to expect. An explanation should precede each suctioning. The patient should be told that breathing will be impossible for a short period but that the patient will soon be connected to oxygen and receive ventilation. The patient should be told that suctioning often stimulates coughing. If the patient has severe coughing during suctioning, ventilation should be done with slow, small-volume breaths using the MRB. Large volumes of air are avoided because they may overdistend the lungs and reflexly stimulate further coughing episodes. The patient with an incision or who has sustained trauma may experience pain during suctioning when coughing is induced. This patient should be premedicated with narcotics and incisions splinted before suctioning.

Closed tracheal suctioning (CTS), in which a suction catheter is enclosed in a plastic sleeve connected directly to the patient's artificial airway and ventilator, is used in many ICUs (Fig. 63-14). With CTS, suctioning can be accomplished without disconnecting the ventilator or opening the system. The nurse follows the usual suctioning procedures by preoxygenating the patient, then activating the suction during inspiration. CTS is designed to prevent loss of positive end-expiratory pressure (PEEP) and minimize hypoxemia during suctioning. There is some cost saving related to decreased need for suction sets and less opportunity for external contamination using this system. Staff members are protected from the patient's secretions, and suctioning can be performed more quickly.

Mouth Care and Endotracheal Tube Repositioning

Meticulous care is required to prevent skin breakdown or pressure sores on the lips and tongue as a result of adhesive tape or pressure from the tube, bite block, or tube holder. For the orally intubated patient, the outer layer of adhesive tape is removed every shift and the tube is moved to the other side of the mouth. The tube must be retaped to the cheeks and not to the jaw. If the jaw moves, the ET tube will also move, causing tracheal irritation and possibly damage. If a tube holder is used, the straps can be loosened, the area under the straps massaged, and the straps reapplied. Mouth care and shaving can be done at this time. Because ET tube position may change during mouth care, whenever the tube is untaped, during repositioning, or when the straps are adjusted, two nurses are needed for these procedures. The presence of bilateral breath sounds should always be confirmed after completion of any of these procedures.

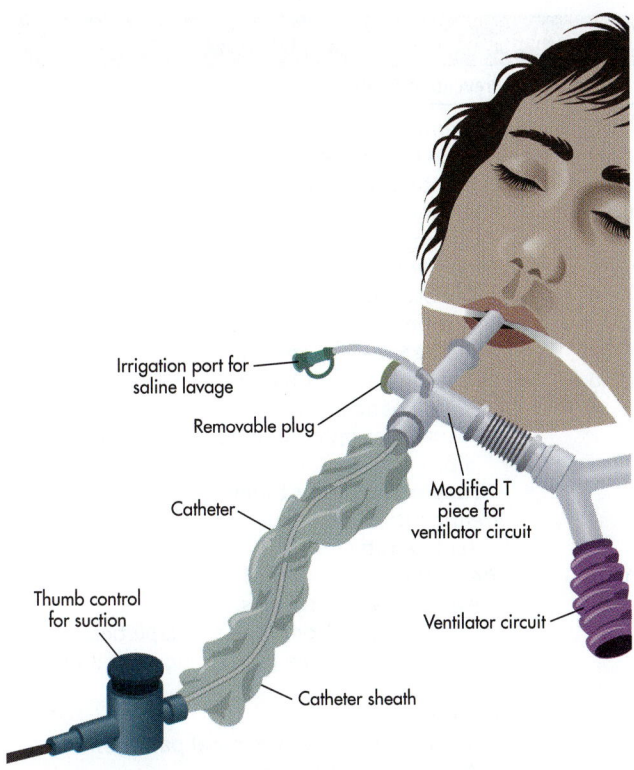

Irrigation port for saline lavage

Removable plug

Catheter

Thumb control for suction

Modified T piece for ventilator circuit

Ventilator circuit

Catheter sheath

To vacuum source

Fig. 63-14 Closed tracheal suction system.

Because the patient's mouth is always open when an oral ET tube is in place, lips and mouth should be moistened with saline or water swabs to prevent mucosal drying. Mouth care, including cleaning of teeth and gums, should be performed every 4 to 8 hours as a comfort measure and to prevent injury to the gums and plaque accumulation. Mouthwash containing alcohol should not be used because these preparations dry the mucosa, predisposing it to cracking and creating sites for infection.

■ Fostering Comfort and Communication

The discomfort associated with ET intubation and mechanical ventilation may make it necessary to sedate the patient or administer an analgesic until the ET tube is no longer required.

Communicating with the intubated patient can be a frustrating experience. To communicate more effectively, the nurse should have available a variety of methods. A magic slate or pad and pencil should be provided if the patient can use her or his hands. Additional options for communication include an alphabet board, flash cards, photo boards, lip reading, and hand signals.

Extubation

Extubation (tube removal) should be performed as soon as possible. The health care team should assess the patient's status each day to determine whether (1) the underlying condition has improved so that intubation is no longer required, (2) spontaneous respiration can be maintained without the ventilator, and (3) the patient can cough, clear secretions, and protect the airway.

Extubation should be attempted only by trained persons. Once the tube is removed, the patient is encouraged to cough to clear secretions. The mouth is suctioned and humidified oxygen is administered through a face mask. The patient is observed at frequent intervals for signs of laryngospasm (e.g., stridor, dyspnea) and respiratory distress (e.g., restlessness, irritability, tachycardia, tachypnea). A pulse oximeter should be used to monitor oxygen saturation. If the patient cannot tolerate extubation, immediate reintubation may be necessary.

Complications of Endotracheal Intubation

The major complications of ET intubation result from injury to the hypopharynx, larynx, and trachea and are related to the pressure exerted on upper airway structures by the tube and cuff. Improper tube placement, aspiration, oral and nasal pressure sores, and accidental extubation are also potential problems. Table 63-12 summarizes complications seen in patients with ET tubes.

Improper Tube Placement and Accidental Extubation. Improper tube placement is a potential hazard of ET intubation. If the tube is not inserted deeply enough, the cuff can damage the larynx or the tube can slip out of the trachea. If the tube is inserted too deeply, it might extend into the right mainstem bronchus, resulting in the ventilation of the right lung only. It is also possible with too deep a tube placement that the distal orifice could rest against the carina or tracheal wall, causing airway obstruction.

A chest x-ray should be taken immediately after intubation and whenever there is a question of improper ET tube placement. The tube should be repositioned as needed by a health care provider who is able to reintubate if necessary. The ET tube tip should be seen on chest x-ray at least 2 cm above the carina. Chest auscultation should be done immediately after intubation and before securing the tube to determine the presence of bilateral equal breath sounds. Auscultation of breath sounds is performed regularly at least every 4 hours. The tube must be well secured to prevent slipping or accidental extubation. Accidental extubation can be a catastrophic event. The nurse is responsible for preventing its occurrence through the use of soft wrist restraints and sedation. It is wise to mark the tube with india ink at the teeth or nose level or note the centimeter mark closest to the teeth or nose level and chart it on the care plan or flowchart. This mark provides a quick reference point to check proper tube placement.

The ET tube should not extend more than 1.5 to 2 in (3.8 to 5 cm) out of the patient's nose or mouth because the added length can cause additional pressure to be exerted on structures. Once ET tube position has been verified by chest x-ray, the tube can be cut and the adapter reapplied.

Aspiration. Aspiration is a potential hazard for the patient with an ET tube. The ET tube passes through the epiglottis, splinting it open. Thus the intubated patient cannot protect the airway from aspiration. The cuff cannot totally prevent the trickle of oral or gastric secretions into the trachea. Furthermore, secretions accumulate above the cuff. When the cuff is deflated those secretions move into the lungs. Oral intubation increases salivation yet swallowing is difficult, so the mouth must be suctioned frequently. The posterior pharynx should always be suctioned before cuff deflation. This may be performed by the patient with a Yankauer (tonsil-tip) suction catheter. Other factors causing aspiration

Table **63-12**	Complications of Endotracheal Tubes and Nursing Management

Complications	Causes	Prevention/Treatment

▪ Tube obstruction	Patient biting tube
	Tube kinking during repositioning
	Cuff herniation
	Dried secretions, blood, or lubricant
	Tissue from tumor
	Trauma
	Foreign body
		Prevention:
		  Place bite block.
		  Sedate patient prn.
		  Suction prn.
		  Humidify inspired gases.
		Treatment:
		  Replace tube.

▪ Tube displacement	Movement of patient's head
	Movement of tube by patient's tongue
	Traction on tube from ventilator tubing
	Self-extubation
		Prevention:
		  Secure tube to upper lip.
		  Restrain patient's hands.
		  Sedate patient prn.
		  Ensure that only 2 in of tube extend beyond
		    lip.
		  Support ventilator tubing.
		Treatment:
		  Replace tube.

▪ Sinusitis and nasal injury	Obstruction of paranasal sinus drainage
	Pressure necrosis of nares
		Prevention:
		  Avoid nasal intubations.
		  Cushion nares from tube and tape/ties.
		  Ensure proper tube positioning and stabiliza-
		    tion.
		Treatment:
		  Remove all tubes from nasal passages.
		  Administer antibiotics.

▪ Tracheoesophageal fistula	Pressure necrosis of posterior tracheal wall
	  resulting from overinflated cuff and rigid
	  nasogastric tube
		Prevention:
		  Stabilize airway.
		  Inflate cuff with minimal amount of air
		    necessary.
		  Monitor cuff pressures q8hr.
		  Use small-bore feeding tube for enteral
		    feeding.
		Treatment:
		  Position cuff of tube distal to fistula.
		  Place gastrostomy tube for enteral feedings.
		  Place esophageal tube for secretion
		    clearance proximal to fistula.

▪ Mucosal lesions	Pressure at tube and mucosal interface	*Prevention:*
		  Inflate cuff with minimal amount of air
		    necessary.
		  Monitor cuff pressures q8hr.
		  Use appropriate size tube.
		Treatment:
		  May resolve spontaneously.
		  Perform surgical intervention.

▪ Laryngeal or tracheal stenosis	Injury to area from end of tube or cuff,
	  resulting in scar tissue formation and
	  narrowing of airway
		Prevention:
		  Inflate cuff with minimal amount of air
		    necessary.
		  Monitor cuff pressures q8hr.
		  Suction area above cuff frequently.
		Treatment:
		  Perform tracheostomy.
		  Place laryngeal stent.
		  Perform surgical repair.

▪ Cricoid abscess	Mucosal injury with bacterial invasion	*Prevention:*
		  Inflate cuff with minimal amount of air
		    necessary.
		  Monitor cuff pressures q8hr.
		  Suction area above cuff frequently.
		Treatment:
		  Perform incision and drainage of area.
		  Administer antibiotics.

From Thelan LA and others, editors: *Critical care nursing: diagnosis and management,* ed 3, St Louis, 1998, Mosby.

Table 63-13   Indicators for Mechanical Ventilation and Weaning

	Measurement and Significance	Normal Values*	Mechanical Ventilation Indicated*	Weaning Feasible*
Tests of Ventilatory Reserve or Mechanical Ability				
V_T	Amount of air exchanged during normal breathing at rest	7-9 ml/kg	<5 ml/kg	>5 ml/kg
Respiratory rate per minute		12-20	<10 or >35	12-20
Forced vital capacity (FVC)	Maximal inspiration and then measurement of air during maximal forced expiration; determination of whether patient can sigh deeply enough to avoid atelectasis; best indicator of ventilatory reserve; patient's cooperation necessary	65-75 ml/kg	<10-15 ml/kg	>10-15 ml/kg
Peak inspiratory pressure, negative inspiratory force	Complete occlusion of anaeroid manometer attached to airway or mouth for 10-20 sec while negative inspiratory efforts of patient noted; useful index of neuromuscular strength; less patient cooperation necessary	−75 to −100 cm H_2O	>−25 cm H_2O	<−20 cm H_2O
Forced expiratory volume in 1 sec (FEV_1)	Volume of air measured in first second of exhalation of forced vital capacity maneuver; use in patients with COPD to determine degree of obstruction	50-60 ml/kg	<10 ml/kg	>16 ml/kg
Resting minute ventilation	Multiplication of tidal volume by respiratory rate for 1 min, general indication of patient's total ventilation	5-10 L/min	>10 L/min	<10 L/min
V_D/V_T	Estimation from V_T; accurate calculation requiring $PaCO_2$ and partial pressure of CO_2 in mixed expired gas; measurement of portion of each breath that does not participate in gas exchange; indication of lungs' efficiency in removing CO_2	0.25-0.40	>0.6	<0.5-0.6
$PaCO_2$	Indication of lungs' efficiency in removing CO_2 and reflection of body's acid-base status	35-45 mm Hg	>55 mm Hg (acute)	<45 mm Hg
Tests of Oxygenation Capability				
PaO_2/FIO_2	Provision of evidence of lung's ability to oxygenate arterial blood; couples PO_2 with amount of oxygen given	350-400	<200	>300

*These parameters are only guidelines and must be related to the individual patient's status (e.g., patients with severe COPD may have a normal $PaCO_2$ of 60 mm Hg and values lower than normal for FEV_1, VC, MV, and maximal voluntary ventilation).
COPD, chronic obstructive pulmonary disease.

include cuff leak, tracheal distention, and tracheoesophageal fistula. The patient with an ET tube is at risk for aspiration of gastric contents. Even when the cuff is inflated, the nurse must take precautions to avoid emesis, which can lead to aspiration. The head of the bed should be elevated when the patient is receiving tube feedings.

MECHANICAL VENTILATION

Mechanical ventilation is the process by which room air or oxygen-enriched air is moved into and out of the lungs mechanically. Mechanical ventilation is not curative. It is a means of supporting patients until they recover the ability to breathe independently. Indications for mechanical ventilation are listed in Table 63-13.

Patients with chronic pulmonary disease who are managed by pulmonary health care specialists on a continuous, long-term basis and their families should be given the opportunity to decide the issue of mechanical ventilation before terminal respiratory disease develops. Other patients with chronic disease should also be encouraged to discuss the subject. It is much easier for the physician, patient, and family to decide not to institute ventilatory support initially than it is to remove the support system once it has been initiated. The decision to use mechanical ventilation must be made carefully, respecting the informed wishes of the patient and family.

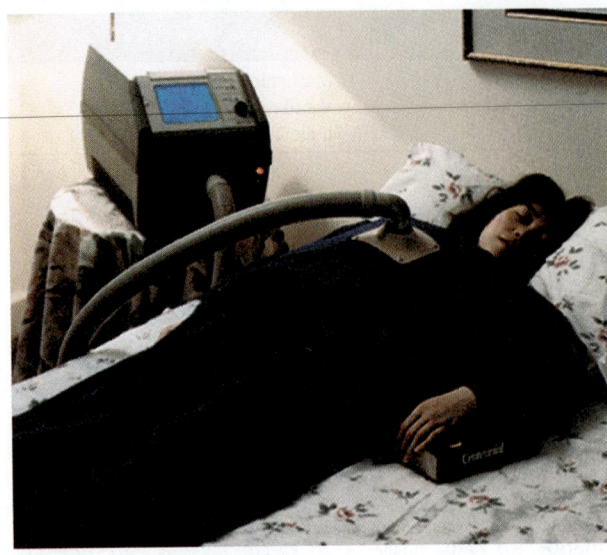

Fig. 63-15   Negative pressure ventilator.

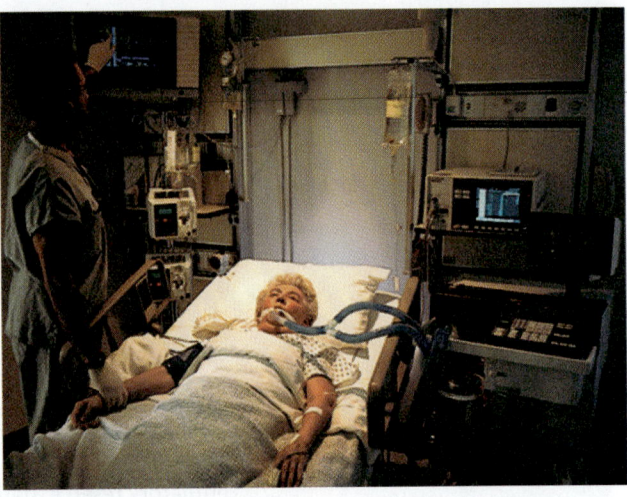

Fig. 63-16   Patient receiving mechanical ventilation.

Types of Mechanical Ventilators

There are two major types of mechanical ventilators: negative pressure and positive pressure ventilators.

Negative Pressure Ventilators. Negative pressure ventilators are composed of chambers that encase the chest or body and surround it with intermittent subatmospheric or negative pressure. Intermittent negative pressure around the chest wall causes the chest to be pulled outward. This reduces intrathoracic pressure. Air rushes in via the upper airway, which is outside the sealed chamber. Expiration is passive; the machine cycles off, allowing chest retraction. This type of ventilation is similar to normal ventilation in that inspiration is produced by decreased intrathoracic pressures and expiration is passive. An artificial airway is not required.

Negative pressure ventilators include the Poncho (Puritan Bennett, Emerson) and Pulmowrap (Lifecare). These ventilators are made of a flexible nylon cover that fits over the head, ties at the neck with drawstrings, and fastens to the arms or wrists and upper legs with elastic (Fig. 63-15).

New developments in negative pressure ventilation enable both control and assist-control ventilation modes. Lightweight, portable negative pressure ventilators are used in the home for patients with neuromuscular diseases, central nervous system (CNS) disorders, diseases and injuries of the spinal cord, and severe COPD. Negative pressure ventilators are not used extensively for acutely ill patients. However, because cardiac output is enhanced and not diminished during inspiration, negative pressure ventilation has been used successfully in those with heart disease.[26]

Positive Pressure Ventilators.   Positive pressure ventilation is the primary method used with acutely ill patients. During inspiration the ventilator pushes air into the lungs under positive pressure. Unlike spontaneous ventilation, intrathoracic pressure is raised during lung inflation rather than lowered. Expiration occurs passively as in normal expiration. The three types of positive pressure ventilators are (1) volume-cycled or volume-limited ventilators, (2) time-cycled or time-limited ventilators, and (3) pressure-cycled or pressure-limited ventilators. Each type is classified by the physical parameter that ends

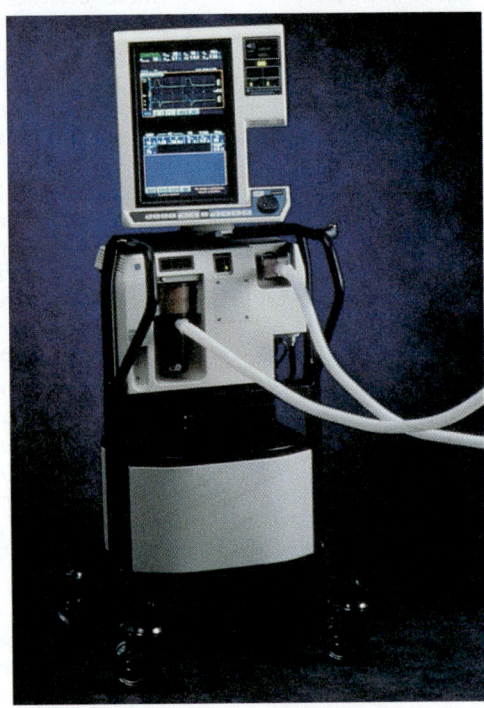

Fig. 63-17   Typical positive pressure ventilator.

the inspiratory cycle. Mechanical ventilators are illustrated in Figs. 63-16 and 17.

Volume-cycled or volume-limited ventilators. Volume-cycled ventilators are the most common type used for intubated adults. Inspiration is terminated when a preset volume of gas is delivered through the ventilator circuit. Volume-cycled ventilators have built-in pressure-limiting valves to prevent excess pressure in the lungs. Once the pressure limit is reached, the remainder of the tidal volume is vented to the outside air. With volume-cycled ventilators, volume delivery remains constant despite lung resistance and compliance changes (unlike pressure-cycled ventilators). Inspired oxygen concentration remains consistent. An example is the Siemens Servo 900. Some ventilators (e.g., Monoghan 225) can be adapted to function as pressure-cycled, time-cycled, or volume-cycled ventilators.

Table 63-14	Settings of Mechanical Ventilation
Parameter	**Description**
Respiratory rate (f)	Number of breaths the ventilator delivers per minute; usual setting is 4-20 breaths/min
Tidal volume (V_T)	Volume of gas delivered to patient during each ventilator breath; usual volume is 5-15 ml/kg
Oxygen concentration (FIO_2)	Fraction of inspired oxygen delivered to patient; may be set between 21% and 100%; usually adjusted to maintain PaO_2 level greater than 60 mm Hg or SaO_2 level greater than 90%
I:E ratio	Duration of inspiration to duration of expiration; usual setting is 1:2 to 1:1.5 unless IRV is desired
Flow rate	Speed with which the tidal volume is delivered; usual setting is 40-100 L/min
Sensitivity/trigger	Determines the amount of effort the patient must generate to initiate a ventilator breath; it may be set for pressure triggering or flow triggering; usual setting for a pressure trigger is 0.5-1.5 cm H_2O below baseline pressure and for a flow trigger is 1-3 L/min below baseline flow
Pressure limit	Regulates the maximal pressure the ventilator can generate to deliver the tidal volume; when the pressure limit is reached, the ventilator terminates the breath and spills the undelivered volume into the atmosphere; usual setting is 10-20 cm H_2O above peak inspiratory pressure

From Thelan LA and others, editors: *Critical care nursing: diagnosis and management,* ed 3, St Louis, 1998, Mosby.
IRV, inverse ratio ventilation.

Time-cycled or time-limited ventilators. Time-cycled ventilators terminate inspiration and switch to expiration at a preset time. The amount of gas delivered with each breath (tidal volume) is regulated by adjusting inspiratory duration and flow rate of the pressurized gas. The tidal volume and inspiratory pressure delivered to the patient may vary from breath to breath. The Siemans 900-C is an example of a time-cycled ventilator for adults. Time-cycled ventilators have fail-safe pressure limits beyond which the ventilator ceases to push gas into the lungs, thus preventing lung overdistention and barotrauma.

Pressure-cycled or pressure-limited ventilators. Pressure-cycled ventilators terminate inspiration when a preselected airway pressure is achieved. The volume of gas delivered to the patient and duration of delivery vary according to airway resistance, pulmonary compliance, and ventilator circuit integrity. When there is obstruction (such as secretions) or when the patient breathes out of synchrony with the ventilator, the pressure limit is reached quickly and the volume of gas delivered is small. Because tidal volume is dependent on the airway resistance, tidal volume is checked frequently when the patient is receiving pressure-cycled mechanical ventilation. Pressure-cycled ventilators are common in acute care. They are indicated in patients at risk for barotrauma and are also used for home therapy, for short-term ventilation, or in a patient whose lungs are relatively free of diseases involving altered resistance and compliance.

Settings of Mechanical Ventilators

Mechanical ventilator settings regulate the rate, depth, and other characteristics of ventilation (Table 63-14). Settings are based on the patient's status (ABGs, body weight, level of consciousness, muscle strength). The ventilator is tuned as finely as possible to match the patient's ventilatory pattern. Settings are evaluated and adjusted frequently until the patient achieves optimal ventilation. Some settings serve as a fail-safe, alerting staff to problems with ventilation. It is important that the nurse en-

sure and document that all ventilator alarms are turned on at all times. Alarms sense potentially dangerous situations of mechanical malfunction, apnea, or patient asynchrony with the ventilator. On many ventilators the alarms can be temporarily bypassed or silenced for up to 2 minutes for suctioning or testing. After that period of time, the alarm system automatically becomes functional again.

Modes of Volume-Cycled Ventilation

The term *mode* refers to the manner in which the breath is initiated and the volume controlled, either by the mechanical ventilator or the patient. Mode is selected based on the patient's ventilatory status, including respiratory drive and ABGs. The three basic modes of mechanical ventilation are (1) controlled mechanical ventilation (CMV), (2) assist-control ventilation (ACV), and (3) synchronized intermittent mandatory ventilation (SIMV). These modes are compared in Table 63-15.

Controlled Mechanical Ventilation. With CMV, breaths are delivered regularly and independent of the patient's ventilatory efforts. Although CMV is infrequently used, it is used when the patient has no drive to breathe (e.g., the anesthetized patient) or is unable to breathe spontaneously (e.g., the paralyzed patient). With CMV the normal processes of regulation of ventilation are not operating. Thus the patient's ability to adjust ventilation to changing demands has been lost.

Assist-Control Mechanical Ventilation. With ACV, the ventilator is set so that it delivers a preset tidal volume at a preset frequency, but the patient is able to initiate a breath by attempting to inhale. The ventilator senses a decrease in intrathoracic pressure and then delivers the preset tidal volume. The patient can ventilate faster than the preset rate but not slower. This mode has the advantage of allowing the patient some control over ventilation while providing support. ACV is used in patients with a variety of conditions, including neuromuscular disorders (e.g., Guillain-Barré syndrome), pulmonary edema, and acute respiratory distress syndrome. The

Table **63-15**	Modes of Mechanical Ventilation		
Description	Advantages	Disadvantages	Uses
Controlled Mechanical Ventilation (CMV)			
Machine delivers preset number of breaths/min at preset volume. Patient cannot trigger breathing.	Breathing is totally controlled by ventilator.	Does not allow patient to initiate breathing or respiratory rate to change with varying patient needs. Airway pressure always positive during inspiration, compromising venous return. Provides limited use of respiratory muscles.	Apnea secondary to brain damage, respiratory muscle paralysis, drug overdose, sedation
Assist-Control Ventilation (ACV)			
Delivery of breath is triggered by inspiratory effort of patient after preselected time interval has elapsed. If patient fails to initiate breathing, ventilator cycles as in controlled ventilation.	Patient can initiate own breathing, use respiratory muscles, and alter respiratory rate according to need. Intrathoracic pressure decreases transiently before inspiratory phase, decreasing the venous return and suppression of cardiac output.	Problems of overventilation and underventilation are possible and can occur in anxious patients or in those with low lung compliance.	Wide range of situations in which patients are spontaneously breathing but have ventilatory failure or gas exchange inefficiency
Synchronized Intermittent Mandatory Ventilation (SIMV)			
Patient breathes spontaneously at own Vᴛ and rate. Ventilator is synchronized to patient's ventilatory rate. Machine set to give certain number of breaths and is triggered by patient's inspiration.	Ventilator does not compete with patient's breathing.	Allows maintenance of even minor spontaneous excursions. Respiratory muscles remain in use. Ventilator augments patient's own efforts.	Wide range of situations in which patients need ventilatory support, method of weaning

patient with ACV mode has the potential for hypoventilation and hyperventilation. The spontaneously breathing patient can easily be overventilated, resulting in hyperventilation. If the volume or minimum rate is set low and the patient is apneic or weak, the patient will be hypoventilated. Thus these patients require vigilant assessment and monitoring of ventilatory status, including ABGs. It is important that the amount of negative pressure required to initiate a breath is appropriate to the patient's condition. If it is too difficult to initiate a breath, the work of breathing is increased. If it is too easy, the patient will be at risk for overventilation and respiratory alkalosis.

Synchronized Intermittent Mandatory Ventilation. With SIMV, the ventilator delivers a preset tidal volume at a preset frequency in synchrony with the patient's spontaneous breathing. Between ventilator-delivered breaths, the patient is able to breathe spontaneously through the ventilator circuit. Thus the patient receives the preset inspired oxygen concentration during the spontaneous breaths but self-regulates the rate and depth of those breaths. This mode of ventilation differs from ACV, in which all breaths are of the same preset volume. SIMV is the most common mode of ventilatory support. It is used during continuous ventilation and during weaning from the ventilator. Potential benefits of

SIMV include avoidance of respiratory alkalosis, minimizing the patient "fighting" the ventilator, lower mean airway pressure, more uniform intrapulmonary gas distribution, and prevention of muscle atrophy.[25]

SIMV has advantages over other modes with respect to cardiovascular effects. Spontaneous inspiration decreases intrathoracic pressure, reduces mean intrathoracic pressure, and enhances venous blood return to the heart. Thus the patient with an extracellular fluid volume deficit is better able to maintain CO. Because of the lower mean intrathoracic pressure, higher levels of PEEP may be used with SIMV than with other modes of volume-controlled ventilation.

Weaning patients from ventilators can be accomplished using SIMV. Instead of abruptly removing patients from ventilators and letting them breathe totally on their own, SIMV allows a smooth transition to spontaneous ventilation by gradually decreasing the ventilator rate as patients assume an increasing percentage of the total work of breathing.

There are disadvantages with SIMV. If spontaneous breathing decreases when the rate is low, ventilation might not be adequately supported. Low-rate SIMV should be used only in patients with regular, spontaneous breathing. Weaning with SIMV demands close monitoring and may take longer because the rate of breathing is gradually reduced. Patients being weaned with SIMV may become fatigued, especially during the night.

Other Ventilatory Maneuvers

Positive End-Expiratory Pressure.

PEEP is a ventilatory maneuver in which positive pressure is applied to the airway during exhalation. Normally during exhalation airway pressure drops to zero, and exhalation occurs passively. With PEEP exhalation remains passive, but pressure falls to a preset level greater than zero, often 3 to 20 cm H_2O. With PEEP lung volume during expiration and between breaths is greater than normal. Thus PEEP increases functional residual capacity (FRC). This often improves oxygenation. The mechanisms by which PEEP increases FRC and oxygenation include increased distention of already patent alveoli, prevention of alveolar collapse, and aeration of previously collapsed alveoli.[25] PEEP often allows the fraction of inspired oxygen (FIO_2) to be reduced, thus lowering the risk of oxygen toxicity.

PEEP is prescribed in increments of 2 to 5 cm H_2O. The amount of PEEP selected is determined by the amount that improves oxygenation without decreasing blood pressure and CO. This is termed *best* or *optimal PEEP*. Often 5 cm H_2O PEEP (so-called physiologic PEEP) is used prophylactically to replace the glottic mechanism, help maintain a normal FRC, and prevent alveolar collapse. Clinical studies vary regarding the benefits of physiologic PEEP. PEEP of 5 cm H_2O is also used for patients with a history of alveolar collapse during weaning. PEEP has demonstrated improvements in gas exchange, vital capacity, and inspiratory force when used during weaning.

Inspiratory pressure increases when expiratory pressure is added. The most common mode of PEEP delivery is with SIMV. The decreased mean airway pressure that occurs during spontaneous breathing is enough to prevent some of the adverse effects produced by the increased pressures.

In general, the major purpose of PEEP is to maintain adequate oxygenation while limiting risk of oxygen toxicity. PEEP is also used to prevent atelectasis. PEEP is thought to be useful in pulmonary edema, providing a counterpressure opposing fluid extravasation. PEEP is indicated in lungs with diffuse disease, severe hypoxemia unresponsive to FIO_2 greater than 0.5 (50% oxygen), and loss of compliance or stiffness. The classic indication for PEEP therapy is acute respiratory distress syndrome (ARDS) characterized by a reduced FRC and hypoxemia that is refractory to oxygen therapy. PEEP is generally contraindicated or used with extreme caution in patients with highly compliant lungs (e.g., COPD), unilateral or nonuniform disease, hypovolemia, and low CO. In these situations the adverse effects of PEEP may outweigh any benefits.

Continuous Positive Airway Pressure.

Continuous positive airway pressure (CPAP) is the use of PEEP in a spontaneously breathing patient. With CPAP there is a constant flow of gas at a rate greater than the patient's spontaneous inspiratory flow rate. Thus the patient's airway pressure never falls to zero. For example, if CPAP is 5 cm H_2O, during exhalation airway pressure is 5 cm H_2O; during inspiration, 1 to 2 cm H_2O of negative pressure is generated, reducing airway pressure to 3 or 4 cm H_2O. The patient receiving SIMV with PEEP receives CPAP when breathing spontaneously. CPAP is often used in infants. It is also commonly used in the treatment of obstructive sleep apnea. CPAP can be administered by a tight-fitting mask or an ET or tracheal tube. CPAP increases work of breathing because the patient must forcibly exhale against the CPAP.

Pressure Support Ventilation.

With pressure support ventilation (PSV), positive pressure is applied to the airway only during inspiration and is used in conjunction with the patient's spontaneous respirations. A preset level of positive airway pressure is selected so that the gas flow rate is greater than the patient's inspiratory flow rate. As the patient initiates a breath, the machine senses the spontaneous effort and supplies a rapid flow of gas, supporting the inspiratory effort. With PSV the patient determines inspiratory length, flow rate, and respiratory rate. Tidal volume depends on the pressure level and airway compliance. PSV is used with continuous ventilation and is especially helpful in combination with SIMV during weaning. PSV is not used as a sole ventilatory support during acute respiratory failure because of the risk of hypoventilation. Advantages to PSV include increased patient comfort, decreased work of breathing (because inspiratory efforts are augmented), decreased oxygen consumption (because inspiratory work is reduced), and increased endurance conditioning (because the patient is exercising respiratory muscles).[26]

Inverse-Ratio Ventilation.

With inverse-ratio ventilation (IRV), inspiration is prolonged and expiration shortened. The I/E ratio is the ratio of duration of inspiration (I) to the duration of expiration (E). This value is normally less than 1. With IRV the I/E ratio approaches 1. With IRV a prolonged positive pressure is applied, increasing inspiratory time. IRV progressively expands collapsed alveoli. The short expiratory time has a PEEP-like effect, preventing alveolar collapse. Because IRV imposes a nonphysiologic breathing pattern, the patient requires sedation or paralysis. IRV is indicated for patients with ARDS who continue to have refractory hypoxemia despite a PEEP of 15 cm H_2O or more. Not all patients with poor oxygenation respond to IRV.

High-Frequency Ventilation.

High-frequency ventilation (HFV) involves delivery of a small tidal volume (usually 1 to 5 ml/kg body weight) at rapid respiratory rates (100 to 300 breaths per minute). HFV can minimize some complications attributed to conventional mechanical ventilation because mean airway pressure is lower. Use of HFV is limited to severely ill patients. HFV is used in patients with bronchopleural fistulas because lower peak airway pressures can prevent worsening of this condition. Some patients with ARDS and acute respiratory failure may benefit from HFV, although results of clinical trials do not indicate many advantages or improvement in mortality rates over conventional forms of mechanical ventilation. HFV is more commonly used in neonatal patients.

Complications of Mechanical Ventilation

Although mechanical ventilation may be essential to maintain ventilation and oxygenation, it can cause adverse effects. It is often difficult to distinguish complications of mechanical ventilation from the underlying disease.

Cardiovascular System.

Positive pressure mechanical ventilation can cause circulatory problems because of transmission of increased mean airway pressure to the thoracic cavity. With increased intrathoracic pressure, thoracic vessels are compressed. This results in decreased venous return to the heart, decreased left ventricular end-diastolic volume (preload), decreased CO, and lowered blood pressure. Mean airway pressure is further increased with PEEP.

If the lungs are noncompliant (as in ARDS), airway pressures are not as easily transmitted to the heart and blood vessels. Thus effects of mechanical ventilation on CO are reduced. Conversely, with compliant lungs (e.g., emphysema), there is increased danger of transmission of high airway pressures and CO may decrease.

Compromise of venous return by positive pressure ventilation is exaggerated by hypovolemia (e.g., hemorrhage, multiple trauma) and decreased venous tone (e.g., sepsis, spinal shock). Restoration and maintenance of the circulating blood volume is important in minimizing cardiovascular complications.

Some studies have found improved cardiac performance after the initiation of mechanical ventilation in patients with poor left ventricular function.[27] It is postulated that positive pressure ventilation decreases right-sided heart preload by its increase in intrathoracic pressure. The increased airway pressure may restrict left ventricular filling by mechanical compression. These effects may improve the failing left ventricle by optimizing ventricular end-diastolic volume.

Sodium and Water Balance. Progressive fluid retention often occurs after 48 to 72 hours of mechanical ventilation. Positive pressure ventilation, especially with PEEP, is associated with decreased urinary output and increased sodium retention. Fluid balance changes may be due to decreased CO, which in turn results in diminished renal perfusion. Renin release is stimulated, which increases aldosterone secretion and subsequent sodium and water retention. It is also possible that pressure changes within the thorax are associated with decreased release of atrial natriuretic peptide, also causing sodium retention. Mild water retention is also associated with mechanical ventilation. There is less insensible water loss via the airway, because inspired gases are saturated with water at body temperature. In addition, as with all stressed patients, release of antidiuretic hormone may be increased, causing water retention.

Pulmonary System

Barotrauma. As lung inflation pressures increase, risk of pneumothorax, pneumomediastinum, and subcutaneous emphysema increases. Patients with compliant lungs (e.g., COPD) are at greater risk because the increased airway pressure readily distends the lungs and may rupture alveoli or emphysematous blebs. Patients with stiff lungs (e.g., ARDS), who are given high inspiratory pressures and high levels of PEEP, and patients with suppurative lung abscesses resulting from necrotizing organisms (e.g., staphylococci) are also susceptible to barotrauma.

Air can escape into the pleural space from alveoli or interstitium, accumulate, and become trapped. Pleural pressure increases and collapses the lung, causing pneumothorax. (Clinical manifestations of pneumothorax are discussed in Chapter 26.) The lung receives air during inspiration but cannot expel it during expiration. Respiratory bronchioles are larger on inspiration than expiration. They may close on expiration, and air becomes trapped. With positive pressure breathing, a simple pneumothorax can become a life-threatening tension pneumothorax. With tension pneumothorax, the mediastinum and contralateral lung are compressed, compromising CO. Immediate treatment of the pneumothorax is required.

Pneumomediastinum usually begins with rupture of alveoli into the lung interstitium; progressive air movement then occurs into the mediastinum and subcutaneous neck tissue. This is commonly followed by pneumothorax. Occurrence of new, unexplained subcutaneous air is an indication for immediate chest x-ray. Pneumomediastinum and subcutaneous emphysema in the neck may be too small to be detected radiographically or clinically before the development of a pneumothorax.

Subcutaneous emphysema may occur after a tracheotomy as a result of leakage of air around the surgical site, or it may occur around the site of a chest tube for pneumothorax. In the latter case, subcutaneous emphysema is usually caused by the passage of gas from the pleural space into the chest tube wound, indicating that the space is not being adequately drained. Chest tube patency must be maintained to prevent a further increase in the pneumothorax.

Alveolar hypoventilation. Hypoventilation can be caused by inappropriate ventilator settings, leakage of air from the ventilator tubing or around the ET tube or tracheostomy cuff, lung secretions or obstruction, and low ventilation/perfusion ratio. Low tidal volume or respiratory rate decreases minute ventilation, causing hypoventilation. A leaking cuff or tubings that are not secured may cause air leakage, lowering the delivered tidal volume. Too low a SIMV rate in a patient who is unable to produce adequate spontaneous ventilation causes hypoventilation, respiratory acidosis, and additional problems related to acidosis such as cardiac arrhythmias. Excess lung secretions can cause hypoventilation. This can be alleviated by turning the patient every 1 to 2 hours, providing chest physical therapy to lung areas with increased secretions, encouraging deep breathing and coughing, and suctioning as needed. Atelectasis may develop. Increasing the tidal volume, adding small increments of PEEP, and sighing the patient lessens the likelihood of atelectasis. Frequent position change also helps.

Alveolar hyperventilation. Respiratory alkalosis can occur if the rate or tidal volume is set too high (mechanical overventilation) or if the patient receiving assisted ventilation is hyperventilating. Hyperventilation means that the $PaCO_2$ tension is less than 35 mm Hg. The patient or the ventilator is blowing off CO_2 too rapidly.

It is easy to overventilate a patient on mechanical ventilation. Particularly at risk is the patient with chronic alveolar hypoventilation and CO_2 retention (e.g., the COPD patient). This patient may have a chronic arterial CO_2 elevation and compensatory bicarbonate retention by the kidneys. When the patient is ventilated, the patient's "normal" rather than standard normal values should be the therapeutic goal. If the COPD patient is returned to a standard normal arterial CO_2 tension, the patient will develop alkalosis because of the retained bicarbonate. Such a patient could move from compensated acidosis to serious metabolic alkalosis. The presence of alkalosis makes weaning from the ventilator difficult. Alkalosis, especially if the onset is abrupt, can have additional serious consequences, including hypokalemia and hypocalcemia, predisposing the patient to arrhythmias. Neuromuscular irritability, seizures, coma, and death can occur.

To prevent alkalosis, mechanical ventilation should be initiated and should remain at a level that will not dramatically lower the arterial CO_2 level ($PaCO_2$). ABGs must be assessed 15 to 30 minutes after mechanical ventilation begins and after each ventilator change, serially thereafter, and whenever changes in the patient's clinical status occur. The $PaCO_2$ tension should be gradually lowered only to the patient's baseline (before acute illness) level. Usually patients with COPD on the ventilator do better with a short inspiratory and longer expiratory time.

If the hyperventilation is spontaneous, it is important to determine the cause and treat it. Causes might include hypoxemia, pain, fear, anxiety, or compensation for metabolic acidosis. Patients who fight the ventilator or breathe out of synchrony may be anxious or in pain. If the patient is anxious and fearful, sitting with the patient and verbally coaching the patient to breathe with the ventilator may help. If these measures fail, manually bagging the patient slowly with the MRB connected to an oxygen source may slow breathing enough to bring it in synchrony with the ventilator. The patient may require morphine, lorazepam (Ativan), or other sedatives.

Ventilator-associated pneumonia. Ventilator-associated pneumonia (VAP) is common because normal upper airway defenses have been bypassed by the ET or tracheostomy tube, increasing the patient's risk for infection. In addition, poor nutritional state, immobility, and the underlying disease process (e.g., immunosuppression, organ failure) make the patient more prone to infection.

In patients receiving prolonged mechanical ventilation, sputum cultures often grow gram-negative bacteria such as *Pseudomonas, Serratia,* and *Klebsiella.* These are abundant in the hospital environment and the patient's gastrointestinal tract. Organisms can spread in a number of ways, including contaminated respiratory equipment, inadequate hand washing, adverse environmental factors such as poor room ventilation and high traffic flow, and decreased patient ability to cough and clear secretions. Colonization of the oropharynx tract by gram-negative organisms is a predisposing factor in the development of gram-negative pneumonia.

Infection can be minimized by using strict aseptic technique while suctioning or handling the artificial airway. Frequent hand washing is imperative. The nurse should wear latex or other impermeable gloves when in contact with the patient or equipment and change gloves between procedures (such as bathing the patient and administering an intravenous medication).

Oral and nasal care are important, as well as frequent turning to promote mobilization of secretions. Condensation collecting in the ventilator tubing should be drained away from the patient as it collects. Instillation of normal saline into the endotracheal tube, a common practice thought to facilitate the removal of secretions with suctioning, is to be discouraged. It is not effective and may actually wash microbes lining the ET tube back into the lungs.

Keeping the head of the bed elevated, especially in patients receiving tube feedings, may help decrease aspiration. Frequent suctioning of the oropharynx will remove pooled secretions. A new type of ET tube is available that has a port above the vocal cords. Suction to the port is thought to evacuate pooled secretions and could reduce aspiration. Chest physical therapy, adequate humidification of inspired gases, and sterile suctioning may help prevent infection by eliminating secretion accumulation.

Clinical evidence suggesting VAP includes fever, elevated white blood cell count, purulent sputum, sputum odor, auscultation that reveals crackles or rhonchi, and pulmonary infiltrates noted on chest x-ray. The patient is treated with antibiotics after appropriate cultures are taken by tracheal suctioning or bronchoscopy and when infection is evident.

Neurologic System. In patients with head injury, positive pressure ventilation, especially with PEEP, can impair cerebral blood flow. This is related to increased intrathoracic positive pressure impeding venous drainage from the head, as evidenced by jugular venous distention. As a result of the impaired venous return and increase in cerebral volume, the patient may exhibit increases in intracranial pressure. Elevating the head of the bed may decrease the effects of PEEP.

Gastrointestinal System. Patients receiving mechanical ventilation are often stressed because of serious illness, immobility, and discomforts associated with the ventilator. Thus the ventilated patient is at risk for developing stress ulcers and gastrointestinal (GI) bleeding. Patients with a preexisting ulcer or those receiving corticosteroid therapy are at an especially increased risk. Direct visualization of the stomach via endoscopy demonstrates that gastric and duodenal mucosal changes occur in many critically ill patients. Any kind of circulatory compromise, including reduction of CO caused by mechanical ventilation, may contribute to ischemia of the intestinal mucosa and possibly increase the risk of translocation of GI bacteria.[28]

Prophylactic administration of antacids to maintain a gastric pH greater than 5 and enteral tube feedings reduce the occurrence of upper GI bleeding. Specially designed feeding tubes with a pH-sensitive probe allow for the measurement of gastric pH. Other methods of assessment include checking the pH of gastric aspirates. Prophylactic use of histamine H_2-receptor blockers (cimetidine [Tagamet] and ranitidine [Zantac]), administered intravenously or orally, decrease gastric acidity and diminish the risk of stress ulcer and hemorrhage.

Gastric and bowel dilation may occur as a result of gas accumulation in the GI tract mainly by being swallowed into the stomach. The irritation of an artificial airway may cause excessive air swallowing and subsequent gastric dilation. Gastric or bowel dilation may put pressure on the vena cava, decrease CO, and prohibit adequate diaphragmatic excursion during spontaneous breathing. Elevation of the diaphragm as a result of paralytic ileus or bowel dilation leads to compression of the lower lobes of the lungs, which may cause atelectasis and compromise respiratory function. Decompression of the stomach can be accomplished by the insertion of a nasogastric tube. Some clinicians routinely insert nasogastric tubes prophylactically when mechanical ventilation is initiated. A nasogastric tube may also be inserted to decrease aspiration if the patient is in danger of vomiting.

Immobility, sedation, circulatory impairment, decreased oral intake, use of opioid pain medications, and stress contribute to decreased peristalsis. The patient's inability to exhale against a closed glottis may make defecation difficult. As a result the ventilated patient could be predisposed to constipation. With the early use of enteral nutrition, constipation is usually not a problem.

Musculoskeletal System. Maintenance of muscle strength and prevention of the problems associated with immobility are important. Exercise tolerance is enhanced by adequate analgesia and adequate nutrition. Progressive ambulation of patients receiving long-term ventilation can be attained without interruption of mechanical ventilation. The ventilator can be pushed around the room, or the patient can be ventilated with an oxygenated MRB while ambulating. Passive and active exercises, consisting of movements to maintain muscle tone in the upper and lower extremities, should be done in bed. Simple maneuvers such as leg lifts, knee bends, quadriceps setting, or arm circles are appropriate. Prevention of contractures, pressure ulcers, footdrop, and external rotation of the hip and legs by proper positioning is important.

Psychologic Effects. The patient receiving mechanical ventilation may experience physical and emotional stress. In addition to the problems related to critical care patients discussed at the beginning of this chapter, the patient on a mechanical ventilator is unable to speak, eat, move, or breathe normally. Tubes and machines may cause pain, fear, and anxiety. Ordinary functions such as eating, elimination, and coughing are complicated.

Patients receiving mechanical ventilation usually require some type of sedation (e.g., propofol [Diprivan]) or paralyzing agent (e.g., pancuronium [Pavulon]) to facilitate optimal ventilation. Before initiating sedation or paralysis in the mechanically ventilated patient who is agitated, it is important to assess for the cause of agitation. Common problems that can result in patient agitation include ET tube malposition, pain, hypoxemia, pulmonary embolism, drug reaction, and emotional distress. The treatment should be explained to the patient. If the patient is paralyzed, the nurse should remember that the patient can hear, see, think, and feel. Sedative and pain medications are commonly administered as continuous infusions and must be given if neuromuscular blocking agents are used. Many patients have few memories of their time in the ICU, whereas others remember in vivid detail. Although appearing to be asleep, sedated, or paralyzed, patients may be aware of their surroundings and should always be addressed as though awake.

It is important that the patient have a means to communicate. This may be as simple as eye blinking or head motion, or a computer, paper and pencil, an alphabet, word or picture boards, or a magic slate might be provided if the patient does not require wrist restraints. In some instances tracheostomy tubes that allow speech can be used. The nurse should be attuned to the patient's body language and facial expressions, but this should not be allowed to substitute for providing the patient an opportunity for verbal expression if at all possible.

Measures to make the ventilated patient's environment more restful include efficient scheduling of care to reduce interruptions and a calm, reassuring approach. Especially helpful to the patient is the presence of a loved one or significant family member. This person may have a calming, restful effect on the patient by merely being in the room. The nurse should assess family members and recruit those who have a therapeutic role.

The patient receiving long-term ventilation should be moved to an area with a window to better appreciate night and day and the outside world. Even if the patient is unable to converse, the patient should be addressed. The nurse should discuss the patient's interests and explain in simple terms what the different tubes and equipment are and what progress is being made. Reassuring the patient honestly about progress and allowing the patient as much control as possible may ease the frustration of dependence. Deciding when to bathe or wash hair, which direction to turn, or what to eat may be the patient's only way of maintaining control.

Machine Malfunction or Disconnection. Mechanical ventilators may malfunction or become disconnected. When turned on and operative, alarms alert the nurse to problems. Most deaths from accidental ventilator disconnections occur while the alarm is turned off, and most accidental disconnections in critical care settings are discovered by alarm activation. The most frequent site for disconnection is between the tracheal tube and the adapter. The nurse should ascertain that alarms are set at all times and should chart that this is the case. Alarms should be paused (not inactivated) during suctioning or removal from the ventilator. If alert, the patient should be provided a call bell to bring attention to problems. Connections should be pushed together and then twisted to secure more tightly. The patient's bedside should be arranged so that an MRB with tubing sufficient to reach the patient is set up and functional at all times. Before placing the patient in a chair, the nurse should make sure that the MRB is accessible and functional and that the tubing will reach the patient in the event of an emergency. Although most institutions have emergency generators in the event of a power failure, the nurse should always consider the possibility that power will fail and have a plan for manually ventilating all the patients who are dependent on a ventilator.

Nutritional Therapy: Patient Receiving Mechanical Ventilation

Mechanical ventilation and the hypermetabolism associated with critical illness can contribute to inadequate nutrition. Presence of an ET tube eliminates the normal route for eating. Although patients who are nasotracheally intubated may be allowed liquid and semiliquid feedings orally, it is difficult to ingest sufficient calories, protein, and fat. A patient with a tracheostomy can eat normally once the stoma has healed. When a tracheostomy tube is present, the patient should tilt the head slightly forward to facilitate swallowing and to prevent aspiration. Often, soft foods (e.g., puddings, ice cream) are more easily swallowed than liquids.

Patients likely to be without food for 3 to 5 days should have a nutritional program initiated. Inadequate nutrition makes the patient receiving prolonged mechanical ventilation more prone to poor oxygen transport secondary to anemia and to poor tolerance of minimal exercise. Disuse of respiratory muscles and poor nutrition result in decreased respiratory muscle strength. In addition, the hypermetabolism associated with critical illness, trauma, and surgery and the presence of anxiety, pain, and increased work of breathing greatly increase caloric expenditure. Serum protein levels (e.g., transferrin, prealbumin) are usually decreased. Inadequate nutrition can delay weaning, decrease the speed of recovery, and decrease resistance to infection. Enteral feeding is the preferred method to meet caloric needs.

A concern regarding the nutritional support of patients on mechanical ventilation is the carbohydrate content of the diet. Metabolism of carbohydrates results in high levels of CO_2 production. The resulting CO_2 load results in a higher required minute ventilation. This in turn can cause an unnecessary increased effort to breathe. Decreasing carbohydrate content in the diet lowers CO_2 production. Preparations such as Pulmocare, which are high in protein and fat but low in carbohydrate content, may be beneficial in ventilated patients. A dietician can provide useful consultation for the ventilated patient.

The ventilated patient receiving enteral feedings should have the head of the bed elevated. A soft, flexible, small-bore feeding tube should be used. When the tube is initially placed, the position of the tube is verified by x-ray. (Procedures for tube feedings are discussed in Chapter 38.)

Tube feedings should be stopped for at least 30 minutes before placing the patient in a head-down position for postural drainage. Residuals should be checked periodically. Elevated residuals indicate that the feeding is not moving through the GI system. Other indications of feeding problems include bloating, nausea, vomiting, and abdominal distention. The tube feeding should be temporarily stopped and the physician notified. The patient must be observed closely for signs of hypoglycemia if the tube feedings are discontinued for long periods of time. Food coloring in the feedings can help identify the presence of feedings in secretions suctioned from the trachea. The presence of a positive glucose reaction on a dipstick of tracheal secretions may indicate aspiration of feedings into the trachea. If there is evidence that aspiration may have occurred, the tube feeding should be stopped immediately and the physician notified.

Manual Resuscitation Bag and Suction Equipment

All patients receiving mechanical ventilation should have an MRB along with a mask attached to oxygen and suctioning equipment ready and available at the bedside. The MRB should contain a reservoir to sequester oxygen so that oxygen concentrations of 90% to 95% can be delivered. The slower the bag is deflated and inflated, the higher the oxygen concentration that will be delivered. The Ambu (air mask bag unit) is a well-known self-inflatable bag. This unit consists of a bag fitted to a face mask or a tracheal tube attachment. In the event the patient self-extubates, ventilation is maintained with the MRB and mask.

Weaning from Mechanical Ventilation

The process of reducing ventilator support and resuming spontaneous ventilation is termed *weaning*. Weaning may be of varying length, ranging from a few hours in postoperative open heart patients to weeks in the patient with chronic pulmonary disease. Patients likely to require prolonged mechanical ventilation generally are those with underlying lung disease who develop respiratory failure because of surgical procedure, trauma, or infection. Preparations for weaning begin well in advance of the event. These preparations include maintaining nutrition, fluid-electrolyte and acid-base balances, CO, pulmonary, and psychologic status.

Readiness for weaning depends on many factors.[29] Criteria vary, depending on prior lung status and ventilatory reserve. For weaning to be successful, the patient should be as stable as possible. Respiratory parameters should demonstrate a patent airway, adequate ventilatory muscle strength, and an effective cough. Oxygenation should be adequate, and the lungs should be reasonably clear on auscultation and chest x-ray. It is important to have an alert, well-rested patient relatively free from pain who will readily take deep breaths to obtain optimum

alveolar ventilation and prevent atelectasis. This does not mean complete withdrawal from sedatives or analgesics. Instead, medications should be titrated to relieve pain without causing excessive drowsiness.

A variety of weaning methods are available, and no one method is superior. All methods can be delivered with the patient remaining connected to the ventilator circuit. The patient on SIMV can have the ventilator breath frequency gradually reduced as the patient's ventilatory status permits. CPAP or PSV can be added to SIMV. Another method involves PSV, CPAP, or both delivered without SIMV. PSV is thought to provide gentle, slow respiratory muscle conditioning and may be especially beneficial for patients who are deconditioned or have cardiac problems. Some patients may be weaned by simply providing humidified oxygen (T-piece or flowby method).

The patient might be allowed spontaneous ventilation for 10 minutes each hour and receive ventilator support for 50 minutes, with the ratio of spontaneous ventilation to ventilation support gradually increasing. Regardless of method used, it is important to allow the patient's respiratory muscles adequate rest between weaning trials. Once the respiratory muscles become fatigued, they may require 12 to 24 hours to recover.

With all methods, patients usually require a 10% increase in FIO_2 to maintain arterial oxygen tension. This is because tidal volume usually drops with spontaneous respiration, and carbon dioxide tension may increase. Weaning is usually carried out during the day, with the patient ventilated at night until there is sufficient spontaneous ventilation without excess fatigue.

The patient being weaned should be provided continuing psychologic support. The weaning process should be explained and the patient informed of progress. The patient should be placed in a sitting or semirecumbent position and made comfortable. Respiratory parameters are measured to provide a baseline with which serial determinations can be compared. The tidal volume, respiratory rate, negative inspiratory force, and vital capacity are measured. ABGs are drawn at baseline and at specified intervals during weaning.

The patient must be monitored closely for signs of respiratory distress, including shallow breathing, use of accessory respiratory muscles, restlessness, tiring, somnolence, tachycardia, decrease or increase in blood pressure, tachypnea or bradypnea, ECG changes, drop in SpO_2, and secretion buildup with a need for frequent suctioning. Statements from the patient regarding weaning tolerance are important.

When the patient is ready for extubation, the mouth and oropharynx should be thoroughly suctioned and the cuff deflated. An oxygen mask or cannula should be set up and ready for use. The patient should be told to expect to cough when the tube is removed. The nurse should be prepared to manage copious secretions. Once the patient has been extubated and stabilized with oxygen delivered by mask or nasal cannula, care of the mouth and nares should be provided. ABGs are obtained 20 to 30 minutes after extubation. The patient must be monitored for respiratory distress caused by the underlying lung problems and also because laryngeal or tracheal edema may develop. Manifestations of laryngeal and tracheal edema include symptoms of acute upper airway obstruction. Measures to ensure pulmonary toilet (e.g., coughing, deep breathing, turning, and suctioning [if necessary]) must be continued.

Home Mechanical Ventilation

Mechanical ventilators are no longer limited to the ICU, but are now a part of home health care. Families can be taught to care for the person receiving mechanical ventilation as an alternative to prolonged hospitalization.[30,31] The emphasis on controlling hospital health care costs has increased the early discharge of patients and the need to provide highly technical care such as mechanical ventilation in home settings.

Home mechanical ventilation has several advantages. Having the patient in the home eliminates the strain that the hospital setting may impose on family dynamics. The feeling of helplessness by family members when they first hear about the necessity for long-term mechanical ventilation is frequently countered by the ability of the family to participate fully in the patient's care in the home setting. At home the patient may be able to participate more in activities of daily living around a more individualized schedule and, because of the smaller size of the home ventilator, be more mobile.[32] Another advantage of home mechanical ventilation is the reduction in the patient's risk of nosocomial infection. Disadvantages include problems related to reimbursement, equipment, caregiving, and the complex needs of these patients. Ventilated patients are usually dependent, requiring extensive nursing care. In one study it was found that an average of 8 hours of care per day was required.[30] Disposable products may be nonreimbursable. Financial resources must be carefully assessed when arranging home mechanical ventilation. Another disadvantage of home mechanical ventilation is its potential impact on the family. Family members may seem enthusiastic about caring for their loved one in the home but may be motivated by guilt. They may lack understanding of the potential sacrifices they may have to make financially and in time and commitment.

Both negative pressure and positive pressure (volume) ventilators can be used in the home. Negative pressure ventilators are frequently the ventilator of choice because they do not require an artificial airway and are less complicated to use. Small, portable volume ventilators that can be attached to a wheelchair or placed on a bedside table are available. Settings and alarms on these ventilators are similar to the larger ones used in ICUs. Some home ventilators have IMV capability.

NURSING MANAGEMENT: MECHANICAL VENTILATION

Nursing management of the patient receiving mechanical ventilation is presented in NCP 63-2.

INTRACRANIAL PRESSURE MONITORING

Intracranial pressure (ICP) is the hydrostatic force measured in the brain cerebrospinal fluid (CSF) compartment. ICP may become elevated because of head trauma, stroke, subarachnoid hemorrhage, brain tumor, inflammation, or brain tissue damage from other causes (see Table 54-4). Any patient who becomes acutely unconscious, regardless of the cause, is managed as if there were actual or potential increased ICP. Patients with or at risk for elevated ICP are usually cared for in an ICU and often receive invasive ICP monitoring. As with other invasive ICU measures, ICP monitoring is provided to those who may benefit from treatment and in whom the underlying process is thought to be self-limiting. Patients with irreversible pathology or advanced neurologic decline caused by primary or metastatic lesions usually do not receive ICP monitoring. Nursing management goals in elevated ICP include preservation of function, early identification of neurologic changes, and prevention of complications. Patients may require intensive physical care and emotional support.

Increased Intracranial Pressure

ICP is important because it influences cerebral perfusion. When evaluating cerebral perfusion, it is important to consider systemic blood pressure, ICP, blood flow, vascular resistance, and blood volume. Mean arterial pressure (MAP) provides the driving force for brain blood flow. ICP, reflecting the pressure within the brain tissue and CSF, opposes blood flow. Thus cerebral perfusion pressure (CPP), which equals MAP minus ICP, is the clinically relevant variable that must be considered. Cerebral blood flow, expressed in milliliters of blood per minute, must be maintained at a relatively high rate because of the high and continuing metabolic needs of brain tissue. Cerebral vascular resistance, generated by the arterioles within the cranium, links CPP and blood flow as follows:

$$CPP = Flow \times Resistance$$

The volume of blood within the cranium (intracranial blood volume) is important because it affects ICP. Cerebral blood flow and increased intracranial pressure are discussed in Chapter 54.

Elevated ICP is clinically significant because it diminishes CPP, causing brain ischemia or infarction. Also, brain structures can be compressed and damaged or irreversibly destroyed. Death can occur. High ICP causes herniation of brain tissue, that is, extrusion into abnormal spaces. Cerebral hemispheres can shift across the midline. Brainstem and cerebral hemispheres can herniate through the tentorium cerebelli. The cerebellum can herniate through the foramen magnum (tonsillar herniation; herniation is discussed in further detail in Chapter 54). These complications are generally fatal.

A slow increase in ICP, as with an enlarging brain tumor, is tolerated better than a rapid increase, as in primary brain injury. If an elevated pressure is evenly distributed throughout the brain, it is better tolerated. Crucial to preservation of tissue is preservation of cerebral blood flow. With slower, distributed rises in ICP, blood flow tends to be preserved.

CPP is useful in evaluating brain blood flow. Normal CPP is 70 to 100 mm Hg. At least 50 to 60 mm Hg is necessary for adequate cerebral perfusion. CPP less than 50 mm Hg is associated with ischemia and neuronal death. It is of paramount importance to maintain MAP when ICP is elevated. It should be remembered that CPP might not reflect perfusion pressure in all parts of the brain. There may be local areas of swelling and compression. Thus a higher CPP may be needed for these patients to prevent localized tissue damage.

Intracranial Pressure Measurement and Line Management

Technical Apparatus. ICP monitoring is used regularly to guide therapy in patients with suspected increased ICP. Some invasive ICP monitoring systems are similar to invasive blood pressure monitoring systems in that a fluid-filled tube couples

63-2 NURSING CARE PLAN PATIENT ON MECHANICAL VENTILATION

Expected Patient Outcomes   Nursing Interventions and *Rationales*

NURSING DIAGNOSIS **Risk for injury** *related to* possible machine malfunction, accidental disconnection, inability to breathe unassisted, asynchrony with ventilator, and settings unsuitable to maintain adequate ventilation.

- ABGs within normal range for patient.
- Early detection of signs and symptoms of decreased PaO_2 and increased $PaCO_2$.
- Breathe synchronously with ventilator.
- Early detection, correction, or prevention of complications associated with mechanical malfunction or disconnection.

- Monitor for risk factors such as hypoxemia, hypercapnia, tachycardia, tachypnea, increase in BP, agitation, confusion, headache, lethargy, cyanosis; respiratory pattern asynchronous with machine's pattern of ventilation; machine malfunction or disconnection *to determine presence of risk factors and plan for intervention.*
- Begin mechanical ventilation slowly (especially in patients with COPD); lower $PaCO_2$ only to patient's baseline level *to prevent alkalosis, especially in patient with compensated respiratory acidosis.*
- Assess patient for possible causes of hyperventilation such as retained secretions, hypoxemia, pain, fear, and anxiety.
- Check ventilator settings (FIO_2, respiratory rate, tidal volume, O_2 flow rate, PEEP, airway pressure, thermistor temperature, and I:E ratio) *to determine if appropriate to clinical situation.*
- Keep manual resuscitation bag connected to O_2 source at bedside *for use in case of an emergency.*
- If patient is fighting ventilation, slowly bag for three to six breaths and verbally coach patient to breathe *to help synchronize patient with ventilator.*
- Determine and treat cause of asynchrony.
- Turn all alarms on; pause but do not turn off alarms during suctioning and disconnections.
- Respond immediately to alarm *because potentially dangerous situations of mechanical malfunction or patient asynchrony with the ventilator may be present.*
- Check cuff for leaks *to prevent loss of ventilation gas and to prevent aspiration of oral secretions.*
- Monitor ventilator tubing q1-2hr for condensed water and drain when water present *to prevent aspiration of accumulated fluid.*

NURSING DIAGNOSIS **Decreased cardiac output** *related to* impeded venous return by positive pressure ventilation *as manifested by* decreased BP, increased heart rate, decreased urine output, presence of arrhythmias, mental confusion.

- BP and cardiac output within normal range.
- Adequate urinary output.

- Monitor vital signs and level of consciousness q2-4hr.
- Observe and monitor for clinical manifestations of decreased cardiac output *to identify decreased venous return to the heart, decreased left ventricular end-diastolic volume, and lowered blood pressure.*
- Monitor direct measurement of cardiac output by thermodilution, especially when >10 cm H_2O PEEP is used *to anticipate need for plasma expanders, vasopressors, and IV fluids as ordered because hemodynamic complications of decreased venous return induced by positive pressure ventilation are exaggerated by hypovolemia.*

NURSING DIAGNOSIS **Ineffective airway clearance** *related to* presence of artificial airway, problems with positioning, accumulation of secretions, and immobility *as manifested by* presence of abnormal breath sounds, absent cough, presence of thick or copious secretions.

- Normal breath sounds.
- Thin and easily removed secretions.

- Change patient's position q2hr *to prevent pooling of secretions in the lungs.*
- Have patient cough and, if feasible, deep breathe q2hr *to remove secretions and to prevent hypoventilation.*
- Perform tracheobronchial suctioning *to remove retained secretions and improve oxygenation.*
- Auscultate breath sounds q2-4hr *to monitor effectiveness of interventions.*

Continued

63-2   NURSING CARE PLAN   PATIENT ON MECHANICAL VENTILATION
—continued

Expected Patient Outcomes	Nursing Interventions and *Rationales*

NURSING DIAGNOSIS   Impaired physical mobility *related to* restricted movement *as manifested by* inability to perform active range-of-motion exercise.

- Normal range of motion of joints.

- Perform active and passive range-of-motion exercises (e.g., leg lifts, knee bends, quadriceps setting, arm circles) *to maintain patient's joint and muscle functioning and improve circulation.*
- Prevent contractures and external rotation of hips by proper positioning *to prevent musculoskeletal complications resulting from bed rest.*
- Use footboard, high-top sneakers, and frequent foot flexion *to prevent footdrop.*
- Provide progressive ambulation for patients receiving long-term ventilation *to prevent "pulmonary crippling."*

NURSING DIAGNOSIS   Anxiety *related to* diagnosis and clinical condition, pain, possible machine malfunction or disconnection, inability to communicate, ICU environment, possibility of death, and fear of suffocation and choking *as manifested by* expression of feelings of anxiety, anxious appearance, rigid body posture.

- Communication of feelings and anxieties.
- Absent or manageable anxiety level.

- Assess patient's behavior for clues of handling stressful situation *to determine a plan for interventions.*
- Give simple, honest explanations regarding care and progress *to foster a realistic understanding and help patient make informed decisions.*
- When possible, allow patient to make decisions regarding all aspects of care *to increase patient's sense of control.*
- Provide for diversion and occupational therapy as needed and tolerated *to relieve anxiety.*
- Refer to psychiatric clinical nurse specialist, psychiatrist, or hospital chaplain when appropriate *to offer additional counseling and support.*
- Be available to family; offer support and help *to lessen their anxiety and increase their cooperation.*

NURSING DIAGNOSIS   Sleep pattern disturbance *related to* frequent awakenings, anxiety, depression, and ICU environment *as manifested by* insomnia, restlessness, irritability, disorientation, morning headaches.

- Rested on awakening.
- Minimal number of awakenings for treatments.

- Perform bedtime preparations (e.g., wash patient's face and hands, rub back, provide oral care) *to promote relaxation and facilitate sleep.*
- Turn off lights at night *to preserve usual sleep-wake cycle.*
- Provide drug therapy intervention as ordered *to promote sleep.*
- Provide relaxation techniques and tapes *to promote relaxation.*
- Schedule activities so that patient gets at least 2 hours of uninterrupted time to sleep.

NURSING DIAGNOSIS   Dysfunctional ventilatory weaning response *related to* too-rapid pacing of the weaning process, insufficient knowledge of the weaning process, and anxiety *as manifested by* restlessness, tachypnea, fatigue, increased blood pressure, shallow breathing, use of accessory muscles, tachycardia, skin color changes (e.g., pallor or cyanosis), agitation.

- Achievement of progressive weaning goals.
- Remain extubated.
- Communication of increased comfort during weaning.
- Less tired from work of weaning.

- Assess respiratory parameters (e.g., inspiratory effort, minute ventilation, vital capacity, effective cough) *to determine patient's weaning ability.*
- Explain the weaning process *so patient understands what is expected.*
- Jointly negotiate progressive weaning goals *to involve patient in establishing the plan.*
- Adopt a weaning pace that will ensure success and minimize setbacks *to maintain patient confidence.*
- Draw ABGs at specified periods during the weaning *to monitor patient's ventilatory status.*
- Deflate cuff totally or partially during weaning *since tracheal tubes add to airway resistance.*
- Monitor for respiratory distress and place patient back on ventilator if observed *to ensure adequate ventilation.*
- If the weaning process is discontinued, explain rationale and revised plan to patient *to minimize frustration and disappointment and enhance cooperation.*

Continued

63-2 **NURSING CARE PLAN** **PATIENT ON MECHANICAL VENTILATION**
—continued

| Expected Patient Outcomes | Nursing Interventions and *Rationales* |

NURSING DIAGNOSIS **Risk for infection** *related to* exposure to environmental pathogens, presence of artificial airway, decreased resistance secondary to debilitated state and prolonged immobility.*

NURSING DIAGNOSIS **Altered nutrition: less than body requirements** *related to* inability to take in nourishment orally and increased caloric demands secondary to clinical condition and need for mechanical ventilation *as manifested by* loss of 10% of body weight.[†]

COLLABORATIVE PROBLEMS

| Nursing Goals | Nursing Interventions and *Rationales* |

POTENTIAL COMPLICATION

- Performance of abdominal assessment.
- Report deviations from expected findings.

Gastric distention *related to* improper ET tube placement, GI bleeding, or ileus.

- Assess for abdominal distention, tympany, and bowel sounds and measure abdominal girth *to detect signs of bowel dilation.*
- Test stools and gastric drainage for occult blood *since the patient is at risk of developing stress ulcers and GI bleeding.*
- Check for gastric air on chest x-ray.
- Administer antacids, H_2-receptor blocker, and tube feedings as ordered *to reduce the occurrence of GI bleeding and to decrease the acidity of gastric secretions.*
- If abdominal distention is present, elevate head of bed to allow for optimal diaphragmatic excursion.
- Obtain order and place nasogastric tube or, if present, confirm patency by irrigating *to relieve gastric tension.*
- Confirm correct position of nasogastric tube *to prevent aspiration and the accumulation of GI fluids.*

POTENTIAL COMPLICATION

- Monitor for signs of pneumothorax.
- Report positive findings.
- Carry out appropriate medical and nursing interventions.

Pneumothorax or pneumomediastinum *related to* barotrauma caused by positive pressure ventilation.

- Observe for sudden increase (by 5 cm H_2O or more) in peak inspiratory pressure, sudden patient agitation or coughing, frequent activation of high-pressure alarm, decrease in static and effective compliance, palpable subcutaneous emphysema over neck and anterior chest areas, deterioration in ABGs and BP, decrease or absence of breath sounds, hyperresonance on percussion; pneumothorax on chest x-ray *to detect signs of pneumothorax.*
- Bag ventilate with O_2 using tidal volume *to reduce airway pressures until a chest tube can be inserted.*
- Notify physician and set up for chest tube insertion immediately *because pneumothorax can convert to a life-threatening tension pneumothorax.*
- Check and record ventilator settings q2hr.
- Record level of peak inspiratory pressure to establish baseline data *to evaluate changes in lung compliance.*[‡]

*Interventions for this nursing diagnosis are presented in the nursing care plan for the patient with an artificial airway (NCP 63-1).
[†]Interventions for this nursing diagnosis are presented in the nursing care plan for the patient with acute respiratory failure (NCP 62-1).
[‡]This assessment is especially important in patients receiving PEEP because they are at more risk of barotrauma.
PAD, pulmonary artery pressure—diastolic; *PAS,* pulmonary artery pressure—systolic; *PAWP,* pulmonary artery wedge pressure.

an internal space to an external transducer. Devices include intraventricular catheters, subarachnoid bolts or screws, and subdural catheters (Fig. 63-18). Table 63-16 outlines advantages and disadvantages of such devices. As with fluid-coupled blood pressure monitoring systems, signals can be distorted by excessive tube length or bubbles in the line. In these systems, the transducer is external and its position must remain constant

with respect to the patient's head to produce pressures that can be compared.

With a second type of technology, the sensor is placed within the cranium. For example, with the fiberoptic catheter the transducer is within the catheter tip. Other, less commonly used transducers include pneumatic systems and intracranial strain gauges. These systems produce excellent quality waveforms and

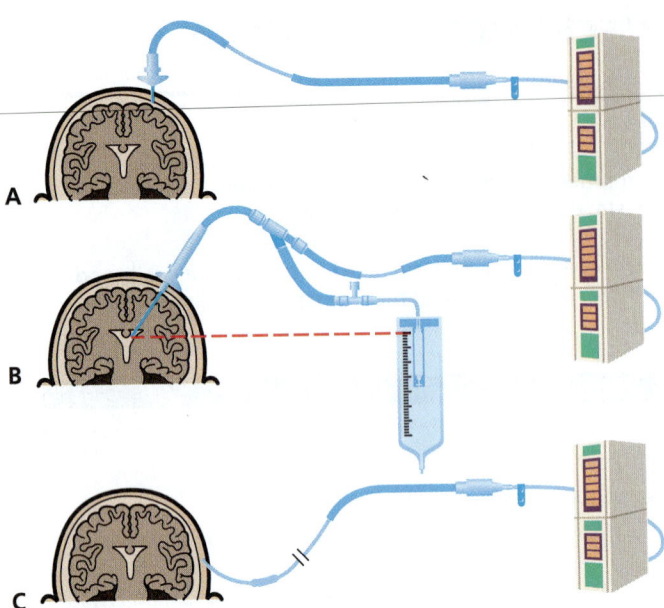

Fig. 63-18 **A,** Subarachnoid pressure monitoring system. **B,** Ventricular pressure monitoring system. **C,** Subdural placement of a sensor.

do not require repositioning with patient movement. They usually cannot be rezeroed.

Infection is a serious consideration with ICP monitoring. Rates are highest in fluid-coupled systems, with reports ranging from 1% to 22% of patients developing infections.[33] Prophylactic systemic antibiotics such as nafcillin (Unipen), cephalothin (Keflin), and gentamicin (Garamycin) have been administered with mixed results.[34]

Intracranial Pressure Waveform. ICP should be measured at end expiration as a mean pressure. The strip recording should be inserted into the record at least every 4 hours. The normal ICP waveform is shaped somewhat like an arterial pressure tracing (Fig. 63-19), although the pressures are in a much lower range. This is because arterial pressure is transmitted to the choroid plexus and then to the CSF in the ventricular and subarachnoid spaces. When the waveform is monitored so that components in synchrony with the cardiac cycle can be visualized, three peaks are noted:

- P1: initial peak, reflecting transmission of systolic arterial pressure from the choroid plexus
- P2: "tidal wave" ends in the dicrotic notch
- P3: third wave follows the dicrotic notch and may reflect venous pressure

Table **63-16**	Comparison of Intracranial Pressure Monitoring Systems		
System	**Description**	**Advantages**	**Disadvantages**
Ventricular catheter	External transducer system; soft, radiopaque Silastic tube inserted via stylet, usually through a twist drill hole into anterior horn of lateral ventricle of nondominant hemisphere	Accurate (can level and zero) CSF can be tapped to reduce ICP and sample CSF Compliance can be tested Contrast media can be inserted for diagnostic tests	Infection risk Hemorrhage risk Difficult to place in patient with small ventricles or intracranial shift Transducer must be repositioned with head movement
Subarachnoid screw or bolt	External transducer system; hollow metal shaft or screw, threaded at one end; threaded end is inserted through a hole drilled into bone through dura into subarachnoid space; placed over frontal area of nondominant hemisphere so that same site can be used for subsequent placement of ventricular catheter if needed.	Simple insertion procedure Useful if ventricle is small or shifted No disruption of neuron tissue of brain Less risk of infection, hemorrhage	Leaks can limit accuracy Obstruction by blood or brain tissue can distort readings Some risk of infection (less than ventriculostomy) Intact skull is required Not useful for draining CSF Not useful for compliance testing If made of metal, patient cannot have MRI performed Transducer must be repositioned with head motion
Fiberoptic devices	Intracranial transducer system; catheter consists of a mobile mirrored diaphragm; fiberoptic signal is bounced off diaphragm and sensed by another fiberoptic cable within the same catheter; usually has CSF sampling port; can be placed into ventricle, subdural, subarachnoid space, or brain parenchyma	Versatile regarding site Insertion possible through subarachnoid bolt Irrigation not necessary Detailed, artifact-free waveform produced If intraventricular, CSF can be tapped to reduce ICP and sample CSF No need to modify equipment with head movement	Catheter fragile Once positioned, rezeroing not possible Unique monitoring system required (but couples to most oscilloscopes) Expensive

CSF, cerebrospinal fluid; *ICP,* intracranial pressure; *MRI,* magnetic resonance imaging.

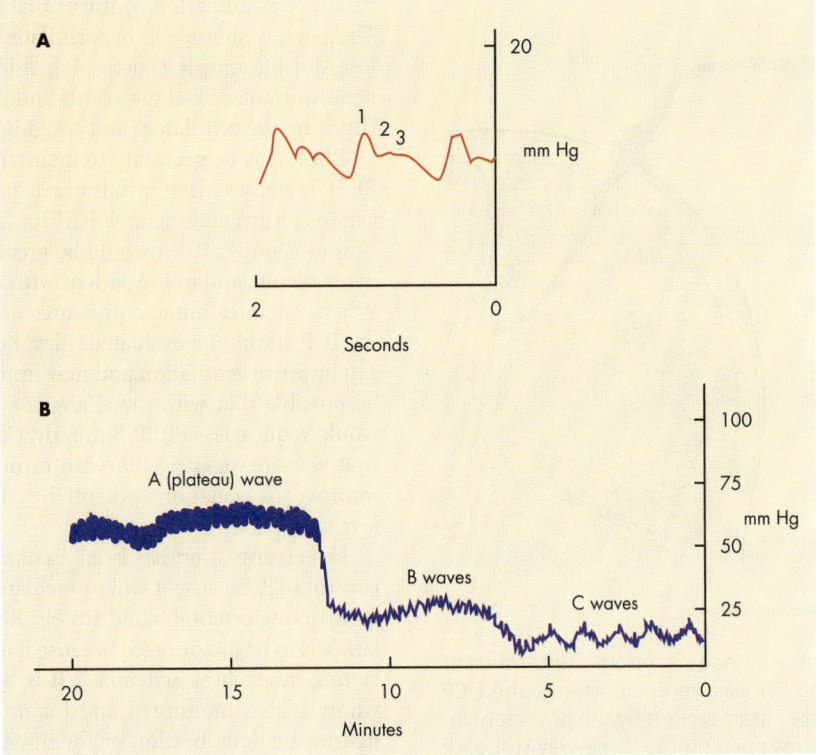

Fig. 63-19   **A,** Intracranial pressure (ICP) waveform as noted on a fast time scale recording. *1, 2, 3* indicate P1, P2, P3 (see text). **B,** Pathologic ICP waves as noted on a slow time scale recording.

Three types of pathologic waves might be seen when ICP is elevated (see Fig. 63-19). Visualization of these requires monitoring with a slowly moving strip recorder.

- A waves: Plateau waves seen with ICP elevations of 50 to 100 mm Hg; last 5 to 20 min; associated with a fall in CPP to less than 40 mm Hg; associated with severe cerebral ischemia; signal a neurologic emergency and must be treated promptly to avoid irreversible brain damage
- B waves: sharp, rhythmic pressure elevations of 20 to 40 mm Hg; frequency of one per 30 to 120 seconds; seen with changes in the respiratory pattern; may be precursors of A waves
- C waves: transient rhythmic pressure elevations of less than 20 mm Hg; frequency of one every 4 to 8 minutes; significance not determined

It is important that the nurse monitor ICP waveform, as well as mean pressure. It has been noted that when the height of P2 is higher than P1, the intracranial space may be noncompliant and the patient is at risk for development of elevated ICP.[35] The patient must be monitored for pathologic waves. In addition to noting pressure measurements and waveform morphology, it is important to consider the rate at which changes occur and the patient's clinical condition. It is important to note that neurologic deterioration might not occur until ICP elevation is pronounced and sustained.[34,35] If A or B waves are noted, the physician must be informed immediately.

In fluid-coupled systems, the waveform should be inspected for damping, which could indicate the presence of bubbles in the line or that the line is obstructed with tissue or blood clots. Inaccurate ICP readings can be caused by CSF leaks around the monitoring device, obstruction of the intraventricular catheter or bolt, difference in the height of the bolt and the transducer, kinks in the tubing, and Valsalva's maneuver.

Cerebrospinal Fluid Drainage. With the ventricular catheter and certain fiberoptic systems, it is possible to control ICP by removing CSF. To do this, a Y-connector or stopcock is inserted in the line (Fig. 63-20). A closed system should be used to decrease infection risk. ICP and drainage volume are controlled by the height of the drainage bag or drip chamber relative to the patient reference point. Typically, a point 15 cm above the ear canal is selected as a reference point. Raising the system diminishes drainage; lowering the system increases drainage volume. Careful monitoring of volume of CSF drained is essential, keeping in mind that normal adult CSF production is about 20 to 30 ml per hour, with a total CSF volume of 90 to 150 ml within the ventricles and subarachnoid space. The amount of fluid to be drained, frequency of drainage, and the height of the highest point in the system should be ordered by the physician.

Ventricular collapse, a major complication of this type of drainage system, occurs when fluid is removed too rapidly. Another complication of rapid decompression is development of a subdural hematoma. To ensure that fluid is not removed too rapidly, intermittent drainage with close observation is used. With this method the line typically is opened only to drain when ICP reaches a preset level and then closed when ICP drops.

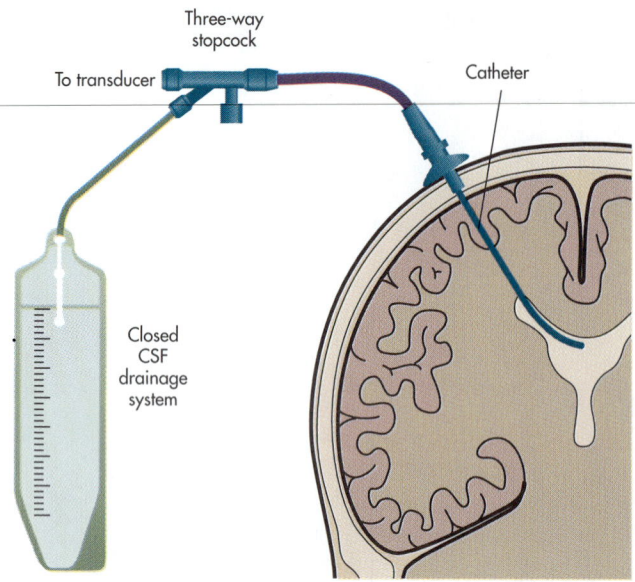

Three-way stopcock

To transducer

Catheter

Closed CSF drainage system

Intraventricular catheter

Fig. 63-20 Intermittent drainage system. Intermittent drainage involves draining CSF via a ventriculostomy when ICP exceeds the upper pressure parameter set by the physician. Intermittent drainage involves opening the three-way stopcock to allow CSF to flow into the drainage bag for brief periods (30 to 120 seconds) until the pressure is below the upper pressure parameters.

NURSING AND COLLABORATIVE MANAGEMENT: INCREASED INTRACRANIAL PRESSURE

Care of the patient with actual or potential increased ICP is similar to that described for the patient with primary brain injury or the unconscious patient (see Chapter 54). Specific therapies are directed at maintaining CPP through manipulating ICP and MAP. Therapies to decrease ICP include CSF drainage, diuresis, oxygenation, neuromuscular blockade, and positioning. Therapies to maintain MAP include fluid resuscitation, positioning, and vasopressors. Intensive monitoring is required, including vital signs, heart rate and rhythm, ventilation, oxygenation, fluid balance, mental status and level of consciousness, ICP, CPP, cranial nerve function, peripheral movement, and sensation.

■ Oxygenation and Ventilation

Patients with elevated ICP or compromised CPP are likely to have a reduced level of consciousness with inadequate ventilatory effort and airway maintenance. Measures taken early in the patient's care include airway control by ET intubation and mechanical ventilation to ensure adequate oxygenation and breathing. Arterial oxygen tensions greater than 100 mm Hg are recommended.

The ET tube must be secured without ties around the neck. Neck ties impede venous return, thus elevating ICP. In patients with normal ICP, ET suctioning is usually well tolerated. In patients with elevated ICP, suctioning can lead to dangerous ICP increases. Three factors associated with suctioning might contribute to ICP elevation: hypercapnia, hypoxemia, and stress. Suctioning should be performed in all patients only when aus-

cultatory examination confirms that suctioning is necessary.[36] The patient should be hyperinflated and preoxygenated before, during, and after suctioning. Additional measures include neuromuscular blocking agents and heavy sedation to prevent "bucking the ventilator" and coughing during suctioning.

PEEP may be necessary to maintain oxygenation. However, PEEP increases mean intrathoracic pressure, so it may impede venous return and increase ICP. It is anticipated that suppression of venous return would be greatest in the patient who is hypovolemic and in the patient with a highly compliant chest. Whenever intrathoracic pressures are changed, the effect on the ICP should be evaluated. Elevation of the bed 30 degrees can improve ventilation and may improve oxygenation. It may be possible that with the change of bed position the patient would require less PEEP. Similarly, relief of abdominal distention via a nasogastric tube can promote lung expansion and improve oxygenation, potentially allowing decreased PEEP levels.

Hyperventilation has been a commonly used treatment to control ICP, because it will immediately decrease ICP by vasoconstricting cerebral blood vessels. Routine use of hyperventilation is to be discouraged because it is possible to overdo it, resulting in cerebral ischemia.[37] It is best used only in patients whose ICP is monitored and for immediate management of neurologic deterioration or for those who do not respond to sedation, paralysis, CSF drainage, and diuresis.[38]

■ Cerebrospinal Fluid Drainage

CSF drainage is an early intervention. However, it can be used only if the ICP device includes an intraventricular catheter. Patients with acute ICP elevation have their CSF drained intermittently when the ICP reaches a specified limit (e.g., 15 mm Hg). The requirement for increasing frequency of CSF drainage is considered a sign of worsening neurologic status.

■ Volume Resuscitation

Volume resuscitation is important in the patient with increased ICP. Hypotension has been identified as a major factor in elevated ICP because it decreases blood pressure and thus CPP. Intravenous fluids are infused to maintain the CPP at greater than 70 mm Hg. Normally a MAP of 90 mm Hg would be judged adequate. However, if the ICP is over 20 mm Hg, the CPP will be less than 70 mm Hg. If fluid infusion is ineffective, vasoactive agents such as norepinephrine (Levophed), dopamine (Intropin), or phenylephrine (Neo-Synephrine) may be used. Pulmonary artery or at least CVP monitoring is used to monitor fluid management. The patient with underlying hypertension presents a special problem because a higher MAP may be required. In this case a higher CPP is the goal of therapy.

■ Diuresis

Diuresis is a cornerstone in the treatment of increased ICP. Osmotic diuresis pulls water out of brain tissue into the systemic circulation and then fluid is removed by the kidneys. Mannitol is the agent most commonly used. Bolus doses are thought to be more effective than continuous infusions because a continuous infusion is thought to encourage accumulation of mannitol in the brain, which could cause a reverse osmotic shift and increase swelling and ICP. When using diuretics, care must be taken to prevent a drop in CPP through volume loss. Serum osmolality and sodium must also be monitored.[39]

■ Sedation

Sedation, pain control, and sometimes neuromuscular blockers are used to control surges in ICP associated with agitation, ventilator asynchrony, and coughing. This therapy also prevents patients who are confused and combative from seriously harming themselves by self-extubation or pulling out lines and catheters. Therapy is usually maintained by continuous infusions of the various agents. A problem with this therapy is the loss of clinical markers for changes in neurologic status. Some clinicians prefer propofol (Diprivan) as a sedative because it is rapidly dissipated once discontinued, and the underlying level of neurologic functioning can be rapidly determined, with the patient then being quickly resedated if needed.

Long-term use of these agents can lead to problems. Prolonged neuromuscular blocker use is associated with a risk of significant residual muscle weakness, and effects from toxicity are poorly understood. Patients on neuromuscular blockers should be closely monitored for achievement of therapeutic effect with the minimal amount of drug necessary. If the patient requires narcotic and sedative administration, gradual weaning of the drugs is needed to prevent withdrawal.[40]

The ultimate in sedation is achieved through the use of barbiturate coma. This treatment is used only when the patient is refractory to other previously mentioned therapies. Barbiturates can reduce cerebral metabolism by as much as 50%, causing a significant reduction in cerebral blood flow. The patient's electroencephalogram is monitored continuously. Problems associated with this therapy include hypotension, hypothermia, and a possible risk for infection because of immune suppression.

■ Temperature Control

Temperature control is important. Hypothermia is induced in some patients to control cerebral metabolic rate and thereby control cerebral blood flow. An elevated temperature will increase cerebral metabolic rate by as much as 7% for each degree centigrade. Elevations in temperature should be reduced in the patient with elevated ICP by means of antipyretics. Cooling blankets can induce shivering, which may require additional medications to control.

■ Positioning

Positioning can affect ICP. Usually patients are placed in a semirecumbent position (30 to 45 degrees) to facilitate jugular venous drainage. Additionally, the head should be maintained in midline position to prevent kinking of the blood vessels, and the ET tube should not be taped circumferentially, because it could restrict venous drainage. However, elevating the head of the bed could lower CPP. Therefore patients who have a reduced CPP may respond better to being flat. Trendelenburg's position should be avoided because it could increase ICP by impeding venous drainage.

CRITICAL THINKING EXERCISES

CASE STUDY

Critical Care and Mechanical Ventilation

Patient Profile

Mr. R., a 55-year-old man, was found lying on the street by the police. He was unconscious on admission and has not regained consciousness. He has an endotracheal tube in place and is receiving mechanical ventilation. It is 24 hours after admission.

Subjective Data

- None; is unresponsive to painful stimuli

Objective Data

- Blood pressure 100/75; heart rate 120; temperature 102° F (38.8° C); SpO2 98%
- CVP 3 mm Hg
- Purulent secretions from ET tube
- Breath sounds: many rhonchi bilaterally, decreased breath sounds on the right

Diagnostic Studies

- Chest x-ray reveals right lower lung consolidation
- ABGs: pH 7.48, PaO_2 100 mm Hg, $PaCO_2$ 30 mm Hg, HCO_3^- 22 mEq/L

Collaborative Care

- Ventilator settings: assist control at 14 breaths per minute; tidal volume 900 cc; FIO_2 0.6

- Enteral nutrition at 25 ml/hr via small-bore feeding tube
- Indwelling urinary catheter to bedside drainage
- Chest physical therapy every 4 hours
- Gentamycin (Garamycin) 80 mg IV q8hr
- Ceftriaxone (Rocephin) 1 g IV q12hr
- D_5NS with KCl 20 mEq/L at 100 ml/hr

Critical Thinking Questions

1. What are two reasons for intubation and mechanical ventilation in Mr. R.?
2. What do Mr R.'s ABGs demonstrate, and what ventilator setting(s) should be changed and why?
3. What is his PaO_2/FIO_2 ratio, and what does it signify?
4. How can the nurse decrease Mr. R.'s chances of aspiration?
5. What clinical signs would the nurse expect to see if Mr. R.'s condition worsens?
6. What clinical signs would the nurse expect to see if Mr. R.'s pulmonary condition improves?
7. As Mr. R. begins to regain consciousness, what psychosocial aspects of his care will change and why?
8. Given Mr. R.'s vital signs, what effect might be expected if he were placed on 10 cm of PEEP and why?
9. Based on the assessment data presented, write one or more appropriate nursing diagnoses. Are there any collaborative problems?

Table **63-17**	Cross-References to Other Critical Care Content	
Topic		**Discussed in Chapter**
Acute congestive heart failure		33
Acute myocardial infarction		32
Acute respiratory distress syndrome		62
Acute respiratory failure		62
Advanced cardiac life support		34
Burns		23
Cardiac arrhythmias		34
Cardiac pacemakers		34
Cardiac surgery		33
Cardiopulmonary resuscitation		34
Emergencies		64
Head injury		54
Multiple organ dysfunction syndrome		61
Oxygen delivery		27
Pulmonary edema		33
Renal dialysis		44
Shock		61
Systemic inflammatory response syndrome		61
Total parenteral nutrition		38
Tracheostomy		25
Trauma		64

■ Environmental Control

Controlling the patient's environment and exercising judgment in nursing interventions have been shown to affect ICP. Each patient should be managed individually by observing the effects of nursing interventions and tailoring care accordingly. Suctioning, turning, and painful procedures are all possible factors that increase ICP. The nurse should space interventions that have an adverse effect and allow the patient's ICP to recover between nursing interventions. The nurse should watch the patient's ICP and hemodynamic parameters for changes when family members interact with the patient. Those individuals with a soothing effect should be included in simple care and comfort measures. Noise, lighting, and other noxious stimuli (identified at the beginning of this chapter) should be controlled. Conversation in the patient's room should not be loud. The nurse should speak quietly and address comments to the patient as though the patient were awake and participating in his or her care.

OTHER CRITICAL CARE CONTENT

Table 63-17 lists additional critical care content presented in other chapters of this text.

REVIEW QUESTIONS

The number of the question corresponds to the same-numbered objective at the beginning of the chapter.

1. The critical care unit is
   a. the best place for dying patients to be cared for.
   b. a special care unit found only in large metropolitan hospitals.
   c. where all patients requiring mechanical ventilation must be placed.
   d. best used for patients who have sustained (or are at risk for) life-threatening illness or injury.

2. Certification in critical care nursing by the American Association of Critical Care Nurses indicates that a nurse
   a. is master's prepared to provide advanced critical care.
   b. has demonstrated clinical competency in caring for critically ill patients.
   c. is an advanced practice nurse specialist in the care of acutely ill patients.
   d. may practice independently to provide symptom management for the critically ill.

3. An appropriate nursing intervention for the patient with delirium in the ICU is
   a. using tranquilizers to establish normal sleep patterns.
   b. identifying the factors contributing to the patient's confusion and irritability.
   c. sedating the patient with psychotropic drugs to protect the patient from harmful behaviors.
   d. silencing all alarms, overhead paging, and conversations around the patient.

4. The critical care nurse recognizes that an ideal plan for family involvement includes
   a. a family member at the bedside at all times.
   b. allowing family at the bedside at preset, brief intervals.
   c. an individually devised plan with family involved with care and comfort measures.
   d. prohibition of visiting in the ICU because the environment is too threatening to visitors.

5. To establish hemodynamic monitoring for a patient, the nurse zeros
   a. pressure monitoring systems to the level of the catheter tip.
   b. cardiac output monitoring systems to the level of the left ventricle.
   c. pressure monitoring systems to the level of the left atrium, identified as the phlebostatic axis.
   d. pressure monitoring systems to the level of the right atrium, identified as the midaxillary line.

6. A patient with a ventricular assist device (VAD) is assessed for complications that include
   a. bleeding.
   b. cardiogenic shock.
   c. aortic valve insufficiency.
   d. severe pulmonary disease.

7. The hemodynamic changes the nurse expects to find after successful initiation of an intraaortic balloon pump in a patient in cardiogenic shock include
   a. $\downarrow$ PAWP and $\uparrow$ CO.
   b. $\downarrow$ CVP and $\uparrow$ right atrial pressure.
   c. $\downarrow$ SVR and $\downarrow$ stroke volume.
   d. $\uparrow$ diastolic BP and $\downarrow$ systolic BP.

8. When caring for a patient with an endotracheal tube, the nurse is assessing for the development of
   a. accidental extubation.
   b. a negative inspiratory force.
   c. increased intracranial pressure.
   d. positive end-expiratory pressure.

9. The nursing management of a patient with an artificial airway includes
   a. routine suctioning of the tube at least every 2 hours.
   b. observing for cardiac arrhythmias during suctioning.
   c. maintaining endotracheal tube cuff pressure at 30 cm H_2O.
   d. preventing tube dislodgment by limiting mouth care to lubrication of the lips.

10. The nurse monitors the patient with positive pressure mechanical ventilation for
    a. paralytic ileus because pressure on the abdominal contents affects bowel motility.

b. diuresis and sodium depletion because of increased release of atrial natriuretic peptide.

c. signs of cardiovascular insufficiency because pressure in the chest impedes venous return.

d. respiratory acidosis in a patient with COPD because of alveolar hyperventilation and increased PaO_2 levels.

11. In a patient with intracranial pressure monitoring the nurse identifies a normal waveform as
   a. plateau waves.
   b. a P3 wave following the dicrotic notch.
   c. sharp, rhythmic elevations of 20 to 40 mm Hg lasting 30 seconds to 2 minutes.
   d. rhythmic pressure elevations of less than 20 mm Hg at a frequency of one every 4 to 8 minutes.

12. While caring for a patient with increased intracranial pressure the nurse recognizes that
   a. the MAP should be maintained below 60 mm Hg.
   b. hypoxemia decreases cerebral blood volume and ICP.
   c. ICP may be decreased by draining cerebrospinal fluid.
   d. the head should be flexed to the right to facilitate venous return from the head.

References

1. Nightingale F: *Notes on hospitals,* ed 3, Longman, 1863, Roberts-Green.
2. Goldhill DR, Summer A: Outcome of intensive care patients in a group of British intensive care units, *Crit Care Med* 26:1337, 1998.
3. Wong DT and others: Evaluation of predictive ability of APACHE II system and hospital outcome in Canadian intensive care unit patients, *Crit Care Med* 23: 1175, 1995.
4. Nasraway SA and others: American College of Critical Care Medicine of the Society of Critical Care Medicine. Guidelines on admission and discharge for adult intermediate care units, *Crit Care Med* 26: 607, 1998.
5. Clark S, Fontaine D, Simpson T: Recognition, assessment, and treatment of anxiety in the critical care setting, *Crit Care Nurse* 14(suppl):2, 1994.
6. Schelling G and others: Health-related quality of life and posttraumatic stress disorder in survivors of the acute respiratory distress syndrome, *Crit Care Med* 26:651,1998.
7. Tess MM: Acute confusional states in critically ill patients: a review, *J Neurosci Nurs* 23:398, 1991.
8. Geary S: Intensive care unit psychosis revisited: understanding and managing delirium in the critical care setting, *Crit Care Nurs Q* 17:51, 1994.
9. Kahn DM and others: Identification and modification of environmental noise in an ICU setting, *Chest* 114:535, 1998.
10. Fontaine DK: Measurement of nocturnal sleep patterns in trauma patients, *Heart Lung* 18:402, 1989.
11. Meyer TJ and others: Adverse environmental conditions in the respiratory and medical ICU settings, *Chest* 105:1211, 1994.
12. Richards KC, Bairnsfather L: A description of night sleep patterns in the critical care unit, *Heart Lung* 17:35, 1988.
13. Grozinger M, Kogel P, Roschke J: Effects of lorazepam on the automatic online evaluation of sleep EEG data in healthy volunteers, *Pharmacopsychiatry* 31:55, 1998.
14. Simpson T: The family as a source of support for the critically ill adult, *AACN Clin Issues Crit Care Nurs* 2:229, 1991.
15. Daly K and others: The effect of two nursing interventions on families of ICU patients, *Clin Nurs Res* 3:414, 1994.
16. Woods SL, Grose BL, Laurent-Bopp D: Effect of backrest position on pulmonary artery pressures in acutely ill patients, *Cardiovasc Nurs* 18:19, 1982.
17. Davidson J and others: Intra-aortic balloon pump: indications and complications, *J Natl Med Assoc* 90:137, 1998.
18. Busch T and others: Vascular complications related to intraaortic balloon counterpulsation: an analysis of ten years experience, *Thorac Cardiovasc Surg* 45:55, 1997.
19. Tatar H and others: Vascular complications of intraaortic balloon pumping: unsheathed versus sheathed insertion, *Ann Thorac Surg* 55:1518, 1993.
20. Oz MC and others: Screening scale predicts patients successfully receiving long-term implantable left ventricular assist devices, *Circulation* 92:II169, 1995.
21. Antonelli M and others: A comparison of noninvasive positive-pressure ventilation and conventional mechanical ventilation in patients with acute respiratory failure, *N Engl J Med* 339:429, 1998.
22. Luce JM, Pierson DJ, Tyler ML: *Intensive respiratory care,* Philadelphia, 1993, Saunders.
*23. Stone KS: Ventilator versus manual resuscitation bag as the method for delivering hyperoxygenation before endotracheal suctioning, *AACN Clin Issues Crit Care Nurs* 1:289, 1990.
24. Shekerdemian LS and others: Cardiopulmonary interactions after Fontan operations: augmentation of cardiac output using negative pressure ventilation, *Circulation* 96:3934, 1997.
25. Sassoon CS: Positive pressure ventilation: alternate modes, *Chest* 100:1421, 1991.
26. Burns SM: Advances in ventilator therapy, *Focus Crit Care* 17:227, 1990.
27. Wright SE, Heffner JE: Positive pressure mechanical ventilation augments left ventricular function in acute mitral regurgitation, *Chest* 102:1625, 1992.
28. Schoeffel U and others: The influence of ischemic bowel wall damage on translocation, inflammatory response, and clinical course, *Am J Surg* 174:39, 1997.
29. Daly BJ, Thomas D, Dyer MA: Procedures used in withdrawal of mechanical ventilation, *Am J Crit Care* 5:331, 1996.
*30. Sevick MA and others: Home-based ventilator-dependent patients: measurement of the emotional aspects of home caregiving, *Heart Lung* 23:269, 1994.
*31. Smith CE and others: Caregiver learning needs and reactions to managing home mechanical ventilation, *Heart Lung* 23:157, 1994.
32. Czarnik B: Home care for the patient receiving mechanical ventilation, *Home Healthc Nurse* 15:777, 1997.
33. Doyle DJ, Mark PWS: Analysis of intracranial pressure, *J Clin Monit* 8:81, 1992.
34. Hickey JV: Intracranial pressure: theory and management of increased intracranial pressure. In Hickey JV, editor: *The clinical practice of neurological and neurosurgical nursing,* ed 4, Philadelphia, 1997, Lippincott.
35. McNair ND: Intracranial pressure monitoring. In Clochesy J and others, editors: *Critical care nursing,* ed 2, Philadelphia, 1996, Saunders.
36. Kerr ME and others: Head-injured adults: recommendations for endotracheal suctioning, *J Neurosci Nurs* 25:86, 1993.
*37. Kerr ME, Brucia J: Hyperventilation in the head injured patient: an effective treatment modality? *Heart Lung* 22:516, 1993.
38. Bullock R and others: Guidelines for the management of severe head injury, Brain Trauma Foundation, *Eur J Emerg Med* 3:109, 1996.
39. Bullock R: Mannitol and other diuretics in severe neurotrauma, *New Horizons* 3:448, 1995.
40. Prielapp RC, Coursin DB: Sedative and neuromuscular blocking drug use in critically ill patients with head injuries, *New Horizons* 3:456, 1995.

*Nursing research-based articles.

Resources

American Association of Critical Care Nurses (AACN)
One Civic Plaza, Suite 330
Newport Beach, CA 92660
714-644-9310
http://www.aacn.org

Anesthesia and Critical Care Website
University of Chicago
5841 S. Maryland
MC 4028
Chicago, IL 60637
773-702-6700
Fax: 773-702-3535
http://dacc.uchicago.edu/

For additional Internet resources, see the website for this book at www.mosby.com/MERLIN/medsurg_lewis

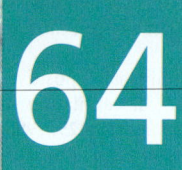

NURSING MANAGEMENT
64 Emergency Care Situations

Lorene Newberry

www.mosby.com/MERLIN/medsurg_lewis

LEARNING OBJECTIVES

1. Describe the sequential steps in the assessment of a patient in an emergency situation.
2. Explain the pathophysiology, assessment, and collaborative care of select environmental emergencies related to thermoregulation, near drowning, and animal bites.

3. Discuss the pathophysiology, assessment, and collaborative care of select toxicologic emergencies.

Most patients with life-threatening or potentially life-threatening problems enter the hospital through the emergency department (ED). Visits to the ED have increased significantly because of the lack of health insurance, increased violence, and inability to access health care. Emergency nurses care for patients of all ages and with a variety of problems. However, some EDs specialize in certain patient populations or conditions, such as pediatric ED or chest pain ED.

Specific emergency management of patients with various medical, surgical, and traumatic emergencies are presented throughout this book where the disorders are discussed. Tables that highlight emergency management of specific problems are presented throughout the book. Table 64-1 lists each emergency management table by title, number, and page location. This chapter focuses on initial assessment and management of the trauma patient and emergency conditions not addressed elsewhere in this book, including heat- and cold-related emergencies, near drowning, bites, stings, and poisonings.

CARE OF THE EMERGENCY PATIENT

Recognition of life-threatening illness or injury is one of the most important aspects of emergency care. Before a diagnosis can be made, recognition of dangerous clinical signs and symptoms with initiation of interventions to reverse or prevent a crisis is essential. This process begins with the first patient contact. The emergency nurse is usually confronted with multiple patients who have a variety of problems. Prompt identification of patients requiring immediate treatment and determination of appropriate treatment area are essential in a busy ED.[1]

A triage system identifies and categorizes patients so the most critical are treated first. *Triage* is a French word meaning "to sort."[2] The process is based on the premise that patients

with a threat to life, vision, or limb should be treated before other patients. The ED may use a system of words, color coding, numbers for triage acuity, or the ED may use international codes (Table 64-2).

The emergency nurse must complete an initial assessment to determine the presence of actual or potential threats to life and then rapidly initiate interventions appropriate for the patient's condition.[3] A history is obtained simultaneously. A systematic approach to the initial patient assessment decreases the time required to identify potential threats and minimizes the risk of missing a life-threatening condition. Two systematic approaches, a primary and secondary survey, were initially developed for use with the trauma patient, but these can be easily applied to assessment of any emergency patient.

PRIMARY SURVEY

The primary survey (Table 64-3) focuses on airway, breathing, and circulation and serves to identify life-threatening problems so that appropriate interventions can be initiated.[4] Life-threatening problems related to the airway (Table 64-4), breathing (Table 64-5), or circulation (Table 64-6) may be identified during the primary survey and appropriate interventions started immediately.

A = Airway with Cervical Spine Immobilization

Nearly all immediate trauma deaths occur because of airway obstruction. Saliva, bloody secretions, vomitus, direct trauma, laryngeal trauma, facial trauma, fractures, and the tongue can obstruct the airway. Medical patients at risk for airway compromise include those who have seizures, near drowning, anaphylaxis, foreign body obstruction, or are in cardiopulmonary arrest. If an airway is not maintained, obstruction of air flow occurs and hypoxia, acidosis, and death result.

Signs and symptoms of a compromised airway are presented in Table 64-4. Airway maintenance should progress rapidly from the least to the most invasive method. Treatment

Reviewed by Darlene F. Schelper, RN, MSN, CEN, RNC, Clinical Nurse Educator of Emergency Services, Hershey Medical Center, Penn State Geisinger Health System, Hershey, Penn.

includes suctioning of secretions, jaw thrust maneuver (avoiding hyperextension of the neck) (Fig. 64-1, p. 1962), insertion of a nasopharyngeal or oropharyngeal airway (will cause gag if patient is conscious), forward sitting position if no cervical spine injuries are present, and intubation. If unable to intubate because of airway obstruction, an emergency surgical cricothyrotomy or tracheotomy should be performed (see Chapter 25).

Any patient with significant upper torso injuries or face, head, or neck trauma should always be suspected of cervical spine trauma. The cervical spine must be kept in alignment and immobilized during assessment of the airway. The cervical spine is immobilized with a stiff immobilization collar, soft rolls are taped to a backboard on either side of the head, and the patient's forehead is taped to the backboard. Sandbags should not be used because the weight of the bags could move the head if the patient must be turned.

B = Breathing

Adequate air flow through the upper airway does not ensure adequate ventilation. Breathing alterations are caused by many conditions, including fractured ribs, pneumothorax, penetrating injury, allergic reactions, pulmonary emboli, and asthma attacks (see Table 64-5). Every injured or ill patient has an increased metabolic and oxygen demand and should have supplemental oxygen. Life-threatening conditions such as tension pneumothorax, open pneumothorax, and flail chest can compromise ventilation. Treatment for a nonbreathing patient includes bag valve mask ventilation with 100% oxygen, intubation, and treatment of the underlying cause.

C = Circulation

An effective circulatory system includes the heart, intact blood vessels, and adequate blood volume. (Life-threatening circulation problems are presented in Table 64-6.) Uncontrolled bleeding places a person at risk for hemorrhagic shock. The patient's carotid or femoral pulse should be checked because peripheral pulses may be absent as a result of direct injury or vasoconstriction. Delayed capillary refill (longer than 3 seconds) and altered mental status are the most significant signs of shock. Care must be taken when evaluating capillary refill in cold environments because cold delays refill.

IV lines are inserted into veins in the upper extremities unless contraindicated, such as in a massive fracture or an injury that affects limb circulation. Two large-gauge IV catheters should be inserted and aggressive fluid resuscitation initiated using lactated Ringer's solution or normal saline. Direct pressure with a sterile dressing should be applied to obvious bleeding sites. Blood samples are obtained for a type and crossmatch; electrolyte, glucose, blood urea nitrogen, and creatinine levels; complete blood cell count; and coagulation studies. Blood samples may also be obtained for alcohol or drug levels or liver or cardiac enzyme levels. The patient should be monitored by electrocardiogram (ECG) for arrhythmias. Type-specific packed red blood cells should be administered if needed.

+ EMERGENCY MANAGEMENT

Table 64-1 Emergency Management Tables

Title	Number	Page
Abdominal trauma	40-14	1149
Acute abdomen	40-13	1146
Acute soft-tissue injury	59-2	1764
Anaphylactic shock	12-12	226
Arrhythmias	34-5	924
Chemical burns	23-5	529
Chest pain	32-11	857
Chest trauma	26-21	644
Cocaine toxicity	10-9	165
Diabetic ketoacidosis	46-21	1395
Drug overdose	10-7	164
Electrical burns	23-7	530
Eye injury	20-4	450
Fractured extremity	59-7	1779
Head injury	54-11	1627
Hyperthermia	64-10	1966
Hypothermia	64-11	1968
Inhalation injury	23-6	529
Near drowning	64-12	1970
Sexual assault	51-7	1530
Shock	61-8	1879
Skin wound	22-7	506
Snakebite	64-13	1973
Spinal cord injury	57-4	1727
Stroke	55-5	1654
Thermal burns	23-8	530
Thoracic injuries	26-22	645
Tonic-clonic seizures	56-8	1682
Unconscious patient	54-6	1617

Table 64-2 Triage Acuity Systems

	Emergent	Urgent	Nonurgent	Expectant
Colors	Red	Yellow	Green	Black
Numbers	Priority I	Priority II	Priority III	Priority 0
Urgency	Life-threatening; needs immediate attention	Needs treatment in 20 minutes to 2 hours	Can wait hours or days	Dying or dead
Example	Trauma, chest pain, respiratory distress, chemicals in the eyes, arm or leg amputation, shock	Fever >104° F (40° C), diastolic blood pressure >130 mm Hg, kidney stone, simple fracture	Sprain, minor laceration, flulike symptoms, rash, chronic headache	Massive head trauma, cardiopulmonary arrest

Table **64-3** Primary Survey of an Emergency Patient

Assessment	Intervention
Airway with Cervical Spine • Clear and open airway • Assess for obstructed airway • Assess for respiratory distress • Check for loose teeth or foreign objects • Assess for bleeding, vomitus, or edema	• Suction • Jaw thrust • Nasal or oral airway, endotracheal tube, cricothyrotomy • Cervical spine immobilization using collar, backboard, soft rolls; tape forehead

Breathing
• Assess ventilation
  Look for chest movements associated with breathing
  Note use of accessory muscles or abdominal muscles
  Listen for air being expired through nose and mouth
  Feel for air being expelled
• Observe and count respiratory rate
• Note color of nail beds, mucous membranes, skin
• Auscultate lungs
• Assess for jugular venous distention and position of trachea
	• Ventilate with bag-valve mask with 100% O_2
	• Prepare to intubate if respiratory arrest
	• Have suction available
	• Give supplemental oxygen via appropriate delivery system
	• If head trauma, hyperventilate with 100% O_2
	• If absent breath sounds, perform needle thoracostomy and prepare for chest tube insertion

Circulation • Check carotid or femoral pulse • Assess color, temperature, and moisture of skin • Assess level of consciousness • Check capillary refill • Assess for external bleeding	• If absent pulse, begin chest compressions • If shock symptoms or hypotensive, start IVs with at least two large-bore (14-16 gauge) IV catheters with normal saline or lactated Ringer's solution • Administer blood products if ordered • Consider autotransfusion if isolated chest trauma • Obtain blood samples for type and crossmatch • Control bleeding with direct pressure
Disability • Assess level of consciousness • Assess response to verbal and painful stimuli • Assess extremity movement (all four) • Perform Glasgow Coma Scale (Table 54-2) • Check pupil response to light	• Periodically reassess level of consciousness

Table **64-4** Life-Threatening Airway Problems

Problem	Signs and Symptoms	Interventions
Airway obstruction (complete or partial)	• Dyspnea, labored respirations • Decreased or no air movement • Cyanosis • Presence of foreign body in airway • Trauma to face or neck	Airway opening maneuvers • Jaw thrust • Chin lift • Suction Airway adjuncts • Nasal airway • Oral airway • Endotracheal tube (ET) Surgical airway • Cricothyrotomy • Tracheostomy
Inhalation injury	• History of enclosed space fire, unconsciousness, or exposure to heavy smoke • Dyspnea • Wheezing, rhonchi, crackles • Hoarseness • Singed facial or nasal hairs • Carbonaceous sputum • Burns to face or neck	• Provide high-flow oxygen (100%) via non-rebreather mask or bag-valve device • Prepare for endotracheal intubation as soon as possible

From Kidd PS, Stuart P: *Mosby's emergency nursing reference,* St Louis, 1996, Mosby.

Table 64-5	Life-Threatening Breathing Problems

Problem	Signs and Symptoms	Interventions
Tension pneumothorax	■ Dyspnea, labored respirations ■ Decreased or absent breath sounds on affected side ■ Unilateral chest rise and fall ■ Tracheal deviation away from affected side ■ Cyanosis ■ Jugular venous distention ■ Tachycardia and hypotension ■ History of chest trauma or mechanical ventilation	■ Provide high-flow oxygen (100%) via non-rebreather mask or bag-valve device ■ Rapid chest decompression by needle thoracostomy on affected side ■ Chest tube placement on affected side
Pneumothorax	■ Dyspnea, labored respirations ■ Decreased or absent breath sounds on affected side ■ May have unilateral chest rise and fall ■ May have visible wound to chest or back ■ History of chest trauma	■ Provide high-flow oxygen (100%) via non-rebreather mask or bag-valve device ■ Chest tube placement on affected side ■ Place occlusive dressing over any open chest wound and secure on three sides with tape
Hemothorax	■ Dyspnea, labored respirations ■ Decreased or absent breath sounds on affected side ■ May have unilateral chest rise and fall ■ Tachycardia and hypotension ■ May have visible wound to chest or back ■ History of chest trauma (usually penetrating)	■ Provide high-flow oxygen (100%) via non-rebreather mask or bag-valve device ■ Chest tube placement on affected side ■ Consider autotransfusion
Sucking chest wound	■ Dyspnea, labored respirations ■ Visible, sucking wound to chest or back ■ Decreased or absent breath sounds on affected side	■ Provide high-flow oxygen (100%) via non-rebreather mask or bag-valve device ■ Cover wound with occlusive dressing and secure on 3 sides with tape ■ Watch for signs of tension pneumothorax and remove dressing during exhalation if they are noted
Flail chest	■ Dyspnea, labored respirations ■ Paradoxical chest wall movement ■ Chest pain ■ Tachycardia	■ Provide high-flow oxygen (100%) via non-rebreather mask or bag-valve device ■ Prepare for intubation and mechanical ventilation

Modified from Kidd PS, Stuart P: *Mosby's emergency nursing reference,* St Louis, 1996, Mosby.

Table 64-6	Life-Threatening Circulation Problems

Problem	Signs and Symptoms	Interventions
External hemorrhage	■ Obvious bleeding site	■ Direct pressure ■ Elevation of extremity
Shock	■ Tachycardia ■ Weak, thready pulses ■ Cool, pale, clammy skin ■ Tachypnea ■ Altered mental status ■ Delayed capillary refill ■ Oliguria or anuria	■ Provide high-flow oxygen (100%) via non-rebreather mask or bag-valve device ■ Place two large-bore IV lines with warm isotonic crystalloid solution (lactated Ringer's or 0.9% NaCl) ■ Administer fluid bolus (2 L in adults) ■ Prepare to administer blood

From Kidd PS, Stuart P: *Mosby's emergency nursing reference,* St Louis, 1996, Mosby.

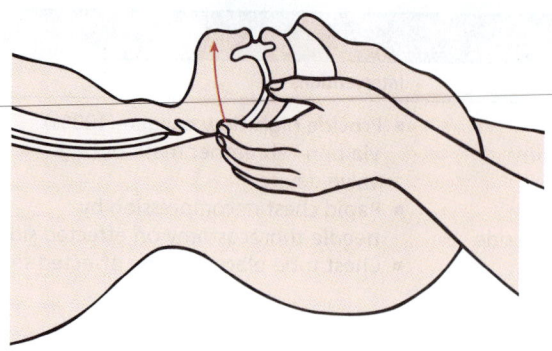

Fig. 64-1 Jaw-thrust maneuver is the only widely recommended procedure for use on an unconscious patient with possible neck or spinal injuries. The patient should be lying supine with the rescuer kneeling at the top of the head. The rescuer should carefully reach forward and gently place one hand on each side of the patient's chin at the lateral angles of the lower jaw. The patient's head should be stabilized with the rescuer's forearms, then the jaw pushed forward while pressure is applied with the index fingers.

D = Disability

A brief neurologic examination should follow the primary survey. Level of consciousness and pupil size and reactivity to light should be assessed. A simple mnemonic to remember is AVPU: A = alert, V = responds to verbal stimuli, P = responds to painful stimuli, and U = unresponsive. Extremities should be observed for spontaneous movement and assessed for sensation. A Glasgow Coma Scale score is calculated (see Chapter 54, Table 54-2).

E = Expose

All trauma patients should have their clothes removed so that a thorough physical assessment can be performed. The patient should be covered with warm blankets to prevent hypothermia.

SECONDARY SURVEY

The secondary survey should not be done until the primary survey is complete. During the primary survey, life-threatening airway, breathing, or circulation problems are corrected as quickly as possible. Once this has been accomplished, a secondary survey is initiated. The secondary survey involves obtaining a history, identifying all injuries, and performing a head-to-toe assessment, including an evaluation of the patient's back (Table 64-7).

F = Fahrenheit

The patient is kept warm with warm IV fluids, warm blankets, and overhead warming lights. Trauma patients and ill medical patients are at risk for hypothermia caused by hypovolemia and environmental exposure.

G = Get Vital Signs

A complete set of vital signs, including blood pressure, heart rate, respiratory rate, temperature, and oxygen saturation, should be obtained after the patient is exposed. The patient's heart rate and rhythm should be monitored.

H = History and Head-to-Toe Assessment

The history of the incident, accident, or illness provides clues to the cause of the crisis and suggests specific assessment needs.

The patient may be unable to give a history, but family, friends, and witnesses can frequently provide information. An experienced ED team can complete a history within 5 minutes of the patient's arrival. If the patient is emergently ill, a thorough history is obtained from the friends or family after the patient is taken to the treatment area. The history should include the following questions:

1. What is the chief complaint? What caused the person to seek attention?
2. How long ago did the accident or incident occur? How long ago did the patient become ill?
3. Where did the accident or incident occur? Where did the patient become ill?
4. Describe the accident, incident, or illness. How did it happen? Details of the incident are extremely important because the mechanism can indicate specific injuries. For example, a front seat passenger with a lap belt may have a head injury from hitting the windshield; knee, femur, or hip fractures or dislocation from striking the dashboard; and an abdominal injury from the lap belt. If other victims were dead at the scene, the patient has a high chance of significant injury.

   Patients who jump from buildings or bridges may have bilateral calcaneal fractures, bilateral wrist fractures, lumbar spine compression fractures, and be at risk for aortic tears. Older patients who have climbed ladders and fallen may have had a cerebrovascular accident or myocardial infarction that led to the fall. Bullets can ricochet in the body if they strike bone. It is essential to determine the number of shots fired and to look for entry and exit wounds. A patient shot in the abdomen may have a bullet lodged in the right shoulder. The bullet trajectory may have gone through the liver and lung en route to the shoulder.

5. What has happened since the onset of the illness or injury?
   a. Has the patient been moved?
   b. What emergency care was started at the scene of the incident?
   c. What are the patient's subjective complaints?
   d. What are witnesses' (if any) descriptions of the patient's behavior since the onset?
6. What is the patient's health care history? The mnemonic AMPLE assists the nurse in remembering what to ask:

   A   Allergies
   M   Medications (current medications that the patient is taking)
   P   Past health history (especially cardiac and respiratory conditions and diabetes), pregnancy status
   L   Last meal
   E   Events preceding illness or injury

Head, Neck, and Face. The patient should be assessed for general appearance, skin color, and temperature. The eyes should be evaluated for extraocular movements. A disconjugate gaze is an indication of neurologic damage. Raccoon eyes or periorbital ecchymosis is usually caused by a basilar skull fracture. The tympanic membranes and external canal are checked for blood and cerebrospinal fluid. Drainage from the ear should not be stopped.

The throat and airway are assessed for bruising, foreign bodies, bleeding, edema, loose or missing teeth, difficulty swal-

Table **64-7**	**Secondary Survey of an Emergency Patient**
Parameter	**Assessment**
Expose	■ Remove clothing for adequate examination.
Fahrenheit	■ Keep patient warm with warm blankets, IV fluids, overhead lights
Get Vital Signs	■ Blood pressure ■ Pulse, cardiac rhythm ■ Respiratory rate and effort ■ Temperature ■ Oxygen saturation ■ Urinary catheter if not contraindicated ■ Gastric tube ■ Laboratory studies for presenting condition
History and Head-to-Toe Assessment	
History	■ Length of time since incident occurred ■ Accident type, location, and patient's position in accident ■ Description of accident, incident, or illness ■ Allergies ■ Medications ■ Past health history, pregnancy ■ Last meal ■ Events leading to accident, incident, or illness
Head, Neck, Face	■ Examine face and scalp for lacerations, bone or soft tissue deformity, tenderness, bleeding, and foreign objects ■ Examine eyes, ears, nose, and mouth for bleeding, foreign bodies, drainage, pain, deformity, ecchymosis, lacerations ■ Examine head for depressions of cranial or facial bones, contusions, hematomas, areas of softness, bony crepitus ■ Examine neck for stiffness, pain in cervical vertebrae, tracheal deviation, distended neck veins, bleeding, edema, difficulty swallowing, bruising, subcutaneous emphysema, bony crepitus
Chest	■ Rate, depth, and character of breathing ■ Anterior and posterior chest wall movement ■ Palpate for bony crepitus, subcutaneous emphysema ■ Use of accessory muscles ■ External signs of injury: petechiae, bleeding, cyanosis, bruises, abrasions, lacerations, old scars
Abdomen and Pelvis	■ Symmetry of external abdominal wall and bony structures ■ External signs of injury: bruising, abrasions, lacerations, punctures ■ Assess for masses, guarding, femoral pulses ■ Type and location of pain ■ Bowel sounds ■ Rigidity or distention of abdomen ■ Assess genitalia for blood at the meatus, priapism, ecchymosis, rectal bleeding, anal sphincter tone
Extremities	■ Signs of external injury: deformity, ecchymosis, abrasions, lacerations, swelling ■ Pain ■ Movement and strength in arms and legs ■ Sensation in each limb ■ Color skin ■ Presence and quality of peripheral pulses
Back	■ Log-roll and inspect and palpate back for deformity, bleeding, lacerations, bruising

lowing, movement of the palate, and ability to open the mouth. Neck examination includes palpation and visualization of the trachea to determine that it is in the midline. A deviated trachea may signal a life-threatening tension pneumothorax. Subcutaneous emphysema may indicate laryngotracheal disruption. A stiff or painful cervical spine area may signify a fracture of a cervical vertebra. The cervical spine *must* be protected using a rigid collar, backboard, towel rolls or other soft rolls on either side of the head, and the forehead should be taped to the backboard.

Chest. The chest is examined for paradoxical chest movements and large sucking chest wounds. The sternum, clavicles, and ribs are palpated for deformity and point tenderness. The chest is assessed for pain on palpation, respiratory distress, decreased breath sounds, distant heart sounds, and distended neck veins. In addition to tension pneumothorax and open

Table **64-8** Prophylaxis Against Tetanus in Wound Management

History of Tetanus Toxoid (Doses)	Type of Wound			
	Tetanus-Prone Wound		Non–Tetanus-Prone Wound	
	Td	TIG*	Td	TIG
Unknown to fewer than three	Yes	Yes	Yes	No
Three or more[†]	No[‡]	No	No[§]	No

*When TIG and Td are administered concurrently, separate sites and syringes must be used.
[†]If only three doses of fluid toxoid have been received, a fourth dose of toxoid, preferably absorbed toxoid, should be given.
[‡]Yes, if more than 5 years since last dose.
[§]Yes, if more than 10 years since last dose.
Td, tetanus and diphtheria toxoid absorbed (for adult use); *TIG*, tetanus immunoglobulin (human).

pneumothorax, the patient should be evaluated for rib fractures, pulmonary contusion, myocardial contusion, and simple pneumothorax. A 12-lead ECG should be obtained, particularly on an older patient or a patient with suspected heart disease. The ECG should be done to detect arrhythmias (e.g., bradycardia).

Abdomen and Pelvis. The abdomen is more difficult to assess. Frequent evaluation for subtle changes in the abdominal examination is essential. Blunt trauma can be caused by motor vehicle collisions and assaults. Penetrating trauma tends to injure specific organs. Decreased bowel sounds may indicate a temporary paralytic ileus. Bowel sounds in the chest may indicate a diaphragmatic rupture. The abdomen is percussed for gastric distention and peritoneal irritation. A dull sound indicates blood or fluid. The pelvis is gently palpated. If pain is elicited, it may indicate a pelvic fracture. The genitalia are inspected for bleeding and obvious injuries. A rectal examination is performed to check for blood, a high-riding prostate, and loss of sphincter tone.

Extremities. The upper and lower extremities are assessed. Injured extremities are splinted above and below the injury to decrease further soft tissue injury and pain. Grossly deformed, pulseless extremities should be realigned and splinted. Pulses are checked before and after movement of an extremity. The extremities are palpated for point tenderness, crepitus, and abnormal movements. Injured extremities should be elevated and ice packs applied. Prophylactic antibiotics are administered for open fractures. Patients with fractures should receive analgesia.

Back. The trauma patient should always be turned (using spinal precautions) to inspect the back. The back is inspected for ecchymosis, abrasions, puncture wounds, cuts, and obvious deformities. The entire spine is palpated for misalignment, deformity, and pain.

INTERVENTION AND EVALUATION

Regardless of the patient's chief complaint, a thorough assessment and an accurate history are critical in an emergency situation. Once the secondary survey is complete, all findings are recorded. Additional interventions may include placement of a nasogastric tube to decrease gastric distention. The contents of the nasogastric drainage should be checked for blood. A nasogastric tube should not be placed in the nares in a patient suspected of having a basilar skull fracture because the tube might enter the brain; rather, it should be placed orally. An indwelling catheter is inserted and urinary output monitored. Urine output should be at least 0.5 ml/kg/hr. An indwelling catheter

should not be inserted if a urethral tear is suspected. Patients with pelvic injuries, blood at the meatus, or men with high-riding prostates are at risk for a urethral tear. A urethrogram should be obtained before a catheter is inserted. The urine should be checked for blood and a urine pregnancy test performed on women. All trauma patients should receive tetanus prophylaxis if the tetanus status is unknown (Table 64-8).

Depending on the patient's injuries, the patient is transported for diagnostic tests such as a CT scan, x-ray, or MRI or admitted to a general or intensive care unit. The emergency nurse is responsible for monitoring the trauma patient during transport and notifying the trauma team should the patient's condition change from baseline.

DEATH IN THE EMERGENCY DEPARTMENT

Unfortunately, there are a number of emergency patients who do not benefit from the skill, expertise, and technology available in the ED. It is important for the emergency nurse to be able to deal with feelings about sudden death so that the nurse can help families and significant others begin the grieving process.

The emergency nurse should recognize the importance of certain hospital rituals in preparing the bereaved to grieve, such as collecting the belongings, arranging for an autopsy, viewing the body, and making mortuary arrangements. The death must seem real so that the significant others can begin to grieve and accept the death. The emergency nurse cannot afford to forget the surviving loved ones after a death in the ED. Family members may benefit from observing resuscitation of a loved one. Should a family member request to be present, it is essential that a member of the team explain care rendered and be available to answer questions.

ENVIRONMENTAL EMERGENCIES

Increased interest in outdoor activities such as running, hiking, cycling, skiing, sailing, and swimming has increased the number of environmental emergencies seen in the ED. Illness or injury may be caused by the activity, exposure to weather, or attack from various animals. Specific environmental emergencies discussed include heat stress and cold stress, drowning and near drowning, bites, and stings.

HEAT-RELATED EMERGENCIES

Brief exposure to intense heat or prolonged exposure to less intense heat leads to heat stress when thermoregulatory mechanisms such as sweating, vasodilation, and increased respirations cannot compensate for exposure to increased ambient

ETHICAL DILEMMAS

Brain Death

SITUATION

The emergency nurse receives a radio call from emergency medical technicians about a young male who has been involved in a motorcycle crash. The patient was not wearing a helmet and has a large open skull fracture with obvious gray matter oozing from the area. Transport from the accident scene was delayed by 45 minutes as a result of downed power lines. En route to the hospital the patient experiences cardiopulmonary arrest. Estimated arrival at the hospital is an additional 45 minutes as a result of severe weather. EMS personnel request permission to stop resuscitation efforts.

DISCUSSION

Degree of trauma and extent of brain damage in this patient has been complicated by delay in providing basic life support. Description of the patient's injuries associated with cardiopulmonary arrest suggest brain death. There is a slight chance that the patient's heart can be resuscitated; however, the likelihood that the patient's brain will survive is minuscule. A hospital is not obligated to continue futile medical care for a brain dead patient who cannot survive even with mechanical intervention.

ETHICAL AND LEGAL PRINCIPLES

The definition of brain death was originally made in 1968 by a Harvard Medical School ad hoc committee in response to technology that kept the heart and lungs functioning—even without brainstem activity.

- When a brain dead patient is maintained on mechanical support, the heart and lungs eventually cease functioning. It is medically futile to continue treatment of a brain dead patient.
- Brain death criteria do not address patients in a permanent vegetative state or anencephalic infants, since the brainstem in these patients is adequate to maintain function of the heart and lungs.

Table 64-9 Risk Factors for Heat-Related Emergencies

Age
Elderly
Infants

Environmental Conditions
High environmental temperature
High relative humidity
Low wind

Preexisting Illness
Cardiovascular disease
Previous stroke or other CNS lesion
Obesity
Diabetes
Cystic fibrosis
Skin disorders (e.g., large burn scars)

Prescription Drugs
Anticholinergics
Phenothiazines
Butyrophenones
Tricyclic antidepressants
Antihistamines
Antispasmodics
Diuretics
Antiparkinsonian drugs
β-Adrenergic blockers

Street Drugs
Lysergic acid diethylamide (LSD)
Jimsonweed
Amphetamines
Phencyclidine (PCP)
Alcohol

From Newberry L, editor: *Sheehy's emergency principles and practice*, ed 4, St Louis, 1998, Mosby.

temperatures.[5] Ambient temperature is a product of environmental temperature and humidity. (See Chapter 11 for discussion of thermoregulation.) Strenuous activities in hot or humid environments, clothing that interferes with perspiration, high fevers, and preexisting illnesses predispose individuals to heat stress (Table 64-9). Effects can be mild (heat rash and heat edema) or severe (heat exhaustion and heat stroke). Heat stress is a leading cause of death in athletes. Specific heat emergencies are heat rash, heat edema, heat cramps, heat syncope, heat exhaustion, and heat stroke (Table 64-10).

Heat rash (miliaria or prickly heat) is a fine, red, papular rash that occurs on the torso, neck, and skin folds.[6] The rash occurs when sweat ducts are obstructed and become inflamed so sweat excretion does not occur. The rash usually occurs in warm weather, but has also been reported in cold weather as a result of clothing.

Heat syncope is associated with prolonged standing and heat exposure. Manifestations include dizziness, orthostatic hypo-

tension, and syncope. Inadequate vasomotor tone associated with aging place the elderly at greater risk for heat syncope.

Heat edema is characterized by swelling of the hands, feet, and ankles, usually in nonacclimatized individuals as a result of prolonged standing or sitting. Swelling usually resolves in days with rest, elevation, and support hose. Diuretics are not recommended as this condition is self-limiting and requires no additional treatment.

Heat cramps are severe cramps in large muscle groups fatigued by heavy work. Cramps are brief, intense, and tend to occur during rest after exercise or heavy labor. Nausea, tachycardia, pallor, weakness, and profuse diaphoresis are often present. The condition is seen most often in healthy, acclimated athletes with adequate fluid intake. Profuse sweating and ingestion of water or other salt-poor solutions deplete sodium and lead to hyponatremia. Cramps resolve rapidly with rest and oral or parenteral replacement of sodium and water. Elevation, gentle massage, and analgesia minimize pain associated with heat cramps. The patient should avoid strenuous activity for 12 hours after discharge. Education should emphasize salt replacement during strenuous exercise in hot, humid environments. Commercially prepared electrolyte solutions such as Gatorade, Powerade, and All Sport are recommended.

✚**EMERGENCY MANAGEMENT**

Table **64-10**   **Hyperthermia**

Etiology	Assessment Findings	Interventions
Environmental Lack of acclimatization Prolonged exposure to extreme temperatures Hot tubs Physical exertion **Trauma** Head injury **Metabolic** Thyrotoxicosis Diabetes Dehydration **Drugs** Sympathomimetic drugs β-Adrenergic blockers Diuretics Cocaine Alcohol Antihistamines Tranquilizers **Other** Cardiovascular disease CNS lesions	**Heat Rash** ■ Rash on torso, neck, skin folds **Heat Edema** ■ Edema of hands, feet, ankles **Heat Cramps** ■ Severe muscle contractions **Heat Syncope** ■ Syncope ■ Dizziness ■ Hypotension **Heat Exhaustion** ■ Fatigue, weakness ■ Profuse sweating ■ Anxiety, irritability ■ Headache ■ Nausea and vomiting ■ Hypotension ■ Tachycardia ■ Weak, thready pulse ■ Hypotension ■ Cold, clammy skin ■ Altered level of consciousness ■ Rectal temperature ≥104° F (40° C) **Heat Stroke** ■ Headache ■ Chills ■ Nausea, vomiting ■ Ataxia ■ Hot, dry skin ■ Altered mental status ■ Hypotension ■ Tachycardia ■ Seizures ■ Coma ■ Rectal temperature >105° F (40.6° C)	**Initial** ■ Ensure patent airway. ■ Refer to text for treatment of heat rash, heat edema, heat cramps, and heat syncope. ■ Establish IV access and begin rapid fluid replacement for significant heat injury. ■ Remove patient's clothing and begin cooling procedures by placing wet sheets over patient with ice packs in groin, neck, and torso. ■ Obtain serum electrolytes, ECG, and CBC. ■ Insert urinary catheter. ■ Cool rapidly. Use cooling blanket if temperature does not decrease with evaporative measures. **Ongoing Monitoring** ■ Monitor vital signs, level of consciousness, cardiac rhythm, oxygen saturation, electrolytes, and urinary output. ■ Monitor urine for development of myoglobinuria secondary to muscle breakdown.

Heat Exhaustion

Prolonged exposure to heat over hours or days leads to heat exhaustion, a clinical syndrome characterized by fatigue, lightheadedness, nausea, vomiting, diarrhea, and feelings of impending doom (see Table 64-10). Tachypnea, hypotension, tachycardia, elevated body temperature, dilated pupils, mild confusion, ashen color, and profuse diaphoresis are also present. Orthostatic hypotension and mild to severe temperature elevation (98.6° F to 105° F [37° C to 40.6° C]) are due to dehydration.[7] Heat exhaustion usually occurs in individuals engaged in strenuous activity in hot, humid weather, but it also occurs in sedentary individuals.

Treatment begins with placement of the patient in a cool area and removal of constrictive clothing. Oral fluid and electrolyte replacement is initiated unless the patient is nauseated. Salt tablets are not recommended because of potential gastric irritation and hypernatremia. A 0.9% normal saline solution is initiated intravenously when oral solutions are not tolerated. An initial fluid bolus may be used to correct hypotension. However, fluid replacement should be correlated to clinical and laboratory parameters. A moist sheet placed over the patient de-

creases core temperature through evaporative heat loss. Hospital admission is considered for the elderly, chronically ill, or those who do not improve within 3 to 4 hours.

Heat Stroke

Heat stroke, the most serious form of heat stress, is common when excessive environmental temperature and high humidity occur over 3 or more days. Table 64-9 lists risk factors for heat-related emergencies, especially heat stroke. Increased sweating, vasodilation, and increased respiratory rate (the body's attempt to lower temperature) deplete fluids and electrolytes. Eventually, sweat glands stop functioning, so core temperature increases rapidly. The patient presents with core temperature greater than 105° F (40.6°C), altered mentation, absence of perspiration, and circulatory collapse. The skin is hot, dry, and ashen. The brain is extremely sensitive to thermal injuries so a range of neurologic symptoms occur, such as hallucinations, loss of muscle coordination, and combativeness. Cerebral edema and hemorrhage may occur as a result of direct thermal injury to the brain and decreased cerebral blood flow.

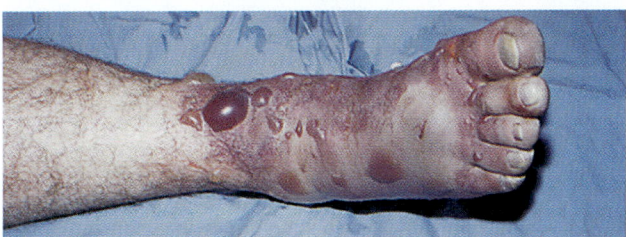

Fig. 64-2   Edema and blister formation 24 hours after frostbite injury occurring in an area covered by a tightly fitted boot.

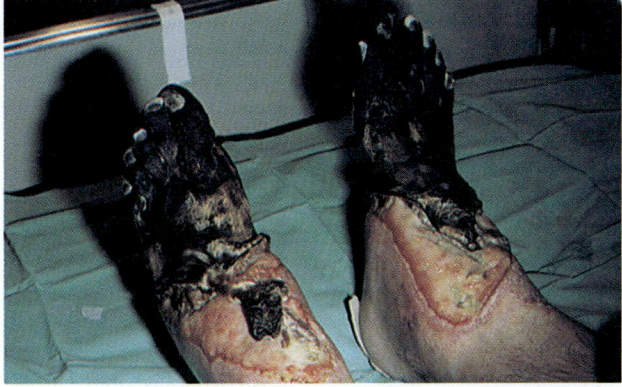

Fig. 64-3   Gangrenous necrosis 6 weeks after the frostbite injury shown in Fig. 64-2.

Mortality with heat stroke approaches 70%.[8] Prognosis is related to age, health, and length of exposure. Older adults and individuals with diabetes mellitus, chronic renal disease, cardiovascular disease, pulmonary disease, or other physiologic compromise are particularly vulnerable.

Collaborative Care

Treatment of heat stroke focuses on rapid reduction of core temperature and treatment of subsequent complications. Administration of 100% oxygen compensates for the patient's hypermetabolic state. Intubation and ventilation with a bag valve mask may be required. Hypovolemia is usually not present. Therefore fluid resuscitation with 1 to 2 L of 0.9% normal saline solution over the first 4 hours is usually adequate. Lactated Ringer's solution is not recommended because the ischemic liver cannot metabolize lactate to bicarbonate.

Conventional cooling methods include tepid water mist, fans, and ice packs to the head, groin, axillae, and neck. Ice baths, alcohol rubs, and antipyretics should not be used. More aggressive cooling techniques are implemented when conventional techniques fail. Ice water immersion is not recommended, since the massive peripheral vasoconstriction that occurs can interfere with cooling. Cooling blankets are used. However, cooling from wet skin is 25 times more effective than cooling from dry skin.[9] Ice water lavage, cold water peritoneal dialysis, and cardiopulmonary bypass are used in extreme cases of hyperthermia.

Cooling efforts are complicated by shivering, since associated muscle activity increases core temperature. Chlorpromazine (Thorazine) IV is the drug of choice to suppress shivers. Aggressive temperature reduction should continue until core temperature reaches 102° F (38.8°C). Additional therapy includes corticosteroid therapy with methylprednisolone for cerebral edema and mannitol when urinary output is less than 0.5ml/kg/hr. Antipyretics are not recommended. Muscle breakdown associated with hypothermia leads to myoglobinuria, which places the kidneys at risk. Therefore urine should be carefully monitored for color, amount, pH, and hemoglobin.

COLD-RELATED EMERGENCIES

Cold injuries may be localized (frostbite) or systemic (hypothermia). Contributing factors include age, duration of exposure, environmental temperature, preexisting conditions (e.g., diabetes), medications that suppress shivering (narcotics, heroin, psychotropic agents, and antiemetics), and alcohol intoxication, which causes peripheral vasodilation, increases sensations of warmth, and depresses shivering. Smokers have an increased risk of cold-related injury as a result of the vasoconstrictive effects of nicotine.

Frostbite

Peripheral vasoconstriction in response to cold exposure decreases blood flow. Average cutaneous blood flow in a 70-kg person is 200 to 250 ml/min. Heat stress increases this rate to as much as 7000 ml/min, whereas cold-related vasoconstriction may decrease cutaneous blood flow to ≤50 ml/min. As cellular temperature decreases and ice crystals form in intracellular spaces, intracellular sodium and chloride increase, the cell membrane is destroyed, and organelles are damaged. Depth of frostbite is the result of ambient temperature, length of exposure, type and condition (wet or dry) of clothing, and contact with metal surfaces. Other factors that affect severity include skin color (dark-skinned people are more prone to frostbite), lack of acclimatization, previous episodes, exhaustion, and poor peripheral vascular status.[10]

Superficial frostbite involves skin and subcutaneous tissue, usually the ears, nose, fingers, and toes. The skin is pale, waxy, and feels crunchy and frozen. The patient may complain of tingling, numbness, or a burning sensation. Injured tissue is easily damaged so the area should be handled carefully and never squeezed, massaged, or scrubbed. Clothing and jewelry should be removed because they may constrict the extremity and decrease circulation. The affected area should be elevated and warm soaks (104°-110° F [40°-43° C]) applied. The nurse should not attempt to warm the area by application of snow or ice or use of flame. The patient often experiences a warm, stinging sensation as tissue thaws. Blisters form within a few hours (Fig. 64-2). The blisters should be debrided and a sterile dressing applied. Heavy blankets and clothing should be avoided as friction and weight can lead to sloughing of damaged tissue. Rewarming is extremely painful. Residual pain may last weeks or even years. Analgesia should be administered and tetanus prophylaxis should be given as appropriate (see Table 64-8). The patient should be evaluated for systemic hypothermia.

Deep frostbite involves muscle, bone, and tendon. The skin is white, hard, and insensitive to touch. The area has the appearance of deep thermal injury with mottling gradually progressing to gangrene (Fig. 64-3). The affected extremity is submersed in a circulating water bath (104° F to 108° F [40° C to

✚ EMERGENCY MANAGEMENT

Table **64-11**   Hypothermia

Etiology	Assessment Findings	Interventions
Environmental Prolonged exposure to cold Prolonged immersion Excessive perspiration Inadequate clothing for environmental temperature **Physiologic** Head injury Hypoglycemia **Iatrogenic** Cold IV fluids Blood administration Inadequate warming in the ED or surgery **Other** Drugs Ethanol	▪ Shivering ▪ Sleepiness ▪ Apathy ▪ Listlessness, areflexia ▪ Coma ▪ Cyanosis ▪ Decreased respiratory rate, pulse rate, temperature, blood pressure ▪ Blue, white, or frozen extremities ▪ Arrhythmias: bradycardia, asystole, ventricular fibrillation ▪ Intoxication ▪ History of exposure	**Initial** ▪ Remove patient from cold environment. ▪ Ensure patent airway. ▪ Administer oxygen via nasal cannula or non-rebreather mask. ▪ Establish IV access with two large-bore catheters and infuse warmed normal saline or lactated Ringer's solution. ▪ Assess for other injuries. ▪ Remove patient's wet clothing and apply warm blankets. ▪ Initiate passive warming with warm humidified oxygen. ▪ Keep patient's head covered with warm, dry towels, or stocking cap. ▪ Warm slowly (1° C/hr) to avoid cardiac irritability from sudden return of cold blood to the heart. ▪ Treat patient gently to avoid increased cardiac irritability. ▪ Do not rub areas of suspected frostbite. ▪ Anticipate intubation for diminished or absent gag reflex. ▪ Anticipate aggressive rewarming techniques if patient does not respond to warm blankets, warm IV fluids, and warmed humidified oxygen. Techniques include warm gastric lavage, thoracotomy, cardiopulmonary bypass, peritoneal lavage, esophageal rewarming, pleural rewarming, and bladder lavage. **Ongoing Monitoring** ▪ Monitor vital signs, level of consciousness, oxygen saturation, cardiac rhythm, temperature. ▪ Loss of ability to shiver indicates severe hypothermia. ▪ Do not give IM medications.

42° C]) until distal flush occurs. Significant edema may begin within 3 hours, with blistering in 6 hours to days. Parenteral analgesia is required in severe frostbite because of the pain associated with tissue thawing. Amputation may be required if the injured area is untreated or treatment is unsuccessful. The patient is admitted to the hospital for observation over 24 to 48 hours with bed rest, elevation of the injured part, and prophylactic antibiotics if the wound is at risk for infection.

Hypothermia

Environmental exposure to freezing temperatures, cold winds, and wet, damp terrain in the presence of physical exhaustion, inadequate clothing, and/or inexperience predispose individuals to hypothermia. Near drowning and water immersion are also associated with hypothermia. The elderly are more prone to hypothermia resulting from decreased mobility, diminished energy reserves, decreased basal metabolic rate, decreased shivering response, decreased sensory perception, chronic medical conditions, and medications that alter body defenses. Hypothermia mimics cerebral or metabolic disturbances causing ataxia, confusion, and withdrawal, so the patient may be misdiagnosed.

Hypothermia, defined as a core temperature less than 95° F (35°C), occurs when heat produced by the body cannot compensate for heat lost to the environment. Fifty-five to sixty percent of all body heat is lost as radiant energy with the greatest loss from the head, thorax, and with each breath.[11] Peripheral vasoconstriction is the body's first attempt to conserve heat. Wet clothing increases evaporative heat loss five times greater than normal and immersion in cold water increases heat loss by a factor of 25. Wind increases heat loss by lowering environmental temperature through conduction. The body produces heat largely through caloric intake. As cold temperatures persist, shivering and movement are the body's only mechanisms for producing heat. Death usually occurs when core temperature falls below 78° F (25.6° C). However, survival has been reported at a core temperature of 64° F (17° C).

Core temperature below 87° F (30.5° C) is severe and potentially life-threatening. Assessment findings in hypothermia are variable and dependent on core temperature (Table 64-11).[11] Patients with *mild hypothermia* (90° F to 95° F [33° C to 35° C]) have shivering, lethargy, confusion, rational to irrational behavior, and minor heart rate changes. Shivering disappears at temperatures less than 92° F (32° C). *Moderate*

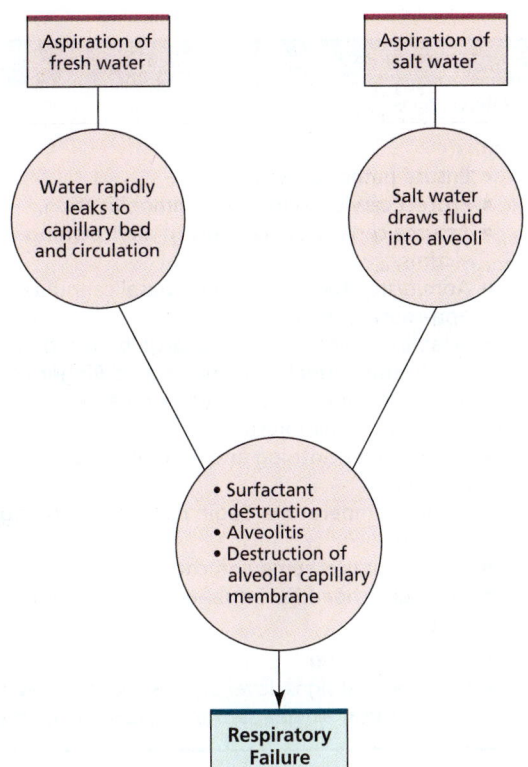

Fig. 64-4 Pulmonary effects of water aspiration.

hypothermia (87° F to 90° F [31° C to 33° C]) causes rigidity, bradycardia, slowed respiratory rate, blood pressure obtainable only by Doppler, metabolic and respiratory acidosis, and hypovolemia.

As core temperature drops by 18° F (10° C), basal metabolic rate decreases two or three times. The cold myocardium is extremely irritable so any movement can precipitate ventricular fibrillation. Decreased renal blood flow decreases glomerular filtration rate, which impairs water reabsorption and leads to dehydration. The hematocrit increases as intravascular volume decreases. Cold blood becomes thick and acts as a thrombus, placing the patient at risk for stroke, myocardial infarction, pulmonary emboli, acute tubular necrosis, and renal failure. Decreased blood flow leads to lactic acid accumulation from anaerobic metabolism and subsequent metabolic acidosis.

Profound hypothermia (<87° F [30.5° C]) makes the person appear dead. Metabolic rate, heart rate, and respirations are so slow they may be difficult to detect. Reflexes are absent and the pupils fixed and dilated. Profound bradycardia, asystole, or ventricular fibrillation may be present. Every effort is made to warm the patient to ≥90° F (32° C) before the person is pronounced dead. The cause of death is usually refractory ventricular fibrillation.

Collaborative Care

Treatment of hypothermia focuses on rewarming the patient, correcting dehydration and acidosis, maintaining patent airway, and treating cardiac arrhythmias (see Table 64-11). *Passive rewarming* is used for mild hypothermia. The patient is moved to a warm, dry place, damp clothing removed, and warm blankets placed on the patient. Gentle handling is essential to prevent stimulation of the cold myocardium.

Active external rewarming with warming blankets, radiant heat lamps, hot water bottles, and hot water baths are used for moderate hypothermia. The patient should be closely monitored for marked vasodilation and hypotension. *Active core rewarming* refers to heat applied directly to the core. Techniques include heated, humidified oxygen 105° F to 115° F (40.5° C to 46.1° C) and installation of heated fluids via IV infusions, bladder lavage, gastric lavage, peritoneal dialysis, hemodialysis, heart-lung bypass, and mediastinal lavage via thoracotomy.

The patient with hypothermia is at risk for ventricular fibrillation when core temperature falls below 82° F (28° C). Ventricular fibrillation does not respond to conventional therapy at low core temperatures, so only one defibrillation attempt is recommended. Only essential IV medications are given; no IM injections are given because of poor perfusion and drug absorption.

Core temperature should be carefully monitored during rewarming procedures. Warming places the patient at risk for rewarming shock, a drop in core temperature, which occurs as cold peripheral blood returns to the central circulation. Rewarming should be discontinued once the core temperature reaches 93° F (34° C). The temperature should not be increased more than 1° C per hour. Fluid resuscitation using warmed IV fluids should be correlated to hemodynamic and respiratory status.

Discharge teaching focuses on teaching the patient how to avoid future problems. Essential information includes dressing in layers for cold weather, covering the head, carrying high-carbohydrate foods for extra calories, and developing a plan for survival should an accident occur. Homeless individuals should be sheltered until fully recovered.

DROWNING AND NEAR DROWNING

Drowning accounts for approximately 9000 deaths annually in the United States with an additional 50,000 near drowning cases reported. Drowning is the third leading cause of death, with 40% of the victims under 5 years of age. Drowning occurs five times more often in men.[11] Alcohol is a significant factor in 60% of all adolescent drownings.

Drowning is death from suffocation after submersion in water or other fluid medium. *Near drowning* is defined as survival from potential drowning. *Immersion syndrome* occurs with immersion in cold water, which leads to stimulation of the vagus nerve and potentially fatal arrhythmias.

Death from drowning is caused by hypoxia secondary to aspiration or airway obstruction. The majority of all drowning victims aspirate water into the pulmonary tree and develop pulmonary edema. Those victims that do not aspirate fluid develop intense bronchospasm and airway obstruction, the cause of death in dry drowning. Regardless of what fluid is aspirated into the pulmonary tree, the ultimate result is pulmonary edema. The osmotic gradient caused by aspirated fluid causes fluid imbalances in the body. Hypotonic fresh water is rapidly absorbed into the circulatory system through the alveoli. Fresh water may be contaminated with chlorine, mud, and algae, causing the breakdown of lung surfactant, fluid seepage, and pulmonary edema. Hypertonic salt water draws fluid from adjacent capillaries into interstitial tissue and the alveoli causing hemoconcentration and hypovolemia. Figure 64-4 shows the pulmonary effects of water aspiration.

✚**EMERGENCY MANAGEMENT**

Table **64-12**   Near Drowning

Etiology	Assessment Findings	Interventions
Exhaustion while swimming Loss of control or support in water Entrapment or entanglement with objects in water Loss of ability to move secondary to cervical spine injury Poor judgment resulting from alcohol or drugs Seizure while in water	**Pulmonary** ■ Ineffective breathing ■ Dyspnea ■ Respiratory distress ■ Respiratory arrest ■ Crackles, rhonchi ■ Cough with pink-frothy sputum **Cardiac** ■ Tachycardia ■ Bradycardia ■ Arrhythmia ■ Cardiac arrest **Other** ■ Panic ■ Exhaustion ■ Coma ■ Cervical spine injury ■ Hypothermia	**Initial** ■ Ensure patent airway. ■ Protect cervical spine with immobilization. ■ Assume cervical spine injury in all drowning victims. ■ Administer 100% oxygen via nasal cannula or non-rebreather mask. ■ Establish IV access with two large-bore catheters and infuse normal saline or lactated Ringer's solution to maintain hemodynamic status. ■ Assess for other injuries. ■ Remove wet clothing and cover with warm blankets. ■ Obtain temperature. Begin passive rewarming if needed. ■ Obtain cervical spine and chest x-rays. ■ Anticipate need for intubation if gag reflex is absent. **Ongoing Monitoring** ■ Monitor vital signs, level of consciousness, respiratory status, oxygen saturation, cardiac rhythm.

The body attempts to compensate for hypoxia by shunting blood to the lungs, which increases pulmonary pressures and worsens the respiratory status. More and more blood is shunted through alveoli. However, the blood is not adequately oxygenated so the hypoxemia worsens. Anaerobic metabolism develops, which leads to metabolic acidosis.

The assessment findings of a patient with near drowning are listed in Table 64-12. Core temperature may be slightly elevated or below normal depending on water temperature.

Near drowning victims have recovered with no long-term effects after being submerged in cold water up to 40 minutes.[12,13] Aggressive resuscitation efforts and the mammalian diving reflex improve survival.[14] Cold water lowers the body's metabolic rate and oxygen demand. The mammalian diving reflex causes apnea, bradycardia, peripheral vasoconstriction, and further decreases metabolic rate. Blood flow is redistributed to the heart, lungs, and brain.

Collaborative Care

Treatment focuses on correcting hypoxia, acid-base imbalances, and fluid imbalances; supporting basic physiologic functions; and rewarming when hypothermia is present. Initial evaluation involves assessment of airway, cervical spine, breathing, and circulation. Other interventions are listed in Table 64-12.

Mechanical ventilation with positive end-expiratory pressure or continuous positive airway pressure may be used to improve gas exchange across the alveolar-capillary membrane when significant pulmonary edema is present. Ventilation and oxygenation are the primary techniques used to treat acidosis. Mannitol or furosemide (Lasix) may be given to decrease free water and treat cerebral edema.

Deterioration in neurologic status suggests cerebral edema, increased hypoxia, or profound acidosis. Near drowning victims may also have head injuries that cause prolonged alterations in level of consciousness. All victims of near drowning should be observed in a hospital for a minimum of 4 to 6 hours. Delayed pulmonary edema (also called secondary drowning), pneumonia, and cerebral edema have been reported in patients who were essentially free of symptoms immediately after the near drowning episode.

Education needs to focus on water safety and minimizing the risks for drowning. Swimming pool gates should be locked, life jackets should be used on all water craft, including inner tubes and rafts, and water survival skills, that is, swimming lessons, should be a priority. The dangers of combining alcohol and drugs with swimming and other water sports should be taught.

BITES AND STINGS

Animals, spiders, and insects cause injury and even death by biting or stinging. Morbidity is a result of either direct tissue damage or lethal toxins. Direct tissue damage is a product of animal size, characteristics of the animal's teeth, and strength of the jaw. Tissue may be lacerated, crushed, or chewed while toxins released through teeth, fangs, stingers, spines, or tentacles have local or systemic effects. Mortality associated with animal bites is due to blood loss, allergic reactions, or lethal toxins. Injuries caused by insects, spiders, scorpions, ticks, snakes, dogs, cats, rodents, and humans are described below.

Hymenoptera Stings

The *Hymenoptera* family includes bees, yellow jackets, hornets, and wasps. Stings can cause mild discomfort or life-threatening anaphylaxis. Venom may be cytotoxic, hemolytic, allergenic, or vasoactive. Symptoms may begin immediately or be delayed up to 48 hours. Reactions are more severe with multiple stings. Most hymenopterans sting repeatedly. However, the honeybee stings only once, usually leaving the stinger in the skin so that release of venom continues. A scraping motion with a finger-nail, knife, or needle is recommended for removing the stinger. Tweezers squeeze the stinger and cause more venom release.

Manifestations vary from stinging, burning, swelling, and itching to edema, headache, fever, syncope, malaise, nausea, vomiting, wheezing, bronchospasm, laryngeal edema, and hypotension. Treatment depends on the severity of the reaction. Mild reactions are treated with elevation, cool compresses, antipruritic lotions, and oral antihistamines. Rings, watches, and restrictive clothing are removed. More severe reactions require IM or IV antihistamines (diphenhydramine [Benadryl]), SC epinephrine (0.3 to 0.5 ml 1:1000), and corticosteroids. Allergic reactions and anaphylaxis are discussed in Chapter 12.

Spider Bites (Arachnid)

Although there are 20,000 species of venomous spiders in the world, only 50 species cause illness. Two venomous spiders found in the United States are the black widow spider and the brown recluse spider. Their venom can cause a localized reaction or systemic anaphylaxis. Tarantulas appear more dangerous than they are, as their bite causes only localized stinging and pain. Other types of spiders release venom when they bite and may cause allergic reactions in some individuals, but they are not considered poisonous.

Black Widow Spiders. *Black widow spiders* have a black body with a bright red hourglass shape on the abdomen. The spider is usually found in damp, cool places under rocks or in woodpiles. The black widow spider venom is neurotoxic. The patient has a tiny, red bite mark associated with pain out of proportion to the size of the bite. Systemic reactions develop over 24 to 48 hours and include nausea, vomiting, elevated temperature, diaphoresis, respiratory distress, hypertension, headache, syncope, and weakness. Symptoms usually peak 2 to 3 hours after onset; however, muscle spasms and hypertension can recur for 12 to 24 hours. Chest and abdominal pain, seizures, and shock can also occur. Bites on the lower body cause abdominal rigidity whereas bites on the upper body lead to chest, back, and shoulder rigidity. A black widow spider bite is not prominent and can be easily missed. Patients not aware of the bite can be misdiagnosed, since symptoms mimic a perforated ulcer, appendicitis, pancreatitis, or other abdominal emergency.

Treatment includes cooling the area to slow the action of the neurotoxin. The wound should be cleaned and tetanus prophylaxis given as appropriate. Muscle spasms are treated with calcium gluconate, methocarbamol (Robaxin), or diazepam (Valium). Severe pain may require narcotic analgesia. Antivenin is used for severe reactions, young children, or adults with hypertension or cardiac disease.

Brown Recluse Spiders. *Brown recluse spiders* are usually found in dark areas such as garages, closets, and boxes. The spider, common in the southeastern, south central, and southwestern United States, is a light brown color with a characteristic dark brown fiddle shape that extends from the eyes down the back. The venom is cytotoxic, so local tissue effects can be dramatic. Stinging, burning, and itching start almost immediately with severe pain several hours later. A bleb (blister), bluish ring around the bite, and erythema eventually progress to necrosis by the third or fourth day. An open sore may persist for days or even weeks. Systemic manifestations, although rare, include fever, myalgia, rash, hemolysis, pe-

techia, joint pain, seizures, shock, hemorrhage, and pulmonary edema. Hemolysis may lead to hemoglobinuria, renal failure, and death.

Treatment depends on severity of the reaction. Treatment is necessary when there is bleb or bullae formation, intense pain, and signs of rapidly progressive ischemia and necrosis. Initial interventions include cool compresses, elevation, and resting of the affected extremity. Analgesia, tetanus prophylaxis, antihistamines, corticosteroids, and antibiotics for prevention of secondary infection may also be required. Surgical debridement with grafting is necessary for some patients. Dapsone, a polymorphonuclear leukocyte inhibitor, has been used for patients with deep crater wounds. Patients with systemic manifestations are hospitalized and monitored for hemolysis, disseminated intravascular clotting, and acute renal failure.

Tick Bites

Ticks inhabit various parts of the country, but they are most common in the Rocky Mountain region and the Northwest. Emergencies associated with tick bites include Rocky Mountain spotted fever, Lyme disease, and tick paralysis. Disease is caused by an infected tick or by the release of neurotoxin. Ticks release a neurotoxic venom as long as the tick head is attached to the body. Therefore, removal of the attached tick is essential for effective treatment. Forceps may be used to safely remove the tick by grasping at the point of entry and pulling upward in a steady motion. Covering the tick with alcohol, mineral oil, petroleum jelly or ether causes the tick to release from the skin. These methods work because the tick breathes through the skin in which they are embedded.

Rocky Mountain spotted fever, caused by *Rickettsia rickettsii,* has an incubation period of 2 to 14 days. A pink, macular rash appears on the palms, wrists, soles, feet, and ankles within 10 days of exposure. Other symptoms include fever, chills, malaise, myalgias, and headache. Treatment is antibiotic therapy.

Lyme disease is the most common arthropod-borne disease in the United States, with 12,000 to 16,000 new cases reported each year.[15] Symptoms appear within 3 to 30 days of exposure to the spirochete *Borrelia burgdorferi,* found on the *Ixodes* tick. Lyme disease occurs most often in the northeastern, north central, and mid-Atlantic regions.[16] The initial stage of this disease is characterized by flulike symptoms and a characteristic bull's eye rash—an expanding circular area of redness of 5 cm diameter or more. Neurologic, cardiac, and musculoskeletal problems such as meningitis, hepatitis, neuropathies, and cardiomyopathies occur days or weeks later. Chronic arthritis and peripheral radiculopathy characterize later stages of the disease, which lasts months or years. Treatment includes antibiotic therapy; however, controversy exists over what the most effective regimen should be. (Lyme disease is discussed in Chapter 60.)

Tick paralysis occurs 5 to 7 days after exposure to the wood tick or dog tick. Classic symptoms are flaccid ascending paralysis, which develops over 1 to 2 days. Without tick removal, the patient dies as respiratory muscles become paralyzed. Tick removal leads to return of muscle movement, usually within 48 to 72 hours.

Snakebite

Only 375 of the 3000 species of snakes in the world are poisonous. Poisonous snakes indigenous to the United States are

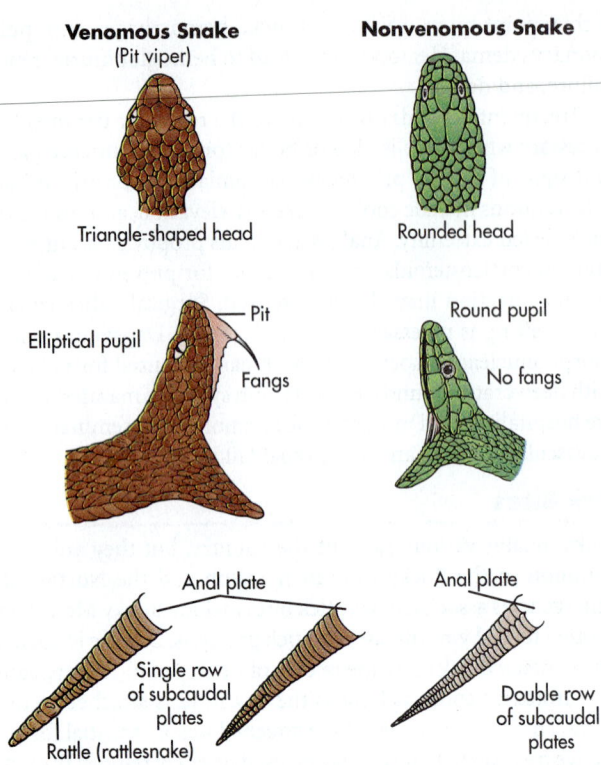

Venomous Snake (Pit viper)

Triangle-shaped head

Elliptical pupil — Pit

Fangs

Anal plate

Single row of subcaudal plates

Rattle (rattlesnake)

Nonvenomous Snake

Rounded head

Round pupil

No fangs

Anal plate

Double row of subcaudal plates

Fig. 64-5 Venomous and nonvenomous snakes.

members of the *Crotalid* and *Elapid* family. *Crotalids,* or pit vipers, include rattlesnakes, copperheads, and water moccasins. Coral snakes belong to the *Elapid* family. Other poisonous snakes in the *Elapid* family not indigenous to the United States are the cobra and the mamba. Figure 64-5 highlights differences between poisonous and nonpoisonous snakes.

Venom from the pit viper is hemolytic, whereas coral snake venom is neurotoxic. Envenomation occurs in approximately 75% to 80% of all snakebites. If swelling does not occur within 30 minutes after the bite, envenomation is unlikely. Local reaction is characterized by 1 or 2 fang marks associated with pain, bruising, edema within 36 hours of injury, petechiae, ecchymosis, and erythema. Loss of function and necrosis of the affected limb may occur 16 to 36 hours after the bite. Systemic reactions include nausea and vomiting, dizziness, tachycardia, muscle fasciculations, gastrointestinal bleeding, and respiratory problems. The patient may experience a metallic or rubber taste. Neurologic symptoms such as constricted pupils, drowsiness, weakness, fasciculations, muscle weakness, and seizures occur with neurotoxic venom. Life-threatening problems associated with systemic envenomation include severe hemorrhage, renal failure, and hypovolemic shock.

Treatment focuses on preventing the spread of venom (Table 64-13). Rings, watches, and restrictive clothing should be removed, and then the affected limb should be immobilized at the level of the heart. Ice and tourniquets are not recommended. Incision of the wound is controversial. If done within 3 minutes of injury, 25% to 30% of the venom may be removed. Caffeine, alcohol, and smoking increase the spread of venom and should be avoided.

ED management includes vascular access with a large gauge catheter and administration of crystalloids to maintain blood pressure. Diagnostic tests include complete blood count, urinalysis, coagulation studies, blood urea nitrogen, creatinine, creatine kinase, and electrolytes. Other measures include assessment of extremity swelling, usually through documentation of circumference every 30 to 60 minutes. Pain should be treated with acetaminophen. Aspirin and nonsteroidal antiinflammatory drugs should be avoided because they may cause bleeding; narcotics may cause respiratory depression. Tetanus prophylaxis should be administered as needed (see Table 64-8). Secondary infection caused by microorganisms in the snake's mouth or other contaminants may require antibiotic therapy. Debridement or fasciotomy is necessary in some patients. Antivenin therapy is used only for life-threatening envenomation because of the high incidence of allergic reactions.[17] A skin test is done before administration of antivenin. The amount of antivenin required depends on the amount of envenomation (Table 64-14). Incomplete dosage is the most common cause of treatment failure so antivenin is administered until symptoms subside. Serum sickness develops in most patients who receive more than 10 vials of antivenin. (Serum sickness is described in Chapter 12.)

Animal Bites

Approximately 500,000 to 2 million animal bites are reported each year in the United States. Children are at greatest risk. The most significant problems associated with animal bites are infection and mechanical destruction of the skin, muscle, tendons, blood vessels, and bone. The bite may cause a simple laceration or be associated with crush injury, puncture wound, or tearing or avulsion of tissue. The severity of injury depends on animal size, victim size, and anatomical location of the bite. Dog bites account for 75% to 90% of reported cases whereas domestic cats are the cause in 10%.[18] Wild or domestic rodents are ranked behind cats and dogs as the third most frequent offenders in reported animal bites. Bite injury secondary to humans, squirrels, ferrets, monkeys, lions, tigers, horses, cows, sheep, goats, camels, and swine also occur. Skull fractures have been reported after camel bites.

Cat bites cause a greater incidence of infection than dog bites. *Pasteurella multocida* occurs in the majority of healthy cats. Cat bites cause deep puncture wounds that can involve tendons and joint capsules. Septic arthritis, osteomyelitis, and tenosynovitis have been reported in cat bites.

Dog bites usually occur on the extremities; however, facial bites are common in small children. Most victims own the dogs that bite them. Dog bites may involve significant tissue damage, with fatalities reported, usually in children. Skull fractures with intracranial injury and death occur in children less than 2 years old. Disfiguring wounds of the face should be evaluated by a plastic surgeon.

Collaborative Care

Treatment of animal bites includes cleaning and irrigation with copious amounts of saline, debridement, tetanus prophylaxis, and analgesics as needed. Prophylactic antibiotics are used for human bites and animal bites at risk for infection such as wounds over joints, those greater than 6 to 12 hours old, puncture wounds, and bites of the hand or foot. Individuals at greatest risk of infection are infants, older adults, immunosup-

✚ **EMERGENCY MANAGEMENT**

Table 64-13 Snakebite

Etiology	Assessment Findings	Interventions
Pit Vipers Rattlesnake Copperhead Water moccasin **Other** Coral snake	■ Fang marks ■ Progressive swelling at site ■ Nausea and vomiting ■ Headache ■ Dizziness ■ Paresthesia ■ Burning pain ■ Ecchymosis, erythema ■ Decreased distal pulses ■ Respiratory compromise ■ Muscular weakness, paralysis ■ Pit viper venom is hemolytic and can be neurotoxic. ■ Severity of injury is due to amount of envenomation.	**Initial** ■ Ensure airway, breathing, and circulation. ■ Reassure patient to decrease panic. ■ Immobilize affected part at heart level. ■ Reduce physical activity. ■ Remove rings, bracelets, and other constricting items on the bitten extremity. ■ Do not put injured part in ice or apply ice packs. ■ Administer oxygen via nasal cannula or non-rebreather mask. ■ Establish IV access in unaffected limb with two large-bore catheters and infuse normal saline. ■ Obtain clotting studies, CBC, electrolytes, BUN, serum creatinine, creatine kinase, urinalysis, and type and crossmatch. ■ Anticipate administration of antivenin. ■ Administer tetanus prophylaxis as appropriate. **Ongoing Monitoring** ■ Monitor vital signs, level of consciousness, oxygen saturation, cardiac rhythm. ■ Monitor for respiratory compromise or hemorrhage.

Table 64-14 Antivenin Snakebite Treatment

Envenomation	Signs and Symptoms	Number of Vials of Antivenin*
None	Fang marks, no local swelling, hemorrhage, or paresthesia	No antivenin. Tetanus prophylaxis, observation
Minimal	Fang marks, local swelling of hands or feet, no systemic reactions	3-5 vials
Moderate	Fang marks, progressive swelling beyond bite, mild systemic reaction	6-10 vials
Severe	Multiple fang marks, progressive swelling, pronounced systemic reaction, hypotension, twitching, clotting abnormalities	15+ vials

*Depends on type of snakebite, body surface area, and age. Skin testing should be done before injection of antivenin.

pressed patients, alcoholics, diabetics, and people taking corticosteroids. Puncture wounds are left open while lacerations are loosely sutured.

Consideration of rabies prophylaxis is an essential component in management of animal bites. Rabies is caused by a neurotoxic virus found in the saliva of some mammals. The condition is fatal in humans. Approximately 35,000 deaths are reported worldwide with one or two cases in the United States.[19] Rabies exposure should be considered if an animal attack was not provoked, involved a wild animal, or involved a domestic animal not immunized against rabies. Rabies prophylaxis is always given when the animal cannot be found or the bite is caused by a carnivorous wild animal. Approximately 25,000 persons receive rabies prophylaxis each year in the United States. Rabies prophylaxis uses an initial injection of rabies immune globulin (RIG) to provide passive immunity, and a series of five injections of human diploid cell vaccine (HDCV) on days 0, 3, 7, 14, and 28 is used to provide active immunity. Dosage is based on the patient's weight.

Human Bites

Human bites carry a high risk of infection from oral bacterial flora, most commonly *Staphylococci aureus* and streptococci. Human bites can cause more tissue destruction than other animal bites. Hands, fingers, and noses are the most common sites of injury with infection rates greatest in wounds of the hands. Boxer's fracture, fracture of the fifth metacarpal, is often associated with an open wound when the knuckles impact teeth. The human jaw has great crushing ability causing laceration, puncture, crush injury, soft tissue tearing, and even amputation. More than 40 potential pathogens found in the human mouth account for an infection rate of approximately 50% in cases where victims did not seek medical intervention within 24 hours of injury.

Initial treatment includes cleaning with copious irrigation, debridement, prophylactic antibiotics, and tetanus prophylaxis. Wounds over joints are splinted; however, initial closure is reserved only for facial wounds. The patient is admitted for IV antibiotic therapy when an infection is present. There is an increased incidence of cellulitis, osteomyelitis, and septic arthritis in these patients. Human bites must be reported to the police in some states.

POISONINGS

A poison is any chemical that harms the body. More than 1 million cases of poisonings occur each year in the United States. Poisonings can be accidental, occupational, recreational, or intentional.[20] Natural or manufactured toxins can be ingested, inhaled, injected, splashed in the eye, or absorbed through the skin. Common poisons are reviewed in Table 64-15. Other poisonings related to the use of illegal drugs such as amphetamines, narcotics, and hallucinogens are discussed in

Chapter 10. Poisoning may also be due to toxic plants or contaminated foods. (Food poisoning is discussed in Chapter 39.)

Severity of the poisoning depends on type, concentration, and route of exposure. Toxins can affect every tissue of the body, so symptoms can be seen in any body system. Specific management of toxins involves decreasing absorption, enhancing elimination, and implementation of toxin-specific interventions.

Options for decreasing absorption of poisons include emesis, gastric lavage, activated charcoal, dermal cleansing, and eye irrigation. Ipecac (15 to 45 ml for adults) followed by 250 to 500 ml water is used to induce emesis. This process is most effective if used within 1 hour of ingestion. Use of Ipecac has lost favor over the past decade for a variety of reasons. Onset of action is delayed and unpredictable, overall rate of drug return is low, and Ipecac is not effective with drugs that are rapidly absorbed such as alcohol.[21] Other problems associated with induced emesis include fluid losses, electrolyte abnormalities, and acid-base disturbances secondary to protracted vomiting.

Table **64-15** **Common Poisons**

Poison	Manifestations	Treatment
▪ Acetaminophen (Tylenol)	Nausea and vomiting, anorexia, malaise, diaphoresis, liver abnormalities	Activated charcoal, *N*-acetylcysteine
▪ Acids and alkalis *Acids:* toilet bowl cleaners, antirust compounds; *alkalis:* drain cleaners, dishwashing detergents, ammonia	Excess salivation, dysphagia, epigastric pain, pneumonitis, burns of mouth, esophagus, and stomach	Immediate dilution (water, milk), corticosteroids (for alkali burns), contraindication for induced vomiting
▪ Aspirin and aspirin-containing medications	Increased respiratory rate, respiratory alkalosis, headache, vertigo, tinnitus, sweating, nausea, electrolyte imbalances	Gastric lavage, activated charcoal, alkaline diuresis, supportive care
▪ Bleaches	Irritation of lips, mouth, and eyes, superficial injury to esophagus; chemical pneumonia and pulmonary edema	Washing of exposed skin and eyes, dilution with water and milk, gastric lavage, prevention of vomiting and aspiration
▪ Carbon monoxide	Dyspnea, headache, tachypnea, confusion, impaired judgment, cyanosis, respiratory depression	Removal from source, administration of 100% oxygen
▪ Cyanide	Headache, faintness, vertigo, tachycardia, hypertension, nausea and vomiting, almond odor to breath	Amyl nitrate, sodium nitrate, sodium thiosulfate, oxygen
▪ Ethylene glycol	Sweet aromatic odor to breath, nausea and vomiting, slurred speech, ataxia, lethargy, respiratory depression	Gastric lavage, activated charcoal, supportive care
▪ Iron	Vomiting (often bloody), diarrhea (often bloody), fever, hyperglycemia, lethargy, hypotension, seizures, coma	Gastric lavage, chelation therapy (deferoxamine)
▪ Nonsteroidal antiinflammatory drugs	Gastroenteritis, abdominal pain, drowsiness, nystagmus, hepatic damage	Gastric lavage, activated charcoal, cathartics
▪ Tricyclic antidepressants (e.g., amitriptyline, imipramine)	In low doses: anticholinergic effects, agitation, hypertension, tachycardia; in high doses: central nervous system depression, respiratory depression, seizures, hypotension	Activated charcoal, gastric lavage, supportive care, contraindication for induced emesis
▪ Alcohol, barbiturates, benzodiazepines, cocaine, hallucinogens, stimulants	See Chapter 10	See Chapter 10

Gastric lavage involves oral insertion of a large diameter (36F to 40F) gastric tube for installation of copious amounts of saline. The head of the bed should be elevated or the patient placed on the side to prevent aspiration. Patients with an altered level of consciousness or diminished gag reflex are intubated before lavage. Lavage is contraindicated in patients who ingested caustic agents. Problems associated with lavage include epistaxis, esophageal perforation, and aspiration.

The most effective intervention for management of poisonings is administration of activated charcoal orally or via a gastric tube. Toxins adhere to charcoal and are excreted through the GI tract rather than absorbed into the portal circulation. Adults receive 50 to 100 g of charcoal. Activated charcoal can absorb a number of poisons from the GI tract, but it does not absorb ethanol, alkali, iron, boric acid, lithium, methanol, or cyanide. Contraindications to charcoal administration are diminished bowel sounds, ileus, ingestion of a substance poorly absorbed by charcoal, or previous administration of N-acetylcysteine (NAC). Charcoal inactivates NAC, the antidote used for acetaminophen toxicity.

Dermal and ocular decontamination involve removal of toxins from eyes and skin using copious amounts of water. With the exception of mustard gas, most toxins can be safely removed with water. Water mixes with mustard gas and releases chlorine gas. As a general rule, dry substances should be brushed from the skin and clothing before water is used. Powdered lime should not be removed with water; it should just be brushed off. Protective clothing (gloves, gowns, and goggles) should be worn for decontamination to prevent secondary exposure. Decontamination procedures are usually done by those specially trained in hazardous material decontamination before the patient arrives at the hospital. Decontamination takes priority over all interventions except basic life support techniques.

Elimination is increased through administration of cathartics, whole-bowel irrigation, repeat-dose activated charcoal, forced diuresis, hemodialysis, charcoal hemoperfusion, oxygen inhalation, surgical removal, and administration of chelating agents. Cathartics such as sorbitol, magnesium citrate, or magnesium sulfate are given together with activated charcoal to stimulate intestinal motility and increase elimination. Multiple doses of cathartics should be avoided because of potentially fatal electrolyte abnormalities. Whole-bowel irrigation involves administration of an isotonic polyethylene glycol and electrolyte solution (GoLYTELY) to flush heavy metals, enteric coated medications, or slowly dissolving tablets. This process is also effective for swallowed objects such as cocaine-filled balloons or condoms.

Repeat-dose activated charcoal (administration of charcoal every 2 to 4 hours) is indicated for theophylline, phenobarbital, salicylates, antidepressants, and carbamazepine (Tegretol).[22] Forced diuresis is used for removal of ethanol, methanol, isopropyl alcohol, and ethylene glycol. Large amounts of IV saline are infused to flush toxins through the kidneys. Mannitol or furosemide (Lasix) may be used to enhance the process. Hemodialysis and hemoperfusion are used for patients when ingestion is associated with severe acidosis.

Other interventions include alkalinization and antidote administration. Sodium bicarbonate administration raises the pH ($\geq$7.5), which is particularly effective for phenobarbital and salicylates. Vitamin C may be added to IV fluids to enhance excretion of amphetamines and quinidine. A limited number of true antidotes are available and many of these recommended agents are themselves toxic.

Education for toxic emergencies focuses on how the poisoning occurred. Patients who experience poisoning because of a suicide attempt or related to substance abuse should be evaluated by a mental health counselor and then admitted for alcohol or drug detoxification or scheduled for follow-up with a mental health professional. Poisoning related to an occupational hazard should be evaluated by the Department of Occupational Safety and Health Administration.

CRITICAL THINKING EXERCISES

CASE STUDY

Trauma

Patient Profile

A 42-year-old male trauma patient is brought to the ED in an ambulance. He was the driver in a motor vehicle collision and was not wearing a seat belt. The passenger in the car was dead at the scene. The paramedics stated that there was significant damage to the car on the passenger side.

Subjective Data

- Is awake
- Complains of shortness of breath and abdominal pain

Objective Data

Physical Examination
- 4-cm head laceration
- Badly deformed right lower leg without pulses
- Unequal pupils
- Decreased breath sounds on left side of chest
- Asymmetric chest movement
- Vital signs: BP 90/40, HR 130 beats/min, respiratory rate 36 breaths/min
- O₂ saturation 82%

Critical Thinking Questions

1. What life-threatening injury does this patient probably have?
2. What is the priority of care?
3. What intervention is needed immediately?
4. What other interventions should the nurse consider?
5. How should the nurse approach the family?
6. Based on assessment data presented, write one or more nursing diagnoses. Are there any collaborative problems?

REVIEW QUESTIONS

The number of the question corresponds to the same-numbered objective at the beginning of the chapter.

1. During triage of patients in an emergency department, the person that the nurse should treat first is
   a. A 2-year-old child with scalp laceration who is awake and crying
   b. An 85-year-old woman with crushing chest pain who is pale and diaphoretic
   c. A 32-year-old complaining of recent onset of fever, aches, and chills after a camping trip
   d. A 34-year-old woman who has raspy breathing and facial and neck edema from a wasp sting

2. An elderly male arrives at the ED disoriented, breathing rapidly, and has hot, dry skin. The priority for treatment is to
   a. Assess his airway, breathing, and circulation
   b. Obtain a detailed medical history from his family
   c. Determine the kind of insurance he has before treating him
   d. Start oxygen administration and have the ED physician see him

3. Which of the following interventions is most effective in decreasing absorption of an ingested poison?
   a. Gastric lavage
   b. Ipecac administration
   c. Activated charcoal
   d. Milk dilution

References

1. Kelly SJ: *Pediatric emergency nursing,* ed 2, Norwalk, Conn, 1994, Appleton & Lange.
2. Rund DA, Rausch TS: *Triage,* St Louis, 1981, Mosby.
3. Brackin JE. In Newberry L, editor: *Sheehy's emergency nursing principles and practice,* St Louis, 1998, Mosby.
4. Kidd PS, Sturt P: *Mosby's emergency nursing reference,* St Louis, 1996, Mosby.
5. Tintinalli JE, Ruiz E, Krome RL, editors: *Emergency medicine: a comprehensive study guide,* ed 4, New York, 1996, McGraw-Hill.
6. Davis LL: Environmental heat-related illnesses, *MEDSURG Nurs* 6:3, 1997.
7. Morris J. In Newberry L, editor: *Sheehy's emergency nursing principles and practice,* St Louis, 1998, Mosby.
8. Simon HB: Hyperthermia and heatstroke, *Hosp Pract* 29:65, 1994.
9. Rosen P, Barkin R: *Emergency medicine concepts and clinical practice,* ed 4, St Louis, 1998, Mosby.
10. Auerbach P, Geehr E: *Management of wilderness and environmental emergencies,* ed 3, St Louis, 1995, Mosby.
11. Emergency Nurses Association: *Emergency nursing core curriculum,* ed 5, Philadelphia, 1999, WB Saunders.
12. Glankler DM: Caring for the victim of near drowning, *Crit Care Nurse* 13:25, 1993.
13. Siebake H and others: Survival after 40 minutes submersion without cerebral sequelae, *Lancet* 1:1275, 1975.
14. DeBoer SL: Neurologic outcomes after near drowning, *Crit Care Nurse* 17:4, 1997.
15. Massachusetts Medical Society: Lyme disease—United States, 1995, *MMWR* 45:481, 1996.
16. Briant C, Roye K, Hutscher AH: Pericarditis as a manifestation of Lyme disease, *J Emerg Nurs* 23:525, 1997.
17. Soski JE: *Snakebite assessment and treatment in the eastern United States,* ed 2, Midway, Fla, 1994, Snakebite Publishing.
18. Strange G, Towns D: Environmental emergencies. In Strange GR and others, editors: *Pediatric emergency medicine: a comprehensive study guide,* New York, 1996, McGraw-Hill.
19. Chonel BB: The modern epidemiological aspects of rabies in the world, *Comp Immunol Microbiol Infect Dis* 16:11, 1993.
20. Kitt S and others: *Emergency nursing: a physiologic and clinical perspective,* ed 2, Philadelphia, 1995, WB Saunders.
21. Criddle LM. In Newberry L, editor: *Sheehy's emergency nursing principles and practice,* St Louis, 1998, Mosby.
22. Johnson D and others: Effect of multiple-dose activated charcoal on the clearance of high-dose intravenous aspirin in a porcine model, *Ann Emerg Med* 26:671, 1995.

Resources

American Association of Emergency Physicians
PO Box 81020
Chicago, IL 60681-0020
800-449-4237
fax: 312-819-1103
http://www.aep.org

American College of Emergency Physicians
PO Box 619911
Dallas, TX 75261-9911
972-550-0911
800-798-1822
fax: 972-580-2816
http://www.acep.org

American Red Cross
8111 Gatehouse Road, 6th Floor
Falls Church, VA 22042
703-206-7090
800-HELP-NOW
http://www.redcross.org

American Trauma Society
8903 Presidential Parkway, Suite 512
Upper Marlboro, MD 20772
301-420-4189
800-556-7890
http://www.amtrauma.org/

Emergency Nurses Association
216 Higgins Road
Park Ridge, IL 60068-5736
708-698-9400
fax: 708-698-9406
http://www.ena.org/

On Emergency Medicine
http://nj5.injersey.com/~pscott/

For additional Internet resources, see the website for this book at www.mosby.com/MERLIN/medsurg_lewis

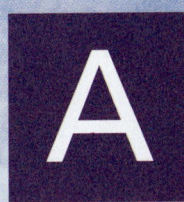

A Nursing Diagnoses

ALPHABETICAL LISTING

Activity Intolerance
Activity Intolerance, Risk for
Adaptive Capacity: Intracranial,
   Decreased
Adjustment, Impaired
Airway Clearance, Ineffective
Anxiety
Aspiration, Risk for
Body Image Disturbance
Breastfeeding, Effective
Breastfeeding, Ineffective
Breastfeeding, Interrupted
Breathing Pattern, Ineffective
Cardiac Output, Decreased
Caregiver Role Strain
Caregiver Role Strain, Risk for
Communication, Impaired Verbal
Confusion, Acute
Confusion, Chronic
Constipation
Constipation, Colonic
Constipation, Perceived
Constipation, Risk for
Coping, Defensive
Coping, Ineffective Community
Coping, Ineffective Individual
Coping, Potential for Enhanced
   Community
Death Anxiety
Decisional Conflict
Denial, Ineffective
Dentition, Altered
Development, Risk for Altered
Diarrhea
Disuse Syndrome, Risk for
Diversional Activity Deficit
Dysreflexia
Dysreflexia, Risk for Autonomic
Energy Field Disturbance
Environmental Interpretation
   Syndrome, Impaired
Failure to Thrive, Adult
Family Coping, Ineffective:
   Compromised
Family Coping, Ineffective: Disabling
Family Coping: Potential for Growth
Family Processes, Altered

Family Processes, Altered: Alcoholism
Fatigue
Fear
Fluid Volume Deficit
Fluid Volume Deficit, Risk for
Fluid Volume Excess
Fluid Volume Imbalance, Risk for
Gas Exchange, Impaired
Grieving, Anticipatory
Grieving, Dysfunctional
Growth, Altered: Risk for
Growth and Development, Altered
Health Maintenance, Altered
Health-Seeking Behaviors (Specify)
Home Maintenance Management,
   Impaired
Hopelessness
Hyperthermia
Hypothermia
Incontinence, Bowel
Incontinence, Functional Urinary
Incontinence, Reflex Urinary
Incontinence, Risk for Urinary Urge
Incontinence, Stress
Incontinence, Total
Incontinence, Urge
Infant Behavior: Disorganized
Infant Behavior, Disorganized: Risk for
Infant Behavior, Potential for
   Enhanced Organized
Infant Feeding Pattern, Ineffective
Infection, Risk for
Injury, Risk for
Knowledge Deficit
Latex Allergy Response
Latex Allergy Response, Risk for
Loneliness, Risk for
Management of Therapeutic
   Regimen, Effective: Individual
Management of Therapeutic
   Regimen, Ineffective: Community
Management of Therapeutic
   Regimen, Ineffective: Families
Management of Therapeutic
   Regimen, Ineffective: Individuals
Memory, Impaired
Mobility, Impaired: Bed
Mobility, Impaired: Physical

Mobility, Impaired: Wheelchair
Nausea
Noncompliance
Nutrition, Altered: Less than Body
   Requirements
Nutrition, Altered: More than Body
   Requirements
Nutrition, Altered: Risk for More
   Than Body Requirements
Oral Mucous Membrane, Altered
Pain
Pain, Chronic
Parent/Infant/Child Attachment, Risk
   for Altered
Parental Role Conflict
Parenting, Altered
Parenting, Altered: Risk for
Perioperative Positioning Injury, Risk
   for
Peripheral Neurovascular
   Dysfunction, Risk for
Personal Identity Disturbance
Poisoning, Risk for
Post-Trauma Syndrome
Post-Trauma Syndrome, Risk for
Powerlessness
Protection, Altered
Rape Trauma Syndrome
Rape Trauma Syndrome: Compound
   Reaction
Rape Trauma Syndrome: Silent
   Reaction
Relocation Stress Syndrome
Role Performance, Altered
Self-Care Deficit, Bathing/Hygiene
Self-Care Deficit, Dressing/Grooming
Self-Care Deficit, Feeding
Self-Care Deficit, Toileting
Self-Esteem, Chronic Low
Self-Esteem Disturbance
Self-Esteem, Situational Low
Self-Mutilation, Risk for
Sensory/Perceptual Alterations
   (Specify: Visual, Auditory,
   Kinesthetic, Gustatory, Tactile,
   Olfactory)
Sexual Dysfunction
Sexuality Patterns, Altered

Skin Integrity, Impaired
Skin Integrity, Impaired: Risk for
Sleep Deprivation
Sleep Pattern Disturbance
Social Interaction, Impaired
Social Isolation
Sorrow, Chronic
Spiritual Distress (Distress of the
    Human Spirit)
Spiritual Distress, Risk for
Spiritual Well-Being, Potential for
    Enhanced
Suffocation, Risk for
Surgical Recovery, Delayed
Swallowing, Impaired
Temperature, Risk for Altered Body
Thermoregulation, Ineffective
Thought Processes, Altered
Tissue Integrity, Impaired
Tissue Perfusion, Altered
    (Specify Type: Renal,
    Cerebral, Cardiopulmonary,
    Gastrointestinal, Peripheral)
Transfer Ability, Impaired
Trauma, Risk for
Unilateral Neglect
Urinary Elimination, Altered
Urinary Retention
Ventilation, Inability to Sustain
    Spontaneous
Ventilatory Weaning Response,
    Dysfunctional
Violence, Risk for: Directed at
    Others
Violence, Risk for: Self-Directed
Walking, Impaired

GROUPED BY FUNCTIONAL HEALTH PATTERNS

HEALTH PERCEPTION–HEALTH MANAGEMENT PATTERN

Development, Altered: Risk for
Energy Field Disturbance
Growth, Altered: Risk for
Health Maintenance, Altered
Health-Seeking Behaviors
Infection, Risk for
Injury, Risk for
Management of Therapeutic
    Regimen, Ineffective
    (Community)
Management of Therapeutic
    Regimen, Ineffective (Family)
Management of Therapeutic
    Regimen, Ineffective
Noncompliance
Poisoning, Risk for
Protection, Altered
Suffocation, Risk for
Surgical Recovery, Delayed
Trauma, Risk for

NUTRITIONAL-METABOLIC PATTERN

Aspiration, Risk for
Breastfeeding, Effective
Breastfeeding, Ineffective
Breastfeeding, Interrupted
Dentition, Altered
Fluid Volume Deficit
Fluid Volume Deficit, Risk for
Fluid Volume Excess
Fluid Volume Imbalance, Risk for
Hyperthermia
Hypothermia
Infant Feeding Pattern, Ineffective
Latex Allergy Response
Latex Allergy Response, Risk for
Nausea
Nutrition, Altered: Less than Body
    Requirements
Nutrition, Altered: More than Body
    Requirements
Nutrition, Altered: Risk for More than
    Body Requirements
Oral Mucous Membrane, Altered
Skin Integrity, Impaired
Skin Integrity, Impaired: Risk for
Swallowing, Impaired
Temperature, Risk for Altered Body
Thermoregulation, Ineffective
Tissue Integrity, Impaired

ELIMINATION PATTERN

Constipation
Constipation, Colonic
Constipation, Perceived
Constipation, Risk for
Diarrhea
Incontinence, Bowel
Incontinence, Functional Urinary
Incontinence, Reflex Urinary
Incontinence, Stress
Incontinence, Total
Incontinence, Urge
Urinary Elimination, Altered
Urinary Retention

ACTIVITY-EXERCISE PATTERN

Activity Intolerance
Activity Intolerance, Risk for
Airway Clearance, Ineffective
Breathing Pattern, Ineffective
Cardiac Output, Decreased
Disuse Syndrome, Risk for
Diversional Activity Deficit
Dysreflexia
Dysreflexia, Risk for Autonomic
Energy Field Disturbance
Failure to Thrive
Fatigue
Gas Exchange, Impaired
Growth and Development, Altered
Home Maintenance Management,
    Impaired

Infant Behavior, Disorganized
Infant Behavior, Potential for
    Enhanced Organized
Infant Behavior, Risk for
    Disorganized
Mobility, Impaired: Bed, Physical,
    Wheelchair
Perioperative Positioning Injury, Risk
    for
Peripheral Neurovascular
    Dysfunction, Risk for
Self-Care Deficit, Bathing/Hygiene
Self-Care Deficit, Dressing/Grooming
Self-Care Deficit, Feeding
Self-Care Deficit, Toileting
Surgical Recovery, Delayed
Tissue Perfusion, Altered
Transfer Ability, Impaired
Ventilation, Inability to Sustain
Ventilatory Weaning Response,
    Dysfunctional
Walking, Impaired

SLEEP-REST PATTERN

Sleep Deprivation
Sleep Pattern Disturbance

COGNITIVE-PERCEPTUAL PATTERN

Adaptive Capacity, Decreased,
    Intracranial
Confusion, Acute
Confusion, Chronic
Decisional Conflict
Environmental Interpretation
    Syndrome, Impaired
Knowledge Deficit
Memory, Impaired
Nausea
Pain
Pain, Chronic
Sensory-Perceptual Alterations
Thought Processes, Altered
Unilateral Neglect

SELF-PERCEPTION– SELF-CONCEPT PATTERN

Anxiety
Body Image Disturbance
Death Anxiety
Fear
Hopelessness
Personal Identity Disturbance
Powerlessness
Self-Esteem, Chronic Low
Self-Esteem Disturbance
Self-Esteem, Situational Low
Self-Mutilation, Risk for

ROLE-RELATIONSHIP PATTERN

Caregiver Role Strain
Caregiver Role Strain, Risk for
Communication, Impaired Verbal

Family Processes, Altered
Grieving, Anticipatory
Grieving, Dysfunctional
Parental Role Conflict
Parenting, Altered
Parenting, Altered: Risk for
Relocation Stress Syndrome
Role Performance, Altered
Social Interaction, Impaired
Social Isolation
Violence, Risk for: Directed at Others
Violence, Risk for: Self-Directed

SEXUALITY-REPRODUCTIVE PATTERN

Rape Trauma Syndrome
Rape Trauma Syndrome: Compound Reaction

Rape Trauma Syndrome: Silent Reaction
Sexual Dysfunction
Sexuality Patterns, Altered

COPING–STRESS-TOLERANCE PATTERN

Adjustment, Impaired
Coping, Defensive
Coping, Ineffective Community
Coping, Ineffective Individual
Coping, Potential for Enhanced Community
Denial, Ineffective
Failure to Thrive, Adult
Family Coping, Ineffective: Compromised
Family Coping, Ineffective: Disabling

Family Coping: Potential for Growth
Post-Trauma Syndrome
Post-Trauma Syndrome, Risk for
Sorrow, Chronic

VALUE-BELIEF PATTERN

Spiritual Distress (Distress of Human Spirit)
Spiritual Well-Being, Potential for Enhanced

Modified from *NANDA nursing diagnosis: definitions and classification 1999-2000,* North America Nursing Diagnosis Association; and Gordon M: *Manual of nursing diagnoses,* St Louis, 1997, Mosby.

B Laboratory Values

Cecilia C. Dail, Sally Sperry Steen, and Lee Danielson

The tables in this appendix list some of the most common tests, their normal values, and possible etiologies of abnormal values. Laboratory values may vary with different techniques or different laboratories. Possible etiologies are presented in alphabetic order. Abbreviations appearing in the tables are defined as follows:

<	=	less than
>	=	greater than
L	=	liter
mEq	=	milliequivalent
ml	=	milliliter
dl	=	deciliter
mm Hg	=	millimeter of mercury
fl	=	femtoliter
mm	=	millimeter

g	=	gram
mg	=	millogram (10^{-3})
μg	=	microgram (one millionth of a gram) (10^{-6})
ng	=	nanogram (one billionth of a gram) (10^{-9})
pg	=	picogram (one trillionth of a gram) (10^{-12})
μU	=	microunit
μl	=	microliter
IU	=	international unit
mOsm	=	milliosmole
U	=	unit
mmol	=	millimole
μmol	=	micromole
nmol	=	nanomole
pmol	=	picomole
kPa	=	kilopascal
μkat	=	microkatal

Table **B-1** Serum, Plasma, and Whole Blood Chemistries

Test	Normal Values		Possible Etiology	
	Conventional Units	SI Units	Higher	Lower
Acetone			Diabetic ketoacidosis, high-fat diet, low-carbohydrate diet, starvation	
Quantitative	0.3-2.0 mg/dl	52-344 μmol/L		
Qualitative	Negative	Negative		
Albumin	3.5-5.0 g/dl	35-50 g/L	Dehydration	Chronic liver disease, malabsorption, malnutrition, nephrotic syndrome, pregnancy
Aldolase	1.0-7.5 U/L	0.02-0.13 μkat/L	Skeletal muscle disease	Renal disease
α-1-Antitrypsin	78-200 mg/dl	0.78-2.0 g/L	Acute and chronic inflammation, arthritis, stress syndrome	Chronic lung disease (early onset), malnutrition, nephrotic syndrome
α-1-Fetoprotein	<15 ng/ml	<15 μg/L	Cancer of testes and ovaries, carcinoma of liver	
Ammonia	30-70 μg/dl	17.6-41.1 μmol/L	Severe liver disease	
Amylase	0-130 U/L (method dependent)	0-2.17 μkat/L	Acute and chronic pancreatitis, mumps (salivary gland disease), perforated ulcers	Acute alcoholism, cirrhosis of liver, extensive destruction of pancreas
Ascorbic acid	0.4-1.5 mg/dl	23-85 μmol/L	Excessive ingestion of vitamin C	Connective tissue disorders, hepatic disease, renal disease, rheumatic fever, vitamin C deficiency
Bicarbonate	20-30 mEq/L	20-30 mmol/L	Compensated respiratory acidosis, metabolic alkalosis	Compensated respiratory alkalosis, metabolic acidosis
Bilirubin			Biliary obstruction, impaired liver function, hemolytic anemia, pernicious anemia, prolonged fasting	
Total	0.2-1.3 mg/dl	3.4-22.0 μmol/L		
Indirect	0.1-1.0 mg/dl	1.7-17.0 μmol/L		
Direct	0.1-0.3 mg/dl	1.7-5.1 μmol/L		
Blood gases*				
Arterial pH	7.35-7.45	Same as conventional units	Alkalosis	Acidosis
Venous pH	7.35-7.45	Same as conventional units		
Arterial PCO_2	35-45 mm Hg	4.67-6.00 kPa	Compensated metabolic alkalosis	Compensated metabolic acidosis
Venous PCO_2	42-52 mm Hg	5.60-6.93 kPa	Respiratory acidosis	Respiratory alkalosis
Arterial PO_2	75-100 mm Hg	10.0-13.33 kPa	Administration of high concentration of oxygen	Chronic lung disease, decreased cardiac output
Venous PO_2	30-50 mm Hg	4.0-6.67 kPa		
Calcium	9-11 mg/dl (4.5-5.5 mEq/L)	2.25-2.74 mmol/L	Acute osteoporosis, hyperparathyroidism, vitamin D intoxication, multiple myeloma	Acute pancreatitis, hypoparathyroidism, liver disease, malabsorption syndrome, renal failure, vitamin D deficiency

Continued

Table **B-1** Serum, Plasma, and Whole Blood Chemistries—cont'd

Test	Normal Values		Possible Etiology	
	Conventional Units	SI Units	Higher	Lower
Calcium, ionized	4-4.6 mg/dl (2-2.3 mEq/L)	1.0-1.15 mmol/L		
Carbon dioxide (CO₂ content)	20-30 mEq/L	20-30 mmol/L	Same as bicarbonate	
Carotene	10-85 µg/dl	0.19-1.58 µmol/L	Cystic fibrosis, hypothyroidism, pancreatic insufficiency	Dietary deficiency, malabsorption disorders
Chloride	95-105 mEq/L	95-105 mmol/L	Metabolic acidosis, respiratory alkalosis, corticosteroid therapy, uremia	Addison's disease, diarrhea, metabolic alkalosis, respiratory acidosis, vomiting
Cholesterol	140-200 mg/dl (age dependent)	3.6-5.2 mmol/L	Biliary obstruction, hypothyroidism, idiopathic hypercholesterolemia, renal disease, uncontrolled diabetes	Extensive liver disease, hyperthyroidism, malnutrition, corticosteroid therapy
HDL (high-density lipoproteins)				
Male	>45 mg/dl	>1.2 mmol/L		
Female	>55 mg/dl	>1.4 mmol/L		
LDL (low-density lipoproteins)	<130 mg/dl	<3.4 mmol/L		
Cholinesterase (RBC)	0.65-1.00 pH	Same as conventional units	Exercise	Acute infections, insecticide intoxication, liver disease, muscular dystrophy
Pseudocholinesterase (plasma)	5-12 U/ml	Same as conventional units		
Copper	80-150 µg/dl	12.6-23.6 µmol/L	Cirrhosis, female on contraceptives	Wilson's disease
Cortisol	8 AM: 5-25 µg/dl	0.14-0.69 µmol/L	Cushing's syndrome, pancreatitis, stress	Adrenal insufficiency, panhypopituitary states
	8 PM: <10 µg/dl	<0.28 µmol/L		
Creatine	0.2-1.0 mg/dl	15.3-76.3 µmol/L	Active rheumatoid arthritis, biliary obstruction, hyperthyroidism, renal disorders, severe muscle disease	Diabetes mellitus
Creatine kinase (CK)			Musculoskeletal injury or disease, myocardial infarction, severe myocarditis, exercise, numerous intramuscular injections, brain damage	
Male	15-105 U/L	0.26-1.79 µkat/L		
Female	10-80 U/L	0.17-1.36 µkat/L		
CK-MB (CK-2)	0-9 U/L	<0.1 µkat/L	Acute myocardial infarction	
Creatinine	0.5-1.5 mg/dl	44-133 µmol/L	Severe renal disease	
Ferritin (serum)			Siderablastic anemia, Anemia of chronic disease (infection, inflammation, liver disease)	Iron deficiency anemia
Male	20-300 ng/ml	20-300 µg/L		
Female	10-120 ng/ml	10-120 µg/L		
Folic acid (folate)	3-25 ng/ml	7-57 nmol/L	Hypothyroidism	Alcoholism, hemolytic anemia, inadequate diet, malabsorption syndrome, megaloblastic anemia
Gamma-glutamyl transpeptidase (GGT)	0-30 U/L	0-0.5 µkat/L		Liver disease, infectious mononucleosis

Continued

Table B-1 Serum, Plasma, and Whole Blood Chemistries—cont'd

Test	Normal Values		Possible Etiology	
	Conventional Units	SI Units	Higher	Lower
Glucose, fasting	70-120 mg/dl	3.89-6.66 mmol/L	Acute stress, cerebral lesions, Cushing's disease, diabetes mellitus, hyperthyroidism, pancreatic insufficiency	Addison's disease, hepatic disease, hypothyroidism, insulin overdosage, pancreatic tumor, pituitary hypofunction, postgastrectomy dumping syndrome
Glucose tolerance (GTT)			Diabetes mellitus	Hyperinsulinism
Fasting	70-120 mg/dl	3.89-6.66 mmol/L		
30 min	30-60 mg/dl above fasting	1.67-3.33 mmol/L		
60 min	20-50 mg/dl above fasting	1.11-2.78 mmol/L		
120 min	5-15 mg/dl above fasting	0.28-0.83 mmol/L		
180 min	Fasting level or lower	Fasting level or lower		
Haptoglobin	26-185 mg/dl	260-1850 mg/L	Infectious and inflammatory processes, malignant neoplasms	Hemolytic anemia, mononucleosis, toxoplasmosis, chronic liver disease
Insulin	4-24 μU/ml	29-172 pmol/L	Acromegaly, adenoma of islet cells, untreated mild case of type 2 diabetes	Diabetes mellitus, obesity
Iron, total	50-150 μg/dl	9.0-26.9 μmol/L	Excessive RBC destruction	Iron-deficiency anemia, anemia of chronic disease
Iron-binding capacity	250-410 μg/dl	45-73 μmol/L	Iron-deficient state, oral contraceptives, polycythemia	Cancer, chronic infections, pernicious anemia, uremia
Lactic acid	5-20 μg/dl	0.56-2.2 mmol/L	Acidosis, congestive heart failure, shock	
Lactic dehydrogenase (LDH)	50-150 U/L	0.83-2.5 μkat/L	Congestive heart failure, hemolytic disorders, hepatitis, metastatic cancer of liver, myocardial infarction, pernicious anemia, pulmonary embolus, skeletal muscle damage	
Lactic dehydrogenase isoenzymes				
LDH_1	20-35%	0.20-0.35	Myocardial infarction, pernicious anemia	
LDH_2	30-40%	0.30-0.40	Pulmonary embolus, sickle cell crisis	
LDH_3	15-25%	0.15-0.25	Malignant lymphoma, pulmonary embolus	
LDH_4	0-10%	0-0.10	Lupus erythematosus, pulmonary infarction	
LDH_5	4-12%	0.04-0.12	Congestive heart failure, hepatitis, pulmonary embolus and infarction, skeletal muscle damage	

Continued

Table **B-1**   Serum, Plasma, and Whole Blood Chemistries—cont'd

| Test | Normal Values | | Possible Etiology | |
	Conventional Units	SI Units	Higher	Lower
Lipase	0-160 U/L	0-2.66 μkat/L	Acute pancreatitis, hepatic disorders, perforated peptic ulcer	
Magnesium	1.5-2.5 mEq/L	0.62-1.03 mmol/L	Addison's disease, hypothyroidism, renal failure	Chronic alcoholism, hyperparathyroidism, hyperthyroidism, hypoparathyroidism, severe malabsorption
Osmolality	285-295 mOsm/kg	285-295 mmol/kg	Chronic renal disease, diabetes mellitus	Addison's disease, diuretic therapy
Oxygen saturation (arterial)	95-98%	0.95-0.98 saturated	Polycythemia	Anemia, cardiac decompensation, respiratory disorders
pH	See blood gases			
Phenylalanine	0-2 mg/dl	0-121 μmol/L	Phenylketonuria	
Phosphatase, acid	0-5.5 U/L	0-90 nkat/L	Advanced Paget's disease, cancer of prostate, hyperparathyroidism	
Phosphatase, alkaline	30-120 U/L	0.5-2.0 μkat/L	Bone diseases, marked hyperparathyroidism, obstruction of biliary system, rickets	Excessive vitamin D ingestion, hypothyroidism, milk-alkali syndrome
Phosphorus, inorganic	2.8-4.5 mg/dl	0.90-1.45 mmol/L	Healing fractures, hypoparathyroidism, renal disease, vitamin D intoxication	Diabetes mellitus, hyperparathyroidism, vitamin D deficiency
Potassium	3.5-5.5 mEq/L	3.5-5.5 mmol/L	Addison's disease, diabetic ketosis, massive tissue destruction, renal failure	Cushing's syndrome, diarrhea (severe), diuretic therapy, gastrointestinal fistula, pyloric obstruction, starvation, vomiting
Prostate-specific antigen (PSA)	<4 ng/mL	<4 μg/L	Prostate cancer	
Proteins			Burns, cirrhosis (globulin fraction), dehydration	Congenital agammaglobulinemia, liver disease, malabsorption
Total	6.0-8.0 g/dl	60-80 g/L		
Albumin	3.5-5.0 g/dl	35-50 g/L		
Globulin	2-3.5 g/dl	20-35 g/L		
Albumin/globulin ratio	1.5:1-2.5:1	Same as conventional units	Multiple myeloma (globulin fraction), shock, vomiting	Malnutrition, nephrotic syndrome, proteinuria, renal disease, severe burns
Renin			Renal hypertension, volume decrease (e.g., hemorrhage)	Increased salt intake, primary aldosteronism
Supine position	1.4-2.9 ng/ml/hr	0.39-0.81 ng/L·sec		
Upright position	0.4-4.5 ng/ml/hr	0.11-1.25 ng/L·sec		
Sodium	135-145 mEq/L	135-145 mmol/L	Dehydration, impaired renal function, primary aldosteronism, corticosteroid therapy	Addison's disease, diabetic ketoacidosis, diuretic therapy, excessive loss from gastrointestinal tract, excessive perspiration, water intoxication

Continued

Table **B-1**   Serum, Plasma, and Whole Blood Chemistries—cont'd

Test	Normal Values		Possible Etiology	
	Conventional Units	**SI Units**	**Higher**	**Lower**
Testosterone				
Male	300-1200 ng/dl	10.4-41.6 nmol/L		Hypofunction of testes
Female	25-90 ng/dl	0.87-3.1 nmol/L	Polycystic ovary, viriliz-ing tumors	
T$_4$ (thyroxine), total	5-12 µg/dl	64-154 nmol/L	Hyperthyroidism, thy-roiditis	Cretinism, hypothy-roidism, myxedema
T$_4$ (thyroxine), free	0.8-2.3 ng/dl	10-30 pmol/L		
T$_3$ uptake	25-35%	0.25-0.35	Hyperthyroidism, metastatic neoplasms	Hypothyroidism, pregnancy
T$_3$ (triiodothyronine)	110-230 ng/dl	1.7-3.5 nmol/L	Hyperthyroidism	Hypothyroidism
Thyroid-stimulating hormone (TSH)	0.3-5.4 µU/ml	0.3-5.4 mU/L	Myxedema, primary hypothyroidism, Graves' disease	Secondary hypothy-roidism
Transaminases				
Serum glutam-icoxaloacetic (SGOT) or aspartate aminotrans-ferase (AST)	7-40 U/L	0.12-0.67 µkat/L	Liver disease, myocar-dial infarction, pul-monary infarction, acute hepatitis	
Serum glutamate pyruvate (SGPT) or alanine aminotrans-ferase (ALT)	5-36 U/L	0.08-0.6 µkat/L	Liver disease, shock	
Triglycerides	40-150 mg/dl	0.45-1.69 mmol/L	Diabetes mellitus, hy-perlipidemia, hy-pothyroidism, liver disease	Malnutrition
Urea nitrogen (BUN)	10-30 mg/dl	1.8-7.1 mmol/L	Increase in protein ca-tabolism (fever, stress), renal disease, urinary tract infection	Malnutrition, severe liver damage
Uric acid			Gout, gross tissue de-struction, high-protein weight reduction diet, leukemia, renal failure, eclampsia	Administration of uri-cosuric drugs
Male	4.5-6.5 mg/dl	149-327 µmol/L		
Female	2.5-5.5 mg/dl	268-387 µmol/L		
Vitamin A	15-60 µg/dl	0.52-2.09 µmol/L	Excess ingestion of vit-amin A	Vitamin A deficiency
Vitamin B$_{12}$	200-1000 pg/ml	148-738 pmol/L	Chronic myeloid leukemia	Strict vegetarianism, malabsorption syn-drome, pernicious anemia, total or par-tial gastrectomy
Zinc	50-150 µg/dl	7.6-22.9 µmol/L		Alcoholic cirrhosis

*Because arterial blood gases are influenced by altitude, the value for PO$_2$ decreases as altitude increases. The lower value is normal for an altitude of 1 mile.
RBC, red blood cell.

Table **B-2** Hematology

Test	Normal Values		Possible Etiology	
	Conventional Units	SI Units	Higher	Lower
Bleeding time (Simplate)	3.0-9.5 min	180-570 sec	Defective platelet function, thrombocytopenia, von Willebrand's disease, aspirin ingestion, vascular disease	
Activated partial thromboplastin time (APTT)	30-45 sec*	Same as conventional units	Deficiency of factors I, II, V, VIII, IX and X, XI, XII; hemophilia, liver disease, heparin therapy	
Prothrombin time (Protime, PT)	10-14 sec*	Same as conventional units	Warfarin therapy, deficiency of factors I, II, V, VII, and X, vitamin K deficiency, liver disease	
Fibrinogen	200-400 mg/dl	2.0-4.0 g/L	Burns (after first 36 hr), inflammatory disease	Burns (during first 36 hr), DIC, severe liver disease
Fibrin split (degradation) products	<10 μg/ml	Same as conventional units	Acute DIC, massive hemorrhage, primary fibrinolysis	
D-Dimer	Negative	Negative	DIC, myocardial infarction, deep vein thrombosis, unstable angina	
Erythrocyte count[†] (altitude dependent)			Dehydration, high altitudes, polycythemia vera, severe diarrhea	Anemia, leukemia, posthemorrhage
Male	$4.5\text{-}6.0 \times 10^6/\mu L$	$4.5\text{-}6.0 \times 10^{12}/L$		
Female	$4.0\text{-}5.0 \times 10^6/\mu L$	$4.0\text{-}5.0 \times 10^{12}/L$		
Mean corpuscular volume (MCV)	82-98 fl	Same as conventional units	Macrocytic anemia	Microcytic anemia
Mean corpuscular hemoglobin (MCH)	27-33 pg	Same as conventional units	Macrocytic anemia	Microcytic anemia
Mean corpuscular hemoglobin concentration (MCHC)	32-36%	0.32-0.36	Spherocytosis	Hypochromic anemia
Erythrocyte sedimentation rate (ESR), Westergren			Moderate increase: acute hepatitis, myocardial infarction; rheumatoid arthritis; marked increase: acute and severe bacterial infections, malignancies, pelvic inflammatory disease	Malaria Severe liver disease Sickle cell anemia
Male <50 yr	<15 mm/hr	Same as conventional units		
>50 yr	<20 mm/hr	units		
Female <50 yr	<20 mm/hr	Same as conventional units		
>50 yr	<30 mm/hr	units		

Continued

Table **B-2** Hematology—cont'd

Test	Normal Values		Possible Etiology	
	Conventional Units	SI Units	Higher	Lower
Hematocrit (altitude dependent)[†]			Dehydration, high altitudes, polycythemia	Anemia, hemorrhage, overhydration
Male	40-54%	0.40-0.54		
Female	38-47%	0.38-0.47		
Hemoglobin (altitude dependent)[†]			COPD, high altitudes, polycythemia	Anemia, hemorrhage
Male	13.5-18.0 g/dl	135-180 g/L		
Female	12.0-16.0 g/dl	120-160 g/L		
Hemoglobin, glycosylated	4.0-6.0%	Same as conventional units	Poorly controlled diabetes mellitus	Sickle cell Chronic renal failure Pregnancy
Red cell distribution width (RDW)	10.2-14.5%	Same as conventional therapy		Anisocytosis, macrocytic anemia, microcytic anemia
Platelet count (thrombocytes)	150-400 × 10³/µl	150-400 × 10⁹/L	Acute infections, chronic granulocytic leukemia, chronic pancreatitis, cirrhosis, collagen disorders, polycythemia, postsplenectomy	Acute leukemia, DIC, thrombocytopenic purpura
Reticulocyte count (manual)	0.5-1.5% of RBC	Same	Hemolytic anemia, polycythemia vera	Hypoproliferative anemia, macrocytic anemia, microcytic anemia
White blood cell count[†]	4.0-11.0 × 10³/µl	4.0-11.0 × 10⁹/L	Inflammatory and infectious processes, leukemia	Aplastic anemia, side effects of chemotherapy and irradiation
WBC differential				
Segmented neutrophils	50-70%	0.50-0.70	Bacterial infections, collagen diseases, Hodgkin's disease	Aplastic anemia, viral infections
Band neutrophils	0-8%	0-0.08	Acute infections	
Lymphocytes	20-40%	0.20-0.40	Chronic infections, lymphocytic leukemia, mononucleosis, viral infections	Corticosteroid therapy, whole body irradiation
Monocytes	4-8%	0.04-0.08	Chronic inflammatory disorders, malaria, monocytic leukemia, acute infections, Hodgkin's disease	
Eosinophils	0-4%	0-0.04	Allergic reactions, eosinophilic and chronic granulocytic leukemia, parasitic disorders, Hodgkin's disease	Corticosteroid therapy
Basophils	0-2%	0-0.02	Hyperthyroidism, ulcerative colitis, myeloproliferative diseases	Hyperthyroidism, stress
Sickle cell solubility test	Negative	Negative	Sickle cell anemia	

*Values depend on reagent and instrumentation used.
[†]Components of complete blood count (CBC).
COPD, chronic obstructive pulmonary disease; *DIC*, disseminated intravascular coagulation; *WBC*, white blood cell.

Table B-3 Serology-Immunology

Test	Normal Values		Possible Etiology	
	Conventional Units	SI Units	Higher	Lower
Antinuclear anti-body (ANA)	Negative or titer <1:10	Same as conventional units	Chronic hepatitis, rheumatoid arthritis, scleroderma, systemic lupus erythematosus	
Anti-DNA antibody	Negative or titer <1:10 or <20% binding	Same as conventional units	Systemic lupus erythematosus	
Anti-RNP	Negative	Negative	Mixed connective tissue disease, rheumatoid arthritis, systemic lupus erythematosus, Sjögren's syndrome, scleroderma	
Anti-Sm (Smith)	Negative	Negative	Systemic lupus erythematosus	
Antistreptolysin-O (ASO)	≤166 Todd units or ≤1:85	Same as conventional units	Acute glomerulonephritis, rheumatic fever, streptococcal infection	
C-reactive protein (CRP)	Negative or ≤1.2 mg/dl	Same as conventional units	Acute infections, any inflammatory condition, widespread malignancy	
Carcinoembryonic antigen (CEA)	≤2.5 ng/ml	≤2.5 µg/L	Carcinoma of colon, liver, pancreas; chronic cigarette smoking; inflammatory bowel disease; other cancers	
Complement components				
C1q	11-21 mg/dl	0.11-0.21 g/L		Acute glomerulonephritis, systemic lupus erythematosus, rheumatoid arthritis, subacute bacterial endocarditis, serum sickness
C3	80-180 mg/dl	0.8-1.8 g/L		
C4	15-50 mg/dl	0.15-0.5 g/L		
Direct antihuman globulin test (DAT) or direct Coombs	Negative	Negative	Acquired hemolytic anemia, hemolytic disease of the newborn, drug reactions, transfusion reactions	
Fluorescent treponemal antibody absorption (FTAAbs)	Nonreactive	Negative	Syphilis	

Continued

Table B-3 Serology-Immunology—cont'd

Test	Normal Values		Possible Etiology	
	Conventional Units	SI Units	Higher	Lower
Hepatitis A antibody	Negative	Negative	Hepatitis A	
Hepatitis B surface antigen (HB$_s$Ag)	Negative	Negative	Hepatitis B	
Hepatitis C antibody Immunoglobulin	Negative	Negative	Hepatitis C	
IgA	90-400 mg/dl	0.9-4.0 g/L	IgA myeloma, chronic liver disease, chronic infection, rheumatoid arthritis, autoimmune disorders	Burns, hereditary telangiectasia, malabsorption syndromes
IgD	0.5-12 mg/dl	5-120 mg/L	Chronic infection, connective tissue disease	
IgE	<1 mg/dl	<10 mg/L	Anaphylactic shock, atopic disease (allergies), parasite infections	
IgG	650-1800 mg/dl	6.5-18.0 g/L	Infections—acute and chronic, hepatitis, IgG monoclonal gammopathy, systemic lupus erythematosus	Congenital deficiencies, acquired deficiencies, nephrotic syndromes, burns, immunosuppression
IgM	55-300 mg/dl	0.5-3.0 g/L	Acute infections, rheumatoid arthritis, liver disease	Congenital and acquired antibody deficiencies, lymphocytic leukemia, protein-losing enteropathies
Monospot or monotest	Negative	Negative	Infectious mononucleosis	
Rheumatoid factor (RA factor)	Negative or titer <1:20	Same as conventional units	Rheumatoid arthritis, Sjögren's syndrome, systemic lupus erythematosus	
RPR	Nonreactive	Same as conventional units	Syphilis, systemic lupus erythematosus, rheumatoid arthritis, leprosy, malaria, febrile diseases, IV drug abuse	
VDRL	Nonreactive	Same as conventional units	Syphilis	
Thyroid antibodies	≤1:10 titer	Same as conventional units	Hashimoto's thyroiditis, thyroid carcinoma, early hypothyroidism, pernicious anemia, systemic lupus erythematosus, Graves' disease	

CSF, colony-stimulating factor; *RNP,* ribonuclear protein; *RPR,* rapid plasma reagin test; *VDRL,* Venereal Disease Research Laboratory test.

Table **B-4** Urine Chemistry

Test	Specimen	Normal Values		Possible Etiology	
		Conventional Units	SI Units	Higher	Lower
Acetone	Random	Negative	Negative	Diabetes mellitus, high-fat and low-carbohydrate diets, starvation states	
Aldosterone	24 hr	1-80 μg/day (depends on urinary sodium)	2.7-222 nmol/day	Primary aldosteronism: adrenocortical tumors; secondary aldosteronism: cardiac failure, cirrhosis, large dose of ACTH, salt depletion	ACTH deficiency, Addison's disease, corticosteroid therapy
Amylase	24 hr	1-17 U/hr	Same as conventional units	Acute pancreatitis	
Bence Jones protein	Random	Negative	Negative	Multiple myeloma, biliary duct obstruction	
Bilirubin	Random	Negative	Negative	Hepatitis	
Calcium	24 hr	100-250 mg/day	2.5-6.3 mmol/day	Bone tumor, hyperparathyroidism, milk-alkali syndrome	Hypoparathyroidism, malabsorption of calcium and vitamin D
Catecholamines	24 hr			Pheochromocytoma, progressive muscular dystrophy, heart failure	
Epinephrine		<20 μg/day	<118 nmol/day		
Norepinephrine		<100 μg/day	<591 nmol/day		
Chloride	24 hr	110-250 mEq/day	110-250 mmol/day	Addison's disease	Burns, excess perspiration, vomiting, diarrhea, menstruation
Copper	24 hr	<30 μg/day	<0.5 μmol/day	Cirrhosis, Wilson's disease	
Coproporphyrin	24 hr	50-200 μg/day	76-305 nmol/day	Lead poisoning, oral contraceptive use, poliomyelitis	
Creatine	24 hr	<100 mg/day	<763 μmol/day	Carcinoma of liver, hyperthyroidism, diabetes, Addison's disease, infections, burns, muscular dystrophy, skeletal muscle atrophy	Hypothyroidism
Creatinine	24 hr	0.8-2.0 g/day	7.1-17.7 mmol/day	Anemia, leukemia, muscular atrophy, salmonellae	Renal disease
Creatinine clearance	24 hr	85-135 ml/min	1.42-2.25 ml/sec		Renal disease
Estrogens	24 hr				
Female				Gonadal or adrenal tumor	Agenesis of ovaries, endocrine disturbance, ovarian dysfunction, menopause
Ovulation peak		28-100 μg/day	104-370 nmol/day		
Luteal peak		22-80 μg/day	81-296 nmol/day		
Pregnancy		Up to 45,000 μg/day	Up to 166,455 nmol/day		
Menopause		1.4-19.6 μg/day	5.2-72.5 nmol/day		
Male		5-18 μg/day	18-67 nmol/day		
Glucose	Random	Negative	Negative	Diabetes mellitus, low renal threshold for glucose resorption, physiologic stress, pituitary disorders	

Continued

Table B-4 Urine Chemistry—cont'd

Test	Specimen	Normal Values Conventional Units	Normal Values SI Units	Possible Etiology Higher	Possible Etiology Lower
Hemoglobin	Random	Negative	Negative	Extensive burns, glomerulonephritis, hemolytic anemias, hemolytic transfusion reaction	
5-Hydroxyindolea-cetic acid (5-HIAA)	24 hr	2-9 mg/day	10.5-47.1 μmol/day	Malignant carcinoid syndrome	
Ketone bodies	24 hr	20-50 mg/day	0.34-0.86 mmol/day	Marked ketonuria	
Lead	24 hr	<100 μg/day	<0.48 μmol/day	Lead poisoning	
Metanephrine	24 hr	<1.3 mg/day	<7.1 μmol/day	Pheochromocytoma	
Myoglobin	Random	Negative	Negative	Crushing injuries, electric injuries, extreme physical exertion	
pH	Random	4.0-8.0	Same as conventional units	Chronic renal failure, compensatory phase of alkalosis, salicylate intoxication, vegetarian diet	Compensatory phase of acidosis, dehydration, emphysema
Phenylpyruvic acid	Random	Negative	Negative	Phenylketonuria	
Phosphorus, inorganic	24 hr	0.9-1.3 g/day	29-42 mmol/day	Fever, hypoparathyroidism, nervous exhaustion, rickets, tuberculosis	Acute infections, nephritis
Porphobilinogen	Random 24 hr	Negative <2.0 mg/day	Negative <9 μmol/day	Acute intermittent porphyria, liver disorders	
Protein (dipstick)	Random	Negative	Negative	Congestive heart failure, nephritis, nephrosis, physiologic stress	
Protein (quantitative)	24 hr	<150 mg/day	<0.15 g/day	Cardiac failure, inflammatory processes of urinary tract, nephritis, nephrosis, toxemia of pregnancy	
Sodium	24 hr	40-250 mEq/day	40-250 mmol/day	Acute tubular necrosis	Hyponatremia
Specific gravity	Random	1.003-1.030	Same as conventional units	Albuminuria, dehydration, glycosuria	Diabetes insipidus
Titratable acidity	24 hr	20-50 mEq/day	Same as conventional units	Metabolic acidosis	Metabolic alkalosis
Uric acid	24 hr	250-750 mg/day	1.5-4.5 mmol/day	Gout, leukemia	Nephritis
Urobilinogen	24 hr	0.5-4.0 EU/day	Same as conventional units	Hemolytic disease, hepatic parenchymal cell damage, liver disease	Complete obstruction of bile duct
	Random	<1.0 Erhlich unit	Same as conventional units		
Uroporphyrins	Random	Random	Same as conventional units	Porphyria	
Vanillylmandelic acid	24 hr	1-8 mg/day 1.5-7 μg/mg creatine	5-40 μmol/day	Pheochromocytoma	

ACTH, adrenocorticotropic hormone; *EU,* Ehrlich unit.

Table B-5 Gastric Analysis

| Test | Normal Values | | Possible Etiology | |
	Conventional Units	SI Units	Higher	Lower
Basal				
Free hydrochloric acid	0.30 mEq/L	Same as conventional units	Hypermotility of stomach	Pernicious anemia
Total acidity	15-45 mEq/L	Same as conventional units	Gastric and duodenal ulcers, Zollinger-Ellison syndrome	Gastric carcinoma, severe gastritis
Poststimulation				
Free hydrochloric acid	10-130 mEq/L	Same as conventional units		
Total acidity	20-150 mEq/L	Same as conventional units		

Table B-6 Fecal Analysis

| Test | Normal Values | | Possible Etiology | |
	Conventional Units	SI Units	Higher	Lower
Fecal fat	<6 g/24 hr	Same as conventional units	Chronic pancreatic disease, obstruction of common bile duct, malabsorption syndrome	
Urobilinogen	30-220 mg/100 g of stool	51-372 μmol/100 g of stool	Hemolytic anemias	Complete biliary obstruction
Mucus	Negative	Negative	Mucous colitis, spastic constipation	
Pus	Negative	Negative	Chronic bacillary dysentery, chronic ulcerative colitis, localized abscesses	
Blood*	Negative	Negative	Anal fissures, hemorrhoids, malignant tumor, peptic ulcer, inflammatory bowel disease	
Color				
Brown			Various color depending on diet	
Clay			Biliary obstruction or presence of barium sulfate	
Tarry			More than 100 ml of blood in gastrointestinal tract	
Red			Blood in large intestine	
Black			Blood in upper gastrointestinal tract or iron medication	

*Ingestion of meat may produce false-positive results. Patient may be placed on a meat-free diet for 3 days before the test.

Table **B-7** Cereobrospinal Fluid Analysis

Test	Normal Values		Possible Etiology	
	Conventional Units	SI Units	Higher	Lower
Pressure	60-150 mm H_2O	Same as conventional units	Hemorrhage, intracranial tumor, meningitis	Head injury, spinal tumor, subdural hematoma
Blood	Negative	Negative	Intracranial hemorrhage	
Cell count (age dependent)				
WBC	0-5 cells/μl	0.5×10^6/L	Inflammation or infections of CNS	
RBC	0	0×10^6/L		
Chloride	100-130 mEq/L	100-130 mmol/L	Uremia	Bacterial infections of CNS (meningitis, encephalitis)
Glucose	40-75 mg/dl	2.5-4.2 mmol/L	Diabetes mellitus, viral infections of CNS	Bacterial infections and tuberculosis of CNS
Protein				
Lumbar	15-45 mg/dl	0.15-0.45 g/L	Guillain-Barré syndrome, poliomyelitis, traumatic tap	
Cisternal	15-25 mg/dl	0.15-0.25 g/L	Syphilis of CNS	
Ventricular	5-15 mg/dl	0.05-0.15 g/L	Acute meningitis, brain tumor, chronic CNS infections, multiple sclerosis	

CNS, central nervous system.

Table B-8   Toxicology of Common Drugs

Drug	Therapeutic Level		Toxic Level	
	Conventional Units	SI Units	Conventional Units	SI Units
Acetaminophen (Tylenol)	0.2-0.6 mg/dl	13-40 μmol/L	>5 mg/dl	>330 μmol/L
Barbiturates				
Short acting	1-2 mg/dl	Dependent on composition of mixture	>5 mg/dl	
Intermediate acting	1-5 mg/dl		>10 mg/dl	
Long acting	15-35 mg/dl		>40 mg/dl	
Carbon monoxide (carboxyhemoglobin)				
Normal values	<5% saturation of hemoglobin	<0.05	Symptoms with >20% saturation	>0.20
Urban nonsmokers	<5% saturation of hemoglobin	<0.05		
Rural nonsmokers	0.5-2% saturation of hemoglobin	0.005-0.02		
Smokers	5-9% saturation of hemoglobin	0.05-0.09		
Heavy smokers	>9% saturation of hemoglobin	>0.09		
Chlordiazepoxide (Librium)	0.05-5.0 mg/L	2-17 μmol/L	>10 mg/L	>33 μmol/L
Chlorpromazine (Thorazine)	0.5 μg/ml	1.6 μmol/L	>2.0 μg/ml	>6.3 μmol/L
Diazepam (Valium)	0.10-0.25 mg/L	0.35-0.88 μmol/L	>1.0 mg/L ≥2.0 mg/L (lethal)	>3.5 μmol/L
Digitalis preparations				
Digoxin	0.8-2.4 ng/ml	1.0-3.1 nmol/L	>2.5 ng/ml	>2.6 nmol/L
Digitoxin	14-30 ng/ml	18-39 nmol/L	>30 ng/ml	>39 nmol/L
Dilantin	10-20 mg/L	40-80 μmol/L	>30 mg/L	>120 μmol/L
Gentamicin (Garamycin)				
Peak	4-10 mg/L	9-22 μmol/L	>10 mg/L	>22 μmol/L
Trough	<2 mg/L	<4 mmol/L	>2 mg/L	>4 μmol/L
Propranolol (Inderal)	50-100 ng/ml	192-386 nmol/L	>200 ng/ml	>771 nmol/L
Salicylates	10-20 mg/dl	0.724-1.45 mmol/L	>20 mg/dl	>1.45 mmol/L
Alcohol (ethanol)*			>60 mg/dl (lethal)	>4.34 mmol/L

*See Table 10-10.

C Answer Key to Review Questions

Chapter 1
1. d
2. c
3. d
4. c
5. b
6. c
7. b
8. b

Chapter 2
1. d
2. d
3. b
4. a

Chapter 3
1. d
2. d
3. b
4. d
5. a
6. c

Chapter 4
1. a
2. a
3. c
4. b
5. d
6. b
7. c
8. c
9. a
10 b
11. a
12. c

Chapter 5
1. d
2. c
3. a
4. b
5. c
6. b

Chapter 6
1. c
2. b
3. c
4. d
5. e
6. c
7. b
8. a

Chapter 7
1. b
2. a
3. a
4. c
5. d
6. d
7. a
8. d

Chapter 8
1. b
2. c
3. a
4. a
5. c
6. c
7. c
8. d
9. b

Chapter 9
1. b
2. c
3. c
4. c
5. b
6. b
7. c
8. b
9. d

Chapter 10
1. a
2. d
3. c

4. b
5. b
6. b
7. d
8. c
9. c
10. d
11. b
12. b

Chapter 11
1. b
2. a
3. b
4. d
5. b
6. b
7. d
8. c
9. d

Chapter 12
1. b
2. b
3. c
4. a
5. d
6. a
7. d
8. b
9. c
10. d
11. a
12. a

Chapter 13
1. a
2. b
3. d
4. a
5. c
6. d
7. c
8. a
9. c

Chapter 14
1. b
2. d
3. d
4. a
5. d
6. b
7. c
8. b
9. c
10. d
11. b
12. c
13. c
14. d
15. d
16. a

Chapter 15
1. c
2. a
3a. d
3b. b
3c. c
3d. c
3e. a
3f. b
3g. c
4. a

Chapter 16
1. d
2. c
3. c
4. a
5. b
6. c
7. a
8. d

Chapter 17
1. c
2. c
3. c
4. a
5. d

6. d
7. c
8. b
9. c

Chapter 18
1. d
2. b
3. d
4. a
5. c
6. a

Chapter 19
1. c
2. d
3. c
4. a
5. c
6. d
7. a

Chapter 20
1. b
2. d
3. c
4. c
5. d
6. b
7. a
8. a
9. a
10. b
11. b

Chapter 21
1. c
2. a
3. c
4. a
5. d
6. a
7. c
8. a
9. a

Chapter 22
1. b
2. a
3. d
4. a
5. d
6. d
7. c
8. b
9. d
10. a
11. c

Chapter 23
1. c
2. a

3. c
4. d
5. c
6. c
7. b
8. a
9. b
10. b
11. b

Chapter 24
1. a
2. c
3. a
4. b
5. b
6. c
7. c
8. a
9. d
10. a
11. d

Chapter 25
1. a
2. b
3. a
4. c
5. b
6. d
7. a
8. d

Chapter 26
1. a
2. d
3. c
4. a
5. c
6. d
7. c
8. d
9. c
10. a
11. c
12. d
13. c
14. b

Chapter 27
1. a
2. a
3. b
4. d
5. c
6. c
7. d

Chapter 28
1. b
2. c
3. b

4. a
5. a
6. c
7. a
8. b

Chapter 29
1. a
2. b
3. d
4. c
5. c
6. a
7. a
8. c
9. c
10. d
11. d
12. c
13. c
14. a
15. c
16. d
17. d

Chapter 30
1. c
2. c
3. d
4. d
5. b
6. d
7. a
8. b
9. c
10. a
11. b

Chapter 31
1. d
2. b
3. d
4. b
5. d
6. d
7. a
8. b

Chapter 32
1. c
2. a
3. a
4. b
5. c
6. c
7. c
8. b
9. c

Chapter 33
1. b
2. b

3. a
4. a
5. b
6. b
7. a

Chapter 34
1. d
2. b
3. d
4. a
5. a
6. c
7. b
8. d

Chapter 35
1. a
2. b
3. a
4. a
5. c
6. c
7. b
8. c
9. c
10. b

Chapter 36
1. a
2. c
3. c
4. c
5. b
6. a
7. c
8. b
9. a
10. d
11. d
12. c

Chapter 37
1. d
2. b
3. b
4. a
5. c
6. c
7. b
8. a
9. b

Chapter 38
1. c
2. d
3. a
4. c
5. b
6. a
7. d
8. d

Chapter 39
1. a
2. d
3. a
4. c
5. d
6. c
7. c
8. c
9. b
10. c
11. a
12. d
13. a
14. d
15. b

Chapter 40
1. d
2. a
3. c
4. b
5. b
6. d
7. c
8. d
9. a
10. a
11. a
12. b
13. b
14. c
15. a
16. c

Chapter 41
1. d
2. b
3. b
4. b
5. d
6. a
7. d
8. d
9. c
10. c
11. b

Chapter 42
1. d
2. b
3. d
4. b
5. a
6. a
7. b
8. d

Chapter 43
1. d
2. a

3. b
4. a
5. d
6. a
7. d
8. d
9. b
10. a
11. b
12. d

Chapter 44
1. b
2. a
3. c
4. c
5. d
6. c
7. d
8. c
9. a
10. d
11. b

Chapter 45
1. b
2. c
3. a
4. d
5. a
6. c
7. d
8. c
9. a

Chapter 46
1. b
2. d
3. c
4. c
5. d
6. d
7. c

Chapter 47
1. b
2. b
3. c
4. a
5. d
6. d
7. d
8. a
9. c

Chapter 48
1. c
2. c
3. d
4. b
5. d

6. b
7. a
8. b

Chapter 49
1. d
2. d
3. c
4. a
5. c
6. c
7. d
8. b

Chapter 50
1. c
2. a
3. c
4. d
5. d
6. c
7. a

Chapter 51
1. d
2. b
3. c
4. d
5. d
6. c
7. a
8. c
9. d
10. c
11. b
12. b
13. c
14. a
15. d

Chapter 52
1. b
2. d
3. b
4. a
5. c
6. b
7. c

Chapter 53
1. c
2. a
3. d
4. c
5. d
6. c
7. d
8. a
9. c
10. a
11. b

Chapter 54
1. c
2. d
3. c
4. d
5. b
6. b
7. b
8. c
9. a
10. a
11. c
12. d
13. a
14. b

Chapter 55
1. d
2. c
3. d
4. a
5. d
6. c
7. b
8. c
9. b

Chapter 56
1. c
2. a
3. b
4. c
5. a
6. d
7. d

Chapter 57
1. c
2. d
3. c
4. c
5. c
6. b
7. c
8. b

Chapter 58
1. c
2. b
3. d
4. d
5. c
6. d
7. c
8. d
9. a

Chapter 59
1. d
2. b
3. d
4. c
5. d
6. b
7. b
8. a
9. d
10. a
11. d
12. c
13. a
14. b

Chapter 60
1. a
2. a
3. c
4. c
5. c
6. d
7. b
8. c
9. b
10. d

Chapter 61
1. c
2. a

3. b
4. a
5. a
6. d

Chapter 62
1. b
2. a
3. d
4. a
5. c

Chapter 63
1. d
2. b

3. b
4. c
5. c
6. b
7. a
8. a
9. b
10. c
11. b
12. c

Chapter 64
1. d
2. a
3. c

ILLUSTRATION CREDITS

Chapter 37

37-1, 37-3, From Thibodeau GA, Patton KT: *Anatomy and physiology,* ed 4, St Louis, 1999, Mosby; 37-9, from Doughty DB, Jackson DB: *Gastrointestinal disorders,* St Louis, 1993, Mosby.

Chapter 38

38-1, From *Human nutrition information service: making health food choices,* Washington, DC, 1993, USDA; 38-2, redrawn from Mahan LK, Arlin M: *Krause's food, nutrition, and diet therapy,* ed 4, 1992, Saunders; 38-7, copyright 1978 by George A. Bray, MD; 38-8, from Fortunato N, McCullough S: *Plastic and reconstructive surgery,* St Louis, 1998, Mosby.

Chapter 39

39-1, From Thibodeau GA, Patton KT: *Anatomy and physiology,* ed 4, St Louis, 1999, Mosby; 39-3, from Murray PR and others: *Medical microbiology,* ed 2, St Louis, 1994, Mosby; 39-4, courtesy RA Weinstein, Denver, CO; 39-6, 39-10, 39-12, 39-17, redrawn from Price SA, Wilson LM: *Pathophysiology: clinical concepts of disease processes,* ed 5, St Louis, 1997, Mosby; 39-8, from Doughty DB, Jackson DB: *Gastrointestinal disorders,* St Louis, 1993, Mosby; 39-13, from McCance KL, Huether SE: *Pathophysiology: the biologic basis for disease in adults and children,* ed 3, St Louis, 1998, Mosby; 39-14, from Damjanov I, Linder J, editors: *Anderson's pathology,* ed 10, St Louis, 1996, Mosby. In McCance KL, Huether SE: *Pathophysiology: the biologic basis for disease in adults and children,* ed 3, St Louis, 1998, Mosby; 39-17, redrawn from Price SA, Wilson LM: *Pathophysiology: clinical concepts of disease processes,* ed 5, St. Louis, Mosby.

Chapter 40

40-2, From Damjanov I, Linder J, editors: *Anderson's pathology,* ed 10, St Louis, 1996, Mosby; 40-5, 40-15, from Stevens A, Lowe J: *Pathology,* London, 1995, Mosby; 40-8, from McCance KL, Huether SE: *Pathophysiology: the biologic basis for disease in adults and children,* ed 3, St Louis, 1998, Mosby. Courtesy David Bjorkman, MD, University of Utah School of Medicine, Department of Gastroenterology; 40-10, from McCance KL, Huether SE: *Pathophysiology: the biologic basis for disease in adults and children,* ed 3, St Louis, 1998, Mosby; 40-12, redrawn from Meeker MH, Rothrock JC: *Alexander's care of the patient in surgery,* ed 9, St Louis, 1991, Mosby; 40-13, redrawn from Hampton BG, Bryant RA: *Ostomies and continent diversions,* St Louis, 1992, Mosby.

Chapter 41

41-1, From Kamal A, Brockelhurst JC: *Color atlas of geriatric medicine,* ed 3, St Louis, 1991, Mosby–Year Book–Europe; 41-4, from Damjanov I, Linder J, editors: *Anderson's pathology,* ed 10, St Louis, 1996, Mosby; 41-6, adapted from Doughty DB, Jackson DB: *Gastrointestinal disorders,* St Louis, 1993, Mosby; 41-11, 41-13, 41-15, from Stevens A, Lowe J: *Pathology,* London, 1995, Mosby.

Chapter 42

42-7, From Brundage DJ: *Renal disorders,* St Louis, 1992, Mosby; 42-8, from Price S, Wilson L: *Pathophysiology: clinical concepts of disease processes,* ed 5, St Louis, 1997, Mosby; 42-10, courtesy Circon Corporation, Santa Barbara, Calif.

Chapter 43

43-3, 43-5, Courtesy Harborview Medical Center, University of Washington, Seattle; 43-6, From Brundage DJ: *Renal disorders,* St Louis, 1992, Mosby; 43-9, 43-11, 43-12, courtesy Lynda Brubacher, Virginia Mason Hospital, Seattle.

Chapter 44

44-2, From United States Data System, Washington, DC, 1998, Dept of Health and Human Services; 44-7, 44-8, 44-9, 44-10, copyright 1994 Baxter Healthcare Corp; 44-12A, courtesy Quinton Instrument Co, Seattle; 44-14, modified from Thelan L, Davie JK, Urden JD: *Textbook of critical care nursing: diagnosis and management,* ed 3, St Louis, 1998, Mosby; 44-15, copyright Baxter Healthcare Corporation.

Chapter 45

45-1, 45-3, 45-4, From Thibodeau GA, Patton KT: *Anatomy and physiology,* ed 4, St Louis, 1999, Mosby; 45-6, from McCance KL, Huether SE: *Pathophysiology: the biologic basis for disease in adults and children,* ed 3, St Louis, 1998, Mosby; 45-9, from Seeley R, Stephens T, Tate P: *Anatomy and physiology,* ed 3, New York, 1995, McGraw-Hill, Carlyn Iverson, artist; 45-10, from Thompson JM, Wilson SF: *Health assessment for nursing practice,* St Louis, 1996, Mosby.

Chapter 46

46-3, From *Diabetes mellitus,* Indianapolis, Eli Lilly, Inc; 46-4, 46-5, from American Diabetes Association: *Maximizing the role of nutrition in diabetes management,* Alexandria, Va, American Diabetes Association, 1994; 46-10, 46-12, redrawn from McCance KL, Huether SE: *Pathophysiology: the biologic basis for disease in adults and children,* ed 3, St Louis, 1998, Mosby; 46-13, from Thelan L, Davie JK, Urden JD: *Textbook of critical care nursing: diagnosis and management,* ed 3, St Louis, 1998, Mosby.

Chapter 47

47-1, Courtesy Linda Haas, Seattle; 47-3, redrawn from Thelan L, Davie JK, Urden JD: *Textbook of critical care nursing: diagnosis and management,* ed 2, St Louis, 1994, Mosby; 47-4, 47-5, redrawn from Thelan L, Davie JK, Urden JD: *Textbook of critical care nursing: diagnosis and management,* ed 3, St Louis, 1998, Mosby; 47-6, redrawn from Seidel HM and others: *Mosby's guide to physical examination,* ed 4, St Louis, 1999, Mosby; 47-7, from Besser GM, Cudworth AG: *Clinical endocrinology: an illustrated text,* London, 1987, Gower Medical Publishing; 47-8, from Williams GH, Dluhy RG: *Diseases of the adrenal cortex.* In Isselbacher K and others, editors: *Harrison's principles of internal medicine,* ed 14, St Louis, 1998, Mosby.

Chapter 48

48-1, 48-5, From Seeley R, Stephens T, Tate P: *Anatomy and physiology*, ed 2, New York, 1992, McGraw-Hill; 48-3, 48-6, from Thibodeau GA, Patton KT: *Anatomy and physiology*, ed 4, St Louis, 1999, Mosby; 48-8, from Seeley R, Stephens T, Tate P: *Anatomy and physiology*, ed 3, New York, 1995, McGraw-Hill.

Chapter 49

49-2, From Powell DE, Stelling CB: *The diagnosis and detection of breast disease*, St Louis, 1993, Mosby; 49-5, from Fortunato N, McCullough SM: *Plastic and reconstructive surgery*, St Louis, 1998, Mosby. Courtesy Brian W. Davies, MD; 49-6, modified from Beare PG, Myers JL: *Adult health nursing*, ed 3, St Louis, 1998, Mosby, and Fortunato N, McCullough SM: *Plastic and reconstructive surgery*, St Louis, 1998, Mosby.

Chapter 50

50-4, 50-5, Courtesy USPHS, Washington, DC; 50-6, 50-7, reproduced with permission of Glaxo Wellcome, Inc, Research Triangle Park, NC.

Chapter 51

51-1, From Gowan ADT, Hodge C, Callender R: *Gynecology illustrated*, ed 3, New York, 1985, Churchill Livingstone; 51-4, from Bobak I, Jensen M, Zalar M: *Maternity and gynecologic care*, ed 5, St Louis, 1993, Mosby; 51-6, from Mishell DR and others: *Comprehensive gynecology*, ed 3, St Louis, 1997, Mosby; 51-7, redrawn from Novak ER, Woodruff JD, editors: *Novak's gynecologic and obstetric pathology*, ed 6, Philadelphia, 1967, Saunders. In McCance KL, Huether SE: *Pathophysiology: the biologic basis for disease in adults and children*, ed 3, St Louis, 1998, Mosby; 51-8, 51-12, redrawn from Seidel HM and others: *Mosby's guide to physical examination*, ed 4, St Louis, 1999, Mosby; 51-9, from Phipps WJ, Sands JK, Marek JF: *Medical-surgical nursing: concepts and clinical practice*, ed 6, St Louis, 1999, Mosby; 51-11, from Seidel HM and others: *Mosby's guide to physical examination*, ed 3, St Louis, 1995, Mosby.

Chapter 52

52-5, From Seidel HM and others: *Mosby's guide to physical examination*, ed 4, St Louis, 1999, Mosby, modified from Burroughs-Wellcome Co, 1989; 52-7, courtesy of *Mayo Clinic Health Letter* with permission from Mayo Foundation for Medical Education and Research, Rochester.

Chapter 53

53-1, 53-4, 53-5, 53-10, 53-11, 53-14, 53-15, 53-20, From Thibodeau GA, Patton KT: *Anatomy and physiology*, ed 4, St Louis, 1999, Mosby; 53-6, 53-13, from Seeley R, Stephens T, Tate P: *Anatomy and physiology*, ed 3, New York, 1995, McGraw-Hill; 53-12, from McCance KL, Huether SE: *Pathophysiology: the biologic basis for disease in adults and children*, ed 3, St Louis, 1998, Mosby; 53-19A, from Elkin MK, Perry AG, Potter PA: *Nursing interventions and clinical skills*, ed 2, St Louis, 1999, Mosby; 53-19B, from Chipps E, Clanin N, Campbell V: *Neurologic disorders*, St Louis, 1992, Mosby.

Chapter 54

54-1, From Wong J, Wong S, Dempster JK: Care of the unconscious patient: a problem-oriented approach, *Am Assoc Neurosci Nurses* 16:145, 1984; 54-5, redrawn from McCance KL, Huether SE: *Pathophysiology: the biologic basis for disease in adults and children*, ed 3, St Louis, 1998, Mosby; 54-7, from Thelan LA and others: *Textbook of critical care nursing: diagnosis and management*, ed 2, St Louis, 1994, Mosby; 54-8, redrawn from Kinney MR and others, editors: *AACN's clinical reference for critical care nursing*, St Louis, 1993, Mosby; 54-11, redrawn from Barker E: *Neuroscience nursing*, St Louis, 1994, Mosby; 54-12, from Bingham BJG, Hawke M, Kwok P: *Clinical atlas of otolaryngology*, St Louis, 1992, Mosby; 54-13, from Price SA, Wilson LM: *Pathophysiology: clinical concepts of disease processes*, ed 5, St Louis, 1997, Mosby; 54-14, from Okazaki H, Scheithauer BW: *Atlas of neuropathology*, Gower Medical Publishing, 1988; 54-16, from Perkin GD and others: *Atlas of clinical neurology*, ed 2, London, 1993, Wolfe Publishing.

Chapter 55

55-8, Modified from Hoeman SP: *Rehabilitation nursing*, ed 2, St Louis, 1995, Mosby; 55-10A-C, courtesy Sammons Preston.

Chapter 56

56-2, 56-7, From Damjanov I, Linder J, editors: *Anderson's pathology*, ed 10, St Louis, 1996, Mosby; 56-5, from McCance KL, Huether SE: *Pathophysiology: the biologic basis for disease in adults and children*, ed 3, St Louis, 1998, Mosby; 56-6, redrawn from Rudy E: *Advanced neurological and neurosurgical nursing*, St Louis, 1984, Mosby; 56-8, redrawn from Barker E: *Neuroscience nursing*, St Louis, 1994, Mosby.

Chapter 57

57-1, From Thibodeau GA, Patton KT: *Anatomy and physiology*, ed 4, St Louis, 1999, Mosby; 57-2, courtesy Joe Rothrock, Media, Pa; 57-3, redrawn from Chipps E, Clanin N, Campbell V: *Neurologic disorders*, St Louis, 1992, Mosby; 57-4, redrawn from Marciano FF and others: *BNI Q* 11:6, 1995. In McCance KL, Huether SE: *Pathophysiology: the biologic basis for disease in adults and* children, ed 3, St Louis, 1998, Mosby; 57-8, courtesy Michael S Clement, MD, Mesa, Ariz; 57-9, 57-13, from Barker E: *Neuroscience nursing*, St Louis, 1994, Mosby; 57-10, courtesy Kinetic Concepts, Inc, San Antonio, Texas; 57-11, courtesy Acromed Corporation, Cleveland; 57-12, courtesy CLG Photographics, St Louis.

Chapter 58

58-1, 58-4, 58-6, From Thibodeau GA, Patton KT: *Anatomy and physiology*, ed 4, St Louis, 1999, Mosby; 58-2, from Seeley R, Stephens T, Tate P: *Anatomy and physiology*, ed 3, New York, 1995, McGraw-Hill; 58-7, 58-9, from Mourad LA: *Orthopedic disorders*, St Louis, 1991, Mosby; 58-8, modified from De Lisa J, Gans B: *Rehabilitation medicine principles*, ed 2, Philadelphia, 1993, JB Lippincott.

Chapter 59

59-1, Redrawn from Price SA, Wilson LM: *Pathophysiology: clinical concepts of disease processes,* ed 5, St Louis, 1997, Mosby; 59-2, 59-15, from Thompson J and others: *Mosby's manual of clinical nursing,* ed 4, St Louis, 1997, Mosby; 59-3, Jobe FW and others, editors: *Operative techniques in upper extremity sports injuries,* St Louis, 1996, Mosby; 59-4, from Thibodeau GA, Patton KT: *Anatomy and physiology,* ed 4, St Louis, 1999, Mosby; 59-8, redrawn from Long BC, Phipps WJ, Cassmeyer VL: *Medical-surgical nursing: a nursing process approach,* St Louis, 1993, Mosby; 59-10, courtesy Howmedica, Inc; 59-17, redrawn from Mourad L: *Orthopedic disorders,* St Louis, 1992, Mosby; 59-19, from Hunter JM and others: *Rehabilitation of the hand,* ed 4, St Louis, 1995, Mosby.

Chapter 60

60-2, From Kamal A, Brockelhurst JC: *Color atlas of geriatric medicine,* ed 2, St Louis, 1991, Mosby. In *Mosby's medical, nursing, and allied health dictionary,* ed 5, 1998, Mosby; 60-3, from Shipley M: *A colour atlas of rheumatology,* ed 3, London, 1993, Mosby–Year Book–Europe; 60-7, reprinted from the Clinical Slide Collection on the Rheumatic Diseases, copyright 1991, 1995, 1997. Used by permission of the American College of Rheumatology. In Seidel HM and others: *Mosby's guide to physical examination,* ed 4, St Louis, 1999, Mosby; 60-9, from Habif TP: *Clinical dermatology: a color guide to diagnosis and therapy,* ed 3, St Louis, 1996, Mosby; 60-11, from Zitelli BJ, Davis HW: *Atlas of pediatric physical diagnosis,* ed 3, St Louis, 1997, Mosby–Wolfe; 60-12, 60-13, courtesy Zimmer, Inc, Warsaw, Ind.

Chapter 61

61-2, 61-3, 61-4, 61-5, From Thelan LA and others: *Critical care nursing: diagnosis and management,* ed 3, St Louis, 1998, Mosby.

Chapter 62

62-6, From Richmond TS: The patient with a cervical spinal cord injury, *Focus on critical care* 12:27, 1985; 62-7, Courtesy Respironics, Inc, Pittsburgh.

Chapter 63

63-1, 63-16, Courtesy Spacelabs Medical, Redmond, Wash; 63-2, redrawn from Gardner PE: *Hemodynamic pressure monitoring,* Redmond, Wash, 1994, Spacelabs Medical; 63-3, redrawn from Flynn JBM, Bruce NP: *Introduction to critical care skills,* St Louis, 1993, Mosby; 63-4, 63-6, 63-7, 63-11, 63-20, from Thelan LA and others, editors: *Critical care nursing: diagnosis and management,* ed 3, St Louis, 1998, Mosby; 63-5, courtesy Edwards Critical Care Division, Baxter Healthcare Corporation, Santa Ana, Calif; 63-9, courtesy Datascope Corporation, Fairfield, NJ; 63-12A, from Beare PG, Myers JL: *Adult health nursing,* ed 3, St Louis, 1998, Mosby; 63-14, from Sills JR: *Respiratory care certification guide: the complete review resource for the entry level exam,* ed 2, St Louis, 1994, Mosby. In Thelan LA and others, editors: *Critical care nursing: diagnosis and management,* ed 3, St Louis, 1998, Mosby; 63-15, courtesy Lifecare, Westminster, Colo; 63-17, courtesy Mallinckrodt, Inc, Carlsbad, Calif; 63-18, courtesy Camino Laboratories, San Diego.

Chapter 64

64-2, 64-3, Courtesy Cameron Bangs, MD, from Auerbach P, editor: *Wilderness medicine: management of wilderness and environmental emergencies,* ed 3, St Louis, 1995, Mosby; 64-5, redrawn from Rosen P and others: *Emergency medicine,* vol 1, ed 2, St Louis, 1988, Mosby.

INDEX

Note: Disorder names are in **bold face.** Entries in **bold face** indicate main discussions. Page numbers followed by *f, t,* and *b* indicate figures, tables, or boxed material, respectively.

Alopecia—cont'd
in radiation therapy and chemotherapy, 291*t*
ALP. *See* Alkaline phosphatase
Alphagan. *See* Bromonidine
Alpha-glucosidase inhibitors
blood glucose level effects, 1381*t*
for diabetes mellitus, 1379, 1380*t*
Alpha-hydroxy acids, 512
Alpha-Nine, 761*t*
Alport's syndrome, 1281
ALT. *See* Argon laser trabeculoplasty
Altace. *See* Ramipril
Alteplase (Activase)
in advanced cardiac life support, 944*t*
for myocardial infarction, 871*t*
Alternative healers, 1425*b*
Alternative therapies, **107-125,** 108*t*-110*t*
nursing role in, 121-122, 122*f*
Alu-Cap, 1116*t*
Aludrox, 1116*t*
Aluminum carbonate, 1116*t*
Aluminum hydroxide, 1116*t*
Aluminum phosphate, 1116*t*
Alupent. *See* Metaproterenol
Alveolar edema, 655
Alveolar hyperventilation, 1944-1945
Alveolar hypoventilation, 1897
with mechanical ventilation, 1944
Alveolar macrophages, 193*t*, 561
Alveoli
and hypercapnia, 1898
pulmonary, 555, 555*f*, 556*f*
Alzheimer's disease, 1702-1708
characteristics of, 1703*t*
clinical manifestations of, 1703
collaborative care, 1704
diagnostic studies, 1703-1704
drug therapy for, 1704, 1704*t*
etiology, 1702-1703
nursing assessment of, 1704, 1704*t*
nursing care plan for caregiver of patient with, 1707*b*-1708*b*
nursing care plan for patient with, 1705*b*-1706*b*
nursing diagnoses, 1704
nursing evaluation, 1708
nursing implementation for, 1706-1708
nursing management of, **1704-1708**
goals, 1706
nursing planning for, 1706
pathologic changes in, 1702, 1703*f*
pathophysiology, 1702-1703
Amantadine (Symmetrel), 1697, 1697*t*
Amaryl. *See* Glimepiride
Ambient air pollution, 683
Amblyopia, 443
Ambu (air mask bag unit), 1947
Ambulation
early postoperative, 400
with fractures, 1783
weight-bearing, 1783
Ambulatory care, 18*t*, 25, 25*f*. *See also specific disorders*
blood pressure monitoring, 824
ECG monitoring, 806*t*, 811-812
Ambulatory liquid oxygen system, 698*f*
Ambulatory peritoneal dialysis, continuous, 1323-1324
Ambulatory surgery
discharge, 399
criteria for, 399*t*
outpatient follow-up, research, 400*b*
AMD. *See* Age-related macular degeneration
Amenorrhea

causes of, 1524, 1525*t*
primary, 1525
secondary, 1525
American Anorexia/Bulimia Association, 1046
American Association of Critical Nurses (AACN)
Certification Corporation, 1915
definition of critical care nursing, 1914
American Burn Association, 527-528, 528*t*
American Cancer Society, 640, 1472
American College of Allergy, Asthma, and Immunology (ACAAI), 364
American College of Cardiology (ACC)/AHA Practice Guidelines, 866
American Diabetes Association, 1390
"ADA" diet, 1372
position statement regarding DCCT, 1393
American Foundation for the Blind, 448
American Heart Association, 1669
"Heart Walk," 848
Practice Guidelines, 866
American Hospital Association, 26*t*
American Joint Committee on Cancer (AJCC), 1482, 1482*t*
American Lung Association, 628, 640, 681
American Nurses' Association, 4
American Parkinson's Disease Association, 1698
American Rheumatism Association, 1830*t*
American Society of Perianesthesia Nursing (ASPAN), 391
American Thoracic Society, 613, 613*t*
American Urological Association (AUA), 1553, 1555*t*
Americans with Disabilities Act (ADA), 262
Amethopterin. *See* Methotrexate
Amidate. *See* Etomidate
Amikacin
nephrotoxicity, 1247*t*
for tuberculosis, 626*t*
Amiloride (Midamor)
for cirrhosis, 1211*t*
for hypertension, 827*t*
Amino acids, 741*t*
Aminoglutethimide (Cytadren)
mechanism of action, 297*t*
toxic side effects, 303*t*
Aminoglycosides
for hospital-acquired pneumonia, 614*t*
for inflammation, 202*t*
Aminophylline, 671*t*, 675*t*
Aminosalicylic acid (Pamisyl, PAS), 727*t*
Aminotransferases, 1197*t*
Amiodarone (Cordarone)
classification of, 934*t*
photosensitivity, 495*t*
Amitriptyline (Elavil)
for Alzheimer's disease, 1704*t*
for headache, 1675*t*
pharmacokinetics, 140*t*
photosensitivity, 495*t*
Amlodipine (Norvasc), 830*t*
Ammonia salt encrustation, 1293, 1296*f*
Amobarbital (Amytal), 161*t*
Amodrine, 675*t*
Amoxicillin
for *H. pylori* infection, 1103*t*, 1115*t*
for infective endocarditis, 951*t*
Amphetamines (Benzedrine), **160**
cancers related to, 273*t*
characteristics of, 160
collaborative management of, 160
complications of, 160
effects of use, 160, 161*t*
and heat-related emergencies, 1965*t*
signs and symptoms of overdose and withdrawal, 163*t*
Amphojel, 1117
Amphojet, 1116*t*
Amphotericin B (Fungizone)
hematologic effects, 727*t*
nephrotoxicity, 1247*t*
Ampicillin, 951*t*
Amprenavir (Agenerase), 251*t*

Amputation, 1798-1802
acute intervention for, 1799-1801
ambulatory and home care for, 1801-1802
clinical indications for, 1798
collaborative care, 1798*t*, 1798-1799
diagnostic studies, 1798
gerontologic considerations, **1802**
guillotine, 1799
health promotion in, 1799
levels of, 1799*f*
nursing assessment in, 1799
nursing diagnoses, 1799
nursing evaluation, 1802
nursing implementation for, 1799-1802
nursing management of, **1799-1802**
goals, 1799
nursing planning, 1799
open, 1799
patient teaching guide after, 1801*t*
postoperative management of, 1800-1801
preoperative management of, 1799-1800
residual limb bandaging for, 1801, 1801*f*
upper-limb, special considerations, **1802**
Amrinone (Inocor)
in advanced cardiac life support, 944*t*
for congestive heart failure, 895*t*
Amsacrine (m-AMSA)
mechanism of action, 297*t*
toxic side effects, 303*t*
Amsler grid test, 431*t*
A-M-T, 1116*t*
Amylase
serum, 1032*t*
in acute pancreatitis, 1221, 1222*t*
urinary, in acute pancreatitis, 1221, 1222*t*
Amyotrophic lateral sclerosis, 1709
pathogenesis of, 1709, 1710*f*
and restrictive lung disease, 653*t*
Amytal. *See* Amobarbital
Anabolic steroids
blood glucose level effects, 1381*t*
cancers related to, 273*t*
hepatotoxicity, 1021*t*
Anacin Caplets/Tablets, 757*t*
Anacin Maximum Strength Tablets, 757*t*
Anadrol-50. *See* Oxymethalone
Anaerobes, 614*t*
oral, 612*t*
Anafranil. *See* Clomipramine
Anal fissure, 1187
Analexin. *See* Phenyramidol
Analgesia
for burns, 539*t*
patient-controlled, 143-144
Analgesics
adjuvant, 141
administration routes, 141-144
epidural, 142-143
intrathecal, 142-143
intravenous, 142-143
oral, 141
recommended, 141-145
rectal, 141-142
subcutaneous, 142-143
sublingual, 141
transdermal, 142
transmucosal, 141-142
transnasal, 141
for burns, 538-539
combinations, for headache, 1675*t*
equianalgesic dose, 137
infusions, 142-144, 144
injections, 144
ladder, 138, 138*f*, 138-141, 319, 320*f*
narcotic, for rheumatic disorders, 1822*t*
nonnarcotic
for headache, 1675*t*
for rheumatic disorders, 1822*t*
recommended drugs, 141-145
scheduling doses, 137-138
selecting, 138

Note: Disorder names are in **bold face.** Entries in **bold face** indicate main discussions. Page numbers followed by *f, t,* and *b* indicate figures, tables, or boxed material, respectively.

Note: Disorder names are in **bold face.** Entries in
bold face indicate main discussions. Page numbers followed by *f, t,* and *b* indicate figures, tables,
or boxed material, respectively.

Note: Disorder names are in **bold face**. Entries in **bold face** indicate main discussions. Page numbers followed by *f*, *t*, and *b* indicate figures, tables, or boxed material, respectively.

Note: Disorder names are in **bold face**. Entries in
bold face indicate main discussions. Page numbers followed by *f*, *t*, and *b* indicate figures, tables, or boxed material, respectively.

Note: Disorder names are in **bold face.** Entries in **bold face** indicate main discussions. Page numbers followed by *f*, *t*, and *b* indicate figures, tables, or boxed material, respectively.

Note: Disorder names are in **bold face.** Entries in **bold face** indicate main discussions. Page numbers followed by *f, t,* and *b* indicate figures, tables, or boxed material, respectively.

Note: Disorder names are in **bold face**. Entries in **bold face** indicate main discussions. Page numbers followed by f, t, and b indicate figures, tables, or boxed material, respectively.

Note: Disorder names are in **bold face.** Entries in **bold face** indicate main discussions. Page numbers followed by *f, t,* and *b* indicate figures, tables, or boxed material, respectively.

Note: Disorder names are in **bold face**. Entries in
bold face indicate main discussions. Page numbers followed by *f*, *t*, and *b* indicate figures, tables, or boxed material, respectively.

Note: Disorder names are in **bold face**. Entries in **bold face** indicate main discussions. Page numbers followed by *f*, *t*, and *b* indicate figures, tables, or boxed material, respectively.

Note: Disorder names are in **bold face.** Entries in **bold face** indicate main discussions. Page numbers followed by *f, t,* and *b* indicate figures, tables, or boxed material, respectively.

Note: Disorder names are in **bold face.** Entries in **bold face** indicate main discussions. Page numbers followed by f, t, and b indicate figures, tables, or boxed material, respectively.

Note: Disorder names are in **bold face.** Entries in **bold face** indicate main discussions. Page numbers followed by *f*, *t*, and *b* indicate figures, tables, or boxed material, respectively.

Note: Disorder names are in **bold face.** Entries in **bold face** indicate main discussions. Page numbers followed by *f*, *t*, and *b* indicate figures, tables, or boxed material, respectively.

Note: Disorder names are in **bold face**. Entries in
bold face indicate main discussions. Page numbers followed by *f, t,* and *b* indicate figures, tables,
or boxed material, respectively.

Nausea and vomiting—cont'd
  nursing implementation for, 399, 1092
  nursing management of, **399, 1090-1092**
    goals, 1090-1092
    nursing planning for, 1090-1092
  nutritional therapy for, 1089-1090
  pathophysiology of, 1088-1089
  postoperative, **399**
    etiology, **399**
  in radiation therapy and chemotherapy, 291*t*
Navelbine. *See* Vinorelbine
Near drowning, 1969-1970
  collaborative care, 1970
  emergency management of, 1970*t*
Nearsightedness. *See* Myopia
Nebulizers, 694-695
Neck. *See also* Head and neck
  assessment of, 1359
  physical examination of, 77*t*, 566
  secondary survey, 1962-1963, 1963*t*
Neck breathers, emergency identification of, 607, 607*f*
Neck pain, 1810
Neck surgery, radical dissection, 601, 602*f*, 608, 1086
  acute intervention for, 1087
  nursing care plan for patient having, 604*b*-605*b*
  nutritional therapy after, 602-603
Neck veins, distended, 803*t*
Necrosis
  aseptic bone, 1339
  caseous, 623
  cell, 190
  fat, 1475*t*
  postpartum pituitary, 1409-1410
  types of, 190, 193*t*
  wave front of, 866
Necrotizing pneumonia, 613
Necrotizing ulcerative gingivitis, 1084*t*
Nedocromil (Tilade)
  for allergic rhinitis and sinusitis, 227*t*, 585*t*
  for asthma, 670*t*, 672
Needle biopsy, transbronchial, 575*f*
Nefazodone (Serzone), 140*t*
Negative inotropes, 1918
Negative inspiratory force (NIF), 577*t*
Negative pressure ventilators, 1940
Neisseria, 192*t*
Neisseria gonorrhoeae, 1496*t*, 1532*t*, 1534
Nelfinavir (Viracept), 251*t*
Nembutal. *See* Pentobarbital
Neomycin
  for cirrhosis, 1211*t*
  nephrotoxicity, 1247*t*
  oral anticoagulant interactions, 999*t*
Neoplastic disorders. *See also* Tumors
  of urinary tract, **1282-1284**
Neoral. *See* Cyclosporine
Neostigmine (Prostigmine), 1689*t*
Neo-Synephrine. *See* Phenylephrine
Nephrectomy
  bilateral, indications for, 1331
  laparoscopic, 1291
Nephritis. *see* Pyelonephritis
Nephrons, 1241, 1241, 1242*f*
  blood supply of, 1242, 1243*f*
  destruction in acute renal failure, 1300, 1301*f*
  functions of segments of, 1243*t*
Nephropathy
  diabetic, 1400
  HIV-associated, 1272
Nephrosclerosis, 1280
  in hypertension, 823
Nephrostomy, 1291*t*
Nephrostomy tubes, 1290

Nephrotic syndrome, 1271-1272
  clinical manifestations of, 1271-1272
  collaborative care, 1272
  etiology, 1271*t*, 1271-1272
  with HIV infection, 1272
  nursing management of, **1272**
Nephrotomography, 1253*t*
Nephrotoxic agents, 1247*t*
Neptazane. *See* Methazolamide
Nerve blocks, 147
Nerve conduction studies, 1606
Nerve impulse, 1582-1584
Nerve tissue, 196, 198*t*
Nerves
  cranial, 1587*f*, 1588, 1590*t*
    gerontologic differences in, 1594*t*
  regeneration of, 1582
  spinal, 1588, 1590*f*
    gerontologic differences in, 1594*t*
Nervous system. *See* Neurologic system
Nervous tissue tumors, 279*t*
Neuroblastoma
  classification of, 279*t*
  radiosensitivity, 286*t*
Neuroendocrine system, 1349-1350
Neurofibroma, 1630*t*
Neurogenic bladder, 1285
  areflexic, flaccid, 1737
  collaborative care, 1738*t*
  hyperreflexic, spastic, 1737
  after spinal cord injury, 1737-1739
  types of, 1738*t*
Neurogenic shock, 1723, 1867
  collaborative care, 1878*t*, 1883
  hemodynamic effects of, 1867*t*
  pathophysiology of, 1867, 1867*f*
  precipitating factors, 1866*t*, 1867
Neuroglia, 1581-1582
Neurohypophysis. *See* Posterior pituitary gland
Neuroleptics, 1704*t*
Neurologic clinical flow sheets, 1618, 1619*f*
Neurologic disorders, 1709-1710
  dermatologic manifestations, 514*t*
  opportunistic diseases associated with AIDS, 247*t*
Neurologic system, **1581-1607**
  age-related changes, 47*t*
  in anemia, 738*t*
  assessment abnormalities, 730*t*, 1601*t*-1602*t*
  assessment of, **1594-1602**
    functional categories in, 1602*t*
    gerontologic differences in, 1594*t*
    important health information, 1594-1595
    key questions to ask, 1596*t*
    nursing approach to, 1601-1602
    objective data, 1597-1602
    preoperative, 363
    subjective data, 1594-1597
  autonomic nervous system, 1588-1589
    effects on blood vessels, 797
    effects on heart, 797
    gerontologic differences in, 1594*t*
    pain mechanisms, 127, 128*t*
    regulation of cardiovascular system by, 797
  cells of, 1581-1582
  central nervous system, 1584-1587
    autoimmune diseases of, 231*t*
    effects of chronic alcohol abuse on, 168*t*
    effects of cocaine use, 164*t*
    failure of, clinical evidence of, 1891*t*
    gerontologic differences in, 1594*t*
    and hypercapnia, 1898
    lesions of, 653*t*, 1965*t*
    lymphomas, 247*t*
    problems in systemic lupus erythematosus, 1843
    projection to, 129
    and restrictive lung disease, 653*t*
    side effects of biologic therapy on, 313*t*
  in chronic renal failure, 1309
  complications of burns, 541
  complications of mechanical ventilation, 1945
  control of hormonal secretion by, 1349

  dangers of unrelieved acute pain, 133, 133*t*
  diagnostic studies, **1602-1607,** 1603*t*-1604*t*
  effects of aging on, 1593
  enteric, 1013
  gerontologic considerations, **1593**
  late effects of radiation and chemotherapy on, 310, 310*t*
  neurochemical links with endocrine and immune systems, 96, 96*f*
  parasympathetic nervous system
    effects of, 1591*t*
    gerontologic differences in, 1594*t*
  peripheral nervous system, 1588-1589
    effects of chronic alcohol abuse on, 168*t*
    gerontologic differences in, 1594*t*
    pain mechanisms, 127, 128*t*
    problems, **1713-1744**
  physical examination of, 1597-1601
    with herniated intervertebral disk, 1809*t*
    outline for, 75*t*
    recording, 78*t*, 1600*t*
  postoperative care, 983
  postoperative complications of, **397-398, 409-410**
    etiology, 397, 409
    nursing assessment of, 397, 409-410
    nursing diagnoses, 397-398, 410
    nursing implementation for, 398, 410
    nursing management of, **397-398, 409-410**
  problems of
    caused by radiation therapy and chemotherapy, 292*t*
    chronic, **1672-1712**
  protective structures, 1591-1593
  response to stress, 96-98
  in shock, 1873*t*, 1885-1887
  signs of protein-calorie malnutrition, 1047, 1048*t*
  in sodium and volume imbalances, 334
  in stroke, acute intervention for, 1662
  structures and functions of, **1581-1593**
Neuroma, 476, 1630*t*
Neuromotor function deficits
  problems associated with, 1650
  of stroke, 1650-1651
Neuromuscular blockade, reversal of, 385, 385*f*
Neuromuscular blocking agents, 385-386
Neuromuscular junction, 1749, 1749*f*
Neuromuscular system
  and hypercapnia, 1898
  and restrictive lung disease, 653*t*
Neuronitis, 475
Neurons, 1581
  characteristics of, 1581
  motor
    lower, 1585
    upper, 1585
  structural features of, 1581, 1582*f*
Neurontin. *See* Gabapentin
Neuropathy
  diabetic, 1400-1402, 1401*f*
  peripheral, in cirrhosis, 1204
Neurosyphilis, 1722
Neurotransmitters, 1583-1584
Neurotrophic ulcerations, 1401, 1401*f*
Neurovascular assessment
  five Ps method, 1778
  in fractures, 1778
  after hip fracture surgery, 1789
Neutralizing agents, 1114, 1115*t*
Neutropenia, 766-768
  causes of, 766*t*
  clinical manifestations, 766-767
  collaborative care, 767*t*
  definition, 766
  diagnostic studies, 767
  nursing and collaborative management of, **767-768**
  nursing care plan for patient with, 769*b*
Neutrophils, 191
Nevirapine (Viramune), 251*t*
Nevus(i)
  dysplastic nevus syndrome, 503*t*, 504
  melanocytic (*see* Moles)
  spider, 729*t*, 1204

Note: Disorder names are in **bold face**. Entries in **bold face** indicate main discussions. Page numbers followed by *f*, *t*, and *b* indicate figures, tables, or boxed material, respectively.

Note: Disorder names are in **bold face**. Entries in **bold face** indicate main discussions. Page numbers followed by *f*, *t*, and *b* indicate figures, tables, or boxed material, respectively.

O

Note: Disorder names are in **bold face**. Entries in
bold face indicate main discussions. Page numbers followed by *f*, *t*, and *b* indicate figures, tables, or boxed material, respectively.

Note: Disorder names are in **bold face**. Entries in **bold face** indicate main discussions. Page numbers followed by f, t, and b indicate figures, tables, or boxed material, respectively.

Note: Disorder names are in **bold face.** Entries in
bold face indicate main discussions. Page numbers followed by *f, t,* and *b* indicate figures, tables,
or boxed material, respectively.

Note: Disorder names are in **bold face**. Entries in **bold face** indicate main discussions. Page numbers followed by *f*, *t*, and *b* indicate figures, tables, or boxed material, respectively.

Q

R

Note: Disorder names are in **bold face.** Entries in **bold face** indicate main discussions. Page numbers followed by f, t, and b indicate figures, tables, or boxed material, respectively.

Note: Disorder names are in **bold face**. Entries in **bold face** indicate main discussions. Page numbers followed by *f*, *t*, and *b* indicate figures, tables, or boxed material, respectively.

Note: Disorder names are in **bold face.** Entries in **bold face** indicate main discussions. Page numbers followed by f, t, and b indicate figures, tables, or boxed material, respectively.

Note: Disorder names are in **bold face.** Entries in **bold face** indicate main discussions. Page numbers followed by f, t, and b indicate figures, tables, or boxed material, respectively.

U

Note: Disorder names are in **bold face.** Entries in **bold face** indicate main discussions. Page numbers followed by *f, t,* and *b* indicate figures, tables, or boxed material, respectively.

Note: Disorder names are in **bold face.** Entries in **bold face** indicate main discussions. Page numbers followed by *f*, *t*, and *b* indicate figures, tables, or boxed material, respectively.